Textbook of Pharmacology
An Integrated Approach

As per CBME 2024 Curriculum

Jagminder Kaur Bajaj
MBBS, MD (Pharmacology), ACME, PG Diploma in Maternal and Child Health
Professor and Head, Department of Pharmacology
Punjab Institute of Medical Sciences, Jalandhar

Satinderjit Singh Bajaj
MBBS, MS (General Surgery), Diploma in Minimal Access Surgery
Medical Superintendent and DNB Coordinator, S.B.L.S. Civil Hospital, Jalandhar

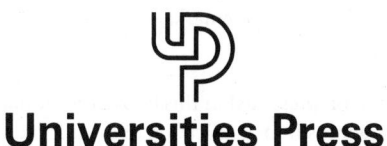

Universities Press

All rights reserved. No part of this book may be (i) modified, reproduced or utilised in any form, or by any means, electronic or mechanical, including photocopying, recording or by any information storage and retrieval system, in any form of binding or cover other than in which it is published, without permission in writing from the publisher; or (ii) used or reproduced in any manner for the purpose of training, development or operation of artificial intelligence (AI) technologies and systems, including generative AI technologies, without permission in writing from the copyright holder.

TEXTBOOK OF PHARMACOLOGY: AN INTEGRATED APPROACH
UNIVERSITIES PRESS (INDIA) PRIVATE LIMITED

Registered Office
3-6-747/1/A and 3-6-754/1, Himayatnagar, Hyderabad 500 029, Telangana, India
info@universitiespress.com; www.universitiespress.com

Distributed by
Orient Blackswan Private Limited

Registered Office
3-6-752, Himayatnagar, Hyderabad 500 029, Telangana, India

Other Offices
Bengaluru / Chennai / Guwahati / Hyderabad / Kolkata,
Mumbai / New Delhi / Noida / Patna

© Universities Press (India) Private Limited 2026
First published 2026

ISBN 978-93-49750-43-2

Cover and book design
© Universities Press (India) Private Limited 2026

Typeset in Minion Pro 10.5/12.5 by
e-Leaf Technologies, Chennai 600 011

Printed at
SDR Printers, Tronica City, Ghaziabad, U.P. 201 103

Published by
Universities Press (India) Private Limited
3-6-747/1/A & 3-6-754/1, Himayatnagar
Hyderabad 500 029, Telangana, India

All product and company names are trademarks™ or registered® trademarks of their respective holders. Use of them does not imply any affiliation with or endorsement by them.

Care has been taken to confirm the accuracy of information presented in this book. The author and the publisher, however, cannot accept any responsibility for errors or omissions or for consequences from application of the information in this book and make no warranty, express or implied, with respect to its contents.

Contents

Competency Mapping   v
Foreword   ix
Preface   x

1 General Pharmacology

1. Introduction to Pharmacology and Pharmacotherapeutics   1
2. Routes of Drug Administration   11
3. Pharmacokinetics   29
4. Pharmacodynamics   50
5. Adverse Drug Reactions   66
6. Variability in Drug Response and Therapeutic Drug Monitoring   76

2 Drugs Acting on the Autonomic and Peripheral Nervous Systems

7. Cholinergic Drugs   89
8. Anticholinergic Drugs   104
9. Adrenergic Drugs   116
10. Antiadrenergic Drugs: α Blockers   132
11. Antiadrenergic Drugs: β Blockers and Drugs for Glaucoma   140
12. Skeletal Muscle Relaxants   154
13. Local Anesthetics   168

3 Drugs Acting on the Central Nervous System

14. General Anesthetics   181
15. Sedative-Hypnotics and Anxiolytics   197
16. Antiepileptic Drugs   210
17. Drugs for Neurodegenerative Disorders   228
18. Antipsychotic Drugs   245
19. Drugs for Mood Disorders   259
20. Alcohols   276
21. Drugs of Abuse and CNS Stimulants   285
22. Opioid Analgesics and Antagonists   297

4 Autacoids and Related Drugs

23. Non-Steroidal Anti-Inflammatory Drugs (NSAIDs)   311
24. Drugs for Gout   329
25. Drugs Used in the Treatment of Rheumatoid Arthritis   339
26. Histamine and Antihistaminics   348
27. Drugs for the Management of Migraine   356

5 Drugs Acting on the Respiratory System

28. Drugs Used in Cough and Bronchial Asthma   367

6 Drugs Acting on the Kidneys

29. Diuretics   385

7 Drugs Acting on the Cardiovascular System

30. Drugs Modulating the Renin-Angiotensin-Aldosterone System (RAAS)   399
31. Calcium Channel Blockers   409
32. Antihypertensive Drugs   416
33. Drug Therapy of Congestive Heart Failure (CHF)   434
34. Drugs for Ischemic Heart Disease   450
35. Drugs for Peripheral Vascular Disease (PVD) and Management of Shock   466
36. Antiarrhythmic Drugs   478

8 Drugs Affecting Blood

37. Coagulants and Anticoagulants   497
38. Antiplatelet and Fibrinolytic Drugs   515
39. Hypolipidemic Drugs   523
40. Hematinics   535

9 Drugs Affecting the Endocrine System

41. Anterior Pituitary Hormones   548
42. Drugs for Thyroid Disorders   557
43. Insulin and Antidiabetic Drugs   570
44. Corticosteroids   588
45. Female Sex Hormones and Antagonists   602

46. Hormonal Contraceptives — 616
47. Drugs Acting on the Uterus — 624
48. Male Sex Hormones and Their Analogues — 632
49. Drugs for Infertility and Erectile Dysfunction — 640
50. Drugs for Osteoporosis — 648

10 Chemotherapeutic Drugs

51. General Principles of Chemotherapy — 658
52. Antimicrobial Agents (AMAs) — 670
53. Drugs Used in UTIs and STDs — 690
54. Antitubercular and Antileprotic Drugs — 699
55. Antifungal Drugs — 725
56. Antiviral Drugs — 734
57. Antiretroviral Drugs — 745
58. Antimalarial Drugs — 755
59. Antiamoebic Drugs — 768
60. Anthelmintics — 777
61. Anticancer Drugs — 790

11 Drugs Acting on the Gastrointestinal System

62. Drugs for Diarrhea, IBD, and Constipation — 810
63. Antiemetic and Prokinetic Drugs — 827
64. Drugs for Acid Peptic Diseases — 834

12 Miscellaneous Topics

65. Immunomodulator Drugs — 846
66. Toxicology — 863
67. Drugs Used in Dermatological Conditions and Germicidal Drugs — 877
68. Evidence-Based Medicine and New Drug Development — 889

13 Applied Pharmacology

69. Pharmacovigilance — 900
70. Practical Pharmacology: Essential Drugs, DPL, Legal Aspects — 907
71. Practical Pharmacology – Prescriptions, Prescription Errors, P-Drug, Dosage Calculation and Drug Interactions — 913

14 AETCOM

72. Attitude, Ethics, and Communication — 927

Index — 936

Competency Mapping

Mapping of *Textbook of Pharmacology: An Integrated Approach* to the CBME 2024 Curriculum

Number	Competency description	Chapter number	Page number
General Pharmacology			
PH1.1	Describe the principles of pharmacology, pharmacotherapeutics and define various terms in pharmacology.	1	1
PH1.2	Describe evidence-based medicine and rational use of drugs and discuss why these are relevant to therapeutics.	68	889
PH1.3	Describe nomenclature of drugs, i.e., generic, branded and scheduled drugs, explaining the utility of the nomenclature, cost effectiveness and use.	1	1
PH1.4	Identify the common drug formulations and drug delivery systems; demonstrate their use and describe their advantages and disadvantages.	2	11
PH1.5	Describe various routes of drug administration, their advantages and disadvantages and demonstrate administration of SC, IV, IM, SL, rectal, spinal, sublingual, intranasal sprays and inhalers.	2	11
PH1.6	Describe salient features of absorption, distribution, metabolism and excretion of drugs with emphasis on various routes of drug administration.	3	29
PH1.7	Describe various principles of mechanism of action of drugs.	4	50
PH1.8	Demonstrate the mechanism of action and effects of common prototype drugs on human body using computer assisted learning.	4	50
PH 1.9	Select rational drug combinations based on the pharmacokinetics/pharmacodynamic (PK/PD) parameters with emphasis on synergism, antagonism, 'therapeutic efficacy', risk benefit ratio.	6	76
PH1.10	Describe changes in pharmacology of drugs in geriatric, pediatric and special situations such as pregnancy, lactation, hepatic and renal disorders and adjust the drug treatment accordingly.	6	76
PH 1.11	Define adverse drug reactions (ADRs) and their types. Identify the ADRs in the given case scenario and assess causality.	5	66
PH1.12	Define pharmacovigilance its principles and demonstrate ADR reporting.	69	900
PH1.13	Identify and describe the management of drug interactions.	71	913
Autonomic and peripheral nervous system, Autacoids			
PH2.1	Describe types, salient pharmacokinetics, pharmacodynamics, therapeutic uses, adverse drug reactions of adrenergic and antiadrenergic drugs.	9, 10, 11	116, 132, 140
PH2.2	Describe types, salient pharmacokinetics, pharmacodynamics, therapeutic uses, adverse drug reactions of cholinergic and anticholinergic drugs and demonstrate OPC poisoning management.	7, 8	89, 104
PH 2.3	Explain the rationale and demonstrate the emergency use of various sympathetic and parasympathetic drug agonists/antagonists (like noradrenaline/ adrenaline/dopamine/ dobutamine, atropine) in case-based scenarios.	35, 71	466, 913
PH2.4	Explain salient pharmacokinetics, pharmacodynamics, therapeutic uses, adverse drug reactions of skeletal muscle relaxants.	12	154
PH2.5	Explain types, salient pharmacokinetics, pharmacodynamics, therapeutic uses, adverse drug reactions of local anesthetics (LA) and demonstrate various methods of administration of LA.	13	168
PH2.6	Explain types, salient pharmacokinetics, pharmacodynamics, therapeutic uses, adverse drug reactions of antihistaminics and explain management of common cold and allergic rhinitis.	26	348
PH2.7	Define pain and enumerate drugs used for pain. Explain salient pharmacokinetics, pharmacodynamics, therapeutic uses, adverse drug reactions of analgesics including NSAIDs (except opioids).	23	311
PH2.8	Devise management plan for a case of gout, arthritis and migraine using appropriate drugs.	24, 25 27	329, 339, 356

Central nervous system

PH3.1	Describe types, salient pharmacokinetics, pharmacodynamics, therapeutic uses, adverse drug reactions of general anaesthetics, and pre-anaesthetic medications.	14	181
PH3.2	Describe types, salient pharmacokinetics, pharmacodynamics, therapeutic uses, adverse drug reactions of different sedative and hypnotic agents and explain pharmacological basis of selection and use of different sedative and hypnotic agents.	15	197
PH3.3	Describe types, salient pharmacokinetics, pharmacodynamics, therapeutic uses, adverse drug reactions of drugs used in epilepsy and devise management plan for a case of uncontrolled seizure.	16	210
PH3.4	Describe types, salient pharmacokinetics, pharmacodynamics, therapeutic uses, adverse drug reactions of drugs of opioid analgesics and explain the special instructions for use of opioids.	22	285
PH3.5	Describe types, salient pharmacokinetics, pharmacodynamics, therapeutic uses, adverse drug reactions of drugs used for depression and psychosis; devise management plan for depressive and psychotic disorders.	18, 19	245, 259
PH3.6	Describe types, salient pharmacokinetics, pharmacodynamics, therapeutic uses, adverse drug reactions of drugs used in anxiety disorders. Discuss about general goals of pharmacotherapy for the management of above disorders.	15	197
PH3.7	Explain types, salient pharmacokinetics, pharmacodynamics, therapeutic uses, adverse drug reactions of drugs used for Parkinsonism and other neurodegenerative disorders. Write a prescription to manage a case of drug induced parkinsonism.	17	228
PH3.8	Identify and manage methanol poisoning and chronic ethanol intoxication.	20	276
PH3.9	Describe the drugs that are abused and cause addiction (dependence, addiction, stimulants, depressants, psychedelics, drugs used for criminal offences). Explain the process and steps for management of drug de-addiction.	21	285

Cardiovascular system and Blood

PH4.1	Explain types, salient pharmacokinetics, pharmacodynamics, therapeutic uses, adverse drug reactions of drugs used for different anemias and thrombocytopenia.	40	535
PH4.2	Explain types, salient pharmacokinetics, pharmacodynamics, therapeutic uses, adverse drug reactions of drugs acting on coagulation system (coagulants/anticoagulants) and devise a plan to monitor therapy and management of adverse effects.	37	497
PH4.3	Describe types, salient pharmacokinetics, pharmacodynamics, therapeutic uses, adverse drug reactions of fibrinolytics and antifibrinolytic agents.	38	515
PH4.4	Explain types, salient pharmacokinetics, pharmacodynamics, therapeutic uses, adverse drug reactions of Antiplatelets agents.	38	515
PH4.5	Explain types, salient pharmacokinetics, pharmacodynamics, therapeutic uses, adverse drug reactions of Diuretics, antidiuretics- vasopressin and analogues.	29	385
PH4.6	Explain salient pharmacokinetics, pharmacodynamics, therapeutic uses, adverse drug reactions of drugs modulating renin angiotensin aldosterone system.	30	399
PH4.7	Explain types, salient pharmacokinetics, pharmacodynamics, therapeutic uses, adverse drug reactions of drugs used for the management of hypertension Devise plan for pharmacologic management of hypertension with diabetes, pregnancy-induced hypertension and hypertensive emergency and urgency.	32	416
PH4.8	Describe types, salient pharmacokinetics, pharmacodynamics, therapeutic uses, adverse drug reactions of drugs used for the management of ischemic heart disease (stable, unstable angina and myocardial infarction), peripheral vascular disease and devise management plan for a patient of acute myocardial infarction.	34, 35	450, 466
PH4.9	Explain salient pharmacokinetics, pharmacodynamics, therapeutic uses, adverse drug reactions of drugs used for the management of heart failure. Devise management plan for heart failure patients and describe the strategies to prevent long term complications of heart failure.	33	434
PH4.10	Explain salient pharmacokinetics, pharmacodynamics, therapeutic uses, adverse drug reactions of drugs used for cardiac arrhythmias. Devise a plan to manage a patient with supraventricular, ventricular arrhythmias, cardiac arrest and fibrillations.	36	478
PH4.11	Explain salient pharmacokinetics, pharmacodynamics, therapeutic uses, adverse drug reactions of drugs used for the management of dyslipidaemias and enumerate drugs leading to dyslipidaemias.	39	523

Respiratory system			
PH5.1	Devise management of various stages of bronchial asthma, COPD. Explain salient pharmacokinetics, pharmacodynamics, therapeutic uses, adverse drug reactions of drugs used for the management of bronchial asthma, COPD and rhinitis.	28	367
PH5.2	Explain types, salient pharmacokinetics, pharmacodynamics, therapeutic uses, adverse drug reactions of drugs used for cough management. Describe management of dry & productive cough.	28	367
Gastrointestinal system			
PH6.1	Explain types, salient pharmacokinetics, pharmacodynamics, therapeutic uses, adverse drug reactions of drugs used in acid peptic diseases, including peptic ulcers, GERD and devise a management plan for a case of peptic ulcer.	64	834
PH6.2	Describe types, salient pharmacokinetics, pharmacodynamics, therapeutic uses, adverse drug reactions of prokinetics & drugs used for emesis and antiemetics.	63	827
PH6.3	Describe salient pharmacokinetics, pharmacodynamics, therapeutic uses, adverse drug reactions of drugs used for the management of diarrhea and devise pharmacotherapeutic plan to manage acute and chronic diarrhea in adults and children.	62	810
PH6.4	Describe salient pharmacokinetics, pharmacodynamics, adverse drug reactions of drugs used for the management of constipation and devise management plan for a case of constipation.	62	810
PH6.5	Describe salient pharmacokinetics, pharmacodynamics, adverse drug reactions of drugs used for the management of inflammatory bowel disease and irritable bowel disorders.	62	810
Endocrine system			
PH7.1	Describe the types, kinetics, dynamics, adverse drug reactions of drugs used in diabetes mellitus and devise management for an obese and non-obese diabetic patient and also comment on prevention of complications of the diabetes.	43	570
PH7.2	Describe the types, kinetics, dynamics, therapeutic uses, adverse drug reactions of drugs used in osteoporosis and devise management plan for a female and male patient with osteoporosis.	50	648
PH7.3	Describe the types, kinetics, dynamics, adverse drug reactions of drugs used in thyroid disorders and devise a management plan for a case with thyroid disorder.	42	557
PH7.4	Describe the types, mechanisms of action, adverse effects, indications and contraindications of the drugs which modify the release of anterior pituitary hormones.	41	548
PH7.5	Explain the types, kinetics, dynamics, adverse effects, indications and contraindications of corticosteroids and communicate to patient the appropriate use of corticosteroids.	44	588
PH7.6	Describe the types, kinetics, dynamics, adverse effects, indications and contraindications of androgens and drugs used of erectile dysfunction.	48, 49	632, 640
PH7.7	Explain the types, kinetics, dynamics, adverse effects, indications and contraindications of drugs which modify female reproductive functions including contraceptives. Explain the important instruction for use of female and male contraceptives.	45, 46	602, 612
PH7.8	Explain the types, kinetics, dynamics, adverse effects, indications and contraindications of uterine relaxants and stimulants.	47	624
PH7.9	Describe drugs used for treatment of Infertility.	49	
Chemotherapy			
PH8.1	Discuss general principles of chemotherapy with emphasis on antimicrobial resistance.	51	658
PH8.2	Discuss rational use of antimicrobials and describe antibiotic stewardship program of your institute.	51	658
PH8.3	Explain the kinetics, dynamics, adverse effects, indications of the following antibacterial drugs: Sulphonamides Quinolones, Beta-lactams, Macrolides, Tetracyclines, Aminoglycosides, and newer antibacterial drugs.	52	670
PH8.4	Devise a pharmacotherapeutic plan for UTI and STDs and explain to patient the instructions and adherence to treatment.	53	690
PH8.5	Explain the types, kinetics, dynamics, therapeutic uses and adverse effects of drugs used in tuberculosis. Devise management plan for tuberculosis treatment in various categories.	54	699
PH8.6	Discuss the types, kinetics, dynamics, adverse effects for drugs used for leprosy and outline management of Lepra reactions.	54	699
PH8.7	Discuss the types, kinetics, dynamics, adverse effects of drugs used for following protozoal /vector borne diseases: amoebiasis, kala-azar, malaria, filariasis.	58, 59, 60	755, 768, 777

PH8.8	Explain the types, kinetics, dynamics, adverse effects of drugs used for fungal infections.	55	725
PH8.9	Discuss the types, kinetics, dynamics, adverse effects of drugs used for intestinal helminthiasis.	60	777
PH8.10	Discuss the types, kinetics, dynamics, adverse effects, indications and contraindications of drugs used for viral diseases, including HIV.	56, 57	734, 745
PH8.11	Describe the types, kinetics, dynamics, adverse effects, indications and contraindications of anti-cancer drugs. Devise plan for amelioration of anticancer drug induced toxicity.	61	790
Miscellaneous			
PH9.1	Describe the types, kinetics, dynamics, therapeutic uses, adverse drug reactions of immunomodulators.	65	846
PH9.2	Describe management of common drug poisonings, insecticides, common stings and bites.	66	863
PH9.3	Describe chelating agents and make a plan for management of heavy metal poisoning.	66	863
PH9.4	Describe basics of vaccine use and types of vaccines.	65	846
PH9.5	Describe types, precautions and uses of antiseptics and disinfectants.	67	877
PH9.6	Describe drugs used in various skin disorders like acne vulgaris, scabies, pediculosis, psoriasis including sunscreens.	67	877
PH9.7	Describe drugs used in glaucoma and other ocular disorders including topical (ocular) drug delivery systems.	11	140
Applied Pharmacology			
PH10.1	Compare and contrast different sources of drug information and update on latest information on drugs.	70	907
PH10.2	Perform a critical evaluation of the drug promotional literature and interpret the package insert information contained in the drug package.	70	907
PH10.3	Prepare and explain a list of P-drugs for a given case/condition.	71	913
PH10.4	Describe parts of a correct, rational and legible prescription and write rational prescriptions for the provided condition (examples of conditions to be used are given with other relevant competencies).	71	913
PH10.5	Identify and apply the legal and ethical regulation of prescribing drugs, especially when prescribing for controlled drugs, off-label medicines, and prescribing for self, close family and friends.	70	907
PH10.6	Perform a critical appraisal of a given prescription and suggest ways to improve it.	71	913
PH10.7	Describe pharmacogenomics and pharmacoeconomics and manage genomic and economic issues in drug use and find out the price of given medication(s).	6, 68	76, 889
PH10.8	Describe essential medicines, fixed dose combination, over-the-counter drugs and explain steps to choose essential medicines.	70	907
PH10.9	Calculate the dosage of drugs for an individual patient, including children, elderly, pregnant and lactating women and patients with renal or hepatic dysfunction.	6	76
PH10.10	Identify when therapeutic drug monitoring is considered for a particular patient, determine timing of sampling and calculate revised dose.	6	76
PH10.11	Identify and apply drug regulations principles, acts and legal aspects related of drug discovery and clinical use.	68	889
PH10.12	Describe overview of drug development including phases of clinical trials and Good Clinical Practice and reflect on the role of research in developing new drugs.	68	889
PH10.13	Demonstrate how to optimize interaction with pharmaceutical representative/media to get/disseminate authentic information on drugs.	70	907
PH10.14	Communicate with the patient regarding optimal use of a drug therapy using empathy and professionalism, e.g., oral contraceptives, anti TB drugs, etc.	46	616
PH10.15	Describe methods to improve adherence to treatment and motivate patients with chronic diseases to adhere to the prescribed pharmacotherapy.	70	907
PH10.16	Demonstrate an understanding of the caution in prescribing drugs likely to produce dependence and recommend the line of management.	22	297
PH10.17	Demonstrate ability to educate public and patients about various aspects of drug use including drug dependence and OTC drugs.	70	907
Module 2.2 - Foundations of bioethics; **Module 2.3** - Healthcare as a right; **Module 2.5** - Patient autonomy and decision making:		72	927

Foreword

The study of pharmacology is pivotal for every medical student. It is the science that empowers future physicians with the knowledge to utilise drugs safely and effectively for the benefit of patients. With the advent of new therapeutic agents and ever-expanding indications, understanding the principles of pharmacodynamics, pharmacokinetics, drug interactions, and rational prescribing is more crucial than ever. As the field of medicine continues to evolve, pharmacology remains a cornerstone of medical education, serving as the vital bridge between the core sciences and their extrapolation to clinical practice.

The National Medical Commission (NMC) has emphasised competency-based medical education (CBME), shifting the focus from rote memorisation to an integrated and application-oriented approach. This book has been designed to align fully with these guiding principles. It has been meticulously crafted to address not only the academic and regulatory requirements but also the practical needs and aspirations of future medical practitioners in accordance with the latest regulations set forth by the NMC.

The correlation with anatomy, physiology, and biochemistry will help strengthen the basics. Explanation of drug action based on pathophysiology, the use of mnemonics for easy recall, concept maps, and concise chapter summaries will support students, employing newer learning methods to build stronger memory traces.

The disease-specific pharmacotherapy and patient management strategies, along with flowcharts to aid recall of therapeutics, coupled with clinical scenario-based MCQs, place the application of knowledge in the right perspective and reflect current treatment trends in Indian settings.

May this book serve not only as preparation for your university examinations, but also as a stepping stone towards your lifelong commitment to patient care and medical excellence. May it also be a useful aid to the faculty for fostering deeper student learning.

Best wishes and happy learning!

Dr Sandeep Kaushal
MD, FRCP (Edin), FCP (ACCP), FIMSA, MAMS, MBPhS
Dean Academics
Professor and Head, Department of Pharmacology
Dayanand Medical College and Hospital, Ludhiana, India
Former Secretary General, Indian Society for Rational Pharmacotherapeutics
Former Vice President, Medical Pharmacologists Society

Preface

The subject of Pharmacology is no longer studied in isolation; it serves as a bridge between basic biomedical and clinical sciences for rationalising pharmacotherapeutics. A sound understanding of pharmacological concepts is essential for safe and effective use of drugs. In addition, the potential risks associated with drug use—such as adverse drug reactions, toxicity, interactions with food/environmental pollutants/concurrently administered medications—as well as the cautions and contraindications, need to be considered while prescribing.

The ever-expanding classification of drugs, the complexity of their mechanisms at the cellular and molecular levels, and the exhaustive listings of therapeutic uses and ADRs makes learning pharmacology an overwhelming experience for students. This book has been crafted with these challenges in mind. Our endeavour has been to integrate fundamental concepts from anatomy and physiology with disease pathogenesis, helping learners connect drug actions with disease processes. This approach is expected to stimulate critical thinking and make learning more immersive and engaging.

This textbook is fully aligned with the revised Competency-Based Medical Education (CBME) Curriculum 2024, with careful consideration given to both horizontal and vertical integrations. To facilitate effective learning and easy recall, this textbook incorporates a variety of learning tools—innovative flowcharts to aid memorisation of drug classifications, colourful and simplified diagrams to clarify mechanisms of action, and concept maps and chapter summaries to support quick revision. Additionally, the book features engaging mnemonics, often drawn from relatable everyday situations, to enhance retention of drug classifications, therapeutic uses, and adverse drug reactions. Management guidelines, as recommended by competent professional bodies, are also included to reinforce evidence-based practice. In recent years, there has been a strong emphasis on 'early clinical exposure', competency-based assessment and the certification of core competencies, as mandated by National Medical Commission. These reforms aim to ensure that an Indian Medical Graduate (IMG) is well-equipped to function effectively as a physician of first contact, while being globally relevant. To fulfill these expectations from a medical graduate, each chapter includes clinical scenario-based MCQs designed not only to reinforce factual knowledge but also to promote its clinical application. Hints, reasoning strategies, and justifications for drug selection or contraindication in specific conditions are provided to enhance analytical thinking. We believe that such features will encourage active recall, break the monotony of continuous text, and help consolidate previously acquired knowledge in a meaningful and engaging way.

This text is the result of the teamwork of all those who believed in us, walked with us and blessed us on our journey. With deep humility and gratitude, we express our thanks to the Almighty for guiding and blessing us in this endeavour. A heartfelt tribute to our parents, whose blessings and belief in us laid the foundation for this work. We are indebted to our teacher and mentor Dr Prem Parkash Khosla for inspiring us to conceptualise this project. We express our heartfelt gratitude to our family and our children, Mehreet Singh and Prabharjun Singh, for their unwavering support, patience, and love throughout this journey. Our warmest thanks go to Dr Sukhminder Kaur for her constant motivation, encouragement, and unwavering moral support during challenging times. A very special mention and sincere appreciation of Mr. Rupinder Singh Walia, whose creativity gave form and colour to our imagination. The beautiful, simple, yet technically sound diagrams, flowcharts, and concept maps in this book owe their life to his artistic and scientific finesse.

We express gratitude to the team of reviewers, illustrators, copy editors and managers at Universities Press, Hyderabad, who have worked with us for nearly 6 years on this project. We are grateful to Mr Ravi Vishwakarma, whose belief in our vision was instrumental in bringing this project to life. We are fortunate to have had the manuscript reviewed by Dr Alpa Agrawal and Dr Sudha Ganesan, who provided valuable academic inputs to improve it. Our sincere thanks to Ms Sreelatha Menon and Dr Rohini Mani for editing the manuscript and for ensuring that the final text reflects the spirit and intent of the book. We are also deeply grateful to Mr Madhu Reddy, Director of Universities Press, for his steadfast support and guidance through all stages of publication.

Finally, we extend our sincere thanks to the faculty of the Department of Pharmacology at PIMS Jalandhar for their valuable inputs, and to our students, whose honest questions, enthusiasm, and curiosity have helped us to understand better the expectations of today's learners from a pharmacology textbook. We hope this book will serve not only as a source of knowledge but also as a trusted companion on your journey toward becoming a competent clinician.

Dr Jagminder Kaur Bajaj
Dr Satinderjit Singh Bajaj

SECTION 1 General Pharmacology

1 Introduction to Pharmacology and Pharmacotherapeutics

PH 1.1 Describe the principles of pharmacology, pharmacotherapeutics and define various terms in pharmacology.
PH 1.3 Describe the nomenclature of drugs, i.e., generic, branded and scheduled drugs, explaining the utility of the nomenclature, cost effectiveness and use.

Learning objectives

A student of MBBS phase II should be able to:
- Define the terms pharmacology and drug.
- Describe drug nomenclature.
- Differentiate various drugs based on generic and brand names.
- Describe the pros/cons of prescribing drugs by generic/brand names.
- Suggest required changes for reducing the treatment cost.
- Describe the important aspects of pharmacology—pharmacokinetics, pharmacodynamics, pharmacoeconomics, pharmacoepidemiology, toxicology, etc.
- Define pharmacotherapeutics.
- Describe the rational prescribing process.
- Recognise common irrationalities in prescribing.
- Describe measures to promote rational prescribing.

PHARMACOLOGY

The term 'pharmacology' is derived by combining two Greek words—'*pharmakon*', which means drug and '*logos*', which means study.

Pharmacology is the study of all aspects of drugs, especially those relevant to their safe and effective use as medicines. The most important branches of pharmacology deal with the following:

- What the drug does to the body (**pharmacodynamics**)
- How the drug is handled by the body (**pharmacokinetics**)
- How the drug is used for various disease conditions (**pharmacotherapeutics**)
- What could be the possible harmful effects (**toxicology**)

Pharmacology also covers drug development, clinical pharmacology, drug manufacturing (pharmaceutics) and compounding or dispensing (pharmacy).

DRUG

The term 'drug' is derived from the French word '*drogue*' meaning 'a dry herb'.

The World Health Organization (WHO) defines a drug as "any substance or product that is used or is intended to be used to modify or explore physiological systems or pathological states for the benefit of the recipient".

Q. What can act as a drug?	A. **Any substance** or product.
Q. What is the use of a drug?	A. It is a substance that is used or intended to be used to **modify or explore physiological systems** or pathological states.
Q. What should be the result of drug use?	A. It should **benefit the recipient**.

General Characteristics of Drugs

- All drugs are **chemical substances**. The majority are xenobiotics, i.e., chemicals that are foreign substances for the body. Some drugs are endogenous substances, e.g., hormones, autacoids, neurotransmitters and endorphins.
- Most drugs are **weak organic acids or bases**. Some are non-electrolytes. Only a few drugs like lithium, iron preparations and calcium preparations are inorganic substances.
- Most drugs are **solids. Liquids and gaseous substances** are also sometimes used as drugs, e.g., alcohol, volatile liquids and N_2O.
- The molecular weight of drugs generally ranges from **10 to 1000 D**, except for some very small substances (e.g., lithium ions) or very large substances (heparin, antibodies, enzymes, etc.).
- The majority of drugs are derived from **plants**, e.g., oils, alkaloids, gums, resins, tannins and glycosides. Some

are derived from **animals**, e.g., hormones, antisera and vaccines. **Microorganisms** like fungi, bacteria and actinomyces are sources of antimicrobial agents. Nowadays, almost all drugs are **synthesised chemically**. Synthetic processes of drug manufacturing offer the advantages of preparing desired quantities of drugs and developing a variety of congeners of natural products with favourable properties.

Nomenclature of Drugs

Drug nomenclature refers to the systematic naming of drugs, especially pharmaceutical drugs. For any drug, there are three types of names:

1. Chemical name
2. Non-proprietary name or pharmacological name
3. Proprietary name or trade or brand name

1. Chemical name

This is the name of a drug based on its **chemical structure**. Chemical names follow the rules established by the **International Union of Pure and Applied Chemistry (IUPAC).**

- The advantage of the chemical name is that it provides accurate information about the molecular structure of a drug. For example, the chemical name for adrenaline is (R)-4-(1-hydroxy-2-(methylamino)ethyl)benzene-1,2-diol.
- The disadvantage of chemical names is that they are very long and complex, and thus difficult to remember. Therefore, in clinical practice as well as for marketing, the chemical names of drugs are not used.

2. Non-proprietary name

When a chemical substance is found to have potential for use as a medicine, it is given a non-proprietary name by competent scientific authorities like the **United States Adopted Name (USAN)** Council, the **British Approved Name (BAN)** Council and the **World Health Organisation (WHO)**, which assign the **Recommended International Non-proprietary Name (rINN)**.

In the past, different names were sometimes given to the same chemical entity by the USAN and BAN, e.g., what the USAN refers to as epinephrine and norepinephrine are called adrenaline and noradrenaline, respectively, by the BAN. For newer drugs, the WHO recommends use of the same names throughout the world to avoid confusion. These names become official names after their inclusion in the official pharmacopoeia and are also called **pharmacological generic names**.

- **Advantages**
  - These are identical across the world.
  - An element of categorisation exists in non-proprietary names, which hints towards their pharmacological classification, e.g.:
    - β-blockers end with 'lol' (propranolol, atenolol, carvedilol).
    - Proton pump inhibitors end with 'prazole' (omeprazole, rabeprazole, pantoprazole)
    - ACE inhibitors end with 'pril' (enalapril, perindopril, lisinopril)

Thus, it becomes convenient to learn and practice with non-proprietary names.

3. Proprietary name

This is also called the trade name or brand name. Proprietary names are selected by pharmaceutical companies that manufacture the drug.

- **Advantages**
  - These names are usually small, catchy, and easy to spell and pronounce.
  - Sometimes, the trade name hints at the action of the drug, e.g., timolol eye drops have brand names like 'Glucomol' (which loosely indicates a β-blocker effective against glaucoma); sumatriptan tablets for migraine treatment are available under the brand name 'Headset'. These names are, therefore, easy to remember. These characteristics help in marketing these drugs for prescription.
- **Disadvantages**
  - There are many proprietary names for a single drug, which makes prescription by brand names non-uniform and less comprehensible.
  - Moreover, since manufacturers spend on marketing their brand, branded drugs are much costlier than generic drugs.

4. Pros and cons of generic prescription

Generic drugs must meet high standards to be approved by the US Food and Drug Administration (FDA), which is a guarantee that a certain generic drug is equivalent to its branded counterparts in providing clinical benefits.

The biggest advantage of generic drugs is that they are substantially less expensive than their branded equivalents. According to the FDA, generics can cost up to 85% less than their branded counterparts. Such significant differences in the cost of branded and generic drugs are due to the costs involved in the lengthy process of drug research, development, manufacturing, and marketing. The pharmaceutical company that introduces a drug into the market for the first time is given an exclusive right called a '**patent**' to manufacture the drug for 20 years. The patent helps the company to recover the costs incurred on the research and development of the drug. However, the company can sell its patents to other manufacturers.

When regulatory agencies ask for the promotion of prescription by generic names, they probably intend for doctors to prescribe drugs under their pharmacological names. This circumvents the problem of a **pharma–physician nexus**; physicians are forbidden from prescribing a brand of their choice. Unfortunately, this offers negligible economic benefit to patients. This is because the prescription of a pharmacological generic by the physician provides liberty to pharmacists to dispense the version of their choice, which is likely to be the one that offers them the maximum margin of profit. Hence, the effort to break the pharma–physician nexus for the benefit of patients threatens to **favour the development of a pharma–pharmacist nexus**.

The problem is compounded by the **uncertain quality control** and **quality assurance** of generic products and the availability of **spurious medicines** in the market. In such a situation, if a patient develops adverse drug reactions or fails to respond to the treatment, it becomes difficult to fix responsibility for the same.

Another disadvantage of generic prescription is that the consequent banning or control of branded drugs leaves multinational companies with no reason to manufacture their brands in India. This will result in branded drugs becoming unavailable even for patients who can afford them. The pharmaceutical industry may collapse in such circumstances.

> **Box 1.1 Generic versus brand prescription— The controversy**
>
> The prescription of drugs by brand or generic names is a matter of great controversy. The high cost of medicines is a major concern, especially for patients from lower socioeconomic brackets and patients who have chronic conditions (such as diabetes mellitus, hypertension, epilepsy and multiple sclerosis) that require long-term (sometimes lifelong) treatment. Patients often succumb to diseases simply because medicines become unaffordable. To control this situation, regulatory agencies issue orders to promote the practice of prescription by generic names. However, the solution to this problem is not so simple.
>
> In developed countries, there is no confusion about branded and generic drugs. A drug marketed by the company holding its patent (even after the patent period) is called a 'branded drug' and the remaining versions of the same drug manufactured by other companies are called 'generics'. In contrast, in India, there is no clear-cut definition of either term. Various terminologies are used in popular practice, creating confusion about branded and generic drugs:
>
> 1. **Branded drug**
>   - It is marketed with a trade name.
>   - It is manufactured by the **company holding the patent** (even after the expiry of the patent period).
>   - It is promoted among doctors by medical representatives hired by the pharmaceutical company.
>   - A branded drug is usually subjected to strict quality control and assurance measures.
>   - It is costlier than all other versions of the same drug.
> 2. **Branded generic drug**
>   - This is the same as a branded drug, except that it is **manufactured by companies other than the one holding the patent** after the expiry of the same.
>   - This version offers a higher profit margin to pharmaceutical companies.
>   - In Indian pharmaceutics, branded generics are the **most dominant versions** of drugs, probably due to the relative lack of original research and innovation.
>   - This is also costly on account of expenses incurred on promoting drugs to doctors through medical representatives.
>   - The quality control is good.
> 3. **Nominally branded generic drug**
>   - It is the version of a branded generic that is **not promoted** to doctors by medical representatives but is supplied directly to distributors and retailers.
>   - It costs much lesser than the first two varieties but offers more profit to retailers.
>   - The active ingredients are the same as in the first two varieties, but quality control may not always be the same.
> 4. **Pharmacological generic drug**
>   - It is marketed under the pharmacological name.
>   - This version is **usually supplied to hospitals** in bulk.
>   - Such a drug is sometimes called a generic.

The weighing of generic drugs against branded variants is a complicated problem, requiring attention and action on the part of government regulatory authorities. Some of the strategies that can be adopted to tackle this problem are as follows:

- The mention of the pharmacological name of a drug along with its brand name should be made mandatory (see also Box 1.1). This allows patients who can afford the branded drugs to access the same while also allowing patients who cannot afford branded drugs to access generic alternatives that meet predefined quality assurance criteria. '*Jan Aushadi*' (meaning 'drugs for the masses') stores are established to allow for this accessibility.
- Government agencies must ensure strict and continued quality control over pharmacological generics.
- Strict action in the form of fines and other punishments should be taken against defaulting pharmaceutical companies, pharmacists, and doctors.

BRANCHES OF PHARMACOLOGY

The important aspects or branches of pharmacology are pharmacokinetics, pharmacodynamics, pharmacotherapeutics, clinical pharmacology, toxicology, pharmacoepidemiology, pharmacogenomics, pharmacoeconomics and pharmacy. The salient features of these concepts are briefly described below.

Pharmacokinetics

The Greek word '*kinesis*' means movement and '*pharmaco*' refers to drugs. Thus, the word pharmacokinetics refers to the study of the manner in which a drug moves in the body and what happens to the drug during its movement in, through and out of the body or simply, what the body does to the drug. Once a drug is administered (ingested/

applied/injected), it undergoes various pharmacokinetic processes. The four most important pharmacokinetic processes of a drug are absorption, distribution, metabolism, and elimination—referred to as its ADME. These pharmacokinetic processes determine the dose–concentration relationship of the drug.

- **Absorption** refers to the movement of the drug from the site of administration to the systemic circulation. It can occur by passive diffusion, facilitated diffusion, active transport, or endocytosis. The rate and extent of drug absorption depend upon the characteristics of the drug, the absorbing surface, and the route selected for administration. Some portion of an orally administered dose gets metabolised during its movement through the intestinal wall and liver before reaching the systemic circulation. This is called the 'pre-systemic or first-pass metabolism of the drug'.

  The fraction of the administered dose that reaches the systemic circulation in the unchanged form is called **bioavailability**. It depends upon the rate and extent of absorption and first-pass metabolism. The greater the first-pass metabolism of a drug, the lesser is its oral bioavailability. The term **bioequivalence** refers to a comparison of the bioavailability of two different preparations of the same drug (from different manufacturers/different batches produced by the same manufacturer) that contain the same amount of the drug.

- **Distribution** is the reversible movement of the drug from the systemic circulation to tissues along the concentration gradient. It continues until equilibrium is attained between the unbound drug (drug not bound to plasma proteins) in the plasma and tissue fluid.

  The fluid volume that would accommodate the whole of the dose administered intravenously (assuming that concentration throughout body fluids is the same as that in plasma) is called the '**apparent volume of distribution**' of the drug. It depends on the ionisation, lipid solubility of the drug, its affinity for binding proteins and regional blood flow. Different drugs have different levels of affinity for binding plasma and tissue proteins. Binding to plasma proteins provides a temporary store for the drug, restricts its volume of distribution and prolongs its duration of action. On the other hand, drugs with an affinity for specific **tissue proteins** get sequestrated in tissues and have a large volume of distribution (even larger than the total water content in the body).

  Tight inter-endothelial junctions of the capillaries of the brain constitute the **blood–brain barrier**. Only highly lipid-soluble, unionised drugs can cross this barrier. Such drugs produce central effects. The **placental barrier**, constituted by a layer of trophoblastic cells in the chorionic villi, is an incomplete barrier easily crossed by lipid-soluble, unionised drugs. Some water-soluble, ionised drugs can also cross the placental barrier when the maternal–fetal concentration gradient is sufficiently high. Thus, certain drugs, when given to women during pregnancy, may cross the placenta and adversely affect fetal organogenesis, growth and development. These harmful effects on the fetus are called **teratogenic** effects. All drugs should be considered teratogenic (unless proven safe) and prescribed cautiously during pregnancy.

- **Biotransformation or metabolism** ('bio' means living and 'transformation' means alteration) refers to the chemical alteration of the drug by the body. It plays an important role in terminating drug action. Biotransformation occurs at some point between the drug's absorption into circulation and its renal excretion. The **liver is the main site of metabolism**. However, other tissues like the gastrointestinal tract, lungs, skin, kidneys and brain also have considerable ability to metabolise drugs. Most drugs are inactivated by metabolism, but some drugs produce active metabolites too. A few drugs are administered in their inactive form and get activated by metabolic reactions in the body. Such drugs are called **prodrugs**.

  Metabolic reactions are of two types—**phase I** and **phase II reactions**, sometimes called non-synthetic and synthetic reactions, respectively. The enzymes that catalyse drug metabolism are of two types, **microsomal and non-microsomal enzymes**. These enzymes differ in their distribution in the body, the types of reactions they catalyse and their affinity for enzyme inducers. Some drugs undergo spontaneous reorganisation without the catalytic effect of any enzyme. Such elimination is called **Hofmann elimination.**

- **Excretion** is the last pharmacokinetic process. Here, the drug or its metabolites are passed out of the body through **urine, feces, exhaled air, saliva, sweat, or even milk**. All the water-soluble substances are excreted by the kidney through glomerular filtration, tubular reabsorption and tubular secretion. Unabsorbed drugs are excreted through feces or secreted in bile. Gases, volatile liquids and particulate matter are exhaled out of the body through the lungs. Only some drugs like lithium, potassium iodide (KI) and heavy metals are excreted in saliva and sweat. The excretion of drugs in milk may affect the suckling infant. So, drugs should be prescribed to lactating women only when absolutely indicated.

Clinical problem-based questions and MCQs

1. The 'pharmacological generic name' of a drug is same as its:
   a. Chemical name
   b. Non-proprietary name
   c. Brand name
   d. Proprietary name

2. The non-proprietary names of drugs have all the following advantages EXCEPT:
   a. Are convenient to use in practice
   b. Are the same across the world
   c. Have some element of categorisation
   d. Are small, catchy and easy to pronounce

3. The pharmaceutical company that introduces a drug into the market for the first time is given an exclusive right to manufacture this drug for 20 years.
   i. What is this right called?
      a. Patent   b. License
      c. Registration   d. Commercial
   ii. What is the need for such an exclusive right to be given to the drug developing company?

4. In India, a drug preparation manufactured by companies other than the one holding the patent, after the expiry of the patent and promoted to doctors through medical representatives is known as a:
   a. Generic drug
   b. Branded drug
   c. Branded generic drug
   d. Pharmacological generic drug

5. The fraction of a drug that reaches the systemic circulation in its unchanged form is called:
   a. Bioavailability
   b. Bioequivalence
   c. Extent of absorption
   d. Volume of distribution

6. The volume of distribution of a drug depends upon all of the following factors EXCEPT:
   a. Regional blood flow
   b. Affinity for plasma proteins
   c. Tissue sequestration
   d. Pre-systemic metabolism

7. A 34-year-old woman, who is a known case of hypertension, was on enalapril therapy. She presented with amenorrhea for 3 weeks. The urine pregnancy test was positive. The prescribing doctor changed her antihypertensive medicine to prevent harm to the fetus. What is the term used for harmful effects of drugs on fetus in utero?
   a. Mutagenic effect   b. Teratogenic effect
   c. Idiosyncratic effect   d. Organogenic effect

8. Drugs and their inactive metabolites are mainly excreted through urine. However, some drugs are excreted in sweat and saliva also. Identify the drug that can be excreted through these secretions.
   a. Lithium   b. Streptomycin
   c. Thiopentone sodium   d. All the above

Pharmacodynamics

Once the drug reaches its site of action, it exerts its effect through a series of intermediate steps. Pharmacodynamics is the study of the biological effects of drugs and how these effects are exerted, i.e., what the drug does to the body.

Mechanism of action of a drug

No drug is capable of imparting any new function to any organ system or tissue. All drugs exert their actions by **modifying the ongoing functions of cells, tissues, or organ systems.** Drugs can cause stimulation/inhibition of bodily function, irritation of epithelial or connective tissues, cytotoxicity on selective cells (cancer cells/microorganisms) or replacement of deficient hormones or natural metabolites, etc.

- Drugs may produce effects on account of their **physical properties** (mass, opacity, radioactivity, adsorptive or osmotic activity) or **chemical properties** (neutralisation, complex formation, or oxidising activity).

- The majority of drugs produce their effects by interacting with specific macromolecules called 'receptors', that are present on the target cell membrane or inside it called 'receptors'. **Receptors** serve as a binding site for the drug and initiate a series of steps resulting in a response. The ability of a drug to bind to receptors is called its '**affinity**'; the ability of a drug to produce a conformational change in the receptors to bring about the response is called its '**intrinsic activity**'. The interaction of a drug with its receptors is not an all-or-none type of response; submaximal or partial responses are also seen. Based on these two properties (affinity and intrinsic activity), a drug can act as an **agonist, partial agonist, antagonist, or inverse agonist** at a particular receptor. All drugs have an affinity for their respective receptors. Drugs that exhibit maximal or submaximal intrinsic activity are called agonists and partial agonists, respectively. On the other hand, drugs that lack intrinsic activity are called antagonists. The intrinsic activity of inverse agonists is in a direction opposite to that of an agonist.

- **Antagonism** can be of four types—physical, chemical, physiological, and receptor antagonism. Physical antagonism is based on the adsorptive effect of drugs, like charcoal. Chemical antagonism involves simple chemical reactions like acid–base neutralisation. Physiological antagonists have diagonally opposite effects on body functions, e.g., histamine and adrenaline have opposing effects on the bronchi and vascular smooth muscles. Receptor antagonism can be further classified into two types—competitive and non-competitive.

- Drug–receptor binding produces a conformational change in receptors, initiating complex multistep processes that amplify and integrate various intracellular and extracellular signals. These are called **transduction mechanisms.** These mechanisms include GTP-activated protein-coupled receptors (GPCR), receptors with intrinsic ion channels, transmembrane receptors linked to tyrosine kinase enzyme/Janus kinase (JAK), signal transducers and activators of transcription (STAT) and receptors regulating gene expression.

- The continuous presence of an agonist or antagonist alters the level of ongoing activity, resulting in **receptor regulation**. This becomes clinically important during the discontinuation of drug therapy—the sudden discontinuation of a drug may be associated with hazardous effects and needs to be properly managed.
- Certain drugs alter the pace of ongoing reactions by **stimulating or inhibiting key enzymes**, increasing or decreasing the rate of the reactions catalysed by them. The enzyme inhibitors may compete with the natural substrate for the catalytic site (competitive inhibition) or bind to an adjacent site on the enzyme (non-competitive inhibition).
- A few drugs act by modulating specific ligand-gated, voltage-sensitive, or stretch-sensitive **ion channels**.
- Some drugs interfere with the **functioning of transporter proteins**, altering the movement of neurotransmitters, autacoids or other endogenous substances across membranes.
- The **dose–response curve (DRC)** is the bridge linking pharmacokinetics and pharmacodynamics. The dose–concentration part depends on pharmacokinetic processes and the concentration–response part depends on the pharmacodynamic characteristics of the drug. DRC is important for estimating the potency, efficacy, selectivity and margin of safety of drugs.

Clinical Pharmacology

This is a branch of pharmacology dealing with the scientific study of the effect of drugs on humans. Data on the potency, efficacy, dose and safety of new drugs are generated to practice '**evidence-based medicine**' **(EBM)**. In this approach, the best 'course of action' is chosen from amongst several available alternatives based on scientifically credible evidence.

There exists a hierarchy of study designs which generates different levels of evidence. Human research can be conducted with or without a comparison group, referred to as **analytical** or **descriptive**, respectively. In some study designs, the investigator does not intervene in the ongoing treatment process but only observes the exposure and outcomes (**observational** study); in others, the investigator assigns a diagnostic/preventive/therapeutic intervention and measures the response (**interventional** studies). Randomised controlled trials (RCTs) are considered the gold-standard and generate evidence of the highest level.

Toxicology

The literal meaning of toxicology is the 'study of toxins'. **Toxins** are harmful chemicals that are produced biologically within a cell or organism. '**Poisons**' are substances that cause harm when ingested, inhaled, or absorbed into circulation by any route. Thus, it can be inferred that all poisons are not toxins; however, these terms are often used interchangeably.

- In the context of pharmacotherapeutics, toxicology deals with the **harmful effects of drugs** on humans. Every drug is a poison in a large dose, though drugs can cause harmful or adverse effects even at therapeutic doses. An **adverse drug reaction** (ADR) is any noxious change, suspected to be caused by a drug, occurring at doses normally used in humans. It may require dose reduction, treatment, or caution for use in future. ADRs can be of **five types**—A, B, C, D, or E. Type A reactions are augmented pharmacological effects of a drug. Type B reactions are bizarre and cannot be predicted from pharmacological actions of drugs, e.g., drug allergies. Type C reactions are associated with chronic use. Type D are delayed effects that occur a long time after the use of the drug. Type E reactions are associated with the end of the use of the drug, i.e., withdrawal from the drug.
- ADRs are an additional burden on the health system. They can be prevented and managed if they are detected early. **Pharmacovigilance** involves detecting, documenting and reporting adverse events/reactions associated with drug use to regulatory authorities. The WHO–Uppsala monitoring scale is generally used for causality assessment of reported ADRs. On this scale, the association between the reported reaction and the drug is rated as certain, probable, possible, unlikely, conditional, or unclassifiable. These reports of ADRs guide necessary action by regulatory authorities, such as ban of a drug, modification of a package insert, changes in labelling, restrictions in the use, or precautions or warnings and information dissemination through drug alerts, medical letters, advisories, etc.

Pharmacoeconomics

This involves identifying, measuring and comparing the costs and consequences of pharmaceutical products and services from the perspective of patients/providers/payers and society. It helps in making a fully informed decision regarding the appropriate use of drugs and in allocating scarce resources. Pharmacoeconomic studies include the comparison of generic versus branded medicines for **cost minimisation analysis**; measurement of outcomes such as the number of cases cured/lives saved for **cost-effectiveness analysis**; calculation of the ratio of benefit to cost for **cost–benefit analysis**; and assessment of costs in comparison to outcomes (expressed as the quality of life) for **cost–utility analysis**. Pharmacoeconomics helps in enhancing the quality of patient care and clinical practice as it strengthens the evaluation process.

Pharmacoepidemiology

This entails the study of drug use among certain populations, involving thousands or even millions of people. These studies aim at ensuring the safety, efficacy and quality of drugs. Epidemiological principles are applied to the use of drugs. Global patterns of prescription of drugs, adherence to prescribed medicines, appropriateness of prescribed drugs, drug–drug interactions, and ADRs are studied in large populations. Various descriptive and interventional study designs are used for pharmacoepidemiologic studies.

Pharmacogenetics

The response of every individual to a drug is not the same. There are significant inter-individual variations in drug response. The study of genetic factors that results in variations in drug response among individuals in a population is called pharmacogenomics. It is a broad term involving the investigation of variations at the genomic level by sequencing of the human genome and testing genome-wide variants for associations with drug response. **Pharmacogenetics**, which involves the study of variations in a targeted gene or group of functionally related genes, is a part of pharmacogenomics.

These studies guide appropriate changes to be made while choosing a drug and dose for a particular patient and form the basis of 'genome medicine' or 'personalised medicine'.

Pharmacy

Pharmacy is the art and science of compounding, preparing and dispensing drugs. It involves identifying, selecting, collecting, purifying, isolating and standardising medicines.

> ### Clinical problem-based questions and MCQs
>
> 9. A drug that produces a biological response similar to that of an endogenous ligand after binding to the receptors is known as:
>   a. Partial agonist   b. Agonist
>   c. Inverse agonist   d. Functional agonist
>
> 10. A patient diagnosed with severe deep vein thrombosis (DVT) is being managed with heparin IV infusion. Patient develops features of heparin overdose in the form of hematuria and thrombocytopenia. Protamine sulphate is injected intravenously to neutralise heparin and control its toxic effects. The use of protamine in heparin toxicity is an example of:
>   a. Competitive antagonism
>   b. Non-competitive antagonism
>   c. Chemical antagonism
>   d. Physiological antagonism
>
> 11. A 36-year-old female patient with a lower respiratory tract infection was given amoxicillin (penicillin). After a few minutes of the first dose, the patient developed rashes and itching. What type of adverse drug reaction is this?
>   a. Type A   b. Type B
>   c. Type C   d. Type D
>   e. Type E
>
> 12. Pharmacovigilance involves all of the following activities EXCEPT:
>   a. Detecting, documenting, and reporting adverse drug reactions
>   b. Dosage calculation for different age groups
>   c. Causality assessment
>   d. Information dissemination
>
> 13. Which of the following concepts serves as a bridge between pharmacokinetics and pharmacodynamics?
>   a. Drug–receptor binding
>   b. Volume of distribution
>   c. Dose–response curve
>   d. Bioavailability
>
> 14. The concept of personalised medicine is based on:
>   a. Pharmacogenetic studies
>   b. Pharmacoeconomic studies
>   c. Cost–utility analysis
>   d. Cost–effectiveness analysis
>
> 15. In which of the following studies is there a comparison of costs to outcomes expressed as quality of life?
>   a. Cost–effectiveness analysis
>   b. Cost–benefit analysis
>   c. Cost–utility analysis
>   d. Cost–minimisation analysis

PHARMACOTHERAPEUTICS

Pharmacotherapeutics is concerned with the **use of drugs for the prevention, diagnosis and treatment of diseases**. It also includes the use of drugs for the **alteration of physiological functions**, such as oral contraceptives for the prevention of pregnancy.

Pharmacotherapeutics links the pharmacokinetics/pharmacodynamics of drugs with the biochemical/pathophysiological/microbiological features of a disease to make informed decisions about the clinical use of drugs for desired beneficial outcomes with minimal adverse effects. The study of all possible factors that can alter drug response qualitatively or quantitatively is important for optimum therapy.

Rational Use of Medicines

The rational use of medicines is defined by WHO as "patients receiving medication appropriate to their clinical needs, in doses that meet their individual requirements, for an adequate period of time and at the lowest cost to them and their community".

Rational prescribing is one of many **steps comprising the rational use of medicines** like selection, procurement, prescription, dispensing, monitoring, and feedback. Rational prescribing involves the following:

- Choice of the **correct drug** to treat/manage the disease.
- **Sound medical basis** to justify the use of a drug in a particular condition.

- Appropriate **dose, route** of administration, and **duration** of treatment for the individual patient, considering his/her specific features.
- Ensuring the **acceptability** of a drug by ruling out any contraindication for its use in a particular patient and minimising chances of adverse effects.
- Proper **dispensing** and **instructions** to patients about the correct use of a drug.
- Follow-up to check the patient's **compliance** with instructions and to monitor improvement of the disease or the development of adverse effects.

Irrational Drug Use

Any use of medication that is not in accordance with the above-mentioned criteria is deemed irrational. The common irrationalities in drug use are as follows.

a. Overuse of drugs

Sometimes drugs are prescribed in situations where they are not needed. Some of these situations are described below.

- **Antibiotics** are frequently prescribed to treat viral diarrheas, especially in children although rational therapy for this indication comprises the maintenance of fluid–electrolyte balance.
- **Antimicrobials** are prescribed for non-bacterial infections or for prophylaxis in patients undergoing clean, elective surgeries. Empirically, broad-spectrum antimicrobial agents are given before diagnosing the exact cause of infection.
- The practice of prescribing **too many medicines** to every patient also contributes to the overuse of drugs, e.g., drugs for decreasing gastric HCl secretion (**proton pump inhibitors, histamine H_2 receptor blockers,** etc.) prescribed to patients receiving analgesics or other drugs which have the potential to cause a gastric irritant effect.
- Vitamins and other **nutritional supplements** are also prescribed very commonly without any clear indication for their use.
- Another factor is the inappropriate self-medication of **'over-the-counter' drugs** by patients themselves, especially antiallergic drugs, analgesics, etc.

b. Inappropriate choices

Sometimes, the drug chosen is not the most appropriate one for a particular condition. Sound knowledge of drug actions and disease condition, the factors affecting drug action, their kinetics and the presence of any contraindications is a must for choosing the most appropriate drug in a particular situation.

- **Underuse of drugs**—the dose and frequency of administration of a drug is not adequate sometimes. The prescriber must know the various patient factors that can alter the dose required. Antibiotics, in particular, are often given in **inadequate dosage/frequency for inadequate duration**. This plays a detrimental role by favouring the development of drug-resistant microbial strains.
- **Inappropriate route of administration** is also considered irrational, e.g., prescribing a drug for parenteral administration when oral administration is possible or prescribing drugs (especially corticosteroids) to patients with bronchial asthma or COPD by the oral or parenteral route when inhalational administration is feasible and will have fewer systemic adverse effects.
- The selection of **costly, branded** drugs over equi-efficacious generic drugs is also irrational and poses an extra burden on the patient's pocket.
- Sometimes, because of the patient load and resulting time constraints, adequate instructions for using the drug and information regarding the warning signs of possible adverse effects are not provided to patients or their attendants. This lack of information about **appropriate drug use,** dose adjustments and regular follow-up is also considered irrational. This is especially important in the case of patients suffering from chronic diseases like diabetes, hypertension, epilepsy, etc., which need long-term (or even lifelong) treatment.

Implications of irrational use of drugs

Irrationalities in drug use as mentioned above are associated with many adverse consequences such as:

- Non-responsiveness or worsening of the condition for which the patient sought treatment in the first place and poor treatment outcomes.
- Increased risk of adverse effects of drugs, drug–drug interactions (DDI) and drug–food interactions.
- The emergence of drug-resistant strains that pose a serious challenge.
- Increased economic burden on the patient because of the worsening of the disease, which may cause or prolong hospitalisation, increase the treatment cost, additional loss of work hours, etc.
- Wastage of meagre resources and deviation of funds from necessary expenditure.

Rational Prescribing

Rational prescribing is a **stepwise process** in which there is a logical flow from one step to the next. Caution is exercised at each step to avoid common errors. The process is said to be complete when pre-decided therapeutic goals (cure/symptom relief/prevention/palliation) are achieved. Steps of rational prescribing include the following:

- Establishing the diagnosis based on history, clinical signs and interpretation of appropriate investigations.
- Defining therapeutic problems, deciding goals to be achieved and selecting drugs appropriate to achieve the same. The selection of drugs appropriate for

a particular clinical situation involves a thorough consideration of numerous drug-related, patient-related and environmental factors.
- **Drug-related factors:** Suitable route of administration, frequency of administration, treatment duration, need for monitoring, potential to cause ADRs/interactions, cost, etc.
- **Patient-related factors:**
  o Indication for drug use
  o Age, weight, renal/hepatic status, etc.
  o Presence of co-morbidities that may contraindicate a drug
  o Other simultaneously administered drugs (including over-the-counter drugs, substances of abuse, AYUSH drugs, etc.)
  o Educational, economic and mental status of the patient to ensure compliance with prescribed drugs
  o Pregnancy and lactational status in the case of female patients to prevent risk to the fetus/suckling infant
  o It must be ensured that patients' beliefs, concerns and expectations are taken into consideration.
- **Environmental factors:** Food, environmental pollutants and surroundings may alter the pharmacokinetics of a drug (e.g., enzyme induction/inhibition).
- Once drugs are selected, the **appropriate route, dose, dosage interval and duration** of treatment are decided.
- After prescribing, all the important **information about the correct use** of the medicine and warning signs and expected side effects should be provided to patients in a language easily comprehensible to them.
- Follow-up should be planned to **monitor the patient's adherence** to the prescribed regimen, development of any **ADRs,** and to ascertain the extent to which the therapeutic goal is achieved. If the result of the treatment is not as expected, appropriate changes and modifications should be made to the selected drugs, their dose, or the frequency of administration.
- Any adverse effects, if detected, should be promptly treated and reported.

Measures to promote rational drug use
- Physicians should be made aware of essential drugs, drug formulary, and standard treatment guidelines.
- A drugs and therapeutics committee should be constituted in hospitals to ensure the safe, rational use of drugs.
- Supervisions and prescription audits can enhance rational practices.
- Efforts should be made to continuously update the knowledge of healthcare professionals to keep them abreast with recent developments in their field of specialisation.
- There should be a coordinated effort to increase public awareness regarding rational medication and essential drug concepts.
- Sufficient funds should be available within the public health system for procurement.

CHEMOTHERAPY

It is a branch of pharmacotherapeutics that deals with the use of chemical substances for reducing the rate of multiplication of microorganisms in the human body (static effect, e.g., bacteriostatic, fungistatic) or for the killing of microorganisms (cidal effect, e.g., tuberculocidal, bactericidal). As cancer or tumour formation also involves uncontrolled cell multiplication that causes harmful effects inside the body, drugs that stop the growth of cancer cells or selectively kill them are also considered chemotherapy.

In both these situations, drugs that have a selective effect on pathogenic organisms or cancer cells and spare the normal host cells are more useful and less toxic.

Summary
- Pharmacology is study of drugs. Drugs are substances used to modify or explore physiological systems or pathological states for the benefit of the patient.
- Its important branches are pharmacokinetics, pharmacodynamics, pharmacotherapeutics, clinical pharmacology, pharmacy, toxicology and chemotherapy.
- Pharmacokinetic processes involve the movement of drugs in, through and out of body by four processes, i.e., absorption, distribution, metabolism and excretion.
- Pharmacodynamics deals with mechanism of action and effects of drugs.
- Pharmacotherapeutics is the application of pharmacology information for prevention and treatment of diseases.
- Rational use of drugs is a stepwise process to ensure that patients are receiving medication appropriate to their clinical needs, in doses that meet their individual requirements, for an adequate period of time and at the lowest cost to them and their community.
- Clinical pharmacology involves pharmacokinetic/pharmacodynamic investigations in humans to evaluate safety and efficacy of drugs.
- Pharmacy deals with the compounding and dispensing of drugs.
- Toxicology is the study of harmful effects of drugs and poisons.
- Chemotherapy is the use of drugs for infectious and malignant diseases.

Questions for practice

1. Define the following:
   a. Pharmacogenomics
   b. Pharmacokinetics
   c. Pharmacodynamics
   d. Chemotherapy
2. Enumerate:
   a. Various activities included in pharmacovigilance
   b. Steps of rational prescribing

Hints for problem-based questions and MCQs

1. b. Non-proprietary name
2. d. Are small, catchy, and easy to pronounce; this is the advantage of proprietary names.
3. i. a. Patent
   ii. A patent is given to a manufacturer to help them recover the costs incurred on the research and development of the drug.
4. c. Branded generic drug
5. a. Bioavailability
6. d. Presystemic metabolism affects the bioavailability of the drug but not its volume of distribution.
7. b. Teratogenic effect
8. a. Lithium
9. b. Agonist
10. c. Chemical antagonism—heparin is acidic and protamine is basic in nature; hence protamine neutralises heparin.
11. b. Type B or bizarre—amoxicillin is an antimicrobial drug; rashes and itching are allergic reactions that cannot be predicted from its pharmacological actions.
12. b. Dosage calculation for different age groups is not included in pharmacovigilance.
13. c. The dose–response curve is a bridge between pharmacokinetics and pharmacodynamics.
14. a. Pharmacogenetic studies guide personalised or genome medicine.
15. c. Cost–utility analysis

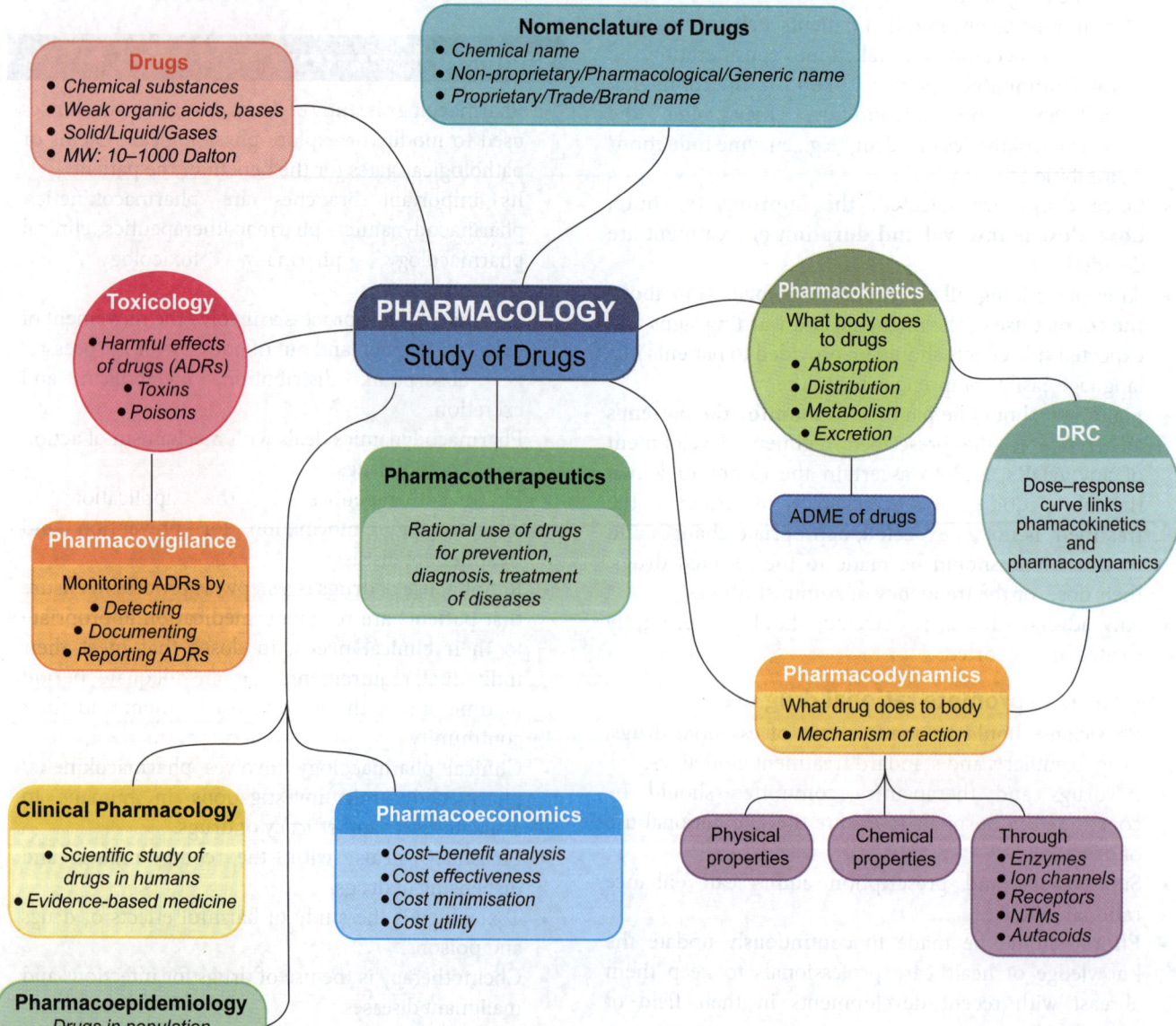

SECTION 1   General Pharmacology

2   Routes of Drug Administration

PH 1.4 Identify the common drug formulations and drug delivery systems, demonstrate their use and describe their advantages and disadvantages.
PH 1.5 Describe various routes of drug administration, their advantages and disadvantages and demonstrate administration of SC, IV, IM, SL, rectal, spinal, intranasal sprays and inhalers.

Learning objectives

A student of MBBS phase II should be able to:
- Enumerate the factors that determine the route of administration of a drug.
- Enumerate the various routes of administration of drugs.
- Describe the frequently used routes of drug administration (oral, sublingual, intravenous, intramuscular, subcutaneous) and enumerate their advantages and disadvantages.
- Describe drug formulations specific for different routes.
- Demonstrate the correct administration of various dosage forms in a simulated environment.
- Enumerate various drug delivery systems.
- Describe the correct use of various drug delivery systems.

Drugs can be administered by various routes such as oral, topical and parenteral. The route to be used in a particular situation depends on numerous drug-/patient-/disease-related factors. Drug molecules are delivered to their site of action within the body by vehicles called **dosage forms/ drug formulations/ pharmaceutical formulations**. There are specific dosage forms for different routes. A dosage form contains pharmaceutical excipients in addition to active ingredients.

Dosage forms are classified based on their physical characteristics and the route through which they are administered.

FACTORS DETERMINING THE ROUTE OF ADMINISTRATION

Drugs can be administered to human beings by different routes. Several drug-, patient-, and disease-related factors are considered before deciding the most suitable route of drug administration in a particular situation.

Drug-Related Factors
This includes **physical and chemical properties of drugs such** as:
- **Physical state** (solid/liquid/gas): Gaseous drugs can be given only by the inhalational route.
- The **pKa** and degree of ionisation of the drug: The unionised form of a drug easily crosses biological membranes, but not its ionised form.
- **Polar or non-polar** nature: Non-polar drugs readily cross membranes, whereas polar ones do not.
- The **aqueous and lipid solubility, stability, irritant, or non-irritant** nature of the drug also matters while deciding the route of its administration. Highly lipid-soluble drugs can cross even intact skin; drugs with irritant effects are usually administered by the intravenous route.
- **Pharmacokinetic characteristics** of the drug such as the rate and extent of absorption from various sites, the effect of digestive enzymes, the extent of first-pass metabolism, and route of excretion, are also important considerations.

Patient- and Disease-Related Factors
- **Rapidity with which a response is required:** In an **emergency**, when an immediate response is required, the intravenous route is preferred.
- **Condition of the patient:** Whether the patient is conscious or not and cooperative or not and whether they have symptoms such as vomiting have bearing on the route of administration; e.g., the oral route is not feasible for a patient who is vomiting or unconscious.
- **Site of desired action:** Whether the site is accessible or not accessible; e.g., for action on the skin and mucous membranes, drugs can be applied topically, whereas for action on the internal organs, drugs must be administered by the systemic routes.

ROUTES OF DRUG ADMINISTRATION

Based on the **extent of action desired**, routes of drug administration can be broadly divided into two groups, **local** and **systemic**.

LOCAL ROUTES

These routes are chiefly used when drug action is required **locally, at an accessible site**. Drug use by local routes allows **minimal absorption** into systemic circulation, so that the drug attains maximum concentration at the desired site of action without affecting other parts of the body. Thus, the greatest advantage of local routes is **negligible systemic toxicity**. Drugs can be conveniently administered using this route without any need for assistance in most cases.

The disadvantage of local drug administration is that these routes are **not suitable for systemic effects** except in the case of a few highly lipid-soluble drugs used as transdermal patches, e.g., glyceryl trinitrate and nicotine patches.

The various local routes are discussed below.

I. Topical Routes

These involve the administration/application of the drug on the surface of:

1. **Skin:** Drug absorption from local sites depends on the thickness of the skin; absorption is maximum at the posterior auricular area, followed by the scrotal skin, scalp, dorsum of the hand and plantar area. Dosage forms like ointment, paste, cream, lotion, paint, liniment, gel, dusting powder, and spray are administered by this route.
2. **Mucous membranes:** These include the oral mucosa, nasal mucosa, anal canal, urethra, vagina, eyes, and ear canal. Important dosage forms for each site are:
   - Mucous membrane of the oral cavity: rinses, mouthwash, gargles, gel, paint, lozenges
   - Nasal mucosa: nasal drops, spray, ointment
   - Eyes and ears: eye drops, ointment, ear drops
   - Rectal/anal canal: suppository
   - Urethra: jellies
   - Vagina: cream, pessaries
   - Bladder: irrigation fluids
   - Gastrointestinal mucosa: oral administration of drugs that do not get absorbed and act locally, e.g., sucralfate, oxetacaine and neomycin

Dosage forms for administration via skin and mucous membranes

1. **Ointments** are **semi-solid, greasy preparations** intended for external application on the skin and mucous membranes. An ointment has a base which acts as a vehicle for the active drug and contains **less than 10% of the powdered ingredients**. The base acts as an emollient to apply the suspended/dissolved medications on the skin and mucous membranes. Ointments are applied on the affected part and rubbed in for therapeutic effect. The presence of an occlusive dressing increases the duration of drug action and maintains hydration of the skin. Ointments can be of **three types,** based on the degree of their penetration into the skin:
   - **Epidermic ointments** penetrate the skin poorly and act only on its surface, e.g., astringents and antiseptics.
   - **Endodermic ointments** partially penetrate the skin, e.g., analgesics and counter-irritants.
   - **Diadermic ointments** are absorbed through the skin to exert a systemic effect, e.g., nitroglycerine ointment.
2. **Pastes** are ointments with a high **powdered content** (> 10%). They are less penetrating, generate less heat, and are stiffer than ointments and **non-greasy**. They are used as protective barriers against the sun and are suitable for use on oozing/moist lesions. A **poultice** is a soft, pasty, viscous preparation that supplies warmth to inflamed parts of the skin.
3. **Creams** are **semisolid emulsions**, i.e., a mixture of oil and water. They can be of two types: oil-in-water or water-in-oil. They are **less greasy than ointments** and hence more acceptable, e.g., cold cream and shaving cream.
4. **Lotions** are **liquid suspensions** applied gently on the skin or mucous membrane without rubbing. They may have soothing, cooling, astringent, antiseptic, and protective effects.
5. **Paints** are liquid preparations that contain **active ingredients in semisolid solvents such as liquid paraffin.** They are applied on the skin or mucous membranes, e.g., povidone–iodine.
6. **Liniments** are **liquid preparations** with an **oil/soap base**. They are rubbed or massaged on the skin for counter-irritant, rubefacient, or astringent effects. They should not be used on bruised or wounded skin.
7. **Gels** consist of a **liquid phase contained within a 3D polymeric matrix** of natural or synthetic gum. These are appropriate for use on hairy parts of the body.
8. **Gargles and mouthwashes** are **aqueous solutions** of povidone–iodine, betahexidine, or saline. They are used for oral hygiene and extend a soothing effect when used for throat infections.
9. **Drops** are solutions, emulsions, or suspensions administered in small volumes.
10. **Dusting powders** are free-flowing, **fine powders** with particle size < 150 μm. They are intended for external use, e.g., talc, neomycin powder and sulfadiazine powder, and are sprinkled from an airtight container through a perforated lid.

11. **Lozenges** are **solid** formulations **containing sugar and gum** that allow the drug to dissolve slowly in the mouth, e.g., cough lozenges.
12. **Pastilles** are softer than lozenges and contain gelatin, sugar, or glue. They dissolve slowly in the mouth, releasing the drug slowly, e.g., fruit pastilles or jellies.
13. **Dental cone** is a form of tablet that contains antibiotics or antiseptics, which is placed in the empty socket after tooth extraction.
14. **Rectal dosage forms**
    - **Suppository** is a cone-shaped, solid, medicated mass that melts at body temperature upon insertion into the rectum, e.g., diazepam in children diagnosed with status epilepticus. Such administration causes unpredictable levels, local irritation and is inconvenient.
    - **Enema** is a liquid dosage form that is administered into the rectum and colon via the anus. An evacuation enema is used for bowel clearing, while a retention enema is used for local and systemic effects.
15. **Vaginal dosage forms**
    - **Pessaries or vaginal tablets** are ovoid tablets with a rounded apex. These are molded and compressed tablets that are inserted into the vagina with an applicator to produce a local effect, e.g., clotrimazole vaginal tablets.
16. **Irrigations** are solutions used for washing surgical wounds and body cavities, e.g., sodium chloride irrigation.
17. **Douches** are aqueous solutions used for antiseptic or cleansing effects.
18. **Intrauterine devices** may be medicated or non-medicated, e.g., CuT and progestasert.

II. Inhalational Route

Inhalation is used both for local as well as systemic effects. The biggest advantage of the inhalational route for local effect in the lungs is the lack of systemic adverse effects. For local effects in the bronchi, devices such as nebulisers, rotahalers, pressurised metered dose inhalers and spacers are used.

1. A **rotahaler** (Fig. 2.1) consists of a **reservoir** or container that has a raised hole for loading the capsule and a **mouthpiece**. Prior to use, the device is first assembled from the two pieces by twisting the barrel in one direction until it stops. Then, one '**rotacap**' (a capsule made specifically for use in a rotahaler) is inserted into the raised hole. The lower end of the device is then turned in the opposite direction as much as possible to break the shell of the rotacap.

    The mouthpiece is held tightly between the lips to ensure a complete air seal. Then, the user takes a quick,

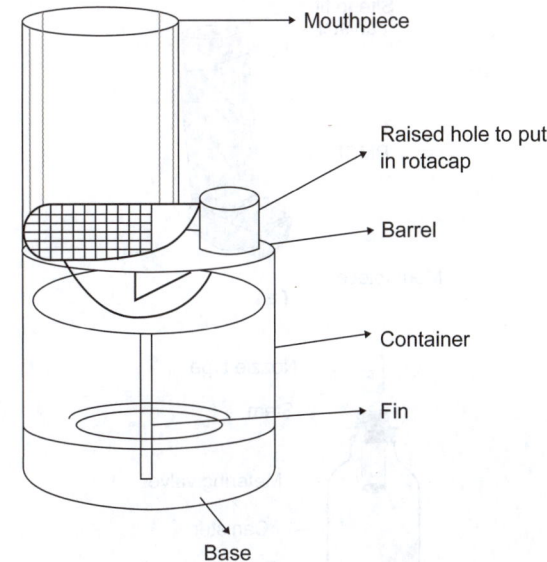

Fig. 2.1 Rotahaler

deep breath through the mouth, holds breath for as long as possible, and then slowly exhales. The microfine particles of the active drug get deposited in the lungs, whereas the larger carrier particles remain in the oropharynx. Therefore, the patient should rinse mouth after using the rotahaler.

2. **The pressurised metered dose inhaler** (PMDI, Fig. 2.2), also known as a hydrofluoroalkane inhaler, is a **handheld device** that works like a spray can. When pushed, it produces a fine mist of pressurised aerosols that **administers a predefined dose of the drug in each puff**. Therefore, it is called the 'metered dose' inhaler.

    A PMDI consists of a handheld plastic pump, a mouthpiece (Fig. 2.2a), and a pressurised metal canister that contains the drug solution. The canister is equipped with a valve to regulate the amount of drug delivered per puff (Fig. 2.2b).

    Detailed instructions must be given to patients to ensure the correct use of this device. The inhaler should be shaken well before removing the dust cap over the mouthpiece. First, the patient should sit in a comfortable position and exhale slowly. Holding the device upside down and with head tilted slightly backwards, the patient should hold the mouthpiece tightly with lips and breathe slowly while pressing down on the metal canister (Fig. 2.2c). Both these processes must be simultaneous for proper drug administration. The patient should then remove the mouthpiece and hold breath for 10 seconds or as long as possible. There should be a gap before taking the next puff.

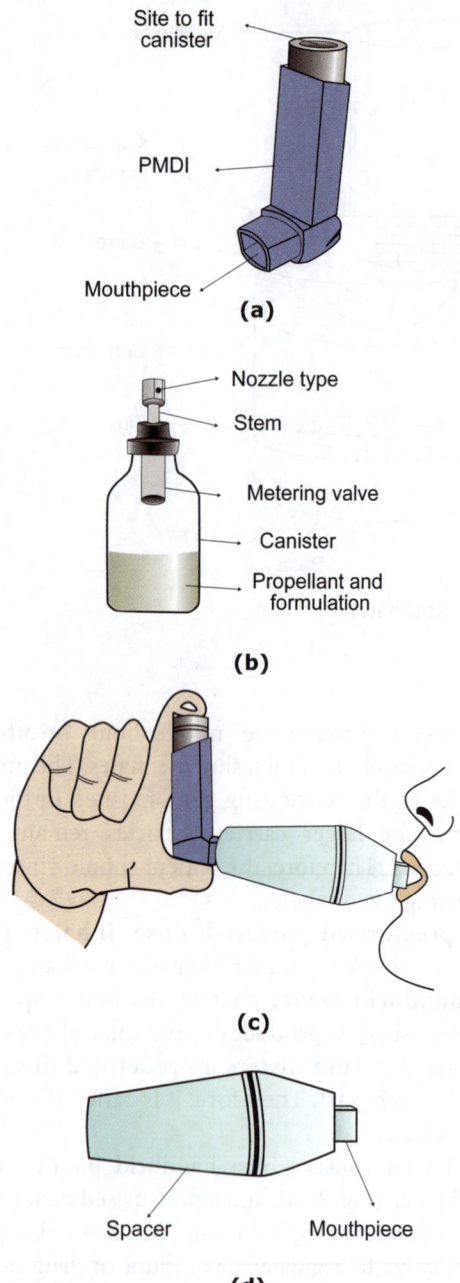

Fig. 2.2 PMDI and spacer

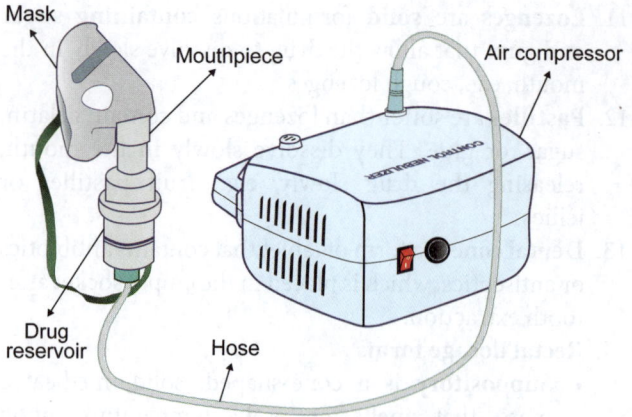

Fig. 2.3 A nebuliser

inhale deeply through their mouth from the spacer and hold their breath for a few seconds before breathing out slowly. The same process can be repeated with a gap of 1–2 minutes, if another puff is required.

4. **Nebulisers** (Fig. 2.3) are used for the **delivery of a drug solution to the bronchioles in the form of a mist**. Nebulisation is indicated during severe attacks of asthma. A nebuliser consists of an **air compressor** (which helps to turn the drug solution into fine droplets of uniform size), **a reservoir** for the drug solution, **a mask, a mouthpiece and a hose**. The patient is instructed to wash hands with soap and water before putting the drug/respirator solution into the reservoir. More than one drug may be added to the reservoir at the same time. Parts of the nebuliser are assembled so that the hose connects the air compressor with the drug reservoir, the other end of which is connected to the mouthpiece.

The patient should place the mouthpiece in their mouth. Then, after **switching on the air compressor, they should breathe slowly and deeply through the mouth** until all of the drug solution in the reservoir is used up. This may take up to 20 minutes. If it is difficult for the patient to use the mouthpiece, the mask is connected to the drug reservoir and the patient is instructed to cover nose and mouth with the mask and breathe through it. Care should be taken to properly wash and dry the drug reservoir and mouthpiece/mask after every use.

3. **Spacers** (Fig. 2.2d): These are **tube-like** or **large-volume devices** provided with an inhaler for convenience of use by children and elderly and dyspneic patients who face difficulty in coordinating inspiration with the pushing of the plastic pump. Spacers allow the movement of the drug from the PMDI to the lungs.

To use the spacer, the two parts of the spacer are first fitted together firmly. Then, the mouthpiece of the inhaler is fixed to the narrow end of the spacer and the mouthpiece cap is placed over its other end. The metal canister of the inhaler is pushed down once to release one puff dose into the spacer. After removing the cap, the mouthpiece is held tightly between the lips, ensuring complete sealing. The patient is asked to

III. Local Injections

Injections given in the deeper tissues for localised action, e.g., intra-articular, retrobulbar, and intrathecal injections are also considered local administration routes, as the drug exerts an action at the site of administration.

Clinical case-based questions and MCQs

1. A 30-year-old male patient presented with expiratory dyspnea and wheezing. On auscultation, bilateral rhonchi were present. The patient was

diagnosed with acute exacerbation of bronchial asthma. Salbutamol was prescribed to be given by the inhalational route.
   i. The inhalation of salbutamol in this case is an example of which of the following routes of drug administration?
      a. Local route
      b. Systemic route
      b. Both
      d. None of these
   ii. What is the advantage of administering the drug by the inhalational route in this case?
   iii. Enumerate the various devices that can be used for salbutamol administration in this case.

2. A 65-year-old female patient with osteoarthritis of the knees was given corticosteroids by intra-articular injection. Is this considered local or systemic administration? Describe the advantage of intra-articular injection in this case.

3. Oral neomycin was given to a patient with hepatic encephalopathy to suppress intestinal flora to reduce blood NH_3 levels.
   i. Is the oral use of the drug in this case considered local or systemic?
   ii. Justify your answer.

4. Which of the following injections represents a local route of administration of drugs?
   a. Intramuscular
   b. Intra-articular
   b. Intradermal
   d. Subcutaneous

5. Some drugs exert systemic effects after administration by local routes.
   i. Which of the following is the most desirable characteristic of drugs for such systemic effects after local administration?
      a. High lipid solubility
      b. High aqueous solubility
      c. High stability
      d. High pKa
   ii. Give two examples of such drugs.

6. A young HIV-positive male patient complaining of painless bleeding with defecation is diagnosed with hemorrhoids. The patient is not willing to undergo surgical treatment. Which route is the most suitable for drug administration in this case?
   a. Transdermal
   b. Intramuscular
   c. Rectal
   d. Oral

SYSTEMIC ROUTES

For the vast majority of drugs, systemic routes of administration are used as their effects are exerted at inaccessible sites. Systemic routes include the following:
1. **Enteral routes:** oral, sublingual and rectal routes
2. **Parenteral routes:** intramuscular, intravenous, transdermal, subcutaneous and sublingual routes
3. **Others:** cutaneous, nasal and inhalational routes

I. Enteral Routes

In enteral routes, the drug is absorbed from the gastrointestinal mucosa into the bloodstream before exerting actions. These include:

A. Oral route

It involves the ingestion of the drug so that it is delivered to the gastrointestinal mucosa for absorption into systemic circulation.

Advantages

- The oral route is the oldest and **most frequently used** route of drug administration, especially for non-hospitalised patients.
- Oral administration is especially useful for patients with **chronic diseases** requiring long-term or sometimes, lifelong treatment.
- It is a very **safe and convenient** route for patients.
- Drug administration is painless, as this is a **non-invasive** route.
- No assistance or special equipment or sterilisation is required. Therefore, the **cost of management is less** than that associated with parenteral routes.
- **Compliance** with orally administered drugs is maximum because of the ease of use.

Disadvantages

- For oral ingestion of the drug, the patient needs to be conscious. Oral administration is **not possible in unconscious** patients.
- It is difficult to administer a drug by the oral route when the patient is **uncooperative**.
- If a patient is **vomiting**, any orally administered drug will be expelled from the body before it is absorbed. Thus, systemic absorption and systemic effects are not obtained.
- Orally administered drugs have to be absorbed through the gastrointestinal mucosa. This process causes a **delay in the onset of drug action**. Therefore, the oral route is not suitable for emergencies.
- Some drugs may interact with food. Thus, patients should be cautioned regarding the ideal interval between the ingestion of the drug and the consumption of food. Some drugs are to be administered on an empty stomach, e.g., proton pump inhibitors, whereas others are meant to be taken with food, e.g., antidiabetic drugs. In contrast, some drugs cannot be taken on an empty stomach because of their gastric irritant action, e.g., NSAIDs.
- The oral route cannot be used for the administration of the following types of drugs:
  - **Polar drugs** are not absorbed from the GI mucosa as they are highly ionised, e.g., amphotericin B, aminoglycosides (although neomycin, an aminoglycoside, is sometimes administered by the oral route for its effect in the GIT only, as in the case of patients with hepatic encephalopathy and for gut sterilisation before surgery).
  - Drugs that are broken down by gastrointestinal juices and enzymes cannot be administered by this route, e.g., drugs like insulin, which are **protein** in nature.

- Drugs that have a **very high first-pass metabolism,** e.g., hydrocortisone, testosterone, and lignocaine, are not suitable for this mode of administration. Most of the orally administered dose gets metabolised during the drug's first pass through the liver. As a result, adequate plasma concentration is not achieved
- It is difficult to administer **irritant and unpalatable drugs** orally.

Dosage forms for oral administration include **solid** (Fig. 2.4) **and liquid forms**.

i. Solid dosage forms

Solid dosage forms (Fig. 2.4) for oral administration include:

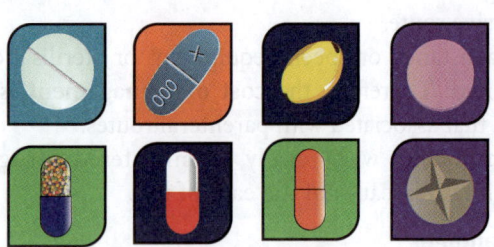

Fig. 2.4 Various solid dosage forms

a. Tablets

A **tablet** is a **hard, compressed dosage form** that comes in different shapes—rounded, discoid, oval or square. A tablet contains an **active pharmaceutical ingredient/ (API),** i.e., active drug/s and **excipients** as binders, glidants (flow aids), lubricants, disintegrants, flavouring/sweetening agents, etc. Binders, glidants and lubricants ensure the proper formation of the tablet. Disintegrants ensure that the tablet breaks up in the digestive tract. Flavouring or sweetening agents mask the bad smell or taste of APIs. Pigments are added to improve the appearance of uncoated tablets.

There are different types of tablets—compressed tablets, moulded tablets, and special tablets. Examples of each are given in Box 2.1.

Box 2.1 Different types of tablets		
Compressed	**Molded**	**Special**
Dispersible	Hypodermic	Sublingual
Effervescent	Dispensing	Buccal
Chewable		Rectal
Coated		Vaginal
Enteric-coated		
Sustained-release		

1. **Compressed tablets**
   - *Dispersible tablets (DT)* are either uncoated or film-coated tablets that should be dissolved in water and then ingested. This decreases the chances of local toxicity in the stomach and esophagus, e.g., doxycycline.
   - *Effervescent tablets* are uncoated tablets containing citric/tartaric acid and carbonates/bicarbonates that quickly react in water to release carbon dioxide. They are very rapidly dispersed, and hence absorbed very quickly and are pleasant to taste, e.g., disprin (dispersible aspirin tablet).
   - *Chewable tablets* are designed for use by children. They disintegrate on chewing and are suitable for administering large doses. These tablets have a smooth texture and are pleasant to taste upon disintegration, e.g., vitamin C tablets.
   - *Coated tablets* are coated with substances such as sugars, resins, polymers, gums, and waxes to:
     - Mask the taste, odour, or appearance of the APIs
     - Make the surface smooth so that the tablet can be easily swallowed
     - Protect APIs or active ingredients from air, moisture, and light and extend their shelf life
   - *Enteric-coated tablets* are coated to make the dosage form resistant to the gastric pH so that the drug disintegration starts only upon reaching the small intestine. This is useful for drugs that can get inactivated by the acidic pH of the stomach or can damage the gastric mucosa, e.g., enteric-coated tablets of diclofenac and aspirin.
   - *Sustained-release or retard tablets* consist of aggregated drug particles that have individual coatings of different inert resins that dissolve at different times. Such tablets provide a slow, sustained release of the active drug for 10–12 hours and have fewer side effects, e.g., diclofenac SR and nifedipine retard, etc.

   Uncoated tablets are sometimes **scored**, i.e., they have break marks to divide one tablet into equal parts.

2. **Molded tablets**
   - *Hypodermic tablets* are water-soluble tablets that readily dissolve in water to form an injectable solution, e.g., apomorphine hydrochloride and morphine sulphate.
   - *Dispensing tablets* contain a large amount of a clinically effective active drug. These are not intended for consumption by humans. It was used previously for preparing bulk solutions of germicidal chemicals, e.g., mercury bichloride tablets containing 100 g of compound for preserving grains.

3. **Special tablets**
   - *Buccal and sublingual tablets* are molded or compressed tablets that are placed in the mouth between the gum and cheek or under the tongue.

b. Capsules

- In capsules, the active ingredients (API) in powdered form are contained in a gelatin container. Capsules can be:
  - Hard-shelled: for powdered ingredients, e.g., amoxicillin capsules. Each capsule has two parts, a capsule body and a cap. The gelatin container helps

to mask the unpleasant taste or odour of the active ingredients.
- Soft-shelled, fully sealed capsules: for oils and suspensions, e.g., vitamin E capsules.
- Modified-release capsules: can be prepared in both these varieties (hard- and soft-shelled) by adding specific excipients or using specific techniques. These can be gastro-resistant enteric capsules and prolonged-release capsules.

c. Spansules

Spansules contain granules instead of powder in a gelatin container, e.g., iron formulations.

d. Granules

Granules are solid, dry aggregates of powered active ingredients held together by starch or an alcoholic spray. They are available as single-dose sachets. They are swallowed as such with water or dissolved in water and swallowed, e.g., vitamin D_3 granules.

e. Powders

Powders for internal use are bulk powders, which are solid, loose, dry particles. These powders are dispersed or dissolved in water before consumption, e.g., aspirin powder and sodium bicarbonate powder. In some powders, drugs are mixed with sodium bicarbonate and citric or tartaric acid for effervescence, e.g., ENO fruit salt.

ii. Liquid dosage forms

These include oral solutions, elixirs, suspensions, and emulsions.

a. **Solutions** are **clear liquid preparations** meant for oral use. A solution contains one or more active ingredients dissolved in a **suitable solvent** (water/sugar solution/ glycerol). Orally used solutions include liquors, syrup, and linctuses. A **liquor** is a solution of a pure substance in water. A **syrup** is a concentrated aqueous solution of a sugar, usually sucrose. It helps to mask the bad taste of the drug, e.g., vitamin syrup and cough syrup. A **linctus** is a viscous and syrupy liquid preparation that is rich in glycerol and possesses demulcent action. A linctus should be sipped slowly without dilution for a soothing effect on sore throat.
b. An **elixir** is clear liquid preparation in which the active drug is **dissolved in alcohol** to mask disagreeable odours, e.g., cough elixirs and vitamin elixirs.
c. **Suspensions** have one or more **insoluble active ingredients, homogeneously dispersed in a suitable vehicle** called a suspending agent like gum, methylcellulose, honey, mucilage, and polyvinyl alcohol.
d. **Emulsions** have two or more **immiscible liquids dispersed together in an emulsifying agent** like gelatin, pectin, egg yolk, gum acacia and gum tragacanth, magnesium hydroxide, magnesium trisilicate, aluminum hydroxide, and benzalkonium chloride. There are two types of emulsions:

- *Water-in-oil emulsion*: in which oil is the continuous phase and water is the dispersed phase. It is waxy and translucent, e.g., butter.
- *Oil-in-water emulsion*: in which water is the continuous phase and oil is the dispersed phase. It is milky white in colour, e.g., milk. These dosage forms need to have suitable preservatives to prevent microbial contamination. The packaging of these emulsions should carry a secondary label that says 'Shake well before use'.

Correct administration of oral formulations

- Tablets and capsules are **swallowed with water while the patient is sitting upright**. Drugs that have a gastric irritant action should never be taken in the recumbent posture because of the risk of esophagitis.
- Chewable tablets must be **chewed** properly before swallowing.
- Powders and dispersible tablets should be **dissolved in water** and taken while sitting upright. Effervescent tablets should be dissolved in a glass of water and ingested quickly, while the effervescence is present.
- Bottles of liquid preparations such as syrups and elixirs should be **properly capped and stored** after use.
- Suspensions and emulsions should be properly **shaken before use** for homogeneous distribution of the active ingredients.

B. Sublingual/buccal route

In sublingual administration (sub: below; lingual: tongue), the tablet or pellet containing the drug is **placed below the tongue. Highly lipid-soluble** drugs are administered by this route. Examples of drugs given sublingually include glyceryl trinitrate (GTN), steroids (estradiol), opioids (like buprenorphine and fentanyl), bronchodilator (fenoterol), prochlorperazine, hydrazine, and peptides (oxytocin).

Advantages

- The drug dissolves in the aqueous buccal fluids; it gets quickly absorbed through the floor of the mouth and the ventral surface of the tongue into the systemic circulation.
- Absorption is fast because of the rich vascularity and thinner epithelium in the sublingual region. Thus, the **effects of the drug appear quickly**. For example, glyceryl trinitrate (GTN) is used sublingually to control angina pain quickly. Similarly, opioids are administered sublingually to control postoperative pain after dental procedures.
- The drug gets absorbed into systemic circulation directly, bypassing the liver and thus avoiding first-pass metabolism. Therefore, the **bioavailability of the drug is high** as compared to the oral route.
- Once the desired effect is obtained, the remaining part of the tablet, which is still in the mouth, **can be spat out to limit the unwanted or adverse effects.**
- The sublingual route is convenient for use in patients with dysphagia. It is especially useful for pediatric, geriatric, and psychotic patients.

Disadvantages

Though it is quite easy to keep the tablet below the tongue, the sublingual route is considered **less convenient than oral ingestion** or injections by some.

- Sublingual administration is not possible if the patient is uncooperative.
- This mode interferes with eating, drinking and talking.
- The sublingual route is not suitable when a prolonged effect is desired.
- It is **not suitable for administering irritant and non-lipid-soluble drugs.**
- Smoking can reduce drug absorption after sublingual administration because it causes vasoconstriction. Therefore, the patient should be instructed to avoid smoking.

Dosage forms for sublingual administration are tablets (molded or compressed), films and sprays.

In the **buccal route of administration**, the dosage form is kept between the cheek and the gums to allow continuous absorption, resulting in a sustained effect for up to 4–6 hours.

C. Rectal route

The rectum is the part of the large intestine that extends from the colon to the anal sphincter. Drugs administered by the rectal route are intended for both local and systemic effects.

Advantages

- Rectal administration is suitable for **drugs that have an unpleasant taste,** especially in **pediatric patients**.
- Rectal administration is useful for **patients with nausea, vomiting,** diseases of the upper GIT that affect drug absorption, and unconscious patients.
- There is **no effect of food** or gastric emptying time on drug absorption after administration by the rectal route.
- Rectal administration allows for the **rapid onset** of action and circumvents the need to inject the drug.

Disadvantages

- Drug absorption after rectal administration is **erratic and unpredictable** due to the following factors:
  - The rectal epithelium consists of non-keratinised cells without villi. Thus, the surface area available for drug absorption is smaller as compared to the intestinal mucosa available for absorption after oral administration.
  - Usually, the rectum contains a few millilitres of viscous fluid containing mucin, with a pH of 6–8 and no buffer capacity. This may interfere with the drug dissolution process.
  - The rectum is drained by upper, middle, and lower hemorrhoidal or rectal veins. The upper or superior hemorrhoidal vein drains into the liver through the mesenteric and portal veins. However, the middle and lower or inferior hemorrhoidal veins drain into the inferior vena cava through hypogastric veins. Thus, a part of the drug going through the superior rectal vein gets exposed to first-pass metabolism in the liver; the parts absorbed through the middle and lower veins bypass the liver.
  - Defecation may interfere with drug absorption, especially for irritant drugs.
- This route is not suitable after rectal or anal surgery.
- Patient **compliance is lower** due to the embarrassment associated with this route. It is also **inconvenient**.
- **Assistance is required** for administration of drugs by the rectal route.

Thus, the rectal route is less popular and less frequently used as compared to other enteral routes. The rectal route is used when local effects are required but is not popular for systemic effects.

Clinical problem-based questions and MCQs

7. A 63-year-old male patient comes to the hospital for a routine follow-up examination. He has been a known hypertensive for the last 7–8 years and has been taking one tablet of lisinopril 5 mg once a day, orally. On examination, his BP is well within the normal limits and he is advised to continue the same treatment.
    i. Why is the oral route selected for drug administration in this case?
    ii. What are the advantages of oral drug administration?
    iii. Enumerate conditions in which the oral route is not suitable for administering drugs.
    iv. Enumerate the dosage forms given by the oral route?

8. Which of the following types of drugs cannot be given by the oral route?
    a. Non-polar drugs
    b. Peptide drugs
    c. Non-irritant drugs
    d. Unionised drugs

9. A 45-year-old female patient complains of severe pain in the presternal region radiating to the left arm along with sweating and anxiety. The patient is diagnosed with angina and it is decided that she should be given glyceryl trinitrate (GTN) for quick symptom relief.
    i. Which of the following is the most suitable route for the administration of GTN in this case?
    a. Intravenous
    b. Inhalational
    c. Sublingual
    d. Subcutaneous
    ii. What are the advantages of the selected route of drug administration in this case?
    iii. Give two examples of drugs given by the selected route.

10. Which of the following drugs is used by the sublingual route?
    a. Streptomycin
    b. Insulin
    c. Fentanyl
    d. Pantoprazole

11. Drugs given by the rectal route can have local as well as systemic effects. However, this is not a popular route of drug administration. Explain.

II. Parenteral Routes

Parenteral refers to the routes in which drug absorption occurs from **sites other than the gastrointestinal mucosa**. So, in a broad sense, it includes all the systemic routes excluding the ones described under enteral routes. Commonly, the routes involving drug administration by injection are called parenteral routes, e.g., intravenous, intramuscular, intradermal and subcutaneous injections.

A. Intravenous route

Aqueous solutions of the drugs are injected or infused into the superficial veins using a needle/cannula, syringe and infusion set.

Advantages

- As the aqueous solution of the drug is injected directly into the systemic circulation, no time is lost in the disintegration, dissolution, and absorption of the drug. The drug reaches its site of action quickly. Thus, the onset of drug action is very fast (almost immediate), making this route **suitable for emergency** situations. For drugs having an easily measurable response and a short duration of action like sodium nitroprusside, the **dose can be easily titrated**.
- In intravenous administration, there are no membrane barriers to be crossed by the drug to reach the systemic circulation. Hence, the **bioavailability of the drug is 100%**, i.e., the entire administered amount is in the systemic circulation in its unchanged form.
- The intravenous route is **suitable for the administration of irritant drugs** because the intimal layer of blood vessels is insensitive. Moreover, the drug quickly flows away from the site of injection with blood and thus gets diluted.
- There is no risk of interaction with food, unlike in the oral route.
- Large volumes of fluids can be infused intravenously, as in cases of fluid replacement therapy to treat shock. Oxytocin drips are used to augment labour. Other examples of drugs given by IV infusion include sodium nitroprusside, nicardipine, and cancer chemotherapy drugs.

Disadvantages

- Self-administration by the intravenous route is not possible. The patient **needs the assistance** of a qualified, skilled professional.
- Since the superficial vein is pricked with a needle, this is an **invasive** procedure causing pain at the site of injection.
- All **aseptic precautions** are mandatory to avoid complications. Solutions to be injected, needles, and syringes must be sterilised.
- Intravenous injections are **costlier** than oral medication as the cost of sterilisation and assistance add to the cost of the drug.
- Extravasation of the drug due to the puncturing of the vein during injection may cause necrosis and intense pain.
- Irritant drugs can cause **thrombophlebitis**, e.g., drugs used for cancer chemotherapy frequently cause inflammation and necrosis of the injected vein. It is recommended to change the site of drug administration in each cycle of chemotherapy.
- If the person administering the intravenous injection is not competent, **complications** like counter-puncture, multiple pricks, infection, and even air embolism may occur.
- A high concentration of the drug achieved after intravenous administration can adversely affect vital organs like the heart and brain. So, in general, intravenous drugs are **injected slowly**, over a few minutes. Such complications can be reduced by infusing the drug **diluted** with intravenous fluids.
- The IV route is not suitable for injecting suspensions because large drug particles may cause embolisms. There are no depot preparations for IV administration.

Administering drugs by the IV route

Injections are dosage forms that are filled in a syringe and administered into the body by piercing the skin with a needle. An injection anywhere on the body—e.g., a muscle/vein/skin layer/below the skin is an invasive procedure. Hence, all aseptic precautions must be observed.

a. Filling the syringe

Injections are dispensed in **ampoules or vials**. After washing the hands properly, the syringe and needle are taken out from their disposable packing, taking care not to touch the naked end of the syringe.

- **Filling from an ampoule:** The ampoule is tapped gently to move the solution downwards from its neck. The top of the ampoule is broken by filing (in the case of a glass ampoule) or twisting (in the case of a plastic ampoule). The solution is aspirated into the syringe using a filter needle by slightly tilting the ampoule.
- **Filling from a vial:** The protective covering over the vial is removed. The top of the vial is cleaned with a cotton swab soaked in disinfectant for 15 seconds and allowed to air dry. The needle is uncovered, and air is sucked into the syringe. The needle is inserted into the vial through the vial cap till it is immersed in the fluid. The plunger is then pressed to push out air to create a pressure that helps in aspirating the solution from the vial into the syringe. After aspirating the required amount of solution from the vial, the needle is removed from the vial.

- **From vials containing sterile powder for reconstitution:** Just before injection, the syringe is filled with the solvent from an ampoule as mentioned above. Then, the needle of this filled syringe is inserted into the vial containing the powder. The whole assembly is then held upright. An amount of air equal to the amount of solvent in the syringe is sucked in, and the solvent is pushed into the vial. The powder is mixed properly with the solvent by shaking the vial upside down. Then, air is injected, and the mixture is sucked into the syringe.

b. Technique of injecting

Washing hands before and after each procedure should be a habit for medical professionals. After filling the syringe from the vial or ampoule, it is important to **remove air** from the syringe by holding it with the needle upwards and tapping it gently with one finger. Once air reaches near the tip of the syringe, the plunger is slightly pushed to remove air. Proper **asepsis** should be maintained. The used needle, syringe, vials, swabs, etc., should be appropriately disposed of.

i. Intravenous injection (bolus)

The patient can be sitting or lying down. Before injecting, the patient should be reassured and informed about the steps of the procedure in a language that can be understood.

Site

The ideal vein for IV injection should be round, firm, full, and flexible. The vein should be palpated with one or two fingers and gently pressed to check refilling. IV injections can be given in the veins of the upper or lower extremities.

- The upper extremity veins are usually preferred as the chances of complications like thrombo-embolism are fewer and because the IV line is more durable than in the lower extremity veins. The metacarpal veins, median antebrachial veins, basilic vein, and cephalic vein are the preferred sites for IV drug administration.
- However, the veins of the lower extremities can be used if those of the upper extremities are not accessible due to conditions like dehydration, shock, IV substance abuse and for chemotherapeutic drugs.
- In neonates, IV drugs/fluids can even be administered in the scalp veins.
- During acute conditions, IV administration is usually done through the median cubital vein as it is easily accessible. However, care should be taken to avoid injection into the radial artery, which lies very close to the median cubital vein.

Procedure

- The arm is uncovered, a tourniquet is tied on the upper arm and the patient is asked to make a tight fist.
- When a sufficient length of the vein becomes prominent, the overlying skin is wiped with a disposable antiseptic swab in circular/back-and-forth motions.
- The skin overlying the selected vein is slightly pulled longitudinally with the left hand to stabilise the vein.
- The needle used for IV injection is usually a **14–24 gauge**—the smallest effective needle should be used. The important factors determining the needle size are age-related or disease-related changes in the vessel size, viscosity of the solution to be injected, and hydration status of the patient. A catheter or butterfly catheter may be preferred over a needle for IV administration. Larger IV catheters are required in acute situations like hypovolemia and shock, when a large amount of fluid is to be administered quickly.
- The loaded syringe and needle are held in the right hand with the bevelled end of the needle pointed upwards. The needle is inserted through the skin **at an angle of 5–30°** and passed gently into the vein. The angle at which the needle is inserted is lesser for superficial veins.
- The plunger is pulled slightly to ensure that the needle is inside the vein. When blood enters the syringe, the drug is **slowly injected** over a few minutes by pushing the plunger slowly while holding the syringe steady.
- If no blood appears in the syringe on pulling the plunger, it indicates that the needle has not yet entered the vein. Then, the needle is slightly withdrawn, and an attempt is made to insert it into the vein. After injecting the drug, the needle is removed, and the opening is compressed with a sterile swab and adhesive tape is applied over it.

Complications

There may be pain, redness, swelling, counter-puncture, extravasation, bruising, infection, thrombophlebitis, necrosis, nerve damage, etc.

ii. Setting up an IV drip or infusion

- First, the drip rate of the prescribed medicine is carefully calculated.
- For this procedure, an infusion set, cannula and fluid bag (Fig. 2.5) are required.
- The spiked end of infusion set is inserted into the port provided for it on fluid bag. The fluid bag is held upside down and hung on the IV stand.

- The roller clamp of the IV set is released to allow fluid to flow through the tubing, so that there is no air left in it. Once the IV set is primed with fluid, the roller clamp is closed.
- The IV cannula has a thin plastic tube enclosing a needle. It is inserted into the vein using the given procedure for IV bolus injections. After ensuring that the cannula is in the vein, its needle is gently removed and plastic tubing is secured in position using adhesive tape.
- The needle free port of the cannula is then attached to the lower end of the infusion set tubing.
- The roller clamp is released gradually to ensure the correct infusion drop rate.

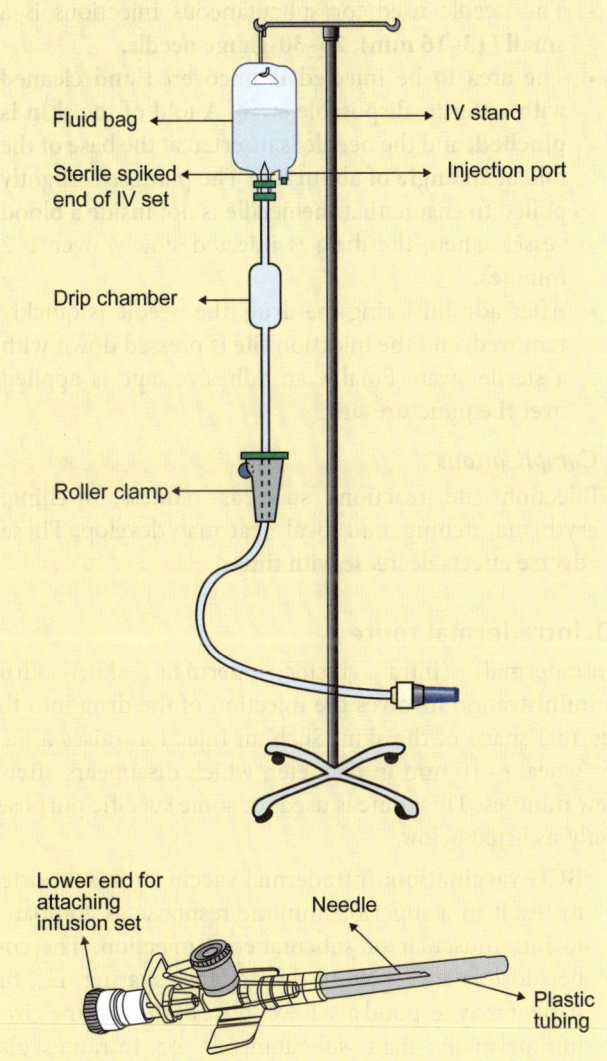

Fig. 2.5 Infusion set and IV cannula

B. Intramuscular route

It involves the injection of the drug into a large skeletal muscle like the deltoid, gluteus maximus, rectus femoris or triceps.

Advantages
- The vascularity of skeletal muscles is high. So, the drug gets absorbed quickly and uniformly as compared to the oral route. Hence, the **onset of action is fast**.
- The sensory nerve supply is comparatively lesser in skeletal muscles than in subcutaneous tissue. Hence, **mild irritant drugs can be injected** intramuscularly but not subcutaneously.
- Intramuscular administration is possible for **both aqueous solutions as well as oily preparations**. The rate of absorption of aqueous preparations is greater than that of oily preparations, which can be given as **depot injections** for a slow, sustained response.
- Gastric factors and first-pass metabolism are bypassed. Hence, the **bioavailability of the drug is better with this route than with the oral route**.

Disadvantages
- Only a limited amount of the drug solution **up to 10 mL** can be injected intramuscularly.
- Since the drug needs to be injected deep inside the muscle, a skilled professional needs to perform the procedure.
- The drug solution, needle, syringe, etc., need to be sterilised. Because of the above two factors, administration by the intramuscular route is **costlier** than the oral route.
- If asepsis is not observed, **complications** like infection, abscess, and nerve damage may occur.
- Anticoagulants given intramuscularly carry the risk of producing local hematoma.

Administering drugs by intramuscular injection

Site

IM injection can be given into the ventrogluteal muscle, the deltoid—about 2.5 cm below the acromion process, the rectus femoris, the vastus lateralis, etc.

Technique
- The patient is reassured, and the procedure is explained using simple words. The patient's privacy should be ensured before administering the injection.
- The patient is asked to lie on their side in such a way that the muscles at the site selected for injection are relaxed. The area is uncovered and the skin overlying the lateral upper quadrant is wiped with a sterile, disposable swab using back and forth motions and allowed to air dry for 30 seconds (recent evidence suggests that scrubbing of skin at the injection site is unnecessary for patients in good health).
- The filled syringe with a **long 21–23-gauge needle** in place is held in the right hand. The needle is quickly

inserted at an angle of **75–90°**. The plunger is slightly pulled to ensure that the needle is not inside a blood vessel. If blood appears on pulling the plunger, the needle should be slightly readjusted to ensure that it is in the muscle.
- The drug is **administered slowly** by gently pushing the plunger at a rate of 1 mL every 10 seconds. After waiting 10 seconds for the drug to diffuse, the needle is quickly removed in a smooth motion and disposed of.
- The **'Z' technique** is used to prevent backtracking and leakage from the injection site. In this technique, the skin overlying the injection site is pulled 2–3 cm with the left hand to displace the subcutaneous tissue. The needle is then inserted, and the drug is injected while holding the skin. After administering the drug, the needle is removed in a swift movement and the skin is released to allow it to return to normal. This ensures that the drug gets trapped in the muscle.
- The site of injection is pressed with a sterile swab and an adhesive tape is applied over it.

Complications
There may be pain at the injection site, injury to the nearby blood vessels or nerves, inadvertent injection into a vein, infection, abscess formation, cellulitis, etc.

C. Subcutaneous route

In the subcutaneous route (sub: below; cutaneous: skin), the drug is deposited by injection or dermojet or as a pellet/implant just below the skin in the loose subcutaneous tissue.

Advantages
- In the case of subcutaneous injection or the use of a dermojet, **self-administration is possible** since deep penetration is not required. This route is widely used by diabetics for insulin administration. Because diabetes requires long-term or even lifelong insulin therapy, patients or their attendants can be taught to administer the medication fairly easily.
- Special dosage forms like dermojets, pellets, and implants (biodegradable or non-biodegradable) are used by the subcutaneous route for **slow and sustained action.**

Disadvantages
- The vascularity of subcutaneous tissue is lesser than that of skeletal muscles. Consequently, the rate of absorption is **lower** than that of the intramuscular route.
- This route is **not suitable for irritant drugs** because the subcutaneous tissue has a rich nerve supply. As a result, an irritant drug given by the subcutaneous route can cause intense pain.
- This route is not suitable for emergency situations because of the slow absorption.
- Subcutaneous administration is **not suitable for patients in shock** because intense vasoconstriction occurs as a compensatory mechanism. Drug absorption is, therefore, not adequate.

Administering drugs by subcutaneous injection
Site
A subcutaneous injection is given in the loose layers of skin below the dermis and epidermis, commonly on the outer part of the upper arm, front of the thigh, upper buttock, above or below the waist, etc.

Technique
- The needle used for subcutaneous injections is a **small (13–16 mm), 26–30-gauge** needle.
- The area to be injected is uncovered and cleaned with a sterile, disposable swab. A fold of the **skin is pinched,** and the needle is inserted at the base of the fold at an **angle of about 45°**. The plunger is slightly pulled to ensure that the needle is not inside a blood vessel. Then, the drug is injected slowly, over 1–2 minutes.
- After administering the drug, the needle is quickly removed, and the injection site is pressed down with a sterile swab. Finally, an adhesive tape is applied over the puncture site.

Complications
Injection site reactions such as redness, swelling, erythema, itching, and local heat may develop. These adverse effects decrease with time.

D. Intradermal route

Intradermal (intra: inside; dermal: skin) drug administration involves the injection of the drug into the dermal space of the skin. Such an injection raises a bleb or wheal 6–10 mm in diameter, which disappears after a few minutes. This route is used for some specific purposes only, as listed below.

- **BCG vaccination**: Intradermal vaccination is reported to result in a superior immune response as compared to intramuscular or subcutaneous injection. The cost per dose is also reduced due to 'dose sparing', i.e., the patient may respond at a lower dose of the vaccine given intradermally than subcutaneous or intramuscular injection. This helps to conserve the supply of limited/costly antigens.
- **Sensitivity testing for penicillin:** The 'tuberculin test' for the screening and confirmation of tuberculosis involves the intradermal administration of the tuberculin reagent. For screening purposes, a Heaf test is done, which uses a multiple-puncture technique. An injector applicator coated with the dried tuberculin

reagent is pressed into the skin, and the test is read after 48–72 hours. The **Mantoux test** is more frequently used for screening as well as confirming. In a **Heaf test**, 0.1 mL or 5 TU (tuberculin units) of a purified protein derivative (PPD) is injected intradermally. The test is read after 48–72 hours to look for induration of the skin.

Disadvantages

- Intradermal injection **needs expertise** in technique and practice. During Mantoux testing, if the injection goes deep into the subcutaneous tissue instead of the dermal space, the reagent will be rapidly washed out of the area before it can produce a reaction. On the other hand, if the injection is too superficial, the reagent leaks into the skin; as a result, the amount delivered intradermally is not sufficient (< 5 TU) for the development of a reaction.
- Variations in the thickness of skin can alter the dose delivered.

> **Administering an intradermal injection**
> For intradermal injection, a tuberculin syringe, calibrated as 10th and 100th of a milliliter, is used. The needle is 25–27 gauge and has a length of 1/2 to 1/4th of an inch. The needle is placed almost flat against the skin at an **angle of 5–15°**, with its bevelled side up. It is then **inserted about one-fourth of an inch** and the plunger is pushed to inject the drug. This raises a **bleb**.

III. Other Systemic Routes

A. Cutaneous route

Skin is permeable to **highly lipid-soluble** and **unionised drugs** applied over its surface. Such drugs get absorbed into the systemic circulation. Absorption can be increased if the drug has an oily base (e.g., an ointment) and is rubbed over the skin. Rubbing increases the blood circulation in that area. The use of occlusive dressing also improves cutaneous absorption by increasing hydration.

Advantages

- As the drug is absorbed slowly, the onset of action is **slow**, but its effects last for 1–3 days.
- It is easy and **convenient** to use drugs by the cutaneous route. As a result, patient compliance is good.
- **Smooth plasma levels** of the drug are achieved.
- **First-pass metabolism is negligible**. Thus, inter-individual variations are minimal.
- No assistance is required for this route of administration.

Disadvantages

- Transdermal therapeutic patches used for cutaneous drug administration are **expensive**.
- These patches may cause **local irritation and contact dermatitis** at the site of application. Therefore, the patch should be applied at a different site each time.
- The patch may get detached from the skin due to a change in temperature (heat/cold), perspiration, swimming, bathing, etc. A new patch is required in such cases, which causes a wastage of the previous patch still containing the drug.
- Permeation through the skin decreases with age.
- This route is useful only for highly lipid-soluble drugs.

Dosage form for cutaneous administration

Transdermal therapeutic systems are drug-delivery devices designed to regulate the rate of drug absorption to achieve slow, sustained action. These are adhesive patches **measuring 5–20 cm^2** (Fig. 2.6).

- The drug is delivered into the blood through the stratum corneum at a constant rate from a **drug reservoir**, which is fully encapsulated in a shallow compartment between an impermeable metallic plastic laminate (backing film) and a rate-limiting micropore membrane. The backing film prevents leakage of the drug to the other side.
- The **micropore membrane** is made up of polymer matrices of either natural polymers (like cellulose derivatives, gelatin, waxes, gums, shellac, or rubber starch) or synthetic polymers (like polyvinyl chloride [PVC], polyethylene, polypropylene and polyurea). The size of the pores in the micropore membrane is such that the membrane delivers drug particles to the skin surface at a rate lower than the slowest rate of absorption across the skin. Thus, a **constant rate of absorption** is ensured, irrespective of the site of application.
- In front of the micropore membrane lies an **adhesive layer containing a priming dose** of the drug. The adhesive should be non-irritant and easily removable. It should not leave any unwashable residues on the skin surface and should be chemically compatible with the active ingredients.
- In addition to polymer matrices and the active drug, these transdermal patches also contain **permeation enhancers** (like oleic acid, dioctyl sulfosuccinate and

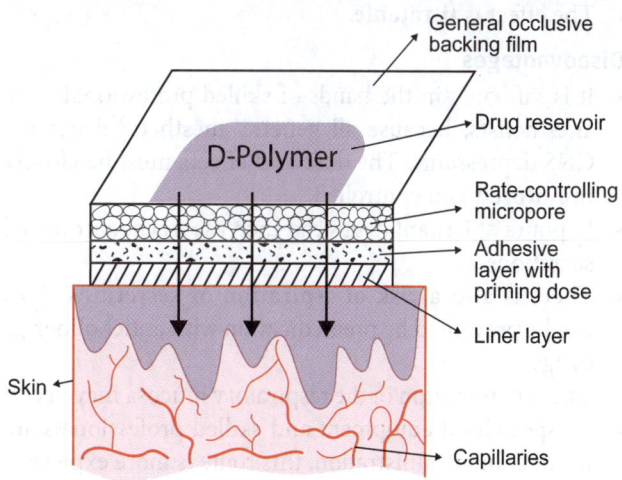

Fig. 2.6 Transdermal patch

sodium taurocholate) which alter the barrier function of the skin and promote permeability.
- The adhesive layer is covered with a **protective film** or liner layer that should be removed just before application.

Site of application
The patch is usually applied over the surface of the skin in the mastoid area, chest, abdomen, upper arm, lower part of the back, and or the buttocks. Examples of drugs available as transdermal patches are glyceryl trinitrate, isosorbide dinitrate, nicotine, estradiol, clonidine, hyoscine, and fentanyl.

B. Nasal route
The nasal mucosa has **good vascularity**. Drugs can be absorbed into systemic circulation through the nasal mucous membrane, whereby they **bypass the first-pass** metabolism in the liver. Examples of drugs given as nasal spray for systemic effects include calcitonin, desmopressin and gonadotropin-releasing hormone agonist (nafarelin). Insulin administration through the nasal route is also being tried.

C. Inhalational route
The inhalational route is useful for local as well as systemic effects. For systemic effects, **volatile liquids and gases** can be administered by the inhalational route for systemic effects. Such drugs are administered through **general anesthesia devices**. The drug gets absorbed into systemic circulation very quickly from the vast alveolar epithelial surface area. General anesthetic drugs rapidly cross the blood–brain barrier to exert an anesthetic effect. On stopping administration, the drug diffuses back from the brain into epithelial circulation and the lungs and is exhaled with the same quickness. Thus, drug administration can be titrated with the desired action.

Advantages
- Quick absorption and **fast onset and offset** of action.
- The effect is **titratable**.

Disadvantages
- It is safe only in the hands of skilled professionals, i.e., anesthetists, because all general anesthetic drugs are CNS depressants. The dose and effects must be **closely monitored** and controlled.
- Vapours of irritant drugs can increase tracheobronchial secretions.
- There is also a **risk of aspiration of secretions**. This can be prevented by premedication with anticholinergic drugs.
- The inflammation of the respiratory mucosa may occur.
- As specialised equipment and skilled professionals are needed for administration, this route is more expensive than other routes.

Clinical problem-based questions and MCQs

12. Drugs can be given by the enteral and parenteral routes based on the condition of the patient and the characteristics of the drug. Enumerate the various parenteral routes of drug administration.

13. A 9-year-old boy with insulin dependent diabetes mellitus (IDDM) who is on insulin therapy fell unconscious during an athletic competition in school and is brought to the emergency. A finger prick test shows a random blood sugar level of 530 mg/dL.
    i. Which route is most suitable for the management of this case to bring down blood glucose levels?
       a. Intramuscular   b. Intravenous
       c. Subcutaneous   d. Oral
    ii. Enumerate the advantages and disadvantages of the route of administration selected in part i of this question.

14. i. Which route of drug administration is used if the drug prescribed is irritant in nature.
       a. Inhalational   b. Oral
       c. Subcutaneous   d. Intravenous
    ii. Justify your choice.

15. A 55-year-old patient, presents to the emergency with headache, anxiety, and irritability. His BP is 220/124. There are no signs of target organ damage. The patient is diagnosed with 'hypertensive urgency'. Nicardipine is given as an intravenous infusion at the rate of 5 mg/hour.
    i. Why is the drug being given by the intravenous infusion in this case?
    ii. Describe the technique of drug administration by IV infusion.
    iii. Give examples of clinical situations in which drugs are given by the IV route.

16. i. Identify the route most suitable for the administration of oily preparations.
       a. Intravenous route
       b. Intramuscular route
       c. Subcutaneous route
       d. Intradermal route
    ii. Describe the technique of drug administration by the route selected in the first part of this question.
    iii. Enumerate the advantages of the chosen route.

17. i. Name the therapeutic systems designed to regulate the rate of drug absorption through intact skin to achieve slow, sustained action.
    ii. Describe the function of various layers of the above-mentioned therapeutic system.

18. Which of the following is NOT given by the intradermal route?
    a. Test dose of drugs   b. Insulin
    c. BCG vaccine   d. Mantoux test

19. i. Which of the following routes of drug administration is used for both local as well as systemic effects?
    a. Intravenous   b. Intramuscular
    c. Subcutaneous   d. Inhalational
   ii. Give one example each of a drug used by the chosen route for local and systemic effects
20. i. Which of the following parenteral routes allows the self-administration of the drug?
    a. Intravenous   b. Intramuscular
    c. Subcutaneous   d. Intradermal
   ii. Describe the technique of administering drugs by the selected route.
   iii. Enumerate the advantages and disadvantages of the selected route.

DRUG DELIVERY SYSTEMS

Drug delivery systems are designed to improve the delivery of the drug at the target site in the active form. The advantages of newly developed drug delivery systems include the following:

- Better patient compliance
- Better drug response
- Prolonged drug action

Some examples of drug delivery systems are discussed below.

Prodrug

A prodrug is an **inactive precursor** that gets converted into its active form by metabolism inside the body.

Prodrugs have **favourable pharmacokinetics** as compared to the active form of the drug and help in the **delivery of the active drug at the site of action**. For example, **levodopa** is a prodrug for dopamine. It is given to correct dopamine deficiency in the basal ganglia of brain in patients suffering from parkinsonism. Dopamine is a quaternary amine that cannot cross the blood–brain barrier, whereas its prodrug, levodopa, crosses the blood–brain barrier easily and then gets converted into dopamine to relieve features of parkinsonism.

Similarly, **dipivefrin** is a pivalic acid ester of adrenaline used topically as 0.1% eye drops to treat glaucoma. It easily penetrates the cornea and gets hydrolysed by esterases into adrenaline, which lowers the intraocular tension by improving the uveoscleral outflow and reducing aqueous humor production.

The ACE inhibitor drug **enalapril** is also a prodrug. It has good oral absorption and is not affected much by food and other intraluminal factors. In the liver, it gets de-esterified to form the active form of the drug 'enalaprilat', which exerts an inhibitory effect on the angiotensin-converting enzyme. Enalaprilat itself has poor oral absorption.

Sulfasalazine is split by colonic bacteria to release sulfapyridine and 5-aminosalicylic acid, which exerts a beneficial anti-inflammatory effect in inflammatory bowel disease, ulcerative colitis, and Crohn's disease.

Prodrugs may help to **prolong the duration of action** of drugs like procaine penicillin, an ester of penicillin G that gets hydrolysed slowly to release penicillin in a sustained fashion to ensure longer lasting action.

Some other examples of prodrugs are α-methyldopa, prednisone, clopidogrel, cyclophosphamide, and 6-mercaptopurine.

Transdermal Therapeutic Systems (TTS)

These are adhesive patches of varying sizes and shapes (refer to Fig. 2.6). These patches contain a polymer-bound drug in a reservoir held between an occlusive film and a rate-controlling micropore membrane. The drug is delivered at a slow, controlled rate into the systemic circulation via the stratum corneum. It ensures a constant, predictable rate of drug absorption and minimises individual variations in the rate of absorption.

Transdermal patches of fentanyl, glyceryl trinitrate, estradiol, and nicotine are available. The patch can be applied over the chest, lower back, abdomen, buttocks, mastoid region, or upper arm. The adhesive smeared on the undersurface of the micropore membrane may sometimes cause mild local irritation and erythema.

Technique of use

The patient is instructed to apply the transdermal patch after washing hands with soap and water. They should choose a hairless, dry, and clean area of skin to apply the patch. A separate site should be chosen everyday to avoid local irritant effects. The skin at the chosen site should be cleaned with warm water and soap and dried. Then, the patch should be applied after tearing the protective covering over it, taking care not to touch the sticky surface of the patch.

Drug-Releasing Implants

To ensure the delivery of the drug only to the target organ, the implant is coated with the drug and placed in the target organ. It slowly releases minute quantities of the drug to exert a prolonged effect. Examples of such implants include the following:

- **Progestaserts** are intrauterine contraceptive devices impregnated with progestins, which provide contraceptive effects for long periods of up to 5 years.
- **Ocuserts** or ocular inserts are placed in the lower cul-de-sac to provide weekly doses of pilocarpine.

Devices to Deliver Inhalational Drugs

Drug administration by inhalation can be achieved by various methods such as the following:

- Volatile liquids/gases can be inhaled from the air or with oxygen through a mouthpiece, face mask, endotracheal tube, general anesthesia devices, etc.
- For the inhalation of solids having fine particles and non-volatile liquids, the drug is aerosolised using devices such as a rotahaler or spinhaler, a metered dose inhaler, or a jet nebuliser (Figs. 2.1 and 2.2).

Liposomes

These are nanovesicles made up of lecithin or other biodegradable phospholipids. They contain non-lipid-soluble drugs. After intravenous administration, they are taken up by the liver, spleen, and some malignant cells before being delivered to the target tissue. For example, **amphotericin B** is available as a liposomal preparation for use in systemic mycosis and kala-azar. Such targeted delivery of amphotericin decreases its nephrotoxicity.

Computerised Miniature Pumps

These are meant for the delivery of the drug at a predetermined definite rate. This is especially useful for hormone administration. Insulin is released continuously at a rate determined by glucose sensors attached to these pumps. Such replacement closely resembles physiological secretion. Such pumps are also available for the release of gonadotrophin-releasing hormone (GnRH) in a pulsatile manner.

Other Insulin Delivery Devices

These are designed with the motive of improving the convenience of insulin administration. These include pen devices, jet injectors, and prefilled syringes refer to Chapter 43, page 575).

Monoclonal Antibodies (MAbs)

These are antibodies that are produced against a single antigenic determinant by using the **'hybridoma' technique**. Hybridomas are obtained by the fusion of specific B lymphocytes with mouse myeloma cells. Hence, they have the characteristics of both, i.e., they produce antibodies (like B lymphocytes) and multiply endlessly (like myeloma cells). The monoclonal antibodies (MAbs) obtained from rodents have a risk of producing allergic reactions. To avoid this, they can be partly **humanised**; such MAbs are known as 'chimeric Abs'. Totally humanised MAbs are obtained by **DNA recombinant technology**.

A monoclonal antibody serves the purpose of **carrying specific antibodies to attack targeted antigens** present on viruses or the tumour cell surface.

The name of a monoclonal antibody is suffixed with 'mab'. The letter 'o' precedes 'mab' in murine antibodies (omab); 'xi' is the prefix for chimeric antibodies (ximab); 'zu' signifies humanised antibodies (zumab); and 'u' refers to totally human antibodies.

The names thus arrived at are further prefixed with 'tu' to indicate use for tumours, 'vi' is used for MAbs used for viral infections, and 'ci' for circulation, e.g., cetuximab, omalizumab, rituximab, and trastuzumab.

Clinical problem-based questions and MCQs

21. Which of the following is not a prodrug?
    a. Sulfasalazine
    b. Diazepam
    c. Prednisone
    d. Dipivefrin
22. Which drug delivery device is useful to reduce the nephrotoxicity of amphotericin B?
    a. Prodrug
    b. Transdermal patch
    c. Liposomes
    d. Drug-releasing implant
23. Monoclonal antibodies can be prepared by various techniques. Enumerate the important techniques to prepare monoclonal antibodies for clinical use.
24. The suffix 'mab' is used in the names of all monoclonal antibodies. 'Xi' preceding mab indicates:
    a. Murine antibodies
    b. Chimeric antibodies
    c. Fully humanised antibodies
    d. None of the above
25. Monoclonal antibodies carry specific antibodies to attack targeted antigens present on:
    a. Tumour cells
    b. Viruses
    c. Circulation
    d. All of the above

Summary

- The choice of the route of drug administration depends upon numerous drug-/disease-/patient-related factors.
- Routes can be local or systemic based on the extent of the effect desired.
- **Local routes** require the action of a drug in the vicinity of the site of administration and involve topical and deep injections. **Topical routes** are used for the administration of drugs at accessible sites like the skin or mucous membranes for local action. **Deep injections** like intra-articular and retrobulbar, are used to produce local effects at inaccessible sites like joint spaces and the retrobulbar space. The greatest advantage of local routes is that adverse systemic effects are reduced.
- **Systemic routes** of drug administration can be enteral—through the gastrointestinal tract—or parenteral.

- The most common **enteral route** is **oral**, i.e., the ingestion of drugs. This is the safest, easiest, and cheapest route. However, the bioavailability of the drug is less than unity. Thus, this route is not suitable for all patients and all drugs.
- Other enteral routes include **sublingual and rectal**, both of which bypass the liver. The sublingual route is good when quick onset of action of the drug is required in an emergency situation, e.g., NTG in acute angina.
- **Parenteral routes** include intravenous, intramuscular, subcutaneous, and intradermal injections. Each route has its own unique advantages and limitations.
- The **intravenous route** is suitable in emergency situations for 100% bioavailability and quick-onset effects.
- The **intramuscular route** is suitable both for aqueous as well as oily preparations of drugs.
- The **subcutaneous** route is widely used for the self-administration of insulin in diabetics.
- **Special dosage forms** like dermojets, pellets and implants are used by subcutaneous route for slow and sustained action.
- Some drugs can be used as a **transdermal patch** for systemic effects after absorption through intact skin at a regulated rate for a slow, sustained effect.

Questions for practice

1. Why are some drugs given by the sublingual route?
2. Enumerate the advantages and limitations of drug administration by the following routes:
   a. Intravenous route
   b. Inhalational route
   c. Subcutaneous route
3. Why is the oral route the most frequently used for drug administration?
4. Write short notes on:
   a. Transdermal patch
   b. Liposomes
   c. Prodrugs

Hints for problem-based questions and MCQs

1. i. a. Local route: Since the drug effect is desired only at the site of administration, i.e., the bronchi
   ii. Minimal adverse systemic effects
   iii. Rotahaler, PMDI, and nebuliser (refer to page 13)
2. Local route, because the effect of the drug is desired at the site of its administration; the advantage of this route is that it is associated with the least systemic toxicity of the drug (refer to page 14).
3. i. Because orally given neomycin affects only the microbial flora in the gastrointestinal tract, this is a local or topical use of the drug;
   ii. Neomycin is used by the oral route in hepatic encephalopathy for suppressing the intestinal flora so that NH_3 production by bacteria decreases and blood NH_3 levels come down.
4. b. Intra-articular
5. i. a. High lipid solubility
   ii. Hyoscine, glyceryl trinitrate, and nicotine transdermal patches
6. c. Rectal route: being topical, it is the most suitable route for this case.
7. i. The oral route is selected because it is the most suitable for the management of chronic disease on account of the convenience of its use, the choice of self-administration, and the fact that it is the most non-invasive.
   ii. Refer to page 15
   iii. Refer to page 15
   iv. Refer to solid and liquid dosage forms, page 16, 17
8. b. Peptide drugs, as they are broken down by digestive juices
9. i. c. Sublingual
   ii. Refer to page 17
   iii. Examples of drugs given sublingually are glyceryl trinitrate (GTN), steroids (estradiol), opioids (like buprenorphine and fentanyl), bronchodilator (fenoterol), prochlorperazine, hydrazine, and peptides (oxytocin).
10. c. Fentanyl
11. Refer to page 18. (Disadvantages of rectal route)
12. It includes intramuscular, intravenous, transdermal, subcutaneous and sublingual routes.
13. i. b. Intravenous (intramuscular, subcutaneous and oral routes are not suitable for emergency situations. Moreover, drugs cannot be given orally because the patient is unconscious).
    ii. Refer to page 19
14. i. d. Intravenous
    ii. Vascular intima non-sensitive; drug dilution on IV administration (refer to page 19).
15. i. The onset of action is very fast (almost immediate). For drugs with an easily measurable response like the lowering of BP, in this case, and a short duration of effects (like nicardipine, in this case), the dose can be easily titrated.
    ii. Refer to page 20, 21
    iii. In emergency situation, to give large volume, to give irritant drugs
16. i. b. Intramuscular route
    ii. Refer to page 21
    iii. Refer to page 21
17. i. Transdermal therapeutic system
    ii. Refer to page 23
18. b. Insulin is given by the subcutaneous or intravenous routes
19. i. d. Inhalational
    ii. Drugs given by the inhalational route for local effects include salbutamol and corticosteroids (triamcinolone) for bronchial asthma. Drugs given by the inhalational route for a systemic effect include halothane, isoflurane, and other volatile liquids for general anesthesia.
20. i. c. Subcutaneous
    ii. Refer to page 22
    iii. Refer to page 22.
21. b. Diazepam
22. c. Liposomes
23. Hybridoma technique, humanisation of murine antibodies, and recombinant DNA technique
24. b. Chimeric antibody
25. d. All of the above. Monoclonal antibodies can be directed against antigens on tumour cells, viruses, and circulating antigens.

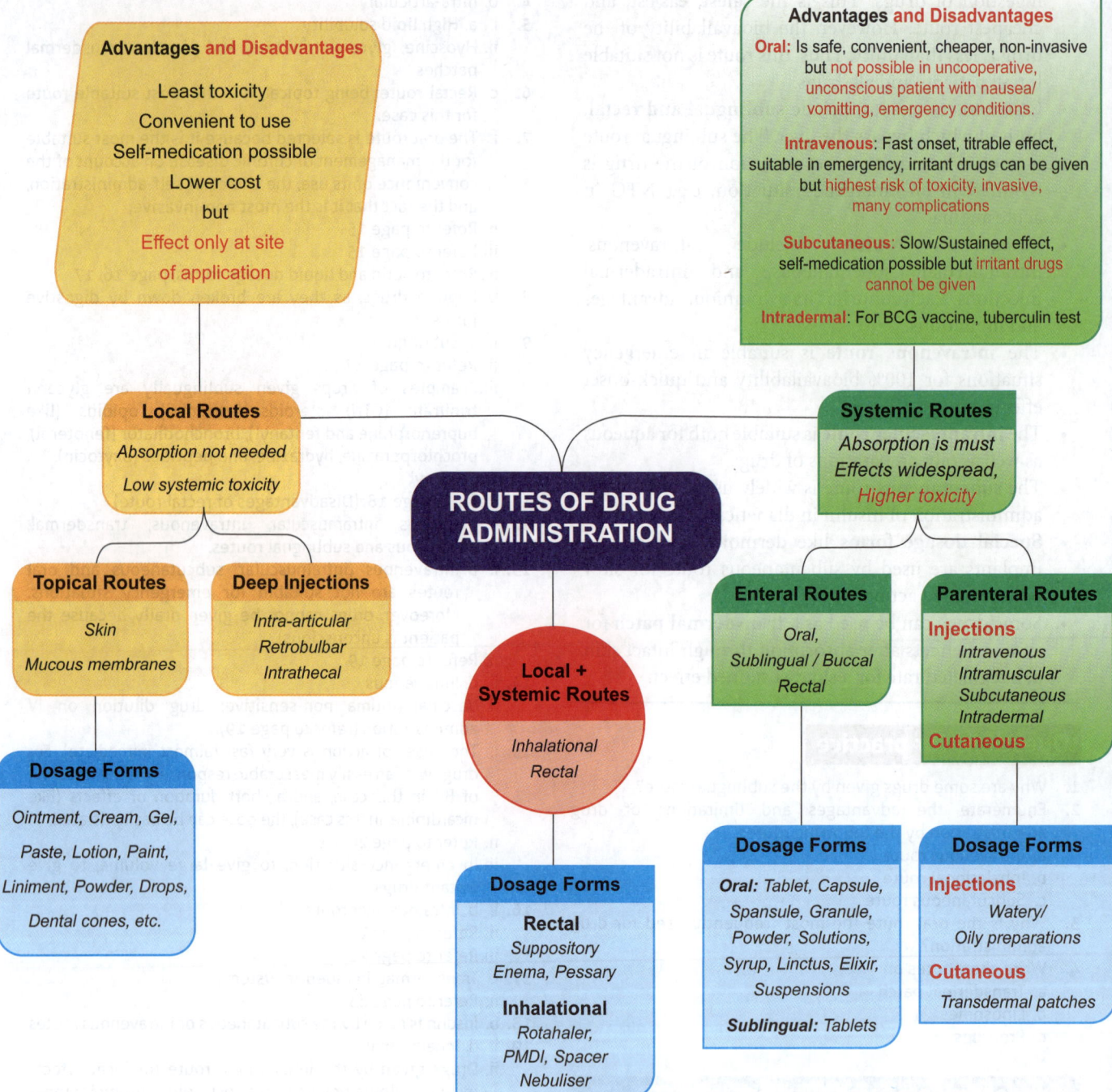

SECTION 1 General Pharmacology

3 Pharmacokinetics

PH 1.6 Describe salient features of absorption, distribution, metabolism and excretion of drugs with emphasis on various routes of drug administration.

Learning objectives

A student of MBBS phase II should be able to:
- Define pharmacokinetics and the stages of drug disposition.
- Describe the processes involved in absorption of drugs and the factors affecting them.
- Explain the terms bioavailability and bioequivalence and enumerate the factors affecting them.
- Describe the clinical importance of bioavailability and bioequivalence.
- Describe volume of drug distribution and the factors affecting it.
- Describe the factors determining the passage of drugs across the blood–brain barrier and the placental barrier.
- Describe the clinical importance of plasma protein binding.
- Describe phase I and phase II reactions of drug metabolism.
- Describe enzyme induction and inhibition and their clinical implications.
- Describe the clearance of drugs through various routes.
- Describe the half-life of a drug.
- Differentiate between first- and zero-order kinetics.
- Describe the plateau principle of drug kinetics.

The term 'pharmacokinetics' is derived from the Greek words '*pharmacon*', meaning 'drug', and '*kinesis*', meaning 'movement'.

Pharmacokinetics is the study of **how a drug moves in the body after administration and what the body does to the drug during its passage**, i.e., the body's response to the drug. It **refers to the movement of the drug through the body, the alteration of the drug by the body and the movement of the drug out of the body**. It includes **four pharmacokinetic processes** or stages of drug disposition:

- Absorption
- Distribution—binding/storage/localisation
- Biotransformation or metabolism
- Excretion of the drug

Pharmacokinetics is thus often summarised by the acronym 'ADME', referring to absorption, distribution, metabolism, and excretion of drugs.

Therapeutics aims to achieve a desired beneficial effect and avoid adverse effects as far as possible. The principles of pharmacokinetics and pharmacodynamics are used to clearly understand the dose–response relationship. The pharmacokinetic processes of absorption, distribution, metabolism, and excretion determine the concentration achieved with a given dose (the dose–concentration relationship). The pharmacodynamic concepts of maximum response and sensitivity determine the effect produced by a particular plasma concentration (the concentration–effect Fig. 3.1). Thus, the **dose-response curve (DRC)** serves as a bridge between pharmacokinetics and pharmacodynamics.

TRANSLOCATION OF DRUG MOLECULES

During pharmacokinetic processes, drug molecules move in the body and across cell membranes in two ways:

1. **Bulk-flow transfer**: It occurs in the **bloodstream**. The cardiovascular system provides a **very fast, long-distance** bulk flow transfer system. The transfer of drugs by bulk flow is not affected by their chemical nature.
2. **Diffusional transfer**: It is the **molecule-by-molecule transfer of drugs over short distances**. Diffusional characteristics of different drugs differ markedly. Drug diffusion is of two types—aqueous and non-aqueous.
   a. *Aqueous diffusion*: This mode of diffusion delivers drug molecules at the non-aqueous barriers and also carries them away from non-aqueous barriers. The rate of aqueous diffusion of a drug varies inversely with its molecular size; the diffusion coefficient is inversely proportional to the molecular weight, i.e., **larger molecules diffuse more slowly than smaller ones**.
   b. *Non-aqueous diffusion*: This occurs across lipid cell membranes and determines '**where, and for how long, will a drug be present**'. Drugs may have to cross the epithelial and endothelial linings or other barriers in the body. Epithelial barriers like the

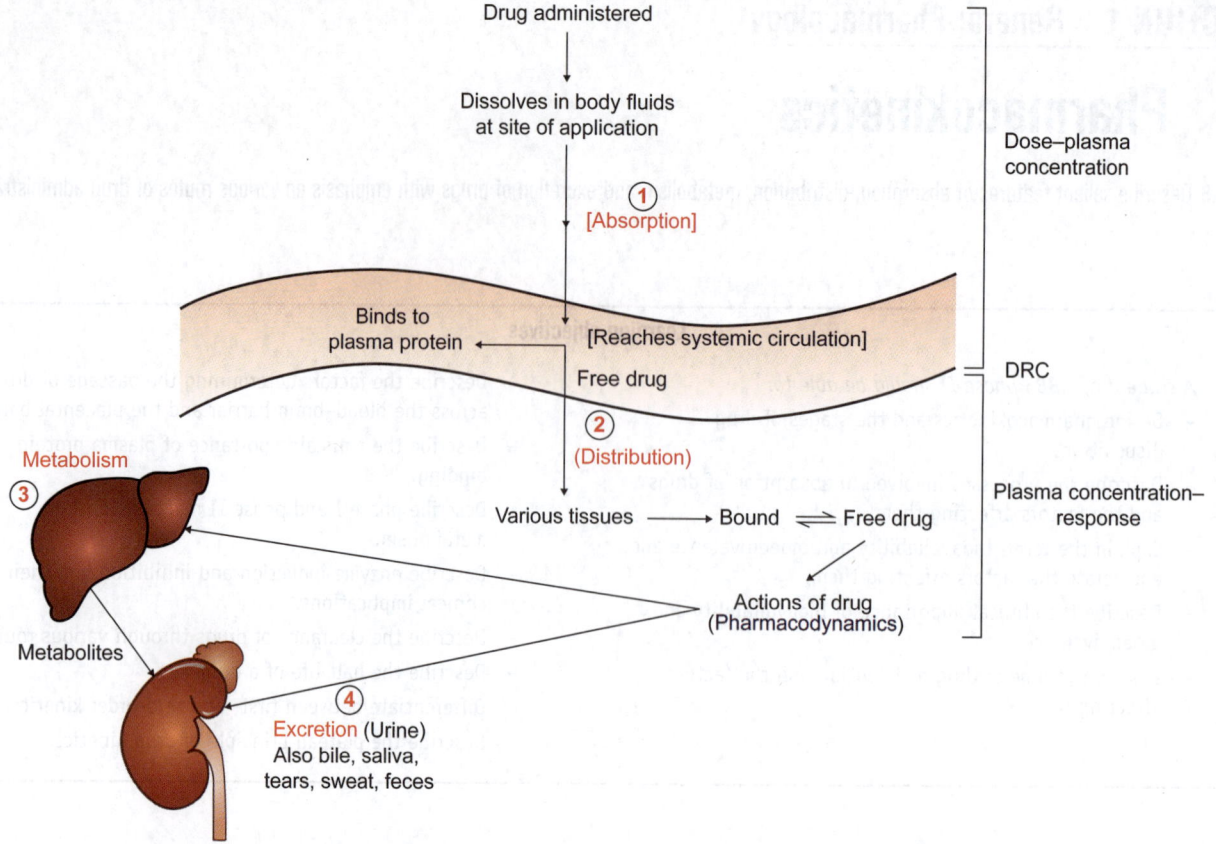

Fig. 3.1 Pharmacokinetics and pharmacodynamics linked by the dose–response relationship

gastrointestinal or renal tubular epithelium consist of a layer of cells tightly connected to each other. Thus, drug molecules must traverse at least two cell membranes (inner and outer) to pass from one side of the epithelial lining to the other.

However, in the vascular endothelium, the gaps between endothelial cells are packed with a loose protein matrix, which act as a filter, retaining the larger molecules and allowing smaller ones to pass. The cut-off molecular size is not exact. Particles with a MW of 80,000–100,000 Daltons transfer very slowly.

The permeability of the vascular endothelium varies from tissue to tissue. Blood vessels, especially those of the **CNS and placenta have tight junctions between endothelial cells.** To penetrate these, the drug molecule must cross the endothelial cell membrane. In contrast, in other organs like the liver and spleen, the endothelium is discontinuous, allowing free passage of molecules.

Movement of Drugs Across Cell Membranes

All pharmacokinetics processes involve the movement of drug molecules across cell membranes.

- The majority of drugs move across cell membranes either by **diffusing** directly through lipid bilayers or by **carrier-mediated transport**.
- Aqueous pores in cell membranes are too small (0.4 nm in diameter) to allow drug molecules, most of which are more than 1 nm in size. However, capillaries (except those in the brain) have large pores (40 Å), allowing drugs (even albumin) to be **filtered** through.
- Drugs with very large molecules move across membranes by the process of **pinocytosis**, which involves the invagination of a part of the cell membrane and the entrapment of a small vesicle with the drug molecule, which is then released within the cell.

A. Diffusion through lipids

All biological membranes consist of a bilayer of phospholipids and cholesterol molecules, with the polar groups oriented at the two surfaces and the nonpolar hydrocarbon chains embedded in the matrix (Fig. 3.2). Drugs diffuse passively across the membrane in the direction of their concentration gradient. The two most important factors affecting the rate of drug diffusion across the cell membrane are **lipid solubility** and **degree of ionisation** of the drug.

1. *Lipid-soluble drugs* get dissolved in the lipoidal matrix of the membrane for diffusion. The rate of transport is directly proportional to the lipid:water partition coefficient of the drug. A more lipid-soluble drug diffuses quickly and attains a higher concentration. The greater the lipid solubility of a drug → the faster is its diffusion → and the higher is the concentration achieved on the other side of the membrane.

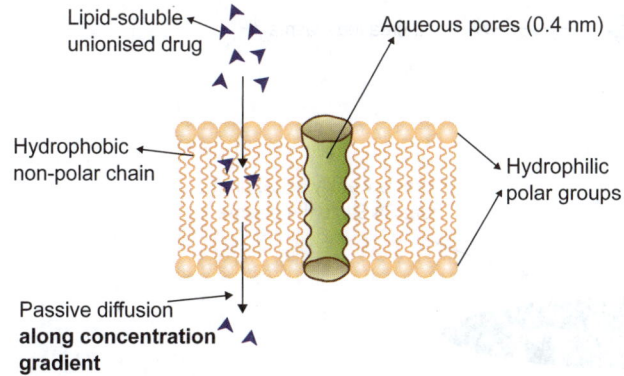

Fig. 3.2 Passive diffusion through the lipid bilayer cell membrane

2. *Unionised (non-polar) drugs:* This form of a drug is more lipid-soluble and hence quickly transferred across membranes. In contrast, the ionic forms of drugs are lipid-insoluble and, therefore, do not diffuse easily across membranes.

Most drugs are weak electrolytes. Thus, the extent of their ionisation depends upon the pH of the medium. The pKa (the negative logarithm of the acidic dissociation constant of a weak electrolyte) is numerically equal to the pH at which it is 50% ionised. The difference between the pH and pKa determines the degree of ionisation. A change in the difference between pH and pKa changes the fraction of the ionised and unionised forms of the drug, as shown in Table 3.1.

Weakly acidic drugs like phenobarbitone, sulfadiazine, and aspirin remain unionised in the acidic pH of the stomach, and hence, their absorption starts in the stomach. The un-ionised form of acidic drugs first crosses the membrane of gastric mucosal cells on the luminal side. These cells have a pH of 7.0, which is much higher than the pH of the gastric cavity, resulting in ionisation of the drug molecules. Then, the ionised form of the drug can only slowly pass into the extracellular fluid. This is called **ion trapping** and might contribute to the gastric mucosal cell damage caused by aspirin.

In contrast, **acidic drugs** are more ionised in the alkaline pH of the intestine, and their absorption slows down. However, **pH partition** is not the main determinant of the site of drug absorption from the GIT. This is because the enormous absorptive surface area of the villi and microvilli in the ileum plays a major determining role in the absorption of drugs.

Acidic drugs like aspirin and barbiturates get more ionised in alkaline urine. Ions cannot be reabsorbed from the lumen of renal tubules and hence, get excreted in the urine. Thus, the **alkalnisation of urine hastens the excretion of acidic drugs.**

In contrast, **basic drugs** like atropine sulphate, and chloroquine phosphate, get ionised in gastric acidic pH. Hence, their **absorption starts only when they reach the intestines**.

Basic drugs attain a higher concentration intracellularly, where the pH is lower (7.0) than plasma pH 7.4. Therefore, the basic drug remains unionised in plasma, but after entering the cell, it encounters a comparatively lower pH. Here, the drug gets ionised and becomes less lipid-soluble, making it difficult for it to move out of the cell. This results in the **intracellular accumulation of the basic drug**.

The excretion of the basic drugs can be hastened by the **acidification of urine.** However, this method is **not useful clinically** in cases of basic drug poisoning, as acidosis itself can worsen the condition and induce cardiotoxic effects.

Table 3.2 compares the effects of pH on acidic and basic drugs.

Table 3.1 Effect of pH of medium on drug ionisation

Nature of drug	pH of medium	Difference between pH and pKa	Ionised fraction of the drug	Unionised fraction of the drug
Acidic	Acidic	Zero	50%	50%
		One	10%	90%
		Two	1%	99%
		Three	0.1%	99.9%
Acidic	Basic	One	90%	10%
		Two	99%	1%
		Three	99.9%	0.1%

Table 3.2 Comparison of the effects of pH on acidic and basic drugs

Parameters	Acidic drugs	Basic drugs
Absorption	Starts in the stomach	Starts in the intestine
Ion trapping	Occurs when they move from low pH (gastric lumen) to high pH (inside gastric mucosal cells)	Occurs when they move from high pH (plasma) to low pH (inside the cells)
Consequences of ion trapping	May be a contributing factor for drug-induced gastric mucosal damage	Causes intracellular drug accumulation
Method to hasten excretion	Alkalinisation of urine interferes with renal tubular reabsorption, resulting in faster excretion. NaHCO₃ is used clinically for the treatment of poisoning with acidic drugs. NaHCO₃ corrects the acidosis and helps in controlling cardiac arrhythmias caused by tricyclic antidepressant drugs, e.g., imipramine, amitriptyline, and nortryptyline.	Acidification of urine increases the excretion of basic drugs but is not useful clinically in cases of poisoning with basic drugs as acidosis can cause cardiotoxicity

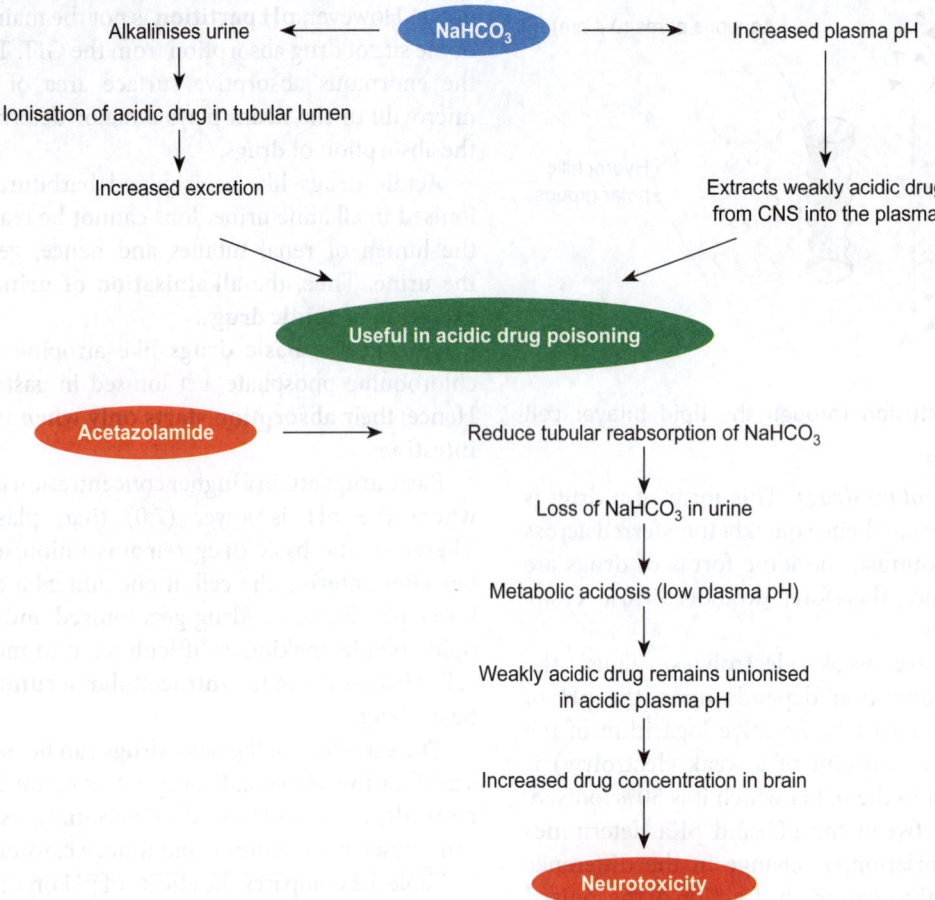

Flowchart 3.1 Choice of urinary alkaliniser

Flowchart 3.1 presents urinary alkalinisers used in cases of acidic drug poisoning. This has practical consequences in choosing the means to alkalinise urine in treating aspirin overdose. While bicarbonate as well as acetazolamide cause alkalinisation of urine, bicarbonate is used in salicylate poisoning because it reduces the distribution of salicylate to the CNS. Carbonic anhydrase inhibitors, which cause acidosis and increase concentration of acidic drugs in the brain, are not suitable for this indication.

B. Carrier-mediated transport

Many cell membranes possess **specialised transport mechanisms** that regulate the entry and exit of physiologically important molecules such as sugars, amino acids, and neurotransmitters. Generally, such transport systems involve a **carrier molecule**, usually a transmembrane protein. The carrier protein binds to one or more drug molecules or ions on one side of the membrane, changes conformation and then releases the drug molecules on the other side of the membrane. Such substances that facilitate the movement of ions across membranes are called **ionophores**. Carrier-mediated transport is:

- **Specific:** for a particular substance.
- **Saturable:** the maximal rate of transport depends on the rate constant (K_m), which is the density of the transporter (in a membrane) and substrate concentration required to achieve half the maximal transport rate. Thus, at higher substrate/ligand concentrations, the carrier sites become saturated, and the rate of transport does not increase beyond this point.
- **Competitively inhibited:** the presence of a second ligand transported by the same carrier protein can cause the competitive inhibition of carrier-mediated transport.

Types

Carrier-mediated transport is further classified into two types:

a. **Facilitated diffusion** (Fig. 3.3): It proceeds more **rapidly than simple passive diffusion**. It can **translocate even non-diffusible substrates along their concentration gradient**. Therefore, it does **not need energy**. For example, glucose is transported into myocytes and adipocytes through glucose transporter 4 (GLUT 4). The antidiabetic drug pioglitazone enhances the expression of this carrier protein, resulting in increased uptake of glucose in the tissues.

b. **Active transport** (Fig. 3.4): It occurs **against the concentration gradient** and therefore needs energy. This process may be **coupled with an energy source**,

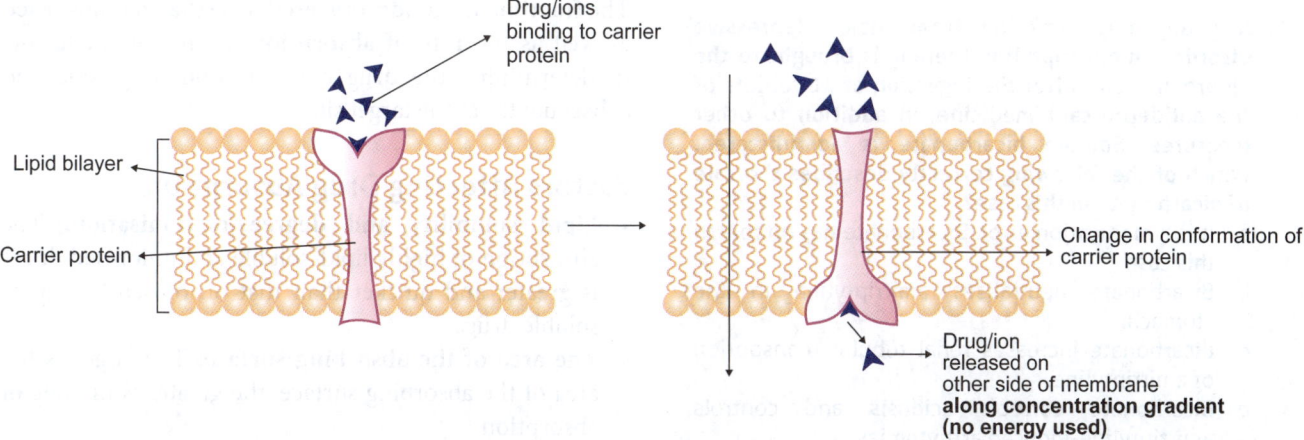

Fig. 3.3 Facilitated diffusion

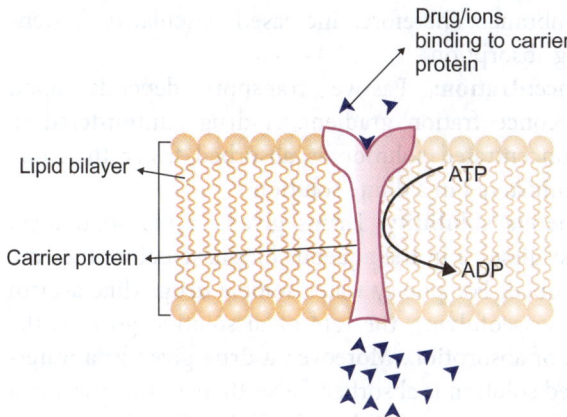
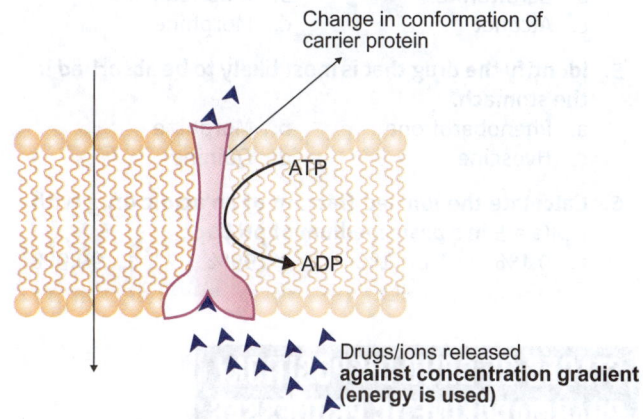

Fig. 3.4 Active transport

either directly (ATP hydrolysis) or indirectly (the electrochemical gradient of another species such as Na⁺). As active transport occurs against the concentration gradient, it results in the **selective accumulation of the substance on one side of the membrane**. This form of transport is inhibited by metabolic poisons.

Carrier-mediated drug transport is important for drug movement in some tissues like the renal tubule, biliary tract, blood–brain barrier, and GIT. P-glycoprotein (P-gp) is a drug transporter present in the renal tubular brush border, bile canaliculi, astrocyte foot processes of brain micro vessels, and GIT. **P-glycoprotein-associated reverse transportation** actively pumps out the drug from the cells of the gut wall into the lumen, resulting in multidrug resistance in neoplastic cells. If P-glycoprotein is inhibited (as by grapefruit juice), the drug absorption increases.

Clinical problem-based questions and MCQs

1. **The long-term use of aspirin (acetylsalicylic acid) is associated with the risk of gastric mucosal damage.**
   i. Explain how the acidic nature of a drug contributes to gastric mucosal damage.
   ii. Which of the following is used to hasten the excretion of aspirin in the case of poisoning?
      a. Sodium bicarbonate   b. Acetazolamide
      c. Citric acid   d. Glucose
   iii. Provide a pharmacological basis to justify your choice.

2. **All pharmacokinetic processes involve the movement of drug molecules across cell membranes, which are lipid bilayers.**
   i. Which of the following statements is correct about drug transport across membranes?
      a. The ionised form of a drug crosses biological membranes more easily than its unionised form.
      b. Lipid-soluble drugs diffuse passively across the membrane against their concentration gradient.
      c. Facilitated diffusion translocates non-diffusible substrates across membranes against their concentration gradient.
      d. Active transport causes the selective accumulation of the drug on one side of the membrane.
   ii. Enumerate the factors favouring the transport of a drug across membranes.

3. A young boy suffering from major depressive disorder on amitriptyline therapy is brought to the emergency unit after the ingestion of 10 tablets of the antidepressant medicine. In addition to other measures, Sodium bicarbonate is administered. Which of the following correctly describes the role of bicarbonate in this case?
   a. It is a medication error. Bicarbonate has no role in this case.
   b. Bicarbonate neutralises amitriptyline in the stomach.
   c. Bicarbonate increases renal tubular reabsoption of amitriptyline.
   d. Bicarbonate corrects acidosis and controls amitriptyline-induced arrhythmias.

4. The alkalinisation of urine is useful in the case of poisoning by:
   a. Barbiturates   b. Amphetamine
   c. Alcohol   d. Morphine

5. Identify the drug that is most likely to be absorbed in the stomach.
   a. Phenobarbitone   b. Morphine
   c. Hyoscine   d. Quinine

6. Calculate the ionised fraction of an acidic drug with a pKa = 5 in a basic medium of pH 8.
   a. 0.1%   b. 1%   c. 99%   d. 99.9%

STAGES OF DRUG DISPOSITION/ PHARMACOKINETIC PROCESSES

I. ABSORPTION OF DRUGS

Absorption is defined as the passage or **movement of a drug from its site of administration into the systemic circulation.** Therefore, it is important for all routes of administration except the intravenous route. Systemically administered drugs must enter plasma before reaching their site of action.

A few drugs can exert their effects without absorption as defined above. For example:
- Bronchodilator aerosols are inhaled to treat asthma.
- Vancomycin, which has very poor oral absorption, is given orally to eradicate the toxin-producing *Clostridium difficile* from the gut lumen, in patients with pseudomembranous colitis.
- Mesalazine is a formulation of 5-aminosalicylic acid in a pH-dependent acrylic coating that gets degraded in the terminal ileum and proximal colon. It is used to treat inflammatory bowel diseases affecting the distal part of the gut.
- Olsalazine is a dimer of 5-aminosalicylic acid (ASA), which is not absorbed from the gut. In the distal bowel, it gets cleaved by colonic bacteria and exerts anti-inflammatory action there. Thus, it is useful in the treatment of distal colitis.

The **fraction of the administered dose that gets absorbed** as well as the **rate of absorption** are important factors in determining the drug concentration in plasma and subsequently, at the target site.

Factors Affecting Drug Absorption

- **Lipid solubility and degree of ionisation:** The absorption of highly lipid-soluble and unionised drugs is greater and quicker than that of ionised/less lipid-soluble drugs.
- **The area of the absorbing surface:** The larger is the area of the absorbing surface, the greater is the rate of absorption.
- **Vascularity of the absorbing surface**: Blood circulation removes the drug from the site of absorption and maintains a concentration gradient across the membrane. Therefore, increased vascularity hastens drug absorption.
- **Concentration**: Passive transport depends upon the concentration gradient. A drug administered in a concentrated solution is absorbed faster than one administered in a dilute solution.
- **Aqueous solubility**: Drugs given in the solid form must dissolve in the aqueous biophase before they are absorbed. For poorly water-soluble drugs (like aspirin and griseofulvin), the rate of dissolution governs the rate of absorption. Moreover, a drug given as a water-based solution is absorbed faster than a drug given in a solid form or as an oil-based solution.
- **Route-specific factors**: Different routes of drug administration have their own peculiarities, which affect drug absorption.
  a. **Oral route**
     - **Gastrointestinal motility** alters the rate and extent of drug absorption. Many disorders (e.g., diabetic neuropathy) cause gastric stasis and slow down the drug absorption. Drugs like muscarinic receptor blockers can reduce motility. In contrast, some drugs increase GI motility, e.g., metoclopramide and other prokinetic drugs.
     - The **presence of food** in the gut also influences drug absorption. A drug taken after a meal is often more slowly absorbed because its progress to the small intestine is delayed. Some drugs form poorly absorbed complexes with food, e.g., tetracycline with milk. In sharp contrast, some drugs such as propranolol reach a higher plasma concentration when taken after meals, probably because food increases the splanchnic blood flow. The decreased splanchnic blood flow, as in hypovolemic states, slows down drug absorption.
     - **Particle size and formulation** have major effects on absorption. Capsules remain intact for some hours after ingestion and delay absorption.

Tablets may have a resistant coating to delay absorption. Small differences in pharmaceutical formulation can make a large difference to the extent of absorption for poorly soluble drugs like digoxin.
- **Physicochemical factors** affect drug absorption by influencing the state of the drug in the intestine. Tetracyclines bind to calcium in milk, which prevents their absorption. Cholestyramine (bile acid-binding resin) binds with several drugs (e.g., warfarin and thyroxine) and decreases their absorption.

b. **Subcutaneous, intramuscular route**—drugs are deposited directly in the vicinity of the capillaries
   - Lipid-soluble drugs readily cross the capillary wall.
   - Very large molecules are absorbed through the lymphatics.
   - Application of heat and muscular exercise accelerate drug absorption by increasing blood flow.
   - A vasoconstrictor (adrenaline) injected with a drug retards its absorption.
   - The incorporation of hyaluronidase facilitates drug absorption from the subcutaneous route by promoting the spread of the drug over a larger surface area.

c. **Topical routes** involve drug administration through the skin, mucous membrane, and cornea
   - Lipid solubility is very important for systemic absorption after topical application. Only few drugs (e.g., nitroglycerine, hyoscine, clonidine, and estradiol) significantly penetrate intact skin and are used topically for systemic effects.
   - Absorption can be promoted by increasing the hydration of skin with an occlusive dressing or by rubbing the drug on the skin. For such application, the drug should be incorporated in an oleaginous base.
   - Drugs are readily absorbed from abraded surfaces, e.g., tannic acid applied over burnt skin may cause hepatic necrosis.
   - The cornea is permeable to lipid-soluble, unionised drugs (like physostigmine) but not to neostigmine. Similarly, the mucous membranes of the mouth, rectum, and vagina allow the absorption of lipophilic drugs.

Bioavailability

The US Food and Drug Administration (FDA) defines bioavailability as "the rate at which and the extent to which the active concentration of the drug is available at the desired site of action" (or, more practically speaking, in the bloodstream). It is represented by the area under concentration–time curve (AUC). In other words, bioavailability is the fraction of unchanged drug reaching the systemic circulation after administration by any route.

Bioavailability for different routes

- For intravenous administration, bioavailability is 100% since the drug is administered in the systemic circulation itself.
- For intramuscular, subcutaneous, and transdermal administration, bioavailability is ≤ 100%, possibly due to the local binding of the drug.
- For oral, rectal, and the inhalational route too, the bioavailability is < 100%. To reach the systemic circulation from the lumen of the gut upon oral administration, the drug has to:
  - Penetrate the mucosa (which is determined by the **extent of absorption**).
  - Encounter the enzymes that may inactivate it in the gut wall and liver (**first-pass metabolism**).

Oral bioavailability may be less than 100% for two main reasons:

- **Incomplete absorption:** Some drugs are not completely absorbed due to their hydrophilic or lipophilic nature. Drugs like atenolol are too hydrophilic. These drugs fail to cross the lipid cell membrane. Some other drugs like acyclovir are too lipophilic and hence, not soluble enough in an aqueous medium to cross the water layer adjacent to the cell. Some drugs get metabolised within the intestine, e.g., digoxin; they are also incompletely absorbed.
- **First-pass metabolism:** After absorption across the gut wall, the drug reaches the liver through the portal blood before entering systemic circulation. Some amount of the drug may get metabolised during its passage through the gut wall, portal blood, and liver. This is called first-pass metabolism or pre-systemic metabolism, i.e., metabolism of the drug when it passes through the liver for first time, before reaching systemic circulation. Some amount of the drug may get excreted in the bile from the liver.

The effect of first-pass metabolism is known as the **extraction ratio** (ER) and is calculated as shown.

$$ER = \frac{CL_{liver}}{Q} \quad (1)$$

where CL_{liver} is the drug clearance by the liver and Q is the hepatic blood flow (normally 90 L/hour in an adult weighing 70 kg).

Systemic bioavailability (F) depends upon the extent of absorption (f) and the extraction ratio (ER) and is calculated by the equation below.

$$F = f \times (1 - ER) \quad (2)$$

Combining equations 1 and 2, we get:

$$F = f \times (1 - \frac{CL_{liver}}{Q}) \quad (3)$$

To calculate the oral bioavailability, the AUC of plasma concentration–time curve after oral administration is compared to that after intravenous administration.

C_{max} is the maximum plasma concentration that can be attained. The AUC (area under the plasma concentration–time curve) represents the extent of drug absorption. T_{max} is the time needed to reach maximum plasma concentration, which reflects the rate of drug absorption.

Though the **rate of absorption** is not considered in the calculation of bioavailability, it influences the clinical effectiveness of the drug. For example, if a drug is completely and rapidly absorbed, it will reach a much higher peak plasma concentration (and have a more dramatic effect) than if it were absorbed slowly.

If a drug preparation 'Y' is more slowly absorbed than preparation 'X', Y may not produce the therapeutic effect, although ultimately, both are absorbed to the same extent (i.e., the area under the curve is same; Fig 3.5). A preparation 'Z' of the same drug which is absorbed more slowly and to a lesser extent has a lower bioavailability than the other two.

Factors affecting bioavailability

Various pharmaceutical and pharmacological factors that affect the bioavailability of drug are described below.

1. Pharmaceutical factors

- **Type of formulation**: The bioavailability from different formulations in descending order is:
  Solution > Suspension > Tablet > Coated tablet > Capsule
- **Rate of disintegration and dissolution** depend on factors mentioned below:
  - Particle size: microfine preparations have higher bioavailability, due to better dissolution.
  - Salt form: salts of weakly acidic drugs are highly water-soluble and have higher bioavailability, e.g., sodium tolbutamide has better bioavailability than tolbutamide.
  - Crystal form: amorphous forms have more bioavailability than crystalline forms, e.g., amorphous chloramphenicol palmitate dissolves faster and has better bioavailability than its crystalline form
  - Nature of excipients/adjuvants, manufacturing process.
  - Degree of ionisation: highly polar drugs like streptomycin, acetylcholine, and neostigmine are not absorbed orally, and have low bioavailability

2. Pharmacological factors

- **Route of drug administration**: Bioavailability is 100% only after intravenous administration and is lesser for other routes. Various factors affect the rate and extent of absorption after administration by different routes, e.g., GI motility/gastric emptying time, GIT diseases, the presence of food, local tissue binding, and area and vascularity of the absorbing surface.
- **First-pass metabolism**: Drugs with high first-pass metabolism have a lower bioavailability since a greater amount of the drug gets metabolised before reaching the systemic circulation (extraction ratio, ER).
- **Drug–drug interactions**: Drugs given simultaneously may affect each other's bioavailability. This is due to **changes in the rate and extent of absorption** of one drug by another simultaneously administered drug like cholestyramine or a prokinetic drug. There may be **reduced first-pass metabolism** (and resulting high oral bioavailability) of one drug, if another drug competing with it for metabolising enzymes is given simultaneously, e.g., chlorpromazine and propranolol can alter each other's hepatic extraction.
- In patients with severe **hepatic disease**, the extent of first-pass metabolism decreases, resulting in higher oral bioavailability and toxicity with the usual doses.

Bioequivalence

The oral formulation of the same drug from different manufacturers or even from different batches produced by the same manufacturer may be chemically equivalent (i.e., contain the same amount of drug) but biologically inequivalent (i.e., do not yield the same blood levels).

> **The History of Bioequivalence**
>
> The term bioequivalence came into existence through an unusual incidence of phenytoin toxicity in Australia in 1968. The pharmaceutical firm marketing 'Dilantin sodium' capsules used calcium sulphate as the inert diluent in the preparation. Stocks of calcium sulphate were exhausted, and the manufacturers used lactose as a substitute, thinking that this minor change in inert diluents would be inconsequential. However, with the reformulated product, the plasma concentration of phenytoin reached higher levels (30 mg/mL) than

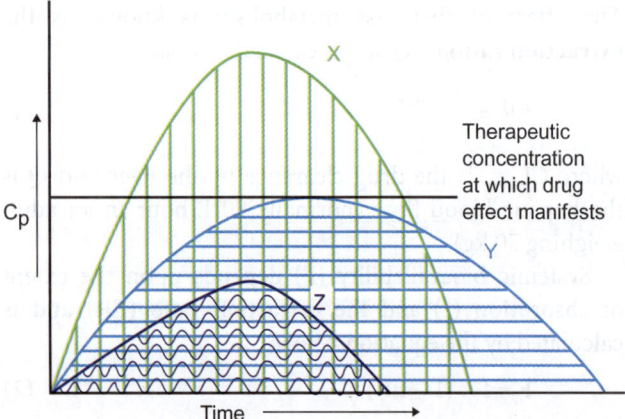

Fig. 3.5 The bioavailability of different preparations of the same drug

required, leading to toxicity. This occurred because lactose dissolved more easily, resulting in quicker absorption and higher plasma concentration, ultimately causing toxicity.

Differences in bioavailability were also observed with different digoxin formulations in 1971.

Causes of bioinequivalence
The bioavailability from different formulations of the same drug may be different because of differences in the rates of disintegration and dissolution.

Disintegration
A drug given as a solid dosage form by the oral route must break (disintegrate) into individual particles of the active drug. Tablets and capsules contain several materials such as diluents, stabilising agents, binders, and lubricants, besides the active moiety. The nature of these substances as well as the details of manufacturing process—e.g., the force used in compressing the tablet—may affect the rate of disintegration. Drug formulations that have **lower rates of disintegration will be absorbed more slowly** and may not reach the same peak plasma concentration as formulations that disintegrate fast.

Dissolution
After disintegration, the released drug must dissolve in the aqueous gastrointestinal contents. Aqueous solubility is an important factor for the movement of a drug 'to' and 'from' lipid barriers (i.e., before crossing the lipid barrier, a drug must reach near it by dissolving in the aqueous medium around; similarly, after crossing the lipid membrane, the drug is carried away from it by dissolving in the aqueous medium). The **rate of dissolution depends upon the inherent solubility, particles size, crystal form, and other physical properties of the drug.**

Clinical Significance of Bioequivalence
- The differences in the bioavailability of different preparations are more frequently observed with poorly soluble, slowly absorbed drugs like aspirin, griseofulvin, spironolactone, etc. A reduction in particle size (**microfining**) increases the rate of absorption of such drugs.
- Practically, bioavailability variations are important for drugs with a **low safety margin** (e.g., digoxin) and **steep DRC**, which need precise dosage control (e.g., oral hypoglycemics and oral anticoagulants).
- Bioavailability variations may be also responsible for the **success or failure of an antimicrobial** regimen.

Bioavailability is an absolute term. It requires a measurement of both the rate and extent of the drug that reaches the systemic circulation from administered dosage form. However, **bioequivalence is a relative term** that implies a comparison of the bioavailability of different branded formulations of the same drug. For two preparations to be labelled as bioequivalent, the difference in their bioavailabilities should be less than 20%.

Clinical problem-based questions and MCQs

7. The rate of drug absorption can be increased by various 'route-specific' factors. Enumerate the factors that may alter the rate of drug absorption after each of the following:
   i. Oral administration
   ii. Intramuscular administration
   iii. Subcutaneous administration

8. A patient of supraventricular tachyarrhythmia requires emergency treatment with a β blocker. Propranolol was given initially intravenously, and later, oral therapy was instituted. The oral dose of propranolol was about 40 times higher than the intravenous dose, due to low oral bioavailability.
   i. Define the term 'bioavailability'.
   ii. What are the factors affecting oral bioavailability?
   iii. Explain the reason for the low oral bioavailability of propranolol.

9. The route of drug administration affects its bioavailability. Which of the following routes achieves the maximum bioavailability?
   a. Subcutaneous route   b. Intramuscular route
   c. Intravenous route   d. Oral route

10. There are historical reports in literature of two formulations of phenytoin that contain the same amount of the drug but yield different blood levels.
    i. What is this phenomenon called? Differentiate the phenomenon involved from bioavailability.
    ii. Explain the cause of different plasma concentrations obtained with the two formulations.
    iii. Describe the clinical implications of the phenomenon involved.

11. The differences in the bioavailability of two bioequivalent preparations having the same drug, dose and dosage form should be:
    a. < 5%   b. < 10%   c. < 15%   d. < 20%

12. Which of the following results in reduced drug bioavailability?
    a. High first-pass metabolism
    b. Increased absorption
    c. IV drug administration
    d. High lipid solubility

II. DISTRIBUTION OF DRUGS
The process of drug absorption takes the drug from the site of administration to systemic circulation. From there, the drug must reach its site of action. This is achieved by the second pharmacokinetic process known as 'distribution'. A drug gets distributed from systemic circulation to various

tissues until the unbound drug achieves an equilibrium between its concentrations in the plasma and the tissue fluid. The extent of drug distribution is indicated by the '**apparent volume of distribution**' **(aV_d)**. This is an important pharmacokinetic parameter for the calculation of the appropriate loading dose of a drug. It is a theoretical value depicting how extensively a drug gets distributed throughout the body and is represented as litre/kilogram of body weight (L/kg).

The volume of distribution (aV_d) is defined as 'the **volume that would accommodate all the drug that is present in the body (Q), if the concentration throughout is assumed to be same as in the plasma**'. Hence, it depicts the relationship between the total amount of the drug in the body and its concentration in plasma/blood or the concentration of the unbound drug in body water, if concentration throughout the body is same as in plasma/blood/body water.

$$V_d = \frac{\text{Amount of the drug in the body (Q)}}{\text{Plasma concentration }(C_p)} \quad (4)$$

The apparent volume of distribution (aV_d) is not real; it is an apparent value because it is calculated based on the assumption that the body is a single homogeneous compartment (which it is not). The total body water is distributed into extracellular, intracellular, and transcellular compartments. However, to calculate the apparent volume of distribution, the body is considered as a single compartment. Thus, the word 'apparent' always precedes V_d.

Factors Affecting the aV_d

The aV_d of a drug depends on several factors such as:

1. Degree of ionisation and lipid solubility of drug

Ionised or polar drugs like vecuronium and aminoglycosides have relatively low lipid solubility. Such drugs fail to enter cells and remain in the extracellular fluid (ECF). Thus, their aV_d is approximately the same as the ECF volume. In contrast, lipid-soluble drugs such as ethanol and phenytoin are widely distributed and their aV_d is equal to that of total body water.

2. Affinity for tissue proteins

Drugs that have a greater affinity for tissue proteins get sequestrated in tissues. Such drugs, which are not homogeneously distributed, attain much higher concentrations in extravascular tissues. Thus, for these drugs, the denominator in Equation 4 (Q/C_p) decreases. Hence, such drugs have a very high aV_d, which exceeds any physical volume, e.g., 6 L/kg for digoxin. For drugs that have high affinity for tissue proteins, the volume of distribution exceeds the total body water, e.g., 1300 L for chloroquine.

3. Affinity for plasma proteins

Drugs that have a high plasma protein-binding (PPB) ability are retained within the vascular compartment and have low aV_d, which is approximately equal to the blood volume, e.g., 0.15 L/kg for warfarin. **Plasma protein binding is a reversible process.**

Acidic drugs have an affinity for albumin and basic drugs for α_1-acid glycoprotein. Examples of acidic drugs that bind to albumin include barbiturates, benzodiazepines, phenytoin, valproate, NSAIDs, penicillins, sulphonamides, and tetracyclines. Basic drugs that are highly bound to α_1-acid glycoprotein include verapamil, lignocaine, bupivacaine, quinidine, disopyramide, and beta blockers.

The fraction of the total drug in plasma that will bind to proteins depends upon the **number of binding sites, affinity of the drug for plasma proteins, and drug concentration.**

Consequences of a high PPB

- Drugs that are strongly bound to plasma proteins are restricted to the vascular compartment. Hence, their **aV_d is low** (equal to the plasma volume). For example, warfarin is 90% plasma protein-bound with aV_d = 0.15 L/kg.
- PPB serves as a temporary storage site for drugs and **increases the duration of drug action**.
- Since dialysis cannot filter proteins, which are large molecules, the excretion of highly plasma protein-bound drugs cannot be enhanced by dialysis. Therefore, dialysis has **no role in toxicity of highly plasma protein-bound drugs**.
- The simultaneous administration of two drugs with high affinity for the same binding site may cause **displacement reactions.** However, such displacements are not clinically very relevant because the displaced portion of the drug gets easily metabolised and excreted.

4. Differences in regional blood flow

Some highly lipid soluble drugs, when administered by IV or the inhalational route exhibit a phenomenon of **redistribution** due to differences in regional blood flow to various organs. These drugs get distributed first to highly vascular organs like the brain, kidney, and heart, and then move quickly to less vascular but more bulky tissues like the skeletal muscles and adipose tissues. For drugs whose target site lies in highly vascular tissues, drug action starts quickly and is terminated quickly because of redistribution.

For example, after IV injection, the ultrashort-acting barbiturate thiopentone sodium gets rapidly distributed to the CNS, resulting in a rapid onset of anesthesia within minutes. However, this action is short-lived because the drug gets redistributed to less vascular sites, and its action in the CNS is terminated. Therefore, thiopentone sodium has a quick but brief effect, and is preferred for the induction of anesthesia.

Later on, the drug is slowly withdrawn from the bulky tissues, metabolised, and eliminated. The repeated administration of such drugs can saturate these low-perfusion, high-capacity sites, making the drug more long-acting.

5. Disease states

V_d is altered by some disease states like **cirrhosis, uremia, and congestive heart failure** owing to changes in the distribution of body water, binding proteins, and membrane permeability.

6. Drug movement across the blood–brain barrier

The capillary endothelial cells in the brain have tight junctions without any paracellular spaces. Further, these capillaries are covered by neural tissue. These **tight junctions and covering neural tissues** together constitute the blood–brain barrier (BBB). Similarly, in the choroid plexus, there exists a blood–CSF barrier constituted by **tight junctions of choroidal epithelium lining the capillaries**. An enzymatic blood–brain barrier is constituted by **enzymes** such as monoamine oxidase (MAO) and cholinesterase present in the **capillary-lining cells**.

The passage of drugs **across the BBB** depends on lipid solubility of drug. **Only lipid-soluble drugs can penetrate** these barriers. In case of an **inflammation of the meninges** or brain as in meningitis or encephalitis, the permeability of the BBB is increased. However, the exit of the drug from the brain is independent of lipid solubility and occurs with the bulk flow of CSF through the arachnoid villi into the blood.

7. Drug movement across the placental barrier

The movement of drugs across the placental barrier depends on lipid solubility. However, the placenta is an **incomplete barrier,** and some amount of non-lipid-soluble drugs can also cross it if present in the maternal blood for a long time or in high concentration. Thus, most drugs given to pregnant women can gain access to the fetus and harm it. For this reason, drugs should be prescribed very cautiously during pregnancy.

Clinical Implications of V_d

If the V_d is high, it indicates a greater concentration of the drug in the tissues than in the blood. Therefore, to achieve the same plasma concentration, the dosage should be higher for drugs that have a high V_d (the V_d of chloroquine is the highest, 1300 L). Such a high dosage is called a 'loading dose'. Thus, **V_d determines the loading dose**.

Drugs that have a low V_d are restricted to the vascular compartment, and can be easily removed by dialysis.

Clinical problem-based questions and MCQs

13. A 34-year-old female patient suffering from vulvovaginitis is on oral fluconazole 100 mg, single-dose therapy. Such a dose results in a peak plasma concentration of 25 μg/mL.
    i. Calculate the apparent volume of distribution of fluconazole in this patient.
        a. 0.5 L   b. 1 L   c. 50 L   d. 4 L
    ii. Define the volume of distribution. Why is it considered an apparent value?
    iii. Enumerate the factors affecting the volume of distribution of a drug.
    iv. Name some diseases that may alter the V_d of drugs.

14. Identify the drug with the highest volume of distribution.
    a. Aspirin   b. Tolbutamide
    c. Chloroquine   d. Warfarin

15. In a pharmacokinetic study, the volume of distribution of digoxin is calculated to be 6 L/kg, which exceeds any physical volume.
    i. Explain the cause for such a high V_d.
    ii. Describe the clinical implications of high volume of distribution.

16. Dialysis is useful for drug with:
    a. High V_d and high PPB
    b. High V_d and low PPB
    c. Low V_d and high PPB
    d. Low V_d and low PPB

17. i. A drug that has high PPB will:
        a. Have a very short-lived effect.
        b. Be filtered quickly by the glomerulus.
        c. Have lower chances of drug interactions.
        d. Have low volume of distribution.
    ii. Enumerate drugs that have an affinity for plasma albumin and α_1-acid glycoprotein.
    iii. What are the clinical implications of a high PPB?

18. Thiopentone sodium is an ultra-short-acting barbiturate, used for the induction of anesthesia. The central action of thiopentone gets terminated within a few minutes due to redistribution.
    i. Describe the phenomenon of redistribution.
    ii. What happens if a drug showing redistribution is given repeatedly in quick succession?

19. Redistribution is a characteristic of drugs that have:
    a. High lipid solubility
    b. High aqueous solubility
    c. High volume of distribution
    d. High plasma protein-binding

III. DRUG METABOLISM/BIOTRANSFORMATION

Once the drug reaches its site of action, the pharmacodynamic processes begin and drug action is exerted through different types of receptors/enzymes, etc. The next objective is to eliminate the drug from the body.

The kidney is the main organ for drug excretion. It can **excrete hydrophilic, ionised drugs as such.** On the other hand, lipophilic, unionised drugs get reabsorbed in the renal tubules. Such drugs need to be changed into a form that can be readily excreted by the kidney. This process of **converting lipid-soluble, non-polar (unionised) drugs into lipid-insoluble, ionised forms in the body is called biotransformation or metabolism.**

Sites of Drug Metabolism

In the human body, the principal organ of drug metabolism is the **liver**. A few biotransformations can occur in the **intestines (lumen, wall), lungs, skin, and kidneys** also.

After absorption from the small intestine, drugs first reach the liver through portal circulation. In the liver, a drug can be metabolised to variable extents, and the remaining portion of the drug reaches the systemic circulation. This is known as **pre-systemic metabolism** (i.e., the metabolism that occurs before the entry of the drug into the systemic circulation) or **first-pass metabolism** (i.e., the metabolism that occurs when a drug passes through the liver for the first time). Therefore, some part of the orally given drug administered is lost or fails to reach the systemic circulation in its unchanged form. This is called the first-pass effect. **Metabolism of some drugs by gastric juices, digestive enzymes, intestinal wall enzymes, and intestinal microorganisms also contribute to this effect.**

Drugs like testosterone, morphine, isoprenaline, lignocaine, and hydrocortisone have a **very high first-pass metabolism**, which makes them ineffective upon oral administration. These drugs are, therefore, **not used orally.** Drugs like propranolol, alprenolol, verapamil, salbutamol, nitroglycerine, methyltestosterone, and pethidine also have a **high first-pass metabolism.** Thus, their bioavailability after oral administration is low. Such drugs have **high oral:parenteral or sublingual dose ratio.** In other words, their oral dosage is much higher than the parenteral dose to compensate for the loss due to first-pass metabolism.

Biotransformation Reactions

Metabolic reactions are categorised as phase I and phase II reactions.

Phase I reactions

These are **non-synthetic** reactions involving the **introduction or unmasking of –OH, –SH or –NH₂ groups,** which converts a drug into a more polar form that is readily excretable. The **metabolites may be inactive or, sometimes, active.** Active metabolites subsequently undergo phase II reactions.

Important reactions in phase I include oxidation, reduction, and hydrolysis.

- Cytochrome P450 (CYP450)-dependent chemical reactions include oxidation, hydroxylation, oxidative dealkylation, deamination, desulfuration, and dechlorination.
- CYP450-independent reactions involve dehydrogenation and oxidation.

Table 3.3 presents examples of drugs metabolised by phase I reactions.

Table 3.3 Examples of drugs metabolised by phase I reactions

Name of reaction	Examples of drugs metabolised
1. Oxidation	
CYP450-dependent oxidation	- Phenobarbital, secobarbital - Phenytoin, carbamazepine, thiopental - Morphine, ethyl morphine, codeine - Ibuprofen, phenylbutazone, acetaminophen - Chlorpromazine, thioridazine, amphetamine, diazepam, caffeine, nicotine - Propranolol, parathion
CYP450-independent oxidation	Amitriptyline, nortriptyline, desipramine, propylthiouracil, methimazole
2. Reduction	Chloramphenicol, clonazepam, dantrolene, methadone, naloxone
3. Hydrolysis	Procaine, lignocaine, procainamide, aspirin, indomethacin, succinylcholine

Phase II reactions

These are **synthetic** reactions involving the **conjugation of an endogenous substrate** like glucuronide, sulphate, amino acid (glycine), acetate, and methyl, with a drug or its phase I metabolite. For some drugs, phase II reactions **may precede** phase I reactions, e.g., isoniazid is first acetylated (phase II reaction) and then hydrolysed (phase I reaction).

Conjugation reactions are often **faster** than phase I reactions. The metabolites of phase II reaction are **mostly inactive**, but sometimes, reactive species are formed, e.g., in the glucuronidation of NSAIDs, the acetylation of isoniazid, and the sulphation of minoxidil. Table 3.4 presents examples of drugs metabolised by phase II reactions.

Table 3.4 Examples of drugs metabolised by phase II reactions

Name of reaction	Examples of drugs metabolised
Acetylation	Isoniazid, sulphonamides, dapsone, hydralazine, procainamide
Methylation	Adrenaline, dopamine, histamine
Glucuronide conjugation	Diazepam, digoxin, digitoxin morphine, meprobamate
Glutathione conjugation	Acetaminophen, ethacrynic acid
Glycine conjugation	Cholic acid, deoxycholic acid nicotinic acid
Water conjugation	Leukotriene A_4, carbamazepine,
Sulfation	Methyldopa, acetaminophen

Drug-metabolising enzymes

1. Microsomal enzymes

These are present in the endoplasmic reticulum of the liver and other tissues. Most important among the microsomal enzymes are mixed-function oxidases (MFOs) or monooxygenases. Two microsomal enzymes that play a key role in oxidation–reduction processes are:

- Flavoprotein NADPH cytochrome P450 reductase
- Hemoprotein cytochrome P450

NADPH and molecular oxygen are also required for drug oxidation.

The oxidation of drugs by microsomal enzymes occurs in a stepwise manner (Fig. 3.6).

- In the first step, NADPH transfers an electron e^- to flavoprotein. This reaction is catalysed by cytochrome P450 reductase.
- In the second step, the reduced form of the flavoprotein, in turn, reduces the oxidised P450–drug complex.
- In the third step, there is a transfer of another e^- through the same P450 reductase to convert molecular O_2 to activated oxygen, which forms a complex with the P450–drug complex.
- In the fourth step, the activated oxygen gets transferred to the drug.

Drug oxidations catalysed by P450 are slow. Highly lipid-soluble drugs and chemicals are metabolised by this enzyme, e.g., phenytoin, phenobarbitone, thiopentone, carbamazepine, morphine, and chlorpromazine. CYP exists in many isoforms, of which the following play important role in drug metabolism:

- CYP1A2
- CYP2A6, 2B6, 2C8, 2C9, 2C19, 2D6, 2E1
- CYP3A4

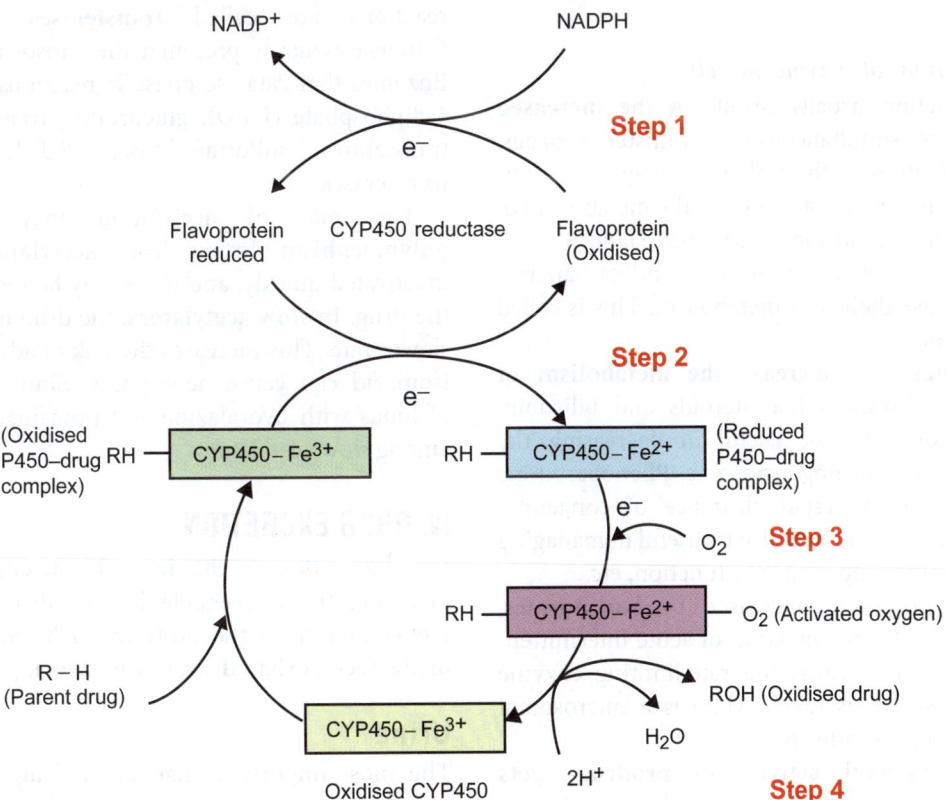

Fig. 3.6 Drug oxidation reaction

CYP3A4 alone catalyses the oxidation of more than half of the prescription drugs that get metabolised in the liver.

Enzyme induction

The synthesis of microsomal enzymes, especially **cytochrome P450 and glucuronyl transferase,** can be induced by a variety of drugs, environmental pollutants, etc. As the **synthesis of the enzyme protein increases**, induction takes about 4–14 days to reach its peak and is maintained as long as the inducing agent continues to be administered. The enzyme levels return to their original value after 1–3 weeks of stopping the inducing agent.

Examples of enzyme inducers:

- CYP450 enzymes can be induced by a variety of chemically dissimilar agents.
- CYP1A2 is induced by the proton-pump inhibitor omeprazole, cruciferous vegetables, and smoking.
- CYP2A6, 2B6, 2C8, 2C9, and 2C19 are induced by barbiturates and rifampicin.
- CYP 2E1is induced by ethanol and isoniazid.
- CYP3A4 is induced by rifampicin, mifepristone carbamazepine, macrolides, phenobarbitone, phenytoin, and atorvastatin.
- CYP4A is induced by lipid-lowering drugs like fenofibrate and gemfibrozil.

The induction of the enzyme mostly involves the increased synthesis of enzyme protein. In some cases, the reduced degradation of enzyme protein may be responsible, e.g., clotrimazole induces CYP3A4 and ethanol induces CYP2E1.

Clinical implications of enzyme induction

- Enzyme induction usually results in the **increased inactivation** of simultaneously administered drugs, causing a reduction of their pharmacological activity. For example, rifampicin can increase the metabolism of oral contraceptives, causing contraceptive failure.
- Some inducing drugs like rifampicin and carbamazepine can increase their own metabolism. This is called **autoinduction.**
- Inducing drugs may **increase the metabolism of endogenous substances** like steroids and bilirubin. Thus, phenytoin may be useful in decreasing the manifestations of Cushing syndrome. Phenobarbitone can bring about the rapid clearance of congenital hemolytic jaundice, and may also be useful in managing chronic poisoning, impaired liver function, etc.
- **Porphyrin synthesis** is increased by **barbiturates**, which results in the precipitation of acute intermittent porphyria. This is because the rate-limiting enzyme of porphyrin synthesis (delta ALA) is a microsomal enzyme, and thus, is inducible.
- The pharmacological **activity of prodrugs gets accentuated** by enzyme induction. Prodrugs, which are given in their inactive form, are activated inside body by enzymatic metabolism.

Enzyme inhibition

Some drugs have the potential to cause the inhibition of the CYP450 enzyme. For example:

- **Imidazole drugs** (ketoconazole, cimetidine, macrolides, etc.) bind to the heme iron of CYP450 and **competitively inhibit** the metabolism of co-administered drugs.
- Drugs like chloramphenicol, steroids (ethinyl estradiol, norethindrone, and spironolactone), carbon disulfide, grapefruit, furanocoumarins, selegiline, phencyclidine, ticlopidine, clopidogrel, ritonavir, and propylthiouracil bind to P450 apoprotein or heme by covalent bonds, resulting in **irreversible enzyme inhibition.** Such inhibitors are called **suicide inhibitors**.
- The mechanism of inhibition of CYP450 by drugs like tamoxifen, raloxifene, and mifepristone is not understood,

2. Flavin monooxygenase or Ziegler's enzyme, amine oxidase and dehydrogenases

These enzymes catalyse CYP450-independent oxidation reactions, e.g., oxidation of amitriptyline, nortriptyline, desipramine, propylthiouracil and methimazole.

3. Esterases and amidases

These enzymes catalyse hydrolysis reactions, e.g., lignocaine, procaine, aspirin, and indomethacine.

4. Conjugases

The enzymes responsible for phase II or conjugation reactions are called **transferases or conjugases**. Conjugases may be present in the cytosol or in microsomes. Enzymes that catalyse phase II reactions include uridine 5-diphosphate (UPD), glucuronosyltransferase, N-acetyl transferases, sulfotransferases (SULTs), and methyl transferases.

The rate of acetylation may show **genetic polymorphism**. In rapid/**fast acetylators**, the drug is inactivated quickly, and there may be reduced efficacy of the drug. In **slow acetylators**, the drug is inactivated at a slower rate. This increases the risk of adverse effects, e.g., isoniazid can cause neuropathy. Similarly, the chances of lupus with hydralazine and procainamide are greater among slow acetylators.

IV. DRUG EXCRETION

Drug excretion is the **last pharmacokinetic process**, involving the irreversible loss of drug or its inactive metabolites from the body through various routes like **urine, feces, exhaled air, sweat, saliva,** and **milk**.

Urine

The most important channel of drug excretion is the kidney. It excretes all **water-soluble** drugs or their inactive metabolites by glomerular filtration, tubular reabsorption, and tubular secretion (Fig. 3.7)

- *Glomerular filtration*: all **non-bound** drugs are excreted by glomerular filtration. It does not depend on lipid solubility, but on renal blood flow and the extent of plasma protein-binding of the drug.
- *Tubular reabsorption*: it depends on **lipid solubility and the degree of ionisation** of the drug, which is determined by urinary pH and the pKa of the drug.
- *Tubular secretion*: it is the **active transport of organic acids and bases** by two separate non-specific mechanisms operating in the proximal convoluted tubule (PCT) of kidney. It is not affected by lipid solubility or plasma protein binding.

Drug interactions at the tubular secretory site

Drugs or endogenous substances that use the same secretory site in the renal tubules compete for the tubular secretory site. The **direction of movement in tubular secretion is from the blood to the lumen for drugs or exogenous substances and the opposite (from the lumen to blood) for endogenous substances** (Fig. 3.7).

When probenecid competes with penicillin (exogenous substance) for renal tubular secretory sites, it reduces the excretion of penicillin. Thus, the duration of the action of penicillin gets prolonged. In contrast, when probenecid competes with uric acid (endogenous substance) for tubular secretion, it inhibits the movement of uric acid from the lumen to the blood. Thus, probenecid increases the excretion of uric acid. Due to this, probenecid has uricosuric action, which is useful in the management of gout.

Feces

The portion of orally administered drugs that is not absorbed or is secreted in the bile is removed from the body through feces. A few drugs may show '**enterohepatic circulation**' like **ampicillin, tetracyclines, erythromycin, oral contraceptives,** and **rifampicin**. The glucuronide conjugates of these drugs are actively transported by the liver into bile. The intestinal bacteria deconjugate these substances, and the drug is absorbed again from the intestine. This makes the drug longer-acting. Such a drug is finally excreted in urine.

Exhaled Air

Some **volatile liquids and gases** like general anesthetics get eliminated from the body through exhaled air. The rate of elimination depends mainly on the partial pressure of the drug.

Saliva, Sweat, and Milk

These are minor routes of drug excretion. Drugs like **lithium, heavy metals, rifampicin, and potassium iodide** are secreted in saliva and sweat. Drug secretion in milk may harm the breastfed infant.

KINETICS OF ELIMINATION

The three most important parameters affecting the kinetics of drug elimination are—**bioavailability, volume of distribution, and clearance.**

a. Bioavailability

As discussed earlier in this chapter, bioavailability (F) is the fraction of unchanged drug that reaches the systemic circulation after administration by any route. It is represented by the 'area under the curve' (AUC) of the blood concentration–time curve. It is calculated as shown:

$$F = f \times (1 - ER)$$
$$F = f \times (1 - CL_{liver}/Q)$$

b. Volume of distribution

The apparent volume of distribution (aV_d) of a drug is defined as the volume that would accommodate all the drug present in the body (Q) if the concentration throughout the body is the same as plasma concentration (C_p).

$$aV_d = Q/C_p$$

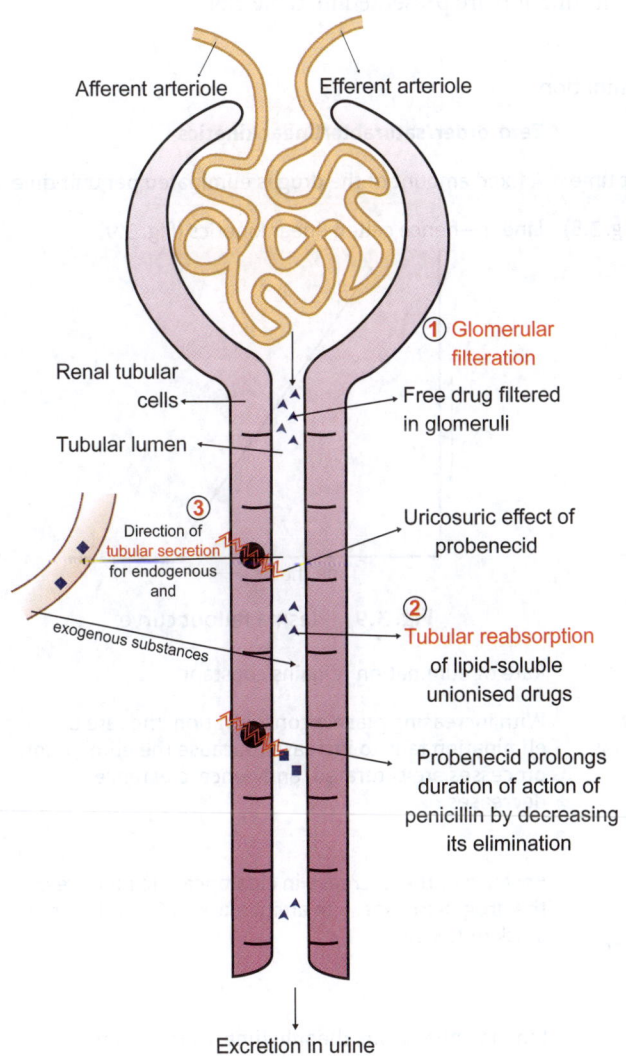

Fig. 3.7 Drug excretion through the kidney

Suppose 5 g of sugar is dissolved in a fixed volume of water and the concentration of this solution measured. If the concentration is 0.2 g/mL, then the volume of water present in glass is 5 g/ 0.2 g/mL, which is 25 mL.

Similarly, knowing the amount of a drug given intravenously (Q) and measuring its plasma concentration (C_p), allows us to calculate the apparent volume of distribution of the drug. However, this is only a rough estimation because body water is not homogenously distributed.

c. Clearance (CL)

Clearance is a measure of the body's ability to eliminate a drug. It predicts the rate of elimination in relation to the drug concentration. Clearance is defined as **the theoretical volume of plasma that is completely cleared of the drug in unit time, and calculated as shown.**

$$CL = \frac{\text{Rate of drug elimination}}{C_p}$$

Most drugs follow **non-saturable or first-order kinetics** and elimination processes are not saturated over the therapeutic range. Here, the clearance remains constant.

For drugs following first-order kinetics, the first part of this equation, i.e., clearance, remains constant. It is implied that CL can remain constant only if the rate of elimination increases with a rise in plasma concentration. This indicates that a fixed fraction (f for first, f for fraction) of drug is eliminated per unit time. Thus, a change in plasma concentration will not change the half-life of the drug.

In contrast, for some drugs, e.g., phenytoin, warfarin, and theophylline, the kinetics of elimination gets saturated over the therapeutic range. In other words, it changes from first-order to **zero-order kinetics**. Zero-order kinetics is characterised by a constant rate of elimination of the drug, irrespective of plasma concentration. It implies that a fixed amount (not a fraction) of the drug is eliminated per unit time (as CL = Rate of elimination/C_p).

A fixed rate of elimination indicates that an increase in plasma concentration, C_p (denominator), will bring about a fall in clearance (as the numerator, i.e., the rate of elimination, remains constant). The half-life of such drugs increases with increased plasma concentration.

Differences between the two types of kinetics of elimination are presented in Table 3.5.

Table 3.5 Differences between the two types of kinetics of elimination

Parameter	First-order/non-saturable/exponential kinetics	Zero-order/saturable/linear kinetics
Definition	A fixed fraction of the drug is eliminated per unit time	A fixed amount of the drug is eliminated per unit time
Plasma fallout curve in which the drop in plasma concentration is plotted against time	Exponential—hence called exponential kinetics (Fig. 3.8) Fig. 3.8 Plasma fallout curve	Linear—hence called linear kinetics (Fig. 3.9) Fig. 3.9 Plasma fallout curve
Constant	Clearance remains constant	Rate of elimination remains constant
Effect of raised plasma concentration on clearance	With increasing plasma concentration, the rate of elimination also increases so that clearance remains constant $$CL = \frac{\text{Rate of drug elimination}}{C_p} = \text{Constant}$$	With increasing plasma concentration, the rate of elimination fails to increase (because the elimination processes are saturated) and hence, clearance decreases
Effect of increased plasma concentration on half-life	$$t_{½} = \frac{0.693 \times V_d}{CL}$$ Because of the constant clearance, the half-life also remains constant, with an increase in C_p	Because of the decrease in clearance, the half-life of the drug **increases** with an increase in C_p, and there is a risk of toxicity
Examples	Most drugs follow first-order kinetics	Ethanol, phenytoin, theophylline, warfarin, etc.

d. Plasma half-life

It is defined as 'the time in which the plasma concentration of a drug is reduced to half of the original value'.

$$t_{1/2} = 0.693/K$$

'K' in this equation is **elimination rate constant.** It is the fraction of the total amount of the drug in the body that is removed per unit time.

Mathematically,

$$K = CL/V_d.$$

So, $t_{1/2} = 0.693 \times V_d/CL$.

Thus, a **decrease in CL causes increase in the half-life of a drug.** It takes a time equal to about 5 half-lives for near-complete elimination of a drug as shown in Box 3.1 below.

Box 3.1 Time for the complete elimination of a drug

Let the total amount of drug present in body = 100 mg
In the first half-life, the amount of drug eliminated

$$= \frac{100}{2} \text{ mg} = 50 \text{ mg}$$

Therefore, the amount of the drug left in the body = 50 mg
In the second half-life, the drug eliminated

$$= \frac{50}{2} = 25 \text{ mg}$$

The total amount eliminated = 50 + 25 = 75 mg
The amount left in the body = 50 – 25 = 25 mg
In the third half-life, the amount of the drug eliminated

$$= \frac{25}{2} = 12.5 \text{ mg}$$

Total amount eliminated = 50 + 25 + 12.5 = 87.5 mg
Amount left = 12.5 mg
90% drug is eliminated in 3.3 half-lives.
In the fourth half-life, the amount of drug eliminated

$$= \frac{12.5}{2} = 6.25 \text{ mg}$$

Total eliminated = 50 + 25 + 12.5 + 6.25 = 93.75 mg
Amount left = 6.25 mg
In the fifth half-life, the amount of the drug eliminated

$$= \frac{6.25}{2} = 3.125 \text{ mg}$$

Total eliminated = 50 + 25 + 12.5 + 6.25 + 3.125 = 96.875 mg
≈ 97 mg.
So, in five half-lives, approximately 97% of the drug present in the body gets eliminated. Half-life thus helps in determining the dosing rate for the calculation of the maintenance dose of a drug.

Plateau principle (Fig. 3.10)

It takes about 4–5 half-lives to completely eliminate a drug from the body. Therefore, if a constant dose of the drug is repeated before four half-lives have passed, a higher peak concentration is achieved. This is because some remanent of the previous dose is present in the body. This continues with further successive doses until the plasma concentration plateaus because, for drugs following first-order kinetics, an increase in plasma concentration causes an increase in the rate of elimination. Such an increasing rate of elimination balances the amount of the drug administered over the dose interval; thus, the plasma concentration plateaus and keeps fluctuating around an average steady-state level. This is called '**steady-state plasma concentration**'(C_{pss}).

$$C_{pss} = \text{Dose rate}/CL$$

Therefore, if C_{pss} and CL of drug are known, its dose rate can be calculated.

$$\text{Dose rate} = C_{pss} \times CL$$

After adjusting for bioavailability, the dose rate can be calculated as given below.

$$\text{Dose rate} = C_{pss} \times CL/F$$

Further, there occur vast inter-individual variations in steady-state plasma concentration. Thus, it becomes important to constantly monitor plasma levels and make desired adjustments in the dosage regimen to achieve and maintain target levels within the therapeutic range.

$$\text{New dose rate} = \frac{\text{Previous dose rate} \times \text{Target } C_p}{C_p}$$

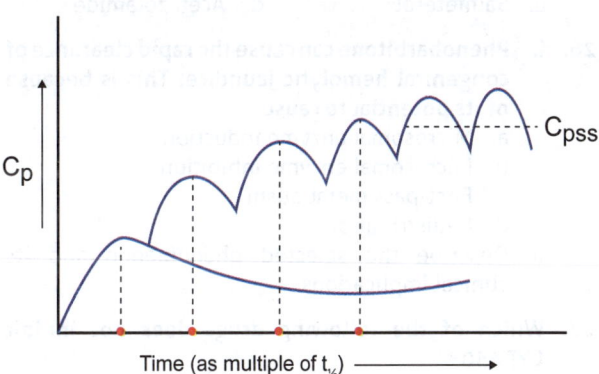

Fig. 3.10 Plasma concentration—time (as multiples of $t_{1/2}$) curve to show C_{pss} and the plateau principle

Clinical problem-based questions and MCQs

20. i. Explain the need for the metabolism of drugs.
    ii. What are phase I and phase II metabolic reactions?
    iii. Identify correct statement about phase I reactions.
       a. These reactions are faster than phase II reactions.
       b. Metabolites of phase I reactions are always inactive.
       c. They commonly involve oxidation–reduction reactions.
       d. Enzymes responsible for phase I reactions show genetic polymorphism.

21. i. Which of the following is a phase II reaction?
       a. Oxidation   b. Acetylation
       c. Dealkylation   d. Hydroxylation
    ii. Name two drugs metabolised by selected reaction.

22. Which of the following chemical reactions is CYP450-independent?
    a. Hydroxylation
    b. Dehydrogenation
    c. Oxidative dealkylation
    d. Dechlorination

23. i. Which of the following is NOT metabolised by acetylation?
       a. Isoniazid   b. Dapsone
       c. Procainamide   d. Metoclopramide
    ii. Describe the terms rapid and slow acetylators and the clinical implications of each with a suitable example.

24. Pre-systemic metabolism is implicated in making some drugs ineffective by the oral route.
    i. What is pre-systemic metabolism?
    ii. Give examples of drugs that are ineffective orally owing to pre-systemic metabolism.

25. Identify a prodrug from the following drugs.
    a. Enalapril   b. Clonidine
    c. Salmeterol   d. Acetazolamide

26. i. Phenobarbitone can cause the rapid clearance of congenital hemolytic jaundice. This is because of its potential to cause:
       a. Microsomal enzyme induction
       b. Microsomal enzyme inhibition
       c. First-pass metabolism
       d. Redistribution
    ii. Describe the selected phenomenon and its clinical implications.

27. Which of the following drugs does not inhibit CYP450?
    a. Cimetidine   b. Ketoconazole
    c. Phenobarbitone d. Erythromycin

28. The kidney is the main site of drug excretion through processes of glomerular filtration, tubular reabsorption, and tubular secretion.
    i. Which of the following can be excreted easily by the kidney?
       a. Drugs with high plasma protein binding
       b. Drugs with a polar nature
       c. Drugs with high lipid solubility
       d. Drugs with a high first-pass metabolism
    ii. Which of the following competes with penicillin for tubular secretion?
       a. Uric acid   b. Probenecid
       c. Cephalosporins   d. Creatinine
    iii. Identify the pharmacokinetic process that is affected by the lipid solubility of a drug.
       a. Glomerular filtration
       b. Tubular reabsorption
       c. Tubular secretion
       d. All of these

29. i. Identify the drug that exhibits enterohepatic circulation.
       a. Erythromycin
       b. Methyltestosterone
       c. Thiopentone sodium
       d. Cimetidine
    ii. Describe the phenomenon of enterohepatic circulation.

30. For drugs following first-order kinetics, clearance and half-life remain constant with an increase in plasma concentration.
    i. Define the terms clearance, half-life, and first-order kinetics.
    ii. Explain why clearance remains constant for drugs following first-order kinetics.

31. The antiepileptic drug phenytoin is eliminated by saturable kinetics.
    i. What is the other name for saturable kinetics?
    ii. How do clearance and half-life change with plasma concentration in saturable kinetics?
    iii. Differentiate between saturable and unsaturable kinetics.
    iv. Give two more examples of drugs showing saturable kinetics and its clinical implications.

32. A 34-year-old male patient with a genitourinary infection was put on antimicrobial drug treatment. He complained of a metallic taste in his mouth because the drug was excreted in his saliva. Identify the drug prescribed.
    a. Tetracycline   b. Ampicillin
    c. Metronidazole   d. Cefotaxime

33. A patient with a urinary tract infection is prescribed cotrimoxazole to be taken twice daily. The half-life of the drug is 12 hours. How long will it take for 90% of the drug to be eliminated from the body?
    a. 24 hours   b. 36 hours
    c. 40 hours   d. 48 hours

34. A person with a history of myocardial infarction is on clopidogrel therapy. Which equation is used to calculate the maintenance dose of clopidogrel?
    a. Dose = $0.693/CL$ b. Dose = Q/C_p
    c. Dose = $C_p \, CL/F$ d. Dose = Q/V_d

Summary

- Pharmacokinetics is study of how the drug moves inside, through and out of a body. Drugs cross cell membranes by passive diffusion and carrier-mediated transport along the concentration gradient (facilitated diffusion) or against the concentration gradient (active transport).
- The pharmacokinetic processes are absorption, distribution, metabolism, and excretion.
- **Absorption** of a drug is movement of the drug into systemic circulation from site of administration. The rate of absorption depends on lipid solubility, the degree of ionisation of the drug based on its pKa, and the pH of the medium. The vascularity and area of the absorbing surface are also important in addition to many route-specific factors like the presence of food/other drugs, GI motility in the oral route, application of heat and muscular exercise in the IM route, and the increased spread of the drug by hyaluronidase in the subcutaneous route.
- **Bioavailability** is the fraction of a given dose that reaches systemic circulation in its unchanged form. It depends on the extent of absorption and first-pass metabolism. Drugs with a very high first-pass metabolism are not effective orally, e.g., methyltestosterone. Some drugs like propranolol can be administered orally in a higher dose.
- The bioavailability of different preparations of the same drug may be different due to a variety of pharmaceutical and pharmacological factors. This is called **bioinequivalence** and is a relative term as compared to bioavailability.
- From systemic circulation, the drug is **distributed** to various tissues based on its lipid solubility, ionisation, and affinity for plasma proteins or tissue proteins.
- The volume of distribution is the volume that would accommodate all the drug present in the body, assuming that the concentration throughout is the same as that in plasma. V_d is low for drugs having high plasma protein binding and very high for drugs sequestrated in tissues.
- Some highly lipid-soluble drugs like thiopentone exhibit a phenomenon of **redistribution** after IV or inhalational use. Such drugs are distributed first to the highly vascular organs and then to less vascular, bulky tissues.
- After exerting its action, the drug is eliminated by the body. Metabolism and excretion are methods of drug elimination. The main site of **metabolism** of drugs is the liver.
- Two types of metabolic reactions phase I and phase II are catalysed by a variety of microsomal enzymes like CYP450 and conjugases. Drug metabolites can be active or inactive. Some drugs given in their inactive form which are activated by hepatic metabolism are called **prodrugs.**
- Some amount of orally given drugs gets metabolised before reaching systemic circulation and is lost. This is called **first-pass or pre-systemic metabolism** and reduces the oral bioavailability of drugs.
- Drugs are **excreted** mainly by the kidney through glomerular filtration, tubular reabsorption, and tubular secretion. Competition between various drugs secreted through the same site can cause interactions.
- The majority of drugs follow first-order kinetics, in which, the rate of elimination increases with increase in concentration, while CL remains constant.
- Some drugs like phenytoin, ethanol, and theophylline follow zero-order kinetics, in which the rate of elimination remains constant and CL decreases as plasma concentration increases and the risk of toxicity also increases.

Questions for practice

1. Write short notes on:
   a. Carrier-mediated transport
   b. Factors affecting drug absorption
   c. Enzyme induction
   d. Redistribution of drugs
   e. Prodrugs
   f. First-pass metabolism
   g. Enterohepatic circulation
2. Differentiate between:
   a. Bioavailability and bioequivalence
   b. Phase I and phase II reactions of drug metabolism
   c. First-order and zero-order kinetics
3. Explain why:
   a. Alkalinisation of urine is useful in cases of poisoning with weakly acidic drugs
   b. The oral dose of propranolol is 40 times higher than its IV dose
   c. Some drugs are not effective when given by the oral route
   d. Chances of toxicity are more with drugs following saturable kinetics
   e. Volume of distribution is more than the total body water for some drugs
   f. Highly plasma protein-bound drugs have a longer half-life

Hints for problem-based questions and MCQS

1. i. Due to ion trapping (refer to page 31)
   ii. a. Sodium bicarbonate
   iii. Urine is alkalinised to hasten the excretion of acidic drugs like aspirin. Citric acid and glucose have no role. Although acetazolamide alkalinises urine, it may increase neurotoxicity (refer to page 32).

2. i. d. Active transport causes the selective accumulation of a drug on one side of the membrane, because drug moves against its concentration gradient.
   ii. Factors favouring drug movement across biological membranes are lipid solubility, unionised or non-polar forms, and transmembrane carrier proteins like GLUT 4 P-glycoproteins cause reverse transportation.
3. d. Bicarbonate corrects acidosis and controls amitriptyline-induced arrhythmias.
4. a. Barbiturates, because they are acidic; the other three options are basic drugs, and the acidification of urine increases their excretion
5. a. Phenobarbitone, being weakly acidic, remains unionised in the acidic pH of the stomach, and so, is likely to be absorbed. The other three are weakly basic drugs, and their absorption is greater in the basic medium of the intestines.
6. d. 99.9%—the drug is acidic and the medium is basic. The drug exist more in its ionised form. The difference between pH and pKa is 3. Thus, the ionised fraction is 99.9% and the unionised fraction is 0.1%. Refer to Table 3.1, page 31.
7. i. Gastrointestinal motility is affected by various diseases or drugs, the presence of food or other drugs, the nature and size of drug particles (refer to page 34).
   ii. Application of heat, muscular exercise, and the use of vasoconstrictors. Refer to page 35.
   iii. The incorporation of hyaluronidase. Refer to page 35.
8. i. Refer to page 35.
   ii. Refer to page 35, 36.
   iii. The high first-pass metabolism of propranolol results in its low oral bioavailability
9. c. The intravenous route has maximum bioavailability as the drug is given directly into systemic circulation through a vein.
10. i. The phenomenon involved is 'bioequivalence'. Refer to page 37 for differences between bioequivalence and bioavailability;
    ii. The use of different diluents (refer to page 36)
    iii. The clinical significance of bioinequivalence—microfining of aspirin, griseofulvin, and spironolactone increases their rate of absorption. Bioavailability variations are important for drugs with low safety margins, steep DRC requiring precise dose control, and antimicrobial therapy. Refer to page 37.
11. d. < 20%
12. a. High first-pass metabolism reduces oral bioavailability
13. i. d. 4 L; Q = 100 100 µg; C_p = 25 µg/mL; V_d = Q /C_p = 4000 mL = 4 L.
    ii. Refer to page 38. This value is not real but apparent as it is calculated based on an assumption that the body is a single homogeneous compartment (which it is not);
    iii. Vd depends on lipid solubility, degree of ionisation, affinity for plasma proteins, tissue proteins, and regional blood flow and disease states. Refer to page 38.
    iv. Cirrhosis, uremia, congestive heart failure, etc. Refer to page 39.
14. c. Chloroquine has highest V_d (1300 L)
15. i. Due to its high affinity for tissue proteins. Refer to page 38
    ii. Cannot be removed by dialysis (refer to page 39).
16. d. Drugs with low V_d, low PPB.
17. i. d. The drug will have low volume of distribution.
    ii. Refer to page 38.
    iii. Low aV_d, longer duration of action, and higher risk of drug–drug interactions. Refer to page 38.
18. i. Refer to page 38
    ii. Repeated administration can saturate low perfusion, high-capacity sites and make the drug longer acting.
19. a. High lipid solubility
20. i. To change a drug into a readily excretable form. Refer to page 40.
    ii. Refer to page 40.
    iii. c. Phase I reactions commonly involve oxidation–reduction reactions
21. i. b. Acetylation is a phase II reaction;
    ii. Isoniazid, dapsone, and sulphonamides
22. b. Dehydrogenations is CYP 450-independent Refer to page 40.
23. i. d. Metoclopramide;
    ii. In rapid acetylators, reduced efficacy of drug; in slow acetylators, increased risk of adverse effects. Refer to page 42.
24. i. Pre-systemic metabolism is that which occurs before the entry of drug into systemic circulation. Refer to page 40.
    ii. Testosterone, morphine, isoprenaline, lignocaine, hydrocortisone, etc.
25. a. Enalapril is a prodrug and is activated to form enalaprilat in the body.
26. i. a. Microsomal enzyme induction;
    ii. The synthesis of microsomal enzymes, especially cytochrome P450 and glucuronyl transferase, can be induced by a variety of drugs, pollutants, etc. Refer to page 42.
27. c. Phenobarbitone is an enzyme inducer, whereas the others are inhibitors.
28. i. b. Drugs with a polar nature;
    ii. b. Probenecid;
    iii. b. Tubular reabsorption
29. i. a. Erythromycin ;
    ii. Refer to page 43.
30. i. Refer to page 44, 45.
    ii. $CL = \dfrac{\text{Rate of drug elimination}}{C_p}$

In drugs following first-order kinetics, an increase in plasma concentration is accompanied by an increase in the rate of elimination. So, CL remains constant.
31. i. Saturable kinetics is also called zero-order kinetics;
    ii. In saturable kinetics, with an increase in plasma concentration, CL decreases and half-life increases.
    iii. See Table 3.5, page 44
    iv. Ethanol, warfarin, and theophylline also show zero-order kinetics
32. c. Metronidazole
33. c. 40 hours. In the first half-life (12 hours) – 50% of the drug is eliminated; in two half-lives (24 hours) – 75%; in three half-lives (36 hours) – 87.5%; in 3.3 half-lives (12 3.3 = 39.6 hours) 90% elimination occurs
34. c. Maintenance dose = $Cp \dfrac{CL}{F}$

Chapter 3 Pharmacokinetics

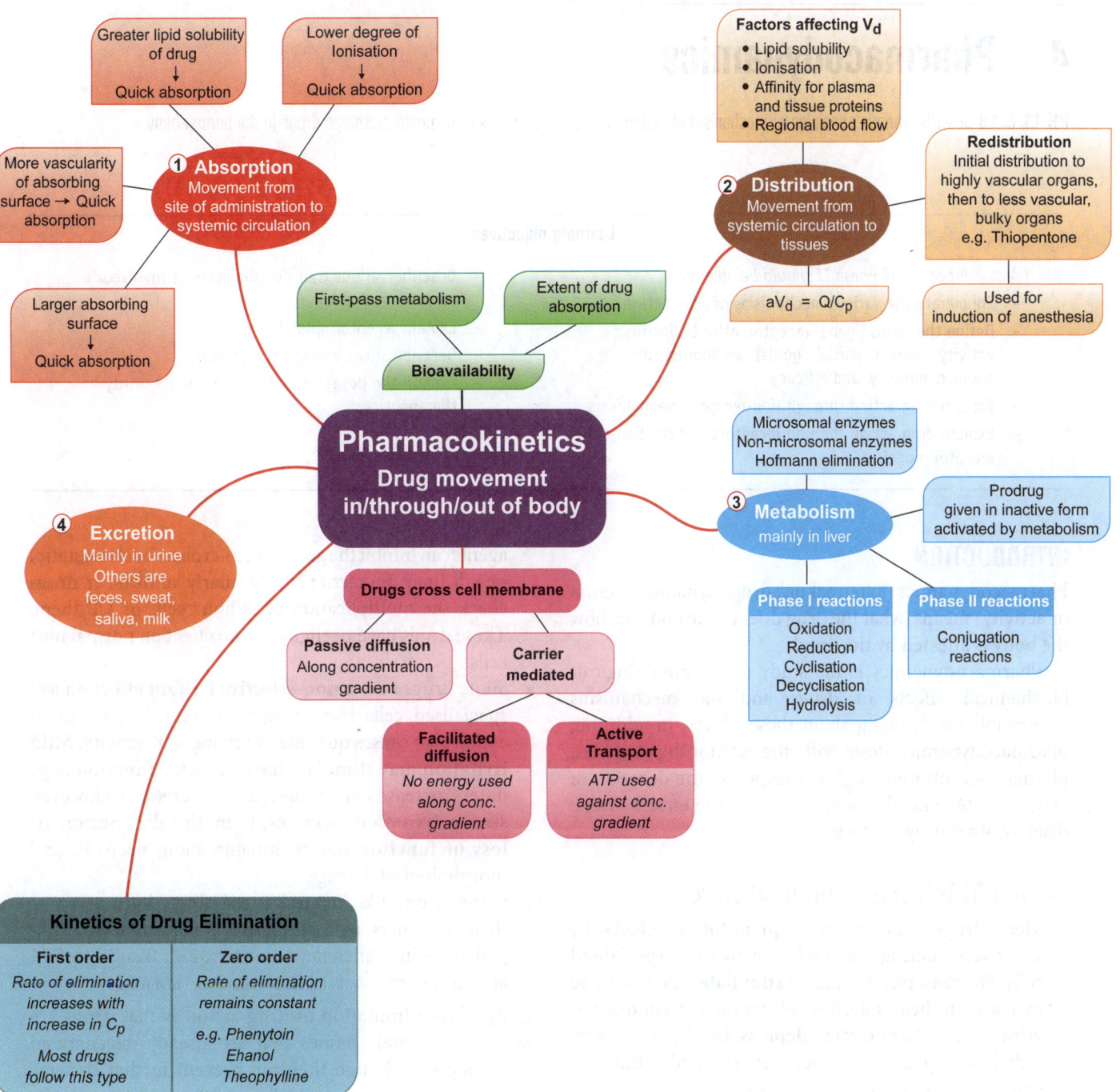

SECTION 1 General Pharmacology

4 Pharmacodynamics

PH 1.7 & 1.8 Describe various principles of mechanism of action of drugs and effects of common prototype drugs in the human body.

Learning objectives

A student of MBBS Phase II should be able to:
- Enumerate the various mechanisms of drug action.
- Define the terms ligand, receptor, affinity, intrinsic activity, agonist, partial agonist, antagonist, inverse agonist, potency, and efficacy.
- Explain drug action through non-receptor mechanisms.
- Explain drug action through receptors and the two-state receptor model.
- Describe various transduction systems involved in receptor activation.
- Explain receptor regulation.
- Describe silent and spare receptors.
- Explain the dose–response curve and its utility in therapeutics.

INTRODUCTION

Pharmacodynamics ('pharmakon': drug; 'dynamics': action or activity) means 'what the drug does to the body' or how the body is affected by the drug.

Pharmacodynamics is the study of the physiological/biochemical effects of drugs and the mechanisms responsible for bringing about these effects. In addition, pharmacodynamics deals with the relationship between plasma concentration (C_p) and response, the duration of action (DOA) and the modification of the effects of one drug by other drugs or factors.

BASIC PRINCIPLES OF DRUG ACTION

- Most drugs produce only **quantitative effects** by selectively altering the level of activity of specialised cells. For example, adrenaline **stimulates** the heart and increases the heart rate, force of contraction, conduction velocity, etc. Barbiturates **depress** the CNS, causing sedation, hypnosis, anesthetic effects, and ultimately, coma, with increasing concentration.
- Physiological **functions usually get suppressed after excessive stimulation**. For example, picrotoxin in high doses causes convulsions followed by coma and respiratory depression.
- Further, a drug may **stimulate one type of cell, but depress another type**. For example, acetylcholine stimulates intestinal smooth muscles, causing increased peristaltic activity and simultaneously depresses the heart, resulting in decreased heart rate, force of contraction, conduction velocity, etc.
- Some drugs have a **selective cell-killing or cytotoxic effect** on invading organisms like bacteria, viruses, parasites, and cancer cells. For example, antimicrobial agents can inhibit the growth of microbes (bacteriostatic) or kill them (bactericidal). Similarly, anticancer drugs check the multiplication of tumour cells or kill them. These drugs have negligible or no effect on normal host cells.
- Some drugs have a **non-selective irritant effect** on less specialised cells like epithelial tissues. Their irritant action also causes quantitative changes in activity. **Mild irritation may stimulate the associated function** (e.g., bitters increase salivary and gastric secretion). However, **strong irritation may result in the diminution or loss of function** due to inflammation, necrosis, and morphological damage.
- Some drugs like natural metabolites, hormones, or their congeners act by the principle of **replacement** in patients with deficiency disorders, e.g., insulin in DM and iron in microcytic, hypochromic anemia.

A significant limitation of drug action is that drugs are not able to repair tissues that are already degenerated or damaged, although they can prevent further damage to some extent, e.g., ACE inhibitors decrease the microvascular complications of diabetes and disease-modifying antirheumatoid drugs (DMARDs) can decrease the disease progression rate in rheumatoid arthritis.

SITES OF DRUG ACTION

Drugs may exert their effects at different extracellular/cellular/intracellular sites, following the above-mentioned basic principles.

- **Extracellular sites**
  - Antacids neutralise gastric acid in the lumen of the stomach through simple chemical reactions.

- Magnesium sulphate (MgSO$_4$) is not absorbed from the intestinal lumen. It increases osmotic pressure and retains water in the gut lumen, resulting in purgative action.
- **Cellular sites**
  - Acetylcholine causes skeletal muscle contraction by acting on nicotinic (Nm) receptors present on the motor end plate.
  - Digoxin exerts a positive inotropic effect by inhibiting membrane-bound Na$^+$/K$^+$-ATPase.
- **Intracellular sites**
  - Methotrexate inhibits the enzyme dihydrofolate reductase and interferes with the conversion of dihydrofolate to tetrahydrofolate, leading to cell death.
  - 5-Fluorouracil (5-FU) gets incorporated into mRNA instead of uracil and exerts a cytotoxic effect.

MECHANISMS OF DRUG ACTION

The terms 'drug effect' and 'drug action' are often used interchangeably. However, drug effect is the net response produced by a drug, while drug action is the term used to explain the series of steps/changes/mechanisms that bring about the net response. Drugs can exert their effects by the following mechanisms of action:

A. Non-receptor-mediated mechanisms
B. Receptor-mediated mechanisms
C. Specific genetic changes

A. Non-Receptor-Mediated Mechanisms

These include drug action due to various physical/chemical properties of the drug and the stimulation or inhibition of enzymes/immune response. Some drugs act as protoplasmic poisons, while others may have a placebo effect. Various non-receptor-mediated mechanisms of drug action are described below.

1. Drug action due to physical properties

Some drugs exert their effect due to one of their physical properties like **mass, adsorptive activity, osmotic effect, radioactivity,** and **radiopacity**. Drugs that act because of their physical properties include:

- Bulk purgatives contain unabsorbable constituents such as cellulose, lignins, and pectins, which absorb water in the intestinal lumen and swell up. Thus, fecal mass increases, feces is softened, and can be easily passed out.
- Activated charcoal is processed carbon with multiple small, low-volume pores that increase its surface area. This allows it to adsorb various ingested poisons and prevent their absorption.
- Mannitol given in a large quantity increases the osmolarity of plasma, which favours the extraction of water from brain parenchyma, CSF, and the anterior chamber of the eye. Thus, it is useful in reducing raised intracranial and intraocular tension.
- I^{131} is a radioactive isotope of iodine. It gets concentrated in thyroid follicles and emits β-particles that penetrate up to 0.5–2 mm of thyroid tissue, causing necrosis and fibrosis. This physical property of radioactivity of I^{131} is utilised in the treatment of toxic nodular goitre.
- Barium sulphate and urografin are valuable in imaging studies because of their radiopacity.

2. Drug actions due to chemical properties

Some drugs owe their effects to their chemical properties. The following are some examples:

- Antacids neutralise hydrochloric acid (HCl) in the stomach lumen and are used to relieve symptoms associated with peptic ulcers, gastro-esophageal reflux disease (GERD), etc.
- Calcium disodium edetate has a high affinity for heavy metals like lead, zinc, and copper. It exchanges its calcium with these metals and helps in their excretion. Such chelating agents are useful in cases of heavy metal poisoning.
- Sodium bicarbonate (NaHCO$_3$) increases the pH of renal tubular fluid. Weakly acidic drugs like aspirin get ionised in alkaline pH, resulting in reduced tubular reabsorption. Thus, in cases of acidic drug poisoning, urinary excretion can be enhanced by the alkalinisation of urine.

3. Drug action through effect on enzymes

Many drugs act by stimulating or inhibiting the catalytic activity of various enzymes.

a. Enzyme stimulation

Some drugs **increase the affinity** of the enzyme for its substrate, resulting in **raised V$_{max}$** (maximal reaction velocity), **lowering the rate constant (k$_M$)** of a reaction. Rate constant (k$_M$) represents the concentration of the substrate required to achieve half the maximal reaction velocity (Fig. 4.1).

Examples of enzyme stimulation:

- Adrenaline stimulates adenylyl cyclase → Increase in cAMP levels, which further stimulates hepatic glycogen phosphorylase enzyme
- Pyridoxine is a cofactor → Increases decarboxylase activity

The induction of enzyme synthesis by various drugs also apparently increases enzyme activity; V$_{max}$ is increased, but k$_M$ is not reduced (Fig. 4.1).

b. Enzyme inhibition

This is a common mode of drug action. **There are two broad types** of enzyme inhibition—specific and non-specific.

52 Section 1 General Pharmacology

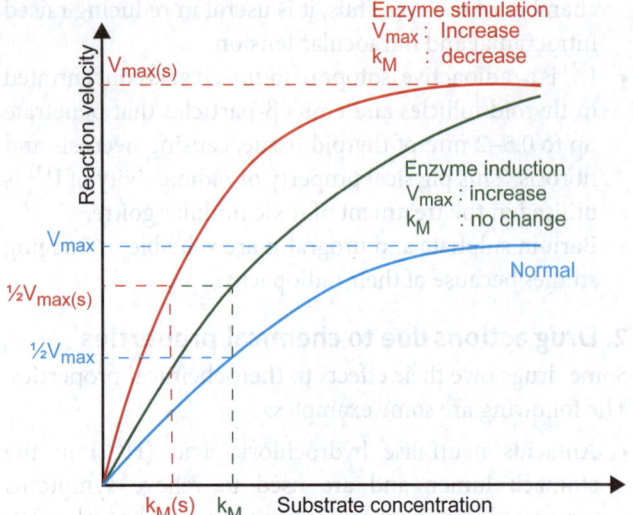

Fig. 4.1 Substrate concentration–reaction velocity curve for enzyme stimulation and induction

- **Specific enzyme inhibition** occurs when a drug inhibits a **particular enzyme** without affecting other enzymes. It is of two types—competitive and non-competitive. Competitive inhibition is further categorised into the equilibrium and non-equilibrium types. Table 4.1 presents the differences between these types of enzyme inhibition.

- **Non-specific inhibition** is brought about by drugs or chemicals that alter the tertiary structure of **any enzyme** with which they come in contact because the drug is capable of **denaturing proteins**, e.g., heavy metal salts, phenol, alcohol, strong acids, formaldehyde, and alkalis. Such drugs that act non-specifically against all enzymes may act as protoplasmic poisons and cause the death of microorganisms; these are used as antiseptics/disinfectants.

4. Immune response
Some drugs like vaccines produce their effects by **stimulating the immune mechanisms** of the body and inducing the formation of antibodies (Abs), e.g., vaccines against smallpox and cholera (both of which provide active immunity); anti-tetanus serum (ATS) and anti-diphtheritic serum (ADS) provide passive immunity.

5. Placebo action
Sometimes, the act of medication rather than the medicine itself brings about a response. This is called **placebo action.** The word placebo means 'I shall please you'. It is a pharmacologically inert and harmless substance that is given in a dosage form resembling the actual medicament in size, shape, colour, smell, taste, etc. Usually, starch or lactose is used as placebos in solid dosage forms, and

Table 4.1 Differences between competitive and non-competitive enzyme inhibition by drugs

	1. a. Competitive enzyme inhibition (Equilibrium type)	2. Non-competitive enzyme inhibition
Binding site	The drug competes with the normal substrate or coenzyme for the catalytic site of the enzyme. It is further of two types–equilibrium and non-equilibrium type.	The drug reacts with the enzyme at an adjacent site and not with the catalytic site. However, this alters the enzyme protein in such a way that it loses its catalytic property.
Effect on rate constant	Drugs increase the k_M (Michaelis–Menten constant), i.e., a higher concentration of the substrate is required to achieve half the maximal reaction velocity.	k_M is unchanged.
Effect on V_{max}	V_{max} remains unchanged, i.e., the same maximal reaction velocity can be achieved (Fig. 4.2). 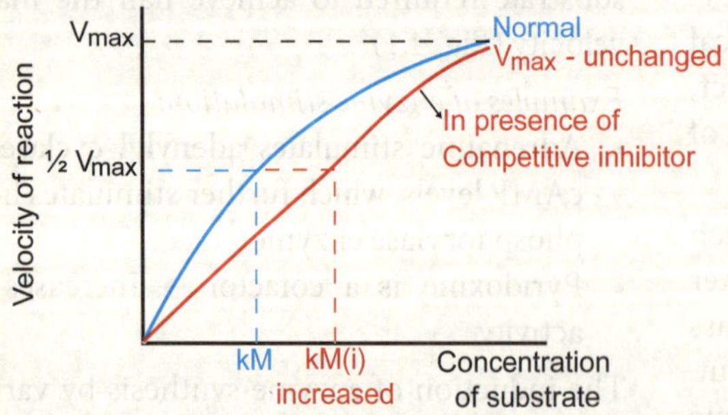 **Fig. 4.2** Substrate concentration–reaction velocity curve	V_{max} is reduced (Fig. 4.3). 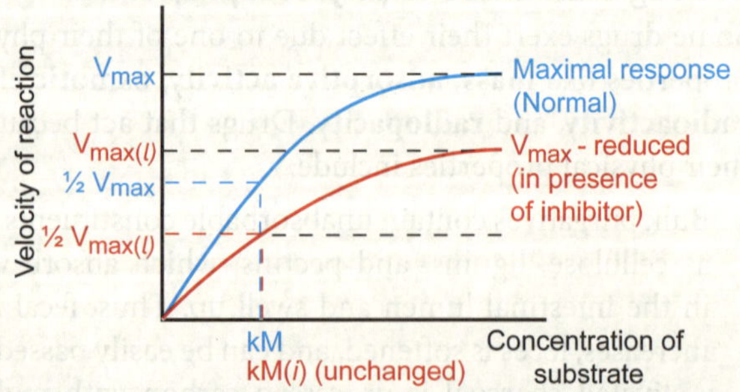 **Fig. 4.3** Substrate concentration–reaction velocity curve
Reversibility	It is **reversible** or surmountable, i.e., if the substrate concentration is sufficiently increased, it can displace the drug from the catalytic site.	It is mostly **irreversible**, as the drug cannot be displaced from the binding site even by a high concentration of the substrate.

(Continues)

Table 4.1	(Continued)	
Examples	- **Sulphonamides** compete with PABA for folate synthase enzyme - **NSAIDs except aspirin** compete with arachidonic acid for cyclooxygenase enzyme - **Allopurinol** competes with hypoxanthine for xanthine oxidase enzyme - **Physostigmine** competes with acetylcholine (ACh) for cholinesterase enzyme [A mnemonic for examples of competitive enzyme inhibitors is **SNAP**—sulphonamides, NSAIDs, allopurinol, and physostigmine.]	**Disulfiram** inhibits aldehyde dehydrogenase - Aspirin acetylates and inhibits cyclooxygenase irreversibly - **Digoxin** inhibits Na^+/K^+–ATPase However, while acetazolamide is a non-competitive inhibitor of carbonic anhydrase enzyme, it causes reversible inhibition. [A mnemonic for examples of non-competitive irreversible enzyme inhibitors is **DADA**—i.e., disulfiram, aspirin, digoxin, acetazolamide.]

I. b. In **competitive non-equilibrium inhibition**, the drug binds **at the catalytic site** and either forms **strong covalent bonds** or has such **high affinity** for the enzyme that the normal substrate is not able to displace the drug. In such cases, k_M increases but V_{max} is reduced. Such inhibition is irreversible. Examples include:
- Organophosphates (OPCs) inhibit acetylcholinesterase
- Methotrexate inhibits dihydrofolate reductase

distilled water in injectable form. If the physician earns significant confidence in the patient, even a placebo can provide dramatic relief from the subjective symptoms associated with psychological problems (e.g., anxiety, insomnia, headache, anorexia, and tremors). Such a patient is called a **placebo reactor**.

The placebo effect is not mediated through any receptor action. However, placebo-induced pain relief may involve the release of endogenous opioids like endorphins.

Placebos are also commonly used in double-blind clinical trials of new drugs to distinguish the real pharmacodynamic effect of a drug from the personal influence of the investigator. The use of placebo control groups on patients in clinical trials reduces chances of false-positive/false-negative results.

Clinical problem-based questions and MCQs

1. Identify the correct statement about mechanisms of action of drugs:
   a. The laxative effect of magnesium sulphate is associated with its adsorptive action.
   b. Antacids act intracellularly to neutralise gastric acid.
   c. All antimicrobials have a bactericidal effect on sensitive microorganisms.
   d. Some drugs stimulate one type of cells but inhibit the other type.

2. Which of the following actions is due to the physical properties of a drug?
   a. Acid neutralisation by antacids
   b. Urinary alkalinisation by $NaHCO_3$
   c. Anti-thyroid effect of I^{131}
   d. Heavy metal chelation by calcium disodium edetate

3. In which type of enzyme inhibition does the rate constant (k_M) increase and V_{max} decrease?
   a. Non-equilibrium type
   b. Equilibrium type
   c. Irreversible type
   d. Non-specific type

4. i. Identify the drug that acts by non-competitive enzyme inhibition.
   a. Digoxin
   b. Sulphonamides
   c. Allopurinol
   d. Physostigmine
   ii. Name the enzyme inhibited by the drug selected in part I and describe the effect on V_{max} and k_M.

5. Match the drug with the characteristic changes in enzymes/V_{max}/k_M caused by it.
   a. Physostigmine 1. Denaturing of proteins
   b. Disulfiram   2. k_M increased, V_{max} reduced
   c. Organophosphates 3. k_M raised, V_{max} unchanged
   d. Phenol   4. V_{max} reduced, k_M unchanged

6. NSAIDs are used in various inflammatory conditions as they reduce prostaglandin synthesis. All NSAIDs cause competitive inhibition of cyclooxygenase except aspirin. Differentiate between competitive and non-competitive enzyme inhibition.

7. Both physostigmine and OPCs are competitive cholinesterase enzyme inhibitors. However, the effect of physostigmine is reversible, while that of OPCs is irreversible. Explain the pharmacological basis of this statement.

B. Receptor-Mediated Mechanism of Action

Most drugs act through specific macromolecular components of the cell, which regulate critical cellular functions like enzyme activity, permeability, template functions, and structural features. These macromolecules or the sites on them which bind and interact with the drug are called 'receptors'. Thus, a **receptor** is defined as a **binding site with functional correlates**.

- **Nature:** Receptors are regulatory macromolecules; they are generally **proteins**, though some are **nucleic acids**.
- **Location:** Receptors are situated **on the surface or inside** the effector cell.
- **Structure:** The structure of the receptor resembles the three-dimensional configuration of the 'lock and key' arrangement.

Drug–receptor binding

The binding of a drug(D) with its receptor(R) results in the formation of a D–R complex, which is responsible for triggering a biological response.

Drug + Receptor ⟶ Drug–receptor complex ⟶ Response

This binding of a drug with its receptors is usually **reversible** because it is held together by weak bonds like hydrogen/Van der Waals/electrostatic bonds. **Drugs that bind to their receptors through weak bonds are more selective** because electrostatic interaction needs a precise fit of the drug to its binding site. In certain cases, the drug–receptor binding is irreversible through the formation of covalent bonds.

Ligands

The ligands for some receptors are **physiological**, i.e., **endogenous substances**, e.g., neurotransmitters, hormones, autacoids, and endogenous mediators. Other receptors exist only for binding to drugs (exogenous substances). There is no physiological ligand for these receptors in the body. These are **true drug receptors**, e.g., benzodiazepine receptors, thiazide receptors, and cardiac glycoside receptors.

Evidence favouring drug action through receptors

- **Structural specificity** is the association of a specific chemical structure with a particular action. It points towards drug–receptor interaction, and supports the theory of drug action through receptors.
- Similarly, the **stereospecificity** of the action of some drugs indicates the interaction of these drugs with specific biomolecules, e.g., levo-noradrenaline is ten times more potent than dextro-noradrenaline. Levo-propranolol is 100 times more potent than dextro-propranolol.
- **Competitive antagonism** between a specific agonist and antagonist also indicates that both of them bind/interact with the same receptor site in the cell.
- Clark demonstrated the maximal effect of acetylcholine on a frog heart while occupying only 1/6,000th of the cell surface of the heart, indicating that special regions of reactivity to such drugs must be present.

Clark's 'receptor occupation theory'

Clark established a fundamental concept in 1937. He stated that the pace of a cellular function can be altered by the interaction of receptors with drugs. The interaction between D and R is governed by the law of mass action. Effect (E) is a direct function of the D–R complex formed.

Drug + Receptor $\underset{K_2}{\overset{K_1}{\rightleftharpoons}}$ Drug–Receptor complex ⟶ Effect (E)

- The intensity of the response is proportional to the fraction of receptors occupied by the drug. Maximal response occurs when all receptors are occupied.
- Drugs exert an **'all-or-none'** action, i.e., either a receptor is fully activated or not activated at all. There is no partial activation.
- A drug and its receptor have **complementary structural features** and form a rigid 'lock and key' arrangement.

Ariens and Stephenson's theory

Postulates of Clark's theory were modified in the 1950s by Ariens and Stephenson, yielding the following:

- All receptors need not be occupied for maximal response. For example, adrenaline and histamine can produce maximal response even when > 99% of receptors are occluded by non-competitive antagonists, i.e., a large number of **spare receptors** are present.
- The 'all-or-none' action is not necessary. Instead, Ariens and Stephenson introduced the concept of '**affinity**' and **intrinsic activity** or 'efficacy'.

As different drugs have different capacities to induce a response, it can be inferred that they occupy different fractions of the available receptors, which means that it is possible to activate a receptor sub-maximally.

Therefore, drugs can occupy different fractions of the available receptors sub-maximally. Ariens and Stephenson postulated that S (strength of the stimulus imparted to a cell by the activation of the receptor) could be strong or weak.

Drug + Receptor $\underset{K_2}{\overset{K_1}{\rightleftharpoons}}$ Drug–Receptor complex ⟶ Strength of stimulus (S) ⟶ Effect (E)

Partial agonists stimulate receptors sub-maximally because they are capable of bringing about an intermediate degree of conformational changes in the receptor.

- Receptors cannot be considered to have a rigid conformation, as a **drug could induce changes in the receptor** to make it more or less favourably aligned to combine with the drug.
- The overall effect of a drug is thus attributable to two factors:

- **Affinity:** This is the ability of a drug to form a complex with its receptor, i.e., the key must fit into the levers of the lock to fit into the keyhole.
- **Intrinsic activity (IA):** This refers to the ability of a drug to trigger the pharmacological response (induce a conformational change in the receptor) after forming the D-R complex, i.e., the key, after entering the keyhole, should be able to open the lock.

Based on affinity and IA, drugs can be broadly classified as agonists, antagonists, partial agonists, and inverse agonists.

- **Agonist:** This term refers to a drug that has **both affinity and maximal IA** (IA = 1). An agonist activates the receptors to produce maximal effect. For example, adrenaline is an agonist at α and β receptors; acetylcholine is an agonist at muscarinic and nicotinic receptors; and morphine is an agonist at μ, k, and δ opioid receptors.
- **Antagonists:** These are drugs that have an **affinity for receptors and no intrinsic activity** (IA = 0). An antagonist (as it occupies the receptor and makes it unavailable for the agonist) prevents the action of an agonist on a receptor but has no effect of its own. For example, propranolol is an antagonist at β receptors, phentolamine at α receptors, atropine at muscarinic receptors, and naloxone at opioid receptors.
- **Partial agonists:** These are drugs that **have an affinity for receptors but submaximal IA** (IA between 0 and 1). Thus, they are only partly as effective as agonists. Partial agonist drugs exert their submaximal effect, occupying the receptors and consequently blocking pure agonists. For example, pentazocine and nalorphine are partial agonists at opioid receptors.
- **Inverse agonist:** They have affinity, but their intrinsic activity (IA) is between 0 and −1. They bind to the receptor and produce an effect opposite to that of an agonist, e.g., β carbolines (DMCM [dimethoxyethyl-carbomethoxy β carboline]) act as inverse agonists at benzodiazepine receptors and produce effects like anxiety, sleeplessness, and seizures, which are the opposite of the effects of agonists like diazepam (antianxiety, sedation, anticonvulsant). Antihistaminic drugs like chlorpheniramine, promethazine, and cetirizine, act as inverse agonists at H_1 receptors and decrease the constitutive activity of histamine.

Two-state receptor model

A receptor exists in two states—R_a (active) & R_i (inactive). Even in the absence of an agonist, some **constitutive activity** occurs as some part of the receptor pool always exists in the R_a state.

$$R_a \rightleftharpoons R_i$$

- An **agonist (Ago)** like morphine binds preferentially to receptors in the R_a state and shifts the equilibrium in such a way that R_a predominates, and a response is generated. Intrinsic activity is the maximum for agonists.

$$R_a Ago + R_a \rightleftharpoons R_i$$

- A **partial agonist (PAgo)** like nalorphine has only slightly more affinity for R_a than R_i. Therefore, only a modest shift in equilibrium occurs towards R_a, and the response is submaximal. Intrinsic activity is between 0 and 1.

$$R_a PAgo + R_a \rightleftharpoons R_i + R_i PAgo$$

- A **competitive antagonist (comp antg)** like naloxone binds to R_a and R_i with equal affinity. Therefore, there is no change in equilibrium, and no response occurs. As a result, a competitive antagonist has no effect on its own and it blocks the effect of the agonist by leaving only a few R_a for binding.

$$R_a \text{ comp antg} + R_a \rightleftharpoons R_i \text{ comp antg} + R_i$$

- An **inverse agonist (IAgo)** has a higher affinity for R_i, and hence produces a response opposite to that of the agonist. An IAgo shifts the equilibrium towards R_i and reduces the constitutive activity.

$$R_a \rightleftharpoons R_i I Ago + R_i$$

Examples: At the $GABA_A$–Cl^- channel receptor:

Agonist: benzodiazepines exert a sedative, hypnotic effect.

Antagonist: flumazenil blocks the effect of the agonist, i.e., benzodiazepine.

Inverse agonist: β carbolines exert effects like anxiety and agitation.

- **Silent receptors** bind to ligands but do not produce any response. These are known as **drug acceptors or sites of loss,** e.g., the binding of drugs to plasma proteins causes temporary storage of the drug; the bound part of the drug is not available for exerting action, for metabolism, or for excretion. Hence, **plasma proteins** can be considered as silent receptors.

Action–effect sequence

The terms '**drug action**' and '**drug effect**' are often loosely used interchangeably, but they are not synonymous.

- **Drug action:** It is the initial combination of the drug with its receptor, which results in a conformational change or the prevention of a conformational change (for an agonist and antagonist, respectively).
- **Drug effect:** It is the net change in biological function brought about through a series of intermediate steps (transducer mechanisms). It is the consequence of drug action.

Transduction systems/receptor types

Transduction mechanisms **involve the translation of receptor activation into a functional response.** The mechanisms linking the occupation of receptors by the drug with its response are commonly known as '**coupling systems**'. Receptors serve two key functions:

- Recognition of a specific ligand molecule
- Transduction of a signal into a response

For these two distinct functions, each receptor molecule has a ligand-binding and an effector domain that undergoes a conformational change to generate a response. The receptor occupancy by a full or pure agonist is more efficiently coupled to the response than a partial agonist. The relation between the number of receptors occupied and the response coupling can be linear or non-linear depending upon the transduction system involved.

Based on the molecular structure and the nature of the transduction mechanism for response effectuation, receptors are classified into four major types:

1. G protein-coupled receptors (GPCR)
2. Receptors with an intrinsic ion channel
3. Enzymatic receptors
4. Receptors regulating gene expression

1. G protein-coupled receptors (GPCR)

These receptors are a large family of serpentine or heptahelical **seven-turn** transmembrane receptors that are linked to the effectors through one or more GTP (**guanine triphosphate**)-activated proteins, called G proteins, for response effectuation. There are three **major effector pathways for G protein-coupled receptors**—the adenylyl cyclase (cAMP) pathway, the phospholipase (PLC)–inositol triphosphate (IP_3)–diacylglycerol (DAG) pathway, and channel regulation.

a. **Adenylyl cyclase (cAMP) pathway (Fig. 4.4):** The G protein has **three subunits—α, β, and γ**. In the inactive state, guanine diphosphate (GDP) is bound to it. Activation leads to the displacement of GDP by GTP. The active α subunit carrying GTP dissociates from the other two subunits and activates (G_s) or inhibits (G_i) the effector. The bound GTP is slowly hydrolysed to GDP. Then, the α subunit rejoins the β and γ subunits.

- G_s → Stimulates adenylyl cyclase → Increase in cAMP (e.g., $β_1$, adenosine$_2$ and D_1 receptors)
- G_i → Inhibits adenylyl cyclase → Decrease in cAMP (e.g., M_2, $α_2$, and D_2 receptors)
- cAMP acts as a second messenger and phosphorylates protein kinases which alter the function of many enzymes, ion channels, carriers, and structural proteins. Some important examples of cAMP-mediated responses are as follows:
  - Catecholamine-induced mobilisation of stored energy by the **metabolism of carbohydrates** in hepatic cells and **triglycerides** in adipocytes
  - Catecholamine-induced **positive inotropic and chronotropic** effects
  - **Smooth muscle relaxation** through the phosphorylation (inactivation) of myosin light chain kinase (MLCK)
  - ACTH-induced **synthesis of adrenal steroids**
  - FSH-induced synthesis of **sex steroids**
  - Vasopressin-mediated **water conservation** in the kidney
  - Parathormone-mediated Ca^{2+} **homeostasis**

b. **Phospholipase C (PLC)–inositol triphosphate (IP_3)–diacylglycerol (DAG) pathway (Fig. 4.5):** The enzyme phospholipase C is activated by G_q. It converts phosphatidyl inositol biphosphate (PIP_2) into inositol triphosphate (IP_3) and diacylglycerol (DAG). Inositol triphosphate (IP_3) mobilises Ca^{2+} from intracellular organelles, and diacylglycerol (DAG) enhances the activation of phosphokinase C (PKC) by Ca^{2+}. This is followed by the formation of the Ca^{2+}–calmodulin complex which regulates the activity of other enzymes and Ca^{2+}-dependent protein kinases.

Examples of G_q-linked receptors are M_1, $α_1$, and M_3 receptors.

c. **Channel regulation:** G proteins can open or close ionic channels specific for Ca^{2+}, K^+, or Na^+ and bring about hyperpolarisation/depolarisation of membranes by changing the intracellular ion concentration.

- G_s opens Ca^{2+} channels on $β_1$ receptor stimulation
- G_i opens K^+ channels on M_2, $α_2$, and D_2 receptor stimulation
- G_i also closes Ca^{2+} channels on D_2, opioid, and $GABA_B$ receptor stimulation

The responses mediated through G protein-coupled receptors reach a peak initially and then diminish over the next few seconds to minutes, even if the agonist is still present. This is because of the **rapid desensitisation of GPCRs** due to the reduced ability of the receptor to interact with G_s and the endocytosis of the receptor. However, this is reversed upon the removal of the agonist.

cAMP, Ca^{2+}, and IP_3/DAG act as second messengers. However, in G_q-linked receptors, Ca^{2+} acts as the third messenger.

2. Receptors with intrinsic ion channels (Fig. 4.6)

These receptors on the cell surface enclose ion-selective channels, e.g., Na^+, K^+, Ca^{2+}, and Cl^- within the molecule.

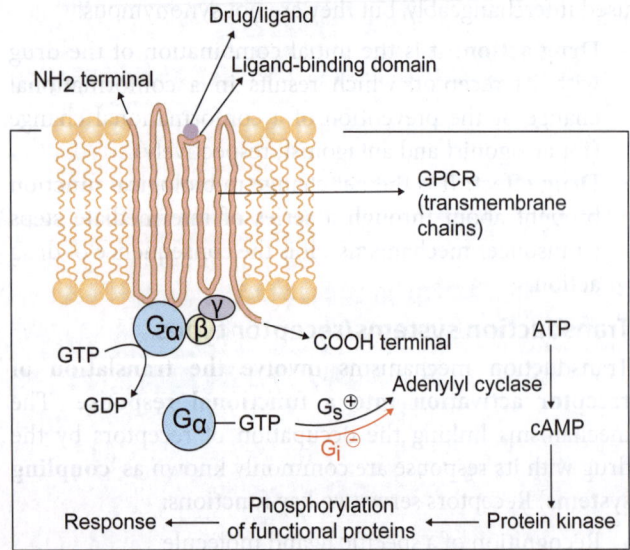

Fig. 4.4 Effector pathways for GPCR (G_s, G_i)

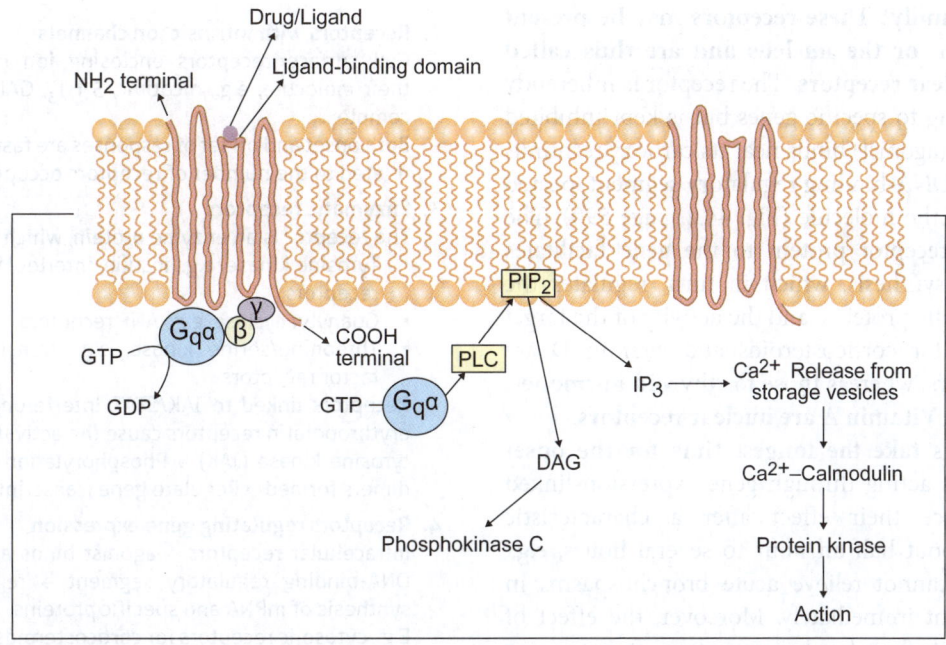

Fig. 4.5 The phospholipase C (PLC)–inositol triphosphate (IP$_3$)–diacylglycerol (DAG) pathway

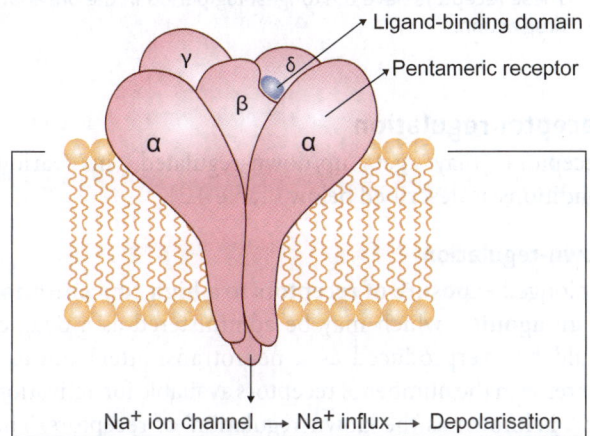

Fig. 4.6 Receptors with intrinsic ion channels

Agonist binding opens the channel. For example, nicotinic receptors for acetylcholine enclose the Na$^+$ channel. Other examples are glycine, NMDA, and 5-HT$_3$ receptors as well as the GABA$_A$–Cl$^-$ channel complex.

The onset and offset of biological responses mediated through this class of receptors is the **fastest** and is **linearly related** to the number of receptors occupied because ion channels are directly operated by agonists, without the intervention of any coupling protein or seconds messengers.

3. Enzymatic receptors

a. **Receptor as an enzymatic protein:** The agonist binding site and the catalytic site lie on the outer and inner face of the plasma membrane, respectively. These two domains are interconnected by a single transmembrane stretch of peptide chain.

In most cases, the enzyme is **tyrosine kinase**, e.g., **insulin receptor, nerve growth factor (NGF), epidermal growth factor (EGF), and interleukin receptors**. The binding of the agonist to the extracellular ligand-binding site results in the formation of receptor dimers and the activation of tyrosine kinase intracellularly. This, in turn, causes the phosphorylation of tyrosine residues, which further phosphorylates SH$_2$-containing substrate proteins, triggering a cascade of phosphorylations and resulting in the regulation of numerous cellular functions (Fig. 43.2, page 572).

The response effectuation is then followed by the internalisation of the receptor into the cell and its degradation by lysosomes.

Other enzymes that are linked with receptors include **guanylyl cyclase in atrial natriuretic peptide (ANP) receptors and threonine or serine kinase in transforming growth factor (TGF-β) receptors.**

b. **JAK/STAT kinase:** Some enzyme-linked, receptors do not have an intracellular catalytic domain. The binding of the drug to the receptor produces a conformational change in the intracellular domain, increasing its affinity for a **cytosolic tyrosine kinase, known as JAK** (a protein tyrosine kinase of the Janus kinase family, refer to Fig. 41.3, page 550). JAK gets activated and causes the phosphorylation of the **tyrosine residues of the receptor, which then bind to another free-moving protein—STAT** (signal transducers and activators of transcription) → JAK phosphorylates STAT → dimers of STAT are formed → get transferred into the nucleus and regulate gene transcription → produce responses, e.g., **interferon, cytokines, GH, and erythropoietin receptors**, are JAK/STAT linked receptors.

4. Receptors regulating intracellular gene expression

In contrast to the above three classes, these are **intracellular receptors**, and are considered to be a part of the 'nuclear receptor superfamily'. These receptors may be present in the cytoplasm or the nucleus and are thus called **cytosolic or nuclear receptors**. The receptor is inherently capable of binding to specific genes but is kept inhibited till the hormone (agonist) binds near its carboxy terminus and exposes the DNA-binding regulatory segment located in the middle of the molecule (Fig. 44.2, page 590). The binding of the receptor protein to the gene facilitates specific mRNA synthesis, which in turn, regulates the synthesis of specific proteins, and the activity of the target cells. Receptors for corticosteroids and vitamin D are cytosolic receptors, whereas those for **thyroid hormones, sex steroids, and Vitamin A are nuclear receptors**.

Such receptors **take the longest time for the onset of action**. Drugs acting through gene expression-linked receptors produce their effect after a characteristic **lag period** of about half an hour to several hours, e.g., glucocorticoids cannot relieve acute bronchospasms in an asthma patient immediately. Moreover, the effect of such drugs persists for a few hours or days after stopping the drug due to the slow metabolism of the synthesised proteins.

Box 4.1 summarises various transduction systems for various drug receptors.

> **Box 4.1 Transduction systems for different drug receptors**
>
> 1. **G-protein coupled receptors (GPCR)**
>   a. **Adenylyl cyclase (cAMP) pathway**
> G_s → Stimulates adenylyl cyclase → Increase in cAMP (e.g., β_1, adenosine$_2$, and D_1 receptors)
> G_i → Inhibits adenylyl cyclase → Decrease in cAMP (e.g., M_2, α_2, and D_2 receptors)
>   b. **Phospholipase C (PLC)–inositol triphosphate (IP$_3$)–diacyl glycerol (DAG) pathway**
> G_q → Activates phospholipase C → Converts phosphatidyl inositol biphosphate (PIP$_2$) into inositol triphosphate (IP$_3$) and diacyl glycerol (DAG)
>   IP$_3$ → Mobilises Ca^{2+} from intracellular organelles
>   DAG → Enhances the activation of phosphokinase C (PKc) by Ca^{2+}
> M_1, α_1, and M_3 receptors are G_q-linked receptors.
>   c. **Channel regulation**
>   G proteins can cause depolarisation/hyperpolarisation of the membrane by changes in intracellular ion concentration
>   *For example,*
> G_s opens Ca^{2+} channels in β_1 stimulation
> G_i opens K$^+$ channels in M_2, α_2, and D_2 stimulation
> G_i closes Ca^{2+} channels in D_2, opioid, and GABA$_B$ stimulation
>
>   **Mnemonic for examples of GPCR**
> G_s-linked—**BAD** (β_1, adenosine$_2$, and D_1 receptors)
> G_i-linked—**MAD** (M_2, α_2, and D_2 receptors open K$^+$ channels)
>   **DOG** (D_2, opioid, and GABA$_B$ receptors close Ca^{2+} channels)
> G_q-linked—**MAM** (M_1, α_1, and M_3 receptors)
>
> 2. **Receptors with intrinsic ion channels**
>   Cell surface receptors enclosing ion channels within their molecule, e.g., nicotinic, 5-HT$_3$, GABA$_A$–Cl$^-$ channel complex.
>   Both onset and offset of responses are fastest and linearly related to the number of receptors occupied.
>
> 3. **Enzymatic receptors**
>   The receptor is an enzyme protein, which can be:
>   - Tyrosine kinase, e.g., insulin, interleukin, NGF, and EGF receptors
>   - Guanylyl cyclase, e.g., ANP receptors
>   - Threonine/serine kinase, e.g., transforming growth factor receptors
>
>   Receptors linked to JAK/STAT: Interferon, cytokines, GH, erythropoietin receptors cause the activation of cytosolic tyrosine kinase (JAK) → Phosphorylation of STAT → STAT dimers formed → Regulate gene transcription
>
> 4. **Receptors regulating gene expression**
>   Intracellular receptors → agonist binds and exposes the DNA-binding regulatory segment → regulation of the synthesis of mRNA and specific proteins.
>   E.g., cytosolic receptors for corticosteroids, vitamin D, and nuclear receptors for thyroid hormone, vitamin A, and sex hormones.
>   These receptors have the longest lag period in the onset of drug action.

Receptor regulation

Receptors may get up/down-regulated in various conditions as described below (Table 4.2).

Down-regulation

Prolonged **exposure of receptors to a high concentration of an agonist** (which may be administered as a drug or could be overproduced as a neurotransmitter) causes a decrease in the number of receptors available for activation. This is known as the 'down-regulation' of receptors. This occurs due to:

- **Endocytosis/masking/internalisation** of receptors from the cell surface, so that it becomes inaccessible to the agonist; refractoriness develops and also fades away quickly
- **Decreased synthesis or increased destruction** of the receptor—refractoriness develops over weeks or months and recedes slowly

For example, the down-regulation of receptors may be **responsible for diminished effects** of β_2-selective agonists like salbutamol in severe asthma. Similarly, the efficacy of levodopa decreases upon long-term usage in parkinsonism.

Up-regulation

On the other hand, prolonged **deprivation of the agonist** (by denervation or the continued use of an antagonist or a drug that reduces input) results in the up-regulation of receptors. The up-regulation of α1 receptors is responsible

Table 4.2 Differences between up- and down-regulation of receptors

Receptor regulation	Up-regulation	Down-regulation
Cause	Prolonged deprivation of the agonist (by denervation or the continued use of an antagonist or a drug that reduces input)	Prolonged exposure to a high concentration of the agonist (which may be administered as a drug or is overproduced as a neurotransmitter)
Mechanism	- Unmasking of receptors - Proliferation of receptors - Accentuation of signal amplification by the transducer	- Endocytosis/masking/internalisation of receptors from the cell surface - Decreased synthesis or increased destruction of the receptor
Clinical implication	- Clonidine and CNS depressant/opioid withdrawal syndromes - Sudden discontinuation of propranolol in angina pectoris	-

for hypertensive crises in cases of clonidine withdrawal syndrome Similarly, sudden discontinuation of beta-blockers in angina patients causes the worsening of angina due to the up-regulation of β₁ receptors.

Up-regulation occurs due to the unmasking or proliferation of receptors and the accentuation of signal amplification by the transducer.

Spare receptors

All the receptors of a cell or a tissue need not be occupied to elicit the maximal response from the drug. This means that each tissue or cell has spare receptors (**receptor reserve**).

For example, the maximal positive inotropic effect of catecholamines can be elicited when less than 10% of the receptors on the myocardium are occupied. This indicates the presence of a high proportion of spare receptors. **The more the spare receptors available, the more the sensitivity of the tissue.**

C. DRUG ACTION THROUGH SPECIFIC GENETIC CHANGES

Hereditary disease are caused by mutations in the genome; transfer of normal genes to patients having monogenic disorders seems to be the most logical treatment option.

Important strategies for genetic medicine include the transfer of DNA, RNA, and somatic stem cells for modifying gene expression, so as to compensate for abnormal phenotypes. While there is no change in the DNA, there is a change in gene expression, the effect of which lasts till the life of that cell.

For example:

- Bone marrow stem cell transplantation in immunodeficiencies and hemoglobinopathies.
- RNA modification therapies targeting mRNA to suppress mRNA/correct or add function to mRNA.

FDA-approved drug therapies for hereditary diseases include:

- Coagulation factor IX (recombinant) for hemophilia B/Christmas disease
- Rilonacept for familial cold auto-inflammatory syndrome and recurrent pericarditis
- Cerliponase Alfa for neuronal ceroid lipofuscinosis type 2 (CLN-2)
- Rufinamide for controlling seizures in Lennox–Gastaut syndrome
- Aztreonam inhalational solution for chronic lung infection in cystic fibrosis
- Exagamglogene autotemcel for sickle cell disease.

In addition, repeated acute use of cocaine induces gene expression changes that result in transition of patients from use to dependence and drug abuse. Similarly, in alcoholics with heavy and binge drinking, a gene modification process called methylation' has been implicated in causing chronic alcoholism.

Dose–response curve (DRC)

Dose refers to the amount of the drug administered to elicit a certain response from a patient. **Response** refers to the change in the activity of the cells or tissues produced by a selected dose of the drug.

Components of DRC

There are two components of the dose–response relationship.

- The dose–plasma concentration relationship, which is determined by various pharmacokinetic factors
- The plasma concentration–response relationship, which is determined by pharmacodynamic factors

The observed effect at a given dose 'D' is:

$$E = \frac{E_{max} \times D}{K_D + D}$$

Where E_{max} signifies maximal effect and K_D is the dissociation constant of the drug–receptor complex; K_D is a measure of the affinity of the drug for receptors and is equal to the dose at which half the maximal response ($E_{max}/2$) is produced.

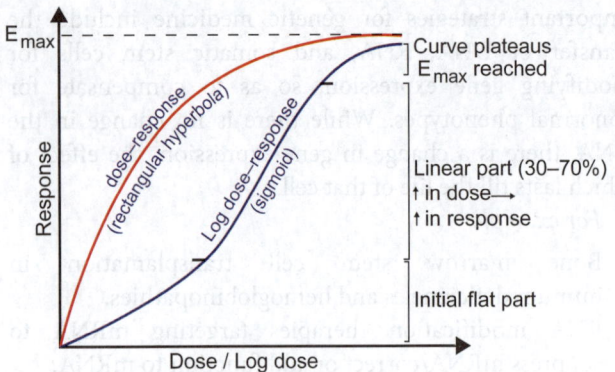

Fig. 4.7 DRC and log DRC

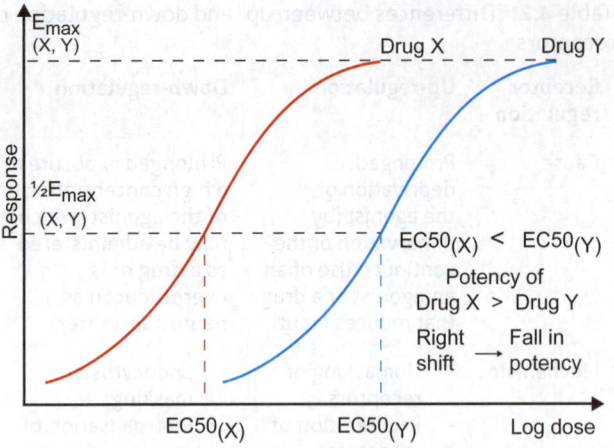

Fig. 4.8 Comparison of drug potency using a log DRC

In the DRC, dose is plotted on the X-axis against the measured response on the Y-axis (Fig. 4.7). The resulting graph is a **rectangular hyperbola** because drug–receptor interactions follows the law of mass action, i.e., the intensity of the response increases as the dose increases.

If **log dose** is plotted against the response, the curve becomes **sigmoid**. Initially, the line is flat because the amount of the drug given is not enough to initiate the response.

In the **intermediate portion (30–70%)**, with each increase in the dose, the response increases and the curve rises steadily. There is a **linear relationship** between the dose and response.

In the **last phase**, the DRC **plateaus** as further increase in the dose has no incremental effect on the response (as maximal efficacy has already been achieved).

On a log DRC, a wide range of drug doses can be displayed, making it possible to compare agonists and study antagonists.

The log dose–response curve of vitamins and essential metals is 'U'-shaped because these cause adverse effects at very high concentrations as well as at very low concentrations.

Utility of DRC in therapeutics

a. **The position of the DRC along the dose axis** is a measure of the **potency** of the drug, which is defined as 'the amount of the drug needed to produce a particular response'. Potency depends upon the affinity of the drug for the receptor and the efficiency of the coupling of the drug–receptor interaction with the response.

The DRC of a drug with lower potency is positioned more towards the right than a drug with higher potency (Fig. 4.8). The relative potency of two drugs is determined by comparing the doses of the two that produce half the maximal response (EC50). For example, the analgesic effect of 10 mg of morphine is equivalent to that of 100 mg of pethidine. In other words, morphine is 10 times more potent as an analgesic than pethidine.

b. **The upper limit of the DRC,** i.e., the maximal response that can be elicited by a drug (E_{max}) is a measure of its

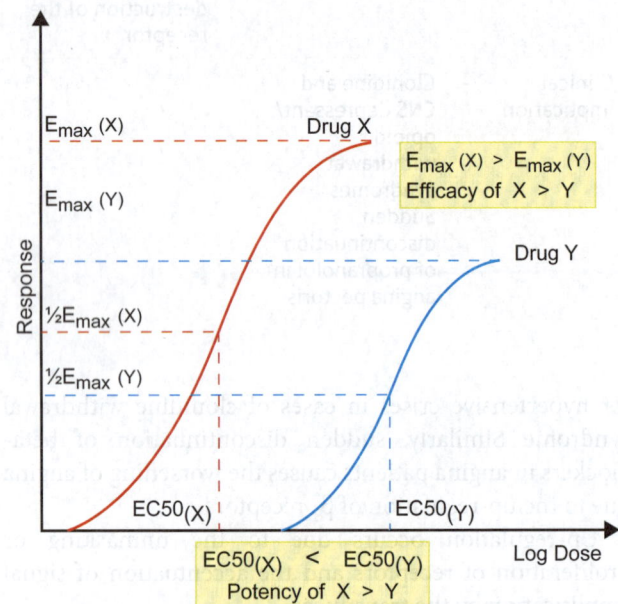

Drug X is more potent and more efficacious than drug Y.

Fig. 4.9 Comparison of drug efficacy using a log DRC

efficacy (Fig. 4.9). It may depend on the IA, i.e., mode of interaction of the drug with its receptors or the characteristics of the effector system involved.

Clinically, drugs with both higher and lower efficacy are desired under different circumstances. For example, moderate-efficacy thiazide diuretics are preferred over high-efficacy loop diuretics in the treatment of mild–moderate hypertension. On the other hand, high-ceiling diuretics are preferable in the treatment of congestive heart failure and other edematous conditions. Table 4.3 summarises the differences between potency and efficacy of drugs.

c. The **efficacy of partial agonists is lower than that of full agonists.** However, a partial agonist acts as an antagonist in the presence of an agonist because

Table 4.3 Difference between potency and efficacy

	Potency	Efficacy
Definition	The amount of the drug needed to produce a particular response	The maximal response that can be elicited by a drug
Depends on	- The affinity of the receptor for the drug - The efficiency of the coupling of the drug–receptor interaction with the response.	- Intrinsic activity of drug i.e. the mode of interaction of the drug with its receptors - The characteristics of the effector system involved.
Method of measuring	- Measured by the position of DRC on dose axis. - Rightward shift of DRC indicates lower potency (Fig. 4.8).	- Represented by the upper limit of the DRC - The DRC of a drug with lower efficacy achieves lesser maxima than a drug with higher efficacy (Fig. 4.9).
Effect of antagonists	Potency is reduced by competitive antagonists resulting in rightward shift of the DRC. However, the same efficacy is attainable with a larger dose of the agonist. (Fig. 4.10)	Potency and efficacy are reduced by non-competitive antagonists, which cause rightward shift and reduced maxima of the DRC. (Fig. 4.10)
Utility in practice	Relative potency of two drugs is determined by comparing the doses required to produce half the maximal response (EC50).	- Partial agonists have lesser efficacy than full agonists. - Drugs with both higher and lower efficacy are desired under different circumstances
Example	The analgesic effect of 10 mg of morphine is equivalent to that of 100 mg of pethidine. Thus, morphine is 10 times more potent than pethidine.	Moderate-efficacy thiazide diuretics are preferred in mild-to-moderate hypertension, whereas high-efficacy loop diuretics are preferred in congestive heart failure.

it competes with the agonist for a finite number of binding sites.

d. Competitive **antagonists** occupy the ligand-binding sites on the receptors, resulting in a decrease in the affinity of the agonist for the receptor. This is depicted in Fig. 4.10 as reduced potency and a rightward shift of the DRC.

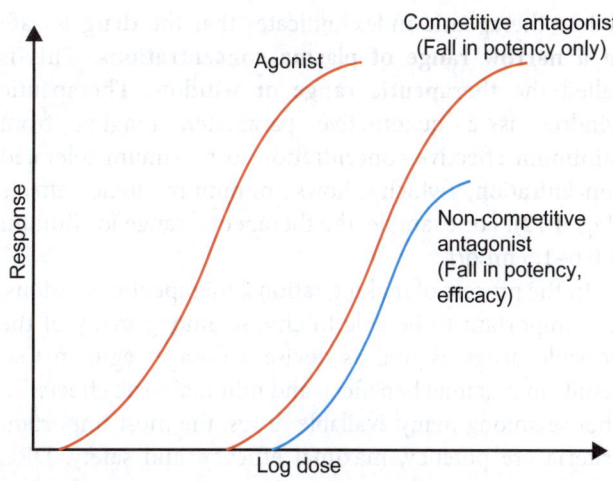

Fig. 4.10 Competitive and non-competitive antagonism on the log DRC

However, the same efficacy is attainable with a larger dose of the agonist. In contrast, the non-competitive antagonists cause reduced potency as well as efficacy.

e. **The slope of the DRC** indicates a change in the response per unit dose. Drugs with a **steeper dose–response curve are more toxic** than drugs with a flat DRC. **Individualisation** of the dose is required for such drugs as the margin of safety is narrow. For example, the slope of the DRC for CNS depression is steeper for barbiturates than for benzodiazepines.

Thus, the **therapeutic index or margin of safety** is a qualitative parameter. It is determined by comparing the DRCs for therapeutic effects and adverse effects. If two curves are close, the drug is more toxic or has a low therapeutic index/narrow margin of safety. For example, the gap between the DRC for sedation and coma is lesser for barbiturates than it is for benzodiazepines (BZDs). Hence, barbiturates have a narrow margin of safety as compared to benzodiazepines (Fig. 4.11).

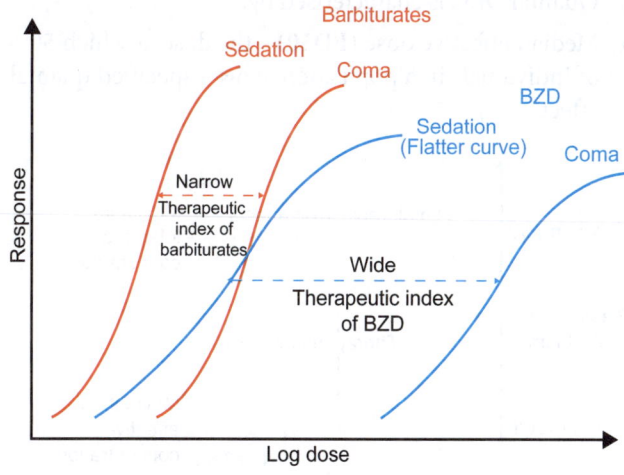

Fig. 4.11 Therapeutic index or margin of safety

A low therapeutic index indicates that the **drug is safe in a narrow range of plasma concentrations.** This is called the **therapeutic range or window.** Therapeutic window is a quantitative parameter, ranging from minimum effective concentration to maximum tolerated concentration, which shows minimum toxic effects (Fig. 4.12). For example, the therapeutic range for lithium is 0.6–1.5 mEq/L.

In the process of making rational therapeutic decisions, it is important to be able to choose among many of the possible drugs as well as devise a dosage regimen that results in maximal beneficial and minimal toxic effects. To choose among many available drugs, the most important criteria are potency, maximal efficacy, and safety. DRC helps in making therapeutic choices by comparing the pharmacological profile (potency, efficacy, and safety) of different drugs. The clinical effectiveness of a drug depends on its efficacy and pharmacokinetic factors. On the other hand, potency is useful for determining the dose of a chosen drug and the comparison of equi-effective doses of two drugs.

A graded DRC is a graphical representation of the relationship between the dose of the drug and the effect it achieves in a patient. In therapeutics, it is **difficult to construct a graded DRC for a patient** because the dose producing the maximal beneficial and minimal toxic effect is chosen and administered to the patient. The dose cannot be further changed for fear of losing effectiveness or producing toxicity. Furthermore, a graded DRC constructed for one individual may not apply to others, owing to variability in the severity of the disease and responsiveness to drugs among individuals. Therefore, **quantal DRCs** are more useful. In a quantal DRC, the dose of a drug required to produce a specified magnitude of a particular effect **in a population** is determined, and the cumulative frequency distribution of responders is plotted against the log dose. In it, the **rate of response occurrence in the population is plotted against the drug dose.**

Quantal DRC is characterised by:

- Median effective dose (**ED50**)—the dose at which 50% of individuals in a population show a specified quantal effect.

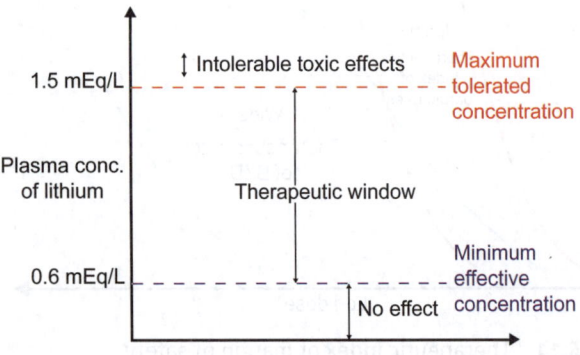

Fig. 4.12 Therapeutic window/range

- Median toxic dose (**TD50**)—the dose required to produce particular toxic effects in 50% of the subjects

Quantal curves indicate the therapeutic index or margin of safety of a drug. **Therapeutic index** is a measure that relates the dose of a drug producing a desired effect to the dose producing an undesired effect. It is calculated as the **ratio of TD50 to ED50 in animal experiments.** However, in humans, the therapeutic index is calculated as the **ratio of maximum tolerated to minimal effective dose.**

Both graded and quantal DRC provide information about the potency and selectivity of a drug. The graded curve provided information about maximal efficacy, whereas the quantal curve indicates a variability of response to a drug among individuals.

Clinical problem-based questions and MCQs

8. A middle-aged male patient was brought to the emergency with bleeding from the nose (epistaxis). Nasal packing with adrenaline-soaked swab controlled the bleeding.
   i. Identify the mechanism of action of adrenaline in this case.
      a. Nerve stimulation b. Enzyme inhibition
      c. Adsorptive effect d. Receptor activation
   ii. Explain the mechanism of action of adrenaline with the help of a suitable diagram.

9. All of the following GPCRs are linked to G_i proteins EXCEPT:
   a. M_2 receptors b. α_2 receptors
   c. β_1 receptors d. D_2 receptors

10. Identify G_q-linked receptors among the following:
    a. M_2 receptors b. α_1 receptors
    c. β_1 receptors d. D_2 receptors

11. The enzyme protein linked with the receptors of all of the following drugs is tyrosine kinase, EXCEPT in the case of:
    a. Atrial natriuretic peptide
    b. Epidermal growth factor
    c. Interleukin
    d. Nerve growth factor

12. All of the following act through JAK/STAT protein-linked receptors EXCEPT:
    a. Interferon b. Cytokines
    c. Interleukin d. Erythropoietin

13. i. Insulin is injected subcutaneously daily in a 9-year-old boy who is a known case of IDDM. It acts through insulin receptors, which are:
       a. Gene-linked receptors
       b. Tyrosine kinase receptors
       c. G protein-coupled receptors
       d. Ion channel receptors
    ii. Describe the transduction mechanism of insulin receptors with the help of a suitable diagram.

14. Identify guanylyl cyclase-linked receptors.
    a. EGF receptors b. ANP receptors
    c. TGF receptors d. GH receptors

15. i. Which of the following receptors has the fastest action?
    a. Gene-linked receptors
    b. Tyrosine kinase receptors
    c. G protein-coupled receptors
    d. Ion channel receptors
    ii. Enumerate drugs acting through the receptors selected in part i.

16. i. Which of the following receptors has the slowest action?
    a. Gene-linked receptors
    b. Tyrosine kinase receptors
    c. G protein-coupled receptors
    d. Ion channel receptors
    ii. Enumerate the drugs that act through the receptors selected in part i.
    iii. Describe the transduction system for the receptors selected in part i with the help of a suitable diagram.

17. Which of the following act through cytosolic receptors?
    a. Corticosteroids   b. Vitamin A
    c. Thyroxine   d. Estrogens

18. The ratio of the drug dose producing toxic effect to that producing beneficial effects is called its therapeutic index. Identify the drug with the largest value for therapeutic index among following drugs.
    a. Lithium   b. Digoxin
    c. Diazepam   d. Theophylline

19. i. Define the potency of a drug.
    ii. Which of the following drugs is the most potent?
        a. Drug X that has EC50 = 5
        b. Drug Y that has EC50 = 50
        c. Drug Z that has EC50 = 75
        d. All three are equipotent
    iii. In which direction does DRC move with increasing potency?
        a. Upward   b. Downward
        c. Towards the right d. Towards the left

20. DRC is a plot of the response on the Y axis against the dose/log dose on the X axis.
    i. Explain the advantage of using a log dose in DRC.
    ii. Explain the utility of DRC with respect to making therapeutic decisions.

21. A 60-year-old female patient with manic depressive psychosis is on lithium therapy. Therapeutic drug monitoring is carried out as lithium is known to have a narrow therapeutic index.
    i. Identify the INCORRECT statement about the therapeutic index of lithium.
        a. The ratio of TD50 to ED50 in quantal DRC in experimental animals is less than one.
        b. It is the ratio of the maximum tolerated to the minimum effective dose.
        c. DRCs of therapeutic and toxic effects are very close.
        d. DRC is steeper.

22. A middle-aged woman who is a known case of bronchial asthma was on salbutamol therapy for the past 4–5 years. The patient has developed refractoriness to salbutamol therapy and her physician is looking for alternatives.
    i. Identify the cause of refractoriness to salbutamol therapy.
        a. Receptor hypersensitivity
        b. Receptor supersensitivity
        c. Receptor depolarisation
        d. Receptor down-regulation
    ii. Describe the term selected in part (i).

Summary

- Drugs act by receptor-mediated or non-receptor-mediated mechanisms.
- Non-receptor-mediated mechanisms are attributed to certain physical/chemical properties of the drug, enzyme stimulation/inhibition, immunostimulation/immunosuppression, or placebo effects.
- The physical properties of drugs are responsible for their action, e.g., the mass of bulk purgatives, the adsorption property of activated charcoal in poisoning, radioactivity of I^{131} in thyroid disorders, osmotic pressure of mannitol in raised IOT, ICT and the radiopacity of barium sulphate in barium meal and barium enema.
- Some chemical properties that result in drug action are acid neutralisation by antacids, protamine sulphate in heparin toxicity, and chelating agents in heavy metal poisonings.
- Enzyme stimulation increases V_{max} and reduces k_M.
- Enzyme inhibition can be competitive (equilibrium/non-equilibrium types) or non-competitive.
- Competitive enzyme inhibition is reversible. The drug competes with its normal substrate for the catalytic site. k_M increases but V_{max} remains unchanged. Examples are sulphonamides, NSAIDs (except aspirin), allopurinol and physostigmine [Mnemonic: SNAP].
- Non-competitive enzyme inhibition is irreversible. Here, the drug binds to a site adjacent to the catalytic site. V_{max} is reduced but k_M is unchanged. Examples are disulfiram, aspirin, digoxin, and acetazolamide [Mnemonic: DADA].
- Drug action through receptors is based on affinity and intrinsic activity (IA). The agonist has affinity and full IA=1. A partial agonist has affinity, but IA is <1. It blocks the effect of the full agonist. An inverse agonist has affinity, but its IA is in the opposite direction, i.e., IA = –1. Antagonists have affinity but no IA, i.e., IA =0. They occupy receptors and block the effect of agonists.

- Receptors are of four types based on their transduction or coupling mechanism. GPCR, enzyme-linked (TK-linked or JAK/STAT-linked), ion channel-linked and gene expression-regulating receptors.
- GPCR can act through adenylyl cyclase stimulation (G_S—e.g. β_1, adenosine$_2$, and D_1 receptors) or inhibition (G_i—e.g., M_2, α_2, and D_2 receptors open K^+ channels and D_2, opioid, and $GABA_B$ receptors close Ca^{2+} channels). G_s and G_i-linked receptors cause raised or lowered cAMP levels, respectively. G_q-linked receptors act through the IP_3–DAG pathway (e.g., M_1, α_1, and M_3 receptors). Mnemonics for GPCR-linked mechanisms are BAD, MAD, DOG, MAM.
- Enzyme-linked receptors may be linked to tyrosine kinase (e.g., insulin, interleukin, NGF, EGF receptors) or guanylyl cyclase. (ANP receptors) or threonine/serine kinase (transforming growth factor beta receptors). Some enzyme-linked receptors are linked to JAK/STAT, e.g., interferon, cytokines, GH, and erythropoietin receptors cause the activation of cytosolic tyrosine kinase (JAK) → phosphorylation of STAT → STAT dimers formed → regulate gene transcription.
- Receptors enclosing ion channels have the fastest onset and a linear relationship as no second messengers are involved. For example, nicotinic cholinergics enclosing the Na^+ channel and $GABA_A$/benzodiazepine receptors enclosing the Cl^- channel.
- Receptors regulating gene expression have the slowest onset after a lag period. These intracellular receptors are responsible for the action of thyroid hormone, steroidal hormones, sex steroids and vitamins A and D.
- Continuous exposure to an agonist causes down-regulation leading to refractoriness to treatment. For example, salbutamol in bronchial asthma and levodopa in parkinsonism. Continuous exposure to an antagonist/the absence of an agonist causes up-regulation of receptors, causing the worsening of angina in patients on propranolol therapy on withdrawal and hypertensive crisis on clonidine withdrawal.
- When response is plotted on the Y axis and dose/log dose on the X axis, the resulting curve is called the dose–response curve or the DRC. It is used to compare the potency and efficacy of drugs. A rightward shift represents a decrease in potency. A downward shift of the maxima represents reduced efficacy. EC50 is the concentration that produces half the maximal response. The therapeutic index or margin of safety and competitive/non-competitive antagonism can also be depicted in the DRC.

Questions for practice

1. Write short notes on:
   i. GPCR
   ii. Receptor regulation
   iii. Gene regulating receptors
2. Explain why:
   i. Sudden clonidine withdrawal causes a hypertensive crisis
   ii. Patients on levodopa therapy for long periods stop responding to treatment
   iii. Asthmatics become refractory to salbutamol after responding for some time
   iv. Partial agonists block the effects of full agonists
3. Differentiate between:
   i. Enzyme stimulation and enzyme induction
   ii. Drug action and drug effects
   iii. Competitive and non-competitive enzyme inhibition
   iv. Potency and efficacy of drugs
   v. Up-regulation and down-regulation of receptors
   vi. Silent and spare receptors

Hints for problem-based questions and MCQs

1. d. Some drugs stimulate one type of cells, but inhibit another type, e.g., acetylcholine stimulates peristalsis, inhibits heart.
2. c. The anti-thyroid effect of I^{131} is because of its radioactivity, which is a physical property.
3. a. In the non-equilibrium type of competitive enzyme inhibition, V_{max} is reduced whereas k_M increases.
4. i. a. Digoxin
   ii. It inhibits the Na^+/K^+-ATPase enzyme. V_{max} is reduced but k_M does not change.
5. a–3; b–4; c–2; d–1.
6. Refer to page 52
7. Physostigmine causes the equilibrium subtype of competitive enzyme inhibition, but OPCs cause the non-equilibrium subtype (refer to page 52).
8. i. d. Receptor activation of α_1 receptors present in the blood vessels of the nasal mucosa causes vasoconstriction and controls epistaxis.
   ii. G_q-linked GPCRs (refer to page 56, Fig. 4.5).
9. c. β_1 receptors are G_s-linked, and the rest are G_i-linked.
10. b. α_1 receptors. Refer to page 58, Box 4.1.
11. a. Atrial natriuretic peptide receptors are linked to guanylyl cyclase. Refer to page 57.
12. c. Interleukin acts through tyrosine kinase-linked receptors.
13. i. b. Tyrosine kinase-linked receptors
    ii. Refer to page 57, Fig. 43.2, page 572.
14. b. ANP receptors
15. i. d. Ion channel receptors
    ii. Nicotinic cholinergics, $GABA_A$–Cl^- channel complex containing barbiturate, and benzodiazepine receptors.
16. i. a. Gene-linked receptors
    ii. Thyroid hormones, steroidal hormones, and vitamins A and D
    iii. Refer to page 58, Fig. 44.2, page 590.
17. a. Corticosteroids act through cytosolic receptors. All the others act through nuclear receptors.
18. c. Diazepam
19. i. The amount of drug that produces a particular response (usually half the maximal response EC50). Refer to page 60.

ii. a. Drug X that has EC50 = 5
iii. d. DRC moves towards the left with an increase in potency.
20. i. Wide range of doses can be displayed (refer to page 60).
ii. Refer to page 60.
21. a. The ratio of TD50 to ED50 in the quantal DRC in experimental animals is less than one. TD50 cannot be lower than ED50 for clinically used drugs.
22. i. d. Receptor down-regulation
ii. Refer to page 58.

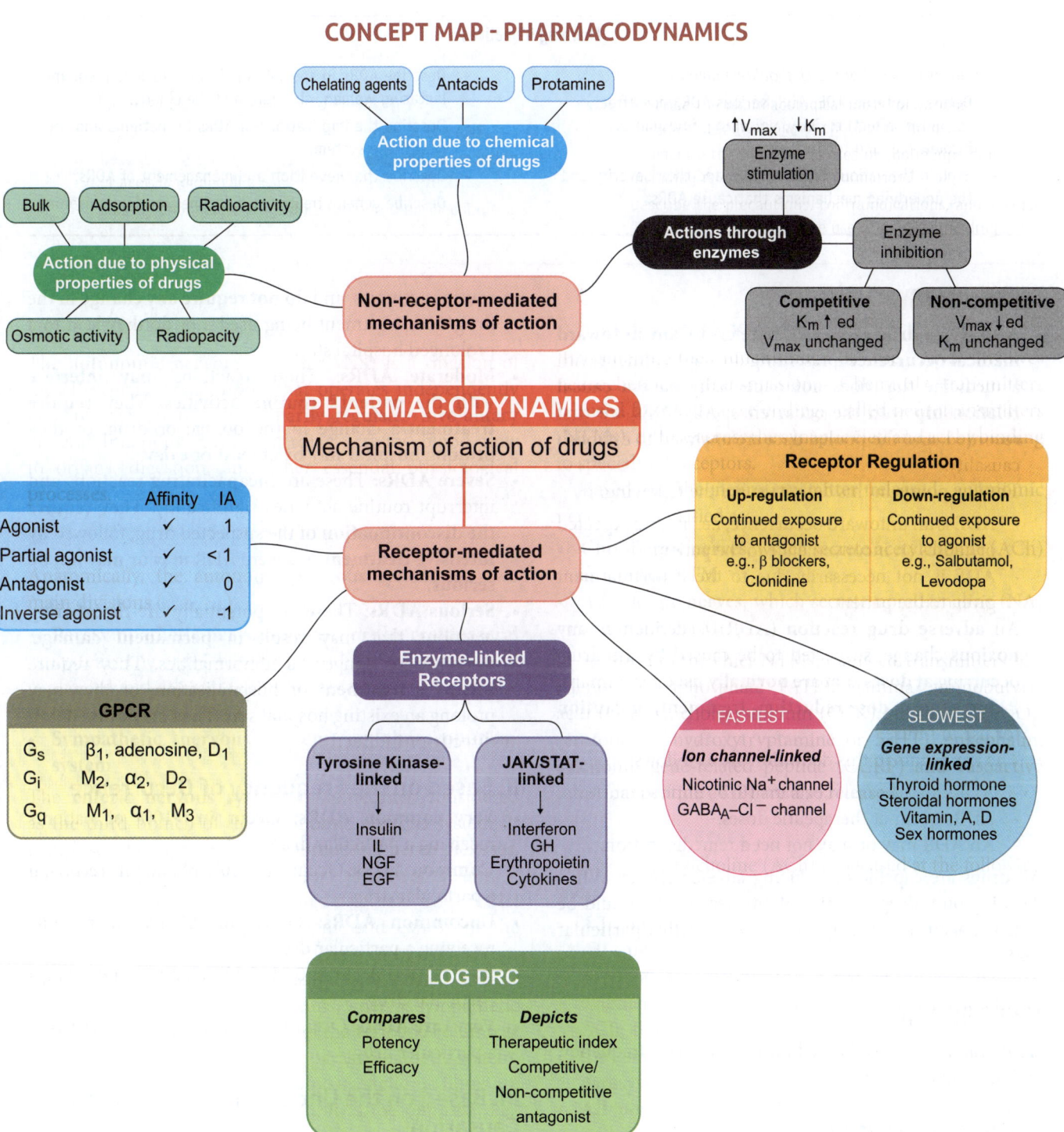

SECTION 1 General Pharmacology

5 Adverse Drug Reactions

PH 1.11 Define adverse drug reactions (ADRs) and their types. Identify the ADRs in the given case scenario and assess causality.

Learning objectives

A student of MBBS phase II should be able to:
- Define the terms ADE, ADR, serious ADR, side effect, secondary effect, toxicity, poisoning, idiosyncrasy, intolerance, and teratogenicity.
- Explain the various types of ADRs and their severity and the underlying mechanisms that cause ADRs.
- Describe ADRs in special populations such as pregnant/lactating women, children, and the elderly.
- Describe the implications of ADRs for patients and the healthcare system.
- Describe the prevention and management of ADRs.
- Describe general treatment guidelines for drug poisoning.

TERMINOLOGY

- An **adverse drug event (ADE)** refers to '**any untoward medical occurrence**' presenting during treatment with a medicine that does **not necessarily have a causal relationship** with the occurrence. All ADEs are first recorded, and the pooled data are analysed to establish causality.

  The key points in this definition are the following:
  - ADE is an untoward occurrence, i.e., it is unexpected or causes an inconvenience to the patient.
  - ADE is not necessarily due to the drug/treatment given to the patient.

- An **adverse drug reaction** (ADR) is defined as any **noxious** change, suspected to be caused by the drug, occurring **at doses that are normally used** for humans. It **may require dose reduction, treatment, or caution** for use in future.

  The key points in this definition are as follows:
  - ADRs are noxious, i.e., harmful or unpleasant.
  - ADRs occur at therapeutic doses.
  - An ADR may or may not need remedial action.

All drugs are capable of inducing adverse effects. While deciding on a drug, the risk of adverse effects should be weighed against its therapeutic benefits in that particular case.

TYPES OF ADRs

ADRs can be classified based on their severity, frequency, and underlying mechanisms.

I. Based on Severity

- **Minor/mild ADRs**: The patient is aware of the symptoms, and the signs can be elicited. The symptoms/signs, however, are **transient**, do not interfere with routine activities, and **do not require any change** in the drug/dose/treatment being used, nor do they lead to a prolonged hospital stay.
- **Moderate ADRs**: These reactions **may interfere with the patient's routine** activities. They **require treatment/a change** in the dosage or drug, or they **prolong hospital stay by at least one day**.
- **Severe ADRs**: These are **incapacitating** reactions and interrupt routine activities significantly. They **require the discontinuation** of the suspected drug, followed by **intensive treatment**. A severe ADR **may or may not be serious**.
- **Serious ADRs**: These are potentially **life-threatening** reactions that may result in **permanent damage**, disability, or congenital abnormalities. They require **intensive treatment** or hospitalisation, or they may prolong an existing hospital stay. They may cause **death** directly or indirectly.

II. Based on the Frequency of Occurrence

- **Very common ADRs**: Occur in >10% of patients receiving a particular drug
- **Common ADRs**: Occur in 1–10% of patients receiving a particular drug
- **Uncommon ADRs**: Occur in 0.1–1% of patients receiving a particular drug
- **Rare ADRs**: Occur in 0.01–0.1% of patients receiving a particular drug
- **Very rare ADRs**: Occur in <0.01% of patients receiving a particular drug

III. Based on the Underlying Mechanism of Causation

a. Type A or augmented reactions

These are based on the pharmacological properties of a drug. They are qualitatively same as the normal response to the drug, but usually, the response is augmented. These reactions have the following properties:

- **Predictable**: They can be predicted based on the pharmacological actions of a drug.
- **Dose-related**: Their occurrence increases with dosage.
- **Preventable**: They can be prevented by selecting the appropriate dose for an individual patient.
- **Reversible**: They can be corrected by reducing the dose or stopping the causative drug.
- **Common**: They are very common because they are dose-related, and dosage errors are quite frequent.

They include side effects, secondary effects, toxic effects, and consequences of drug withdrawal.

(i) Side effects

These are **unwanted but often unavoidable** pharmacodynamic effects.

- These occur at the **therapeutic dose** and can be predicted from the pharmacological actions of the drug.
- Sometimes, the 'therapeutic action' of a drug is responsible for side effects as well. For example, the anticholinergic drug atropine causes dryness of the mouth when used to reduce tracheobronchial secretions as a pre-anesthetic medication.
- In some other situations, side effects are due to the actions of a drug other than its therapeutic action. For example, antihistaminic drugs used for their antiallergic effects can cause sedation as a side effect.
- In certain situations, one particular effect may be therapeutic in one setting and a side effect in another. For example, atropine decreases exocrine secretion. This is a therapeutically required effect when atropine is used for pre-anesthetic medication. However, when atropine or other anticholinergic drugs are used for other indications such as spasms/bronchial asthma, the reduced exocrine secretions cause dryness of the mouth, skin, eyes, etc., as side effects. Similarly, constipation is the therapeutic effect of codeine in traveller's diarrhea but becomes a side effect when the same drug is used for cough suppression. **Side effects can usually be controlled by dose reduction.**

(ii) Secondary effects

These are the **indirect consequences of a primary action** of the drug. For example, broad-spectrum antibiotics like tetracyclines reduce the multiplication of a large spectrum of bacteria including the normal bacterial flora. This increases susceptibility to superinfection. Similarly, corticosteroids or other immunosuppressant drugs weaken the host defense mechanism, resulting in the activation of latent tuberculosis or other opportunistic infections.

(iii) Toxic effects

These are the extensions of the pharmacological actions of a drug that occur due to **overdose or prolonged use**. Overdose may be of the following types:

- **Absolute**—wherein an excess dose has been taken. It can be accidental, suicidal, or homicidal.
- **Relative**—wherein the usual dose of a drug is taken, but it causes toxic effects due to an individual's specific condition or susceptibility; for example, gentamicin in renal function impairment.

Toxicity can also occur due to **tissue damage or functional alteration.**

The manifestations of toxicity can be predicted from the known pharmacological actions of the drug. For example, oral hypoglycemic drugs used in the treatment of DM can cause hypoglycemia if the dose is increased or a meal is missed/delayed or the person engages in an unaccustomed degree of activity. Sedative hypnotics, when taken in excess, can cause coma as a result of excessive CNS depression. Anticoagulant drugs like heparin or warfarin can cause bleeding tendencies.

Sometimes, an action of the drug other than its therapeutic action may be responsible for toxicity manifestations. For example, morphine causes respiratory depression; aminoglycosides cause vestibular damage; and paracetamol overdose causes hepatic necrosis.

Poisoning

Poisoning refers to the harmful, toxic effects of drugs/chemicals on biological systems. It may occur because of:

- The consumption of **very large doses** of drugs, usually **intentionally** (because the only parameter that distinguishes a drug from a poison is the 'dose').
- Household, environmental, and industrial **chemicals, insecticides,** etc., are frequently responsible for poisoning

The **treatment of poisoning** involves general detoxification and supportive measures as described below.

- **Maintenance of vitals (ABC—airways, breathing, and circulation)**: This includes the maintenance of the airways, adequate ventilation, O_2 inhalation, and maintenance of BP with intravenous infusion, pressor agents, cardiac stimulation, pacing, etc. It is important to monitor and maintain temperature, blood glucose levels, electrolyte balance, and physiological pH.
- **Decontamination:** In cases of inhaled poisoning, the patient is kept in **fresh air**. Contaminated clothes are changed, and the skin and eyes are washed with soap and plenty of water (poison can be absorbed from the skin, as in the case of insecticides).
- For ingested poisons, **vomiting is induced** or **gastric lavage** is performed to remove any unabsorbed poison. However, these measures may not be beneficial if the patient presents > 2 hours after the ingestion of the poison. It should be noted that emesis should not be induced for kerosene/corrosive/CNS-stimulant poisoning and for comatosed or hemodynamically unstable patients as there is a high risk of aspiration. The absorption of an ingested poison can be prevented

by the administration of **activated charcoal** 1g/kg body weight in 200 mL of water. It can decrease drug absorption because of its adsorptive properties. However, charcoal cannot adsorb strong acids, alkalis, hydrocarbons, alcohol, cyanide, and other organic solvents. It is not used if the patient reports after > 2 hours of ingestion or has intestinal obstruction or a paralytic ileus.

- **Hastening the elimination of the poison from the body:** Poisons can be eliminated by increasing urine output (diuresis) using drugs like furosemide or mannitol. However, hemodialysis is a more effective method. Alkalinisation of urine helps to clear acidic drugs like aspirin. If a specific antidote exists, it should be given.

(b) Type B or bizarre reactions

These are called bizarre reactions because these are **not the usual actions** of the drug. Type B ADRs are usually **unpredictable** and **not dose-related**. Some type B reactions can be predicted and prevented if their genetic basis is known. Some characteristics of type B reactions are as follows:

- They are **based on peculiarities in patients** and not on the known actions of the drug.
- They are less common than type A ADRs but more serious.
- They require drug discontinuation and active treatment.
- The future use of the causal drug should be contraindicated for that patient.

Type B reactions include hypersensitivity reactions, idiosyncratic reactions, intolerance, and photosensitivity.

(i) Hypersensitivity reactions

- These are immunologically-mediated reactions to drugs and may appear even with a small dose in a particular individual but cannot be produced in other individuals at any dose.
- The drug or its metabolite acts as an antigen or hapten (incomplete Ag, which becomes antigenic only after combining with some endogenous proteins) and induces the production of antibodies or sensitised lymphocytes, resulting in different types of allergic symptoms.
- The presenting symptoms and severity of allergic reactions may vary from drug to drug.
- Hypersensitivity reactions can be of type I, II, III, or IV.

Type I (anaphylactic) reactions

These are brought about by IgE-mediated histamine release. Other mediators like 5-hydroxytryptamine (5-HT), leukotrienes (LT), prostaglandins (PG), and platelet-activating factor (PAF) are also released. These can cause itching, urticaria, angioedema, bronchospasm, rhinitis, paresthesia, flushing, lip swelling, palpitation, wheezing, syncope, and anaphylactic shock. Symptoms appear within minutes to a few hours of drug use. Because of the short reaction time, these reactions are called **immediate hypersensitivity reactions**. An intradermal skin sensitivity test may warn against type I sensitivity but is not completely reliable.

The **treatment** of type I reactions comprises the following measures:

- The offending drug is immediately stopped.
- Antihistamines are given to block the effects of histamine, which is the most prominent mediator of hypersensitivity reactions. Antihistamines relieve itching, urticaria, rhinitis, lip swelling, etc.
- Corticosteroids are useful because of their immunosuppressant effect. They are useful in severe or recurrent cases, especially in prolonged reactions in asthma patients. Hydrocortisone intravenous 200 mg is used.
- **Adrenaline is life-saving in severe anaphylactic reactions** as it is a physiological antagonist of histamine. Histamine released in response to the Ag–Ab reaction causes bronchoconstriction resulting in dyspnea and vasodilatation, which manifests as hypotension and shock. Adrenaline has just the opposite effects on the bronchi and blood vessels. It brings about bronchodilatation and vasoconstriction. Thus, it reverses both respiratory as well as hemodynamic features of anaphylactic shock. Adrenaline 0.5 mL, of a 1:1000 solution, is administered via the IM route and is repeated every 5–10 minutes till the patient improves. Adrenaline should not be used by the IV route unless the shock is immediately life-threatening. For intravenous use, adrenaline is diluted to a 1:10,000 (or even 1:100,000) solution, and infused slowly with constant monitoring.
- Supportive measures like the reclining position, O_2 inhalation, and cardiopulmonary resuscitation (CPR) are also required in the management of anaphylactic shock.

Type II hypersensitivity reactions

These are **complement-mediated cytolytic** reactions like aplastic anemia, hemolysis, agranulocytosis, systemic lupus erythematosus (SLE), organ damage, etc.

Type III hypersensitivity reactions

These are retarded **Arthus reactions**, e.g., serum sickness, Stevens–Johnson syndrome, polyarteritis nodosa.

Type IV or delayed hypersensitivity reactions

These are **cell-mediated immune reactions (CMI) that are brought about by T lymphocytes**, which release cytokines. This results in inflammation which manifests as contact dermatitis, rashes, photosensitisation, etc.

The only effective treatment for hypersensitivity reaction types II, III, and IV is the administration of **glucocorticoids**.

Common offending drugs
Hypersensitivity reactions are seen with penicillins, sulphonamides, tetracyclines, cephalosporins, metronidazole, aspirin, indomethacin, angiotensin-converting enzyme inhibitors, hydralazine, etc.

(ii) Idiosyncrasy
It is a **genetically-determined**, **abnormal reactivity** to a drug. The drug interacts with a unique feature of the individual (a feature that is not seen in the majority of the population) and produces an abnormal reaction or discontinuous variation. Such reactions occur in individuals with a particular genotype. Examples of idiosyncratic reactions include prolonged apnea with succinylcholine in pseudocholinesterase deficiency and hemolysis with primaquine in G6PD deficiency (refer to Chapter 6).

(iii) Intolerance
Normally, most drug effects show continuous variations and have a Gaussian 'bell-shaped' frequency distribution. However, some subjects fall on the extreme left side of this curve for sensitivity to the drug. In such individuals, the **characteristic toxic effects of the drug appear even with therapeutic doses**, i.e., such a person has a low threshold for the effects of the drug. This is the opposite to tolerance. For example, in some patients, a single tablet of chloroquine causes vomiting and abdominal pain and a single dose of triflupromazine can induce muscle dystonias. Similarly, a few doses of carbamazepine can cause ataxia in some patients.

(iv) Photosensitivity
This refers to drug-induced sensitisation of the skin to ultraviolet radiation resulting in cutaneous reactions. These reactions are of two types.
- **Phototoxic reactions:** The drug or its metabolite accumulates in the skin and absorbs ultraviolet light (wavelength 290–320 nm). The resulting photochemical and photobiological reactions lead to local tissue damage, which manifests as sunburn characterised by erythema, edema, vesicular eruptions, blister formation, hyperpigmentation, or desquamation. The larger the dose of the drug, the greater is the severity of the reaction.

  Common drugs that cause such phototoxic reactions are tetracyclines (especially demeclocycline), tar products, thiazides, fluoroquinolones, phenothiazines, dapsone, sulfones, etc.

  The treatment of phototoxic reactions involves measures such as:
  - Avoiding sun exposure and using sunscreens with SPF 15–60.
  - Soothing lotions such as calamine and wet dressings for symptomatic relief.
  - Mild topical steroids may be used.
- **Photo-allergic reactions:** These involve a cell-mediated immune response induced by the drug or its metabolites. On exposure to long wavelengths of 320–400 nm, a papular rash or contact dermatitis-like patch develops. Sometimes, antibodies may mediate photo-allergy as an immediate wheal-and-flare reaction to sun exposure.

  Common drugs that cause such reactions are sulphonamides, sulphonylureas, chloroquine, chlorpromazine, carbamazepine, etc. Treatment requires strong topical steroids or systemic steroids.

(c) Type C or continuous reactions
These reactions result from the **long-term/chronic/continuous use** of a drug. The following are some examples of this type of reaction:
- The prolonged use of analgesics can cause nephropathy.
- Tardive dyskinesia can occur with the long-term use of antipsychotic drugs.
- After the long-term use of levodopa in parkinsonism, patients show response fluctuations such as 'on–off phenomenon' or the 'end-of-dose phenomenon'.
- The chronic use of the antiepileptic drug phenytoin is associated with coarsening of facial features, gum hyperplasia and megaloblastic anemia, etc.

(d) Type D or delayed reactions
These are delayed reactions, which occur a long time after the patient has used the drug. These reactions involve mutagenesis and carcinogenesis.

Mutagenicity and carcinogenicity refer to the ability of a drug to cause genetic defects and cancer, respectively. The oxidation of drugs produces reactive intermediates that affect genes and may bring about **structural changes in the chromosomes**. Covalent interaction with DNA **modifies DNA** and induces mutations which may translate into a **heritable** defect. If the modified DNA codes for factors regulating cell growth and proliferation (proto-oncogenes), it may result in cancer. Some chemicals (drugs) can **promote malignant changes in genetically damaged cells** even without interacting directly with DNA. Chemical carcinogenesis generally takes **10–40 years** to develop.

Such ADRs are reported with anticancer drugs, radioisotopes, tobacco, estrogens, etc. Drugs with mutagenic or carcinogenic potential are not approved for marketing unless they are needed in life-threatening conditions.

(e) Type E or end-of-use reaction

These are like **rebound reactions** that occur due to the sudden withdrawal of a drug after continued use. For example,

- **Clonidine withdrawal** causes rebound hypertension, tachycardia, anxiety, palpitation, etc.
- The sudden **withdrawal of corticosteroids** after chronic use can cause the suppression of the hypothalamic–pituitary–adrenal axis (HPAA). This is characterised by fever, malaise, anorexia, and postural hypotension or the reactivation of the disease for which the drug was being used.
- Discontinuation of beta-blocker therapy can precipitate or worsen angina.

(f) Type F or failure of therapy

This is also considered a type of ADR. For example, the non-responsiveness of infecting microbes to antimicrobial drugs due to the development of resistance is a type F ADR. **Antimicrobial resistance** can develop because of the synthesis of a drug-metabolising enzyme by the organism, or alteration in the target site of the organism, or reduced concentration of the drug (decreased influx or excessive efflux of the drug) in organisms. P-glycoprotein (Pgp) causes efflux of drugs in the intestine and decreases its bioavailability. The efflux of antimicrobial drugs from the microbial cell as mediated by Pgp causes treatment failure. For example, digoxin and rifampicin are Pgp substrates. Microsomal inducers are Pgp inducers as well, while macrolides are Pgp inhibitors. Pgp inducers can cause treatment failure, while inhibitors can cause toxicity.

IV. ADRs in Special Populations

Pregnant and lactating women, elderly individuals, and children are considered special groups or populations prone to peculiar types of ADRs as described below.

(a) Pregnant women

The ability of a drug to cause fetal abnormalities on administration to a pregnant woman is called '**teratogenicity**' (Box 5.1). The embryo is the most dynamic biological system, constantly undergoing rapid growth, differentiation, and complex developmental changes. Hence, the effects of a drug on it are often irreversible. The type of deformities or malfunctioning caused by a drug in a fetus depends on the drug and the stage at which the exposure occurs. Drugs can affect the fetus during the following **three stages**:

- **Stage of fertilisation and implantation:** It lasts from conception till the 17th day after conception. During this phase, drugs can cause failure of pregnancy, which manifests as a delayed period and often goes unnoticed.
- **Stage of organogenesis:** It lasts from day 18–55 of conception. Drug use in this stage is most dangerous, as structural deformities may occur upon drug exposure.
- **Stage of growth and development:** It lasts from the 56th day of conception till term. Drug exposure in this stage can cause developmental and functional abnormalities.

Box 5.1   Teratogenic effects of drugs

- **Thalidomide:** Originally used as an antiemetic to manage morning sickness, thalidomide was later found to cause phocomelia, a severe limb deformity where fetal limbs resemble seal-like flippers. The widespread birth defects affected hundreds of fetuses, drawing attention towards this phenomenon of teratogenicity.
- **Angiotensin-converting enzyme inhibitors:** These are known to cause hypoplasia of organs, growth retardation, and fetal loss.
- **Aspirin/indomethacin:** These cause the premature closure of the ductus arteriosus.
- **Alcohol:** Fetal alcohol syndrome, growth retardation, and low IQ are some effects of alcohol on the fetus.
- **Antiepileptics:** Phenytoin causes hypoplastic phalanges, cleft lip/palate, and microcephaly.
- **Carbamazepine and valproate:** These drugs cause neural tube defects like spina bifida.
- **Antithyroid drugs:** Causes fetal goitre and hypothyroidism.
- **Androgens:** These drugs cause the virilisation of the female fetus.
- **Progestins:** These may also cause virilisation.
- **Stilbesterol:** Causes vaginal carcinoma in female offspring during adolescence.
- **Tetracyclines:** They cause retarded bone growth and discoloured, deformed teeth.

Drug categories

The USFDA has categorised drugs into five classes based on the risk of birth defects—A, B, C, D, and X.

- **Category A** drugs show no risk to the fetus in animal studies and well-controlled human studies, e.g., folic acid, pyridoxine, doxylamine, and levothyroxine.
- **Category B** drugs are those which:
  - show no evidence of risk in animal studies, but for which well-controlled human studies are not available, or
  - show some risks in animal studies but not in well-controlled human studies.

  Examples of category B drugs are penicillins, cephalosporins, macrolides, metronidazole, nitrofurantoin, ondansetron, and metoclopramide.

- **Category C** drugs are those for which risk cannot be ruled out. Drugs not listed in any other category are assigned to this category.

(In pregnancy, safety of drugs in category **A > B > C**.))

- **Category D** drugs are those for which there is evidence of teratogenicity, e.g., aminoglycosides, tetracyclines, ACE inhibitors, angiotensin receptor blockers, aspirin, lithium, phenytoin, carbamazepine, and corticosteroids.
- **Category X** drugs are highly teratogenic and are absolutely contraindicated in pregnancy, e.g., thalidomide, isotretinoin, methotrexate, and griseofulvin.

(b) Lactating mothers

Drugs given to a lactating mother may affect the suckling infant if secreted in the breast milk, e.g., antipsychotics, antianxiety, and antidepressant drugs. The dosage of these drugs should be to limit the amount of the drug absorbed by the infant. Care should be taken to administer the drug immediately after feeding the baby. Some drugs like anticancer drugs, amphetamines, lithium, and radioactive substances are contraindicated in lactating women.

(c) Pediatric population

Children are susceptible to the adverse effects of drugs because:
- Many drugs have the potential to affect growth, development and maturation. For example, corticosteroids can cause early epiphyseal closure, resulting in short stature. This adverse effect only occurs in children and is not seen in adults, who have already attained their full height at the time of the use of the drug. Similarly, sex steroids can cause precocious puberty and growth hormone can cause gigantism only in children.
- Genetic polymorphisms, polypharmacy, the use of over-the-counter (OTC) tonics/nutritional supplements, etc., without prescription and immature drug-eliminating mechanisms (hepatic/renal) are other risk factors that predispose the pediatric population to the harmful effects of drugs.
- During pre-marketing clinical trials, children are usually excluded. Therefore, adequate pharmacokinetic and safety data for the pediatric population is not available when the drug is introduced as a medicine for use in humans.

Therefore, spontaneous reporting of adverse effects by pediatricians and phase IV clinical studies on the pediatric population in the post-marketing phase become even more important to ensure the safe use of drugs in children.

(d) Geriatric population or elderly individuals

The elderly are more prone to drug-related problems like ineffectiveness or decreased efficacy, poor adherence or compliance to prescribed drugs, adverse effects of drugs, drug–disease/drug–drug interactions and underdosage/overdosage. The rate of hospitalisation due to adverse effects of drugs is also higher among the elderly. Commonly reported adverse effects in elderly individuals are confusion, hallucinations, excessive sedation, bleeding tendencies, falls, etc.

The drug groups most frequently known to cause ADRs in the elderly are sedative–hypnotics, antipsychotics, antidepressants, insulin, oral hypoglycemics, anticoagulants, and antiplatelet drugs.

The reasons for the **higher susceptibility of elderly patients** to ADRs include the following:
- **Polypharmacy**: The elderly have multiple chronic illnesses, for which they take multiple drugs. In addition, the use of non-prescription drugs like herbal medicines, nutritional supplements, and vitamin preparations is also very frequently observed in this age group. Thus, the risk of **drug–drug interactions** and **drug–disease interactions** is high. For example, patients taking Ginkgo biloba extract have an increased risk of warfarin toxicity resulting in a bleeding tendency. Moreover, the use of more than one drug having a similar toxicity profile may be harmful. Some drugs with the potential to inhibit CYP450 enzymes can result in the toxicity of concurrently used drugs.
- **Age-related changes in drug elimination mechanisms and drug actions:** The renal clearance of drugs is reduced, which predisposes the elderly to toxic effects with normal therapeutic doses. Thus, the doses of renally excreted drugs should be adjusted on the lower side. Some subtle drug effects may be indistinguishable from the symptoms of common diseases or ageing changes. This may result in a '**prescribing cascade**'. For example, a hypertensive patient on calcium channel blocker (CCBs) therapy may be well-controlled for the condition, but may develop peripheral edema as an adverse effect of CCBs. The ideal approach for this patient should be to reduce the dose of CCBs or switch to some other antihypertensive drug. If ADRs are not suspected, however, a prescription cascade can start at this point—for instance, adding diuretics to control peripheral edema; the diuretics in turn cause hypokalemia, which further needs potassium supplementation.
- **Inadequate communication with healthcare providers**: This could be due to poor comprehension or reduced hearing, language problems, dementia, etc. As a result, the patient may not understand the drug regimen properly and may either underdose or overdose.

Such medication errors and harmful effects of drugs can be **prevented** by the following measures:
- Proper communication, taking detailed medication history, periodic follow-ups and close monitoring for new symptoms/signs/lab findings can help in ensuring the safe use of drugs in the elderly. A high index of suspicion is helpful. Any new symptom arising during treatment should be considered as an adverse drug reaction rather than a new disease.
- The American Geriatric Society has prepared a list of '**potentially inappropriate drugs in older adults**'. Some of the drugs included in this list are freely available as over-the-counter preparations, e.g., oral NSAIDs and

diphenhydramine. Patients should be warned against the use of OTCs and self-medication.

V. Iatrogenic Diseases

These are **drugs-induced or physician-induced diseases** that occur because of functional disturbances caused by drugs and persist even after stopping the offending drug, e.g., NSAIDs induce peptic ulcer disease; phenothiazines induce extra-pyramidal symptoms and parkinsonism; hydralazine causes disseminated lupus erythematosus (DLE); and isoniazid causes hepatitis.

IMPLICATIONS OF ADRs

ADRs are harmful to the patient, the healthcare system, and society.

Implications for the Patient

- Increased discomfort and suffering
- Prolonged treatment and/or prolonged hospitalisation
- Increased cost of treatment and/or hospitalisation
- Economic losses due to more days of work lost
- Reduced compliance with therapy
- Poor outcomes

Implications for the Healthcare System

Adverse drug reactions result in increased OPD consultations and increased or prolonged admissions in hospitals for ADRs, which are easily preventable. ADRs thus unnecessarily overburden the healthcare system and result in the diversion of scarce healthcare resources.

PREVENTION OF ADRs

A large majority of ADRs are easily preventable by dealing with the patient meticulously.

- Care should be taken to **elicit an accurate medication history** from every patient. This may prevent many hypersensitivity reactions and drug–drug interactions. Some patients, e.g., those with glucose-6-phosphate dehydrogenase deficiency (G6PD), have a list of contraindicated drugs.
- A **proper diagnosis** should be made after ruling out differential diagnoses systematically.
- The majority of risk factors for the occurrence of ADRs are patient-specific, e.g., extremes of age, compromised hepatic or renal function, overweight or underweight, the presence of co-morbidities, or the concurrent use of other medications. Before prescribing a drug, **extreme caution must be exercised in looking for the presence of risk factors** and in weighing the risk of ADRs against the benefits (therapeutic/preventive) of the drug.
- Drugs should be **prescribed rationally**, taking utmost care to avoid common prescription errors. The writing on the prescription should be clearly legible and preferably in capital letters.
- The patient should be **instructed in detail** about the correct route, dose, time, frequency, duration, and precautions (if any) of prescribed medicines.
- Treatment should be **thoroughly monitored**.

MANAGEMENT OF ADRs

The most important factor in managing ADRs is **early and prompt detection**. The science and activities relating to detection, assessment, understanding and prevention of adverse effects and other drug-related problems is called 'pharmacovigilance'. It involves detection, causality assessment as per the WHO-UMC scale, and reporting of adverse effects to enhance appropriate, timely action. (refer to Chapter 69). One must suspect ADRs to detect and control them at the earliest. Any new or unusual sign/symptom during drug therapy should raise the suspicion of an ADR.

- Mild ADRs are easily tackled with **patient education** and **reassurance** alone. For example, the red discolouration of urine by clofazimine may alarm a patient. In this case, explaining this reaction to the patient and providing reassurance is usually sufficient.
- Some adverse reactions need **supportive treatment** without discontinuing the causative drug. For example, diarrhea associated with antibiotics is managed by maintaining hydration and giving probiotics while the causative drug is continued until the full course is completed.
- Some situations warrant an **adjustment of the dose/time of administration** of the offending drug. For example, daytime sedation associated with the use of antihistamines can be controlled by giving the drug at bedtime. Similarly, excessive sedation associated with sedative–hypnotics may require dose reduction.
- When the ADR is severe, it may require the **replacement of the offending drug** with some other suitable drugs. For example, a dry, brassy cough in a hypertensive patient on ACE inhibitor therapy is an indication to stop and substitute the latter with angiotensin receptor blockers (ARBs), which share the therapeutic (blood-pressure lowering) effect, but not the adverse reactions associated with ACE inhibitors.
- Some ADRs such as serious hypersensitivity reactions indicate the **immediate withdrawal of the offending drug** and the **active management of adverse reactions**. For example, in patients who develop anaphylactic shock with penicillin, the drug should be immediately stopped and the anaphylaxis should be managed with adrenaline, hydrocortisone, and supportive measures. Such adverse effects contraindicate the offending drug for future use.

Clinical problem-based questions and MCQs

1. A 35-year-old patient is diagnosed with cholelithiasis. The patient must undergo laparoscopic cholecystectomy under general anesthesia. The anesthetist injects the anticholinergic drug glycopyrrolate as pre-anesthetic medication to reduce tracheobronchial secretions. Postoperatively the patient complains of dryness of the mouth and difficulty in talking.
   i. What is the type of adverse drug reaction in this case?
      a. Type A　　　　　b. Type B
      b. Type C　　　　　d. Type D
   ii. Describe the selected type of adverse drug reaction.

2. A patient suffering from respiratory tract infection was on amoxicillin therapy 250 mg thrice daily. After four days of taking the medicine as prescribed, the patient complained of loose stools. Which of the following correctly describes this adverse effect?
   a. Toxic effect　　　　b. Side effect
   c. Drug allergy　　　　d. Secondary effect.

3. A farmer who was spraying insecticide (malathion) in his fields suddenly falls unconscious. He is brought to the emergency with pinpoint pupil, increased lacrimation, salivation, and rhinorrhea. A diagnosis of OPC poisoning is made.
   i. How is poisoning different from toxicity?
   ii. Describe the general principles of management in a poisoning case.

4. Inducing vomiting is useful in cases of poisoning by ingestion as it removes the portion of the drug that is yet unabsorbed. However, in some conditions, emesis is CONTRAINDICATED.
   i. Identify the type of poisoning in which the induction of emesis is HARMFUL.
      a. Morphine poisoning
      b. Kerosene poisoning
      c. Paracetamol poisoning
      d. All of the above
   ii. What is the danger of emesis induction in the selected poisoning?

5. A 25-year-old patient diagnosed with 'subacute bacterial endocarditis' is given injection penicillin G 10MU by the intravenous route. Immediately, the patient develops difficulty in breathing and angioedema and had a sudden drop in BP. Injection adrenaline 1:1000 is given intramuscularly, after which, the symptoms improve.
   i. What type of adverse reaction has occurred in this case?
      a. Type A　　　　　b. Type B
      c. Type D　　　　　d. Type F
   ii. What is the role of adrenaline in this case?
   iii. What precaution could have prevented such a severe reaction?

6. A patient with deficient pseudocholinesterase status is at the risk of developing which of the following adverse effect with succinylcholine?
   a. Hemolysis
   b. Fasciculations
   c. Headache
   d. Apnea

7. Which of the following drugs can cause hemolysis in a patient with G6PD deficiency?
   a. Phenobarbitone
   b. Procainamide
   c. Halothane
   d. Chloramphenicol

8. A 45-year-old female patient who is a known case of mild hypertension is on hydrochlorothiazide 25 mg once daily. On sun exposure, the patient develops vesicular eruptions with blisters. The patient is diagnosed with 'phototoxic reaction' to thiazides.
   i. At what wavelength of light is phototoxicity caused?
      a. < 290 nm　　　　b. 290–320nm
      c. 320–400 nm　　　d. > 400 nm
   ii. Enumerate the drugs that may cause phototoxic reactions.

9. The oxidation of drugs is known to produce reactive intermediates that may cause modifications in DNA and structural changes in chromosomes.
   i. What are the adverse effects described above called?
      a. Carcinogenicity　　b. Oncogenicity
      c. Teratogenicity　　　d. Mutagenicity
   ii. What type is the above-mentioned adverse effect?
      a. Type A　　　　　b. Type B
      c. Type C　　　　　d. Type D

10. Great care should be exercised while prescribing medicines to pregnant women.
    i. What is the pharmacological basis of such recommendations?
    ii. Describe the drug categorisation of medicines based on their safety for pregnant women with two examples of each.

11. A 24-year-old patient was using a vitamin A-based acne control medication (isotretinoin). She conceived and visited a gynecologist for her antenatal advice and checkup, but didn't mention the acne medication, considering it unimportant.
    i. What is the risk in this case?
    ii. Isotretinoin falls in which of the following categories?
       a. Category A　　　b. Category B
       c. Category D　　　d. Category X

12. i. Explain why elderly individuals have a higher risk of medication-related problems.
    ii. What measures can be taken to reduce this risk?

Summary

- A noxious change, suspected to be drug-related, occurring at doses normally used in humans, which may require modification of therapy or treatment, and may also contraindicate future use of the drug is called an adverse drug reaction.
- ADRs can be mild, moderate, severe, or serious.
- Based on their incidence, ADRs are classified as very common (in > 10% of drug users), common (in 1–10% of users), uncommon (0.1–1%), rare (0.01–0.1%), and very rare (< 0.01%).
- Based on the underlying cause, ADRs are classified into six classes—A, B, C, D, E, and F.
- Type A (augmented) ADRs are dose-related, predictable and usually reversible—side/secondary/toxic effects.
- Type B ADRs are bizarre, unpredictable, and not dose-related—these include hypersensitivity, photosensitivity, intolerance, and idiosyncratic reactions. Adrenaline is life-saving in type I hypersensitivity, i.e., anaphylactoid reactions, as it is a physiological antagonist of the mediator of anaphylaxis 'histamine'. Type II, III, and IV hypersensitivity reactions respond to corticosteroids.
- Type C ADRs occur due to prolonged drug use.
- Type D ADRs are delayed effects like carcinogenic and mutagenic effects of drugs.
- Type E ADRs occur at the end of therapy and Type F indicate failure to respond to drug therapy.
- Special populations like pregnant/lactating women, children, and elderly individuals are more prone to adverse effects.
- Extreme caution should be exercised before prescribing medicines to pregnant women as some drugs can cause structural and developmental defects in the fetus in utero. These effects are known as teratogenic effects.
- The elderly are prone to over/underdosage, non-adherence to the regimen, and frequent adverse effects due to polypharmacy, lack of suspicion of ADR resulting in a prescribing cascade, and age-related changes in pharmacokinetic processes.
- The majority of ADRs can be easily prevented by careful history-taking and diagnosis, being vigilant about risk factors, and close, periodic monitoring.
- Some ADRs are managed only with reassurance. Some may need a change in the dosage/the offending drug or supportive treatment/drug treatment based on the severity of the case.

Questions for practice

1. Differentiate between:
   a. Adverse drug event and adverse drug reaction
   b. Type A and type B adverse drug reactions
   c. Drug toxicity and poisoning
   d. Hypersensitivity and intolerance
   e. Iatrogenic and idiosyncratic reactions.
2. Explain why:
   a. Sensitivity testing is recommended before giving penicillins
   b. Drugs should be prescribed cautiously in pregnancy
   c. Geriatric patients are more prone to harmful drug-related effects
   d. Succinylcholine causes prolonged apnea in some patients
   e. Corticosteroids should not be stopped abruptly
3. Write short notes on:
   a. Phototoxicity
   b. Clonidine withdrawal

Hints for problem-based questions and MCQs

1. i. a. Type A;
   ii. Refer to page 66.
2. d. Secondary effect
3. i. Toxicity occurs as an extension of the pharmacological actions of a drug due to overdose or prolonged use. Poisoning refers to the harmful effects of a very large dose of drug (usually intentional) or household/environmental/industrial chemicals. Refer to page 67
   ii. Refer to page 67.
4. i. b. Kerosene poisoning
   ii. The risk of aspiration of vomitus
5. i. b. Type B ADR
   ii. Adrenaline is a physiological antagonist of histamine. Refer to page 68.
   iii. Sensitivity testing and eliciting detailed history could have prevented such an event (refer to page 68
6. d. Apnea
7. b. Procainamide
8. i. b. 290–320 nm; ii. Refer to page 69.
9. i. d. Mutagenicity
   ii. d. Type D
10. i. To prevent the teratogenic effect of drugs
    ii. Categories A, B, C, D, and X; for examples, refer to page 70.
11. i. Risk of teratogenic effects
    ii. d. Category X
12. i. Refer to page 71.
    ii. Refer to page 71.

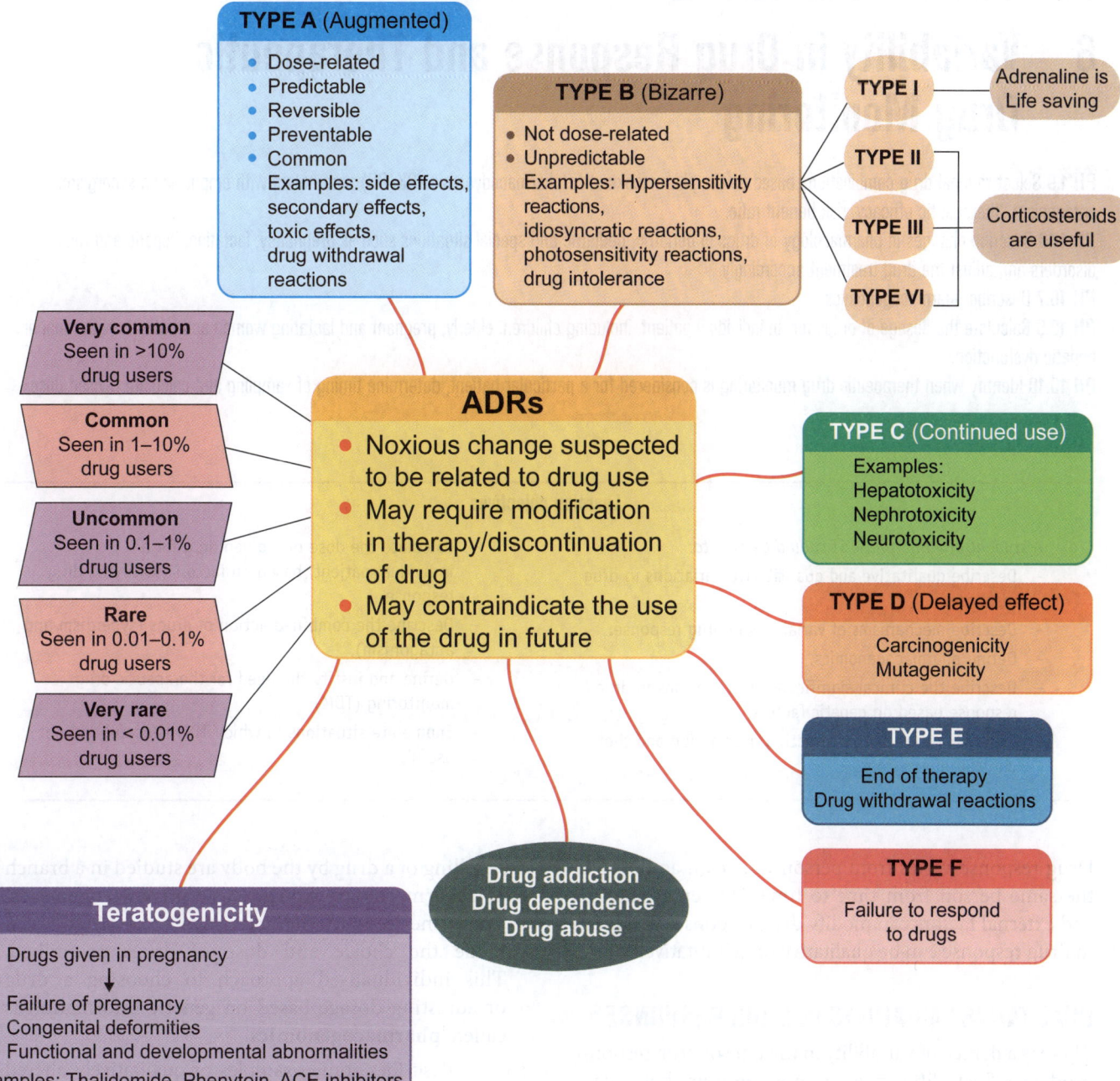

SECTION 1 General Pharmacology

6 Variability in Drug Response and Therapeutic Drug Monitoring

PH 1.9 Select rational drug combinations based on the pharmacokinetics/pharmacodynamic (PK/PD) parameters with emphasis on synergism, antagonism, 'therapeutic efficacy', risk benefit ratio.
PH 1.10 Describe changes in pharmacology of drugs in geriatric, pediatric and special situations such as pregnancy, lactation, hepatic and renal disorders and adjust the drug treatment accordingly.
PH 10.7 Describe pharmacogenomics.
PH 10.9 Calculate the dosage of drugs for an individual patient, including children, elderly, pregnant and lactating women and patients with renal or hepatic dysfunction.
PH 10.10 Identify when therapeutic drug monitoring is considered for a particular patient, determine timing of sampling and calculate revised dose.

Learning objectives

A student of MBBS phase II should be able to:
- Describe qualitative and quantitative variations in drug response.
- Describe mechanisms of variations in drug response.
- Define pharmacogenomics.
- Describe the clinical significance of variations in drug response based on genetic factors.
- Explain various factors affecting drug action and their clinical implications.
- Calculate the dose of a given drug for an individual patient, based on factors modifying drug response
- Describe the combined action of drugs (synergism and antagonism).
- Define and justify the need for therapeutic drug monitoring (TDM).
- Enumerate situations in which TDM is useful and not useful.

Drug response varies from person to person and even in the same person from time to time. Numerous internal and external factors can modify drug response. Variations in drug response can be qualitative or quantitative.

QUALITATIVE VARIATIONS IN DRUG RESPONSE

There is a degree of variability in the type of drug response produced. Such differences are **not common**, but usually contraindicate future use of the drug in that particular patient. Important **factors** responsible for qualitative variations in drug response are as follows:

1. **Immunological factors**: Some patients develop immune-mediated allergic reactions to drugs, such as itching, rashes, urticaria, fixed drug eruptions, or laryngeal edema. In some cases, reactions may be very severe and life-threatening, such as anaphylactic shock, exfoliative dermatitis, and Stevens–Johnson syndrome.
2. **Genetic factors**: An abnormal drug response may sometimes be attributable to a particular genetic factor. The genetic basis of altered drug response and/or the handling of a drug by the body are studied in a branch of pharmacology known as '**pharmacogenetics**'. Thus, the genetic characteristics of a person can guide the choice and dose of drugs prescribed. This individualised approach to choosing a drug or adjusting dosage based on genetic information is called '**pharmacogenomics**'.

Box 6.1 describes some examples of qualitatively altered drug responses due to genetic factors.

Box 6.1 Examples of qualitative variations in drug response due to genetic factors

- In patients who have a genetic defect that affects porphyrin synthesis, barbiturates can precipitate **acute intermittent porphyria.**
- The deficiency of **glucose-6-phosphate dehydrogenase** enzyme (G6PD deficiency) due to an X-linked trait is associated with a risk of dose-dependent hemolysis with many drugs such as:
  - Antimalarial drugs—primaquine, chloroquine, quinine, proguanil, and pyrimethamine

- Antimicrobial drugs—sulphonamides, cotrimoxazole, fluoroquinolones, chloramphenicol, nalidixic acid, and nitrofurantoin
- Other drugs like dapsone, aspirin, thiazides, hydralazine and procainamide.
• In certain patients, excessive calcium release from the sarcoplasmic reticulum—triggered by the general anesthetic halothane—can lead to **malignant hyperthermia**.
• Patients who have a narrow iridocorneal angle may develop acute **angle closure glaucoma** with mydriatics.
• Barbiturates are CNS depressants that normally have a sedative-hypnotic effect. However, in some patients, they may produce an unusual response in the form of excitement and mental confusion.

3. **Route of administration**: Some drugs may produce qualitatively different responses when administered by different routes. For example,
   • Magnesium sulphate administered intravenously causes hypotension and CNS depression, but when it is administered via enteral route, it has a purgative effect.
   • N-acetylcysteine given by intravenous infusion replenishes glutathione stores and is useful in cases of acute paracetamol poisoning. The same drug, when administered through bladder irrigation, facilitates the detoxification and elimination of acrolein—a toxic metabolite of the anticancer drug cyclophosphamide—and helps prevent hemorrhagic cystitis.

4. **Age**: Some drugs produce qualitatively different responses in children. The following are some examples:
   • Tetracyclines cause the discolouration of teeth.
   • Steroidal hormones (corticosteroids and sex hormones such as androgens/estrogens) result in the early closure of the epiphysis of the long bones, resulting in growth stunting in children.
   These drugs do not cause such effects in adults.

5. **Gender**: Drugs may have different effects in males and females. For example, estrogens cause gynecomastia, reduced libido, and feminisation in males. However, no such effect is seen in females with the use of estrogens. In contrast, androgens cause virilisation, hirsutism, and menstrual irregularities only in females.

Clinical problem-based questions and MCQs

1. A 45-year-old female patient diagnosed with acute gouty arthritis is prescribed diclofenac 50 mg BD (a NSAID). The patient reports within a few hours with complaints of itching all over the body, swelling of lips, and urticaria. What is the cause of the patient's symptoms?
   a. Reduced absorption of diclofenac
   b. Excessive distribution of the drug to the skin
   c. Genetically determined variable response
   d. All of the above

2. A 10-year-old boy presents with fever with rigors, chills, and dysuria. Urine analysis shows numerous pus cells in urine. A diagnosis of urinary tract infection is made. After sending a urine sample for culture sensitivity, a decision is made to start an antimicrobial agent empirically. The boy's mother gives a list of drugs (provided by the family doctor), which cannot be prescribed to her son because he has a G6PD enzyme deficiency.
   i. The given list would contain all of the following drugs EXCEPT:
      a. Nitrofurantoin   b. Nalidixic acid
      c. Clarithromycin   d. Cotrimoxazole
   ii. What is the harm of prescribing any of the drugs mentioned in the above list?

3. Which of the following drugs can precipitate acute intermittent porphyria in genetically predisposed individuals?
   a. Phenobarbitone   b. Ethosuximide
   c. Valproate   d. Lorazepam

4. Halothane, a general anesthetic agent, may cause malignant hyperthermia in some genetically predisposed individuals. What is the cause of this uncommon adverse effect?
   a. Excessive Ca^{2+} release from the sarcoplasmic reticulum
   b. Increased metabolic rate and heat generation
   c. Reduced heat dissipation due to vasoconstriction
   d. All of the above

5. i. Drug toxicities can be prevented by some specific measures. Which of the following measures can prevent cyclophosphamide-induced hemorrhagic cystitis?
      a. Urinary alkalinisation with $NaHCO_3$
      b. Acidification of urine with NH_4Cl
      c. Bladder irrigation with $KMNO_4$
      d. Bladder irrigation with N-acetylcysteine
   ii. Justify the use of the selected measure.

QUANTITATIVE VARIATIONS IN DRUG RESPONSE

The action of a drug is enhanced or diminished under different conditions. Such variations in drug response are **more frequently encountered** than qualitative variations and necessitate appropriate **dosage adjustments**.

Factors Causing Quantitative Variation in Drug Response

Variations in the magnitude of drug effects may be associated with changes in plasma concentrations achieved at the site of action or the continued use of drugs resulting in pharmacodynamic changes (such as receptor regulation/cumulation/tolerance/dependence/resistance) or by combined use of drugs. The mechanisms responsible for quantitative variations in drug responsiveness are discussed below.

A. Pharmacokinetic differences in rate of drug absorption, distribution, and elimination

Such differences can be predicted from factors like age, sex, body weight, hepatic/renal dysfunction, presence of diseases like CHF, hypothyroidism, and environmental and genetic variations.

i. Factors causing alterations in drug absorption

Numerous factors alter the rate and extent of drug absorption across membranes. These must be kept in mind while deciding the appropriate dose for a particular patient.

1. **Age:**
   - In **newborn** babies, drug absorption is slow because of low intestinal motility and gastric acid secretion.
   - In **infants and young children**, many drugs can be absorbed through topical application as the skin is thin and more permeable. Rectal absorption is also faster and more predictable than in adults.
   - In the **elderly**, gut motility slows down, and blood flow reduces. This decreases the rate of oral absorption of drugs.
2. **Pregnancy:** Oral absorption of drugs slows during pregnancy due to reduced GI motility.
3. **Disease states:** Some gastrointestinal ailments can cause complex changes in the rate and extent of drug absorption—e.g., malabsorption syndrome, achlorhydria, and gastrointestinal stasis. In patients with congestive heart failure, oral absorption of some drugs gets reduced owing to mucosal congestion.
4. **Food and other drugs:** Drug absorption may be affected by food and other drugs used simultaneously; these variations are a result of complex formation, adsorption, alterations in gut motility, gastric pH, etc.

ii. Factors causing altered drug distribution

The distribution of drugs in various fluid compartments can get disturbed under the following conditions:

1. **Changes in levels of plasma proteins:** Alterations in the levels of drug-binding proteins for any reason can affect the concentration of the bound and free drug, which in turn, affects the volume of distribution. For example, plasma protein binding of drugs is reduced in elderly individuals, hypoproteinemia, liver disease, renal disease (causing albuminuria, uremia) and the concomitant use of two highly bound drugs.

   In pregnancy, plasma albumin decreases, but glycoprotein increases. Thus, the binding of acidic drugs is reduced while that of basic drugs is enhanced.
2. **Disturbances in fluid distribution:** The fluid distribution in various compartments of the body may be disturbed due to old age, pregnancy, dehydration, congestive heart failure, reduced tissue perfusion, or brisk diuresis. This, in turn, can alter the volume of distribution of drugs.
3. **Permeability of the blood–brain barrier:** In newborns and infants, the blood–brain barrier is not well-formed, allowing most drugs to reach the CNS. Inflammation of the meninges also favours the penetration of drugs into the CNS.
4. **Placental barrier:** This is an incomplete barrier which allows the entry of lipid-soluble drugs. However, non-lipid soluble drugs may also cross the placenta to some extent, when drug levels are high in maternal blood for a long time. Thus, the fetus gets exposed to the damaging effects of drugs used by mother.

iii. Factors altering drug metabolism

There are inter-individual differences in the rate of drug metabolism from two- to thirty-fold. Important factors responsible for these variations in the metabolism of drugs include:

1. **Genetic polymorphisms in drug metabolism:** Genetic variations in enzyme levels result in important differences in the rate of drug metabolism among individuals. Some examples of genetically determined quantitative variations in drug response are described in Box 6.2.

> **Box 6.2 Examples of quantitative variation in drug response due to genetic factors**
>
> - There is genetic polymorphism in the **rate of acetylation**. Decreased levels of N-acetyl-transferase-2 enzyme occur due to an autosomal recessive disorder and result in slow acetylator status. Such persons are at a high risk of developing the adverse effects of drugs, e.g., peripheral neuropathy and hepatotoxicity with isoniazid and a lupus erythematosus-like syndrome with hydralazine.
> - The depolarising neuromuscular blocker succinylcholine can cause prolonged apnea in persons with a deficiency of atypical **pseudocholinesterase enzyme**.
> - **Glucuronide conjugase** polymorphism can cause hyperbilirubinemia.
> - **Deficiency of CYP2D6** is inherited as autosomal recessive trait known as **debrisoquine–sparteine oxidative polymorphism.** It leads to impaired oxidation of debrisoquine, leading to orthostatic hypotension. Codeine metabolism also gets reduced, affecting its analgesic activity.
> - **Polymorphism of CYP2C19** decreases the metabolism of drugs like warfarin, phenytoin, tolbutamide and losartan, resulting in toxicity Poor metabolisers lack the ability to hydroxylate mephenytoin, which in turn, gets demethylated to form an inactive metabolite 'nirvanol'. Such patients develop excessive sedation and ataxia with normal therapeutic doses.

2. **Environmental factors:** Several environmental pollutants like pesticides, polychlorinated biphenyls used in plasticisers/insulating material, polycyclic hydrocarbons in charcoal broiled meat, and tobacco smoke can induce the CYP1A enzyme, which increases the rate of metabolism of many drugs.

3. **Diet:** Cruciferous vegetables and charcoal broiled foods induce CYP1A enzyme, increasing the rate of metabolism of drugs like caffeine, theophylline and warfarin. In contrast, grapefruit juice inhibits the CYP3A enzyme, resulting in an increased risk of adverse effects of drugs like verapamil, diltiazem, diazepam and triazolam.
4. **Age:** The drug metabolising capacity of body is compromised at the extremes of age. Therefore, neonates, children, and the elderly are more prone to the adverse/toxic effects of drugs in comparison to adults.
5. **Sex:** Differences in rates of metabolism of some drugs between males and females are well documented in rats. In humans too, drugs like estrogens, propranolol, and ethanol are metabolised somewhat faster in males than in females.
6. **Temperature:** Hypothermia may affect drug metabolism in a complex, but yet poorly understood manner.
7. **Disease states:**
   - The rate of metabolism of some rapidly metabolised drugs like propranolol, alprenolol, morphine, meperidine, pentazocine, and propoxyphene is altered by a reduction in hepatic blood flow as in cardiac diseases.
   - Chronic liver diseases like alcoholic liver disease, cirrhosis, acute viral hepatitis, cholestasis, and drug-induced liver damage decrease the rate of drug metabolism, especially for drugs that are metabolised by microsomal enzymes. For example, diazepam can cause coma in patients with cirrhosis or viral hepatitis.
   - The hydrolysis of drugs like procainamide and procaine is impaired in patients with chronic respiratory insufficiency.
   - The rate of metabolism of some drugs is altered by thyroid status. For example, the metabolism of digoxin, beta-blockers, and methimazole is reduced in hypothyroidism and increased in hyperthyroidism.
8. **Presence of other drugs:** Some drugs may induce or inhibit certain enzymes, resulting in enhanced or diminished metabolism, respectively, of other co-administered drugs. Different drugs may compete for conjugation with endogenous substances like glucuronyl and glutathione. This results in the depletion of endogenous substances and drug toxicities.

iv. Factors affecting drug excretion

Renal excretion is the major route of elimination of drugs and their inactive metabolites from the body. It is affected by many physiological and pathological states that have the potential to cause prolonged drug effects and toxicity.

1. In the **extremes of ages**, the renal excretory system is not fully functional. In newborns, glomerular filtration and tubular transport are not yet fully mature. On the other hand, renal function keeps on declining gradually after 50 years of age, due to the loss of intact nephrons. Thus, the dose of drugs that are excreted unchanged by the kidney (e.g., aminoglycosides) should be reduced to prevent toxic effects.
2. In **pregnant women**, renal blood flow is increased, thus enhancing the glomerular filtration and excretion of polar drugs.
3. In patients with **chronic renal disease**, the excretion of drugs like phenobarbitone, aminoglycosides, and digoxin is reduced, predisposing to prolonged effects and toxicity. As the maintenance dose depends on drug clearance (maintenance dose = target concentration × CL), the dose rate/dose must be appropriately adjusted according to clearance. In general, nephrotoxic drugs are contraindicated in patients with impaired creatinine clearance, as they may worsen the existing condition.
4. **Simultaneously used drugs** may also alter drug elimination, e.g., probenecid reduces the renal tubular secretion of penicillin and cephalosporins, increasing their duration of action. Probenecid also interferes with renal tubular secretion of uric acid and exerts uricosuric effect.

v. P-glycoprotein

In addition to the above pharmacokinetic factors, the concentration of drug achieved at the target site can be altered by multi-drug resistance (MDR) genes coding for membrane transporters (P-glycoproteins [Pgp]) that cause a **reduced influx or increased efflux or pumping out of the drug from the target cells,** resulting in resistance to certain anticancer drugs like vinca alkaloids, taxanes, etc.

B. Pharmacodynamic differences

Alterations in the number of receptors and the efficiency of the receptor–effector coupling system with the continued use of drugs may cause variations in the drug response as described below.

i. Change in the number of receptors

Changes in the number of receptors can occur due to:
- Hormonal effects—for example, the thyroid hormone increases the number and sensitivity of cardiac β receptors
- Variations in the concentration of endogenous agonists—for example, in individuals with raised circulating catecholamine levels as in pheochromocytoma, the cardiodepressant effects of β blockers are more pronounced (in contrast, β blockers have negligible cardiac effect in athletes as such individuals have low circulating catecholamines)
- Down-regulation/up-regulation of receptors (refer to Chapter 4, page 58)

ii. Variations in the biochemical processes of the target cell

Variations in the receptor–effector system distal to the drug receptor affect drug activity.

iii. Alterations in drug response due to continued use

The long-term or chronic use of drugs can cause cumulative toxicity and development of tolerance.

- **Cumulative toxicity** is more frequently encountered with drugs that have slow rates of elimination and high affinity for some tissues

  When used for a prolonged period as a disease-modifying anti-rheumatic drug (DMARD), chloroquine can accumulate in melanin-containing tissues, resulting in the greying of hair, retinal damage and corneal opacity.

  Amiodarone, an antiarrhythmic drug, can cause sunburn-like skin pigmentation and corneal microdeposits, leading to headlight dazzle effect during night-time driving.

- **Drug tolerance** refers to reduced responsiveness to a drug. There are many types of tolerance—natural/acquired, pharmacokinetic/pharmacodynamic, or cellular, homologous/heterologous, cross-tolerance, tachyphylaxis, homeostatic adaptation, etc. The important features of different types of tolerance are detailed in Box 6.3.

> **Box 6.3 Types of tolerance**
>
> 1. **Natural tolerance:** Some individuals are inherently or naturally less sensitive to the effects of a drug. For example:
>   - In Afro-Caribbean hypertensive patients, a less marked fall in BP is observed with the use of β-blockers.
>   - People of African origin need higher doses of mydriatics like atropine and ephedrine than whites.
>   - Chloramphenicol-induced aplastic anemia and quiniodochlor-induced subacute myeloptic neuropathy (SMON) are not common among Indians.
> 2. **Acquired tolerance:** It involves decreased responsiveness to a drug **with repetitive use** in a person who was initially responding. It is commonly seen with CNS depressant drugs. Tolerance develops **unequally for different actions** of a drug. For example, tolerance to the analgesic, euphoric action of morphine develops quickly but not to its miotic and constipating effects. The underlying mechanisms of the development of acquired tolerance are **pharmacokinetic or pharmacodynamic**.
> - **Pharmacokinetic mechanisms:** These result in a reduced concentration of the drug at the site of action with repeated use. For example, some enzyme-inducing drugs like barbiturates and carbamazepine increase their own metabolism (**autoinduction**), resulting in the development of tolerance.
> - **Pharmacodynamic mechanisms:** The drug concentration at the target site is not altered, but the responsiveness of the target tissue is diminished. Hence, this type of tolerance is called **cellular tolerance**. The underlying cause may be the desensitisation of receptors, which can be homologous or heterologous.
> - **Homologous desensitisation** involves:
>   - The internalisation or masking of receptors so that they are not accessible to the drug; tolerance develops rapidly in such cases, and responsiveness is regained quickly on discontinuing the drug
>   - The increased destruction or decreased synthesis of receptors, i.e., down-regulation; such tolerance develops and recovers slowly, taking a few weeks to months after stopping the drug
>   - Impairment of receptor–transducer coupling
> - **Heterologous desensitisation:** It is exhibited by different drugs producing the same effect through different receptors. With prolonged exposure to one drug, tolerance also develops to the effect of the other due to the reduced efficiency of response effectuation. For example, tolerance develops to the gastrointestinal smooth muscle contracting action of histamine after prolonged exposure to acetylcholine and vice versa.
> 3. **Cross-tolerance:** This refers to the phenomenon of development of tolerance to the effects of a drug after exposure to a pharmacologically related drug. This is common among CNS depressants, e.g., alcohol and opioids show cross-tolerance, which can be complete or partial.
> 4. **Tachyphylaxis** (*tachy*: fast or rapid)**:** This refers to rapidly developing tolerance to the effects of a drug with just a few doses given in quick succession. For example, the indirectly-acting sympathomimetic drug ephedrine exerts its action through the release of catecholamines. With quick repetition of this drug, the catecholamine stores get depleted (as the rate of synthesis fails to match the rate of release.
> - **Compensatory homeostatic adaptation:** The tolerance that develops to the hypotensive action of hydralazine is due to compensatory mechanisms (like tachycardia and rennin release) evoked by decreased total peripheral resistance because of its vasodilator action.

C. Combined effect of drugs

The simultaneous administration of two drugs may enhance or diminish their response. Such an alteration in the magnitude of drug effects may be due to a pharmacokinetic or pharmacodynamic interaction between drugs; synergism or antagonism can occur.

i. Synergism

When one drug enhances the effect of another drug, this effect is called synergism. This effect can be either additive or supra-additive.

- **Additive** synergism is the simple addition of the same therapeutic effect of two simultaneously administered drugs. For example, the cardioselective β-blocker atenolol is combined with the calcium channel blocker amlodipine for its antihypertensive effect. The blood pressure-lowering effect of these two drugs, although obtained by different mechanisms, adds up.

Similarly, the bronchodilator effects of ephedrine and theophylline add up in the treatment of asthma. The two drugs of a synergistic pair are from different groups and have different mechanisms of actions and adverse effects. Such combinations are useful as the dose of an individual drug is reduced, thereby reducing the risk/intensity of its adverse effects.
- In **supra-additive** synergism, the combined effect of two simultaneously administered drugs is greater than the sum of their individual effects. It is also known as the '**potentiation**' of the effect of one drug by the other. One of the drugs in the pair may be inactive when used alone.

For example, **levodopa and carbidopa** are used in combination for parkinsonism. Carbidopa is a 'peripheral dopa decarboxylase inhibitor'. It has no dopaminergic activity of its own, but it prevents the conversion of levodopa to dopamine in the periphery. So, more levodopa is available to cross the blood–brain barrier to reverse central dopamine deficiency and relieve parkinsonian symptoms. The addition of carbidopa reduces the dose of levodopa many-folds. The peripheral adverse effects of levodopa are also reduced owing to the reduced formation of dopamine in the periphery.

Another useful combination that exhibits supra-additive synergism is that of **sulphamethoxazole and trimethoprim**. These two drugs inhibit two sequential steps in bacterial folate metabolism. Sulphamethoxazole inhibits the conversion of para-aminobenzoic acid (PABA) to dihydrofolic acid (DHFA) by inhibiting bacterial folate synthase enzyme. Trimethoprim further interferes with the reduction of dihydrofolic acid into tetrahydrofolic acid (THFA) by inhibiting the enzyme dihydrofolate reductase (DHFRase). When used alone, both trimethoprim and sulphamethoxazole (components of cotrimoxazole) have bacteriostatic effects, but their combination, cotrimoxazole, exerts a bactericidal effect against many organisms. Thus, the **effect of the combination is much greater than the sum of their individual effects.**

(ii) Antagonism

Antagonism involves the diminution of the effect of one drug by another simultaneously given drug. One drug can antagonise the other by various mechanisms based on its physical, chemical, physiological, and pharmacological actions. Antagonism of drug action is useful in some situations, while in others, it may be harmful. Some examples of each type of antagonism are as follows:
- **Physical antagonism:** Activated charcoal is used as a universal antidote as it adsorbs many poisonous substances and decreases their absorption, thus antagonising their actions.
- **Chemical antagonism:** One drug may antagonise the effect of another on account of its chemical properties. For example:
  - Potassium permanganate is used for gastric lavage in cases of poisoning with alkaloids, as it oxidises and neutralises the poison.
  - Disodium edetate and other chelating agents form complexes with heavy metal ions and are useful in heavy metal poisoning.
  - Calcium present in milk and antacid preparations can form non-absorbable complexes with tetracyclines and diminish their effect. For this reason, while prescribing, the patient is advised against taking tetracyclines with milk.
  - Sometimes, chemical reactions can occur in vitro, e.g., succinylcholine chloride and thiopentone sodium or penicillin G sodium should not be mixed in the same syringe for injection because they react chemically.
- **Physiological antagonism** occurs when the effects of two drugs on a physiological function are in opposite directions. The mechanism of action of two drugs in an antagonistic pair may be different, but one drug cancels the effect of other. For example:
  - Histamine is released from mast cells during immunological reactions like anaphylactic shock. It causes bronchoconstriction (through H_1 action) and vasodilatation (through its early, short-lasting H_1 action and slow, persistent H_2 action). Thus, the patient develops dyspnea, hypotension, and shock which is life-threatening. All these symptoms improve dramatically with adrenaline, which has just the opposite effects on bronchial and vascular smooth muscles, i.e., adrenaline is a physiological antagonist of histamine and causes bronchodilatation through $β_2$ receptors and vasoconstriction through $α_1$ receptors. Thus, although histamine and adrenaline act through different receptors, their effects are antagonistic.
  - Potassium-sparing diuretics like spironolactone antagonise the potassium-losing effect of thiazides or loop diuretics. Thus they are combined with thiazides and loop diuretics to prevent hypokalemia associated with prolonged diuretic therapy in patients with hypertension and congestive heart failure.
- **Receptor antagonism:** A drug that has affinity for certain receptors only but no intrinsic activity binds to the receptors, blocks them, and prevents the action of the agonist. Receptor antagonism can further be of two types—competitive and non-competitive—based on the site of binding of the antagonist. Competitive antagonism can further be of two types—the equilibrium and non-equilibrium types. Table 6.1 presents the differences between competitive and non-competitive antagonism.

Table 6.1 Differences between competitive and non-competitive antagonism

Competitive receptor antagonism (equilibrium type)	Non-competitive receptor antagonism
The antagonist has **structural similarities** with the agonist. It competes with the agonist for the **ligand-binding site** of the receptor molecule.	The drug has **no structural similarity** with the agonist; it binds with the receptor at an **allosteric site** and alters the receptor in a way that agonist fails to bind at the ligand-binding site.
There is a **decrease in the potency** of the agonist, but its maximal efficacy remains unchanged.	The potency of the agonist is unchanged, but **maximal efficacy is reduced.**
There is a **rightward shift in the dose–response curve (DRC)** (Fig. 6.1).	There is a **flattening** of the DRC with reduced maxima (Fig. 6.2).
It is **reversible** or surmountable, i.e., if the agonist concentration is sufficiently increased, it can displace the antagonist from the ligand-binding site.	The antagonist cannot be displaced from the binding site by any concentration of the agonist. So, it is **irreversible** or unsurmountable.
Examples: Atropine competes with ACh for muscarinic receptors, naloxone competes with morphine for opioid receptors.	Example: Ketamine is a non-competitive antagonist at NMDA-glutamate receptors.

In the **non-equilibrium type** of competitive antagonism, the antagonist binds with the receptor by strong covalent bonds or dissociates from the receptor very slowly so that the agonist cannot displace it from the binding site. In such cases, potency as well as maximal efficacy are reduced. There is flattening as well as a rightward shift of the DRC (Fig. 6.3). For example, phenoxybenzamine forms an ethylene-immonium metabolite that causes an irreversible blockade of α receptors.

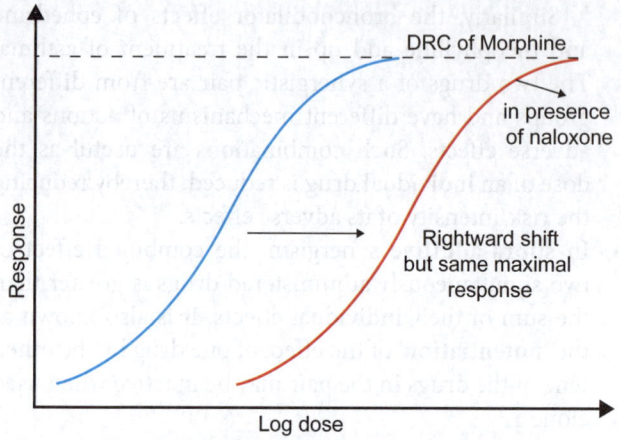

Fig. 6.1 Competitive (equilibrium type) antagonism

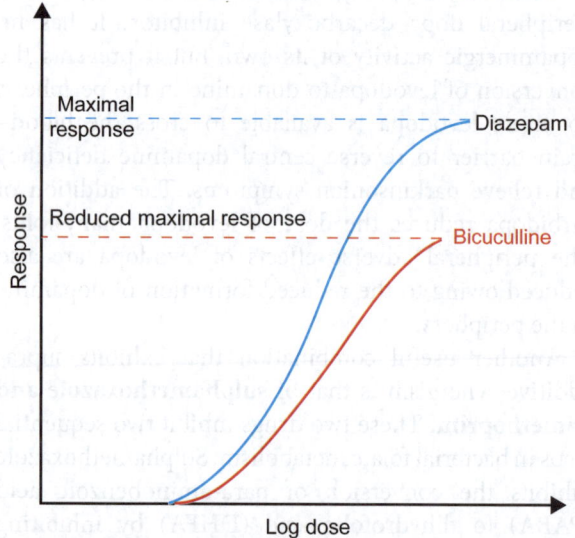

Fig. 6.2 Non-competitive antagonism

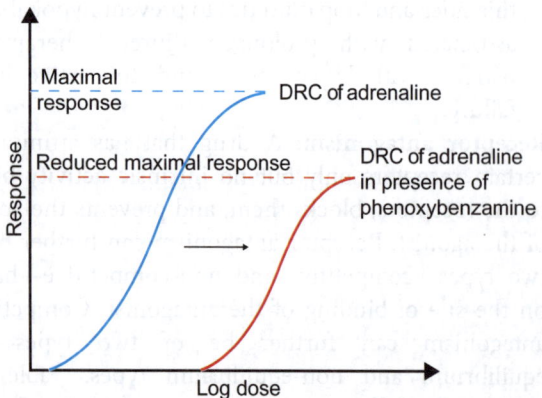

Fig. 6.3 Competitive antagonism (Non-equilibrium type)

Clinical problem-based questions and MCQs

6. Some groups of patients are considered special groups in clinical practice, like patients at the extremes of ages and pregnant women.
   i. Explain why the patient groups mentioned are special groups.
   ii. What are the various changes in the pharmacokinetics and dynamics of drugs in these special groups?

7. Hyperbilirubinemia can occur due to genetic polymorphism of a metabolic enzyme. Identify the enzyme responsible:
   a. Glucuronide conjugase
   b. CYP2D6
   c. CYP2C19
   d. Pseudocholinesterase

8. Genetic polymorphism of which of the following enzymes is responsible for prolonged apnea with succinylcholine?
   a. Glucuronide conjugase
   b. CYP2D6

c. CYP2C19
d. Pseudocholinesterase

9. Identify the drug that may cause lupus erythematosus in slow acetylators.
   a. Isoniazid   b. Rifampicin
   c. Hydralazine   d. Succinylcholine

10. Excessive sedation and ataxia with mephenytoin occurs due to the genetic polymorphism of which of the following enzymes?
    a. Glucuronide conjugase
    b. CYP2D6
    c. CYP2C19
    d. Pseudocholinesterase

11. Overexpression of Pgp is implicated in resistance to anticancer drugs. Explain the role of Pgp in drug resistance.

12. Sulphamethoxazole and trimethoprim are bacteriostatic drugs, but their combination is bactericidal. This beneficial interaction between two drugs is an example of:
    a. Additive effect
    b. Potentiation
    c. Partial agonistic effect
    d. Pharmacokinetic interaction

13. A 45-year-old male patient, a known case of congestive heart failure is on loop diuretics therapy. Hypokalemia caused by loop diuretics can be managed by the addition of spironolactone.
    i. Which of the following correctly describes the underlying mechanism of this beneficial interaction?
       a. Synergism
       b. Chemical antagonism
       c. Physiological antagonism
       d. Tolerance
    ii. Describe the phenomenon involved.

14. All of the following are competitive antagonists EXCEPT:
    a. Naloxone   b. Atropine
    c. Prazosin   d. Ketamine

CLINICAL IMPLICATIONS OF FACTORS MODIFYING DRUG RESPONSE

Drug therapy involves a complex interplay of patient-related, drug-related, and environmental factors. Therefore, while prescribing, all these factors must be kept in mind, and an appropriate change in the choice or dose should be made to minimise the adverse effects and maximise the benefits. Some frequently needed dose adjustments are based on the following factors:

1. **Age, body weight, body surface area**: Children have many physiological differences from adults, and cannot be thought of as smaller adults. Ideally, child doses should be learned as such, especially for drugs with low safety margins. Though formulae are available to calculate dosages based on age—e.g., Young's formula and Dilling's formula—it is more practical to use body weight based calculations. Adult dosages are calculated for patients of average build. For extreme cases, i.e., very lean or grossly obese, dosage adjustment is required.

   Individual dose = [Body weight (kg) × Average adult dose]/70

   Body surface area (BSA) is a better parameter than body weight and is used for calculating the dose of more toxic drugs like anticancer drugs. The body surface area is calculated from a person's height and weight using the Dubois formula:

   BSA (m^2)= [Bodyweight(kg)]$^{0.425}$ × [Height(cm)]$^{0.725}$ × 0.007184

   This involves complex calculations, which can be circumvented by using slide-rule nomograms. Then, dose is calculated using the following formula:

   Individual dose = [BSA (m^2) × average adult dose]/1.7

2. **Co-morbidities:**
   - **Hepatic and renal function**—As most drugs use hepatic metabolism and renal excretion for elimination from the body, the functional capacity of these two organs should be carefully considered before choosing appropriate drugs for a particular patient.

     In patients who have **abnormal liver function tests (LFT),** it is better to avoid or adjust the dose/dose interval on the lower side for drugs that are:
     - Inactivated by liver, e.g., morphine and propranolol
     - Highly bound to albumin, e.g., diclofenac and aspirin
     - Have high first-pass metabolism, e.g., verapamil and glyceryl trinitrate
     - Hepatotoxic, e.g., pyrazinamide (prferably avoided)

     Prodrugs that are dependent on hepatic metabolism for activation should be avoided, or a dose adjustment should be made on the higher side.

     In patients having reduced creatinine clearance because of **renal function impairment:**
     - It is better to avoid nephrotoxic drugs like amphotericin B, aminoglycosides, tetracyclines and nitrofurantoin. Alternatives should be looked for and used preferentially.
     - Some polar drugs are excreted unchanged by the kidney. These drugs should be avoided in severe renal dysfunction. If they are used, dosage adjustment must be done based on creatinine clearance.

The extent of renal function impairment is determined by the Cockroft–Gault equation for creatinine clearance (CLCr):

$$CLCr = \frac{[140 - \text{age (in years)}] \times \text{Weight (in kg)} \times 1.23}{\text{S. creatinine (in } \mu\text{mol/L)}}$$

However, this equation is not reliable in pregnancy, catabolic state, acute renal failure, acute dehydration, or sepsis.

A rough guide for dose reduction based on creatinine clearance is presented in Table 6.2.

Table 6.2 Dose reduction based on creatinine clearance

Creatinine clearance (mL/minute)	Percentage of usual dose allowed
50–70	70%
30–50	50%
10–30	30%
5–10	20%

Some drugs may worsen renal disease and should be avoided, e.g., tetracyclines may worsen uremia because of their anti-anabolic effect. Thiazides worsen uremia by reducing GFR. Similarly, potassium-sparing diuretics may cause hyperkalemia and NSAIDs enhance fluid retention.
- **Cardiac diseases**: Drug handling by the body is altered at nearly every stage—absorption, distribution, metabolism, and excretion (ADME)—in congestive heart failure. Cardiac patients are, therefore, more prone to adverse drug effects. Thus, they should be closely monitored, and appropriate changes in the drug or dose should be made, as and when needed.
- **Thyroid function**: The functioning of the thyroid gland can affect the action of drugs like morphine, central depressants, and digoxin.
- **Injury**: Patients with **head injury** can develop respiratory failure even with normal doses of morphine.
- **Myasthenia gravis**: This condition may be aggravated by quinine and skeletal muscle relaxants.
- **Benign prostatic hypertrophy**: In patients who have this condition, urinary retention may occur with drugs having anticholinergic side effects, e.g., tricyclic antidepressants.
- **AIDS**: People living with AIDS are more prone to develop adverse reactions with cotrimoxazole.

3. **Concomitant medicines**: Drug–drug interactions may occur when more than one drug is administered; the risk increases with an increase in the number of drugs prescribed. Sometimes, herbal medicines and over-the-counter drugs may cause serious interactions with prescribed drugs.
- A detailed medication history must be elicited from the patient or their relatives to be aware of the totality of treatment.
- Readjustment in the dose of chronically administered drugs may be required when new drugs are prescribed for an acute illness. For example, a patient on anticoagulant therapy with warfarin may develop toxic effects if broad-spectrum antimicrobials are given for an intercurrent infection. This is because the gut flora is reduced by antimicrobial drugs, which results in a decrease in vitamin K production. As a result, the effect of warfarin is enhanced. So, the dose of warfarin needs to be adjusted on the lower side.

4. **Miscellaneous factors** (social/personal/psychological):
- **Compliance** to prescribed drugs may be lower in some patients, e.g., those with psychiatric problems, low affordability, poor comprehension of instructions, or cultural beliefs, resulting in the failure of therapy. These factors must be considered while prescribing a drug for the first time or making changes in the dose or drug.
- **Psychological factors** play an important role. A good doctor–patient relationship, gentle, empathetic behaviour of the prescriber, and proper communication with the patient in easily understandable language also improves the compliance as well as response (especially of subjective effects) to prescribed drugs.

Clinical problem-based questions and MCQs

15. An anticancer drug 'X' is to be given to a patient with carcinoma rectum. The patient is very lean with a BSA of 1.3 m². The adult dose of the drug is 200 mg. What is the correct dose of x in this case?
    a. 100 mg b. 125 mg
    c. 150 mg d. 175 mg

16. All of the following need dose reduction in a patient with abnormal liver function tests (LFT) EXCEPT:
    a. Morphine b. Diclofenac
    c. Verapamil d. Enalapril

17. The average adult dose of drug 'A' is 500 mg. Calculate the dose for a grossly obese person weighing 125 kg.

18. A 65-year-old male patient is suffering from multiple sclerosis. His creatinine clearance is 40 mL/minute. What is the correct dose of drug 'X' if the adult dose is 250 mg?
    a. 200 mg b. 175 mg
    c. 150 mg d. 125 mg

19. All of the following drugs are CONTRAINDICATED in renal failure EXCEPT:
    a. Amphotericin B   b. Aminoglycosides
    c. Thiazides   d. Verapamil
20. Urinary obstruction may occur in an elderly male having benign prostatic hypertrophy with all the following drugs EXCEPT:
    a. Hyoscine   b. Imipramine
    c. Neostigmine   d. Dicyclomine

THERAPEUTIC DRUG MONITORING (TDM)

For safe and effective use, drugs need to be given in a dose that achieves a plasma concentration sufficient to produce the desired response with minimal or no harmful effects. The dosage of drugs having easily quantifiable effects (e.g., antihypertensives) can be adjusted by monitoring the therapeutic response. In sharp contrast, many drugs have non-quantifiable responses, e.g., antiepileptics and antipsychotics. The dose of such drugs is adjusted to attain a '**target plasma concentration**' proven to be in the therapeutic range, i.e., a concentration range in which the drug is already proven to be effective. This requires repeatedly measuring or monitoring drug concentrations in plasma and is known as '**therapeutic drug monitoring (TDM)**'.

So, TDM involves the repeated measurement of plasma concentrations of a drug, in an effort to maintain the same in the defined therapeutic range. It is a process of optimising the dose in an individual.

Parameters for Devising Dosage Regimens

Rational dosage regimens are devised on the basis of the kinetics of elimination of drugs. The bioavailability, volume of distribution and clearance of a drug are important parameters for determining its dosage regimen.

- **Bioavailability (F):** The fraction of the given amount of drug that reaches the systemic circulation in the unchanged form is called the bioavailability of a drug.

$$F = f(1 - ER)$$

where F is bioavailability, f the extent of absorption and ER the extraction ratio in the liver.

$$ER = CL_{liver}/Q$$

where Q is the hepatic blood flow. It helps in deciding the appropriate route of drug administration and the oral: parenteral dose ratio.

- **Volume of distribution (V_d):** This refers to the volume that can accommodate the entire quantity of the drug present in the body, provided the concentration throughout is the same as in plasma.

$$aV_d = \frac{\text{Total amount of drug present in body }(Q)}{\text{plasma concentration }(Cp)}$$

V_d is an important pharmacokinetic parameter for calculating the loading dose of the drug.

If the loading dose is considered to be equal to the amount of the drug in the body immediately after administering the loading dose (Q), then:

$$\text{Loading dose or } Q = V_d \times C_p$$
[from the above equation]

In routes other than intravenous, adjustment for bioavailability is done such that:

$$\text{Loading dose or } Q = \frac{V_d \times C_p}{F}$$

- **Clearance (CL):** The theoretical volume of plasma from which the drug is completely removed in unit time is called the clearance. It can be calculated by dividing the rate of elimination with plasma concentration.

$$CL = \frac{\text{Rate of elimination}}{\text{Plasma concentration }(C_p)}$$

A steady-state plasma concentration (Cp_{ss}) is achieved when the rate of elimination balances the amount of drug administered over a suitable dosage interval. Thus, the rate of elimination in the above equation can be substituted with 'dose rate':

$$CL = \text{Dose rate}/C_p$$

By rearranging this equation, we obtain the dose rate:

$$\text{Dose rate} = CL \times C_p$$

For routes other than intravenous, adjustment for bioavailability is done:

$$\text{Dose rate} = [CL \times C_p] / F$$

Thus, 'dose rate' for maintaining plasma concentration at steady state (Cp_{ss}) depends on clearance and is called the '**maintenance dose**'.

It is important to note that loading dose is determined by the volume of distribution and the maintenance dose is determined by clearance. Further, pharmacokinetic variables exhibit **interindividual variations** that determine plasma concentration at steadystate. The individual differences in bioavailability, volume of distribution, and clearance can cause vast differences in the steady state plasma concentration (C_p). Thus, it becomes important to constantly monitor plasma levels and make desired adjustments in the dosage regimen to achieve and maintain target levels lying within the therapeutic range.

$$\text{New dose rate} = \frac{\text{Previous dose rate} \times \text{Target } C_p}{\text{Measured } C_p}$$

The correct **time of blood sample collection** after drug administration varies based on the purpose of the TDM:

- If TDM is being performed for dosage adjustment, the blood sample should be drawn just before the next scheduled dose to measure the trough plasma concentration of long-acting drugs. For short-acting drugs, the therapeutic levels are achieved only intermittently. So, the peak concentration should be measured by drawing blood samples in the immediate post-absorptive phase, i.e., 1–2 hours after oral/IM administration.
- In the case of poisoning, a blood sample should be drawn as soon as possible after stabilising the vitals. Repeat samples should be taken to monitor the patient's recovery.
- In a case of a compliance check, random blood samples can be taken.
- Sample for TDM should be collected only after steady-state plasma concentration is achieved, i.e., after 4–5 half-lives have elapsed. For example, if the half-life of a drug is 24 hours, the results of TDM will be reliable only if the sample is taken after 5 days (4–5 × 24 hours) of starting the drug.

Indications and Applications of TDM

- TDM is essentially required in some situations and futile in others. TDM should be performed only if the effect (beneficial or harmful) has a good correlation with the plasma concentration of the drugs.
- Some drugs have effects that are **not easily quantifiable**, e.g., anticonvulsants, lithium, antidepressants, and antiarrhythmics. Moreover, these drugs have a **low margin of safety**. This makes it very important to keep the plasma concentration of these drugs within the defined therapeutic range. This is called '**target level strategy**'. For such drugs, the plasma concentration needs to be measured repeatedly.
- Therapeutic drug monitoring is extremely useful for **drugs with a narrow therapeutic index** or safety margin. For these drugs, the dose–response curve (DRC) of the therapeutic effect is not far from that of the toxic effects. For example, digoxin, anticonvulsant drugs, lithium, theophylline, and antiarrhythmic drugs.
- If a patient has **renal function impairment** and their clinical condition warrants the use of potentially nephrotoxic drugs, e.g., vancomycin, amphotericin B, and aminoglycosides.
- Drugs for which large **inter-individual variations are known to exist,** e.g., lithium and antidepressants.
- In cases of **poisoning** with a drug, it becomes necessary to monitor the plasma concentration to check the patient's progress during recovery.
- Sometimes, the plasma concentration of drug is monitored **to confirm the patient's compliance to the treatment regimen**. This becomes especially important for patients with psychiatric problems who are on antipsychotics and antidepressant drugs.
- When there is a **failure of antimicrobial therapy** without any apparent reason, TDM is indicated.
- In contrast, there are some situations in clinical practice in which TDM is not at all required, i.e., **TDM is futile**:
  - If the effect of a drug can be easily appreciated and measured as for antihypertensives, anticoagulants antidiabetics, diuretics, etc., TDM is not required.
  - Monitoring plasma levels is not useful for irreversibly acting drugs like organophosphates and phenoxybenzamine.
  - For drugs whose actions last longer than their plasma concentration, like MAO inhibitors and omeprazole, there is no benefit of TDM. Such drugs are called hit and run drugs.
  - The same applies to prodrugs that get converted to their active form in the body, e.g., levodopa.

TDM is an important step of **target concentration strategy** and involves the following measures:

1. First, the target concentration is selected.
2. The volume of distribution and clearance are predicted using standard population values. Adjustment for weight, liver and kidney functions, etc., are made.
3. The dose is calculated based on the calculated pharmacokinetics values, and the selected target concentration is administered. For long-acting drugs, a loading dose may also be required.
4. After the optimum time, the patient's response is observed, and plasma concentration is measured.
5. Based on the measured concentration, the volumes of distribution and clearance are recalculated.
6. The dose is readjusted.

These steps can be repeated as many times as needed till the optimum response is achieved.

Clinical problem-based questions and MCQs

21. A 20-year-old male patient is brought to the emergency with a history suggestive of generalised tonic–clonic seizures. The patient is put on carbamazepine therapy and followed-up regularly. During each follow-up examination, a blood sample is collected to monitor drug levels.
    i. Is therapeutic drug monitoring useful in this case?
    ii. Enumerate all the conditions in which TDM is justifiable.
22. In which of the following drugs, is TDM NOT indicated?
    a. Lithium   b. Digoxin
    c. Phenytoin   d. Lisinopril
23. TDM has NO role in monitoring therapy with which of the following drugs?
    a. Antidiabetic drugs   b. Antipsychotic drugs
    c. Cardiac glycosides   d. Antimicrobials

24. i. Which pharmacokinetic parameter is important to calculate the loading dose of a drug?
    a. Clearance
    b. Volume of distribution
    c. Hepatic blood flow
    d. Degree of ionisation
    ii. Define the selected pharmacokinetic parameter and its relationship with the loading dose.

25. i. Which pharmacokinetic parameter is important to calculate the maintenance dose of a drug?
    a. Clearance
    b. Volume of distribution
    c. Hepatic blood flow
    d. Degree of ionisation
    ii. Define the selected pharmacokinetic parameter and its relationship with the maintenance dose.

Summary

- Multiple patient-related, disease-related, and route-related factors can cause variability in drug response.
- Variations in drug response can be qualitative or quantitative.
- **Qualitative** differences in drug response lead to a different type of response. These may be due to immune response, genetic factors, age, gender, or the route of drug administration.
- **Quantitative** differences in drug response include increased/reduced response due to multiple factors affecting pharmacokinetic and pharmacodynamics of drugs, e.g., genetic polymorphisms, age, sex, pregnant state, hepatic/renal/cardiac diseases, environmental influences, and the use of other concomitant drugs.
- **Combined effect of drugs** can manifest as synergism (additive/supra-additive) or antagonism (physical/chemical/physiological/pharmacological).
- Receptor antagonism can be competitive or non-competitive depending on the site of binding of the antagonist. Competitive antagonism is further of the equilibrium and non-equilibrium types.
- For the safe use of medicines, drug choice and drug dose need to be adjusted after considering all these factors.
- Dose adjustment is more important at the extremes of ages due to immature/impaired drug eliminating systems. Formulae based on body weight and BSA are used for deciding individualised doses, especially for toxic drugs.
- In cases of hepatic or renal dysfunction, dose adjustment is done on the lower side, or some drugs are contraindicated. Cardiac diseases alter all four pharmacokinetic processes.
- **Tolerance** refers to reduced responsiveness to drugs with continued use. Various types of tolerance are natural/acquired, pharmacokinetic/pharmacodynamic, homologous/heterologous, cross tolerance, tachyphylaxis, etc.
- **Cumulative toxicity** can occur with the continued use of drugs having slow rates of elimination and high affinity for some tissues.

Questions for practice

1. Explain why:
   a. Some drugs need dose reduction in patients with impaired LFT.
   b. Patients at the extremes of age are more prone to adverse drug effects.
   c. Succinylcholine can cause prolonged apnea in some patients.
   d. Primaquine is contraindicated in a patient with G6PD deficiency.
2. Differentiate between the following:
   a. Competitive and non-competitive antagonism
   b. Physical and physiological antagonism
3. Write short notes on:
   a. Drug tolerance   b. Pharmacogenetics
   c. Tachyphylaxis

Hints for problem-based questions and MCQs

1. c. Genetically determined variable response due to immunological factors
2. i. c. Clarithromycin;
   ii. Hemolysis can occur
3. a. Phenobarbitone
4. a. Excessive Ca^{2+} release from the sarcoplasmic reticulum
5. i. d. Bladder irrigation with N-acetylcysteine.
   ii. N-acetylcysteine detoxifies and excretes the active metabolite (acrolein) of cyclophosphamide
6. i. Because these patient groups are prone to ineffectiveness or toxicity/peculiar adverse effects of drugs, the drug and dose should be decided upon carefully
   ii. Refer to page 78, 79 for pharmacokinetic/dynamic changes in children, elderly patients, and pregnant women
7. a. Glucuronide conjugase
8. d. Pseudocholinesterase
9. c. Hydralazine
10. c. CYP2C19
11. Reduced influx or increased efflux of the drug from cancer cells (Refer to page 79)
12. b. Potentiation
13. i. c. Physiological antagonism
    ii. Refer to page 81.
14. d. Ketamine
15. c. 150 mg (Adult dose × 1.3/1.7). Refer to page 83.
16. d. Enalapril. It is a prodrug, so its dose needs to be adjusted on the higher side for patients with hepatic function impairment. Morphine (which is metabolised by the liver), diclofenac (which greatly binds to albumin), and verapamil (which has a high first-pass effect) need dose reduction.
17. 900 mg (125 × 500/70 = 892). Refer to page 83.
18. d. 125 mg (50% dose reduction needed if creatinine clearance is 30–50 mL/minute). Refer to Table 6.2, page 84.
19. d. Verapamil

20. c. Neostigmine; the remaining options are drugs that have anticholinergic effects
21. i. TDM is useful as the effect of carbamazepine is not easily quantifiable
  ii. Refer to page 86.
22. d. Lisinopril, as it lowers BP, which can be easily measured
23. a. Antidiabetic drugs Lower blood glucose, which is monitored; there is no need to monitor drug levels
24. i. b. Volume of distribution
  ii. Refer to page 85.
25. i. a. Clearance
  ii. Refer to page 85.

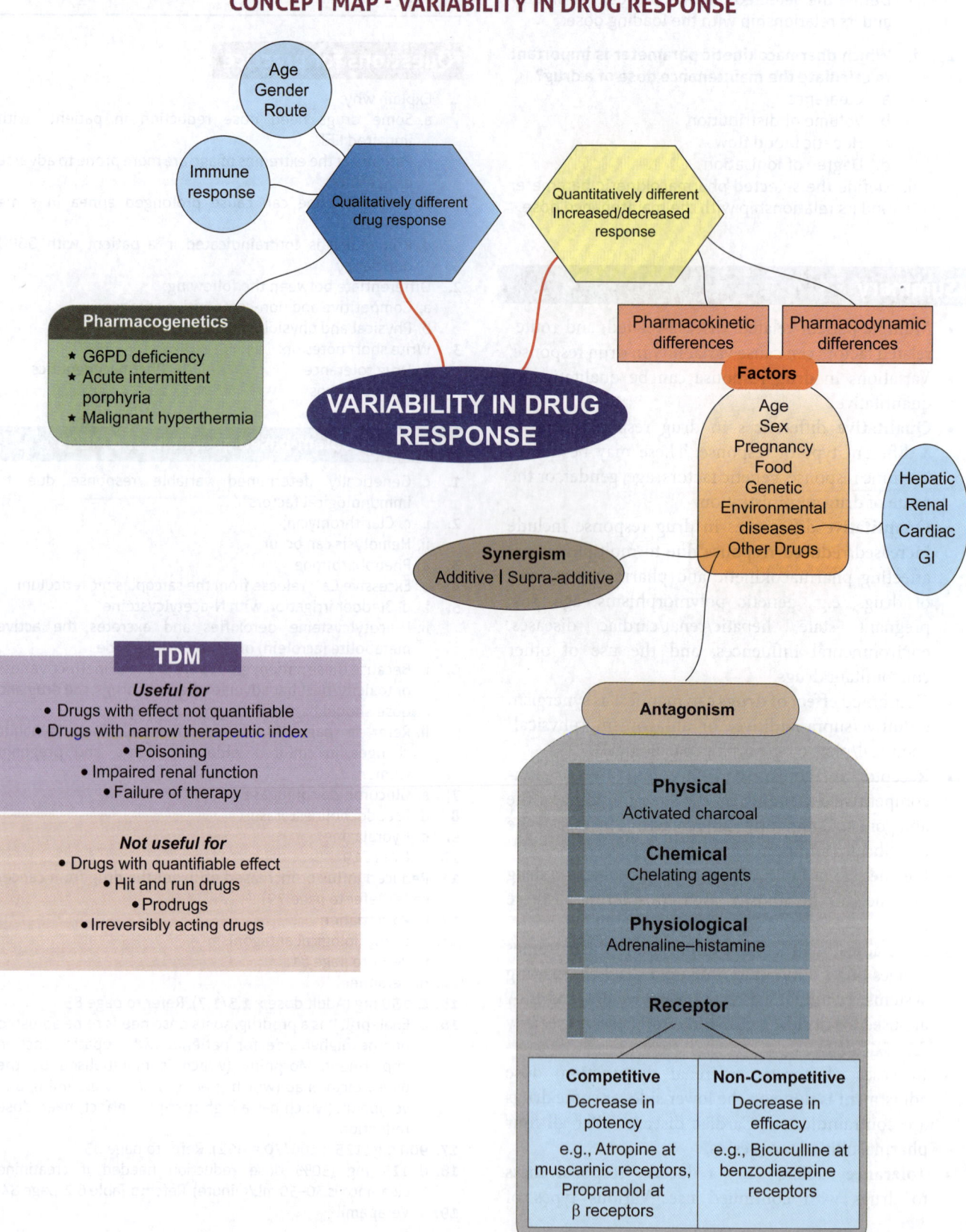

SECTION 2   Drugs Acting on ANS and PNS

7 Cholinergic Drugs

PH 2.2 Describe types, salient pharmacokinetics, pharmacodynamics, therapeutic uses, adverse drug reactions of cholinergic drugs and demonstrate OPC poisoning management.

Learning objectives

A student of MBBS phase II should be able to:
- Explain the process of neurotransmission in the ANS.
- Describe the synthesis, storage, release, and degradation of acetylcholine (ACh) and the drugs that affect it.
- Classify cholinergic drugs and describe their mechanisms of action.
- Describe the pharmacological basis for various therapeutic indications of cholinergic drugs.
- Enumerate the therapeutic uses of cholinergic drugs, including relevant dosage information.
- Describe the precautions, contraindications, and adverse effects associated with the use of cholinergic drugs.

THE AUTONOMIC NERVOUS SYSTEM

The **autonomic nervous system (ANS)** is a division of the efferent nervous system that operates independently of conscious control. It primarily regulates involuntary visceral functions such as cardiac activity, blood flow to organs, digestion, and other essential physiological processes.

Divisions of the ANS

Anatomically, the autonomic nervous system has two main divisions (Fig. 7.1).

- **Parasympathetic nervous system or the craniosacral system**: The 3rd, 7th, 9th and 10th cranial nerves, and the 3rd and 4th sacral nerves contain parasympathetic fibres.
- **Sympathetic nervous system or thoracolumbar system**

The **enteric nervous system** is sometimes considered as the third branch of the autonomic nervous system. It comprises the myenteric and submucosal nerve plexuses. It controls the motility and secretory activity of the gut.

Preganglionic, autonomic fibres originate from nuclei within the central nervous system, and exit from the brainstem or spinal cord. These fibres end in the motor ganglia. The parasympathetic ganglia are located near or within the walls of innervated organs, whereas sympathetic ganglia are located on both sides of the vertebral column as sympathetic chains. Thus, in the parasympathetic system, preganglionic fibres are long and postganglionic fibres are short. In the sympathetic system, it is the opposite, i.e., preganglionic fibres are short and postganglionic fibres are long (Fig. 7.1).

Neurotransmission in the ANS

In general, the functioning of the ANS involves neurochemical transmission. Chemical transmitters released from the nerve endings, called neurotransmitters (NTMs), diffuse across the synaptic cleft and act by binding to specialised receptors.

Based on the neurotransmitter released, autonomic nerves are classified as:

- **Cholinergic nerves**, which secrete acetylcholine (ACh) as a major NTM
- **Adrenergic nerves**, which secrete noradrenaline (NA) as a major NTM.

In addition to the chief NTMs, many co-transmitters like adenosine triphosphate (ATP), gamma aminobutyric acid (GABA), cholecystokinin (CCK), nitric oxide (NO), serotonin (5-hydroxytryptamine or 5-HT), enkephalin, calcitonin gene-related peptide (CGRP) and vasoactive intestinal peptide (VIP) are also released.

Cholinergic Nerves

The NTM acetylcholine (ACh) is released at the following sites:

- **Adrenal medulla**
- **All preganglionic nerves** (sympathetic as well as parasympathetic): the NTM at all the ganglia, whether they are parasympathetic or sympathetic, is ACh; thus, ACh or drugs simulating its actions cause the simultaneous stimulation of sympathetic and parasympathetic ganglia.
- **All postganglionic, parasympathetic nerves** release ACh to exert parasympathetic actions (through muscarinic and nicotinic receptors)

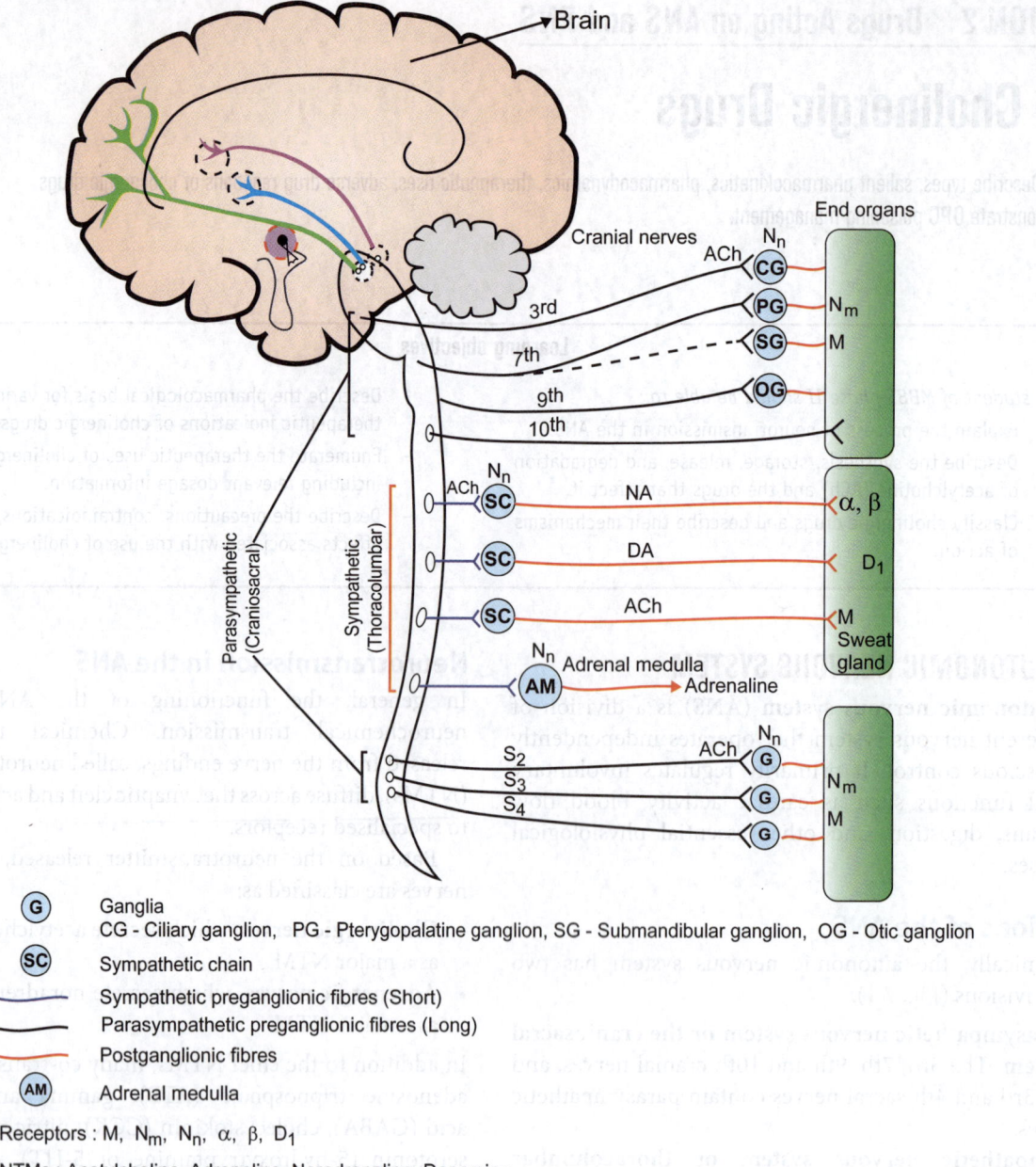

Fig. 7.1 The autonomic nervous system

- **Somatic motor nerves:** the amount of ACh secreted with each action potential is more than that released by the autonomic nerves. These are responsible for the contraction of skeletal muscles
- **Some postganglionic sympathetic nerves,** like those supplying eccrine sweat glands and skeletal muscle blood vessels, also release ACh

Because all parasympathetic nerves (preganglionic as well as postganglionic) release ACh, the term cholinergic is considered synonymous with parasympathetic.

Adrenergic Nerves
The NTM released is noradrenaline (NA), sometimes called norepinephrine (NE). Nerves that secrete NA are called adrenergic (and not noradrenergic) nerves, even though the NTM is noradrenaline. **Most postganglionic sympathetic nerves** are adrenergic in nature and are considered synonymous with the adrenergic system.

DRUGS AFFECTING THE CHOLINERGIC SYSTEM
ACh Synthesis
Acetyl coenzyme A (Acetyl-CoA) is synthesised (Fig. 7.2) by the mitochondria in nerve terminals and 'choline' is transported from the extracellular fluid (ECF) into nerve endings by a sodium-dependent transporter. In the cytoplasm of cholinergic nerve endings, acetyl-CoA and choline combine in the presence of the enzyme 'choline

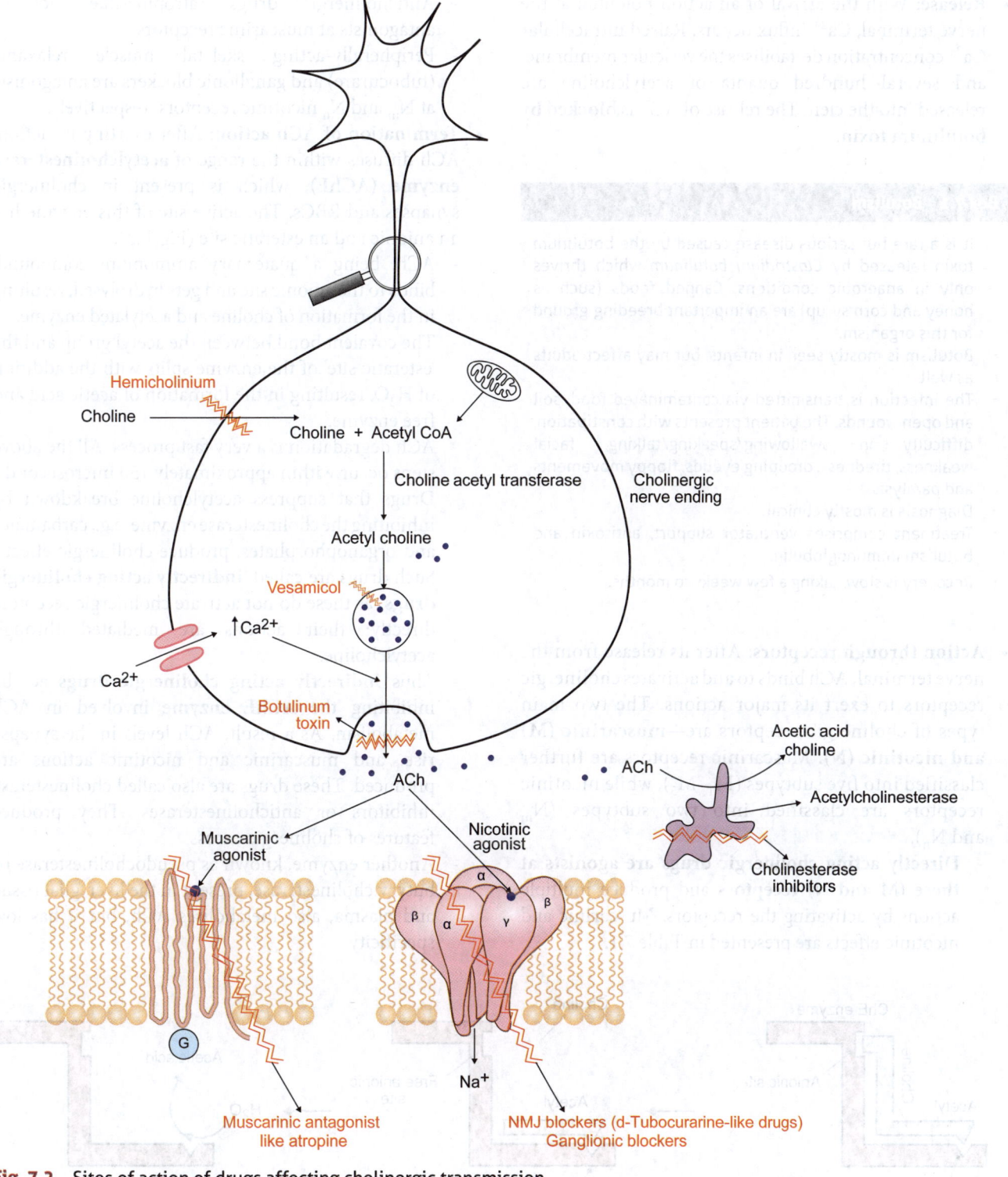

Fig. 7.2 Sites of action of drugs affecting cholinergic transmission

acetyltransferase', resulting in the synthesis of acetylcholine (ACh). This process is fast and efficient, to support a high turnover rate of ACh.

$$\text{Acetyl-CoA + Choline} \xrightarrow{\text{Choline acetyltransferase}} (\text{ACh})$$

The transport of choline from extracellular fluid into the nerve ending is blocked by the **hemicholinium**.

- **Storage:** After synthesis in the cytoplasm, ACh is transported into the vesicles by an antiporter that removes protons (H^+) and packs 1,000–50,000 molecules of ACh in each vesicle. This process is blocked by **vesamicol**.

- **Release:** With the arrival of an action potential at the nerve terminal, Ca^{2+} influx occurs. Raised intracellular Ca^{2+} concentration destabilises the vesicular membrane, and several hundred quanta of acetylcholine are released into the cleft. The release of ACh is **blocked by botulinum toxin**.

> **Box 7.1 Botulism**
> - It is a rare but serious disease caused by the botulinum toxin released by *Clostridium botulinum* which thrives only in anaerobic conditions. Canned foods (such as honey and corn syrup) are an important breeding ground for this organism.
> - Botulism is mostly seen in infants, but may affect adults as well.
> - The infection is transmitted via contaminated food, soil and open wounds. The patient presents with constipation, difficulty in swallowing/speaking/talking, facial weakness, tiredness, drooping eyelids, floppy movements and paralysis.
> - Diagnosis is mostly clinical.
> - Treatment comprises ventilator support, antitoxin and botulism immunoglobulin.
> - Recovery is slow, taking a few weeks to months.

- **Action through receptors**: After its release from the nerve terminal, ACh binds to and activates cholinergic receptors to exert its major actions. The two main types of cholinergic receptors are—**muscarinic (M) and nicotinic (N)**. Muscarinic receptors are further classified into five subtypes (M_1–M_5), while nicotinic receptors are classified into two subtypes (N_m and N_n).
  - **Directly acting cholinergic drugs are agonists at these (M and N) receptors** and produce multiple actions by activating the receptors. Muscarinic and nicotinic effects are presented in Table 7.1.
  - Anticholinergic drugs (atropine-like) act as antagonists at muscarinic receptors.
  - Peripherally-acting skeletal muscle relaxants (tubocurare) and ganglionic blockers are antagonists at N_m and N_n nicotinic receptors, respectively.
- **Termination of ACh action:** After exerting its action, ACh diffuses within the range of **acetylcholinesterase enzyme (AChE)**, which is present in cholinergic synapses and RBCs. The active site of this enzyme has an anionic and an esteratic site (Fig. 7.3).
  - ACh, being a quaternary ammonium compound, binds to the anionic site and gets hydrolysed, resulting in the formation of choline and acetylated enzyme.
  - The covalent bond between the acetyl group and the 'esteratic site' of the enzyme splits with the addition of H_2O, resulting in the formation of acetic acid and free enzyme.
  - ACh degradation is a very fast process. All the above steps occur within approximately 150 microseconds.
  - Drugs that suppress acetylcholine breakdown by inhibiting the cholinesterase enzyme, e.g., carbamates and organophosphates, produce cholinergic effects. Such drugs are called '**indirectly acting cholinergic drugs**', as these do not activate cholinergic receptors directly; their actions are mediated through acetylcholine.
  - Thus **indirectly acting cholinergic drugs** act by inhibiting the **AChE enzyme** involved in ACh metabolism. As a result, ACh levels in the synapse rise, and muscarinic and nicotinic actions are produced. These drugs are also called cholinesterase inhibitors or anticholinesterases. They produce features of cholinergic excess.
  - Another enzyme, known as pseudocholinesterase or butyrylcholinesterase, present in the liver, glial tissue and plasma, also metabolises ACh, but it has low specificity.

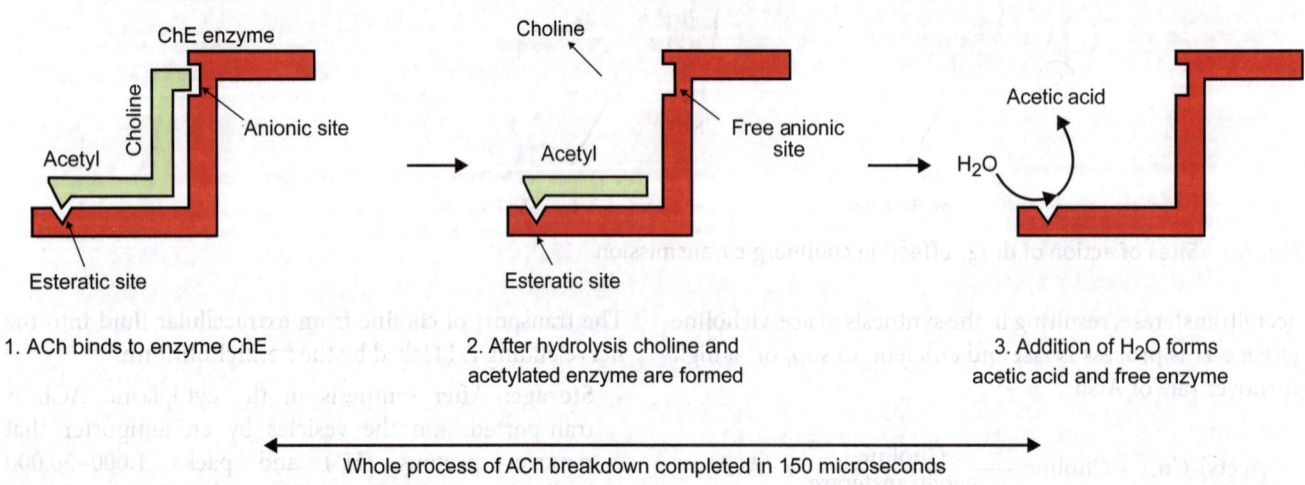

Fig. 7.3 Termination of acetylcholine

CLASSIFICATION OF CHOLINERGIC DRUGS

Cholinergic drugs can be classified based on their mechanism of action into **directly acting drugs** and **indirectly acting drugs**.

Directly acting drugs include choline esters and naturally occurring alkaloids, while indirectly acting drugs are cholinesterase inhibitors that have reversible or irreversible inhibitory action on enzyme cholinesterase (Flowchart 7.1).

DIRECTLY ACTING CHOLINERGIC DRUGS

These include choline esters and natural alkaloids.

a. Choline Esters

Acetylcholine, methacholine, bethanechol and carbachol are some directly acting cholinergic drugs.

Mechanism of action

Directly acting cholinergic drugs act as agonists at muscarinic and/or nicotinic receptors. The effects of individual drugs vary depending on their affinity for different types of receptors e.g.,

- Acetylcholine activates both muscarinic and nicotinic receptors equally.
- Methacholine and bethanechol activate only the muscarinic receptors.
- Carbachol also activates both receptor types (muscarinic and nicotinic), but its nicotinic effects are more prominent.

All muscarinic receptors are G protein-coupled receptors (GPCRs). M_1, M_3 and M_5 (odd-numbered) receptors are G_q protein-coupled and cause the activation of enzyme phospholipase C (PLC), which generates IP_3 and DAG from PIP_2 and increases cytosolic Ca^{2+} levels. M_2 and M_4 (even-numbered) receptors are G_i-coupled. Their activation inhibits adenylyl cyclase, reducing cAMP levels and causes the opening of K^+ channels, leading to hyperpolarisation of the membrane. Both subtypes of nicotinic receptors are ion channel-linked. Their activation opens up Na^+ channels, leading to the depolarisation of the membrane.

Table 7.1 presents the distribution of cholinergic receptors and the effects of agonists.

Pharmacological actions of cholinergic drugs

The pharmacological actions of cholinergic drugs are produced through the activation of cholinergic receptors.

1. **Central effects**: Cholinergic transmission in the brain plays an important role in memory, learning and cognition. A deficit in cholinergic activity in certain specific areas of the brain is responsible for short-term memory loss and cognitive defects in patients of Alzheimer disease.

   ACh and other choline esters cannot be used in the management of Alzheimer disease, as these substances contain a quaternary NH_4^+ group which renders them highly polar and unable to penetrate the blood–brain barrier.

2. **CVS:**
   - **Heart:** Cholinergic drugs exert an inhibitory effect on the heart through M_2 receptors. As a result, the heart rate decreases (negative chronotropic effect), the force of contraction reduces (negative inotropic effect), and atrio-ventricular conduction slows down (negative dromotropic effect). However, in the atria, acetylcholine-induced hyperpolarisation activates additional Na^+ channels, thereby increasing atrial conduction. Thus, the action potential duration is reduced and atrial refractory period is abbreviated.
   - **Blood vessels:** Activation of endothelial M_3-receptors leads to the release of the endothelium-derived relaxing factor (EDRF; chemically, nitric

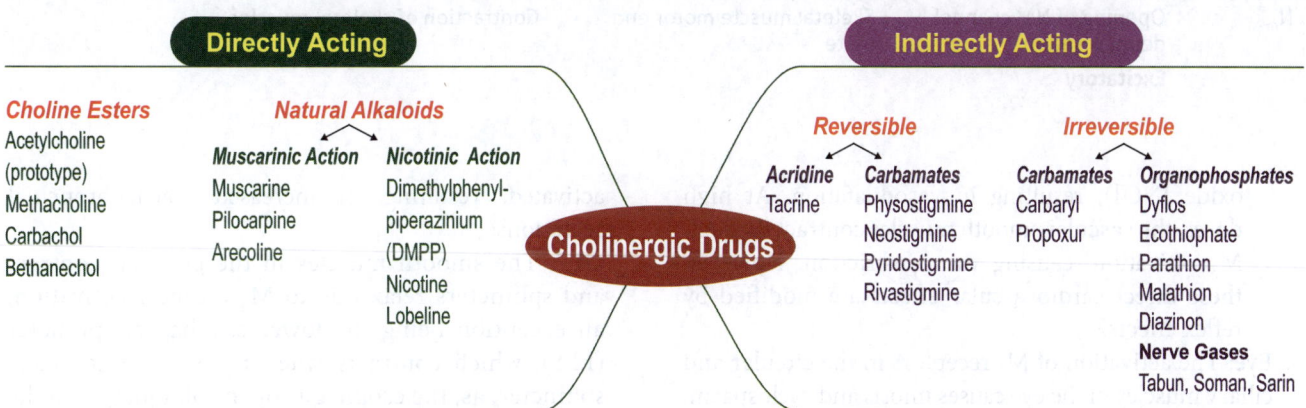

Flowchart 7.1 Classification of cholinergic drugs

Table 7.1 Distribution of cholinergic receptors and effects of agonists

Name of receptor	Transduction system and nature of receptors	Distribution	Clinically relevant organ system effects
Muscarinic M_1	IP_3–DAG → increased Ca^{2+} **Excitatory**	Gastric gland	Increased gastric acid secretion
		CNS	Role in memory, learning, cognitive and motor activity
		Presynaptically on autonomic ganglia	Increased ACh secretion
M_2	Inhibits adenylyl cyclase enzyme → reduced cAMP opens K^+ channels → hyperpolarisation **Inhibitory**	Heart	Decreases heart rate, contractility and atrio-ventricular conduction (negative chronotropic, inotropic and dromotropic effects, respectively) Abbreviation of the atrial refractory period*
M_3	IP_3–DAG → increased Ca^{2+} **Excitatory**	Exocrine glands	Increased secretion of lacrimal, salivary, nasopharyngeal, tracheobronchial and sweat glands
		Smooth muscles as in	
		Eye (circular and ciliary muscles)	Miosis, cyclospasm
		Bronchi	Bronchoconstriction
		GIT and genitourinary tract	Contraction of the wall and relaxation of the sphincters in the GIT and genitourinary tract (except lower esophageal sphincter [LES], which contracts**)
		Vascular smooth muscles	Vasoconstriction at high doses
		Endothelium	EDRF# release and vasodilatation
M_4	Inhibits adenylyl cyclase → reduced cAMP **Inhibitory**	CNS	Regulate release of other NTMs
M_5	IP_3–DAG, increased Ca^{2+} **Excitatory**	CNS	Regulate release of other NTMs

NOTE: Receptor subtypes with even numbers are inhibitory in nature, e.g., M_2, M_4
*Abbreviation of atrial refractory period and **Contraction of the LES are the only two actions that cannot be predicted from the nature of the receptors, i.e., they seem paradoxical.
#EDRF - Endothelium-derived relaxing factor

Nicotinic N_n	Opening of Na^+ channel → depolarisation **Excitatory**	- Postganglionic neurons	Ganglionic stimulation
		- Adrenal medulla	Increased release of catecholamines
		- Somatic motor nerves	Increased release of ACh
N_m	Opening of Na^+ channel → depolarisation **Excitatory**	Skeletal muscle motor end plate	Contraction of skeletal muscles

oxide [NO]), resulting in vasodilatation. At high doses, the vascular smooth muscles contract through M_3 activation, causing vasoconstriction. However, these direct cardiovascular effects are modified by reflex effects.

3. **Eye:** The activation of M_3 receptors in the circular and ciliary muscles in the eye causes miosis and cyclospasm, respectively.

4. **Bronchi:** M_3-receptor activation in the bronchial smooth muscles causes bronchoconstriction. The M_3 receptors in the tracheobronchial glands are also activated, resulting in increased tracheobronchial secretions.

5. **GIT:** The smooth muscles in the gut wall contract and sphincters relax due to M_3-receptor activation, an exception being the lower esophageal sphincter (LES), which contracts (the LES is a physiological sphincter; as, the esophagus opens obliquely into the stomach to prevent the reflux of gastric contents). Cholinergic action thus facilitates bowel evacuation. Gastric acid secretion increases due to M_1-receptor activation.

6. **Genitourinary tract:** M_3-receptor activation causes the contraction of the detrusor muscle and the relaxation of the sphincter and trigone, facilitating the voiding of urine.
7. **Exocrine glands:** M_3 receptors of the exocrine glands are excitatory in nature. Thus, cholinergic drugs cause an increase in lacrimal, nasopharyngeal, tracheobronchial, salivary and sweat gland secretions. However, pancreatic and intestinal secretions are not much affected.
8. **Nicotinic effects:**
   - The activation of the N_m receptors present at the motor end plate causes depolarisation leading to skeletal muscle contraction.
   - N_n-receptor activation causes ganglionic stimulation (of both sympathetic and parasympathetic ganglia), and increased release of acetylcholine at somatic nerve terminals and catecholamines in the adrenal medulla.

Pharmacokinetics of choline esters

The choline esters, ACh, carbachol, methacholine and bethanechol, have a quaternary ammonium group (NH_4^+), as a result of which these substances are partly absorbed and poorly distributed into the CNS (as they cannot cross the blood–brain barrier). Different choline esters vary in their susceptibility to the cholinesterase enzyme.

- Acetylcholine is very rapidly metabolised (in 150 microseconds). Thus, large amounts must be administered by intravenous infusion to achieve detectable effects.
- Methacholine is three times more resistant to hydrolysis by the cholinesterase enzyme than acetylcholine.
- Carbachol and bethanechol are extremely resistant to this enzyme. Hence, their duration of action is comparatively longer.

Therapeutic uses

The use of choline esters is limited in current clinical practice.

1. **Acetylcholine is not used therapeutically** for any indication for the following reasons:
   - It has evanescent or very short-lasting action, and is very rapidly metabolised by cholinesterase enzyme. Thus, large doses must be given by intravenous infusion for any detectable effects.
   - It is non-selective and acts on all muscarinic and nicotinic receptors resulting in many adverse effects.
2. **Carbachol** may be used topically as eye drops for its miotic action in **glaucoma**.
3. **Bethanechol** can be used for the following indications:
   - Postoperative or postpartum paralytic ileus
   - Congenital megacolon
- Gastro-esophageal reflux disease (GERD)
- Non-obstructive urinary retention
- Neurogenic bladder
- Xerostomia

Adverse drug reactions

Choline esters are **not popular** as they produce many adverse effects like belching, colicky pain, abdominal cramps, involuntary urination or defecation, flushing, sweating, fall in BP and bronchospasm.

They may also cause excessive salivation, lacrimation, rhinorrhea, headache, loss of accommodation, weakness and paralysis of skeletal muscles.

Before prescribing cholinergic drugs, it is essential to rule out any mechanical obstruction in the gastrointestinal or genitourinary tract. These drugs stimulate smooth muscle contraction and are beneficial only in paralytic conditions; in the presence of an obstruction, they may worsen the condition.

Contraindications

- Bronchial asthma and COPD are contraindications as these drugs cause bronchoconstriction.
- Choline esters should not be prescribed in peptic ulceration because they increase gastric secretions.
- Choline esters are contraindicated in coronary artery disease as they further compromise coronary flow due to their hypotensive action.
- Choline esters can induce atrial fibrillation in a hyperthyroid patient. Hence, these are contraindicated in hyperthyroidism.

Clinical problem-based questions and MCQs

1. **A 48-year-old female patient had an abdominal surgery after which she developed postoperative urinary retention.**
   i. Which of the following drugs is most suitable for relieving symptoms in this case?
      a. Acetylcholine b. Pilocarpine
      c. Bethanechol d. Muscarine
   ii. Describe the pharmacological basis for the use of the selected drug.
   iii. What caution should be exercised while prescribing this drug?
   iv. Enumerate the other therapeutic uses and adverse effects of the selected drug.

2. **Acetylcholine released from cholinergic nerve endings acts on all the subtypes of cholinergic receptors and has many useful effects on organ systems, but still has no therapeutic indication.**
   i. Explain the pharmacological basis for the above statement.
   ii. Name the cholinergic receptors.
   iii. Enumerate the major muscarinic effects of ACh.

b. Natural alkaloids
(i) Pilocarpine
Pilocarpine is a tertiary amine with predominant muscarinic actions. It is too toxic for systemic use. It is used only topically as **eye drops (0.5–4%)** to produce the following effects:
- Miosis for counteracting the effect of mydriatics.
- In alternation with mydriatics to prevent or break adhesions/synechia between the cornea and lens in patients with inflammatory conditions of the eye.
- As a third-line drug for open-angle glaucoma.
- Rarely, it is used in patients who have xerostomia (decreased salivation and dryness of mouth) that may occur as a symptom of Sjogren's syndrome (Box 7.2) or after laryngeal surgery and radiotherapy. Pilocarpine **oral lozenges** can be used as a sialagogue; bethanechol is an alternative to pilocarpine for this indication

ADRs: Adverse effects are the same as those of bethanechol. Topical administration of pilocarpine causes a stinging sensation in the eye and painful spasm of accommodation, resulting in brow pain.

> **Box 7.2   Sjogren's syndrome**
>
> It is a chronic, slowly progressing autoimmune disease involving lymphocytic infiltration of the exocrine glands, resulting in extreme dryness of the eyes, mouth and skin. It can occur alone or may be secondary to other autoimmune diseases like SLE, scleroderma, rheumatoid arthritis or other connective tissue disorders.
>
> Patients commonly present with xerostomia (dry mouth), accompanied by burning sensation, difficulty in swallowing and speaking, and an increased risk of dental caries. Ocular manifestations include a sandy or gritty sensation in the eyes, reduced tear production, thick secretions at the inner canthus, itching, and progressive damage to the corneal and conjunctival epithelium, ultimately leading to keratoconjunctivitis sicca.
>
> The diagnosis is confirmed by sialometry, sialography, ultrasound/MRI/biopsy of the salivary glands.
>
> Treatment is symptomatic and includes artificial tears, sialogogues in the form of pilocarpine lozenges, and immune suppression with corticosteroids and monoclonal antibodies.

(ii) Muscarine
Muscarine is only of toxicological importance. It is present in poisonous mushrooms of the *Amantia* and *Inocybe* species. The three types of mushroom poisoning are **early mushroom poisoning, late mushroom poisoning** and the **hallucinogenic** type (refer to Chapter 8, page 108). Early mushroom poisoning has features of muscarinic excess like bradycardia, excessive exocrine secretions, colicky pain and diarrhea, which are managed with atropine.

(iii) Nicotine
- It acts as an agonist at both N_m and N_n subtypes of nicotinic receptors.
- N_m action: nicotine activates the motor end plate in skeletal muscles, causing contraction.
- N_n action: nicotine activates both sympathetic as well as parasympathetic ganglia. However, larger doses cause persistent depolarisation, and ganglionic blockade.
- In clinical practice, nicotine is useful for short-term therapy for **smoking cessation** (Box 7.3).
- It is clinically relevant on account of its presence in cigarettes and tobacco. Nicotine dependence makes it difficult to quit smoking and chewing tobacco.

> **Box 7.3   Smoking cessation**
>
> - **Psychotherapy** provides counselling and motivates smokers to quit.
> - **Pharmacotherapy** decreases the craving for nicotine and suppresses withdrawal symptoms like anxiety, irritability, tremors, restlessness, aggression, lack of concentration and depression. The following drugs are used for this purpose:
>   a. **Short-term nicotine replacement therapy:**
>   - **Transdermal nicotine patches** measuring 10, 20, and 30 cm², release 7, 14, and 21 mg of nicotine, respectively, in 24 hours. The application of such patches is effective in controlling withdrawal symptoms as well as suppressing cravings to some extent.
>   - Nicotine **chewing gum** is also available in doses of 1, 2 and 4 mg. The dose is kept in the mouth and chewed for about 30 minutes to satisfy the urge to smoke. The maximum number of pieces allowed daily should not exceed 15.
>   - Nasal sprays and inhalers are also available.
>   - The duration of treatment can be 12 weeks at the most, after which it is tapered off.
>   - Adverse effects of nicotine replacement therapy are abdominal cramps, diarrhea, insomnia, headache and flu-like symptoms. It is contraindicated in cardiac arrhythmias and ischemic heart disease.
>   b. **Varenicline:** Nicotine is addictive because it has a rewarding effect, mediated through a specific subtype of neuronal nicotinic receptors in the mesolimbic area—the $\alpha_4\beta_2$ nicotinic receptors. Varenicline is a partial agonist at $\alpha_4\beta_2$ receptors. It provides some substitution of nicotinic action, but blocks the reward effect of smoking.
>   The recommended dosage of varenicline is 0.25 mg BD orally, increased slowly up to a maximum of 1 mg BD, as per the requirement. The **duration of treatment should** not exceed **12 weeks.** Adverse effects include altered mood, behaviour, taste and sleep disturbances.
>   c. **Bupropion:** It is an atypical anti-depressant drug that inhibits the reuptake of dopamine and noradrenaline. Its efficacy in controlling cravings and withdrawal symptoms is the same as that of nicotine replacement therapy, but it is better tolerated.

Clinical problem-based questions and MCQs

1. **A 36-year-old male who had been a chain smoker for the last 5–6 years presented with cough and difficulty in breathing. Investigations did not suggest lung carcinoma, but the chest specialist advised him to stop smoking to reduce the risk of malignant disease in the future and prescribed him nicotine.**
   i. Which is the most appropriate route for the administration of nicotine?
      a. Oral b. Subcutaneous
      c. Cutaneous d. Intravenous
   ii. The patient wondered why nicotine was being prescribed to treat his smoking habit, considering that cigarettes contain nicotine. What is the rationale for using nicotine for smoking cessation?
   iii. What is the dose and duration of treatment with nicotine in smoking cessation?
   iv. What other drugs are used for smoking cessation?

2. **Pilocarpine eye drops (0.5%) were administered to a 10-year-old boy following refraction testing. The patient complained of brow pain and a stinging sensation in his eyes.**
   i. Explain the pharmacological basis for the use of pilocarpine eye drops in this patient.
   ii. Explain the cause of brow pain associated with pilocarpine eye drops.

3. **A 55-year-old woman presented with dryness of the mouth and inability to eat properly. She has a history of dryness of the eyes along with a sandy, gritty sensation in her eyes. On examination, her parotid and submandibular salivary glands were enlarged and oral hygiene was poor with diffuse black pigmentation of the buccal mucosa. Her ESR was raised and serum immunoglobulin test for Sjogren's syndrome was positive. An exocrine gland biopsy showed lymphocytic infiltration.**
   i. Which of the following drugs can be used as a sialagogue for symptomatic relief?
      a. Pilocarpine b. Atropine
      c. Nicotine d. Acetylcholine
   ii. Describe the pharmacological basis for your selection.

- The NH_4^+ group of ACh has an affinity for the anionic site of the enzyme and its acetoxy group has an affinity for the esteratic site of the enzyme.
- After binding, choline is released and the enzyme gets acetylated.
- The acetylated enzyme then reacts with H_2O and undergoes rapid hydrolysis; acetic acid is released, and the enzyme is free to bind to next molecule of acetyl choline.

Instead of ACh, when carbamates react with cholinesterase, the enzyme gets carbamylated. This **carbamylated enzyme** reacts comparatively **slowly** with water, and takes about **30 minutes** for the active site of the enzyme to get free.

- Cholinesterase enzyme undergoes phosphorylation on reaction with organophosphates. The reaction of the **phosphorylated enzyme with water is extremely slow**, even longer than the time required for the synthesis of new enzyme. For this reason, organophosphates are called irreversible enzyme inhibitors. The loss of an alkyl group from the phosphorylated enzyme makes it completely resistant to hydrolysis. This is called the **ageing** of the **enzyme–phosphate bond**.
- **Acridine (tacrine)** and **edrophonium** (Fig. 7.4) attach to the cholinesterase enzyme only at the anionic site. The enzyme is reactivated when the drug diffuses away from the enzyme. This reaction does not involve hydrolysis; thus, drugs have a short duration of action.

Pharmacological actions

The inhibition of cholinesterase enzyme interferes with acetylcholine metabolism. The pharmacological actions of cholinesterase inhibitor drugs are, therefore, because of the accumulation of ACh at cholinergic sites.

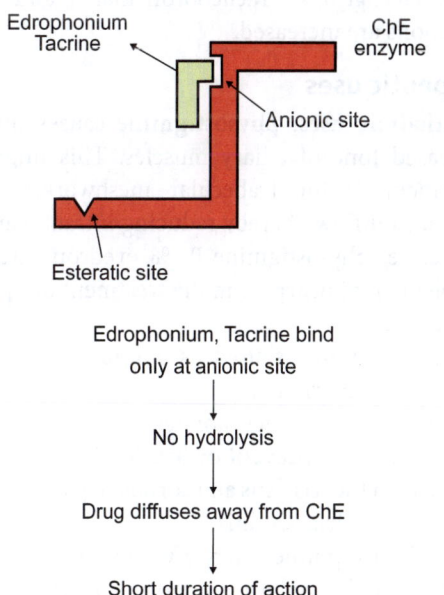

Fig. 7.4 Mechanism of action of edrophonium

INDIRECTLY ACTING CHOLINERGIC DRUGS

Indirectly acting cholinergic drugs are also known as cholinesterase inhibitors (ChEIs) or anticholinesterases. These include carbamates and organophosphates (Flowchart 7.1).

Mechanism of action

As discussed earlier in this chapter, the cholinesterase enzyme has an anionic and an esteratic site.
- Acetylcholine combines with cholinesterase (ChE) by electrostatic attraction.

Nicotinic effects
- The excessive stimulation of N_n receptors causes ganglionic stimulation. Later on, the persistent depolarisation results in the blockade of transmission.
- The activation of N_m receptors present on the motor end plate increases the force of contractions of skeletal muscles in myasthenia gravis and partially curarised muscle. Because ACh is not metabolised, it binds again to the same receptors, and diffuses to bind to the neighbouring receptors too. Therefore, repetitive firing, twitching and fasciculations occur. However, a high dose of these drugs is counterproductive, resulting in persistent depolarisation and blockade of neurotransmission resulting in muscular weakness and paralysis. This condition is known as 'cholinergic crisis' and warrants a reduction in the dosage of cholinesterase inhibitors. Neostigmine possesses some direct action also on the motor end plate.

Muscarinic effects
- **CVS:** Cholinesterase inhibitors have complex effects on the cardiovascular system due to their muscarinic effects (through M_2 receptors), ganglionic stimulation (through N_n receptors), and medullary-cardiovascular centre stimulation followed by depression and reflex effects.
- **Smooth muscles:** M_3-receptor activation results in the contraction of the smooth muscles, causing miosis, cyclospasm, bronchoconstriction, increased peristaltic activity, abdominal cramps and bowel evacuation. However, the tone of LES is increased. The contraction of the detrusor in the bladder wall and the relaxation of the trigone and sphincter favour voiding.
- **Exocrine secretions:** Salivary, sweat, lacrimal, nasopharyngeal, tracheobronchial and gastric secretions are increased.

Therapeutic uses
1. **Ophthalmic uses: physostigmine** causes miosis and increased tone of ciliary muscles. This improves the alignment of the trabecular meshwork, facilitating aqueous outflow, thereby reducing intraocular tension. Therefore, physostigmine 0.1% eyedrops are used to supplement pilocarpine in the treatment of **open-angle glaucoma**.
   - Physostigmine is used as a **miotic** to reverse the effect of mydriatics.
   - Sometimes, miotics are used in alternation with mydriatics to **prevent or break adhesions/synechia** between the iris, lens and cornea in patients suffering from iritis/iridocyclitis.

   Physostigmine, tertiary amine, is absorbed through the cornea on topical ocular application, potentially leading to systemic adverse effects.

2. Physostigmine can be used as a last resort measure in cases of **atropine poisoning** to reverse peripheral as well as central effects. Generally, only supportive measures are used in atropine poisoning, as physostigmine itself can cause arrhythmias, hypotension and central side effects.

3. **Myasthenia gravis** is an autoimmune disease, involving the formation of antibodies against N_m receptors. The number of N_m receptors decreases to one-third of the normal value or even less. This structural damage and reduced neurotransmission at the neuromuscular junction results in weakness and easy fatigability, which is relieved upon resting.
   - Cholinesterase inhibitors like **neostigmine, pyridostigmine, edrophonium and ambenonium** allow acetylcholine released from nerve endings to accumulate and act on N_m receptors over a larger area. Neostigmine also possesses a direct depolarising action on the motor end plate. Being quaternary ammonium compounds, these drugs do not cross the blood–brain barrier and hence, are free of central side effects and are preferred over physostigmine for this indication. Treatment of myasthenia gravis is initiated with oral neostigmine at a dose of 15 mg administered every six hours. The dosage and frequency are then adjusted based on the individual patient's clinical response. Adverse effects arising from the muscarinic actions of accumulated acetylcholine can be managed by co-administration of an antimuscarinic agent, such as atropine.
   - Edrophonium has a very short duration of action.

   Myasthenia gravis is diagnosed by the **edrophonium test**. Edrophonium 2 mg intravenous is administered as a test dose. If it is tolerated, 8 mg more is given after a few minutes. If there is an improvement in muscle strength, it confirms the diagnosis of myasthenia and rules out other muscular dystrophies.
   - Edrophonium also helps to **distinguish between myasthenic crisis** (due to more severe disease) **and cholinergic crisis** (due to an overdose of cholinesterase inhibitors). If symptoms improve upon administration of IV edrophonium, a diagnosis of myasthenic crisis is made. Conversely, if the symptoms worsen, cholinergic crisis is diagnosed.

   Myasthenic crisis is managed by tracheal intubation and mechanical ventilation for respiratory support and plasmapheresis to remove antibodies. Neostigmine therapy is stopped for 2–3 days and then gradually reintroduced. Methylprednisolone is given intravenously, whereas supportive treatment and neostigmine dose adjustment are needed to tide over cholinergic crisis.

- Corticosteroids are useful in severe cases of myasthenia that do not respond adequately to cholinesterase inhibitors. Corticosteroids act by inhibiting the production of antibodies against N_m receptors and may even increase the synthesis of Nm receptors. Prednisolone 30–60 mg per day is given to induce remission, and 10 mg is given daily or on alternate days for maintenance therapy. Other drugs that may be useful because of their immunosuppressive action include azathioprine and cyclosporine.
- Sometimes, plasmapheresis is required to remove excessive antibodies.
- Thymectomy is advised for younger patients, especially those who have a thymoma. It is effective because the thymus may have modified muscle cells bearing N_m receptors on their surface, which may serve as antigens for the production of autoantibodies against N_m receptors. Thus, thymectomy may help in controlling myasthenic symptoms.
4. **Postoperative decurarisation** is needed to reverse muscular paralysis caused by competitive neuromuscular junction (NMJ) blockers, i.e., tubocurare and similar drugs. Neostigmine intravenous 0.5–2 mg is effective. Muscarinic side effects are blocked by co-administering atropine.
5. In case of a **cobra bite,** neostigmine and atropine are given along with anti-snake venom to prevent respiratory paralysis.
6. **Postoperative urinary retention** due to bladder atony and **paralytic ileus** can be relieved with neostigmine given subcutaneously after ruling out organic obstruction.
7. **Alzheimer's disease** is a neurodegenerative disorder that chiefly affects the cholinergic neurons. Increasing cholinergic transmission in the CNS improves symptoms. Cholinesterase inhibitors with relatively cerebro-selective action (e.g., rivastigmine, donepezil and galantamine) are used for this purpose.

In addition to the above-mentioned therapeutic uses, malathion and diazinon are extensively used as **insecticides** and tabun, soman and sarin as **nerve gases.**

Adverse drug reactions

Most of the adverse reactions of cholinesterase inhibitors are due to cholinergic excess at muscarinic and nicotinic receptors.

- Increased salivary, sweat, lacrimal and tracheobronchial secretions and dyspepsia due to increased gastric secretion
- Abdominal cramps, diarrhea and involuntary micturition may occur.
- Bronchospasm and dyspnea, especially in asthmatics
- Bradycardia, fall in BP
- Muscular weakness and paralysis

OPC poisoning

Organophosphates like parathion, malathion and diazinon are extensively used as insecticides in agriculture. Exposure to large doses of OPCs can be accidental, suicidal or even homicidal.

Clinical features

These are direct extensions of cholinergic actions and include the following:

- Excessive secretions, lacrimation, rhinorrhea, sweating and tracheobronchial secretions are common in organophosphate (OPC) poisoning. Aspiration of these secretions has led to the description that such patients appear to be 'drowning in their own secretions.'
- Miosis, spasm of accommodation and blurring of vision.
- Abdominal cramps, colic pain, involuntary defecation and micturition.
- Bronchospasm and dyspnea; respiratory failure is a common cause of death.
- Skeletal muscle weakness and fasciculations followed by paralysis.
- Cardiac rhythm disturbances, hypotension and cardiovascular collapse may occur.
- Ataxia, disorientation, convulsions, coma and death.

Treatment

OPC poisoning is an acute emergency. It requires supportive as well as specific therapy.

a. **Supportive treatment** includes the following:
   - **Prevention of further exposure to the drug**—the patient should be shifted to fresh air and skin should be washed with a liberal amount of water and soap. If the drug is ingested, gastric lavage is done to remove the unabsorbed portion of the drug from the stomach.
   - Maintaining **ABC, i.e., patent airways, breathing and circulation,** is of prime importance as in any other poisoning.
   - Some patients have **convulsions,** which need to be treated with **diazepam.**
b. **Specific treatment:** The specific antidote for OPC poisoning is atropine.

Atropine

Atropine can reverse the muscarinic symptoms. However, it does not relieve the paralysis of skeletal muscles. Atropine is administered by the IV route in a dose of 2 mg, repeated every 10 minutes till the pupil starts dilating or till signs of atropinisation appear. The maximum dose can be up to 200 mg.

Because the inhibition of cholinesterase by organophosphates is irreversible and ChE enzyme activity

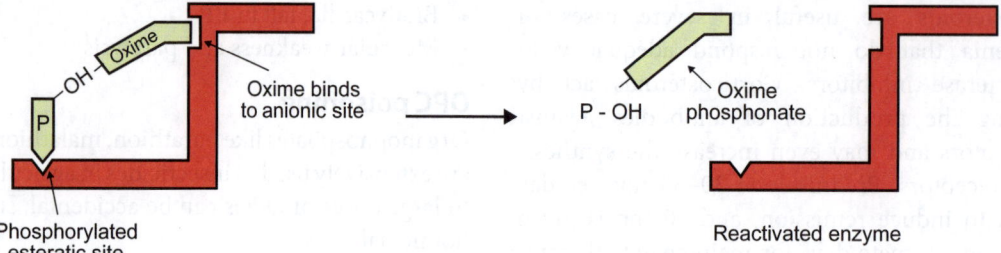

Fig. 7.5 Mechanism of action of oximes in OPC poisoning

is restored only after the biosynthesis of the new enzyme, maintenance treatment with atropine should be continued for 12 weeks.

Oximes

Oximes (pralidoxime, obidoxime and diacetylmonoxime (DAM)) are reactivators of enzyme. Cholinesterase reacts very slowly with water after phosphorylation, taking hundreds of hours. The reactivation of the enzyme depends on speeding up this reaction. When pralidoxime is administered, its quaternary nitrogen attaches to the anionic site of cholinesterase enzyme. The highly reactive OH group of oxime, reacts with the phosphate at the esteratic site of the enzyme, resulting in the formation of oxime phosphonate, which diffuses away, and the enzyme gets reactivated (Fig. 7.5).

Pralidoxime (1–2 g) is given as a slow intravenous injection. The dose is repeated based on need. A maximum of 12 g can be given in the first 24 hours. The treatment is continued for 1–2 weeks. Treatment should be initiated as early as possible, because the phosphorylated enzyme undergoes ageing with time by losing its alkyl group and the bond between the phosphate group and enzyme becomes resistant to hydrolysis.

The reactivation of cholinesterase with oximes is more effective at skeletal muscle motor end plates than at muscarinic sites. However, oximes cannot cross the blood–brain barrier and hence, are unable to reactivate central cholinesterase enzyme.

Oximes are not useful in the management of carbamate toxicity, where the anionic site of the enzyme is not vacant to bind with oximes. Moreover, oximes have a weak cholinesterase-inhibiting effect of their own.

Clinical problem-based questions and MCQs

6. A 52-year-old woman presented with double vision, difficulty in chewing food, easy fatigability and muscular weakness on continued activity. The symptoms are relieved with rest. On examination, the patient had drooping eyelids and weakness of the limbs. On investigation, antibodies against N_m receptors were present and the edrophonium test was positive.
    i. What is the likely diagnosis in this case?
    ii. Describe the edrophonium test.
    iii. Which of the following is the most suitable drug for the treatment of this patient?
        a. Tacrine   b. Neostigmine
        c. Edrophonium   d. Physostigmine
    iv. Describe the mechanism of action of the selected drug and the pharmacological basis of your choice.

7. A patient with myasthenia gravis who is on neostigmine therapy reports with sudden-onset extreme weakness and worsening of the existing condition.
    i. Which of the following drugs can be used to determine the cause of the worsening of his condition?
        a. Tacrine   b. Neostigmine
        c. Edrophonium   d. Pilocarpine
    ii. What is the differential diagnosis for his condition? How will you proceed to confirm the diagnosis?
    iii. Describe the management of this patient.

8. A 76-year-old patient presented with progressive dementia and was diagnosed with Alzheimer's disease.
    i. Identify the most effective strategy for symptom relief in this case.
        a. Inhibiting acetylcholine release in the brain
        b. Blocking cholinergic receptors in the brain
        c. Inhibiting cholinesterase enzyme in the brain
        d. Reactivating cholinesterase enzyme in the brain
    ii. Describe the pharmacological basis for your answer.
    iii. Enumerate the drugs that can be used in this case.

9. A farmer working in his fields suddenly developed excessive rhinorrhea, lacrimation, breathing difficulty, colicky pain in the abdomen and extreme weakness. His family brought him to the Emergency. His history revealed that he had planned to spray his fields with insecticides that day. On examination, the patient had lacrimation, excessive salivation and rhinorrhea; his pulse and BP were low, and his pupils were constricted.
    i. What is the probable diagnosis?
    ii. Explain the possible reasons for the constricted pupils and low pulse and BP in this patient.
    iii. How will you manage this patient?

10. What is the correct dosage of atropine to manage OPC poisoning?
    a. 0.5 mg repeated every 5 minutes
    b. 1 mg repeated every 10 minutes
    c. 2 mg repeated every 10 minutes
    d. 4 mg repeated every 30 minutes
11. i. Pralidoxime is NOT indicated in the case of poisoning with which one of the following drugs?
       a. Propoxur   b. Parathion
       c. Ecothiophate   d. Nerve gases
    ii. Explain the pharmacological basis of your choice.
12. Pancuronium was used for skeletal muscle relaxation in a patient undergoing total knee replacement surgery. To speed up the recovery of the skeletal muscles in the postoperative period, a combination of neostigmine and atropine was administered.
    i. Describe the pharmacological basis for the use of neostigmine to reverse the effect of pancuronium.
    ii. Justify the use of atropine along with neostigmine in this case.

Summary

- Hemicholinium blocks the transport of choline to nerve endings; vesamicol blocks the storage of ACh in vesicles, and the botulinum toxin blocks the release of ACh.
- Acetylcholine is not used clinically because of its non-selectivity and extremely short duration of action.
- Directly acting cholinergics are agonists at M and N receptors.
- The muscarinic actions of ACh include increased gastric secretion, inhibitory effect on the heart, bronchoconstriction, contraction of the smooth muscles in the walls of the gastrointestinal/genitourinary tract, and relaxation of the sphincters that favour defecation and voiding. Exocrine secretions are increased.
- The nicotinic actions of ACh include ganglionic stimulation and skeletal muscle contraction.
- Pilocarpine is used topically as a miotic in the treatment of glaucoma. An adverse effect associated with this drug is brow pain. Pilocarpine is also used in the form of lozenges as a sialagogue in Sjogren's syndrome.
- Bethanechol is useful in postoperative/postpartum paralytic ileus, urinary retention and congenital megacolon. However, mechanical obstruction of the tract must be ruled out.
- Indirectly acting cholinergics inhibit cholinesterase enzyme. These include carbamates and organophosphates.
- Reversible cholinesterase inhibitors include, pyridostigmine, neostigmine, rivastigmine, galantamine, donepezil, and tacrine.
- Neostigmine is useful in the treatment of myasthenia gravis, postoperative decurarisation, cobra bite, etc. Being a quaternary ammonium compound, it does not cross the blood–brain barrier and is free of central adverse effects. Atropine is combined with it to control muscarinic adverse effects.
- Edrophonium is short-acting, and hence is the preferred drug for the diagnosis of myasthenia gravis or for differentiating myasthenic crisis from cholinergic crisis.
- Donepezil, rivastigmine and tacrine improve symptoms of Alzheimer's disease.
- Organophosphates are irreversible cholinesterase inhibitors and are widely used as pesticides. Poisoning with OPCs is associated with a characteristic excess of secretions (rhinorrhea, lacrimation and salivation), pinpoint pupils, colic, bronchospasm, hypotension and shock. It is managed with supportive measures and specific antidote drug atropine 2 mg intravenous, repeated every 10 minutes until the pupil starts dilating, up to a maximum of 200 mg.
- Oximes are reactivators of cholinesterase and should be used within 24 hours of poisoning for maximal benefit. They have no role in carbamate poisoning.

Questions for practice

1. Explain why:
   a. Acetylcholine is not used clinically.
   b. Neostigmine is preferred over physostigmine for the management of myasthenia gravis.
   c. Edrophonium is used for the diagnosis of myasthenia gravis.
   d. Oximes are useful in OPC poisoning but not in carbamate poisoning.
   e. Atropine is combined with neostigmine for postoperative decurarisation.
   f. Obstruction of the genitourinary tract is ruled out before using cholinergic drugs.
2. Enumerate the therapeutic uses and adverse effects of cholinesterase inhibitors.
3. Describe the drugs used to achieve smoking cessation.
4. Write short notes on:
   a. Pilocarpine
   b. Mushroom poisoning
   c. OPC poisoning

Hints for problem-based questions and MCQs

1. i. c. Bethanechol
   ii. Through M_3 excitatory receptors, contraction of the wall and relaxation of the sphincters occur, relieving postoperative urinary retention
   iii. Rule out any mechanical obstruction of the genitourinary tract
   iv. Refer to page 95.

2. i. ACh is not useful clinically because of its very short duration of action and non-selectivity.
   ii. Refer to page 93.
   iii. Refer to Table 7.1, page 94.
3. i. c. Cutaneous
   ii. To control withdrawal symptoms and suppress cravings to some extent
   iii. Refer to page 96.
   iv. Bupropion and varenicline
4. i. To counteract the effect of the mydriatic after refraction testing
   ii. Brow pain occurs due to cyclospasm caused by pilocarpine
5. i. a. Pilocarpine
   ii. Pilocarpine increases salivary secretion due to the agonistic effect on M_3 receptors
6. i. Myasthenia gravis
   ii. Edrophonium 2 mg intravenous is administered as a test dose. If it is well-tolerated, 8 mg more is given after a few minutes. Edrophonium is a short-acting cholinesterase inhibitor as it binds to the anionic site of the cholinesterase enzyme and inhibits the degradation of ACh. As a result, ACh accumulates and acts on N_m receptors over a larger area, resulting in improved muscle power in myasthenia
   iii. b. Neostigmine
   iv. Refer to page 98.
7. i. c. Edrophonium, as it has a very short duration of action
   ii. Myasthenic crisis or cholinergic crisis
   iii. Refer to page 98.
8. i. c. Inhibiting cholinesterase in the brain
   ii. Increased cholinergic transmission in the CNS improves symptoms of Alzheimer's disease
   iii. Tacrine, rivastigmine, donepezil and galantamine are useful
9. i. OPC poisoning
   ii. Excess accumulation of ACh causes the symptoms mentioned
   iii. Atropine, oximes; refer to page 99.
10. i. c. 2 mg repeated every 10 minutes
11. i. a. Propoxur
    ii. Propoxur is a carbamate and the rest of the drugs mentioned are organophosphates. In carbamate poisoning, the anionic site is not free to allow pralidoxime binding (refer to page 100).
12. i. Pancuronium is a competitive antagonist of ACh at the N_m receptors on the motor end plate. Postoperatively, its effect can be reversed by increasing the concentration of ACh at the motor end plate with the help of a cholinesterase inhibitor like neostigmine.
    ii. To prevent cholinergic muscarinic adverse effects of neostigmine.

CONCEPT MAP - VARIABILITY IN DRUG RESPONSE

CHOLINERGIC DRUGS

1. Classification

Directly Acting Drugs
Acetylcholine, Pilocarpine, Carbachol, Bethanochol

Indirectly Acting Drugs

Reversible:
- **Carbamates:** Neostigmine, Pyridostigmine, Physostigmine, Rivastigmine, Donepezil, Galantamine
- **Acridine:** Tacrine

Irreversible:
- **Carbamates:** Carbaryl, Propoxur
- **Organophosphates:** Ecothiophate, Diazinon, Parathion, Malathion, Nerve gases

2. Mechanism of Action

- Agonists at Muscarinic receptors (M_1–M_5) Nicotinic receptors (N_n, N_m)
- Inhibit cholinesterase enzyme

Major Pharmacological Actions

Muscarinic actions
- Negative ino/chrono/dromotropic
- Increased exocrine secretions
- Miosis, Bronchoconstriction
- Smooth muscle contraction, Sphincter relaxation in GIT and Urinary tract

Nicotinic actions
- Skeletal muscle contraction
- Ganglionic stimulation

3. Therapeutic Uses

- **ACh:** Not used clinically because of non-selective and very-short-lasting action
- **Pilocarpine:** Glaucoma, Sjogren syndrome
- **Bethanechol:** Post-operative paralytic ileus, Urinary retention, Congenital megacolon
- **Physostigmine:** As miotic
- **Neostigmine:** Myasthenia gravis, Post operative decrurarisation, Cobra bite
- **Donepezil / Rivastigmine:** Alzheimer disease
- **OPC:** As insecticides and nerve gases for chemical warfare

4. ADRs

- Increased salivary, sweat, lacrimal, and tracheobronchial secretion
- Dyspepsia due to increased gastric secretion, Abdominal cramps, Diarrhea
- Involuntary micturition
- Bronchospasm & dyspnea, especially in asthmatics
- Bradycardia, hypotension
- Muscular weakness & paralysis, etc.

OPC poisoning

Clinical features: Increased secretions (rhinorrhea, lacrimation, salivation), pin-point pupil, colic, hypotension, bronchospasm, shock.
Treatment: Supportive, Atropine, Oximes

5. Caution/Contraindications

- Rule out mechanical obstruction of GIT, Urinary tract
- Bronchial asthma, COPD
- Peptic ulcer
- Coronary artery disease
- Hyperthyroidism

SECTION 2 Drugs Acting on ANS and PNS

8 Anticholinergic Drugs

PH 2.2 Describe types, salient pharmacokinetics, pharmacodynamics, therapeutic uses, adverse drug reactions of anticholinergic drugs.

Learning objectives

A student of MBBS phase II should be able to:
- Classify anticholinergic drugs.
- Describe the mechanism of action of anticholinergic drugs.
- Describe the pharmacological basis for various therapeutic indications of anticholinergic drugs.
- Enumerate therapeutic uses of anticholinergic drugs, mentioning important doses and their adverse effects.
- Describe contraindications to the use of atropine.

Cholinergic receptors are of two main types: **muscarinic** and **nicotinic**. Drugs blocking these receptors include:
- Muscarinic receptor antagonists, usually called antimuscarinic or anticholinergic drugs.
- Nicotinic receptor antagonists, which
    - at N_n receptor are called ganglionic blockers
    - at N_m receptor are called neuromuscular junction blockers.

ANTICHOLINERGIC/ANTIMUSCARINIC DRUGS
Classification of Antimuscarinic Drugs

Loosely called anticholinergic, this class of drugs includes natural alkaloids, their semisynthetic derivatives and synthetic compounds (Flowchart 8.1).

In addition to muscarinaic receptor blocking drugs, **hemicholium** (which decreases the uptake of choline into cholinergic nerve ending), **vesamicol** (which decreases the

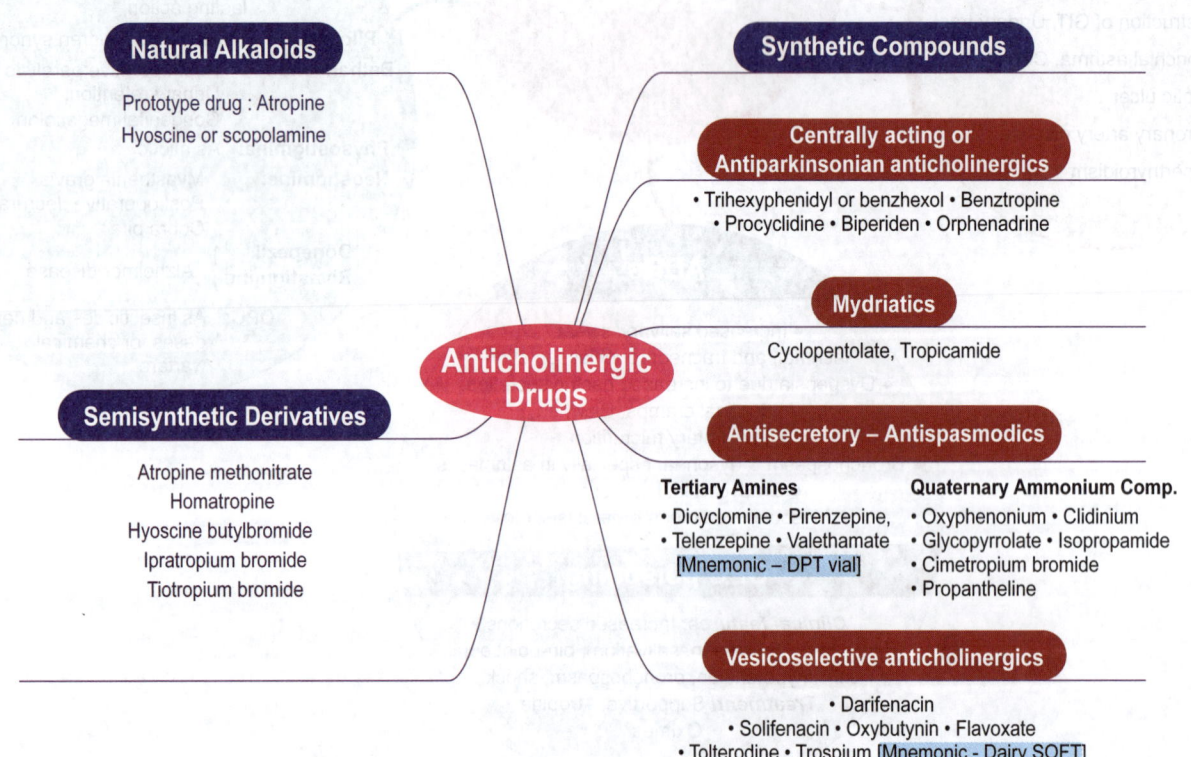

Flowchart 8.1 Classification of anticholinergic drugs

uptake of formed acetylcholine into vesicles) and **botulinum toxin A, B** (which decrease the release of acetylcholine from nerve ending) also exert anticholinergic actions.

Clinically Relevant Pharmacokinetic Features

- Natural alkaloids (atropine, hyoscine) and tertiary amines (dicyclomine, pirenzepine, telenzipine, valethamate) are rapidly absorbed after oral administration.
- Hyoscine can cross intact skin and has good penetration into CNS. As a result, it can be used as transdermal patch for motion sickness.
- Quaternary ammonium compounds are absorbed to a limited extent, typically ranging from 10–30%, and due to their polar nature, they are unable to cross the blood–brain barrier.
- Atropine is partly metabolised and partly excreted unchanged by kidney. Its half-life is 2 hours, but its effect lasts for about 72 hours in the eye. Hence, shorter-acting atropine substitutes such as tropicamide are preferred for ophthalmic uses.

Clinical problem-based questions and MCQs

1. i. **Identify the anticholinergic drug that can cross the intact skin:**
   a. Ipratropium b. Oxybutynin
   c. Hyoscine d. Clidinium
   ii. What is the clinical implication of such transdermal absorption of drugs?

2. **Which of the following drugs is a tertiary amine?**
   a. Clidinium b. Valethamate
   c. Oxyphenonium d. Isopropamide

3. **Tropicamide is preferred over atropine for ophthalmic uses because of its**
   a. Higher selectivity
   b. Lower toxicity
   c. Shorter duration of action
   d. Wider margin of safety

4. **Identify the drug with vesicoselective anticholinergic activity:**
   a. Flavoxate b. Trihexyphenidyl
   c. Ipratropium d. Dicyclomine

Mechanism of Action

Atropine is a muscarinic blocker that exhibits no significant activity at other receptor types. It is a **competitive antagonist of acetylcholine at all subtypes of muscarinic receptors,** i.e., it blocks M_1, M_2, M_3, M_4 and M_5 receptors. Hyoscine and ipratropium bromide are also non-selective drugs. However, certain synthetic agents exhibit some selectivity for specific muscarinic receptor subtypes, such as

M_1**-selective** – Pirenzepine, Telenzipine
M_2**-selective** – Gallamine, Tripitramine
M_3**-selective** – Oxybutynin, Darifenacin, Tolterodine

Different **tissues vary in their sensitivity to atropine**'s actions.

- Salivary glands, sweat glands and bronchial glands are the most sensitive.
- Myocardium and smooth muscles exhibit intermediate sensitivity to atropine.
- Gastric parietal cells are the least sensitive.

Pharmacological Actions

Most of the pharmacological actions of atropine can be predicted easily from its property to block all subtypes of muscarinic receptors. Table 8.1 shows the clinically relevant actions of atropine produced by antagonising ACh action at various subtypes of muscarinic receptors.

1. Central nervous system

- Low doses of anticholinergic drugs (except hyoscine) do not produce significant central effects.
- **Hyoscine** has depressant action on the CNS and reduces vestibular excitation This effect is **useful in motion sickness.** It also causes amnesia and drowsiness. This effect induces a 'twilight sleep'-like mental state, which has historically been utilised as a so-called 'truth serum' during **lie detection** procedures conducted on suspects.
- **Atropine** has dose-dependent central actions. Therapeutic doses have mild **CNS stimulant action** (especially on vagal, vasomotor and respiratory centre), followed by slowly developing but longer lasting sedative action. CNS stimulant action of higher doses of atropine manifests as excitement, agitation, restlessness, disorientation, delirium, hallucinations and psychosis. [Mnemonic for one important feature of atropine toxicity is, 'mad as hatter', suggestive of insanity. The description hints at the dementia-like symptoms experienced by hat makers owing to their long-term exposure to mercury products used in hat making.]
- Centrally acting anticholinergic drugs like **benzhexol, benztropine, procyclidine,** and **biperiden** improve the balance of dopaminergic and cholinergic transmission in parkinsonism. They reduce tremors and rigidity, which is especially **beneficial in parkinsonism** induced by typical antipsychotic drugs. In such cases levodopa is not effective, as D_2 receptors are already blocked by the offending drug.

2. Cardiovascular system

Atropine administration causes transient **initial bradycardia, followed by tachycardia**.

Initial bradycardia is probably due to:

- Central stimulant effect on vagal centre
- Blockade of presynaptic muscarinic autoreceptors present on vagal postganglionic fibres in SA node, which enhances ACh release.

Table 8.1 Clinically relevant actions of atropine as an antagonist of ACh action

Receptor name and nature	Distribution	Effect of acetylcholine or agonist	Effect of atropine or muscarinic antagonist or blocker	Clinical implications
M_1 receptors **Excitatory**	Gastric glands	Increased gastric secretion	Decreased gastric secretion (acid, pepsin as well as mucus secretions are decreased)	May be useful in peptic ulcer but less efficacious than H_2 blockers
M_2 receptors **Inhibitory**	Heart	Decreased heart rate	Tachycardia	Useful in bradyarrhythmias
		Decreased AV conduction	Increased AV conduction and reduced PR interval	Useful in partial heart blocks
		*Atrial refractory period abbreviated	(Prolongs atrial refractory period)	*Useful in atrial flutter and fibrillation, as muscarinic effects are blocked in atria
M_3 receptors **Excitatory**	Exocrine glands	Increased secretions	Decreased secretions from:	
			Salivary and sweat glands	**Dryness** of mouth, dry skin, decreased sweating, atropine fever
			Lacrimal glands	Dry, sandy eyes
			Tracheobronchial glands	Thickening and inspissation of bronchial secretions are typical anticholinergic side effects
	Smooth muscles	Contraction of smooth muscles	Relaxation of smooth muscles	
	Eye	Miosis Cyclospasm	- Passive mydriasis - Cycloplegia	Useful in fundoscopy, testing refractory errors, inflammation of eye. Because of the mydriatic effect, atropine is **contraindicated in glaucoma**. ADRs: blurring of visions, photophobia
	Bronchi	Bronchoconstriction	Bronchodilatation	Useful in **bronchial asthma and COPD**
	GIT Genitourinary	Contraction of wall and relaxation of sphincters in GIT and genitourinary tract	Spasmolytic action	Useful as antispasmodic drugs in hypermotility; useful in common traveller's diarrhea **but risk of urinary retention** in elderly males

*Abbreviation of atrial refractory period by ACh cannot be predicted from the nature of receptors, which is paradoxical.

[Muscarinic autoreceptors are inhibitory in nature. ACh reduces its own release by binding to these receptors. Thus, the blockade of these receptors by atropine augments ACh release.]

Thereafter, the blockade of M_2 receptors present in heart leads to cardio-stimulant action causing

- Increased heart rate, i.e., tachycardia.
- Improved conduction – **reduced PR interval,** which is useful in partial heart blocks.
- Blockade of effect of ACh on atria prolongs atrial refractory period and makes it useful in atrial flutter and fibrillation.
- Blockade of EDRF release from endothelium in response to cholinergic drugs.
- Blockade of vasodilation of skeletal muscle blood vessels, mediated through sympathetic cholinergic fibres.
- Through an unknown mechanism, high doses of atropine cause cutaneous vasodilatation especially in blush area and upper body

[Mnemonic for atropine toxicity due to this cutaneous vasodilatation: Red as beet]

3. Eye

Atropine has a slow-developing but longer-lasting effect in the eyes. Although the half-life of atropine is 2 hours, its effect in eye persists for 72 hours.

- Blockade of M_3 receptors in circular muscles of iris leads to **passive mydriasis** due to unopposed dilator action of the sympathetic system (Fig. 8.1). [It is called passive, because the circular muscles of the iris do not contract or are passive. In contrast, mydriasis resulting from contraction of the dilator pupillae muscle, mediated by sympathetic stimulation, is referred to as active mydriasis.]
- This may be useful in fundoscopic examination and for prevention and breaking of adhesions/synechia in eye by alternating it with a miotic. However, the mydriatic effect of anticholinergic drugs may be risky in patients with narrow iridocorneal angle, where acute attack of glaucoma can be precipitated due to reduced aqueous drainage.
- M_3 blockade in ciliary muscles causes **cycloplegia**. This effect makes atropine useful for diagnosis of refractory errors. Long-lasting ophthalmic effect of atropine is also utilised to relieve painful spasm of intraocular

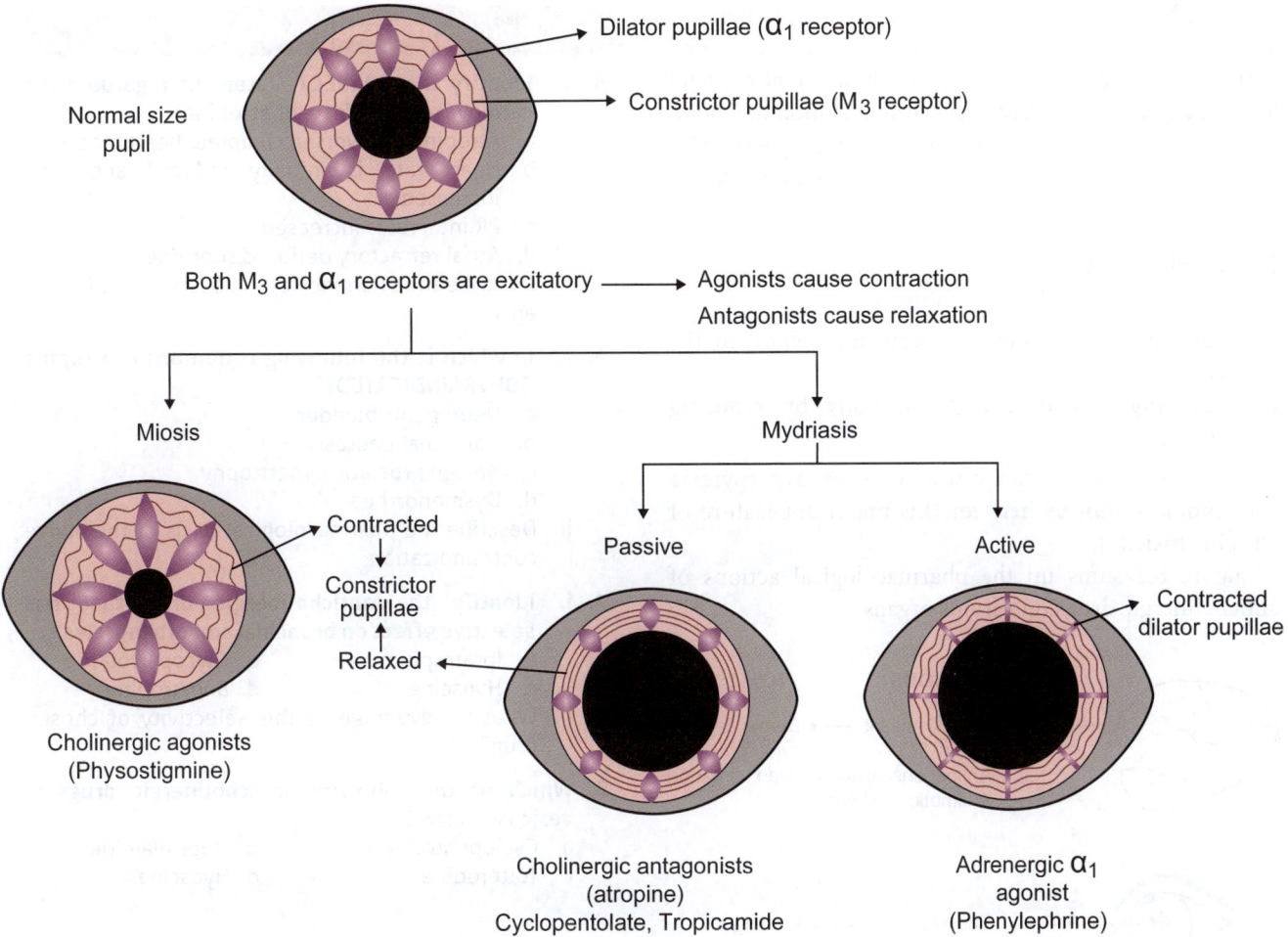

Fig. 8.1 Effect of autonomic drugs on pupil size

muscles in inflammatory conditions of the eye such as iritis, iridocyclitis and keratitis.
- The drawback of cycloplegic effect is the loss of ability to accommodate for near vision leading to **blurring of vision, abolition of light reflex and photophobia**. Thus, blurring of vision is also one of the characteristic features of atropine toxicity. [Mnemonic: **blind as bat**]
- M_3 blockade in exocrine glands causes **reduced lacrimal secretions** resulting in dry or 'sandy' eyes as an adverse effect.

4. Respiratory system
- The blockade of M_3 receptors by atropine in bronchial smooth muscles leads to **bronchodilator** effect, wherein the airway resistance gets reduced. The effect is beneficial in patients with bronchial asthma and chronic obstructive pulmonary disease (COPD).
- Atropine also **reduces mucociliary clearance** by bronchial epithelium.
- **Tracheobronchial secretions are reduced**, and become thick, inspissated.

Ipratropium bromide, a semisynthetic derivative, is preferred over atropine for regular prophylaxis in asthma patients, because **ipratropium has selective action on bronchial smooth muscles,** resulting in bronchodilatation. It has no effect on the volume or consistency of tracheobronchial secretions and mucociliary clearance.

5. Gastrointestinal effects
Atropine has **spasmolytic** action in the GIT, as it reduces the tone as well as amplitude of contraction of smooth muscles. However, peristalsis is not completely suppressed because ACh is not the only transmitter responsible for peristaltic activity of gut. Other NTMs like 5-HT, enkephalins and local reflexes are also involved.

Due to visceral smooth muscle relaxing action, anticholinergic drugs are useful in conditions such as irritable bowel syndrome and intestinal/ biliary colic, but they can cause constipation as an adverse effect.

Anticholinergic drugs **decrease the volume of gastric juice** by reducing acid, pepsin and mucus secretion, but the effect on pH of gastric secretions is not marked. The effect on intestinal and pancreatic secretions is lesser.

6. Genitourinary tract
Atropine exerts **spasmolytic** action in the genitourinary tract also, and is useful in ureteric colic, urinary incontinence, overactive neurogenic bladder and nocturnal

enuresis. Vesicoselective anticholinergics like darifenacin and flavoxate can relieve urinary urgency, frequency and dysuria associated with lower UTI. These are also useful for dysmenorrhea and hasten cervical dilatation in labour.

In elderly males with benign prostatic hypertrophy, anticholinergic drugs may cause urinary retention. Hence, they are contraindicated in such cases.

7. Miscellaneous

Atropine can raise body temperature by:
- Stimulating the temperature regulating centre in the brain
- Decreasing loss of heat from body by reducing sweating

High or toxic doses can cause fever or hyperpyrexia [Mnemonic – 'hot as hen' for this important feature of atropine toxicity].

Figure 8.2 sums up the pharmacological actions of anticholinergic drugs on various organs.

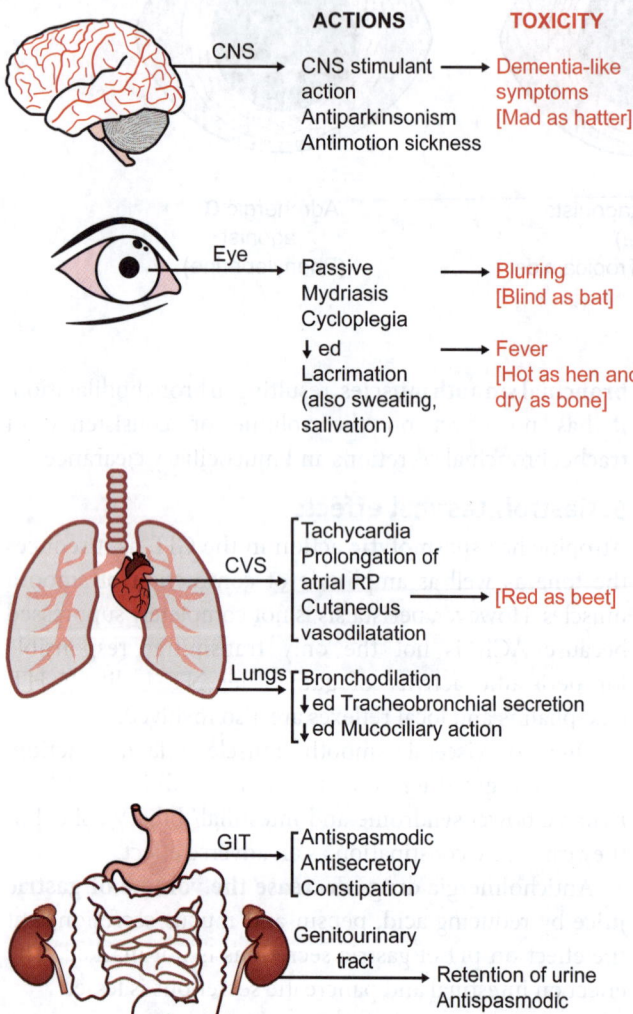

Fig. 8.2 *Pharmacological actions of anticholinergic drugs*

Clinical problem-based questions and MCQs

5. i. Identify the CORRECT statement regarding the cardiovascular effects of atropine:
   a. Atropine can worsen complete heart blocks
   b. Heart rate is initially reduced and then increased
   c. PR interval is increased
   d. Atrial refractory period is shortened.
   ii. Describe the pharmacological basis to justify your answer.

6. i. In which is the following conditions is atropine CONTRAINDICATED?
   a. Neurogenic bladder
   b. Nocturnal enuresis
   c. Benign prostatic hypertrophy
   d. Dysmenorrhea
   ii. Describe the pharmacological basis of the above contraindication.

7. i. Identify the anticholinergic drug that has selective effect on bronchial smooth muscles.
   a. Ipratropium   b. Glycopyrrolate
   c. Hyoscine   d. Benztropine
   ii. What is advantage of this selectivity of chosen drug?

8. Which of the following anticholinergic drugs is vesicoselective?
   a. Cyclopentolate   b. Isopropamide
   c. Tolterodine   d. Hyoscine

THERAPEUTIC USES OF ANTICHOLINERGIC DRUGS

A. Natural Drugs

Atropine has been superseded by its congeners or other drugs for most of the indications, but it is still useful in the following conditions.

- Atropine is a lifesaving drug in **organophosphate poisoning**. It acts as a specific antidote by blocking muscarinic receptors. **Atropine is given in a dose of 2 mg intravenously and can be repeated after every 10 minutes**, till the pupil starts dilating. Atropine is continued for about a week, till new cholinesterase enzyme is synthesised, and takes over the function of ACh degradation.

- Atropine is used to relieve symptoms of **early mushroom poisoning** called mycetism (Box 8.1).

Box 8.1 Types of mushroom poisoning

Mushroom poisoning can be of three types based on species of mushrooms ingested.

a. *Early mushroom poisoning* caused by *Inocybe* and *Clitocybe* species: Symptoms of muscarinic excess like bradycardia, excessive exocrine secretions, colicky pain,

and diarrhea occur within half an hour of ingestion of mushrooms of these species. These can be reversed by atropine.
b. *Hallucinogenic poisoning* caused by *Amantia muscaria* species: Ingestion of mushrooms of this species causes restlessness, ataxia, delirium, hallucinations, etc., which can be worsened by central effects of atropine. So, atropine is contraindicated in such poisoning.
c. *Late mushroom poisoning* caused by *Amantia phalloides* and *Galerina* species: These mushrooms contain amatoxins, which interfere with mRNA synthesis resulting in hepatic and renal function impairment. Atropine has no role in such cases. Treatment is mainly supportive. Thioctic acid, silibinin and penicillin may have some role.

- Atropine is also used as '**pre-anesthetic medication**' to reduce tracheobronchial secretions before giving irritant inhalational anesthetics However, glycopyrrolate is preferred for this indication as it is free from central side effects.
- In **pulmonary embolism**, atropine is used to reduce reflexly evoked respiratory secretions.
- Atropine can be used for relief of ocular pain and spasm in **inflammatory conditions of the eye** such as iritis, keratitis, iridocyclitis and corneal ulcers. The long duration of ocular action (72 hours) of atropine is an advantage in these conditions. It can be alternated with a miotic to prevent the formation of adhesion/synechia between the iris, lens and cornea or to break the adhesions formed secondary to inflammation. It is also used topically as ophthalmic ointment for **refraction testing in children**.
- Atropine is useful in **partial heart blocks** and **bradyarrhythmias** due to raised vagal tone in patients of myocardial infarction and digoxin toxicity.
- It is combined **with neostigmine** to prevent muscarinic adverse effects in conditions like decurarisation or myasthenia gravis.

Hyoscine is effective in preventing **motion sickness** due to its central anticholinergic action. It readily crosses intact skin and is administered as a transdermal patch applied behind the pinna prior to travel. It is also used **as 'truth serum'** in lie detection tests.

B. Semisynthetic Drugs

Hyoscine butylbromide is longer acting than atropine. It is widely used for **intestinal colic** in a dose of 20–40 mg via oral route.

Ipratropium bromide has a slowly-developing bronchodilator effect, which is maximum after 40–60 minutes of administration, and lasts for 4–6 hours. So, it is more useful for **regular prophylaxis in bronchial asthma and COPD** rather than for relieving acute attack. It is administered via the inhalational route in a dose of 20–40 micrograms per puff. Two puffs are inhaled through a metered dose inhaler, thrice a day.

- The efficacy of ipratropium is greater in COPD than in bronchial asthma as it blocks increase in parasympathetic tone, which is an important contributing factor in COPD.
- Ipratropium nasal spray can be used for symptomatic relief in **perennial rhinitis and common cold**.
- **Ipratropium is preferred over atropine for respiratory conditions,** as atropine suppresses mucociliary function and causes thickening and inspissations of respiratory tract secretions. These secretions may form a mucus plug that is difficult to clear when the mucociliary function is suppressed. In contrast, ipratropium causes selective bronchial smooth muscle relaxation. It has no effect on the mucociliary function of bronchial epithelium or the consistency of tracheobronchial secretions.
- **Tiotropium bromide** is a congener of ipratropium with higher selectivity of bronchial action. It is also used via the inhalational route using a rotahaler. Its effect lasts longer than ipratropium and thus, one dose daily is sufficient.

C. Synthetic Drugs
a. Centrally acting anticholinergics

Centrally acting anticholinergics like trihexyphenidyl and benztropine are useful in relieving the tremors and rigidity of **parkinsonism**. They also reduce excessive sweating and salivation in parkinsonism. They are less efficacious than levodopa, but are better tolerated.

- These drugs are useful in drug-induced parkinsonism, in which levodopa is not effective as D_2 receptors are blocked by the offending drug.
- They are also useful in patients in whom levodopa is contraindicated, e.g., patients with psychotic, liver and kidney disease, ischemic heart disease, and glaucoma.
- In severe cases of parkinsonism, central anticholinergics can be used as adjuvants to levodopa for reducing its dose and restoring balance between dopaminergic and cholinergic transmission.
- The dose of trihexyphenidyl and orphenadrine is 2–10 mg by oral route. Their effect lasts for 4–8 hours. Therapy is started with the lowest dose, and gradually increased.

b. Mydriatics
- Mydriatics like cyclopentolate and tropicamide are useful for dilatation of pupil and to cause cycloplegia for **diagnostic purposes**. Tropicamide has a rapid onset of ocular action, typically within 20–40 minutes, with effects lasting for approximately 3–6 hours. Thus, tropicamide is preferred over atropine for diagnostic purpose in **refraction testing** and **fundus examination** with an ophthalmoscope, as photophobia and blurring lasts for a shorter time (3–6 hours only, in comparison to 72 hours with atropine)
- Cyclopentolate 0.5% and 1% eyedrops are preferred to block accommodation during refraction testing,

especially in children. Atropine, having more potent and longer lasting cycloplegic effect in eye (for about 72 hours), is used as 1% ointment for refraction testing in children as their tone of ciliary muscles is higher. Atropine ointment is applied topically in eye twice (24 hours and 2 hours) before testing for refractory errors.

c. Antispasmodic drugs

- **Dicyclomine** has anticholinergic, antiemetic and direct smooth muscle relaxant actions. It is useful in **morning sickness, motion sickness, dysmenorrhea and irritable bowel syndrome**. It is given via oral route or intramuscular route in a dose of 20–40 mg. Dicyclomine is very frequently used in spasmodic conditions in children as 10 mg/mL drops in a dose of 5–10 mg.
- M_1 selective blockers **pirenzepine** and **telenzepine** were previously used in peptic ulcer, but nowadays, proton pump inhibitors and H_2 blockers are preferred.
- **Valethamate** is useful in **urinary, biliary and intestinal colic**. It is also used for cervical dilatation to shorten the first stage of labour and to minimise **cervical dystocia**. Valethamate 8 mg IM can be repeated after half-hour intervals up to a maximum of three doses.
- Drugs such as **clidinium, cimetropium bromide** and **isopropamide** do not cross the blood–brain barrier because of the quaternary ammonium group present in their structure. So, there are no central adverse effects. These drugs are used in **irritable bowel syndrome (IBS), abdominal colic, and nervous dyspepsia**. The most common side effect is dryness of mouth. The dose of clidinium is 2.5–5 mg oral; isopropamide is also 5 mg oral and cimetropium is 50 mg, 2–3 times daily.
- **Glycopyrrolate**, another potent rapid-acting quaternary ammonium compound, is used exclusively for **pre-anesthetic medication** in a dose of 0.2–0.4 mg, given intramuscularly. It is preferred over atropine as it has no central side effects.

d. Vesicoselective drugs

- Anticholinergics such as **darifenacin, solifenacin, oxybutynin, flavoxate** and **tolterodine** have higher affinity for muscarinic receptors present in the urinary bladder, resulting in fewer adverse effects. These are useful in:
  - Controlling urinary urgency, frequency and urge incontinence
  - Neurogenic bladder (Box 8.2)
  - Nocturnal enuresis
  - Postoperative vesical spasm in prostatectomy
  - Symptomatic relief of dysuria in lower UTI.
- **Oxybutynin** has the shortest and **solifenacin** the longest duration of action among vesicoselective drugs.

- **Fesoterodine**, a prodrug of tolterodine, is also useful.
- **Trospium** is a quaternary amine that fails to cross the blood–brain barrier. So, it is free of central adverse effects and is safe for use in elderly people.

Box 8.2   Neurogenic bladder

Neurogenic bladder is characterised by a loss of voluntary bladder control resulting from impaired neural regulation of bladder function. It is classified into the following three types:

- **Spastic type** (overactive bladder): Also known as hyperactive bladder, characterised by increased frequency and/or urgency of urination due to hyperstimulation of the bladder's nerves and muscles. It is commonly associated with conditions such as stroke, multiple sclerosis, Parkinson's disease, Alzheimer's disease, and spinal cord injuries.
- **Flaccid type** (underactive bladder): Characterised by weak or absent bladder contractions, this type leads to incomplete emptying, increased post-void residual volume, overflow incontinence, and recurrent urinary tract infections (UTIs). It typically results from damage to peripheral nerves, as seen in diabetic neuropathy, benign prostatic hypertrophy (BPH), pelvic surgeries, and postmenopausal changes.
- **Mixed type:** In this form, patients exhibit features of both overactive and underactive bladder—such as urinary frequency, urgency, and retention—often observed in severe spinal injuries and advanced multiple sclerosis.

Management of neurogenic bladder

- In case of overactive bladder, initial non-pharmacological measures include behavioural therapy, bladder training, pelvic floor exercises, and fluid management.
- Drug therapy is tried only after exhausting the above mentioned measures. Vesicoselective anticholinergics such as darifenacin, solifenacin, and flavoxate help relieve urgency and incontinence.
- Mirabegron, a selective β_3-adrenoceptor agonist, is approved for overactive neurogenic bladder.
- Intravesical injection of botulinum toxin A is used in refractory cases, particularly in patients with persistent symptoms despite medical therapy. (Botulinum toxin A is approved for some other conditions like glabellar lines, blephrospasm, squint and cervical dystocia.)

Drotaverine

Drotaverine is another smooth-muscle relaxing drug frequently useful in spasmogenic conditions like renal, intestinal and biliary colic and IBS. It does not block cholinergic receptors. It acts by inhibition of phosphodiesterase 4 enzyme (PDE-4) in smooth muscles, resulting in raised cAMP/cGMP levels and smooth muscle relaxation (spasmolysis). It can be used via the oral route in a dose of 40–80 mg, thrice a day. IV injection is useful in severe pain. Drotaverine is free of typical anticholinergic adverse effects, but it may cause headache, dizziness, flushing and fall in BP with IV use. The therapeutic uses of anticholinergic drugs are summed up in Box 8.3.

Box 8.3 Therapeutic uses of anticholinergic drugs

1. Central uses
   - Motion sickness: Hyoscine
   - Drug-induced parkinsonism: Centrally acting anticholinergic agents such as benztropine, trihexyphenidyl (benzhexol), and biperiden
2. Partial heart block and bradyarrhythmias: Atropine is used
3. Ophthalmic uses:
   - Diagnostic - For inducing mydriasis and cycloplegia during refraction testing and fundus examination: Tropicamide, cyclopentolate preferred.
   - Therapeutic: In alternation with miotics to prevent or break synechia between iris, lens and cornea and to prevent painful ocular spasm in inflammatory conditions of the eye. Atropine is used, as the effect is required for a longer time.
4. For pre-anesthetic medication and in pulmonary embolism patients to reduce respiratory secretions: Glycopyrrolate and atropine are used.
5. For regular prophylaxis in bronchial asthma and COPD: Ipratropium bromide is preferred over atropine.
6. In conditions of muscarinic excess like OPC poisoning, early mushroom poisoning, along with neostigmine in decurarisation and myasthenia gravis: Atropine is used.
7. Useful in morning sickness, motion sickness, dysmenorrhea and irritable bowel syndrome: Dicyclomine is most frequently used.
8. Used in intestinal/ biliary/ ureteric colic: Synthetic antispasmodic drugs clidinium and isopropamide are used.
9. Used for cervical dilatation to shorten the first stage of labour and for minimising cervical dystocia: Valethamate
10. For controlling urinary urgency, frequency and urge incontinence in neurogenic bladder, nocturnal enuresis, postoperative vesical spasm in prostatectomy: Vesicoselective drugs like darifenacin, and flavoxate are preferred.
11. For symptomatic relief of dysuria in lower UTI: Flavoxate is useful.

Clinical problem-based questions and MCQs

9. A 42-year-old patient presents with a history of long-term smoking. He ceased smoking four years ago following a diagnosis of chronic obstructive pulmonary disease (COPD). He was prescribed an inhalational drug for preventing acute exacerbation of symptoms.
   i. Identify the inhalational drug preferred for regular prophylaxis of COPD:
      a. Valethamate   b. Dicyclomine
      c. Ipratropium   d. Atropine
   ii. Describe the rationale for preferring the chosen drug over the other options given.
   iii. State the dose of this drug used by MDI.

10. i. Select the most appropriate drug used prior to refraction tests in children:
      a. Cyclopentolate   b. Atropine
      c. Tropicamide   d. Isopropamide
    ii. Describe pharmacological basis to justify your choice.

11. A 55-year-old patient with a history of heavy smoking for nearly 35 years is suffering from cardiac disease and chronic obstructive pulmonary disease. The patient frequently has episodes of bronchospasm and dyspnea.
    i. Which of the following bronchodilators is most suitable for regular prophylaxis in this case, keeping in mind both COPD and heart disease?
       a. Salbutamol   b. Aminophylline
       c. Isoprenaline   d. Ipratropium
    ii. Describe the pharmacological basis to justify your choice.

12. A 38-weeks pregnant, primigravida presents in the OBG OPD with labour pains. She was shifted to the labour room. Oxytocin drip was started. The patient showed poor progress of labour, had cervical dystocia and was in first stage for about 10 hours. Valethamate 8 mg was injected intramuscularly.
    i. Identify the drug class to which valethamate belongs.
       a. Selective β2 agonist
       b. Muscarinic antagonist
       c. Phosphodiesterase-4 inhibitor
       d. α antagonist
    ii. Describe the pharmacological basis of injecting valethamate in the patient
    iii. After how long it may be repeated in case of non-responsiveness?

13. A 45-year-old male patient, a known case of schizophrenia, was on antipsychotic drug treatment. The patient presented with extrapyramidal symptoms like tremors, bradykinesia and rigidity as an adverse effect of the antipsychotic drug.
    i. Identify most suitable drug for control of extrapyramidal symptoms in this case.
       a. Diazepam   b. Levodopa
       c. Selegiline   d. Trihexyphenidyl
    ii. Describe the pharmacological basis for use of chosen drug in this patient.
    iii. Enumerate the adverse reactions of the chosen drug.

14. A 22-year-old woman presenting with visual disturbances underwent refraction to assess for refractory error. Prior to the procedure, she was administered eyedrops to facilitate evaluation.
    i. Identify the drug given as eyedrops in this patient:
       a. Physostigmine   b. Tropicamide
       c. Atropine   d. Carbachol
    ii. Describe the pharmacological basis for using the chosen drug for refraction testing.
    iii. Why is the chosen drug is preferred over other options?

15. A 30-year-old male patient with intestinal colic was given intravenous drotaverine.
    i. Identify the correct mechanism of action of drotaverine.
        a. Phosphodiesterase 4 inhibition
        b. 5-HT$_3$ antagonism
        c. M$_3$ antagonism
        d. D$_2$ blockade
    ii. Describe the mechanism of spasmolytic action of drotaverine.
    iii. What is the advantage of drotaverine over anticholinergic antispasmodics?
    iv. What are the possible adverse reactions (ADRs) with intravenous drotaverine?

16. A 38-year-old obese female patient presented with nausea and pain in the right hypochondrium. USG examination revealed multiple small stones in the gall bladder. A diagnosis of cholelithiasis was made and laparoscopic cholecystectomy was advised. On the day of surgery, injection glycopyrrolate, 0.4 mg/kg body-weight, was administered before anesthetising the patient.
    i. Classify glycopyrrolate.
    ii. Describe the pharmacological basis for using glycopyrrolate before anesthesia.
    iii. Why is glycopyrrolate preferred over atropine for this indication?

17. A 65-year-old male patient suffering from severe UTI complains of dysuria.
    i. Select the most suitable drug for symptomatic relief in this case.
        a. Flavoxate   b. Clidinium
        c. Dicyclomine   d. Valethamate
    ii. Give reasons to justify your answer.

ADVERSE EFFECTS OF ANTICHOLINERGIC DRUGS

The following are the most commonly encountered adverse effects of anticholinergic drugs.

- Dryness of mouth is most frequent ADR. It results in difficulty in swallowing, talking, etc.
- Dry, sandy eyes
- Dry, hot and flushed skin. Flushing occurs especially in blush area of face and Atropine fever may occur.
- Photophobia and blurring of vision
- Palpitation
- Weak, rapid pulse
- Difficulty in passing urine. In elderly patients with benign prostatic hypertrophy (BPH), it may cause urinary retention.
- Constipation

Atropine Toxicity

Atropine toxicity [Mnemonic: **dry as bone, blind as bat, red as beet, hot as hen and mad as hatter**] is characterised by

- Excitement, agitation, restlessness, psychosis, convulsions (Mad as hatter)
- Fever and hyperpyrexia (Hot as hen)
- Reduced exocrine secretions (Dry as bone)
- Cutaneous vasodilation (Red as beet)
- Blurred vision (Blind as bat)
- Tachycardia

Toxic doses of atropine may cause coma, respiratory depression and cardio vascular collapse.

Treatment is mainly symptomatic.

- Maintenance of airways, breathing and circulation is of prime importance, as in any other poisoning.
- Gastric lavage is done with tannic acid, as KMnO$_4$ cannot oxidise atropine. If toxicity is due to ingestion, gastric lavage with tannic acid can prevent further absorption of drug.
- As the patient is likely to be agitated, he should be kept in a dark room with quiet surroundings.
- IV diazepam may be required to control convulsions.
- Hyperpyrexia is controlled by cold sponging. Injection paracetamol is also useful.
- Physostigmine may be used as a last resort measure to reverse both central and peripheral effects of atropine. It is preferred over neostigmine for this indication because it is a tertiary amine and can cross blood–brain barrier to reverse central effects of atropine.

Cautions/Contraindications of Atropine

Anticholinergic drugs should be avoided or used with caution in the following cases.

1. Elderly male patients with **benign prostatic hypertrophy**, as they may cause retention of urine
2. In **gastric peptic ulcer**, because they cause gastric stasis due to smooth muscle relaxant action. So, the gastric ulcers get exposed to acidic contents for a longer period of time. Although anticholinergic drugs decrease the secretion of gastric acid, pepsin and mucus, they do not have any marked effect on the pH of gastric contents.
3. In patients with **narrow iridocorneal angle**, the mydriatic effect of atropine further interferes with the drainage of aquous humor and raises intraocular tension which can precipitate an acute attack of glaucoma.

Clinical problem-based questions and MCQs

18. A 54-year-old female patient presented in a confused and agitated state with convulsions, high grade fever, dry mouth, difficulty in talking, swallowing, difficulty in micturition and blurring of vision a couple of hours after eating berries of the belladonna plant. On examination, her pupil was found dilated and tongue and skin were dry. Her temperature was 104°F; PR was 134 per minute.
    i. What is the diagnosis?
        a. OPC poisoning

    b. Mushroom poisoning
    c. Atropine poisoning
    d. Opioid poisoning
  ii. Explain the cause of tachycardia and high temperature in this patient.
  iii. Describe management of this case.
19. Select the condition in which atropine is contraindicated:
    a. Pulmonary embolism
    b. Partial AV block
    c. Glaucoma
    d. Bronchial asthma

    Justify for your answer.
20. Explain why atropine is contraindicated in gastric peptic ulcer.

Summary

- Atropine is a competitive blocker at all subtypes of muscarinic receptors.
- Salivary/sweat and bronchial glands are the most sensitive to atropine, followed by myocardium, smooth muscles and gastric parietal cells in that order.
- Atropine has been superseded by its semisynthetic or synthetic congeners or other drugs for most of the indications. However, atropine is still preferred over all its congeners as sapecific antidote in OPC poisoning and early mushroom poisoning, because in these cases the effect of poison needs to be counteracted at all sites.
- Hyoscine can cross intact skin and has better penetration across blood–brain barrier, causing drowsiness and amnesia. It is used in motion sickness as a transdermal patch, and in lie detection test as truth serum.
- Ipratropium has a slowly-developing bronchodilator effect and is used via the inhalation route for regular prophylaxis in bronchial asthma and COPD. It lacks depressant effect on mucociliary function and tracheobronchial secretions. Its efficacy is greater in COPD compared to bronchial asthma.
- Cyclopentolate and tropicamide, having faster onset and shorter duration of ophthalmic action than atropine, are preferred over atropine for diagnostic ophthalmic indications.
- For relieving painful spasm of intraocular muscles in inflammatory conditions of the eyes, the longer-lasting ophthalmic effect of atropine (about 72 hours) is more desirable.
- Synthetic anticholinergics with their prominent antisecretory and antispasmodic activity are useful in intestinal, biliary and ureteric colic as well as cervical dystocia in labour.
- Quaternary ammonium compounds are free of central side effects.
- Some drugs like darifenacin, tolterodine and flavoxate have vesicoselective action and are useful in controlling urinary urgency, frequency and urge incontinence, in neurogenic bladder and for symptomatic relief of dysuria in lower UTI.
- Synthetic anticholinergics like trihexyphenidyl and benztropine, with their prominent central effects, are useful in relieving extrapyramidal symptoms or drug-induced parkinsonism.
- Typical anticholinergic adverse effects include dry mouth, dry/sandy eyes, dry hot and flushed skin, photophobia, blurring of vision, palpitation, weak, rapid pulse, constipation and difficulty in passing urine.
- In elderly patients with benign prostatic hypertrophy (BPH), anticholinergic drugs may cause urinary retention.
- Anticholinergic drugs are contraindicated in patients with narrow iridocorneal angle due to the risk of precipitating acute glaucoma.
- Atropine toxicity manifests as tachycardia, confusion, agitation, hyperpyrexia and convulsions. It is managed with supportive measures.

Questions for practice

1. Classify anticholinergic drugs.
2. Explain the pharmacological basis for:
   a. Use of injection glycopyrrolate in pre-anesthetic medication.
   b. Use of flavoxate in lower urinary tract infection.
   c. Use of trihexyphenidyl in schizophrenic patients on antipsychotic drug therapy.
   d. Use of hyoscine transdermal patch before journey
3. Write short notes on:
   a. Vesicoselective anticholinergics
   b. Antisecretory antispasmodics
   c. Drotaverine
   d. Ipratropium bromide
4. Enumerate the therapeutic uses of atropine-like drugs.
5. Enumerate the adverse effects and contraindications of anticholinergics.

Hints for problem-based questions and MCQs

1. i. c. Hyoscine
   ii. Hyoscine can be used as transdermal patch for motion sickness.
2. b. Valethamate
3. c. Shorter duration of action
4. a. Flavoxate
5. i. b. Heart rate is initially reduced and then increased by atropine
   ii. Refer to page 105, 106.

6. i. c. Benign prostatic hypertrophy
   ii. Refer to page 108.
7. i. a. Ipratropium
   ii. Refer to page 107.
8. c. Tolterodine
9. i. c. Ipratropium
   ii. Valethamate and dicyclomine are mainly antispasmodics. Ipratropium has a selective, slowly-developing bronchodilator effect, and is thus more useful for regular prophylaxis in bronchial asthma and COPD. Ipratropium has no effect on mucociliary function of bronchial epithelium and consistency of tracheobronchial secretions, unlike atropine.
   iii. It is administered by the inhalational route in a dose of 20–40 micrograms per puff. Two puffs are inhaled through a metered dose inhaler, thrice a day.
10. i. b. Atropine
    i. Refer to page 110.
11. i. d. Ipratropium
    iii. Salbutamol is a selective β_2 agonist; isoprenaline is a selective β agonist; aminophylline is a phosphodiesterase inhibitor. All have bronchodilator effects. β agonists are more useful in aborting acute attack of bronchial asthma. Aminophylline has a cardiac stimulant action, which can cause tachycardia and may be harmful in such patients. The efficacy of ipratropium is more in COPD than in bronchial asthma as it blocks increase in parasympathetic tone, an important contributing factor in COPD.
12. i. b. Muscarinic antagonist
    ii. The antispasmodic action of valethamate is used for cervical dilatation to shorten the first stage of labour and minimise cervical dystocia.
    iii. Valethamate, 8 mg IM, can be repeated at half-an-hour intervals and a maximum of three doses can be administered.
13. i. d. Trihexyphenidyl
    ii. Antipsychotic drugs such as chlorpromazine act as D_2 receptor antagonists, leading to an imbalance between dopaminergic and cholinergic activity in the basal ganglia. This disruption can result in extrapyramidal symptoms, including drug-induced parkinsonism. Levodopa will not be effective in this case, as D_2 receptors are blocked by the offending drug.
    iii. Trihexyphenidyl can cause typical anticholinergic or atropinic adverse effects. Refer to page 112.
14. i. b. Tropicamide
    ii. Tropicamide is an anticholinergic drug having mydriatic and cycloplegic action, that is required for refraction testing to knock out the effect of accommodation.
    iii. Tropicamide has fast onset of ocular action within 20–40 minutes and effect lasts for 3–6 hours only. Thus, tropicamide is preferred over atropine Both the remaining options (physostigmine and carbachol) are miotics and miosis is undesirable before refraction testing.
15. i. a. Phosphodiesterase-4 inhibition
    ii. Refer to page 110.
    iii. Refer to page 110.
    iv. Refer to page 111.
16. i. Anticholinergic antispasmodic, quaternary ammonium compound.
    ii. Glycopyrrolate is used exclusively for 'pre-anesthetic medication' to reduce tracheobronchial secretions before giving inhalational anesthetics through IM injection in a dose of 0.2–0.4 mg.
    iii. Unlike atropine, it has no central side effects because it is a quaternary ammonium compound and is rapidly acting.
17. i. a. Flavoxate
    ii. Flavoxate is a vesicoselective anticholinergic, so it will have minimal adverse effects.
18. i. c. Atropine poisoning
    ii. Tachycardia in case of atropine toxicity occurs due to blockade of M_2 receptors present in the heart. Hyperpyrexia is due to decreased sweating due to blockage of M_3 receptors in the sweat glands and decreased heat loss.
    iii. Management is mainly supportive; refer to page 112.
19. c. Glaucoma
    Atropine can further obliterate iridocorneal angle leading to dangerous rise in intraocular tension.
20. Refer to page 112

CONCEPT MAP – ANTICHOLINERGIC DRUGS

1. Classification

Natural Alkaloids: Atropine, Hyoscine

Semisynthetic drugs:
Atropine, Methonitrate, Homatropine, Hyoscine butylbromide, Ipratropium, Tiotropium

Synthetic drugs:

Centrally acting
Benztropine, Benzhexol, Trihexyphenidyl, Biperidin, Procyclidine

Antisecretory, Antispasmodic
Tertiary amines - Dicyclomine, Pirenzipine, Telenzipine, Valethamate
Quaternary amm. compds: Clidinium, Glycopyrrolate, Isopropamide

Vesicoselective
Darifenacin, solifenasin, Oxyphenonium, Flavoxate, Tolterodine

2. Mechanism of Action

Competitive antagonists at muscarinic receptors

Major Pharmacological Actions

Tachycardia
Decreased exocrine secretions
Smooth muscle relaxation
↓
Bronchodilatation, Mydriasis
Constipation
Urinary retention

ANTICHOLINERGIC DRUGS

3. Therapeutic Uses

Atropine: OPC poisoning, Early mushroom poisoning, Pre-anesthetic medication, Pulmonary embolism, Partial heart blocks, Bradyarrythmias, Ocular inflammatory conditions, with neostigmine to counteract muscarinic adverse effects.

Hyoscine: Motion sickness as transdermal patch

Ipratropium: In regular prophylaxis of bronchial asthma & COPD.

Centrally acting drugs: In 'Drug-induced Parkinsonism' Post operative decurarisation, Cobra bite

Mydriatics: In fundoscopic examination and refraction testing. Atropine used in inflammatory eye conditions.

Antispasmodics: In intestinal, biliary, ureteric colics, cervical dystocia (Valethamate), Pre-anesthetic medication (glycopyrrolate)

Vesicoselective drugs: In urinary urgency, dysuria in UTI, neurogenic bladder, nocturnal enuresis

Ipratropium preferred over atropine because of its selectivity for bronchial smooth muscles→no effect on mucociliary clearance and tracheobronchial secretions

5. Cautions/Contraindications

Narrow iridocorneal angle
Elderly males with prostatic hypertrophy
Gastric peptic ulcer

4. ADRs

Dry mouth, dry sandy eyes, dry hot and flushed skin, photophobia, blurring of vision, palpitation, weak, rapid pulse, difficulty in passing urine, constipation

Atropine toxicity

Tachycardia, confusion, agitation, hyperpyrexia, convulsions and is managed by supportive measures

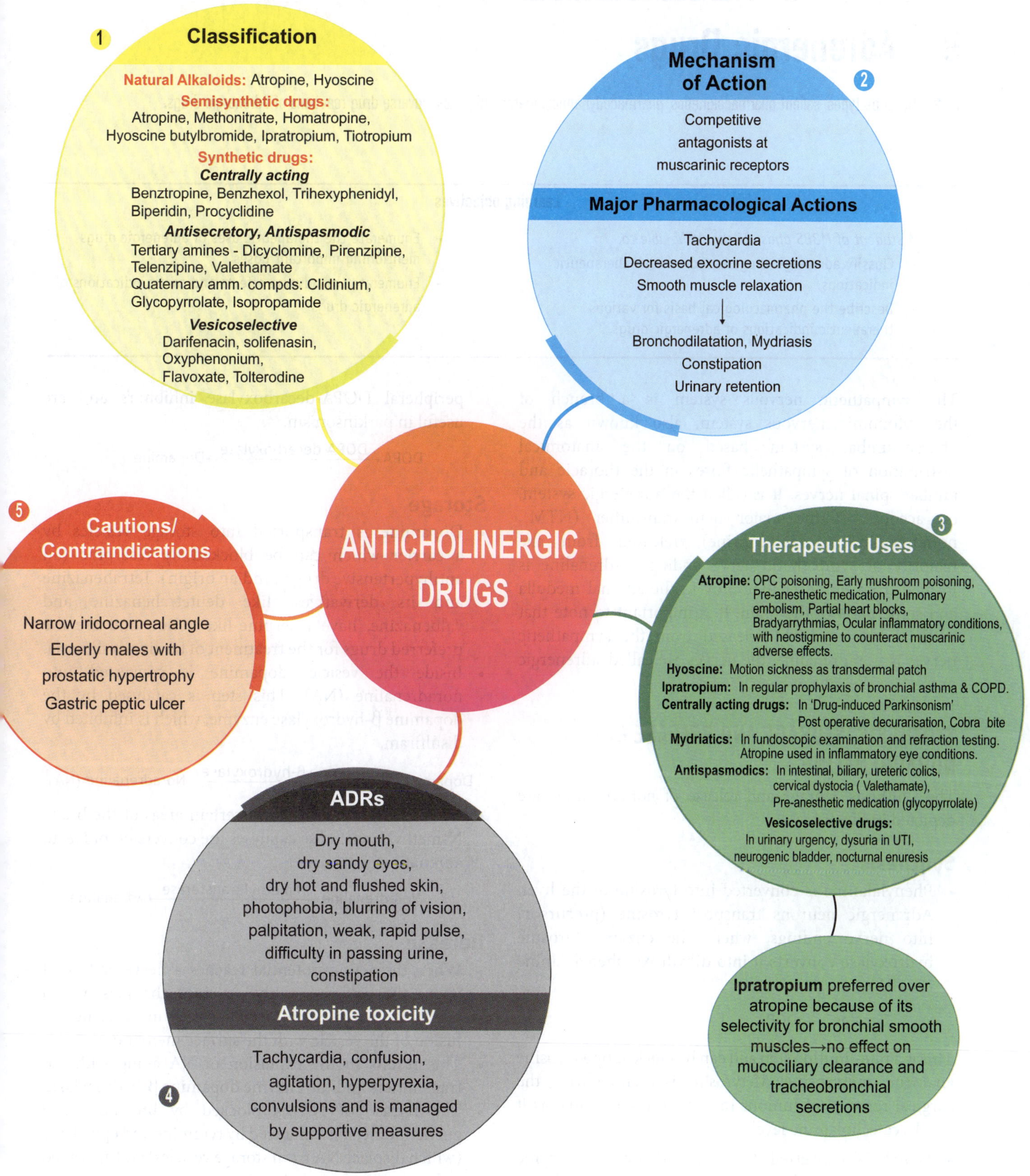

SECTION 2 Drugs Acting on ANS and PNS

9 Adrenergic Drugs

PH2.1 Describe types, salient pharmacokinetics, pharmacodynamics, therapeutic uses, adverse drug reactions of adrenergic drugs.

Learning objectives

A student of MBBS phase II should be able to:
- Classify adrenergic drugs based on their therapeutic indications
- Describe the pharmacological basis for various therapeutic indications of adrenergic drugs
- Enumerate the therapeutic uses of adrenergic drugs mentioning important doses
- Enumerate the adverse effects and contraindications of adrenergic drugs

---

The sympathetic nervous system is a branch of the autonomic nervous system, also known as the 'thoracolumbar system' based on the anatomical distribution of sympathetic fibres in the thoracic and lumbar spinal nerves. It is called the 'adrenergic system', on account of the major neurotransmitter (NTM), noradrenaline (norepinephrine), released from the majority of sympathetic nerve endings. Adrenaline is formed from noradrenaline only in the adrenal medulla and some parts of the brain. It is important to note that while the major NTM released from the sympathetic nerves is noradrenaline, the nerves are called 'adrenergic nerves' for the sake of convenience.

SYNTHESIS, STORAGE AND RELEASE OF NORADRENALINE

The synthesis, storage and release of noradrenaline are depicted in Fig. 9.1.

Synthesis

- Phenylalanine is converted into tyrosine in the liver. Adrenergic neurons transport tyrosine (precursor) into nerve endings, where the enzyme tyrosine hydroxylase converts it into dihydroxy phenylalanine (DOPA).

$$\text{Tyrosine} \longrightarrow \text{DOPA}$$

This is a rate-limiting step and can be blocked by a tyrosine analogue, **metyrosine**; Metyrosine is useful during the surgical removal of tumour in pheochromocytoma, as it checks catecholamine levels.

- DOPA is converted to dopamine by the enzyme DOPA-decarboxylase. Carbidopa and benserazide are peripheral DOPA-decarboxylase inhibitors and are useful in parkinsonism.

$$\text{DOPA} \xrightarrow{\text{DOPA-decarboxylase}} \text{Dopamine}$$

Storage

- Dopamine is transported into storage vesicles by a carrier which can be blocked by reserpine (an antihypertensive drug of Indian origin). Tetrabenazine and its derivatives, like deutetrabenazine and valbenazine, have reserpine-like action and are the preferred drugs for the treatment of tardive dyskinesia.
- Inside the vesicle, dopamine is converted into noradrenaline (NA). This step is catalysed by the dopamine β-hydroxylase enzyme, which is inhibited by disulfiram.

$$\text{Dopamine} \xrightarrow{\text{Dopamine β-hydroxylase}} \text{Noradrenaline (NA)}$$

- In the adrenal medulla and certain areas of the brain, N-methyl transferase catalyses the conversion of NA to adrenaline.

$$\text{Noradrenaline} \xrightarrow{\text{N-methyl transferase}} \text{Adrenaline}$$

Release

- When the action potential reaches a nerve ending, it opens the voltage-sensitive calcium channels, which results in increased intracellular calcium, causing the fusion of the vesicle with the surface membrane.
- This results in the expulsion of NA along with co-transmitters and the enzyme dopamine β-hydroxylase.
- The release of NA is blocked by bretylium and guanethidine; it is enhanced by tyramine and ephedrine (which displace NA from storage vesicles) and are called indirect-acting sympathomimetics.

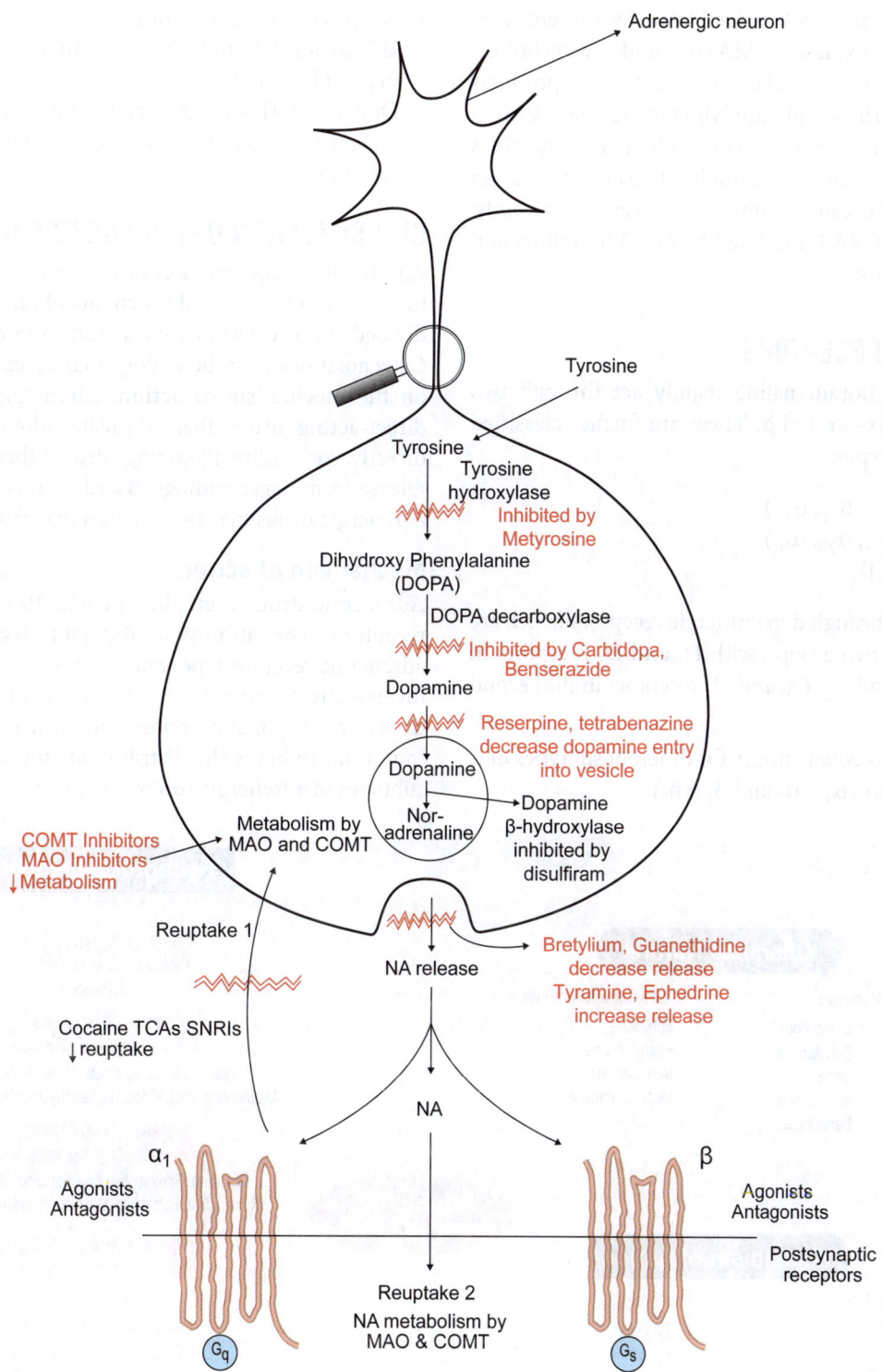

Fig. 9.1 Synthesis, storage and release of noradrenaline (norepinephrine)

- After release, NA acts on the adrenergic receptors present pre- or post-synaptically to produce all the sympathetic effects.

Termination of Action

- The action of NA is terminated by the following routes:
  - Diffusion out of the synaptic cleft, followed by metabolism
  - Transportation into cytoplasm of nerve endings—known as **reuptake 1**—followed by metabolism; reuptake 1 is blocked by cocaine and tricyclic antidepressants (TCA), and serotonin and noradrenaline reuptake inhibitors (SNRIs).
  - Transportation into the post-junctional cell—known as **reuptake 2** is followed by metabolism.

- The metabolism of NA is facilitated by the enzymes monoamine oxidase (MAO) and catechol-O-methyltransferase (COMT). The metabolic products are metanephrines and vanillylmandelic acid (VMA), which are excreted in urine. The levels of metanephrines and VMA in a 24-hour sample of urine provide an estimate of the catecholamine turnover in the body. Metabolism of NA is inhibited by MAO inhibitors and COMT inhibitors.

ADRENERGIC RECEPTORS

Adrenaline and noradrenaline mainly act through two types of receptors—α and β. These are further classified into various subtypes:

- α – α_1 (α_{1A}, α_{1B}, α_{1D})
  α_2 (α_{2A}, α_{2B}, α_{2C})
- β – β_1, β_2, β_3

Dopamine acts through dopaminergic receptors which are categorised into two groups, with **D_1 and D_5** receptors in the first group, and **D_2, D_3, and D_4** receptors in the second group.

- Adrenaline has equal affinity for different subtypes of α and β receptors ($\alpha_1 = \alpha_2$ and $\beta_1 = \beta_2$).
- NA has equal affinity for α_1 and α_2 ($\alpha_1 = \alpha_2$), but more affinity for β_1 than β_2 ($\beta_1 \gg \beta_2$). In other words, NA has negligible β_2 action.
- Dopamine (DA) has equal affinity for D_1 and D_2 receptors, which is more than affinity for β and α receptors. $D_1 = D_2 \gg \beta \gg \alpha$.

CLASSIFICATION OF ADRENERGIC DRUGS

Adrenergic drugs can be classified in multiple ways (refer to Flowchart 9.1). Based on **chemical structure**, they are divided into catecholamines and non-catecholamines. Catecholamines can be endogenous or exogenous. Based on the **mechanism of action**, adrenergic drugs can be direct-acting drugs that stimulate adrenergic receptors directly, or indirectly-acting drugs that enhance NA release from nerve endings. Based on **receptor selectivity** adrenergic drugs may be non-selective or selective.

Mechanism of action

Adrenergic drugs exert their actions through adrenergic receptors. The affinity of different drugs for various adrenergic receptor types and subtypes varies, resulting in diverse effects. Sometimes, the effects of two adrenergic drugs are diagonally opposite to each other. Thus, it is important to know the distribution and nature of various subtypes of adrenergic receptors (Table 9.1).

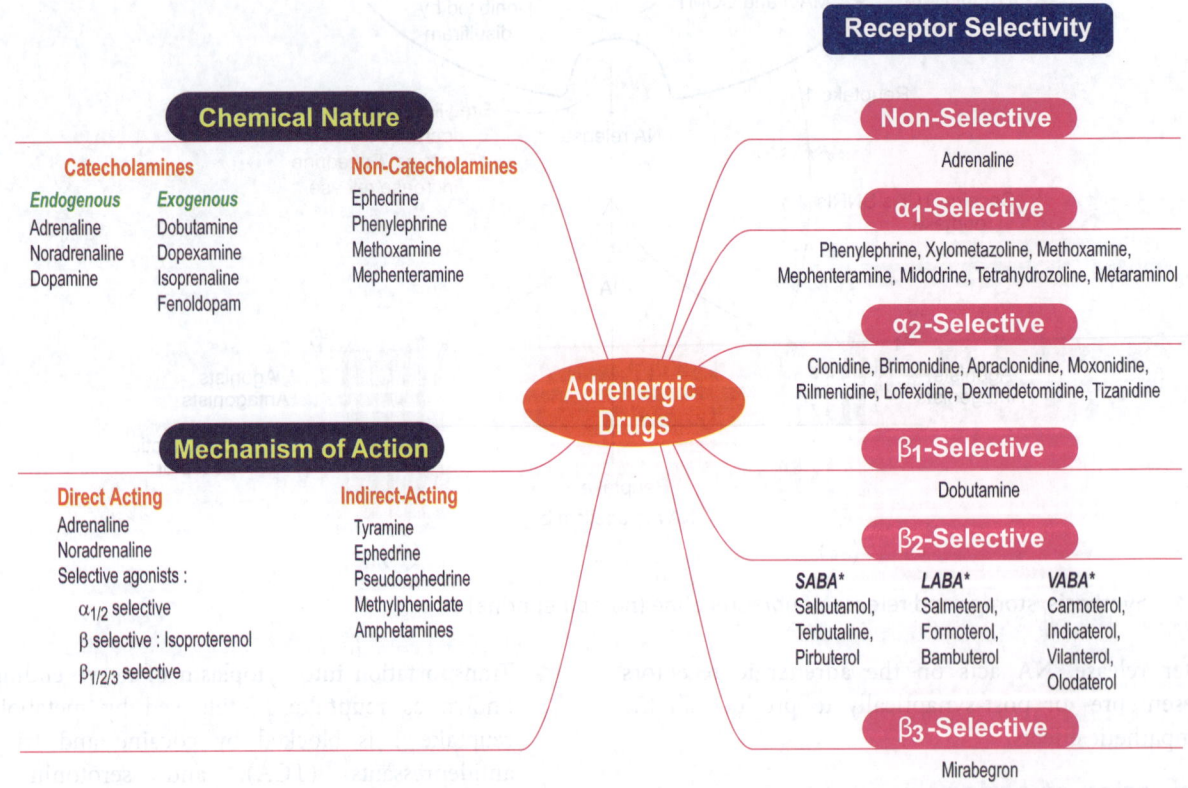

Flowchart 9.1 Classification of adernergic drugs

Table 9.1 Distribution and actions mediated through adrenergic receptors

Name	Transduction system & nature	Distribution	Action	Implications
α$_1$	IP$_3$–DAG → increased Ca^{2+} **Excitatory**	**Smooth muscles as in:**	Contraction of smooth muscles	
		• Radial muscles of iris	Mydriasis	Used as mydriatic for fundus examination and in alternation with miotics for prevention and treatment of adhesions
		• Vascular smooth muscles predominantly in blood vessels of skin, mucous membrane, splanchnic and renal vessels.	Vasoconstriction	Used as nasal decongestants and pressor agents in hypotension and shock
		• GIT & genitourinary tract sphincters	Contraction	Used in stress incontinence
		• Pilomotor muscles	Contraction	Causes goose flesh in anxiety due to sympathetic stimulation
α$_2$	Inhibition of adenylyl cyclase → reduced cAMP, opening of K$^+$ and closing of Ca^{2+} channels **Inhibitory**	**Presynaptic on adrenergic nerve endings**	Reduced NA release	α$_2$ receptor agonists are used in hypertension and glaucoma
		Platelets	Platelet aggregation	
		Lipocytes	Inhibit lipolysis	
β$_1$	Stimulation of adenylyl cyclase → raised cAMP levels **Excitatory**	**Heart**	Increased heart rate, contractility, conduction velocity, increased ectopic activity	Useful in sudden cardiac arrest, Stokes–Adams syndrome, acute cardiac decompensation, AV blocks
		Lipocytes	Stimulate lipolysis	
		Presynaptic on nerve endings	Facilitate NTM release	
β$_2$	Stimulation of adenylyl cyclase → raising cAMP levels. cAMP causes phosphorylation of myosin light chain kinase enzyme (MLCK), which is the inactive form, causes Ca^{2+} expulsion, resulting in a **relaxing effect on the smooth muscles*** **Excitatory**	**Smooth muscles as in:**	Relaxation of smooth muscles	
		• GIT & Genitourinary tract wall	Relaxation	
		• Uterine smooth muscles	Uterine relaxant	Agonists used in premature labour
		• Bronchi	Bronchodilatation	Agonists used in bronchial asthma
		• Skeletal muscle blood vessels, coronaries	Vasodilatation	
		Liver	Gluconeogenesis glycogenolysis	
		Ciliary epithelium	Increased secretion of aqueous humor	
β$_3$	Stimulation of adenylyl cyclase → raised cAMP levels **Excitatory**	**Lipocytes**	Stimulate lipolysis	

*β$_2$ receptors are excitatory in nature, but in smooth muscles relaxation occurs owing to inactivation of MLCK.

PHARMACOLOGICAL ACTIONS OF ADRENERGIC DRUGS

The actions exerted by adrenergic drugs vary due to the variable affinity of different drugs for various receptor types and subtypes. The prominent, clinically relevant actions of adrenergic drugs are as mentioned below:

1. Central Action

The central action of drugs varies based on their ability to cross the blood–brain barrier.

- **Catecholamines** like adrenaline, noradrenaline and dopamine do not cross the blood–brain barrier. Hence, they do not have central effects at therapeutically used doses. However, at high rates of infusion, certain subjective central effects may occur. These resemble effects of sympathetic stimulation like nervousness, anxiety, restlessness, and feelings of impending disaster (as if something very wrong is going to happen).

- Certain **synthetic adrenergic drugs** with high central:peripheral actions ratio like amphetamine, dexamphetamine, and methamphetamine have prominent central stimulant action but weak cardiovascular effects. The central action of amphetamine is due to:
  - Increased release of NA from adrenergic neurons in the brain
  - Increased release of dopamine and serotonin
  - Inhibition of reuptake of dopamine

At therapeutic doses, amphetamine produces a mild alerting effect. It increases an individual's attention span and ability to concentrate on repetitive or monotonous tasks. This effect produces paradoxical quietening and improves performance in hyperkinetic children with **attention deficit disorder**. Work capacity and athletic performance is improved and fatigue and boredom are reduced. The ascending reticular activating system (RAS), which causes wakefulness and postpones sleep, is activated. Euphoria and mood elevation also occur because of improved performance.

However, larger doses of amphetamine may cause excessive central stimulation, resulting in anxiety, dysphoria, restlessness, agitation, insomnia, anorexia, panic, confusion, delirium and psychotic behaviour.

Amphetamine has the potential for misuse by players and athletes, and their presence is routinely screened in anti-doping tests. Methamphetamine has a high abuse potential. It is commonly called 'crystal meth'. The use of methamphetamine is associated with 'drug-seeking behaviours' and the development of tolerance to the subjective effects of the drug. However, there is no dependence and withdrawal syndrome with these drugs.

2. Cardiovascular Actions

Adrenergic drugs have **direct and reflex effects** on the Important terms used in the context of cardiovascular actions are explained in Box 9.1.

a. Heart

Direct effects

Drugs exert direct effects on the heart through β_1-mediated cardiac stimulation.

- Positive chronotropic effect is due to the increased automaticity of the SA node as well as ectopic sites.
- Conduction velocity in the AV node is increased, resulting in reduced 'effective refractory period' (ERP).
- Contractility is increased, and relaxation is accelerated. Thus, intraventricular pressure rises and falls quickly. Though the contraction is more forceful, the ejection

> **Box 9.1 Terms used in the context of cardiovascular effects**
>
> **Chronotropic effect:** This represents the effect of a drug on the heart rate. Drugs that increase the heart rate are said to have a positive chronotropic effect and ones that reduce it are said to have a negative chronotropic effect.
>
> **Inotropic effect:** This represents an increase (positive) or decrease (negative) in the force of contractions of myocardial cells.
>
> **Dromotropic effect:** This represents an increase (positive) or decrease (negative) in atrio-ventricular conduction.
>
> **Bathmotropic effect:** This represents an increase (positive) or decrease (negative) in the excitability of the cardiac muscle membrane and the ease with which the action potential can be generated.
>
> **Reflex effects:** These occur as compensatory response to alteration in BP. An increase in BP evokes the baroreceptor reflex, leading to central vagal stimulation, in an effort to reduce the raised BP. Conversely, a decrease in BP evokes central sympathetic stimulation in an attempt to raise the lowered BP.
>
> **Blood pressure:** This refers to systolic blood pressure (SBP) and diastolic blood pressure (DBP). SBP largely depends on cardiac output (COP).
>
> **Cardiac output (COP):** COP is the volume of blood pumped out by the heart in one minute. It is a product of stroke volume (SV) and hear rate (HR). SV is the amount of blood pumped out by the heart in one contraction. Multiplying it with heart rate gives the COP, i.e., the amount of blood pumped out per minute.
>
> $$COP = SV \times HR$$
>
> Thus, an increase in the force of contractions will increase SV and hence, COP. Similarly, an increase in HR can also increase COP;
>
> When HR is more, it means the heart has to contract and relax more times in one minute. Therefore, the diastolic time (relaxation time between two consecutive contractions) gets reduced. As the filling of the heart occurs only during the diastolic phase, the volume of blood entering the heart—called end diastolic volume (EDV)—will be less if diastolic time is less. Further, the heart can pump only as much as it has received. Thus, a reduction in EDV can reduce the SV, and in turn, COP.
>
> Diastolic blood pressure (DBP) chiefly depends upon peripheral vascular resistance (PVR) or total peripheral resistance (TPR). Vasoconstriction of the resistance vessels (arterioles) increases PVR and hence, DBP. Vasoconstriction of the capacitance vessels (capillaries) pushes out blood from the capillaries into the venules and veins, which send it to the heart. Thus, venous return increases, which in turn, raises the EDV and SV.

time decreases. Direct effects thus increase heart rate, cardiac output, contractility and conduction.

Reflex effects

Adrenergic drugs that have a prominent α_1-mediated vasoconstrictor effect cause an increase in BP. Raised blood pressure activates the baroreceptor reflex, leading to a rise in vagal tone, which brings down the heart rate.

b. Blood vessels

Adrenergic drugs have complex effects on blood pressure because blood vessels have two types of receptors—α_1-mediating vasoconstriction and β_2-mediating vasodilatation.

- Blood vessels of the skin, mucous membranes and splanchnic bed have α_1-receptors. The blood vessels of the upper respiratory tract mucosa contain α_1 receptors. Their activation causes decongestion by mucosal vasoconstriction.
- Renal and skeletal muscle blood vessels have both α_1 and β_2 receptors.
- In addition, renal, splanchnic, coronary, and cerebral blood vessels have D_1 receptors, which mediate vasodilatation.

c. Blood pressure

The effects of different adrenergic drugs on BP varies depending on variations in affinities of the drugs for receptor subtypes.

- **Adrenaline** is a non-selective drug that acts at α as well as β receptors. Vascular β_2 **receptors are more sensitive to adrenaline than** α_1 receptors. Thus, α_1 action is seen at high concentration as these receptors are less sensitive to adrenaline (e.g., immediately after a rapid IV injection). On the other hand, β_2-mediated vasodilation persists longer because these receptors are more sensitive to adrenaline, and hence, they respond even to low concentrations of the drug.

  The rapid IV injection of **adrenaline produces a biphasic response** (Fig. 9.2) because:
  - β_1-mediated cardiac stimulation → increase in SBP
  - α_1-mediated vasoconstriction (prominent at high concentration) → increase in PVR and DBP
  - β_2-mediated vasodilatation (more persistent effect) → marked fall in DBP

  Sir Henry Dale demonstrated that if α_1-mediated vasoconstriction is blocked by an α-blocker like dihydroergotamine, the biphasic response to NA changes into a depressor response. This is called **Dale's reversal phenomenon**.

- **Noradrenaline** ($\alpha_1 = \alpha_2$; $\beta_1 >> \beta_2$) has a negligible β_2 effect, i.e., NA acts equally on α_1 and α_2 receptors.
  - α_1-mediated vasoconstriction → increase in PVR → increase in DBP and in venous return
  - α_2-mediated reduction in NA secretion → fall in BP
  - β_1-mediated cardiac stimulation → along with increased venous return due to vasoconstriction of capacitance vessels → increase in cardiac output → increase in SBP
  - As NA has negligible β_2 effect → no vasodilatation/minimal vasodilatation. Thus, NA causes a rise in SBP, DBP, and mean BP, and is useful as a pressor agent.

- **Isoproterenol** is selective for β receptors, i.e., $\beta_1 = \beta_2 >> \alpha$.
  - β_1-mediated cardiac stimulation → increase in SBP
  - β_2-mediated vasodilatation → marked fall in DBP
  - No α_1-mediated vasoconstriction

3. Respiratory System

Adrenaline causes bronchodilatation by β_2 action. This action is more marked when bronchi are constricted.

Selective β_2 agonists are preferred for this effect as they have minimal cardiovascular adverse effects at therapeutic doses. Selective β_2 agonists are classified into three types based on their duration of action:

- **Short-acting selective β_2 agonists (SABA)** are salbutamol and terbutaline. Their effect lasts for only 2–4 hours. These are highly selective for β_2 receptors. They achieve adequate bronchodilatation and relieve symptoms of asthma exacerbation with minimal cardiovascular effects.
- **Long-acting selective β_2 agonists (LABA)** include bambuterol, salmeterol and formoterol. Bambuterol is a prodrug of terbutaline. It is hydrolysed slowly by pseudocholinesterase enzyme to release terbutaline for about 24 hours. Salmeterol has a slow onset and longer duration of action than salbutamol. Formoterol, like salmeterol, has a duration of action lasting up to 12 hours. These long-acting β_2 agonists are useful along with inhalational steroids as 'relievers' in acute episodes of asthma.
- **Very-long-acting β_2 agonists (VABA)** include drugs like carmoterol, indicaterol, olodaterol and vilanterol, which continue to act for up to 24 hours. These are used in COPD only through the inhalational route.

Drugs like ritodrine and isoxsuprine are selective agonists at β_2 receptors, especially in the uterine muscles. They are useful for the treatment of premature labour, dysmenorrhea, threatened abortion, etc.

4. Gastrointestinal Tract

The smooth muscles of the visceral wall relax through β_2 stimulation, whereas sphincters contract through α_1 stimulation.

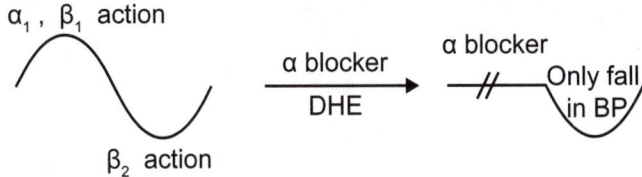

Fig. 9.2 The biphasic response of adrenaline

Selective α_2 agonists decrease muscle activity indirectly by reducing the release of noradrenaline.

5. Genitourinary System

The activation of β_2 receptors causes the relaxation of uterine muscles and bladder wall muscles. The activation of α_1 receptors present in the bladder base, urethral sphincter and prostate leads to contraction of the smooth muscles, thereby promoting urinary continence.

6. Ocular Actions

The contraction of the radial muscles of the iris mediated through α_1 receptors causes mydriasis. This effect is minimal after the topical instillation of adrenaline, which being a catecholamine, crosses the cornea poorly. Dipivefrine, a prodrug formed by the esterification of adrenaline with pivalic acid, has better corneal penetration. Adrenaline has complex effects on aqueous humor dynamics (Fig. 9.3).

a. α_1-mediated vasoconstriction of ciliary vessels → decrease in aqueous humor formation
b. α_2-mediated decrease in NTM release → decreased secretory activity of ciliary epithelium (less NTM → less β_2 stimulation → less secretion of aqueous humor)
c. β_2 receptors in ciliary epithelium activated → enhanced secretory activity of ciliary epithelium
d. Even though adrenaline is a mydriatic, it increases uveoscleral outflow by a poorly understood mechanism → decrease IOT.

Owing to actions (**a, b, d**) mentioned above, the intraocular tension falls, especially in patients suffering from wide-angle glaucoma. The blockade of effect (**c**) mentioned above by β-blockers is also useful in glaucoma. Selective agonists of α_2-receptors also reduce IOT through action (b) mentioned above and are useful in glaucoma.

7. Exocrine and Endocrine Glands

Exocrine glands

- Clonidine causes dryness of the mouth by an unknown mechanism.
- Non-thermoregulatory sweating from the apocrine sweat glands located on the palms of the hands increases. This type of sweating is typically associated with psychological stress-induced sympathetic stimulation and has no role in regulating body temperature.

Endocrine glands

- The activation of β receptors stimulates insulin and renin secretion, whereas α_2 activation inhibits the same.
- Metabolic actions—β_1 and β_3 receptor activation increases lipolysis, resulting in increased levels of free fatty acids (FFA) in plasma and calorigenesis.
- β_2 activation causes glycogenolysis (the breakdown of glycogen into glucose) and gluconeogenesis (the synthesis of glucose from non-carbohydrate sources). Both these actions cause hyperglycemia. Hyperlactacidemia may also occur.

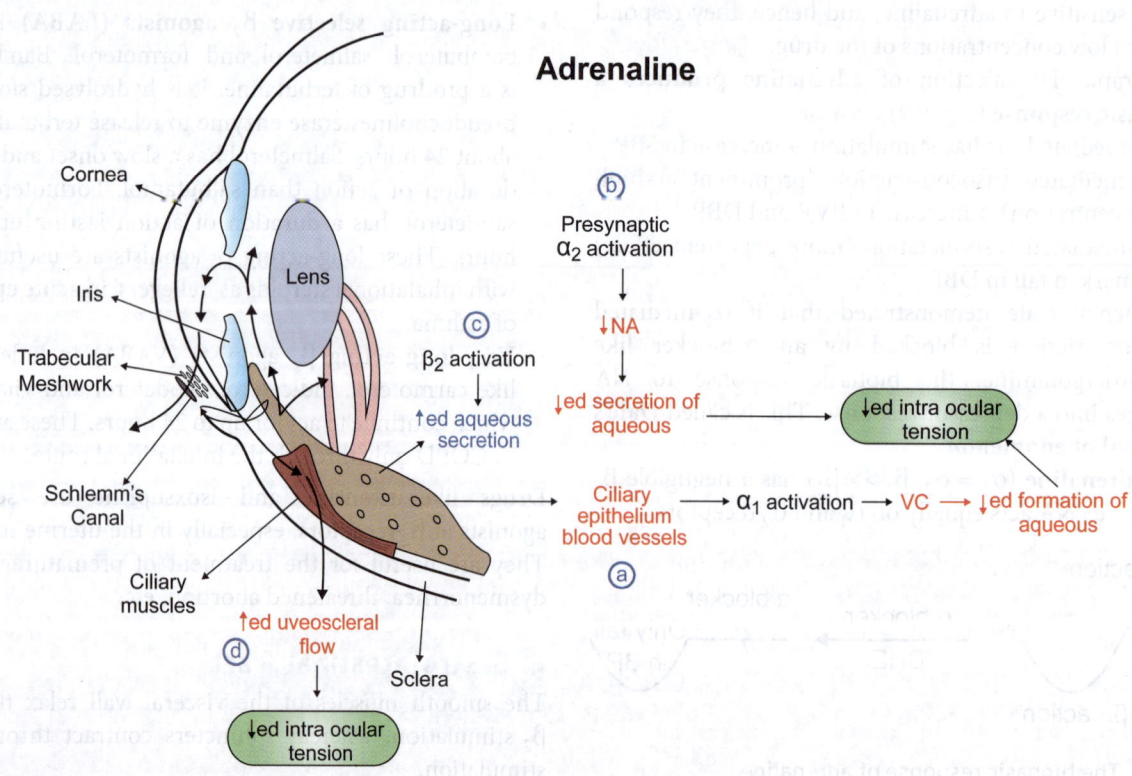

Fig. 9.3 Effect of adrenaline on intra ocular tension

- β_2-receptor activation also increases K^+ uptake into the cells, leading to a fall in extracellular K^+ levels. This mechanism helps in preventing a dangerous rise in plasma K^+ level during exercise.

Fig. 9.4 presents the major pharmacological actions of adrenergic drugs.

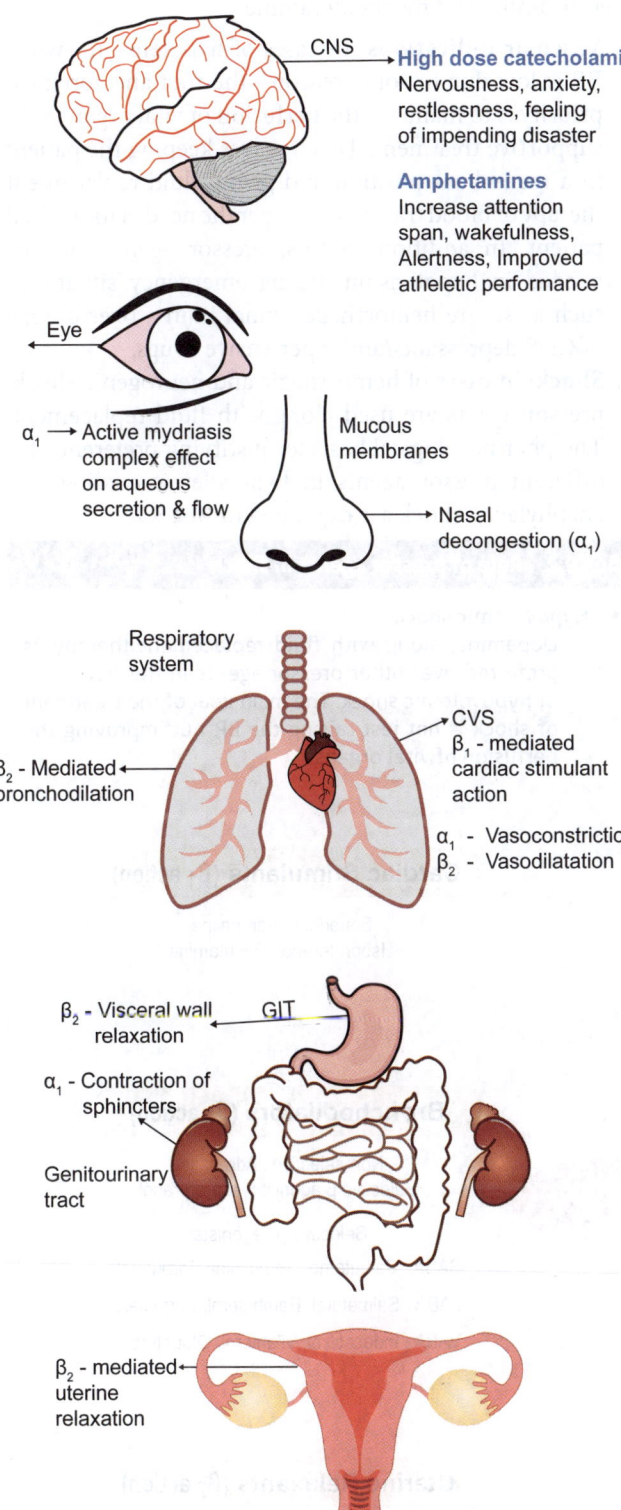

Fig. 9.4 Major pharmacological actions of adrenergic drugs

Clinical problem-based questions and MCQs

1. The parents of a 7-year-old boy complain that their son demonstrates restless and confrontational behaviour, constantly runs around, is defiant, does not listen to instructions, and frequently gets upset on not getting attention. He has normal physical and social activity and interacts well with children of his age group, but gets easily influenced or led by others. His teachers think that the boy seems to have academic potential, but has difficulty in focusing, sitting still in class, and sustaining attention. His academic grades are not good, but sometimes, while pursuing activities of his interest, he is extremely focused. The boy's mother also gives a history of the boy having trouble falling asleep as an infant, saying that he used to stay awake at night for hours together. The boy is diagnosed with attention deficit disorder (ADD).
   i. Which of the following drugs can improve this child's behaviour and performance?
      a. Dexamphetamine   b. Sibutramine
      c. Xylometazoline   d. Phenylephrine
   ii. Describe the role of the selected drug in this case.
   iii. Enumerate the adverse effects of the selected drug.

2. A 19-year-old boy is admitted to the trauma centre after sustaining multiple injuries in a road accident. His BP is 80/30. CT abdomen rules out any visceral injury. He is put on IV adrenaline drip to maintain his BP and heart rate. After starting treatment, a blood sample sent for routine investigations shows blood glucose levels of 430 mg/dL.
   i. Explain the cause of the abnormally raised blood glucose levels with adrenaline.
   ii. Describe the other metabolic esffects of adrenaline.

3. The administration of a rapid IV injection of adrenaline has a biphasic effect on BP. Pre-treatment with dihydroergotamine changes this response into a depressor one.
   i. Name the phenomenon involved.
   ii. Explain the cause of biphasic BP response to adrenaline given intravenously.
   iii. Explain the change in response with dihydroergotamine.

4. A 48-year-old male presented with history of gradual, painless vision loss. On examination, the unaided visual acuity was counting fingers at one metre with the left eye and 6/60 with the right eye. Both corneas were clear, and intraocular tension (IOT) was raised in both eyes, more so in the left eye than in the right. Gonioscopy revealed open angles in both eyes. The patient was prescribed timolol (β-blocker) and dipivefrine eye drops and called for a follow-up after one week.
   i. What is the likely diagnosis?
   ii. What is dipivefrine? Explain its role in this case.
   iii. Describe the rationale of prescribing β-blockers and dipivefrine in this patient.

5. i. Which of the following is the most suitable drug for the regular prophylaxis of bronchial asthma?
   a. Salbutamol
   b. Salmeterol
   c. Ritodrine
   d. Budesonide
   ii. Describe the pharmacological basis of your choice.
6. Which of the following is short acting selective β_2 agonist?
   a. Salbutamol
   b. Salmeterol
   c. Formoterol
   d. Bambuterol
7. i. Select the receptors mediating the vasoconstrictor effect of adrenergic agonists.
   a. α_1
   b. α_2
   c. β_1
   d. β_2
   ii. Name two selective agonists of the receptors mediating vasoconstrictor activity.
   iii. What are the clinical uses of the agonists?
8. Which of the following adrenergic drugs acts selectively on the heart?
   a. Salbutamol
   b. Dobutamine
   c. Adrenaline
   d. Dopamine
9. i. Identify the adrenergic drug constricting the nasal mucosal blood vessels.
   a. Naphazoline
   b. Salbutamol
   c. Ritodrine
   d. All of the above
   ii. Describe the clinical use of the above-mentioned action.

THERAPEUTIC USES OF ADRENERGIC DRUGS

Adrenergic drugs are divided into seven therapeutic groups based on their therapeutic uses, i.e., pressor agents, nasal decongestants, CNS stimulants, anorectics, cardiac stimulants, bronchodilators and uterine relaxants (Flowchart 9.2). The uses of adrenergic drugs are described next, group-wise.

I. Pressor Agents

Pressor agents include drugs with α_1 vasoconstrictor action, such as noradrenaline, ephedrine, phenylephrine, methoxamine and mephenteramine.

1. **Vascular indications**: In cases of hypotension—when BP is low due to some reason—the first and foremost priority is to maintain the perfusion of vital organs with supportive treatment. This involves keeping the patient in a recumbent position and giving fluid replacement therapy or blood transfusion as per the need of individual patient. In addition to this, pressor agents may be needed in hypotension during emergency situations, such as severe hemorrhage, spinal injury, over-dosage of CNS depressants/antihypertensive drugs.
2. **Shock:** in cases of hemorrhagic and neurogenic shock, pressor agents are used along with fluid replacement. The pharmacological basis for justifying preference for different pressor agents in hypovolemic/cardiogenic/anaphylactic shock are explained in Box 9.2.

Box 9.2 Role of pressor agents in shock

- **Hypovolemic shock**
  - Dopamine, along with fluid replacement therapy, is preferred over other pressor agents in the treatment of hypovolemic shock. The main goal of the treatment of shock is not just raising the BP, but improving the perfusion of vital organs.

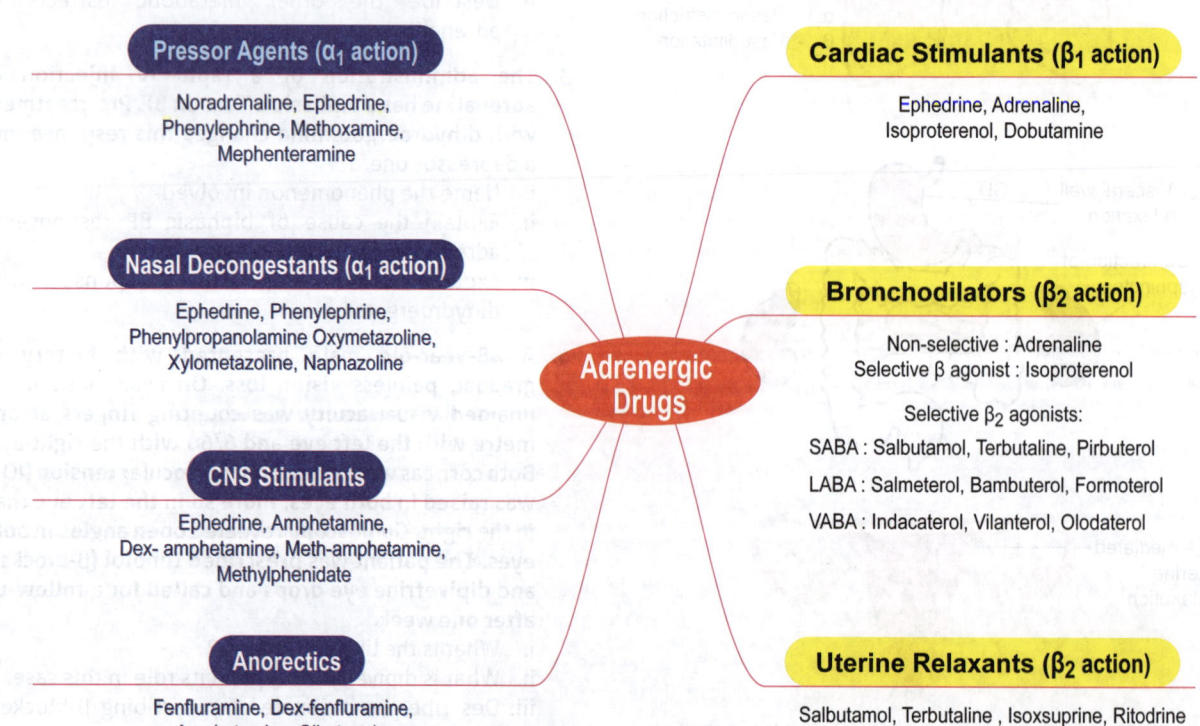

Flowchart 9.2 Therapeutic classification of adernergic drugs

- Dopamine is a catecholamine that has a prominent effect on D_1 and D_2 receptors, followed by β and α receptors. Hence, dopamine has $D_1 = D_2 \gg β \gg α$ action.
- The potency series of dopamine indicates that D_1 receptors are most sensitive to dopamine and hence respond to low doses of dopamine (2–5 mcg/kg/minute). D_1 receptors are present prominently in renal and mesenteric blood vessels. These are inhibitory in nature, and thus cause vasodilatation, resulting in improved renal and mesenteric perfusion. Increased renal blood flow (RBF), in turn, improves the glomerular filtration rate (GFR) and Na^+ excretion.
- D_2 receptors present pre-synaptically on adrenergic nerve endings are also inhibitory in nature. D_2 activation by dopamine reduces NA release, which may contribute to the D_1 effect (by preventing $α_1$-mediated vasoconstriction).
- When the rate of dopamine infusion is increased to 5–20 mcg/kg/minute, β action also manifests. $β_1$-mediated cardiac stimulation improves cardiac output and systolic BP. $β_2$-mediated vasodilatation is also useful to maintain the perfusion of vital organs.
- But with further increase in dopamine infusion rate at >20 mcg/kg/minute, the least sensitive $α_1$ receptors also get activated. Consequently, $α_1$-mediated vasoconstriction occurs. This increases the PVR and hence, DBP. Vasoconstriction of the renal vascular bed occurs, resulting in reduced renal blood flow that compromises renal function, which could be dangerous.

In contrast, NA has prominent $α_1$ action, which causes vasoconstriction. BP may be raised, but the perfusion of vital organs is compromised. **Therefore, dopamine is preferred over NA in hypovolemic shock.** The infusion rate should be low (2–5 mcg/kg/minute) so that tissue perfusion is maintained.

- **Cardiogenic shock** is managed by mechanically-assisted perfusion, volume replacement, administration of dobutamine, and treatment of the underlying cause. Pressor agents are not very useful in these cases.
- **Anaphylactic shock** is managed with adrenaline 1:1000 (1 mg/mL) given subcutaneously in a dose of 0.3–0.5 mL. It is life-saving because adrenaline is a physiological antagonist of histamine (which is one of the important mediators of anaphylaxis). Histamine and adrenaline have opposite effects on physiological functions. Histamine released during anaphylaxis causes bronchoconstriction leading to dyspnea, and vasodilatation leading to a fall in BP and shock.

Adrenaline, being a non-selective drug on adrenergic receptors, can reverse both of these prominent effects of histamine. Activation of $β_2$ receptors by adrenaline causes bronchodilatation, thus relieving dyspnea, and $α_1$ receptor-mediated vasoconstriction restores BP to normal levels.

3. **Along with local anesthesia:** Pressor agents are commonly co-administered with local anesthetics such as lignocaine. Adrenaline (1:100,000) or phenylephrine (1:20,000) is frequently used for this purpose. These drugs cause $α_1$-mediated vasoconstriction, which reduces blood supply at the site of injection of the local anesthetic. This reduces the systemic absorption of lignocaine from the site of administration, providing a dual benefit in the form of prolonged local action and lesser adverse effects. This is because of reduced absorption of lignocaine into systemic circulation, allowing more of it to remain at the local site, producing a prolonged effect. There are fewer systemic adverse effects of lignocaine due to lesser absorption.
4. **Facial, oral or nasopharyngeal surgery:** Pressor agents or vasoconstrictors are useful during these surgeries to reduce regional blood flow and achieve hemostasis.
5. **Epistaxis:** A cotton swab soaked in 1:10,000 adrenaline or 1% phenylephrine can be inserted into the nasal cavity for control of epistaxis. $α_1$-mediated vasoconstriction arrests bleeding from the nasal mucosa. Such use can control local bleeding in surgery, trauma and even gastric erosions.

In contrast to the above-mentioned vascular uses based on $α_1$-mediated vasoconstrictor action, the $β_2$-mediated vasodilator effect of selective $β_2$-agonists like isoxsuprine may offer some relief in cases of peripheral vasospastic diseases (PVDs) such as Buerger disease, frostbite, Raynaud disease, etc. The response, however, is not remarkable as ischemia itself is an important cause of compensatory vasodilatation in the affected areas.

II. Nasal Decongestants

These include ephedrine, phenylephrine, oxymetazoline, xylometazoline and naphazoline. In inflammatory conditions involving the upper respiratory tract, like common cold, rhinitis, sinusitis, Eustachian tube blockade, etc., there is vasodilatation of the blood vessels of the nasal mucosa resulting in nasal stuffiness. This can be controlled by the vasoconstriction of mucosal blood vessels. Drugs like pseudoephedrine and phenylephrine are used orally, whereas oxymetazoline, xylometazoline and naphazoline are used topically as nasal drops. These drugs cause vasoconstriction by $α_1$ stimulation, resulting in nasal decongestion.

However, frequent and habitual use of topical nasal decongestants in allergic conditions carries the risk of rebound congestion and atrophy of the nasal mucosa. Orally used nasal decongestants like phenylephrine and pseudoephedrine do not cause much after-congestion, but there is a risk of rise in BP, especially when these drugs are combined with MAO inhibitors.

III. Cardiac Stimulants

Drugs that have cardio-stimulant activity via $β_1$-receptor activation have several uses:

- In cardiac arrest secondary to drowning, electrocution, or Stokes–Adam syndrome, intravenous adrenaline 1:10,000 is administered in the central vein along with other emergency life-saving measures like cardiac massage.
- In partial or complete atrio-ventricular block, isoproterenol is useful as a temporary measure as it

improves atrio-ventricular conduction through β_1 activation.
- In patients with acute cardiac decompensation due to severe resistant chronic heart failure (CHF), myocardial infarction (MI), or those undergoing cardiac surgery, the short-term intravenous infusion of drugs having β_1-agonistic action, like dopamine or dobutamine, helps to tide over the crisis. This measure should be used only during crisis, as these drugs have no place in routine treatment of CHF or MI.

IV. CNS Stimulants

Amphetamines are useful in the following conditions:
- In cases of narcolepsy, to control daytime sleepiness; however, there is a risk of tolerance and abuse due to their subjective actions (refer to Box 9.3).
- The CNS stimulant effect of amphetamines can be used to counter the sedative effect of anti-epileptics.
- Amphetamines can improve the mood and rigidity in parkinsonism.
- Amphetamines can be useful in nocturnal enuresis for symptomatic relief.
- Hyperkinetic children with attention deficit disorder feel calmer and have an improved attention span with the use of these drugs.

Box 9.3   Narcolepsy

It is a chronic sleep disorder characterised by extreme daytime drowsiness/sleepiness and a strong tendency to fall asleep irrespective of the surroundings and circumstances. It may be accompanied by a sudden loss of tone of skeletal muscles, (cataplexy), vivid/frightening hallucinations during sleep or on waking, obstructive sleep apnea, restless leg syndrome, and insomnia.

The exact cause of narcolepsy is not clearly understood, but probably involves disturbances in the **rapid eye movement** (REM) phase of sleep due to some alterations in the chemicals signalling sleep and wake cycles. Although no definitive cure exists for this condition, symptomatic relief can be achieved through non-pharmacological measures such as avoiding alcohol, smoking, caffeine, and heavy meals. Schedules for sleep, meals and exercise should be fixed and followed regularly.

Pharmacological measures include the following:
- CNS stimulants like amphetamine to check daytime sleepiness. However, these have subjective effects, and risk of tolerance, abuse potential and behavioural disturbances.
- Modafinil is a better option than amphetamine, but it also has some abuse potential.
- Pitolisant is an inverse agonist at H_3 receptors; it increases the synthesis and release of wake-promoting NTMs in the brain.
- Solriamfetol, which inhibits the reuptake of dopamine and NA, is also used to stay awake for longer periods.
- Antidepressants are also used to treat REM sleep problems.
- Sodium oxybate or gamma-hydroxybutyrate (GHB), a CNS depressant, can control cataplexy.

V. Anorectics

In cases of obesity, drugs like fenfluramine, dexfenfluramine, mazindol, etc., maybe used on short-term basis to help control appetite in patients who find it difficult to control their dietary intake. However, obesity being a lifestyle problem, can be controlled or reversed effectively only with lifestyle modifications like caloric restriction and increased physical activity.

VI. Bronchodilators

In **bronchial asthma**, short-acting selective β_2-agonists like salbutamol and terbutaline have been used to abort attacks. These drugs achieve adequate bronchodilatation and relieve symptoms of asthma exacerbation within five minutes of administration by the inhalational route and their effect lasts for 2–4 hours. Current GINA guidelines recommend low dose inhalational corticosteroids with formoterol as a reliever in acute attack of asthma.

Salbutamol is given in a dose of two puffs (100 mcg per puff) through a metered dose inhaler. Terbutaline is inhaled in a dose of 250 mcg at the beginning of the attack to terminate it. Care should be taken to avoid the continuous presence of these drugs at the receptor site; this causes the down-regulation of receptors and results in reduced responsiveness and worsening of bronchial hyper reactivity. Therefore, patients who have frequent asthma episodes and require daily bronchodilator therapy should be put on inhaled corticoids (ICS).

Long-acting selective β_2-agonists drugs like salmeterol and formoterol have a slow onset and a longer duration of action than salbutamol. These drugs were mainly used for the prevention of acute exacerbation of asthma. However, current GINA guidelines recommend the use of formoterol as 'reliever' along with low-dose inhalational corticosteroids (ICS) in case of an acute attack of asthma. The dosage is two puffs of 25 mcg each, taken through a metered dose inhaler, twice a day.

VII. Uterine Relaxants

- Selective β_2 agonists like salbutamol, isoxsuprine and ritodrine cause the relaxation of uterine muscles and are used in the management of premature labour to delay labour pains, thereby allowing more time for fetal growth and lung maturation.
- Threatened abortion, dysmenorrhea—calcium channel blockers are preferred over selective β_2 agonists for these indications because they have better tolerability.
- These drugs may alleviate symptoms of stress incontinence.

VIII. Other Uses of Adrenergic Drugs

In addition to above-mentioned uses, adrenergic drugs are also used for the following indications.

Ocular uses

- Phenylephrine eye drops can be used as mydriatics for fundus examination.

- The vasoconstrictor action of phenylephrine can be used to reduce allergic hyperemia of the conjunctiva.
- Dipivefrin, a prodrug of adrenaline, and selective α_2-agonists like apraclonidine and brimonidine are useful as second-line drugs in wide-angle glaucoma.

Insulin-induced hypoglycemia

Adrenaline can be used as an expedient measure to rapidly reverse insulin-induced hypoglycemia. The condition is routinely treated with IV glucose and IM glucagon administration.

Clinical problem-based questions and MCQs

10. A 60-year-old patient is brought to the emergency ward with a history of ischemic heart disease (IHD) since the last three years. He has oliguria and altered sensorium. Positive findings in examination include cold, clammy skin, low BP of 60/unrecordable. IV fluid therapy is started.
    i. Along with IV fluids, which of the following is the best choice for immediate management in this case?
        a. Dopamine   b. Noradrenaline
        c. Isoprenaline   d. Digoxin
    ii. Describe the rationale behind your choice.
    iii. Mention the dose and route of administration of the chosen drug.

11. A 35-year-old male, victim of a severe road accident, presented to the Emergency with disorientation, fracture in the right leg, and multiple injuries with severe blood loss. On examination, his BP is 80/50. A blood transfusion is ordered, but some delay is expected due to the non-availability of matching blood in the hospital blood bank.
    i. Which of the following is the most suitable initial management in this case?
        a. Injection hydrocortisone
        b. Pressor agents
        c. Rapid infusion of normal saline
        d. Management of fracture
    ii. Describe the rationale behind your choice.

12. A 10-year-old girl was brought to the Emergency with a history of something pricking her feet while she was participating in a water sport event at the beach. Her face was swollen and she had an erythematous rash and intense pruritis all over her body along with breathlessness, extreme anxiety, and tachycardia. Her BP was 90/60.
    i. What is the most likely diagnosis in this case?
    ii. Which of the following drugs is life-saving in this case?
        a. Phentolamine   b. Adrenaline
        c. Prednisolone   d. Atropine
    iii. Describe the rationale behind your choice.
    iv. Mention the dose and route of administration of the chosen drug.

13. A 50-year-old male presented to the Emergency with hypotension and severe dyspnea immediately after an intramuscular injection of penicillin.
    i. Which of the following drugs is life-saving in this case?
        a. Phentolamine   b. Adrenaline
        c. Prednisolone   d. Atropine
    ii. Describe the rationale behind your choice.
    iii. Mention the dose and route of administration of the chosen drug.

14. A 58-year-old woman presents with a 4-day history of cough, runny nose, nasal congestion, and mild headache.
    i. Which of the following may be considered by physicians for symptomatic relief in this patient?
        a. Phenylephrine   b. Noradrenaline
        c. Salbutamol   d. Atropine
    ii. Which important clinical condition may be worsened by the chosen drug?
        a. Diarrhea   b. Hypertension
        c. Epistaxis   d. Constipation
    iii. Describe the rationale behind your choices in the above two questions.

15. A 36-year-old patient reports to the emergency department with an acute asthma attack.
    i. Which of the following is the most suitable drug to abort an acute attack?
        a. Omalizumab   b. Salbutamol
        c. Montelukast   d. Theophylline
    ii. Describe the pharmacological basis for using the chosen drug for aborting an acute attack of asthma.
    iii. Mention the dose and route of administration of the chosen drug.
    iv. Enumerate the adverse effects of the chosen drug.

16. i. Phenylephrine 1:20,000 combined with lignocaine prolongs its local anesthetic action. The underlying mechanism involves:
        a. A decrease in the absorption of lignocaine
        b. An increase in plasma protein binding of lignocaine
        c. Decreased metabolism of lignocaine
        d. Slow excretion of lignocaine
    ii. Describe the pharmacological rationale and advantages and limitations of the above combination.

17. i. Choose the correct dose of dopamine infusion for a patient presenting with hypovolemic shock.
        a. 1–2 mcg/kg/minute
        b. 2–5 mcg/kg/minute
        c. 5–20 mcg/kg/minute
        d. >20 mcg/kg/minute
    ii. Describe the pharmacological basis for choosing this dosage.

ADVERSE DRUG REACTIONS OF ADRENERGIC DRUGS

- α_1-mediated vasoconstriction can cause:
  - A marked rise in BP, which may be dangerous, leading to cerebral hemorrhages, pulmonary edema, etc.

- Extravasation of NA during an IV injection can cause severe local vasospasm, resulting in ischemia and intense pain. This can be reversed by immediate administration of the α-blocker, phentolamine.
- β_1 receptor-mediated cardiac stimulation may cause:
  - Sinus tachycardia
  - Ventricular arrhythmias
  - Increased oxygen demand due to cardiac stimulant action, which may worsen angina
  - Myocardial infarction
- Central stimulant action can cause restlessness, tremors, anxiety, feelings of impending disaster, insomnia, paranoid delusions, etc.

CONTRAINDICATIONS TO ADRENERGIC DRUGS

- Hypertension is a contraindication because α_1-mediated vasoconstriction can worsen the situation by further increasing the PVR and BP.
- Adrenergic drugs can cause a dangerous increase in the BP of patients on β-blockers as α_1-mediated vasoconstriction becomes unopposed in such patients.

> It is interesting to note here that clonidine, a selective agonist at α_2 receptors, is used in the treatment of hypertension. This seems paradoxical. Although clonidine is an agonist at adrenergic receptors, it elicits an anti-adrenergic response because of the inhibitory nature of α_2 receptors and reduces the release of NA from adrenergic nerve endings. This helps in lowering the raised BP. For this reason, clonidine is better described as an antihypertensive drug rather than an adrenergic drug.

- Adrenergic drugs are not used in patients with hyperthyroidism as thyroxine sensitises the myocardium to catecholamines.
- Adrenergic drugs are contraindicated in patients who have angina as they can worsen the condition by further increasing oxygen demand through their cardio-stimulant activity.
- Adrenergic drugs can cause arrhythmias in patients receiving halothane, a general anesthetic.

Clinical problem-based questions and MCQs

18. i. In which of the following conditions is the use of adrenergic drugs contraindicated?
    a. Bronchial asthma
    b. Stokes–Adam syndrome
    c. Hypovolemic shock
    d. Angina pectoris
    ii. Describe the pharmacological basis for the above contraindication.

SALIENT POINTS FOR OTHER ADRENERGIC DRUGS

I. Exogenous Catecholamines

These include dobutamine, dopexamine and fenoldopam.

- Dobutamine is a selective β_1-receptor agonist, used as an inotropic agent in patients who have acute congestive heart failure.
- Dopexamine is an agonist at D_1 and β_2 receptors. Both actions lower the peripheral vascular resistance and BP.
- Fenoldopam is an agonist at D_1 and α_2 receptors. Both actions lower BP. For this reason, it is useful in hypertensive emergencies.
- Isoprenaline is selective for β receptors. β_1-agonistic action is useful in AV node blocks and bradycardia. β_2-agonistic action is used in bronchial asthma.
- Droxidopa, a prodrug of noradrenaline, is useful in patients with postural hypotension.

II. Selective Agonists

Selective α_1-receptor agonist: Phenylephrine, xylometazoline, tetrahydrozoline, midodrine, methoxamine, mephentermine, metaraminol, etc. α_1 receptors are excitatory in nature. The major actions of these drugs are vasoconstriction and nasal decongestion.

- Phenylephrine is mainly used for nasal decongestion and to normalise BP in anesthetic-induced hypotension.
- Metaraminol is the preferred drug for the management of hypotension associated with spinal anesthesia.
- Midodrine is useful for the management of postural hypotension.
- Methoxamine is useful as a pressor agent in patients with shock.

Selective α_2-receptor agonists: Clonidine, brimonidine, apraclonidine, moxonidine, rilmenidine, lofexidine, dexmedetomidine, tizanidine, etc.

- Clonidine decreases noradrenaline secretion as α_2 autoreceptors are inhibitory in nature. It is useful in hypertensive urgency, diarrhea due to diabetic neuropathy involving the autonomic nerves, migraine prophylaxis, attention deficit disorder in children, to control symptoms of alcohol/ nicotine/opioid withdrawal, and in Tourette's syndrome. The most disturbing limitation of clonidine use is the **clonidine withdrawal** reaction. Clonidine reduces only the release of noradrenaline, not its synthesis. Thus, the sudden withdrawal of clonidine causes an excessive release of catecholamines, manifesting as a hypertensive crisis. This can be managed by α_1-receptor blocker phentolamine, given intravenously.
- Moxonidine and rilmenidine are useful in resistant cases of hypertension and neuropathic pain.

- Apraclonidine and brimonidine are useful in reducing raised intraocular tension in open-angle glaucoma.
- Tizanidine acts as a centrally-acting muscle relaxant and is useful in amyotrophic lateral sclerosis.
- Lofexidine is used in opioid dependence.

Selective β-receptor agonists:

- Isoprenaline, an exogenous catecholamine, acts equally at $β_1$ and $β_2$ receptors but lacks α actions. Cardiostimulant $β_1$-agonistic action is useful in bradycardia and AV nodal blocks, whereas $β_2$-agonistic action causing bronchodilatation is useful in bronchial asthma.
- Selective $β_1$- and $β_2$-agonists are described earlier in this chapter (refer to page 121)
- The selective $β_3$-agonist mirabegron is being tried in patients with CHF and urge incontinence. It can cause hypotension and headache as adverse effects.

Summary

- Adrenergic drugs can be classified based on their chemical structure (catecholamines/non-catecholamines), mechanism of action (direct/indirect), and their therapeutic uses (pressor agents, nasal decongestants, bronchodilators, uterine relaxants, cardiac stimulants, central stimulants and anorectics).
- Adrenergic receptors are of two types—α and β. α has two subtypes—$α_1$ and $α_2$, whereas β has three subtypes—$β_1$, $β_2$ and $β_3$.
- $α_1$-excitatory receptors are present in the vascular smooth muscles of the blood vessels of the skin, mucous membrane, skeletal muscles and splanchnic vessels. $α_1$-mediated vasoconstrictor action forms the basis of the use of adrenergic drugs as pressor agents and nasal decongestants.
- Pressor agents are useful in the treatment of hypotension and shock in emergencies such as severe hemorrhage, spinal injury, etc.
- In hypovolemic shock, low-dose dopamine is preferred over noradrenaline as its prominent D_1-agonistic action helps to maintain renal blood flow and GFR.
- Adrenaline, being a physiological antagonist of histamine, is useful in the management of anaphylactic shock. Dipivefrine, a prodrug of adrenaline, is useful in wide-angle glaucoma.
- $α_1$ agonists are used along with lignocaine to prolong its local anesthetic action and reduce systemic toxicity, to control bleeding in epistaxis/facio-oral surgery, and as a nasal decongestant for cough/colds.
- $α_2$ receptors are inhibitory in nature. Agonists reduce the release of noradrenaline from adrenergic nerve endings. The $α_2$ agonist clonidine is useful in the treatment of hypertension. Apraclonidine and brimonidine are used as add-on drugs to reduce IOT in open-angle glaucoma.
- The selective $β_1$ agonist dobutamine is useful in cardiogenic shock along with fluid therapy. Adrenergic drugs should not be used in routine treatment of CHF, as they increase oxygen demand and may precipitate angina. They may, however, be given as an expedient measure in acute cardiac decompensation.
- Selective $β_2$-agonists cause bronchodilatation and uterine relaxation. Short-acting drugs (salbutamol and terbutaline) are widely used to abort acute attacks of bronchial asthma. Currently, inhalational corticosteroids and formoterol combination is recommended as 'relievers' in acute attack. Long-acting drugs (salmeterol and formoterol) are used to prevent acute attacks. However, the down-regulation of receptors with continued use may decrease responsiveness. $β_2$-agonists like ritodrine and isoxsuprine are used for their uterine relaxant action in dysmenorrhea and premature onset of labour.
- Adrenergic drugs with higher central:peripheral actions, e.g., amphetamine, improve attention and performance in hyperkinetic children with attention deficit disorder. Also useful in narcolepsy, and reducing rigidity in parkinsonism. However, these drugs improve athletic performance and may be abused by athletes. Hence, they are included in **dope tests**.
- The adverse effects of adrenergic drugs include worsening of hypertension, angina and pulmonary edema. Tachyarrhythmias may occur. Central adverse effects include anxiety, tremors, restlessness, insomnia, etc.
- Adrenergic drugs are contraindicated in hyperthyroidism, hypertension and angina.

Questions for practice

1. Describe the therapeutic classification of adrenergic drugs.
2. Enumerate the therapeutic uses and adverse effects of adrenergic drugs.
3. Explain why:
   a. Dipivefrine is useful in wide-angle glaucoma.
   b. Adrenaline is combined with local anesthetics.
   c. Adrenaline-soaked swabs are used to control epistaxis.
   d. Adrenaline is used in cases of anaphylactic shock.
   e. Catecholamines are not used for the routine treatment of CHF.
   f. Dopamine low-dose infusion is preferred over noradrenaline in hypovolemic shock.
   g. Adrenergic drugs are contraindicated in angina.
   h. Terbutaline is used to abort an acute attack of asthma.
   i. Isoxsuprine is used in premature labour.

4. Write short notes on:
   a. Selective β₂-agonists   b. Nasal decongestants
   c. Amphetamines   d. Cardiac stimulants
   e. Dale's reversal phenomenon
5. Describe the management of:
   a. Anaphylactic shock   b. Cardiogenic shock

Hints for problem-based questions and MCQs

1. i. a. Dexamphetamine
   ii. Refer to page 120
   iii. Refer to page 120
2. i. Refer to page 122
   ii. Refer to page 122
3. i. Dale's reversal phenomenon
   ii. This is because adrenaline is a non-selective agonist at adrenergic receptors
   iii. Refer to page 121
4. i. Wide-angle glaucoma
   ii. Adrenaline has complex effects on aqueous humor dynamics (refer to page 122)
   iii. Refer to page 122
5. i. a. Salmeterol
   ii. Longer-acting selective β₂-agonist
6. a. Salbutamol
7. i. a. α₁
   ii. Phenylephrine and methoxamine
   iii. Nasal decongestion, control of epistaxis, combined with local anesthetic, and used as a pressor agent.
8. b. Dobutamine
9. i. a. Naphazoline
   ii. Used as a nasal decongestant
10. i. a. Dopamine
    ii. Refer to Box 9.2, page 125
    iii. The infusion rate of dopamine should be low (2–5 mcg/kg/minute) so that tissue perfusion is maintained.
11. i. c. Rapid infusion of normal saline
    ii. The main goal of treatment in shock is not just to raise the BP but to improve perfusion of vital organs. Until blood is arranged for transfusion, rapid IV fluids can be used. Tissue ischemia itself causes vasoconstriction. For this reason, pressor agents may be combined in emergency situations only when BP is not being maintained with fluid therapy alone.
12. i. Anaphylactic shock
    ii. b. Adrenaline
    iii. Refer to page 125
    iv. Adrenaline 1:1000 (1 mg/mL) given subcutaneously in a dose of 0.3–0.5 mL.
13. i. b. Adrenaline
    ii. See question 12.iii.
    iii. See 12.iv.
14. i. a. Phenylephrine
    ii. b. Hypertension
    iii. Phenylephrine is used for its nasal decongestant action as it causes vasoconstriction in the blood vessels of the nasal mucous membrane and relieves nasal stuffiness. Hypertension is worsened due to α₁-mediated vasoconstriction caused by phenytephrine.
15. i. b. Salbutamol
    ii. Refer to page 126
    iii. Salbutamol is given in a dose of 2 puffs (100 mcg per puff) through a metered dose inhaler
    iv. Muscle tremors and down-regulation of receptors leading to non-responsiveness to treatment and worsening of condition.
16. i. a. A decrease in the absorption of lignocaine
    ii. Refer to page 125
17. i. b. 2–5 mcg/kg/minute
    ii. Refer to page 125
18. i. d. Angina pectoris
    ii. Refer to page 128

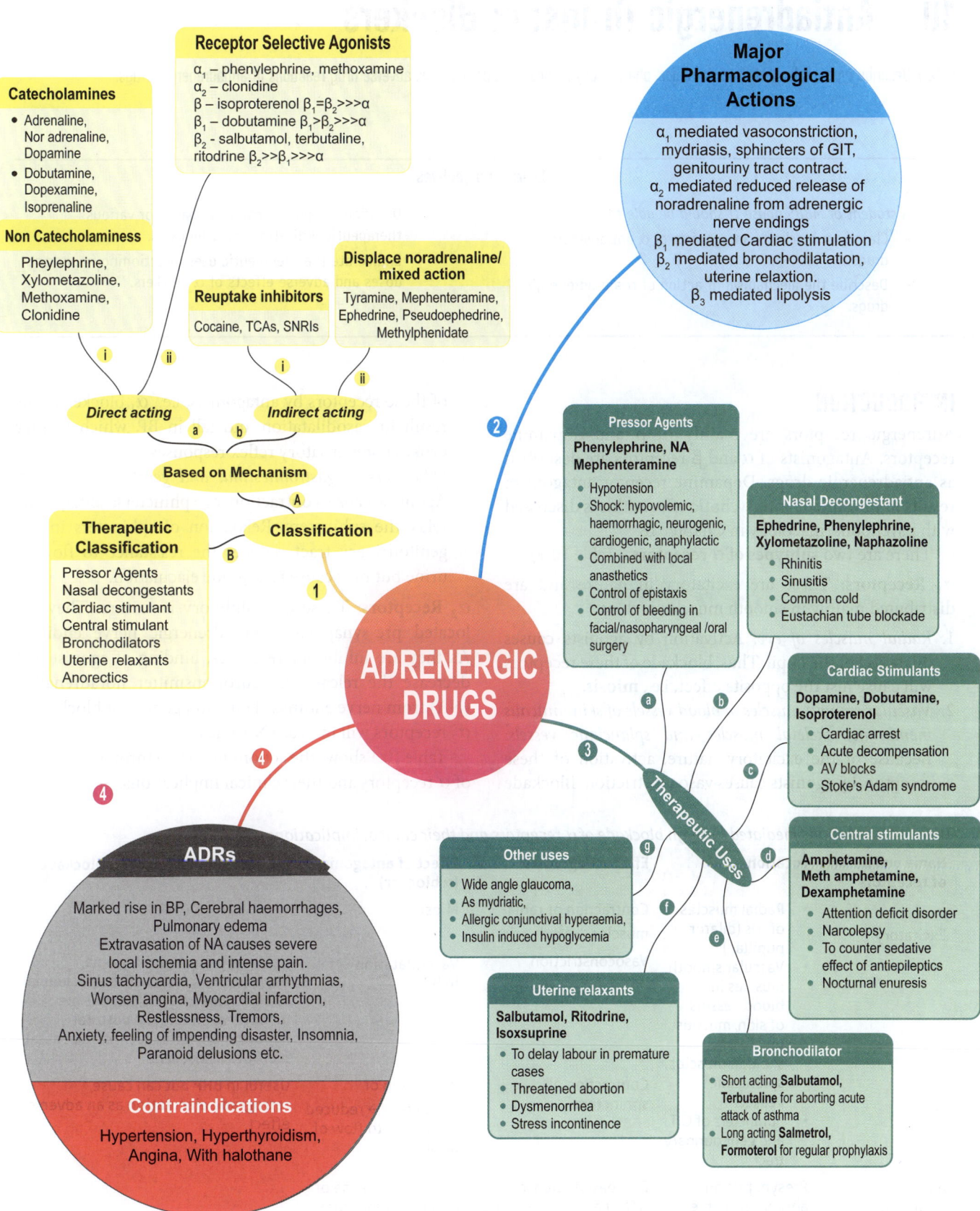

SECTION 2 Drugs Acting on ANS and PNS

10 Antiadrenergic Drugs: α Blockers

PH2.1 Describe types, salient pharmacokinetics, pharmacodynamics, therapeutic uses, adverse drug reactions of antiadrenergic drugs.

Learning objectives

A student of MBBS phase II should be able to:
- Classify α blockers/ antagonists or α antiadrenergic drugs.
- Describe the mechanism of action of α antiadrenergic drugs.
- Describe the pharmacological basis for various therapeutic indications of α blockers.
- Enumerate the therapeutic uses, mentioning important doses and adverse effects of α blockers.

INTRODUCTION

Adrenergic receptors are mainly α, β and dopamine receptors. Antagonists of α and β receptors are described as antiadrenergic drugs. Dopamine receptor antagonism results in prominent antipsychotic effects; this is discussed with psychopharmacology in Chapter 18.

There are **two subtypes of α receptors.** (Table 10.1).

α_1 **Receptors:** These are excitatory in nature and are distributed mainly in smooth muscles such as

1. *Radial muscles of eye*: Activation by agonists causes dilatation of the pupil. Thus, blockade of these receptors will cause just the opposite effect, i.e., **miosis.**
2. *Vascular smooth muscles in blood vessels of skin, mucous membrane, skeletal muscles and splanchnic vessels*: Because of the excitatory nature, activation of these receptors by agonists causes vasoconstriction. Blockade of these receptors by antagonists, i.e., α_1 blockers, thus result in vasodilatation and fall in BP, which further evokes compensatory reflex responses.
3. *Sphincters of gastrointestinal and genitourinary tract*: Agonists cause contraction of sphincters; antagonists relax the sphincters. Relaxation of sphincters in the genitourinary tract reduces the resistance to flow of urine but may cause retrograde ejaculation.

α_2 **Receptors:** These are inhibitory in nature. They are located pre-synaptically on adrenergic nerve endings. As they are inhibitory receptors, binding of agonist will decrease the release of neurotransmitter noradrenaline (NA) from nerve endings. Thus, antagonists or blockers of α_2 receptors will increase NA release.

Table 10.1 shows the actions mediated through blockade of α receptors and their clinical implications.

Table 10.1 Actions mediated through blockade of α receptors and their clinical implications

Name and nature of receptors	Location	Effect of agonists	Effect of antagonist (α blocker)	Clinical implications of α blockade
α_1 Excitatory	• Radial muscles of iris (dilator pupillae)	Contraction of radial muscles → Mydriasis	Miosis	–
	• Vascular smooth muscles in blood vessels of skin, mucous membrane, skeletal muscles, splanchnic vessels	Vasoconstriction	Vasodilatation → fall in BP	Useful in **pheochromocytoma, hypertension, reverse tissue ischemia**, but the same effect is responsible for adverse effects like **postural hypotension, reflex tachycardia, nasal stuffiness, headache**
	• Sphincters of GIT and genitourinary tract	Contraction of sphincters	Relaxation of sphincters → reduced resistance to flow of urine	Useful in **BHP** but can cause **retrograde ejaculation** as an adverse effect
α_2 Inhibitory	Presynaptic on adrenergic nerve endings	Decreased release of NTM, i.e., noradrenaline from adrenergic nerve endings	Increased release of noradrenaline from nerve endings	

CLASSIFICATION OF α BLOCKERS

Alpha blockers can be divided on the basis of their **mechanism of action** into irreversible and reversible blockers. Based on selectivity, alpha blockers can be non-selective or selective for various subtypes as shown in Flowchart 10.1.

MECHANISM OF ACTION OF α BLOCKERS

The interaction of some α blockers with receptors is irreversible. Drugs like phenoxybenzamine and dibenzylchlorethylamine (dibenamine) form a reactive ethylene immonium intermediate compound in the body that binds covalently with α receptors. Thus their effect lasts longer for about 3–4 days till new receptors are synthesised.

Drugs such as phentolamine, prazosin and their congeners interact with receptors in a reversible manner. They dissociate from receptors after some time, and hence their duration of action depends on the half-life of the drug and the rate of its dissociation from receptors. It is shorter compared to irreversible blockers.

PHARMACOLOGICAL ACTIONS OF α BLOCKERS

1. Cardiovascular effects

Alpha blockers have direct as well as reflex effects on CVS.

Direct effects

Blockade of excitatory α_1 receptors, present in vascular smooth muscles in blood vessels of skin, mucous membranes, skeletal muscles and splanchnic vessels → Vasodilatation → Fall in peripheral vascular resistance → **Fall in BP**.

Thus, in the presence of α blockers:

- Pressor effect of pure α_1 agonists is prevented.
- Biphasic response of BP to adrenaline is converted to only depressor response. (Dale's reversal phenomenon was demonstrated in presence of dihydroergotamine, which is an α blocker.)

With drugs such as **phenoxybenzamine and phentolamine,** the *vasodilator effect is more prominent on veins than on arterioles*. So, in patients taking these drugs, a change in posture—such as rising from a seated position—can lead to blood suddenly pooling in the leg veins that are dilated under the effect of α blockers. This results in a sudden drop in blood pressure, known as **postural hypotension**, which may cause dizziness, a sensation of faintness, or even syncope. Episode of postural hypotension and syncope seen with the initiation of α blocker therapy is called ' first-dose phenomenon', which can be prevented by starting the therapy with a low dose of the drug at bedtime.

Prazosin and its congeners have **more prominent dilator effect on arterioles than on veins**. Hence, postural hypotension is less marked.

Reflex effects

A fall in BP secondary to vasodilatation caused by α blockers results in baroreceptor-mediated sympathetic stimulation → β_1 stimulation → tachycardia.

This **reflex tachycardia is more prominent with non-selective α blockers** because

- α_1 Block → Vasodilatation → Fall in BP → Baroreceptor reflex → sympathetic stimulation → Increased NA levels → Excessive β_1 stimulation → Tachycardia.
- α_2 Block → Increased NA release → More β_1 stimulation of heart → Tachycardia.

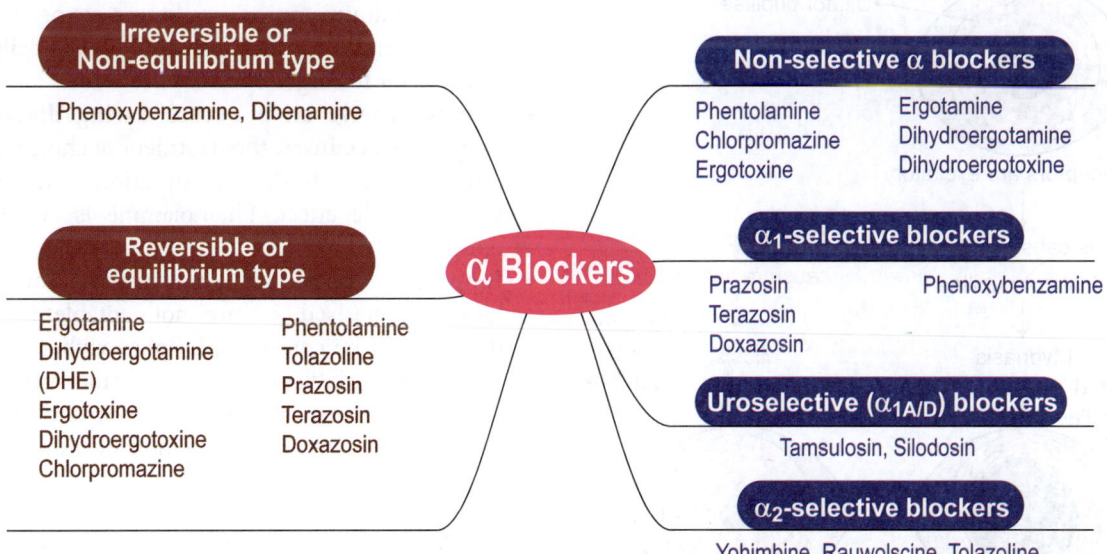

Flowchart 10.1 Classification α blockers

Chronic use of α blockers causes **compensatory rise in blood volume**. It is because:

- Hypotension caused by α blockers → Fall in renal blood flow (RBF) → Decreased glomerular filtration rate → More complete reabsorption of Na^+ and water in renal tubules → Expansion of blood volume.
- In addition, hypotension caused by α blockers → Reflex increase in renin release mediated through $β_1$ receptors → RAAS stimulation → Increased aldosterone → Na^+ water retention → Expansion of blood volume.

2. Ocular effects

As α receptors present in radial muscles are excitatory in nature, their stimulation causes mydriasis. Thus, α blockade in radial muscles causes miosis (Fig. 10.1).

3. Other actions of α blockers

- $α_1$ Blockade in blood vessels of nasal mucosa → Vasodilation → **Nasal stuffiness**
- **Headache** due to vasodilatation
- **Improved urinary flow:** $α_1$ Blockade in genitourinary tract reduces resistance to the flow of urine, as the tone of the bladder trigone, sphincter, and prostate is decreased This effect relieves urinary symptoms in elderly males with benign hypertrophy of prostate. **Retrograde ejaculation** occurs as an adverse effect of this action.
- Terazosin and doxazosin, longer-acting congeners of prazosin, **promote apoptosis in prostatic tissue** in addition to their $α_1$-adrenergic blocking activity. They thus contribute to reducing disease progression in benign prostatic hyperplasia (BPH).

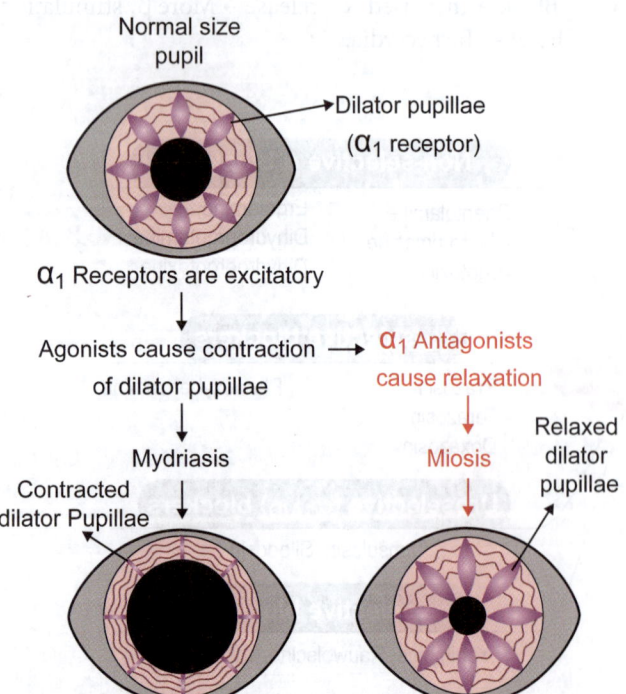

Fig. 10.1 Effect of $α_1$ agonists and blockers on pupil size

- Adrenergic sweating decreases.
- Intestinal motility increases.

THERAPEUTIC USES OF α BLOCKERS

1. Pheochromocytoma

Pheochromocytoma is a tumour of adrenal medulla, which releases a mixture of catecholamines such as adrenaline and noradrenaline. Excess circulating catecholamines activate adrenergic receptors, and patient presents with hypertension, tachycardia and arrhythmia.

Alpha blockers have a role in:

- **Diagnosis of pheochromocytoma**: Phentolamine infusion is a diagnostic test for pheochromocytoma. Phentolamine, being an α blocker, causes fall in BP as it blocks constrictor effect of catecholamines on blood vessels. The hypotensive effect is seen in normal individuals also, but is more prominent, when catecholamines are contributing more to the vascular tone, such as in pheochromocytoma. Hence a **fall in BP greater than 35 mm of Hg in SBP and 25 mm of Hg in DBP with phentolamine infusion** is considered diagnostic of pheochromocytoma. Other techniques for the diagnosis of pheochromocytoma include assessing the levels of circulating catecholamines, measuring 24-hourly urinary excretion of catecholamine metabolites, namely metanephrine, normetanephrine and vanillylmandelic acid (VMA) and imaging studies. These techniques are safer than phentolamine infusion in confirming the diagnosis of pheochromocytoma.
- **Definitive treatment of pheochromocytoma** is surgical resection, but there is risk of release of stored catecholamines during **surgical handling of tumour**. This may precipitate hypertensive crisis due to explosive rise in BP, which has its own set of complications. Such complications during surgery can be prevented by oral administration of longer-acting α blocker phenoxybenzamine in a dose of 10–20 mg daily, for few weeks prior to surgery.
- If **hypertensive crisis occurs during diagnostic or surgical procedures**, the treatment of choice is sodium nitroprusside. It has a short duration of action and an easily titrable effect. Phentolamine is an alternative option.
- **Inoperable cases of pheochromocytoma** which have metastasised, or are not suitable for surgical therapy, can be controlled by phenoxybenzamine and metyrosine. Metyrosine is a tyrosine analogue that causes competitive inhibition of tyrosine hydroxylase enzyme and interferes with the rate limiting step of catecholamine synthesis.

2. Hypertensive emergencies

Alpha blockers such as phentolamine and tolazoline are useful in hypertensive emergencies secondary to enhanced $α_1$ action such as:

- Surgical handling of pheochromocytoma (as mentioned earlier).
- **Clonidine withdrawal** – Clonidine, an agonist at α_2 receptors, reduces the release of NTM (noradrenaline) from adrenergic nerve endings. However, the synthesis of NTM continues. Hence, under the influence of clonidine, the nerve endings are loaded with NTM. Moreover, continuous deficiency or absence of neurotransmitter or agonist may cause up-regulation of post synaptic receptors. Sudden withdrawal of clonidine causes explosive release of noradrenaline from nerve endings, which causes excessive α_1 action, resulting in hypertensive crisis. Thus, α blocker phentolamine can control clonidine withdrawal phenomenon.
- **Overdosage of sympathomimetic drugs** causes excessive α_1 action, resulting in hypertensive emergency, which can be managed with α blockers.
- **Cheese reaction** is due to the intake of tyramine-rich foods in patients receiving non-selective MAO inhibitors. Tyramine causes excessive release of neurotransmitter (NA) from nerve endings, but its metabolism is blocked by concurrently administered MAO inhibitors. Therefore, symptoms of adrenergic excess and hypertensive crisis occur, which are managed with phentolamine..

3. Chronic hypertension

For treatment of **mild to moderate hypertension**, selective α_1 blockers like prazosin are useful. The main drawback with use of α blockers is postural hypotension, which is more disturbing with the first dose. This 'first-dose' phenomenon can, however, be prevented by starting therapy with a small dose given at bed time and then increasing the dose gradually. Selective α_1 blockers have a favourable effect on lipid profile as they reduce LDL and raise HDL. Therefore, these drugs are preferred in hypertension coexisting with dyslipidemia and benign prostatic hypertrophy.

4. Peripheral vasospastic diseases

In peripheral vasospastic diseases such as **Raynaud's phenomenon and acrocyanosis**, vasospasm is a prominent contributing factor. α Blockers such as phenoxybenzamine, prazosin and tolazoline provide symptomatic relief. However, calcium channel blockers are the preferred drugs for these conditions.

5. Intense local vasospasm and ischemia

This may occur secondary to **inadvertent leaking of noradrenaline** or other α agonists in subcutaneous tissue during IV injection. It can be reversed by α blockers like phentolamine.

6. PIPE therapy

This is a 'papaverine/phentolamine-induced penile erection' therapy for males with erectile dysfunction and impotence. Local injection of papaverine alone or with phentolamine into corpus cavernosum can improve **erectile function**. However, this should be reserved only for severe cases not responding to other therapies, because intracavernosal injection may be associated with complications such as painful persistent erection called **priapism, penile hematoma/infection/fibrosis and deviation**.

7. Scorpion sting

Selective α_1 blockers like **prazosin** are useful in scorpion sting. The venom of scorpion probably opens voltage-sensitive sodium, potassium, calcium and chloride channels, resulting in membrane depolarisation, calcium entry and catecholamine release. Dangerous rise in BP and acute pulmonary edema occurs in severe cases. α_1 Blocker prazosin dilates veins and arterioles, reducing BP, preload and afterload, and thereby, pulmonary edema is reversed. Thus prazosin acts as a physiological and pharmacological antidote for scorpion sting. In addition to prazosin, analgesics such as acetaminophen, antihistamines are also useful for controlling symptoms like pain, swelling, itching and redness at the site of the sting. Midazolam, a short-acting benzodiazepine with fast onset of action, is used to control central excitation caused by scorpion sting. In some patients the heart rate is slowed, which can be reversed by the anticholinergic drug atropine.

8. Angiography

Tolazoline is used **during angiography** as it allows better visualisation of smaller vessels due to its peripheral vasodilator effect.

9. Benign prostatic hypertrophy (BPH)

In elderly males, urinary obstruction may occur owing to benign hypertrophy of prostate. There are two components of such urinary obstruction: static and dynamic. The static component is due to enlarged size or hypertrophy of prostate, whereas the dynamic component is due to increased tone of bladder neck and the smooth muscles of prostate.

Symptoms of BPH are:

- Voiding symptoms like hesitancy, narrowing of urine stream, dribbling and increased residual urine volume.
- Irritative symptoms of BPH are frequency of micturition, feeling of urgency and nocturia.

The **definitive treatment** is surgical, but drugs are used for symptomatic improvement. Drugs useful in benign prostatic hypertrophy include:

- 5-α-reductase inhibitors like **finasteride** and **dutasteride** interfere with the conversion of testosterone into dihydrotestosterone and arrest further growth of prostate. Finasteride mainly improves the static component in BPH, and may reduce prostate size. Clinical improvement occurs late, approximately after 6 months of starting therapy.

- Alpha blockers like α_1-selective blocker **prazosin**
- α_{1A}/α_{1D}-selective or uroselective α blockers like **tamsulosin** and **silodosin** are used. These drugs act by relaxing the bladder trigone, prostate and prostatic part of urethra, leading to increased urinary flow rate and more complete emptying of the bladder. Voiding symptoms of BPH are improved better than the irritative symptoms. Thus, α blockers improve the dynamic component of urinary obstruction and clinical improvement occurs quickly within 2 weeks of starting therapy.

Limitations of α blockers therapy in BPH include the following.

- They have no effect on prostate size, and therefore, the effect lasts only till therapy is continued. Rather, the symptomatic benefit provided may diminish with continued therapy after few years, as the disease continues to progress.
- Alpha blockers usually do not have much effect on disease progression. However, terazosin and doxazosin have some apoptosis-promoting effect on prostate. These are longer acting than prazosin and are suitable for once-a-day administration.
- Uroselective α blocker tamsulosin has minimal vascular adverse effects.

Silodosin is another uroselective α blocker, with a longer duration of action than tamsulosin.

Finasteride and tamsulosin are combined in BPH in an effort to improve the static and dynamic components, respectively.

Clinical problem-based questions and MCQs

1. A 75-year-old patient presents with thinning of urine stream, dribbling, frequency and urgency of micturition. On per rectal physical examination, prostate is seen enlarged and nodular. The patient is a known case of heart failure and shows signs of fluid retention.
   i. Which of the following drugs is most suitable for providing symptomatic relief?
      a. phenoxybenzamine   b. phentolamine
      c. tolazoline   d. tamsulosin
   ii. Explain the pharmacological basis to justify your choice.
   iii. Which drug can be combined with the above chosen drug and why?

2. Which of the following drugs improve static component of BPH?
   a. tamsulosin   b. silodosin
   c. dutasteride   d. phentolamine

3. Which of the following α blockers promote apoptosis in prostate?
   a. phentolamine   B. phenoxybenzamine
   c. terazosin   d. dibenaine

4. i. Select α_{1A}/α_{1D} blocker from the following drugs.
      a. terazosin   b. tamsulosin
      c. tolazoline   d. rawolscine
   ii. What is the indication for use of α_{1A}/α_{1D} blocker?

5. A 49-year-old hypertensive patient was well controlled with clonidine 0.2 mg, twice a day. He went to attend a wedding in a remote area in a village and forgot to carry his medicine box. Clonidine was not available in the local market over there. On the 3rd day of his stay, he had pounding headache, irritability and anxiety. BP was 200/130.
   i. What is the cause of his symptoms?
      a. Excessive catecholamine synthesis
      b. Excessive catecholamine release
      c. Reduced metabolism of catecholamines
      d. Reduced affinity of adrenergic receptors
   ii. Which of the following drugs is most suitable in the management of this case?
      a. prazosin   b. phentolamine
      c. propranolol   d. hydrochlorthiazide
   iii. Describe the pharmacological basis for patient's symptoms and use of the chosen drug in this case.

6. A 53-year-old male patient presents with episodic headache, tremors and palpitation that lasts for about 15–20 minutes. The patient gives a history of experiencing such episodes since the last 3–4 years, but now these episodes occur more frequently, twice or thrice a week. The patient has no other significant medical or drug history. On examination, HR was 120 beats per minute, BP was 170/100, and respiration rate 20 breaths per minute. No other positive signs were elicited. On investigating, there was
   - sinus tachycardia in ECG
   - significant rise in 24-hour urinary metanephrine levels (1300 mcg/24 hours; normal range 45–290 mcg/24 hours)
   - Chest X ray showed mild left ventricular hypertrophy
   - Abdominal CT scan showed left adrenal gland mass approximately 3.5 cm in diameter.
   i. What is the most probable diagnosis?
   ii. Which drug can be used to confirm this diagnosis and how?
   iii. What is the definitive and conservative treatment for this patient?

7. i. Identify the α blocker suitable in a patient with mild hypertension:
      a. dihydroergotamine b. prazosin
      c. phentolamine   d. tamsulosin
   ii. Describe the pharmacological basis to justify your choice.

8. A 40-year-old male patient diagnosed with mild hypertension was put on prazosin therapy. The patient, on taking his first dose after breakfast felt dizzy and had a fainting fit (syncope). On examination, BP was 90/60.
   i. What is the cause of the symptoms?
   ii. How can such attack be prevented?

ADVERSE EFFECTS OF α BLOCKERS

1. Postural hypotension and first-dose phenomenon. This is more prominent with phenoxybenzamine and phentolamine than prazosin because of their prominent dilator effect on venules than arterioles.
2. Reflex tachycardia, arrhythmia and angina may be precipitated in susceptible patients. This adverse effect is also seen more with non-selective α blockers than prazosin group.
3. Phentolamine has some agonistic effect on H_1 receptors. Thus, gastric acid secretion is increased.
4. Vasodilatation caused by α blockers may lead to headache and nasal stuffiness.
5. Phenoxybenzamine can cross the blood–brain barrier and cause central adverse effects like nausea, fatigue, and sedation.
6. Retrograde ejaculation may occur.
7. With PIPE therapy, there is risk of painful, persistent erection called priapism, penile hematoma/ infection/ fibrosis and deviation with repeated injections.
8. Alpha blockers may cause 'floppy iris syndrome' during cataract surgery. This is due to reduced radial muscle tone in iris resulting in miosis, fluttering and bellowing of iris stroma. The iris may prolapse towards the incisions.

Cautions/Contraindications to Using α Blockers

These drugs should be cautiously used in patients with a history of postural hypotension or syncopal attacks.
- Heart failure and fluid retention, as vasodilatation favours further fluid retention.
- Urinary incontinence.

Clinical problem-based questions and MCQs

9. i. **Which α blocker has more risk of causing postural hypotension?**
   a. Phenoxybenzamine
   b. Prazosin
   c. Doxazosin
   d. Tamsulosin
   ii. **Describe pharmacological basis to justify your answer.**

10. i. **Which α blocker has more risk of causing tachycardia?**
    a. Non-selective α blockers
    b. $α_1$-selective blockers
    c. $α_2$-selective blockers
    d. $α_{1A}$-selective blockers
    ii. **Describe the pharmacological basis to justify your answer.**

11. i. **Identify the drug used as antidote in case of scorpion sting.**
    a. Phentolamine
    b. Prazosin
    c. Dopamine
    d. Timolol
    ii. Describe pharmacological basis to justify your choice.
    iii. Name other drugs useful in cases of scorpion sting.

12. **A psychiatric patient on non-selective MAO inhibitor therapy attended a wedding and consumed wine. Shortly afterward, he became anxious and irritable and complained of a severe headache. He was rushed to the hospital, where his blood pressure was found to be 200/110 mmHg.**
    i. What is the likely cause of the patient's symptoms?
    ii. Name the drug that is useful in the management of this condition.

Summary

- Alpha receptors are of two types, $α_1$ and $α_2$.
- $α_1$ receptors are excitatory in nature. Their blockade causes miosis, vasodilatation and relaxation of sphincters in GIT and genitourinary tract.
- $α_2$ receptors are inhibitory in nature. Their blockade increases the release of noradrenaline from nerve endings.
- Vasodilation caused by blockade of $α_1$ receptors lowers BP and causes postural hypotension. Reflex response to hypotensive effect results in tachycardia.
- Alpha blockers are useful in mild to moderate hypertension, hypertensive emergencies, diagnosis/treatment of pheochromocytoma and as intracavernosal injection in erectile dysfunction due to their vasodilator effect.
- Their sphincter relaxing effect is useful to relieve symptoms of benign hypertrophy of prostate. Uroselective blockers like tamsulosin are preferred for this indication and are usually combined with finasteride, a 5α-reductase inhibitor that decreases the disease progression in BPH.
- Reflex tachycardia is more prominent with non-selective blockers.
- Postural hypotension is more prominent with phentolamine and phenoxybenzamine due to their greater vasodilatory effect on venules than arterioles. It may cause syncopal attack as an adverse effect, especially after the first dose, which can be prevented

- by initiating therapy with low dose and administering the drug at bed time.
- Vasodilator effect can also cause headache and nasal stuffiness as adverse effects.
- Retrograde ejaculation may occur. Intracavernosal injections may cause priapism, penile infection hematomas and penile fibrosis; deviation may also occur.

Questions for practice

1. Enumerate the therapeutic uses and adverse effects of α blockers.
2. Write short notes on
   i. Tamsulosin
   ii. Uroselective α blockers
   iii. Management of pheochromocytoma
   iv. Medical management of BPH
   v. PIPE therapy in erectile dysfunction
3. Explain why
   i. Reflex tachycardia is more with non-selective α blockers.
   ii. Postural hypotension is more with phentolamine than prazosin.
   iii. Phenoxybenzamine is used preoperatively in pheochromocytoma.
   iv. Finasteride and tamsulosin are combined in treatment of benign hypertrophy of prostate.
   v. Alpha blockers cause expansion of blood volume.

Hints for problem-based questions and MCQs

1. i. d. Tamsulosin
   ii. The patient has fluid retention due to heart failure, which may be worsened by vasodilator effect of α blockers. So, tamsulosin having uroselective action and negligible cardiovascular effects is preferred for this patient.
   iii. 5-α reductase inhibitors, such as finasteride and dutasteride, inhibit conversion of testosterone to DHT, thereby preventing further growth of prostate. They improve the static component of BPH.
2. c. Dutasteride
3. c. Terazosin
4. i. b. Tamsulosin
   ii. Benign prostatic hypertrophy
5. i. b. Excessive catecholamine release
   ii. b. Phentolamine
   iii. Clonidine only reduces the release of NA, not its synthesis. So, in patients on clonidine therapy, the nerve endings are loaded with NA. Moreover, post-synaptic receptors are up-regulated. Sudden withdrawal of clonidine causes explosive release of catecholamines and hypertensive crisis. Phentolamine is useful due to its α_1 blocking effect.
6. i. Pheochromocytoma
   ii. b. Phentolamine test is used to diagnose pheochromocytoma. Fall in BP caused with phentolamine is more in such patients as compared to normal adults. A fall of > 35 mm of Hg in SBP and > 25 mm of Hg in DBP is diagnostic of pheochromocytoma.
   iii. Definitive treatment - surgical resection of tumour; conservative treatment is with irreversible α blocker, phenoxybenzamine.
7. i. b. Prazosin
   ii. α_1 selective action. Reflex tachycardia and postural hypotension is more with non-selective drugs (dihydroergotamine, phentolamine). Tamsuosin is uroselective, so not much effect on BP.
8. i. Postural hypotension (first-dose phenomenon)
   ii. Can be prevented by starting therapy with a low dose and giving the drug at bed time.
9. i. Phenoxybenzamine
   ii. It causes more dilatation of venules than arterioles. Refer to page 133
10. i. a. Non-selective α blocker
    ii. Fall in BP due to blockade of α_1 receptors → reflex sympathetic stimulation → tachycardia. Increased NA release due to α_2 blockade → tachycardia.
11. i. b. Prazosin
    ii. Scorpion venom opens voltage sensitive channels. Catecholamine release → Dangerous rise in BP and acute pulmonary edema → Blockade of α_1 receptors with Prazosin causes vasodilation → Fall in BP reduces preload, after-load, reverses pulmonary edema.
    iii. Analgesics, antihistamines and benzodiazepines are useful in cases of scorpion stings.
12. i. Cheese reaction. Tyramine-rich substances like cheese, wines and pickles cause catecholamine release. In patients on non-selective MAO inhibitor therapy, these catecholamines are not metabolised. So, intense vasoconstriction and hypertensive crisis occur.
    iii. Phentolamine is useful.

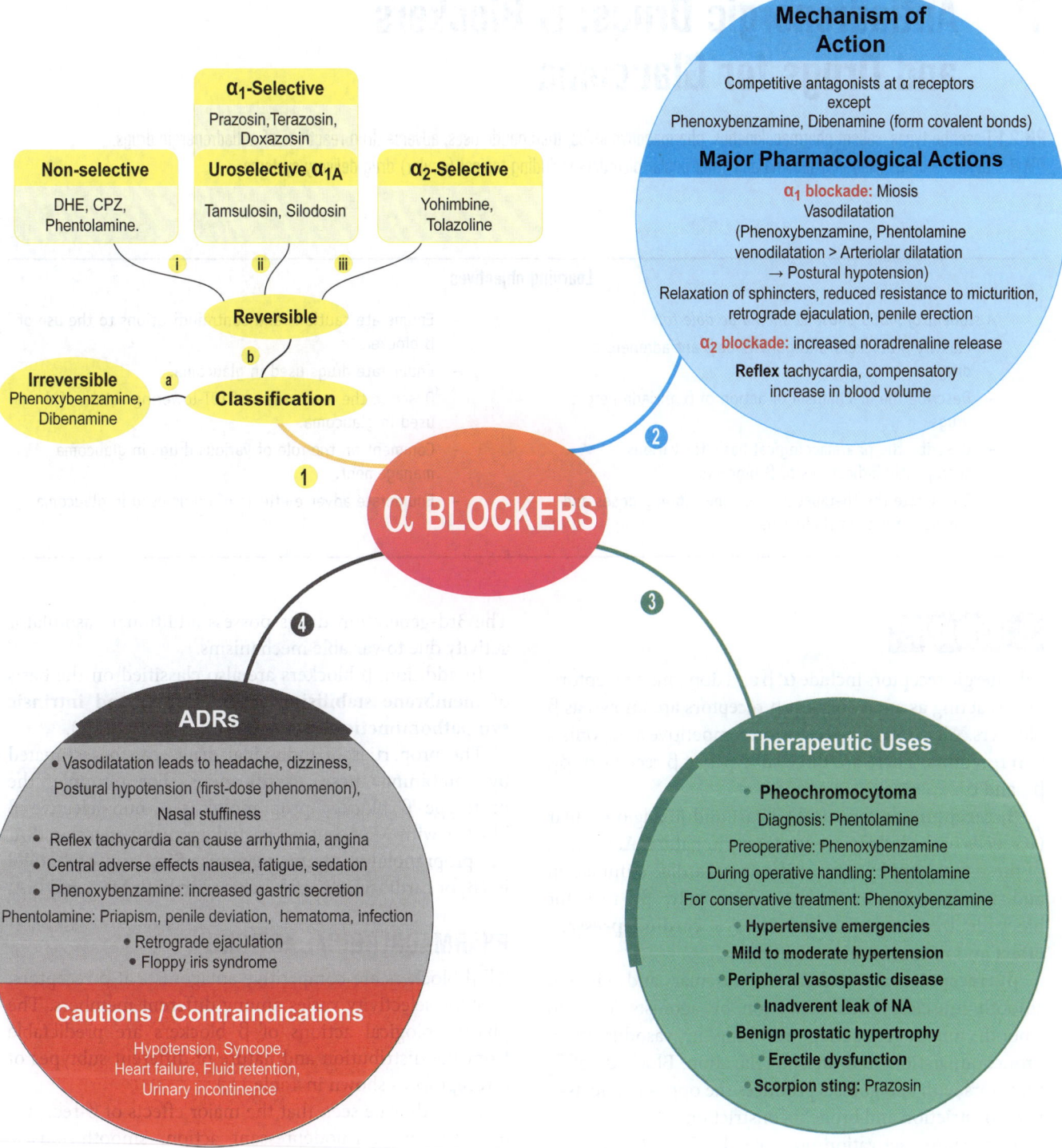

SECTION 2   Drugs Acting on ANS and PNS

11 Antiadrenergic Drugs: β Blockers and Drugs for Glaucoma

PH 2.1 Describe types, salient pharmacokinetics, pharmacodynamics, therapeutic uses, adverse drug reactions of antiadrenergic drugs.
PH 9.7 Describe drugs used in glaucoma and other ocular disorders including topical (ocular) drug delivery systems.

Learning objectives

A student of MBBS phase II should be able to:
- Classify β blockers/antagonists or β antiadrenergic drugs.
- Describe the mechanism of action of β antiadrenergic drugs.
- Describe the pharmacological basis for various therapeutic indications of β blockers.
- Enumerate the therapeutic uses, mentioning doses and adverse effects of β blockers.
- Enumerate cautions and contraindications to the use of β blockers.
- Enumerate drugs used in glaucoma.
- Describe the mechanism of IOT-lowering action of drugs used in glaucoma.
- Comment on the role of various drugs in glaucoma management.
- Enumerate adverse effects of drugs used in glaucoma.

β BLOCKERS

Adrenergic receptors include α, β and dopamine receptors. Drugs acting as antagonists at β receptors are known as β blockers. All drugs of this class are competitive antagonists at β receptors. There are three subtypes of β receptors: $β_1$, $β_2$, and $β_3$.

$β_1$ **receptors** present in the heart and juxtaglomerular (JG) cells of the kidney are excitatory in nature. Activation of these receptors by agonists leads to cardiac stimulation and increased renin release. Conversely, $β_1$ receptor blockade by antagonists produces a **cardiodepressant effect and reduces renin secretion**.

$β_2$ **receptors** are present in vascular and visceral smooth muscles. Their activation by agonists leads to smooth muscle relaxation, resulting in vasodilatation, bronchodilatation, and uterine relaxation. Blockade of $β_2$ receptors with antagonists produces the opposite effects—vasoconstriction and bronchoconstriction.

$β_3$ **receptor** activation promotes lipolysis. Conversely, $β_3$ blockade inhibits lipolysis (Table 11.1).

CLASSIFICATION OF β BLOCKERS

β Blockers are classified into 3 generations based on **selectivity of their action**. The first-generation drugs are non-selective, blocking all 3 subtypes of β receptors. The 2nd-generation drugs antagonise only the $β_1$ subtype. These are also called $β_1$-selective or cardioselective drugs. The 3rd-generation drugs possess additional vasodilator activity due to variable mechanisms.

In addition, β blockers are also classified on the basis of **membrane stabilising action (MSA) and intrinsic sympathomimetic activity (ISA)** (Flowchart 11.1).

The properties of individual drugs can be estimated by combining these classifications. For example, the prototype β blocker propranolol is a non-selective β blocker with MSA but no partial agonistic effect or ISA, i.e., propranolol is a pure antagonist. Similarly, acebutolol is a $β_1$ or cardioselective β blocker with both MSA and ISA.

PHARMACOLOGICAL ACTIONS

All β blockers are competitive antagonists at β receptors. Subtype selectivity varies among different members. The pharmacological actions of β blockers are predictable from the distribution and nature of different subtypes of β receptors as shown in Table 11.1.

It can thus be seen that the major effects of β-receptor blockade are cardiodepressant action, smooth muscle contraction and inhibition of lipolysis.

1. Cardiovascular Effects
Heart

$β_1$ Receptors present in the heart are excitatory in nature. Their activation has a cardio-stimulant action. Therefore, blockade of $β_1$ receptors in the heart by β blockers (non-selective as well as cardioselective drugs) causes the following effects:

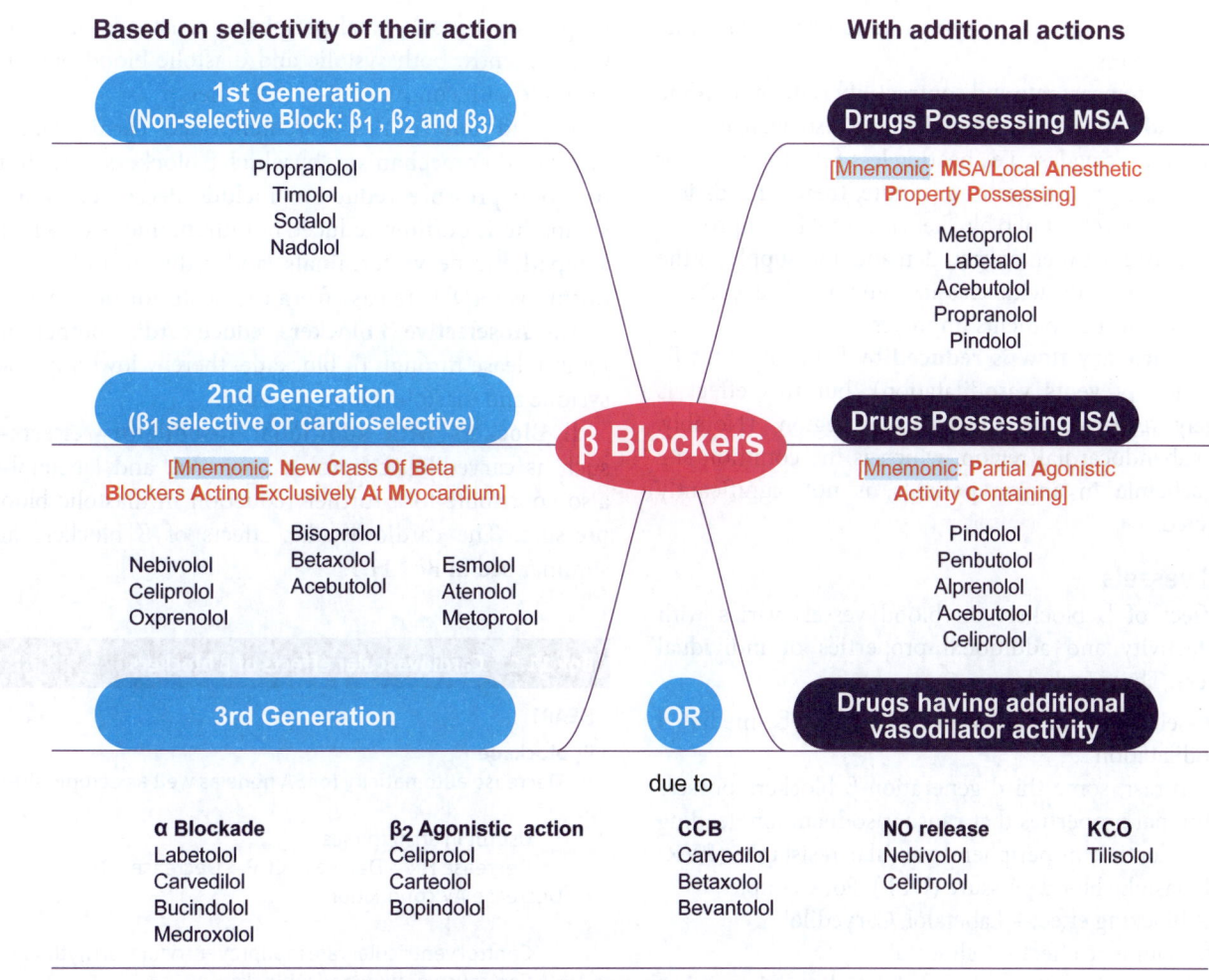

Flowchart 11.1 Classification of β blockers
[CCB: Calcium channel blockade; KCO: Potassium channel opener]

Table 11.1 Pharmacological actions of β blockers

Receptor name and nature	Distribution	Effect of β agonist	Effect of β blocker
β₁ (excitatory)	- Heart - Juxtaglomerular cells in kidney	- Cardiac stimulant effect - Increased renin secretion	- Cardiac depressant effect - Decreased renin secretion
β₂ (inhibitory in smooth muscles)	- Vascular muscles - Visceral smooth muscles - Liver	- Vasodilatation - Relaxation of smooth muscles (bronchodilatation) - Glycogenolysis	- Block vasodilatation - Contraction of smooth muscles (bronchoconstriction) - Inhibit glycogenolysis
β₃ (excitatory)	Lipocytes	Promote lipolysis	Inhibit lipolysis

- **Decrease in automaticity leading to decreased heart rate**: This effect can be useful in the treatment of tachyarrhythmias (rhythm disturbances with faster heart rate).
- Decrease in the rate of diastolic depolarisation in ectopic sites: This **reduces the automaticity at ectopic sites** and is useful in treatment of arrhythmias.
- **Decrease in atrio-ventricular conduction**: This effect is useful in controlling ventricular rate when the atrial rate is very high.
- **Decrease in force of contraction** (this effect occurs at a higher dose)
- **Decrease in cardiac output** occurs secondary to reduced heart rate and force of contraction.

The above-mentioned effects of β blockers are not prominently seen in resting condition but manifest more evidently in states of sympathetic overactivity like stress, exercise, and anxiety. In other words, rather than saying 'β blockers decrease heart rate', it is more appropriate to say that β blockers prevent a rise in heart

rate under situations of sympathetic overactivity like fear and stress.
- Decrease in heart rate and contractility **reduces cardiac work and hence, the oxygen demand** also decreases. (If heart is working less, i.e., beating less forcefully and for lesser number of times in a minute, then it needs less oxygen) This effect of β blockers is useful for improving the balance between oxygen demand and supply to the heart in patients with classical angina. The exercise tolerance of such patients improves.
- **Total coronary flow is reduced** by β blockers (as $β_2$ blockade prevents vasodilatation), but this effect is largely restricted to subepicardial region. (Notably, the subendocardial region, which is the common site of ischemia in angina patients, is not significantly affected.)

Blood vessels

The effect of β blockers on blood vessels varies with the selectivity and additional properties of individual members. These include:

- Non-selective β blockers: Prevent $β_2$-mediated vasodilatation
- In contrast, some third-generation β blockers possess additional properties that cause vasodilatation, leading to a reduction in peripheral vascular resistance (PVR) and diastolic blood pressure (DBP). For example:
  - α-blocking effect – Labetalol, Carvedilol
  - $β_2$-agonistic effect – Celiprolol
  - NO-releasing effect – Nebivolol, Celiprolol
  - Calcium channel-blocking effect – Carvedilol

Blood pressure

The effect of different β blockers on BP varies depending on their vascular effects. Upon initiating therapy with non-selective β blockers:

- $β_1$ Blockade causes reduced cardiac output, leading to a fall in systolic blood pressure (SBP).
- $β_1$ Blockade also decreases renin release, which in turn reduces RAAS activity, leading to a decrease in blood volume and peripheral vascular resistance (PVR), and consequently, a fall in diastolic blood pressure (DBP).
- $β_2$ Blockade leads to increased peripheral vascular resistance and hence, rise in DBP.

Thus, it can be seen that the **acute use of β blockers has a negligible net effect on blood pressure**. Upon continued use, however, cardiac output remains low due to $β_1$ blockade, but **resistance vessels gradually adapt to the chronically reduced cardiac output**. Normally, reduced cardiac output evokes reflex vasoconstriction, but in the continuous presence of β-blockers, the blood vessels do not constrict in response to the lowered cardiac output. As a result, total peripheral resistance decreases. Consequently, both systolic and diastolic blood pressure decrease with continued β-blocker therapy.

In addition to the aforementioned cardiovascular effects, other mechanisms by which β blockers contribute to blood pressure reduction include decreased central sympathetic outflow, reduced noradrenaline release from sympathetic nerve terminals, and reduced antidiuretic hormone (ADH) release from the posterior pituitary.

Cardioselective β blockers reduce cardiac output and renin release through $β_1$ blockade, thereby lowering both systolic and diastolic blood pressure.

β Blockers with additional vasodilatory effects—such as carvedilol, celiprolol, nebivolol, and labetalol—also contribute to a further reduction in diastolic blood pressure. The cardiovascular effects of ß blockers are summarised in Box 11.1.

Box 11.1 Cardiovascular effects of β blockers

HEART

$β_1$ blockade
- Decrease automaticity (of SA node as well as ectopic site)
  ↓
  - Useful in arrhythmias
  - Decrease HR → Decrease COP → Decrease SBP
- Decrease AV conduction
  ↓
  - Control ventricular rate in supraventricular arrhythmias
  - Can cause or worsen AV blocks
  - Should not be used in combination with other drugs that decrease cardiac conduction, such as verapamil
- Decrease force of contraction (high concentration)
  ↓
  - Contributes to reduced COP → Fall in systolic BP (SBP)
  - Decrease myocardial oxygen demand due to reduced HR and force of contraction
  ↓
  Improves demand–supply balance and exercise tolerance; useful in angina

$β_2$ blockade
Prevents $β_2$-mediated vasodilatation
  ↓
- Total coronary flow is reduced; however, subendocardial region not much affected
- PVR rises initially, but later, **vessels adapt to the chronically reduced COP** and resistance decreases → Fall in PVR and DBP

Additional effects
- Blockade of $α_1$ receptors by carvedilol, labetalol, bucindolol
- $β_2$ agonism by celiprolol, carteolol
- NO release by nebivolol, celiprolol.
- Calcium channel blockade by carvedilol, betaxolol
- Potassium channel opening by tilisolol All these mechanisms result in **vasodilatation** → Fall in PVR and DBP

2. Effect on Respiratory System

Beta blockers prevent $β_2$ receptor-mediated bronchodilatation, thereby causing **bronchospasm**, which increases airway resistance, especially in patients suffering from bronchial asthma. Hence, **β blockers should be avoided in patients prone to asthmatic attacks**. If use of β blockers is absolutely indicated, cardioselective β blockers and those with ISA are better suited than non-selective ones.

3. Effect on Central Nervous System

β blockers that cross the blood–brain barrier can cause **forgetfulness, increased dreaming, nightmares and behavioural change**s. Anxiety associated with sympathetic stimulation is controlled by β blockers through their peripheral actions. Non-thermoregulatory sweating and tremors are important symptoms associated with anxiety. These are mediated through sympathetic stimulation and have a reinforcing effect, i.e., anxiety manifests as tremors/sweating. These symptoms, in turn, lead to more anxiety. Beta blockers are useful in **reducing anxiety by controlling peripheral symptoms** like tremors and sweating.

4. Ocular Effects

Beta blockers **reduce aqueous humour production** from ciliary epithelium, resulting in reduction in intraocular tension (Fig. 11.1). This effect makes them useful in the treatment of wide-angle glaucoma. **Timolol and betaxolol** are the most suitable drugs for this indication, as they do not have MSA or local anesthetic action, which could otherwise be dangerous. If the cornea loses sensitivity to touch or pain due to MSA, it becomes more prone to injury. Therefore, for topical ocular use, drugs lacking MSA are preferred.

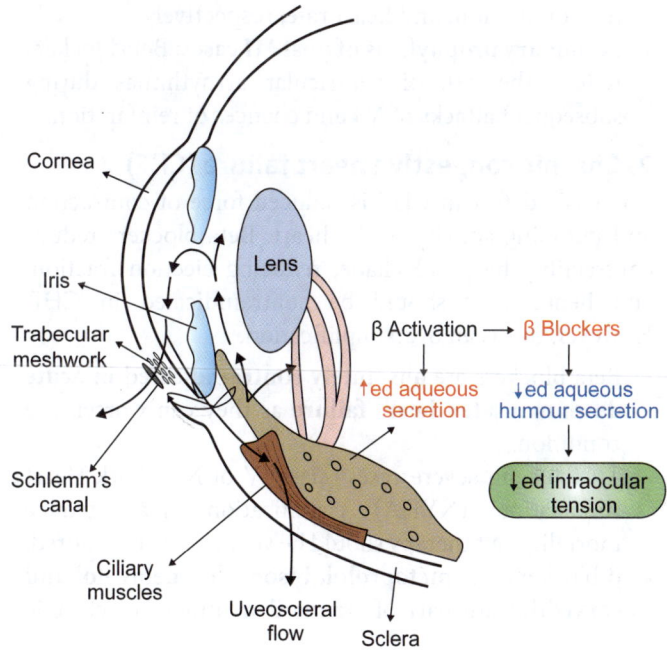

Fig. 11.1 Effect of β blockers on intraocular tension

5. Metabolic Effects

Lipid metabolism

β blockers inhibit lipolysis through $β_3$ blockade. As a result, triglyceride and VLDL levels increase, while HDL levels decrease. These **changes in lipid profile are unfavourable** and increase the risk of coronary artery disease. The unfavourable effect on lipid profile is less marked with β blockers having ISA or partial agonistic effect, like pindolol, penbutalol, alprenolol, acebutolol and celiprolol.

Carbohydrate metabolism

Beta blockers inhibit glycogenolysis. They can therefore delay recovery from hypoglycemia, as glycogen breakdown is an important compensatory mechanism in hypoglycemia. Hence, β blockers should be carefully used in patients of type I DM on insulin therapy. Not only do β blockers delay the recovery from hypoglycemia, they mask the warning symptoms suggestive of hypoglycemia (e.g., tremors and palpitation), so that the patient goes into severe hypoglycemia without experiencing any warning symptoms. Hence, β blockers should be used very cautiously in diabetics. The risk of such metabolic complications is reported to be lower with cardioselective β blockers. Third generation β blockers, in fact, have favourable metabolic effects like decreased levels of insulin, decreased blood glucose levels, reduction in LDL and raised HDL.

6. Local Anesthetic or MSA

Some β blockers like metoprolol, labetalol, acebutolol, propranolol, pindolol, and carvedilol possess local anesthetic action, but they are not used for this property because of their irritant nature. Membrane stabilising effect is maximum with propranolol and minimum with betaxolol. Drugs which have MSA are contraindicated in glaucoma.

7. Intrinsic Sympathomimetic Action

Beta blockers possessing ISA or partial agonistic effect include acebutolol, pindolol, penbutalol, labetolol, celiprolol and carteolol. They have some intrinsic sympathomimetic activity, because of which the risk of bradycardia is lower with these drugs. However, such drugs are contraindicated in migraine prophylaxis and MI.

PHARMACOKINETIC CONSIDERATIONS

The prototype β blocker, propranolol, is well absorbed orally; however, its bioavailability is low due to extensive first-pass metabolism. Therefore, a high oral dose is required. In fact, the oral dose of propranolol is approximately 40 times greater than its parenteral dose. Most β blockers are metabolised in the liver and excreted by the kidneys.

Some β blockers are lipid-insoluble and are excreted unchanged by the kidneys. These drugs have a long duration of action. Examples include nadolol, sotalol, atenolol, acebutolol, betaxolol, bisoprolol, and celiprolol. Such drugs are contraindicated in patients with renal failure due to the risk of accumulation and toxicity

Esmolol has the shortest and nadolol the longest duration of action among β blockers.

Clinical problem-based questions and MCQs

1. **A 45-year-old female hypertensive patient with history of myocardial infarction 2 years back is receiving enalapril and metoprolol therapy.**
   i. Describe the mechanism of the blood pressure lowering effect of β blockers.
   ii. What is the advantage of selecting metoprolol over prototype β blocker- propranolol?

2. **A 36-year-old female patient presented with complaints of polyuria, polydipsia, and polyphagia. On investigation, her fasting blood sugar (FBS) was 186 mg/dL and HbA_{1c} was 7.2%. She was diagnosed with diabetes mellitus and initiated on sulfonylurea therapy. The patient was also receiving propranolol for migraine prophylaxis. Following a road traffic accident, her blood glucose levels became uncontrolled with oral sulphonylureas alone, necessitating the addition of insulin (8 units, twice daily, subcutaneously). Upon initiating insulin therapy, propranolol was temporarily discontinued.**
   i. Why was propranolol therapy stopped during initiation of insulin therapy?
   ii. Describe the metabolic effects of β blockers.

3. **A 46-year-old male diabetic patient needs to be put on ß blocker therapy.**
   i. Which of the following β blockers is safest for this patient?
      a. Labetalol   b. Sotalol
      c. Metoprolol   d. Propranolol
   ii. Give pharmacological basis to justify your choice.

4. **A 25-year-old IT engineer is scheduled to give a presentation of his project in front of a large audience that includes his superiors and distinguished guests. Before the presentation, he felt extremely nervous and experienced palpitations; his anxiety had kept him awake the night before. This had never happened to him in the past, so, before heading to the venue, he consulted a doctor. On examination, the young man exhibited signs such as tachycardia, tremors, and sweaty palms. The doctor prescribed him β blockers.**
   i. What is possible cause of symptoms in this case?
   ii. Describe the pharmacological basis for prescribing β blockers.

5. **Which of the following drugs is a cardioselective β blocker?**
   a. Sotalol   b. Timolol
   c. Nadolol   d. Metoprolol

6. **Which of the following β blockers possesses additional α blocker effect?**
   a. Carvedilol   b. Sotalol
   c. Timolol   d. Propranolol

THERAPEUTIC USES

Beta blockers are commonly used drugs for a variety of cardiovascular and other related indications. They are indicated in some extracardiac conditions also. Important indications for use include the following.

1. Ischemic heart disease

Ischemic heart disease can present as angina and in very severe cases as myocardial infarction. Beta blockers are useful in:

- **Classical angina**, as they improve the myocardial oxygen demand–supply ratio by **reducing demand through their cardiodepressant action**. Exercise tolerance improves and frequency of angina attacks is reduced. However, they can **worsen vasospastic/variant/Prinzmetal angina**, as they block $β_2$-mediated vasodilatation of coronaries. Hence, β blockers are contraindicated in variant angina.
- **Myocardial infarction:** In patients of MI, β blockers administered intravenously within 4–6 hours of attack can **limit the size of infarcted area and prevent rhythm disturbances**. However, patients must be selected very carefully. β blockers should be administered only to patients who are not in shock or experiencing cardiac failure, do not have more than first-degree AV block, and have a heart rate greater than 50 beats per minute. This is important because β blockers can worsen these conditions by further decreasing cardiac contractility, AV conduction, and heart rate, respectively.
- **Secondary prophylaxis of post MI cases:** Beta blockers reduce the risk of ventricular arrhythmias during subsequent attacks of MI and chances of reinfarction.

2. Chronic congestive heart failure (CHF)

The basic defect in CHF is reduced force of contraction and pumping activity of the heart. Beta blockers reduce contractility by $β_1$ blockade, reducing ejection fraction, and hence they should be contraindicated in CHF. However, this is an oversimplification.

- Beta blockers are **absolutely contraindicated in acute decompensated heart failure** as they can worsen the condition.
- Their use in severe cases (class IV of New York Heart Association (NYHA) classification) may reduce mortality, but therapy should be very closely monitored.
- β blockers like **metoprolol, bisoprolol, nebivolol and carvedilol** are part of standard treatment of chronic

CHF along with other groups of drugs like ACE inhibitors and diuretics in:
- **Mild-to-moderately severe CHF** (classes II and III of NYHA)
- Patients of **dilated cardiomyopathy with systolic dysfunction.**

Although initial hemodynamic effects of β blockers are not favourable in CHF, β blockers introduced gradually and maintained for long term **control the disease progression rate, reduce mortality and improve survival** in CHF.

The mechanism underlying these beneficial effects is not well understood, but may involve blocking of the reflex sympathetic overactivity by β blockers resulting in reduced ventricular wall stress, which in turn reduces pathological remodelling and prevents dangerous arrhythmias.

Dose: The starting dose should be very low to prevent negative inotropic effect and worsening of heart failure. The dose is then slowly built up. The maximum dose of metoprolol is 200 mg/day; carvedilol is 50 mg /day; and bisoprolol is 10 mg/day. If the patient's condition worsens with introduction of β blocker therapy, these should be discontinued and contraindicated for future use.

3. Hypertension

Beta blockers are mild antihypertensives. While they were among the first choice drugs for mild-to-moderate hypertension, currently, they are considered **inferior to thiazides, ACE inhibitors/ARBs and CCBs for initial treatment of hypertension.**

However, β blockers like metoprolol (25–100 mg), carvedilol (12.5–25 mg), and nebivolol (2.5–5 mg) are used along with ACE inhibitors or ARBs in **hypertensive patients with stable heart failure and a history of MI.** Esmolol may be used for quick reduction of BP in **hypertensive urgency** because of its rapid onset and short duration of action. It is administered intravenously as a loading dose of 0.5 mg/kg, followed by IV infusion of 0.05–0.2 mg/kg/minute.

4. Cardiac arrhythmias

Beta blockers are useful in the treatment of tachyarrhythmias and extrasystole. Esmolol is an alternative drug for paroxysmal supraventricular tachycardia (PSVT). In atrial flutter and fibrillation, β blockers control the ventricular rate by decreasing AV conduction.

5. Obstructive hypertrophic cardiomyopathy

Beta blockers decrease the resistance to left ventricular outflow under conditions of sympathetic overactivity like stress and exercise and are the drugs of choice in hypertrophic cardiomyopathy.

6. Dissecting aortic aneurysm

Beta blockers decrease aortic pulsation by decreasing cardiac contractility.

7. Fallot's tetralogy and mitral valve prolapse

β blockers are useful in emergency management of **Fallot's tetralogy of heart** and **prolapsed mitral valve.**

8. Pheochromocytoma

Beta blockers are used to control tachycardia and arrhythmias in pheochromocytoma after α blockers. They also suppress catecholamine-induced cardiomyopathy.

9. Thyrotoxic states

Beta blockers like propranolol provide symptomatic relief by reducing anxiety, tremors, palpitation, sweating, etc. They also inhibit the activation of thyroxine (T_4) to liothyronine (T_3). They are useful in managing thyroid storm or crisis, and in thyrotoxicosis patients due for surgery of thyroid gland or while waiting for response to antithyroid drugs/radioactive iodine to set in.

10. Anxiety

Beta blockers relieve symptoms like fear or panic of examination or public presentation associated with performance anxiety by controlling peripheral symptoms such as tremors, sweating and palpitation.

11. Essential tremors

Essential tremors are relieved by non-selective β blockers, but tremors associated with parkinsonism are not. Non-selective β blockers are effective in akathisia also.

12. Alcohol and opioid withdrawal symptoms

These may be relieved by β blockers.

13. Migraine prophylaxis

Propranolol is very useful in chronic prophylaxis of migraine. Initially, a dose of 40 mg, twice daily, is given. It may be increased up to 160 mg, twice a day, as per individual requirement.

14. Glaucoma

Beta blockers reduce intraocular tension (IOT) by decreasing the production of aqueous humour from the ciliary epithelium. This effect is useful in wide-angle glaucoma. Timolol is the preferred agent, as it has no MSA or ISA. However, after topical administration in the eye, it gets absorbed into systemic circulation, resulting in adverse effects on cardiovascular and respiratory systems. Other β blockers for topical use in glaucoma are betaxolol, carteolol and levobunolol.

15. Portal hypertension

β blocker are useful in the **prophylaxis of bleeding in portal hypertension.**

Therapeutic uses of beta blockers are summarised in Box 11.1.

Box 11.1 Therapeutic uses of beta blockers

Cardiovascular uses
- Ischemic heart disease
  - Classical angina
  - Myocardial infarction, within 4–6 hours IV for myocardial salvage
  - Secondary prophylaxis in post-MI cases
- mild-to-moderate CHF, especially dilated cardiomyopathy with systolic dysfunction
- Obstructive hypertrophic cardiomyopathy
- mild-to-moderate hypertension
- Rhythm disturbances: PSVT, tachyarrhythmias, to control ventricular rate in atrial flutter and fibrillation
- Dissecting aortic aneurysm
- Pheochromocytoma after alpha blockers
- Emergency management of Fallot's tetralogy and mitral valve prolapse

Extracardiac uses
- Thyrotoxicosis
- Anxiety
- Essential tremors
- Migraine prophylaxis
- Wide-angle glaucoma
- Alcohol and opioid withdrawal
- Prophylaxis of bleeding in portal hypertension

Clinical problem-based questions and MCQs

7. A 30-year-old female patient reports experiencing precordial pain that radiates to her left shoulder whenever she walks for about 400 meters. However, the pain subsides with rest. She has been prescribed tablet metoprolol 25 mg to be taken once daily, which has provided significant relief from her symptoms.
   i. What is this patient suffering from?
   ii. What is the rationale behind prescribing metoprolol to this patient?
   iii. Can the same treatment be given if patient had precordial pain unrelated to physical activity? Give pharmacological basis for your answer.

8. i. Which of the following β blockers possesses selectivity for $β_1$ receptors?
      a. Atenolol   b. Propranolol
      c. Sotalol   d. Timolol
   ii. What is the advantage of cardioselectivity of β blockers?

9. A 54-year old male patient reports in emergency in a semiconscious state. His BP is 180/120 and pulse is weak.
   i. Which of the following β blockers is most suitable in this patient for quick control of high BP?
      a. Propranolol   b. Metoprolol
      c. Esmolol   d. Labetalol
   ii. Give pharmacological basis to justify your choice.

10. A 52-year-old male patient with chronic hypertension was on propranolol 40 mg BD therapy. His BP was well within normal limits with this treatment, but on examination, resting heart rate was recorded as 50 beats per minute.
    i. Explain the mechanism of BP lowering effect of propranolol.
    ii. Explain the reason of slow heart rate with propranolol.
    iii. Which of the following drugs can be a better choice in this patient?
       a. Pindolol   b. Metoprolol
       c. Labetalol   d. Esmolol
    iv. Give pharmacological basis to justify your choice.

11. A 49-year-old female patient visited an ophthalmologist with chief complaints of frontal headache and decreased vision. On examination, refraction was normal but IOT was raised in both the eyes. The doctor asked for any past history of wheezing and dyspnea. There was no such history and the patient was prescribed 0.5% timolol eyedrops, twice a day.
    i. Explain the pharmacological basis of prescribing timolol in this patient.
    ii. Name other β blockers that can be used in this patient.
    iii. Why did the doctor specifically ask about a history suggestive of bronchial asthma?

12. i. Which of the following β blockers has no ISA and MSA?
       a. Penbutolol   b. Celiprolol
       b. Timolol   d. Acebutolol
    ii. What are clinical implications of ISA and MSA?

13. A 5-year-old girl presented with a history of increased appetite, tiredness, weight loss and excessive sweating for the past one month. There is a swelling in her neck and her eyes are prominently protruding (exophthalmos). On examination, HR is found to be 120 per minute, extremities are warm, BP is raised and a small smooth goitre is palpable. Investigations showed raised thyroxine and thyroid peroxidase levels. The patient is prescribed carbimazole 20 mg, once a day, and propranolol 10 mg, three times a day, and called for a follow-up after one week. The symptoms are more than half resolved at the follow-up visit.
    i. What is the child suffering from?
    ii. Describe pharmacological basis for prescribing propranolol.

ADVERSE EFFECTS OF β BLOCKERS

1. Beta blockers can worsen acute CHF by blocking sympathetic support to the failing heart.
2. Bradycardia: HR reduces to less than 60 beats per minute. Patients with sick sinus syndrome are more prone to β blocker-induced bradycardia.
3. Variant angina may become worse due to coronary vasospasm.
4. Conduction defects may be worsened.

5. Chronic obstructive pulmonary disease (COPD) and bronchial asthma may be exacerbated due to bronchospasm.
6. Carbohydrate tolerance is impaired, especially in prediabetics.
7. Unfavourable changes occur in lipid profile. Raised TG, VLDL and reduced HDL increase the risk of coronary artery disease.
8. Fatigue, decreased capacity to exercise
9. Forgetfulness, lack of drive, nightmares, increased dreaming
10. Cold hand/feet, worsening of peripheral vasospastic diseases may occur.
11. Gastrointestinal upset may occur.

Precautions and Contraindications
- Variant angina
- Acute decompensated heart failure
- Severe atrio-ventricular conduction defects
- Bronchial asthma
- Peripheral vasospastic disease
- IDDM

Beta blockers should not be combined with calcium channel blocker verapamil because both drugs suppress AV conduction. Given together, the additive effect will result in dangerous heart blocks.

SALIANT FEATURES OF INDIVIDUAL DRUGS

1. Cardioselective or β₁-Selective Blockers
Examples: Nebivolol, Celiprolol, Bisoprolol, Betaxolol, Acebutolol, Esmolol, Atenolol, Metoprolol [Mnemonic: **N**ew **C**lass of **B**eta **B**lockers **A**cting **E**xclusively **A**t **M**yocardium]

Their selectivity for $β_1$ receptors is only relative and is lost at higher doses.

Advantage: The risk of $β_1$-selective blockers causing bronchospasm and inhibition of glycogenolysis and lipolysis is lower than that for non-selective drugs. ADRs like cold hand, feet, impaired exercise capacity, and fatigue are also comparatively less. So, if it is essential to give β blockers to a patient with bronchial asthma or diabetes, cardioselective or $β_1$-selective blockers are preferred over non-selective drugs.

Limitation: These drugs are not effective in relieving essential tremors. Some cardioselective β blockers like nebivolol and celiprolol have additional effects.

Nebivolol
This is a highly cardioselective β blocker with additional stimulant effect on nitric oxide synthase. Thus, nebivolol does not block $β_2$-mediated vasodilatation and causes vasodilatation through increased NO synthesis. Hence, the BP-lowering effect of nebivolol is fast in onset compared to other β blockers. It is useful in hypertension and CHF.

Celiprolol
It causes $β_1$ blockade, $β_2$ agonism and nitric oxide (NO) production. It is safer in asthma patients due to the $β_2$ agonistic effect. Vasodilatation caused by $β_2$ agonism and nitric oxide adds to its BP-lowering action.

Esmolol
This is a cardioselective β blocker with no ISA or MSA. It has rapid onset of action on IV infusion. Because it is metabolised by esterases, it is short acting, with action lasting for just 10–15 minutes. Thus, it is useful for fast reduction of BP in case of hypertensive emergencies and terminating episodes of atrial flutter, fibrillation and supraventricular tachycardia.

2. Drugs Possessing ISA
Examples: **C**eliprolol, **P**indolol, **P**enbutolol, **A**lprenolol, **A**cebutolol [Mnemonic: **C**ontaining **P**artial **A**gonistic **A**ctivity]

Advantages:
- These drugs have partial agonistic effect and therefore lower risk of bradycardia. Hence, these are more useful in patients with 'sick sinus syndrome' and in elderly individuals who are prone to bradycardia. Changes in lipid profile are also less marked.
- The continued presence of antagonist causes supersensitivity of receptors. Thus, the sudden withdrawal of β blockers causes worsening of the primary condition (e.g., hypertension or angina) for which the β blocker drug was being used. However, the use of β blockers possessing ISA or partial agonistic activity prevents the development of receptor supersensitivity. Therefore, sudden withdrawal of these drugs carries a lower risk of worsening hypertension or angina.

Limitation: Drugs with intrinsic sympathomimetic activity (ISA) dilate cerebral blood vessels and are therefore are not suitable for migraine prophylaxis.

3. Sotalol
The levo isomer of sotalol is a non-selective β blocker with additional potassium channel blocking effect, whereas its dextro isomer has only K^+ channel blocking effect. In cardiac muscle fibres, potassium (K^+) efflux is involved in repolarisation. So, a blockade of K^+ channels causes prolonged repolarisation. This, in turn, prolongs the action potential duration (APD). AV conduction is delayed and ERP increases. Due to these effects, sotalol is effective in treating ventricular tachyarrhythmias, maintaining sinus rhythm, and controlling ventricular rate in patients with atrial flutter or fibrillation.

Limitation: Prolongation of APD can cause dose-dependent torsade de pointes, especially in patients with prolonged QT interval. So, sotalol is contraindicated if QT is prolonged.

4. β Blockers without ISA and MSA

Timolol is a non-selective β blocker. It is preferred for ocular use as it lacks corneal anesthetic activity.

5. Combined α and β Blockers

Drugs that have α_1, β_1, and β_2 blocking effect include labetalol and carvedilol.

Labetalol causes α_1, β_1, and β_2 blockade and weak agonistic effect on β_2 receptors. It has more potent blocking effect on β receptors than on α. So, while the actions of a low dose of labetalol are similar to those of propranolol, at higher doses, its actions resemble those of a combination of propranolol and prazosin. α_1 and β_1 blockade and β_2 agonism contribute to its hypotensive action. Labetalol is useful in pheochromocytoma, clonidine withdrawal and hypertensive emergencies. It is safe in pregnancy-induced hypertension or pre-eclampsia as well.

Carvedilol causes α_1, β_1, and β_2 blockade. It has additional calcium channel blocking and antioxidant actions. It is used in stable cases of CHF for its cardioprotective action in a dose of 3.125 mg, twice a day, for few days. If no adverse effects occur, the dose can be increased slowly. It is also used in angina and hypertension.

Clinical problem-based questions and MCQs

14. **Which of the following drugs cannot be combined with β blockers and why?**
    a. Nifedipine b. Losartan
    c. Verapamil d. Ramipril

15. **In which of the following patients, β blockers are contraindicated and why?**
    a. Moderate CHF
    b. Post myocardial infarction
    c. Acute decompensated heart failure
    d. Hypertension with stable heart failure

16. i. **In which of the following conditions, ß blockers are contraindicated and why?**
       a. Essential tremors
       b. Ventricular extrasystoles
       c. Thyrotoxicosis
       d. Chronic obstructive pulmonary disease
    ii. **If it is absolutely necessary to give ß blockers in the contraindicated condition identified above, which of the following is chosen and why?**
       a. Carvedilol b. Propranolol
       c. Celiprolol d. Nebivolol

17. **A 32-year-old primigravida has pre-eclampsia. Which ß blocker is most suitable in this patient?**
    a. Carvedilol b. Labetalol
    c. Celiprolol d. Nebivolol

18. **A 55-year-old male patient with stable congestive heart failure is to be put on ß blocker therapy. Select the most suitable drug possessing cardioprotective effect in CHF:**
    a. Carvedilol b. Labetalol
    c. Celiprolol d. Nebivolol

19. **One of the following β blockers activates nitric oxide synthesis in the endothelium. Identify the drug.**
    a. Carvedilol b. Labetalol
    c. Sotalol d. Nebivolol

20. **Identify the β blocker that has additional potassium channel blocking activity.**
    a. Carvedilol b. Labetalol
    c. Sotalol d. Nebivolol

DRUG TREATMENT OF GLAUCOMA

Glaucoma is a condition involving progressive optic nerve damage of unknown etiology, causing loss of vision. Intraocular tension (IOT) is raised (> 21 mm of Hg) in most of the cases. However, in few cases, IOT may be normal or even low.

Physiology of Aqueous Humour Synthesis and Drainage

Aqueous humour is synthesised in the ciliary body epithelium.

- Carbonic anhydrase enzyme present in epithelial cells of the ciliary body produces HCO_3^- ions for secretion into aqueous humour.
- Activation of β_2-adrenergic receptors present on ciliary epithelium increases aqueous production via cAMP generation. β_2-Mediated vasodilatation also favours aqueous humour production.
- In contrast, α_1-adrenergic receptor activation causes vasoconstriction and reduces blood flow to ciliary epithelium. Thus, it opposes aqueous humour production.
- α_2 Activation reduces release of catecholamines, resulting in decreased β_2 action on ciliary epithelium. Thus, aqueous humour production is reduced.

Ninety percent of the aqueous humour released from the ciliary body passes from the posterior chamber of the eye into the anterior chamber through the space between the iris and lens. From the anterior chamber, it drains out through the trabecular meshwork and 'canal of Schlemm' at the iridocorneal angle. The remaining drainage (10%) occurs through uveoscleral route into episcleral (Fig. 11.1).

The **important risk factors for glaucoma** include: genetic predisposition, narrow iridocorneal angle, shallow anterior chamber and use of mydriatics.

Types of Glaucoma

Glaucoma is of 2 types:

a. **Chronic simple glaucoma**, also known as **open- or wide-angle glaucoma**, is a degenerative disease occurring in genetically predisposed individuals, usually in the middle age. It involves progressive reduction

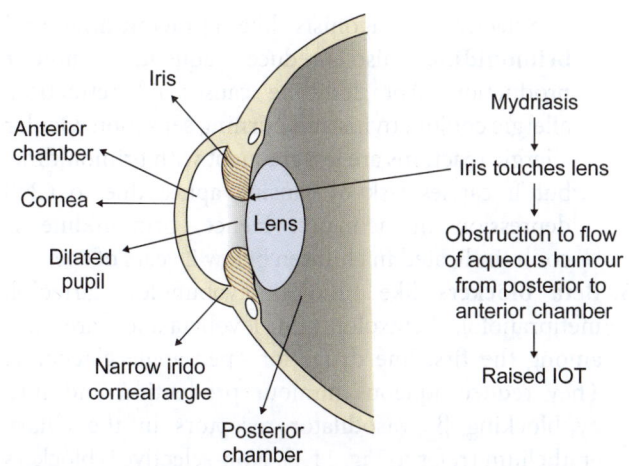

Fig. 11.2 Mydriatics precipitate glaucoma

in the patency of trabecular meshwork, resulting in slowly-rising IOT. It is managed with drug therapy.

b. **Acute congestive glaucoma**, also known as **angle-closure glaucoma**, affects individuals with narrow iridocorneal angle and shallow anterior chamber. Use of mydriatics in such individuals causes contact of iris and lens, blocking the movement of aqueous humour from the posterior to anterior chambers. Pressure caused by aqueous humour causes bulging of the iris that obliterates iridocorneal angle and obstructs trabecular outflow (Fig. 11.2). This causes a sudden marked rise in IOT, up to 60 mm of Hg, congestion in eyes (red eye) and severe headache. It is an emergency condition requiring vigorous drug therapy, followed by definitive surgical management.

Management of Glaucoma

Reduction in IOT has been shown to reduce the progression of optic nerve damage in all cases of glaucoma including those with normal or low IOT at baseline. Therefore, the main strategy for management of glaucoma is reduction of IOT that can be achieved with drugs and peripheral iridectomy by laser or surgery. Drugs reduce intraocular tension by either decreasing synthesis of aqueous humour or by increasing its drainage.

CLASSIFICATION OF DRUGS USED IN GLAUCOMA

Drugs beneficial in reducing IOT include autonomic drugs, carbonic anhydrase inhibitors and prostaglandin analogues (Flowchart 11.2).

Drugs for Glaucoma

Chronic simple glaucoma is managed with drug treatment only. In current clinical practice, treatment of chronic simple glaucoma is initiated as monotherapy with prostaglandin analogues or topical β blockers. If the response is not adequate, a combination of the two or an alternative drug is tried. If prostaglandin analogues and β blockers are contraindicated, only then adrenergic agonists like brimonidine or carbonic anhydrase inhibitor dorzolamide are considered. However, they can be used as 'add-on' drugs to supplement the action of first-line drugs.

Prostaglandin analogues

$PGF_{2\alpha}$ analogues like latanoprost, bimatoprost and unoprostone increase permeability of ciliary body tissues and episcleral vessels. This improves uveoscleral outflow, resulting in decreased intraocular tension. Trabecular outflow is also increased somewhat. $PGF_{2\alpha}$ analogues are the drugs of choice in glaucoma.

These drugs can cause excessive growth of eyelashes as an adverse effect. However, this effect is useful in patients with hypotrichosis. Iris pigmentation can also occur in some cases. In aphakics, it can cause macular edema.

Autonomic drugs that lower IOT

These include cholinergic, adrenergic and antiadrenergic drugs.

1. **Cholinergic drugs** like pilocarpine, physostigmine and ecothiophate cause miosis by activation of M_3

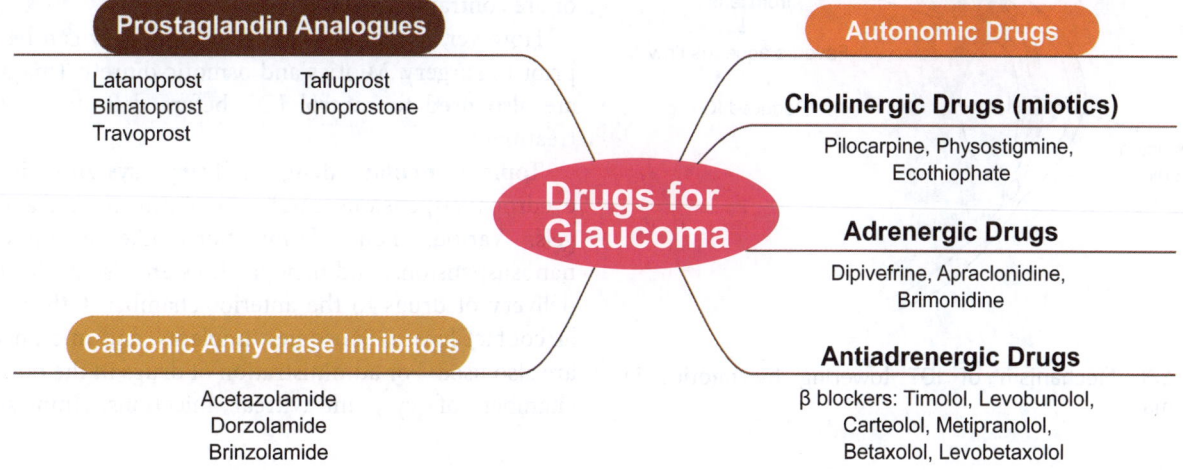

Flowchart 11.2 Drugs for glaucoma

receptors in constrictor papillae. Miosis pulls the iris away from the lens, allowing flow of aqueous humour from the posterior to anterior chamber (Fig. 11.3). They also increase the tone of ciliary muscles, resulting in improved patency of the trabecular meshwork.

2. **Adrenergic agonists:** Though it seems paradoxical, both adrenergic and antiadrenergic drugs are useful in glaucoma. Non-selective adrenergic agonist adrenaline has a complex effect on aqueous humour production and drainage as described below (refer to Fig 9.3, page 122).
   - α_1 Agonism leads to vasoconstriction of blood vessels in the ciliary epithelium, which reduces aqueous humour production.
   - α_2 Agonism reduces catecholamine release. This reduces activation of β_2 receptors on ciliary epithelium, which, in turn, decreases aqueous humour production. This effect is selectively shown by α_2 agonists such as apraclonidine and brimonidine.
   - β_2 Agonism increases cAMP production, which leads to vasodilatation of ciliary blood vessels. This increases aqueous humour production. (This effect is counterproductive in glaucoma and can be blocked by β blockers.)
   - β_2 Agonism favours aqueous outflow by increasing hydraulic conductivity of the filtering cells in trabeculae, leading to decreased IOT.
   - Adrenergic drugs increase uveoscleral outflow by an unknown mechanism, which decreases IOT.

   Dipivefrine, a prodrug of adrenaline, crosses the cornea and gets hydrolysed to release adrenaline, which is oxidised to produce adrenochrome that may cause blackening of the conjunctiva. This causes a burning sensation in the eyes, and is therefore used infrequently and only as an 'add-on' drug.

   Selective α_2 agonists like **apraclonidine and brimonidine** also reduce aqueous humour production. Apraclonidine causes lid retraction, allergic conjunctivitis and burning sensation. Ocular allergic reactions are less frequent with brimonidine, but it carries risk of causing apnea due to CNS depression in neonates. Hence, brimonidine is contraindicated in children below 2 years of age.

3. **Beta blockers** like timolol, levobunolol, carteolol, metipranolol, betaxolol and levobetaxolol are also among the first-line drugs for open-angle glaucoma. They reduce aqueous humour production and IOT by blocking β_2 vasodilator receptors in the ciliary epithelium (refer to Fig. 11.1). Non-selective β blockers like timolol, levobunolol, carteolol, metipranlol are approved for ocular use. **Timolol** lacks ISA and MSA, and therefore does not affect corneal sensations. Ocular action is quick and well sustained.

   These drugs can cause mild transient burning, stinging sensation and allergic blepheroconjunctivitis upon ocular use. Absorption of non-selective beta blockers through nasolacrimal duct may cause systemic adverse effects. This can be prevented by asking patients to lightly press the inner canthus of the eyes for few minutes after the instillation of eyedrops. This prevents entry of the drug into nasolacrimal duct.

   Betaxolol and **levobetaxolol** are β_1 selective blockers; they are less efficacious than non-selective drugs, but safe for use in glaucoma patients who have coexistent bronchial asthma.

Carbonic anhydrase inhibitors

Carbonic anhydrase inhibitors such as acetazolamide, dorzolamide and brinzolamide decrease aqueous humour secretion by reducing HCO_3^- ion production. Acetazolamide is given orally, whereas both brinzolamide and dorzolamide are used topically. Frequent adverse effects upon topical use include ocular allergy and corneal edema. These are considered for use in open-angle glaucoma only when the first-line drugs are not effective or are contraindicated.

However, in closed-angle glaucoma, they can be used prior to surgery. Miotics and osmotic diuretic (mannitol) are also used to control IOT before definitive surgical treatment.

Topical ocular drug delivery systems include eyedrops, suspensions, emulsions, ointments, and aqueous gels. Various nano formulations like nanomicelles, nanosuspensions, and nanoparticles are also available for delivery of drugs to the anterior chamber. Others, such as contact lenses, liposomes, implants, and microneedles are also used. For administration of drugs in the posterior chamber of eye, intravitreal injections, trans-scleral

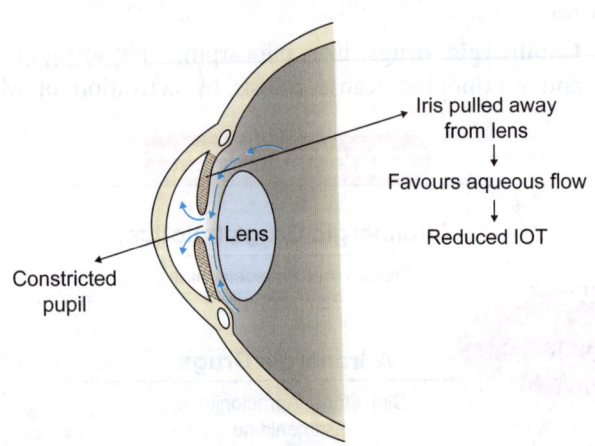

Fig. 11.3 Mechanism of IOT lowering by miotics in glaucoma

delivery through periocular injections, or systemic administration are effective.

Clinical problem-based questions and MCQs

21. **A 65-year-old male patient presents with headache and progressive decrease in vision. On tonometry, IOT is raised. The patient is diagnosed with chronic simple glaucoma.**
    i. Identify the drug of choice in this case.
       a. Brimonidine   b. Latanoprost
       c. Dipivefrin   d. Dorzolamide
    ii. Describe the mechanism of useful effect of the selected drug and its adverse effects.
    iii. Enumerate all the drugs that may be useful in this condition.

22. **Which of the following is safer in a patient of glaucoma with co-existent asthma?**
    a. Levobunolol   b. Carteolol
    c. Levobetaxolol d. Timolol

Summary

- β Receptors are of 3 types: $β_1$, $β_2$, $β_3$.
- Beta blockers can be non-selective, cardioselective or those having additional properties like ISA, MSA.
- β receptors present in heart are excitatory in nature. Their blockade with β blockers has a cardio-depressant effect.
- Decreased heart rate with β blockers is useful in anxiety and tachyarrhythmias but manifests as an adverse effect when β blockers are used for other indications. If bradycardia is disturbing, β blockers with intrinsic sympathomimetic activity (ISA) like pindolol and celiprolol are a better choice.
- Reduced conduction through AV node is beneficial for control of ventricular rate in atrial fibrillation, but it can worsen preexisting AV blocks. β Blockers should not be combined with CCB verapamil as both drugs reduce AV conduction and may cause complete AV block.
- Reduced cardiac work improves cardiac oxygen demand–supply ratio, making these drugs useful in classical angina. While the total coronary flow is reduced, the subendocardial region, which is a common site for ischemia, is not significantly affected. β blockers are also used in MI for primary salvage and chronic prophylaxis. However, in variant angina, β blockers are contraindicated as they may worsen coronary vasospasm.
- Beta blockers like carvedilol are also useful in certain cases of CHF, but they are contraindicated in acute decompensated heart failure.
- Beta blockers have a BP-lowering effect. SBP is lowered due to cardio-depressant action and reduced cardiac output. Vascular effect through $β_2$ blockade prevents vasodilatation, but with chronic use of β blockers, blood vessels adapt to the chronically reduced COP resulting in a fall in PVR and DBP. Currently, β blockers are not among the first-choice drugs for hypertension, but they can be used along with other drugs in patients with stable heart failure and a history of MI.
- Rapid-acting drug esmolol is useful in quick control of heart rate in tachyarrhythmias and BP in hypertensive urgencies.
- Blockade of $β_2$ receptors prevents vasodilatation and causes contraction of visceral smooth muscles, resulting in bronchospasm. Thus, β blockers should be avoided in asthmatics. However, if it is absolutely necessary to give β blockers, cardioselective or $β_1$-selective blockers like atenolol and metoprolol are preferred.
- Blockade of $β_3$ receptors inhibits lipolysis and has an unfavourable effect on the lipid profile. Inhibition of glycogenolysis delays the recovery from hypoglycemia and masks warning symptoms of hypoglycemia; hence, they should be used with caution in diabetic patients. However, β blockers with ISA have fewer unfavourable metabolic effects.
- In addition, β blockers relieve symptoms of thyrotoxicosis, anxiety, alcohol withdrawal and essential tremors. They reduce intraocular tension in glaucoma. Drugs lacking MSA are preferred for topical use in glaucoma.
- Important adverse effects of β blockers are bradycardia, worsening of acute CHF, variant angina, AV blocks, COPD, bronchial asthma, carbohydrate tolerance and lipid profile.
- Beta blockers are contraindicated in bronchial asthma, COPD, PVD, AV conduction blocks and insulin-dependent diabetes.
- Glaucoma involves progressive optic nerve damage, usually associated with raised IOT. The major types are chronic simple or wide-angle glaucoma, and acute congestive glaucoma.
- The treatment of glaucoma aims at reducing IOT by reducing secretion or increasing drainage. In chronic simple glaucoma, $PGF_{2α}$ analogues like latanoprost are the drugs of choice. Beta blockers like timolol, betaxolol and levobunolol are also first-line drugs. In patients who do not respond to these drugs, other drugs like dipivefrin and apraclonidine are tried. In acute congestive glaucoma, surgical or laser peripheral iridectomy is the definitive treatment. Miotics and carbonic anhydrase inhibitors may be used as initial measures prior to surgery.

Questions for practice

1. Classify β blockers. Enumerate the therapeutic uses of β blockers.
2. Comment on the current status of β blockers in the treatment of:
   a. Hypertension
   b. CHF
3. Enumerate the adverse effects of β blockers.
4. Explain why:
   a. β Blockers are contraindicated in variant angina.
   b. β Blockers are used cautiously in IDDM.
   c. Carvedilol is used in CHF.
   d. β Blockers are used in myocardial infarction.
   e. Propranolol should not be combined with verapamil.
   f. β Blockers can be given after α blockers in the treatment of pheochromocytoma.
   g. β Blockers are used in anxiety.
   h. β Blockers are used in thyrotoxicosis.
5. Write short notes on:
   a. Cardioselective β blockers
   b. Carvedilol
   c. Esmolol

Hints for problem-based questions and MCQs

1. i. Refer to page 142.
   ii. The advantage of selective $β_1$ blockers is safety in patients with coexistent bronchial asthma or COPD. These drugs, like metoprolol, reduce cardiac output and renin release through $β_1$ blockade. Thus, systolic as well as diastolic BP is reduced. In this patient, metoprolol exerts antihypertensive effect as well as prophylactic effect to prevent reinfarction.
2. i. This patient is type II DM on sulphonylureas that have the potential to cause hypoglycemia as an adverse effect. After the stress due to road accident, diabetes was poorly controlled with oral drugs alone, requiring addition of insulin. The addition of insulin further increases the risk of hypoglycemia. Beta blockers can delay recovery from hypoglycemia and mask the warning symptoms suggestive of hypoglycemia.
   ii. Refer to page 143.
3. i. c. Metoprolol
   ii Metoprolol is a cardioselective β blocker; the risk of metabolic effects causing hypoglycemia is reported to be lesser with cardioselective blockers.
4. i. The cause of symptoms is anxiety as the person has to present to a large audience.
   ii. Refer to page 143.
5. d. Metoprolol
6. a. Carvedilol
7. i. The patient has classical angina.
   ii. Refer to page 144.
   iii. If the patient develops symptoms unrelated to physical activity, the cause can be coronary vasospasm, i.e., vasospastic angina. β blockers block the $β_2$-mediated vasodilatation of coronaries. So, β blockers are contraindicated in variant angina.
8. i. a. Atenolol
   ii. Cardioselective β blockers pose a lower risk of precipitating bronchial asthma or COPD in predisposed individuals. Metabolic adverse effects are also reported to be less than with non-selective blockers.
9. i. c. Esmolol
   ii. Esmolol has rapid onset and short duration of action, so is suitable in emergency situations.
10. i. Refer to page 142.
    ii. Bradycardia is due to blockade of $β_1$ receptors, resulting in reduced automaticity of SA node.
    iii. a. Pindolol
    iv. Out of the given choices, pindolol is the most suitable as its ISA reduces the risk of cardio-depression and bradycardia.
11. i. This patient has raised IOT and is suffering from glaucoma. Timolol is a β blocker with no ISA or MSA. It is useful in glaucoma as it decreases secretory activity of ciliary epithelium. Aqueous humour production decreases and IOT falls. The lack of MSA in timolol is beneficial as the sensitivity of cornea will be maintained.
    ii. Betaxolol, carteolol, and levobunolol are other β blockers useful in glaucoma.
    iii. The doctor specifically asked for symptoms suggestive of asthma before prescribing timolol eyedrops, as it may get absorbed from eye and cause bronchospasm by $β_2$ blockade in susceptible individuals.
12. i. c. Timolol has no ISA and MSA.
    ii Agents with ISA have partial agonistic effects. Risk of cardio-depressant adverse effects is lower with these agents. MSA of β blockers is not used clinically as they have irritant property. However, lack of MSA is a beneficial property for ocular use of β blockers.
13. i. Symptoms and investigations suggest that the patient has hyperthyroidism/thyrotoxicosis.
    ii. Propranolol provides symptomatic relief by reducing anxiety, tremors, palpitation, sweating, etc. Activation of thyroxine (T_4) to liothyronine (T_3) is also inhibited.
14. c. Verapamil cannot be combined with β blockers because the combination causes additive cardio-depressant effect and AV blocks.
15. c. Acute decompensated heart failure
    CHF involves reduced force of contraction and pumping activity of the heart. Beta blockers reduce contractility by $β_1$ blockade, reducing ejection fraction. Beta blockers are absolutely contraindicated in acute decompensated heart failure, as they can worsen the condition.
16. i. d. Chronic obstructive pulmonary disease can be worsened due to bronchospasm caused by $β_2$ blockade.
    iii. c. Celiprolol is safer in asthma patients due to its $β_2$ agonistic effect.
17. b. Labetalol
18. a. Carvedilol
19. d. Nebivolol
20. c. Sotalol
21. i. b. Latanoprost
    ii. Refer to page 149.
    iii. Refer to page 149.
22. c. Levobetaxolol, as it is $β_1$-selective.

Chapter 11 Antiadrenergic Drugs: β Blockers and Drugs for Glaucoma

CONCEPT MAP - β BLOCKERS AND DRUGS FOR GLAUCOMA

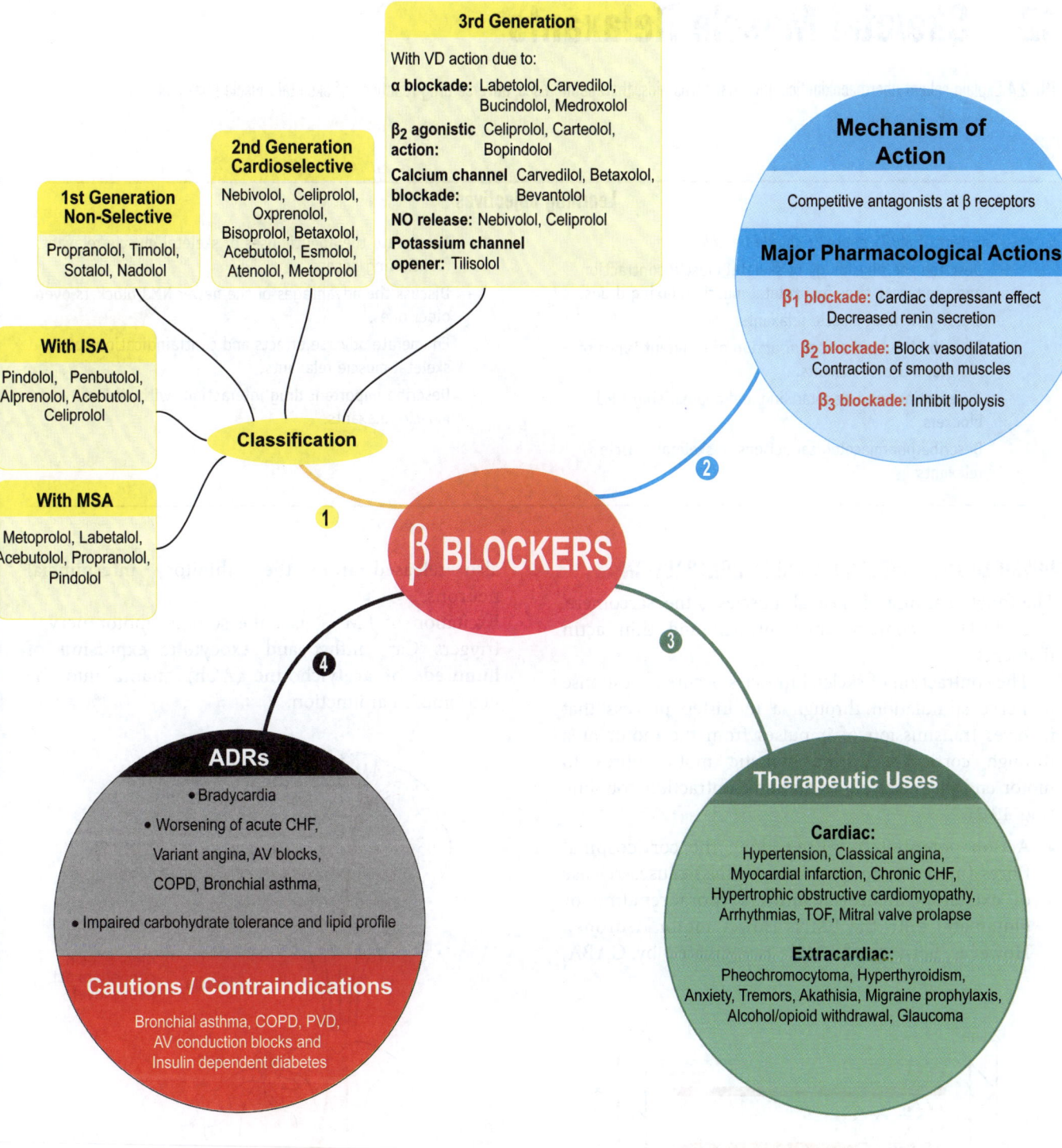

Drugs for Glaucoma

Prostaglandin analogues: Latanoprost, Bimatoprost, Travoprost, Tafluprost, Unoprostone

Miotics: Pilocarpine, Physostigmine, Ecothiophate

Adrenergic drugs: Dipivefrine, Apraclonidine, Brimonidine

β blockers: Timolol, Levobunolol, Carteolol, Metipranolol, Betaxolol, Levobetaxolol

Carbonic anhydrase inhibitors: Acetazolamide, Dorzolamide, Brinzolamide

SECTION 2 Drugs Acting on ANS and PNS

12 Skeletal Muscle Relaxants

PH 2.4 Explain salient pharmacokinetics, pharmacodynamics, therapeutic uses, adverse drug reactions of skeletal muscle relaxants.

Learning objectives

A student of MBBS phase II should be able to:
- Describe the physiology of skeletal muscle contraction and the target sites for skeletal muscle relaxing drugs.
- Classify skeletal muscle relaxants.
- Describe the mechanism of action of different types of skeletal muscle relaxants.
- Differentiate non-depolarising and depolarising NMJ blockers.
- Describe pharmacological actions of skeletal muscle relaxants.
- Enumerate therapeutic uses of skeletal muscle relaxants mentioning doses.
- Discuss the advantages of the newer NMJ blockers over older ones.
- Enumerate adverse effects and contraindications of skeletal muscle relaxants.
- Describe important drug interactions with skeletal muscle relaxants.

PHYSIOLOGY OF SKELETAL MUSCLE CONTRACTION

The functional unit of skeletal muscles is the 'sarcomere' (Fig. 12.1). It contains thick myosin and thin actin filaments.

The contraction of skeletal muscles occurs in response to nerve stimulation through a multistep process that involves transmission of impulses from the motor area through corticospinal and somatic motor fibres to motor end plate causing excitation–contraction coupling (Fig. 12.2).

- Action potential travelling along the corticospinal fibres (upper motor neurons, UMNs) causes release of excitatory neurotransmitters (noradrenaline or glutamate) onto the LMNs (lower motor neurons). However, activity of LMNs is regulated by GABA, also released from the inhibitory internuncial neurons.
- Excitation of LMNs, i.e., the somatic motor nerves, triggers Ca^{2+} influx and exocytotic **expulsion of hundreds of acetylcholine (ACh) quanta** into the neuromuscular junction.

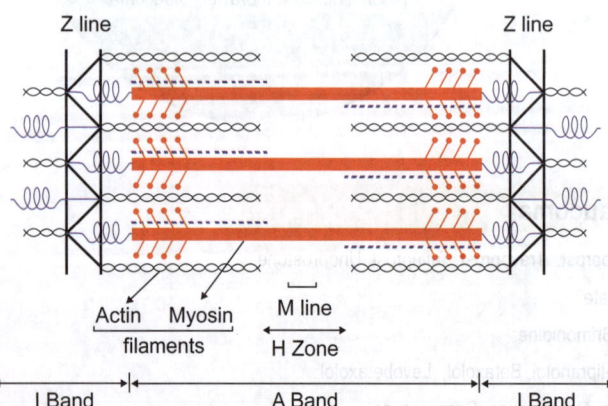

Fig. 12.1 Sarcomere in relaxed muscle

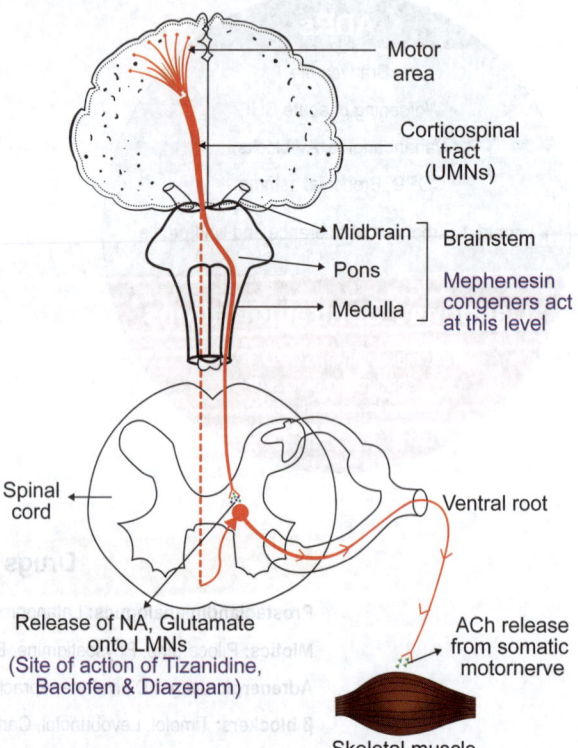

Fig. 12.2 Site of action of centrally acting muscle relaxants

- Acetylcholine activates neuromuscular nicotinic (Nm) receptors causing rapid Na⁺ influx and end plate depolarisation. Thus, action potential is generated and conducted (Fig. 12.3).
- The arrival of action potential at skeletal muscle fibre causes Ca^{2+} influx through L-type Ca^{2+} channels → increased intracellular calcium → sequestration of calcium into sarcoplasmic reticulum (SR) → interaction of Ca^{2+} with ryanodine receptor on sarcoplasmic reticulum → **Ca^{2+} released from sarcoplasmic reticulum** in the vicinity of actin-troponin-tropomyosin complex → transient increase in Ca^{2+} concentration → exposure of actin binding sites → formation of crossbridges and **sliding of actin filaments over myosin filaments** → **muscle contraction** (Fig. 12.3).

A brief contraction followed by relaxation in response to single action potential is known as 'muscle twitch'. There is a time gap of 2 milliseconds between the start of **action potential and the twitch response**.

Acetylcholine's effects are rapidly terminated through diffusion and enzymatic breakdown by local acetylcholinesterase. Another enzyme, **butyrylcholinesterase** (also known as pseudocholinesterase), found in the plasma, liver, and glial tissue, is primarily responsible for metabolising succinylcholine, although it has low specificity for acetylcholine.

CLASSIFICATION OF SKELETAL MUSCLE RELAXANTS

Skeletal muscle relaxation can be achieved by interrupting the physiological processes involved in muscle contraction at various levels. Based on their site of action, skeletal muscle relaxants are classified into three main categories: **centrally acting, peripherally acting,** and **directly acting agents**, as illustrated in Flowchart 12.1.

- **Centrally acting drugs** modulate motor control by acting at the level of the brainstem or at the synapses between upper and lower motor neurons (Fig. 12.2).
- **Peripherally acting drugs** inhibit neuromuscular transmission at the junction between somatic motor neurons and skeletal muscle fibers. These agents, known as neuromuscular junction (NMJ) blockers, are further subdivided into **non-depolarising agents (NDAs)** and **depolarising agents (DAs)**.
- **Directly acting drugs** exert their effect on the **sarcoplasmic reticulum (SR)** of skeletal muscle cells, interfering with calcium release and thus inhibiting contraction.

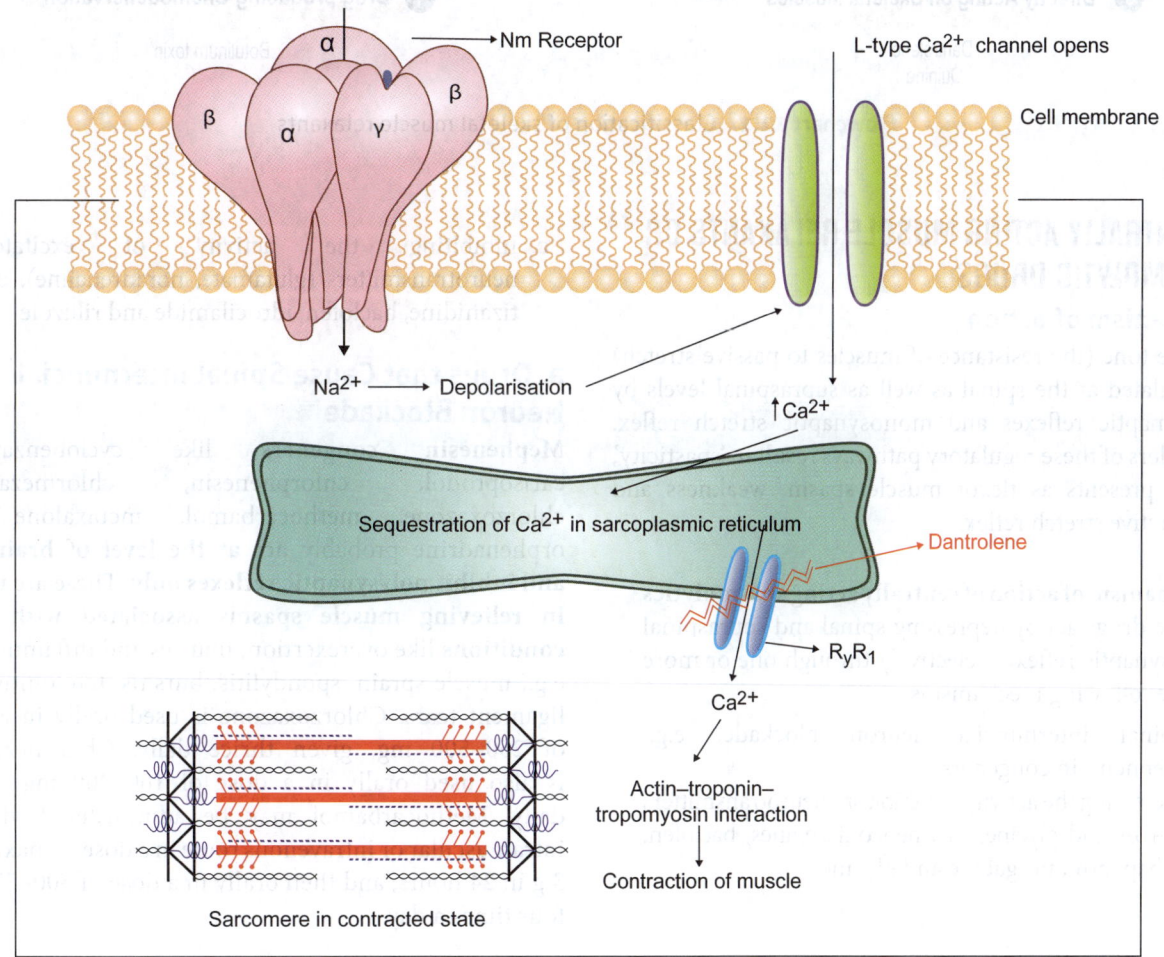

Fig. 12.3 Mechanism of contraction of skeletal muscle

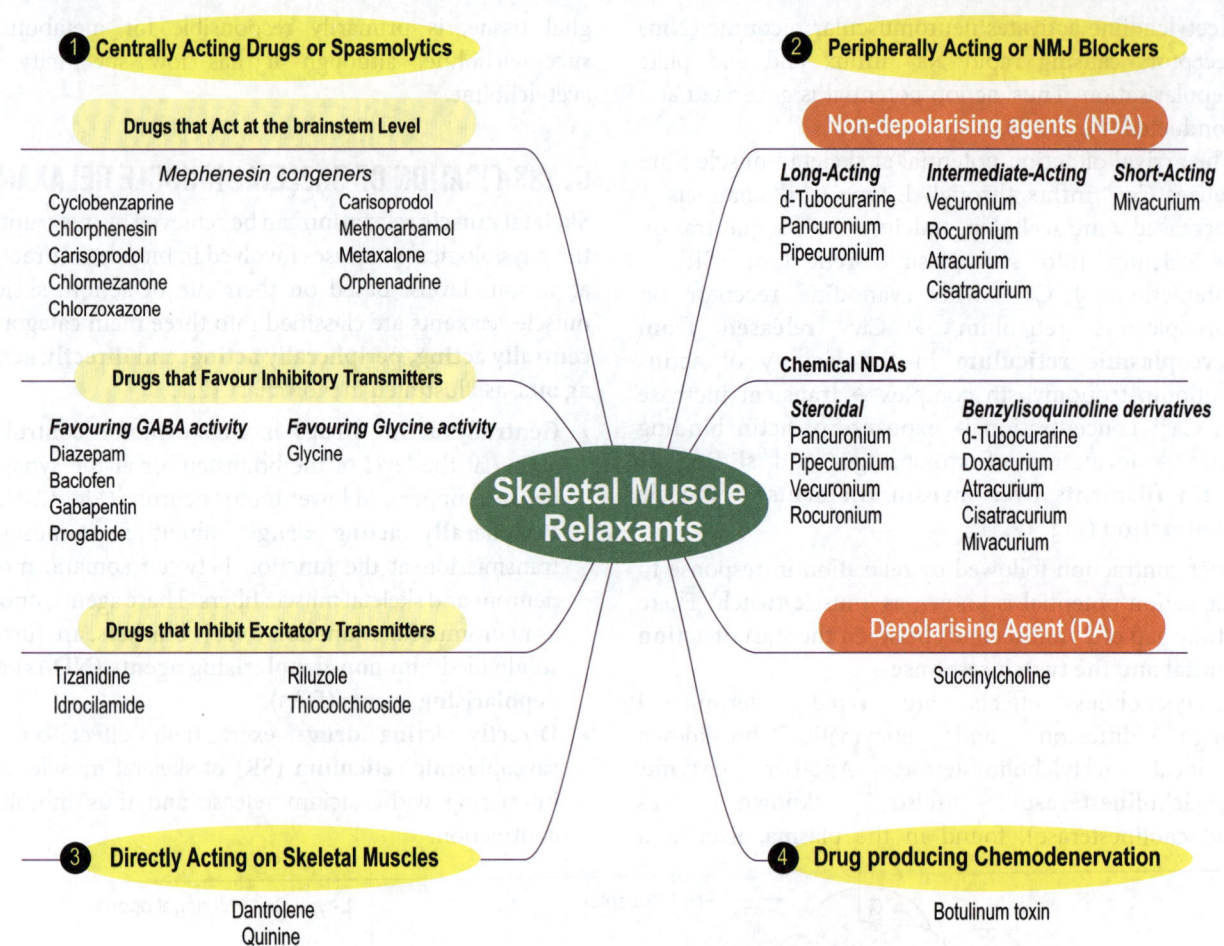

Flowchart 12.1 Classification of skeletal muscle relaxants

1. CENTRALLY ACTING MUSCLE RELAXANTS OR SPASMOLYTIC DRUGS

Mechanism of action

Muscle tone (the resistance of muscles to passive stretch) is regulated at the spinal as well as supraspinal levels by polysynaptic reflexes and monosynaptic stretch reflex. Disorders of these regulatory pathways result in 'spasticity', which presents as flexor muscle spasm, weakness and hyperactive stretch reflex.

> **Mechanism of action of centrally acting spasmolytics**
> These drugs act by depressing spinal and supraspinal polysynaptic reflexes selectively through one or more of the following mechanisms:
> a. Spinal internuncial neuron blockade, e.g., mephenesin congeners
> b. Increasing the activity of inhibitory neurotransmitters GABA and glycine, e.g., benzodiazepines, baclofen, gabapentin, progabide and glycine
> c. Inhibiting the activity of excitatory neurotransmitters (glutamate, noradrenaline), e.g., tizanidine, baclofen, idrocilamide and riluzole

a. Drugs that Cause Spinal Internuncial Neuron Blockade

Mephenesin congeners like cyclobenzaprine, carisoprodol, chlorphenesin, chlormezanone, chlorzoxazone, methocarbamol, metaxalone and orphenadrine probably **act at the level of brainstem and inhibit polysynaptic reflexes only.** These are **useful in relieving muscle spasms associated with local conditions** like overexertion, injuries and inflammation, e.g., muscle sprain, spondylitis, bursitis, tendonitis, and ligament tears. Chlorzoxazone is used orally in a dose of 250–500 mg, given thrice daily. Chlormezanone is also used orally in a dose of 100–200 mg, thrice daily. Methocarbamol may be administered via the intramuscular or intravenous route in a dose of maximum 3 g in 24 hours, and then orally in a dose of 500–750 mg four times a day.

b. Drugs that Increase Activity of Inhibitory Neurotransmitters

Drugs such as benzodiazepines, baclofen, gabapentin, progabide, and glycine exert their effects by enhancing the activity of inhibitory neurotransmitters, primarily GABA (gamma-aminobutyric acid) and glycine (Fig. 12.4).

- Diazepam and other benzodiazepines augment GABA action by binding to $GABA_A$ receptors at LMNs, resulting in increased Cl^- permeability and hyperpolarisation. Thus, the frequency of action potentials travelling to muscles through LMNs is reduced.

    Diazepam can be used for relieving muscle spasm of any origin, e.g., tetanus, spinal injuries, local muscle injuries, and rheumatic diseases, and in patients undergoing electroconvulsive therapy (ECT). Diazepam is given orally in a dose of 5 mg thrice a day. In tetanus patients, the dose can be 10–40 mg, given intravenously. The dose and frequency of administration of diazepam varies depending on the response and extent of respiratory depression.
- Baclofen acts on $GABA_B$ receptors located presynaptically on UMNs and postsynaptically on LMNs. Baclofen exerts its action both presynaptically and postsynaptically. Presynaptically, it reduces the release of excitatory neurotransmitters from UMNs. Postsynaptically, it acts on LMNs to increase K^+ conductance, leading to membrane hyperpolarisation and reduced neuronal excitability.
- Progabide acts as an agonist at $GABA_A$ as well as $GABA_B$ receptors.
- Gabapentin and pregabalin act by increasing GABA concentration in the brain.
- Glycine is an inhibitory neurotransmitter which readily crosses blood brain barrier after oral administration

These drugs are useful in relieving spasticity and hyperreflexia associated with UMN lesions, such as hemiplegia, paraplegia, and generalised conditions like multiple sclerosis, cerebral palsy, spinal cord injuries and amyotrophic lateral sclerosis. They can also reduce decerebrate rigidity. Baclofen is given in a dose of 10 mg orally, twice a day. The dose can be increased as per need in individual cases up to a maximum of 25 mg, thrice a day.

c. Drugs that Inhibit Activity of Excitatory Neurotransmitters

The spasmolytic activity of drugs like tizanidine, baclofen, idrocilamide and riluzole is a result of the inhibition of excitatory neurotransmitters in the brain. For example:

- Tizanidine acts as an agonist at presynaptic α_2 receptors on UMNs and decreases the release of excitatory neurotransmitters like noradrenaline and glutamate (Fig. 12.4). Tizanidine reduces both monosynaptic and polysynaptic reflex activity. It is effective in relieving spasticity associated with multiple sclerosis, amyotrophic lateral sclerosis and spinal diseases. Tizanidine is used orally, in a dose of 2 mg thrice a day; the total daily dose should not exceed 24 mg.
- Baclofen also decreases the release of excitatory neurotransmitters by binding to $GABA_B$ receptors.
- Idrocilamide and riluzole inhibit glutamatergic transmission in the brain.

Thiocolchicoside

The mechanism of muscle relaxant action of this drug is not well understood; it is thought to involve nicotinic receptor antagonism. In addition to its muscle relaxant properties, it also exhibits analgesic and anti-inflammatory effects. Its proconvulsant potential is likely due to a competitive antagonistic effect on $GABA_A$ and glycine receptors, which diminishes inhibitory neurotransmission. Therefore, it is contraindicated in individuals with epilepsy.

> **Therapeutic uses**
>
> Centrally acting skeletal muscle relaxants are used in:
> - Painful musculoskeletal conditions.
> - Acute muscle spasm associated with overexertion, sprain, bursitis, tendonitis, ligament tears, etc.
> - To relieve spasticity and hyperreflexia associated with UMN lesions, such as in hemiplegia, paraplegia, and generalised conditions like multiple sclerosis, cerebral palsy, spinal cord injuries and amyotrophic lateral sclerosis.
> - To reduce decerebrate rigidity.
> - Diazepam is used for tetanus and in patients on electroconvulsive therapy (ECT).
> - Centrally acting relaxants are useful in orthopedic procedures like fracture reduction and correction of dislocations.

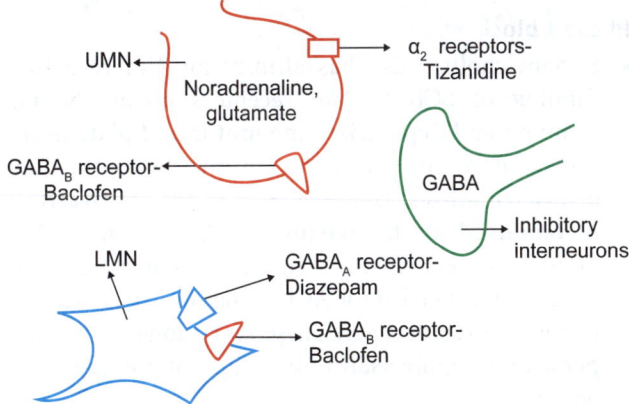

Fig. 12.4 Mechanism of action of centrally acting muscle relaxants

ADRs

Central side effects
- Dizziness, lightheadedness, fatigue, and muscular weakness are common with mephenesin congeners.
- Sedation occurs with mephenesin congeners and benzodiazepines.
- Sudden withdrawal of baclofen may increase seizure activity.
- Tizanidine may cause dryness of mouth, dizziness, drowsiness and hypotension.

Clinical problem-based questions and MCQs

1. A 42-year-old female patient presented in neurology clinic with a long-standing history of heat intolerance, stumbling gait, spasm in leg muscles and frequent falls. Her problem is worsened with stress, fatigue, etc. She also has low visual acuity, bladder incontinence and vertigo. After a thorough neurological examination and MRI, she is diagnosed with multiple sclerosis. Tab tizanidine 2 mg, thrice daily, is prescribed.
   i. Which of the following describes the mechanism of action of tizanidine?
      a. α_2 receptor agonist
      b. $GABA_B$ receptor agonist
      c. $GABA_A$ receptor agonist
      d. Nm receptor antagonist
   ii. Describe the role of tizanidine in multiple sclerosis.
   iii. Enumerate the therapeutic uses and adverse effects of spasmolytic drugs.

2. Match the drug with its mechanism of action.

a.	Diazepam	1.	Inhibits glutaminergic transmission
b.	Chlorzoxazone	2.	Augments GABA action by binding to $GABA_A$ receptors at LMNs
c.	Riluzole	3.	Agonist at presynaptic and postsynaptic GABA receptors
d.	Baclofen	4.	Spinal internuncial neuron blockade

3. Drugs can relax skeletal muscles by acting either centrally at the level of CNS, peripherally at the neuromuscular junction or directly at the muscle. Identify the drug acting at the level of brainstem.
   a. Methocarbamol   b. Pancuronium
   c. Dantrolene   d. Succinylcholine

2. PERIPHERALLY ACTING MUSCLE RELAXANTS OR NMJ BLOCKING DRUGS

The drugs in this category fall in two major groups based on their mechanism of action, viz., depolarising and non-depolarising agents.

Mechanism of Action

All neuromuscular junction (NMJ) blockers have structural resemblance to acetylcholine, and hence have affinity for Nm receptors at the motor end plate.

a. Non-Depolarising Agents (NDAs)

d-Tubocurarine is the prototype of this class. Other commonly used NDAs include pancuronium, pipecuronium, rocuronium, vecuronium, atracurium, cisatracurium, and mivacurium.

- These agents act as **competitive antagonists at nicotinic (Nm) receptors** on the motor end plate. By occupying these receptors, they **prevent depolarisation in response to acetylcholine (ACh)**, thereby inhibiting neuromuscular transmission (see Fig. 12.5).
- This **competitive blockade** can be **reversed** by increasing ACh concentration at the NMJ by administering **cholinesterase inhibitors** such as neostigmine, pyridostigmine, or edrophonium. These drugs **inhibit the breakdown of ACh**, allowing it to accumulate and displace the NDA from Nm receptors.
- This principle is used clinically to **reverse residual neuromuscular blockade** caused by NDAs, following surgery—a process known as **decurarisation**—by using drugs like **neostigmine**.
- Because cholinesterase inhibitors also increase ACh at muscarinic receptors (e.g., in the heart and GI tract), **antimuscarinic agents** (such as **atropine** or **glycopyrrolate**) are co-administered to **counteract muscarinic side effects**.
- At higher doses, NDAs may enter the pore of ionic Na^+ channels, further weakening nerve–muscle transmission. At this stage, blockade cannot be reversed by cholinesterase inhibitors.

b. Depolarising Agents (DAs)

Succinylcholine (SCh) is the only drug in this group. It causes dual block in two phases – phase 1 and phase 2 (Fig. 12.6).

Phase 1 block

- Succinylcholine also has affinity for Nm receptors. Binding of SCh to Nm receptors opens the ion channels and **depolarises the motor end plate** in the same way as ACh, resulting in muscle contractions or **fasciculations**. However, SCh is **not as effectively metabolised at the synapse as ACh** (it takes 5–8 minutes to metabolise SCh in comparison to only a few milliseconds needed for ACh metabolism). Hence, the membrane remains depolarised for a longer time. i.e., **persistent depolarisation** or failure of repolarisation occurs.
- End plate repolarisation or repriming and repetitive firing is necessary for maintaining muscle tone.

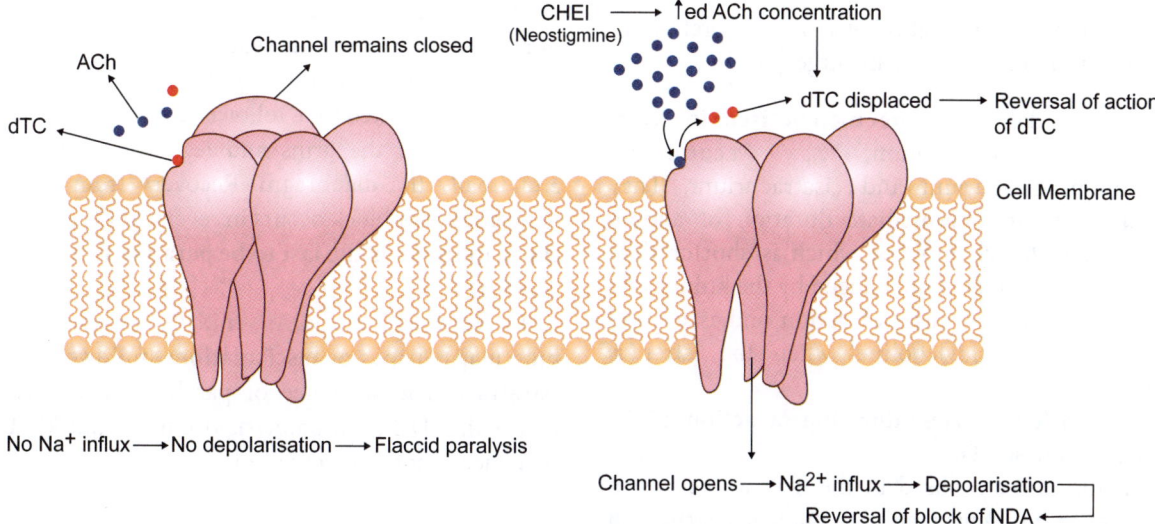

Fig. 12.5 Mechanism of action of NDAs and reversal by neostigmine

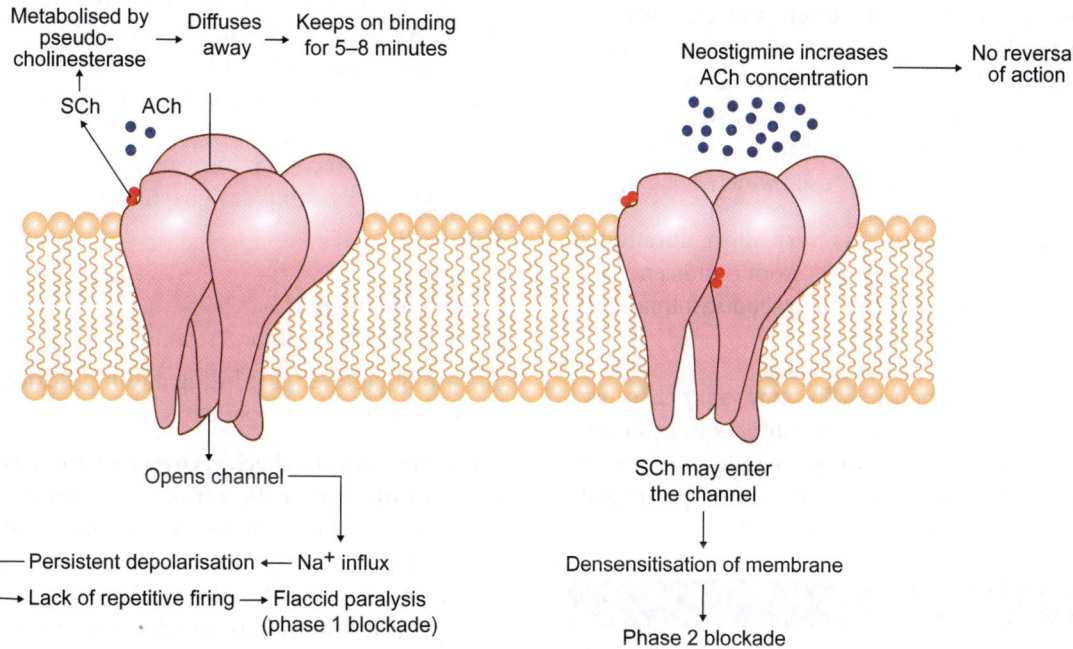

Fig. 12.6 Mechanism of the action of DA and failure of reversal by neostimine

Persistently depolarised membrane thus fails to respond to further stimuli, resulting in **lack of repetitive firing** and **flaccid paralysis**. This is a phase 1 block. It cannot be reversed by cholinesterase inhibitors.

Phase 2 block
- On prolonged exposure to SCh, though the membrane gets slowly repolarised, it fails to depolarise again in response to action potential. This is because of **desensitisation of receptors**. While the exact mechanism of desensitisation is not clearly delineated, SCh likely enters pores of the ion channel so that the channels seem to be in a prolonged closed state. This **failure of depolarisation** is called **phase 2 or desensitisation block**. It shows some of the characteristics of non-depolarising blockers.

Clinically Relevant Pharmacokinetic Characteristics of NMJ Blockers

All NMJ blockers contain quaternary ammonium groups, which make them highly polar and ionised compounds. They do not readily cross membranes. Thus, they are ineffective by oral route and are always administered parenterally.

The duration of drug action depends on its elimination half-life.

NDAs
- **Certain NDAs are excreted unchanged by the kidneys**, e.g., d-tubocurarine, pancuronium, pipecuronium and doxacurium. Such drugs are **long-acting** (duration of action > 60 minutes).

Drugs that have a long duration of action are preferred in prolonged surgeries, e.g., neurosurgery.

- Certain steroidal NDAs are **metabolised in liver/plasma** by hydroxylation, e.g., vecuronium, rocuronium, atracurium and cisatracurium. They typically have an intermediate duration of action, lasting about 20–40 minutes, which is shorter than that of drugs eliminated unchanged by the kidneys.
- Rocuronium has fast onset of action and is a good alternative to succinylcholine, when the latter is contraindicated.
- **Mivacurium has shortest duration of action** 15–30 minutes) amongst NDAs.
- **Atracurium** is metabolised in the liver as well as in plasma by a non-enzymatic spontaneous structural reorganisation called 'Hofmann elimination'.

Laudanosine, one of the **metabolites of atracurium,** can cross the blood–brain barrier and **cause central adverse effects.** It precipitates seizure activity upon prolonged atracurium administration in ICU settings. Cisatracurium, however, is less likely to produce such adverse central reactions and is used widely.

- **Depolarising agent** SCh has very short duration of action (5–8 minutes). It diffuses from motor end plate into ECF and is metabolised by pseudocholinesterase into succinic acid and choline.

The ability to metabolise SCh may vary because of **genetic variations in pseudocholinesterase.** In patients who have abnormal genetic variants of pseudocholinesterase, SCh may cause prolonged neuromuscular blockade and apnea.

Box 12.1 The Paradox of SCh

At the Nm receptor, SCh is said to be responsible for producing persistent depolarisation for a prolonged period because it slowly diffuses away from the receptors for metabolism by pseudocholinesterase enzyme. At the same time, SCh is said to have very short duration of action, i.e., only 5–8 minutes.

It is a fact that SCh is a short-acting drug; it takes only 5–8 minutes for its metabolism at the synapse. However, when compared to ACh which gets metabolised in a few milli seconds, the process is very slow. Therefore, the 5–8 minutes of SCh action is labelled as persistent depolarisation of the motor end plate.

Pharmacological Actions of NMJ Blockers
1. Skeletal muscles

The action of NMJ blockers on skeletal muscles is therapeutically useful. **NDAs** produce **muscular weakness, which progresses to flaccid paralysis.** Paralysis of muscles occurs in a set sequence as shown in Fig. 12.7. Small muscles such as those of the fingers and extraocular muscles are affected first, followed by muscles of the hands and feet, then the arms and legs, intercostal muscles, and finally the diaphragm. Recovery from competitive neuromuscular block occurs in reverse order. **Fortunately, the diaphragm is the last to be paralysed and the first to recover.**

In contrast, the **DAs** initially produce transient muscular twitches or **fasciculations, followed by flaccid paralysis.** The sequence of paralysis is different from that with NDAs, but paralysis occurs so quickly that the sequence is not well perceived.

Recovery from NM block

The time to recover from neuromuscular blockade by NDAs depends upon the elimination half-life of the drug. Drugs excreted by the kidney have a longer duration of action than drugs metabolised in liver/plasma.

Clinically, recovery from neuromuscular blockade is indicated by simple signs like the ability of the patient to

- open eyes
- stick out tongue
- lift and hold head for 5 seconds

In case of children, leg lifting and hip flexion indicate recovery from muscle paralysis.

Other methods to check recovery of muscles

- **Train-of-four (ToF) ratio:** This method involves comparing the single twitch responses of the thumb muscles following transcutaneous stimulation of the ulnar nerve. An electrical stimulus at 2 Hz is applied to the thumb muscles, four times in quick succession and the response is recorded. The **ToF ratio** is calculated by dividing the strength of the fourth twitch by that of the first.
- NDAs decrease the ToF ratio during induction of paralysis; the effect is called **fade response.** However, because SCh diminishes all four responses equally, the ToF ratio remains constant.
- **Tetanic stimulation:** A high-frequency (typically 50 Hz) continuous stimulation is used to assess neuromuscular transmission. In the presence of NDAs, fade is observed here as well.
- **Post-tetanic count (PTC)** is also used sometimes (when there is no response to ToF or tetanic stimulation) to gauge the level of recovery from neuromuscular blockade.

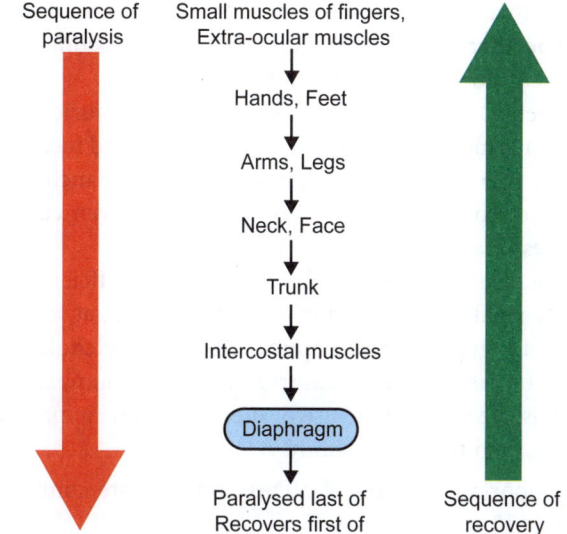

Fig. 12.7 Sequence of paralysis and recovery with NDAs

Recovery from blockade **is hastened by a combination of neostigmine and atropine**. Neostigmine reverses the action of NDAs by increasing local concentration of acetylcholine at Nm receptors, and atropine controls muscarinic manifestations of raised ACh. **Sugammadex** can quickly reverse the effect of vecuronium and rocuronium by forming inactive complexes (chelates) that get subsequently excreted.

2. GIT
The use of NDAs during surgery may cause **post-operative paralytic ileus.**

3. Ganglia
d-Tubocurarine produces some degree of ganglionic blockade. This effect is minimal with other steroidal NDAs. SCh causes initial transient ganglionic stimulation, followed by blockade.

4. CVS
Some NMJ blockers like **d**-tubocurarine, **a**tracurium, **m**ivacurium and **s**uccinylcholine [Mnemonic: **DAMS**] have histamine releasing effect which may cause vasodilatation, flushing, hypotension, bronchospasm and dyspnea.

Blood pressure
- A **significant fall in blood pressure** occurs with **d-tubocurarine**. This is due to the combined effect of histamine release, ganglionic blockade and reduced venous return because of the relaxation of skeletal muscles in the limbs. Newer agents of the non-depolarising group, however, do not have much effect on blood pressure and heart rate.
- **SCh** has significant cardiovascular effects. It causes initial bradycardia due to vagal ganglionic stimulation, followed by tachycardia and a rise in blood pressure due to sympathetic ganglionic stimulation.

> Cardiac arrhythmias and even cardiac arrest may occur upon SCh administration in patients with severe burns, soft tissue injuries and tetanus because of severe, dangerous hyperkalemia. Therefore, SCh is contraindicated in such cases.
>
> **Rocuronium** is a good alternative to SCh (owing to fast onset of muscle relaxant action) in such conditions where SCh is contraindicated.

Therapeutic Uses of NMJ Blockers
1. As adjuvants to general anesthetics
The main indication for use of NMJ blockers is as **adjuvants to general anesthetics** in abdominal, thoracic, orthopedic and other prolonged surgical procedures.

> **Role of NMJ blockers in anesthetic practice**
> NMJ blockers are used as **adjuvants in anesthetic practice** because they;
> - Facilitate surgical manipulations by relaxing skeletal muscles.
> - Prevent reflex muscle contraction in operative area.
> - Improve safety during general anesthesia by allowing lower dose of anesthetic drug.
> - Maintain adequate gas exchange and prevent aspiration by controlled ventilation.
>
> **Selection of drug:** The drug for a particular procedure is chosen by matching the expected duration of procedure with the onset and duration of action of the drug. For example, for brief procedures like reduction of fractures/dislocations, bronchoscopy, esophagoscopy, and endotracheal intubation, short-acting drugs like mivacurium (shortest-acting NDA with effect lasting for 15–30 minutes) and succinylcholine (duration of action only 5–8 minutes) are used because their effect wears off by the time the procedure is completed. Succinylcholine is given as intravenous injection in a dose of 1 mg/kg of body weight.
>
> **For longer procedures** like intracavitary surgery in thoracic or abdominal cavity, orthopedic procedures like joint replacement surgery, longer-acting NDAs such as pancuronium, pipecuronium and doxacurium are preferred.

In addition, patient factors must also be considered while selecting the drug. For example, in patients with impaired hepatic or renal function, drugs like atracurium and cisatracurium, which are metabolised spontaneously by Hoffman elimination, are preferred.

2. In critically ill patients

In intensive care units, NMJ blockers are commonly used for improving the outcome. They reduce chest wall resistance and improve ventilator synchrony in ICU patients on ventilator. Continuous infusion of competitive NMJ blockers, especially vecuronium, is used for this indication.

3. In psychiatric practice

In psychiatric practice, electroconvulsive therapy (ECT) is indicated in severe refractory schizophrenia and mood disorders that do not respond to other therapies. It involves risk of injuries, and even fractures secondary to excessive convulsions. These complications associated with ECT can be prevented by centrally acting muscle relaxant **diazepam combined with DA succinylcholine**.

4. Other indications

NMJ blockers can be used in combination with diazepam to control the spasm and convulsions in conditions like tetanus, local anesthetic toxicity and status epilepticus.

ADRs of NMJ Blockers

- The adverse effect of NMJ blockers, which is a direct extension of its therapeutic effects, is **prolonged respiratory paralysis and apnea**. Recovery in case of NDAs can be hastened by cholinesterase inhibitors.
- **Histamine release** is seen with benzylisoquinoline NDAs like d-tubocurarine, doxacurium, atracurium, cisatracurium and mivacurium, resulting in flushing, vasodilatation, hypotension, asthma precipitation and sometimes, cardiovascular collapse.
- Succinylcholine causes postoperative **soreness of muscles and myalgias** because of the initial muscle twitches or fasciculations.
- Succinyl choline has potential to produce **malignant hyperthermia** in some patients receiving halothane or other fluorinated anesthetics.
- Patients with severe burns, soft tissue injuries, and tetanus may develop severe hyperkalemia and increased heat rate with succinylcholine, thereby enhancing the risk of rhythm disturbances; sometimes, even **cardiac arrest** may occur.
- Patients with genetically determined deficiency or abnormality of pseudocholinesterase are at risk of developing **prolonged apnea with succinylcholine**. It can be predicted by measuring 'dibucaine number'. It is advisable to avoid the use of succinylcholine in patients with such history in family.

The important features of NDAs and DAs are compared in Table 12.1.

Cautions/Contraindications and Drug–Drug Interactions

Drugs/conditions that enhance the effect of NMJ blockers

1. Myasthenia gravis is an autoimmune disease characterised by weakness of skeletal muscles. So, the effect of muscle relaxants gets augmented.
2. Advanced age leads to reduced clearance of drugs, which prolongs the duration of their action. Therefore, the dose should be reduced in patients above 70 years of age.
3. General anesthetics, especially ether, isoflurane and antimicrobial agents like aminoglycosides, tetracyclines, clindamycin and lincomycin, enhance the effect of NDAs, whereas calcium channel blockers can potentiate both NDAs as well as DAs.

Table 12.1 A comparison of features of DAs and NDAs

	NDAs	DAs
Drugs included	d-Tubocurarine, pancuronium, rocuronium, atracurium, doxacurium, mivacurium, etc	Succinylcholine
Mechanism of action	Bind to Nm receptors and prevent action of ACh. No depolarisation occurs.	In phase1, bind to Nm receptors resulting in persistent depolarisation followed by lack of repetitive firing and flaccid paralysis. In phase 2, desensitisation of receptors
Reversal	Cholinesterase inhibitor neostigmine can hasten recovery	Neostigmine cannot hasten recovery
Metabolism and duration of action	By liver. Atracurium shows Hoffman elimination as well. Duration of action varies. May be long, intermediate, short	Metabolised by pseudocholinesterase. Very short duration of action
Uses	Adjuvants to anesthesia for intracavitary surgery, neurosurgery, and ICU settings to decrease chest wall resistance	Preferred for brief procedures and during ECT

Drugs/conditions that diminish the effect of NMJ blockers

1. The effect of NDAs can be reversed postoperatively by neostigmine, edrophonium and other cholinesterase inhibitors. Prior administration of atropine or glycopyrrolate checks hypotension, bronchospasm and other features of muscarinic excess with neostigmine-like drugs.
2. Patients with upper motor neuron (UMN) diseases and severe burns are resistant to non-depolarising agents (NDAs) because of the proliferation of extra-junctional receptors. Hence, the dosage should be increased.
3. Sugammadex is a gamma cyclodextrin that can form inactive chelate with vecuronium and rocuronium, which subsequently gets excreted in urine. The effect of vecuronium and rocuronium, therefore, can be reversed postoperatively within few minutes by administering sugammadex intravenously in a dose of 2–4mg/kg.
4. Thiopentone sodium and succinylcholine can react chemically. Therefore, these two should not be mixed in the same syringe prior to administration.

Other cautions

1. Succinylcholine can cause dangerous hyperkalemia, arrhythmias and even cardiac arrest in conditions such as severe burns and tetanus.
2. Succinylcholine has the potential to induce phase-2 block and malignant hyperthermia when co-administered with fluorinated anesthetics, especially halothane and isoflurane.
3. Succinylcholine carries the risk of causing hyperkalemia in patients with muscle and nerve disorders. Hence, it is not used in patients suffering from Guillain–Barre syndrome, hemiplegia/paraplegia, myasthenia gravis, muscular dystrophy, rhabdomyolysis, etc.
4. Succinylcholine has the potential to increase blood pressure, intracranial pressure and intraocular tension. Hence, it is contraindicated in hypertension, head injury and glaucoma. Intragastric pressure is also raised leading to adverse effects like nausea, vomiting.

Clinical problem-based questions and MCQs

4. **Neostigmine was administered postoperatively to a 30-year-old patient. He complained of abdominal cramps, diarrhea, excessive salivation, lacrimation and difficulty in breathing.**
   i. Describe the rationale behind the use of neostigmine in the postoperative period.
   ii. Explain the causes of the patient's symptoms.
   iii. Describe management of this patient.
5. **A patient with severe burns (70%) is to be intubated.**
   i. Name the muscle relaxant to be avoided in this patient.
   ii. Explain the rationale for this caution.
6. **A 32-year-old woman is brought to trauma ward with severe soft tissue injury. Emergency intubation is ordered to prevent aspiration of gastric contents.**
   i. Which is the most suitable skeletal muscle relaxant in this case?
      a. Baclofen   b. Succinylcholine
      c. Rocuronium   d. Methocarbamol
   ii. Explain the rationale of your choice.
7. **Identify the drug that can cause malignant hyperthermia when co-administered with succinylcholine.**
   a. Aminoglycosides
   b. Calcium channel blockers
   c. Fluorinated anesthetics
   d. Thiopentone sodium
8. **Identify the skeletal muscle relaxant having the potential to induce seizures.**
   a. d-Tubocurarine   b. Atracurium
   c. Vecuronium   d. Succinylcholine

NMJ Blockers in Current Clinical Practice

d-Tubocurarine: Prototype competitive NMJ blocker, but **not used much nowadays** because of (i) its long duration of action which necessitates postoperative reversal of action, (ii) large number of adverse effects such as hypotension and bronchospasm (due to its histamine-releasing and ganglion-blocking action)

Doxacurium has maximum potency and longest duration of action.

Pancuronium is a long-acting NDA used for protracted surgeries like neurosurgery. Its adverse effects are less because of its lower ganglion-blocking and histamine-releasing potential. However, sometimes, rapid injection may cause vagal block, resulting in tachycardia.

Vecuronium: It has an intermediate duration of action due to rapid distribution and hepatic metabolism. So, postoperative recovery from blockade occurs spontaneously. Hence it is one of the **most commonly-used neuromuscular blockers** for routine surgical procedures and in ICU setting. Histamine-releasing and ganglionic effects are milder than that of d-tubocurarine. Hence, **cardiovascular effects are not troublesome.**

Rocuronium: It has **very fast onset** of action (within 1–2 minutes) and intermediate duration of action. Hence, recovery occurs spontaneously. ADRs are also mild, and therefore it is also commonly used for routine surgeries, in ICU settings, and also as an alternative to succinylcholine for intubations.

Atracurium is an intermediate-acting NDA. In addition to hepatic metabolism, it undergoes Hofmann elimination in the plasma, i.e., spontaneous molecular reorganisation resulting in its inactivation. Hence, it is safe for use in patients with hepatic or renal dysfunction. One of the hepatic metabolites, **laudanosine**, has the ability to cross the blood–brain barrier. This results in central toxic effects in the form of seizures, especially in ICU patients receiving prolonged atracurium infusion.

Cisatracurium: This is a newer intermediate-acting NDA. It is a potent isomer of atracurium with slow onset but the same duration of action. It has negligible hepatic metabolism and hence less laudanosine is formed. Thus, it is devoid of central toxic effects. Its histamine-releasing potential is also very low, and therefore, it is widely used clinically. It is safe for use in the elderly, and in patients with compromised hepatic and renal function.

Mivacurium: It is the shortest-acting NDA with duration of action 15–30 minutes. Reversal of neuromuscular action is not needed. Rapid injection may cause histamine release, resulting in transient flushing and fall in blood pressure. **Gantacurium** is the fastest and shortest-acting NDA in the investigational stage.

Succinylcholine: It is the only drug that causes depolarising blockade. It is the most preferred drug for intubation and other short procedures like bronchoscopy, laryngoscopy, and esophagoscopy.

Clinical problem-based questions and MCQs

9. NMJ blockers used in anesthetic practice as adjuvants to general anesthetics relax skeletal muscles by either preventing or causing depolarisation at the motor end plate. Differentiate between these two types of NMJ blockers.

10. i. Cisatracurium and atracurium both have same duration of action, but for routine surgical procedures, cisatracurium is preferred over atracurium. Explain.
    ii. Succinylcholine is a depolarising agent used for brief procedures. Explain why it should not be mixed with thiopentone sodium in the same syringe.

11. Identify the skeletal muscle relaxant useful in:
    i. Neurosurgery
        a. Dantrolene   b. Pancuronium
        c. Succinylcholine d. same
    ii. Short diagnostic procedures
        a. Pipecuronium   b. Dantrolene
        c. Succinylcholine d. Baclofen
    iii. Justify your choice in both conditions.

---

3. DIRECTLY ACTING MUSCLE RELAXANTS

Drugs included in this group include dantrolene and quinine.

a. Dantrolene
Mechanism of action

Dantrolene interferes with excitation–contraction coupling by blocking **ryanodine receptor1 (RyR1) calcium channels** in the sarcoplasmic reticulum of skeletal muscles, thereby inhibiting the release of activator calcium. As a result, depolarisation gets uncoupled from muscle contraction. Rapidly contracting muscles are more sensitive to the relaxing effect of dantrolene than the slow-contracting, antigravity muscles.

The ryanodine receptor in cardiac and smooth muscles is of a different type (RyR2), which is not susceptible to block by dantrolene. As a result, dantrolene has no relaxing effect on cardiac and smooth muscles.

Therapeutic uses

- Dantrolene is used to relieve the **spasticity associated with UMN lesions**, cerebral palsy, multiple sclerosis, paraplegia, hemiplegia. It is given orally in a dose varying from 25 mg once daily to 100 mg four times a day.
- A very important indication for the use of dantrolene is **malignant hyperthermia**. The condition is characterised by persistent Ca^{2+} release from the sarcoplasmic reticulum in susceptible individuals, typically precipitated by agents such as succinylcholine and fluorinated anesthetics, including halothane. This excessive release of activator calcium causes massive contraction resulting in lactic acidosis and hyperthermia. The treatment involves control of acidosis, body temperature and sarcoplasmic calcium release. Dantrolene, 1 mg/kg body weight, given intravenously is the drug of choice in this condition.
- Dantrolene is effective in the management of **'malignant neuroleptic syndrome'** induced by high doses of potent antipsychotic agents. The syndrome is characterised by marked rigidity, immobility, tremors, hyperthermia, fluctuating BP and pulse. Dantrolene used intravenously and bromocriptine are useful in this condition.

ADRs

- Muscular weakness is a dose-limiting adverse effect.
- Diarrhea may occur.
- Dantrolene may cross the blood–brain barrier, resulting in central side effects like sedation, light headedness, and generalised malaise.
- Long-term use results in hepatic toxicity.

b. Quinine

It is an anti-malarial drug that decreases response to repetitive nerve stimulation by increasing the refractory period of motor end plates.

Therapeutic uses

- Quinine can reduce muscle tone in myotonia congenita.
- A single 300 mg dose at bedtime may help in decreasing nocturnal leg cramps.

ADRs

Quinine is associated with several intolerable adverse effects, including nausea, vomiting, and diarrhea. These are primarily due to its irritant action on the gastric mucosa and stimulation of the chemoreceptor trigger zone (CTZ). Headache, vertigo, confusion, hearing and visual defects, marked muscular weakness and hypoglycemia are some other important adverse effects. Thus, the risks outweigh the benefits with use of quinine.

4. DRUG CAUSING CHEMICAL DENERVATION: BOTULINUM TOXIN

It is a neurotoxin that acts by blocking the release of ACh from the somatic motor nerves by interfering with the fusion of vesicular membrane with that of the nerve terminal. Thus, it results in chemo-denervation and local paralysis.

Uses: Botulinum toxin is given as local facial injection in the treatment of **ageing-associated wrinkles** around the eyes and mouth.

Local injections are useful in general **spastic disorders and dystonias**. A single injection provides relief lasting for several weeks to months. It is approved for **chronic migraine** and **urinary incontinence** due to overactive bladder.

ADRs: Muscular weakness, which may lead to falls is a common **adverse effect**. Fever, respiratory infections and immune reactions may occur. To minimise the risk of immunogenic reactions, repeat injections should be avoided at least for 3 months.

Clinical problem-based questions and MCQs

12. i. Identify the drug causing chemical denervation
    a. Sugammadex   b. Botulinum toxin
    c. Succinylcholine   d. d-Tubocurarine
    ii. Enumerate the therapeutic uses and adverse effects of the chosen drug.

13. i. Select the ryanodine receptor blocker among the following:
    a. Neostigmine   b. Pancuronium
    c. Succinylcholine   d. Dantrolene
    ii. Describe the therapeutic uses and adverse effects of the chosen drug.

14. Quinine is an anti-malarial drug. Comment on its role as a skeletal muscle relaxant.

15. A 50-year-old patient developed hyperthermia and lactic acidosis postoperatively. Halothane was used to anesthetise the patient for the procedure. The patient is diagnosed with malignant hyperthermia and dantrolene is given intravenously.
    i. Explain the pharmacological basis to justify the use of dantrolene in this case.
    ii. Select the correct dose of dantrolene for this indication.
       a. 1 mg/kg body weight
       b. 10 mg/kg body weight
       c. 25 mg OD
       d. 100 mg QID

Summary

Skeletal muscle relaxants can be centrally-, peripherally- or directly acting drugs.
- Centrally acting drugs (spasmolytics) act by
  - Internuncial neuron blockade at (i) the level of brainstem (mephenesin congeners), (ii) by favouring inhibitory neurotransmitters (benzodiazepines), (iii) by inhibiting excitatory neurotransmitters (tizanidine).
  - They are used for muscle spasm due to sprain or overexertion and spasticity of cerebral palsy, multiple sclerosis, amyotrophic lateral sclerosis, spinal cord injuries, etc.
  - Adverse reactions include dizziness, light-headedness, fatigue, weakness, and sedation. Tizanidine causes dryness of mouth, hypotension and dizziness.
- Peripherally acting drugs cause blockade at the level of NMJ. They can be depolarising agents (DA) or non-depolarising agents (NDA).
- DA succinylcholine (SCh) produces dual block.
  - Phase 1 block is due to persistent depolarisation at Nm receptors. It cannot be reversed by neostigmine. Phase 2 block is due to desensitisation of receptors.
  - It is the drug of first choice for brief procedures like bronchoscopy, laryngoscopy, esophagoscopy and intubations because of its short duration of action (5–8 minutes).
  - ADRs occur due to initial twitching, histamine release and K^+ efflux.
  - It may precipitate malignant hyperthermia in genetically predisposed persons receiving fluorinated anesthetics.
  - Prolonged apnea may occur in genetic deficiency of pseudocholinesterase.
- NDAs include long-, intermediate- and short-acting drugs.
  - They cause competitive blockade at Nm receptors; their effect can be reversed postoperatively by neostigmine. Atropine or glycopyrrolate are added to check muscarinic stimulation by excess ACh. Sugammadex is a gamma cyclodextrin, which can form an inactive chelate with vecuronium and rocuronium and reverse their action.
  - Pancuronium is used for long procedures like neurosurgery due to its long duration of action.
  - Intermediate-acting drugs like vecuronium, rocuronium, atracurium and cisatracurium

are most frequently used for routine surgical procedures as adjuvants to general anesthetics and to decrease chest wall resistance in ICU patients.
- ADRs include prolonged respiratory paralysis and apnea, potential for seizures with atracurium due to an active metabolite laudanosine, histamine-release causing flushing, hypotension, and bronchospasm.
• DA dantrolene acts by inhibiting the release of activator calcium from sarcoplasmic reticulum through blockade of ryanodine receptor (RyR1).
- It is useful in the treatment of malignant hyperthermia and spasticity of UMN lesions. It causes muscular weakness and central side effects.

Questions for practice

1. Differentiate between depolarising and non-depolarising NMJ blockers.
2. Describe the mechanism of action of succinylcholine.
3. Enumerate the therapeutic uses and adverse effects of NMJ blockers.
4. Explain why:
    a. Cisatracurium is preferred over atracurium.
    b. NMJ blockers are always administered parenterally.
    c. Atropine/glycopyrrolate and neostigmine are used in decruarisation or reversal of neuromuscular blockade.
    d. SCh causes prolonged apnea in some patients.
    e. SCh should not be mixed with thiopentone in the same syringe.
    f. Dantrolene is used in malignant hyperthermia.
    g. Dantrolene has no effect on smooth and cardiac muscles.
5. What is malignant hyperthermia? Describe its treatment.
6. Write short notes on:
    a. Cisatracurium

b. Hofmann elimination
c. centrally acting muscle relaxants
d. tizanidine
e. baclofen
f. dantrolene

Hints for problem-based questions and MCQs

1. i. a. α_2 receptor agonist
   ii. Refer to page 157.
   iii. Refer to page 157, 158.
2. a–2; b–4; c–1; d–3.
3. a. Methocarbamol
4. i. To reverse effect of NDAs. Refer to page 161.
   ii. Muscarinic excess caused by neostigmine
   iii. Atropine / glycopyrrolate. Refer to page 161.
5. i. Succinylcholine is to be avoided.
   ii. Risk of hyperkalemia. Refer to page 162.
6. i. c. Rocuronium
   ii. Fast onset of action of rocuronium, SCh may cause hyperkalemia
7. c. Fluorinated anesthetic like halothane and isoflurane
8. b. Atracurium. Refer to page 160.
9. Refer to Table 12.1, page 162.
10. i. Refer to page 164.
    ii. They react chemically. Refer to page 163.
11. i. b. Pancuronium
    ii. c. Succinylcholine
    iii. Pancuronium is long-acting; succinylcholine is short-acting.
12. i. b. Botulinum toxin
    ii. Refer to page 165.
13. i. d. Dantrolene
    ii. Refer to page 164.
14. Refer to page 164.
15. i. Refer to page 164.
    ii. a. 1 mg/kg body weight

CONCEPT MAP - SKELETAL MUSCLE RELAXANTS

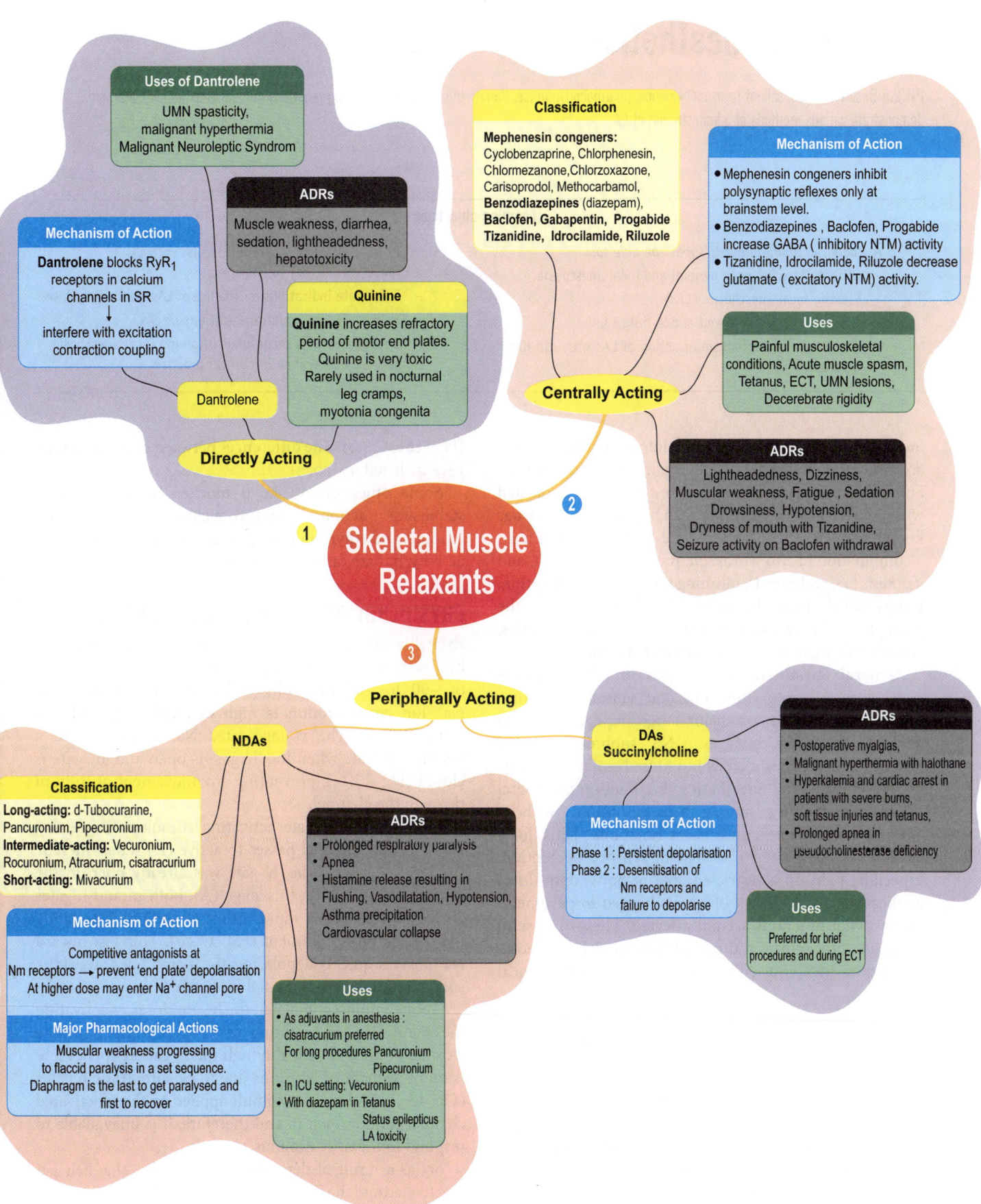

SECTION 2 Drugs Acting on ANS and PNS

13 Local Anesthetics

PH 2.5 Describe types, salient pharmacokinetics, pharmacodynamics, therapeutic uses. adverse drug reactions of local anesthetics (LAs) and demonstrate various methods of administration of LA.

Learning objectives

A student of MBBS phase II should be able to:
- Differentiate between general and local anesthesia.
- Classify local anesthetics (LAs).
- Compare ester-linked and amide-linked LAs.
- Illustrate the mechanism of action of LAs with suitable diagram.
- Explain rationale of combining LA with VC (vasoconstrictor) substances.
- Enumerate indications for the use of LAs mentioning doses.
- Enlist ADRs and contraindications of LAs.
- Describe various techniques of giving local anesthesia and their relevance in clinical practice.

Surgical procedures involve cutting into skin, subcutaneous and other tissues that are richly supplied by sensory nerves. Surgical procedures, therefore, are invariably associated with the sensation of pain. This can be prevented by drugs known as anesthetics. The term anesthetic is derived from a combination of two words: *an*, meaning absence of, and *aesthesis* (a Greek word), meaning sensation or perception. Drugs which have the potential to knock down the perception of sensations temporarily are called anesthetics. Anesthetics are of two types – **general** and **local**.

General anesthetics act at level of CNS, suppress consciousness, motor functions and sensory functions. These are preferred for major surgical procedures. As general anesthesia involves CNS suppression, vital functions need to be carefully monitored and maintained.

In contrast, **local anesthetics (LAs)** act on peripheral nerves, suppressing mainly the sensations, without altering consciousness and motor functions. Thus, local anesthetics cause reversible loss of sensory perception, especially pain, in a restricted area of body, upon local application. As the effect of LAs is limited to peripheral nerves, vital functions are not affected. These are useful in minor procedures and are administered by different techniques involving either topical application or local injections.

CLASSIFICATION OF LOCAL ANESTHETICS

Local anesthetics can be classified based on the method of their administration as surface and injectable anesthetics. Surface anesthetics are further of two types based on their solubility, while injectable anesthetics are divided into three types based on their potency and duration of action. Local anesthetics can also be divided based on their chemical structure into esters and amides (Flowchart 13.1). The differences between ester and amide LAs are listed in Table 13.1.

Some other drugs like β blockers with membrane stabilising action, chlorpromazine, antihistamines, quinine, and ethyl chloride spray also have local anesthetic activity, but are rarely used for this action.

PHYSIOLOGY OF NEURONAL ACTION POTENTIAL

Excitable membranes of nerve axons and neuronal cell bodies maintain a resting membrane potential (RMP) of –90 to –60 millivolts (mV). In the resting state, Na^+ ion concentration is high extracellularly and low intracellularly. The voltage-gated Na^+ channel is in a resting (R) state when the 'h' gate is open and 'm' gate is closed (Fig. 13.1a), preventing any movement of sodium through the channel.

With an appropriate activating stimulus, the resting (R) state Na^+ channel passes to active (A) state, whereby the 'm' gate opens; the 'h' gate was already open in the resting state. Thus, in this stage (A), both m and h gates are open, allowing a rapid influx of sodium ions along the concentration gradient (Fig. 13.1b). This fast inward Na^+ current quickly depolarises the membrane toward the sodium equilibrium potential (+ 40 mV).

About a millisecond later, the h gate closes, inactivating the channel (IA) and shutting off the Na^+ current. So, in the IA state of the channel, although the m gate is open, there is no movement of Na^+ ions due to closure of the h gates (Fig. 13.1c). Additional stimuli applied to the inactivated channel cannot open it, and therefore, it is unavailable to respond to the next stimulus.

So, as a result of depolarisation, the Na^+ channels get inactivated and the K^+ channels open up. The concentration of K^+ is high intracellularly. Hence, the opening of the

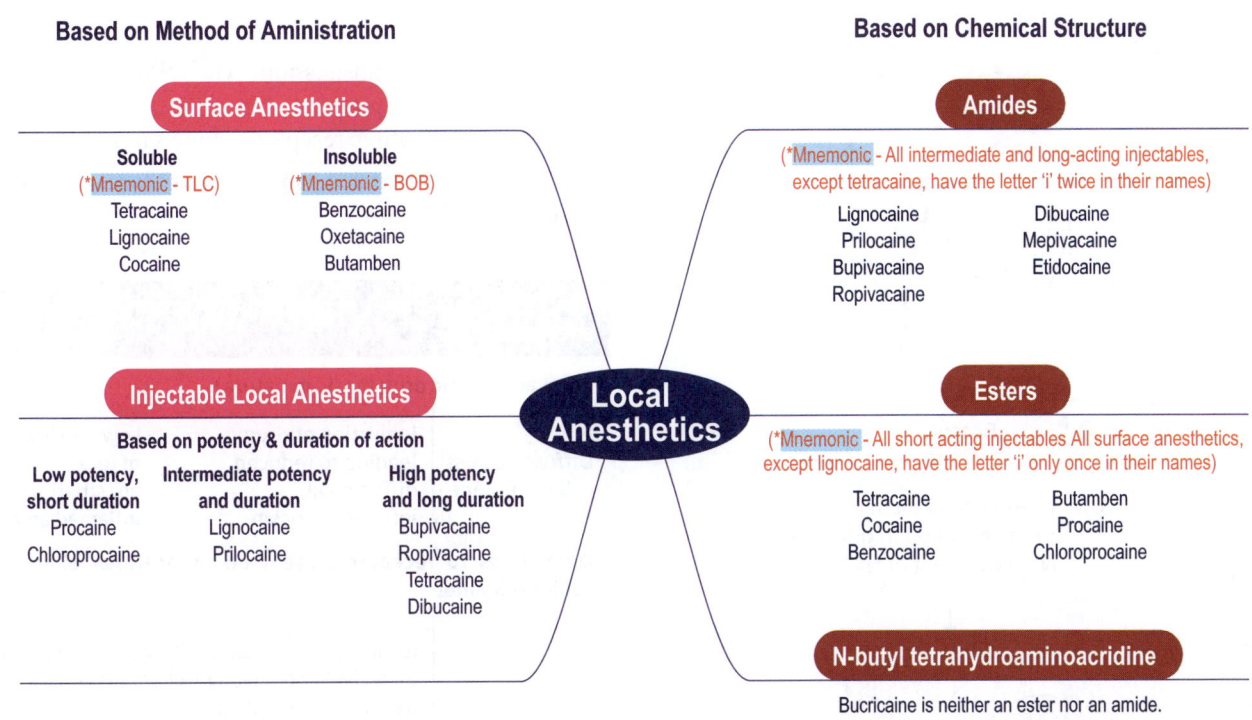

Flowchart 13.1 Classification of local anesthetics

Table 13.1 A comparison of ester and amide LAs

Esters	Amides
Drugs include:	
Benzocaine, cocaine, tetracaine, butamben, procaine, chloroprocaine	Lignocaine, prilocaine, ropivacaine, bupivacaine, dibucaine, etidocaine, mepivacaine, etc.
Pharmacokinetics	
- Metabolised very rapidly by pseudocholinesterase in plasma - Very short half-life	- Bind to α_1 acid glycoprotein in plasma, - Metabolised in liver by CYP450; hence, risk of toxicity in liver disease - Longer half-life
Hypersensitivity reactions	
Common	Rare, no cross-sensitivity with esters

K^+ channels begins an outward flow of K^+ along its concentration gradient, resulting in repolarisation of the membrane towards the potassium equilibrium potential (–95 mV).

As the membrane repolarises, i.e., returns towards RMP, the Na^+ channels also return to the resting (R) state. This is called the 'recovery' of Na^+ channels from the inactive (IA) state to resting (R) state with closed m gate and open h gate. At this stage, the Na^+ channel can respond to the next stimulus.

Mechanism of action of local anesthetics (Fig. 13.1)
Local anesthetic drugs cross the cell membrane, bind to receptors near the intracellular end of the Na^+ channel and slow down recovery of the channel from the IA to R state, i.e., channels remain in IA state for longer times.

The voltage-dependent Na^+ channels are blocked in a time- and voltage-dependent manner. Refractory period is lengthened and generation and conduction of nerve impulse is blocked, leading to membrane-stabilising action. Channels in the 'activated/inactivated' state have a much higher affinity for local anesthetics than channels in the 'resting' state. Such blockade is called "use-dependent blockade". It means that channels that are used more frequently are blocked more effectively by LAs. Therefore, the effect of a given concentration of local anesthetics is more marked in rapidly firing neurons.

Thus, with progressively increasing concentrations of a local anesthetic applied to a nerve fibre, the threshold for excitation increases, slowing down conduction. The rate of rise of action potential and its amplitude decreases. Finally, the nerve fibres lose their ability to generate action potential. These **progressive effects result from the binding of the local anesthetics to more and more of Na^+ channels with increasing concentration.** When the sodium current over a critical length of the nerve gets blocked, propagation of impulse across the blocked area stops.

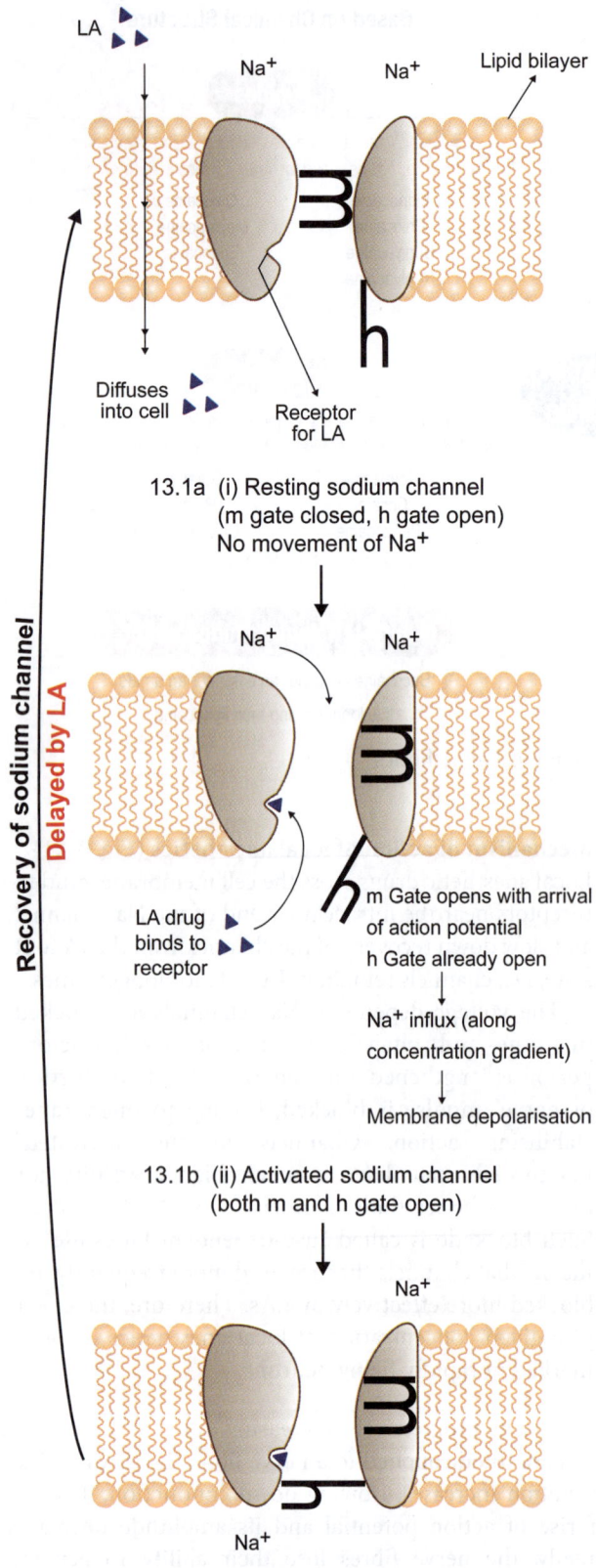

Fig. 13.1 Mechanism of action of local anesthesia

In addition to blockade of Na^+ channels, LAs also cause
- Inhibition of transmission via NMDA, AMPA, neurokinin-1 receptors.
- Blockade of nicotinic receptor channels in spinal cord.

The key features of mechanism of action of local anesthetic are summarised in Box 13.1.

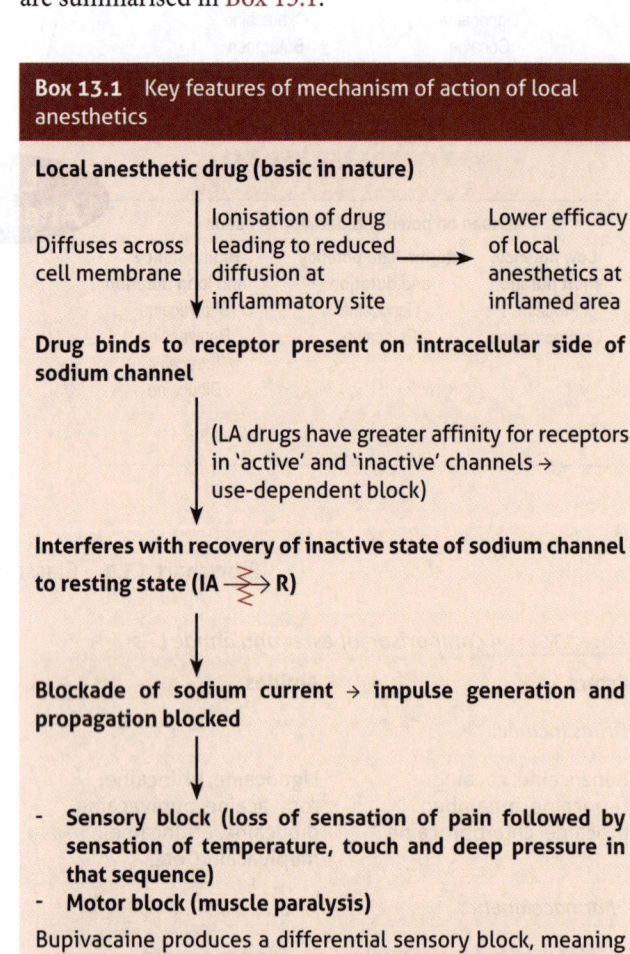

Box 13.1 Key features of mechanism of action of local anesthetics

CLINICALLY RELEVANT PHARMACOKINETICS

Absorption and Distribution

LAs are weak bases that exist in the body in two forms. In the unionised base form, they can rapidly cross the cell membrane and reach intracellular receptor sites.

- Once the drug enters the cell, it becomes ionised into its cationic form due to the lower intracellular pH (around 7.0) compared to the blood pH (7.4). This cationic form is more active at the receptor site and is less likely to diffuse out of the cell.

If the LA is injected at an infected site, where extracellular pH is acidic, more of the basic drug gets ionised. Thus, less of it is able to cross the membrane (as the ionised form is less lipid soluble). In addition, vasodilation and high blood flow at site of inflammation removes the drug quickly. Thus, the efficacy of LA decreases. Therefore, local anesthetics are not effective at the site of inflammation.

- Local anesthetic drugs are usually administered via injection into the area of the nerve fibres to be blocked. Hence, absorption and distribution are not important in determining the onset of their effect. These pharmacokinetic processes rather determine the rate of offset of the anesthesia and the likelihood of central and cardiac toxicity. However, topically applied local anesthetics require absorption for both onset and offset of effect.

Factors affecting systemic absorption of injected local anesthetics

These include dosage, site of injection, drug–tissue binding, presence of vasoconstrictor substances and physicochemical properties of the drug.

- **Site of injection**: Local anesthetic given at highly vascular areas such as tracheal mucosa results in rapid absorption and higher blood levels than if the drug was injected in a poorly vascular area like a tendon.

  For regional anesthesia involving blockade of large nerves, the maximum blood levels of LA required depend on site to be blocked. Highest blood level of LA is required for blocking intercostal nerves followed by caudal, epidural, brachial plexus and sciatic nerve in that order. (Intercostal > caudal > epidural > brachial plexus > sciatic).

- **Drug–tissue binding**: Drugs like bupivacaine become long-acting because of their high tissue binding property. Vasoconstrictors (VCs) are not very effective in prolonging the effects of such tissue bound drugs.

- **Presence of vasoconstrictors**: As LAs are intended for action at the local site of application/ injection, systemic absorption takes the drug away from site of action and reduces its duration of action at the local site. Thus, to prolong the duration of local effect, systemic absorption is decreased by reducing local tissue perfusion. This is achievable by combining LAs with vasoconstrictor substances like adrenaline or phenylephrine. Adrenaline is usually combined with LA in a ratio of 1:80000 and phenylephrine as 1:20000.

  The **benefits/advantages** of combining vasoconstrictors with LAs are as follows.

  - Reduced systemic absorption, with reduced systemic adverse effects.
  - Higher levels of LAs at local site, resulting in enhanced neuronal uptake and prolonged duration of action of LA.
  - Reduced blood loss as vasoconstriction provides a bloodless field for surgery.
  - When used in spinal anesthesia, adrenaline prolongs and enhances effect of LAs. This is due to a α_2-mediated reduction in the release of substance-P and sensory neuron firing. Recognition of this concept has led to the use of α_2-agonists clonidine and dexmedetomidine to produce analgesia and augment the effect of local anesthetics.

  However, there are some **drawbacks/limitations** of combining vasoconstrictors with LAs, such as:
  - Injection becomes more painful.
  - Chances of subsequent local tissue edema, necrosis and delay in wound healing increase.
  - Adrenaline may increase BP and cause arrhythmias in susceptible patients.

  LA combined with a vasopressor is **contraindicated** for use in regions like toes, fingers, pinna of ear and nose, because these locations have terminal arteries that lack anastomosis. Use of vasoconstrictor in such regions may result in irreversible ischemia, necrosis and even gangrene. It is also not suitable for intravenous regional anesthesia (Bier's block). Such combinations should not be used in patients with hypertension, myocardial ischemia and hyperthyroidism.

  In patients suffering from cardiovascular diseases, the use of adrenaline is risky. For such cases, lignocaine is combined with a vasopressin analogue, felypressin.

Lignocaine combined with adrenaline 1: 80,000–1,00,000 (vasoconstrictor)

Advantages

- Prolonged duration of LA action
- Enhanced LA action
- Reduced systemic toxicity
- Reduced blood loss during surgery

Disadvantages

- Injection more painful
- Tissue edema, damage, necrosis
- Delayed healing
- Risk of hypertension and arrhythmias in susceptible persons
- *Contraindicated* in regions with end arteries (e.g., toes, fingers, nose, and pinna for risk of ischemia, necrosis, gangrene) myocardial infarction, hypertension, hyperthyroidism and in IVRA or Bier's block

Clinical problem-based questions and MCQs

1. All surgical procedures involve cutting through tissues that are richly supplied by sensory nerves leading to sensation of pain. This can be prevented by either general or local anesthesia.
   i. Differentiate between general and local anesthesia.
   ii. Classify drugs used as local anesthetics.

2. Most of the local anesthetic agents are esters or amides in nature.
   i. Enumerate the differences between ester- and amide-linked LAs.
   ii. Identify the LA that is neither an ester nor an amide.
      a. Ropivacaine
      b. Benzocaine
      c. Bucricaine
      d. Tetracaine
   iii. What is the advantage of the chosen drug over prototype LA lignocaine?

3. A 45-year-old obese female is diagnosed with chronic cholecystitis with cholelithiasis. She is operated laparoscopically under spinal anesthesia. Lignocaine in combination with adrenaline 1:80000 is injected between L_2–L_3 in the subarachnoid space for anesthesia.
   i. Explain the pharmacological basis of combining adrenaline with lignocaine.
   ii. What are the drawbacks of this combination?
   iii. Name two alternatives of adrenaline for this combination.
   iv. What are the contraindications to use of such a combination?

4. Dexmedetomidine is used in clinical practice to augment the effect of local anesthetics. Explain the pharmacological basis for the same.

PHARMACOLOGICAL ACTIONS

1. Local Actions

Clinically used local anesthetics have no or minimal local irritant action.

- They block the structures like sensory nerve endings, nerve trunks, NMJ, ganglionic synapse or receptors, which function through increased Na^+ permeability.
- They decrease release of acetylcholine (ACh) from motor nerve endings.
- When injected around a mixed nerve, they cause anesthesia of skin and paralysis of voluntary muscles supplied by that nerve.
- Sensory and motor fibres are equally blocked by LAs. Thus, LAs cause sensory loss and exert good analgesic effect in well-defined parts of the body, depending upon the site of administration.

> Local anesthetics first block the sensation of pain, followed by temperature (cold sensation is blocked before heat) → touch → deep pressure and proprioception, in that order.

- Paralysis of the muscles supplied by nerve around which LA is injected is useful during surgery, but sometimes it may interfere with the ability of the patient to follow commands, e.g., bearing down (pushing down by voluntary contraction of abdominal muscles during uterine contraction) during child birth. In such cases, bupivacaine epidural is a better choice because **bupivacaine causes differential sensory block**, i.e., the sensory block occurs earlier, at a lower concentration than motor block. In this situation, the patient is relieved of labour pain due to sensory block, but can effectively bear down due to the absence of motor blockade. Such differential sensory block is also used in postoperative epidural analgesia to achieve pain relief as well as early ambulation after joint replacement surgery.
- Blockade of conduction in autonomic nerves by LAs causes hypotension, impaired respiration and urinary retention.

> **The sensitivity of different type of fibres to blockade by local anesthetics varies**
> - Smaller diameter fibres (types B and C) are more sensitive than larger diameter fibres (type A). Thus, the sequence of blockade by local anesthetics is type B followed by C, Aδ, Aβ, Aγ and Aα.
> - Myelinated fibres are more sensitive than non-myelinated fibres.
> - Autonomic fibres are more sensitive than somatic fibres. Autonomic fibres are blocked at first, followed by sensory fibres and motor fibres, in that order.
> - Recovery occurs in reverse sequence, i.e., motor fibres recover first, followed by sensory and autonomic fibres.

2. Systemic Actions

Any local anesthetic, injected or applied, is ultimately absorbed and can produce systemic effects depending on its concentration.

CNS

All local anesthetics are capable of producing a sequence of stimulation followed by depression. The apparent stimulation seen initially is due to the inhibition of inhibitory neurons. Subsequent depression occurs because all neurons are inhibited at high concentrations.

At high doses, lignocaine can cause numbness—particularly around the mouth (circumoral area) and tongue, along with symptoms such as tinnitus, blurred vision, lethargy, and drowsiness. A very high dose can cause seizures followed by flattening of all EEG waves, inhibition of all neuronal activity and coma.

CVS

Heart: Lignocaine has quinidine-like effects on the heart. It reduces excitability, contractility, and conduction rate at high doses. It reduces the 'effective refractory period'. These effects of lignocaine and procainamide are used in the treatment of ventricular arrhythmias (refer to Chapter 36, page 488).

Bupivacaine has more cardiotoxic effects than other LAs.

Blood vessels: All local anesthetic agents except cocaine cause vasodilatation. Generally, LAs cause hypotension due to sympathetic blockade and arteriolar dilatation. At toxic doses, cardiovascular collapse can occur.

Smooth muscles

Intestinal, bronchial and vascular smooth muscles are relaxed by local anesthetics.

- **Cocaine** is the only exception to the above-mentioned actions of local anesthetics. It is a powerful CNS stimulant that causes euphoria, excitement, confusion, restlessness, tremors, muscle twitching, convulsion, unconsciousness or even death due to respiratory failure in a dose-dependent manner.
- Cocaine interferes with re-uptake of adrenaline and noradrenaline into nerve endings, resulting in vasoconstriction, mydriasis, increased heart rate and blood pressure.
- Cocaine is never used by IV route or with adrenaline.
- It is a drug with potential for abuse and is not used in anesthetic practice nowadays.

Clinical problem-based questions and MCQs

5. Sensory block is the most prominent action of lignocaine. Identify the sensation that is blocked first of all.
   a. Touch
   b. Pain
   c. Temperature
   d. Deep pressure

6. Which of the following is most sensitive to block by local anesthetics?
   a. Larger nerves
   b. Nonmyelinated nerves
   c. Somatic nerves
   d. Autonomic nerves

7. Which of the following local anesthetics is most suitable for painless delivery?
   a. Lignocaine
   b. Bupivacaine
   c. Ropivacaine
   d. Procaine

8. Identify the local anesthetic that causes a rise in blood pressure
   a. Lignocaine
   b. Ropivacaine
   c. Cocaine
   d. Bupivacaine

9. Identify the local anesthetic with powerful central stimulant action
   a. Lignocaine
   b. Ropivacaine
   c. Cocaine
   d. Bupivacaine

THERAPEUTIC USES OF LAS

1. Used in surface/infiltration/conduction block /spinal/epidural/regional anesthesia and analgesia.
2. Lignocaine and procainamide are used in cardiac arrhythmias (refer to Chapter 36).

A. Surface Anesthesia

It involves application of the anesthetic agent on mucous membranes or abraded skin. Sensory loss occurs in superficial layers without any motor paralysis. Fig. 13.2 depicts some of the sites for surface anesthesia and the dosage forms used.

For example,

- Proparacaine and tetracaine eyedrops are used for ocular surgery and tonometry (measuring IOT).
- Lignocaine and tetracaine are used in nasal and ear drops for painful lesions, polyps, etc., in nose and ears.
- Lignocaine and benzocaine lozenges or rinsing solutions are useful for sore throat, painful ulcers in mouth and stomatitis.

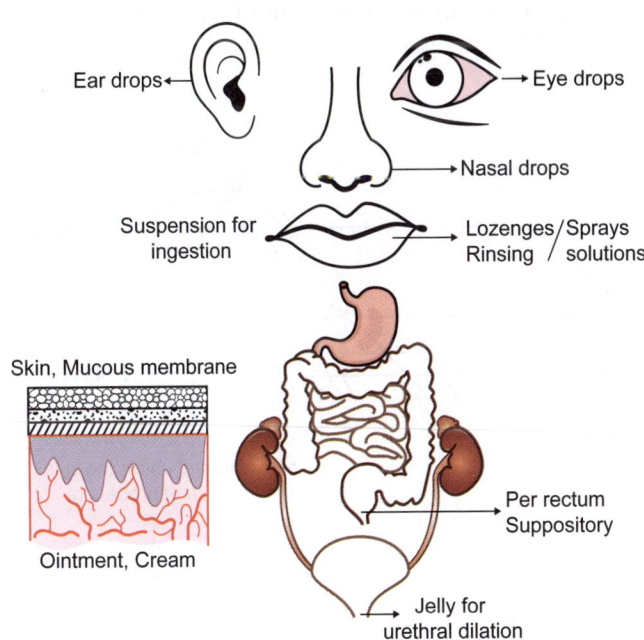

Fig. 13.2 Dosage forms for surface anesthesia

- Lignocaine spray into pharynx, larynx and trachea is used during endotracheal intubation, endoscopy, etc.
- Oxethazaine suspension can relieve symptoms of gastritis and esophagitis.
- Lignocaine jelly is applied in urethra for catheterisation and urethral dilatation.
- Lignocaine or dibucaine cream, ointment, suppository, etc., are applied per rectum for painful piles, fissure in ano and during proctoscopy.
- For ulcers, burns or itchy dermatitis on abraded skin, tetracaine, benzocaine, butamben cream, ointment, dusting powder, etc. are used.

For anesthetising intact skin, a **eutectic mixture of local anesthetics (EMLA)** is effective. This is a mixture of lignocaine and prilocaine in equal proportion (2.5% each), with a lower melting point than either drug alone. Thus, it is in liquid form at room temperature, which allows better skin penetration. It is applied as a cream under occlusive dressing at least an hour before the procedure. Anesthesia of intact skin is needed in procedures like IV cannulation or split-skin graft harvesting surgery.

B. Infiltration Anesthesia

For minor operations like incision, excision, hydrocoele, and herniorrhaphy, when area to be anesthetised is small, a dilute solution of lignocaine/bupivacaine is infiltrated under the skin in the area of operation (Fig. 13.3).

This blocks the sensory nerve endings almost immediately without any effect on muscles, and the action lasts for about 1–3 hours. Adrenaline can be combined with lignocaine in infiltration anesthesia to prolong the duration of anesthesia and check systemic adverse effects.

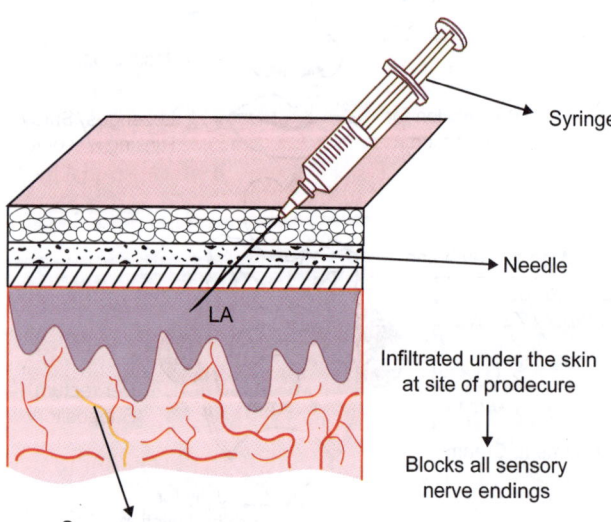

Fig. 13.3 Infiltration anesthesia

C. Conduction Block

This technique involves injection of LA around major nerve trunks, resulting in both sensory and motor blockade in the region distal to the injection site. It can be performed using two approaches:

a. **Field block:** In case of operation on limbs, appendicectomy, hernia repair or dental procedures, local anesthetic is injected subcutaneously such that it blocks all nerves coming to that particular field. A larger area can be anesthetised with lesser drug using this technique, in comparison to infiltration anesthesia.

b. **Nerve block** of the celiac/cervical/ brachial plexus, stellate ganglion and trigeminal/ facial/ lingual/ phrenic/intercostal/ulnar/sciatic/femoral/ilioinguinal/ iliohypogastric nerves can be produced by injecting local anesthetic around anatomically localised nerve trunks or plexuses. A larger area is anesthetised/ paralysed, and the effect of nerve block lasts longer than infiltration or field block using the same amount of drug. This technique is used during surgery on limbs, ribs, abdominal wall, eye and dental procedures.

The most dangerous complication associated with brachial plexus block is pneumothorax.

D. Spinal Anesthesia

This involves injection of local anesthetic in the subarachnoid space in the cauda equina, below the lower end of spinal cord, i.e., between L_2–L_3 in adults or L_4–L_5 in children (because the spinal cord terminates at level of L_1 in adults and L_3 in children). To reach the subarachnoid space, the needle passes sequentially through the skin, subcutaneous tissue, supraspinous ligament, interspinous ligament, ligamentum flavum, dura mater, and arachnoid mater from the outside inward (Fig. 13.4).

Higher segments get exposed to progressively lower concentration of local anesthetic. Spinal anesthesia results in a zone of differential blockade. The autonomic fibres (being most sensitive) are blocked two segments higher than sensory fibres, whereas the motor blockade is two segments lower than the sensory block. The level of anesthesia depends on many factors such as specific gravity of the injected solution, posture of the patient, and volume of drug injected. The nerve roots absorb the drug quickly from the CSF and retain it, leading to a rapid decline in CSF drug concentration after injection. As a result, the level of anesthesia remains unaffected by changes in posture beyond 10 minutes post-administration.

The duration of anesthesia varies from 1–2 hours based on the drug used and its concentration. Anesthetic action can be further augmented and prolonged by addition of adrenaline. Drugs used for spinal anesthesia are lignocaine 1.5–5%, bupivacaine 0.5% and ropivacaine 0.75%.

Chloroprocaine is the shortest-acting local anesthetic. It is contraindicated in spinal anesthesia, because it

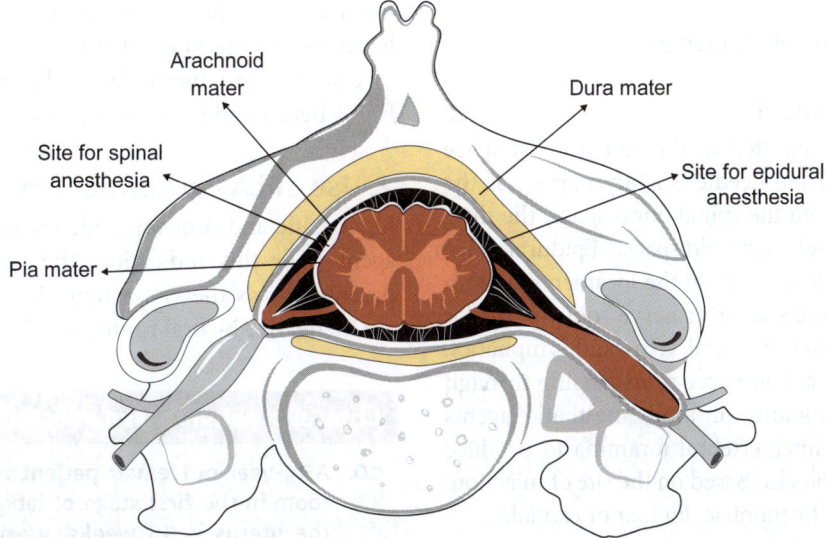

Fig. 13.4 Site of injection for epidural and spinal anesthesia

contains sodium metabisulphite as preservative, which is neurotoxic and can cause paraplegia.

Advantage of spinal anesthesia over GA
- Spinal anesthesia is safer than GA.
- Adequate analgesia and muscle relaxation are achieved without loss of consciousness.
- Comorbid conditions like cardiac, pulmonary and renal diseases are less of a problem during spinal anesthesia than in GA.

Complications of spinal anesthesia
- **Headache** occurs very frequently because of seepage of CSF through the hole in the dura mater. This is labelled as 'post-dural puncture headache' (PDPH). Pain is usually reported in the occipital region after 12–24 hours of spinal anesthesia. It worsens in sitting or standing position. This can be prevented by using small bore needles of 25 gauge. PDPH is managed by maintaining a supine position for 24 hours, ensuring adequate hydration, using abdominal compression to raise venous pressure, and, if needed, sealing the dural puncture site with an epidural blood patch.
- **Pain** and **paresthesia** in lower limbs and back is experienced by some patients for a few days.

> **Hypotension** may result from sympathetic blockade and venous pooling, which reduce venous return to the heart. Paralysis of the skeletal muscles of lower limbs may also contribute to reduced venous return. Prior loading with crystalloids or colloids can help prevent drop in blood pressure. Additionally, measures like administration of sympathomimetic agents such as ephedrine or mephentermine and elevating the foot end of the bed (Trendelenburg position) promote venous return and thereby overcome hypotension.

- **Respiratory paralysis**: If there is paralysis of intercostal and external abdominal muscles, coughing out the sputum becomes less effective and pulmonary complications may occur.

  Respiration is usually maintained by diaphragmatic contractions, even if intercostal muscles are paralysed. Rarely, respiratory failure may occur due to hypotension, which, in turn, results in ischemia of respiratory centre.
- **Urinary retention**, **cranial nerve paralysis** (most common is 6th nerve) **meningitis**, and **arachnoiditis** may occur.
- **Cauda equina syndrome** is a a rare neurological complication resulting from compression of nerves in the lumbar region. The patient develops prolonged loss of control over bowel and bladder sphincters, as well as sensory and motor deficit in one or both lower limbs. This may be because of traumatic damage to nerve roots/chronic arachnoiditis/neurotoxicity of the LA. Treatment is mainly surgical decompression of the nerves to prevent permanent damage. High doses of corticosteroids may relieve symptoms by reducing inflammation. Antibiotic therapy may be useful in infective causes.
- After abdominal operation under spinal anesthesia, patients may have **nausea** and **vomiting** due to reflexes initiated by traction on abdominal viscera.

Contraindications to spinal anesthesia
- Uncooperative, mentally ill patients
- Infants/ children
- Hypotension, hypovolemia, patients in shock
- Kyphosis, lordosis etc.
- Sepsis at injection site
- Septicemia
- Raised intracranial tension..

- Bleeding disorders
- Anticoagulant/thrombolytic therapy

E. Epidural Anesthesia

The local anesthetic is injected in the spinal dural space with a hollow hypodermic needle, slightly curved at the end (Tuohy needle). From the spinal dural space, the drug passes to epidural and subarachnoid spaces. Epidural space is a triangular space extending from the foramen magnum to sacral hiatus. It contains anterior nerve roots, posterior nerve roots, spinal nerves, epidural veins and lymphatics. Local anesthetic agents act on nerve roots passing through these spaces. Small amounts of local anesthetic agents permeate through the intervertebral foramina to produce multiple paravertebral blocks. Based on the site of injection, epidural anesthesia can be thoracic, lumbar or caudal.

- Thoracic epidural injection is used for pain relief after thoracic/ upper abdominal surgeries.
- Lumbar injection has the same indications as spinal anesthesia.
- Caudal injection through sacral hiatus is used in vaginal delivery, operations on genitourinary tract and ano-rectal part of GIT.

Epidural anesthesia, achieved by placing an epidural catheter, is suitable for surgeries of longer duration. PDPH is not a problem as the epidural injection is superficial compared to spinal anesthesia (Fig. 13.4). However, epidural injection is more difficult than spinal anesthesia and therefore it is less reliable.

F. Intravenous Regional Anesthesia (IVRA or Bier's Block)

Local anesthetic injection is administered into a large vein distal to a tourniquet in a tourniquet-occluded limb. The pressure in the tourniquet is kept at 50 mm of Hg above SBP, which allows quick diffusion of the drug in a retrograde manner from the peripheral vascular bed into non-vascular tissues, including nerve endings. The onset of analgesia typically occurs within 3–4 minutes and lasts for 5–10 minutes after deflating the tourniquet.

The tourniquet must not remain inflated for more than one 1 hour to avoid the risk of ischemic tissue damage. This technique is ideal for orthopedic procedures lasting 40–60 minutes, commonly performed on the arm below the elbow or the foot.

At the end of the procedure, the tourniquet should be deflated very gradually over a period of about 15 minutes. Rapid deflation can cause a sudden release of the local anesthetic into systemic circulation, increasing the risk of local anesthetic systemic toxicity (LAST). After deflation, the anesthetic effect typically persists for an additional 5–10 minutes.

Among available agents, prilocaine is preferred for intravenous regional anesthesia (IVRA) due to its high therapeutic index. If prilocaine is unavailable, plain lignocaine (without adrenaline) is a good alternative.

Cocaine and bupivacaine should never be used for IVRA because of their cardiotoxicity.

2. Use of LAs in Cardiac Arrhythmias

Lignocaine and procainamide are used as antiarrhythmic agents. For this indication, they are administered only parenterally as they have high first pass metabolism and are ineffective by oral route (see Chapter 36)

Clinical problem-based questions and MCQs

10. A 24-year-old female patient presents in the labour room in the first stage of labour. On examination, the uterus is 38 weeks, uterine contractions are good and vitals are stable. The fetal heart sounds are normal. Cervix is 2 fingers dilated, soft, effaced. There is no cephalopelvic disproportion or any other indication for LSCS, but the patient insists on painless delivery.
    i. Which of the following is most suitable approach for this case?
        a. Spinal anesthesia
        b. General anesthesia
        c. Epidural anesthesia
        d. Infiltration anesthesia
    ii. Explain the rationale behind your chosen answer.
    iii. Which local anesthetic is most suitable in this situation and why?

11. A 56-year-old male patient underwent herniorrhaphy under spinal anesthesia a month ago. He complains of urinary and bowel incontinence, severe low backache, and numbness in the left leg. MRI shows displacement and compression of spinal nerves.
    i. What is spinal anesthesia?
    ii. What is the cause of the symptoms in the patient? Describe the management of this case.
    iii. Describe the complications and contraindications of spinal anesthesia.

12. Oxethazaine suspension is used as surface anesthetic for
    a. Esophagitis
    b. Nasal polyps
    c. Urinary catheterisation
    d. Burns

13. Which of the following statements is NOT true about conduction block?
    a. LA injection is given around anatomically defined nerves.
    b. Anesthetic effect lasts longer than infiltration anesthesia.
    c. It is the commonly used method for dental procedures.
    d. There is no motor paralysis.

ADVERSE EFFECTS OF LOCAL ANESTHETICS

Local anesthetics possess central, cardiovascular and local adverse effects.

1. Central adverse effects
These include
- Confusion, disorientation
- Light headedness, dizziness
- Visual, auditory disturbances
- Shivering, twitching, tremors, convulsions
- Respiratory depression, coma, death

Central adverse effects can be prevented and treated by diazepam. Cocaine has abuse potential.

2. Cardiovascular Adverse effects
Local anesthetics (except cocaine) can cause bradycardia, hypotension, arrhythmias and cardiovascular collapse. Bupivacaine is the most cardiotoxic local anesthetic, so it is never used for IVRA. It causes slow idioventricular rhythm, characterised by absence of P waves and broad QRS complexes. Ventricular tachycardia may occur. Bretylium is the drug of choice for bupivacaine-induced arrhythmias.

3. Local adverse effects
Local toxicity is low. However, the addition of a vasoconstrictor makes the injection painful, delays wound healing, and may cause local tissue damage and necrosis. This risk is higher in regions having end arteries. So, vasoconstrictor substances should not be added for ring block of hands, feet, finger, toes, pinna, etc. Local tissue irritancy is highest with bupivacaine.

4. **Hypersensitivity reactions:** like rashes, angioedema dermatitis and asthma are more common with ester LAs than amides. Rarely, anaphylaxis may occur.
5. Lignocaine can precipitate **malignant hyperthermia** in susceptible individuals by causing excess calcium release. Procaine is the local anesthetic of choice in such patients.
6. A metabolite of prilocaine (O-toluidine) oxidises hemoglobin to cause **methemoglobinemia**. Lignocaine and benzocaine also have the potential to cause methemoglobinemia.
7. The most potent, longest-acting and most toxic local anesthetic agent is dibucaine.
8. **Local anesthetic systemic toxicity (LAST)** is a life-threatening emergency seen in 0.03% cases of peripheral nerve blocks with local anesthetic agents. It usually occurs immediately after the injection of local anesthetic. The risk of severe systemic toxicity with local anesthetic agents is high at extremes of ages, in pregnancy, and in patients with cardiac, hepatic and renal function impairment. The risk also increases when the LA injection is given at sites of high vascularity and the dose is near the maximal dose. Most cases of LAST are reported from patients undergoing infiltration anesthesia, followed by epidural/caudal central neuraxial blocks and continuous infusion.

Initially, patients usually present with features of CNS stimulation like increased sensations, muscular activation, agitation, confusion and convulsions. Diverse symptoms like perioral paresthesia, audio-visual and taste disturbances, conduction defects, arrhythmias, and myocardial dysfunction are reported. More severe cases develop CNS depression resulting in impaired consciousness, coma, respiratory arrest and asystole.

Management of LA toxicity: This involves immediately stopping the injection of local anesthetic drug, maintenance of airway, breathing and circulation. Acidosis is corrected by $NaHCO_3$ administration. Intravenous lipid emulsion therapy is constituted early, immediately after securing the airway. Lipid emulsion shuttles local anesthetic agent a from highly vascular organs to storage organs like muscle, liver, and adipose tissue. Thus, vascular organs like the heart and brain get detoxified.

20% Intravenous lipid emulsion is administered at the first sign of toxicity.

To control the seizures, benzodiazepines are the drugs of choice. In uncontrolled seizures, succinylcholine or propofol can be used. Cardiac arrhythmias caused by LAs are managed using amiodarone or bretylium.

SALIENT FEATURES OF INDIVIDUAL LAs

Procaine was the first LA to be introduced. It is an ester-type anesthetic that is metabolised rapidly by pseudocholinesterase. It has delayed onset, low potency and short duration of action. Therefore, it is not a preferred agent except in case of infiltration anesthesia for short diagnostic procedures. **Chloroprocaine** has faster onset of action than procaine.

Lignocaine is the prototype amide LA agent. It has intermediate potency, intermediate duration of action and is the most widely used agent for local anesthesia. Vasoconstrictor substances are added to decrease the rate of its systemic absorption. It is also used in ventricular arrhythmias by IV route. Lignocaine nebulisation may provide symptomatic relief in intractable cough, as in bronchogenic carcinoma.

Prilocaine has similar potency and duration of action as lignocaine, but can be used without vasoconstrictor substances. It has the potential to cause methemoglobinemia, especially in neonates.

Bupivacaine has longer duration of action and is preferred over lignocaine in conditions requiring prolonged effect, such as during labour and to control post-operative pain.

Etidocaine has greater effect on motor nerves than bupivacaine, and is hence preferred over bupivacaine in surgeries requiring good muscle relaxation.

Mepivacaine is safer than lignocaine in adults though toxicity is high in neonates.

Bupivacaine and etidocaine are more cardiotoxic than lignocaine, whereas **levobupivacaine** and **ropivacaine** are less cardiotoxic than lignocaine.

Bucricaine is a drug of Indian origin. It is neither an ester, nor an amide in nature; it is N-butyl tetrahydroaminoacridine. It has longer duration of action than lignocaine and some inherent vasopressor activity. Hence, there is no need to combine vasopressor substances like adrenaline with bucricaine. Its central and cardiovascular adverse effects are less than lignocaine. It is suitable for use in patients showing hypersensitivity reactions with lignocaine and other amides.

Dibucaine is very toxic. **Benzocaine** is poorly absorbed and therefore its effect as a surface anesthetic lasts longer. Both these drugs are used only for surface anesthesia.

Oxetacaine (also known as **oxethazaine**) has a low pKa in comparison to other local anesthetic agents. Thus, it remains unionised in the acidic pH of stomach and can penetrate gastric mucosa and exert local anesthetic action in acidic medium. It is used orally for local action on gastric mucosa in patients with esophagitis and drug-induced gastritis.

Tetracaine and **proparacaine** are non-irritant, and thus useful for ocular anesthesia.

Clinical problem-based questions and MCQs

14. A 34-year-old male patient suffering from peptic ulcer disease complains of nausea, belching, pain in epigastrium and bloating sensation. Which of the following local anesthetic agents is used orally for local action on gastric mucosa?
    a. Bupivacaine
    b. Mepivacaine
    c. Oxetacaine
    d. Tetracaine

15. A 62-year-old male patient having corneal ulcers complains of disabling pain and irritation in his right eye.
    i. Which drug is the most suitable ocular anesthetic for this case?
        a. Bupivacaine
        b. Mepivacaine
        c. Oxetacaine
        d. Tetracaine
    ii. Why is the selected LA preferred over others for ocular anesthesia?

16. i. What is EMLA?
    ii. What is indication for use of EMLA?

17. i. Which of the following drugs is LEAST cardiotoxic?
        a. Lignocaine
        b. Bupivacaine
        c. Etidocaine
        d. Ropivacaine
    ii. Describe the cardiovascular adverse effects of local anesthetics.

18. All of the following measures are used for controlling LA systemic toxicity EXCEPT,
    a. Intravenous lipid emulsion for shuttling effect
    b. Injection NaHCO$_3$ to correct acidosis
    c. Injection diazepam for control of convulsions
    d. Injection verapamil for correcting cardiac rhythm disturbances

Summary

- **Local anesthetics** (LA) – the prototype LA is lignocaine.
- Drugs causing reversible loss of sensory perceptions on local application cause blockade of conduction through peripheral nerves. Consciousness /vital functions not affected → **safer as compared to general anesthesia**.
- **Classified** based on their chemical nature into esters and amides. Esters are short-acting and have higher risk of hypersensitivity reactions compared to amides.
- Can be low potency–short duration of action; intermediate potency– intermediate duration of action; and high potency–long duration of action.
- Can be given as surface anesthetics or injectables.
- **Act by delaying recovery of sodium channels from inactive to resting stage** → use-dependent blockade of sodium channels, resulting in blockade of generation and conduction of nerve impulses.
- **Actions:** Sensory and motor fibres equally sensitive to all LAs except **bupivacaine which cause differential sensory block** → useful for epidural analgesia in painless vaginal delivery and post operatively after joint replacement surgery.
- Sensitivity of smaller, autonomic and non-myelinated fibres > larger, somatic and myelinated fibres, respectively.
- All LAs cause CNS stimulation followed by depression, **except cocaine, a powerful CNS stimulant and drug of abuse.**
- Cardiovascular effects include bradycardia, hypotension and cardiovascular collapse at high doses, except **cocaine, which causes rise in pulse rate and BP.**
- **Combination of lignocaine with vasoconstrictors** like adrenaline and phenylephrine prolongs the duration of action, lowers toxicity, reduces blood loss in surgery but not suitable for sites having end arteries like fingers and toes.
- LA is **not effective when given at infected/ inflamed site**, as extracellular pH is acidic → more of the basic drug gets ionised → less is able to cross membrane.

- **Different techniques** are suitable for different indications like spinal, epidural, infiltration and nerve block anesthesia.
- **Spinal anesthesia** involves injection into subarachnoid space between L_2–L_3 or L_3–L_4 → achieves good analgesia and muscular relaxation without affecting consciousness → useful for surgeries of lower limbs, pelvis, lower abdomen, prostate and obstetric procedures.
- For procedures requiring voluntary muscular activity, such as bearing down during vaginal delivery, **epidural anesthesia** with caudal injection is useful. Bupivacaine has more effect on sensory fibres than motor fibres and is suitable for patients desiring painless delivery.
- **Infiltration anesthesia** involves injection of dilute solution under the skin for minor operations.
- **Conduction block** involves injection of LA agent around nerve trunks It can be given as field block or nerve block
- **Adverse effects** include dizziness, light-headedness, disorientation, visual or auditory disturbances, hypotension, bradycardia, rhythm disturbances, and respiratory depression. Hypersensitivity reactions are common with esters.
- In cases of lignocaine allergy, bucricaine, a non-ester, non-amide agent is useful.

Questions for practice

1. Describe the mechanism of action of lignocaine with the help of a suitable diagram.
2. What is spinal anesthesia? What are its advantages and complications? Enumerate conditions in which spinal anesthesia cannot be given.
3. Explain why:
   a. Adrenaline is combined with lignocaine.
   b. Cocaine is not preferred as LA.
   c. LA fail to provide good analgesia in inflamed tissues.
   d. Bupivacaine is preferred in obstetric analgesia.
4. Write short notes on:
   a. Infiltration anesthesia
   b. Conduction block
   c. Epidural analgesia

Solutions for problem-based questions and MCQs

1. i. Refer to page 168.
   ii. Refer to page 169.
2. i. Referto page 169.
   ii. c. Bucricaine is N-butyl tetrahydroaminoacridine.
   iii. Bucricaine is longer acting than lignocaine. Refer to Flowchart 13.1, page 169.
3. i. Refer to page 171.
   ii. Refer page 171.
   iii. Phenylephrine, Felypressin
   iv. Refer to page 171.
4. The α2-mediated decrease in release of Substance P and sensory neuron firing results in analgesia that augments the effect of local anesthetics. Refer to page 171.
5. b. Pain sensation is blocked first of all.
6. d. Autonomic nerves
7. b. Bupivacaine
8. c. Cocaine
9. c. Cocaine
10. i. c. Epidural anesthesia
    ii. In spinal as well as general anesthesia, the patient will not be able to bear down because of motor block. Infiltration anesthesia is suitable for minor operation. In epidural anesthesia, pain sensation is blocked but motor activity persists. So, the patient is able to follow instructions, such as bearing down, to assist in a normal vaginal delivery.
    iii. Bupivacaine causes sensory block earlier, at lower concentrations than motor block → Relief of labour pain but effective bearing down is possible.
11. i. Refer to page 174.
    ii. This patient has developed symptoms suggestive of cauda equina syndrome. Refer to page 175.
    iii. Refer to page 175.
12. a. Esophagitis
13. d. There is no motor paralysis
14. c. Oxetacaine
15. i. d. Tetracaine
    ii. Non-irritant → Thus useful for ocular anesthesia
16. i. EMLA is eutectic mixture of local anesthetics (EMLA). Refer to page 174.
    ii. Refer to page 174
17. i. d. Ropivacaine is less cardiotoxic than lignocaine, whereas bupivacaine and etidocaine are more cardiotoxic than lignocaine.
    ii. Refer to page 176.
18. d. Injection verapamil for correcting cardiac rhythm disturbances.

CONCEPT MAP - LOCAL ANESTHETICS

Classification

Surface Anesthetics
- **Soluble:** Tetracaine, Lignocaine, Cocaine
- **Insoluble:** Benzocaine, Oxetacaine, Butamben

Injectables
- **Short-acting:** Procaine, Chloroprocaine
- **Intermediate:** Lignocaine, Prilocaine
- **Long-acting:** Bupivacaine, Ropivacaine, Tetracaine, Dibucaine

	Esters	Amides
Drugs	Benzocaine, Cocaine, Tetracaine, Butamben, Procaine, Chloroprocaine	Lignocaine, Prilocaine, Ropivacaine, Bupivacaine
Metabolism	In plasma by pseudocholinesterase	In liver by CYP450
Half-Life	Very short	Longer
Hypersensitivity Reactions	Common	Rare

Mechanism of Action

Use-dependent blockade of Na^+ channels
Delays recovery of Na^+ channel from IA to R stage

Major Pharmacological Actions

Equally block motor and sensory nerves.
Loss of sensations: Pain → Temperature → Touch → Deep Pressure.
CNS stimulation → Depression.
Hypotension, Urine retention, Impaired respiration, Smooth muscle relaxation.
Lignocaine: Class I_b antiarrhythmic action.

Bupivacaine: Differential block: Preferred in epidural analgesia and painless delivery.

LOCAL ANESTHETICS

LAST
Perioral numbness, Agitation, Confusion, Seizures, Coma, Hypotension and Arrhythmias
Treatment
Supportive, $NaHCO_3$, Lipid emulsion IV

Techniques of LA

- **Surface:** On abraded skin, Mucous membranes (Eutectic mixture on intact skin)
- **Infiltration:** Injection under the skin
- **Conduction Block:** Field block, Nerve block
- **Intravenous regional injection:** Bier's block
- **Epidural:** Injection in spinal dural space in thoracic/lumbar/caudal area
- **Spinal Anesthesia:** Injection in subarachnoid space in cauda equina

Combination of LA + VC

Advantages
Prolonged duration of LA action
Enhanced LA action
Reduced systemic toxicity
Reduced blood loss during surgery

Disadvantages
Injection more painful
Tissue edema, damage, necrosis
Delayed healing
Risk of hypertension & arrhythmias

Contraindicated in regions with end arteries (eg., toes, fingers, nose, pinna for risk of ischemia, necrosis, gangrene)

Spinal Anesthesia

Advantages Over GA	Complications
Safer	Headache
No loss of consciousness	Pain, paresthesia in lower limbs and back
Fewer problems in patients with Comorbidities	Respiratory paralysis → pulmonary complications
	Hypotension
	Cauda equina syndrome

SECTION 3   Drugs Acting on CNS

14   General Anesthetics

PH 3.1 Describe types, salient pharmacokinetics, pharmacodynamics, therapeutic uses and ADRs of general anesthetics and pre-anesthetic medications.

Learning objectives

A student of MBBS phase II should be able to:
- Describe the concept of balanced anesthesia.
- Classify general anesthetics.
- Describe the characteristics of various stages of general anesthesia.
- Describe factors that determine the rate of induction and recovery from general anesthesia; describe minimal alveolar concentration.
- Explain the mechanism of action and pharmacological actions of general anesthetics.
- Enumerate indications, adverse effects and contraindications of general anesthetics.
- Describe the aim of pre-anesthetic medication (PAM).
- Enumerate the drugs used for pre-anesthetic medication.

BALANCED ANESTHESIA

The state of general anesthesia is characterised by:

- Analgesia
- Amnesia
- Inhibition of autonomic reflexes
- Inhibition of sensory reflexes
- Skeletal muscle relaxation
- Loss of consciousness.

These effects are produced to different extents by different anesthetic agents. Characteristic features of an ideal anesthetic agent are listed in Box 14.1.

Box 14.1   Characteristics of an ideal anesthetic agent

- Rapid and smooth induction (loss of consciousness)
- Prompt recovery when stopped
- Should be potent enough so that oxygenation is not compromised
- Has a wide margin of safety, i.e., a wide gap between doses producing therapeutic and adverse effects
- Has negligible adverse effects
- Should provide adequate analgesia, muscle relaxation and immobility
- Should be non-explosive and non-inflammable to allow the use of electrocautery

A wide variety of general anesthetics is available, administered either intravenously or through the inhalational route. However, none of these drugs possess all the properties of an ideal anesthetic agent. Xenon, a colourless and odourless noble (inert) gas with fast onset and recovery is considered very close to an ideal anesthetic agent. Unfortunately, it is scarcely available, and is very expensive for routine use. Among other available anesthetic agents, some have rapid onset of action but are associated with more adverse effects; other agents are safe but have a slower onset. Therefore, in clinical practice, different drugs are combined strategically to maximise their beneficial effects while minimising adverse reactions. This yields what is called **balanced/multimodal anesthesia**. *Loss of consciousness, analgesia, muscle relaxation and abolition of compensatory reflex responses* are the key features of balanced anesthesia.

The **choice of drugs** for balanced anesthesia depends on the type of procedure being performed (Fig. 14.1).

1. Monitored Anesthesia Care (MAC)

For **minor surgical or diagnostic procedures**, sedation combined with local anesthesia is usually sufficient. This approach is known as **monitored anesthesia care (MAC)**, where profound analgesia is achieved without loss of consciousness. The patient remains responsive to verbal commands and is able to maintain patent airways, spontaneous breathing and airway reflexes. There is no need for tracheal intubation. This technique of 'monitored anesthesia care' typically involves

- Pre-anesthetic medication with IV midazolam, followed by
- Propofol infusion for moderate-to-deep sedation, and
- Opioid or ketamine to reduce pain/discomfort associated with the local anesthetic injection and surgical procedures.
- MAC involves lesser physiological disturbances than GA, and the recovery is faster.

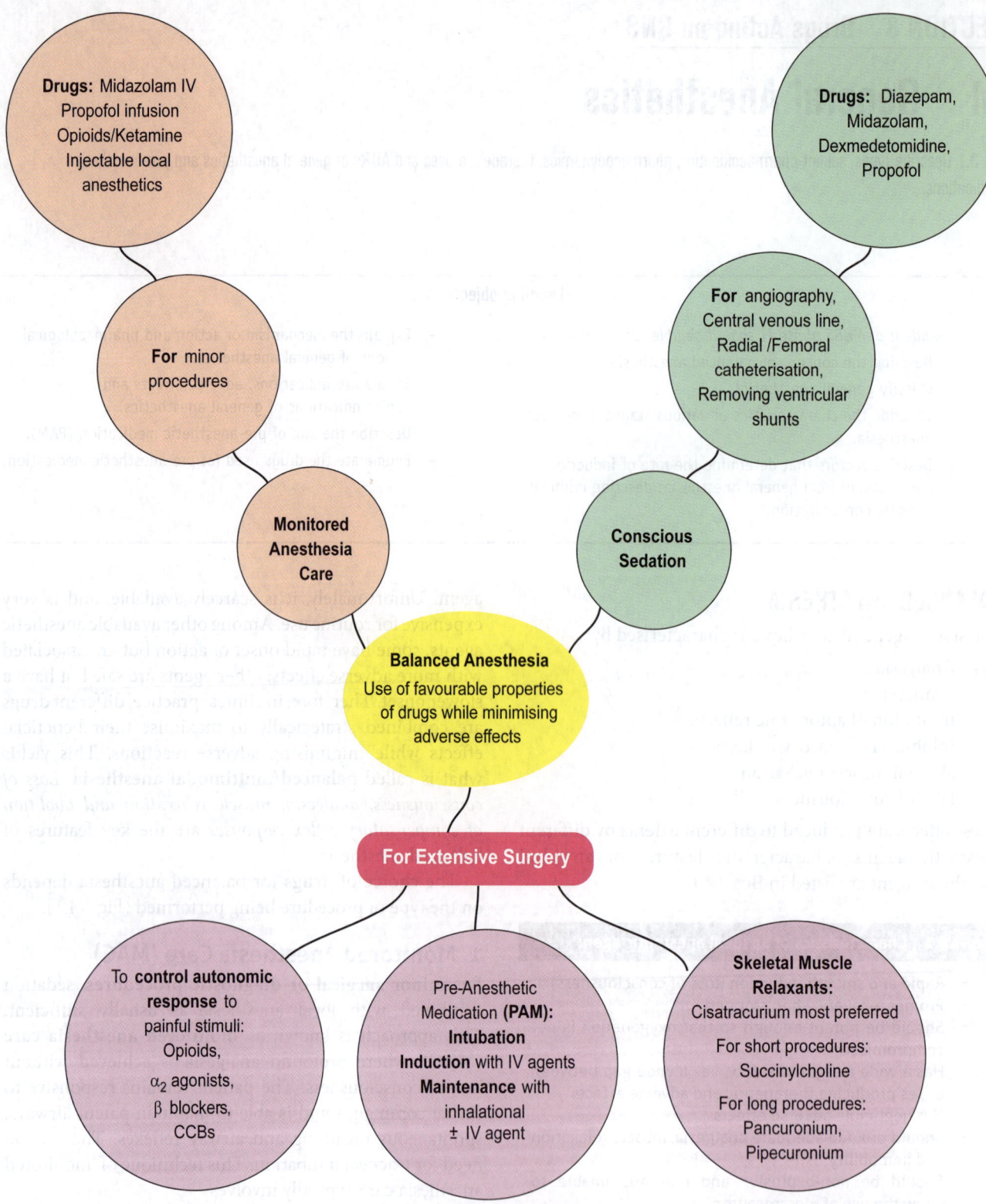

Fig. 14.1 Balanced anesthesia

2. Conscious Sedation

This usually involves administration of drugs to decrease anxiety or pain. Consciousness is altered, but the patient is able to respond to verbal commands. The commonly used drugs include diazepam, midazolam, propofol, and dexmedetomidine. This technique is useful in angiography, placement of central venous line, radial/femoral artery catheterisation, removal of ventricular shunts, etc.

3. Anesthesia for More Extensive Surgical Procedures

a. For more extensive surgical procedures, pre-anesthetic medication is given, followed by induction of general anesthesia, usually with IV anesthetics. Thereafter, anesthesia is maintained for the duration of procedure with inhalational agents alone or in combination with IV drugs. The patient is unconscious and thus unable to respond to commands. Intubation is needed to maintain airway patency.
b. **Skeletal muscle relaxants** The use of skeletal muscle relaxants to facilitate tracheal intubation and orthopedic procedures is an example of balanced anesthesia.
c. **Perioperative analgesia** Before, during, and after surgery, local anesthetics are administered via peripheral nerve blocks or tissue infiltration to manage the associated pain.
d. **Transient autonomic response control** To control transient autonomic responses to painful stimuli during the procedure, opioid analgesics, α$_2$ agonist, β blockers, calcium channel blockers, and other agents may be used, tailored to the individual needs of each patient.

CLASSIFICATION OF GENERAL ANESTHETICS

General anesthetics are divided into **two broad classes** based on the route of their administration: **inhalational** and **intravenous** anesthetics. Inhalational agents include gases and volatile liquids. Intravenous agents are classified based on their onset of action into fast-acting and slow-acting drugs (Flowchart 14.1).

STAGES OF INCREASING DEPTH OF ANESTHESIA

There are four stages of increasing depth of anesthesia, reflecting progressive central nervous system (CNS) depression, as originally described with the traditional, slow-induction agent diethyl ether. The characteristic features of each stage are outlined in Table 14.1. However, in modern anesthetic practice, the clear demarcation between these stages has become obscured due to:

- The introduction and widespread use of anesthetic agents with a rapid onset of action, leading to the merging of clinical signs across different stages.
- Controlled ventilation during induction, which accelerates anesthesia and obscures respiratory signs.
- Administration of pre-anesthetic medications such as opioids and skeletal muscle relaxants, which interfere with stage-specific clinical assessments.

The aim of monitoring the depth of anesthesia is to **reach stage III Plane 1,** i.e., the stage of surgical anesthesia, and **maintain this stage** till the completion of the procedure, without further progression into stage IV of medullary depression. The most reliable indicators of the attainment of stage of surgical anesthesia are **re-establishment of regular respiration** and **loss of purposeful motor and autonomic responses** to specific surgical stimuli. In addition, monitoring of vital signs, automated cerebral monitoring techniques using computer-assisted EEG-derived indices such as bispectral index (BIS), auditory evoked potential (AEP), cerebral state index (CSI), and physical state index (PSI) are used to assess the depth of anesthesia.

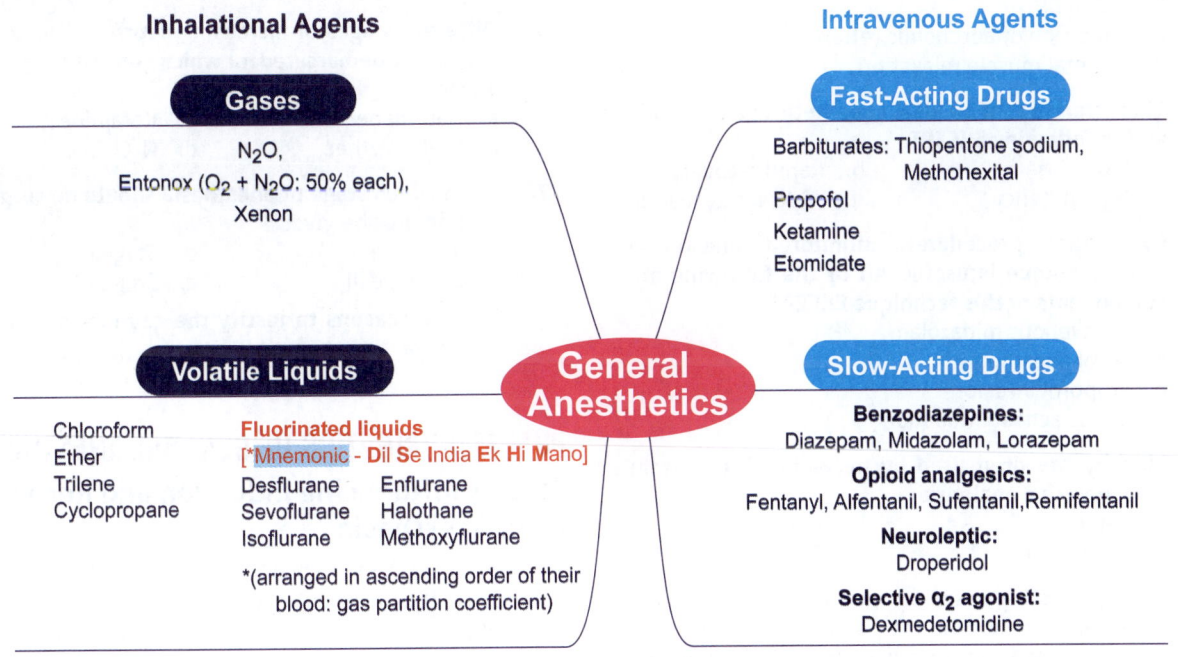

Flowchart 14.1 Classification of general anesthetics

Table 14.1 Stages of anesthesia

Stage of anesthesia	Features	Clinical importance
I Stage of analgesia	- Patient is conscious, responds to verbal commands but amnesia occurs. - Pain is abolished. - Respiration is normal.	Minor procedures, incision and drainage, etc., can be done in this stage.
II Stage of excitement or delirium	- Patient shows features of excitement, may struggle and hold breath. - Muscle tone increases. - Respiration is irregular. - BP and HR increase and pupils dilate because of sympathetic stimulation.	Surgeon must wait for this stage to end; no surgical stimulus should be given at this stage.
III Stage of surgical anesthesia	- Breathing is regular in stage III. However, as the depth of anesthesia increases, respiration rate and depth decreases. - Slowly, the muscle tone decreases. - Pulse is fast but weak. - BP decreases. Stage III is further divided into the following four planes: **Plane 1** - Eyeballs are moving **Plane 2** - Corneal and laryngeal reflexes are lost **Plane 3** - Light reflex is lost and pupil starts dilating **Plane 4** - Pupil is dilated, respiration is abdominal as intercostals paralysis occurs	Most surgeries are done in plane 1 of stage III. Reaching deeper planes is not attempted in modern practice.
IV Stage of medullary depression	- Breathing stops - Failure of circulation - Muscles paralysed - Pulse imperceptible - Pupils dilated - Death	

Clinical problem-based questions and MCQs

1. All of the following are characteristic features of 'balanced anesthesia' EXCEPT:
   a. Analgesia
   b. Fall in BP
   c. Inhibition of autonomic reflexes
   d. Skeletal muscle relaxation

2. Characteristics of an ideal anesthetic agent include all the following EXCEPT:
   a. Slow onset
   b. Rapid recovery
   c. High potency
   d. Wide safety margin

3. For minor procedures, monitored anesthesia care technique is useful. All of the following are components of this technique EXCEPT:
   a. Intravenous midazolam
   b. Local anesthesia
   c. Propofol infusion
   d. Endotracheal intubation

4. Identify the drug used by nerve block to obtain perioperative analgesia.
   a. Ketamine
   b. Propofol
   c. Lignocaine
   d. Thiopentone

5. A 45-year-old patient complains of sudden chest pain. On examination, the patient is anxious, pale and distressed due to severe pain. ECG shows ST elevation. The patient is given GTN sublingual and sent for angiography. Which of the following drugs is suitable for 'conscious sedation' for relief of fear and anxiety associated with the disease and procedure?
   a. Thiopentone
   b. Halothane
   c. Nitrous oxide
   d. Dexmedetomidine

6. Different stages of increasing depth of anesthesia are clearly demarcated for which general anesthetic agent?
   a. Halothane
   b. Ketamine
   c. Diethyl ether
   d. N_2O

7. i. In which stage of anesthesia should no surgical stimulus be given?
   a. Stage I
   b. Stage II
   c. Stage III
   d. Stage IV
   ii. Give reasons to justify the caution mentioned above.

PHARMACOKINETICS OF GENERAL ANESTHETICS

Factors Influencing Induction and Recovery from Anesthesia

The rate of onset of anesthesia (Fig. 14.2) depends upon how rapidly the therapeutic concentration is reached in the CNS, which, in turn, depends upon the following factors:

a. Concentration of inhaled anesthetic in inspired mixture of gases, known as **partial pressure**: The higher the partial pressure of anesthetic in the inspired gas mixture,

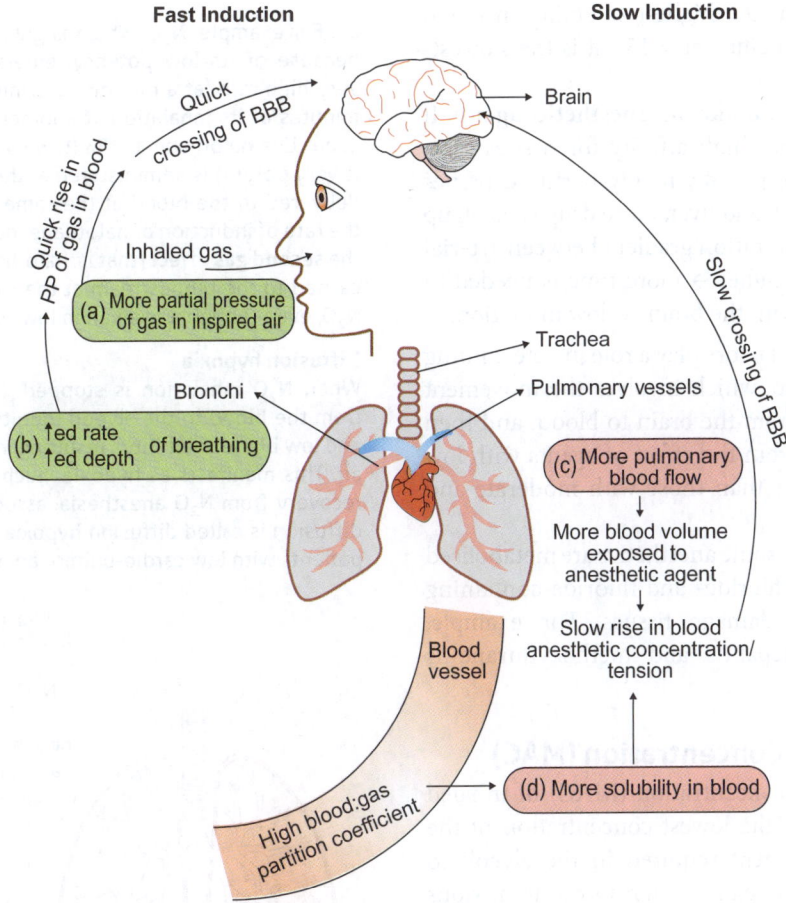

Fig. 14.2 Pharmacokinetic factors affecting the induction of anesthesia

the faster is the rate of transfer of the drug into the blood and then the brain, resulting in an increase in the rate of induction. This is why certain inhaled anesthetics, such as isoflurane (which have moderate blood solubility), are initially administered at higher concentrations (around 1.5%) to achieve rapid induction, and subsequently reduced to 0.75–1% for maintenance.

b. A **higher rate and depth of ventilation** increases the rate of induction with agents which normally have a slow onset like isoflurane and halothane.

c. **Pulmonary blood flow:** If the pulmonary blood flow is increased, a larger volume of blood gets exposed to the anesthetic agent present in the alveoli. Thus, anesthetic tension in blood will rise slowly, reducing the rate of induction. In contrast, **induction rate is high in patients having circulatory shock** due to reduced cardiac output leading to reduced pulmonary blood flow and hyperventilation.

d. **Blood solubility of inhaled anesthetics,** represented by the **blood:gas partition coefficient,** is the relative affinity of a drug for blood as compared to inspired gas. It is the **most important factor** determining the rate of movement of the anesthetic agent from the lungs to blood, then to the brain (during induction) and back in the reverse direction (during recovery).

There is an **inverse relationship** between the **blood solubility** of an anesthetic agent and the **rate of rise of its tension (partial pressure) in arterial blood**. Anesthetics with low blood solubility (low blood:gas partition coefficient) achieve a rapid increase in arterial partial pressure with fewer molecules. Consequently, these anesthetic agents induce anesthesia more quickly than those with high blood solubility. Xenon, with the lowest blood solubility (blood:gas partition coefficient = 0.115), is the fastest-acting anesthetic.

Volatile liquid anesthetics arranged in order of increasing solubility in the blood are: **desflurane, sevoflurane, isoflurane, enflurane, halothane and methoxyflurane** [Mnemonic: Dil Se India Ek Hi Mano]. The blood solubility of gaseous anesthetic agent nitrous oxide is also low. So, the **onset of anesthesia is quick with agents having low solubility in blood,** like desflurane, nitrous oxide and sevoflurane (blood:gas partition coefficients of 0.42, 0.47, and 0.69, respectively).

To increase the rate of induction by agents that have moderate solubility (isoflurane, enflurane, halothane), they are commonly combined with less soluble agents like nitrous oxide.

Methoxyflurane has the highest solubility in blood (blood:gas partition coefficient = 15); it is the slowest-acting agent.

e. **Tissue solubility or uptake of anesthetic agent**: If an anesthetic agent has high affinity for tissues (e.g., volatile anesthetics), especially highly-perfused tissues such as the brain, heart, and liver, more drug is taken up by the tissues → concentration gradient between arterial and venous blood is higher → more time is needed to achieve equilibrium with the brain → slow induction.

All the above-mentioned factors play a role in determining the **rate of recovery** also, which involves the movement of the anesthetic agent from the brain to blood, and then to the lungs. Recovery from the effect of agents with low **blood solubility** is faster than those with moderate and high solubility.

Besides being exhaled, some anesthetics are metabolised in the liver, generating chloride- and fluoride-containing free radicals that can damage tissues. For example, halothane can cause hepatitis and methoxyflurane is nephrotoxic.

Minimum Alveolar Concentration (MAC)

The minimum alveolar concentration (MAC) of inhaled anesthetic is defined as "the lowest concentration of the inhalational anesthetic agent required in the alveoli to cause immobility in 50% of patients in response to noxious stimuli like surgical incision". It is a measure of potency. There exists an inverse relationship between MAC and potency, i.e., a high MAC indicates a low potency. For example, **nitrous oxide which has the highest MAC (= 104) is the least potent anesthetic**. Potency of nitrous oxide is so low that even if 100% nitrous oxide is inspired, complete anesthesia is not achieved. Thus, it is always combined with other agents to achieve surgical anesthesia.

Nitrous oxide is used in high concentration (80% in inhaled air) because of its low potency. Inhalation of such high anesthetic concentration has useful as well as harmful consequences in the form of **second gas effect** and **diffusion hypoxia**, respectively (Box 14.1).

In contrast, methoxyflurane, which has the lowest MAC (= 0.16), is the most potent agent, followed by trilene, halothane, isoflurane, enflurane, sevoflurane and desflurane.

Box 14.1 Second gas effect and diffusion hypoxia

Second gas effect (Fig. 14.3)
When the administration of inhalational anesthetic agents is started, their diffusion gradient from alveoli to blood is high (as the concentration of anesthetic in blood is zero at the time of initiation of the inhalation) → large quantity of anesthetic diffuses into blood from alveoli along the concentration gradient. This effect is further accentuated if the partial pressure of anesthetic is high in the inhaled air. For example, N_2O, which is given as 80% of inhaled air because of its low potency, enters the bloodstream at a very high rate (at a rate of ~ 1 L/min) during the initial few minutes of its inhalation. If another inhalational anesthetic agent like halothane 1–2% (low concentration is used as it is very potent) is administered at the same time, it also gets delivered to the blood at the same high rate as N_2O. Thus, the rate of induction of halothane increases. This is known as the **second gas effect** [that is, halothane, the second gas, gets carried to the bloodstream at the same rate as the first gas N_2O, even though it is given in low concentrations].

Diffusion hypoxia
When N_2O inhalation is stopped, it quickly diffuses back from the blood to the alveoli (due to its high concentration and low blood solubility), resulting in the dilution of alveolar air. This manifests as hypoxia. Such hypoxia at the time of recovery from N_2O anesthesia, associated with high rate of diffusion is called diffusion hypoxia. It may be dangerous in patients with low cardio-pulmonary reserve.

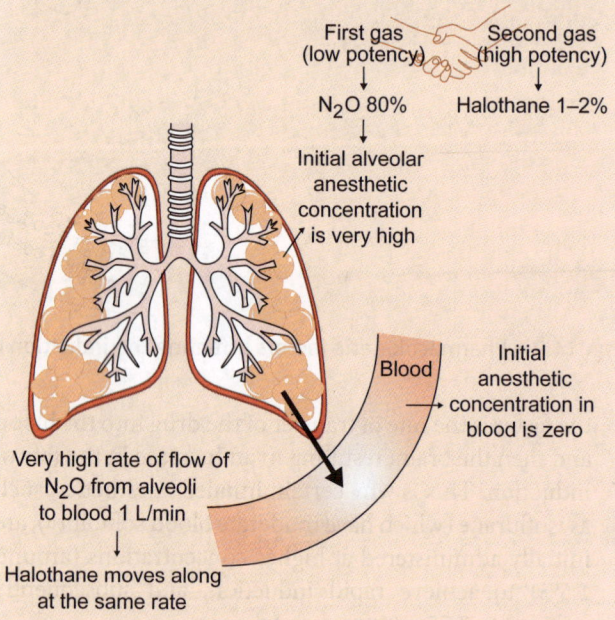

Fig. 14.3 Second gas effect

To prevent this adverse consequence, 100% oxygen should be given for few minutes after discontinuing N_2O inhalation so that alveolar O_2 concentration is maintained.

Diffusion hypoxia is not seen with inhalational agents other than N_2O as they are inhaled in low concentrations (up to 4%) only.

MAC of general anesthetics decreases with increasing age, presence of hypothermia, and the use of IV opioid, analgesics/sedative hypnotics/antiadrenergic drugs as adjuvants. Therefore, the concentration of anesthetic in the inspired gas should be adjusted on the lower side. In contrast, MAC increases in pregnancy, chronic alcoholism and usage of central stimulant drugs such as cocaine and amphetamines, which calls for a higher dose of anesthetic agent.

MECHANISM OF ACTION OF GENERAL ANESTHETICS

General anesthetics **reduce spontaneous as well as evoked neuronal activity** in many regions of the brain by interacting with ligand-gated ion channels. The important targets for general anesthetics include the following (Fig. 14.4):

- **GABA$_A$ receptor–chloride channel complex**: It is a pentameric protein made up of α, β and γ subunits. Inhaled as well as intravenous anesthetics with sedative–hypnotic effects **increase the chloride ion flux** by facilitating the effect of GABA or by directly activating receptors. Barbiturates, benzodiazepines, and propofol act through these receptors.
- **Glycine receptors** may be activated by inhaled anesthetics.
- **Potassium channels linked to NTMs**, like acetylcholine, noradrenaline, dopamine and serotonin may be activated by some general anesthetics causing membrane hyperpolarisation.
- **N$_n$ receptors**: Inhaled anesthetics decrease the duration of the opening of N$_n$ receptor-operated cation channels and prevent membrane depolarisation.
- **NMDA receptors**: Ketamine and nitrous oxide probably act by antagonising the effect of excitatory NTM glutamate on NMDA (N-methyl-D-aspartate) receptors.

The sensitivity of different neuronal pathways to various general anesthetics differ. **The most sensitive pathway is the substantia gelatinosa of the dorsal horn of the spinal cord that blocks the transmission of nociceptive (painful) sensations.** Golgi type II cells, ascending pathways of reticular activating system, spinal reflexes, respiratory and vasomotor centres are inhibited, in that order, with progressively increasing depth of anesthesia.

A. INHALATIONAL AGENTS

Inhalational agents include gases such as nitrous oxide, entonox, and xenon; volatile liquids like ether, chloroform, and cyclopropane; and fluorinated volatile liquids such as desflurane, sevoflurane, isoflurane, enflurane, halothane, and methoxyflurane.

Pharmacological Actions

1. **Action on CNS**

   - General anesthetics produce **dose-dependent progressive CNS depression** leading to anxiolytic → sedative → general anesthesia stages I to IV, in that sequence.
   - Nitrous oxide, trilene, and ether have good analgesic action, whereas fluorinated anesthetics generally have poor analgesic properties.
   - Volatile liquids reduce cerebral vascular resistance, resulting in **increased cerebral blood flow**. It is harmful in patients with raised intracranial tension (ICT). Increase in cerebral blood flow and ICT is least likely with nitrous oxide.

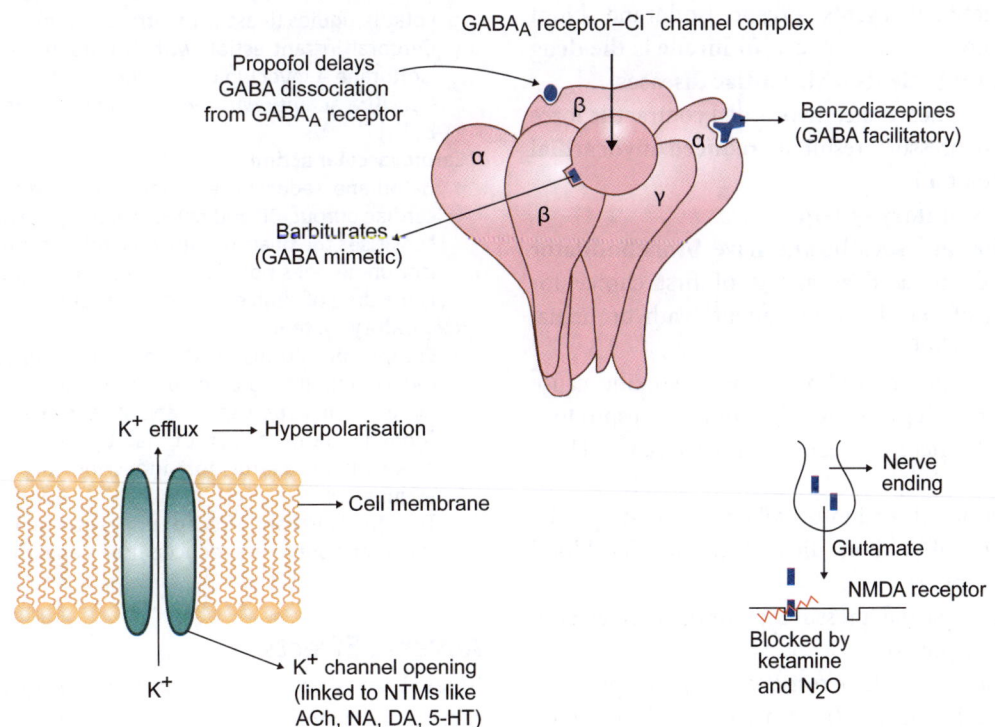

Fig. 14.4 Sites and mechanism of action of general anesthetics

- At high doses, enflurane and sevoflurane have **cerebral irritant** effects causing myoclonic activity and spike and wave pattern in EEG.

2. **Action on CVS**

Some anesthetic agents reduce heart rate, myocardial contractility, BP and oxygen demand of the heart.
- Heart rate: Halothane causes bradycardia by direct vagal stimulation, whereas isoflurane and desflurane increase the heart rate through transient sympathetic stimulation. Moreover, halothane and isoflurane sensitise the myocardium to the effects of catecholamines. This may cause **ventricular arrhythmias** in patients with high catecholamine turnover or on therapy with sympathomimetic drugs.
- Cardiac output: All inhaled agents exert **myocardial depressant** effects in a dose-dependent manner. This effect is greater with halothane and enflurane, resulting in reduced cardiac output. Enflurane causes the maximum fall in cardiac output, whereas myocardial depression is far less with nitrous oxide. The use of nitrous oxide in balanced anesthesia, therefore, reduces the required dose of other agents (**anesthesia sparing effect**) and thereby prevents/reduces their myocardial depressant effect.
- Blood pressure: Volatile anesthetics (e.g., desflurane, sevoflurane, isoflurane) **reduce arterial blood pressure** due to fall in peripheral vascular resistance and reduced cardiac output (enflurane, halothane). However, this fall in BP is attenuated by hypercapnia that stimulates the release of catecholamines.
- All inhalational agents except isoflurane blunt baroreceptor reflexes. Hence, **isoflurane is the drug of choice for patients with cardiac diseases**.
- Reduction in heart rate, myocardial contractile force and blood pressure result in **reduced myocardial oxygen demand**.

3. **Action on respiratory system**
- **Halothane and sevoflurane have bronchodilator effect** and are used as agents of first choice for induction of anesthesia in patients with bronchial asthma and COPD.
- All inhaled anesthetics except nitrous oxide cause **respiratory depression.** Maximum respiratory depressant effect is seen with enflurane. There occurs:
  - Reduction in minute volume, raised partial pressure of carbon dioxide in arterial blood (hypercapnia)
  - Reduced partial pressure of oxygen in arterial blood (hypoxia)
  - In addition, ventilator response to hypercapnia and hypoxia is reduced (maximum with halothane). However, these effects of volatile anesthetics are countered by mechanically assisted or controlled ventilation.
- All inhaled anesthetics (except ether) **suppress mucociliary function** of respiratory mucosa. This can cause mucus pooling, atelectasis, post-operative respiratory infections, etc.
- Desflurane has a pungent smell and **irritates airway mucosa,** causing coughing and breath-holding. Because of this, desflurane is not a preferred drug for induction.

Other Effects
- Hepatic blood flow is temporarily reduced by inhaled volatile drugs but returns to normal afterwards.
- Renal blood flow is also decreased → reduced GFR.
- Inhalational agents, except nitrous oxide, cause profound uterine relaxant action. This may be beneficial for intrauterine fetal manipulations but may increase post-partum hemorrhage.
- Inflammability: Ether and cyclopropane have high inflammability. So, when these are used for induction of anesthesia, cautery should not be used.

The major pharmacological actions of inhalational agents are summarised in Box 14.2.

Box 14.2 Key pharmacological actions of inhalational agents

Central actions
- Dose-dependent progressive CNS depression
- Analgesia and amnesia by nitrous oxide
- Increased cerebral blood flow → increased ICT with volatile liquids (least with nitrous oxide)
- Cerebral irritant action with enflurane, sevoflurane and isoflurane → myoclonic or seizure activity [Mnemonic: ESI - seizure activity with drugs having names starting with E, S, I]

Cardiovascular actions
- Halothane reduces heart rate, myocardial contractility, cardiac output, BP and myocardial oxygen demand, but it sensitises the heart to catecholamines actions.
- Isoflurane does not blunt baroreceptor reflexes, hence it is the drug of choice in cardiac patients.

Respiratory system
- Except for nitrous oxide, all inhalational anesthetics reduce minute volume, blunt ventilatory response to hypoxia and hypercapnia, and increase $PaCO_2$.
- Bronchodilator effect of halothane and sevoflurane make them useful for induction of anesthesia in asthmatics.
- The airway irritant effect of pungent-smelling desflurane is responsible for its reduced use in anesthetic practice.

Adverse Effects

Inhaled anesthetics can cause organ system toxicities such as hepatotoxicity, nephrotoxicity, and malignant hyperthermia; it also increases the risk of abortions in pregnant patients. Operation theatre workers are also at increased risk of cancer and megaloblastic anemia.

1. **Hepatotoxicity** occurs in one in 20,000–35,000 cases exposed to **halothane**. Risk of halothane-induced hepatic dysfunction may be higher in obese patients exposed to halothane more than once in a short span of time. The hepatotoxicity probably occurs due to the formation of reactive metabolites or free radicals and trifluoroacetated proteins (TFA) that can cause hepatocellular damage or initiate an immune response resulting in the formation of autoantibodies against hepatic proteins. No specific treatment exists for halothane-induced hepatotoxicity; liver transplantation is the only solution for most severe cases.

2. **Nephrotoxicity** occurs with **methoxyflurane and enflurane**, as these are partly metabolised by renal β-lyase enzyme, resulting in the formation of fluoride ions in the kidney. These ions cause proximal tubular damage and reduce the concentrating ability of kidneys. Methoxyflurane is highly nephrotoxic and thus not used much in clinical practice.

    Sevoflurane is itself not metabolised in the kidney, but a haloalkene (compound A) formed by its reaction with CO_2 absorbents in the anesthesia machine is metabolised in kidney. Renal metabolism of 'compound A' forms thioacylhalides which may cause proximal tubular damage.

3. **Malignant hyperthermia**: It is a rare autosomal dominant genetic disorder characterised by mutations in genetic loci coding for:
    - Ryanodine receptors on sarcoplasmic reticulum in skeletal muscles → excessive Ca^{2+} release from sarcoplasmic reticulum.
    - α_1-subunit of L-type calcium channels → increased entry of Ca^{2+} into skeletal muscle cell from ECF.

    The raised calcium in the vicinity of actin–troponin–tropomyosin complex results in severe muscle rigidity, hyperthermia, hyperkalemia, tachycardia and hypertension. Halothane can cause malignant hyperthermia in predisposed individuals. It is managed by external cooling and dantrolene, a direct-acting smooth muscle relaxant that acts by inhibiting the release of calcium from sarcoplasmic reticulum.

4. **Occupational hazards**: In pregnant patients and OT workers exposed to inhalant anesthetics, the risk of **abortion** is reported to be high; however, the causal relationship is not established.
    - Increased occurrence of **cancer** in operation theatre workers as they are exposed to trace concentrations of anesthetics.
    - Nitrous oxide can cause **megaloblastic anemia** as an occupational hazard, because it reduces the activity of methionine synthase.

Status of Inhalational Agents in Clinical Practice

Inhalational agents are commonly employed **along with intravenous agents** as a part of balanced anesthesia. Nitrous oxide and volatile anesthetics with low blood solubility, such as desflurane, sevoflurane, and isoflurane, are preferred due to their rapid recovery rates, especially as an increasing number of surgical procedures are now performed on a short-stay basis. However, as desflurane has the disadvantage of a pungent smell, **sevoflurane is more frequently used**. Halothane is still used in pediatric surgeries because of the vast experience with the drug.

The key features of important inhalational agents are given in Box 14.3.

Box 14.3 Salient features of inhalational agents

N_2O
- Gas dispensed in blue cylinders
- Highest MAC (least potent); low blood solubility(fast induction and recovery)
- Good analgesia, but poor skeletal muscle relaxation
- Can cause methemoglobinemia, laryngospasm
- It may produce high pressure in closed cavities, hence contraindicated in volvulus and pneumothorax

Ether
- It is the safest agent in unskilled hands.
- Possesses good analgesic and muscle relaxant action
- Safe in asthmatics
- However, its irritant, pungent smell is a disadvantage.
- Ether is highly inflammable; therefore, the use of cautery is contraindicated during its administration.
- It can cause hyperglycemia and is not safe in diabetics.

Halothane
- Colourless volatile liquid with pleasant smell, dispensed in amber-coloured bottles
- Non-irritant, non-explosive
- Good anesthetic, poor analgesic.
- Causes bronchodilatation and hence a preferred anesthetic agent in asthma and COPD
- Preferred in children for induction of anesthesia
- Its tocolytic effect makes it the drug of choice for internal version to manipulate fetal presentation and for manual removal of placenta.
- However, it carries the risk of postpartum hemorrhage when used in labour.
- Can cause adverse effects like post-operative shivering, malignant hyperthermia, cardiac depression, hypotension and hepatotoxicity.
- It sensitises myocardium to catecholamines, resulting in arrhythmias. Hence, it is contraindicated in condition of high catecholamine levels in the body, i.e., pheochromocytoma.

Isoflurane
- Anesthetic agent of choice in cardiac surgery, neurosurgery for producing controlled hypotension and daycare surgery.
- It is safe in pheochromocytoma as it does not sensitise myocardium to catecholamines.

Methoxyflurane
- In contrast to N_2O, it has the least MAC and highest blood solubility.

- It is not to be used in a closed environment as it may react with the rubber tubing of the insulation. It is hepatotoxic and nephrotoxic.

Sevoflurane
- It is safe for use in children.
- Bronchodilator effect → preferred in asthma
- It produces a nephrotoxic compound when used in closed circuit
- Enflurane, Sevoflurane and Isoflurane [Mnemonic ESI] can precipitate seizures. So, they are contraindicated in epileptics.

Clinical problem-based questions and MCQs

8. Which of the following factors does NOT affect the rate of induction with inhalational general anesthetics?
   a. Depth and rate of ventilation
   b. Cardiac output
   c. Blood gas partition coefficient
   d. Minimum alveolar concentration

9. The rate of induction of general anesthesia using inhalational agents is faster in patients in circulatory shock. Explain the pharmacological basis for this.

10. Arrange the following inhalational agents in ascending order of their onset of anesthetic action.
    a. Methoxyflurane   b. Sevoflurane
    c. Isoflurane   d. Halothane

11. Identify the neurons most sensitive to inhibitory effects of general anesthetics agents.
    a. Dorsal horn of spinal cord
    b. Ascending pathways of reticular activating system
    c. Respiratory centre
    d. Vasomotor centre

12. i. The potency of inhaled general anesthetics is determined by its
       a. MAC
       b. Partial pressure
       c. Blood:gas partition coefficient
       d. Rate of diffusion
    ii. Describe the relationship of potency with the selected factor.

13. Desflurane, a volatile inhalational anesthetic agent with very a fast onset of anesthetic action, is not used in clinical practice for induction of anesthesia. Explain why.

14. Match the drug with the organ system toxicity caused by it.
    a. Halothane   1. Seizures
    b. Methoxyflurane   2. Hepatotoxicity
    c. Sevoflurane   3. Nephrotoxicity

15. A 40-year-old female patient, a known case of bronchial asthma, presents with severe pain in the right hypochondrium, nausea, vomiting and fever. USG of the abdomen shows multiple small calculi in gall bladder and wall thickening. Laparoscopic cholecystectomy is planned under GA.
    i. Which general anesthetic is the most preferable in this case?
       a. Sevoflurane   b. Desflurane
       c. N₂O   d. Methoxyflurane
    ii. Describe the pharmacological basis to justify your choice.

16. i. Which of the following inhalational anesthetic causes diffusion hypoxia?
       a. Sevoflurane   b. N₂O
       c. Diethyl ether   d. Halothane
    ii. Explain the reason for diffusion hypoxia to occur with the drug selected in part (i) of the question.

B. INTRAVENOUS ANESTHETIC AGENTS

These are used alone or in combination with inhalational agents as part of balanced anesthesia.

Advantages of IV Agents

- No need for specialised anesthetic machines
- No need of facilities to dispose off the exhaled gases
- Very fast onset of action of IV drugs, e.g., thiopental, methohexital, etomidate, propofol and ketamine, which makes them beneficial for induction of general anesthesia.
- Fast recovery from effects of IV agents makes them more suitable for daycare surgery or ambulatory surgical procedures.
- The analgesic effect of most IV agents (except opioids) is negligible, but it is sufficient for short surgical procedures, when combined with nitrous oxide or local anesthetics.
- Opioids are used as adjuvants in pre-anesthetic medication/perioperative analgesia. In addition to analgesic effect, opioids provide cardiovascular stability and adequate sedation.
- Benzodiazepines given as pre-anesthetic medication provide sedative, amnesic and anxiolytic effect.

a. Barbiturates

Thiopental and **methohexital** are the commonly used barbiturates in anesthetic practice.

Role in anesthetic practice

- These drugs are used for **induction** of anesthesia. Owing to their high lipid solubility, they cross blood–brain barrier quickly and loss of consciousness occurs in one circulation time.
- Recovery from the effect of thiopentone is very fast as it **gets redistributed** from the brain to less vascular tissues like adipose tissues and skeletal muscles. Later, it is metabolised by liver and excreted by kidney.

- Thiopental does not increase intracranial tension (ICT), so it is beneficial in patients who have raised ICT due to cerebral tumours or head injury.
- **Methohexital is preferred over thiopental for short ambulatory procedures** due to its faster elimination, and **for patients undergoing electroconvulsive therapy (ECT)** as it lowers seizure threshold.

Adverse effects

- Repeated administration of large doses or continuous infusion of barbiturates can cause myocardial and respiratory depressant effects.
- Accidental intra-arterial injection of thiopentone may cause intense vasoconstriction, thrombosis, ischemia and gangrene. It is managed by leaving the needle where it is (in situ) and giving saline to dilute the drug. Inj. papaverine to reverse vasospasm and heparinisation is indicated.
- Glomerular filtration rate (GRF) and hepatic blood flow are reduced by barbiturates.
- Barbiturates can precipitate acute intermittent porphyria in susceptible individuals.

b. Benzodiazepines

Midazolam, **diazepam** and **lorazepam** are commonly used benzodiazepines in anesthetic practice.

Role in anesthetic practice

- Benzodiazepines have sedative, anxiolytic and amnesic effects. So, these are drugs of choice in **pre-anesthetic medication**.
- They are useful as **adjuvants** in procedures done under local anesthesia.
- **Midazolam** is water soluble and has faster onset and recovery than other benzodiazepines. Hence, it is the **most preferred benzodiazepine** for IV administration in daycare surgery. However, as the CNS depressant effect of benzodiazepines given IV develops slowly, it is not sufficient for surgical anesthesia. Hence, IV midazolam is administered before the patient is brought into the operation theatre.

Adverse effects

- Diazepam and lorazepam, are not water soluble. They are dissolved in non-aqueous vehicles, which may cause pain and irritation at the injection site.
- Benzodiazepines can cause anterograde amnesia and respiratory depression.
- Post-anesthetic recovery period is long. Recovery from effect of benzodiazepines can be hastened by giving antagonist flumazenil. It is usually needed in elderly patients or in situations where large doses of longer-acting benzodiazepines like lorazepam, and diazepam have been used.

c. Opioid Analgesics

- Opioids and benzodiazepines given in high dose are combined for general anesthesia in situations when the patient has limited circulatory reserve as in **cardiovascular surgery.**
- Shorter-acting potent opioids like remifentanil and alfentanil have quick onset of action. They can be used as **co-inducing agents along with IV sedative hypnotics.**
- Fentanyl is combined with droperidol to produce a state of neurolept analgesia. If nitrous oxide is also combined, it is a state of **neurolept anesthesia.**
- Low dose of fentanyl and sufentanil are used for **perioperative analgesia** as adjuvants to other IV or inhalational agents.
- Epidural and subarachnoid administration of opioids is useful for **post-operative analgesia.**

Adverse effects

The disadvantage of high dose of opioids is **respiratory depression** and chest wall rigidity, which further impairs ventilation, and leads to increased post-operative morbidity and mortality. To minimise these complications of high dose opioids, **more potent drugs like fentanyl and sufentanil are preferred over morphine.**

d. Propofol

- This is the **most preferred drug among IV agents for ambulatory surgery** because its fast onset of action (as fast as IV barbiturates) and faster rate of recovery from anesthetic effect.
- In post-operative period, the risk of nausea/vomiting is less with propofol. Hence, patients have a better sense of well-being.
- It is used both for induction and maintenance as a part of balanced anesthesia and total IV anesthesia (TIVA) involving the administration of alfentanil and propofol.
- It is the **drug of choice for sedation** in monitored anesthesia in operation theatres for diagnostic procedures and prolonged sedation in critical care units.
- It is the anesthetic drug of choice in patients suffering from malignant hyperthermia.

Adverse effects

- The most common adverse effect is **pain at injection site**, which can be reduced by pre-treatment with lignocaine or using fospropofol, the water-soluble prodrug of propofol.
- It causes dose-related depression of central drive for ventilation. Transient apnea may occur.
- It causes a marked fall in BP due to vasodilator effect and direct negative inotropic effect.

- Prolonged administration can cause delayed arousal, raised serum lipids, severe acidosis, tremors and neurological complications.

e. Etomidate

- It causes **minimum depression of respiratory and cardiovascular function.** Hence, it is preferred over other anesthetics in elderly patients who have low cardiovascular reserve, in cardiac disease and patients undergoing aneurysm surgery. It causes rapid induction without any noticeable effect on heart rate, blood pressure and respiration. However, the recovery rate is slower than with propofol. Redistribution contributes to termination of its anesthetic effect.
- A drawback of etomidate is **lack of analgesic activity**: hence, opioids are usually used in conjunction.
- Adverse effects occur as pain at the site of injection, nausea, vomiting, involuntary muscle movements, and inhibition of steroid synthesis in adrenal cortex. Prolonged infusion in ICU settings can cause oliguria, electrolyte imbalance and hypotension.

f. Ketamine

- It produces a state of **dissociative anesthesia**. In this state, analgesia, amnesia, immobility, light sleep, and a feeling of dissociation from the body and surroundings occurs. Consciousness may or may not be lost.
- It acts as an NMDA glutamate receptor antagonist.
- Among all the IV agents, this is the **only drug which has both analgesic as well as anesthetic actions,** but it lacks muscle relaxant action.
- Ketamine causes central sympathetic stimulation and inhibits reuptake of noradrenaline at sympathetic nerve endings, resulting in dose-related stimulation of the cardiovascular system, increase in heart rate, cardiac output and blood pressure after 2–4 minutes of IV injection. These parameters return to normal in 10–20 minutes. Airway reflexes and tone are usually maintained. Therefore, it is preferred in high-risk elderly patients, cardiogenic/septic shock patients.
- In pediatric patients undergoing short, painful procedures and monitored anesthesia care, ketamine is used along with propofol.
- Due to its bronchodilator effect, it is considered safe for use in asthmatics.
- Ketamine has no depressant effect on pharyngeal and laryngeal reflexes, making it the preferred agent in emergency surgery (While giving anesthesia to a patient who is not in fasting state, the risk of vomiting and aspiration is lower with use of ketamine.)
- Topical ketamine is used for some types of arthritis.
- It is commonly used in low doses of 0.1–0.25 mg/kg of bodyweight along with other IV or inhalational drugs as an alternative to opioids, as it does not suppress ventilation.

Adverse effects

- Ketamine can cause psychiatric symptoms in immediate post-operative period known as **emergence phenomenon,** characterised by vivid dreams, illusions, hallucinations and disorientation. The incidence of emergence reactions is reduced by premedication with diazepam/midazolam or propofol.
- Ketamine can raise cerebral blood flow, oxygen consumption and ICT. It is therefore not suitable for use in patients with head injury, cerebral tumours, etc.
- It increases intraocular tension and is hence contraindicated in glaucoma.

g. Dexmedetomidine

- It is a selective central α_2 receptor agonist, like clonidine.
- It possesses sedative and analgesic actions but not amnesic, anesthetic action. Respiratory depression is minimal.
- It is used as an adjuvant to general anesthetics to reduce their dose.
- It is also used along with regional or spinal anesthesia and in critically ill patients on ventilators for prolonged periods.
- Adverse effects are similar to clonidine i.e., bradycardia, hypotension, and dryness of mouth.

Clinical problem-based questions and MCQs

17. Match the drug with its use in anesthetic practice.
    - a. Thiopentone
    - b. Methohexital
    - c. Midazolam
    - d. Low dose sufentanil

    1. Patient undergoing ECT
    2. Before entering OT
    3. Perioperative analgesia
    4. Induction

18. All of the following are essentially seen in dissociative anesthesia EXCEPT:
    - a. Analgesia
    - b. Amnesia
    - c. Catatonia
    - d. Loss of consciousness

19. A 32-year-old primigravida presents in gynae obstetrics OPD with labour pains and watery vaginal discharge. On PV examination, the patient has good uterine contractions; soft, effaced and fully dilated cervix. Under local anesthesia, right mediolateral episiotomy is done, but uterine contractions become weak and the patient delivers a healthy, live baby after about 20–25 minutes of episiotomy. By the time episiotomy repair is attempted, the effect of the local anesthetic has worn off, causing the patient to experience pain. Injection ketamine at a dose of 1.5 mg/kg is administered to facilitate suturing.
    i. What is the mechanism of action of ketamine?
    ii. What are the adverse effects of ketamine?

20. A 54-year-old female patient presents with epigastric pain, belching and bloating sensation in abdomen. There is a history of chronic pain and swelling of the left knee for past 4–5 months and the patient is using tab. diclofenac 50 mg twice a day on most days of the week. The patient is called for endoscopy. Inj. propofol 2 mg/kg is given IV before starting endoscopy.
    i. Why endoscopy is advised in this patient?
    ii. What is the pharmacological basis for administering propofol?
    iii. What are the adverse effects of propofol?

21. A 45-year-old patient presented with fever, cough, and difficulty in breathing. Oxygen saturation was 82%. CT scan of lungs showed patches of fibrosis in right lung. RT PCR test was positive for COVID19. The patient was given oxygen inhalation, but saturation did not improve, and hence advised mechanical ventilation. Injection dexmedetomidine was given IV in a dose of 0.05 mcg/kg just before endotracheal intubation.
    i. What is the basis for the use of dexmedetomidine in this patient?
    ii. Describe the mechanism of action and adverse effects of dexmedetomidine.

22. Identify the intravenously administered general anesthetic having both analgesic and anesthetic action from the following.
    a. Propofol   b. Sufentanil
    c. Ketamine   d. Etomidate

PRE-ANESTHETIC MEDICATION (PAM)

As the name indicates, this concerns the administration of some drugs **prior to administering general anesthetics** for the safety of the patient.

The **objectives** of giving pre-anesthetic medication (PAM) are:

- To reduce the patient's anxiety and apprehensions about the procedure so that anesthetic induction is smooth and eventless.
- To prevent aspiration of respiratory tract secretions due to irritant anesthetics.
- To prevent vagal stimulation with anesthetic agents.
- To decrease gastric secretions and raise gastric pH in order to lower the risk of aspiration, and if aspirated, their effects are less damaging.
- To prevent the patient from recalling the events before, during and just after the surgery, i.e., perioperative amnesia.
- For the anesthesia-sparing effect (reduction in the dose of anesthetic agent by using drugs that supplement the analgesic effect).
- To reduce nausea and vomiting during and after the procedure.

Drugs for PAM

To achieve these goals, **different groups of drugs are used,** including:

1. **Anticholinergic drugs**

   As blockade of M_3 receptors reduces exocrine secretions, anticholinergic drugs like atropine/glycopyrrolate are helpful in reducing salivary and tracheobronchial secretions. However, nowadays, as most of the anesthetics are non-irritant, increased secretions are not a problem. In modern clinical practice, atropine or related drugs are used **to prevent bradycardia and hypotension secondary to vagal stimulation** associated with surgical manipulations. These drugs also **prevent laryngeal spasm** caused by respiratory secretions. Glycopyrrolate is preferred over atropine for this indication as it is more potent, has fast onset of action and is longer acting than atropine. It is a quaternary amine which cannot cross the blood–brain barrier. Hence, there are no central side effects.

   Dose of glycopyrrolate: 0.4 mg by IM or IV route

2. **Proton pump inhibitors or H_2 antagonists**

   These are used to reduce gastric acid secretion and raise the pH of gastric contents. They are given on the night before the surgery and in the morning of the surgery. Proton pump inhibitors block the final step of gastric acid secretion. Omeprazole 20 mg or pantoprazole 40 mg may be used. H_2 blockers inhibit the basal, nocturnal and meal-stimulated acid secretion in the stomach. The dose of ranitidine is 150 mg, famotidine, 20 mg.

   As the volume of gastric contents decreases, the risk of regurgitation and aspiration decreases. Because pH is raised (or acidity of gastric contents is lowered), the damage caused to respiratory mucosa is less if regurgitation or aspiration occurs. These drugs are frequently used before prolonged procedures.

3. **Benzodiazepines**

   For preventing the recall of perioperative events, i.e., amnesia, **benzodiazepines** are used. Diazepam 5 mg or lorazepam 2 mg are administered an hour before the surgery. They assist in the smooth induction of anesthesia because of their anxiolytic action. The advantage of benzodiazepines is the lower risk of respiratory depression compared to other sedatives and the availability of specific antagonist **flumazenil** to reverse their effect as and when needed. **Midazolam**, which is more potent, fast and short-acting, is well suited for this role.

4. **Opioids**

   Opioids are useful for supplementing analgesic effect and reducing anxiety and apprehension associated with surgery. However, nowadays, the use of opioids in premedication is reserved only for patients with preoperative pain. Fentanyl, being more potent, is preferred over morphine in such patients.

The causes of reduced popularity of opioids in premedication are:
- Risk of respiratory depression
- Risk of hypotension
- Difficulty in assessing the pupillary signs of depth of anesthesia, as opioids cause miosis.
- Post-operative nausea, vomiting, constipation and urinary retention, which may be troublesome
- Possible delay in recovery from anesthetic effect

5. **Antiemetics**

Antiemetics like metoclopramide, ondansetron and domperidone reduce the incidence of post-operative nausea and vomiting. These drugs increase the tone of the lower esophageal sphincter (LES) and enhance peristalsis, promoting forward movement of gastric contents, thereby reducing the risk of reflux, retching, and vomiting.

Metoclopramide, a D_2 receptor antagonist, is administered intramuscularly in doses of 10–20 mg. A potential adverse effect is the development of muscular dystonias, which generally respond well to benzodiazepines. It can also cause extrapyramidal adverse effects. The risk of such ADRs is lower with **domperidone. Ondensetron**, a $5-HT_2$ blocker, is preferred over other drugs nowadays, as it has no central side effects. **Promethazine**, an H_1 blocker, is also useful.

Clinical problem-based questions and MCQs

23. A 56-year-old woman presents with severe pain in the right iliac region, nausea and vomiting. On examination, there is pain at Mcburny's point. Ultrasonography of the abdomen reveals acute inflammation of the appendix. An emergency appendicectomy is advised.
    i. All of the following drugs should be given to the patient before surgical procedure, EXCEPT:
       a. Glycopyrrolate
       b. Pantoprazole
       c. Lignocaine
       d. Midazolam
    ii. Justify the use of the other drugs listed above.

CHOICE OF ANESTHETIC AGENT

The choice of anesthetic agent depends on multiple drug-related, disease-related and patient-related factors. Table 14.2 summarises the various types of surgeries in which a particular anesthetic is preferred in **current clinical practice**.

Table **14.2** *Anesthetic preferences in different types of surgeries*

Drug	Preferred in
Propofol	Daycare surgeries, ICU sedation, malignant hyperthermia [Mnemonic – DIM]
Propofol + Alfentanil	Total IV anesthesia
Ketamine	Emergency surgery (on full stomach), patients in shock, CHF, bronchial asthma, children
Halothane	Asthma patients, COPD, children, for internal versions, manual removal of placenta
Isoflurane	Cardiac surgery, neurosurgery, controlled hypotension
Thiopentone	Inducing agent, preferred in epileptics
Methohexital	ECT
Propofol, midazolam, alfentanil, desflurane, sevoflurane, isoflurane	Daycare surgery

Summary

- Analgesia, amnesia, inhibition of autonomic and sensory reflexes, skeletal muscle relaxation and loss of consciousness are components of GA.
- Different drugs are combined to use their favourable properties and minimise their adverse effects in balanced anesthesia.
- Monitored anesthesia care for minor procedures includes PAM with intravenous midazolam, followed by propofol infusion, opioid/ketamine and local anesthesia.
- Conscious sedation using midazolam, diazepam, propofol, and dexmedetomidine (used for relieving fear and anxiety without altering consciousness), is used for procedures such as arterial/venous catheterisation and angiography.
- More extensive procedures require PAM, induction with IV drug, maintenance of anesthesia with inhalational + IV drugs, and endotracheal intubation. Skeletal muscle relaxants, opioids/local anesthetic for perioperative analgesia, α_2 agonist, β blockers and CCBs for controlling autonomic reflexes are components of balanced anesthesia.
- GA agents are intravenous and inhalational. Inhalational agents are N_2O, desflurane, sevoflurane, isoflurane, enflurane, halothane, and methoxyflurane; intravenous agents are phenobarbitones, benzodiazepines, opioids, propofol, ketamine, etomidate, and dexmedetomidine.

- There are 4 stages reflecting increasing depth of anesthesia. Most surgeries done in plane 1 of stage III.
- For inhalational agents, factors such as the partial pressure of inhaled air, pulmonary blood flow, rate/depth of ventilation, and blood:gas partition coefficient determine the rate of onset and recovery. The lower the blood:gas partition coefficient, the faster is the onset and recovery. It increases from desflurane to sevoflurane, isoflurane enflurane, halothane and methoxyflurane, in that order.
- Inhaled anesthetics cause dose-dependent central depressant action, myocardial and respiratory depressant actions. Halothane and isoflurane sensitises the heart to catecholamines → arrhythmias. Methoxyflurane is nephrotoxic and halothane hepatotoxic. Desflurane is not much used because of its pungent smell → respiratory tract irritant action.
- N_2O shows second gas effect and diffusion hypoxia because of its low potency and low blood solubility.
- Intravenous agents are used alone or with inhalational agents. Thiopentone is preferred for induction and is safe in case of head injuries. Methohexital is preferred over thiopentone for ECT and short ambulatory procedures.
- Midazolam, being water soluble, is short-acting and is most commonly employed before the patient is taken to the OT.
- Opioids are used with benzodiazepines for cardiovascular surgeries. Potent opioids like fentanyl are useful as co-inducing agents with thiopentone. Other uses in anesthetic practice are for neurolept analgesia/anesthesia, perioperative and post-operative analgesia. The most important drawback of opioids is respiratory depression.
- Propofol is the intravenous agent of choice in ambulatory surgery and sedation in operation theatre. ADRs include injection site pain, fall in BP and transient apnea.
- Ketamine is used for dissociative anesthesia. It is preferred in patients with poor cardiopulmonary reserve, but can raise ICT. Hence, it is not good in cases of head injuries. It causes emergence phenomenon as an adverse effect.
- PAM is given to reduce anxiety, apprehension, tracheobronchial secretions, gastric acid secretion and amnesia. Drugs used are anticholinergics, midazolam, proton pump inhibitors and benzodiazepines.

Questions for practice

1. Write short notes on:
   a. Balanced anesthesia
   b. Pre-anesthetic medication
   c. Factors determining rate of induction and recovery with inhalational anesthetics
   d. Second-gas phenomenon
   e. Diffusion hypoxia
2. What are the objectives of pre-anesthetic medication? Name the drugs used in PAM.

Hints for problem-based questions and MCQs

1. b. Fall in BP
2. a. Slow onset
3. d. Endotracheal intubation is not done in 'monitored anesthesia care'
4. c. Lignocaine
5. d. Dexmedetomidine
6. c. Diethyl ether
7. i. b. Stage II
   ii. Stage II is 'stage of stimulation'. Refer to Table 14.1, page 184.
8. d. Minimum alveolar concentration.
9. Circulatory shock → low cardiac output → less pulmonary blood flow → lesser amount of blood exposed to anesthetic agent in alveoli → anesthetic concentration in blood rises rapidly → faster passage into CNS → faster onset. Refer to page 185.
10. b, c, d, a (based on blood solubility). Refer to page 185.
11. Neurons of dorsal horn of spinal cord are most sensitive to general anesthetics, resulting in analgesia.
12. i. a. MAC
    ii. Lower the MAC, Greater is the potency.
13. Due to pungent smell → irritation of airway mucosa → coughing and breath holding may occur with desflurane.
14. a–2; b–3; c–1.
15. i. a. sevoflurane
    ii. Preferred in asthmatic patient due to its bronchodilator effect.
16. i. b. N_2O
    ii. Low potency → use of high concentration. Refer to Box 14.1, page 186.
17. a – 4; b – 1; c – 2; d – 3.
18. d. Loss of consciousness may or may not occur in dissociative anesthesia.
19. i. NMDA antagonist
    ii. Refer to page 192.
20. i. To rule out peptic ulceration due to prolonged use of NSAIDs.
    ii. Propofol is the preferred agent for ambulatory procedures due to its fast onset and recovery, lesser risk of post-operative nausea, vomiting. Refer to page 191.
    iii. Pain at injection site, fall in BP, transient apnea, etc.
21. i. IV agent used for short procedures, having sedative analgesic effect but no anesthetic/amnesic action.
    iii. Selective α_2 agonist Refer to page 192.
22. c. Ketamine
23. i. c. Lignocaine
    iii. Glycopyrrolate is more potent, has fast onset of action and is longer acting than atropine. It does not have central side effects and is used to prevent bradycardia and laryngeal spasm. Pantoprazole is used to reduce gastric acidity, and midazolam for amnesia and antianxiety effect.

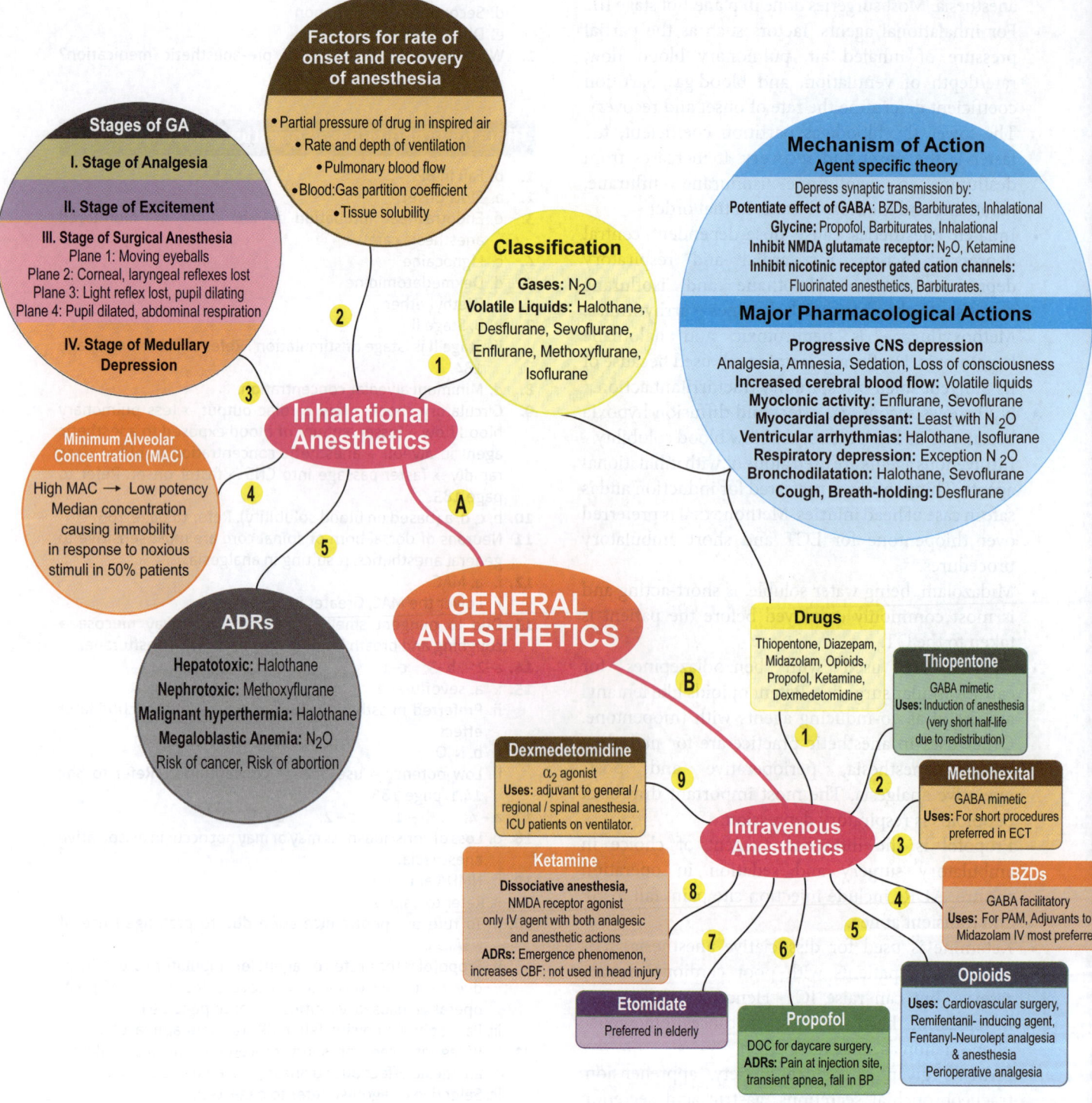

SECTION 3 Drugs Acting on CNS

15 Sedative-Hypnotics and Anxiolytics

PH 3.2 Describe types, salient pharmacokinetics, pharmacodynamics, therapeutic uses, adverse drug reactions of different sedative and hypnotic agents and explain pharmacological basis of selection and use of different sedative and hypnotic agents.
PH 3.6 Describe types, salient pharmacokinetics, pharmacodynamics, therapeutic uses, and adverse drug reactions of drugs used in anxiety disorders. Discuss the general goals of pharmacotherapy for the management of above disorders.

Learning objectives

A student of MBBS phase II should be able to:
- Classify sedative-hypnotic drugs.
- Illustrate the mechanism of action of sedative-hypnotics using suitable examples.
- List the indications of sedative-hypnotics mentioning their doses.
- Enumerate the contraindications and ADRs of sedative-hypnotics.
- Compare benzodiazepines and barbiturates as sedative-hypnotics.
- Describe non-benzodiazepine hypnotics.
- Describe the treatment of anxiety disorders.

Sedative-hypnotics are a class of drugs used in the management of insomnia and related sleep disorders.

Insomnia
Insomnia is the most common of sleep disorders, wherein the subject finds it hard to fall asleep or stay asleep, resulting in a feeling of not being refreshed on waking up and excessive daytime sleepiness.

Etiology
Insomnia can affect anyone, but it is comparatively common among **women and elderly** people. Factors such as **stress, menopause**, and various **medical** or **psychiatric conditions** predispose individuals to insomnia.

Types
Insomnia may be categorised into the following types: acute insomnia, chronic insomnia, onset insomnia, maintenance insomnia, behavioural insomnia of childhood.
- **Acute insomnia:** This is the commonest type of insomnia. It is a short-term condition lasting from a few days to a few weeks and is commonly triggered by stressful life events, unfamiliar sleep environments, noise, light, physical discomfort or illness, medications, or jet lag.
- **Chronic insomnia:** A person is considered to have chronic insomnia when sleep problems occur at least three times a week and last for a month or more.

Chronic insomnia can be **idiopathic** (without obvious cause), or **secondary** to other physical or mental diseases, drugs or lifestyle factors. Diseases like diabetes, hyperthyroidism, parkinsonism and sleep apnea may cause insomnia. Insomnia is also an important symptom in anxiety, depression and attention deficit disorders. Some lifestyle factors such as frequent travel and jet lag, excessive use of caffeine, nicotine, or alcohol, and jack of fixed sleeping routine are significant yet easily modifiable cause of chronic insomnia.

Almost one-fourth of children suffer from **behavioural insomnia**. These children have learnt to fall asleep while being rocked, nursed or listening to a story. In such cases, behavioural changes and self-relaxation techniques can be helpful in resolving the issue.

A patient of insomnia may have difficulty with **onset of sleep** (characterised by a prolonged latency between going to bed and falling asleep) or **staying asleep** for a sufficient duration; some may **wake up frequently in the night** and have trouble falling asleep afterwards.

In some people (usually totally blind), the circadian rhythm is not fixed—it may be less than or more than 24 hours. This is called non-24-hour sleep–wake disorder (N24SWD). Sleeping and waking times shift progressively earlier or later by a few hours in such patients, resulting in complete desynchronisation from daylight hours. Appetite, mood and alertness fluctuate with the shifting circadian rhythm.

SEDATIVE-HYPNOTICS
Sedatives are drugs that reduce excitement, ideation, motor activity and responsiveness to stimuli. In other words, sedatives make a person drowsy but do not induce sleep.

Box 15.1 Sleep cycle

Normal sleep architecture follows a cyclic pattern (Fig. 15.1), although there is considerable individual variation in its duration and structure. Stage 0 represents the awake state, while Stage 1 is a transitional phase between wakefulness and sleep. Stages 2, 3, and 4—representing unequivocal sleep, deep sleep and cerebral sleep, respectively—together constitute non-rapid eye movement (NREM) sleep. This is followed by rapid eye movement (REM) sleep. In a typical adult, the sleep cycle progresses from Stage 0 through Stage 4 and into REM sleep over approximately 90 to 120 minutes. The cycle then repeats, beginning from Stage 1 through Stage 4 to REM sleep.

Sleep Latency
α, β waves
Hypnic jerk
Onset of sleep
Wave activity
starts slowing
0
1
2
3
4
5
Sleep Cycle
REM
NREM
Recallable dreams, Nightmares
Paradoxical
Mixed frequency waves
K not evoked
Easily arousable
Unequivocal sleep
Wave activity continues to slow down
bursts of rapid activity (K complex)
Not easily arousable
Cerebral sleep
Slow δ wave
K not evoked
Slow δ wave
K complex with
strong stimulus
Transition into
deep sleep
Most restorative stages

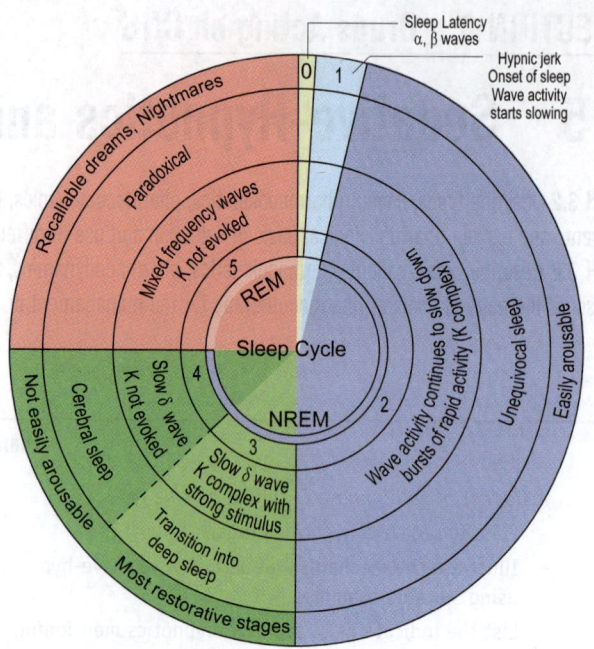

Fig. 15.1 Sleep cycle

Hypnotics are drugs which induce or maintain a state resembling normal arousable sleep. Different sedative-hypnotic drugs affect phases of sleep cycle/sleep architecture in different ways. The stages of sleep cycle are described in Box 15.1 and Table 15.1.

Classification of Sedative-Hypnotics

Sedative-hypnotics include **barbiturates, benzodiazepines (BZDs), non-benzodiazepines**, newer drugs, and **miscellaneous drugs** which cause sedation as an adverse effect, as depicted in (Flowchart 15.1).

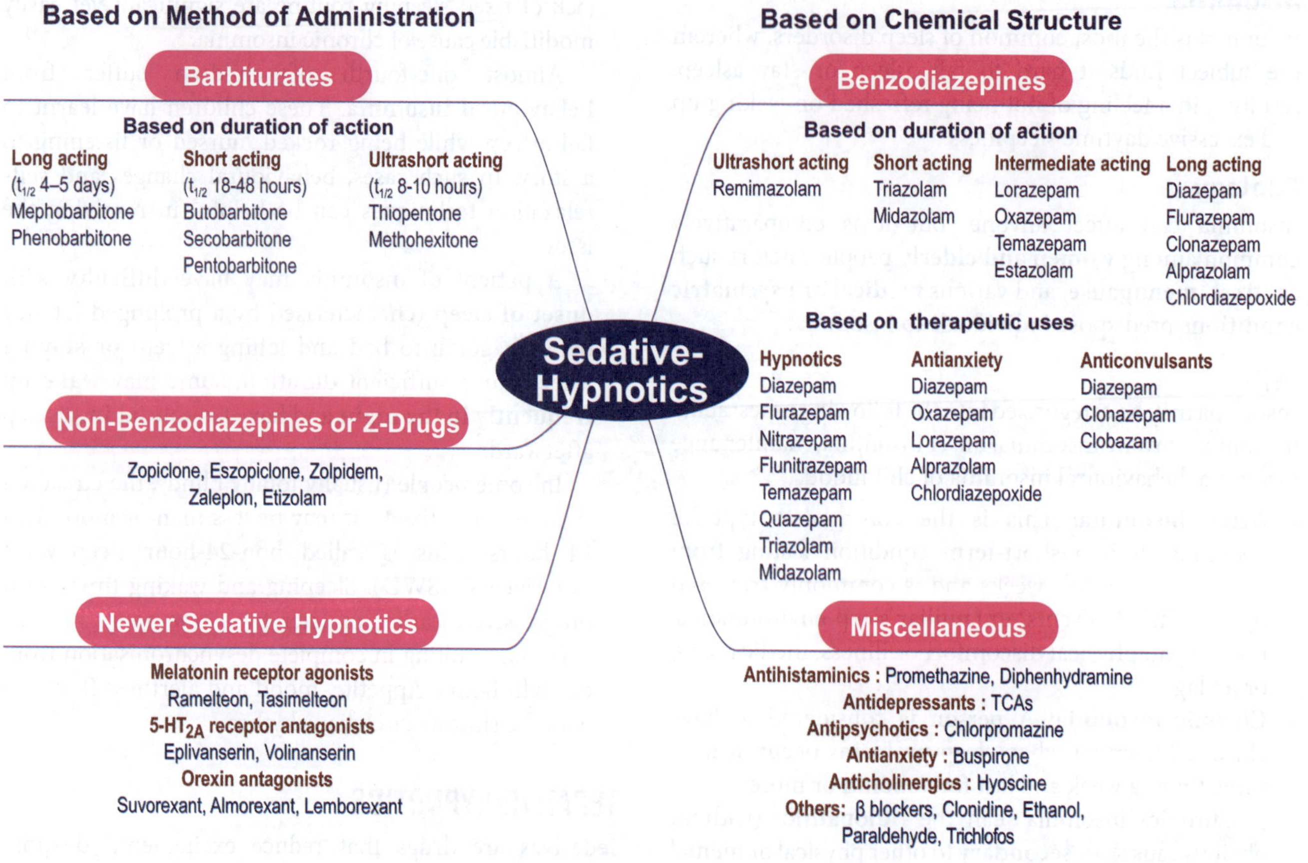

Sedative-Hypnotics
Based on Method of Administration
Barbiturates
Based on duration of action
Long acting
(t1/2 4–5 days)
Mephobarbitone
Phenobarbitone
Short acting
(t1/2 18-48 hours)
Butobarbitone
Secobarbitone
Pentobarbitone
Ultrashort acting
(t1/2 8-10 hours)
Thiopentone
Methohexitone
Non-Benzodiazepines or Z-Drugs
Zopiclone, Eszopiclone, Zolpidem,
Zaleplon, Etizolam
Newer Sedative Hypnotics
Melatonin receptor agonists
Ramelteon, Tasimelteon
5-HT2A receptor antagonists
Eplivanserin, Volinanserin
Orexin antagonists
Suvorexant, Almorexant, Lemborexant
Based on Chemical Structure
Benzodiazepines
Based on duration of action
Ultrashort acting
Remimazolam
Short acting
Triazolam
Midazolam
Intermediate acting
Lorazepam
Oxazepam
Temazepam
Estazolam
Long acting
Diazepam
Flurazepam
Clonazepam
Alprazolam
Chlordiazepoxide
Based on therapeutic uses
Hypnotics
Diazepam
Flurazepam
Nitrazepam
Flunitrazepam
Temazepam
Quazepam
Triazolam
Midazolam
Antianxiety
Diazepam
Oxazepam
Lorazepam
Alprazolam
Chlordiazepoxide
Anticonvulsants
Diazepam
Clonazepam
Clobazam
Miscellaneous
Antihistaminics : Promethazine, Diphenhydramine
Antidepressants : TCAs
Antipsychotics : Chlorpromazine
Antianxiety : Buspirone
Anticholinergics : Hyoscine
Others: β blockers, Clonidine, Ethanol,
Paraldehyde, Trichlofos

Flowchart 15.1 Classification of sedative-hypnotics

Table 15.1 Stages of sleep cycle

Stage	% of sleep time	Characteristics	EEG/brain waves activity
Stage 0 Awake	1–2% of total sleep time	- It lasts from the time an individual lies down to sleep to the time he/she falls asleep (sleep latency) - Irregular eye movements/ slow rolling	- EEG shows α waves when eyes are closed and β waves when eyes are open. - Wave frequency 15–50 Hz and amplitude < 50 μV, i.e., **high-frequency, low-amplitude activity**.
Stage 1 Transition between waking and sleep	3-6% of the total sleep time	- Indicates the **onset of sleep** - Eye movements are reduced, but there occur bursts of rolling. - Neck muscles relax. - Sometimes people feel a sensation of falling or abrupt muscular spasm (hypnic jerk) while drifting into or out of this stage.	- Brain wave activity begins to slow down. - EEG shows α waves interspersed with θ waves. - As sleep progresses, wave **frequency keeps on decreasing and amplitude keeps increasing.** - In this stage, frequency is 4–8 Hz and amplitude 50–100 μV.
Stage 2 Unequivocal sleep	40–60% of the total sleep time	- Slow moving eye rolling discontinues. - HR begins to slow. - Body temperature begins to decrease. - Subject is **easily arousable** by stimulation.	Brain waves continue to slow but there are bursts of rapid activity known as **K complex with spindle activity**, which probably protects the brain from awakening.
Stage 3 Deep sleep transition	5–15% of the total sleep time in adults. This stage is longer in children and adolescents.	- Negligible eye movements. - Subject is **not easily arousable** from this state.	- Slow waves known as δ **waves appear**. - K complex can be evoked only by strong stimulation.
Stage 4 Cerebral sleep	10–20% of the total sleep time	- Eyes are fixed. - Subject is **difficult to arouse**. - Parasomnias-like somnambulism (sleep-walking), somniloquy (sleep talking), night terrors and bed-wetting occur in this stage. - Stages **3 and 4 are the most restorative stages of sleep and are called SWS (slow wave sleep).** Deep sleep triggers the release of growth hormone (GH), which aids in muscle recovery from daily stress, supports the immune system, and rejuvenates the mind for learning and cognitive functioning on the following day. - At the same time, **deep sleep tends to decrease sleep drive.** Hence, a long afternoon nap up to the level of deep sleep results in difficulty in falling asleep at night. - Stages **2, 3 and 4 together constitute non-rapid eye movement (NREM)** sleep. In this, the muscles are relaxed and blood pressure and respiratory rate are steady.	- δ **waves are prominent.** - **K complexes cannot be evoked.**
REM (Rapid eye movement sleep) or dreaming stage or paradoxical sleep	20–25% of the total sleep time	- Marked, irregular, darting eye movements. - Heart rate, blood pressure, and respiratory rate rise. - Breathing is shallow and irregular, body loses some ability to regulate temperature. - Most recallable dreams and nightmares occur in this stage. Muscular atonia occurs, which protects subjects from acting out their dreams. - In male subjects, erection occurs. - The subject can be **easily aroused in REM** stage, but feels overly sleepy on waking up in this stage.	Brain wave activity is **as seen in awake stage.** K complexes cannot be evoked.

Mechanism of Action of Sedative-Hypnotics

Neuronal activity in midbrain reticular activating system (RAS) and limbic system is regulated by numerous inhibitory and excitatory inputs. The main excitatory neurotransmitter (NTM) is glutamate, and inhibitory NTM is gamma-aminobutyric acid (GABA).

GABA exerts its action through $GABA_A$ and $GABA_B$ receptors. **$GABA_A$ receptor** is a hetero-oligomeric glycoprotein consisting of pentameric structure and at least 3 different subunits, α, β and γ (epsilon, delta and rho subunits have also been proposed) that enclose a Cl^- channel (Fig. 15.2). Each subunit has four membrane-spanning domains. GABA binds to receptor sites on the α or β subunits and acts as a major inhibitory neurotransmitter in CNS.

Benzodiazepines, barbiturates, and zolpidem act at different sites on the $GABA_A$ receptor–Cl^- channel complex.

Barbiturates act at a site (on the α or β subunit) other than benzodiazepine receptor binding site and produce:

- GABA **facilitatory action** (i.e., they **increase the duration of Cl^- channel opening induced by GABA**).
- GABA **mimetic action** (i.e., at high concentrations, barbiturates **directly increase the Cl^- conductance, resulting in CNS depression**).
- They also enhance the binding of benzodiazepines to its receptors.
- At high concentrations, they decrease Ca^{2+}-dependent release of excitatory neurotransmitters and glutamate-induced depolarisation of neurons.
- At very high concentrations, Na^+ and K^+ channels are also depressed.

Benzodiazepines bind to a site at or near the γ_2 subunit and potentiate the GABAergic neurotransmission at all levels including the spinal cord, hypothalamus, hippocampus, substantia nigra, cerebral cortex and cerebellar cortex.

- Benzodiazepines do not substitute for GABA; however, they appear to enhance GABA's effects without direct activation of $GABA_A$ receptors or associated Cl^- channels. With benzodiazepines, there is an **increase in the frequency of channel opening events by GABA**. This may be in part due to increased affinity of the receptor for GABA.
- The **GABA facilitatory effect is more at the limbic system than reticular activating system (RAS)**. Hence, benzodiazepines produce anxiolytic effect at a dose that has negligible hypnotic effect.
- Benzodiazepines do not themselves increase Cl^- conductance, i.e., they **do not have GABA mimetic effect**. This explains the low-ceiling CNS depressant effect of benzodiazepines in comparison to barbiturates.
- The sedative-hypnotic, amnesic and anticonvulsant action of benzodiazepines are mediated through benzodiazepine receptors containing α_1 subunits, whereas the anxiolytic and muscle relaxant actions are mediated through benzodiazepine receptors containing α_2 subunits.
- Benzodiazepines have some additional mechanisms of action. At higher concentrations, they **potentiate depressant actions of adenosine** by blocking its uptake. Theophylline can reverse some actions of benzodiazepines by adenosine antagonism.

Drugs acting at different sites of $GABA_A$ receptor–Cl^- channel complex are summarised in Box 15.2.

Box 15.2 Drugs acting at the $GABA_A$ receptor–Cl^- channel complex

1. At $GABA_A$ binding site
   - Agonist: GABA, Muscimol
   - Competitive antagonist: Bicuculline
2. **At benzodiazepine binding site**
   - Agonist: Benzodiazepines
   - Competitive antagonist: Flumazenil
   - Non-competitive antagonist: Bicuculline
   - Inverse antagonist: Dimethyl carbomethoxy β-carbolines (DMCM)
3. At allosteric site
   - Agonist: Barbiturates
4. At Cl^- channel
   - Non-competitive blocker: Picrotoxin

Non-benzodiazepine drugs like zolpidem and zaleplon bind to the α_1 subunit of benzodiazepine receptors on the $GABA_A$ receptor–Cl^- channel complex. They exert amnesic, sedative, and hypnotic effect, but lack anticonvulsant and muscle relaxant actions.

BARBITURATES

Pharmacological Actions
CNS

Barbiturates exert **dose-dependent depressant effects** on CNS, ranging from sedation through hypnotic to anesthetic effect to coma. This may be due to depressant effect on

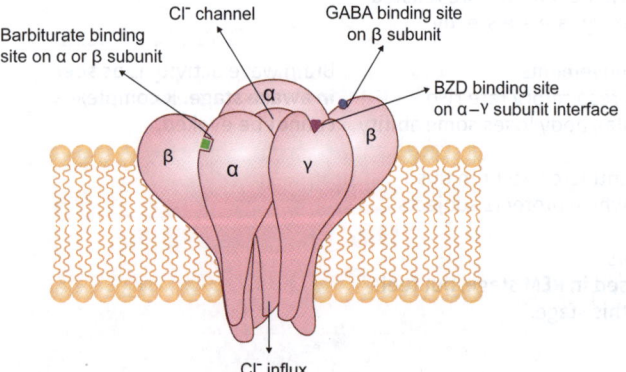

Fig. 15.2 $GABA_A$ receptor–chlorine channel complex

multiple neuronal targets (AMPA receptors, voltage-sensitive Na$^+$, K$^+$ channels) at higher concentrations.

- **Sedative** dose (smaller dose) reduces excitability/anxiety and causes drowsiness, impairment of short-term memory, learning and judgment.
- With higher dose, sleep latency decreases, total duration of sleep increases. The time spent in deep sleep (stage 3, 4) and REM is reduced, whereas, duration of stage 2 is increased. Thus, **barbiturates disturb the REM-NREM sleep cycle**, and after discontinuation of the drug, it takes several days for normal sleep pattern to be restored.
- In the morning, the patient experiences irritability, lethargy, headache and dizziness as hangover of the previous night's dose.
- Phenobarbitone possesses significant **anticonvulsant** effect. It increases the seizure threshold and limits the spread of seizures.

Other actions

Barbiturates may cause hyperalgesia. Higher doses **depress respiratory and cardiovascular function**, reducing contractility, heart rate and blood pressure. However, reflex tachycardia may occur. Toxic doses can cause cardiovascular and respiratory failure and are fatal.

Clinically Relevant Pharmacokinetic Characteristics

After oral administration, barbiturates are **well absorbed and widely distributed**. Individual drugs **cross the blood–brain barrier** at a rate determined by their lipid solubility.

The ultra short-acting barbiturate thiopentone sodium crosses the blood–brain barrier rapidly, exerts central action within one minute after intravenous injection, in the form of induction of anesthesia, and gets **redistributed** to less vascular, bulky tissues like muscle and fat. The redistribution terminates its action quickly, within 5–10 minutes. Later on, metabolism occurs in the liver and the inactive metabolites are excreted by the kidney.

Less lipid-soluble, intermediate-acting drugs like butobarbitone, secobarbitone and pentobarbitone are metabolised by phase I and phase II reactions in the liver. The long-acting drug phenobarbitone is, however, largely excreted unchanged by the kidney; its excretion can be enhanced by urinary alkalinisation.

Barbiturates influence the metabolism of several endogenous substances and simultaneously administered drugs due to the **induction of hepatic microsomal enzymes**. This results in the development of pharmacokinetic tolerance, precipitation of acute intermittent porphyria and interactions with other drugs (warfarin, tolbutamide, theophylline, contraceptives). However, the microsomal enzyme-inducing property of barbiturates is useful in managing congenital non-hemolytic jaundice, Cushing syndrome and chronic poisoning.

Therapeutic Uses

In current clinical practice, barbiturates find limited indications.

1. Phenobarbitone is still used in **generalised tonic-clonic and partial seizures as an 'add-on' drug**. The adult dose is 60 mg TDS.
2. Phenobarbitone may be useful due to its enzyme-inducing action in congenital **non-hemolytic jaundice, chronic poisonings, Cushing syndrome,** etc.
3. Thiopentone sodium 2.5% solution, injected intravenously in a dose of 3–5 mg/kg body weight is used for **induction of anesthesia**.
4. Intravenous thiopentone sodium (20 mg/kg in 10 mL normal saline) is used for active **euthanasia** and **capital punishment** in some countries (Belgium, Netherlands). In India, however, active euthanasia is not legal.

For sedative hypnotic action, barbiturates have been largely **superseded by other safer drugs** such as benzodiazepines and non-benzodiazepines or Z drugs.

Adverse Drug Reactions (ADRs)

- Hangover effects, such as headache, dizziness, and irritability, may occur the following morning after a nighttime dose of barbiturates for hypnotic effect.
- Long-term use (as in epilepsy) can lead to impaired memory, reduced cognitive function, poor judgment, and behavioural disturbances.
- Paradoxically, barbiturates may cause **hyperactivity in children and confusion in elderly people.**
- Both pharmacokinetic and pharmacodynamic **tolerance** develops to barbiturates. **Cross-tolerance** can occur with other CNS depressant drugs. **Dependence and abuse liability** is also seen. Abstinence/withdrawal symptoms occur as tremors, anxiety, nausea, vomiting, weakness, hallucinations, convulsions, and cardiac depression. It may even be fatal.
- Barbiturates can precipitate acute intermittent porphyria in susceptible individuals.
- **Acute poisoning** manifests as bullous eruptions over body, called barbiturate blisters, hypotension, shallow failing respiration, cardiovascular collapse, renal impairment, coma and death. Treatment is mainly supportive, comprising the following:
  - Gastric lavage with activated charcoal to prevent further absorption of drug is useful.
  - If poisoning is with phenobarbitone, alkaline diuresis can enhance renal exertion.
  - Hemodialysis through activated charcoal column is very useful. There is no specific antidote available for barbiturates.

Clinical problem-based questions and MCQs

1. **Barbiturates have been largely superseded by other sedative-hypnotics for sleep disturbances. However, phenobarbitone is still used in clinical practice.**
   i. Identify the indication for use of phenobarbitone.
      a. Partial seizures   b. Chronic insomnia
      c. Alcohol withdrawal   d. Anxiety
   ii. Describe the mechanism of action of phenobarbitone with the help of a suitable diagram.
   iii. Enumerate the adverse effects of phenobarbitone.

2. **Identify the drug having shortest duration of action among the following.**
   a. Secobarbitone   b. Butobarbitone
   b. Pentobarbitone   d. Methohexitone

3. **A 9-year-old boy with nephritic syndrome was treated with glucocorticoids for a long time. The patient reports with a cushingoid face, buffalo hump, thinning of skin. The patient receives phenobarbitone therapy that achieves reversal of symptoms to some extent.** Describe the pharmacological basis for the beneficial effect of phenobarbitone in this case.

4. **Thiopentone sodium is an ultra-short-acting barbiturate, preferred for induction of anesthesia. Identify the statement that correctly explains the reason of short duration of its action.**
   a. Redistribution to less vascular organs
   b. Microsomal enzyme induction, causing quickening of metabolism
   c. Direct effect on GABA receptor–chloride channel complex
   d. Quick excretion through glomerular filtration

5. **A 10-year-old girl presents in pediatrics OPD with pyrexia of unknown origin (PUO). There is no sign, symptom or investigation suggesting hepatitis. HBV and HCV tests are negative. Medication history elicits the use of phenobarbitone for the past 5 years after an attack of generalised tonic–clonic seizures. Routine investigations show pus cells in urine, raised AST and ALT. Serum bilirubin is low. The patient is diagnosed with UTI.**
   What is the cause of raised AST, ALT and low bilirubin?

BENZODIAZEPINES

Pharmacological Actions

CNS

Unlike barbiturates, benzodiazepines are not general depressants of whole of the CNS. The **site of action of individual drugs in CNS determines their prominent effects.**

- Midbrain reticular activating system (**RAS**) maintains wakefulness. GABA facilitatory effect of benzodiazepines at this site brings about the **sedative-hypnotic** effect. They reduce sleep latency and intermittent awakenings. Total sleep time, and duration of stage 2 is increased, whereas stages 3 and 4 become shorter. Duration of REM is also reduced, but more REM cycles occur, so that the net effect on REM sleep is less marked than with barbiturates. Night terrors are reduced and the patient wakes up with a feeling of having had a refreshing sleep. **Tolerance develops** to this action with repeated use. The hypnotic effect is prominent with diazepam, lorazepam, temazepam, flurazepam, nitrazepam, flunitrazepam, midazolam and triazolam.

- **Limbic system** is concerned with thought and mental function. Excessive GABAergic activity at this site results in **anxiolytic action** of benzodiazepines. The anxiolytic action seems to be independent of their sedative action, because with chronic use **tolerance develops to sedative action but not to anxiolytic effect.** This is prominent with diazepam, oxazepam, lorazepam and alprazolam.

- **Muscular relaxation and ataxia** occur due to their action on the medulla and cerebellum, respectively. Clonazepam and diazepam cause centrally-mediated skeletal muscle relaxation without impairing voluntary activity.

- **Anticonvulsant effect** is prominent with diazepam, clonazepam and clobazem. **Tolerance develops** to this action also.

- High dose of benzodiazepines can cause- **anterograde amnesia,** which is an inability to recall events that occurred during the time of the drug effect, though some degree of awareness is maintained.

Other actions

Intravenous diazepam causes analgesia and temporary coronary dilatation. Diazepam also reduces basal gastric secretions.

Pharmacokinetics

Different members of the benzodiazepine group **vary in lipid solubility**, and thus, in the **time course** (duration) of their action (refer to Flowchart 15.1). There are vast differences in the rate of absorption after oral administration, extent of plasma protein binding and duration of central action. They are metabolised in the liver. Formation of **active metabolites** and **enterohepatic circulation** may increase the duration of action of drugs like diazepam and flurazepam.

Therapeutic Uses

Due to variations in receptor selectivity and time course of action, different drugs of this group are employed for distinct clinical indications.

1. Benzodiazepines are **preferred over barbiturates as sedative-hypnotic** for treatment of short-term **insomnia** with anxiety and chronic insomnia. Triazolam (0.125–0.25 mg) and temazepam (10–20 mg) are the preferred drugs in patients having difficulty in falling asleep, and nitrazepam (30 mg), lorazepam

(10–20 mg) diazepam (30–60 mg) in patients with frequent awakenings or difficulty in staying asleep for an adequate period of time.

Benzodiazepines are a better choice than barbiturates because:

i. Benzodiazepines exhibit a **low-ceiling CNS depressant effect**, meaning that even at high doses, they typically do not cause loss of consciousness. At hypnotic doses, they do not produce significant cardiovascular or respiratory depression. Sedation, hypnosis and general anesthesia represent increasing grades of CNS depression. Hypnosis involves more pronounced depression of CNS than sedation. So, the same drug acts as sedatives at low dose, hypnotics at a higher dose and may cause general anesthesia and coma at still higher doses. Drugs with a flat dose–response curve (like benzodiazepines) have a wider margin of safety compared to those with a steep dose–response curve, such as barbiturates (see Fig. 15.3). As a result, benzodiazepines are considered safer and have a higher therapeutic index than barbiturates.

ii. Benzodiazepines cause **less disturbance to sleep architecture** compared to barbiturates.

iii. Upon discontinuation, **rebound phenomena are less marked** with benzodiazepines.

iv. Benzodiazepines **do not have prominent effects on other organ systems.** I/V administration of diazepam may cause fall in BP and coronary dilatation.

v. **Mild tolerance** develops to sedative-hypnotic and anticonvulsant actions. **Dependence, abuse liability and withdrawal symptoms are much lesser** than with barbiturates.

vi. Benzodiazepines **do not have enzyme-inducing property**. So, the chances of pharmacokinetic interactions with other co-administered drugs are lower.

vii. Flumazenil is a **specific antidote** available for benzodiazepine poisoning, whereas for barbiturate poisoning, supportive therapy is the only choice.

2. Diazepam 0.2–0.3 mg/kg body weight (slow I/V) is useful for controlling **status epilepticus and febrile convulsions**. Lorazepam (0.1 mg/kg body weight) is the drug of choice in status epilepticus. Clonazepam can be used for **akinetic epilepsy** and **myoclonic jerks in a dose varying from 0.5–5 mg, thrice a day.** However, tolerance develops soon to their antiseizure action.

3. Benzodiazepines, especially alprazolam(0.25–0.5 mg) is used **as an anxiolytic**; they are uesful in panic disorders as well.

4. Benzodiazepines are useful in **muscle spasms**, spasticity of upper motor neuron lesions, spinal injuries and tetanus.

5. Benzodiazepines are useful in **pre-anesthetic medication** because of their sedative and amnesic effect. **Midazolam 1–2.5 mg IV is preferred** over other benzodiazepines for anesthetic use and as continuous IV infusion (0.02–0.1 mg/kg/hour) in critical care anesthesia due to its rapid onset and short duration of action.

6. Diazepam, midazolam and lorazepam are used for **inducing, maintaining and supplementing anesthesia and for conscious sedation.** For procedures like ECT, endoscopy, cardiac catheterisation and fracture reduction, benzodiazepines are frequently used. Remimazolam is used for sedation in procedures of < 30 minutes duration.

7. Chlordiazepoxide is preferred over clorazepate and diazepam for patients with alcohol dependence. Benzodiazepines control **alcohol withdrawal symptoms** in these patients.

8. They also provide relief in **non-specific dyspepsia**.

Adverse Effects

- They have a **wider margin of safety** compared to barbiturates. However, their hypnotic doses can cause **vertigo, dizziness, disorientation, ataxia and impairment of psychomotor skills.**
- **Hangover** is seen with longer-acting benzodiazepines given in larger doses.
- In some patients, there may be paradoxical **irritability** and nightmares, more frequently observed with flurazepam.
- Flunitrazepam is tasteless and is misused for 'date rape'.
- Slowly, **tolerance** develops to sedative effect. Their abuse liability and potential to cause dependence is low. **Mild withdrawal symptoms** like restlessness, anxiety, insomnia and nightmare may occur. In rare instances, convulsions may occur.
- Use of diazepam during childbirth can cause **respiratory depression in the newborn.**

Cautions/Contraindications

Benzodiazepines should be avoided in pregnancy, liver disease and acute angle closure glaucoma.

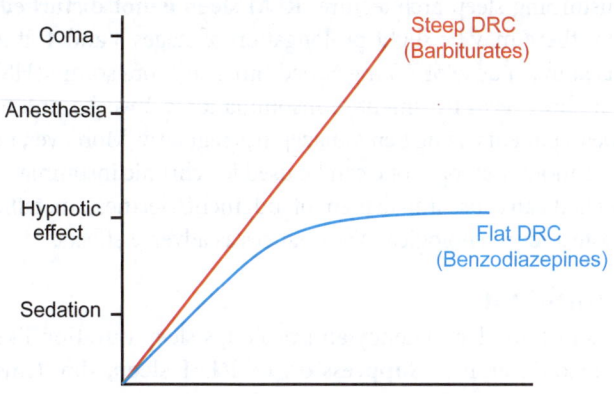

Fig. 15.3 Steep/flat DRC for sedative-hypnotics

Interactions

- Benzodiazepines have additive action with alcohol and other CNS depressants.
- Enzyme inhibitors like ketoconazole, isoniazid and oral contraceptives reduce the metabolism of benzodiazepines and thus, prolong their duration of action.

Flumazenil

Flumazenil is a **competitive antagonist** at benzodiazepine receptors. It blocks sedative-hypnotic, anxiolytic, muscle relaxant, and anti-convulsant actions of benzodiazepines. It has low oral bioavailability and is hence used intravenously in a dose of 0.2 mg/minute in benzodiazepine toxicity. The symptoms are controlled within 5 minutes. The hypnotic effect of Z drugs is also blocked. Adverse effects may occur in the form of **anxiety, agitation, restlessness** and rarely, **convulsions**.

Clinical problem-based questions and MCQs

6. A 36-year-old man with a history of alcohol abuse and chronic anxiety visits medicine OPD with sleeping problems. He complains of inability to sleep after lying in bed for a long time, even when he is tired after a long day's work.
   i. Which of the following drugs is most suitable in this case to reduce sleep latency?
      a. Phenobarbitone   b. Diazepam
      b. Nitrazepam   d. Triazolam
   ii. Give pharmacological basis to justify your choice.

7. Which of the following differences in the mechanism of action of barbiturates and benzodiazepines results in better safety margin of benzodiazepines?
   a. BZDs are more selective than barbiturates on $GABA_A$ receptors.
   b. BZDs are partial agonists but barbiturates are full agonists on $GABA_A$ receptors.
   c. BZDs are GABA facilitatory, but barbiturates are GABA mimetic as well.
   d. Benzodiazepines are GABA mimetic but barbiturates are GABA facilitatory.

8. A 55-year-old male patient visits medicine OPD. He is a known case of peptic ulcer disease, type 2 DM and moderate hypertension. The patient is taking multiple medications for these conditions. Since the last 6 months, diazepam is also being given to reduce his anxiety.
   Which of the following is most expected adverse effect of diazepam?
   a. Loss of ability to taste
   b. Dyspnea
   c. Anterograde amnesia
   d. Muscular dystonia

9. A psychiatrist examines the following four patients of chronic anxiety in his OPD. Benzodiazepines are being considered for managing anxiety.
   In which of the patients is this drug class most suitable?
   a. 25-year-old primigravida who is 12 weeks pregnant
   b. 36-year-old man with history suggestive of gastro-esophageal reflux disease
   c. 60-year-old woman with acute angle closure glaucoma
   d. 50-year-old male with alcoholic liver disease

10. A 16-year-old boy is brought to emergency in unconscious state. His mother informs that the boy was under immense stress because of his medical entrance exam due the next day. She fears that boy has probably ingested all her insomnia prescription pills and shows the empty pill bottle. On examination, RR is 12 breaths per minute.
    i. Identify a drug most suitable for this case.
       a. Amphetamine   b. Adrenaline
       c. Prednisolone   d. Flumazenil
    ii. Describe the mechanism of beneficial effect, dose used and possible adverse effects of the drug chosen for this case.

NON-BENZODIAZEPINES OR 'Z' DRUGS

These include zolpidem, zopiclone, eszopiclone, zaleplon and etizolam.

- These are chemically different from benzodiazepines but act selectively through the α_1 **subunit containing $GABA_A$ benzodiazepine receptors**.
- For this reason, hypnotic and amnesic effects are prominent, but **antianxiety, muscle relaxant and anticonvulsant effects are negligible.**
- Abuse liability is lower.
- Duration of action is shorter as compared to benzodiazepines.

Thus, they are **preferred** nowadays for the treatment of insomnias.

Zopiclone

Like benzodiazepines, it exerts hypnotic effect without disturbing sleep architecture. **REM sleep is not disturbed**, but there may be slight prolongation of stages 3 and 4. It is used in a a dose of 7.5 mg at bed time, i.e., hora somni (HS) for short-term treatment of insomnia for < 2 weeks, and to wean patients using benzodiazepines regularly. Moreover, its enantiomer eszopiclone can be used for chronic insomnia as well. It can cause impairment of judgment/alertness, metallic taste and psychological disturbances as adverse effects.

Zolpidem

It shortens sleep latency and prolongs sleep duration like benzodiazepines. **Suppression of REM sleep, day time** sedation, tolerance and dependence are negligible. There is no rebound phenomenon on stopping the drug. It is useful for sleep onset insomnia and intermittent awakenings, in a dose of 5–10 mg given at bed time. If administered late night, some daytime sedation may occur. It is a very safe drug, with no respiratory depressant action.

Zaleplon

It is rapidly absorbed, rapidly metabolised and has no active metabolites. Because of these pharmacokinetic characteristics, it has brief duration of action and is used **only for patients with difficulty in falling asleep**. It can be taken at late night without any risk of daytime sedation or drowsiness. Inspite of the short duration of action, rebound insomnia or anxiety is not reported with zaleplon. No tolerance or dependence is reported.

Etizolam

A thienodiazepine having sedative, hypnotic, muscle relaxant and anticonvulsant actions, its hypnotic action is 10 times more potent than that of diazepam. As a result, abuse potential is high.

NEWER SEDATIVE-HYPNOTICS

Ramelteon

Melatonin is a hormone secreted by the pineal gland. It maintains a normal circadian rhythm underlying the sleep–wake cycle. Ramelteon has **agonistic effect on melatonin receptors** (MT1 and MT2), without any direct effect on GABAergic transmission. It does not alter sleep architecture. No rebound phenomenon and dependence is reported. Abuse liability is negligible. It is the **drug of choice for sleep onset insomnia, shift workers and jet lag**. Adverse effects like fatigue, dizziness and sleepiness are observed.

Tasimelteon is used for non-24 hour sleep–wake disorder.

Eplivanserin and Volinanserin

These drugs are antagonists at 5-HT$_{2A}$ receptors. They have minimal effect on onset of sleep, but are good for sleep maintenance.

Suvorexant, Daridorexant, Almorexant and Lemborexant

These are dual orexin receptor antagonists (DORA). Orexin or hypocretin is a neuropeptide that regulates wakefulness, arousal and appetite. These are drugs of choice for sleep maintenance. If response is not adequate, Z drugs are tried.

The most important adverse effect associated with the use of DORA is the worsening of depressive disorder and suicidal tendency.

Clinical problem-based questions and MCQs

11. Which Z-drug is used only for sleep latency problem and may be given at late night without risk of daytime drowsiness?
    a. Eszopiclone   b. Zaleplon
    c. Zolpidem   d. None

12. Enumerate Z drugs and their advantages over benzodiazepines.

13. A hypnotic mimicking the effect of an endogenous hormone is prescribed to a medical student facing trouble in falling asleep due to stress of completing his project on time.
    Identify the drug given.
    a. Ramelteon   b. Zopiclone
    c. Temazepam   d. Zolpidem

14. Which of the following drugs is abused for date rape and why?
    a. Thiopentone   a. Zolpidem
    b. Flunitrazepam c. Midazolam

15. All of the following drugs are useful in sleep onset insomnia except
    a. Triazolam   b. Zaleplon
    c. Ramelteon   d. Volinanserin

16. Match the drug with its mechanism of action:
    a. Thiopentone   1. 5-HT$_{2A}$ antagonist
    b. Ramelteon   2. Increased frequency of Cl$^-$ channel opening
    c. Triazolam   3. Dual orexin receptor antagonist
    d. Suvorexant   4. Melatonin receptor agonist
    e. Volinanserin   5. GABA mimetic action

MANAGEMENT OF ANXIETY DISORDERS

Anxiety is a **normal fight-or-flight emotional response to a stressful situation**. As defined by the American Psychological Association (APA), anxiety is "an emotion characterised by feelings of tension, worried thoughts and physical changes like raised BP". It is an **unpleasant** emotional state, characterised by fear, discomfort, uneasiness and somatic symptoms like palpitation, anorexia, and dyspnea. Anxiety commonly occurs in association with phobias, stress, obsessive compulsive disorders and some neurotic disorders.

Anxiety disorders are the **most prevalent psychiatric illnesses**, in which the duration and severity of unpleasant anxious feeling is much more than the normal emotional response to a given trigger or situation that causes distress and marked impairment of performance. Anxiety disorders can occur as generalised anxiety disorder (GAD), panic attacks, phobias, obsessive compulsive disorders (OCD) and stress disorders.

Anxiety disorders are characterised by:
- **Psychological symptoms:** Fear or phobia, tension, apprehension, lack of concentration, feeling of being on the edge and sleep disturbances.
- **Somatic symptoms:** GIT distress, anorexia, gastric hurrying, fatigue, tremors, dizziness, hyperventilation, breathlessness, paresthesias, tightness in the chest, etc.
- **Autonomic symptoms:** Tachycardia, palpitation, sweating
- In addition, patients of generalised anxiety disorder are at high risk of suffering from major depression, dysthymia and substance abuse, especially with alcohol and sedative-hypnotics.

The treatment of anxiety disorder involves **psychotherapy and antianxiety (anxiolytic) drugs**. Psychotherapy is mainstay of treatment in anxiety disorders and is quite effective in cases of recent onset. The aim of psychotherapy is to reassure and encourage patients for adequately adjusting with environment. Patient is reassured and supported to enable them to stay confident while facing new situations, to learn to fight negative thoughts and be comfortable with his/her own presence. Psychological counseling, cognitive therapy, relaxation therapy is useful. Behavioural therapy intends to desensitise the patient to phobic stimulus, in which patients are repeatedly exposed to the situation which precipitates anxiety or panic attacks in a guarded environment, with moral support and reassurance. Drug therapy aims at rapid symptom relief. Anxiolytic effect involves CNS depression of a degree lesser than sedation.

ANTIANXIETY DRUGS
Classification
Antianxiety drugs encompass various groups as depicted in Flowchart 15.2.

1. Benzodiazepines
Benzodiazepines with slow, prolonged action are useful in controlling anxiety when administered in low doses. Drugs in this group vary in their potency, pharmacokinetics (lipid solubility, elimination mode, half-life, presence of active metabolites) and duration of action.
- **Alprazolam** has high potency and slight mood deviating effect. It is used in a dose of 0.25–1 mg, thrice a day for **severe anxiety associated with depression and panic disorders**.
- **Lorazepam** has no active metabolites and is useful in **short-lasting anxiety** states and panic disorders.
- **Diazepam** produces strong initial effect followed by prolonged mild effect. It is useful in **acute panic attacks** as well as anxiety associated with organic diseases in a dose of 5–20 mg.
- **Chlordiazepoxide** has slow absorption and produces active metabolites. Thus, it is suitable for smooth, prolonged effect in **chronic anxiety** states.
- BZDs are sometimes combined with antidepressant drugs for initial weeks and then slowly tapered off. The dose of benzodiazepines is reduced by 10% every one or two weeks; slowly, these are discontinued over 6–12 weeks.

The general rule is to **use benzodiazepines in lowest possible dose for the shortest possible duration.** Short course of benzodiazepines is given on an 'as and when required' basis, depending on symptoms. The duration should not exceed 4–6 weeks.

2. Azapirones
Buspirone, gepirone and ipsapirone are non-benzodiazepines. Their exact mechanism of action is not clear. They have **partial agonistic action at 5-HT$_{1A}$** receptors, and also **D$_2$ blocking** effect.

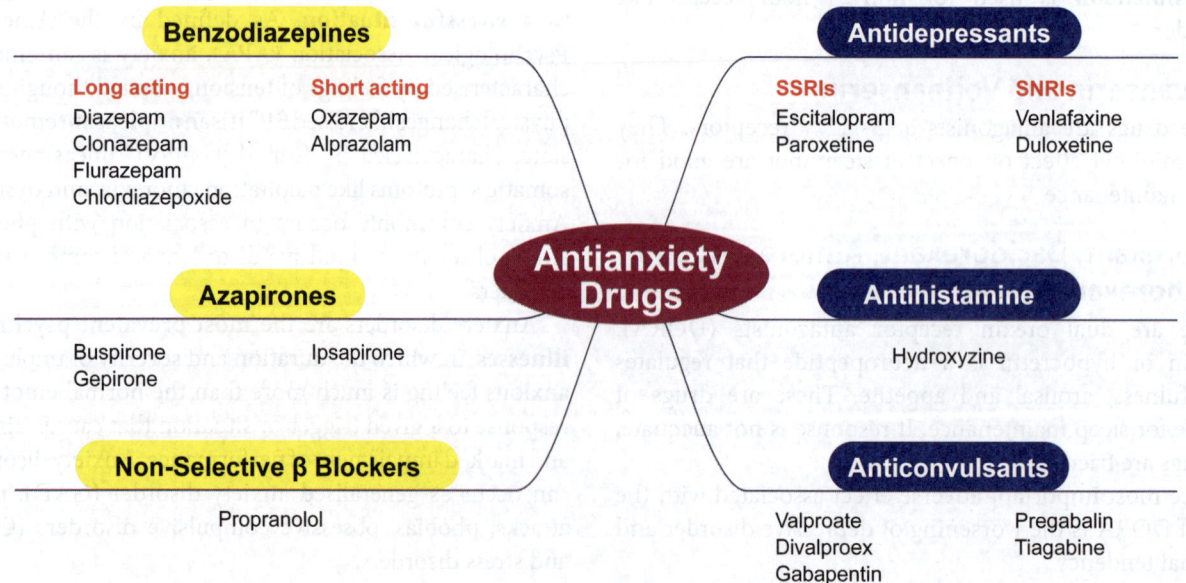

Flowchart 15.2 Classification of antianxiety drugs

As an antianxiety drug, the **efficacy of buspirone is comparable** to benzodiazepines but it **differs in following aspects**:

- Buspirone lacks sedative-hypnotic and generalised CNS depressant effects.
- Does not have additive effect with other CNS depressants like alcohol.
- Does not interfere much with motor functions, hence it is suitable in elderly people.
- Buspirone has no abuse liability.
- It also lacks muscle relaxant and anticonvulsant action.

One of its metabolites is a potent antagonist at α_2 receptors. This may be involved in the rise in BP with buspirone in patients on MAO inhibitor therapy. The effect of buspirone can be reversed by an α_2 agonists like clonidine.

Buspirone is **FDA-approved for short-term as well as long-term treatment of generalised anxiety disorders** in a dose of 5–10 mg, once to thrice daily. It has to be administered for 2–4 weeks before the effect becomes manifest. Hence it is **not effective in 'as needed' treatment** for acute anxiety.

Adverse effects to buspirone occur in the form of nausea, abdominal discomfort, headache, light headedness, dizziness and nervousness.

Gepirone is similar to buspirone. It has negligible D_2 blocking effect. Ipsapirone also has antidepressant and anxiolytic effects.

1. **Role of antidepressants in anxiety disorder:** Selective serotonin reuptake inhibitors (SSRIs) like escitalopram, paroxetine and selective serotonin and norepinephrine reuptake inhibitors (SNRIs) like venlafaxine and duloxetine are extensively used in chronic anxiety. They are the **drugs of choice for GAD, obsessive compulsive disorders, panic attacks and anxiety associated with addiction.** At the onset of therapy, they are combined with benzodiazepines for 4–6 weeks. Once the effect of antidepressants is established, BZD can be slowly tapered off.
2. **Non-selective beta blocker propranolol** relieves peripheral somatic symptoms due to sympathetic overactivity like tremors, tachycardia, palpitation, raised BP and gastric hurrying. These symptoms have an anxiety reinforcing effect, which is controlled by β blockers. The role of β blockers in anxiety is limited as adjuvants to benzodiazepines and in situational anxiety.
3. **Hydroxyzine** is an antihistaminic drug with marked sedative effect. Hydroxyzine is used only for the anxiety cases not responding to other drugs.
4. **Barbiturates** have largely been superseded by other drugs in the treatment of anxiety.
5. **Anticonvulsants** may be useful as alternatives to SSRIs in panic attacks and phobic disorders.

Clinical problem-based questions and MCQs

17. A 24-year-old medical student complained of severe anxiety during public speaking, discomfort in talking to strangers and seniors, and a fear that people would shout at him and embarrass him. He had experienced these symptoms since his teens and consistently avoided such situations. His worst moments frequently flash through his mind during idle times, causing distress and irritability. According to DSM-V criteria, he is diagnosed with social anxiety disorder.
    i. What are the various drugs that may be useful in this patient?
    ii. Describe mechanism of action of buspirone.
    iii. What are the advantages of buspirone over benzodiazepines.
18. A 40-year-old male patient presented with difficulty in breathing, but general physical and chest examinations were inconclusive. There was no medical explanation for the symptoms experienced by the patient. Due to this, he felt stressed, confused, and angry. Careful history taking revealed that several episodes had occurred over the past 4–5 months, during which the patient experienced intense fear of climbing a high peak and falling, accompanied by palpitations, sweating, breathing difficulty, and chest discomfort. During these episodes, he felt that death was imminent. He admitted to constantly worrying about such episodes and had begun avoiding unfamiliar places due to his fear, preferring to stay at home. His wife felt that his behaviour and fear were irrational. He was prescribed tablet escitalopram 10 mg daily.
    i. What is the probable diagnosis?
    ii. What is the role of escitalopram in this patient?
    iii. Describe the mechanism of action of escitalopram.
    iv. Enumerate other drugs that may be useful in this patient.
19. Name the drug of choice in following conditions.
    i. Myoclonic seizures
    ii. Chronic anxiety
    iii. Acute severe anxiety
    iv. Sleep onset insomnia
19. Comment on the role of propranolol in generalised anxiety disorder.

Summary

- Sedation, hypnosis and general anesthesia represent increasing grades of CNS depression. Sedatives make a person drowsy, but do not induce sleep. Hypnotics help in inducing or maintaining sleep.
- Sedative-hypnotics include barbiturates, benzodiazepines, Z drugs, melatonin agonists $5\text{-}HT_{2A}$ and dual orexin receptor antagonists.

- Barbiturates increase the duration of chloride channel opening by GABA (GABA facilitatory) and GABA mimetic actions. They also reduce glutamate release. They are not preferred as sedative-hypnotics but are still used in GTCS, partial seizures (phenobarbitone) and induction of anesthesia (thiopentone sodium).
- Drawbacks of barbiturates include hangover, disturbed REM–NREM sleep cycle; they can cause cardiovascular and respiratory depression at high doses, impaired cognition, memory and judgment, risk of interactions with many drugs due to microsomal enzyme induction, and acute intermittent porphyria in susceptible individuals.
- Benzodiazepines are preferred over barbiturates as hypnotics for insomnia treatment as these have fewer adverse effects, and less abuse potential and dependence. A specific antidote, flumazenil, is available in the case of acute poisoning with BZDs. Alprazolam is the preferred drug in anxiety disorders. Triazolam and temazepam are short-acting drugs useful for reducing sleep latency, whereas diazepam, lorazepam and nitrazepam are useful in patients with frequent night awakenings and difficulty to stay asleep for adequate time.
- BZDs are avoided in liver disease, alcoholism, angle closure glaucoma and along with alcohol/ other CNS depressants.
- Z drugs like zolpidem, zopiclon, zaleplon are preferred nowadays. These act on the α_1 subunit containing $GABA_A$-benzodiazepine receptors. They possess hypnotic and amnesic effects; antianxiety, muscle relaxant and anticonvulsant effects are negligible. They have less abuse liability and shorter duration of action as compared to benzodiazepines.
- Newer sedative-hypnotics include ramelteon (melatonin agonist), epivalserin, volinanserin (5-HT_{2A} antagonist) and suvorexant (orexin receptor antagonist).
- Anxiety is an unpleasant emotional state characterised by fear, discomfort, uneasiness and somatic symptoms like palpitation, anorexia, and dyspnea. These occur as GAD, phobias, panic attacks or OCD. Benzodiazepines, azapirones, antidepressants, propranolol, etc. are used
- Diazepam is used for acute panic attack, anxiety of organic diseases, Aalprazolam for anxiety associated with panic attack and depression, lorazepam for short-lasting anxiety and chlordiazepoxide for chronic anxiety
- Azapirones such as buspirone, ipsapirone, and gepirone act as partial agonists at 5-HT_{1A} receptors. They exhibit **efficacy comparable** to that of benzodiazepines but do not possess sedative-hypnotic, muscle relaxant, and anticonvulsant properties. They do not have abuse liability and generalised CNS depressant effect and do not interfere much with motor functions. These are useful for managing both short-term as well as long-lerm anxiety.
- Propranolol reduces peripheral symptoms of anxiety and antidepressants have a role in panic disorders.

Questions for practice

1. Explain why benzodiazepines are preferred over barbiturates as sedative-hypnotics.
2. Enumerate therapeutic uses and adverse effects of benzodiazepines.
3. Describe the mechanism of action of benzodiazepines.
4. Write short notes on
   a. Flumazenil   b. Non-benzodiazepine sedatives
   c. Ramelteon   d. Azapirones

Hints for problem-based questions and MCQs

1. i. a. Partial seizures
   ii. Refer to Fig. 15.2, page 200
   iii. Refer to page 201.
2. d. Methohexitone
3. Enzyme induction improves metabolism and excretion of corticosteroids.
4. a. Redistribution to less vascular organs quickly terminates the action of thiopentone sodium.
5. Chronic phenobaritone intake causes enzyme induction, and increase in levels of AST and ALT.
6. i. d. Triazolam
   ii. Barbiturates are not preferred for hypnotic effect. Refer to page 203 for reasons. Triazolam is preferred for such cases. Diazepam and nitrazepam are useful in cases with difficulty in staying asleep, but not in the present case.
7. c. BZDs are GABA facilitatory, but barbiturates GABA mimetic as well.
8. c. Anterograde amnesia
9. b. A 36-year-old man with history suggestive of gastro-esophageal reflux disease and chronic anxiety is a suitable patient for prescribing benzodiazepines. For the other three options, BZDs are avoided.
10. i. d. Flumazenil
    ii. Competitive antagonist at BZD receptor. Refer to page 204.
11. b. Zaleplon
12. Refer to page 204.
13. a. Ramelteon
14. c. Flunitrazepam, as it is tasteless.
15. Volinanserin
16. a–5; b–4; c–2; d–3; e–1.
17. i. Refer to page 206 for classification of antianxiety drugs.
    ii. Refer to page 206.
    iii. Refer to page 207.
18. i. Panic disorder
    ii. Refer to page 207 for the role of antidepressants in panic disorders.
    iii. Selective serotonin reuptake inhibitor
    iv. Paroxetine, venlafaxine, duloxetine
19. a. Clonazepam   b. Chlordiazepoxide
    c. Alprazolam   d. Ramelteon
20. Propranolol reduces peripheral symptoms of anxiety. Refer to page 207.

Chapter 15 Sedative-Hypnotics and Anxiolytics

CONCEPT MAP - SEDATIVE HYPNOTICS

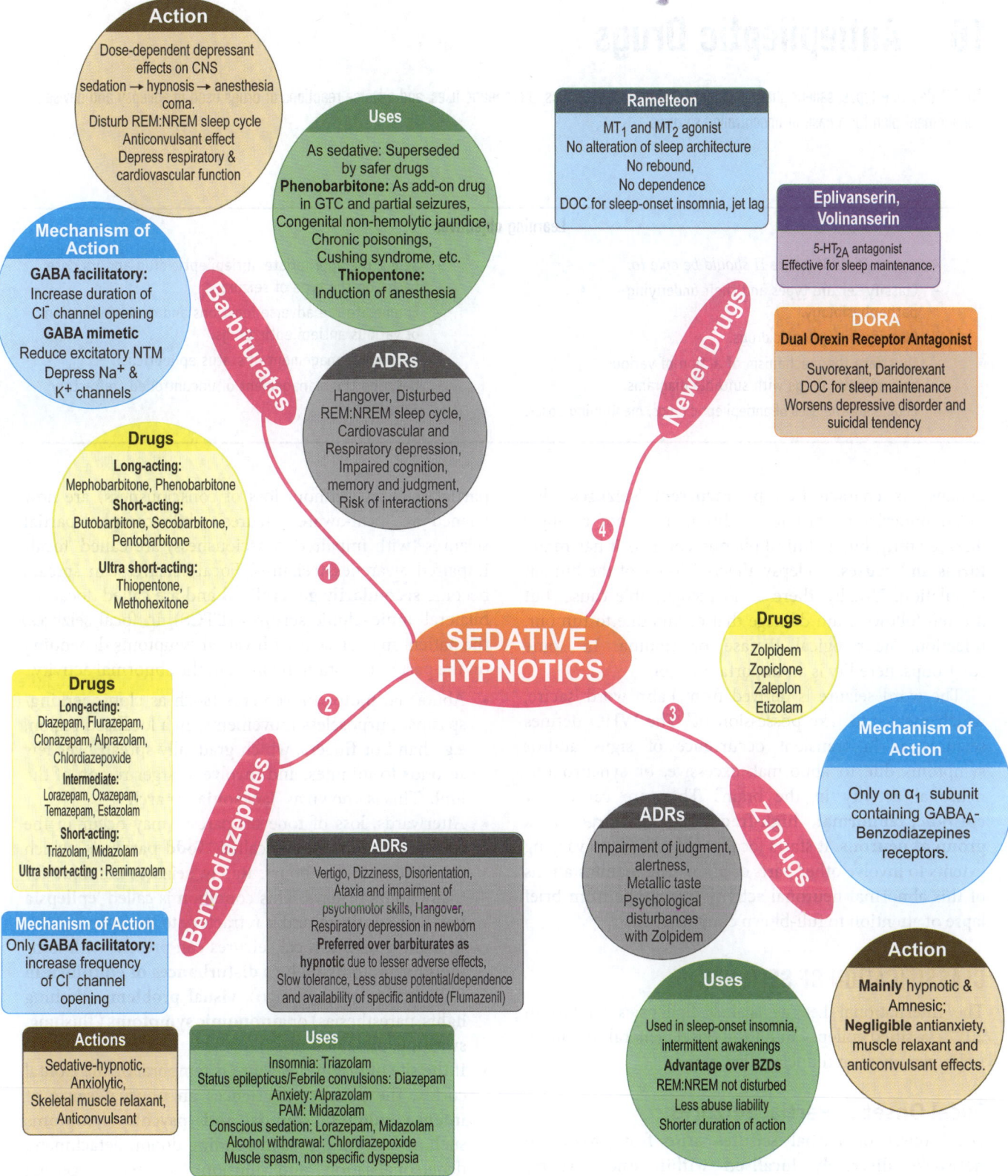

SECTION 3 Drugs Acting on CNS

16 Antiepileptic Drugs

PH 3.3 Describe types, salient pharmacokinetics, pharmacodynamics, therapeutic uses, and adverse reactions of drugs used in epilepsy and devise a management plan for a case of uncontrolled seizures.

Learning objectives

A student of MBBS phase II should be able to:
- Classify seizure types and their underlying pathophysiology.
- Classify antiepileptic drugs.
- Illustrate the mechanism of action of various antiepileptic drugs with suitable diagrams.
- Enumerate the uses of antiepileptic drugs, mentioning doses.
- Select the appropriate antiepileptic drug and its dose based on the type of seizure.
- Enumerate the adverse reactions and contraindications of various antiepileptic drugs.
- Describe management of status epilepticus.
- Describe the management of uncontrolled (refractory) seizures.

Epilepsy is characterised by **recurrent 'seizures'** due to an underlying chronic condition. It is not a single disease entity, but a clinical phenomenon, as it has **many forms and causes**. Epilepsy affects 0.5–1% of the human population. Usually, there is no recognisable cause, but it often follows brain damage that occurs due to tumour, infection, neurological disease or trauma. In some subgroups, heredity is an important factor.

The word seizure is derived from Latin word 'sacire', which means 'to take possession of'. The WHO defines seizures as "a transient occurrence of signs and/or symptoms due to abnormal, excessive, or synchronous neuronal activity in the brain". They are caused by **episodic, abnormal, high-frequency discharge of a group of neurons**. It starts focally and spreads to varying extents to involve other parts of brain. The manifestations of this abnormal neuronal activity may range from brief lapse of attention to full-blown convulsive fit.

CLASSIFICATION OF SEIZURES

The International League against Epilepsies (ILAE) in 2017 classified epilepsy into focal onset, generalised onset, unknown onset, and unclassified types.

Focal Onset or Partial Seizures

Focal onset or partial seizures arise from **neuronal networks discretely localised within one cerebral hemisphere**. Under the new classification system, focal seizures can be further described as those **having motor, sensory, autonomic or psychic symptoms**, with or without **cognitive impairment**. The terms simple and complex partial seizures are no longer in use. Simple partial seizures (without loss of consciousness) are now termed as 'focal-aware seizures', while complex partial seizures (with impaired consciousness) are called 'focal-impaired awareness seizures'. Focal seizures can spread, become **secondarily generalised** and are called 'focal-to-bilateral' tonic–clonic seizures (BTCS). In focal seizures, the patient may present with varied symptoms depending on the part of the brain involved in the abnormal activity.

- Abnormal motor movements (such as clonic jerking/ spasms/ purposeless movements) in a localised region, e.g., hand or fingers, which gradually spread over few seconds to minutes, and involve a larger region of the limb. This is known as '**Jacksonian march**'.
- Afterwards, loss of tone or 'paresis' may occur in the involved region. This is called '**Todd paralysis**', which may last for a few hours. Rarely, seizures continue for many hours or days. This condition is called '**epilepsia partialis continua**' and is refractory to therapy.
- In some patients, focal seizures can present with non-motor symptoms such as **disturbances of equilibrium** (falling sensation, vertigo), **visual problems** (flashing lights, paresthesias) or **autonomic symptoms** (flushing, sweating, piloerection).
- If the site of origin of seizure is temporal or the frontal cortex, the patient experiences an unusual **sense of intense odours, sounds and psychic symptoms** such as fear, feeling of impending doom, detachment, depersonalisation and illusion of objects getting unusually larger (macropsia) or smaller (micropsia).
- In some cases, **cognitive impairment** is also present. The patient does not respond to visual or verbal commands, loses contact with their surroundings, and presents with a 'motionless stare' accompanied by automatism, like

chewing, lip-licking, hand-movements, and running. After the seizure, the patient is confused; recovery occurs in 30–90 seconds.

Generalised Onset Seizures

In generalised onset seizures, the abnormal electrical activity spreads rapidly to **involve neuronal networks in both cerebral hemispheres.** Generalised seizures are further divided into motor and non-motor types:

- **Generalised tonic–clonic seizures (GTCS)** are also known as **'grand mal'** epilepsy or maximal electroshock seizures (MES). The seizure begins abruptly with **tonic contraction** of the muscles of the whole body, lasting for about 10–20 seconds (producing an 'ictal cry' due to tonic contraction of laryngeal muscles, followed by respiratory impairment, pooling of secretions in oropharynx, cyanosis, tongue biting, etc.). The tonic phase is followed by a **clonic phase** after about 15–30 seconds, characterised by massive jerking for about 1–2 minutes. The patient is usually unresponsive or **unconscious and flaccid.** Bladder/bowel incontinence, excessive salivation, stridor, and partial airway obstruction also occur frequently. After few minutes to hours, the patient regains consciousness. In the post-ictal phase, the patient is **confused** and complains of **fatigue, headache or muscular pain,** lasting for several hours.
- **Myoclonic seizures,** also known as juvenile myoclonic epilepsy (JME), involve **sudden but brief contraction of the muscles of one particular body part or the whole body.** It commonly occurs with degenerative diseases, hypoxic brain injury and metabolic diseases.
- **Absence seizures** are generalised onset non-motor seizures, also known as **'petit mal'** epilepsy or pentylenetetrazole (PTZ) seizures. These can be typical or atypical. In **typical absence seizure,** there occurs **sudden, brief lapse of consciousness,** lasting only for few seconds, without loss of postural control. Then, suddenly, consciousness is regained without any postictal confusion. Many seizures (possibly hundreds) may occur in a single day. Subtle motor signs like bilateral rapid eye blinking or clonic hand movements may also occur sometimes. EEG shows a characteristic spike and wave pattern. Absence seizures usually affect young children and spontaneous remission occurs as the child grows up. In **atypical absence seizure,** on the other hand, the lapse of consciousness is less abrupt at the onset and recovery and usually lasts longer. **Mental retardation** and other **motor signs** are also present.
- **Atonic seizures** involve **sudden loss of tone of postural muscles and impaired consciousness** for just about 1–2 seconds and the patient may fall suddenly. There is no confusion after the seizure.

- **Epilepsy syndromes:** These are a constellation of seizure types and EEG/imaging changes, along with defined onset age and comorbidities. These include the **Lennox–Gastaut syndrome,** characterised by onset before 4 years of age, multiple seizure types (tonic and atonic), characteristic EEG pattern, and mental retardation.
- **The Draven syndrome** is characterised by brief, bilateral, recurrent myoclonic jerks of the body with sudden flexion or extension of the limbs and body in the first year of life. Such seizures. usually have genetic basis, are aggravated by fever, impair mental development and are refractory to treatment.

PATHOPHYSIOLOGY

1. GTCS or grand mal epilepsy and juvenile myoclonic seizures (JME) involve the generation of an action potential (AP) in the thalamus due to spontaneous firing of **T-type Ca^{2+} channels**

   The AP propagates in a retrograde manner to the cortex, causing depolarisation of cortical neurons.

   Opening of **Na^+ channels** → Depolarisation of spinal cord segments → Spontaneous muscle contraction

2. **Absence seizures** or petit mal epilepsy occur due to spontaneous firing of **T-type Ca^{2+} channels** in the thalamus causing an AP within the subcortex. The AP does not spread to the cortex and motor centres. Thus, there is **no role of Na^+ channels** in these seizures.

3. **Focal onset seizures** occur due to cortical space occupying lesions such as gliosis, tumours, and neurocysticercosis that cause **Na^+ channel opening** and firing of focal neurons, generating an AP that stimulates specific segments of the spinal cord. Thus, seizures affect only the muscles supplied by that specific spinal segment and Ca^{2+} channels have no role in this type of seizure.

   Thus, it can be seen that GTCS and JME involve Ca^{2+} and Na^+ channels. Absence seizures involve only T-type Ca^{2+} channels and focal onset seizures involve only Na^+ channels. Channels involved in different types of seizures are summarised in Box 16.1. This information helps to decide the drug suitable for a particular seizure type.

Box 16.1	
Seizure type	**Channels involved**
GTC, JME	T-type Ca^{2+}, Na^+
Absence seizures	T-type Ca^{2+}
Focal onset seizures	Na^+

MECHANISM OF SEIZURE INITIATION AND PROPAGATION

Seizures result from an imbalance between excitatory and inhibitory influences in the central nervous system (Fig. 16.1).

The opening of the voltage-gated Na^+ channels in glutamatergic neurons causes membrane depolarisation, which triggers Ca^{2+} influx through high-voltage activated (HVA) Ca^{2+} channels. Raised intracellular calcium brings about the release of glutamate (Fig. 16.2).

Glutamate is a major excitatory neurotransmitter in the brain. It causes Na^+ and Ca^{2+} influx in postsynaptic neurons through activation of AMPA and NMDA receptors, respectively. The low-voltage activated (LVA) channels or T-type channels open in response to small depolarisations.

The **major inhibitory influence is exerted by GABA-ergic neurons.** Gamma-aminobutyric acid (GABA) acts on $GABA_A$ receptors, opening Cl^- channels. The resulting Cl^- influx makes the membrane potential negative inside. Its action is terminated by re-uptake by GABA transporter (GAT) and metabolism by GABA transaminase (GABA-T).

The high-frequency bursts of action potentials in neurons and hyper-synchronisation initiates seizure activity. The sites for antiepileptic action of drugs are depicted in Fig.16.2 (sites 1–9).

CLASSIFICATION OF ANTIEPILEPTIC DRUGS

Antiepileptic drugs reduce seizure activity by **restoring the balance between excitatory and inhibitory NTM activity** by various mechanisms. Drugs can either decrease the excitatory transmission or enhance the inhibitory transmission. They may be classified based on their:

1. Major mechanisms of antiepileptic action
2. Usage

Classification Based on Mechanisms of Antiepileptic Action

As seen in Flowchart 16.1 and Fig. 16.3, many drugs have multiple mechanisms of action, e.g., valproate, divalproex, lamotrigine, and topiramate.

Classification Based on Use

1. Drugs for focal and generalised tonic–clonic seizures
2. Drugs for absence seizures
3. Other drugs

1. Drugs for focal and generalised tonic–clonic (grand mal) seizures

These include the following drugs:

[Mnemonic: Platelet, TLC, LFT. These are the names of common lab investigations. The drug names start with the letters p, t, l, c, l, f, and t].

Platelet: Drugs starting with the letter P and related drugs such as Phenytoin (mephenytoin, ethotoin, fosphenytoin), Phenobarbitone, Primidone, Perampanel

T – Topiramate
L – Lamotrigine
C – Carbamazepine, Oxcarbazepine
L – Lacosamide, (Zonisamide, Rufinamide)
F – Felbamate
T – Tiagabine
V – Valproate, Vigabartin (Valproate is a broad-spectrum antiepileptic drug and is used for both major seizure types, i. e., generalised tonic–clonic and absence seizures.)

2. Drugs for absence seizures

- Valproic acid, Sodium valproate
- Succinimides: Ethosuximide, Phensuximide, Methsuximide
- Oxazolidinediones: Dimethadione, Trimethadione, Paramethadione
- Lamotrigine

3. Others

Benzodiazepines (Diazepam, Clonazepam, Clobazam), Acetazolamide, Magnesium sulphate

---

Clinical problem-based questions and MCQs

1. An 12-year-old boy is brought for neurological evaluation after experiencing complete blanking episodes several times during the past six months. During these episodes, the boy appears confused, has a blank expression on his face, makes chewing and swallowing movements, grunting sounds, does not respond properly to questions and has impaired consciousness. He becomes normal a few minutes after the episode. He is diagnosed with focal-to-BTCS.
   i. Which of the following is a suitable drug for this patient?
      a. Carbamazepine   b. Ethosuximide
      c. Fosphenytoin   d. Lorazepam

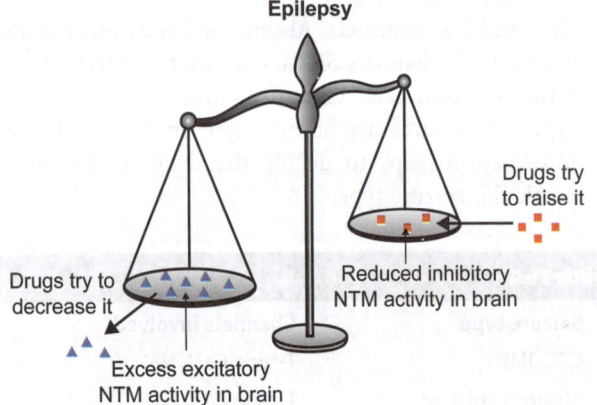

Fig. 16.1 NTM imbalance in CNS → seizures

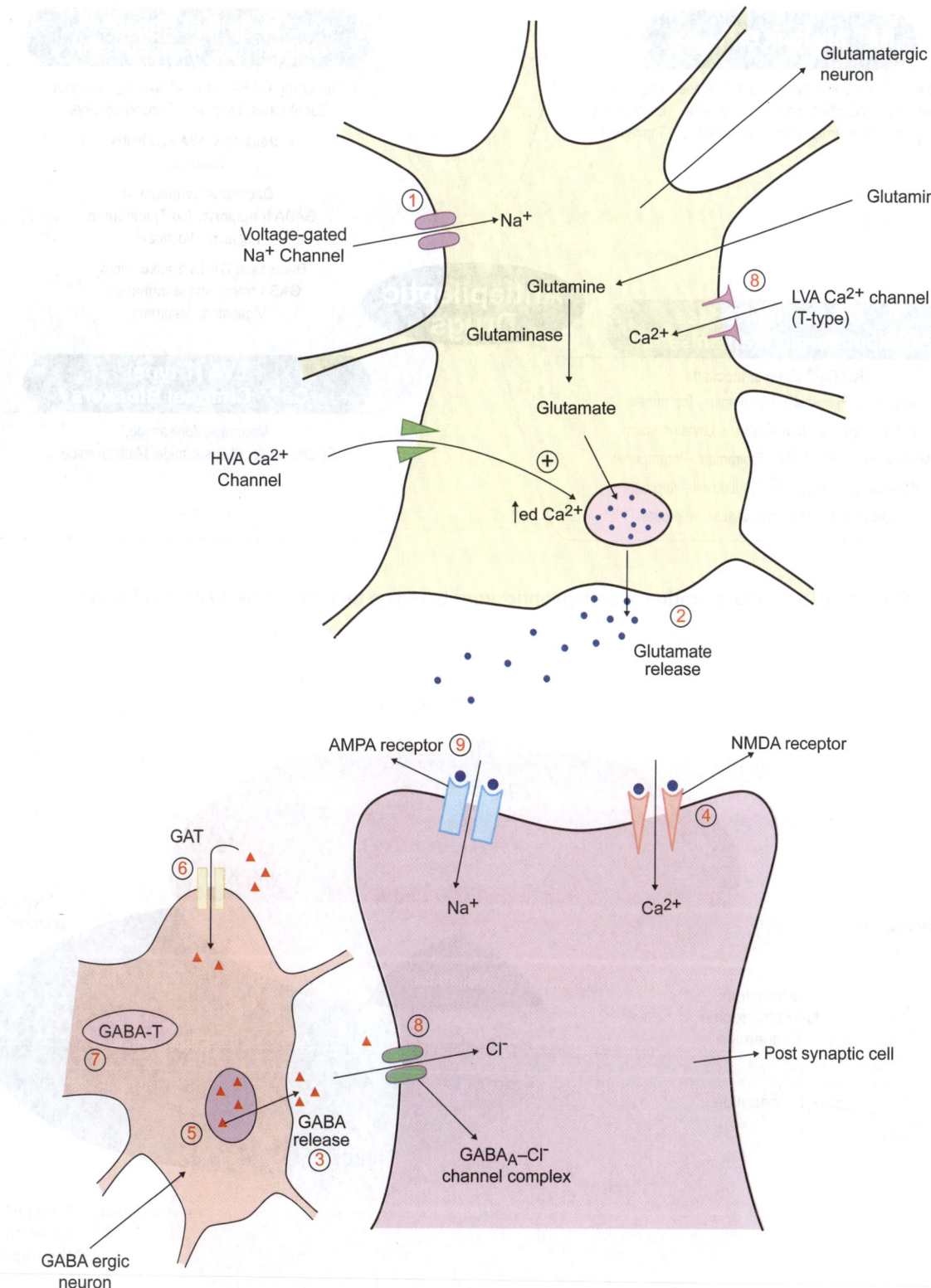

Fig. 16.2 Site of action of various antiepileptic drugs
① Sodium channel blockade; ② Reduced glutamate release; ③ Increased GABA release; ④ NMDA receptor blockade; ⑤ Increased GABA synthesis; ⑥ Reduced reuptake of GABA; ⑦ Reduced GABA degradation; ⑧ T-type calcium channel attenuation; ⑨ AMPA receptor blockade.

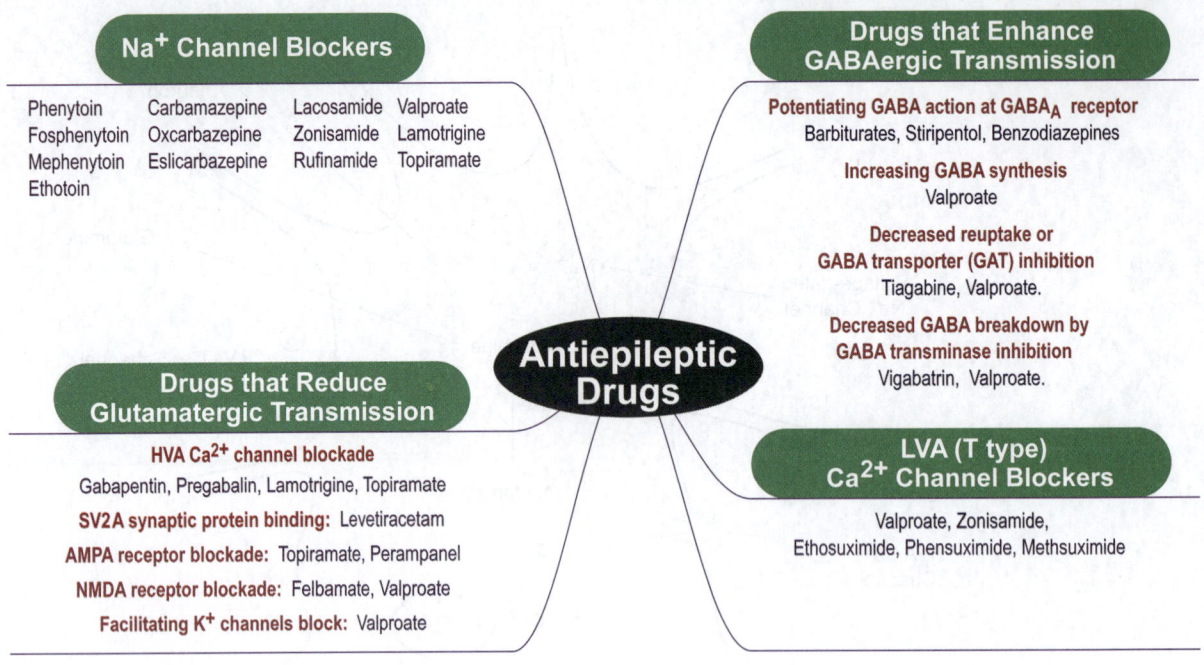

Flowchart 16.1 Classification of antiepileptic drugs based on their major mechanisms of action

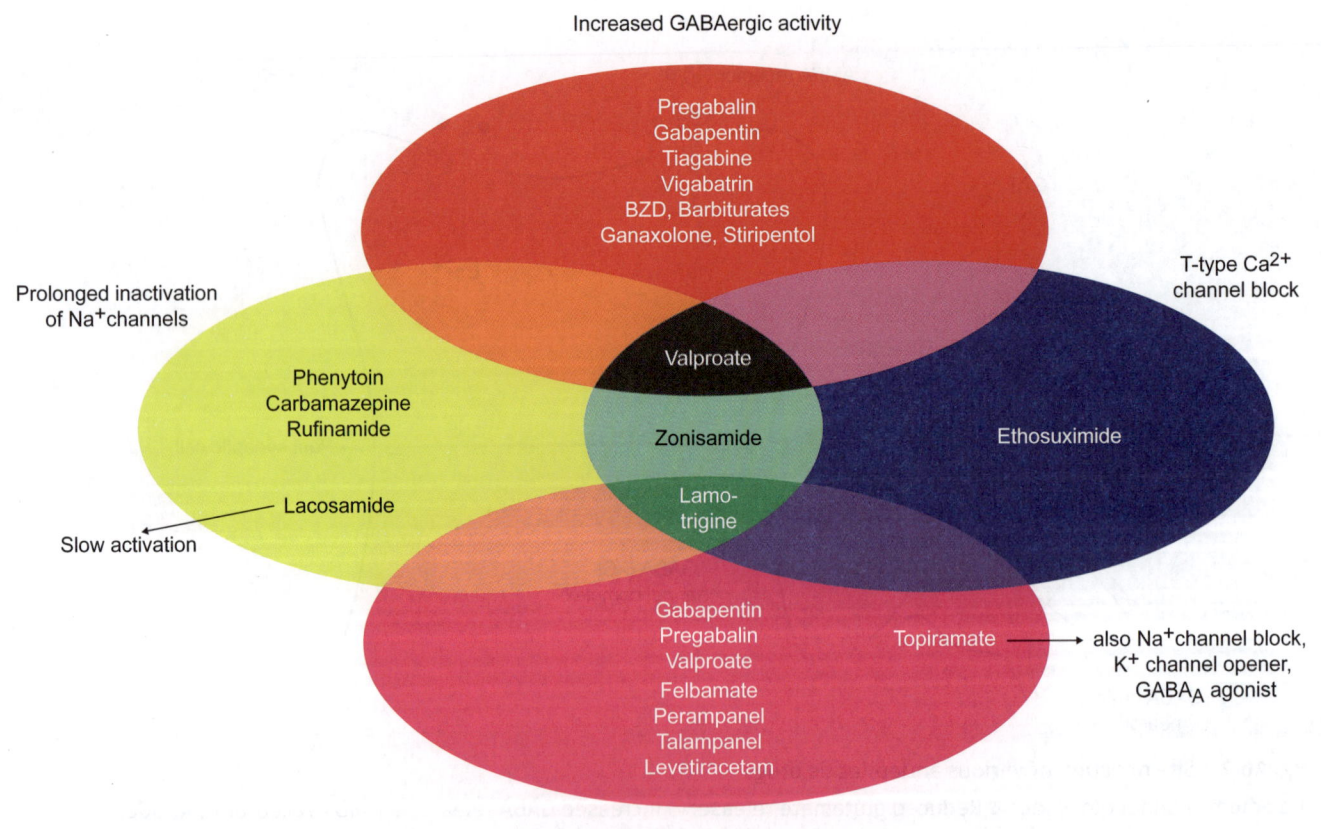

Fig. 16.3 Mechanism of action of various antiepileptic drugs

2. A 10-year-old girl is brought to emergency by her teacher after a seizure-like activity. The teacher notices that she simply kept on staring for about 30–40 seconds and did not respond to verbal commands in that period; she appeared confused for a minute or so and then recovered. Both teacher and mother give a history of a few such episodes having in the past 3–4 months; they are worried and want a complete neurological checkup of the child.
   i. Identify the type of seizure reported in this case.
      a. Absence seizure   b. Jacksonian epilepsy
      c. Myoclonic seizure d. Partial seizure
   ii. Which is the most suitable drug in this case?
      a. Valproate   b. Fosphenytoin
      c. Phenobarbitone   d. Lorazepam

words, channels which are not in the resting phase but are undergoing a cycle of activation–inactivation and recovery back to the resting state are blocked by phenytoin because phenyto in; this is **preferentially binds to the active or inactive state of the sodium channels** and delays the recovery from inactive to resting stage. Hence, the channel is unavailable, which prevents the generation of repetitive action potential.

- Phenytoin also **decreases synaptic release of glutamate** (excitatory NTM) and **enhances that of GABA** (inhibitory NTM) by reducing the permeability of the membrane at high concentrations.

Pharmacokinetics and dosage

The pharmacokinetic parameters of phenytoin are very important for its safe use.

- Absorption of phenytoin is almost complete after oral administration. However, the rate of absorption depends upon factors like the dosage form, particle size, and additives or fillers used. Hence, **bio-inequivalences can occur** on changing the formulation.
- Intramuscular administration of phenytoin is not recommended because some drug precipitation occurs in the muscle and absorption is unpredictable. **Fosphenytoin, a prodrug of phenytoin, is well absorbed intramuscularly**.
- Phenytoin is highly (almost **90%) bound to plasma proteins**. Other highly-bound drugs like sulphonamides and phenylbutazone can displace phenytoin from the binding sites, resulting in a transient rise in free drug levels. **Protein binding decreases in conditions like hypoalbuminemia and renal disease**. The total plasma

DRUGS FOR FOCAL AND GENERALISED TONIC-CLONIC SEIZURES

1. Phenytoin

Mechanism of action

Phenytoin has a combination of actions at several levels.

- The major mechanism of action is **blockade of sodium channels**. Sodium channels exist in three states—resting, active and inactive—based on their 'm' and 'h' gates (Fig. 16.4). From the resting state these channels pass to the active and then to the inactive state. Recovery of channel occurs from the inactive state to resting state. Phenytoin **slows down the recovery of sodium channels**. The blockade of sodium channel caused by phenytoin is **use dependent**, which means that the channels that are used more are blocked more. In other

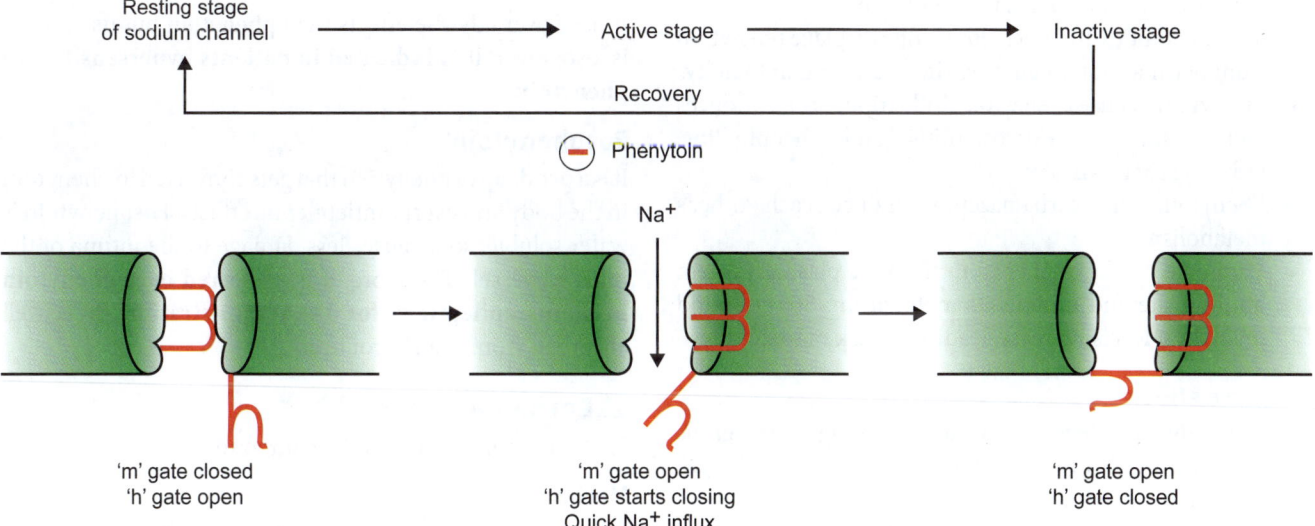

Fig. 16.4 Mechanism of action of phenytoin

concentrations (not free drug levels) are reduced in these situations. If the dose is increased to maintain the total plasma concentration in the therapeutic range, toxicity can result.
- Phenytoin is metabolised by parahydroxylation and glucuronide conjugation. Metabolites are excreted in urine. The elimination **kinetics of phenytoin change from first order to zero order within the therapeutic range**. Thus, the chances of toxicity are higher.

It is very **important to monitor the plasma concentration** of phenytoin to maintain its levels in the therapeutic range (**10–20 mcg/mL**). This is because phenytoin shows bio-inequivalence; the elimination kinetics changes from first order to zero order over the therapeutic range, and phenytoin is a toxic drug with a steep dose–response curve. The usual dose is 300 mg/day. If needed, the dose can be increased gradually by small increments of 25–30 mg only.

- Phenytoin **induces microsomal enzymes**. Hence, the metabolism of concurrently administered drugs like steroids and theophylline increases, resulting in reduced efficacy of these drugs.

Indications
- Phenytoin is used in generalised tonic–clonic and focal seizures. Because of its higher toxicity, it is **only used when better tolerated drugs are not effective**.
- In status epilepticus, phenytoin sodium I/V is used if fosphenytoin is not available.
- It is also useful in trigeminal neuralgias and cardiac arrhythmias.
- Recently, it has been reported to promote wound healing.

Contraindications and interactions
- Phenytoin should not be used in absence and myoclonic seizures as it can worsen the condition.
- Sulphonamides and phenylbutazone displace phenytoin from plasma protein binding sites, resulting in toxicity.
- Phenytoin causes enzyme induction; this induces metabolism of corticosteroids and theophylline, reducing their efficacy.
- Phenytoin and carbamazepine induce each other's metabolism.
- Valproate displaces phenytoin from the plasma-protein binding site and inhibits its metabolism. So, unbound phenytoin levels increase, leading to risk of toxicity.

Adverse effects
- Mild adverse effects like headache, vertigo, nystagmus and loss of extra-ocular pursuit movements do not warrant dose reduction.
- At higher concentrations, mild sedation, confusion and intellectual deterioration occur, which are reversible. Diplopia and ataxia indicate dose reduction.
- Prolonged use is associated with gum hyperplasia due to overexpression of platelet-derived growth factor (PDGF). Hirsutism, coarsening of facial features, acne, megaloblastic anemia, osteomalacia and peripheral neuropathy are also reported.
- Hypersensitivity and idiosyncratic reactions are rare with phenytoin.
- Use of phenytoin in pregnant women causes 'fetal hydantoin syndrome', characterised by microcephaly, mental retardation, hypoplastic phalanges, and cleft lip and palate.

Toxicity of phenytoin
Phenytoin toxicity causes:
- Ataxia, vertigo, diplopia, nystagmus
- Confusion drowsiness, behavioural disturbances, disorientation
- Epigastric pain, nausea, vomiting
- I/V administration can cause vascular intimal damage, thrombophlebitis, fall in BP and arrhythmias. So, I/M fosphenytoin is preferred over I/V phenytoin. If needed, ECG must be monitored.

[Mnemonic for important ADRs of phenytoin: '**P**unjab **G**ovt **H**andled **V**an', i.e., **P**henytoin (**G**um hyperplasia, **O**steomalacia, **V**isual disturbances, **T**eratogenicity, **H**ypocalcemia, **A**nemia, **D**iplopia, **L**ymphadenopathy, **D**yspepsia, **V**ertigo, **A**taxia, **N**eutropenia.]

Mephenytoin
It is metabolised to '**nirvanol**' that has anticonvulsant action; however, it has a **higher incidence of severe reactions** (like dermatitis, hepatitis and agranulocytosis) than phenytoin.

Ethotoin
It has fewer adverse effects than phenytoin but its efficacy is also lower. It **is indicated in patients hypersensitive to phenytoin**.

Fosphenytoin
It is a **prodrug** of phenytoin that gets converted to phenytoin in the body and exerts antiepileptic effects. Fosphenytoin is water soluble, so it causes less damage to the intima of the injected vessel. Therefore, it is **preferred over phenytoin in status epilepticus for IV administration**. It is well absorbed from the IM route as well.

2. Carbamazepine
Carbamazepine is a tricyclic compound.

Mechanism of action
Like phenytoin, carbamazepine **blocks voltage-gated Na$^+$ channels at therapeutic concentration**. High-frequency repetitive firing of neurons is thus inhibited. It also acts

pre-synaptically to decrease synaptic transmission. It binds to adenosine receptor, but the significance of this action is not very clear. Adenosine is an endogenous anti-seizure substance.

Pharmacokinetics and dose
- Oral absorption is almost complete but there are wide inter-individual variations in the rate of absorption.
- It is 70% bound to plasma proteins. Hence, there is no risk of interactions with other drugs due to displacement from binding sites.
- It is completely metabolised, and one of the metabolites, carbamazepine 10,11-epoxide possesses anticonvulsant activity.
- Its clearance is slow and half-life is 36 hours at initiation of therapy. However, it causes microsomal enzyme induction and increases its own metabolism (**autoinduction**) as well as that of other concurrently administered drugs. After prolonged treatment, its half-life decreases to 8–12 hours as a result of autoinduction. The rate of metabolism of other anticonvulsants drug like phenytoin, primidone, valproate and ethosuximide is increased by carbamazepine.

The daily dose of carbamazepine is 1–2 g.

Indications
- It is the **drug of choice in focal (partial) seizures, trigeminal neuralgia, postherpetic neuralgia and glossopharyngeal neuralgia.**
- It is very commonly used in generalised tonic–clonic seizures.
- It is also useful in some patients with bipolar disease
- It may be as effective as ADH in diabetes inspidus.

Adverse effects
- A dose-related adverse effect of carbamazepine is **diplopia**, which may occur during a particular time of the day lasting for less than an hour.
- **Sedation, ataxia, drowsiness**
- Mild gastrointestinal upset
- **Hyponatremia, water intoxication**
- **Hypersensitivity reactions** like erythematous skin rash occurs frequently.
- Mild leukopenia is seen in some patients.
- **Blood dyscrasias** may occur within first 4 months of carbamazepine use, especially in elderly patients with trigeminal neuralgias. Fatal agranulocytosis and aplastic anemia can occur.

[Mnemonic: **CAR Driver Who Sleeps AT Highway Brings Disaster**, i.e., **CAR**bamazepine: Diplopia, Water intoxication, Sedation, Ataxia, Hyponatremia, Blood Dyscrasia]

Oxcarbazepine
Oxcarbazepine resembles carbamazepine in its mechanism of action and indications. The advantage of oxcarbazepine is its **lesser propensity to cause enzyme induction and hypersensitivity reactions.** However, it is **less potent**, and thus requires higher dosages than carbamazepine; **hyponatremia** occurs more commonly with oxcarbazepine.

Eslicarbazepine
It is a **prodrug** that is converted in the liver to an epoxide metabolite, responsible for same therapeutic and adverse effects as oxcarbazepine. It can be given as **once daily dose as an 'add-on' drug in focal seizures** with or without generalisation.

3. Lamotrigine
Lamotrigine is a **broad-spectrum** antiepileptic.

Mechanism of action
- It causes use-dependent **blockade of Na^+ channels** and delays their recovery from the inactive to resting stage. This effect suppresses high-frequency, repetitive firing of neurons. Sensitive Na^+ channels may be blocked directly by lamotrigine.
- Lamotrigine also **inhibits high-voltage-associated Ca^{2+} channels.** Thus, the presynaptic membrane is stabilised and **synaptic release of glutamate is reduced.** Due to this action, lamotrigine is effective in primarily generalised seizures in children, including absence seizure.

Pharmacokinetics and dose
Lamotrigine is well absorbed, completely metabolised and excreted in urine. Enzyme inducers like phenytoin, phenobarbitone and carbamazepine decrease its half-life; valproate, on the contrary, inhibits the metabolism of lamotrigine. The usual adult dose of lamotrigine is 50 mg/day, up to a maximum of 300 mg/day, but the dose should be reduced to half when valproate is added.

Indications for use
- Lamotrigine is a **first-line drug for focal, generalised tonic–clonic seizures and myoclonic seizures.**
- It is used as second choice drug after valproate in **Lennox–Gastaut syndrome.**
- **Absence** seizures also respond.
- It is also effective in depressive phase of **bipolar disease** and **neuralgias**.

Adverse effects
ADRs are mild. It is **better tolerated than carbamazepine**.

- Common adverse drugs reactions with lamotrigine are **headache, nausea, vomiting, dizziness, ataxia, diplopia and somnolence**.
- **Hypersensitivity reactions** to lamotrigine occur in the form of skin rashes. Severe **life-threatening dermatitis** may occur in 1–2% of pediatric population. It may cause Stevens–Johnson syndrome. To prevent it, lamotrigine is started with low dose and increased slowly, and hence, it cannot be used in emergency conditions.

Contraindication

It is **not preferred in children** because of the risk of severe dermatitis.

4. Valproate

This is a **broad-spectrum** antiepileptic drug with **multiple mechanisms of action.** Both valproic acid and sodium valproate are converted to valproate ions at the physiological pH, which exerts anticonvulsant actions.

Mechanism of action

- It **blocks voltage-sensitive Na⁺ channels** and prevents high-frequency repetitive firing of neurons.
- It may also **block NMDA receptor** mediated excitation.
- It **increases GABAergic activity** in the brain by increasing GABA synthesis and reducing its reuptake as well as metabolism by the following mechanisms;
    - Facilitating GABA synthesis by decarboxylation of glutamic acid
    - Decreasing GABA re-uptake by GABA transport (GAT) inhibition.
    - At high concentration, valproate decreases the degradation of GABA by inhibition of GABA transaminase enzyme.
- Valproate also **attenuates low-voltage-associated LVA or T-type Ca²⁺ currents** weakly. This effect may be responsible for its efficacy in absence seizures.

Pharmacokinetics and dose

It is well absorbed orally and is highly plasma protein-bound. Due to its high plasma protein-binding and complete ionisation, its volume of distribution is **confined to extracellular fluid** only.

It is an **inhibitor of microsomal enzymes** and can inhibit metabolism of other antiepileptic drugs like phenytoin, phenobarbitone, carbamazepine and lamotrigine, causing toxic effects.

Dose: 200 mg TDS is the usual starting dose. It can be increased as per need up to 600 mg TDS.

Therapeutic uses

Valproate is a broad-spectrum anticonvulsant effective in **many types of seizures**, such as:

- Juvenile myoclonic seizures, generalised tonic–clonic seizures, mixed seizure syndrome, and rheumatic chorea: it is the drug of choice.
- Absence seizures: it is the preferred drug.
- Focal seizures, atonic seizures

In addition, valproate is also useful in **bipolar disease** and **migraine prophylaxis**.

Adverse effects

It is a well-tolerated drug, although serious idiosyncratic reactions have occurred in small number of patients. It can cause:

- Dose-related **GI upset**, causing anorexia, nausea, vomiting, epigastric pain, and diarrhea. Such effects can be avoided by starting with a lower dose.
- High dose can cause **sedation, ataxia and tremors**. However, cognitive and behavioural impairment is not seen with valproate.
- In some patients, valproate causes **increased appetite, weight gain, curling of hair and hair loss**.
- **Idiosyncratic reaction** can occur as **hepatotoxicity**. Risk of hepatotoxicity is higher in patients < 2 years of age and those taking multiple medications. In some cases, hepatotoxicity may be fatal, especially within the first 4 months of treatment. So, **monitoring of liver function** test is important. If hepatotoxicity occurs, valproate should be stopped and treatment with L-carnitine is recommended. In some patients idiosyncratic reactions can cause increased ammonia, pancreatitis, and thrombocytopenia.
- In pregnant patients it has been reported to cause spina bifida, cardiovascular, orofacial and digital abnormalities in fetus.

[Mnemonic for adverse effects of valproate: **VAL**iant **CAT SAT** o**N LAP** [**VAL**proate: **C**urly hair, **A**lopecia, **T**eratogenicity, **S**edation, **A**taxia, **T**remor, **N**ausea, **L**iver damage, increased **A**mmonia, **P**ancreatitis]

Contraindications

Valproate should be avoided during **pregnancy and in children < 2 years** of age. It should **not be used along with clonazepam** as this combination can precipitate status condition of absence seizures, i.e., absence status.

Divalproex

It is a 1:1 co-ordination compound of sodium valproate and valproic acid. Its mechanism of action and uses are the same as valproate. **Gastrointestinal adverse effects with divalproex are less** than with valproate.

A summary of the features of main drugs for GTC and focal onset seizures is given in Table 16.1.

Chapter 16 Antiepileptic Drugs

Table 16.1 Features of preferred drugs for GTC and partial seizures

Drug	Major mechanism of action (Fig. 16.2)	Status in epilepsy	Characteristic ADRs
Phenytoin	① Blocks voltage-gated Na⁺ channels: Slows down recovery ② Reduced release of glutamate ③ Increased release of GABA	Used only when better tolerated drugs are not effective	[Mnemonic for important ADRs of phenytoin: 'Punjab govt handled van', i.e., phenytoin (gum hyperplasia, osteomalacia, visual disturbances, teratogenicity, hypocalcemia, anemia, diplopia, lymphadenopathy, dyspepsia, vertigo, ataxia, neutropenia).]
Carbamazepine	Same as mechanism ① above	**Drug of choice** for focal seizure, trigeminal neuralgia. Useful in GTCs and bipolar disease	[Mnemonic: Car driver who sleeps at highway brings disaster, i.e., Carbamazepine: diplopia, water intoxication, sedation, ataxia, hyponatremia, blood dyscrasia]
Valproate (broad spectrum)	① Blocks sodium channels ④ Blocks NMDA receptors ⑤ Increased synthesis of GABA ⑥ Reduced neuronal reuptake of GABA ⑦ Reduced degradation of **GABA** ⑧ Attenuates T-type Ca²⁺current	**Drug of choice** for GTCs, mixed seizure syndrome, juvenile myoclonic epilepsy, absence seizures. Useful in focal, atonic seizures, bipolar disease and migraine prophylaxis.	[Mnemonic for adverse effects of valproate: valiant cat sat on lap [Valproate: curly hair, alopecia, teratogenicity, sedation, ataxia, tremor, nausea, liver damage, increased ammonia, pancreatitis]
Lamotrigine	① Blocks sodium channels ② ↓ed release of glutamate	**First-line drug** for focal and generalised tonic–clonic seizures. Also useful in **myoclonic**, absence seizures and neuralgias	**Better tolerated** Headache nausea vomiting, dizziness, ataxia, diplopia and somnolence, etc. **Life-threatening dermatitis in children**

Clinical problem-based questions and MCQs

3. A 30-year-old female patient presents in emergency department in a stuporous condition. The history elicited from her relative is as follows: Around half an hour before, the patient made a shrill cry and fell unconscious, followed by tonic rigidity of all four limbs; this was followed by jerking movements for about 1–2 minutes. The patient had passed urine involuntarily during this episode prior to becoming unconscious. Family history of epilepsy is negative, but there is a past history of head injury in a road accident about 6 months back. Examination reveals findings within normal limits. EEG of the patient shows fast spike and wave activity at 4–5 Hz, which is usually associated with generalised tonic–clonic seizures.
   i. Which of the following is currently a first choice drug for this patient?
      a. Ethosuximide   b. Diazepam
      c. Valproate   d. Pregabalin
   ii. Describe the mechanism of action and adverse effects of the antiepileptic drug chosen.
   iii. Name other drugs that may be used in this case.

4. A 12-year-old boy, a known case of tonic–clonic epilepsy, is on antiepileptic medication for the past 6 months. The patient reports for follow up. He had no seizure in the months after starting therapy, but he complains of excessive fatigue and looks pale. Complete blood count shows megaloblastic anemia. The physician reassured him that it is adverse effect of given medication and advised monitoring plasma concentration of the drug every month.
   i. Identify the antiepileptic drug being used.
      a. Carbamazepine   b. Valproate
      c. Phenytoin   d. Divalproex
   ii. Enumerate all the possible adverse effects.
   iii. Why is repeated monitoring of plasma concentration advised?

5. A 25-year-old girl from a village, a known case of epilepsy, was well controlled with tab. phenytoin 100 mg, given twice a day. She got married and was not willing to have a baby soon after. Her sister advised her to take oral contraceptive pills containing ethinyl estradiol 30 mcg and norgestrel 0.3 mg every day. She started taking these pills regularly, but after 2

months she missed her periods and her urine tested positive for pregnancy.
  i. Describe the mechanism of antiepileptic effect and the adverse effects of phenytoin.
  ii. Explain why oral contraceptive pills failed to prevent pregnancy in this case.
  iii. What information about risk to fetus should be provided to the patient to help her make a decision about continuing the pregnancy and antiepileptic treatment.

6. Which of the following drugs should not be combined with clonazepam?
   a. Phenytoin   b. Carbamazepine
   c. Valproate   d. Lamotrigine

7. i. Which of the following drugs shows reduction in half-life after prolonged use?
      a. Lamotrigine   b. Valproate
      c. Divalprox   d. Carbamazepine
   ii. Explain the cause of reduced half-life with the selected drug.

8. A 24-year-old girl is on antiepileptic drug treatment for about an year. During the whole year, she had no epileptic fit or any other complaints except mild drowsiness. During follow-up visit, the patient complains of blurring of vision and double vision. Complete blood count shows mild leukopenia.
   i. Identify the antiepileptic drug being used here.
      a. Carbamazepine
      b. Valproate
      c. Ethosuximide
      d. Lorazepam
   ii. Describe the mechanism of action, uses and adverse effects of the selected drug.

5. Topiramate

This is also a **broad-spectrum antiseizure drug** because it has multiple mechanisms of action.

- It causes blockade of voltage-gated Na^+ channels like phenytoin and prolongs their inactivation.
- It blocks high-voltage-associated Ca^{2+} channels, thus interfering with glutamate release.
- Topiramate also blocks AMPA receptors and thus inhibits glutamate-induced Na^+ entry into postsynaptic neurons.

Indications

Because of its multiple mechanisms, it is useful in **refractory cases of focal seizures, generalised tonic–clonic seizures** as monotherapy, as well as a supplementing drug. Treatment is started with 25 mg once or twice daily and increased as needed up to a maximum of 200 mg BD.

- It is also effective in **myoclonic and absence seizures** as an add-on drug.
- It can be used for **migraine prophylaxis** in patient where β blockers are not effective or are contraindicated.

Adverse drug reactions

ADRs include sedation, ataxia, confusion, nervousness, increased risk of metabolic acidosis, angle closure glaucoma, renal stones and weight loss.

Table 16.2 summarises the important features of topiramate and other (newer) drugs for GTC and focal seizures.

6. Lacosamide

Mechanism of action

It causes '**slow inactivation**' of Na^+ **channels** as compared to the 'prolongation of inactivation' caused by phenytoin. It causes **no enzyme induction or inhibition**. Thus, it can be used as **add-on** drug for focal seizures with or without generalisation, **without any dose adjustment of the primary drug**. It is used only in patients older than 17 years of age.

Adverse effects are diplopia, ataxia, tremors, headache, dizziness, vertigo and cardiac rhythm disturbances.

7. Zonisamide

It is a sulphonamide derivative that acts on Na^+ **channels and T-type Ca^{2+} channels**. It can be used for **monotherapy or as an add-on** drug in refractory focal seizures with or without generalisation. It may be used in myoclonic seizures and infantile spasms.

Adverse effects are anorexia, headache, dizziness and irritability. Renal stones can occur. It is contraindicated in patients with hypersensitivity to sulphonamides.

8. Rufinamide

Its major mechanism is by **prolonging inactive state of sodium channels**, leading to reduction in sustained high-frequency firing of neurons. It is approved as adjunctive treatment of Lennox–Gastaut syndrome and tonic–clonic seizures in patients older than 4 years of age.

Adverse effects are diarrhea, vomiting, pyrexia and somnolence.

9. Gabapentin

- It is an analogue of GABA but does not act at GABA receptors. Instead, it acts by **decreasing the release of glutamate and increasing the release of GABA.**
- It binds to a subset of high-voltage-associated (HVA) Ca^{2+} channels containing $\alpha_2\delta_{-1}$ subunits and decreases Ca^{2+} influx into presynaptic neurons, which in turn decreases glutamate release.

Indications

- Gabapentin is used as an **add-on drug** in refractory focal and generalised tonic–clonic seizures.
- It is the drug of choice for **neuropathic pain** due to diabetic neuropathy and postherpetic neuralgia; it is also effective in migraine prophylaxis and phobias.

Adverse drug reactions

It is **well tolerated**. Mild sedation, fatigue, ataxia, somnolence, tremors may occur.

It causes **no enzyme induction or inhibition**. Thus, dosage change is not required while adding gabapentin to other first-line antiepileptic drugs.

10. Pregabalin

Pregabalin is similar to gabapentin in its mechanism of action and uses. It is **less sedative than gabapentin** but can cause **allergic reactions** such as rashes.

11. Levetiracetam

Mechanism of action of levetiracetam is unique. It binds to synaptic vesicular protein SV2A and **decreases the release of glutamate**. It probably **alters GABA release also** across the synapse.

Therapeutic uses

- It is effective as monotherapy as well as an adjuvant drug in **resistant focal seizures** with or without generalisation and also in **myoclonic seizures**.
- It is used as second-line add-on drug in **absence seizures**.
- It has **no enzyme-inducing or inhibiting potential**. Thus, no interactions occur on combining levetiracetam with other antiepileptic drugs.

Adverse drug reactions

It is well tolerated. Mild sedation, ataxia, dizziness and somnolence can occur. It is not approved for children < 4 years of age.

12. Tiagabine

It **blocks neuronal reuptake of GABA** by inhibiting GABA transporter 1 (GAT-1). Thus, GABA levels in synapses increase and exert antiseizure effect. It is also used only as an **add-on drug for focal seizures** with or without generalisation, if they are not controlled by first-line drugs.

Adverse effects are confusion, depression, ataxia, dizziness, nervousness, amnesia, etc.

12. Vigabatrin

It exerts antiseizure activity by increasing synaptic GABA concentration by **reducing GABA degradation through inhibition of enzyme GABA transaminase.**

It is a **reserve drug** for patients refractory to other safer drugs, as it causes many **disturbing adverse effects**. Common side effects are weight gain, dizziness and drowsiness. Less common and more troublesome side effects are:

- Confusion, agitation and psychotic behaviour. Thus, it is **contraindicated in patients with pre-existing psychiatric disorders.**
- Irreversible **defects of visual field and colour vision, paresthesias**, etc.

13. Perampanel

This new drug **blocks postsynaptic AMPA receptors** non-competitively, preventing Na^+ influx and repetitive discharge. It is approved as an **adjunctive drug for focal seizures** with or without generalisation in patients > 12 years of age. It is well tolerated. Commonly observed side effects are headache, dizziness, somnolence and rashes. In some patients, however, severe behavioural effects like irritability, hostility and aggression are reported.

14. Felbamate

It exerts anticonvulsant action by **blocking NMDA glutamate receptors** on the postsynaptic membrane. It also has **GABA-potentiating action** like barbiturates. It is effective in **focal epilepsy and Lennox–Gastaut** syndrome. It, however, has the status of a third-line drug for refractory cases because of its potential to cause **aplastic anemia and hepatitis.**

15. Retigabine

It has a unique mechanism of action—it acts by **facilitating K^+ channels**. It is approved as an **adjunctive drug in focalonset seizures**, but can cause many adverse effects that require discontinuation of the drug.

Adverse drug reactions

Dizziness, dysarthria, confusion, blurring of vision and bladder dysfunction can occur. Permanent blue pigmentation of skin and lips, retinal pigmentation and reduced visual acuity are reported and may need discontinuation of treatment. Thus, it is used only in cases where other drugs are not effective or are contraindicated.

16. Stiripentol

It **prolongs the duration of Cl^- channel opening** in $GABA_A$ receptors, similar to barbiturates. It increases the level of GABA in the brain. By enzyme inhibition, it enhances effects of other antiepileptic drugs.

It is combined with valproate and clobazam for treating refractory generalised tonic–clonic seizures in severe myoclonic epilepsy (SME) of infancy.

Adverse effects of valproate and clobazam can get increased by stiripentol because of enzyme inhibition.

DRUGS FOR ABSENCE SEIZURES

17. Valproate

This is the **drug of choice** for absence seizures.

18. Succinimides

Ethosuximide is effective only in absence seizures. It exerts action by **blocking low-voltage-associated (LVA) or T-type Ca^{2+} channels in the thalamocortical system.**

Table 16.2 Salient features of other (newer) drugs for GTC and focal seizures

Drug	Mechanism of action	Use and status in epilepsy	Characteristic ADRs
Topiramate (broad spectrum)	Action 1, 2, 9 from Fig. 16.2, i.e., blocks Na channels, reduces glutamate release, and blocks AMPA receptors	Used in **refractory cases** of GTC and focal seizures. **Add-on** drug in myoclonic, absence seizures, migraine prophylaxis	Ataxia, confusion, nervousness, increased risk of **metabolic acidosis, angle closure glaucoma, renal stones** and weight loss
Lacosamide	Action 1 from Fig. 16.2 but it causes **slow inactivation of Na⁺ channel,** rather than delayed recovery.	An **add-on** drug for focal seizures with or without generalisation. **No change in dose of primary drug required.**	Headache, dizziness, vertigo, diplopia, ataxia, tremors, and **cardiac rhythm disturbances**
Zonisamide	**Actions 1, 8** from Fig. 16.2 (Na⁺, T type Ca²⁺ channels)	An **add-on** drug in refractory focal seizures; May be used in myoclonic seizures and infantile spasms.	Headache, dizziness, anorexia, irritability, **renal stones,** hypersensitivity, **cross sensitivity with sulphonamides**
Rufinamide	Action 1 from Fig. 16.2, i.e., sodium channel blockade	**Adjunctive** treatment of **Lennox–Gastaut syndrome** and GTC seizures in patients > 4 years of age.	Diarrhea, vomiting, pyrexia and somnolence
Gabapentin	**Actions 2, 3** from Fig 16.2, i.e., reduced glutamate and increased GABA release	An **add-on drug** in refractory focal and GTC seizures. **No change in dose of primary drug required** **Drug of choice** for neuropathic pain	Mild sedation, fatigue, ataxia, somnolence and tremors may occur.
Levetiracetam	**Actions 2, 3** from Fig 16.2, i.e., reduced glutamate and increased GABA release	Adjuvant drug in **resistant focal seizures** also in **myoclonic seizures.** 2ⁿᵈ line add-on drug in **absence seizures.** **No change in dose of primary drug required**	Mild sedation, ataxia, dizziness and somnolence
Tiagabine	Action 6 from Fig. 16.2 Blocks neuronal reuptake of GABA	An **add-on drug for focal seizures,** if they are not controlled by first-line drugs.	Confusion, depression, ataxia, dizziness, nervousness, amnesia, etc.
Vigabatrin	Action 7 from Fig. 16.2 Reduces degradation of GABA	**Reserve drug** for patients refractory to other safer drugs	Weight gain, dizziness and drowsiness, confusion, agitation and **psychotic behaviour;** irreversible **defects of visual field and colour vision, paresthesias**
Perampanel	Action 9 from Fig. 16.2 Blocks AMPA receptors	**Adjunctive drug** for focal seizures	Headache, dizziness, somnolence and rashes; irritability, hostility and aggression in some patients

Ethosuximide has no effect on other types of Ca²⁺ or Na⁺ currents. At high concentrations, ethosuximide can inhibit GABA transaminase enzyme responsible for GABA breakdown.

Indication for use is **absence seizures,** even though valproate is preferred nowadays because it is better tolerated. However, ethosuximide is used in children < 2 years of age with absence seizures due to the risk of irreversible hepatic necrosis with valproate. Ethosuximide is also approved for treatment of **myoclonic seizures.**

Adverse effects are gastrointestinal distress, which can be checked by starting therapy with a low dose, 20 mg/kg/day and increasing it gradually. Ethosuximide can also cause headache, dizziness, hiccups, and fatigue or lethargy. Rarely, it causes idiosyncratic reactions such as rashes, thrombocytopenia, leukopenia, pancytopenia, and eosinophilia.

Phensuximide is less efficacious than ethosuximide.
Methsuximide is more toxic than ethosuximide.

19. Oxazolidine Diones
Trimethadione has same the mechanism of action as ethosuximide. It causes marked sedation, and is hence not used much for absence seizures.

OTHER ANTIEPILEPTICS
20. Barbiturates
Phenobarbitone acts by **potentiating the effect of GABA** on $GABA_A$ receptors. It raises the seizure threshold and limits its spread. It is **not a preferred antiepileptic** because of its sedative and enzyme-inducing effects and behavioural disturbances. It may be used **intramuscularly or intravenously in status epilepticus** if other drugs fail to produce response.

Primidone gets converted to phenobarbitone in body. It is **seldom used nowadays** because of its poor tolerability.

21. Benzodiazepines
These bind to the $GABA_A$ receptor–Cl⁻ channel complex and **increase the frequency of channel opening** in response to GABA.

a. Clonazepam
This has prominent anti-seizure activity in pentylenetetrazol-induced generalised seizures at a dose that causes little sedation. It is useful in **absence, myoclonic, atonic or akinetic and infantile** seizures. However, **tolerance** develops to its therapeutic action within six months.

b. Clobazam
This has anticonvulsant activity in a wide variety of seizures like focal, generalised tonic–clonic, absence and atonic seizures. It is used as **adjuvant** to other antiepileptic drugs like valproate, carbamazepine and lamotrigine.

c. Diazepam
Is effective as anticonvulsant but is **not used in long-term treatment** as tolerance develops soon to this action. It is a **first-line drug in status epilepticus, eclampsia, poisoning with convulsant drugs and tetanus.** For these indications, 0.2–0.3 mg/kg is administered slow I/V. It can cause thrombophlebitis of vein.

d. Lorazepam
In emergency situations, 0.1 mg/kg slow I/V is an **alternative to diazepam** as the incidence of thrombophlebitis is lesser than diazepam.

MANAGEMENT OF EPILEPSY
Treatment of epilepsy is always **multimodal,** including:
- Treatment of the underlying disease that might be the cause of seizures.
- Identifying and avoiding the precipitating factors like sleep deprivation, alcohol intake, stress, music, and flashing lights.
- Suppression of recurrent seizures with antiepileptic drugs.
- Taking care of associated psychological and social issues.

The treatment is individualised.

Aim of Antiepileptic Drug Therapy
The aim of antiepileptic drug therapy is to prevent the seizures completely without causing any adverse effects.

Therapeutic Strategy
Therapeutic strategy is designed in a way that:
- A single, most effective and best-tolerated drug is preferred, as **monotherapy** is associated with fewer side effects.
- Because the drug treatment is to be continued for a long time, the dosing schedule should be convenient for the patient.
- Before prescribing the drug, the type of seizures should be ascertained for choosing the most appropriate drug **for the patient's specific needs**.

Any patient suffering from recurrent seizures, where the cause of seizures is not known or cannot be corrected, should be put on antiepileptic drug therapy.

CHOICE OF DRUG
The choice of drug for a particular patient **depends on many factors** such as the type of seizures, characteristics of the drug (dosage schedule, kinetics, toxicity, etc.) and the characteristics of the patient (age, pregnancy, status of liver/renal functions, profession of the patient, etc).

Mostly, **older medications like carbamazepine** and **valproate are preferred as first-line drugs**, because of the vast experiences with these drugs and precise knowledge of their therapeutic levels, pharmacokinetics and characteristic toxicities. Therapeutic drug monitoring is required for drugs like phenytoin. While some new drugs, e.g., lamotrigine, are also in use as first-line monotherapy, they are mostly used as alternatives or add-ons.

Most of the newer drugs have the advantage of fewer drug interactions and easier dosing schedule.

In general, commonly used antiepileptic drugs cause dose-related sedation, ataxia, diplopia or nausea. Patients should be followed up closely to identify and manage the common adverse effects to improve compliance. Idiosyncratic reactions such as rashes, bone marrow suppression (TCP, aplastic anemia, etc.) and hepatitis are rare, but patients should be educated about warning signs of such reactions.

Drugs for particular seizure types are given in Fig. 16.5.

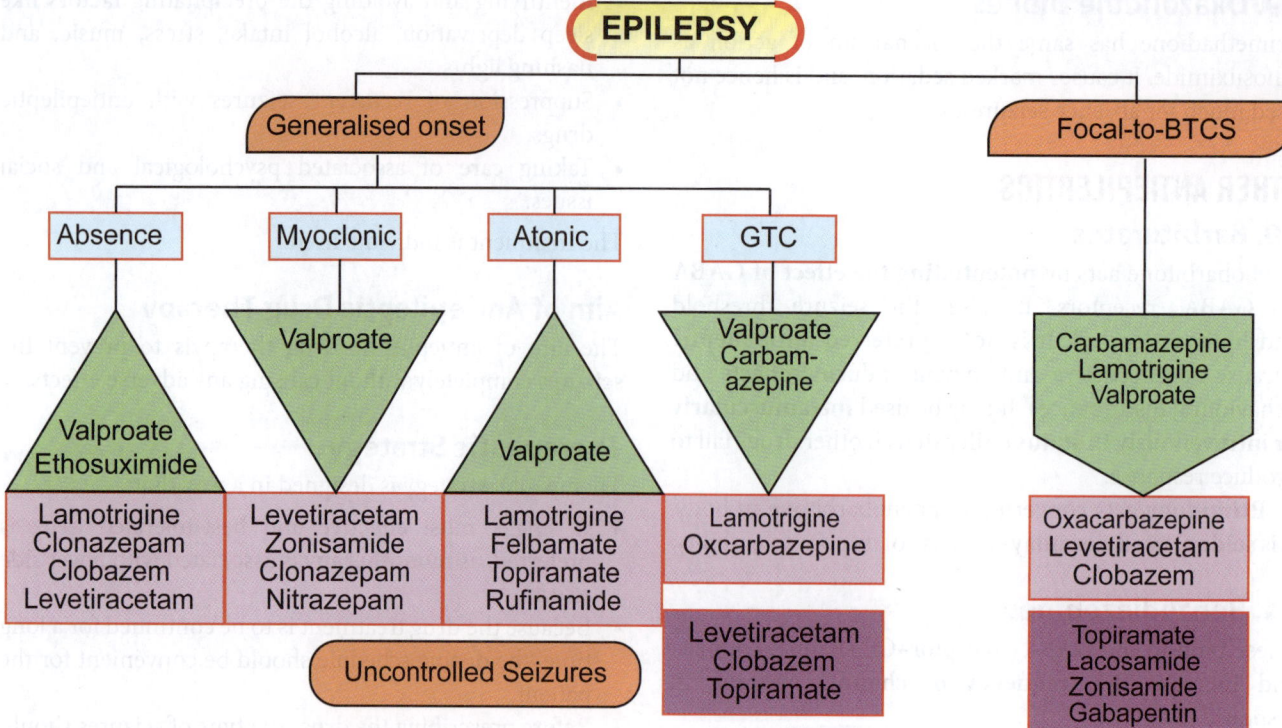

Fig. 16.5 First-line drugs in different seizure types

Drugs for Focal and Focal-to-BTCS

In focal seizures, treatment is initiated with any one of these three drugs, namely carbamazepine, lamotrigine, and valproate. These drugs have similar efficacy and the choice for a particular patient will depend on pharmacokinetics and toxicity factors. Oxcarbazepine, levetiracetam, and clobazam are alternative drugs. In cases of uncontrolled seizures, drugs such as gabapentin, lacosamide, zonisamide, and topiramate may be added.

Drugs for Generalised Onset Seizures

For primary generalised tonic–clonic seizures, valproate and carbamazepine are considered as first-choice drugs. Lamotrigine and oxcarbazepine are alternatives. In cases refractory to these drugs, levetiracetam, clobazam and topiramate are useful.

Drugs for Epilepsy Syndromes

Valproate is effective in tonic, atonic, myoclonic and absence seizures also. So, in patient with generalised epilepsy syndrome of mixed seizures types, valproate is the drug of choice as atonic, absence, or myoclonic seizures may be worsened by phenytoin and carbamazepine. **Lamotrigine** is also effective in epilepsy syndromes like Lennox–Gastaut syndrome with mixed generalised seizures.

For absence seizures, valproate, ethosuximide and clonazepam are very effective. Valproate is commonly the first choice. Ethosuximide is also good for uncomplicated absence seizures but carries the risk of rare bone marrow suppression. So, it is important to monitor blood cell counts periodically. Clonazepam is equally efficacious but marked sedation and development of tolerance to anticonvulsant effect are its drawbacks. So, it is used in refractory cases. Clobazam and levetiracetam are also effective.

For **myoclonic seizures,** valproate produces dramatic relief. Clonazepam and nitrazepam are also effective, but with benzodiazepines, associated sedation is a problem. Zonisamide and levetiracetam are good alternative drugs.

Atonic seizures are difficult to treat and respond to valproate, lamotrigine, felbamate, etc.

Infantile spasms, the cause of which may be inflammatory, respond to intramuscular corticotropin (ACTH) or oral prednisone. These drugs may help by controlling inflammatory process. Clonazepam, nitrazepam are nearly as efficacious as corticosteroids. Vigabatrin is also effective in infantile spasm.

Lennox–Gastaut syndrome usually occurs in children between 2–6 years of age and is characterised by different types of seizures resistant to treatment. Such children also have developmental delay and behavioural and psychological abnormalities. The drugs of choice are valproate, rufinamide and clobazam. Felbamate and topiramate may be used as second-line drugs.

SWITCHING OF DRUGS

Most anticonvulsant drugs are **started at relatively lower dosages** to minimise side effects. **Monitoring of plasma concentration** of drug may be required to achieve appropriate therapeutic benefit. If the patient does not respond adequately, it is necessary to **switch over** to alternative drugs. This is done by **continuing the first drug and adding a second drug**. Dose of the second drug **is adjusted** to achieve seizure control without toxic effects. After that, the **first drug is gradually tapered off over a few weeks**.

DURATION OF TREATMENT

The duration of treatment is usually long. It is appropriate to **attempt drug withdrawal after 2 years of treatment** in patients having complete control of seizures for 1 to 5 years, normal EEG, single seizure type (focal or general) and normal neurological examination including intelligence. The dose of the drug is reduced very gradually over 2 to 3 months. For patients who are refractory to monotherapy, it becomes necessary to try combinations of drugs for seizure control. It is advisable to combine drugs with different mechanisms of action. Initially, drugs of first choice are combined. If no improvement occurs, a third drug may be combined.

Status Epilepticus

Status epilepticus is characterised by **continuous seizure or discrete repetitive seizures** with impaired consciousness in between. It has many subtypes, e.g., generalised convulsive status epilepticus (GCSE) of the tonic–clonic type, nonconvulsive status epilepticus (e.g., persistent absence or focal seizures with partially impaired consciousness).

Status epilepticus is an **emergency** situation requiring immediate respiratory, cardiovascular and metabolic management. I/V diazepam 20–30 mg is the most effective drug. Lorazepam is a good alternative. Once the patient is seizure free, I/V phenytoin 20 mg/kg is given. Fosphenytoin is preferred nowadays over phenytoin for parenteral administration.

If seizures continue, I/V valproate 25 mg/kg body weight is tried. Phenobarbitone 20 mg/kg I/V, propofol or midazolam are tried if seizures are not controlled.

For patients with absence status, benzodiazepines are the drugs of first choice. I/V valproate is given in refractory cases.

Clinical problem-based questions and MCQs

9. A 20-year-old male was brought to medicine department with a history of brief episodes of loss of awareness of his surroundings, each lasting 3–4 minutes and occurring multiple times a day. The patient regains awareness after a short period but has giddiness and blurring of vision afterwards. There is no history of abnormal body movements, vomiting, or urinary or bowel incontinence. Pulse, BP and respiration were within normal range, and general physical, cardiovascular and abdominal examination detected no abnormality. ECG, serum electrolytes and hematology were normal; liver function test and renal function tests were also normal. EEG revealed spike and wave activity at 2–3 Hz, which is usually associated with absence seizures.
    i. All of the following drugs can be used in this patient, EXCEPT:
       a. Topiramate   b. Ethosuximide
       c. Valproate   d. Carbamazepine
    ii. Name the oldest drug effective in absence seizures. Describe its mechanism of action and adverse effects.

10. A 30-year-old male patient of focal epilepsy was on treatment for last three years. He is not responding adequately to treatment.
    i. All the following can be used as an add-on drug, EXCEPT:
       a. Valproate   b. Lacosamide
       c. Ethosuximide   d. Gabapentin
    ii. Which add-on drug mentioned in part (i) will not require dose adjustment of the primary drug and why?

11. i. Name antiepileptic drugs useful for relieving neuropathic pain in a diabetic patient.
    ii. Describe the mechanism of action, uses and ADRs of drugs named in part (i) above.

12. A 36-year-old male patient, a known case of generalised tonic–clonic epilepsy and uncontrolled diabetes, presents in emergency department in unconscious state with a fit that lasted for about 10 minutes.
    i. What is the diagnosis?
    ii. How will you manage this case?

13. Which of the following has NO role in absence seizures?
    a. Gabapentin   b. Lamotrigine
    c. Valproate   d. Levetiracetam

14. The preferred drug for immediate management of status epilepticus is
    a. I/V phenytoin
    b. I/V valproate
    c. I/V propofol
    d. I/V diazepam

15. Which of the following is not effective in infantile spasm?
    a. Vigabatrin
    b. Prednisolone
    c. Gabapentin
    d. Nitrazepam

Summary

- Epilepsy is characterised by episodic, abnormal, high-frequency discharge of a group of neurons causing recurrent seizures.
- Seizures can be focal/partial or generalised onset. Focal seizures may occur as Jacksonian march, Todd paralysis, abnormal intense sensations, autonomic, psychiatric symptoms and cognitive impairment. Generalised seizures include GTCS, absence seizures, atonic, myoclonic, and infantile spasm.
- Seizures occur because of an imbalance between excitatory and inhibitory influences in the central nervous system. Drugs try to restore the balance by decreasing excitatory NTMs and/or increasing inhibitory NTM activity.
- Drugs are classified based on their **mechanism of action** and the **type of seizures** treated. GTCS/focal seizures respond to drugs like phenytoin, phenobarbitone, topiramate, lamotrigine carbamazepine, lacosamide, felbamate, tiagabine, and valproate. Absence seizures respond to valproate, succinimides and oxazolidinones. Diazepam/lorazepam are used for status epilepticus, clonazepam for myoclonic seizures.
- Phenytoin causes use-dependent blockade of Na$^+$ channels, and delays the recovery of channels from the 'inactive' to 'resting' state. However, it is used only when other better tolerated drugs are not available as it has steep DRC, many ADRs (gum hyperplasia, osteomalacia, visual disturbances, teratogenic effects, hypocalcemia, anemia, diplopia, lymphadenopathy, vertigo, ataxia and neutropenia), shows bio-inequivalence and kinetics changes from first order to zero order over the therapeutic range. TDM is required while using phenytoin. Fosphenytoin is a prodrug, preferred over phenytoin for IV use in status epilepticus.
- Carbamazepine is also a sodium channel blocker and is the preferred drug for focal/focal-to-BTCS, GTCS and trigeminal neuralgia. It may cause diplopia, sedation, ataxia, hyponatremia, water intoxication and blood dyscrasias.
- Lamotrigine is a broad-spectrum drug causing Na$^+$ channel block and reduced glutamate release. It is the first-line drug for focal/focal-to-BTCS. It is also useful in absence, myoclonic seizures and neuralgias. It is better tolerated than carbamazepine, but there is a risk of severe dermatitis in young children.
- Valproate is also a broad-spectrum drug with multiple mechanisms of action and is the drug of choice in GTC, juvenile myoclonic seizures, mixed seizure syndrome, partial, absence and atonic seizures as well. ADRs are curly hair, alopecia, teratogenic effects, sedation, ataxia, tremors, nausea, hepatic damage, hyperammonemia and pancreatitis. It is not preferred in children. It should not be combined with clonazepam.
- Adjuvant or add-on drugs for refractory cases of focal, GTC seizures include topiramate, gabapentin, tiagabine, vigabatrin, lacosamide, zonisamide, rufinamide, and levetiracetam.
- Lacosamide, levetiracetam and gabapentin do not cause any induction or inhibition of enzymes, and hence there is no need to change the dose of the primary antiepileptic drug
- For absence seizures, valproate is the first choice. Ethosuximide, which blocks T-type calcium current, is also useful. Lamotrigine, topiramate and levetiracetam are also effective in absence seizures.

Questions for practice

1. Classify antiepileptic drugs.
2. Enumerate the adverse effects of:
   a. Phenytoin
   b. Carbamazepine
   c. Valproate
3. Write short notes on:
   a. Newer antiepileptic drugs
   b. Drugs for absence seizures
   c. Management of status epilepticus

Hints for problem-based questions and MCQs

1. a. Carbamazepine
2. i. a. Absence seizure
   ii a. Valproate.
3. i. c. Valproate
   ii. Refer to page 218.
   iii. Phenytoin, lamotrigine, felbamate, topiramate, tiagabine, carbamazepine
4. i. c. Phenytoin
   ii. Refer to page 216.
   iii. TDM is needed in phenytoin therapy; refer to page 216.
5. i. Refer to page 215.
   ii. Enzyme induction by phenytoin results in contraceptive failure
   iii. Teratogenicity with phenytoin. Refer to page 216.
6. c. Valproate, if combined with clonazepam can cause absence seizure status.
7. i. d. Carbamazepine
   ii. Autoinduction Refer to page 217.
8. i. a. Carbamazepine
   ii. Refer to page 216, 217.
9. i. d. Carbamazepine
   ii. Ethosuximide. Refer to page 221, 222.
10. i. c. Ethosuximide
    ii. Lacosamide, as it does not cause any enzyme induction or inhibition
11. i. Gabapentin, pregabalin
    ii. Refer to page 220, 221.
12. i. Status epilepticus
    ii. Refer to page 225.
13. a. Gabapentin.
14. d. Intravenous diazepam
15. c. Gabapentin

CONCEPT MAP - ANTIEPILEPTIC DRUGS

Mechanism of Action

Na⁺ channel blockade: Phenytoin, Carbamazepine, Rufinamide, Lacosamide, Valproate, Zonisamide, Lamotrigine
T-type Ca²⁺ channel block: Ethosuximide, Valproate, Zonisamide, Lamotrigine.
Increased GABAergic activity: Pregabalin, Gabapentin, Tiagabine, Vigabatrin, BZD, Barbiturates, Ganaxolone, Stiripentol
Decreased glutamatergic activity: Topiramate, Felbamate, Perampanel, Talampanel, Lamotrigine

Seizure Type & First-line Drugs

GTCS: Valproate, Lamotrigine, Carbamazepine
Focal: Carbamazepine, Lamotrigine, Phenytoin, Levetiracetam
Absence: Valproate, Ethosuximide in < 2 years age
Myoclonic: Valproate, Lamotrigine, Topiramate
Worsened by Phenytoin, Carbamazepine
Infantile spasm: Associated with tuberous sclerosis - Vigabatrin
Not associated with tuberous sclerosis - ACTH, steroids
Lennox–Gastaut syndrome (LGS): Valproate, Rufinamide, Clobazam
Status epilepticus: Lorazepam, Diazepam
Eclamptic seizures: Magnesium sulphate

Classification
Based on mechanism of action
Seizure type in which used

ANTIEPILEPTIC DRUGS

GTCS & Focal Seizures

Phenytoin
Uses: GTCS, Focal, Status epilepticus, Neuropathic pain, Arrhythmias

ADRs
Mild: Headache, Vertigo, Nystagmus, Loss of extra-ocular pursuit movements
High dose: Sedation, Confusion, Reversible intellectual deterioration, Diplopia and Ataxia (reduce dose)
Prolonged use: Gum hyperplasia, Hirsutism, Coarsening of facial features, Acne, Megaloblastic anemia, Osteomalacia, Peripheral neuropathy.
Fetal hydantoin syndrome: Microcephaly, Mental retardation, Hypoplastic phalanges, Cleft lip & palate.
Therapeutic drug monitoring needed

Carbamazepine
Uses: DOC in focal seizures, GTCS, Trigeminal neuralgia & Bipolar disease

ADRs
Diplopia, Sedation, Ataxia, Drowsiness, GI upsets, Hyponatremia, Water intoxication, Hypersensitivity reactions, Mild leukopenia, Blood dyscrasias.
Autoinduction → decrease in t½

Zonisamide, Lacosamide
Lacosamide is the only drug that slows activation of Na+ channels
Use: Focal seizures

ADRs
Zonisamide: CA inhibition
Lacosamide: Suicidal tendency, PR prolongation

Rufinamide
Used in LGS

ADRs
Leukopenia, QT shortening

Topiramate (Broad spectrum)
Uses: 2nd-line in GTCS, JME, focal, LGS, Pseudotumor cerebri, Migraine prophylaxis, Bipolar disorder

ADRs
Ataxia, Confusion, Nervousness, CA inhibition (Acidosis, Renal stones, Hypohidrosis), Weight loss

Levetiracetam
Decrease glutamate release by SV2A binding
Use: Adjuvant in resistant focal, Myoclonic seizure.
2nd line drug in absence seizure

ADRs
Sedation, Ataxia, Dizziness, Somnolence

Gabapentin
Decreased release of glutamate and increased release of GABA
DOC in neuropathic pain, add-on drug in refractory focal and GTC seizures

ADRs
Mild sedation, Fatigue, Ataxia, Somnolence, Tremors

Tiagabine
Reduced GABA reuptake
Use: Add-on drug in focal seizures

ADRs
Confusion, Depression, Ataxia, Dizziness, Amnesia

Vigabatrin
Decrease GABA metabolism
Reserve drug because of many ADRs like weight gain, dizziness, drowsiness, visual field defects, psychosis

2nd Line Drugs

Absence Seizures

Valproate (Broad spectrum)
Uses: DOC for GTCS, JME, Focal seizures, Atonic seizures, Absence seizures, Mixed seizure syndrome, Rheumatic chorea, Bipolar disease, Migraine prophylaxis.

ADRs
Dose-related GI upset, Sedation, Ataxia, tremors, Increased appetite, Weight gain, Curling of hair, hair loss, Idiosyncratic reaction, Hepatotoxicity, Pancreatitis and Thrombocytopenia.
Spina bifida, Cardiovascular, Orofacial and Digital abnormalities in fetus.

Ethosuximide
Uses: Absence seizures in children < 2 years of age, myoclonic seizures.

ADRs
Gastrointestinal distress, Headache, Dizziness, Hiccups, Fatigue or Lethargy. Rarely, idiosyncratic reactions such as rashes, thrombocytopenia, leukopenia, pancytopenia, eosinophilia, SLE.

Lamotrigine
Uses: GTCS, JME, Focal, Absence seizure Lennox–Gastaut syndrome, Bipolar disease

ADRs
Headache, Nausea, Vomiting, Dizziness, Ataxia, Diplopia and Somnolence, Stevens–Johnson syndrome
(Dose increased gradually, Not suitable for emergency)

SECTION 3 Drugs Acting on CNS

17 Drugs for Neurodegenerative Disorders

PH 3.7 Explain types, salient pharmacokinetics, pharmacodynamics, therapeutic uses, and adverse effects of drugs used for parkinsonism and other neurodegenerative disorders. Write a prescription to manage a case of drug-induced parkinsonism.

Learning objectives

A student of MBBS phase II should be able to:
- Enumerate drugs used for Alzheimer's disease and describe their mechanism of action.
- Enumerate ADRs and contraindications of drugs used in Alzheimer's disease.
- Classify antiparkinsonian drugs and describe their mechanism of action.
- Comment on the rationale behind combining levodopa and carbidopa in Parkinson's disease, mentioning doses.
- Enumerate ADRs and contraindications of antiparkinsonian drugs.
- Describe the pharmacotherapy of parkinson's disease.
- Write a prescription for drug-induced Parkinsonism.
- Describe the role of drugs in the management of patients with Huntington's disease, amyotrophic lateral sclerosis and multiple sclerosis.

Neurodegenerative disorders are a group of diseases resulting from **progressive** and **irreversible loss of neurons in specific regions of the brain**. It occurs with the **aging** of brain due to oxidative stress and excitotoxicity[1] caused by glutamate, amyloidosis and apoptosis. Many of the brain cells, once damaged, remain dysfunctional forever, resulting in slowly-progressing disorders. Common neurodegenerative diseases include:

1. Alzheimer's disease (AD): involves loss of neurons from the hippocampus and cortex
2. Parkinson's disease (PD): involves loss of neurons in the basal ganglia.
3. Huntington's disease (HD): also involves loss of neurons in the basal ganglia.
4. Amyotrophic lateral sclerosis (ALS): involves degeneration of spinal, bulbar and cortical motor neurons.
5. Multiple sclerosis (MS): an autoimmune disorder involving demyelination of nerves.
6. Other less common neurodegenerative disorders include Batten disease, Friedreich ataxia, Lewy body disease, Prion disease, motor neuron disease, spinocerebellar ataxia and spinal muscular atrophy.

ALZHEIMER'S DISEASE (AD)
Pathophysiology
The basic defect in Alzheimer's disease (AD) is reduced cholinergic activity. The disruption of the neuronal network begins in the transentorhinal region. As the disease progresses, it extends to involve the hippocampus, medial temporal lobes, parietal neocortex, and lateral frontal cortex. The **pathophysiological process** of AD comprises:

- Deposition of extracellular senile amyloid plaques.
- Formation of intracellular neuro-fibrillary tangles made up of abnormally phosphorylated neuronal (tau) protein.
- Marked involvement of cholinergic neurons in the nucleus basalis in forebrain that project on to the frontal cortex and hippocampus. As a result, **marked cholinergic deficiency** occurs in the brain of AD patients, affecting **learning, memory and cognition**.
- **Raised glutamatergic transmission** through NMDA receptors is also implicated.

Risk factors
- Age is the most significant risk factor for Alzheimer's disease. The incidence of disabling memory loss rises with each decade after the age of 50, with approximately 20–40% of individuals over 85 years old developing AD.
- A positive family history suggests genetic predisposition for AD.
- Females are more prone than males.
- Low intake of fruits/vegetables, low activity level, hypercholesterolemia, diabetes, raised homocysteine

---

[1]Excitotoxicity is the excessive activation of neuronal amino acid receptors. The specific type of excitotoxicity triggered by the amino acid glutamate is the key mechanism implicated in the mediation of neuronal death in many disorders.

and reduced folic acid levels are also recognised as risk factors for AD.

Clinical Picture

- The most important symptom of AD is memory loss. Approximately 75% of patients are elderly, with insidious-onset **progressive memory loss over years**.
- The early neuropsychological symptoms to appear are **deficit of verbal or visual episodic memory**. The patient exhibits deficit of visuoconstructive ability and category generation. **Language is impaired**. Initially, naming abilities are affected, followed by impairments in comprehension, and eventually a decline in fluency.
- The patient may have **difficulty driving, managing finances, following instructions, finding words, fluency, and navigating**.
- Early-onset AD may result in seizures. Motor functions are intact till later stages of the disease; however, the patient may face **problems in performing learned sequential motor tasks**.
- As the disease progresses, the patient is easily **lost and confused**, becoming incapable of independent work, and requiring daily supervision. The patient experiences difficulty in eating, dressing, walking, solving simple puzzles, and drawing geometrical shapes due to **visuospatial deficits**.
- Loss of reasoning and judgment, wandering aimlessly, especially at night, a shuffling gait and **generalised marked rigidity (without tremors)** are features that develop slowly.
- Mild **affective symptoms** like depression, social withdrawal, irritability and anxiety are common, but the patient maintains core social skills till the late stages of the disease. In the advanced stages, however, delusions, sleep disturbances and agitation may occur.
- End-stage AD patients become **mute, rigid, incontinent and bed-ridden**, requiring assistance even for dressing, eating, toileting, etc.
- The duration of the disease may vary from 1–25 years, but commonly, it lasts for 8–10 years and the patient usually dies from immobility-related complications like pneumonia and pulmonary embolism.

Diagnosis

The sequence of the appearance of symptoms in AD is different from other neurodegenerative diseases. For example, patients with frontotemporal dementia (FTD) and Huntington's disease (HD) have impaired judgment, and mood and behaviour disturbances, rather than memory loss. Parkinsonism patients develop tremors, which are usually not seen in AD. Such distinctions help in the diagnosis of AD.

CT scan and MRI help to exclude vascular, malignant and other causes of neuronal degeneration such as frontotemporal dementia and Creutzfeldt–Jakob disease.

Management

The management of AD is quite challenging. The aim of the treatment is prevention of long-term behavioural and neurological symptoms.

- **Memory aids** like daily reminders, notebooks, etc., are useful in the early stages of AD.
- The patient should **avoid falls** as far as possible; bathrooms, stairs, kitchen should be made simple and safe for use. The patient should not drive.
- Repeated **reassurances,** communication, adult daycare centers, local support groups, and caregiver alliances are useful in the long-term care of AD patients.

Drugs in the Treatment of AD

The drugs that have a **role in the palliation of symptoms** of AD are shown in Flowchart 17.1.

1. Cholinesterase inhibitors

As there is marked deficiency of cholinergic transmission in the brain in AD, cholinesterase inhibitors **that cross the blood–brain barrier (BBB)** are useful. They block the degradation of acetylcholine and thus increase cholinergic activity in the brain.

- **Tacrine** is a long-acting, reversible inhibitor of cholinesterase enzyme. It also facilitates the release of acetylcholine from nerve endings.
  - Tacrine provides symptomatic relief and improves memory, cognition and general well-being in mild to moderate cases of AD, but is less beneficial after long-term use or in advanced stage of the disease.
  - It is **out of use nowadays due to risk of hepatotoxicity**.
- **Donepezil, rivastigmine** and **galantamine** are reversible cholinesterase inhibitors that can cross the blood–brain barrier.

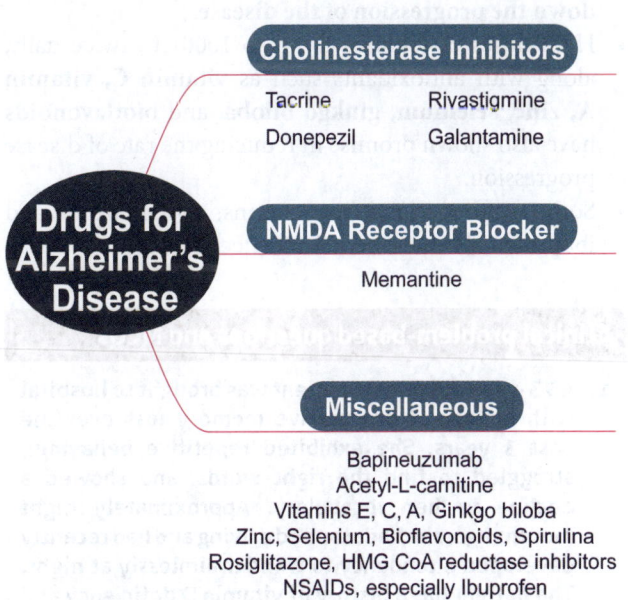

Flowchart 17.1 Drugs for Alzheimer's disease

- They produce modest and temporary relief of symptoms but are **better tolerated and safer than tacrine**.
- The dose of donepezil is 5 mg once daily, up to a maximum of 10 mg.
- Rivastigmine and galantamine are typically administered twice daily. Additionally, rivastigmine is available as transdermal patch for continuous drug delivery.

ADRs
ADRs occur due to excessive cholinergic activity such as

- Nausea, vomiting, diarrhea, increased micturition, etc.
- Abdominal cramps, muscle cramps
- Altered sleep and vivid dreams
- Bradycardia.

2. NMDA receptor blockers
Memantine

Because overactivity of glutamate through NMDA receptors is implicated in AD. **Memantine, a non-competitive blocker of NMDA receptors,** can be used to relieve symptoms in moderate-to-severe AD; dosage is 5–20 mg per day. It has **fewer adverse effects** than cholinesterase inhibitors, in the form of headache, dizziness, confusion, and constipation.

3. Miscellaneous Drugs
- **Bapineuzumab** is an anti-amyloid monoclonal antibody that has shown good results in trials; however, it is **yet to be approved** for treatment of AD. Aducanumab is a β-amyloid inhibitor, beneficial in mild cases of AD.
- **Acetyl-L-carnitine** is a structural analogue of acetylcholine. It **increases cholinergic transmission** in the brain and has **antioxidant** activity as well. It shows promise of **improving AD symptoms** and **slowing down the progression of the disease**.
- High doses of **vitamin E**, up to 1000 IU, twice daily, along with antioxidants such as **vitamin C, vitamin A, zinc, selenium, ginkgo biloba,** and **bioflavonoids** have also shown promise in reducing the rate of disease progression.
- Some studies claim that statins, rosiglitazone and ibuprofen also have beneficial effect in AD.

Clinical problem-based questions and MCQs

1. A 73-year-old female patient was brought to hospital with history of progressive memory loss over the past 3 years. She exhibited repetitive behaviour, struggled to find the right words, and showed a decline in her vocabulary. Approximately eight months ago, she had stopped driving and had recently developed a tendency to wander aimlessly at night. The patient has a history of vitamin D deficiency and hypercholesterolemia, along with a family history of memory disturbances. Her mother had similar symptoms but much later, around the age of 8. Her elder brother also had a few mild symptoms of memory problems at the age of 77. There is no history of any head injury, surgery, smoking or alcoholism. On examination, muscle tone/power is found to be normal for her age; she had no tremors and her gait is also normal. No depressive or psychotic symptoms are seen. MRI scan shows mild generalised cortical atrophy. The patient was prescribed tab donepezil 5 mg once a day.
   i. What is the diagnosis?
   ii. What is the rationale behind prescribing donepezil in this case?
   iii. Enumerate all drugs that may be useful in such a case.
   iv. What other measures are useful in long-term management of such patients?

2. A 75-year-old man with AD has severe symptoms of forgetfulness and disorientation of time/place/persons.
   i. For symptomatic relief in this case, transmission at which of the following receptors may be increased?
      a. GABAergic receptors
      b. Serotonergic receptors
      c. Cholinergic receptors
      d. Dopaminergic receptors

3. A 75-year-old female patient suffering from Alzheimer's disease is brought to OPD for follow-up examination. She is on donepezil therapy. Her caretaker reports that the patient is becoming more forgetful and is not able to recognise people and places and has disoriented sense of time as well. The physician reassures the patient and counsels the caretaker about the slowly progressive nature of the disease for which medicines do not have much of a role in slowing down or arresting the progression of the disease. The doctor adds memantine to the existing regimen of treatment.
   i. Identify the correct mechanism of action of donepezil.
      a. Acetylcholine receptor blocker
      b. Cholinesterase inhibitor
      c. NMDA receptor blocker
      d. Dopamine agonist
   ii. Identify the correct mechanism of action of memantine.
      a. Acetylcholine receptor blocker
      b. Cholinesterase inhibitor
      c. NMDA receptor blocker
      d. Dopamine agonist

4. Rivastigmine provides symptom relief in Alzheimer's disease by altering the levels of NTM at the synapses. Identify the change in NTMs caused by rivastigmine at synapses.
   a. Decrease in synaptic glutamate
   b. Increase in synaptic GABA
   c. Increase in synaptic acetylcholine
   d. Increase in synaptic dopamine.

5. All of the following have shown promising results in slowing down disease progression rate in Alzheimer's disease except
   a. Tacrine
   b. L-carnitine
   c. Ginkgo biloba
   d. Bioflavonoids

PARKINSON'S DISEASE

Parkinson's disease (PD) is the **second most common** neurodegenerative disease after Alzheimer's. It can affect individuals of all genders, races, and occupations worldwide. The mean age at onset of the disease is 60 years.

Etiology

- **Genetic factors** play an important role in 10–15% of patients, especially those with onset of PD at a younger age.
- **Environmental factors** are proposed as being more important in patients > 50 years of age. Those who live in **rural areas**, consume **well water**, and are exposed to **pesticides** are at a higher risk of developing PD.
- MPTP (methyl phenyl tetrahydropyridine) formed during the illicit production of heroin gets transported into the CNS and forms **MPP⁺** (methyl phenylpyridinium cation), which acts as a mitochondrial toxin; it is selectively taken up by dopaminergic neurons and damages them.

In a majority of patients, a **'double hit'** due to a combination of genetic susceptibility and toxic environmental factors is responsible for the increased risk.

Secondary parkinsonism can occur due to **drugs, infection, tumours and exposure to toxins** such as manganese and carbon monoxide. D_2-blocking antipsychotic agents are the most common cause of secondary parkinsonism. Other drugs like metoclopramide, chlorpromazine, lithium, and amiodarone may also cause parkinsonism.

Atypical parkinsonism includes a group of neurodegenerative conditions with **more wide-spread degeneration**. It involves multi-system atrophy, progressive supranuclear palsy and corticobasal ganglionic degeneration. Patients present with **early speech and gait impairment**. Resting tremors are usually not seen. These patients show **poor or no response to levodopa**.

Pathophysiology

The basic defect in parkinsonism is dopamine (DA) deficiency in the corpus striatum, resulting in relative cholinergic excess (Fig. 17.1). Motor function is regulated via a series of neuronal loops, which link the basal ganglia nuclei with the corresponding motor regions in the cortex. The dopaminergic neurons of substantia nigra (SN) normally inhibit the output of GABAergic cells in corpus striatum. In contrast, the cholinergic neurons exert an excitatory effect (Fig. 17.2). A functional balance between dopaminergic and cholinergic transmission is crucial for the maintenance of optimum tone and movement of voluntary muscles.

In idiopathic Parkinson's disease, the **dopaminergic neurons of SN are lost** or deficient, resulting **in an imbalance in the activity of two crucial neurotransmitters in neostriatum**. The resulting increase in GABAergic activity, in turn, suppresses the thalamocortical pathway,

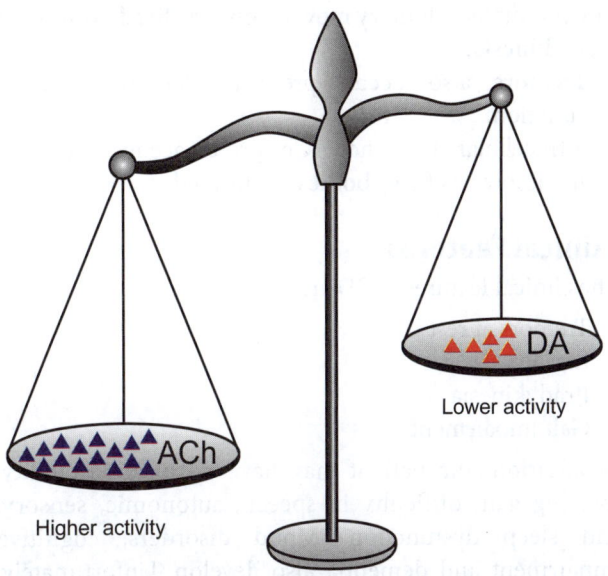

Cholinergic Activity > Dopaminergic Activity

Fig. 17.1 Cholinergic excess in parkinsonism: Cholinergic activity > Dopaminergic activity

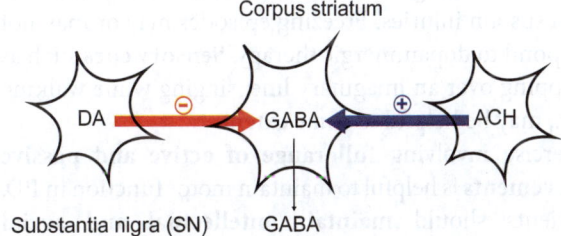

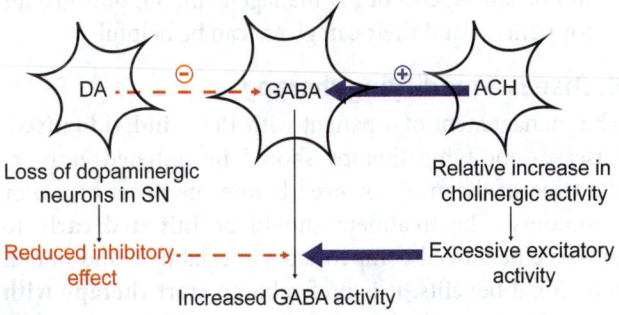

Fig. 17.2 Pathophysiology of parkinsonism

which inhibits voluntary movements, i.e., **bradykinesia** or even **akinesia**.

Tremors also occur, probably due to thalamic dysfunction.

Intracellular DA and ACh proteinaceous inclusion bodies known as **Lewy bodies** are formed.

Clinical Features

The clinical features of PD are:
- Tremors at rest
- Rigidity
- Bradykinesia
- Gait impairment

In addition, the patient may have postural instability, freezing gait, difficulty in speech, autonomic, sensory, and sleep dysfunction. Mood disorders, cognitive impairment and dementia also develop. Unfortunately, these additional features do not respond much to dopaminergic treatment.

Management of PD

It involves non-pharmacological therapy, disease-modifying measures, management of non-dopaminergic/non-motor features, drug treatment and surgical intervention.

I. Non-pharmacological therapy

- Gait disturbance and falls are important disabling factors in PD. In some patients, these features improve with dopaminergic therapy, and become worse during off periods. Walkers and canes are advised to **avoid falls and injuries.**
- Some patients freeze in a place for few seconds to few minutes. During the freeze period, the patient may fall and sustain injuries. Freezing episodes may or may not respond to dopaminergic therapy. **Sensory cues** such as stepping over an imaginary line, singing while walking etc., may be helpful to some extent.
- Exercise involving **full range of active and passive movements** is helpful to maintain motor function in PD.
- Patients should **maintain intellectual and social activities** as much as possible.
- Ensuring home safety, awareness of disease, social services and financial planning are some other important aspects of PD management. Support groups for patients and their caregivers can be helpful.

II. Disease-modifying therapy

The management of a patient with PD is **individualised**. Disease-modifying therapy should be initiated early, at the time of diagnosis or even before the onset of motor symptoms. The treatment should be **initiated early** to preserve beneficial compensatory mechanism and obtain functional benefits. It is preferable to **start therapy with MAO-B** (monoamine oxidase B) **inhibitors and/or dopamine agonists and use levodopa in later stages**, when other drugs fail to control symptoms. However, in elderly patients with **severe disability and cognitive impairment, therapy can be initiated with levodopa** also. Adverse effects of levodopa can be controlled by adjusting its dose and frequency of administration, or combining a dopamine agonist or COMT (catechol-O-methyltransferase) / MAO-B inhibitor with it.

III. Non-motor, non-dopaminergic features of PD

Non-motor, non-dopaminergic features of PD such as freezing, falling, mood disturbances and dementia also need treatment.

- Symptoms like anxiety, depression, sensory problem, sweating and freezing improve with good dopaminergic control and worsen during 'off' periods. In addition, drugs such as short-acting **benzodiazepines for anxiety, SSRIs for major depression, atypical antipsychotics** like clozapine and quetiapine may be used, depending upon the prominent symptoms.
- Dementia is seen in 80% of PD patients, and worsens with aging. Language, memory and calculation are spared, but executive functions and attention are greatly affected. **Dopaminergic drugs can aggravate cognitive impairment**. They should be stopped or their dose reduced to achieve a balance between preservation of cognitive function and control of PD.
- Autonomic disturbances like postural hypotension leading to falls also occur. Measures such as **increased salt in diet, raising the head end of bed** to prevent overnight salt natriuresis and **low-dose fludrocortisone** are useful. **Sildenafil** is useful for improving sexual dysfunction. Patient may also require **mild laxatives** for constipation and low-dose **clonazepam** for sleep disturbances.

IV. Surgical treatment

In severe cases, intervention in the form of **deep brain stimulation (DBS)** is needed. The procedure is more useful for patients suffering from levodopa-induced motor complications.

V. Antiparkinsonian drugs

The optimum tone and movement of voluntary muscles is a result of functional balance between dopaminergic and cholinergic transmission in neostriatum. Degeneration of dopaminergic neurons causes an imbalance, and cholinergic hyperactivity occurs indirectly. Acetylcholine, in turn, has an excitatory effect on GABAergic neurons. Thus, the inhibitory effect of GABAergic transmission on thalamocortical pathway becomes prominent.

The treatment involves **restoring the balance between dopaminergic and cholinergic transmission** for controlling symptoms. This is possible by either increasing the dopaminergic transmission or decreasing the cholinergic transmission (Fig. 17.3).

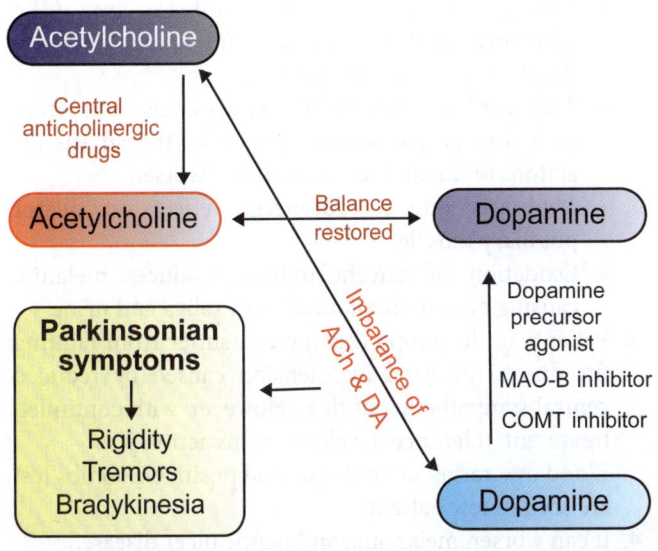

Fig 17.3 Dopaminergic–cholinergic imbalance and drugs effective in PD

ANTIPARKINSONIAN DRUGS

Antiparkinsonian drugs are classified on the basis of their mechanism of action into 2 groups (Flowchart 17.2).

A. Drugs that Increase Dopaminergic Activity

a. Levodopa

Mechanism of action

Levodopa is the **immediate precursor** of the neurotransmitter dopamine. Dopamine fails to cross the blood–brain barrier, and hence its precursor is utilised instead to make up for the deficiency in certain areas of the brain. Only **1–2 % of the administered levodopa crosses the blood–brain barrier**. It gets converted to dopamine in the surviving neurons of SN, and restores the balance between dopaminergic and cholinergic transmission to improve parkinsonism. Both D_1 and D_2 type actions are involved in the therapeutic effect of levodopa. About 95% of levodopa gets decarboxylated to dopamine in the liver and gut, and exerts its action on peripheral organs, resulting in adverse drug reactions.

Pharmacological actions

1. **CNS:** Levodopa brings about **marked improvement in parkinsonian symptoms.** Hypokinesia, rigidity and tremors resolve. The gait, posture, facial expression, speech and mood are also normalised.
   - General **alerting** response is seen. However, levodopa may cause excitement and even frank **psychosis**.
   - A non-specific '**awakening**' effect is seen with levodopa in patients of hepatic coma.
   - **Increased libido and dementia** are troublesome.
   - Dopamine formed centrally **decreases prolactin** secretion.

2. **CTZ:** The chemoreceptor trigger zone is not protected by the blood–brain barrier. Peripherally formed dopamine stimulates the CTZ to cause anorexia, nausea and vomiting. **Tolerance develops to emetic effect** with continued use of the drug. These adverse effects can be reduced by giving the drug in divided doses, with or after meals, increasing the dose slowly and adding carbidopa.

3. **CVS:** A major part (about 95%) of the daily dose of levodopa gets decarboxylated in the periphery, forming catecholamines. It exerts cardiac stimulant action, resulting in **tachycardia, ventricular extrasystole and atrial flutter.**

Levodopa causes postural hypotension, likely through central action (reduced central sympathetic outflow). Dopamine also causes renal vasodilatation and diuresis (D_1 action). This may contribute to its hypotensive action. In contrast, very large doses of levodopa co-administered

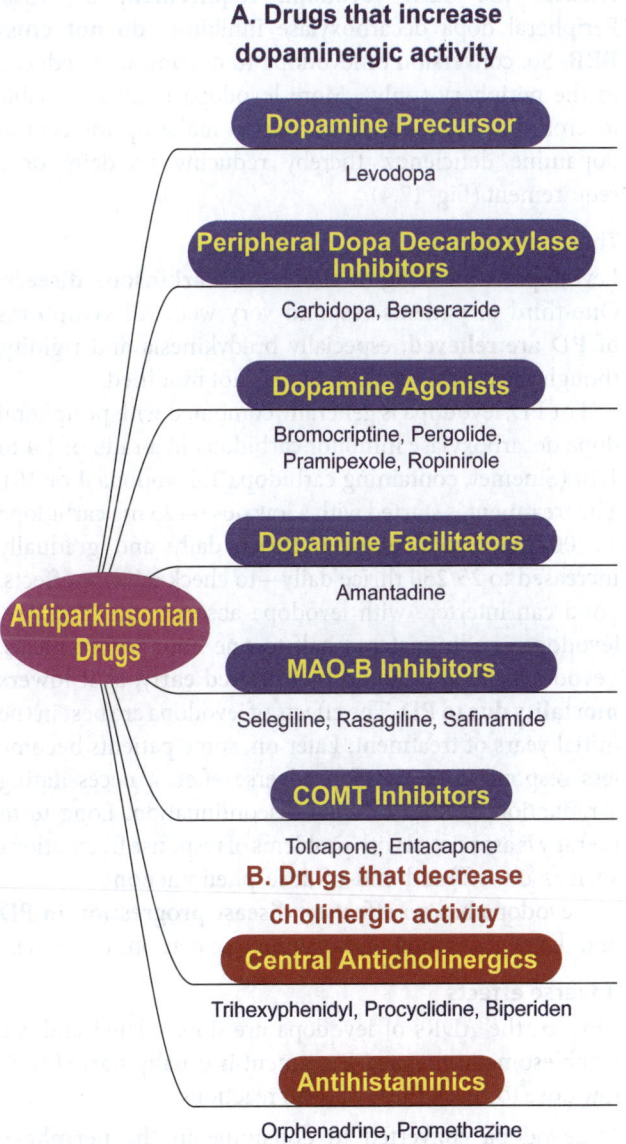

Flowchart 17.2 Classification of antiparkinsonian drugs

with non-selective MAO inhibitors or sympathomimetics can cause hypertension.

Pharmacokinetics

- Levodopa gets **rapidly absorbed** in the intestine through aromatic amino acid active transport sites, but undergoes **high first-pass metabolism** in the gut wall and liver.
- Only **1% of the administered dose crosses the blood–brain barrier** through amino acid carrier-mediated active transport to exert therapeutic action. The rest is decarboxylated to form dopamine that fails to cross the blood–brain barrier and exerts only peripheral actions. Its plasma half-life is 1–2 hours and it is metabolised by MAO-B and COMT; subsequently, the metabolites get conjugated with sulphate/glucuronide and are excreted in urine.

Concomitant administration of a peripheral dopa decarboxylase inhibitor, e.g., **carbidopa, benserazide, reduces the daily levodopa requirement by 75%**. Peripheral dopa decarboxylase inhibitors **do not cross BBB**. So, conversion of levodopa to dopamine is reduced in the periphery (only). More levodopa is thus available to cross the blood–brain barrier to make up for central dopamine deficiency, thereby reducing its daily dose requirement (Fig. 17.4).

Therapeutic uses

Levodopa is the **drug of choice for Parkinson's disease**. One-third of patients respond very well. All **symptoms of PD are relieved,** especially bradykinesia and rigidity, though the course of the disease is not modified.

For PD, levodopa is generally combined with peripheral dopa decarboxylase inhibitor carbidopa in a ratio of 1:4 to 1:10 (Sinemet, containing carbidopa 1: levodopa 4 or 10). The treatment is started with a low dose—25 mg carbidopa + 100 mg levodopa given thrice daily and gradually increased to 25/250 thrice daily—to check adverse effects. Food can interfere with levodopa absorption. Therefore, levodopa is administered half to one hour before meals. Levodopa therapy should be **initiated early,** as it **lowers mortality due to PD**. The effects of levodopa are best in the initial years of treatment. Later on, some patients become less responsive or develop adverse effects, necessitating a reduction of dose or even discontinuation. Long-term therapy is associated with problems of response fluctuations such as 'on–off' and 'end-of-dose' phenomenon

Levodopa has **no effect on disease progression in PD** and the degeneration of dopaminergic neurons continues.

Adverse effects

Most of the ADRs of levodopa are dose-related and are troublesome to manage. Treatment is usually started with low dose to check these adverse reactions.

1. Levodopa converted to dopamine in the **periphery** causes:

   - Nausea, vomiting and anorexia by CTZ (chemoreceptor trigger zone) stimulation. Tolerance develops to this action slowly.
   - Tachycardia, ventricular extrasystoles and even arrhythmias may occur because of the adrenergic actions of dopamine. Angina may worsen.
   - Mydriasis due to adrenergic effect on dilator pupillary muscle.
   - Oxidation of catecholamines produces melanin, causing brown discolouration of saliva and urine.

2. Patients on levodopa therapy can suffer from fainting fits due to postural hypotension caused by reduced central sympathetic out flow. However, with continued treatment, tolerance develops to this action also.

3. Blood dyscrasias, altered taste and positive Coombs test are seen in few patients.

4. It can worsen melanoma and peptic ulcer disease.

5. **Central side effects** are usually seen after prolonged therapy.

   - **Behavioural effects** manifest as depression, anxiety, confusion, psychosis and mood alterations. Overactivity of dopamine in basal ganglia may manifest as visual/auditory hallucinations and abnormal involuntary movements.
   - **Dyskinesias** are important dose-limiting adverse effects of levodopa. These occur in about 80% of patients on levodopa therapy for months, and worsen with time. Dyskinesias are a variety of **abnormal repetitive, involuntary movements of facial, limb and trunk muscles** in the form of grimacing, tongue thrusting, tics and choreoathetoid movements of limbs. In some patients, an episode of dyskinesia is **followed by sudden freezing** of movements known as 'kinesia paradoxa'. Tolerance does not develop to this action of levodopa. It can be **controlled only by dose reduction**, which may, in turn, worsen parkinsonian symptoms. Amantadine and levetiracetam can be useful.
   - **Response fluctuations** occur after 2–5 years of levodopa therapy. The patient may experience **'end of dose'** or **'wearing off'** phenomenon, characterised by improved mobility with each dose and rapid return of rigidity and akinesia before the next dose is due. In this situation, increase in dose and frequency of administration can be tried, but a larger dose is associated with risk of dyskinesias. Addition of COMT inhibitors or D_2 receptor agonists can be useful in such patients. Some patients experience **'on–off response'** fluctuation, in which 'on periods' of good response to levodopa and improved mobility alternate with 'off periods' of lack of levodopa response characterised by increased rigidity and immobility.

6. If levodopa is suddenly stopped, neuroleptic malignant syndrome may be precipitated.

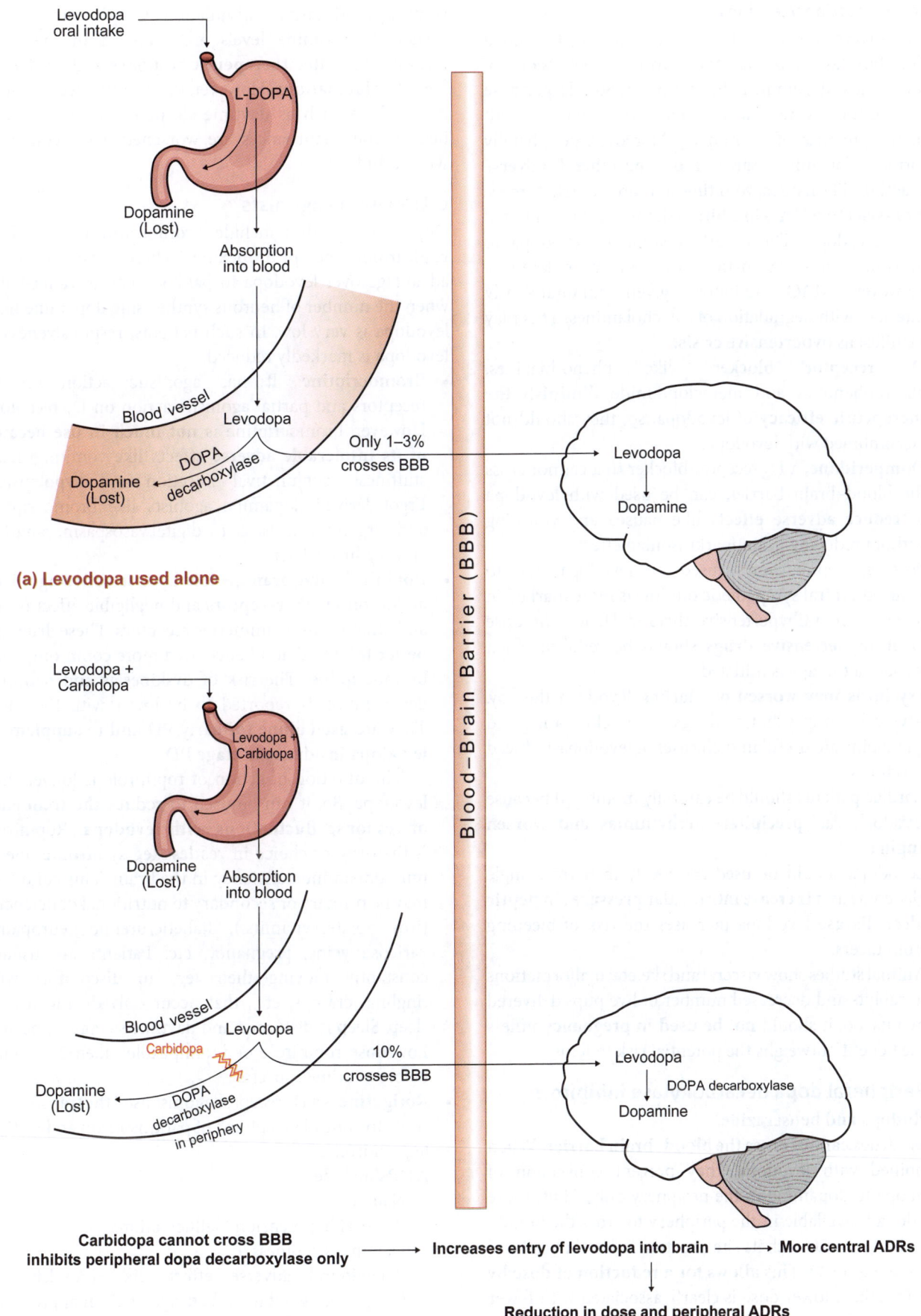

Fig. 17.4 Effect of combining levodopa and carbidopa

Drugs interactions/cautions

1. **Pyridoxine** (vitamin B_6) is a cofactor for dopa decarboxylase enzyme and favours conversion of levodopa to dopamine in the periphery. So, a **larger dose of levodopa is needed** to produce therapeutic benefit in the presence of vitamin B_6. Moreover, peripherally formed dopamine causes **more peripheral adverse reactions** like nausea, vomiting and cardiac arrhythmias.
2. **Non-selective MAO inhibitors** should not be combined with levodopa. The decarboxylation of levodopa to dopamine causes formation of excess catecholamines. However, MAO inhibitors given simultaneously interfere with degradation of catecholamines. This may manifest as **hypertensive crisis.**
3. **D_2 receptor blockers** like phenothiazines, butyrophenones and metoclopramide **diminish the therapeutic efficacy** of levodopa; so, they should not be combined with levodopa.
4. **Domperidone**, a D_2 receptor blocker that cannot cross the blood–brain barrier, can be used with levodopa to **reduce adverse effects** like nausea and vomiting without reducing its antiparkinsonian effect.
5. Postural hypotension caused by levodopa due to reduced central sympathetic outflow is more marked in patients on antihypertensive therapy. Hence, the dose of **antihypertensive drugs** should be reduced when levodopa therapy is initiated.
6. **Psychosis may worsen** on starting levodopa therapy. Atypical antipsychotic drugs like clozapine and quetiapine are useful in such cases of levodopa-induced psychosis.
7. Cardiac patients should be carefully monitored because levodopa can **precipitate arrhythmias and worsen angina.**
8. Levodopa should be used cautiously in narrow angle glaucoma as it **increase intraocular pressure**. In **peptic ulcer disease** levodopa increases the risk of bleeding from ulcers.
9. Animal studies show visceral and skeletal malformations in rabbits and decreased number of live pups delivered by rats. So, it should **not be used in pregnancy** unless the benefit outweighs the potential risk to fetus.

b. Peripheral dopa decarboxylase inhibitors

Carbidopa and benserazide.

These drugs **cannot cross the blood–brain barrier.** When combined with levodopa, they prevent conversion of levodopa to dopamine in the periphery only. Thus, more levodopa is available in the periphery to cross the blood–brain barrier and reach its site of action in basal nuclei and SN (see Fig. 17.4). This **allows for a reduction of dose by one-fourth.** A lower dose is clearly associated with **fewer dose-related adverse effects** of levodopa. Moreover, the amount of dopamine formed in the periphery is smaller, which **reduces peripheral adverse effects** like nausea, vomiting and cardiac stimulation. On the other hand, sustained dopamine levels are achieved in the CNS, resulting in **better therapeutic response** and **control of 'on–off' fluctuations.** However, the central adverse effects of levodopa such as daytime sleepiness, dyskinesia and behavioural disturbances are worsened when combined with carbidopa.

c. Dopamine agonists

Dopamine agonists include **bromocriptine, pergolide, ropinirole,** and **pramipexole.** These drugs have an advantage over levodopa in patients with **advanced PD**, when the number of neurons synthesising dopamine from levodopa is very low. In such patients, responsiveness to levodopa is markedly reduced.

- **Bromocriptine**: It has agonistic action on D_2 receptors and partial agonistic action on D_1 receptors. However, bromocriptine is **not much in use because of its intolerable adverse effects** like vomiting, nasal stuffiness, conjunctival injection and hypotension. Ergot-derived dopamine agonists like bromocriptine and pergolide can also cause digital vasospasm, gangrene and erythromelalgia.
- **Ropinirole and pramipexole** have **selective agonistic action on D_2/D_3 receptors** and negligible effect on D_1 and other non-dopaminergic receptors. These drugs are **better tolerated** and hence used more commonly than bromocriptine. The risk of dyskinesias and neuronal degeneration is reported to be lower with their use. They are **used alone for early PD and to supplement levodopa in advanced stage PD**.

  The duration of action of ropinirole is longer than levodopa. So, it can be used to **reduce the frequency of response fluctuations with levodopa**. Ropinirole is the drug of choice in **restless leg syndrome** due to mild dopamine deficiency in the brain. This condition may be primary or secondary to nutritional deficiencies (iron, folate, vitamins), diabetic/uremic neuropathy, varicose veins, pregnancy, etc. Patients are usually constantly moving their legs in discomfort with tingling, cramps, etc., that occur only during rest or sleep. Sleep is disturbed and daytime sleepiness occurs. Low-dose ropinirole or pramipexole taken 2–3 hours before bedtime is useful.
- **Rotigotine** is a D_2 receptor agonist used the transdermal route to control symptoms of parkinsonism and restless leg syndrome.
  ADRs include:
  - Nausea
  - Postural hypotension, hallucinations
  - Daytime sleepiness
  - Behavioural adverse effects like impulsiveness (shopping, gambling, betting, etc.), inappropriate sexual overactivity
  - **Psychotic adverse effects are more as compared to levodopa.**

d. COMT inhibitors

COMT inhibitors are **entacapone and tolcapone**. When carbidopa and levodopa are combined, the peripheral decarboxylation of levodopa gets inhibited by carbidopa. This levodopa gets diverted to COMT enzyme for metabolism, and 3-O-methyldopa (3-OMD) is formed.

COMT inhibition by entacapone/tolcapone exerts the following actions:

1. Metabolism of levodopa to 3-OMD is inhibited. Thus, more levodopa will be available to cross the BBB and reach its site of action to exert antiparkinsonian effect. Further, 3-OMD can compete with levodopa for active transport to brain. Thus, COMT inhibitors reduce levels of 3-OMD and **improve the entry of levodopa into the brain** (Fig. 17.5).
   Tolcapone can cross the BBB to exert central effects.
2. In the brain, tolcapone prevents conversion of levodopa to 3-OMD; consequently, more levodopa gets decarboxylated to form dopamine and exerts therapeutic action.
3. In addition, tolcapone prevents dopamine degradation to 3-methoxytyramine (3MT) in the brain, and prolongs the therapeutic action of dopamine.

COMT inhibitors are useful in prolonging the duration of the action of levodopa–carbidopa combination in the brain in advanced PD and controlling the 'wearing off' and 'on–off' phenomena.

ADRs include
- Worsening of central ADRs of levodopa (nausea, vomiting, postural, hypotension, hallucinations). The dose of levodopa can be reduced to control these ADRs.
- Diarrhea
- Yellow discolouration of urine.
- Tolcapone is **hepatotoxic** as well, and is banned in some countries.

e. MAO-B inhibitors

Selegiline is a monoamine oxidase B inhibitor that mainly **prevents intracerebral dopamine metabolism**. Thus, dopamine levels rise in the brain resulting in therapeutic effect in early cases of PD. Low doses (10 mg) do not inhibit dietary amine metabolism, but high doses can precipitate hypertensive episodes when co-administered with sympathomimetic amines and levodopa. It is used as an **adjuvant to levodopa therapy** to control the wearing-off effect and motor response fluctuations. However, the beneficial effects of selegiline in PD lasts only for few months.

ADRs with selegiline include:
- Nausea, hypotension, confusion, worsening of psychosis and involuntary movement
- Restlessness, insomnia, agitation, etc., experienced by the patients as selegiline is converted to amphetamines by liver.
- Selegiline **co-administered with pethidine causes formation of norpethidine, resulting in rigidity, hyperthermia, excitement and respiratory depression**

Rasagiline is a new **reversible MOA-B inhibitor**, and is **preferred** over selegiline nowadays. It is more potent than selegiline and its duration of action is longer. So, once-daily-dosing with breakfast is sufficient. It is reported to

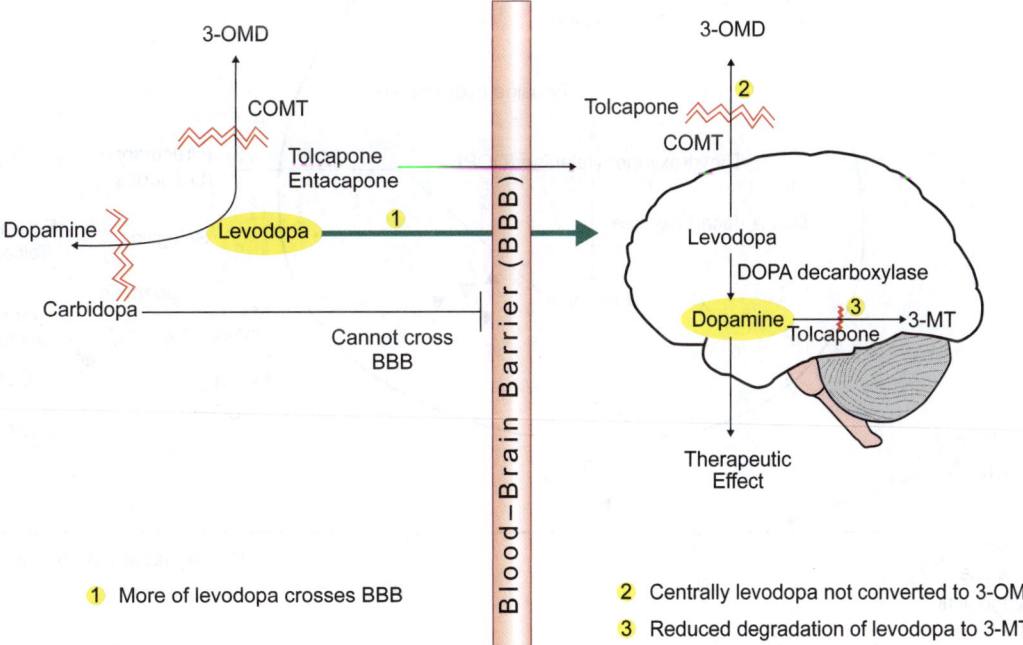

Fig. 17.5 Role of COMT Inhibitors in parkinsonism

have **some neuroprotective effect** also in PD. ADRs like insomnia and excitation are not seen with rasagiline.

Safinamide is also a selective MAO-B inhibitor. It is the drug of choice for young-onset Parkinson's disease. It can be used as **adjuvant to levodopa–carbidopa**.

f. Dopamine facilitator

Amantadine is an antiviral drug that is effective in PD also. Its **efficacy is lower than that of levodopa** and tends to diminish gradually over time due to development of **tolerance**. Its exact mechanism of antiparkinsonian effect is not well understood. Possibly, amantadine **increases the synthesis and release of dopamine in the brain and has antagonist action on NMDA glutamate receptors**.

- It is useful in **mild cases** of PD.
- It can be **added to levodopa in advanced disease** to control abnormal movements and response fluctuations in a dose of 100 mg BD.

ADRs
- Nausea, restlessness, confusion, insomnia. Sometimes, even hallucinations may occur.
- Some anticholinergic adverse effects.
- Bluish discolouration (livedo reticularis) and ankle edema (can occur).

The site of action of different drugs that increase dopaminergic activity is shown in Fig. 17.6.

B. Drugs that Reduce Cholinergic Activity

These include central anticholinergic drugs like trihexyphenidyl, procyclidine and biperiden, and antihistamines like promethazine and orphenadrine.

PD involves reduced dopaminergic activity in the substantia nigra resulting in imbalance between dopaminergic and cholinergic transmission. Anticholinergic drugs with high central-to-peripheral

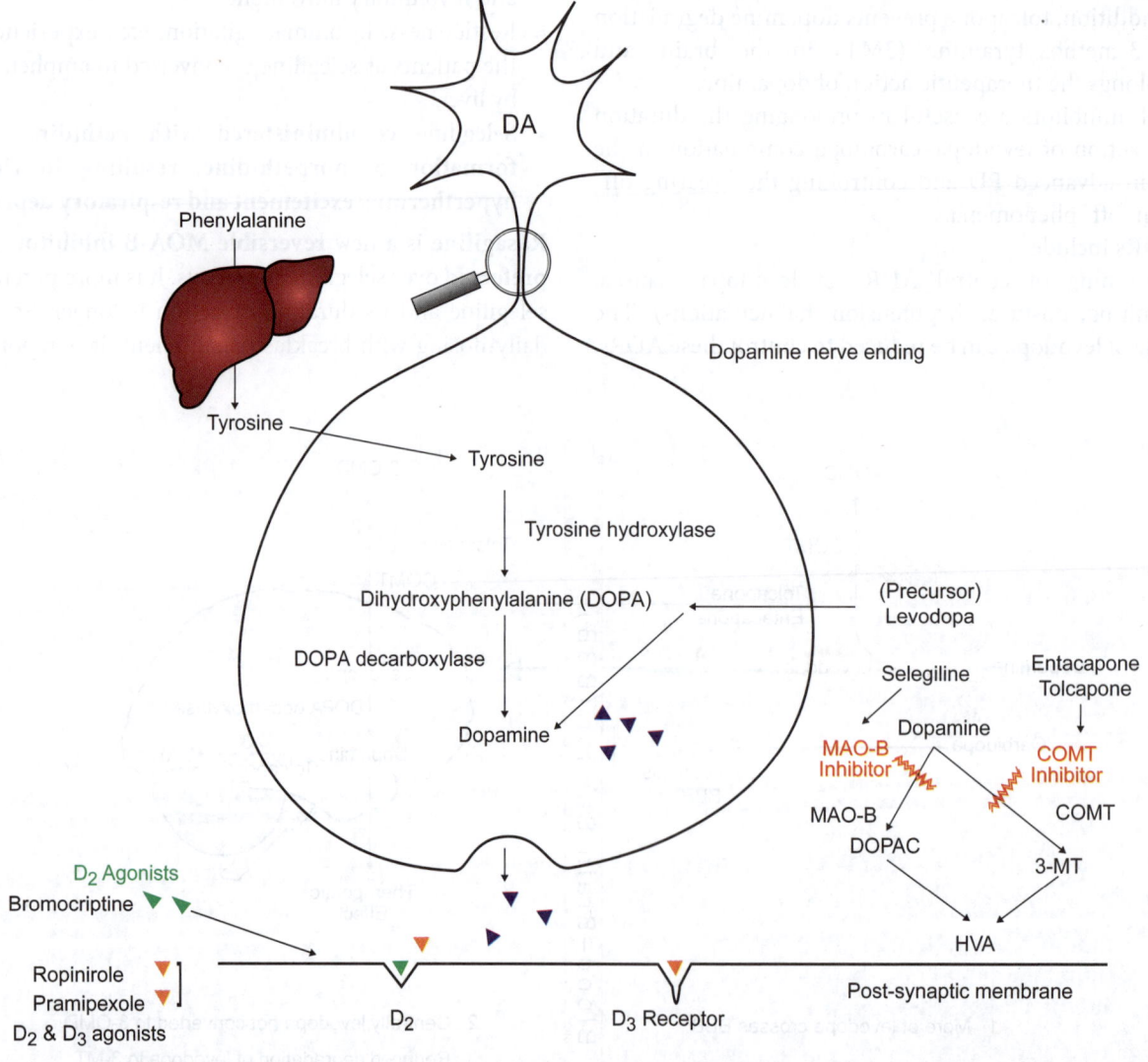

Fig. 17.6 Site of action of different drugs in parkinsonism [DOPAC: 3,4-dihydroxyphenylacetic acid; HVA: Homovanillic acid; 3-MT: 3-methoxytyramine; COMT: Catechol-O-methyl transferase; MAO: Monoamine oxidase]

action can improve this balance by **controlling cholinergic activity in the striatum**. These drugs bring about symptomatic improvement in PD, lasting for about 4–8 hours after drug administration. **Maximum relief is obtained in tremors, followed by rigidity; hypokinesia improves the least**. (Note the difference from levodopa, which causes maximum relief in hypokinesia.)

In PD, the **efficacy of these drugs is less than levodopa**, but **adverse effects and costs are also lower**.

Uses
- They are useful **alone in early PD.**
- Can be combined **with levodopa to decrease its dose**.
- Useful in **drug-induced parkinsonism precipitated by D_2 receptor blockers like phenothiazines**. In such cases, levodopa is not effective, because dopamine formed from levodopa is not able to exert action due to blockade of D_2 receptors by the offending drug. Thus, the balance of dopaminergic and cholinergic activity can be achieved only by using anticholinergic drugs.

ADRs
The ADRs are similar to **anticholinergic** drugs in the form of blurring of vision, xerostomia, confusion, cognitive impairment, and urinary retention (especially in elderly males). Trihexyphenidyl (benzhexol) is given in a dose of 2–10 mg/day. Antihistamines help in PD because of their anticholinergic and sedative actions. **Orphenadrine** has mild euphoriant action also.

HUNTINGTON'S DISEASE

Huntington's disease (HD) is an **autosomal dominant** disorder characterised by progressive cognitive, motor and behavioural dysfunction. The symptoms start between 25–45 years of age.

Pathophysiology
HD involves **progressive atrophy of caudate nuclei.** Later on, **diffuse cortical atrophy** occurs. There is neuronal loss and gliosis in caudate nucleus and putamen. There occurs degeneration of GABAergic neurons in the basal ganglia, resulting in **hyperactivity of dopaminergic neurons.** In addition, choline acetyltransferase enzyme responsible for **ACh synthesis is reduced**. Thus, in HD, the neurotransmitter defect is **just the opposite of PD**.

Clinical Features
- Rapid non-patterned, semi-purposeful, choreiform, **involuntary movements** occur. Initially, these movements are focal/segmental, but later on, multiple regions of the body are involved. **Gait is abnormal**. In advanced stage, choreiform movements decrease but **dystonia** (patterned, sustained or repeated involuntary movements of twisting muscles associated with abnormal posture), **myoclonus, rigidity, spasticity and bradykinesia** develop.
- Patients also develop **behavioural and cognitive dysfunction and dementia.** Behavioural disturbances occur in the form of aggression, depression with suicidal intent and psychosis.
- Insulin-dependent **DM and hypothalamic dysfunction** may also occur.

Management of HD
Patients and their families need neuropsychiatric, medical, social and genetic counseling and support. Choreiform movements can be controlled by D_2 receptor antagonists such as chlorpromazine and haloperidol. **Tetrabenazine** is a dopamine-depleting agent. It is the drug of choice for control of symptoms in HD, but it can induce secondary parkinsonism. Reserpine can also cause dopamine depletion.

Associated depression and anxiety need antidepressants and anxiolytics. Atypical antipsychotics drugs like clozapine and quetiapine may control psychosis.

Nothing much can be done to control the progress of the disease and associated motor and cognitive dysfunction.

Clinical problem-based questions and MCQs

6. An 81-year-old male presented with tremors in his right hand, difficulty maintaining balance, and a general sense of unsteadiness. He reported a decline in confidence while driving and expressed mild embarrassment about his unsteadiness, which has led him to avoid social interactions and gatherings. On examination, he exhibited a slightly masked facial expression, mild kyphotic posture, right-hand tremors, a stiff gait, and dysarthric speech. He walked with small, shuffling steps. Muscle weakness was noted in the back and neck extensors, hip flexors, and quadriceps. Sensory examination was normal, reflexes were intact, and cognitive functions were preserved.
   i. What is the probable diagnosis in this case?
   ii. What are the various non-pharmacological measures to be considered in this patient
   iii. Enumerate the drugs that may be used in this case.

7. A 76-year-old female patient had bradykinesia, rigidity and tremors. She was diagnosed with Parkinson's disease about 6 years ago, and since then she has been taking levodopa 250 mg and carbidopa 25 mg fixed-dose preparations before meals. The patient had adequate symptom relief throughout these years. However, since last week, the patient has been complaining of weakness, stiffness, unsteadiness and tremors before the next dose of the drug is due.
   i. What is the role of levodopa–carbidopa combination in the management of this patient?
   ii. What could be the possible cause of her symptoms expressed before next dose is due?

iii. How should this patient be managed?
iv. Enumerate the adverse effects of levodopa.

8. **Identify the INCORRECT statement about the effect of levodopa in parkinsonism.**
   a. Symptoms are relieved.
   b. Disease progression rate is reduced.
   c. Mortality is reduced.
   d. Dyskinesia occurs after continued use for few months.

9. **All of the following are benefits of combining levodopa with carbidopa EXCEPT:**
   a. Reduced dose-related adverse effects
   b. Increased therapeutic efficacy
   c. Reduced peripheral adverse effects
   d. Reduced central adverse effects like dyskinesia

10. A 60-year-old man, diagnosed with parkinsonism 6 months earlier, is on levodopa–carbidopa therapy. On a follow-up vist to his physician, the patient complains of worsening of his symptoms, with more unstable gait and tremors. The physician decides to add selegiline.
    What is the mechanism of beneficial effect of selegiline?
    a. Agonistic effect at dopaminergic receptors
    b. Inhibition of metabolism of dopamine
    c. Increased conversion of dopamine to noradrenaline
    d. Antagonist at cholinergic receptors.

11. A 46-year-old schizophrenic patient receiving haloperidol therapy for the past 4 months develops parkinsonian symptoms like tremors, rigidity and bradykinesia.
    i. Identify the most suitable drug for this patient.
       a. Levodopa   b. Benztropine
       c. Scopolamine   d. Selegiline
    ii. Describe the pharmacological basis to justify your choice.
    iii. Write a prescription for this patient.

12. An 86-year-old male patient with parkinsonism is on levodopa–carbidopa therapy for last 8 years. His symptoms are worsening. His physician decides to add a drug that prevents metabolism of dopamine, resulting in increased dopaminergic activity.
    i. Identify the drug:
       a. Entacapone   b. Bromocriptine
       c. Amantadine   d. Biperiden
    ii. Describe the status of the chosen drug in parkinsonism.

13. A 45-year-old female patient complains of discomfort, tingling, cramps in her legs during nights only. The patient keeps moving her legs constantly, which disturbs her sleep and causes daytime sleepiness. She is diagnosed as a case of 'restless leg syndrome' due to mild dopamine deficiency in the brain.
    i. Identify most suitable drug for this case
       a. Risperidone   b. Diazepam
       c. Pramipexole   d. Buspirone.
    ii. Enumerate the adverse effects of drug selected.

14. Parkinsonism involves reduced dopaminergic transmission in the brain and is managed with dopamine precursor 'levodopa'. The efficacy of levodopa is reduced by antipsychotic drugs that cause D_2 receptor blockade. However, domperidone, another D_2 receptor blocker, can be combined with levodopa to check the adverse effects without affecting its efficacy.
    Explain the pharmacological basis for the above-mentioned use of domperidone.

15. **Which antiparkinsonian drug is a dopamine facilitator?**
    a. Benserazide   b. Amantadine
    c. Pramipexole   d. Biperiden

16. **Which of the following drugs causes rigidity, hyperthermia, excitement and respiratory depression when combined with selegiline?**
    a. Pethidine   b. Safinamide
    c. Adrenergic drugs d. All of the above

AMYOTROPHIC LATERAL SCLEROSIS (ALS)

ALS is a **progressive motor neuron degenerative disease** involving **both upper and lower motor neurons**. In ALS, the motor neuron cytoskeleton is affected, along with focal enlargements of proximal axons, lipofuscin accumulation and cell shrinkage. It results in denervation and **atrophy of corresponding muscles**. It is because of this muscular atrophy that disease is termed 'amyotrophic'.

Clinical Features

These may vary depending upon which type of motor neurons (upper or lower: UMN or LMN) are affected prominently. In LMN dysfunction, the patient presents with

- Insidiously developing **asymmetric weakness** starting usually distally in the limbs
- **Cramps** with voluntary movements, especially early in the morning
- **Twitching or fasciculation** and progressive **muscle wasting**
- Difficulty in tongue movements swallowing, chewing, etc.
- Paralysis of respiratory muscles that may be fatal

In prominent UMN (corticospinal) dysfunction, patients present with:

- **Spastic resistance** to passive movement of the affected limb
- **Hyperactive tendon jerks**
- **Muscle stiffness** more than muscle wasting
- Dysarthria and possibly exaggerated motor expression of emotions in the form of **excessive weeping or laughing.**

A characteristic feature of ALS is that whether the upper or lower motor neurons are involved initially, both types get involved in the later stages of the disease. However, the **sensory, cognitive, bowel and bladder functions are** well maintained even in late stages of the disease. Ocular motility is also maintained till late stages.

Management

At present there are **no drugs** which can check the underlying degenerative pathology of ALS.

- **Riluzole** is approved to **prolong survival in ALS**. It decreases neurodegeneration and delays disease progression. Its exact mechanism of action is not known. It likely reduces excitotoxicity by **reducing glutamate release**, thereby inhibiting NMDA, kainate receptors and Na$^+$ channels. It is well tolerated. Adverse effects are minor and include nausea, dizziness, weight loss and raised hepatic enzymes levels.
- **Edaravone** has free-radical scavenging action and may reduce neurodegeneration and incidence of acute stroke in ALS. It may cause headache, gait abnormalities and hypersensitivity reactions as adverse effects.
- **Baclofen** is a centrally-acting skeletal muscle relaxant, useful for reducing spasticity in UMN lesions.
- **Ceftriaxone** may augment transport of glutamate in astroglia, and thus prevents excitotoxicity.
- **Tamoxifen and pramipexole** also have some neuroprotective action.
- Patients benefit mainly from **rehabilitative measures** like foot-drop splints, finger extension splints; tracheostomy may be needed for long-term ventilation; cough assist devices can produce artificial cough to clear airways and prevent aspiration pneumonias. Speech synthesisers can augment speech.

MULTIPLE SCLEROSIS

It is an **autoimmune, demyelinating** disease. involving inflammation, demyelination, scarring, gliosis and neuronal degeneration of **different CNS locations at different times**. Remissions and relapses are common in the course of this disease. Myelin-specific autoantibodies are present on the degenerating myelin sheath. Axonal destruction of varying extent may also occur. Cumulative axonal loss results in a **permanent progressive neurologic disability**.

- MS affects **women** more than men. The age of onset is usually between **20–40 years**, but can occur at any age.
- Disease onset may be **abrupt or insidious**.
- Some patients have very mild symptoms like exercise-induced **weakness** in limbs and fatigue, which remain undiagnosed, but in some cases the weakness of limbs is associated with UMN-type symptoms, such as **hyperreflexia, spasticity** and the **Babinski sign**.
- Optic neuritis, blurring of vision, diplopia and **variable sensory symptoms** like paresthesias, tingling sensations and band-like tightness sensation around the torso may be present in some patients, depending on which nerves are involved in the disease pathology.
- Varying degrees of **cognitive dysfunction, bowel and bladder dysfunction and ataxia** may occur.

Treatment of MS

The **aim** of therapy in MS is:
- Control of acute attack
- Disease modification
- Symptom control

1. **Control of acute attack:** During an *acute attack*, **glucocorticoids** are used to decrease severity and duration of the episode. The benefit is short term. I/V methylprednisolone 500–1000 mg/day for 3–5 days is given, followed by oral prednisone 60–80 mg/day, and gradually tapered down over a period of 2 weeks.

   Dalfampridine, a potassium channel blocker can improve walking in MS, but it reduces seizure threshold. Fatigue is improved by **modafinil**.

2. **Disease modification in MS:** The FDA has approved the use of **interferon IFNβ-1a, IFNβ-1b, glatiramer acetate, natalizumab, fingolimod, cladribine, mitoxantrone, etc.,**
   - **Interferon β** has immunomodulatory effects and decreases the attack rate and severity of the disease. It is administered I/M weekly in a dose of 30 mg. Its adverse effects include flu-like symptoms such as fever and chills, myalgias and abnormally elevated LFT (liver function tests). Injection site pain, redness, or necrosis may also occur.
   - **Glatiramer acetate** is a polypeptide made of 4 amino acids (glutamic acid, lysine, alanine and tyrosine). It reduces the attack rate and severity similar to the action of IFN β. It is given as 20 mg subcutaneous injection daily. The injection site reactions are milder. Other adverse effects include chest tightness, dyspnea, palpitations and flushing for 1 hour or so after the injection.
   - **Natalizumab** is a humanised monoclonal antibody against integrin present on the lymphocyte surface. It prevents the entry of lymphocytes into CNS and reduces the attack rate and disease severity. It is given as monthly I/V infusion of 30 mg, which is well tolerated. However, continuous use of the drug for more than 2 years caused progressive multifocal leukoencephalopathy (PML) in 0.2% of patients. Therefore, it is reserved for patients in whom other drugs are not effective. It can be given for 12–18 months when other disease-modifying agents are not effective.
   - **Fingolimod** is an inhibitor of sphingosine-1-phosphate (S1P). It prevents lymphocytes from entering into CNS by trapping them in the periphery. It reduces the attack rate and severity of MS. A dose of 0.5 mg oral is well tolerated. FDA has approved it as the **first-line drug for disease modification in MS**.

Mild lymphopenia, elevated LFT and first-degree heart block can occur. It can cause disseminated varicella–zoster infection.
- **Cladribine** is a purine analogue that inhibits DNA synthesis and repair and has immunosuppressant action. It is effective orally and given only for 2 weeks in a year. However, its long-term safety is questionable.
- **Mitoxantrone** is an immunosuppressant drug; because it is cardiotoxic, it is reserved for use in MS patients with progressive disability who do not respond to other drugs.

3. **Symptom control**: A healthy balanced diet, regular exercise as per the capacity of body and a positive outlook are very important in the management of MS. Dietary supplementation of **omega 3 unsaturated fatty acid** has an immunomodulatory effect. **Physiotherapy** may improve spasms and spastic symptoms. **Baclofen, diazepam, tizanidine and dantrolene** are useful in reducing spasticity.

For the improvement of weakness in lower extremity, potassium channel blockers like **4-aminopyridine** may be useful, though there is a risk of seizures with these drugs. **Anticonvulsants, antidepressants and analgesics** are needed, depending on the symptoms of individual patients.

Clinical problem-based questions and MCQs

17. i. Identify the neurodegenerative disorder in which sensory and cognitive functions are well maintained till late stage disease.
    a. Alzheimer's disease
    b. Amyotrophic lateral sclerosis
    c. Parkinsonism
    d. Huntington's disease
    ii. Describe the clinical features of the selected disease.
    iii. Enumerate the drugs that are useful in the selected disease.

18. Identify the drugs that can reduce incidence of acute stroke in ALS.
    a. Benztropine
    b. Baclofen
    c. Edaravone
    d. All of the above.

19. Identify an autoimmune demyelinating disease.
    a. Alzheimer's disease
    b. Parkinsonism
    c. Multiple sclerosis
    d. Amyotrophic lateral sclerosis

20. Identify the drugs used to reduce severity and duration of acute attack of multiple sclerosis.
    a. Interferons
    b. Glucocorticoids
    c. Riluzole
    d. Fingolimod

Summary

- Neurodegenerative diseases like Alzheimer's disease, parkinsonism, Huntington's disease, amyotrophic lateral sclerosis, and multiple sclerosis involve progressive and irreversible loss of neurons in specific regions of the brain.
- In **Alzheimer's disease (AD),** marked cholinergic deficiency occurs in the nucleus basalis in the forebrain, which project to the frontal cortex and hippocampus, affecting learning, memory and cognition. Raised glutamatergic transmission is also thought to play a role.
  - Patients develop progressive memory loss, language impairment, difficulty in performing learned sequential motor skills, driving, managing financial matters, following instructions, rigidity without tremors and visuospatial deficits.
  - Cholinergic drugs (cholinesterase inhibitors) are used in mild, moderate and even severe cases of AD. The drug of choice is donepezil. Rivastigmine, galantamine and tacrine are also useful.
  - Memantine is an NMDA blocker used as an add-on drug in moderate and severe cases of AD.
  - Aducanumab (a β- amyloid inhibitor), bapineuzumab, vitamins E and C, Zn, selenium, and acetyl-L-carnitine are beneficial in mild cases of AD.
- **Parkinson's disease** or parkinsonism (PD) is due to imbalance between dopaminergic (reduced) and cholinergic (relatively increased) activity in the substantia nigra, resulting in increased GABAergic activity in the corpus striatum.
  - Tremors, rigidity, and bradykinesia are key clinical features.
  - Levodopa is the drug of choice. It is always combined with carbidopa, a peripheral dopa decarboxylase inhibitor in order to reduce dose and systemic peripheral toxic effects of levodopa.
  - ADRs of levodopa include orthostatic hypotension, psychosis, anorexia, nausea, vomiting, mydriasis, dyskinesia and response fluctuations. Levodopa is contraindicated in patients with glaucoma and psychosis.
  - MAO-B inhibitors like selegiline, rasagiline, and safinamide are preferred in early onset parkinsonism and on–off phenomenon.
  - COMT inhibitors such as entacapone, tolcapone and opicapone are used in patients showing on–off phenomenon.
- **Huntington's disease** is caused by NTM defects, just the opposite of PD. Tetrabenazine is useful.
- **Amyotrophic lateral sclerosis** is a progressive motor neuron degenerative disease, affecting UMNs or LMNs. Riluzole is used as it decreases glutamate

release and blocks Na⁺ channels. Edaravone acts as a free radical scavenger. Baclofen, ceftriaxone, tamoxifen and pramipexole are also useful.
- **Multiple sclerosis** is autoimmune demyelination of different CNS locations at different times. Glucocorticoids are useful.
  - Interferon IFNβ-1a, IFNβ-1b, glatiramer acetate, natalizumab, fingolimod, mitoxantrone, etc., also have a disease-modifying role in the management of multiple sclerosis.

Questions for practice

1. Explain why:
   a. Pyridoxine should not be used in patients receiving levodopa therapy.
   b. Dose of antihypertensives needs readjustment on starting levodopa therapy.
   c. Central anticholinergics are drugs of choice in 'drug induced' secondary parkinsonism.
2. Write short notes on:
   a. Role of dopamine agonists in parkinsonism
   b. Dopa decarboxylase inhibitors
   c. COMT inhibitors

Hints for problem-based questions and MCQs

1. i. Alzheimer's disease
   ii. Increases cholinergic activity in the brain. Refer to page 229.
   iii. Refer to Flowchart 17.1, page 229.
   iv. Reassurance, memory aids, avoid falls; refer to page 229.
2. c. Cholinergic receptors
3. i. b. Cholinesterase inhibitor
   ii. c. NMDA receptor blocker
4. c. Increase in synaptic acetylcholine
5. a. Tacrine
6. i. Parkinsonism
   ii. Refer to page 232.
   iii. Refer to page Flowchart 17.2, page 233.
7. i. Refer to page 234.
   ii. 'End-of-dose' phenomenon
   iii. Refer to page 234.
   iv. Refer to page 234.
8. b. Reduces rate of disease progression.
9. d. Reduced central adverse effects like dyskinesia.
10. b. Inhibition of metabolism of dopamine.
11. i. b. Benztropine
    ii. Refer to page 238
    iii. a. Dose reduction of haloperidol is tried in patients with stabilised symptoms.
        b. If dose reduction results in return of psychotic symptoms, replace haloperidol with clozapine (low dose, 150–300 mg/day).
        c. Benztropine 4 mg/day or Amantadine 100 mg/day
12. i. a. Entacapone
    ii. Refer to page 237.
13. i. c. Pramipexole
    ii. Refer to page 236.
14. Domperidone does not cross the blood–brain barrier. So, it does not affect efficacy of levodopa. Domperidone prevents levodopa's effect on CTZ (which lies outside the blood–brain barrier) and checks nausea and vomiting caused by levodopa.
15. b. Amantadine
16. a. Pethidine
17. i. b. Amyotrophic lateral sclerosis
    ii. Features of both UMN and LMN lesions are present. LMN features are asymmetrical muscular weakness, cramps, twitching and fasciculations. UMN features include spastic resistance, hyperactive tendon jerks, and muscle stiffness.
    iii. Drugs cannot check underlying degenerative pathology. Riluzole can prolong survival, Edaravone prevents acute stroke, and baclofen decreases UMN spasticity. Tamoxifen, pramipexole and ceftriaxone have some neuroprotective effect.
18. c. Edaravone
19. c. Multiple sclerosis
20. b. Glucocorticoids

CONCEPT MAP - DRUGS FOR NEURODEGENERATIVE DISORDERS

DRUGS FOR NEURO-DEGENERATIVE DISEASES

Alzheimer's Disease

Memantine
- Add-on drug in moderate and severe cases.
- Less ADRs than ChEIs.

Drugs
- Cholinesterase Inhibitors
- Memantine: NMDA blocker
- Others: Bapineuzumab, Acetyl-L-carnitine, High-dose vitamin E, Vitamin C, Vitamin A, Zinc, Selenium, Ginkgo biloba, Bioflavonoids

ChEI
- DOC: Donepezil
- Rivastigmine, Galantamine also useful
- Tacrine not used: Hepatotoxic

Clinical Features
- Progressive memory loss
- Language impairment
- Rigidity without tremors,
- Visuospatial deficits,
- Difficulty in driving/ managing finances following instructions/finding words/ fluency and navigation.

Pathophysiology
- Marked cholinergic deficiency in nucleus basalis in forebrain
- Raised glutamatergic transmission

Huntington's Disease

Drugs
- Choreiform movements: **Dopamine antagonists**
- **Tetrabenazine**: approved for symptom control → can induce secondary parkinsonism.
- Mood disorders: **Atypical antipsychotics, Antidepressants, Anxiolytics**

Management
- Neuropsychiatric
- Medical
- Social
- Genetic counselling

Clinical Features
- Focal involuntary choreiform movements
- Abnormal gait, Dystonia, Myoclonus
- Rigidity, Spasticity, Bradykinesia
- Behavioural, Cognitive dysfunction
- Dementia

Pathophysiology
- Progressive neuronal loss & gliosis in caudate nuclei → diffuse cortical atrophy
- Hyperactivity of dopaminergic neurons
- Reduced ACh synthesis

Parkinson's Disease

Pathophysiology
- Loss of dopaminergic neurons of SN → imbalance between ACh-DA activity in neostriatum.
- Lewy bodies formed.
- Increase in GABAergic activity → suppression of thalamo-cortical pathway → Bradykinesia or Akinesia.
- Thalamic dysfunction → Tremors

Clinical Features
- Tremors at rest
- Rigidity
- Bradykinesia
- Gait impairment

Classification
- **Drugs increasing dopaminergic activity**: Levodopa, Carbidopa, Benserazide (Dopa decarboxylase inhibitors), dopamine agonists, facilitators, MAO-B inhibitors and COMT inhibitors.
- **Drugs decreasing cholinergic activity**: Central anticholinergics: Trihexyphenidyl, Procyclidine, Biperiden and Antihistamines

ADRs
Nausea, Vomiting, Anorexia, Altered taste, Brown discolouration of saliva and urine. Postural hypotension, Syncope, Arrhythmias, Angina may worsen. Behavioural disturbances, Dyskinesia and response fluctuations (on-off, end of dose)

Levodopa
DOC: Dopamine precursor, Only 1-2 % crosses blood brain barrier → converted to dopamine in SN and restores NTM balance → relieves symptoms lowers mortality in PD.

Carbidopa, Benserazide
Peripheral DOPA decarboxylase inhibitors — reduce daily levodopa requirement by 75%, reduced peripheral ADRs

MAO-B inhibitors
Selegiline, Rasagiline, Safinamide - Preferred in early onset parkinsonism and on-off phenomenon.

COMT inhibitors
like Entacapone, Tolcapone in on-off phenomenon

Multiple sclerosis

Pathophysiology
Autoimmune demyelination of different CNS locations at different times.

Clinical Features
Fatigue, Exercise induced weakness in limbs, Hyper-reflexia, Spasticity, Babinski sign, Optic neuritis, Blurring of vision, Diplopia, Variable sensory symptoms, Cognitive dysfunction, Bowel and Bladder dysfunction, Ataxia.

Drugs
During acute attack Glucocorticoids are useful. Methylprednisolone IV for few days, then oral and tapered down.
For **disease modification** interferon IFNβ-1a, IFNβ-1b, Glatiramer acetate, Natalizumab, fingolimod, Mitoxantrone useful.

Amyotropic Lateral Sclerosis

Drugs
Riluzole reduces excitotoxicity by reducing glutamate release and improves survival duration.
Ceftriaxone, Tamoxifen, Pramipexole some neuroprotective action.

Pathophysiology
Progressive motor neuron degenerative disease, involving both upper and lower motor neurons, resulting in muscular atrophy.

Clinical Features
LMN
Assymetric muscular weakness, Cramps, Twitching, Fasciculations, Wasting
UMN
Spasticity, Hyperactive tendon jerks, Stiffness, Dysarthria.

ADRs Riluzole
Nausea, Dizziness, Weight loss and Raised hepatic enzymes levels.

SECTION 3 Drugs Acting on CNS

18 Antipsychotic Drugs

PH 3.5 Describe types, salient pharmacokinetics, pharmacodynamics, therapeutic uses, adverse drug reactions of drugs used for psychosis. Devise a management plan for psychotic disorders.

Learning objectives

A student of MBBS phase II should be able to:
- Describe the pathophysiology and symptoms of schizophrenia.
- Classify drugs used for schizophrenia.
- Describe the mechanism of action of antipsychotic drugs.
- Enumerate therapeutic uses and adverse effects of typical and atypical antipsychotics.
- Describe the advantages of atypical antipsychotics over typical antipsychotics.
- Devise management plan for a patient with schizophrenia.

Definition

A *psychiatric* or *mental disorder* is the occurrence of a **clinically significant, behavioural or psychological pattern** in an individual, usually **resulting in distress, disability and increased risk of suffering.**

CLASSIFICATION OF MENTAL DISORDERS

The classification of mental disorders is essential for standardising diagnoses and facilitating effective communication between clinicians, patients, caregivers, and peers regarding the prognosis of the disease. In the past, the terms 'psychosis' and 'neurosis' were used in most classifications.

Psychosis is a severe psychiatric illness characterised by distortion in behaviour, perception and thought, **severe enough to cause inability to recognise reality.** It includes a range of disorders such as schizophrenia, mania, depression and bipolar disease. Patients of psychosis fail to meet the demands of routine life.

Neurosis is less serious than psychosis and encompasses conditions such as anxiety neurosis, obsessive compulsive disorders, phobias and hysterical fits. While patients of neurosis experience **extreme suffering, they can still comprehend reality**.

The **two major classifications** of psychiatric disorders used currently are:

ICD 11: International Classification of Diseases and Related Health Problems, 11th edition, released by WHO in June 2018.
DSM-V: Diagnostic and statistical manual of mental disorders, 5th edition, released by American Psychiatric Association in 2013.

The terms psychosis and neurosis are not used in these systems of classification; instead, the term '**dimensional description of symptoms**' is used with focus on the **current clinical presentation**. These systems are more in line with recovery-based approaches to psychiatric rehabilitation.

Dimensional Symptom Description of Psychiatric Disorders

Symptoms are described in **six domains,** viz., positive, negative, depressive mood, maniac mood, psychomotor, and cognitive symptoms.

1. **Positive symptoms** can occur as delusions, hallucinations, illusions, disorganised thinking and behaviour, or experiences of passivity and control. A detailed description of these symptoms is given in Box 18.1.

> **Box 18.1. Positive symptoms in psychiatric disorders**
>
> a. **Delusions are unshakeable beliefs** that are not true or based on reality. Delusion may be **non-bizarre** or **completely bizarre.**
>   Non-bizarre delusions are beliefs in things that may happen in reality, e.g., being followed, poisoned or conspired against.
>   Bizarre delusions are beliefs of things that cannot happen in real life, e.g., being cloned by aliens or inner thoughts being broadcasted on TV.
>   There can be delusions of:
>   - Jealousy: belief of spouse or sexual partner being unfaithful.
>   - Grandiosity: overinflated sense of power, worth, knowledge or identity.
>   - Persecutory delusions: belief of being mistreated or being harmed.

- **Erotomanic delusions:** belief that someone famous or important is in love with him/her.
- **Somatic delusions:** belief of having some physical defect or medical problem.

b. **Hallucinations are false perceptions** of having seen, heard, touched, tasted or smelled something which was not really present.
   - **Auditory hallucinations** are sense of hearing voices coming from inside or outside the mind, talking to each other or telling the patient to do something.
   - **Visual hallucinations** are seeing insects crawl, or flashes of light or bright spots or shapes which are not present.
   - **Olfactory hallucination** is the sense of odour coming from one's own body or something nearby.
   - **Gustatory hallucinations** are false perceptions of taste in the absence of oral stimulus.
   - **Tactile hallucinations** are feelings of being tickled, blast of hot or cold air on face, insects crawling, etc.

c. **Illusions** are misinterpretation of actual sensory stimulus, e.g., considering a rope to be a snake.

d. **Disorganised thinking and behaviour** is evidenced by disorganised speech or inappropriate behaviour, actions or gestures. 'Inappropriate' implies exhibiting incorrect emotional responses for a given context, e.g., crying at a joke or laughing at a funeral.

e. **Experience of passivity and control** is the belief that one's thoughts or actions are influenced or controlled by an external agent or alien.

2. **Negative symptoms** include paucity of speech, interest, emotional responses and drive. For example:
   - **Alogia** or paucity of speech is the inability to speak because of mental defect, confusion or aphasia.
   - **Anhedonia** is the loss of interest in previously enjoyable or rewarding activities such as hobbies, friendship, food, work and sex.
   - **Constricted, blunted or flat affect:** Constricted affect is narrow range of emotional expression, with mildly reduced emotional expressiveness. Blunted affect is more severe than a constricted affect but less severe than a flat affect, where the person has nearly no emotional expression or display of emotions.
   - **Avolition** means lack of initiative for normal behaviours like grooming, dressing, social interaction or goal-directed tasks.

3. **Depressive mood symptoms** include sadness, lack of interest, guilt, apathy, apprehension, hopelessness, crying, eating in excess or eating less, weight gain/loss, sleep disturbance, fatigue and suicidal intent.

4. **Manic mood symptoms** like mood swings, elevated mood, euphoria, anxiety, apprehension, risk-taking behaviours, self-harm, racing and crowded thoughts, hyperactivity, impulsivity, and rapid and frenzied speaking.

5. **Psychomotor symptoms** include:
   - **Psychomotor agitation** refers to engaging in movements that serve no purpose, e.g., pacing around, tapping toes, fidgeting, hand-wringing, moving objects for no reason, and starting and stopping abruptly. It is associated with emotional distress, physical restlessness, talking fast, and racing and crowded thoughts.
   - **Psychomotor retardation** involves slowing down of thought process and sluggish or diminished movements.
   - **Catatonic symptoms** include stiffness of muscles with inability to move (the patient stays still), amnesia, staring spells or muteness, imitation of someone's movements and limited range of emotions.

6. **Cognitive symptoms** include deficits in speed of processing information, attention/concentration, orientation, judgment, abstraction, verbal or visual learning, and working memory.

TREATMENT OF MENTAL DISORDERS

Treatment is mostly **empirical and symptom-oriented** as the exact pathophysiology is not well understood. Psychotropic drugs are named based on their primary indication, e.g., antipsychotics, antidepressants, antimanics, and antianxiety drugs.

The commonly encountered problems in psychiatric practice are anxiety, schizophrenia, and affective disorders like depression, mania and bipolar disease.

Schizophrenia

It is chronic psychosis characterised by specific psychological symptoms that lead to disorganisation of the patient's personality.

Etiology

The etiology of schizophrenia is not clearly understood, though several theories implicate a variety of causative factors such as:

- **Genetic vulnerability** may have a role, as the lifetime morbid risk is higher in first-degree relatives (twins, siblings, children, first cousins) of schizophrenic patients than in normal population. Children born to men older than 60 years of age are also prone to develop this disorder.
- **Neurotransmitter dysfunction** in the form of **dopamine** or **serotonin overactivity, glutamate dysfunction** (hypo/hyperactivity or glutamate-induced neurotoxicity) and **lack of inhibitory GABAergic control** over dopaminergic neurons are implicated in the causation of schizophrenia.
- **Neuro-developmental** hypothesis implicates developmental abnormalities of the brain, especially those involving the amygdala and frontal cortex, due to

gestational complications, viral infections, maternal starvation, etc., in the etiology of schizophrenia.
- In addition, personality disorganisation, stressful life events and socio-cultural factors like social deprivation, migration, and urban environment have also been implicated.

Types
Previously, schizophrenia was classified as Types I and II. **Type I** has acute onset of symptoms that are predominantly positive, respond well to treatment, and has a good patient outcome. **Type II** schizophrenia has insidious onset of symptoms that are predominantly negative, respond poorly to treatment, and has a poor patient outcome.

Clinical features
The prevalence of schizophrenia is 1% in general population. Onset of the disease is **usually insidious** (over a period of several months) but may be acute in some cases (over 2–3 weeks). Variations in type and severity of symptoms may occur over time. There are periods of **acute exacerbations and remission**. The patient has disturbed perception, thought, affect and behaviour. Diagnosis is purely clinical. The patient may present with **positive** and **negative** symptoms.

Positive symptoms
Delusions (persecutory, grandiose, reference or religious): In some patients, the delusions become quite fixed, extensive and tend to determine what the patient does or says. Such delusions are known as **systematised delusions**.

Hallucinations: Auditory hallucinations are the most common symptom reported in schizophrenia. Patients complain of hearing threatening, accusing, insulting, conspiring, and obscene voices. Visual hallucinations are also frequent. However, tactile (touch), olfactory (smell) and gustatory (taste)-related hallucinations are not usual.

Depersonalisation (being a detached observer of oneself), **derealisation** (a feeling that one's surroundings are not real) and **somatic preoccupations** (the patient has no genuine physical disorder but manifests psychological conflicts in a somatic manner).

Negative symptoms
These include affective flattening, (reduced display of emotions), alogia (poverty of speech), avolition (lack of motivation to do any tasks), apathy (detachment/indifference), anhedonia (lack of pleasure), asociality (reduced social initiative) and attention deficit.

Behavioural disturbance
The patient may be agitated, screaming, talkative or completely silent and groomed. Inappropriate emotions, impulsiveness, violent behaviour and suicidal intent are also seen in some schizophrenics.

Psychomotor activity
Psychomotor activity may be decreased or increased. Sometimes, catatonic features may be present.

Thought disturbance
Thought content, form and process are disturbed to varying extent, causing impaired attention, poor abstract thinking abilities, thought blocking, etc.; this is evident from the patient's language (spoken and written) that shows incoherence, derailment, loosening of associations, neologism (coining new words), tangentiality (unrelated content), echolalia (repetition), etc.

Management of schizophrenia
Diagnosis
The diagnosis of schizophrenia is purely clinical. Patient may have positive or negative symptoms or disturbances of thought, behaviour and psychomotor activity for at least one month. Psychometric tests that measure specific aspects of personality, thinking and intelligence are ancillary to clinical assessment.

Treatment
The management of a schizophrenic patient involves antipsychotic drug therapy, electroconvulsive therapy in resistant cases, and patient rehabilitation measures.

1. **Antipsychotic drugs** are the mainstay of treatment. These reduce the severity as well as frequency of symptomatic exacerbations and improve the quality of life. The acute stage of schizophrenia usually lasts for 4–8 weeks. Drugs should be selected for a patient after considering factors such as efficacy, accessibility, availability, affordability, and adverse effects. Currently, conventional antipsychotics, e.g., haloperidol 1–10 mg BD, atypical antipsychotic risperidone 1–3 mg BD, or aripiprazole are commonly prescribed. After initiating therapy, if improvement occurs, the drug is continued for 6 months to stabilise the patient; then a minimal effective dose is continued for about 2 years to prevent relapse. If acute symptoms do not improve after 4–6 weeks of using a drug, a drug from some other class is tried. In refractory cases, clozapine 25–100 mg daily is prescribed.

   The rate of non-compliance is high among schizophrenics (40–50%); this can be checked by using long-acting injectable preparations (such as fluphenazine decanoate and haloperidol decanoate) in the maintenance phase. Relapse of acute exacerbation at any stage needs reinstatement of therapy/increase in dose/change in drug.

2. **Electroconvulsive therapy (ECT)** is required in schizophrenia if acute symptoms are not controlled by drugs, adverse drug reactions occur, or there is uncontrollable catatonic excitement or stupor.

3. **Rehabilitation**: In addition to drugs and ECT, several psychosocial interventions are required to rehabilitate the schizophrenic patients. These include, educating the patients and their families about the nature and course of the disease, training the patient in self-care, hygiene, cognitive behaviour therapy, social skills training, vocational retraining in a new or previous skill, and family therapy to enhance interpersonal communication and decrease stress in the family.

ANTIPSYCHOTIC DRUGS

Broadly speaking, 'antipsychotics' are the drugs used for the **treatment of schizophrenia and other agitated states.** However, all types of psychosis may not respond to these drugs. This term is often used interchangeably with the term '**neuroleptics**'. Previously, they were also called '**major tranquilizers**'.

Classification

Antipsychotic drugs can be classified as (a) **typical** and (b) **atypical agents.** Typical antipsychotics are further classified based on their chemical nature into phenothiazines, butyrophenones and thioxanthenes (Flowchart 18.1).

Mechanism of Action of Antipsychotic Drugs

Dopaminergic and serotonergic overactivity has been implicated in the etiology of schizophrenia. Most of the available antipsychotic drugs affect these two neurotransmitter systems in the brain.

The distribution of dopaminergic pathways and receptors in the brain is described in Box 18.2 and depicted in Fig. 18.1.

Box 18.2 Dopaminergic fibres and receptors

Dopaminergic fibres: The distribution of dopaminergic fibres in the brain is shown in Fig. 18.1. These comprise:

1. The mesolimbic–mesocortical pathways (from brainstem ventral tegmentum to the limbic system and neocortex) are closely related to behaviour and psychosis. **D_2 receptor blockade in this pathway is considered responsible for antipsychotic efficacy of typical agents like chlorpromazine.**
2. The nigrostriatal pathway (from substantia nigra to caudate nucleus and putamen, constituting dorsal striatum) is involved in the coordination of voluntary movements. **D_2 receptor blockade in this pathway leads to extrapyramidal symptoms** like tremors, rigidity and bradykinesia that resemble Parkinson's disease.
   At least 60% of striatal D_2 receptors must be occupied by typical antipsychotic agents for obtaining therapeutically useful effect in psychosis. Extrapyramidal symptoms, however, occur if ≥ 80% D_2 receptors are occupied.
3. Tuberoinfundibular pathway (from arcuate nuclei to pituitary) controls prolactin secretion from anterior pituitary. **D_2 blockade in this pathway results in hyperprolactinemia, galactorrhea, gynecomastia and amenorrhea.**
4. Medullary periventricular and incertohypothalamic pathways appear to regulate **eating and copulatory behaviour**, respectively.

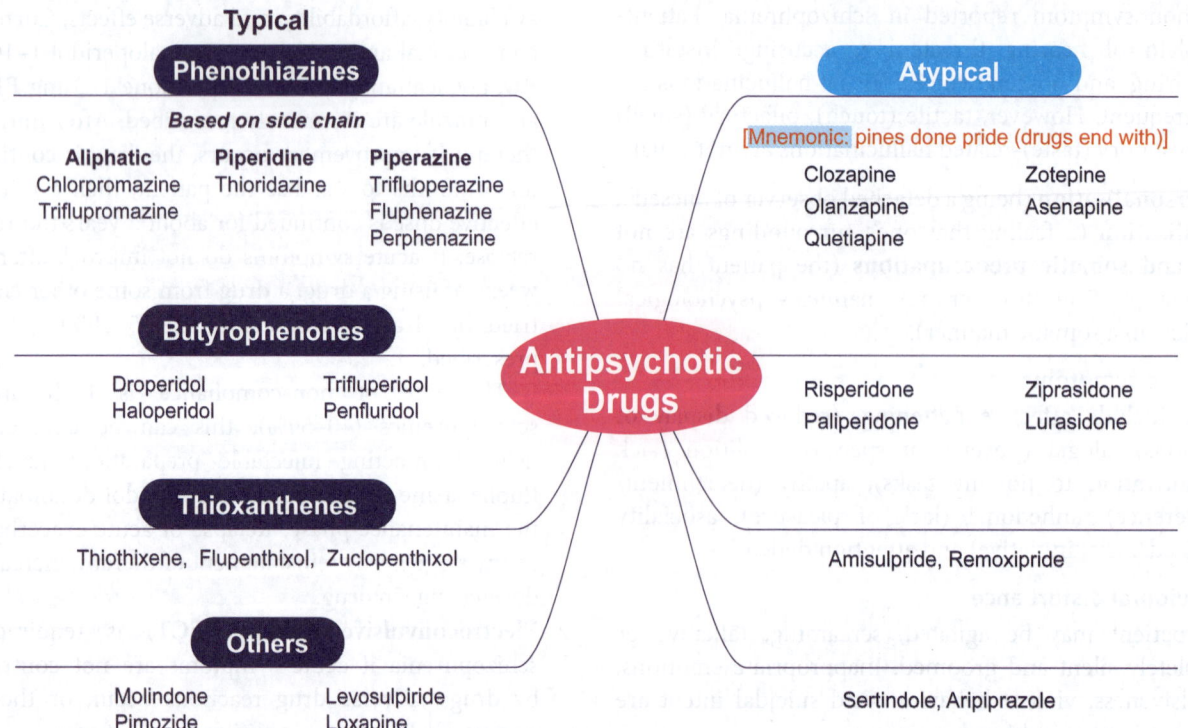

Flowchart 18.1 Classification of antipsychotic drugs

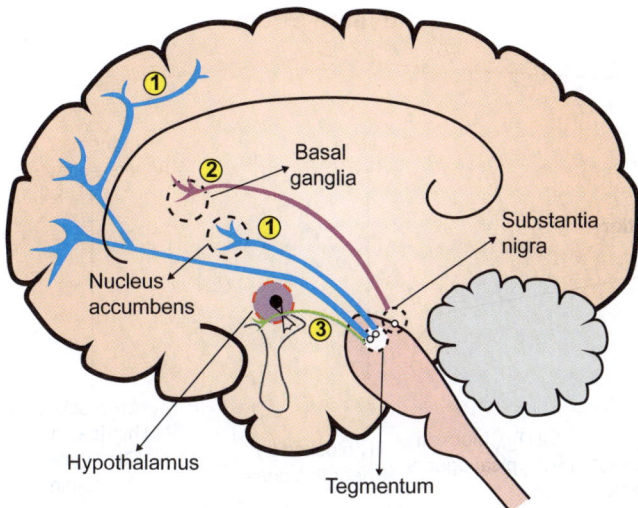

Fig. 18.1 Distribution of dopaminergic fibres in the brain
[① Mesolimbic and mesocortical pathways are concerned with antipsychotic effect. ② Nigrostriatal pathways cause extrapyramidal symptoms on blockade. ③ Tuberoinfundibular fibres raise prolactin levels on blockade.]

Box 18.2 continued

Dopamine receptors are of 5 types, consisting of two separate families: D_1-like and D_2-like.

D_1-like include D_1 and D_5 receptors that are Gs protein-coupled receptors, which activate adenylyl cyclase to increase cAMP levels.
- D_1 receptors are located in putamen, nucleus accumbens, olfactory tubercle and cortex.
- D_5 receptors are located in hypothalamus and hippocampus.

D_2-like receptors include D_2, D_3 and D_4 receptors; these are G_i protein-coupled receptors, which inhibit adenylyl cyclase, resulting in decreased cAMP, inhibition of calcium channels and openning of potassium channels.
- D_2 receptors are located in caudate nucleus, putamen, nucleus acumbens and olfactory tubercle.
- D_3 receptors are in frontal cortex, medulla and midbrain.
- D_4 receptors are mainly in the cortex.

Majority of antipsychotic drugs act by the following mechanisms:

a. **Blocking D_2 receptors to varying extent:** The antipsychotic action of drugs can be partly attributed to blockade of dopamine's inhibitory effect on adenylyl cyclase in the mesolimbic system (Fig. 18.2). For typical antipsychotic drugs, the affinity for D_2 receptors is well correlated with their clinical efficacy and potential to cause extrapyramidal symptoms as adverse effect.

b. Most of the atypical (and some typical) antipsychotic drugs have **5-HT_{2A} receptor antagonistic action** in addition to D_2 blockade. Hence, they show clinically useful effect even when just 30–50% of D_2 receptors are occupied (in comparison to 60% occupancy for typical agents).

c. Aripiprazole is a **partial agonist at D_2 receptors**, and thus, does not cause extrapyramidal symptoms. It also possesses **5-HT_{1A} partial agonistic and 5-HT_{2A} antagonistic** activity.

d. In addition to D_2 and 5-HT_{2A} receptors, these drugs have some action on other receptors also, e.g., $α_1$, H_1, M_1, M_3 **blocking and 5-HT_{1A} partial agonistic** effects.
- $α_1$-Blocking action is prominent with chlorpromazine, triflupromazine, and thioridazine.
- Phenothiazines have prominent H_1-blocking action.
- M_1, M_3 blocking or anticholinergic effect is seen with thioridazine, clozapine, and olanzapine.

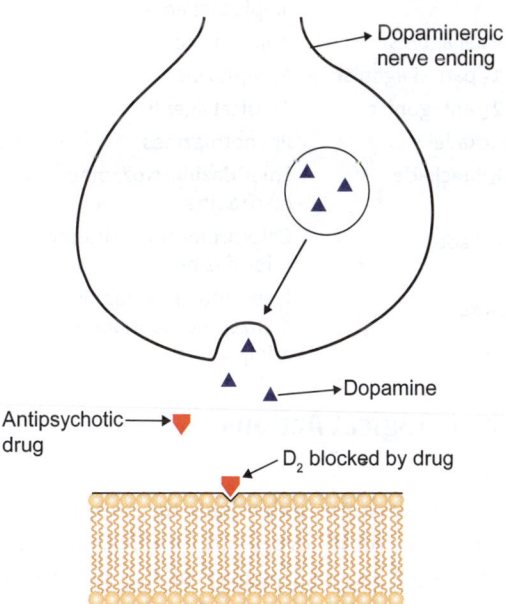

Fig. 18.2 Major mechanism of action of typical antipsychotic drugs

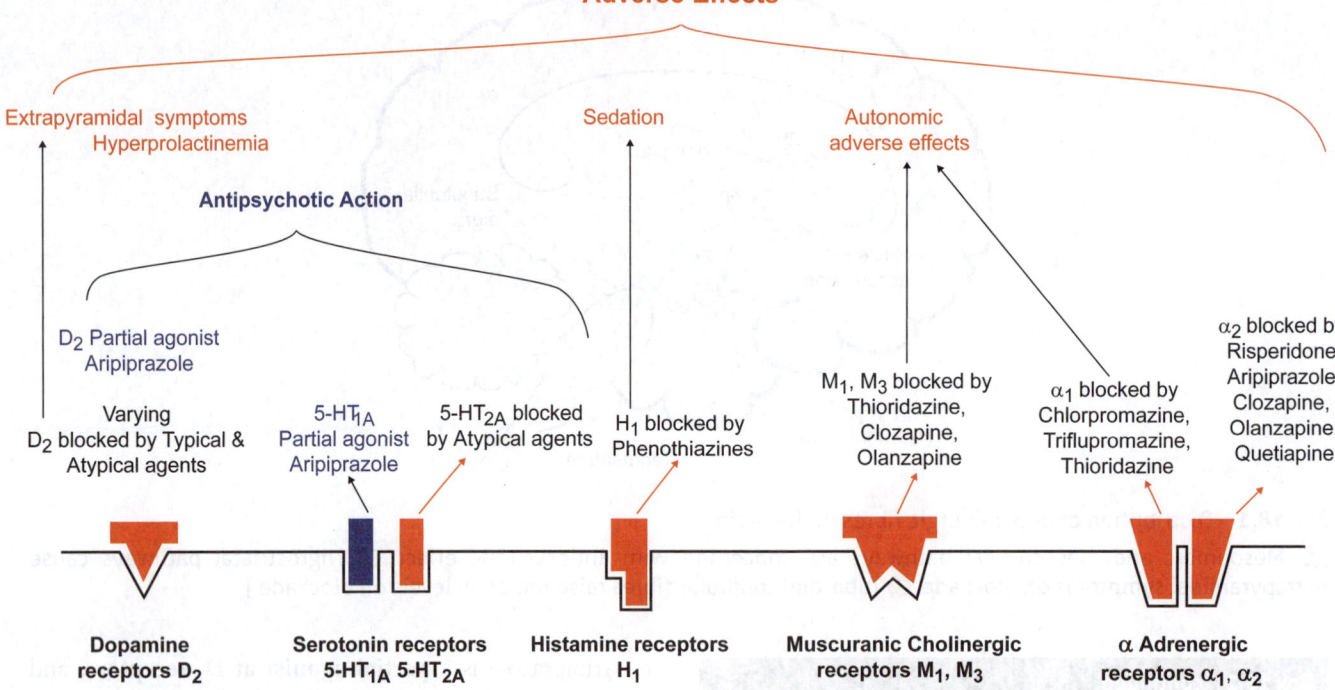

Fig. 18.3 Receptor actions of antipsychotic drugs

- Varying degrees of α_2-blockade are also seen with risperidone, clozapine, olanzapine, quetiapine and aripiprazole.

Receptor actions of antipsychotics are summarised in Box 18.3 and also depicted in Fig.18.3.

Box 18.3	Receptor actions of antipsychotics
D_2 blockade	Typical antipsychotics, atypical agents
D_2 partial agonist	Aripiprazole
5-HT_{1A} partial agonist	Aripiprazole
5-HT_{2A}-antagonist	Atypical agents
H_1 blockade	Phenothiazines
M_1, M_3 blockade	Thioridazine, clozapine, olanzapine
α_1 blockade	Chlorpromazine, triflupromazine, thioridazine
α_2 blockade	Risperidone, clozapine, olanzapine, quetiapine, aripiprazole

Pharmacological Actions

1. CNS

- In a non-psychotic individual, the subjective effects of most of these drugs are **unpleasant**, such as psychomotor slowing, paucity of thought, sleepiness, minimum spontaneous movements and emotional quietening. This is known as **neuroleptic syndrome**. Thus, abuse potential is not seen with these drugs.

- However, in psychotic patients, **symptoms are alleviated and performance improves.** Disturbed perception, thought, behaviour and sleep pattern start normalising slowly. Hallucination, delusions and anxiety are controlled. **Positive symptoms are better controlled than negative symptoms with typical agents.**

All phenothiazines, butyrophenones and thioxanthenes are **equi-efficacious but differ in potency**. Chlorpromazine, triflupromazine and thioridazine are less potent and more sedative. **Sedation** appears to be independent of antipsychotic action because it appears earlier than therapeutic action and tolerance soon develops to it. **Extrapyramidal symptoms,** however, are closely related to antipsychotic action and are more prominent with the higher potency drugs such as fluphenazine, trifluperazine, and haloperidol and least with thioridazine and atypical drugs.

- In addition, chlorpromazine has a propensity to **precipitate seizures** in epileptics; it **knocks off temperature control** and exerts **antiemetic action** through the chemoreceptor trigger zone (CTZ).

2. ANS

- Antimuscarinic or **anticholinergic effect** of neuroleptics is weak. It is seen with thioridazine, clozapine and olanzapine and results in dryness of mouth, blurring of vision, constipation and urinary hesitancy, especially with thioridazine.

- **α₁-blocking action** is maximum with chlorpromazine, triflupromazine and thioridazine and lesser with more potent drugs. It is responsible for adverse effects like postural hypotension, palpitation and ejaculatory dysfunction.

3. CVS
- Antipsychotics cause **hypotension** because of α-blocking action. It is accompanied by **reflex tachycardia** and is more severe in hypovolemic patients.
- ECG changes like **QT prolongation** or abnormality of **ST segment and T wave** are seen especially with **thioridazine** and disappear on stopping the drug. QT prolongation occurs with atypical agents also like sertindole, ziprasidone and quetiapine.

4. Endocrines
- Blockade of dopaminergic activity in the tuberoinfundibular pathway knocks down the inhibitory control over prolactin secretion from anterior pituitary. This results in **amenorrhoeic, galactorrhea, gynecomastia and infertility.**
- Chlorpromazine can **impair glucose tolerance** and **raise triglyceride levels.**

5. Other actions
- Chlorpromazine also possesses potent **local anesthetic** action; however, it is not used for this action as it is an irritant.
- Majority of typical antipsychotics exert **antiemetic action** by D_2 blockade in GIT as well as CTZ.

Tolerance

Fortunately, **tolerance develops soon to sedative and hypotensive actions** of antipsychotics, but not to their antipsychotic action. Hence, maintenance doses need not be increased overtime. There is **no drug-seeking behaviour or dependence** (psychological and physical) with antipsychotics. Withdrawal of antipsychotics may cause **emergent dyskinesia**, but it is not serious or life-threatening.

CLINICALLY RELEVANT PHARMACOKINETICS
- Most antipsychotic drugs are incompletely absorbed after oral administration. They also undergo first pass metabolism, so oral bioavailability is less than unity.
- They are highly bound to plasma proteins as well as tissue proteins, so they have large volumes of distribution.
- Clinically, the duration of action of these drugs is much longer than that estimated from their elimination half-life. This can be attributed to prolonged binding to D_2 receptors and some active metabolites. Once-daily dose is sufficient, which is convenient for patient and improves compliance.
- They are metabolised in liver and excreted in urine. So, there is a risk of drug–drug interactions when they are co-administered with enzyme inhibitors like ketoconazole.
- The average time to recurrence of schizophrenic symptoms after stopping the drugs is approximately 6 months. However, relapse occurs early after discontinuing clozapine.

Therapeutic Uses
Antipsychotic drugs have several psychiatric and some non-psychiatric indications.

a. Psychiatric uses

1. Schizophrenia
Antipsychotic drugs are the mainstay of schizophrenia treatment. They are not curative, but provide relief from variety of psychiatric symptoms. **Positive symptoms are relieved with typical as well as atypical drugs, whereas negative symptoms are relieved better with atypical agents**. Affective symptoms improve significantly but symptoms related to cognition, intellect, memory and judgment, etc. do not benefit as much. Atypical agents are better tolerated and more frequently used nowadays.

Dose: Dose depends on **severity** of the disease and **tolerability** of drug. For example,

- Oral dose of chlorpromazine varies from 10–100 mg, TDS, up to a maximum of 800 mg per day.
- **Haloperidol** is the **most frequently used typical antipsychotic**. Its dose varies from 1–10 mg, twice a day.
- **Risperidone** is atypical antipsychotic and the **drug of choice** in the treatment of schizophrenia. It is used in a dose of 1–3 mg, twice a day.
- **Clozapine** is used only in **refractory cases**, in a dose of 25–100 mg per day, up to a maximum of 300 mg.

The therapeutic benefit is usually evident after 2–4 months of therapy with antipsychotic drugs. A combination of antipsychotic drugs does not offer any advantage.

2. Schizoaffective disorders
Patients show features of both schizophrenia as well as affective disorders. Antipsychotics are **combined with antidepressants or lithium,** depending on the predominant affective symptoms.

- In patients of **bipolar affective disorders:** Severe manic symptoms like agitation associated with schizophrenia and bipolar disorders are controlled quickly within 1–2 hours by intramuscular administration of some antipsychotics like **haloperidol, ziprasidone or aripiprazole.**
- For treatment of **acute phase of mania**, monotherapy with **atypical antipsychotics** for about 4 weeks is effective. These are also effective for maintenance treatment and

prevention of mania in bipolar disease. **Lithium and valproate** are usually started after the acute phase.
- For **depressive disorders**, antipsychotics are used as **adjuvants to antidepressant** drugs. **Olanzapine, quetiapine** and **lurasidone** are approved for treatment of bipolar depression **along with fluoxetine.**

3. Tourette Syndrome
This is characterised by tics (motor or phonic) and responds symptomatically to haloperidol, pimozide, risperidone, aripiprazole and behavioural therapy.

4. Alzheimer's disease
Antipsychotics may be used to treat disturbed behaviour in Alzheimer's disease.

5. Alcoholic hallucinosis and Huntington's disease also improve with antipsychotics.

6. Antianxiety effect is also seen. For this indication, however, benzodiazepines are preferred over antipsychotics.

b. Non-psychiatric indications
Non-psychiatric indications for the use of antipsychotic drugs include the following.

1. Intractable **hiccoughs** respond to chlorpromazine or haloperidol, probably due to dopamine blockade resulting in central suppression of hiccough reflex.
2. Chlorpromazine can be used to relieve **skeletal muscle spasm** in tetanus.
3. As **antiemetic:** Some phenothiazines like **prochlorperazine and promethazine** are used as **antiemetic** but not as antipsychotics. Promethazine has antihistaminic and anticholinergic actions as well and is useful in **motion sickness**.
4. Promethazine is used as a sedative in **pre-anesthetic medication.**
5. **Domperidone (butyrophenone) and metoclopramide** are peripheral dopamine receptor blockers used as **prokinetic drugs**. They have low affinity for mesolimbic receptors and are hence not used as antipsychotics. They can control **drug- and disease-induced vomiting**. However, 5-HT$_3$ antagonists are preferred for this action nowadays.
6. Droperidol is used along with fentanyl (opioid drug) as **neuroleptanalgesia**.

The therapeutic uses of antipsychotics are summarised in Table 18.1.

Table 18.1 Therapeutic uses of antipsychotic drugs

Indications for use of antipsychotic drugs	Preferred drug
Psychiatric indications	
- Schizophrenia	- Atypical agents: Risperidone is the first-choice drug. - Typical agent: Haloperidol is frequently used.
- Schizoaffective disorders	For bipolar disease: - Acute agitation with schizophrenia: **h**aloperidol, **a**ripiprazole, **z**iprasidone by intramuscular route - Depression with psychotic symptoms: **l**urasidone, **o**lanzapine, **q**uetiapine along with fluoxetine
- Tourette syndrome	- **R**isperidone, **a**ripiprazole, **p**imozide, **h**aloperidol
- Alzheimer's disease	- Disturbed behaviour improves with antipsychotics.
- Alcoholic hallucinosis and Huntington's disease	- May also improve with antipsychotic drugs.
- Anxiety	- Benzodiazepines are preferred.
Non-psychiatric indications	
- Intractable hiccough	May be relieved by chlorpromazine or haloperidol
- Skeletal muscle spasm in tetanus	Chlorpromazine
- Antiemetic	Prochlorperazine and promethazine are effective
- Drug- and disease-induced vomiting, motion sickness	Domperidone (butyrophenone) and metoclopramide. Nowadays, 5-HT$_3$ antagonists are preferred.
- In pre-anesthetic medication for sedation	Promethazine is useful for this indication
- Neurolept analgesia	Droperidol along with fentanyl is used.

> **Mnemonic**
> - In case of acute manic agitation with schizophrenia: go for a **HAZ**: **H**aloperidol, **A**ripiprazole, **Z**iprasidone
> - In case of depression along with schizophrenia – try to **LOQ** (i.e., lock) the symptoms with **FLUOXETINE**, i.e., **L**urasidone, **O**lanzapine, and **Q**uetiapine along with **FLUOXETINE**
> - Tics of Tourette syndrome can be controlled by doing a **Rap** with **HALOPERIDOL**, i.e., **R**isperidone, **A**ripiprazole, **P**imozide, **HALOPERIDOL**

Adverse Drug Reactions

In general, **atypical antipsychotics are better tolerated** than typical agents. Typical agents cause central, cardiac, autonomic, endocrine and metabolic adverse effects as extensions of their pharmacological actions. In addition, individual drugs have some characteristic adverse reactions.

1. Central adverse effects

a. Sedation is the prominent adverse effect caused by phenothiazines and thioxanthenes among typical agents, and by clozapine, olanzapine and quetiapine among atypical drugs. So, small doses of drug are given during daytime and the major portion of the daily dose is given at bed time. However, tolerance develops to this action.
b. High doses may cause psychomotor impairment and pseudo-depression because of drug-induced akinesia at higher doses. In such cases, dose reduction can relieve the symptoms.
c. The threshold for seizures is lowered by clozapine and olanzapine. Chlorpromazine can also precipitate seizures in untreated epileptic patients.
d. High doses of chlorpromazine knock off the hypothalamic temperature control mechanism. Patients becomes poikilothermic (the body temperature changes with changes in atmospheric temperature, i.e., body temperature falls during winters and rises in summers.)
e. Phenothiazines, clozapine and olanzapine have prominent anticholinergic action and may cause toxic confusional state.

2. Neurological or extrapyramidal side effects

These are the **dose-limiting adverse effects** of typical antipsychotics. Akathisia, acute muscular dystonias, parkinsonian symptoms and malignant neuroleptic syndrome occur early in treatment, whereas tardive dyskinesia and perioral tremors occur after a year or more of therapy.

a. **Akathisia** is the unexplained **agitation and restlessness without** anxiety in about 20% of patients receiving antipsychotic therapy. It may be mistaken as worsening of psychosis. It needs dose reduction or a change from typical to atypical drugs. **Propranolol and benzodiazepines** can also provide some relief.
b. **Acute muscular dystonias** are spastic retrocollis or torticollis involving linguo-facial muscles resulting in locked jaw, tongue thrusting or grimacing features. These may last for a few hours and can be resolved with **promethazine or diphenhydramine**.
c. **Parkinsonian symptoms** occur because of D_2 blockade in nigrostriatal pathway, disturbing acetylcholine–dopamine balance. Patients may develop symptoms like rigidity, tremors, hypokinesia, mask like expressionless face and defective gait within a month of starting typical antipsychotic drugs.
Symptoms can be controlled by restoring cholinergic-dopaminergic balance in CNS. Levodopa is not effective in this situation as D_2 receptors are already occupied. **Central anticholinergic drugs** such as benztropine, benzhexol, procyclidine or orphenadrine are effective. Dose reduction and a switch to atypical agents may also be beneficial.
d. Rarely, some patients may develop **neuroleptic malignant syndrome (NMS)** with more potent typical agents like fluphenazine and haloperidol. Among atypical agents, only asenapine may cause NMS. It may be because of central D_2 blocking as well as the peripheral neuromuscular effects of neuroleptic drugs. Patients develop tremors, marked rigidity, immobility, hyperpyrexia and fluctuating blood pressure. Muscle damage may occur, raising creatine kinase and myoglobin levels. It requires **stopping the neuroleptic** drug immediately and starting **supportive symptomatic measures** to control hyperpyrexia and maintain blood pressure. Muscular rigidity can be reduced by muscle relaxants and **diazepam. Dantrolene** is useful. In some cases, **bromocriptine**, a dopamine agonist, relieves symptoms. However, central anticholinergics are of no value in this condition.
g. A rare extrapyramidal adverse effect are **perioral tremors or the rabbit syndrome** that may occur after years of therapy with typical antipsychotics. It is characterised by rapid chewing movements similar to a rabbit, and responds well to **central anticholinergic drugs.**
h. **Tardive dyskinesia** is another extrapyramidal adverse effect of prolonged antipsychotic therapy. It may occur because of progressive **neuronal damage and dopamine supersensitivity**. Patients present with choreoathetosis, i.e., **slow, purposeless, involuntary movements of the oral, buccal, lingual and limb muscles,** e.g., constant pouting, puffing, chewing and lip-licking movements.
Central anticholinergics rather worsen the symptoms, probably by further widening the gap between dopaminergic and cholinergic transmission. No satisfactory treatment exists for this syndrome. **Neurolept holidays** involving withdrawal of antipsychotic drug may improve symptoms. Substitution with atypical agents as clozapine or olanzapine may also be beneficial.

3. Autonomic adverse effects

Autonomic adverse effects occur because of muscarinic and α₁ blocking effects.

a. **Anticholinergic side effects** like dryness of mouth, eyes, blurring of vision, constipation and urinary retention are prominent with thioridazine, clozapine and olanzapine.

b. Postural hypotension, tachycardia and retrograde ejaculation occur due to α₁ blockade with chlorpromazine, triflupromazine and thioridazine. Autonomic effects are less with atypical drugs and high potency typical drugs.

4. Endocrinal adverse effects

a. Dopamine receptor blockade in the tuberoinfundibular pathway knocks out the inhibitory control of prolactin inhibitory hormone (PIH or dopamine) on anterior pituitary. The resulting **hyperprolactinemia** manifests as galactorrhea in women and gynecomastia in males. Patient should be shifted to atypical agents. Dopamine agonist cabergoline may be useful

b. In addition, antipsychotic drugs decrease FSH and LH, resulting in amenorrhea, anovulation and infertility.

5. Miscellaneous adverse effects

Adverse effects such **weight gain, hyperglycemia, hyperlipidemia, skin pigmentation, corneal /lenticular opacities, retinal degeneration,** and **hypersensitivity reactions** in the form of **urticaria, jaundice** and **agranulocytosis** may also occur with some antipsychotic drugs, especially, atypical agents.

The important adverse effects of antipsychotic drugs are summarised in Table 18.2.

Table 18.2 Adverse effects of antipsychotic drugs

Adverse effect and the drug causing it	Management of adverse effect

1. Central
 a. **Sedation**
  - Low-potency phenothiazines, thioxanthenes
  - Atypical drugs like clozapine, olanzapine and quetiapine
 b. Psychomotor impairment, **akinesia**, pseudo depression at high dose
 c. **Seizure precipitation** by clozapine, olanzapine, chlorpromazine
 d. **Poikoilothermia** by chlorpromazine
	a. Tolerance develops; major portion of dose given at bedtime.
	
	 b. Dose reduction
	
	 c. Antiseizure drugs – Diazepam
	
	 d. Supportive treatment to maintain temperature

2. Extrapyramidal symptoms	
Most commonly caused by high-potency typical agents such as fluphenazine, trifluoperazine and haloperidol	
a. **Akathisia** b. **Acute muscular dystonia** c. **Parkinsonian symptoms** d. **Neuroleptic malignant syndrome** with fluphenazine and haloperidol, asenapine e. **Perioral tremors** f. **Tardive dyskinesia**: Further worsened by central anticholinergics	a. Dose reduction, propranolol and benzodiazepines b. Promethazine or diphenhydramine c. Central anticholinergics d. Stop drug; supportive: diazepam, dantrolene. No role of central anticholinergics. e. Central anticholinergics f. Neurolept holiday may provide some benefit. No satisfactory treatment available. Central anticholinergics may worsen the condition.
3. Autonomic adverse effects – More with low potency typical agents	
a. **Anticholinergic effects** with thioridazine, clozapine and olanzapine: Dryness of mouth, eyes, blurring of vision, constipation, urinary retention b. **α blockade** with chlorpromazine, triflupromazine, thioridazine: postural hypotension, tachycardia, retrograde ejaculation	Mild, tolerable Shift to atypical agents.
4. Endocrinal a. Hyperprolactinemia b. Impaired glucose tolerance raised triglycerides with chlorpromazine	Shift to atypical drugs, cabergoline
5. Hypersensitivity reactions With clozapine, olanzapine, quetiapine	Reversible upon stopping the drug. Monitor WBC counts and stop clozapine when TLC < 3000 mm³
6. Metabolic side effects like weight gain, hyperlipidemia, diabetes with clozapine, olanzapine and quetiapine	Reversible upon stopping drug
7. ECG changes such as QT prolongation, abnormal ST segment, and abnormal T wave can occur with quetiapine, thioridazine, sertindole, ziprasidone, and amisulpride	

SALIENT FEATURES OF ANTIPSYCHOTIC DRUGS

Typical Antipsychotic Drugs

a. **Phenothiazines** are of three chemical types:
   - Drugs with **aliphatic side chain** (chlorpromazine and triflupromazine) and **piperidine side chain** (thioridazine) are low-potency drugs. In general, the **low-potency drugs have more adverse effects, as sedation and hypotension** occur due to α_1 blocking action. Thioridazine has marked anticholinergic activity resulting in adverse effects. Triflupromazine is mostly used as antiemetic. A common side effect is acute muscular dystonias, especially in children.
   - Drugs with **piperazine side chain**, such as trifluoperazine and fluphenazine, are **high-potency drugs and cause more extrapyramidal side effects** than low-potency drugs.

b. **Butyrophenones**
   Haloperidol is the most commonly used typical antipsychotic drug. It resembles the high potency phenothiazines in its actions and adverse effect profile. It is used for acute schizophrenia, Tourette syndrome and Huntington's disease.
   - Penfluridol is a long-acting drug that is given once a week for chronic schizophrenia.
   - Droperidol is used with fentanyl (opioid) for neurolept analgesia.

c. **Pimozide**
   It is a selective D_2 antagonist.
   - α Blocking, anticholinergic actions and dystonias are negligible but it carries the **risk of causing arrhythmias**.
   - Long half-life makes it suitable for maintenance therapy of schizophrenias as **once-daily administration**. It is also used in Tourette syndrome and tics.

Clinical problem-based questions and MCQs

1. i. Which of the following is considered a first-line drug in schizophrenia?
   a. Droperidol   b. Promethazine
   c. Risperidone   d. Clozapine

2. A 34-year-old female patient on maintenance therapy with haloperidol for schizophrenia, complains of increased secretions from nipple, amenorrhea and failure to conceive. Explain the cause of the patient's symptoms and suggest remedy for the same.

3. Which of the following adverse effects is more commonly associated with haloperidol than chlorpromazine?
   a. Anticholinergic side effects
   b. Extrapyramidal reactions
   c. Risk of postural hypotension
   d. Sedation

4. A patient being treated for schizophrenia developed muscular rigidity, immobility, fluctuating blood pressure and hyperpyrexia. Myoglobin and creatine kinase levels were found to be raised.
   i. What is the cause of these symptoms?
   ii. Which of the following drugs can control these symptoms?
      a. Benztropine   b. Dantrolene
      c. Haloperidol   d. Metoclopramide

5. All of the following drugs are used in Tourette syndrome except
   a. Risperidone   b. Amisulpride
   c. Pimozide   d. Haloperidol

6. A 56-year-old man, a known case of schizophrenia, is on haloperidol therapy. He develops an extrapyramidal adverse effect which becomes worse with central anticholinergic drugs.
   i. Identify the extrapyramidal adverse effect in this case.
      a. Tardive dyskinesia
      b. Perioral tremors
      c. Parkinsonian symptoms
      d. Akathisia.
   ii. Explain the cause of worsening of selected adverse effect with central anticholinergics.

7. Which of the following antipsychotic drugs has the maximum risk of anticholinergic adverse effects?
   a. Thioridazine   b. Aripiprazole
   c. Haloperidol   d. Ziprasidone

Atypical Antipsychotic Drugs

- They have **prominent 5-HT$_{2A}$ blocking** effect, weak D_2 blocking effect.
- They have **fewer adverse effects** than typical antipsychotics.
- They **improve both positive and negative symptoms** of schizophrenia. These include the following:

1. **Clozapine**
   - Receptor activity: It possesses 5-HT$_2$, D$_4$ and α-blocking actions.
   - It improves both positive and negative symptoms. It is the only drug that may decrease the risk of suicide.
   - Clozapine is preferred only **in refractory cases** not responding to typical agents as it has many adverse effects.
   - Clozapine has weak D_2 blocking effect, so it does not cause hyperprolactinemia, tardive dyskinesia and extrapyramidal adverse effects.
   - **Sedation is a prominent** side effect. Incidence of **agranulocytosis and blood dyscrasias** is high. Monitoring of CBC is indicated and drug should be stopped if TLC falls below 3000/mm^3.

- Metabolic complications like **weight gain, hyperlipidemia and diabetes** are common.
- Fluctuating BP, tachycardia and myocarditis may also occur.

2. **Olanzapine**
   - It resembles clozapine in action.
   - It is effective in schizoaffective disorders and mania However, it is not preferred because of many serious adverse effects (like that of clozapine).

3. **Quetiapine**
   - Quetiapine resembles clozapine in most of its actions and adverse effects, but has shown efficacy in bipolar depression and acute mania.
   - It has the potential to prolong QT interval and cause arrhythmias.

4. **Risperidone**
   - Considered as a **first-line drug** in the treatment of schizophrenia.
   - Possesses **D_2, 5-HT_2, H_1, $α_1$, $α_2$ receptor blocking actions**.
   - D_2 blocking effects of risperidone is more than clozapine, hence it has **more propensity to cause extrapyramidal symptoms and prolactin secretion than clozapine**.
   - However, **adverse effects like weight gain, metabolic complications, seizure precipitation are much less than clozapine.**

5. **Ziprasidone**
   - In addition to antipsychotic effect, it also possesses antidepressant, antimanic and anxiolytic activity.
   - Like clozapine, it has low potential to cause extrapyramidal effects and prolactin secretion.
   - Advantage over clozapine is due to its **lower sedative and metabolic adverse effects; anticholinergic effects are also nil.**
   - Commonly seen side effects are nausea, vomiting and dose-related QT prolongation, and **risk of cardiac arrhythmias.**

6. **Amisulpride**
   - Unlike other atypical drugs, amisulpride has a high affinity for blockade of D_2 receptors and low affinity for 5-HT_2 receptors. It is, however, still counted as atypical agent because:
     - Extrapyramidal side effects are negligible, though hyperprolactinemia is common.
     - Both positive and negative symptoms are relieved.
   - It also possesses antidepressant effect.
   - It offers advantage over clozapine since the risk of weight gain and metabolic side effects is lower. QT prolongation, however, may occur in predisposed patients.
   - It can cause insomnia, anxiety and agitation as side effects.

7. **Aripiprazole**
   - Possesses unique receptor actions.
   - It is **partial agoinst at D_2 and 5-HT_{1A} receptor** and **antagonist at 5-HT_2** receptor. Thus, hypotension, hyperprolactinemia and extrapyramidal effects are not disturbing. Sedation is not seen; rather, it **may cause insomnia**. Weight gain, metabolic complications and QT prolongation are also seen only at high doses.
   - Common adverse effects include nausea, dyspepsia, lightheadedness and constipation.
   - It is indicated in **schizophrenia, resistant depression and bipolar diseases.**
   - It has long half-life, so **dose adjustment** should be done periodically and when simultaneous administration of enzyme inducers or inhibitors is there. The dose is doubled when carbamazepine (inducer) is co-administered and halved with ketoconazole and other enzyme inhibitor.

Clinical problem-based questions and MCQs

8. Match the drug with its typical adverse effect
   - a. Clozapine   1. Insomnia
   - b. Aripiprazole   2. Blood dyscrasia
   - c. Amisulpride   3. Extrapyramidal symptoms
   - d. Risperidone   4. QT prolongation

9. i. Identify the drug that acts as partial agonist at D_2 receptors.
   - a. Amisulpride   b. Risperidone
   - c. Aripiprazole   d. Olanzapine

   ii. Enumerate the therapeutic uses and adverse effects of the selected drug.

10. A 56-year-old man, suffering from schizophrenia for past 4 years, has stopped responding to haloperidol and risperisone. The patient is put on clozapine therapy.
    i. The patient should be monitored regularly for development of which adverse effect?
       - a. Pancreatitis   b. Polycythemia
       - c. Visual disturbances   d. Agranulocytosis

    ii. Describe the mechanism of action and adverse effects of clozapine.

11. A 55-year-old male patient of manic depression is on long-term lithium therapy. Due to sudden worsening of his symptoms, his psychiatrist added ziprasidone to his medication.
    i. To which group does ziprasidone belong?
    ii. Which of the following adverse effects should the patient should be warned of?
       - a. Risk of cardiac arrhythmias
       - b. Parkinsonian adverse effects
       - c. Tinnitus
       - d. Urinary retention

Summary

- **Schizophrenia:** It is a chronic, functional psychosis, diagnosed on the basis of clinical features.
- **Antipsychotic drugs** can be classified as typical or classical and atypical antipsychotics.
- Antipsychotic drugs act by blocking D_2 receptors to varying extents. Most atypical (and some typical) drugs have 5-HT_{2A} receptor antagonistic action also.
- Other actions are blockade of $α_1$, H_1, M_1, M_3 receptors and 5-HT_{1A} partial agonistic effects.
- In psychotic patients, the symptoms are alleviated and performance improves. Positive symptoms are better controlled than negative symptoms with typical agents.
- **Therapeutic uses:** Schizophrenia, schizoaffective disorders (bipolar affective disorders, acute phase of mania, depressive disorders), Tourette syndrome, disturbed behaviour in Alzheimer's disease, antianxiety, alcoholic hallucinosis, Huntington disease, antiemetic, intractable hiccough, skeletal muscle spasm in tetanus, sedative in pre-anesthetic medication. Droperidol is used along with fentanyl (opioid drug) as neuroleptanalgesia.
- Chlorpromazine, triflupromazine and thioridazine are **less potent, more sedative and have more $α_1$ blocking action,** whereas fluphenazine, trifluoperazine, haloperidol, etc., are **more potent antipsychotics and have more extrapyramidal side effects.**
- ECG changes like QT prolongation, abnormality of ST segment and T wave are seen, especially with thioridazine, sertindole, zipracidone, and quetiapine.
- **Adverse effects** are sedation, psychomotor impairment, pseudo depression, extrapyramidal side effects (akathisia, acute muscular dystonias, parkinsonian symptoms, neuroleptic malignant syndrome and perioral tremors or rabbit syndrome, and tardive dyskinesia), anticholinergic and $α_1$ blocking effects, and hyperprolactinemia.
- Atypical antipsychotic drugs have prominent 5-HT_2 blocking effect and D_2 blockade is weak. They have fewer extrapyramidal adverse effects than typical antipsychotic drugs. They improve both positive and negative symptoms of schizophrenia.
- Atypical agents cause weight gain, hyperglycemia, hyperlipidemia, skin pigmentation, corneal/lenticular opacities and retinal degeneration; hypersensitivity and agranulocytosis may also occur.
- **Risperidone** is considered as a first-line drug in the treatment of schizophrenia. It has more extrapyramidal symptoms and prolactin secretion but fewer metabolic adverse effects than clozapine.
- **Clozapine** is used only in refractory patients not responding to typical agents because of many metabolic effects, fluctuating BP, tachycardia and myocarditis.
- **Aripiprazole** is a partial agonist at D_2 and 5-HT_{1A} receptor and antagonist at 5-HT_{2A} receptor. Thus, hypotension, hyperprolactinemia and extrapyramidal effects are not a concern. Sedation is not seen; rather, it may cause insomnia.

Questions for practice

1. Classify antipsychotic drugs.
2. Explain why:
   a. Major part of daily dose of chlorpromazine is given at bed time.
   b. Lithium and haloperidol are combined to control acute mania.
   c. Risperidone is the first-choice drug in treatment of schizophrenia.
   d. Clozapine is a reserve drug, only for refractory cases.
3. Write short notes on:
   a. Atypical antipsychotics
   b. Neuroleptic malignant syndrome
   c. Aripiprazole
4. Enumerate:
   a. Therapeutic uses of antipsychotic drugs
   b. Adverse effects of typical antipsychotic drugs

Hints for problem-based questions and MCQs

1. i. c. Risperidone
2. Hyperprolactinemia due to D_2 blockade. Refer to page 253.
3. b. More extrapyramidal adverse effects
4. i Malignant neuroleptic syndrome
   ii. Dantrolene
5. b. Amisulpride
6. i. a. Tardive dyskinesia
   ii. Refer to page 253.
7. a. Thioridazone.
8. a–2; b–1; c–4; d–3.
9. i. c. Aripiprazole
   ii. Refer to page 256.
10. i. d. Agranulocytosis
    ii. Refer to page 255.
11. i. Antipsychotic
    ii. a. Risk of cardiac arrhythmias due to QT prolongation

CONCEPT MAP - ANTIPSYCHOTIC DRUGS

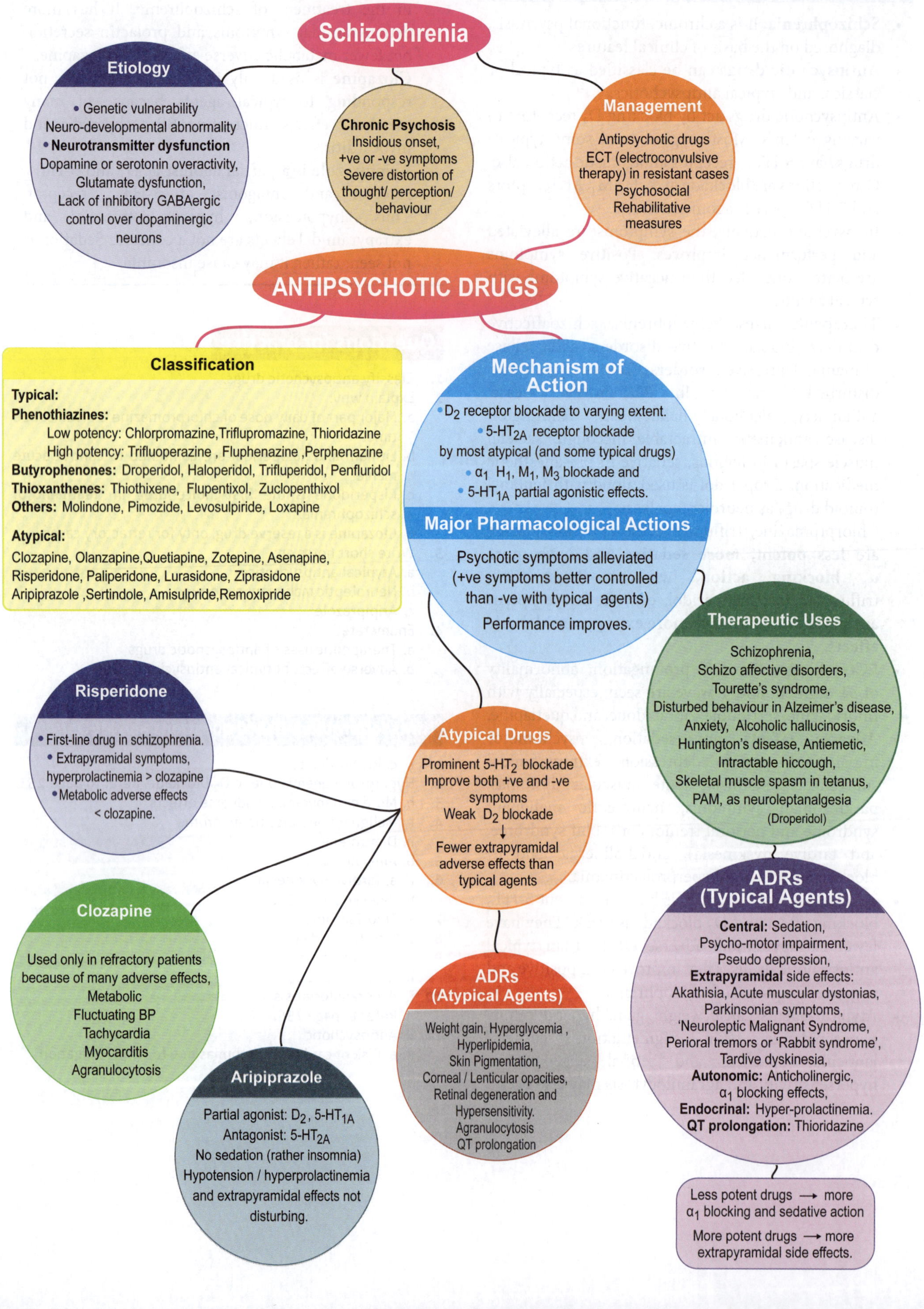

Schizophrenia

Etiology
- Genetic vulnerability
  Neuro-developmental abnormality
- Neurotransmitter dysfunction
  Dopamine or serotonin overactivity,
  Glutamate dysfunction,
  Lack of inhibitory GABAergic control over dopaminergic neurons

Chronic Psychosis
Insidious onset,
+ve or -ve symptoms
Severe distortion of thought/ perception/ behaviour

Management
Antipsychotic drugs
ECT (electroconvulsive therapy) in resistant cases
Psychosocial
Rehabilitative measures

ANTIPSYCHOTIC DRUGS

Classification

Typical:
Phenothiazines:
  Low potency: Chlorpromazine, Triflupromazine, Thioridazine
  High potency: Trifluoperazine, Fluphenazine, Perphenazine
Butyrophenones: Droperidol, Haloperidol, Trifluperidol, Penfluridol
Thioxanthenes: Thiothixene, Flupentixol, Zuclopenthixol
Others: Molindone, Pimozide, Levosulpiride, Loxapine

Atypical:
Clozapine, Olanzapine, Quetiapine, Zotepine, Asenapine,
Risperidone, Paliperidone, Lurasidone, Ziprasidone
Aripiprazole, Sertindole, Amisulpride, Remoxipride

Mechanism of Action
- D_2 receptor blockade to varying extent.
- $5-HT_{2A}$ receptor blockade by most atypical (and some typical drugs)
- α_1, H_1, M_1, M_3 blockade and
- $5-HT_{1A}$ partial agonistic effects.

Major Pharmacological Actions
Psychotic symptoms alleviated (+ve symptoms better controlled than -ve with typical agents)
Performance improves.

Risperidone
- First-line drug in schizophrenia.
- Extrapyramidal symptoms, hyperprolactinemia > clozapine
- Metabolic adverse effects < clozapine.

Clozapine
Used only in refractory patients because of many adverse effects,
Metabolic
Fluctuating BP
Tachycardia
Myocarditis
Agranulocytosis

Aripiprazole
Partial agonist: D_2, $5-HT_{1A}$
Antagonist: $5-HT_{2A}$
No sedation (rather insomnia)
Hypotension / hyperprolactinemia and extrapyramidal effects not disturbing.

Atypical Drugs
Prominent $5-HT_2$ blockade
Improve both +ve and -ve symptoms
Weak D_2 blockade
↓
Fewer extrapyramidal adverse effects than typical agents

ADRs (Atypical Agents)
Weight gain, Hyperglycemia,
Hyperlipidemia,
Skin Pigmentation,
Corneal / Lenticular opacities,
Retinal degeneration and Hypersensitivity.
Agranulocytosis
QT prolongation

Therapeutic Uses
Schizophrenia,
Schizo affective disorders,
Tourette's syndrome,
Disturbed behaviour in Alzheimer's disease,
Anxiety, Alcoholic hallucinosis,
Huntington's disease, Antiemetic,
Intractable hiccough,
Skeletal muscle spasm in tetanus,
PAM, as neuroleptanalgesia
(Droperidol)

ADRs (Typical Agents)
Central: Sedation,
Psycho-motor impairment,
Pseudo depression,
Extrapyramidal side effects:
Akathisia, Acute muscular dystonias,
Parkinsonian symptoms,
'Neuroleptic Malignant Syndrome,
Perioral tremors or 'Rabbit syndrome',
Tardive dyskinesia,
Autonomic: Anticholinergic,
α_1 blocking effects,
Endocrinal: Hyper-prolactinemia.
QT prolongation: Thioridazine

Less potent drugs → more α_1 blocking and sedative action

More potent drugs → more extrapyramidal side effects.

SECTION 3 Drugs Acting on CNS

19 Drugs for Mood Disorders

PH 3.5 Describe types, salient pharmacokinetics, pharmacodynamics, therapeutic uses, adverse drug effects of drugs used for depression and devise a management plan for depression

---

Learning objectives

A student of MBBS phase II should be able to:
- Describe common symptoms of major depressive disorder (MDD).
- Describe neurotransmitter defects underlying depression.
- Classify antidepressant drugs.
- Explain the mechanism of action of tricyclic antidepressants (TCAs) and atypical antidepressants.
- Enumerate the therapeutic uses, adverse effects, and features of toxicity of antidepressant drugs.
- Compare the features of TCAs and selective serotonin reuptake inhibitors (SSRIs).
- Devise a management plan for depressive disorders.
- Enumerate drugs used in treatment of mania.
- Describe mechanism of action and uses of lithium.
- Describe adverse effect and drug–drug interactions caused by lithium.

MOOD DISORDERS

Mood disorders are psychiatric disorders that affect the mood, behaviour, and overall health of an individual and cause serious disruption of routine activities. Three major mood disorders are:

- Major depressive disorder (MDD)
- Secondary depression in association with medical illnesses or alcohol/substance abuse
- Bipolar disorder

The absence of manic episodes differentiates MDD from bipolar disorder.

The prevalence of bipolar disorders is about 1–2% and that of MDD about 5%. Milder forms of depression may affect up to 15–20% of the population.

Etiology
Risk factors for depression

- Depressive disorders are more common among **women** than men.
- **Genetic factors** contribute to the risk of depression. The risk of developing depression two-to threefold higher in offspring of parents who have a history of depression. Heritability for depression is 40–50%.
- Non-genetic factors like **stress, emotional trauma**, some **viral infections** and **abnormalities in brain development** are reported to increase the chances of developing depressive disorders.
- Stress-induced **damage to the hippocampus, nucleus accumbens** and other parts of the limbic system, **reduced hippocampal neurogenesis, deficiency of monoamines** and **up-regulation of pro-inflammatory cytokines** are commonly implicated in causation of affective disorders.
- Raised CRF from the hypothalamus and amygdala causing **raised cortisol levels** is implicated in mood alterations.
- Depressive symptoms may occur because of **functional deficit of NA or 5-HT or both** in certain parts of brain.
- Recent evidence implicates the **deficiency of neurotropic factors like** brain-derived neurotropic factor (BDNF) in the etiology of depression.
- **Reactive depression**: Negative life events like assault, death of dear ones or severe marital discord can contribute to precipitation of depression in susceptible individuals.
- **Secondary depression** occurs due to some general medical illnesses or substance abuse. Depressive symptoms frequently occur in association with cardiovascular, neurological, malignant, endocrine diseases (like diabetes and thyroid dysfunction) and AIDS. Patients suffering from chronic diseases of unknown etiology like fibromyalgia and chronic fatigue syndrome also develop depression and anxiety. Obesity and depression are important risk factors for each other.

Depression is also classified as **typical or atypical depression**. In case of typical depression, mood is constantly depressed. Symptoms like insomnia and loss of appetite are usually present. In atypical depression, however, mood is temporarily elevated in response to some positive life events, along with increased appetite and hypersomnia. Moreover, one form may change to other over time.

Risk factors for bipolar disease and mania
- Bipolar disorder is the **most heritable** psychiatric disease, with a genetic risk of 80%.
- **Stress and disturbed circadian rhythm** can promote manic episodes.
- **Preponderance of noradrenergic (NA)** and **dopaminergic (DA)** activity can exacerbate mania, whereas reduced activity of these neurotransmitters relieves mania symptoms.
- **Increased levels of BDNF** are implicated in mania, whereas levels fluctuate in bipolar disease (see Box 19.2, page 270).

Clinical Features of Affective Disorders
a. Major depressive disorders (MDD)
MDD usually presents in early adulthood and its incidence increases with age. An untreated episode of depression can last for a few months to ≥ 1 year.

Depressive symptoms include:
1. Depressed mood for most of day as reported by the patient or family members.
2. Marked decrease in interest or pleasure in almost all activities.
3. Significant (> 5%) change in body weight (gain or loss) in 1 month or decreased/increased appetite.
4. Insomnia or hypersomnia almost every day.
5. Psychomotor agitation or retardation.
6. Feeling loss of energy or fatigue almost every day.
7. Feeling of guilt or worthlessness.
8. Decreased ability to think, decide, concentrate.
9. Recurrent thoughts or ideation of death/suicide or attempt.

Diagnosis of depressive disorders
The diagnosis of depression is based on a comprehensive assessment, including a detailed history obtained from multiple sources, particularly family members. A thorough physical examination and mental status evaluation are essential components of this process. It is important to identify and appropriately treat any underlying physical or psychiatric conditions that may be contributing to depressive symptoms. Depression secondary to bipolar disorder, substance use, medication, or premenstrual syndrome should be ruled out. The final diagnosis is made in accordance with current diagnostic criteria, as outlined below.

- **Major depressive disorder (MDD):** A patient having **5 or more depressive symptoms daily, for a minimum duration of 2 weeks** is diagnosed as suffering from major depressive disorder (MDD). Significant impairment of routine social and occupational functioning and distress occurs.
- **Minor depression:** The patient has at least **2 depressive symptoms for 2 weeks.**
- **Dysthymic disorder:** Chronic ongoing **mild depressive symptoms** (less distressing and less severe than MDD) persisting **for at least 2 years** are indicative of dysthymic disorder.
- **Double depression:** Dysthymic disorder may co-exist with major depression. **Episodes of major depression can occur in these patients of mild, chronic depression.** Such a condition is called double depression.
- **Seasonal depression:** In some patients, especially women, depressive symptoms like anergy, fatigue, carbohydrate craving, hypersomnia and weight gain occur in a particular season.
- **Pseudodementia** consists of the **cognitive deficits** seen in patients with major depressive disorder, but **without any neurodegenerative component**. As the term signifies, it is a clinical condition that presents as full-blown dementia but is actually a different entity. This condition involves severe depressive episodes leading to psychotic state and cognitive deficit.

b. Bipolar disorders (BPD)/Manic depressive psychosis (MDP)
Bipolar disorder or MDP is characterised by **unpredictable mood swings** varying from mania or hypomania to depression.

A manic episode is associated with increased psychomotor activity, insomnia, talkativeness, impulsivity, impaired judgment, racing/crowded thoughts, inflated self-esteem, paranoid thinking or delusions of grandiose.

Such episode may last for 1 week. Mood disturbance is **severe enough to impair usual social or occupational activities,** calling for hospitalisation. The **manic episodes alternate with periods of depression**. Such mood fluctuations persisting **for at least 2 years** lead to the diagnosis of manic depressive psychosis (MDP) or bipolar disease. The onset of MDP is between 20–30 years of age, with the an equal prevalence among men and women. However, over a lifetime, the likelihood of depressive episodes is higher in women, and that of manic episodes is more among men. The standardised 'mood disorder questionnaire' is useful to differentiate the depressive phase of MDP from unipolar depression.

Management Plan for Depressive Disorders
The aim of treatment of a patient with depression is to:
- Induce remission
- Prevent recurrence

It is achievable by combining **drug therapy, management of co-morbid conditions and psychotherapy**. Majority of the cases of mild-to-moderate depression are treated on out-patient basis in home settings. If the patient has had any previous episodes, their treatment history including drugs used, compliance of patient to treatment regimens, response to treatment, and any adverse drug reactions should be considered while choosing suitable drugs. The patient and caregivers should be involved in the decision making process to ensure compliance to treatment and follow-up regimens. Psychotherapy helps the patient to cope with decreased self-esteem. Patients should be educated about depression, its risks, and benefits of the prescribed drugs. Stress management and cognitive behavioural therapies improve social adjustment of the patient.

Non-compliance to the treatment regimen is a major concern in patients with depressive disorders. Measures that may enhance patient compliance include:

- Devising convenient dosage regimens (preferably once-daily regimens).
- Explain the importance of regular drug intake, the lag period of a few weeks before the beneficial effect of the drug manifests, and the need to continue the drug even after symptoms are relieved.
- Establish a positive therapeutic alliance with the patient.
- Encourage the patient to report any adverse effects with drugs or relapse of symptoms.

Treatment options

Reactive depression, i.e., disproportionate sadness or grief to some life event, is self-limiting and antianxiety drugs given on short-term basis are useful. However, patients of major depressive disorder with suicidal thoughts and intent need treatment with **antidepressant drugs** or **electroconvulsive therapy (ECT)** and hospitalisation. In addition, patients with loss of appetite, severe malnutrition and catatonia also need hospitalisation and intensive treatment. Less frequently used treatment options in depressive disorders include vagal nerve stimulation, transcranial direct/magnetic stimulation, deep brain stimulation, sleep deprivation therapy and light therapy.

ANTIDEPRESSANT DRUGS

Antidepressant drugs **are classified as typical** and **atypical** antidepressants (Flowchart 19.1).

Typical antidepressants include tricyclic antidepressants (TCA), monoamine oxidase (MAO) inhibitors, selective serotonin reuptake inhibitors (SSRIs), and serotonin and noradrenaline reuptake inhibitors (SNRIs).

Mechanism of Action of Antidepressant Drugs

As reduced adrenergic and serotonergic transmission is widely implicated in the etiology of depression, antidepressant drugs exert their action by increasing the activity of these neurotransmitters through different mechanisms (Fig. 19.1). These include:

- TCAs (tricyclic antidepressants), SSRIs (selective serotonin reuptake inhibitors), serotonin and NA reuptake inhibitors (SNRIs), bupropion, trazodone and nefazodone **reduce the reuptake** of neurotransmitters (serotonin and/or noradrenaline) into nerve endings.

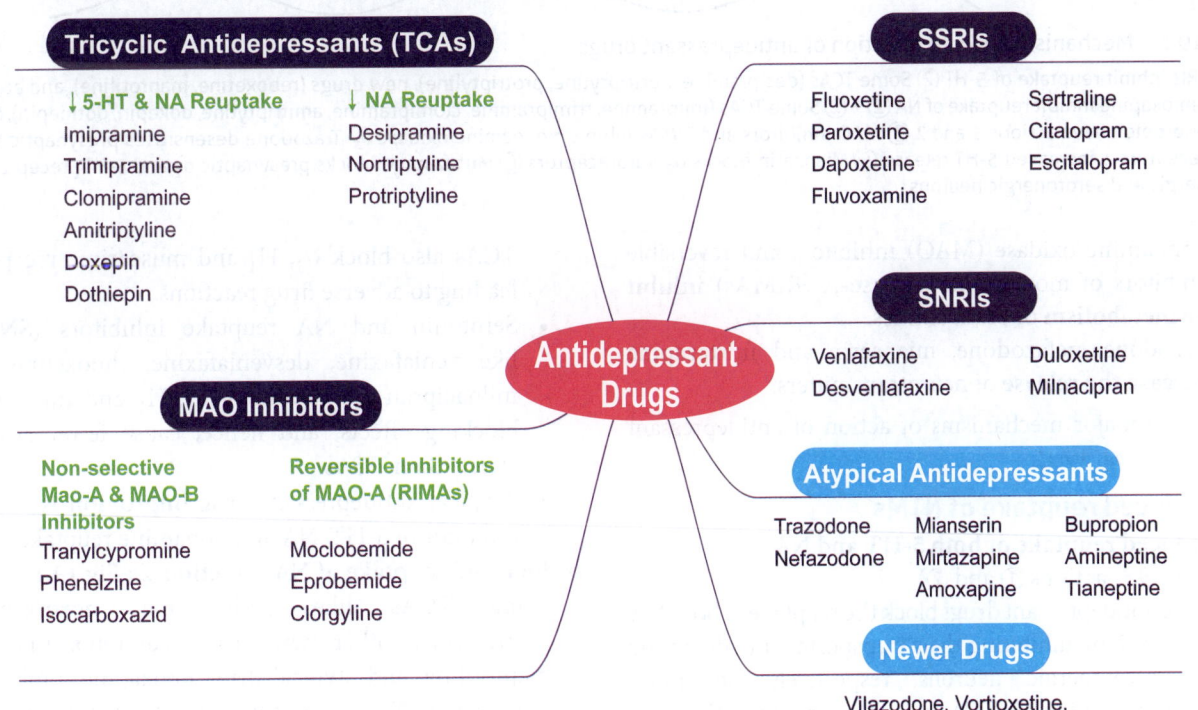

Flowchart 19.1 Classification of antidepressant drugs

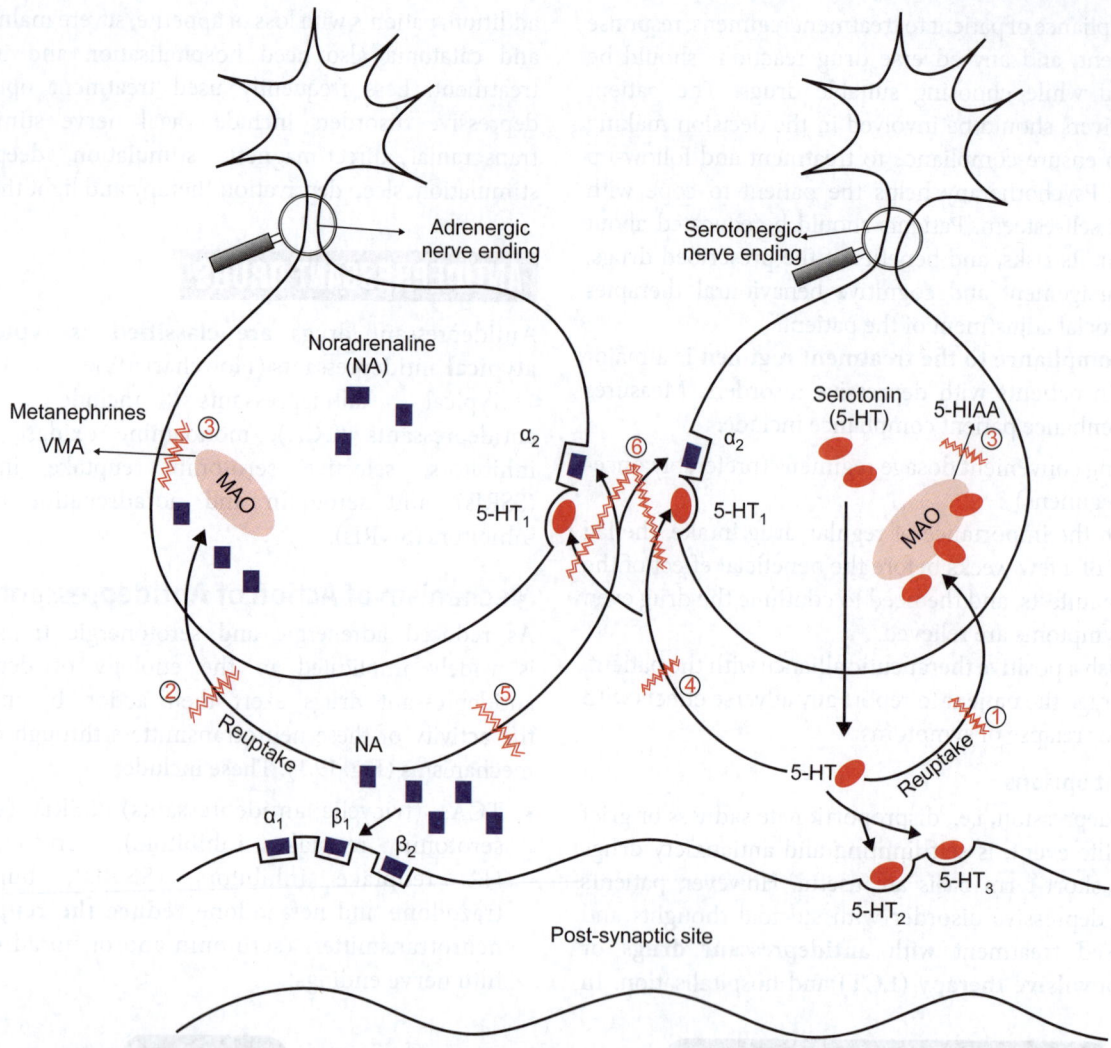

Fig. 19.1 Mechanism and site of action of antidepressant drugs
① SSRIs inhibit reuptake of 5-HT ② Some TCAs (desipramine, nortriptyline, protriptyline), new drugs (reboxetine, maprotiline), and atypical drug amoxapine inhibit reuptake of NA ① + ② Some TCAs (imipramine, trimipramine, clomipramine, amitriptyline, doxepin, dothiepin), SNRIs and bupropion have actions 1 and 2 ③ MAO inhibitors and RIMAs inhibit monoamine oxidase ④ Trazodone desensitises presynaptic 5-HT₁ autoreceptors → increased 5-HT release ⑤ Mianserin blocks α₂ autoreceptors ⑥ Mirtazapine blocks presynaptic α₂ and 5-HT₁ receptors on adrenergic and serotonergic neurons

- Monoamine oxidase (MAO) inhibitors and reversible inhibitors of monoamine oxidase-A (RIMAs) **inhibit the metabolism** of brain amines.
- Trazodone, nefazodone, mianserin and mirtazapine **increase the release** of neurotransmitters.

Thus, the major mechanisms of action of antidepressant drugs are (Fig. 19.1):

(i) Reduced reuptake of NTMs

a. Reduced reuptake of both 5-HT and NA
(Fig. 19.1, actions ① and ②)
Some antidepressant drugs block the reuptake of both NA and 5-HT by inhibiting their transporters in adrenergic and serotonergic neurons, respectively. So, more neurotransmitter (NTM) molecules remain available at receptor sites, for a longer duration. These include:
- **TCAs** (imipramine, trimipramine, clomipramine, amitriptyline, doxepin and dothiepin). However, TCAs also block α_1, H_1 and muscarinic receptors, leading to adverse drug reactions.
- Serotonin and NA reuptake inhibitors (**SNRIs**) like venlafaxine, desvenlafaxine, duloxetine and milnacipran are devoid of α_1, H_1 and muscarinic blocking effects, and hence, cause fewer adverse effects than TCAs.
- Atypical antidepressant drug **bupropion** is a weak inhibitor of 5-HT, NA and dopamine reuptake.

b. Reduced reuptake of NA → (action ②; Fig 19.1)
Some TCAs like desipramine, nortriptyline, protriptyline, other new drugs like reboxetine and maprotiline, and atypical drug amoxapine inhibit the reuptake of NA. Amoxapine has D_2 blocking effect also, resulting in its antipsychotic action. Atomoxetine is a selective NA reuptake inhibitor, useful in attention deficit hyperkinetic disorder.

c. **Reduced reuptake of 5-HT**
(Fig. 19.1, action ①)
SSRIs like fluoxetine, paroxetine, dapoxetine, vortioxetine, fluvoxamine, sertraline, citalopram and escitalopram inhibit only serotonin reuptake. The atypical drugs **trazodone** and **nefazodone** also decrease 5-HT reuptake.

(ii) Inhibition of metabolism of transmitters

(Fig. 19.1, action ③)
Some drugs act by inhibiting the metabolism of brain amines and raising the levels of 5-HT and NA in the vesicular stores available for release, thereby enhancing the action of these NTMs.

- MAO-A is present in the peripheral nerve endings, intestines and liver. It preferentially metabolises 5-HT, NA and dopamine and is inhibited selectively by RIMAs (moclobemide, eprobemide and clorgyline).
- MAO-B is present in the brain, liver and platelets. It metabolises dopamine and is inhibited by selegiline (deprenyl).
- Tranylcypromine, phenelzine and isocarboxazid are irreversible, non-selective MAO inhibitors (inhibit both MAO-A and MAO-B)

(iii) Other mechanisms

Among atypical antidepressants, the mechanism of action varies from drug to drug.

- **Trazadone:**
  - Inhibits 5-HT reuptake
  - Blocks *5-HT$_{2A}$ receptors* leading to its antianxiety and antidepressant effect
  - *Desensitises 5-HT$_1$ autoreceptors* present presynaptically, resulting in increased 5-HT release (Fig. 19.1, action ④).
  - It also causes α_1 block, leading to ADRs like sedation, postural hypotension and erectile dysfunction.
- **Nefazodone** is a congener of trazodone that has fewer side effects
- **Bupropion**: The exact mechanism of action of this drug is not clearly understood. It is a weak inhibitor of 5-HT, NA and DA reuptake. ADRs like sedation, hypotension and anticholinergic effects are minimal.
- **Mianserin** has no effect on reuptake of 5-HT and NA, but acts by *blocking presynaptic α_2 autoreceptors* present on adrenergic nerve endings. Thus, release of NA is increased. (Fig. 19.1, action ⑤)
- **Mirtazapine** blocks both *α_2 and 5-HT$_1$ receptors* present presysnaptically on adrenergic and serotonergic nerve endings. Thus, the release of both NA and 5-HT is increased (Fig. 19.1, action ⑥). It does not exert any effect on 5-HT$_2$ and 5-HT$_3$ receptors. Hence, it has fewer side effects like sexual dysfunction, agitation, and insomnia that are associated with SSRIs. However,

it blocks H$_1$ receptors (causing sedation) and 5-HT$_{2C}$ receptors (causing increased appetite).
- **Vilazodone,** a newer drug, inhibits serotonin reuptake (like SSRIs) and acts as a partial agonist at 5-HT$_{1A}$ receptors (like buspirone).
- **Vortioxetine** inhibits serotonin reuptake (like SSRIs), acts as agonist at 5-HT$_{1A}$, partial agonist at 5-HT$_{1B}$ and antagonist at 5-HT$_3$ and 5-HT$_7$ receptors.

Biological lag

With antidepressant drugs, though the NTM levels are raised immediately, the **onset of clinical effect is delayed for 2–3 weeks**. This biological lag is due to:

- Pharmacokinetic factors like high plasma protein binding and long half-life of drugs.
- Adaptive changes occurring with long-term use of antidepressants. Most important biological adaptation is
  - down-regulation of β_1, β_2 and 5-HT$_{1A}$, 5-HT$_{2A}$, 5-HT$_{2C}$, receptors
  - desensitisation of presynaptic α_2 and 5-HT$_{1A}$ auto receptors.

So, the time interval required for receptor down-regulation (β_1, β_2, 5-HT$_{2A, C}$) and desensitisation (α_2, 5-HT$_{1A}$ autoreceptors) becomes the biological lag period.

Recent evidence indicates significant reduction in levels of a nerve growth factor known as 'brain-derived neurotrophic factor' (BDNF) in depression. The time required for BDNF synthesis is about 2 weeks, which resembles the biological lag period.

Clinical problem-based questions and MCQs

1. A 55-year-old man with a long-standing major depressive disorder on venlafaxine therapy presents for a follow up. His symptoms are well controlled with venlafaxine. Identify the correct mechanism of action of venlafaxine.
   a. Inhibits metabolism of monoamines
   b. Inhibits reuptake of 5-HT and NA
   c. Inhibits reuptake of 5-HT only.
   d. Increases release of 5-HT.

2. All of the following antidepressant drugs cause erectile dysfunction as an adverse effect EXCEPT:
   a. Desipramine   b. Citalopram
   c. Venlafaxine   d. Bupropion

3. Deficiency of monoamines is implicated in the causation of depressive symptoms. Which of the following drugs increase the release of both NA and 5-HT?
   a. Trazodone   b. Nefazodone
   c. Mirtazapine   d. Mianserin

4. Tricyclic antidepressants have multiple actions on receptors. Which of the following statements about receptor action of TCAs is INCORRECT?
   a. Block α_1 receptors
   b. Block β_2 receptors
   c. Block H$_1$ receptors
   d. Block muscarinic receptors

Pharmacokinetics

The oral absorption of most antidepressant drugs is good; however, **bioavailability is variable** because of varying first-pass metabolism.

These drugs are extensively metabolised in the liver resulting in the formation of **active metabolites**, which contribute to their **long half-life**. Later on, inactivation occurs by glucuronide conjugation. The inactive metabolites are excreted in urine over 1–2 weeks.

Because of the long half-life of most antidepressant drugs, steady state is reached slowly. Hence, once daily **(OD) dosing** is adequate for maintenance treatment.

Pharmacological Actions

i. **Antidepressant action**: Though antidepressant drugs have different mechanisms of action and side effects, **all are equally effective**. They **relieve depressive symptoms in 60–70% of patients and prevent recurrence**. The antidepressant effect is because of increased monoaminergic transmission, which, in turn, may promote neurogenesis in critical brain areas. In addition, the **biological lag** of 2–3 weeks suggests some adaptive changes occurring with continued therapy such as down-regulation of post-synaptic receptors (β_1, β_2, 5-HT_{1A}, 5-HT_{2A}, 5-HT_{2C}), desensitisation of presynaptic receptors (α_2, 5-HT_1) and increased synthesis of BDNF and other nerve growth factors.

Imipramine, amitriptyline and nortriptyline exhibit the '**therapeutic window**' phenomenon and exert antidepressant effect over a narrow range of plasma concentration from 50–200 ng/mL.

ii. **Autonomic effects**: Most TCAs have **anticholinergic** action resulting in adverse effects like dryness of mouth, blurring of vision, constipation and urinary retention. Anticholinergic effect is maximum with amitriptyline. Antidepressant drugs **potentiate effects of NA** by inhibiting its reuptake. They also possess **weak α_1 blocking** action.

iii. **Cardiac effects**: TCAs can cause prominent cardiac effects at therapeutic dose.
- **Tachycardia** can occur because of NA-potentiating and anticholinergic actions.
- **Postural hypotension** can occur due to α_1 blockade.
- With overdose, there is a risk of cardiac arrhythmias in the form of **conduction defects**. Arrhythmogenic potential is due to direct myocardial suppressant action. Risk of arrhythmias is higher in older patients. T wave suppression or inversion is seen in ECG.

Therapeutic Indications

Antidepressant drugs are used in psychiatric and some non-psychiatric conditions.

A. Psychiatric indications

i. **Endogenous depression**: The aim of treatment in depression is to relieve the symptoms and prevent recurrence.
- **SSRIs, SNRIs and atypical antidepressants are preferred** over older drugs because of their better safety profile. TCAs are used only in refractory cases. ECT is required in severe depression.
- The only effective drugs in juvenile depression are fluoxetine and sertraline.
- Desipramine relieves depressive symptoms in cocaine-dependent patients.
- In depression with insomnia or erectile dysfunction, atypical drugs like trazodone and mirtazapine are useful.

After controlling an episode of depression, the drug is continued at the same dose for 6–12 months. For discontinuation, the drug is slowly tapered off over 6 weeks to avoid withdrawal symptoms.

ii. **Panic disorders**: SSRIs (paroxetine, fluoxetine, and fluvoxamine) are used with **alprazolam to control panic disorders. [Mnemonic: Panic Fear For Anything]**

iii. **Phobias**: For social phobia and school phobia, **paroxetine** and moclobemide are preferred. In post-traumatic stress, paroxetine along with **alprozolam** are used. Antidepressants, especially SSRIs, are also useful for impulse control in conditions like gambling and kleptomania.

iv. **OCDs**: Obsessive compulsive disorders respond to **f**luvoxamine, **c**italopram, **c**lomipramine, etc. **[Mnemonic: Feeling Continuously Compelled]**

v. **Attention deficit disorder**: Imipramine and desipramine are preferred.

B. Non-psychiatric indications

i. **Enuresis**: Antidepressants with anticholinergic effect, like **imipramine, amitriptyline and desipramine,** are useful, but their effect lasts only while the drug is in use.

ii. **Chronic neuropathic pain** is relieved by TCAs like **imipramine**, **amitriptyline**, and **nortriptyline**. The exact mechanism of the pain-relieving effect is not fully understood, but increased levels of NTMs (that reduce pain signals) in the spinal cord might be responsible. TCAs, SSRIs, and SNRIs may relieve chronic pain and the associated depression.

iii. Milnacipran is useful in **fibromyalgia**.

iv. **Migraine pain** is also relieved by amitriptyline.

v. **Bulimia nervosa** responds to fluoxetine and fluvoxamine.

vi. Bupropion is used in **smoking cessation** and nicotine dependence.

vii. Citalopram **suppresses the desire to drink alcohol**.

viii. Doxepin cream relives itching in **lichen simplex** and **atopic dermatitis**.

ix. SSRIs are useful in **premenstrual syndrome** as well.

The therapeutic uses in various conditions and the drugs preferred for each are summarised in Box 19.1.

Box 19.1	Therapeutic uses of antidepressant drugs	
	Indication for use	**Preferred drugs**
1.	Depressive disorders - Endogenous depression - Refractory cases - Very severe depression - Juvenile depression - Depression with insomnia or erectile dysfunction	- SSRIs, SNRIs, atypical drugs - TCAs - ECT - Fluoxetine, sertraline - Trazodone, mirtazapine preferred
2.	Panic disorders [Mnemonic: **P**anic **F**ear **F**or **A**nything]	Paroxetine, fluoxetine, fluvoxamine with alprazolam
3.	School phobia, social phobia, post-traumatic stress, impulse control	Paroxetine with alprazolam
4.	OCDs [Mnemonic: **F**eeling **C**ontinuously **C**ompelled]	Fluvoxamine, citalopram, clomipramine
5.	Attention deficit disorder	Imipramine, desipramine
6.	Nocturnal bed wetting	Imipramine, desipramine, amitriptyline
7.	Chronic neuropathic pain	Imipramine, amitriptyline, nortriptyline
8.	Fibromyalgia	Milnacipran, duloxetine, etc.
9.	Migraine	Amitriptyline
10.	Bulimia nervosa	Fluoxetine, fluvoxamine
11.	Smoking cessation	Bupropion
12.	Reduce the desire to drink	Citalopram
13.	Lichen simplex	Doxepin
14.	Premenstrual syndrome	SSRIs: Citalopram

Adverse Drug Reactions

a. TCAs

TCAs have lost their status as first-line antidepressant drugs and are used only in severe, refractory cases of depression because of many adverse effects such as:

1. **Sedation** due to H_1 block, mental confusion, likelihood of switch-over to manic phase.
2. They can also cause increased appetite and weight gain.
3. Lowering of seizure threshold and **seizure precipitation**.
4. **Anticholinergic side effects** like dryness of mouth, blurring of vision, constipation, and urinary retention; these are more prominent with imipramine, desipramine and amitriptyline.
5. α_1 **blockade** leading to postural hypotension, tachycardia, palpitation, erectile and ejaculatory dysfunction.
6. **Metabolic acidosis and cardiac arrhythmias**, especially in ischemic heart disease (IHD) patients, which may cause sudden death. Sodium bicarbonate is useful for correcting acidosis. Cardiac conduction defects, QT prolongation and flattening of T wave occur.
7. **Acute TCA poisoning** is common. Patients present with:
   - Excitement, confusion, delirium and other anticholinergic symptoms
   - Muscle spasm
   - Convulsions
   - Coma
   - ECG changes, tachycardia, ventricular arrhythmias, hypotension

   Treatment:
   - Gastric lavage
   - Maintenance of respiration, BP and body temperature
   - I/V diazepam is used to control seizures
   - Propranolol and lignocaine are used to control rhythm disturbances
8. Defects of fetal eyes, ears, face and neck, if used during pregnancy.

b. SSRIs

Adverse effects of SSRIs are much less than those of TCAs. SSRIs do not block α_1, muscarinic and H_1 receptors. Hence, these are preferred over TCAs in treatment of depression. Important adverse effects of SSRIs are:

- **Central**: On starting treatment with SSRIs, 5-HT_2 action in the brain causes **anxiety, agitation, insomnia and vivid dreams**. To prevent these adverse effects, the dose of SSRIs should be preferably given in the morning and increased slowly. Benzodiazepines may be used to control these adverse effects.

- Increased serotonergic tone and 5-HT$_2$ action at the spinal cord level can cause sexual dysfunction in the form of decreased libido, anorgasmia, erectile dysfunction and delayed ejaculation. However, the adverse effect of delayed ejaculation may be useful in premature ejaculation.
- **Gastrointestinal adverse effects:** 5-HT$_3$ action in the gut causes nausea, vomiting and 5-HT$_4$ action causes diarrhea.
- While SSRIs are weight-neutral; paroxetine may cause weight gain.
- Increased incidence of epistaxis and ecchymosis due to impaired platelet function is reported.
- Withdrawal effects like headache, dizziness and paresthesias occur on sudden withdrawal. Such symptoms are maximum with short-acting drugs like paroxetine and sertraline. Fluoxetine is the longest acting SSRI, and has no withdrawal symptoms.
- All typical antidepressant drugs cause erectile dysfunction, while atypical ones do not. Rather, trazodone and mirtazapine are useful in patients with depression along with erectile dysfunction.

c. Atypical antidepressants
- **Trazodone** can cause sedation, nausea, postural hypotension, and priapism.
- Nefazodone is better tolerated, but prolonged use causes hepatotoxicity.
- **Bupropion** can cause agitation, insomnia and risk of seizures. So, it should not be given at bedtime.
- **Mirtazapine** causes sedation due to H$_1$ blocking action and weight gain.
- **Mianserin**
  - Sedation due to H$_1$ block
  - Risk of seizure precipitation at higher dose
  - May cause blood dyscrasias and hepatotoxicity

Drug Interactions
TCAs
- TCAs potentiate the effects of direct-acting sympathomimetics, e.g., cough, cold remedies, lignocaine and adrenaline combination.
- MAOIs with TCAs: Dangerously raised BP, excitement and hallucinations can occur.

SSRIs
SSRIs act as enzyme inhibitors, and when administered concurrently with drugs such as TCAs, warfarin, haloperidol, or clozapine, they can increase the plasma concentrations of these medications, leading to potential toxic effects.

MAO inhibitors + SSRIs
These precipitate '**serotonin syndrome**' characterised by restlessness, agitation, rigidity, hyperthermia, twitching, sweating and convulsions. It can be avoided by delaying SSRI therapy for at least 2 weeks after stopping MAO inhibitors. This provides time for regeneration of MAO enzyme.

This syndrome can be precipitated by tramadol and pethidine as well.

MAO inhibitors
Large quantities of tyramine are present in some wines, beer, cheese, fish, pickled meat, banana, yoghurt, etc. In patients undergoing MAOI therapy, indirectly-acting sympathomimetic amines (such as tyramine) are not metabolised, resulting in the release of large amounts of NA from nerve endings. This results in hypertensive crisis and cerebrovascular accidents, known as the 'cheese reaction'.

Drugs like ephedrine (present in cold, cough remedies), SSRIs, SNRIs and levodopa can also precipitate hypertensive crisis with MAO inhibitors. Cheese reaction is treated with phentolamine, an α blocker. Moclobemide is better tolerated than non-selective MAO inhibitors.

Non-selective MAO inhibitors increase the risk of seizures with pethidine due to generation of the metabolite nor-meperidine which has excitatory effect on neurons.

Clinical problem-based questions and MCQs

5. Which of the following antidepressant drugs show the 'therapeutic window' phenomenon:
   a. Sertraline   b. Amitriptyline
   c. Nortriptyline   d. Imipramine

6. All antidepressants are equally effective, but clinical response starts only after 2–3 weeks of continued once-daily administration. Such lag in clinical response is because of
   a. Down-regulation of presynaptic receptors
   b. Desensitisation of post-synaptic receptors
   c. Time required for BDNF synthesis
   d. High first-pass metabolism of drug

7. A 65-year-old man suffering from benign hypertrophy of prostate develops depressive symptoms due to severe osteoarthritis of the knee joint, which hampers his routine activities.
   i. Which antidepressant drug is CONTRAINDICATED in this case?
      a. Fluoxetine   b. Mirtazapine
      c. Bupropion   d. Amitriptyline
   ii. Why is the selected drug contraindicated?

8. A 60-year-old female patient is a chronic case of MDD for the past 5–6 years. She has stopped responding to SSRIs, SNRIs and atypical drugs. She is prescribed amitriptyline. On follow up, the patient complains of giddiness while getting up from sitting position and palpitations. On examination, her BP is 110/64 in standing position, PR is 120 bpm. What is the cause of fall in BP and tachycardia in this case?

9. The nursing staff of ENT 'in-patient department' (IPD) reports nocturnal bedwetting in a 9-year-old boy admitted for adenoidectomy. His parents are initially hesitant, but later admit that though the boy was toilet trained at the age of 4, he was never able to achieve complete nighttime dryness. They had tried non-pharmacological measures like stopping beverages after dinner, limited fluid intake 2–3 hours before bedtime, and taking the boy to the restroom after a fixed time interval. However, none of the methods provided consistent relief. He was referred to medicine OPD, where he was prescribed tab imipramine 25 mg at bedtime. In follow-up, the patient reported improvement of his symptoms. Explain the pharmacological basis for symptomatic relief in this case.

10. A 60-year-old female patient is very particular about personal hygiene. Her family members reveal that she starts washing her hands with soap every time she touches any object. This is disturbing her sleep and routine activity. She likes remaining isolated in her room for the fear of being touched by something or someone, and does not talk much to anyone. A diagnosis of minor depression with obsessive compulsive disorder is made.
   i. Which of the following is most suitable drug for this patient?
      a. Imipramine   b. Bupropion
      c. Doxepin   d. Citalopram
   ii. Describe the mechanism of action of the drug selected.
   iii. At a follow-up visit, the patient shows no signs of improvement. Which of the following can be tried in this patient next?
      a. Clomipramine   b. Mirtazapine
      c. Mianserin   d. Sertraline

SALIENT FEATURES OF VARIOUS ANTIDEPRESSANT DRUGS

(a) SSRIs

SSRIs like fluoxetine, paroxetine, dapoxetine, fluvoxamine, sertraline, citalopram and escitalopram act by selectively inhibiting membrane-associated serotonin transporter (SERT).

SSRIs have **replaced TCAs as 1st line drugs** in the treatment of depression, because of their better tolerability. In addition, these are used as drugs of first choice in treatment of panic disorders, phobias, OCDs, bulimia nervosa and chronic alcoholism. Citalopram is useful in premenstrual agitation. Drugs preferred in each of these conditions are mentioned in Box 19.1.

SSRIs are preferred as they offer many **advantages over TCAs** such as:
- They have the same efficacy as TCAs in depression.
- They do not cause any sedation or impairment of cognitive and psychomotor function.
- No anticholinergic adverse effects.
- No α_1-blocking side effects.
- No seizure precipitation
- No weight gain, except in case of paroxetine
- No potential to cause cardiac arrhythmias in overdose.

Fluoxetine is the longest-acting SSRI with a half-life of 50 hours. Thus, it has no withdrawal symptoms. In contrast, paroxetine is the shortest-acting SSRI with maximum withdrawal reactions (nausea, paresthesia, insomnia, fatigue and flu-like symptoms). Paroxetine causes sedation due to H_1 blockade, so, it is preferred in depression with insomnia, given at bedtime.

ADRs of SSRIs are due to raised synaptic 5-HT levels.

$5-HT_2$ **actions** → Insomnia, anxiety, vivid dreams, erectile dysfunction, delayed ejaculation

$5-HT_3$ **actions** → Nausea, vomiting

$5-HT_4$ **actions** → Diarrhea

These can also cause akathisia, bleeding and prolongation of QT interval.

(b) SNRIs

SNRIs like venlafaxine, desvenlafaxine, duloxetine, and milnacipran are also preferred over TCAs because:
- These are equally efficacious as TCAs in depression and are effective in some resistant cases as well.
- These are useful in relieving mood changes and hot flashes of menopausal syndrome, eating disorders and social phobias.
- Other uses are in neuropathic pain, fibromyalgia, and stress incontinence.
- SNRIs do not cause sedation, anticholinergic and α blockade side effects.
- Common adverse effects include nausea, dizziness, sweating, anxiety, and impotence.

Venlafaxine is the shortest-acting SNRI with maximum risk of withdrawal reactions and duloxetine is the longest acting. Duloxetine possesses mild sedation and anticholinergic effects, so it is contraindicated in close-angle glaucoma.

(c) Atypical antidepressants

Atypical antidepressants include trazodone, nefazodone, mianserin, mirtazapine and bupropion. Their mechanisms of action are different from typical drugs.

Trazodone and mirtazapine are useful in depression associated with insomnia and erectile dysfunction. These can cause sedation and priapism as adverse effects. Priapism (prolonged penile erection lasting longer than 4 hours) can be reversed by intracavernosal injection of phenylephrine.

Nefazodone is hepatotoxic.

Bupropion is a weak inhibitor of NA, 5-HT and dopamine reuptake. It is **infrequently used** in the treatment of depression. It is also not used in bipolar disease, eating disorders and anxiety as it causes excitatory adverse effects like insomnia, agitation and even seizures at higher dose in susceptible individuals. The main indication for its use is in **smoking cessation** to help control nicotine withdrawal symptoms.

Mianserin relieves anxiety associated with panic attacks, but reports of blood dyscrasias and hepatotoxicity have reduced its use.

Clinical problem-based questions and MCQs

11. i. A 20-year-old college student presents with a persistently low mood, fatigue, social withdrawal, and loss of interest in previously enjoyable activities. These symptoms have been ongoing for the past 1.5 years, with recent worsening marked by isolation and lack of communication. The consultant psychiatrist initiates treatment with fluoxetine. Which of the following is expected adverse effect in this patient?
    a. Sedation
    b. Weight gain
    c. Impotence
    d. Seizure precipitation
    ii. What is the possible harm of fluoxetine in a patient on MAO inhibitor therapy?
    a. Malignant neuroleptic syndrome
    b. Precipitation of acute intermittent porphyria
    c. Malignant hyperthermia
    d. Serotonin syndrome
    iii. How can the above-mentioned interaction between fluoxetine and MAO inhibitors be prevented?

12. A 54-year-old male patient complains of loss of appetite, weight loss, depressed mood and lack of ability to think coherently and concentrate on work. The physician reassures him, prescribes fluoxetine and advises him to take the drug regularly, although he may not get much benefit from it for some time in the beginning.
    i. How long is this time of 'no benefit' in symptoms expected to last?
    a. 12 hours
    b. 4 days
    c. 14 days
    d. 1 month
    ii. What is the cause of this time gap between the start of drug therapy and the clinical benefit it brings?
    iii. Describe the mechanism of action, uses and adverse effects of fluoxetine.

13. A 45-year-old male banker presents with depressive symptoms, including poor concentration during the day and insomnia at night. A detailed history reveals significant occupational stress and chronic neuropathic pain, with a recent diagnosis of fibromyalgia made two months ago. The patient has been excessively researching his condition online, leading to health-related anxiety and fear of disability. He is particularly concerned about the potential loss of his job, as he is the sole breadwinner in his family. He is not able to concentrate at work during the day and is unable to sleep at night.
    i. Which of the following is the most suitable drug for this case?
    a. Mirtazapine
    b. Bupropion
    c. Duloxetine
    d. Sertraline
    ii. Describe the mechanism of action of the selected drug.

14. A 35-year-old housewife complains of excessive fatigue while doing routine activities. She feels gloomy and wants to stay alone. She has even lost interest in painting her hobby since childhood. Her doctor prescribes bupropion as an antidepressant.
    i. Identify the correct mechanism of action of bupropion.
    a. Inhibits reuptake of NTMs
    b. Blocks D_2 receptors
    c. Causes desensitisation of pre-synaptic receptors
    d. Causes up-regulation of post-synaptic receptors
    ii. Identify another common indication for the use of bupropion in clinical practice.
    a. Alcohol withdrawal
    b. Opioid withdrawal
    c. Nicotine withdrawal
    d. All the above

15. A 30-year-old rickshaw puller is a chronic alcoholic. During winter, his income decreases significantly and he struggles to manage his day-to-day expenses. Sometimes, he fails to get his usual quantity of alcoholic drinks, which leaves him with a strong craving for alcohol. He also suffers from seasonal depression every year. The doctor prescribes a medicine that can relieve his depressive symptoms and reduce his craving for alcohol. Identify the drug prescribed.
    a. Fluvoxamine
    b. Imipramine
    c. Amitriptyline
    d. Citalopram

16. i. Which of the following atypical antipsychotic should not be given at bedtime?
    a. Trazodone
    b. Mianserin
    c. Bupropion
    d. Mirtazapine
    ii. Describe the reason for the precaution mentioned above.

CONCEPT MAP - ANTIDEPRESSANT DRUGS

Classification

Typical:
TCAs: Imipramine, Trimipramine, Clomipramine, Amitriptyline, Doxepin, Dothiepin, Desipramine, Nortriptyline, Protriptyline, Maprotiline, Reboxetine
SSRIs: Fluoxetine, Paroxetine, Dapoxetine, Fluvoxamine, Sertraline, Citalopram, Escitalopram
SNRIs: Venlafaxine, Desvenlafaxine, Duloxetine, Milnacipran
MAO inhibitors: Tranycypromine, Moclobemide, Clorgyline

Atypical: Trazodone, Nefazodone, Bupropion, Mianserin, Mirtazipine, Amoxapine, Amineptine, Tianeptine

Newer: Vilazodone, Vortioxetine

Mechanism of Action

Inhibit reuptake of NA and/or 5-HT: TCAs, SSRIs, SNRIs
Inhibit metabolism of NTMs: MAO inhibitors
Increase release of NA and/or 5-HT: Atypical drugs

Major Pharmacological Actions

Central: Relieve depressive symptoms (60–70% cases), Prevent recurrence
Cardiac: Tachycardia, Postural hypotension, Arrhythmogenic.
Other Actions: Anticholinergic, Potentiate effects of NA, Weak α_1 blocking action

Biological Lag
2–3 weeks

- Down-regulation of β_1, β_2, 5-HT$_2$ receptors
- Desensitisation of presynaptic α_2, 5-HT auto receptors
- Time needed for BDNF synthesis

ANTIDEPRESSANT DRUGS

ADRs

TCAs
Central: Sedation, Confusion, Switching over to manic phase, Seizure precipitation
Autonomic: Anticholinergic, Postural hypotension, Tachycardia, Erectile and Ejaculatory dysfunction, Cardiac arrhythmias, Increased appetite and Weight gain
Acute poisoning: Excitement, Delirium, Convulsions, Arrhythmias, Hypotension.
Treatment: Supportive, Diazepam, Propranolol, Lignocaine

SSRIs
Nausea, Diarrhea, Anxiety, Insomnia, Agitation, Sexual dysfunction.
No M, α_1, H$_1$ blocking adverse effects.

Atypical
Better tolerated than TCAs.
Terazodone: Sedation, Nausea, Postural hypotension and Impotence.
Mianserin: Sedation, Weight gain, Blood dyscrasia, Hepatotoxicity
Bupropion: Insomnia, Agitation, Seizure.

Therapeutic Uses

Endogenous depression: SSRIs, SNRIs, atypical preferred. Refractory cases: TCAs, ECT.
Panic Disorders, Phobias: Paroxetine + Alprazolam
OCDs: Fluvoxamine, Citalopram, Clomipramine.
Attention deficit disorder / Nocturnal enuresis: Imipramine, Desipramine
Bulimia nervosa: Fluoxetine, Fluvoxamine
Smoking cessation: Bupropion
Reduce desire to drink: Citalopram
Other Uses: Chronic neuropathic pain, Fibromyalgia, Migraine, Lichen simplex and Premenstrual syndrome.

Advantages of SSRIs over TCAs

No sedation, cognitive and psychomotor function impairment

No anticholinergic, α-blocking adverse effects

No seizure precipitation

No weight gain except with Paroxetine

No potential to cause cardiac arrhythmias in overdose.

DDIs

MAO inhibitors with tyramine-rich foods, cold/cough remedies, SSRIs, SNRIs and levodopa precipitate hypertensive crisis **(Cheese reaction)**

MAOI+SSRIs precipitate **'Serotonin syndrome'** characterised by restlessness, agitation, rigidity, hyperthermia, twitching, sweating, convulsions

ANTIMANIC (MOOD-STABILISING) DRUGS

Acute mania is characterised by inappropriate cheerfulness or irritability, high energy levels, talkativeness, crowded racing thoughts, restlessness, insomnia, inflated self-esteem and violent behaviour. Usually, it occurs as episodes of mania alternating with episodes of depression in the form of bipolar disorder, known as **manic depressive psychosis (MDP)**. Onset usually occurs between 20–30 years of age.

Prevalence of MDP is **higher in men**, in contrast to depression which is more common in women.

DRUGS FOR MANIA
1. **Lithium carbonate** or **lithium citrate**
2. **Anticonvulsants**: Carbamazepine, valproate, lamotrigine
3. **Antipsychotics**: Haloperidol, rispridone, olanzapine, aripiprazole, quetiapine

Lithium
Li^+ is a monovalent cation that is handled by the body the same way as Na^+ ion.

Mechanism of action
Normally, in α-adrenergic and muscarinic transmission, inositol triphosphate (IP_3) and diacylglycerol (DAG) serve as second messengers. IP_3 and DAG are formed by hydrolysis of phosphatidyl inositol biphosphate (PIP_2) via a G_q protein-coupled phospholipase C (PLC) (Fig. 19.2).

- IP_3 diffuses into plasma and causes release of Ca^{2+} from storage vesicles.
- DAG remains in the membrane and activates Ca^{2+}-sensitive protein kinase C and brings about effects of adrenergic and cholinergic transmission.
- IP_3 gets inactivated first to IP_2, then IP_1 and then inositol.
- Inositol, thus formed again serves as a precursor for synthesising phosphatidyl inositides (PI, PIP, PIP_2) which again participate in IP_3–DAG pathway.

In mania, there is overactivity of neuronal circuits leading to higher turnover of IP_3 and DAG. Li^+ selectively inhibits enzyme inositol monophosphatase in overactive neurons. Thus, it **blocks conversion of IP_1 → inositol**, and the supply of inositol to regenerate PIP_2 is reduced; in turn, the generation of IP_3 and DAG also decreases.

> **Box 19.2** Role of BRAIN-derived neurotrophic factor (BDNF) in mood disorders
>
> **BDNF levels in mood Disorders**
> - Increased BDNF levels are implicated in the causation of mania, whereas reduced levels are linked to depressive symptoms.
> - Fluctuating BDNF levels are proposed to cause bipolar disease, i.e., manic depressive psychosis (MDP).
> - Rapid cyclers with more than 4 episodes of hypomania, mania or depression per year also show fluctuating BDNF levels.
>
> **BDNF synthesis** is supported by β-catenin and IP_3–DAG pathway.
> - The activation of G_q-linked receptors increases BDNF levels through IP_3–DAG pathway.

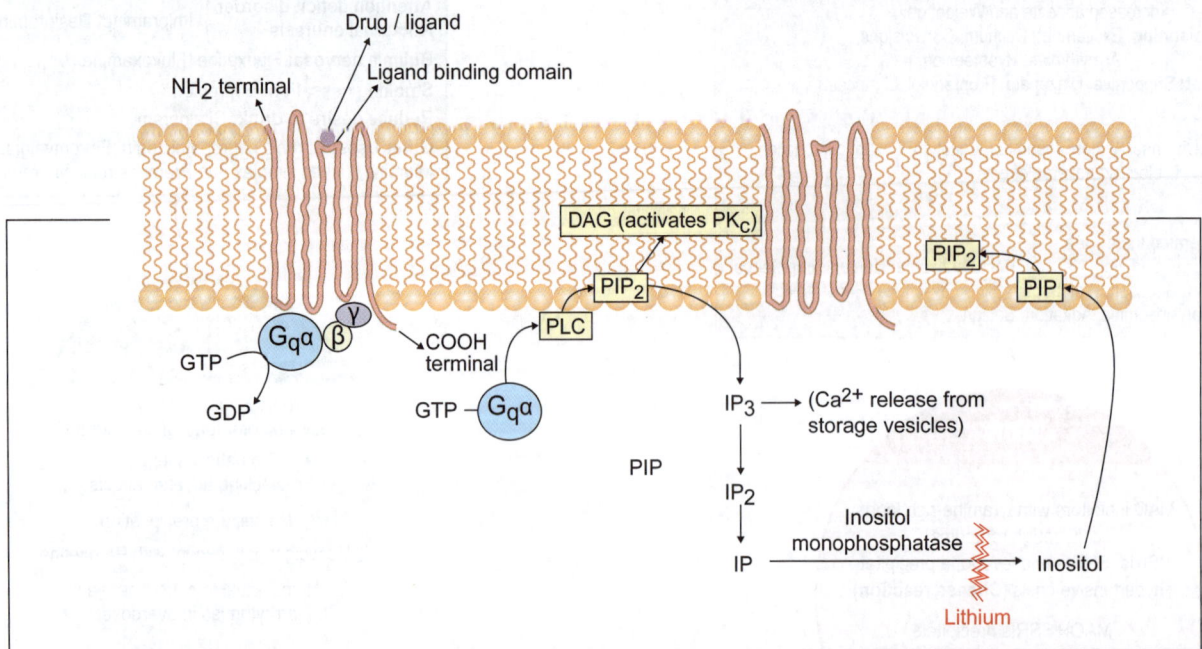

Fig. 19.2 Mechanism of action of lithium
[PLC: phospholipase C; GPCR: G protein-coupled receptor; PIP_2: phosphatidyl inositol biphosphate; IP_3: inositol triphosphate; DAG: diacylglycerol; PK_C: phosphokinase C; IP_2: inositol biphosphate; IP: inositol monophosphate]

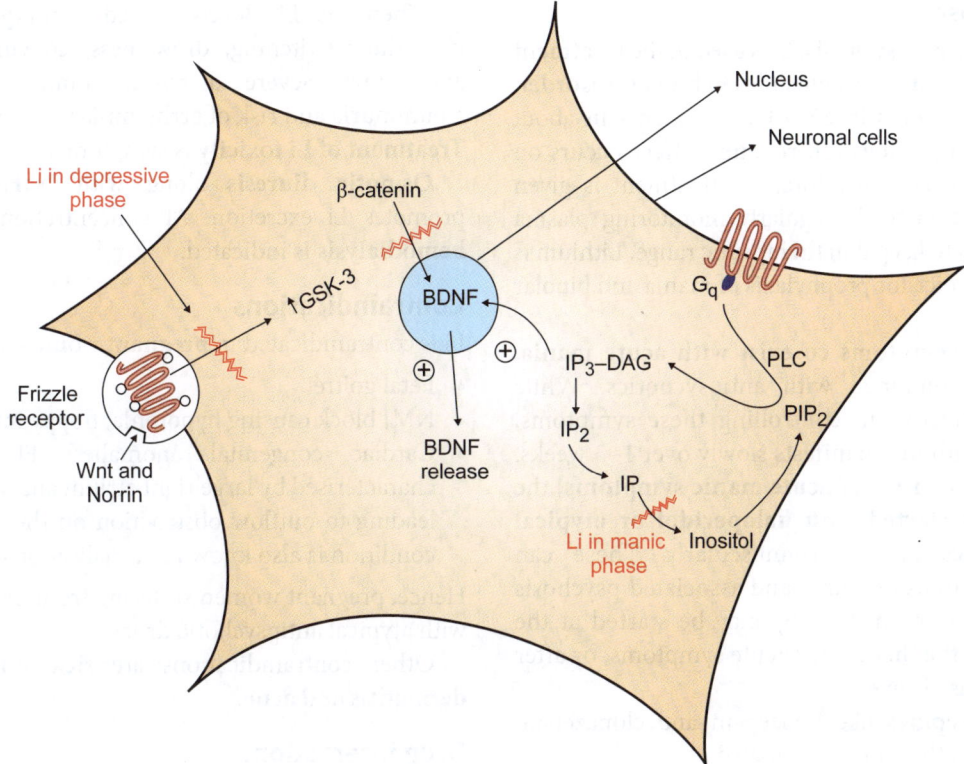

Fig. 19.3 Effect of Li on BDNF release in bipolar disease

- The entry of β-catenin into the neuronal nucleus favours BDNF release. In contrast, glycogen synthase kinase-3 (GSK-3) interferes with the entry of β-catenin into the neuronal nucleus, resulting in reduced BDNF levels. GSK-3 also seems to be involved in BDNF degradation.
- The activation of frizzle receptors [a family of atypical G protein-coupled receptors, by Wnt proteins (derived from wingless Int-1)] stimulates several cellular processes, including raised levels of 'glycogen synthase kinase-3' (GSK-3) enzyme → reduced BDNF.

Effect of drugs on BDNF levels: Lithium is a mood stabiliser. It chooses its mechanism of action based on BDNF levels as (Fig. 19.3).

- Manic phase involves raised BDNF levels. Thus, lithium tries to reduce it by interfering with the IP_3–DAG pathway, by inhibiting inositol monophosphatase enzyme as described earlier.
- Depressive phase involves reduced BDNF levels. Thus, lithium blocks GSK-3 enzyme, so that β-catenin can enter neuronal nucleus and stimulate BDNF release.
- Valproate can also inhibit GSK-3 enzyme, which, in turn, raises BDNF levels.

Pharmacological actions

- **CNS:** Lithium has no actions on normal individuals. Even in patients with bipolar disease/mania, there are **no acute effects** of lithium. Long-term use brings about **mood stabilisation** in bipolar disease. Manic episodes are **gradually controlled in 1–2 weeks.** It normalises reduced sleep time in mania patients.
- **Kidney:** Lithium can **induce nephrogenic diabetes inspidus** by reducing the responsiveness of distal convoluted tubule (DCT) to antidiuretic hormone. It can cause sodium and water retention.
- **Endocrinal effects:** Lithium **inhibits thyroid hormone release**, resulting in raised TSH levels. It also exerts **insulin-like effects** on carbohydrate metabolism.
- **Leukocyte count** is **increased** by lithium.

Pharmacokinetics

Absorption: Li is **readily absorbed** upon oral administration.

Distribution: Li gets distributed **throughout body water.** It does not undergo **plasma protein binding (PPB) and metabolism.** Concentration achieved in CSF is half of the plasma concentration.

Excretion: 96% of the administered Li^+ gets excreted through **urine.** Remaining 4% is excreted in **sweat and saliva.**

As mentioned earlier, Li^+ is handled by the kidney the same way as Na^+, i.e., there is 80% reabsorption in proximal convoluted tubule (PCT). Thus, Na^+ **loading enhances Li^+ excretion and Na^+ depletion promotes Li^+ retention.**

The drug has **low safety margin** and narrow **therapeutic range of 0.5–1.5 mEq/L.** The usual dose is 300–600 mg TDS. However, the dose will need to be individualised by **therapeutic drug monitoring** (TDM) to maintain plasma concentration between 0.8–1.4 mEq/L.

Therapeutic uses

1. **Manic depressive psychosis**: Li is used in the **treatment and prevention of manic episodes in bipolar disorder.** It relieves symptoms in 65–70% of patients in about 10–15 day's time. However, **rebound effect** occurs on stopping the drug. Therefore, the treatment is given over longer term while regularly monitoring plasma concentration to keep it in therapeutic range. Lithium is the drug of choice for prophylaxis of mania and bipolar disease.
2. If **psychotic symptoms co-exist with acute mania**, Li may be combined with antipsychotics. While lithium is effective in controlling these symptoms, the effect of lithium manifests slowly over 1–3 weeks. So, **for rapid control of acute manic symptoms,** the **treatment is started with haloperidol or atypical antipsychotics** given intramuscularly. These can control symptoms of mania and associated psychosis in 1–3 days. Lithium therapy may be started at the same time as the therapy for acute symptoms, or after the acute phase is over.
   - **Benzodiazepines** like lorazepam and clonazepam are added if the patient is agitated.
   - **Antidepressants** like paroxetine and bupropion are required in patients with severe bipolar depression.
3. Lithium is useful in resistant unipolar depression with suicidal tendency.
4. Li increases leukocyte count, and is hence used in **chemotherapy-induced leukocytopenia and agranulocytosis.**
5. Li is also useful in **neuropsychiatric illness and cluster headaches.**

ADRs

- **At therapeutic concentration,** mild ADRs like fine tremors (controllable with propranolol), confusion and slurring of speech occur.
- **Long-term use** of Li^+ is associated with development of subclinical hypothyroidism.
- Nephrogenic diabetes insipidus is induced, which is managed with amiloride and thiazides.
- Edema and weight gain may occur.
- Nausea, vomiting, diarrhea: Diarrhea associated with Li use causes loss of Na^+; depletion of Na^+ favours Li^+ reabsorption. Thus, the patient becomes more prone to develop Li^+-induced diarrhea.
- Acne, folliculitis, alopecia and worsening of psoriasis
- Leukocytosis

Li toxicity

Li toxicity occurs when plasma concentration **exceeds 1.5 mEq/L**, resulting in coarse tremors, giddiness, motor incoordination, ataxia, nystagmus, slurring of speech, confusion and hyperreflexia.

When the Li^+ levels exceed 2 mEq/L, the patient may show twitching, drowsiness, convulsion, delirium and coma. Severe diarrhea, vomiting, hypotension, albuminuria and risk of arrhythmias may also occur.

Treatment of Li toxicity is symptomatic.

Osmotic diuresis along with $NaHCO_3$ **infusion** promotes Li excretion. At concentrations > 4 mEq/L, **hemodialysis** is indicated.

Contraindications

Li is contraindicated in **pregnant women** as it may cause:
- Fetal goitre
- NMJ block causing hypotonia, floppy infant syndrome
- Cardiac congenital anomalies: Ebstein anomaly characterised by large right atrium and small ventricles, leading to outflow obstruction on the right side (The condition is also known as atrialisation of ventricles.)

Hence, pregnant women suffering from mania are treated with atypical antipsychotic drugs.

Other contraindications are **sick sinus syndrome, dermatitis and acne.**

Drug interactions

- **Thiazide diuretics** can cause lithium toxicity by inducing Na^+ loss, as Na^+ depletion favours more reabsorption of lithium. However, osmotic diuretics increase lithium clearance.
- Lithium clearance is reduced by drugs like **ACE inhibitors, NSAIDs and tetracyclines,** which may lead to lithium toxicity.
- Lithium has some NMJ blocking effect, and can thus potentiate the effect of non-depolarising-type of skeletal muscle relaxants. In view of this, it is better to stop lithium 24 hours prior to elective surgery.
- Lithium can **enhance insulin-induced hypoglycemia.**
- In some patients, the combined use of **lithium and haloperidol may cause tremors and rigidity.**

Clinical problem based questions and MCQs

17. **A 40-year-old man is brought to the emergency ward with minor facial and arm abrasions sustained during a fight in a restaurant over a trivial issue. His friends reveal that such episodes of aggressive behaviour are frequent. While his wounds are being dressed, he is noted to be restless, over-talkative, aggressive, and uncooperative. He attempts to persuade nursing staff and nearby patients to invest in his sugar mills, claiming they will become wealthy and powerful due to the "energy from glucose." He also insists that powerful individuals, including the president of the United States, drink milk with sugar to gain strength.**

    Given these grandiose ideas, pressured speech, and behavioural agitation, a psychiatric evaluation

is requested. The psychiatrist initiates treatment with tablet lithium 300 mg and tablet haloperidol 5 mg daily.
   i. What is the diagnosis?
   ii. Explain the rationale of the prescribed combination.

18. The dose of lithium in bipolar disease is individualised by careful monitoring of plasma concentrations.
    i. Explain why therapeutic drug monitoring is important for lithium.
    ii. Enumerate the adverse effects of lithium.
    iii. Describe the features of lithium toxicity and its treatment.

19. Identify the correct action of lithium in the following.
    a. It quickly relieves manic symptoms.
    b. It opposes action of aldosterone in kidney.
    c. Leukocyte count is reduced.
    d. Thyroid hormone release is reduced.

20. At what concentration of lithium is hemodialysis indicated?
    a. 0.8 mEq/L   b. 1.5 mEq/L
    c. 4 mEq/L   d. 10 mEq/L

Summary

Antidepressant drugs

- Deficiency of monoamines such as noradrenaline and serotonin is implicated in the causation of depression. Antidepressants act by varied mechanisms to correct these neurotransmitter defects.
- TCAs act by inhibiting reuptake of NA/5-HT or both at nerve endings. SSRIs inhibit reuptake of serotonin only, whereas SNRIs inhibit uptake of both NA and 5-HT. MAO inhibitors inhibit metabolism of brain amines. Atypical antipsychotics cause increased release of NA and/or serotonin.
- All the above are equally efficacious; there is however, a biological lag of 2–3 weeks because of adaptive changes such as down-regulation of postsynaptic (β_1, β_2 and 5-HT_{1A}, 5-HT_{2A}, 5-HT_{2C}) receptors, desensitisation of presynaptic (α_2 and 5-HT_{1A}) receptors, and increased synthesis of BDNF.
- Psychiatric indications for use include depression, panic disorders, phobias, obsessive compulsive disorders and attention deficit disorder. Non-psychiatric indications include enuresis, chronic neuropathic pain, migraine, lichen simplex, atopic dermatitis, bulimia nervosa, smoking cessation and alcoholism. SSRIs and SNRIs are preferred over TCAs which have many adverse effects and are used only in refractory cases.
- ADRs of TCAs include sedation, confusion, switching over to manic phase, seizure precipitation, anticholinergic adverse effects, postural hypotension, tachycardia, erectile and ejaculatory dysfunction, cardiac arrhythmias, increased appetite and weight gain.
- Acute TCA poisoning causes excitement, delirium, convulsions, ventricular arrhythmias and hypotension. Diazepam, propranolol, lignocaine and supportive treatment are given.
- **SSRIs** do not have α_1-blocking, H_1 blocking and antimuscarinic adverse effects, but they can cause nausea, diarrhea, anxiety, insomnia, agitation and sexual dysfunction. Dose is given in the morning.
- MAO inhibitors can cause serotonin syndrome if co-administered with SSRIs, and hypertensive crisis with tyramine-rich foods and cough/cold remedies.
- Atypical drugs are better tolerated than TCAs. Trazodone and mirtazapine are used in depression with erectile dysfunction. They can cause sedation, nausea, postural hypotension and impotence. Bupropion may cause insomnia, agitation and seizure. Mianserin and mirtazapine may cause sedation due to H_1 blockade. The risk of seizure precipitation, hepatotoxicity and weight gain are also seen with mianserin. Bupropion has a role in smoking cessation.

Antimanic drugs

- Preponderance of noradrenaline, dopamine activity is blamed to exacerbate manic symptoms.
- **Lithium** acts by selectively inhibiting overactive circuits by blocking conversion of IP to inositol so that regeneration of PIP_2 and hence **IP_3–DAG pathway is suppressed.**
- Li is handled in same way as Na^+ by the body, i.e., rapid absorption and distribution through body water, no binding to plasma proteins, no metabolism. Li is excreted through kidney, sweat and saliva. **Na^+ loading enhances Li excretion and vice versa.** Diarrhea can cause Na^+ depletion, which in turn causes Li retention, thus further worsening Li toxicity.
- *Uses:* Long-term treatment with lithium is required in MDP as rebound effect is seen on stopping the drug. Other uses are to build up leukocyte count in patients receiving chemotherapy and in cluster headaches.
- Li has low safety margin. So, it is important to carry out therapeutic drug monitoring to keep plasma concentration between **0.8–1.4 mEq/L.**
- At therapeutic concentration, fine tremors, confusion and slurring of speech may occur. Long-term use causes nausea, vomiting, diarrhea, leukocytosis,

- weight gain, nephrogenic diabetes insipidus and subclinical hypothyroidism.
- At concentrations > 1.5 mEq/L, coarse tremors, giddiness, ataxia, motor incoordination, nystagmus, slurring, confusion and hyperreflexia can occur.
- Concentration up to 2 mEq/L may cause drowsiness, delirium, convulsions, coma, hypotension and rhythm disturbances.
- Treatment of Li toxicity is symptomatic; osmotic diuresis along with sodium bicarbonate infusion and hemodialysis promotes Li excretion.

Questions for practice

1. Enumerate therapeutic uses and ADRs of:
   a. Tricyclic antidepressants
   b. SSRIs
   c. Li carbonate
2. Explain why:
   a. Major part of daily dose of chlorpromazine is given at bed time.
   b. SSRIs are preferred over TCAs in the treatment of depression.
   c. Cough and cold medicines should be avoided in patients taking TCAs.
   d. Patients receiving MAO inhibitors are advised not to take cheese, wine, etc.
   e. Therapeutic drug monitoring is necessary while using lithium.
   f. Lithium-induced diarrhea increases the risk of lithium toxicity.
3. Explain pharmacological basis for the use of:
   a. Antidepressants in chronic pain
   b. Lithium in mania
4. Write short notes on:
   a. SSRLs
   b. Atypical antipsychotics
   c. Venlafaxine

Hints for problem-based questions and MCQs

1. b. Inhibits reuptake of 5-HT and NA
2. d. Bupropion
3. c. Mirtazapine
4. b. Block β_2 receptors
5. a. Sertraline. Refer to page 264.
6. c. Time required for BDNF synthesis results in biological lag. In addition, down-regulation of postsynaptic, desensitisation of presynaptic receptors and high plasma protein binding of drug contribute to a lag of 2–3 weeks in response.
7. i. d. Amitriptyline is contraindicated.
   ii. Amitriptyline has prominent anticholinergic activity, which may cause urinary retention in this patient having benign hypertrophy of prostate (BHP).
8. TCAs have α_1 blocking effect resulting in postural hypotension. NA reuptake is reduced, so its action is augmented causing tachycardia and palpitations. Reflex response to low BP also contributes to tachycardia.
9. Imipramine reduces bedwetting due to its anticholinergic action.
10. i. d. Citalopram
    ii. SSRI
    iii. a. Clomipramine
11. c. Impotence can occur because of erectile dysfunction due to increased serotonergic tone in spinal cord. SSRIs do not cause sedation, rather insomnia is seen. Seizure precipitation and weight gain is also not seen with SSRIs.
12. i. c. 14 days
    ii. Refer to page 263.
    iii. Refer to page 262, 265, 267.
13. i. c. Duloxetine has a role in depression as well as fibromyalgia.
    ii. SNRI; refer to page 262.
14. i. Refer to page 267, 268.
    ii. Smoking cessation
15. d. Citalopram
16. i. c. Bupropion
    ii. It may cause insomnia as an adverse effect.
17. i. Acute mania
    ii. Haloperidol is combined for quick response. Refer to page 271.
18. i. TDM is required in patients on lithium therapy, because lithium has a narrow margin of safety and is effective in a narrow therapeutic range of 0.5–1.5 mEq/L. Further, lithium excretion is reduced by sodium depletion, increasing the risk of toxicity. Refer to page 271.
    ii. ADRs at therapeutic concentrations are mild: confusion, slurring of speech, and fine tremors. Long-term use can cause hypothyroidism, nephrogenic diabetes inspidus, edema, weight gain, diarrhea, acne, folliculitis, leukocytosis etc.
    iii. Lithium toxicity is characterised by muscle incoordination, coarse tremors, ataxia, nystagmus, confusion, slurred speech and hyperreflexia. At concentrations > 2 mEq/L, drowsiness, convulsions, delirium, coma, and rhythm disturbances may occur.
    Treatment is symptomatic, osmotic diuresis, and sodium bicarbonate infusion. At very high concentrations (4 mEq/L), hemodialysis is indicated
19. d. Thyroid hormone release is reduced. Manic symptoms are relieved by lithium in 10–15 days (not quickly). Li increases leukocyte count and opposes action of ADH (not aldosterone) in the kidney.
20. c. 4 mEq/L

CONCEPT MAP - ANTIMANIC DRUGS

Classification
Lithium carbonate or citrate
Anticonvulsants: Carbamazepine, Valproate, Lamotrigine,
Antipsychotics: Haloperidol, Rispridone, Olanzapine, Aripiprazole, Quetiapine

Mechanism of Action
Lithium selectively inhibits overactive circuits by blocking conversion of IP to inositol ⟶ suppresses PIP_2 regeneration & IP_3–DAG pathway ⟶ reduced BDNF release

Major Pharmacological Actions
No acute effects
Gradually controls manic episode in 1–2 weeks time.
Normalises reduced sleep time in mania.
Induces leukocytosis, Nephrogenic diabetes inspidus, Hypothyroidism

Contraindications
Pregnancy: Fetal goitre, Ebstein anomaly in heart
Sick sinus syndrome, dermatitis and acne

Li Toxicity
At concentration > 1.5 mEq/L:
Coarse tremprs, Giddiness, Ataxia, Motor incoordination, Nystagmus, Slurring of speech, Acne, Folliculitis, Alopecia, Worsening of psoriasis, Hyperreflexia, Drowsiness, Delirium, Convulsions, Coma, Hypotension and Arrhythmias.
Treatment: Symptomatic, Osmotic diuresis, $NaHCO_3$ infusion (Na^+ loading enhances Li excretion and vice versa.). Hemodialysis needed at conc. > 4 mEq/L.

ADRs
At therapeutic concentration
Fine tremors, Confusion, Slurring of speech
Long term use
Nausea, Vomiting, Diarrhea, Leukocytosis, Weight gain, Nephrogenic diabetes inspidus, Hypothyroidism

Low safety margin ↓ TDM required to keep plasma concentration between 0.8–1.4 mEq/L

Uses
- Drug of choice for treatment & prophylaxis of mania and manic episode in MDP
Effect of Li manifests in 1–3 weeks, so antipsychotics (Haloperidol, Olanzapine) given with lithium in acute manic episode.
- Resistant unipolar depression with suicidal tendency
- To build up leukocyte count in patients receiving chemotherapy,
- Cluster headaches.

SECTION 3 Drugs Acting on CNS

20 Alcohols

PH 3.8 Identify and manage methanol poisoning and chronic ethanol intoxication.

Learning objectives

A student of MBBS phase II should be able to:
- Describe pharmacokinetics of ethanol.
- Describe pharmacological effects of acute ethanol intake.
- Describe pharmacological effects of chronic ethanol intake.
- Describe management of chronic alcoholism and the principles of alcohol de-addiction.
- Describe the drugs used in alcohol de-addiction.
- Describe the symptoms of acute ethanol poisoning.
- Explain the management of ethanol poisoning.
- Describe the symptoms of methanol poisoning.
- Explain the management of methanol poisoning.

Ethanol, or ethyl alcohol, is the most widely abused substance globally. Studies indicate that at least 30% of hospitalised patients have coexisting alcohol abuse disorders. In cases of **alcohol abuse**, individuals consume alcohol in hazardous situations, such as while driving or alongside other central nervous system depressants, and often continue drinking despite known health risks. Those who are **alcohol-dependent** exhibit compulsive behaviours centered around obtaining and consuming alcohol. They may experience withdrawal symptoms due to the development of physical dependence.

PHARMACOKINETICS OF ETHANOL

To understand the effects of acute and chronic alcoholism, it is important to know its pharmacokinetics.

Absorption
- Ethanol is a small, water-soluble molecule and is therefore **rapidly absorbed** from GIT.
- Peak blood concentration is achieved within half an hour of alcohol ingestion on empty stomach. However, the presence of food delays absorption by slowing down gastric emptying.

Distribution
- Ethanol is **rapidly distributed** and its volume of distribution is approximately equal to the total body water.
- Peak plasma concentrations are more in women than men after ingestion of equivalent amount of alcohol. This may be due to lower total body water content and low first-pass metabolism in women.

- Since brain receives a large proportion of total blood flow and alcohol crosses biological membranes readily, the **concentration of alcohol in CNS rises quickly**.

Metabolism and Excretion
- Ninety percent of alcohol consumed is metabolised in the liver by oxidation, and the remaining is excreted through lungs and urine. The small proportion of alcohol excreted through lungs forms the basis of 'alcohol consumption analysis' by breath analyzers.
- In the liver, ethyl alcohol is mainly metabolised by **alcohol dehydrogenase enzyme to form acetaldehyde** (Fig. 20.1). During this oxidation process, a hydrogen ion (H^+) is shifted from ethanol to nicotinamide

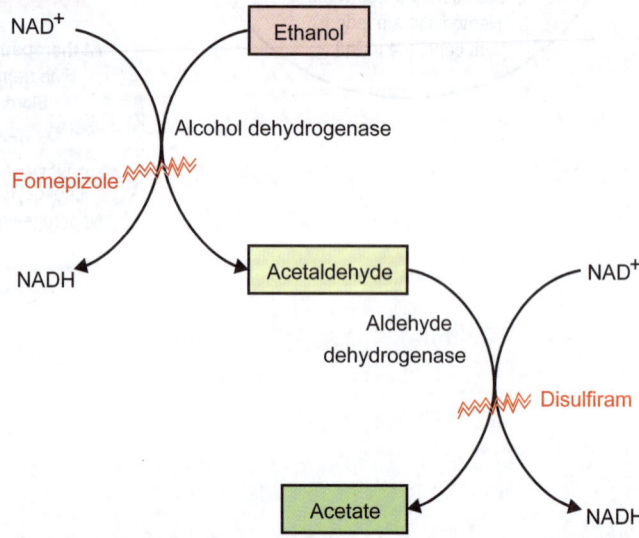

Fig. 20.1 Ethanol metabolism

adenine dinucleotide (NAD$^+$). Thus, ethanol oxidation generates acetaldehyde and NADH. Excess NADH contributes to lactic acidosis and hypoglycemia in acute alcohol poisoning and metabolic disorders in chronic alcoholism.
- Acetaldehyde is further metabolised by NAD$^+$ dependent **aldehyde dehydrogenase enzyme to form acetate and NADH**. Acetate can break into CO_2 and H_2O or it is utilised in the production of acetyl CoA.
- **Fomepizole** inhibits enzyme 'alcohol dehydrogenase' and interferes with production of acetaldehyde. **Disulfiram** is an inhibitor of enzyme aldehyde dehydrogenase. Therefore, alcohol consumption in presence of disulfiram results in acetaldehyde accumulation, which causes an unpleasant reaction called 'aldehyde syndrome' in the form of headache, dizziness, facial flushing, nausea and vomiting. This disulfiram reaction is used as **aversion therapy** to discourage alcohol consumption. Drugs such as metronidazole, cefoperazone, trimethoprim, nitrofurantoin and chlorpropamide can also cause disulfiram-like reaction. Therefore, patients on these drugs are warned about the adverse effects of alcohol consumption.
- Mixed function oxidases (MFOs) are microsomal enzymes that utilise NADPH as a co-factor. The MFOs that oxidise ethanol are called the 'microsomal ethanol oxidising system' and normally play a minor role in alcohol metabolism. However, chronic alcoholism induces the synthesis of MFOs and increases the metabolism of alcohol as well as other drugs metabolised by it. Large amounts of toxic byproducts, free radicals and H_2O_2 are also generated.

Effects of Acute Ethanol Consumption (Fig 20.2)

1. CNS

The exact **mechanism of central actions of alcohol** is not fully understood, but it is believed to affect neurotransmission involving glutamate and gamma-aminobutyric acid (GABA).

- Acute ethanol intake enhances GABAergic activity at $GABA_A$ receptors, which is why its acute effects are potentiated by other drugs acting on these receptors (e.g., benzodiazepines, barbiturates) and attenuated somewhat by the $GABA_A$ receptor antagonist flumazenil.
- Glutamate is the main excitatory neurotransmitter in CNS. Glutamate affects cognitive functions, learning, and memory through its action on N-methyl-D-aspartate (NMDA) receptors. Ethanol **inhibits 'cation channel opening' in response to NMDA receptor activation by glutamate**. This effect might be responsible for the 'blackouts' (periods of memory loss) seen at higher alcohol levels.

- **Central effects** of alcohol vary with plasma concentration.
- **Low to moderate** consumption of alcohol causes relief from anxiety and sedation.
- As **blood alcohol concentration increases**, individuals may exhibit slurred speech, ataxia, an unsteady or 'drunken' gait, disinhibition, mental clouding, impaired judgment, attention deficits, and inhibition of both cognitive and motor skills necessary for operating machinery or driving. These impairments are largely responsible for road accidents involving drunk drivers; it is one of the leading causes of death, particularly among young adults.
- **Very high concentration** (>500 mg/dL) causes respiratory depression, coma and death.

Tolerance develops to central effects of alcohol, and chronic drinkers develop these effects at much higher concentrations.

2. Smooth muscles

- Vasodilation and fall in BP occur in alcohol overdose, especially in cold environment due to depression of central vasomotor centre and acetaldehyde-induced smooth muscle relaxation.
- Uterine smooth muscles are relaxed, but this effect of ethanol cannot be used for suppression of premature labor because of the depressant action on the fetal CNS.

3. Heart

Myocardial depressant effect of ethanol is seen at blood concentration exceeding 100 mg/dL.

4. Diuresis

Acute alcohol intake inhibits ADH, resulting in diuresis, but tolerance develops to this action.

5. Metabolic effects

Acute alcohol intake causes depletion of NAD. This leads to inhibition of gluconeogenesis and hypoglycemia. However, alcohol-induced catecholamine release can cause hyperglycemia.

Effects of Chronic Ethanol Consumption (Fig. 20.2)

Ethanol is a low-potency drug in comparison to other drugs of abuse such as opioids and cocaine and is therefore widely consumed. Chronic alcohol intake has a **tissue-damaging effect** on multiple organ systems, including the liver, gastrointestinal tract, and the cardiovascular, nervous, and immune systems. The tissue damage occurs due to:

- Direct effects of alcohol and its metabolite acetaldehyde.
- A heavy load of metabolic byproducts such as NADH, free radicals and H_2O_2 due to the ingestion of large

amounts of alcohol for a long period of time. This oxidative stress leads to glutathione depletion, cytokine-induced injury, mitochondrial damage and disturbances in the regulation of growth factors.
- Deaths related to chronic alcoholism are often due to hepatic cirrhosis and liver failure, malignancies, psychiatric disorders, suicide, or accidental injuries.

Organ system effects of chronic alcohol intake include the following (Fig. 20.2):

1. Liver
The most commonly encountered consequence of chronic alcoholism is liver disease. **Fatty liver** is the initial stage of alcoholic liver disease (ALD). This is a reversible stage if alcohol intake is stopped. Otherwise, the disease progresses to hepatitis, cirrhosis and hepatic failure. The proposed mechanisms underlying alcohol-induced hepatic damage include:
- Oxidative stress due to accumulation of NADH and free radicals
- Disturbed fatty acid oxidation and synthesis
- Immune system activation
- Increased cytokine production, particularly TNF-α.

Women are more prone to the hepatic complications of alcohol intake than men. Concurrent infections with hepatitis B or C also increase the severity of alcoholic liver disease.

2. GIT
- Chronic alcoholism is the most prominent cause of chronic **pancreatitis**. Alcohol has direct tissue-damaging effect on acinar cells and increases the formation of protein plugs and **calcium carbonate stones in small ducts.**
- Chronic alcoholics are prone to gastritis. Ethanol causes irritation, inflammation, scarring and induration of gut mucosa, resulting in diarrhea, weight loss and malnutrition. Ethanol interferes with the absorption of nutrients, leading to **nutritional deficiencies,** especially that of water-soluble vitamins.
- **Portal hypertension** associated with hepatic changes can cause bleeding (hematemesis) from esophageal varices.

3. Cardiovascular effects
Intake of large amounts of alcohol for a long time is associated with **dilated cardiomyopathy, ventricular hypertrophy and fibrosis.** Cessation of alcohol intake can reduce cardiac size and improve cardiac function. However, response to treatment (with β blockers or ACE inhibitors), and overall outcome remains poor.
- Binge drinking can cause atrial as well as ventricular **arrhythmias.** Dangerous arrhythmias can occur during alcohol withdrawal also.
- More than 3 drinks per day is associated with risk of **hypertension** in the presence of other co-existent factors like obesity, smoking and excessive salt/caffeine intake. However, there is evidence of some protective effect against coronary artery disease, peripheral arterial disease and ischemic stroke with moderate alcohol intake. This preventive effect may be due to raised serum HDL levels, increased production of tissue plasminogen activator (tPA), inhibition of some inflammatory processes by moderate alcohol intake the presence of antioxidants in alcoholic beverages.

4. Nervous system
Alcohol consumption in high doses for long times results in development of **tolerance and dependence**.
- The mechanism for development of tolerance is not well understood but involves both cellular and pharmacokinetic mechanisms. The up-regulation of NMDA receptors, voltage sensitive calcium channels, and down-regulation of $GABA_A$ receptors cause cellular tolerance. Pharmacokinetic tolerance may be due to reduced rate of absorption and enzyme induction.
- Both psychological and physical dependence are seen with chronic alcohol intake. Psychological dependence consists of a compulsive desire to drink and intense craving. Reduction or cessation of alcohol precipitates disturbing withdrawal symptoms such as hyperexcitability, seizures, psychosis and delirium tremens.
- Prolonged, heavy alcohol intake also causes **neurologic deficits**, including generalised, symmetrical peripheral neuropathy with distal paresthesias of hands and feet. There can occur disturbances of gait, ataxia, dementia and in rare cases, demyelination.
- In some patients, chronic alcoholism associated **thiamine deficiency** results in paralysis of extraocular muscles, ataxia, and confusion. Subsequently, it leads to coma and finally, death. This is known as **Wernicke-Korsakoff syndrome**. Symptoms typically improve rapidly with thiamine administration, though residual memory impairment, referred to as Korsakoff psychosis, may persist.
- Bilateral, symmetrical impairment of visual acuity followed by degeneration of optic nerve may also occur.

5. Blood
Metabolic and nutritional effects of chronic alcohol intake inhibit proliferation of all cellular elements in the bone marrow. Mild anemia occurs in almost all alcoholics. In rare cases, hemolysis can occur due to liver disease and hyperlipidemia.

6. Fluid–electrolyte balance and endocrine functions
Chronic alcohol intake causes derangement of steroid hormone balance causing testicular atrophy and

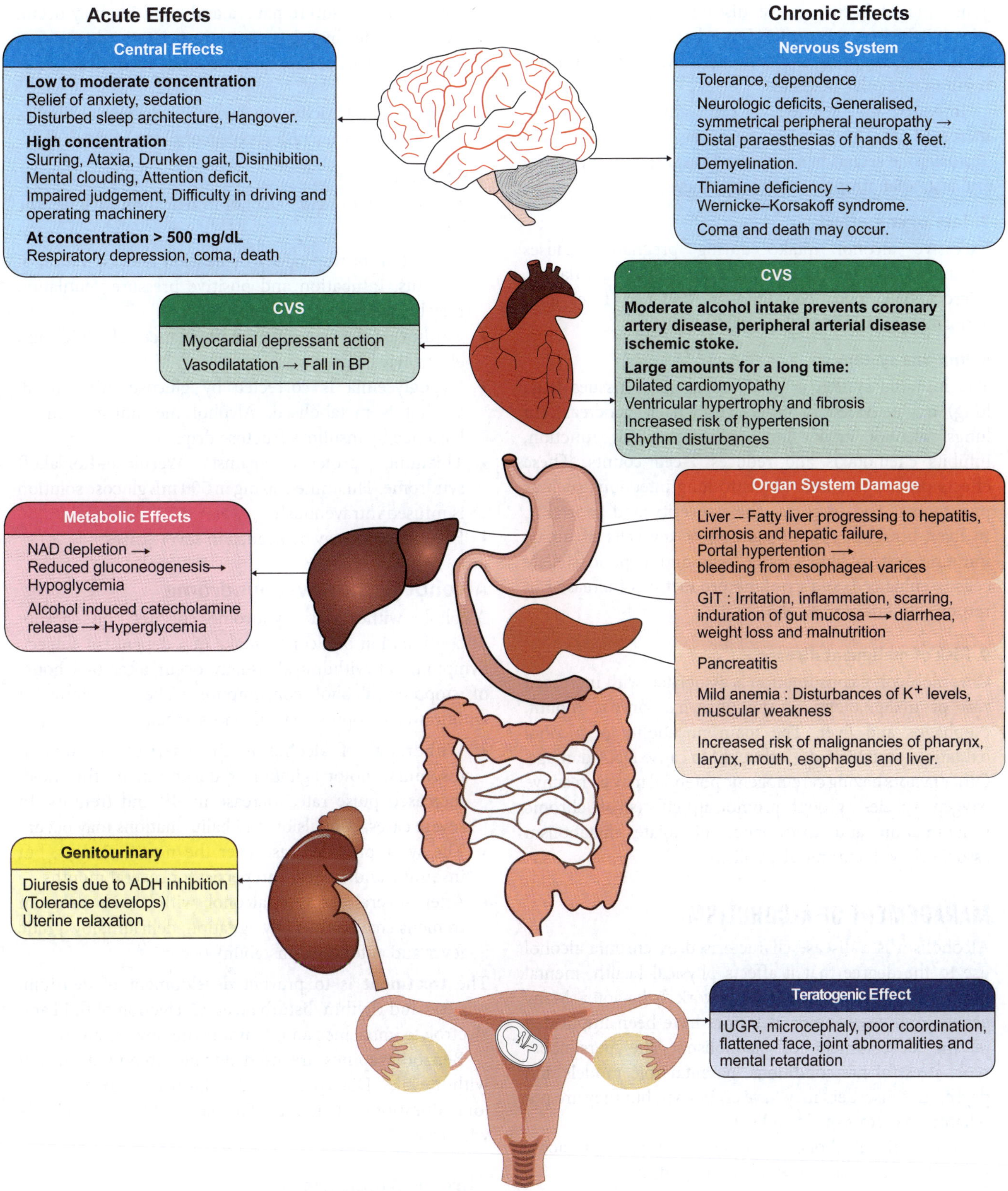

Acute Effects

Central Effects

Low to moderate concentration
Relief of anxiety, sedation
Disturbed sleep architecture, Hangover.

High concentration
Slurring, Ataxia, Drunken gait, Disinhibition, Mental clouding, Attention deficit, Impaired judgement, Difficulty in driving and operating machinery

At concentration > 500 mg/dL
Respiratory depression, coma, death

CVS

Myocardial depressant action
Vasodilatation → Fall in BP

Metabolic Effects

NAD depletion →
Reduced gluconeogenesis →
Hypoglycemia

Alcohol induced catecholamine release → Hyperglycemia

Genitourinary

Diuresis due to ADH inhibition (Tolerance develops)
Uterine relaxation

Chronic Effects

Nervous System

Tolerance, dependence

Neurologic deficits, Generalised, symmetrical peripheral neuropathy → Distal paraesthesias of hands & feet.

Demyelination.

Thiamine deficiency → Wernicke–Korsakoff syndrome.

Coma and death may occur.

CVS

Moderate alcohol intake prevents coronary artery disease, peripheral arterial disease ischemic stoke.

Large amounts for a long time:
Dilated cardiomyopathy
Ventricular hypertrophy and fibrosis
Increased risk of hypertension
Rhythm disturbances

Organ System Damage

Liver – Fatty liver progressing to hepatitis, cirrhosis and hepatic failure,
Portal hypertension → bleeding from esophageal varices

GIT : Irritation, inflammation, scarring, induration of gut mucosa → diarrhea, weight loss and malnutrition

Pancreatitis

Mild anemia : Disturbances of K^+ levels, muscular weakness

Increased risk of malignancies of pharynx, larynx, mouth, esophagus and liver.

Teratogenic Effect

IUGR, microcephaly, poor coordination, flattened face, joint abnormalities and mental retardation

Fig. 20.2 Acute and chronic effects of alcohol

gynecomastia. In chronic liver disease, the patient develops edema, effusions and ascites. Disturbance of K^+ levels due to diarrhea, vomiting and secondary hyperaldosteronism result in muscular weakness.

Impaired gluconeogenesis can cause hypoglycemia, increased ACTH secretion and raised cortisol levels. Testosterone secretion is impaired, resulting in impotence and testicular atrophy on prolonged use.

7. Teratogenic effect
Excessive alcohol intake during pregnancy causes teratogenic effects such as intrauterine growth retardation, microcephaly, poor coordination, flattened face, joint abnormalities and mental retardation.

8. Immune system
The immune system is inhibited in some tissues (e.g., lung) but activated in others (e.g., liver, pancreas). In lungs, alcohol intake impairs alveolar cell function, inhibits chemotaxis and reduces T-cell counts. These effects predisposes individuals to lung infections such as pneumonia, and increases their severity and mortality. In liver, however, the functioning of key cells of innate immune system like Kupffer cells and hepatic stellate cells is enhanced, and cytokine productions increased in response to intake of alcohol.

9. Risk of malignant disease
Chronic alcohol consumption is associated with increased risk of malignancies of the pharynx, larynx, mouth, esophagus and liver. The main metabolite of alcohol oxidation, acetaldehyde, is thought to cause DNA damage. Other factors having carcinogenic potential may be reactive oxygen species, growth-promoting effects of chronic inflammation and disturbance of folate metabolism associated with chronic alcoholism.

MANAGEMENT OF ALCOHOLISM

Alcoholism is a disease characterised by chronic alcohol use to the degree that it affects physical health, mental health, and normal social and work behaviour. Many genetic and environmental factors have been implicated in the development of alcoholism. The personality type, stressful life conditions, parental role models and psychiatric disorders may have an impact, but they are not reliable predictors of alcoholism.

A chronic alcoholic is prone to suffer from acute intoxication and alcohol withdrawal syndrome.

Acute Alcohol Intoxication
- Acute alcohol intoxication occurs in a non-tolerant individual upon consumption of a large amount of alcohol, leading to blood alcohol levels of around 400 mg/dL. The patient is in stupor; vasodilation, hypotension, tachycardia and gastrointestinal irritant effects such as severe nausea and vomiting may occur. Severe acute hypoglycemia, respiratory depression, cardiovascular collapse, coma and even death may occur.
- Severe acute toxicity can occur in chronic alcoholics also, as tolerance to effects of alcohol is not absolute.

Treatment
The treatment for acute alcohol intoxication includes the following.

- Prevention of respiratory depression and aspiration of vomitus. Intubation and positive pressure ventilation may be needed.
- Cardiovascular support, maintenance of fluid and electrolyte balance
- Hypoglycemia is corrected by glucose infusion till alcohol is metabolised. Alcohol metabolism can be hastened by insulin + fructose drip.
- Thiamine protects against Wernicke–Korsakoff syndrome. Thiamine 100 mg in 500 mL glucose solution is infused intravenously.
- Hemodialysis may be needed in severe cases.

Alcohol Withdrawal Syndrome
Alcohol withdrawal syndrome occurs on abrupt discontinuation of alcohol intake in a dependent subject. Symptoms of withdrawal usually occur after 6–8 hours of stopping alcohol consumption. The symptoms of withdrawal are opposite to alcohol's effects.

- Withdrawal of alcohol is characterised by anxiety, insomnia, motor agitation, reduced seizure threshold, increased pulse rate, increase in BP and tremors. In severe cases, convulsion and hallucinations may occur.
- The symptoms decrease over the next 1–2 days, but insomnia and anxiety can persist for several months.
- After several days of alcohol withdrawal, delirium tremens characterised by agitation, delirium, low grade fever and autonomic instability occur.

The **treatment** is to prevent development of delirium, seizures and rhythm disturbances. Correction of fluid and electrolyte imbalance and thiamine therapy are given.

Benzodiazepines are used during attempted alcohol withdrawal. Diazepam and chlordiazepoxide have long durations of action. Thereafter, these are slowly withdrawn.

Chronic Alcoholism
Low degree **tolerance** develops to subjective as well as behavioural effects of ethanol. The **mechanism of tolerance** is both pharmacodynamic and pharmacokinetic.

- Pharmacodynamic or cellular tolerance may be due to up-regulation of NMDA receptors and down-regulation of $GABA_A$ receptors.

- Pharmacokinetic tolerance is because of decreased rate of absorption due to alcohol-induced gastritis. Increased rate of metabolism by MFOs (induced by chronic alcoholism) also contributes to tolerance.
- Psychological dependence manifests as alcohol-seeking behaviour and cravings, and physical dependence manifests as withdrawal symptoms in absence of alcohol intake.
- Nutritional deficiencies are common in chronic alcoholics due to neglect of balanced diet and malabsorption.
- Neurological symptoms like megaloblastic anemia, pellagra, polyneuritis, Wernicke encephalopathy and Korsakoff psychosis may develop. Many neurological symptoms are controlled with thiamine replacement.
- Chronic alcoholics may also develop hypertension, gynecomastia, acute pancreatitis, impotence, infertility, CHF, stroke, cardiomyopathy and cirrhosis of liver.

Treatment

Detoxification involves the substitution of alcohol with a long-acting sedative hypnotic drug (e.g., **diazepam**) and then gradual reduction and tapering off of this substituent drug over several weeks. Restoration of normal neurological function, especially sleep, may take several months after detoxification.

Rehabilitation of the patient is a crucial aspect in the treatment of alcohol dependence. Co-existent psychiatric problems such as anxiety or depression should be appropriately treated, as they increase the risk of relapse in a detoxified alcoholic person. Psychosocial measures such as counselling, acceptance and moral support provided by family and friends help to reduce the relapse rate.

- **Naltrexone** (an opioid antagonist at μ receptors), **disulfiram** (an aversion agent that acts by aldehyde dehydrogenase inhibition), and **acamprosate** (a weak NMDA antagonist and $GABA_A$ agonist) are drugs approved by FDA for adjunctive therapy in alcohol dependence.
- Several other drugs such as $5-HT_3$ antagonist **ondansetron**, antiseizure drug **topiramate** and GABA antagonist **baclofen** aid in maintaining alcohol abstinence and controlling cravings, but these are not FDA approved for this indication.

METHANOL POISONING

Methanol is present in canned meat, fresh fruits, juices, fermented and distilled beverages, etc. Poisoning is often from exposure to methanol-containing products like windshield cleaners, rectified spirit, antifreeze, or other commercial solvents. Poisoning may also result from ingesting methanol as a substitute for ethanol (out of ignorance) or from spurious alcohol.

Pharmacokinetics

Methanol gets absorbed from skin, respiratory and gastrointestinal tract. It is well distributed in body water. It gets oxidised by the same enzymes as ethanol, i.e., alcohol dehydrogenase and aldehyde dehydrogenase, but the metabolites of methanol are different from that of ethanol.

Methanol is oxidised to formaldehyde by enzyme alcohol dehydrogenase, which further forms formic acid with aldehyde dehydrogenase (Fig. 20.3). Formic acid is mainly responsible for toxic effects of methanol. Formic acid is further oxidised to CO_2 and water by folate-dependent systems.

Symptoms of Methanol Poisoning

The development of symptoms may be delayed for up to 6–30 hours after exposure, as the symptoms are not caused by methanol itself, but by its oxidation metabolites. The characteristic features of methanol poisoning are the following.

- The patient appears inebriated and has **formaldehyde odour** in breath and urine.
- The calculated value of serum osmolarity based on serum sodium, glucose and blood urea is usually 280–290 mOsm/litre. Like other alcohols, methanol contributes to measured serum osmolarity. So, in the presence of methanol, the difference between the measured and calculated osmolarity, known as **osmolar gap, increases**.
- Anion gap metabolic acidosis develops. It is usually resistant to treatment and is an indicator of poor prognosis. Anion gap is calculated by subtracting the measured anion sum from that of cations.

$$\text{Anion gap} = (Na^+ + K^+) - (HCO_3^- + Cl^-).$$

Normally, it is 12–16 mEq/litre, but in case of methanol poisoning the anion gap is larger because of the presence of unmeasured anions $HCOO^-$ (formate) and accompanying **metabolic acidosis**.
- The most prominent feature of methanol poisoning is **visual disturbance**. Patients experience sensations similar to being caught in a snowstorm. Blurring of vision with relatively clear sensorium strongly points to exposure to methanol. Retinal damage and blindness may occur in severe cases.
- Headache, vomiting, epigastric pain, dyspnea, tachypnea and hypotension may occur.
- Bradycardia, seizures, acidosis resistant to correction, coma, respiratory failure and death may occur.

Management of Methanol Poisoning

- Methanol levels should be estimated if there is a history and symptoms suggestive of exposure. If methanol levels exceed 20 mg/dL, immediate treatment is indicated. A concentration of 75–100 mg/dL is fatal.

- Serum formaldehyde levels are a better indicator of severity, but such tests are not available widely.
- Decreased serum bicarbonate levels and metabolic acidosis occur.

Treatment
- The patient should be kept in a dark, quiet room.
- Respiratory support and maintenance of BP are life saving as in all cases of poisoning.
- Gastric lavage with $NaHCO_3$ and correction of metabolic acidosis with bicarbonate are needed in most patients.
- As symptoms are from formic acid, the aim of treatment in methanol poisoning is to reduce formate levels. This is achievable with the following methods (Fig. 20.3):
  - **Suppression of methanol metabolism** to prevent formation of toxic metabolites by giving alcohol dehydrogenase inhibitors.
  - **Ethanol and fomepizole:** These compete with methanol for metabolising enzyme alcohol dehydrogenase. Ethanol has a higher affinity for this enzyme than methanol. So, in the presence of ethanol, the metabolism of methanol gets reduced and toxic metabolites (formates) are not formed. Ethanol (10% in water) is given through nasogastric tube as a loading dose of 0.7 mL/kg body-weight and then at 0.15 mL/kg/hour. Blood alcohol levels should be carefully monitored.

  Fomepizole also acts as alcohol dehydrogenase inhibitor. It is approved by the FDA for treatment of methanol and ethylene glycol poisoning. It is given intravenously in a loading dose of 15 mg/kg, followed by 10 mg/kg, 12-hourly, for the first 48 hours. Fomepizole induces its own metabolism rapidly. So, after 48 hours, its dose is increased to 15 mg/kg, 12-hourly, till methanol levels fall below 20 mg/dL. The commonly observed adverse effects of fomepizole are headache, dizziness, nausea and burning at the site of infusion.
  - Folic acid can help oxidation of formates to CO_2 and H_2O. **Calcium leucovorin** 50 mg, 6-hourly, is injected as an adjuvant therapy.
  - Hemodialysis is indicated for quick removal of methanol and its metabolites in severe cases if serum methanol levels exceed 50 mg/dL.

Clinical problem-based questions and MCQs

1. A 35-year-old chronic alcoholic presents at a de-addiction centre wanting to quit the habit.
   i. Enumerate the harmful effects of chronic alcoholism
   ii. Name the drugs having a role in alcohol de-addiction.
   iii. Which of the following can be used as aversion therapy in alcoholics:
      a. Fomepizole
      b. Calcium leucovorin
      c. Disulfiram
      d. Chlordiazepoxide

2. A 35-year-old patient presents with fever and burning micturition. Urine examination reveals numerous pus cells. The patient is diagnosed with UTI and nitrofurantoin is prescribed. The patient reports after 3 days with headache, dizziness, facial flushing, nausea and vomiting. Careful history elicits alcohol intake at a family function.
   i. Explain cause of the patient's symptoms.
   ii. Enumerate other drugs having the risk of such symptoms when taken after consuming alcohol
   iii. How can such episodes be prevented?

3. A 45-year-old farm worker presents in emergency with headache, vomiting, sudden blurring of vision, reduced visual acuity and a feeling like being caught in a snow storm. The patient has clear sensorium and gives history of consuming rectified spirit as a substitute for alcohol. Respiration is elevated: RR=32/min and there is formaldehyde odour in expired air; HR= 58 BPM, BP= 100/60.
   i. What is the probable diagnosis?
   ii. All of the following are useful in this case, EXCEPT:
      a. Ethanol   b. Disulfiram
      c. Calcium leucovorin   d. Fomepizole
   iii. Describe the management of this case.

4. i. Describe central effects of acute alcohol intake.
   ii. Identify the correct mechanism of central effects of alcohol.
      a. Increased glutaminergic activity
      b. Increased adrenergic activity
      c. Increased GABAergic activity
      d. All of the above

5. A 40-year-old man with a long history of alcohol dependence reports intense cravings and inability

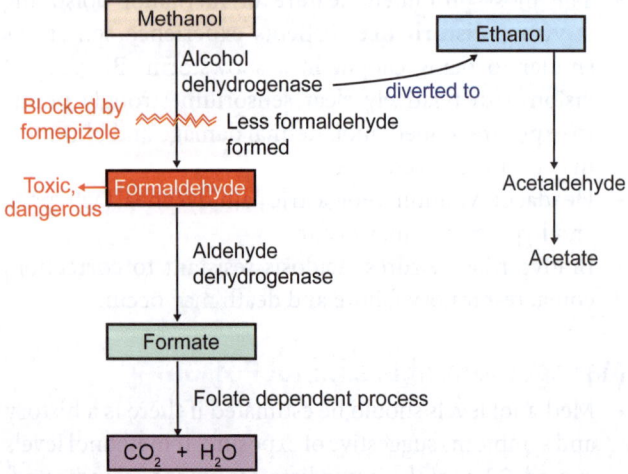

Fig. 20.3 Role of drugs in methanol poisoning

to quit despite strong motivation stemming from immense pressure from his family.
  a. Describe the harmful effects of chronic alcoholism.
  b. Explain the cause of the patient's craving and inability to quit drinking.
  c. Name the drugs that can be used to reduce alcohol craving.

Summary

- Ethanol, also known as ethyl alcohol, is rapidly absorbed and widely distributed throughout the body, including the CNS. It is metabolised primarily by alcohol dehydrogenase into acetaldehyde, which is then further converted to acetate by enzyme aldehyde dehydrogenase.
- Inhibition of aldehyde dehydrogenase by **disulfiram** and other drugs, e.g., cefoperazone, chlorpropamide, metronidazole and nitrofurantoin, causes accumulation of acetaldehyde → aldehyde syndrome characterised by disturbing symptoms like headache, dizziness, facial flushing, nausea and vomiting. Hence, disulfiram can be used as 'aversion therapy' in chronic alcoholics.
- The **mechanism** of central actions of ethanol involves increased GABA action at $GABA_A$ receptors and inhibition of cation channel opening in response to NMDA receptor activation by glutamate.
- **Acute effects** vary with concentration: **low concentration** relieves anxiety and causes sedation; **higher concentration** causes disinhibition, ataxia, slurring of speech, drunken gait, impaired judgement/cognition/motor skills, resulting in accident proneness. Ethanol > 500 mg/dL can cause respiratory depression, coma and death.
- Other acute effects of alcohol are vasodilation, diuresis, fall in BP, myocardial depression, uterine smooth muscle relaxation and inhibition of gluconeogenesis → hypoglycemia.
- **Chronic alcohol intake** has a tissue-damaging effect on several organ systems due to oxidative stress that results in glutathione depletion, cytokine induced injury, mitochondrial damage and disturbance in regulation of growth factors.
- Alcoholic liver disease, nutritional deficiencies (thiamine: Wernicke–Korsakoff syndrome), pancreatitis, portal hypertension, arrhythmias, hypertension, development of tolerance, dependence and withdrawal symptoms may occur. The risk of teratogenic effects and malignant disease is high.
- **Acute ethanol toxicity** results when ethanol in blood exceeds 400 mg/dL in non-tolerant subjects and is mainly managed by supportive treatment.
- **Withdrawal symptoms** like anxiety, insomnia, motor agitation, reduced seizure threshold, increased pulse rate, increase in BP, tremors, convulsion and hallucinations occur 6–8 hours after withdrawal in dependent subject. These can be controlled by benzodiazepines.
- **Chronic alcoholics** are managed with detoxification treatment with benzodiazepines, reduced craving with naltrexone, disulfiram (aversion agent), and acamprosate, and psychosocial rehabilitative measures.
- **Methanol poisoning** due to ingestion of spurious alcohols occurs accidently. Harmful effects are due to its metabolite (formic acid). The patient has formaldehyde odour in breath, increased osmolar and anion gap, visual disturbance, bradycardia, seizures, acidosis resistant to correction, coma, respiratory failure; even death may occur.
- Treatment is supportive and by suppressing methanol metabolism with alcohol dehydrogenase inhibitors ethanol and fomepizole. The metabolism of formate to CO_2 and H_2O is enhanced by calcium leucovorin. Hemodialysis may be needed.

Questions for practice

1. Describe the management of
   a. Acute alcohol intoxication
   b. Chronic alcoholism
   c. Methanol poisoning

Hints for problem-based questions and MCQs

1. i. Refer to page 277
   ii. Refer to page 281
   iii. c. Disulfiram
2. i. Disulfiram reaction with nitrofurantoin.
   ii. Chlorpropamide, cefoperazone, metronidazole, etc.
   iii. Counseling should be done to avoid alcohol in patients receiving these drugs.
3. i. Methanol poisoning
   ii. b. Disulfiram has no role in methanol poisoning. Ethanol and fomepizole reduce formation of formates and calcium leucovorin enhances metabolism of formates to CO_2 and H_2O. Thus all these three reduce the toxic effects of methanol which are mainly due to formic acid.
   iii. Refer to page 282
4. i. Refer to page 277
   ii. c. Increased GABAergic activity
5. i. Refer to page 277
   ii. Patient has craving owing to psychological dependence.
   iii. Naltrexone, acamprosate, topiramate, baclofen may be useful.

CONCEPT MAP – ALCOHOLS

ALCOHOLS (ETHANOL)

Pharmacokinetics
Rapidly absorbed and distributed

Alcohol
↓ *Alcohol dehydrogenase*
Acetaldehyde
↓ *Aldehyde dehydrogenase*
Acetate

Acute effects

CNS:
Low Concentration: Relieves anxiety, sedation.
Higher concentration: Disinhibition, Ataxia, Slurring of speech, Drunken gait, Impaired judgement/ cognition / motor skills, resulting in accident proneness.

Others:
Vasodilation, Diuresis, Fall in BP, Myocardial depression, Uterine relaxation, Inhibition of gluconeogenesis → Hypoglycemia

Acute Intoxication

At 400 mg/dL: Patient is stuporous, hypotension, Tachycardia, Severe Nausea & Vomiting.

> 500 mg/dL: Acute hypoglycemia, Cardiovascular collapse, Respiratory depression, Coma and Death

Management: Supportive, Insulin + Fructose drip, Thiamine IV infusion, Hemodialysis.

Mechanism of Action
Increased GABA action at $GABA_A$ receptors

Inhibits cation channel opening on NMDA receptor activation by glutamate

Chronic Alcoholism
Tissue damaging effect on organ systems due to oxidative stress → glutathione depletion, cytokine induced injury, mitochondrial damage and disturbance in regulation of growth factors.

Alcoholic liver disease, Nutritional deficiencies (Thiamine – Wernicke–Korsakoff syndrome), Pancreatitis, Portal hypertension, Arrhythmias, Hypertension, Withdrawal symptoms, Teratogenicity and Risk of malignancies.

Tolerance, Dependence and Withdrawal
After 6-8 hours of abruptly stopping alcohol in dependent subjects: Anxiety, Insomnia, Motor agitation, Reduced seizure threshold, Increased pulse rate, Increase in BP, Tremors. In severe cases convulsion & hallucinations.

Symptoms decrease over next 1-2 days

After several days of withdrawal Delirium tremens characterised by agitation, delirium, low grade fever and autonomic instability occurs.

Management
Detoxification treatment by substitution of alcohol with long acting BZDs (e.g., diazepam) → gradual reduction and tapering off of this substituent drug over several weeks.

Rehabilitation, psychosocial support Treatment of coexistent psychiatric conditions

Adjunctive therapy:
Naltrexone - μ opioid receptor antagonist, Disulfiram - aldehyde dehydrogenase inhibitor as **aversion agent**
Acamprosate - neuromodulator
Ondansetron, Topiramate, Baclofen, etc., aid in maintaining alcohol abstinence and controlling cravings

Methanol Poisoning
Due to spurious alcohol ingestion, accidental → Formaldehyde odour in breath, increased osmolar gap, anion gap, visual disturbance, bradycardia, seizures, acidosis resistant to correction, coma, respiratory failure and death

Treatment
- Supportive
- Suppression of methanol metabolism by alcohol dehydrogenase inhibitors **(Ethanol and Fomepizole)**.
- Metabolism of formate to CO_2 & H_2O is enhanced by **Calcium leucovorin**.
- **Hemodialysis** may be needed.

SECTION 3   Drugs Acting on CNS

21   Drugs of Abuse and CNS Stimulants

PH 3.9 Describe the drugs that are abused and cause addiction (dependence, addiction, stimulants, depressants, psychedelics, drugs used for criminal offences). Explain the process and steps of management of drug addiction.

Learning objectives

A student of MBBS phase II should be able to:
- Explain the concept of dependence and addiction.
- Classify and describe drugs of abuse as stimulants, depressants, psychedelics, etc.
- Describe prescription drug abuse.
- Describe drugs used for criminal offences.
- Describe the steps in process of drug de-addiction.
- Explain the mechanism of drug de-addiction using suitable examples.

DRUGS OF ABUSE

Terminology
Drug dependence and drug addiction are major health problems throughout world. Numerous overlapping terms have been used for this disorder such as drug/ substance misuse, abuse, habituation, dependence and addiction. Important terms related to substance abuse include the following.

Drug misuse
It involves the inappropriate or indiscriminate use of medications that are not classified as CNS stimulants or depressants, such as antibiotics, laxatives, and proton pump inhibitors.

Drug abuse
This term is used for misuse or **indiscriminate use of CNS stimulant or depressant drugs** for their euphoriant/ calming effects, e.g., opioid abuse. The term also includes the **use of drugs for non-medicinal purposes**, e.g., the use of anabolic steroids for body building.

Drug habituation
This refers to a pattern of drug use that may cause some degree of harm to the individual but does not significantly impact society. It typically involves a psychological desire for the substance without the development of tolerance, intense craving, or distressing withdrawal symptoms. Common examples include habitual consumption of tea or coffee, where the user desires the beverage but does not exhibit harmful or compulsive behaviour to obtain it. However, the term 'habituation' is better avoided, as it merely denotes a mild form of psychological dependence.

Tolerance
Chronic or repeated exposure to addictive drugs causes adaptive changes in the brain, resulting in the development of tolerance to drug effects. As a result, a higher dose is required to get the same effect. Hence, the dose of drug is increased progressively to maintain its effects. Development of tolerance may be considered as the root cause of physical dependence and repetitive drug use.

- Tolerance may not develop to all the actions of a drug, e.g., in the case of opioids, tolerance develops to their analgesic, euphoriant action but not to their constipating, miotic and convulsant actions.
- Numerous pharmacokinetic and/or pharmacodynamic mechanisms are responsible for the development of tolerance.
- Tolerance may or may not be present in psychological dependence, but it is invariably present in physical dependence.
- **Sensitisation** or reverse tolerance is the increased drug effect after repeated administration. It is seen with cocaine.
- **Cross-tolerance** is the development of tolerance to a drug being taken repeatedly/chronically, as well as to other related drugs. For example, tolerance to morphine due to it repeated use causes tolerance to other narcotic analgesics as well.

Addiction/ psychological dependence/ substance abuse
This refers to compulsive and repetitive drug use driven by **cravings**, leading to failure in fulfilling responsibilities, and the use of the substance in situations where it poses serious risks—such as while driving or operating heavy machinery.

- Addiction is a kind of **maladaptive learning**. The patient feels highly motivated to procure and use the drug despite being aware of the negative consequences of its use. In other words, **obtaining and consuming the drug takes precedence over all other considerations**.
- An addict exhibits '**compulsive drug use**' behaviour, i.e., wanting to use the drug without liking to use it.
- Addiction is stubbornly relapsing. **Relapse** is very common among addicts after successful completion of de-addiction (stage at which they are not dependent on the drug anymore). Many factor contribute to relapse of drug addiction, including stress, re-exposure to environments or situations that trigger memories of prior drug use, and renewed accessibility of the drug.
- Psychological dependence **usually develops before physical dependence.** Some drugs/substances show only psychological dependence, e.g., tea, coffee nicotine.

Drug dependence/physical dependence

Repetitive use of a drug causes a **physiological state that requires the continuous presence of the drug for normal functioning**. When the exposure to the drug is terminated or interrupted, **withdrawal reaction** of variable degree/severity manifests. Such a person is said to have developed physical dependence. Thus, presence of withdrawal syndrome on abstinence from the abused drug defines physical dependence. These **withdrawal symptoms are just the opposite of the pharmacological actions of drug**. For example, on abstaining from opioids (which have analgesic, antitussive and miotic effects), the withdrawal symptoms include pain, cough, and mydriasis. This is due to neuroadaptation, secondary to repeated exposure to addicting drug.

In addition to drugs, such dependence has been reported with substances such as **petrol, nail paint remover,** and **liquid petroleum**. So, the term used in the new Diagnostic and Statistical Manual of mental disorders (DSM) is '**substance dependence**', which includes dependence on drugs as well as other substances that do not fall in the category of drugs. The differences between drug addiction and drug dependence are tabulated in Box 21.1

Cross-dependence

This is the ability of a drug to suppress withdrawal symptoms caused by abstinence from another drug. For example, methadone can suppress the symptoms of morphine withdrawal. Such drugs are useful in de-addiction.

In ICD-10 criteria, **drug abuse** is defined as a broad term that includes "mental and behavioural disorders due to psychoactive substance use". It encompasses a variety of disorders associated with the use of one or more psychoactive substances, which may or may not have been medically prescribed. The severity may vary from uncomplicated intoxication and harmful use to obvious psychotic disorders and dementia.

Clinical problem-based questions and MCQs

1. i. Indiscriminate use of drugs other than CNS stimulants/depressants is called as:
   a. Drug abuse b. Drug misuse
   c. Drug resistance d. Drug tolerance
   ii. Give two examples of the term defined above.

2. The term 'drug abuse' includes all of the following EXCEPT
   a. Indiscriminate use of CNS stimulants for euphoriant action
   b. Indiscriminate use of CNS depressants for calming effect
   c. Use of anabolic steroids for body building
   d. Use of antibiotics for trivial viral infections.

Box 21.1 Differences between drug addiction and dependence

	Drug addiction	Drug dependence
Synonyms	Psychological dependence	Physical dependence
Definition	Compulsive repetitive use of the drug triggered by cravings	Presence of withdrawal symptoms on abstinence from the drug
Cause	Maladaptive learning, where obtaining and consuming drug takes precedence over all other activities	Neuroadaptation on repetitive use of drug causes a physiological state which requires continuous presence of drug for normal functioning.
Impact	Compulsive behaviour, where patient uses drug without liking to use it. Relapse is common.	Withdrawal symptoms may be very severe or life-threatening.
Examples	Only psychological dependence. Examples include tea, coffee, nicotine, cocaine	For substances such as opioids, alcohol and tetrahydrocannabinol, psychological dependence develops first, followed by physical dependence.

3. Which of the following drugs shows phenomenon of reverse tolerance?
   a. Morphine   b. Heroine
   c. Cocaine   d. Caffeine

4. Repeated exposure to addictive drugs is known to cause adaptive changes in the brain so that a higher dose is required to get the same effect. Identify the correct name of this phenomenon.
   a. Sensitisation   b. Tolerance
   c. Habituation   d. Resistance

5. A habitual user of diacetylmorphine, who is fully aware of his strained finances, expresses guilt and shame over his inability to provide even basic meals for his family. His wife reports that over the past three years he has repeatedly promised to stop using the drug, but each time he has relapsed, managing to procure and consume it again. Now, with no money left to buy the drug, he presents with complaints of intense abdominal pain and a persistent cough. On physical examination, his pupils are dilated, and multiple needle-prick marks are visible on his limbs.
   i. What is the cause of the patient's symptoms?
   ii. What is the term used for the phenomenon involved?

6. Differentiate between the two commonly used terms – drug addiction and drug dependence.

CLASSIFICATION OF DRUGS OF ABUSE

Drugs of abuse are classified based on their major central effects, mechanisms of mesolimbic dopaminergic activation, and dependence potential (Flowchart 21.1).

Depending upon Major Central Effects

Drugs of abuse can be stimulants or hallucinogens. In addition, alcohol as well as some prescribed drugs may also cause dependence and addiction. The pharmacology of these drug groups is briefly described below.

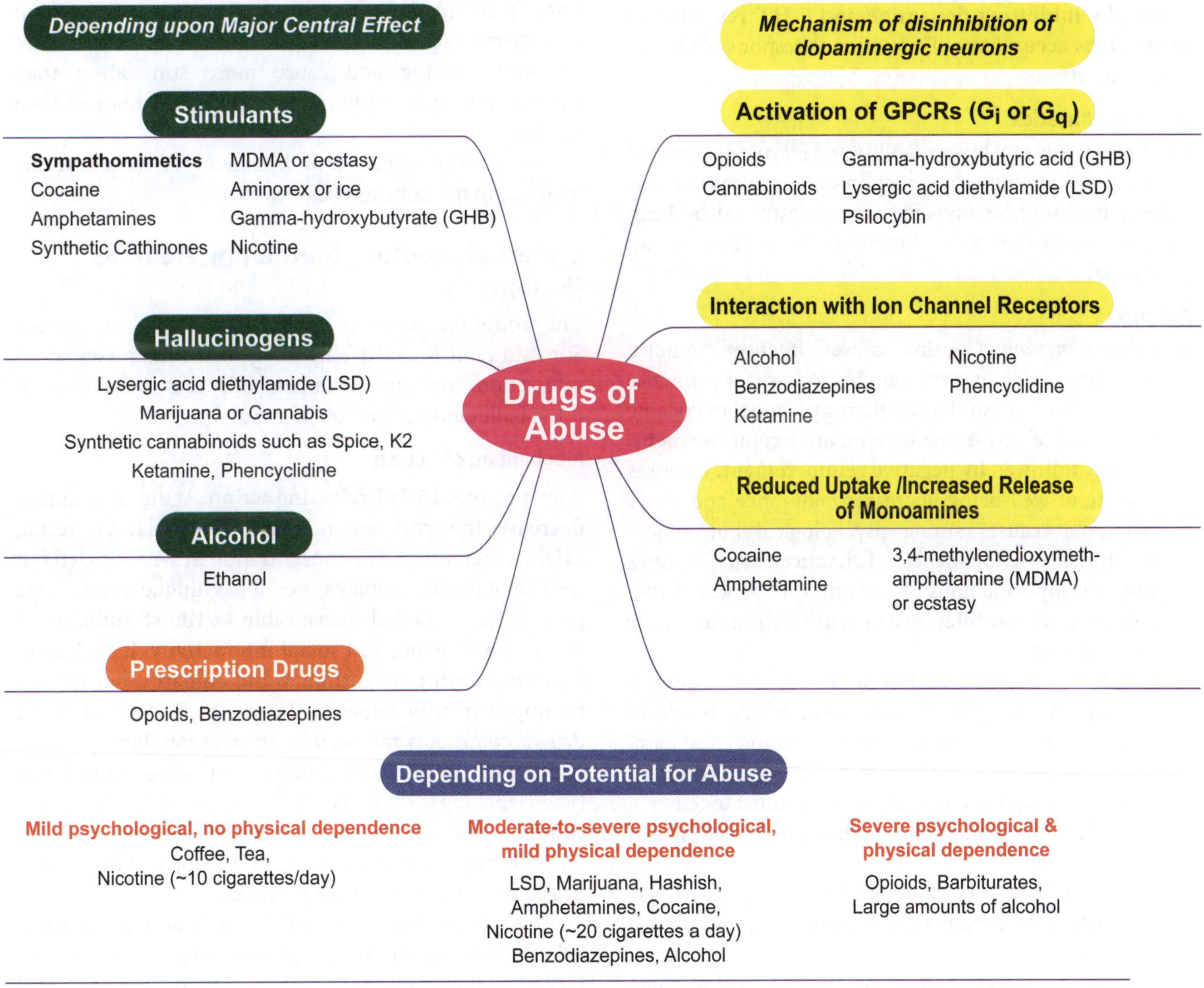

Depending upon Major Central Effect

Stimulants
- Sympathomimetics
- Cocaine
- Amphetamines
- Synthetic Cathinones
- MDMA or ecstasy
- Aminorex or ice
- Gamma-hydroxybutyrate (GHB)
- Nicotine

Hallucinogens
- Lysergic acid diethylamide (LSD)
- Marijuana or Cannabis
- Synthetic cannabinoids such as Spice, K2
- Ketamine, Phencyclidine

Alcohol
- Ethanol

Prescription Drugs
- Opoids, Benzodiazepines

Mechanism of disinhibition of dopaminergic neurons
- Opioids
- Cannabinoids

Activation of GPCRs (G_i or G_q)
- Gamma-hydroxybutyric acid (GHB)
- Lysergic acid diethylamide (LSD)
- Psilocybin

Interaction with Ion Channel Receptors
- Alcohol
- Benzodiazepines
- Ketamine
- Nicotine
- Phencyclidine

Reduced Uptake /Increased Release of Monoamines
- Cocaine
- Amphetamine
- 3,4-methylenedioxymeth-amphetamine (MDMA) or ecstasy

Depending on Potential for Abuse

- **Mild psychological, no physical dependence**: Coffee, Tea, Nicotine (~10 cigarettes/day)
- **Moderate-to-severe psychological, mild physical dependence**: LSD, Marijuana, Hashish, Amphetamines, Cocaine, Nicotine (~20 cigarettes a day) Benzodiazepines, Alcohol
- **Severe psychological & physical dependence**: Opioids, Barbiturates, Large amounts of alcohol

Flowchart 21.1 Classification of drugs of abuse

1. STIMULANTS

These include cocaine, amphetamines, MDMA or ecstasy, aminorex or ice, gamma-hydroxybutyric acid (GHB), synthetic cathinones, and nicotine. The potential to cause physical dependence is maximum with nicotine, followed by amphetamines, cocaine and caffeine, in that order, i.e., **physical dependence potential of nicotine> amphetamines ≥ cocaine > caffeine**.

Sympathomimetics produce a stimulant effect of fight or flight response and have a remarkable ability to produce pleasure.

a. Cocaine

Cocaine is obtained from the coca shrub (*Erythroxylum coca*).

Mechanism of action

It acts by inhibiting the reuptake of noradrenaline into adrenergic nerve endings, leading to increased synaptic noradrenaline levels, resulting in CNS stimulant effect. Cocaine possesses **profound ability to stimulate pleasure centre, by inhibiting dopamine and 5-HT reuptake in the nucleus accumbens.** This action is responsible for its rewarding effects.

Pharmacokinetics

Cocaine has low oral bioavailability and is typically snorted or injected, enabling rapid entry into the central nervous system. It cannot be smoked, as it is destroyed by heat; however, its alkaloid form, known as 'crack cocaine', can be smoked.

Actions

i. *Central action:* Cocaine causes intense euphoria or 'rush', which is very rapidly followed by intense dysphoria or 'crush'. The addicting potential of cocaine is because of this **immediate positive reinforcement, rapidly followed by negative reinforcement.** It causes a sense of well-being, increases endurance and allays fatigue. It causes strong psychological but almost nil physical dependence. **Tolerance usually does not develop** to actions of cocaine with repeated use. However, **reverse tolerance or sensitisation can occur** in some users.
ii. *Cardiac:* Cocaine blocks noradrenaline reuptake, causing **cardiac-stimulant actions**, which result in tachycardia, hypertension, arrhythmias and chest pain. The chest pain is due to vasoconstriction of coronary artery. If alcohol and cocaine are consumed together, a secondary metabolite, coca ethylene, is formed, which is cardiotoxic.
iii. *Peripheral nerves:* Cocaine inhibits voltage-gated Na^+ channels in the peripheral nerves and is a good surface anesthetic.
iv. *Pulmonary:* Effects of cocaine depend on the route of use, dose and frequency of use. Respiratory rate is increased. It may cause airway injury, bronchiolitis, asthma, pulmonary hypertension, edema and pulmonary hemorrhage.

Cocaine toxicity

Large doses cause agitation and convulsions because of its CNS stimulant action. Hyperthermia results due to stimulation of the temperature regulating centre, increased heat production and reduced heat dissipation. Psychiatric symptoms occur in cases of cocaine toxicity. Dyspnea, respiratory failure, coma and even death can occur.

Treatment

Treatment is mainly supportive.
- External cooling
- Benzodiazepines are useful to calm down the agitated patient, and control convulsions. Lorazepam is useful.
- Anticonvulsants are used to control convulsions.
- Antihypertensives to control raised blood pressure.

b. Amphetamines

They act by enhancing the release of biogenic amines from nerve terminals. As a result, the effects of amphetamines are longer-lasting and cause more stimulation than cocaine, but their euphoriant action is less marked than cocaine.

The clinical effects and treatment of amphetamine toxicity are the same as cocaine.

c. Methylenedioxy Methamphetamine (MDMA)

The common name of MDMA is molly or ecstasy. Sometimes, it is called 'empathogen', as it increases social interaction, communication, empathy and social oneness. It is a hallucinogenic amphetamine.

Mechanism of action

It has **profound 5-HT releasing action**. At the same time, it **decreases the synthesis** and reuptake of 5-HT. As a result, MDMA increases 5-HT concentration in synaptic cleft but depletes it in intracellular stores. It has unique serotonergic properties. Users feel **pleasurable tactile stimulation, a sense of well-being and social interactivity**. It appears to foster the **feelings of intimacy and empathy,** but there is no impairment of intellectual capacity. This effect of the drug is commonly **misused by sexual offenders**.

MDMA can cause bruxism (teeth grinding) and trismus (jaw clenching), which is why pacifiers and lollipops are commonly used by ravers to relieve jaw tension.

Withdrawal symptoms occur in the form of depression or aggression lasting for many weeks.

Acute toxic effects of MDMA include hyperthermia, dehydration, serotonin syndrome (marked by altered mental status), autonomic hyperactivity, seizures, and abnormal neuromuscular activity.

Management includes:
- Benzodiazepines to calm agitation and reduce seizures.
- Endotracheal intubation in severe cases to secure the airway.
- Neuromuscular blockers to control severe muscle rigidity.
- Cyproheptadine is useful to control serotonin syndrome. However, it is available only as oral preparation.

d. Aminorex (Ice)

It was introduced in medical practice for its anorexiant (appetite decreasing) action but was withdrawn because of reports of pulmonary hypertension.

The central actions of 'ice' resemble those of amphetamines. It has moderate potential to cause dependence.

e. Synthetic Cathinones

Drugs such as butylone, naphyrone, methcathinone and methylenedioxy pyrovalerone are commonly called **bath salts or pond water cleaner**, but they are snorted, ingested or even injected by addicts.

Similar to cocaine and amphetamines, these drugs **increase the release and reduce reuptake of catecholamines** noradrenaline, adrenaline, and dopamine. They exert rapid-onset, amphetamine-like stimulant and psychotomimetic action of variable duration. Treatment of toxicity is also the same as amphetamines. These are not easily detected in urine samples.

e. Gamma-Hydroxybutyric Acid (GHB)

GHB or sodium oxybate is endogenously produced during GABA metabolism. It was introduced as a general anesthetic but is not in use due to its narrow safety margin and addiction liability.

- It reduces daytime sleepiness and episodes of cataplexy.
- It causes euphoria, feeling of social intimacy/closeness, amnesia and increased sensory perceptions followed by sedation and coma.
- It is a popular 'club drug' commonly known by names such as liquid ecstasy and date rape drug, as it readily dissolves in beverages, is odourless and is used frequently in date rape.

f. Nicotine

Nicotine **addiction is more prevalent than all other addictions.** Smoking, chewing, and snuffing tobacco are the most common methods of consumption. Nicotine acts on nicotinic cholinergic receptors and **enhances cognitive performance.** Nicotinic receptors present on dopaminergic neurons mediate the rewarding effect of nicotine and are responsible for its addiction potential. Nicotine has maximum potential for causing physical dependence among stimulant drugs.

Withdrawal symptoms of nicotine are milder than opioids. Treatment of nicotine addiction is with nicotine itself, administered via chewing, inhalation or transdermal routes. Other drugs useful in the treatment of nicotine addiction are plant extract **cytosine, varenicline and bupropion** (see Chapter 7, page 96)

> **Clinical problem-based questions and MCQs**
>
> 7. i. CNS stimulants have the potential to produce physical dependence. Which of the following has maximum potential for physical dependence?
>   a. Caffeine b. Cocaine
>   c. Amphetamines d. Nicotine
>   i. Describe the mechanism of action and addiction with drug selected in part (i) of question.
>   ii. Name the drugs used for de-addiction from the drug selected.
>
> 8. i. Identify the drug causing immediate positive reinforcement followed by negative reinforcement.
>   a. Nicotine b. Alcohol
>   c. Cocaine d. Morphine
>   ii. Describe features of toxicity of the selected drug and its management.
>
> 9. Match the common name used by drug addicts with pharmacological name of the drug
>   a. Ecstasy   1. Cathinones
>   b. Ice   2. MDMA
>   c. Bath salts   3. Aminorex
>
> 10. MDMA is commonly misused by sexual offenders. What effects of drug favour such misuse. Describe the mechanism of action involved.
>
> 11. i. Identify the popular club drug misused as 'date rape drug'.
>   a. Nicotine
>   b. Cocaine
>   c. Heroine
>   d. Gamma-hydroxybutyric acid
>   ii. Explain the cause of such misuse.

2. HALLUCINOGENS

These include lysergic acid diethylamide (LSD), mescaline, psilocybin, marijuana (*bhang, ganja, charas*), ketamine, phencyclidine, and synthetic cannabinoids such as spike and K2.

a. LSD, Mescaline, Psilocybin

LSD is a partial agonist at $5\text{-}HT_{2A}$ receptors. It produces **psychedelic actions** such as

- Colourful hallucinations
- Mood alterations
- Sleep disturbances
- Anxiety (may occur)

Repetitive exposure causes down-regulation of receptors, leading to the development of rapid tolerance, i.e., **tachyphylaxis**. But **they do not cause dependence or addiction**.

Adverse reactions

LSD has minimal physical effects. It may cause sweating, anorexia, mydriasis, tachycardia, hypertension and hyperthermia. It can cause dizziness, impaired reasoning and loss of judgment. Sometimes, it produces panic state that may lead to trauma as well. Such an episode is named 'bad trip'.

N-BOMe

Commonly known as N-bomb or Smiles, this group of serotonin agonists is often used as a substitute for LSD. They are typically administered in liquid form or absorbed through blotting paper. These can also cause hypertension, seizures and trauma that may be fatal.

b. Marijuana

Marijuana is obtained from the cannabis plant.

- Leaves of *cannabis indica* plant consumed orally are known as ***bhang***.
- Dried resinous extract of leaves and flowering tips smoked with tobacco is known as ***charas***.
- Dried female inflorescence is also smoked. It is known as ***ganja***.

Cannabis sativa is used for psychoactive properties. Among new users, marijuana is the most- frequently used drug. The most important active ingredient in *bhang*, *charas* and *ganja* is **tetrahydrocannabinol (THC)**. It binds to cannabinoid (CB_1) receptors in the brain, and causes physical relaxation, pain relief, conjunctivitis, increases appetite/sensory activity/heart rate, and impairs muscle coordination and skilled motor activity.

Psychological effects **include euphoria followed by drowsiness and relaxed mind and mild hallucinations; short-term memory decreases.** Long-term use causes down-regulation of CB_1 receptors and the patient feels boredom in the absence of drug. **Tolerance and dependence occur.** Withdrawal symptoms of the drug occur in the form of cravings, pain, irritability, insomnia and depression.

Prescription forms of marijuana include nabiximols, nabilone, and dronabinol. These are used as adjuvant therapies for conditions such as chemotherapy-induced nausea and vomiting (CINV), cancer- and AIDS-related cachexia, chronic pain, and multiple sclerosis, among others.

c. Synthetic Cannabinoids

Synthetic cannabinoids such as **Spike** and **K2** are smoked after spraying (dusting) them on plant material. The users of these dustings do not test positive for THC. The effects of spike and K2 are sympathomimetic, i.e., tachycardia, hypertension, extreme hallucinations and psychotic reactions. They can cause convulsions, acute renal injury and even death.

d. Ketamine and Phencyclidine

Both of these drugs were originally introduced as general anesthetics. Ketamine continues to be used for "dissociative anesthesia." Like phencyclidine (PCP), it is also abused as a "club drug" under street names such as **special K, hog,** and **angel dust**.

These substances act as use-dependent competitive antagonists of glutamate at NMDA receptors. Their use can lead to **psychedelic effects, hallucinations,** and **vivid dreams**—particularly during the recovery phase from ketamine anesthesia, known as the **emergence reaction**. Other effects include elevated blood pressure, memory impairment, and visual disturbances.

Abuse routes include oral ingestion, injection, smoking, and snorting. At high doses, users may experience distressing phenomena such as 'out-of-body' sensations or 'near-death' experiences. Although these drugs do not cause **physical dependence or addiction**, prolonged use can induce a psychotic state resembling schizophrenia.

3. ALCOHOL

The most common way in which alcohol is consumed is as a drink, but aerosolised ethanol can also be inhaled.

Mechanism of Action

Alcohol acts by enhancing the effects of inhibitory neurotransmitter GABA, increasing the release of endogenous opioids and altering the levels of dopamine and serotonin.

In habitual drinkers, **tolerance occurs** due to induction of hepatic drug metabolising enzymes, so that more of alcohol is converted to acetaldehyde, leading to tolerance. The acetaldehyde thus formed causes **organ damage** on chronic exposure. Chronic alcoholism or abuse causes cardiovascular, hepatic, pulmonary, hematological, central metabolic and endocrine abnormalities.

In contrast, **hepatic enzymes are inhibited by acute intake** of substantial amount of alcohol, known as binge drinking, and acute toxicity occurs in the form of general CNS depression, respiratory depression and coma. Treatment of acute toxicity is supportive and symptomatic. If levels are very high, dialysis may be needed. Thiamine and folate are also administered.

Dependence develops to alcohol. Abstinence for 6–8 hours leads to the precipitation of withdrawal symptoms such as anxiety, tremors, agitation, tachycardia and sweating. Later, at about 72 hours of abstinence, acute psychotic attack called delirium tremens, hallucinations and even convulsions occur, which may be life-threatening.

Treatment of Addiction

Treatment is symptomatic and supportive. For short-term control of symptoms, benzodiazepines are used. In long term, disulfiram is used to control alcohol addiction.

- **Disulfiram** inhibits enzyme aldehyde dehydrogenase resulting in accumulation of acetaldehyde, which causes disturbing symptoms such as flushing, sweating, hyperventilation, nausea, vomiting, chest pain, dyspnea, tachycardia and hypotension within 5 minutes of alcohol intake. Such unpleasant experience after drinking leads to conditioned avoidance response. In some patients, disulfiram reaction can be very severe, causing convulsions and circulatory collapse. So **disulfiram aversion therapy in alcoholism should always be done in hospital setting.**
- Drugs such as metronidazole, chlorpropamide, cefamandole, procarbazine and griseofulvin can also cause disulfiram-like reactions. Hence, patients on these drugs are warned not to take alcohol.
- **Naltrexone**, when **combined with psychotherapy**, can help reduce cravings for alcohol. Similarly, **acamprosate** also lowers alcohol craving by normalising the neurobiological disturbances caused by chronic alcohol consumption. It serves as a prototype for the neuromodulatory approach in the management of alcohol dependence.

4. PRESCRIPTION DRUGS ABUSE

a. Benzodiazepine

Benzodiazepines are the most commonly used drugs among sedative hypnotics. They are abused for their euphoriant action and ability to check anxiety associated with opioid withdrawal. Barbiturates, though not much in clinical use nowadays, continue to be abused.

Benzodiazepine dependence **is very common**. Withdrawal reaction occurs after a few days of abstaining from the drug in the form of irritability, photophobia, phonophobia, insomnia, muscle cramps, and even seizures and depression. The symptoms may last from few days to several months depending on:

- The particular drug abused, its half-life, etc.
- Dosage, route of administration
- Duration of abuse
- Other concurrent drug abuse
- Other underlying medical or mental disorders.

Severe benzodiazepine withdrawal symptoms may be controlled by phenobarbitone, trazodone (an antidepressant with sedative action), carbamazepine (for control of convulsions) and β blockers (for patients with autonomic symptoms such as tachycardia and hypertension).

b. Opioids

Opioids are also one of the commonly abused prescription drugs. They are highly addictive. Morphine, heroin (diacetyl morphine), codeine, oxycodone, meperidine, etc., are commonly abused opioids. All these drugs have addicting potential as they inhibit GABAergic interneurons, resulting in disinhibition of dopamine neurons.

These drugs have strong tolerance and dependence, inducing potential. Withdrawal symptoms are very severe, such as nausea, vomiting, diarrhea, intense dysphoria, rhinorrhea, lacrimation, mydriasis, yawning, fever, sweating and piloerection.

In case of acute toxicity, opioid antagonist **naloxone** is life-saving, but it can precipitate acute withdrawal syndrome in addicts. De-addiction is by **substitution therapy** with a long-acting opioid such as methadone, administered orally once a day. Buprenorphine is a partial agonist and have some beneficial effects. Withdrawal syndrome of methadone is less dramatic and less severe.

c. Inhalants

Drug abuse by inhalation involves the deliberate breathing in of chemical vapors such as ketones, nitrates, and aromatic hydrocarbons such as benzene and toluene. This is typically done through methods such as sniffing, huffing, or bagging:

- Sniffing involves inhaling the substance directly from an open container.
- Huffing entails soaking a cloth in the volatile substance and inhaling the vapours from it.
- Bagging uses a plastic or paper bag filled with the inhalant fumes, which is then held to the face for inhalation.

Most inhalants produce euphoria. Nitrates cause smooth muscle relaxation and erectile response. Treatment of overdose is only supportive.

DRUG DE-ADDICTION

In spite of the enormous research in the field of de-addiction, the outcome is far from satisfactory, as there are no pharmacological agents available that can completely overcome addiction. The **aim of treatment** in drug addiction is to

- Achieve a drug-free status with pharmacotherapy.
- Prevent the relapse of drug abuse with rehabilitative and psychosocial interventions.

Pharmacotherapy

Drug treatment to obtain a drug-free status in addicts involves the following strategies.

1. Detoxification
This is achieved in the following ways:

a. Substitution therapy
This involves substitution of the abused drug with a similar drug having longer a half-life, e.g., methadone substitution therapy for **morphine and heroin addicts. Methadone** is an agonist at opioid receptors. Its duration of action is longer than morphine, and it is effective by the oral route. In absence of morphine, methadone keeps on occupying opioid receptors for a longer time. Thus, distressing morphine withdrawal symptoms are prevented. Slowly, the dose of methadone is tapered off over a few weeks and then discontinued. Withdrawal symptoms of methadone are less intense and are delayed. Other alternatives for substitution therapy in opioid addicts are **buprenorphine** and **levo-α acetylmethadol (LAAM).** The severity of opioid withdrawal symptoms can be checked by clonidine and lofexidine as well.

In alcohol abuse, diazepam or chlordiazepoxide can be used for substitution therapy. Care should be taken to maintain fluid electrolyte balance and to prevent nutritional deficiencies.

b. Weaning-off
Weaning-off is the process of gradual reduction in dose of the abused drug in such a way that withdrawal symptoms are very mild or do not occur at all. This may take a longer time.

2. Prevention of relapse
This is achievable with:

a. **Antagonism of the abused drug:** Once the patient is detoxified and is opioid-free for at least 10 days, **naltrexone,** an opioid antagonist, is given orally in a dose of 100–150 mg thrice a week to prevent relapse. Naltrexone occupies opioid receptor, but has no effects of its own. As the receptors are occupied, the pleasurable effects of opioids are not experienced when a person, after de-addiction, restarts taking the abused drug due to cravings. In other words, the abused drug no longer gives the patient the desirable central effects, leading to getting rid of the habit. But care should be taken to complete the detoxification process and make the patient drug free, because naltrexone use in opioid-dependent patients can precipitate intense withdrawal symptoms. **Naltrexone and acamprosate** are useful in alcohol addicts to prevent relapse.

b. **Methadone maintenance therapy** can lead to such a high level of opioid tolerance that subsequent administration of morphine may not produce its desirable central effects.

c. Aversion therapy
This involves the administration of a drug that produces disturbing and unpleasant symptoms when given with the abused drug, e.g., disulfiram in alcohol addicts. The patient receiving disulfiram therapy suffers from disturbing aldehyde syndrome on consuming alcohol. This causes an aversion to alcohol.

d. Use of drugs to reduce craving
An example of this strategy is the use of **baclofen,** which can reduce cravings by inhibiting dopaminergic neurons in the reward region. Likewise, varenicline aids in smoking cessation by reducing cravings.

e. Rehabilitative and psychological and social interventions
Such measures must also be applied at the same time as pharmacotherapy to increase the social acceptability of the treated addict and to prevent relapse. Psychological counselling of the patient along with family and friends is important for motivating and supporting the patient to maintain a drug-free status. This will also help in preventing circumstances that contributed to drug addiction in the first place. Counselling is done over several sessions.

Clinical problem-based questions and MCQs

12. i. Which of the following psychedelic drugs has the potential to cause tolerance, addiction, dependence?
    a. Marijuana   b. LSD
    c. Ketamine   d. Phencyclidine
    ii. What are the prescription forms of marijuana and their therapeutic uses?

13. A 35-year-old chronic alcoholic has developed early signs of alcoholic liver disease and sincerely wishes to quit drinking. He is hospitalised for disulfiram aversion therapy.
    i. Describe the pharmacological basis of the therapy in alcohol de-addiction.
    ii. Why it is necessary to hospitalise this patient?
    iii. Identify the drug useful for decreasing alcohol craving
       a. Acamprosate   b. Varenicline
       c. Bupropion   d. Diazepam

14. A 16-year-old boy began snorting heroin for the first time under peer pressure. Initially used occasionally, he soon developed a strong craving for the drug. As his use continued, his academic performance declined. Despite repeated warnings and efforts by his concerned parents to help him quit, he struggled with withdrawal symptoms—including excessive sweating, yawning, goosebumps, abdominal pain, and diarrhea—each

time he attempted to stop, leading him to resume drug use.
  i. What does the history of the boy reflect?
  ii. Explain the cause of development of the symptoms on abstaining from drug.
  iii. Explain the mechanism of development of dependence on drug.

15. The boy mentioned in the above case developed difficulty in breathing after heavy consumption of the drug at a friend's rave party and was admitted to critical care in a stuporous condition. He had cyanosis, pinpoint pupils, shallow breathing and his BP was 94/60. He was given treatment immediately. When he gained consciousness and the acute episode was controlled, he recalled with fear his recent experience and expressed keen desire to quit the habit. He was referred to the drug de-addiction centre.
  i. What was the cause of this patient's acute symptoms?
  ii. What drugs would have been used to control these symptoms?
  iii. What would be a long-term management plan for this patient to help him quit the habit successfully? Describe the steps of the de-addiction process.

CNS STIMULANTS

CNS stimulants are drugs that can cause global stimulation of the central nervous system and improve functions of the brain. These include:

1. **Convulsants** such as picrotoxin, strychnine, bicuculline and pentylenetetrazol (PTZ).
2. **Psychostimulants** such as amphetamines, atomoxetine, modafinil, armodafinil, methylphenidate, cocaine and caffeine.
3. **Analeptics** like doxapram.

Convulsants

These are the drugs used for producing convulsions. They are **useful only for drug testing or for their toxicological importance**. There is no clinical utility of this group of drugs.

- **Strychnine**: Strychnine acts by **inhibiting the effect of glycine** (inhibitory NTM) at post-synaptic receptors and causes **tonic–clonic symmetrical type of convulsions**. Strychnine poisoning is managed in the same way as status epilepticus, with intravenous diazepam, phenytoin, etc.
- **Picrotoxin:** It acts by **inhibiting the effect of GABA** and causes **asymmetrical tonic–clonic convulsions**. Toxicity of picrotoxin can be managed by benzodiazepines e.g., diazepam
- **Bicuculline** also antagonises effect of GABA at the GABA receptor–Cl$^-$ channel complex.
- **Pentylenetetrazol** also acts by interfering with GABA-mediated inhibitory effects. PTZ-induced seizure is **used for testing antiepileptic drugs in experimental animals.**

Psychostimulants

Psychostimulants include drugs such as amphetamines, methylphenidate, atomoxetine, modafinil, armodafinil, cocaine and caffeine.

Amphetamine, dexamphetamine and methamphetamine are sympathomimetics useful in narcolepsy, attention-deficit disorder, etc. (refer to Chapter 9, page 120).

- **Methylphenidate**, like **amphetamines**, promotes the release of the neurotransmitters noradrenaline and dopamine. Methylphenidate is commonly used to treat attention deficit hyperactivity disorder (ADHD) in hyperactive children. It is also used in the management of narcolepsy and attention deficits in adults.

  Adverse effects such as anxiety, sleep disturbance, insomnia, anorexia, bowel upset and growth retardation in children are due to CNS stimulant action. It has no role in elevating mood in patients with depression.

- **Atomoxetine** acts by **inhibiting reuptake only of nor adrenaline**. It is useful for increasing the attention span in hyperkinetic children as well as adults. Important adverse effects of atomoxetine are anorexia, gastrointestinal symptoms, mood swings, growth retardation, etc.

- **Modafinil** is a new drug that reduces reuptake of dopamine. Noradrenaline, glutamate and serotonin concentrations are increased in certain regions of the brain, while GABAergic transmission is reduced. It is used to control daytime sleepiness in **narcolepsy, sleep apnea syndrome** and **shift workers.** It may cause nausea, dyspepsia, headache, insomnia, amnesia, confusion and tremors as adverse effects.

- **Cocaine** is a drug of abuse (see page 287).

- **Caffeine** is a methylxanthine like theophylline. It is used to **allay boredom and fatigue** in the form of a beverage. As a drug, it is useful in **headache, migraine** and **apnea** in infants. Adverse effects of caffeine are mainly gastrointestinal (nausea, vomiting) and central (nervousness, anxiety, insomnia, restlessness and agitation). Heart rate is increased and ectopic beats may occur.

ANALEPTICS

Analeptics such as **doxapram** cause **respiratory stimulation in lower dose and convulsions in higher dose**. In cases of poisoning with CNS depressants, doxapram may be **used as expedient measure to stimulate respiration**. However, because of its low therapeutic index, supportive treatment is preferred to doxapram. Analeptics are not used in clinical practice as well.

COGNITION ENHANCERS

These drugs are called **cerebroactive** or **nootropic drugs** and are **useful in dementia** for short-term effects. Drugs such as **rivastigmine, donepezil, galantine** and **memantine** used in Alzheimer disease are cognition enhancers (refer to Chapter 7, page 99) Others include ginkgo biloba, piracetam, pyritinol, piribedil, citicoline, dihydroergotoxine.

- Piracetam is used for **dementia** in ageing people and **mental retardation** in children, but its benefits are not well documented.
- **Dihydroergotoxine** and **citicoline** are drugs that increase cerebral blood flow and are helpful in dementia. Citicoline improves cerebral blood flow and increases cerebral metabolism. It is **used in head injury and stroke to improve impaired brain function.**
- **Ginkgo biloba**, obtained from a tree native to East Asia, has an action antagonistic to that of platelet activating factor (PAF). It is claimed to be useful in **preventing cerebrovascular insufficiency** as it can check PAF-induced thrombosis and infarction. It improves cognitive performance.
- **Piribedil** improves **memory and concentration** through its dopamine agonistic effect.
- **Pyritinol** increases glucose transport across the blood–brain barrier. It is used in **children with delayed milestones** and in people with **senile changes** and **memory loss**, but its beneficial effect is not well documented.

Clinical problem-based questions and MCQs

16. The drugs inhibiting the effect of inhibitory NTMs produce convulsions. All of the following drugs inhibit GABA EXCEPT
    a. Strychnine b. Pentylenetetrazol
    c. Picrotoxin d. Bicuculline

17. Identify the convulsant drug used to induce seizures in experimental animals for testing the effect of antiepileptic agents.
    a. Strychnine b. Pentylenetetrazol
    c. Picrotoxin d. Bicuculline

18. i. Identify the drug useful in hyperkinetic children with attention deficit disorder.
    a. Picrotoxin b. Methylphenidate
    c. Piracetam d. Donepezil
    ii. Describe the mechanism of action and adverse effects of the selected drug.

19. i. Identify the nootropic drug amongst the following:
    a. Atomoxetine b. Citicoline
    c. Doxapram d. Modafinil
    ii. Describe the mechanism of action and indication for using the selected drug.

20. Identify the CNS stimulant having abuse potential from the following:
    a. Donepezil b. Citicoline
    c. Amphetamines d. Doxapram

Summary

Drugs of abuse

- Indiscriminate use of CNS stimulant/depressant drugs for their euphoriant/calming effect is termed as drug abuse, while that for drugs other than CNS stimulants/depressants is called drug misuse.
- Tolerance is the decreased drug response with repeated use due to numerous pharmacokinetic or dynamic factors. Tolerance does not necessarily develop to all actions of a drug. Cross-tolerance exists between related drugs. Reverse tolerance is shown by cocaine.
- Addiction is maladaptive learning causing compulsive drug use derived by craving. Many of the drugs show psychological dependence only.
- Physical dependence is the altered physiological state requiring continuous presence of a drug for proper functioning. Drug withdrawal causes symptoms opposite to the drug effects.
- Drugs of abuse can be stimulants, hallucinogens, alcohol or prescription drugs.
- **CNS stimulants**, the physical dependence potential is maximum with nicotine, followed by amphetamines, cocaine and caffeine in that order.
- Cocaine causes increased adrenergic and serotonergic activity, resulting in rush and crush effect, central and cardiac stimulant actions, raised respiratory rate, airway injury, bronchiolitis, asthma, pulmonary hypertension, edema and pulmonary hemorrhage. Cocaine is usually snorted or injected; crack cocaine is smoked.
- MDMA, also called molly/ecstasy, increases 5-HT release, decreases reuptake but does not increase synthesis. So, it increases concentration in cleft but depletes intracellular stores. It causes pleasurable tactile stimulation, a sense of well-being, social interactivity, feelings of intimacy and empathy and is hence commonly misused by sexual offenders. MDMA can cause bruxism, so lollipops and pacifiers are popular among the ravers.
- Aminorex (ice), synthetic cathinones such as butylone, naphyrone, methcathinone and methylenedioxypyrovalerone (bath salts) exert amphetamine-like actions of variable duration.
- γ-hydroxybutyric acid (GHB), a popular 'club drug' known as liquid ecstasy or the date rape drug, is odourless and readily dissolves in beverages.
- In addition, modafinil, atomoxetine and methylphenidate are CNS stimulants, useful in attention-deficit disorder, narcolepsy, sleep apnea, etc.
- Other CNS stimulants include convulsants, analeptics and cognition enhancers.
- Convulsants such as strychnine, pentylenetetrazol, picrotoxin, bicuculline are used only in drug testing/have toxicological importance.

- Analeptics also not much used clinically; doxapram may be used as an expedient measure to stimulate respiration in toxicity with CNS depressant drugs.
- Cognition enhancers such as rivastigmine, donepezil, galantine and memantine used in Alzheimer's disease. Piracetam is used for dementia and mental retardation. Dihydroergotoxine and citicoline are used in dementia, head injury, stroke, etc. Ginkgo biloba, Piribedil and pyritinol are some of the other examples.
- **Hallucinogen** Lysergic acid diethylamide (LSD), a partial agonist at 5-HT$_{2A}$ receptors, causes colourful hallucinations, mood alterations, sleep disturbances and anxiety. Tolerance develops quickly, but no dependence occurs.
- Tetrahydrocannabinols (THC) **present in marijuana**, *charas, ganja* and *bhang* cause euphoria followed by drowsiness, mind relaxation, mild hallucination and decreased short-term memory. Addiction and dependence occur. Examples of synthetic cannabinoids are spike, K2, etc.
- Ketamine and phencyclidine abused under names like 'hog' 'special K' and 'angel dust', cause use-dependent competitive antagonism of glutamate actions at NMDA receptors, leading to psychedelic effects, hallucinations and vivid dreams as an emergence reaction.
- **Alcohol** dependence is very common. Disulfiram aversion therapy, naltrexone and acamprosate are used for reducing craving.
- Bupropion, varenicline and nicotine are useful for reducing nicotine cravings and **cessation of smoking**.
- **Prescription drugs** abused commonly include benzodiazepines and opioids.
- **Drug de-addiction** involves reducing the use of abused drug and prevention of relapse. Drug substitution therapy, maintenance therapy, aversion therapy and psychotherapy are the mainstay of de-addiction programme.

Questions for practice

1. Describe
   a. Prescription drug abuse
   b. Drugs for criminal offences
2. Describe aims of de-addiction therapy and drugs used for de-addiction.
3. Describe substitution therapy and aversion therapy in de-addiction with suitable examples.
4. Write short notes on
   a. Tetrahydrocannabinoids
   b. Cocaine
   c. MDMA

Hints for problem-based questions and MCQs

1. i. b. Drug misuse
   ii. Misuse of antibiotics, laxatives
2. d. Use of antibiotics for trivial viral infections. It is called as drug misuse, not abuse.
3. c. Cocaine.
4. b. Tolerance
5. i. Withdrawal symptoms
   ii. Drug dependence
6. Refer to page 286
7. i. d. Nicotine
   ii. Improves cognitive performance by acting on cholinergic nicotinic receptors. Addiction is through reward action on dopaminergic neurons. Refer to Chapter 7, page 96.
   iii. Nicotine, varenicline, bupropion
8. i. c. Cocaine.
   ii. Cocaine toxicity causes agitation, convulsions, psychiatric symptoms and hyperthermia. In severe cases, dyspnea, respiratory failure, coma and death may occur. Treatment includes external cooling to lower the body temperature, lorazepam for calming down the patient and controlling convulsions. Anti-hypertensive drugs are also needed.
9. a–2 b–3 c–1
10. MDMA causes 5-HT release but reduces its synthesis and reuptake. It is misused by sexual offenders due to its ability to induce a sense of well-being, enhance social interactivity, heighten pleasurable tactile stimulation, and foster feelings of empathy and intimacy. Refer to page 288.
11. i. d. Gamma-hydroxybutyric acid
    ii. As it easily dissolves in beverages, is colorless, odourless.
12. i. a. Marijuana (*bhang, charas, ganja*, etc., causes psychedelic effects, addiction, tolerance and dependence)
    ii. Prescription forms of marijuana include nabiximols, nabilone, and dronabinol. These are useful as adjuvants in CINV, cancer/AIDS cachexia, chronic pain and multiple sclerosis. Refer to page 290.
13. i. Inhibition of aldehyde dehydrogenase by disulfiram leads to disturbing symptoms causing aversion.
    ii. Risk of convulsions, circulatory collapse in some cases of disulfiram reaction.
    iii. a. Acamprosate
14. i. Opioid addiction and dependence
    ii. Withdrawal symptoms due to physical dependence
    iii. Opioids have addicting potential as they inhibit GABAergic interneurons resulting in disinhibition of dopamine neurons. Refer to page 291.
15. i. Acute opioid toxicity
    ii. Naloxone
    iii. Methadone substitution therapy, maintenance therapy, psychotherapy, social support, etc. Refer to page 291.
16. a. Strychnine (inhibits glycine, not GABA)
17. b. Pentylenetetrazol
18. i. b. Methylphenidate
    ii. Methylphenidate increases the release of NTMs noradrenaline and dopamine. Adverse effects include anxiety, insomnia, anorexia, growth retardation and bowel disturbances. Refer to page 293.
19. i. b. Citicoline
    ii. Citicoline increases cerebral blood flow and cerebral metabolism and is useful in head injury and stroke for improving brain functions.
20. c. Amphetamines

CONCEPT MAP - DRUGS OF ABUSE

Terms
- **Tolerance**: Decreased drug response with repeated use due to numerous pharmacokinetic or dynamic factors, not necessarily for all actions of drugs, however.
- **Cross-tolerance** exists between related drugs.
- **Addiction** is maladaptive learning causing compulsive drug use derived by craving → psychological dependence.
- **Physical dependence** is altered physiological state requiring continuous presence of drug for proper functioning. Abstinence causes withdrawal symptoms opposite to the drug effects.

Drug De-addiction
- Reducing the use of abused drug
- Prevention of relapse
- Drug substitution therapy
- Maintenance therapy
- Aversion therapy
- Psychotherapy

MDMA (Molly/Ecstasy)
- Increases 5-HT release, decreases reuptake, but does not increase synthesis.
- Pleasurable tactile stimulation, sense of well-being, social interactivity, feelings of intimacy & empathy
- Misused by sexual offenders.
- Can cause bruxism → so lollipops and pacifiers popular among ravers.
- **Toxicity**: Hyperthermia, Dehydration, Serotonin syndrome
- **Treatment**: BZDs, NMJ blockers, Cyproheptadine.

Aminorex (Ice)
Moderate potential for dependence

Synthetic cathinones (Bath salts)
Amphetamine like central actions
Not detected in urine sample.

Gamma-hydroxybutyric Acid (GHB)
- 'Club drug', Liquid ecstasy, Date rape drug,
- Odourless, readily gets dissolved in beverages
- Causes euphoria, feeling of social intimacy / closeness, amnesia and increased sensory perceptions.

Nicotine
- Tobacco smoked, chewed & snuffed
- Enhances cognitive performance
- Most addicting, rewarding action
- Withdrawal symptoms milder than opioids.

Treatment of nicotine addiction
- Nicotine itself given by chewing, inhalation or trans-dermal routes.
- Cytosine, Varenicline and Bupropion

Cocaine
- Snorted/injected. Crack cocaine smoked
- Increased adrenergic, serotonergic activity
- Rush and crush effect
- Stimulate pleasure center in nucleus accumbens → rewarding action → Strong psychological dependence.
- No tolerance, No physical dependence. May show reverse tolerance.
- Raised HR, BP, Arrhythmias, Coronary vasospasm Raised RR, Airway injury, Bronchiolitis, Asthma, Pulmonary hypertension, Pulmonary hemorrhage.
- **Toxicity**: Agitation, Convulsions, Hyperthermia, Respiratory failure, Coma
- **Treatment**: Supportive, Lorazepam, Antihypertensives

Stimulants
Physical dependence potential
Nicotine > Amphetamines > Cocaine > Caffeine

DRUGS OF ABUSE

Tetrahydrocannabinol (THC)
- Present in marijuana, charas, ganja, bhang
- Cause relaxation of mind & body, increased appetite, conjunctivitis, pain control, enhanced sensory activity, euphoria, drowsiness, hallucinations,
- Short-term memory decreases. Muscle coordination and skilled motor activity reduced.
- Addiction and dependence occurs.

Synthetic Cannabinoids
- Spike, K2
- Smoked after spraying (dusting) on plant material.
- Users don't test positive for THC.
- Sympathomimetic effects: Tachycardia, Hypertension, Extreme hallucinations, Psychotic reactions.
- **Overdose**: Convulsions, Renal damage, Death

Hallucinogens

LSD
- Partial agonist at 5-HT$_{2A}$ receptors
- Causes colourful hallucinations, mood alterations, sleep disturbances and anxiety.
- Quick tolerance but no dependence
- N-bomb/ smiles - serotonin agonists used in liquid form/blotting paper for substituting LSD.

Ketamine & Phencyclidine
- 'Hog' 'special K' , 'angel dust'
- Causes use-dependent, competitive antagonism at NMDA receptors
- Psychedelic effects, hallucinations and vivid dreams as emergence reaction

Prescription Drugs Abuse

Benzodiazepines
- Euphoriant, check anxiety of opioid withdrawal.
- Dependence common, withdrawal reactions like irritability, photophobia, phonophobia, insomnia, muscle cramps, seizures and depression after few days of abstinence.
- **Treatment**: Phenobarbitone, Trazodone, Carbamazepine, β blockers

Opioids: Highly addictive
- Morphine, Heroin, Codeine, Oxycodone, Meperidine commonly abused.
- Inhibits GABAergic interneurons → Disinhibition of dopamine neurons → Rewarding action.
- Strong tolerance & dependence inducing potential. Withdrawal symptoms very severe, such as: Nausea, Vomiting, Diarrhea, Dysphoria, Rhinorrhea, Lacrimation, Mydriasis, Yawning, Fever, Sweating, Piloerection.
- **De-addiction** is by substitution therapy with Methadone, Buprenorphine.
- **Acute toxicity**: Opioid antagonist naloxone

SECTION 3   Drugs Acting on CNS

22   Opioid Analgesics and Antagonists

PH 3.4 Describe types, salient pharmacokinetics, pharmacodynamics, therapeutic uses, adverse drug reactions of opioid analgesics and explain the special instructions for use of opioids.

Learning objectives

A student of MBBS phase II should be able to:
- Classify opioid analgesics.
- Describe the mechanism of action of opioids.
- Enumerate therapeutic uses of opioid analgesics and mention doses.
- Enumerate adverse effects and contraindications of opioid analgesics.
- Describe the management of opioid poisoning, opioid dependence and withdrawal.
- Enumerate opioid antagonists.
- Describe therapeutic uses and adverse effects of opioid antagonists.
- Describe endogenous opioid peptides.

OPIOIDS

Algesia or **pain** is the most common symptom evoked by many external or internal noxious stimuli. Drugs that relieve pain selectively without significantly affecting consciousness are called **analgesics**. Analgesics are broadly divided into 2 types.

1. Non-narcotic/Non-opioid/Non-steroidal anti inflammatory drugs (NSAIDs)
2. Narcotic/opioids

CLASSIFICATION OF OPIOIDS

Opioid analgesics is a broad term that includes many natural, semisynthetic and synthetic drugs, along with endogenous peptides (Flowchart 22.1).

a. **Natural and semisynthetic** derivatives of opium poppy known as **opiates**, e.g., morphine, codeine, oxycodone and heroin.
b. **Synthetic drugs** which may be:
   i. Strong agonists
   ii. Mild-to-moderate agonists or partial agonists
   iii. Complex action drugs based on their actions on opioid receptors, are classified as
      - κ Analgesics
      - Partial/weak μ-agonist but κ-antagonists
      - Pure antagonists
   iv. Others
c. **Endogenous opioids** or **opiopeptins**

Nociceptin or orphanin is a newly isolated endogenous peptide that exerts its effects through nociceptin/orphanin-like receptors.

Clinical problem-based questions and MCQs

1. **Identify a drug that is a strong agonist on opioid receptors.**
   a. Codeine
   b. d-Propoxyphene
   c. Meperidine
   d. Diphenoxylate

2. **Identify the CORRECT statement about the action of buprenorphine.**
   a. Antagonist at κ and partial agonist at μ-receptors
   b. Partial agonist at κ-receptors
   c. Strong agonist at all opioid receptors
   d. Antagonist at μ and κ-receptors

3. **All of the following are strong opioid agonists EXCEPT:**
   a. Morphine
   b. Fentanyl
   c. Methadone
   d. Butorphanol

4. **Identify an opioid that acts as an agonist at κ and partial agonist at μ-receptors.**
   a. Meperidine
   b. Buprenorphine
   c. Pentazocine
   d. Nalmefene.

5. **A 54-year-old postmenopausal woman visits her physician for counselling due to significant weight gain since menopause, which has left her feeling depressed.**
   i. What are endorphins?
      a. Antipsychotic drugs
      b. Psychotomimetic drugs
      c. Endogenous opioids
      d. Opioid antagonists
   ii. Name two other members of the class to which endorphins belong.

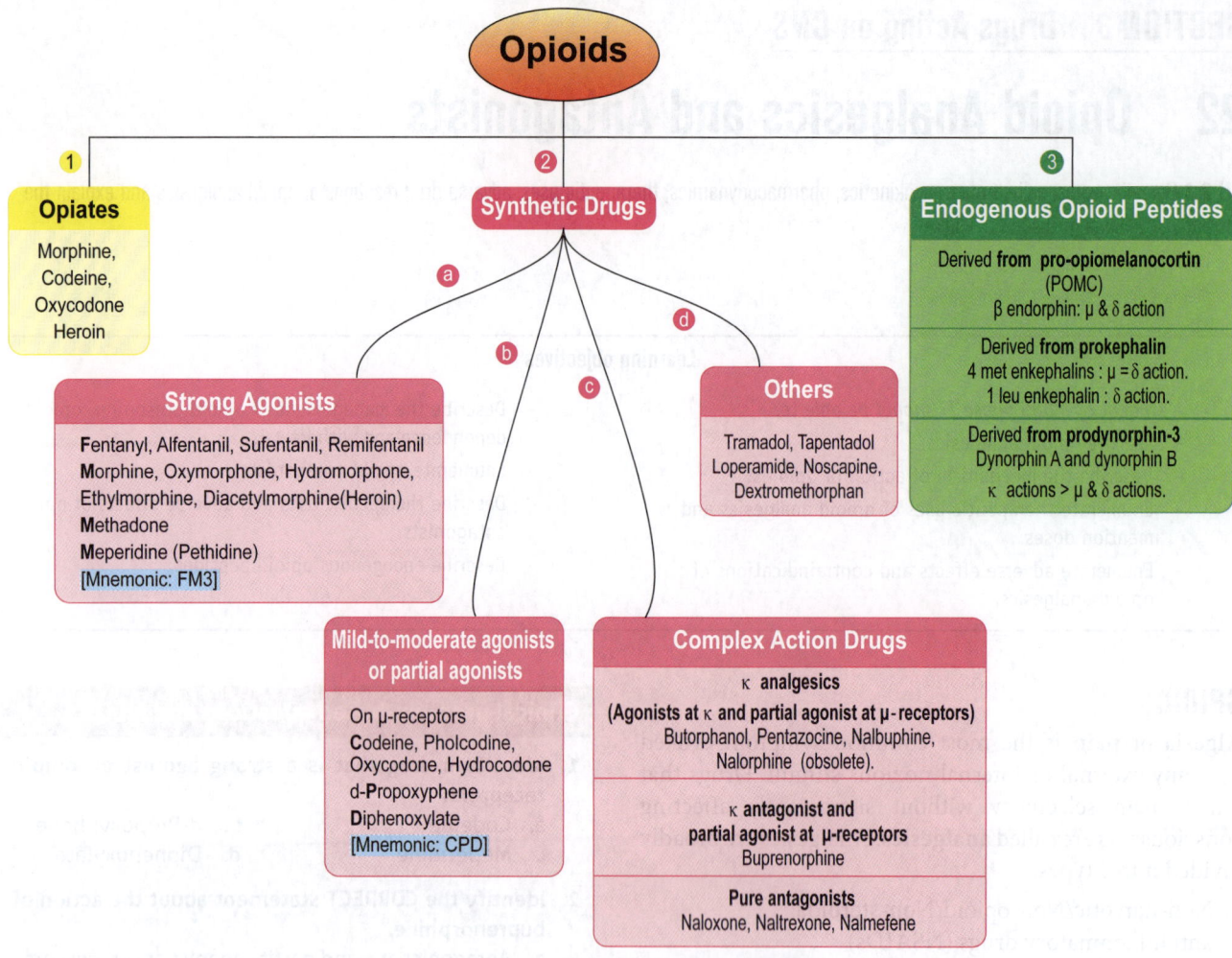

Flowchart 22.1 Classification of opioids

Mechanism of Action

Opioids produce their effects by interacting with opioid receptors, which are G protein-coupled receptors (GPCRs) having G_i protein at the α subunit. Opioids exert the following actions through G_i-linked receptors:

- On presynaptic nerve terminals: Closing of voltage-gated Ca^{2+} channels → Decreased neurotransmitter release of glutamate, ACh, NA, substance P, serotonin, etc.
- On postsynaptic neurons (Fig. 22.1): Decreased cAMP production and opening of K^+ channels → hyperpolarisation → decreased calcium ion influx → reduced intracellular calcium. Activation of kappa receptors also decreases calcium influx through N-type calcium channels.

There are **3 subtypes of opioid receptors,** namely mu (μ), kappa (κ) and δ (delta), distributed at supraspinal, spinal and peripheral sites. Multiple mechanisms contribute to analgesic action of opioids, such as:

- **Supraspinal:** μ Receptors are present on pain-modulating neurons in the periaqueductal grey area, rostral ventral medulla, locus caeruleus and other sites such as the thalamus, nucleus tractus solitarius, nucleus ambiguus and area postrema. Opioids exert inhibitory effect on these neurons, resulting in activation of the descending pathways. The inhibitory descending pathways in turn inhibit *pain transmission neurons* in the spinal cord. δ Receptors mediate affective response to pain. Thus, opioids not only reduce pain transmission, they also modify the emotional response to pain.
- **In the dorsal horn of the spinal cord,** μ-opioid receptors are present on primary afferents Opioids decrease the release of excitatory neurotransmitters from primary afferents and inhibit pain transmission neurons.
- Peripheral μ receptors are present on the terminals of **sensory neurons**. Through these receptors, **opioids decrease sensory neuron activity and transmitter release.** Pain of inflammatory origin seems to be especially responsive to these peripheral actions of opioids. Peripheral μ-receptors are also activated by β-endorphins released from immune cells within injured or inflamed tissues.

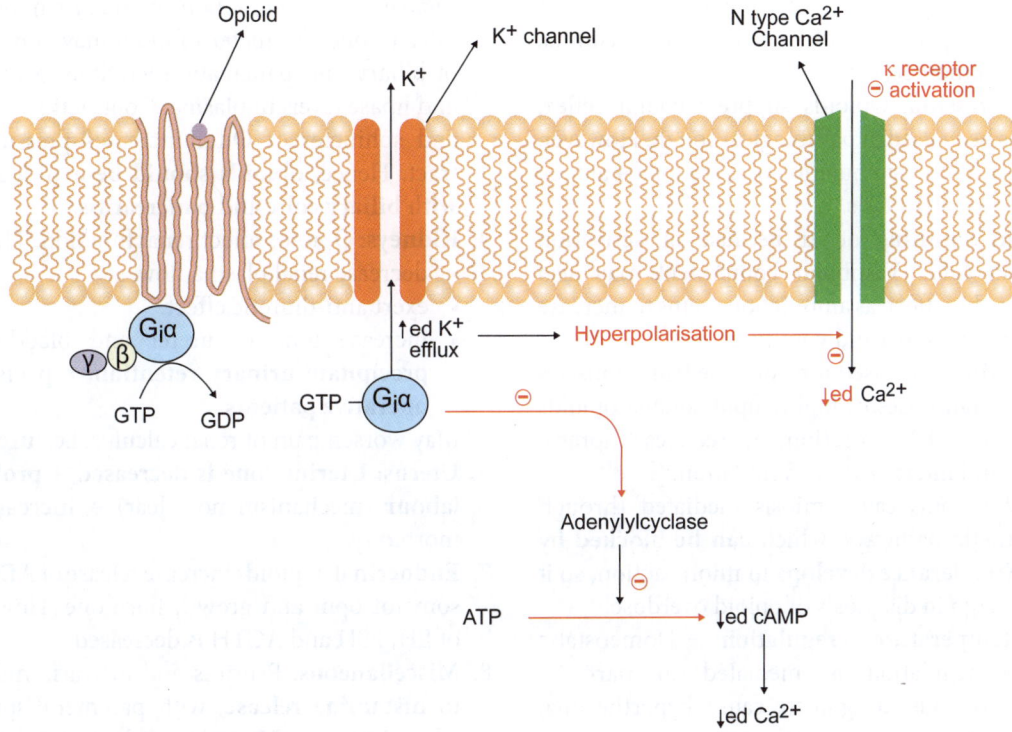

Fig. 22.1 Mechanism of action of opioids

- Exogenous opioids acting at μ receptors **evoke endogenous opioid release,** which in turn act at κ and δ receptors also.

Actions mediated by different types of opioid receptors

1. **μ Receptors** have high affinity for morphine and its congeners. Two subtypes are proposed:
   - μ$_1$: higher affinity for morphine (mediates supraspinal analgesia)
   - μ$_2$: lower affinity for morphine

   [Mnemonic for μ-receptor-mediated actions: **DM CARES** (**D**ependence (physical), **M**iosis, **C**onstipation, **A**nalgesia (spinal), **R**espiratory depression/rigidity (truncal), **E**uphoria, **S**edation.]

2. **κ Receptors** have high affinity for dynorphin A, the endogenous ligand. Subtypes are:
   - κ$_1$: spinal analgesia
   - κ$_3$: lower ceiling supraspinal analgesia

   [Mnemonic for κ actions is **CAPPA**: **C**onstipation, **A**nalgesia, **P**sychotomimetic (dysphoria), **P**ulmonary (respiratory depression), **A**nticonvulsant action]

3. **δ Receptors** mediate spinal analgesia, the affective component of supraspinal analgesia, affective behaviour, convulsions and respiratory depression.

(**Note:** Sigma receptors are no longer considered as opioid receptors as they are neither activated by morphine nor blocked by naloxone.)

Pharmacological Action of Morphine

Morphine exerts central and peripheral actions.

Central actions

Opioids with affinity for μ receptors produce analgesia, euphoria, sedation, cough suppression, miosis, truncal rigidity, nausea/vomiting, alteration of temperature regulation and respiratory depression.

1. **Analgesia:** Opioids reduce both sensory and affective (emotional) components of pain. They are effective in severe, constant pain of any origin.
2. **Euphoria:** Patients or I/V drug users experience pleasant floating sensation, decreased anxiety and distress. However, sometimes dysphoria (unpleasant state characterised by restlessness and malaise) may occur.
3. **Sedation:** Drowsiness, clouding of mentation, little or no amnesia and sleep are induced more frequently in elderly than in young healthy individuals. Patient can be easily aroused from this sleep. However, there is additive effect with other central depressant drugs such as sedative hypnotics. Morphine disrupts REM–NREM sleep patterns.
4. **Respiratory depression:** All opioids cause significant respiratory depression by inhibiting brainstem respiratory mechanisms in a dose-dependent manner. This results in increased alveolar pCO_2 and reduced response to CO_2 challenge. This is tolerated by patients

without prior respiratory impairment but may not be tolerated by patients with increased ICT, asthma, COPD, cor pulmonale, etc.

5. **Cough suppression**: Opioids suppress cough reflex. Codeine has been used in pathological cough. However, opioids may lead to accumulation of secretions → airway obstruction and atelectasis.
6. **Nausea and vomiting** occur because of activation of brainstem CTZ. Vestibular component may also contribute to this effect, as ambulation seems to increase the incidence of nausea and vomiting.
7. **Truncal rigidity**: Increased tone of large trunk muscles occurs with high doses of highly lipid soluble opioids given by rapid I/V injection. It reduces thoracic compliance and interferes with ventilation.
8. **Miosis**: All opioids cause miosis mediated through parasympathetic pathways, which **can be blocked by atropine**. **No tolerance develops** to miotic action, so it is a valuable sign in diagnosis of opioid overdose.
9. **Altered temperature regulation**: Homeostatic temperature regulation is mediated in part by endogenous opioids. μ agonists cause hyperthermia, whereas κ agonists induce hypothermia.

Peripheral actions

1. **CVS:** Most opioids have no significant direct effect on the heart except **bradycardia**. Meperidine is an exception that causes tachycardia because of its antimuscarinic effect. Pentazocine also causes tachycardia due to sympathetic stimulation.

   BP is usually maintained, except in patients with hypovolemia, where central depression of the vasomotor centre and histamine release cause peripheral arterial and venous vasodilatation, leading to **hypotension**.

   Increased pCO_2 because of respiratory depression causes **cerebral vasodilatation** → increased cerebral blood flow → increased Intracranial tension (ICT).
2. **GIT: Constipation** is prominent, to which tolerance **does not develop**. This is because of the effect of opioids on enteric nervous system as well as CNS.

   Stomach: Motility decreases, but the tone of the central portion of stomach may increase. HCl secretion decreases.

   Small intestine: Resting tone is increased with periodic spasms, but amplitude of non-propulsive contraction is decreased.

   Large intestine: Tone increases, but propulsive peristaltic contractions decrease. Thus, passage of fecal matter is delayed → excessive H_2O absorption → constipation. Peripheral opioid antagonist alvimopan is useful in paralytic ileus.
3. **Smooth muscles**

   Bronchi: Bronchoconstriction is not significant at therapeutic dose, but it can **worsen asthma** by causing histamine release.

   Biliary tract: Contraction of biliary smooth muscles → biliary colic. Sphincter of Oddi may constrict → reflux of biliary and pancreatic secretions → raised amylase and lipase levels in plasma. Contraction of gall bladder and sphincter of Oddi increases pressure in biliary tract. Hence, **opioids should be avoided in patients with biliary colic and pancreatitis**.
4. **Kidneys:** Opioids affect renal function. They:
   - decrease renal plasma flow.
   - exert anti-diuretic effect.
   - increase tone of ureter and bladder that may **precipitate urinary retention, especially in post-operative patients**.
5. May worsen pain of renal calculus, i.e., **ureteral colic**.
6. **Uterus:** Uterine tone is decreased → **prolongation of labour** (mechanism not clear) → **increased** neonatal morbidity.
7. **Endocrinal:** Opioids increase release of ADH, prolactin, somatotropin and growth hormone. However, release of LH, FSH and ACTH is decreased.
8. **Miscellaneous:** Pruritus and urticaria may occur due to **histamine release**, with parenteral/spinal/epidural administration. Migration of leukocytes to the site of injury is increased, but cytolytic activity and lymphocyte proliferation in response to mitogens is decreased.

Tolerance develops to most actions of opioids except miosis, constipation and convulsions.

Clinical problem-based questions and MCQs

6. Opioids are widely used in clinical practice as these drugs effectively relieve severe, constant pain.
   i. Which of the following statements about the analgesic effect of opioids is INCORRECT?
      a. Increased sensory neuron activity and transmitter release
      b. Change in sensory as well as affective component of pain
      c. Inhibition of spinal cord pain transmission neurons
      d. Release of endogenous opioids
   ii. Describe the mechanism of analgesic effect of morphine.

7. i. Opioids decrease the tone of which of the following smooth muscles?
      a. Bronchial   b. Biliary
      c. Uterine   d. Ureteral
   ii. What are the implications of the action of opioids on the selected smooth muscles.

8. Morphine exerts many central and peripheral actions. Identify a central action of morphine among the following.
   a. Bradycardia
   b. Miosis
   c. Increased ureteric tone
   d. Worsening of bronchial asthma

9. i. Opioids have high abuse potential as tolerance develops to most of their actions EXCEPT:
   a. Miosis
   b. Sedation
   c. Analgesia
   d. Respiratory depression.
   ii. Describe the clinical implication of the above statement.
10. Match the opioid actions with the receptor mediating the same.
   a. Dependence   1. δ receptors
   b. Dysphoria   2. μ receptors
   c. Affective behaviour 3. k receptors

CLINICALLY RELEVANT PHARMACOKINETIC FEATURES

Most of the opioids are well absorbed by oral, subcutaneous and intramuscular routes. However, because of **high and variable first-pass metabolism**, the oral bioavailability of morphine is only 20 to 40%.

Codeine and oxycodone have low first-pass metabolism and are therefore effective orally.

Other routes such as nasal insufflations (butorphanol), transdermal (fentanyl) and buccal transmucosal (fentanyl) are sometimes used for different opioids.

Different opioids have varying affinity for plasma proteins; however, their blood concentrations reduce rapidly, and they **localise in high concentrations in highly perfused tissues** such as the brain, lungs, liver, kidney and spleen. Concentration in fat and skeletal muscle is lower, but because of greater bulk, these are the main reservoirs. Frequent high doses of fentanyl-like drugs can cause accumulation.

Opioids are **metabolised in the liver by glucuronide conjugation**. Morphine-6-glucuronide is an active metabolite of morphine that is 4–6 times more potent as an analgesic. However, it does not contribute much to the acute effects of morphine because of its polar nature. Morphine-3-glucuronide is an inactive metabolite of morphine with neurotoxic potential. These metabolites may accumulate in patients with renal disease and cause unexpected side effects such as convulsions.

Excretion of glucuronide conjugates is through urine and bile. Some enterohepatic circulation may occur. Half life is 2–3 hours.

Opioids, especially morphine, **cross the placental barrier freely** and can cause respiratory depression in the fetus.

THERAPEUTIC USES OF OPIOIDS

1. As analgesics

Opioids (strong agonists) are effective in relieving **severe, constant pain of any origin**. However sharp, intermittent pain is not controlled that effectively. Opioids provide only symptomatic relief; the cause of pain must be looked into and treated.

- Opioids are useful in:
  - Traumatic pain, burn pain
  - Visceral, ischemic and postoperative pain, MI, internal bleed and abdominal pain. Pain of MI and internal bleeds should be treated promptly to allay anxiety/apprehension and reflex sympathetic stimulation.
  - Severe excruciating pain may cause neurogenic shock and other autonomic effects, and hence must be treated immediately with adequate dose of opioids.
  - For obstetric analgesia, pethidine is more useful as it appears to produce less respiratory depression in neonates than morphine.
  - The pain of renal and biliary colic may be paradoxically worsened by morphine, because of drug-induced increase in smooth muscle tone. However, opioids like pentazocine and buprenorphine have lower potential to aggravate biliary spasms.
  - Pain of cancer or other terminal illnesses must be treated aggressively. They may require continuous use of potent opioid analgesics. Although some degree of tolerance and dependence occurs, this should not be a barrier to provide patients with the best possible care and quality of life.
- A fixed-dose interval administration is shown to be more effective for pain relief than dosing on demand.
- New dosage forms and new routes of administration such as sustained release preparations (e.g., fentanyl transdermal patches) are available, for longer and more stable levels of analgesia; Buccal/transmucosal fentanyl is useful for short episodes of break-through pain. Nasal insufflations of strong opioids and rectal suppositories are also available.
- Patient-controlled analgesia (PCA) is used for treatment of break-through pain. Here, the patient controls a parenteral (usually I/V) infusion device by pressing a button to deliver a pre-programmed dose of opioid as per need. This approach is reported to be quite useful for post-operative pain control. However, care should be taken to prevent overdose and respiratory depression by proper monitoring of vital signs.

2. In acute pulmonary edema

Intravenous morphine significantly reduces pulmonary congestion and relieves dyspnea in left ventricular failure (LVF) with the following effects:

- Decreases anxiety (perception of breathlessness).
- Checks sympathetic stimulation, thereby reducing cardiac workload.
- Causes vasodilation, leading to reduced preload and afterload.

- Tendency to shift blood from pulmonary to systemic circulation because of greater vasodilation in the latter. So, pulmonary congestion and edema decrease.

3. In anesthetic practice
- **Preoperatively**, opioids are frequently used in pre-anesthetic medication (PAM). Because of their sedative effect, they aid in smooth induction and decrease the dose of anesthetic.
  - Anxiolytic effect → reduces anxiety/apprehension of operation.
  - Analgesic effects → produce pre/post-operative analgesia.
- However, because of the risk of respiratory depression, post-operative nausea, vomiting, urinary retention/constipation and dysphoria, use is restricted to:
  - Patients with severe preoperative pain; fentanyl is given just before induction.
  - Those undergoing cardiovascular or other high risk surgery (in which primary goal is to decrease cardiovascular depression).
- **Intraoperatively** also, opioids are used:
  - As adjuvants to other anesthetic agents.
  - As a primary component of the anesthetic regimen in high doses, e.g., 0.02–0.075 mg/kg fentanyl is used as neurolept analgesia and anesthesia.
  - Analgesia: fentanyl and droperidol
  - Anesthesia: fentanyl, droperidol and N_2O
- **Postoperatively**: Epidural/intrathecal injection can produce segmental analgesia for long duration (approximately 12 hours). So, it can be used for long-lasting analgesia with minimal adverse effects. Epidural administration of 3–5 mg morphine is useful as surgical analgesia for abdominal, pelvic and lower limb operations; it can be used post-operatively also. A low dose of local anesthetic along with fentanyl is infused through a thoracic catheter, followed by slow infusion through catheter placed in the epidural space for pain control in patients recovering from thoracic and major upper abdominal surgery.

4. Cough
Cough suppression is achieved at doses lower than the analgesic dose. Codeine and dextromethorphan are useful in pathological cough. Dextromethorphan is likely free of addictive property and is present in over-the-counter (OTC) antitussive preparations. It causes less constipation than codeine but abuse of its purified (powdered) form is reported to cause serious adverse events, including death.

Levopropoxyphene, a stereoisomer of dextropropoxyphene, is devoid of most of other effects except sedation and is used as antitussive. Noscapine also has antitussive action.

5. Diarrhea
Opioids can effectively control diarrhea due to any cause. However, in infective diarrheas, appropriate chemotherapy must be given. Synthetic drugs like diphenoxylate and loperamide that have more GIT effects with little or no CNS effects are used exclusively for this purpose.

6. Shivering
All opioids have the ability to reduce shivering but pethidine (meperidine) has the most pronounced anti-shivering properties, probably due to its action on $α_2$ adrenoreceptor subtypes.

The therapeutic uses of opioids are summarised in Box 22.1.

Box 22.1 Therapeutic uses of opioids

1. As analgesics in severe constant pain of any origin: trauma, burns, visceral, ischemic, post-operative, MI, internal bleeds, obstetric, abdominal pain, pain of cancer or other terminal illnesses.
2. In anesthetic practice:
   - Preoperative: As part of PAM in patients with severe preoperative pain and in patients undergoing cardiovascular or other high-risk surgery.
   - Intra-operative: As adjuvants to other anesthetics as primary component of anesthetic regimen.
   - Post-operative: epidural injection or infusion for segmental analgesia.
3. Cough
4. Pulmonary edema in acute LVF
5. Diarrhea
6. Shivering

ADVERSE EFFECTS AND TOXICITY OF OPIOIDS
Adverse effects of opioids are mainly the extensions of their pharmacological actions.

1. Behavioural: Restlessness, hyperactivity, malaise, dysphoria
2. Respiratory depression → Increased pCO_2 → Cerebral vasodilation → Increased intracranial tension and worsening of cerebral edema.
3. Histamine release: Itching, urticaria (more frequently with spinal and parenteral administration)
   - Bronchospasms can worsen bronchial asthma.
   - Vasodilation leads to orthostatic hypotension. Blood pressure falls, especially in hypovolemic patients.
4. Nausea, vomiting, constipation
5. Urinary retention
6. **Tolerance:** Although development of tolerance starts with the first dose of opioids, it manifests clinically after 2–3 weeks of frequent exposure to therapeutic doses. This is probably because of the failure of morphine to induce endocytosis of μ-receptors for recycling and receptor uncoupling. NMDA receptors also probably play a role in the development of tolerance to opioids, as

ketamine (antagonist at NMDA receptors) can prevent or reverse opioid tolerance.

Tolerance develops to different extents for different actions.
- Marked tolerance develops to analgesic, sedative and respiratory depressant effects.
- Some tolerance develops to emetic, antidiuretic and hypotensive actions also.
- However, there is no tolerance to miotic, constipation and convulsant actions.

[Mnemonic: Tolerance develops to most actions of morphine except **C3**, i.e., **C**onstipation, **C**onstriction of pupil, and **C**onvulsions.]

The rate of appearance and disappearance of tolerance (on withdrawal/ discontinuation) varies among different opioids and even among individuals for the same drug.

7. **Cross-tolerance** is an extremely important characteristic of opioids. Morphine and its congeners show cross- tolerance not only for analgesic, but also for euphoriant, sedative and respiratory effects.

8. **Dependence:** Repeated administration of opioids with μ-agonistic action leads to tolerance and physical dependence. Failure to administer the drug results in **withdrawal syndrome,** characterised by symptoms (mostly opposite of pharmacological actions) such as rhinorrhea, lacrimation, yawning, chills, gooseflesh, hyperventilation, hyperthermia, mydriasis, diarrhea, muscular aches, anxiety and hostility. Administration of the opioid suppresses the symptoms immediately. **Withdrawal symptoms** appear 6–10 hours after the last dose of morphine or diacetyl morphine (heroin); they reach at a peak at 36–48 hours, after which they gradually subside and disappear by 5 days.

Methadone has a less intense syndrome. The peak of signs and symptoms occurs after several days and they subside after about 2 weeks. Methadone along with buprenorphine and clonidine are FDA-approved treatments for opioid analgesic detoxification.

Psychological dependence occurs because of the sedative, euphoriant actions and leads to compulsive use and craving. It persists even after physical dependence is treated.

Acute overdose of morphine

Acute overdose can occur in drug addicts. It can be accidental or suicidal. Lethal dose is 250 mg, but in non-tolerant adults, serious toxic effects can occur at lower doses of 50 mg.

Clinical features of overdose are extension of pharmacological actions in the form of:
- Pinpoint pupil
- Stupor/coma
- Fall in BP, shock
- Respiratory depression (shallow and occasional breathing, cyanosis, pulmonary edema in terminal stages, death due to respiratory failure).

Diagnosis and treatment
- Coma because of opioid overdose is reversed dramatically by I/V naloxone.
- Respiratory support
- Maintenance of BP (intravenous fluids, vasoconstrictions)
- Gastric lavage with $KMnO_4$ to remove unabsorbed drug in oral administration, and even after parenteral administration, to remove the drug which has reached the acidic gastric juice because of pH partition.
- Intravenous naloxone 0.4–0.8 mg, repeated every 2–3 minutes, till respiration picks up. Then, naloxone should be repeated every 1–4 hours, according to the response of the patient.

Precautions/contraindications

1. Morphine is contraindicated in **head injuries,** because:
   - Even the therapeutic dose can cause marked respiratory depression.
   - Increase in pCO_2 leads to cerebral vasodilation, which increases intracranial tension and can worsen cerebral edema.
   - Morphine causes sedation/altered mentation, vomiting and miosis; these actions interfere with assessment of comatose patient's neurological status.
2. **Undiagnosed abdominal pain:** Morphine can worsen the pain in biliary colic, pancreatitis and diverticulitis; inflamed appendix may rupture. Pentazocine and buprenorphine are better tolerated in these conditions.
3. **Impaired pulmonary function**: Morphine-induced respiratory depression can cause acute respiratory failure in patients with impaired respiratory reserve.
4. In patients with **impaired hepatic/renal function** and **hypothyroidism,** the half-life of morphine is longer so, dose reduction is necessary.
5. **Bronchial asthma** may be worsened by morphine because of histamine release. Low-dose fentanyl should be used if the use of opioids in an asthma patient is unavoidable.
6. Elderly patients are more prone to respiratory depression. Elderly males can develop urinary retention.
7. **In pregnancy:** Chronic use in pregnancy may lead to dependence of the baby on opioids in utero. Withdrawal syndrome occurs in neonate soon after birth, and is characterised by diarrhea, irritability, shrill cry and convulsions. If mild, it can be controlled by diazepam. If severe, oral opium tincture or oral methadone is used.

Drug interactions

1. Combining full agonists like morphine with partial agonists like pentazocine may decrease analgesic action or even induce a state of withdrawal. So, such combinations should be avoided.

2. Additive effect with other CNS depressants such as sedative hypnotics and antipsychotics, in the form of increased CNS depression, particularly respiratory depression.
3. Patients on monoamine oxidase (MAO) inhibitors have high incidence of hyperpyrexia, coma and hypertension, if opioids are combined.

Clinical problem-based questions and MCQs

11. A 75-years-old patient was diagnosed with colorectal carcinoma, stage III. Chemotherapy with oxaliplatin and 5-fluorouracil was given. After 9 months of treatment, the patient became refractory to treatment, developed ascites, severe abdominal pain and generalised malaise. Injection morphine is prescribed SOS.
    i. Justify the use of morphine in this case.
    ii. Name the new dosage forms that can decrease the patient's inconvenience caused by repeated injections.

12. A 45-year-old male patient with chronic hypertension and angina is brought to emergency with severe piercing pain in the left side of chest, radiating to the left shoulder and neck, dyspnea, anxiety and cold sweat. Basal crepitations are present on auscultation; ECG shows ST elevation, CPK MB is raised. The patient is diagnosed as ST elevation myocardial infarction (STEMI) with acute pulmonary edema. Comment on the role of opioids in acute MI and pulmonary edema.

13. Identify the opioid drug that is suitable for the treatment of diarrhea.
    a. Diacetyl morphine   b. Oxycodone
    c. Butorphanol   d. Diphenoxylate

14. All of the following opioids are suitable for pathological cough, EXPECT
    a. Dextromethorphan   b. Noscapine
    c. Nalbuphine   d. Levopropoxyphene

15. Opioids are extensively used in current anesthetic practice. Comment on use of opioids in the preoperative, intraoperative and post-operative period.

16. Tolerance develops to some actions of opioids but not to others. Identify the action for which marked tolerance develops:
    a. Respiratory depression   b. Miosis
    c. Constipation   d. Convulsions

17. A 65-year-old patient presents in emergency department after a fall from staircase. He is unable to stand and is experiencing severe pain in the right hip region. Clinical examination and radiography confirm the diagnosis of fracture of right femur. Careful elicitation of history reveals that the patient is a known case of bronchial asthma for the last 30 years. The senior consultant cautions resident doctors about using opioids in this patient.
    i. What is the caution in the use of opioids in this patient?
    ii. What is the pharmacological basis for this caution?
    iii. Which opioid can be used if extremely necessary?

18. A young patient is brought to trauma centre in a semiconscious state following a road accident. Bleeding from the nose and ears is present. BP= 100/60, PR = 120 BPM, RR = 20 per minute, GCS is 9/15. The patient is managed with ringer lactate by intravenous infusion, oxygen inhalation, injection tetanus toxoid and analgesics.
    i. Which of the following analgesics is contraindicated in this patient?
        a. Diclofenac   b. Morphine
        c. Paracetamol   d. Piroxicam
    ii. Explain your choice.

19. A 30-year-old male patient is brought to hospital emergency by police personnel. He was found in a semiconscious condition at the site of a rave party. The patient is unresponsive, has shallow breathing and cyanosis. On examination, patient has pin-point pupils and skin turgidity is poor. Multiple bruises and needle puncture marks are seen on both arms. HR = 106 bpm, BP = 94/64, temperature = 99.6°C, blood glucose = 90 mg/dL.
    i. What is the diagnosis?
    ii. How will you manage this patient? Mention the specific antidote and its dose.

20. A newborn baby girl develops diarrhea, irritability, shrill cry and convulsions. Careful history of her mother shows opioid addiction. Multiple needle prick marks are present.
    i. What is the cause of baby's symptoms?
    ii. How is this case managed?

SALIENT FEATURES OF INDIVIDUAL OPIOID DRUGS

1. Opiates
These are natural and semisynthetic drugs derived from opium poppy, e.g., morphine, codeine, oxycodone and heroin. Morphine is the prototype opioid drug.

2. Synthetic Drugs
Synthetic opioid drugs include the following groups.

a. Strong Agonists
i. Diacetyl morphine or heroin
This is a **highly abused** drug because it is **3 times more potent** than morphine, more lipid soluble → crosses brain–blood barrier → **fast action**. However, the duration of action is same as that of morphine.

- It is m**ore euphoriant** (especially upon intravenous use), less sedative, less hypotensive, has high addictive potential and emetic effect.

- Banned in most countries.
- Offers no therapeutic advantage over morphine.

ii. Meperidine (Pethidine)

Similarities with morphine
- As an analgesic, meperidine and propoxyphene are the **least potent** opioids. However, meperidine and morphine are equi-efficacious.
- Sedative, euphoriant, respiratory depressant actions and abuse potential are similar to morphine.

Differences from morphine
- Because of antimuscarinic activity → pethidine causes **tachycardia**, not bradycardia.
- It reduces shivering after anesthesia due to its action on κ and $α_2$ receptors.
- **Less spasmodic action** on smooth muscles; miosis, constipation and urine retention are less prominent.
- **Histamine release is less,** so it is comparatively safe in bronchial asthma patients.
- Duration of action is shorter → withdrawal syndrome develops rapidly.
- It is mainly metabolised via hydrolysis by MAO enzyme. However, some part (1%) is metabolised by dealkylation, resulting in formation of a neurotoxic metabolite, **norpethidine**, which is responsible for central excitatory effects like tremors, delirium, hyperreflexia, myoclonus and convulsions in overdose or in renal failure patients.

The use of pethidine as analgesic is decreasing in favour of fentanyl group of drugs. Abuse is common, especially among healthcare professionals. However, it is the drug of choice for controlling shivering due to infusion reaction to drugs like amphotericin B and monoclonal antibodies and in the post-operative period.

iii. Methadone

Similarities to morphine
Analgesic, respiratory depressant, emetic, antitussive, constipating, biliary spasm actions are the same as morphine.

Differences
- The most important difference is that it has much **better oral bioavailability** than morphine.
- In addition to μ-receptor agonist effect, it blocks NMDA receptors and monoaminergic reuptake. Thus, it **can relieve cancer pain** and **neuropathic pain in situations** where morphine trial has failed. **Opioid rotation** (i.e., shifting to methadone from morphine when tolerance or intolerable adverse effects develop upon increasing doses of morphine) is widely used.
- Other important pharmacokinetic differences of methadone from morphine include:
  - Strong binding to tissue proteins → cumulation in tissues on repeated administration, leading to progressive increase in duration of action. On chronic

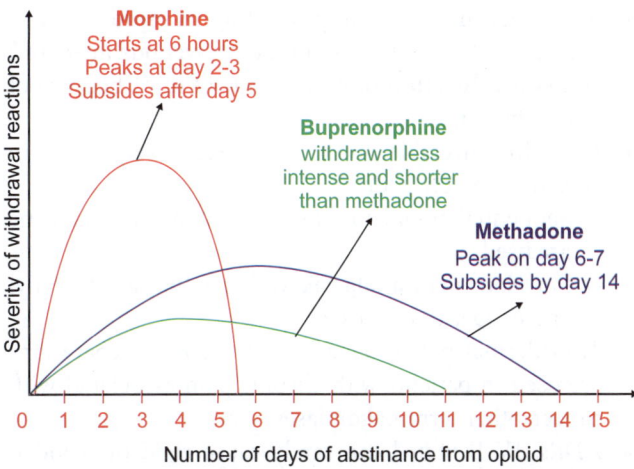

Fig. 22.2 Severity of withdrawal reaction with different opioids

use, **half-life can extend up to 24–36 hours**. Due to this long duration of action, tolerance/dependence develop more slowly with methadone than with morphine, and withdrawal symptoms are milder but more prolonged. These properties make it useful in the treatment of opioid abuse for detoxification and maintenance of chronic relapsing heroin addicts. For the **detoxification of heroin-dependent addicts** → oral methadone is given in a low dose of 5–10 mg, 2–3 times daily for 2 to 3 days and then stopped. The addict will experience milder withdrawal syndrome that is endurable.

- The **withdrawal symptoms** of more potent drugs like morphine and heroin are more severe and appear after about 6–8 hours of abstinence, reaching a peak on day 2 or 3 and subsiding around day 5 (Fig. 22.2). In contrast, methadone withdrawal symptoms are less severe, reach a peak in 6 to 7 days and subside around the 14th day of abstinence. Buprenorphine has withdrawal syndrome less intense and shorter-lasting than methadone. Hence, buprenorphine and methadone are useful in opioid-dependent subjects.

For **maintenance therapy of chronic, relapsing heroin addicts** → 50–100 mg/day oral methadone is given to deliberately produce tolerance to methadone → because heroin has cross-tolerance, even if addicts procure and consume heroin, they do not get the expected pleasant response → so, craving or drug-seeking behaviour decreases.

iv. Fentanyl

This subgroup includes fentanyl, sufentanil, alfentanil and remifentanil.

- Fentanyl is **80–100 times more potent** than morphine in its analgesic and respiratory depressant effects.
- Cardiovascular effects are minimal at analgesic dose.
- Lower potential to cause histamine release.

- It has high lipid solubility resulting in **rapid onset** of analgesic effect (within 5 min of intravenous injection) and **short duration of action** (30–40 min) because of redistribution.
- *Uses:* In injectable form, it is exclusively used in anesthetic practice for:
    - Sequential opioid anesthesia – fentanyl, pentazocine are used.
    - For **Neurolept analgesia and anesthesia** – fentanyl and droperidol are used.
- Transdermal patch, buccal/transmucosal preparations are used in patients with chronic pain associated with cancer/other terminal diseases.
- *ADRs:* IV Fentanyl can rarely cause rigid or wooden chest syndrome (WCS), characterised by rigidity of chest wall muscles, diaphragm and laryngospasms.

v. Sufentanil
Sufentanil is 5–7 times more potent than fentanyl. It is the most potent of opioids available for blocking stress response during laryngoscopy and intubation.

vi. Alfentanil
This is 20 times more potent than morphine. It is used with propofol for total IV anesthesia (TIVA).

vii. Remifentanil
Remifentanil is the shortest and fastest acting drug among opioids. It is used by IV infusion for day-care surgeries.

b. Mild-to-Moderate/Partial Agonists
i. Codeine
Codeine is methyl morphine. It occurs naturally in poppy plant and is partly converted in the body to morphine by demethylation and exerts analgesic effect.
- As an **analgesic,** it is **less potent** (1/10th) and less efficacious than morphine, and can relieve mild-to-moderate pain only.
- It has greater selective cough suppressant action at doses < analgesic doses.
- Good activity by oral route. The effect of oral dose lasts for 4–6 hours.
- Constipation is an important adverse effect; consequently, it has been used in diarrhea.

ii. Others
- **Pholcodine** is similar to codeine, used mainly as an antitussive drug. It is claimed to be less constipating than codeine.
- **Propoxyphene** is the least potent and least efficacious of opioids
- **Diphenoxylate** is used as a fixed-dose combination with atropine for its antidiarrheal effect (refer to Chapter 62 page 814).

c. Complex Action Opioids
i. Kappa analgesics
Nalbuphine, nalorphine: Agonist at κ, receptors antagonist at μ-receptors. These are obsolete.

Butorphanol, pentazocine: Agonist at κ receptors, partial agonist at μ-receptors.

Pentazocine
- It is a strong agonist at κ receptors and partial agonist at μ-receptors.
- Less potent than morphine as an analgesic.
- Causes euphoria in low doses and dysphoria at high doses.
- It is used in moderately severe pain, such as post-operative pain, fractures, burns, trauma and cancer.
- Effective orally but the parenteral-to-oral ratio is 1:3 because of its high first-pass metabolism.
- Causes sympathetic stimulation at high dose resulting in increase in HR and BP, which increases cardiac workload. Hence, pentazocine **should not be given to patients with ischemic heart disease** or myocardial infarction.
- **ADRs:** Tolerance and dependence occur on repeated use. However, its addiction potential is lower than that of morphine.
- Sedation, respiratory depression, biliary spasm and vomiting are less marked than with morphine.

Butorphanol
It is also κ agonist, and has a weak effect on μ-receptors like pentazocine, but is more potent.
- Analgesia and respiratory depression effects are less than that of morphine.
- Sedation and cardiac stimulation are the same as pentazocine but dysphoric effects are less. Withdrawal reaction is mild; abuse potential is low.
- 1–4 mg intramuscular or intravenous is used for postoperative and other short painful conditions but avoided in cardiac ischemia.

ii. κ Antagonist and Partial Agonist at μ-Receptors
Buprenorphine
- Buprenorphine has μ agonistic and κ antagonistic actions. It is **50 times more potent than morphine but less efficacious**. It has a slow onset and longer duration of action (6–8 hours) as it **binds tightly and dissociates slowly** from μ receptors. With repeated dosing, the duration of action may increase upto 24 hours because of accumulation.
- Sedative, emetic, miotic, subjective and cardiovascular effects are the same as morphine, but constipation is less marked.
- Tolerance/dependence is low grade; withdrawal syndrome is milder, delayed and longer-lasting than

morphine. However, in comparison to methadone, withdrawal symptoms are less intense and short-lasting (Fig. 22.2). Thus, buprenorphine can be used as an alternative to methadone for managing opioid withdrawal.
- It binds tightly to μ receptors, so naloxone can prevent its effects but cannot reverse them.
- It is used in long-lasting conditions requiring opioids, e.g., cancer pain, pre-anesthetic medication, post-operative pain and myocardial infarction pain.
- Sometimes, it **may be used sublingually in opioid detoxification and maintenance,** but a high dose can precipitate withdrawal symptoms.

iii. Opioid antagonists

Central opioid antagonists are naloxone, naltrexone and nalmefene. **Peripheral opioid antagonists** are methyl naltrexone, naloxegol, naldemedine and alvimopan.

- These are derivatives of morphine having bulkier substituents at N_{17}.
- They have relatively **higher affinity for μ than δ and κ receptors,** but can reverse the agonistic effect at all three receptor sites.
- They have **no agonistic action** even at high doses.
- If a person has not received any opioid, then these drugs produce no subjective or autonomic effects. But in a patient who has taken morphine, these drugs **antagonise all the actions** of morphine.
- Opioid antagonists can **precipitate acute withdrawal symptoms in dependent subjects.** So, these can be used in the diagnosis of opioid dependence.

Naloxone
- Naloxone reverses opioid-induced analgesia. Respiratory depression is normalised or even stimulated (probably because of sudden sensitisation of the respiratory centre to retained CO_2). Pupils dilate, sedation is less completely reversed.
- **Naloxone** has very high first-pass metabolism, and hence is **not effective orally.** When given intravenously, the effect lasts for 1–2 hours
- It is the drug of choice for morphine poisoning: 0.4–0.8 mg is given intravenously every 2–3 minutes up to a total of 10 mg.
- In a dose of 4–10 mg, it can antagonise actions of pentazocine, nalbuphine, etc., although their psychotomimetic and dysphoric effects are reversed incompletely.
- Buprenorphine binds tightly to receptors and dissociates slowly. So, its effects can be prevented but not reversed effectively.
- Analgesia induced by stress/placebo/acupuncture, which is probably mediated through endogenous opioids, is also blocked by naloxone.
- Respiratory depression caused by non-opioid drugs such as N_2O, alcohol and diazepam is also partly antagonised.
- Adverse reactions are uncommon. It may increase release of catecholamines resulting in hypertension, arrhythmia and pulmonary edema.

Naltrexone
- It is **more potent** than naloxone.
- Orally active and has **long DOA** (1–2 days). Hence, it is suitable for **opioid-blockade therapy** for post addicts (50 mg/day, given orally). If the patient takes their usual shot of opioids after naltrexone, they fail to experience any subjective effects. Therefore, craving subsides.
- It also decreases alcohol craving.
- Adverse effects include headache, nausea; high doses have hepatotoxic potential.

Nalmefene
- It also has high oral bioavailability and long duration of action.
- No hepatotoxic effect is seen.

Peripheral opioid antagonists

Peripheral opioid antagonists such as **naloxegol, naldemedine and methyl naltrexone** cannot penetrate the blood–brain barrier but block peripheral μ actions of opioids. It is **used to reverse constipation** in cancer patients being treated with opioids and in patients on methadone maintenance therapy. **Alvimopan** is used to reverse postoperative ileus.

d. Other Opioids

1. **Tramadol** exerts analgesic effect by acting as weak agonist at μ receptor. It also inhibits 5-HT and NA reuptake. Therefore, the analgesic effect of tramadol can be blocked by 5-HT antagonists.
2. **Tapentadol** also exerts μ-receptor-agonistic and noradrenaline reuptake inhibiting action.
3. **Eluxadoline** is agonist at μ receptor and antagonist at δ receptors. It is useful in irritable bowel syndrome with diarrhea as dominant symptom.

3. Endogenous Opioid Peptides

Endogenous opioids are peptides isolated from the mammalian brain, pituitary, spinal cord and gastrointestinal tract. These exert morphine-like actions by binding to opioid receptors with high affinity. Actions of endogenous opioids are blocked by naloxone.

The endogenous opioid system comprises 3 distinct families:

a. **Endorphins** derived from pro-opiomelanocortin (POMC) act primarily at μ receptors, but some δ activity is also seen.

b. **Enkephalins derived** from pro-enkephalin: There are four methionine enkephalins (met Enk) and one leucine enkephalin (leu Enk); met Enk has equal affinity for μ and δ receptors, while leu Enk prefers δ receptors.
c. **Dynorphins** derived from prodynorphin, which gives leu Enk, dynorphin A and B: These are more potent on κ receptors, but also act on μ and δ receptors.

Actions of endogenous opioids

Endogenous opioid system modulates pain perception, mood, hedonic (pleasure) response, motor behaviour, emesis, pituitary hormone release and gastrointestinal motility. The important actions of endogenous opioids and their roles are given below.

- β endorphins probably have a **neurohormonal** function. They decrease LH and FSH releases but increase release of GH and PRL and have a long half-life.
- Dynorphins and enkephalins have a short $t_{1/2}$. They probably function as **neuromodulators** or neurotransmitters. They regulate pain responsiveness at spinal and supraspinal levels.
- Endogenous opioids are probably **involved in placebo, acupuncture and stress-induced analgesia**.
- They also appear to be involved in **regulation of affective behaviour and autonomic functions**.
- A new peptide, nociceptin, acting on NOP (nociceptin opioid peptide) receptors is believed to play a role in stress response, reward and reinforcing action, learning and memory. It likely has some anti-opioid effects as well.

Clinical problem-based questions and MCQs

21. Which opioid is a less potent and less efficacious analgesic than morphine?
    a. Codeine   b. Pethidine
    c. Diacetylmorphine   d. Fentanyl

22. Which opioid is less potent but equally efficacious analgesic as morphine?
    a. Codeine   b. Pethidine
    c. Diacetylmorphine   d. Fentanyl

23. i. Identify an opioid which is more potent than morphine and is a highly abused drug.
        a. Codeine   b. Pethidine
        c. Diacetyl morphine   d. Diphenoxylate
    ii. Describe the management of an addict of drug selected in part (i) of the question.

24. All the following opioid drugs are more potent than morphine EXCEPT:
    a. Fentanyl   b. Sufentanil
    c. Pentazocine   d. Buprenorphine

25. A 25-year-old heroin addict on maintenance therapy with methadone develops severe constipation. Which of the following drugs is effective in reversing constipation?
    a. Pentazocine   b. Buprenorphine
    c. Methyl naltrexone   d. Nalmefene

Summary

- Opioid analgesics include natural, semisynthetic and synthetic drugs. Synthetic drugs can be strong agonists, mild-to-moderate agonists or complex action drugs.
- These drugs mediate their actions through G_i protein-coupled receptors. Receptors are of μ, κ and δ types.
- μ receptors mediate dependence, miosis, constipation, analgesia, respiratory depression/rigidity, euphoriant and sedative effects. κ receptors mediate constipation, analgesia, psychomimetic, i.e., dysphoric, pulmonary (respiratory depression) and anticonvulsant actions. δ receptors mediate affective, behavioural effects and modulate the release of hormones and NTMs.
- Morphine is the prototype opioid.
- Central effects of opioids include analgesia, sedation, respiratory depression, miosis, nausea/vomiting, euphoria, truncal rigidity and cough suppression.
- Peripheral actions include bradycardia (except pethidine-induced tachycardia due to antimuscarinic action), hypotension in hypovolemic patients, constipation, increased tone of smooth muscles of bronchi, ureter and biliary smooth muscles, and reduced uterine tone.
- Morphine is useful in constant severe pain due to vascular ischemia, trauma, burns, cancer and other terminal illnesses. Other uses are in acute pulmonary edema, as pre anesthetic medication, as analgesic with anesthesia, and for post-operative pain.
- Codeine, dextromethorphan and noscapine are used as antitussive agents.
- Diphenoxylate and loperamide are used in diarrhea.
- Pethidine is useful in shivering.
- ADRs include sedation, drowsiness, constipation, respiratory depression, risk of convulsions, tolerance, dependence, and addiction. Opioids cause histamine release, which can worsen bronchial asthma. Fentanyl and pethidine are preferred to morphine in asthmatic patients.
- Morphine is contraindicated in undiagnosed abdominal pain, head injury, impaired pulmonary, cardiac, hepatic and renal function, pregnancy, and in elderly individuals.
- Opioid dependence can be managed with methadone for detoxification and maintenance therapy.
- Opioid antagonists like naloxone and naltrexone can reverse the effect of agonists. Naloxone is the drug of choice in acute morphine poisoning. Methyl naltrexone is used for reversing constipation in patients on long-term opioid therapy. The effect of buprenorphine is not completely reversed, as it is tightly bound to receptors.

- Endogenous opioids like endorphins, enkephalins and dynorphins modulate pain perception, mood, hedonic (pleasure) response, motor behaviour, emesis, pituitary hormone release, gastrointestinal motility, placebo/stress/acupuncture-induced analgesia, and neurohormone and neuromodulator role.

Questions for practice

1. Classify opioid analgesics.
2. Enumerate therapeutic uses of morphine.
3. Enumerate adverse effects of morphine.
4. Write short notes on:
   a. Opioid antagonists
   b. Endogenous opioids
   c. Opioid tolerance and dependence
   d. Neurolept analgesia
5. Describe pharmacological basis for the use of
   a. Morphine in acute left ventricular failure
   b. Methadone in opium addiction
6. Explain why morphine is contraindicated in
   a. Undiagnosed abdominal pain
   b. Head injury

Hints for problem-based questions and MCQs

1. c. Meperidine (Refer to Flowchart 22.1, page 298 for questions 1–5).
2. a. antagonist at κ and partial agonist at μ-receptors
3. d. Butorphanol
4. c. Pentazocine
5. i. c. Endogenous opioid
   ii. Dynorphins, enkephalins
6. i. a. Increased sensory neuron activity and transmitter release is the incorrect statement (opioids decrease peripheral sensory neuron activity and NTM release → refer page 298)
   ii. Refer to page 298
7. i. c. Uterine
   ii. Prolonged labour and Increased neonatal morbidity (Refer to page 300)
8. b. Miosis (Refer to page 300)
9. i. a. Miosis (no tolerance develops to miotic action of opioids)
   ii. Pin-point pupil indicates opioid overdose
10. a–2; b–3; c–1 (Refer to page 299)
11. i. Refer to page 301
    ii. Sustained-release preparations, transdermal patch, buccal/transmucosal, nasal insufflations of strong opioids, rectal suppositories, etc.
12. Refer to page 301
13. d. Diphenoxylate
14. c. Nalbuphine (Refer page 302)
15. Refer to page 302
16. a. Respiratory depression
17. i. Bronchial asthma can be worsened
    ii. Due to histamine release
    iii. Fentanyl in low dose
18. i. b. Morphine is contraindicated in head injury
    ii. Refer to page 303
19. i. Acute opioid poisoning
    ii. Refer to page 303
20. i. Opioid withdrawal symptoms in neonates
    ii. Diazepam, tincture opium, methadone (Refer page 303)
21. a. Codeine
22. b. Pethidine
23. i. c. Diacetylmorphine
    ii. Methadone for detoxification and maintenance therapy. Refer to page 305
24. c. Pentazocine
25. c. Methylnaltrexone

CONCEPT MAP – OPIOID ANALGESICS AND ANTAGONISTS

OPIOIDS (Prototype: Morphine)

Mechanism of Action
Act through G_i-linked μ, κ, δ-receptors
↓
↓ed sensory neuron activity
↓ed spinal cord pain transmission
↑ed endogenous opioid release

Major Pharmacological Actions
μ actions: dependence, miosis, constipation, analgesia, respiratory depression/rigidity, euphoriant and sedative effects.

κ actions: constipation, analgesia, psychomimetic i.e. dysphoric, pulmonary (respiratory depression) and convulsant action.

δ actions: affective, behavorial effects and modulate release of hormomes and NTMs.

Others: Nausea, Vomiting, Cough suppression, ↑ed ICT, Bronchoconstriction, Contraction of sphincter of Oddi, Urinary retention, Uterine relaxation

Tolerance: To most actions except miosis, convulsions & constipation

Dependence: Psychological & Physical

Contraindications
Bronchial asthma: Fentanyl and pethidine better than morphine.

Undiagnosed abdominal pain (can worsen biliary colic, pancreatitis)

Head injury

Impaired pulmonary, cardiac, hepatic and renal function.

Elderly individuals and Pregnant women.

Therapeutic Uses
Severe, constant pain due to (trauma, burns, visceral, ischemic, MI, post operative, internal bleed, vascular, cancer or terminal illnesses).

Acute pulmonary edema

In anesthetic practice: pre/intra/post operatively.

Cough suppression: Codiene, Dextromethorphan, Noscapine

Diarrhea: Diphenoxylate, Loperamide

Shivering: Pethidine

ADRs
- Drowsiness, Sedation, Behavioural (restlessness, hyperactivity, malaise, dysphoria)
- Histamine release causing bronchospasm, hypotension especially in hypovolemic patients.
- Nausea, vomiting, Constipation, urinary retention.
- Respiratory depression, Risk of convulsions.
- Tolerance, Dependence, Addiction, etc.

Tolerance: Marked tolerance to analgesic, sedative and respiratory depressant actions.
Some tolerance to emetic, anti diuretic and hypotensive actions.
No tolerance to miotic, constipation and convulsant actions

Cross-tolerance among morphine and its congeners for analgesic, sedative, euphoriant and respiratory effects

Psychological dependence leads to craving and abuse potential

Physical dependence causes withdrawal symptoms on abstinence

Acute Toxicity
Accidental or suicidal, Lethal dose 250 mg.

Presents with Pinpoint pupil, stupor/coma, fall in BP, shock, respiratory depression, shallow breathing, cyanosis, pulmonary edema and death.

Management: Supportive
Intravenous naloxone 0.4–0.8 mg, repeated every 2–3 minutes till respiration picks up.

Withdrawal Symptoms
Intense, start in 6–8 hours, peak at 36 hours & subside in 5 days.

Patient presents with: Rhinorrhea, Lacrimation, Yawning, Chills, Gooseflesh, Hyperventilation, Hyperthermia, Mydriasis, Diarrhea, Muscular aches, Anxiety, Hostility

Management: For detoxification and maintenance therapy.
Buprenorphine, Methadone

SECTION 4 Autacoids and Related Drugs

23 Non-Steroidal Anti-Inflammatory Drugs (NSAIDs)

PH 2.7 Define pain and enumerate drugs used for pain. Explain salient pharmacokinetics, pharmacodynamic, therapeutic uses, adverse drug reactions of analgesics including NSAIDs (except opioids).

Learning objectives

A student of MBBS phase II should be able to:
- Define pain.
- Describe the synthesis of prostaglandins and their role in pain, fever, inflammation, and labour.
- Classify NSAIDs based on their chemical nature and cyclooxygenase (COX) selectivity.
- Describe the mechanism of action as well as pharmacological actions of NSAIDs.
- Comment on the status of selective COX-2 inhibitors in current clinical practice.
- Explain indications for the use of NSAIDs, mentioning the doses.
- Enumerate the adverse effects of NSAIDs and the cautions and contraindications for their use.
- Describe the features and management of salicylate poisoning.
- Describe the features and management of paracetamol poisoning.

PAIN

The International Association for the Study of Pain (IASP) defines pain as 'an unpleasant sensory and emotional experience associated with, or resembling that associated with actual or potential tissue damage'. Prostaglandins are important mediators of pain sensation. Therefore, non-steroidal anti-inflammatory drugs (NSAIDs) mainly exert their analgesic action by inhibiting prostaglandin synthesis.

Prostaglandin Synthesis
(Fig. 23.1)

Increased intracellular calcium, after any type of cell injury activates phospholipase A_2, and arachidonic acid is released from membrane phospholipids. Arachidonic acid is acted upon by cyclooxygenase (COX) and lipooxygenase (LOX) enzymes to synthesise prostaglandins and leukotrienes, respectively (Fig. 23.1).

Prostaglandins (PG) are synthesised from arachidonic acid through the catalytic action of enzyme cyclooxygenase (COX), which exists in 2 isoforms, COX-1 and COX-2.

- COX-1 is the constitutive isoform of the enzyme that supports physiological synthesis of prostaglandins.
- COX-2 is inducible by cytokines and provides prostaglandins at the site of inflammation.

Cyclooxygenase generates prostaglandin G_2 (PGG_2) from arachidonic acid, which is then converted into:

- PGD_2, PGE_2, $PGF_{2\alpha}$, by the action of isomerase in the lungs, spleen, and platelets.
- Prostacyclin (PGI_2) by action of prostacyclin synthase in endothelium of blood vessels
- Thromboxane A_2/B_2 (TxA_2, TxB_2) by action of thromboxane synthase in platelets
- Prostaglandins play important role in pain, inflammation, pyrexia, platelet aggregation, gastroprotection and onset of labour (Table 23.1).

Lipooxygenase catalyses the formation of LTA_4 from arachidonic acid, that subsequently changes into LTB_4, LTC_4 and LTD_4. LTB_4 exerts a chemotactic effect, while LTC_4 and LTD_4 act as slow-reacting substances of anaphylaxis (SRS-A) that may precipitate asthma and anaphylactoid reactions in susceptible individuals.

Non-steroidal anti-inflammatory drugs (NSAIDs) are a group of chemically diverse drugs that possess varying degrees of analgesic, anti-inflammatory, antipyretic and anti-aggregatory properties. These are among the most commonly prescribed drugs. Some NSAIDs are available over-the-counter (OTC), i.e., as non-prescription drugs.

CLASSIFICATION OF NSAIDs

NSAIDs are classified into 2 major groups based on their anti-inflammatory activity.

a. Analgesics and anti-inflammatory drugs
b. Analgesics but poor anti-inflammatory drugs

Based on the selectivity for different isoforms of cyclooxygenase (COX), NSAIDs are classified as non-selective, preferential COX-2 and selective COX-2 inhibitors (Flowchart 23.1).

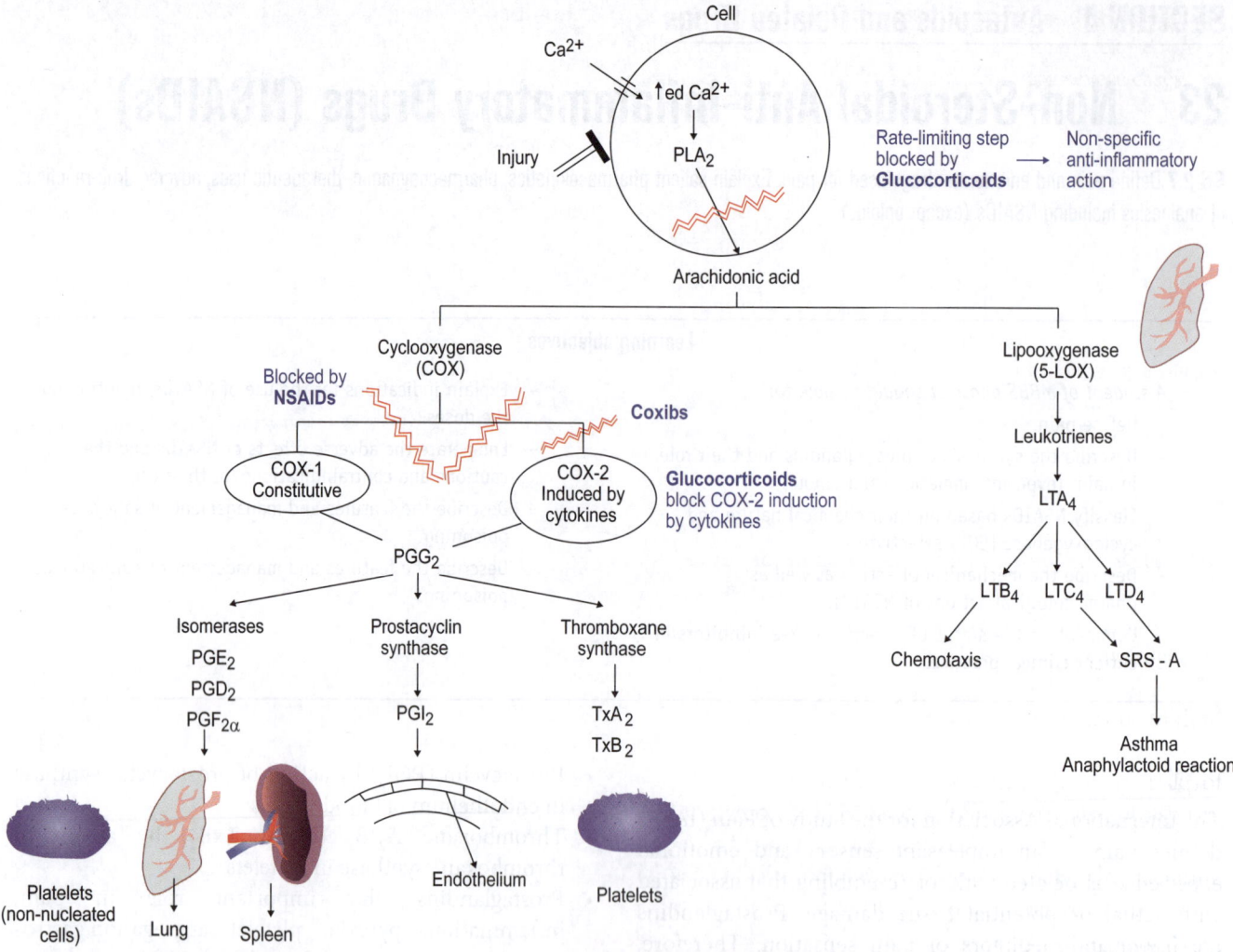

Fig. 23.1 Mechanism of action of NSAIDs

Flowchart 23.1 Classification of NSAIDs

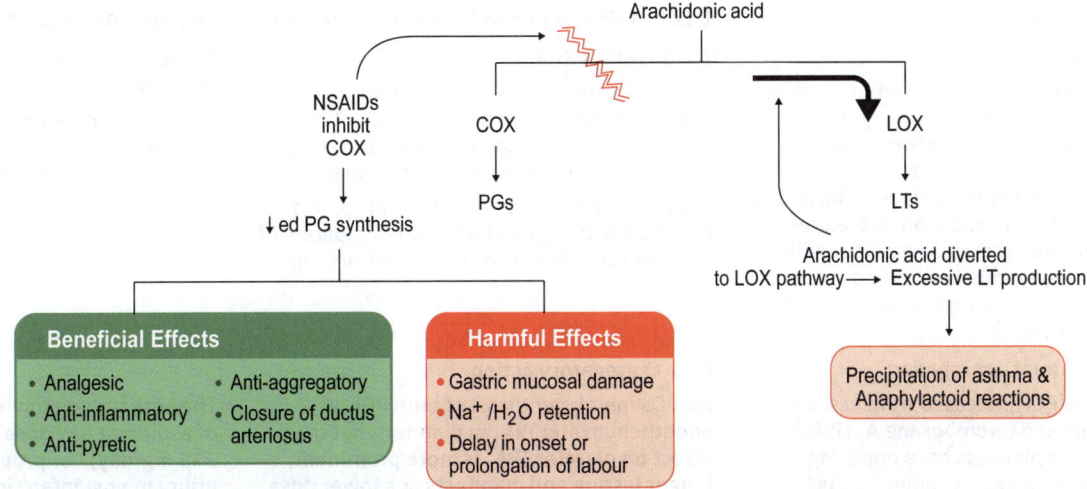

Fig. 23.2 Major actions of NSAIDs

MECHANISM OF ACTION OF NSAIDS

All non-steroidal anti-inflammatory drugs act by **decreasing synthesis of prostaglandins** through cyclooxygenase (COX) inhibition. All NSAIDs cause **competitive, reversible inhibition of cyclooxygenase**, except aspirin, which causes acetylation of COX at the serine residue, resulting in its irreversible inhibition.

Different NSAIDs inhibit COX-1 and COX-2 to different extents, i.e., NSAIDs can be non-selective COX inhibitors, preferential COX-2 inhibitors, or selective COX-2 inhibitors. Inhibition of the COX pathway causes **diversion of arachidonic acid to the LOX pathway**, resulting in excessive production of leukotrienes.

Glucocorticoids exert non-specific anti-inflammatory action by increasing the synthesis of proteins called 'annexins'. These proteins inhibit phospholipase A_2 and **interfere with the release of arachidonic acid from membrane phospholipids**. This is the rate-limiting step of prostaglandin synthesis. Thus, glucocorticoids inhibit the formation of end products of both COX as well as LOX pathways. This is beneficial in bronchial asthma patients. Glucocorticoids also **inhibit induction of COX-2 by cytokines** and other mediators. Thus, prostaglandin synthesis at the site of inflammation is suppressed, contributing to their non-specific anti-inflammatory action.

PHARMACOLOGICAL ACTIONS OF NSAIDS (ASPIRIN PROTOTYPE)

Most of the useful as well as harmful effects of NSAIDs are linked to their major action, i.e., inhibition of PG synthesis (Fig. 23.2).

Table 23.1 describes pathophysiological roles of prostaglandins and correlates the major actions and adverse effects of NSAIDs to inhibition of PG synthesis.

Table 23.1 Major actions and adverse effects of NSAIDs

Action of prostaglandins	Effect of NSAIDs due to PG synthesis inhibition	Therapeutic use/ADR
1. Role in pain Prostaglandins are released in response to bradykinin and cytokines. These cause sensitisation of afferent nerve endings to painful stimuli by lowering the threshold of polymodal nociceptors of C-fibres, leading to hyperalgesia	**Analgesic action** - NSAIDs prevent prostaglandin-mediated sensitisation of nerve endings - Increase pain threshold and exert analgesic effect - Relieves inflammatory, integumental, connective tissue injury pain	Used in aches and pains e.g., headache, backache, toothache, joint pain, myalgia, neuralgia and dysmenorrhea **Analgesic dose of aspirin: 0.3–0.6 g, 6-8 hourly**
2. Role in inflammation Cytokines and other inflammatory mediators induce COX-2, releasing prostaglandins at the site of inflammation. Prostaglandins cause: - Vasodilatation - Increased permeability - Chemotaxis - Pain during inflammation	**Anti-inflammatory action** - PG synthesis inhibition by NSAIDs is the major mechanism of their anti-inflammatory action. - NSAIDs also decrease sensitivity of vessels to other mediators of inflammation like histamine and bradykinin. - Some NSAIDs inhibit adhesion of granulocytes to damaged vasculature, stabilise lysosomes and inhibits migration of leukocytes/macrophages to the inflammatory site.	**Useful in inflammatory conditions** such as acute rheumatic fever, rheumatoid arthritis, acute gout and osteoarthritis - **Anti-inflammatory dose of aspirin is 4–6 g/day. It is higher than the analgesic dose.**

Action of prostaglandins	Effect of NSAIDs due to PG synthesis inhibition	Therapeutic use/ADR
3. Role in fever Conditions such as infection, inflammation, malignancy, tissue damage and graft rejection lead to increased formation of pyrogens like cytokines (IL-1β, IL-6, TNFα, IFα, IF β) → These **cytokines lead to increased synthesis of PGE$_2$ in and around the pre-optic hypothalamic area** → Increase cAMP that resets the hypothalamic temperature regulating centre at a higher temperature, resulting in fever.	**Antipyretic action** NSAIDs interfere with pyrogen induced production of PGE$_2$ in pre-optic area. Thus, these drugs **reduce body temperature only in fever, not in normothermic individuals.** Vasodilatation of superficial blood vessels → profuse sweating and increased dissipation of heat also contributes to antipyretic action.	NSAIDs are **useful in fever of any origin.** **Antipyretic dose of aspirin is same as the analgesic dose, i.e., 0.3–0.6 g, 6–8 hourly.**
4. Role in platelet aggregation Prostacyclin (PGI$_2$) released from vascular endothelium and thromboxane A$_2$ (TxA$_2$) synthesised in platelets have opposing effects on platelet aggregation, i.e., **TxA$_2$ induces platelet aggregation, whereas PGI$_2$ opposes it.**	**Anti-aggregatory action** NSAIDs inhibit synthesis of both PGI$_2$ in endothelium and TxA$_2$ in platelets, but the **effect on platelet TxA$_2$ is more prominent, longer lasting and manifests at a lower dose of aspirin** (as low as 40 mg) → Reduction of pro-aggregatory factor (TxA$_2$) → anti-aggregatory effect → So, there is tendency to prolong bleeding time. Platelets are non-nucleated and are therefore not able to synthesis new enzyme. Thus, once irreversibly inhibited by **aspirin, the effect on platelets persists for their life span of 8–10 days,** till they are replaced by new platelets. Long-term use of aspirin **decreases synthesis of clotting factors,** which contributes to increased bleeding tendency. At higher dose (> 325 mg), PGI$_2$ synthesis in endothelium is also inhibited. As PGI$_2$ has anti-aggregatory and vasodilator activity → decreased PGI$_2$ levels favour platelet aggregation. In other words, **beneficial anti-aggregatory effect of aspirin can be reversed at high doses.** Hence, aspirin is always used in a low dose for its anti-aggregatory effect.	The anti-aggregatory effect of aspirin **at low dose (40–325 mg/day)** has prophylactic utility in **post infarction, post stroke** and **TIA** patients. But owing to their anti-aggregatory potential, NSAIDs are **contraindicated in patients with bleeding tendencies and are stopped one week prior to elective surgery.**
5. Role in patency of ductus arteriosus (DA) PGE$_2$, PGF$_{2α}$, and PGI$_2$ cause vasodilatation, maintain placental blood flow and patency of ductus arteriosus in fetal life. At birth, PG synthesis turns off and DA closes. If DA fails to close after birth, the condition is known as **patent DA (PDA)**	Aspirin or indomethacin inhibit PG synthesis and **close PDA within few hours.** - Sometimes, NSAIDs given in late pregnancy may cause premature closure of DA.	**Used in PDA** NSAIDs should be **avoided in late pregnancy, near term.**
6. Role in labour - PGE$_2$ and PGF$_{2α}$ **increase the tone and amplitude of uterine contractions** in pregnant as well as non-pregnant uterus. - Excessive PG production by endometrium causes uncoordinated uterine contractions, blood vessels compression and uterine ischemia and **dysmenorrhea.** - Release of PG from fetal tissue at term causes **initiation and progress of labour** and makes the cervix soft and more compliant. Due to this effect, PG analogues are used for termination of pregnancy at any stage and induction/augmentation of labour due to their oxytocic action and **cervical priming/ripening action.**	NSAIDs can **prevent uncoordinated contraction** of uterine muscles and relieve pain of dysmenorrhea. NSAIDs inhibit PG synthesis and have a potential for **delaying labour** or decrease its progression rate.	Mefenamic acid is effective in **dysmenorrhea.** NSAIDs are **contraindicated in pregnancy** because of the risk of delayed labour and premature DA closure. Risk of low-birth-weight baby is also reported.

Action of prostaglandins	Effect of NSAIDs due to PG synthesis inhibition	Therapeutic use/ADR
- For induction of labour in patients with eclampsia, pre-eclampsia, cardiac diseases or renal diseases, PG analogues may be considered better than oxytocin as these do not possess antidiuretic effect. - PGs are also useful in post-partum hemorrhage not controlled by oxytocin or ergometrine.		
7. Ulcer-protective role In stomach, PGE_2 and PGI_2 are gastro-protective as they: - Reduce acid secretion, volume of gastric juice, and pepsin content. - Increase mucus secretion - Increase mucosal blood flow PG increases propulsive and secretory activity in intestines and may cause colic pain and diarrhea as important adverse reactions.	**NSAIDs enhance the aggressive factors and suppress defensive factors** in gastric mucosa by inhibiting PG synthesis. So, NSAIDs tend to increase acid secretion, reduce mucus and HCO_3^- secretion and promote mucosal ischemia. Hence they have ulcerogenic potential.	NSAIDs can cause **gastric pain, mucosal erosion, ulceration** and blood loss from ulcer as important adverse effects. NSAIDs are **contraindicated in patients with pre-existing peptic ulcer** disease.
8. Diuretic effect PG causes: - Renal vasodilatation → increase in renal blood flow - Inhibition of tubular reabsorption - Oppose action of ADH All three actions result in diuresis.	NSAIDs cause **Na^+ and H_2O retention** by inhibiting PG synthesis.	The sodium–water retaining effect of NSAIDs is not marked in normal individual but can be **deleterious in CHF, cirrhosis, renal disease and hypertension.**
9. Bronchial muscles PGE_2 and PGI_2 are **bronchodilators.** They reduce histamine release from mast cells, whereas $PGF_{2\alpha}$ and TxA_2 cause bronchoconstriction.	NSAIDs can precipitate asthma and anaphylactoid reactions in susceptible individuals, because of the diversion of arachidonic acid to lipoxygenase pathway after COX inhibition by NSAIDs. Thus, more leukotrienes are produced, resulting in such action.	Precipitation of **asthmatic attack can occur in susceptible patients,** so, caution should be observed.

Aspirin, the prototype member, has important effects on **metabolism, fluid–electrolyte balance, respiration** and **urate levels**.

Metabolic Effects

These are seen at anti-inflammatory doses only.

- Aspirin **increases cellular metabolism,** especially in skeletal muscles. This results in increased glucose utilisation. Thus, **blood glucose levels** may decrease and liver glycogen stores may get depleted, especially in diabetics. However, sympathetic stimulation at toxic doses may cause hyperglycemia.
- Chronic use of large doses of aspirin favours conversion of proteins to carbohydrates, resulting in **negative nitrogen balance**.
- Levels of **free fatty acids and cholesterol** also decrease.
- **Heat and CO_2 production** increases.

Effect on respiration

Aspirin has a **dose-dependent** effect on respiration that disturbs the acid–base balance (Fig. 23.3).

- Respiration is stimulated at anti-inflammatory doses due to:
  - Peripheral actions: Increased CO_2 production because of increased cellular metabolism.
  - Central action: Increased sensitivity of respiratory centre to CO_2.

  As a result, **respiratory stimulation** and hyperventilation occurs → Washing out excess CO_2 → Respiratory alkalosis → HCO_3^- loss in urine compensates this alkalosis. Respiratory alkalosis manifests as vomiting, headache, vertigo and tinnitus.
  - Very high doses cause **respiratory depression**; CO_2 accumulates, leading to acidosis. Other factors contributing to acidosis include salicylic acid formed by deacetylation of aspirin and excessive pyruvic/lactic/acetoacetic acid formed due to increased cellular metabolism. This acidosis remains uncompensated as HCO_3^- ions are already lost in urine. At this stage, the patient presents with dehydration, loss of vision, hyperpyrexia, convulsions and coma. Death may occur due to vasomotor collapse or respiratory failure.

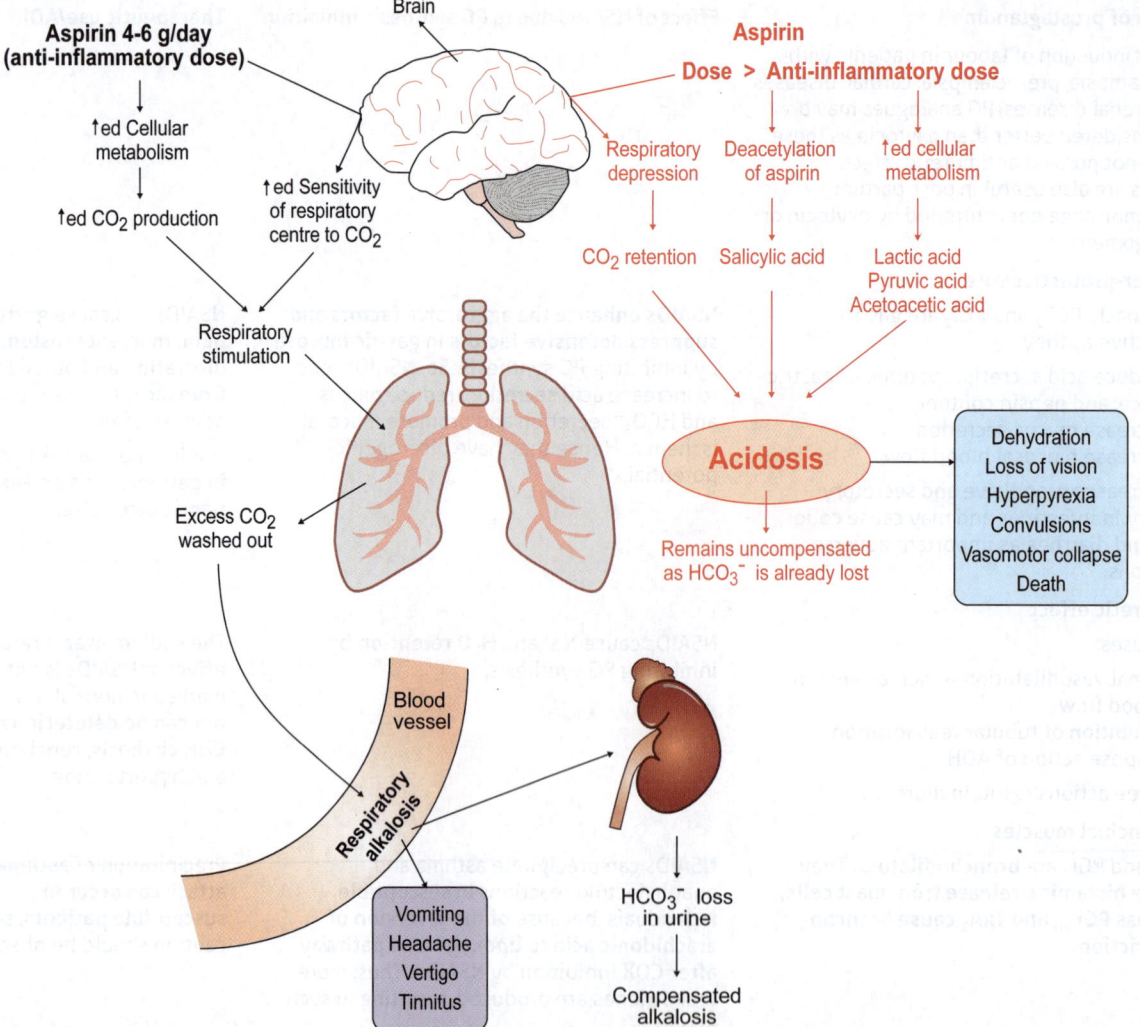

Fig. 23.3 Effect of aspirin on respiration and acid–base balance

Effect on urate excretion

The effect of aspirin on urate excretion is **dose-dependent**.
- Dose lesser than 2 g/day causes urate retention and antagonises other uricosuric drugs.
- There is no significant effect at a dose of 2–5 g/day.
- At high dose > 5 g/day, there is uricosuric effect.

Due to this dose-dependent effect on urate excretion, **salicylates are not used in gout.**

Clinical problem-based questions and MCQs

1. Which of the following drugs possesses almost equal affinity for COX-1 and COX-2?
   a. Valdecoxib
   b. Meloxicam
   c. Acetylsalicylic acid
   d. Aceclofenac

2. Identify the NSAID that has poor anti-inflammatory action.
   a. Indomethacin
   b. Piroxicam
   c. Ibuprofen
   d. Acetaminophen

3. Most of the useful as well as adverse effects of NSAIDs are linked to their inhibitory effect on COX. Identify the adverse effect of NSAIDs not related to COX inhibition.
   a. Peptic ulcer
   b. Fixed drug eruption
   c. Bleeding tendency
   d. Asthmatic symptoms

4. Identify the dose at which aspirin exerts uricosuric effect.
   a. < 1 g/day
   b. 1–2 g/day
   c. 2–5 g/day
   d. > 5 g / day

5. Which of the following correctly describes the metabolic effects of aspirin?
   a. Depletion of hepatic glycogen stores
   b. Hepatic glycogen deposition
   c. Increased protein synthesis
   d. Increased levels of cholesterol

6. Which of the following effects of aspirin is lost at higher dose?
   a. Anti-aggregatory
   b. Analgesic
   c. Anti-inflammatory
   d. Gastric irritant

7. Match the drug to its chemical class.
   a. Ibuprofen   1. Anthranilic acid derivative
   b. Nimesulide   2. Arylacetic acid derivative
   c. Mefenamic acid 3. Sulfonanilide
   d. Aceclofenac   4. Propionic acid derivative

8. A 60-year-old female patient presented with pain, swelling on medial aspect of her left knee, difficulty in climbing stairs and inability to fold her leg completely. On examination, there is redness, swelling and heat at her left knee joint. Crepitus is present. X-ray reveals narrowed joint space, cartilage loss and osteophytes. The patient is diagnosed with osteoarthritis of the left knee.
   i. Comment on the mechanism of beneficial effect of NSAIDs in this case.
   ii. What is the appropriate dose of aspirin in this case?

9. Aspirin being used in the above case of osteoarthritis has the potential to cause respiratory alkalosis as well as respiratory acidosis. Describe the mechanism of respiratory actions of aspirin at different doses.

10. A 50-year-old hypertensive woman's symptoms were well controlled with antihypertensive drugs. She suffered from osteoarthritis concurrently, and naproxen therapy was started. On regular follow-up, her BP control was observed to be worsening. The dose of antihypertensive was increased.
    i. What is role of naproxen in this case?
    ii. Explain the worsening of hypertensive control on starting naproxen.

PHARMACOKINETICS OF NSAIDs

- NSAIDs are well absorbed orally. Aspirin has poor water solubility. Its absorption can be enhanced by **microfining** the drug particles.
- Most of NSAIDs are metabolised by liver. **Metabolic process of aspirin gets saturated over the therapeutic range.**
- Excretion occurs in urine. Varying degree of biliary secretion and entero-hepatic circulation also occurs.

Therapeutic Uses of NSAIDs

1. **Fever**: NSAIDs can relieve fever of any origin. For aspirin, the antipyretic dose is **0.3–0.6 g, given 6–8 hourly. Paracetamol, which has more central-to-peripheral cyclooxygenase inhibitory activity is the preferred drug.** It is especially beneficial in children with viral infections, where aspirin can cause Reye's syndrome. Paracetamol is devoid of anti-aggregatory and gastrointestinal adverse effects.
2. **Pain of musculoskeletal disorders**: NSAIDs are used as analgesics in relieving mild-to-moderate pain of musculoskeletal disorder. They can relive **headache, backache, toothache, myalgia, arthralgia, neuralgia and dysmenorrhea.** Analgesic dose of aspirin is the same as the antipyretic dose.
3. **Inflammatory conditions**: NSAIDs are used to relieve symptoms like pain, swelling and morning stiffness in **rheumatoid arthritis**. They also relieve symptoms of **acute gout, osteoarthritis, ankylosing spondylitis, bursitis and tendonitis.** Anti-inflammatory dose of aspirin is **4–6 g/ day.**

Choice of NSAIDs in current clinical practice

All the NSAIDs have almost equal efficacy; the choice depends on their relative gastric mucosal damaging effect.

- **Aspirin is rarely used** nowadays for analgesic, antipyretic or anti-inflammatory actions. **Other NSAIDs are preferred** because of their better tolerability.
- **Preferential COX-2 inhibitors** like diclofenac, aceclofenac, nimesulide and lornoxicam have much better gastric tolerability than non-selective COX inhibitors, and are more frequently prescribed.
- **Doses of commonly prescribed NSAIDs:**
  - Diclofenac is given in a dose of 50 mg TDS or 75mg BD orally. It can also be used intramuscularly.
  - Dose of aceclofenac is 100 mg BD.
  - Another commonly prescribed NSAID for analgesic action is ibuprofen in a dose of 400–600 mg TDS.
  - Mefenamic acid 250–500 mg TDS is preferred for dysmenorrhea.
  - Sulfasalazine (0.5–1 g/day) can be used along with methotrexate as disease-modifying antirheumatic drug.
- **Topical application** is used to decrease the risk of systemic adverse effects of NSAIDs, e.g.,
  - Ethyl ammonium salt of diclofenac is used for topical application as 1% gel ointment or eye drops.
  - Other topically used NSAIDs are nimesulide 1%, piroxicam 0.5%, ibuprofen 10% gel/ointment.
  - Methyl salicylate or oil of wintergreen is used as counterirritant.
  - Flurbiprofen and ketorolac are used as eye drops in relieving pain associated with ocular surgeries and conjunctivitis.

4. **Migraine**: NSAIDs are used as abortive therapy in **mild-to-moderate migraine**. The treatment is more effective if given early, within 15 minutes of onset of mild headache, with occasional throbbing but no functional impairment. If pain is not relieved by one or two doses of NSAIDs, other drugs like triptans are used.

5. **Post-operative pain**: **Ketorolac** is effective for controlling post-operative pain. It may be combined with opioids to decrease their dose.
6. **Acute rheumatic fever**: Aspirin used in acute rheumatic fever produces dramatic symptom relief. Naproxen can be used as an alternative.
7. **In post-myocardial infarction, post-stroke, transient ischemic attack**: Aspirin is used as a prophylactic to prevent recurrence. It also decreases chances of infarction in new-onset or sudden worsening angina. For anti-aggregatory effect, aspirin is used in **low dose of 75–162 mg/day** (usual dose is 81 mg), because at higher doses the beneficial effect may be lost (due to prostacyclin PGI_2 synthesis inhibition). Anti-aggregatory doses of aspirin* are given after the 12th week in pregnant women prone to **preeclampsia, to decrease the risk of** developing the condition.

> * Some NSAIDs such as **ibuprofen, fenamates, naproxen, nimesulide and piroxicam significantly interfere with the anti-aggregatory effect of aspirin.** Thus, if any of these NSAIDs is to be used in a patient on chronic low-dose aspirin therapy for anti-aggregatory effect, care should be taken to give aspirin at least half an hour before the other NSAID. However, ketorolac, diclofenac and acetaminophen do not interfere with the antiplatelet action of aspirin.

8. Aspirin may have a role in providing symptom relief in **familial colonic polyposis** and **prevention of colonic carcinoma**.
9. Topical application of salicylic acid is useful in treating **acne, corns, calluses and warts**.
10. Sulfasalazine and olsalazine are useful in the treatment of **lower GI inflammatory conditions like ulcerative colitis**.

Clinical problem-based questions and MCQs

11. A 60-year-old male presented in the emergency department with sudden-onset slurred speech, left facial droop, and weakness in the left arm and leg. He has a 3-year history of diabetes and 5-year history of grade II hypertension, which were well-controlled with metformin and thiazides respectively. He is a non-smoker and consumes approximately 10 standard alcoholic drinks per week. On examination, BP was 140/90 mmHg and pulse 76 bpm. Neurological exam revealed left facial droop, 0/5 motor power in the left arm, and 2/5 in the left leg. CT scan showed occlusion of the M1 segment of the right middle cerebral artery, which has caused the acute ischemic stroke. He was treated with IV tissue plasminogen activator and showed significant improvement over 10 days. At discharge, he was started on aspirin 75 mg daily along with his existing medications.
    i. Explain the rationale behind the prescription of aspirin in this patient with a history of stroke.
    ii. Why is the dose of aspirin is kept very low compared to anti-inflammatory dose?

12. A 65-year-old known case of diabetes and grade II hypertension presented in emergency with a history of dyspnea, orthopnea, profuse sweating and severe pain on the left side of chest radiating to left shoulder and left side of the jaw. On examination, BP = 124/86, PR = 78 bpm; ECG shows T wave inversion in lateral leads. The patient responded well to nitrate therapy and oxygen inhalation. At discharge, along with nitrates, aspirin 75 mg once a day was prescribed as drug of first choice.
    i. What is the diagnosis?
    ii. Describe the pharmacological basis for prescribing low-dose aspirin in this case.
    iii. Why other NSAIDS are not preferred for this indication?

13. Aspirin is the prototype NSAID, but other NSAIDs are preferred nowadays for analgesic, antipyretic, anti-inflammatory action.
    i. Explain the cause of disrepute of aspirin.
    ii. Mention the clinical conditions in which aspirin is still preferred.

Adverse Drug Reactions of NSAIDs

Most of the NSAIDs cause qualitatively similar adverse effects as given below (Fig. 23.4).

1. Central adverse effects

- Tinnitus is ringing sensation in ears,
- Dizziness
- Nimesulide can cause ataxia, dizziness, somnolence, etc.
- Indomethacin has the risk of causing mental confusion, hallucinations, depression, psychosis and is contraindicated in patients with pre-existing psychiatric illnesses.

2. Gastrointestinal adverse effects

The common gastrointestinal adverse effects of NSAIDs are nausea, vomiting, dyspepsia, epigastric pain or discomfort, erosions/ulcerations of mucosa and occult blood loss in stools. These are related to gastric mucosal damage caused by NSAIDs. The **ulcerogenic potential** of NSAIDs is due to their ability to suppress prostaglandin (PGE_2, PGI_2) synthesis that knock down the ulcer-protective effect of prostaglandins. Ion trapping of acidic drugs due to pH partition contributes to mucosal damage.

The extent of mucosal damage caused by NSAIDs varies. Relative gastric toxicity is an important factor in the choice of NSAIDs.

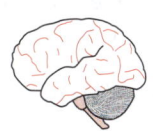

Central
- Tinnitus
- Ataxia, dizziness, somnolence (Nimesulide)
- Psychosis (Indomethacin)

Pulmonary adverse effects
- Risk of precipitating asthma
- Hyperventilation at high dose

Cardiovascular adverse effects
- Na^+ and H_2O retention
- Risk of hypertension, edema, CHF, myocardial infarction
- Increased risk of cardiovascular events with coxibs

Hepatic Effects
- Aspirin: Raised serum transaminase, especially in children with rheumatoid arthritis.
- Hepatic encephalopathy or Reye's syndrome in children with viral infections
- Fulminant hepatic failure especially in children with Nimesulide

Gastrointestinal
- Nausea, vomiting, dyspepsia, gastric pain or discomfort, erosions, ulcerations of mucosa, occult blood loss in stools.
- *Risk*: Maximum with Indomethacin
- Negligible with preferential and selective COX-2 inhibitors and paracetamol.
- Diarrhea (Mefenamic acid, Nabumetone)

Hematological effects
- Increased risk of bleeding with aspirin
- Hemolytic anemia (Mefenamic acid)
- Rarely neutropenia, thrombocytopenia, aplastic anemia

Renal adverse effects
- Fluid retention
- Edema and azotemia (piroxicam).
- Renal insufficiency, Nephritis, Renal failure rarely.

Pregnancy
- Premature closure of ductus arteriosus
- Delayed onset or prolongation of labour.

Hypersensitivity reactions
- Rashes, urticaria, rhinorrhea or fixed drug eruptions
- Rarely, serious angioedema, asthma and anaphylactoid reactions

Fig. 23.4 Adverse drug reactions of NSAIDs

- Aspirin can cause gastric mucosal damage even at analgesic doses (0.3–0.6 g, 6–8 hourly).
- **Indomethacin has very high ulcerogenic potential**. So, it is reserved for refractory cases only, such as Bartter syndrome.
- Mucosal damage is **negligible with preferential and selective COX-2 inhibitors and paracetamol**.
- The extent of irritant effect in lower GIT correlates with the degree of enterohepatic circulation.

- Food does not interfere with absorption of NSAIDs but decreases the risk of gastric irritant actions. Therefore these **drugs should be administered after intake of food**.
- Proton pump inhibitors and prostaglandin analogue **misoprostol, are co-administered** with NSAIDs to counteract their GI toxic effects.
- The anthranilic acid derivative, **mefenamic acid, causes diarrhea** as an important dose-related adverse effect.
- Nabumetone causes **abdominal cramps and diarrhea**.

3. Cardiovascular adverse effects

As NSAIDs block the synthesis of PG in the kidney, they favour Na^+ and H_2O retention.

- Fluid retention is associated with the risk of **hypertension, edema, congestive heart failure, and in rare cases, myocardial infarction.**
- None of the NSAIDs, except low-dose aspirin, show cardioprotective actions.
- NSAIDs **can blunt the antihypertensive action of many drugs**.
- NSAIDs with high COX-2 selectivity increase the risk of cardiovascular events by inhibiting prostacyclin (PGI_2) synthesis.

4. Renal adverse effects

- **Fluid retention** caused by renal action can be risky for patients with congestive heart failure, cirrhosis of liver or renal function impairment.
- Piroxicam has been reported to cause **edema** and **azotemia**.
- Renal **insufficiency, nephritis** and **renal failure** may also occur in rare cases.

5. Hematological effects

- There is increased **risk of bleeding** with aspirin due to decreased platelet aggregation and reduction in synthesis of coagulation factors. Thus, aspirin is contraindicated in patients with bleeding tendencies and is withheld one week prior to elective surgery.
- Mefenamic acid can cause **hemolytic anemia.**
- **Neutropenia, thrombocytopenia and even aplastic anemia** may occur with NSAIDs in rare cases.

6. Hepatic effects

- Aspirin **can raise serum transaminases**, especially in children with rheumatoid arthritis. It is also blamed to cause hepatic encephalopathy or **Reye's syndrome** in children with viral infections like influenza and varicella.
- Nimesulide has the potential to cause **fulminant hepatic failure,** especially in children, and is banned in many countries.

7. Pulmonary adverse effects

Due to blockade of cyclooxygenase pathway by NSAIDs, the arachidonic acid is diverted to the lipoxygenase pathway. This results in production of excess leukotrienes.

NSAIDs, thus, have a risk of **precipitating asthma** in susceptible individuals.

8. Hypersensitivity reactions
Hypersensitivity reactions are not very frequent with NSAIDs, but some patients can develop **rashes, urticaria, rhinorrhea or fixed drug eruptions**. Rarely, serious **angioedema, asthma and anaphylactoid reactions** may occur.

9. Premature closure of ductus arteriosus
This can occur in pregnancy. Given near term, NSAIDs can delay the onset of labour or prolong labour.

10. Salicylism
Salicylism is a syndrome characterised by tinnitus, reversible hearing and visual impairment, confusion, excitement, dizziness, vertigo, hyperventilation and electrolyte imbalance. The syndrome can occur with anti-inflammatory dose (4–6 g/day) of aspirin and thus dose given should be just below the dose at which tinnitus occurs.

11. Acute salicylate poisoning
Also known as aspirin poisoning, this is characterised symptoms such as vomiting, acidotic breathing, hyperventilation, dehydration (due to excessive fluid loss with vomit, with breath and in urine due to HCO_3^- loss), petechial hemorrhages, hyperpyrexia, delirium, restlessness, hallucinations, convulsions and coma. Death occurs due to respiratory or cardiovascular failure.

The fatal dose of aspirin is 15–30 g.

Treatment is mainly supportive to maintain fluid–electrolyte balance, external cooling, gastric lavage, blood transfusion or vitamin K for bleeding tendencies. Forced alkaline diuresis can increase the rate of excretion of aspirin. Hemodialysis is indicated in very severe cases.

Contraindications to the Use of NSAIDs
Aspirin is contraindicated in
- Peptic ulcer
- Bleeding tendency
- Hypersensitivity
- Children with influenza, varicella
- Chronic liver disease: risk of hepatic necrosis
- Pregnancy: risk of low birth weight baby, premature closure of ductus arteriosus, delayed labour
- In asthma patients, selective COX-2 inhibitors are safer than non-selective drugs.

Cautions
- Aspirin administration should be stopped a week prior to surgery.
- High-dose aspirin carries the risk of hemolysis in patients with glucose-6-phosphate dehydrogenase deficiency.
- Congestive heart failure may get worsened due to fluid retention.
- In juvenile rheumatoid arthritis, there is risk of derangement of hepatic enzymes with use of aspirin. Serum transaminase is raised.
- Aspirin should be avoided in diabetics, lactating mothers, and patients with low cardiac reserve.

The therapeutic uses and adverse effects are summarised in Table 23.2.

Table 23.2 Therapeutic uses and adverse effects of NSAIDs

Therapeutic uses of NSAIDs	
- Fever of any origin: paracetamol preferred over aspirin - Headache, toothache, myalgia, neuralgia, arthralgia - Mild-to-moderate migraine - Dysmenorrhea - Acute rheumatic fever - Acute gout, rheumatoid arthritis, osteoarthritis - Ankylosing spondylitis, tendonitis, bursitis	Preferential COX-2 inhibitors are better tolerated than aspirin (Naproxen is commonly used.)
- Post operative pain: ketorolac preferred - Post stroke, post myocardial infarction, transient ischemic attack: low-dose aspirin (75–325 mg) - In high-risk pregnancy to prevent eclampsia: low dose aspirin after 12 weeks of gestation - Familial colonic polyposis: for symptom relief and prevention of carcinoma colon - Acne, corns, calluses and warts: topical salicylic acid used - Lower GI inflammatory diseases like ulcerative colitis: sulfasalazine, olsalazine used	

Adverse effects of NSAIDs	
Central adverse effects	- Dizziness, tinnitus or ringing sensation in ears with **salicylates** - Ataxia, dizziness, somnolence with **nimesulide** - Mental confusion hallucinations, depression, psychosis with **indomethacin**
Gastrointestinal effects	- Gastric mucosal damage, dyspepsia, nausea, vomiting, epigastric pain or tenderness erosions, ulcerations, occult blood loss in stools. **Indomethacin** has maximum ulcerogenic potential. - Abdominal cramps and diarrhea with **nabumetone** and **mefenamic acid**

Adverse effects of NSAIDs	
Hepatic effects	- **Aspirin** can increase serum transaminases, especially in children with rheumatoid arthritis. - It may cause hepatic encephalopathy or Reye's syndrome in children with viral infections like influenza and varicella. - **Nimesulide** has potential to cause fulminant hepatic failure, especially in children. It is banned in many countries.
Renal effects	- Sodium, water retention, which is risky for patients with congestive heart failure, cirrhosis of liver or renal function impairment - Edema and azotemia, especially with **piroxicam** - Occurrence of renal insufficiency, nephritis, renal failure (**rare**)
Cardiovascular effects	- Hypertension, edema, congestive heart failure - Myocardial infarction (**rare**)
Pulmonary effects	- Risk of precipitating asthma in susceptible individuals. - **Nimesulide** is better tolerated by asthmatics than other NSAIDs
Hypersensitivity reactions	- Rashes, urticaria, rhinorrhea or fixed drug eruptions - Occurrence of serious angioedema, asthma and anaphylactoid reactions (rare)
Premature closure of ductus arteriosus	- Can occur in pregnancy
Delay in onset of labour or prolonged labour	- NSAIDs can delay labour when used near term
Salicylism	- Syndrome caused by **aspirin** (Characterised by tinnitus, reversible hearing and visual impairment, confusion, excitement, dizziness, vertigo, hyperventilation and electrolyte imbalance)

Clinical problem-based questions

14. NSAIDS are contraindicated in some conditions.
    i. Which of the following conditions represents a contraindication for use of NSAIDs?
        a. Peptic ulcer
        b. Post-stroke patients
        c. Familial colonic polyposis
        d. Patent ductus arteriosus
    ii. Explain the reason for the contraindication of NSAIDs use in the selected condition.

15. A 35-year-old housemaid had fever and generalised malaise after a hectic day. She took OTC analgesic preparation containing aspirin and paracetamol. Although the fever subsided and body aches were relieved, on the second day she developed severe expiratory dyspnea and wheezing. History revealed several such episodes of dyspnea and wheezing on exposure to dust and pollen. On examination, bilateral rhonchi were present.
    i. What is pharmacological basis for precipitation of symptoms with OTC analgesics in this patient?
    ii. What caution should be observed in future?
    iii. Which analgesics should be preferred over aspirin in this patient in the future and why?

16. A 55-year-old rickshaw puller uses analgesic combination of diclofenac and paracetamol almost daily to allay fatigue. He is a smoker and a habitual drinker. He suffered from a bout of severe epigastric pain with blood-stained vomiting. Upper GI endoscopy revealed hyperemic patches in the gastric mucosa and a small ulcer in the second part of the duodenum.
    i. Explain the role of chronic analgesic use in causation of his signs and symptoms.
    ii. Name the drug that can counteract the GI toxic effects of NSAIDs.

17. A 55-year-old labourer presented in surgery department with a history of swelling in right inguino-scrotal region, which was reducible on lying down. Cough impulse is present. The patient is a known case of atherosclerotic coronary artery disease and is on long-term therapy with aspirin 75 mg daily and nitrates. The surgeon attending him decided to stop aspirin therapy and called him for hernioplasty after one week.
Explain the reason behind the surgeon's decision to stop aspirin therapy.

CHARACTERISTIC FEATURES OF INDIVIDUAL NSAIDs

As selectivity for COX-2 increases, ulcerogenic potential decreases. However, the risk of cardiovascular events (stroke, MI) increases, as shown in Fig. 23.5.

Preferential COX-2 Inhibitors

These drugs have a **20-fold selectivity** for COX-2 over COX-1. They include nimesulide, aceclofenac, diclofenac, etodolac and meloxicam. [Mnemonic – NAMED] They

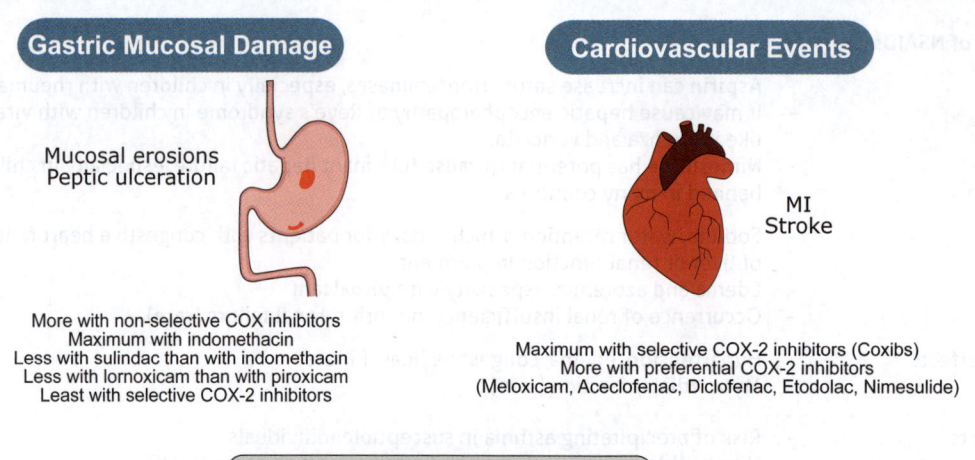

Fig. 23.5 Potential of different NSAIDs for gastrointestinal and cardiovascular adverse effects

are **equally efficacious** as other NSAIDs, but their **gastrointestinal safety is better.**

- **Nimesulide** is a sulfonanilide derivative having some selectivity for COX-2. Its inhibitory effect on PG synthesis is weak, but other mechanisms contribute to its anti-inflammatory action, like free radical scavenging action and inhibition of formation of PAF, TNFα and superoxides.
  - It is useful in **short-lasting conditions,** like sinusitis, bursitis, sports injury, dysmenorrhea, post-operative pain and dental surgery.
  - **Better tolerated by asthmatics** who develop bronchoconstriction with aspirin or other NSAIDs.
  - Due to its **hepatotoxic** potential, it is banned for use in children in many countries including India.
- **Aceclofenac and diclofenac** are both aryl acetic acid derivatives. They are potent anti-inflammatory, analgesic, and antipyretic drugs. These drugs cause preferential COX-2 inhibition and **get accumulated in synovial fluid**. Hence, their therapeutic effect lasts longer than their half-life.
  - In addition, **aceclofenac increases proteoglycan and hyaluronic acid synthesis** in a dose-dependent manner, which may contribute to its anti-inflammatory action.
  - The dose of diclofenac is 50 mg TDS or 75 mg BD, and that of aceclofenac is 100 mg BD.
  - COX-2 selectivity of aceclofenac is higher than that of diclofenac.
  - GI-related adverse effects are fewer than for non-selective COX inhibitors.
  - However, there is a **risk of cardiovascular events**, like stroke and myocardial infarction.
  - Diclofenac has hepatotoxic potential.
- **Meloxicam** is one of the oxicam derivatives that has the same efficacy as piroxicam, but is better than the latter due to lesser gastric adverse effects. Its dose is 7.5–15 mg once a day.
- **Etodolac** (an indole derivative similar to indomethacin) has maximum selectivity for COX-2 after COX-2 inhibitors (also known as coxibs). Hence, gastrointestinal adverse effects are mild. The dose used is 200–400 mg BD for post-operative analgesia and arthritis. It has some uricosuric action in gout.

Selective Cox-2 Inhibitors

These have significant (> **50-fold) selectivity** for COX-2 over COX-1. Drugs included in this category are celecoxib, etoricoxib, parecoxib, and valdecoxib.

Celecoxib is about 375 times more selective for COX-2 than COX-1.

- It is useful in the treatment of rheumatoid arthritis and osteoarthritis.
- The incidence of ulcers is lower than with most other NSAIDs, but as COX-2 inhibition decreases prostacyclin (anti-aggregatory PG) synthesis, the **risk of cardiovascular events like MI or stroke is increased**.
- Celecoxib can also cause abdominal pain or diarrhea as adverse effects.

Etoricoxib is given for ankylosing spondylitis, arthritis or surgical pain in a dose of 60–120 mg once a day. Incidence of GI toxic effects is very low.

Valdecoxib is the shortest-acting drug in this group. **Parecoxib** is a prodrug for valdecoxib and is suitable for parenteral use in post-operative pain. It can cause severe reactions at the injection site. Rofecoxib and valdecoxib have been banned due to risk of myocardial infarction, while lumiracoxib has been banned because of its hepatotoxicity.

NON-SELECTIVE COX INHIBITORS

A. Analgesic, anti-inflammatory

i. Salicylates
- **Aspirin** is the prototype drug. Its actions have been already described in detail
- **Diflunisal** is a fluorinated derivative of salicylic acid. It is more potent than aspirin in anti-inflammatory action, but lacks antipyretic effect due to poor CNS entry. Its antiplatelet effect and GI toxicity are also much lower.
- **Methyl salicylate** or oil of wintergreen is used topically as a counterirritant.
- **Salicylic acid** is used topically in the treatment of acne, warts, corns, calluses.

ii. Oxicam derivatives
Piroxicam is a potent anti-inflammatory drug that has good antipyretic and analgesic effect. Its half-life is long and one daily dose is effective, which is more convenient for patients of chronic arthritis. However, in addition to GI toxicity, it can cause serious skin reactions; hence, it is not considered a first-line drug. Another oxicam derivative, meloxicam, shows some selectivity for COX-2 enzyme, and is described with preferential COX-2 inhibitors.

Lornoxicam is a balanced COX-1 and COX-2 inhibitor; its gastrointestinal adverse effects are comparatively lesser than piroxicam.

iii. Propionic acid derivatives
Ibuprofen is a good analgesic but its anti-inflammatory, anti-aggregatory activity is weaker than aspirin. It is a **very commonly prescribed analgesic in a dose of 400–600 mg TDS.** Rarely, it may cause drug induced aseptic meningitis, blurring of vision and amblyopia as adverse effects.

Ketoprofen is similar to ibuprofen. Additional action of ketoprofen is **stabilisation of lysosomal membrane and bradykinin antagonism.**

Flurbiprofen is fluorinated propionic acid derivative similar to ibuprofen. It is used as 0.03 % eye drops in inflammatory ophthalmic conditions, and for miosis during ocular surgery.

Naproxen has **good anti-inflammatory action** when compared to other propionic acid derivatives. It is useful in osteoarthritis, rheumatoid arthritis, ankylosing spondylitis, bursitis or tendonitis, in a dose of 250 mg BD or TDS.

iv. Indole derivatives
Indomethacin, although more potent than aspirin in anti-inflammatory action, has more incidences of adverse effects. Hence, it is not a first-line drug, but a **reserve drug for refractory cases** like Bartter syndrome related to increased PG synthesis, acute gout and psoriatic arthritis. It causes vasoconstriction which makes it **useful in patent ductus arteriosus.** Indomethacin has high ulcerogenic potential, nephrotoxicity, and carries risk of causing pancreatitis.

Sulindac is a prodrug with fewer GI adverse effects as compared to indomethacin.

Etodolac is a preferential COX-2 inhibitor.

v. Anthranilic acid derivatives
Mefenamic acid has analgesic and antipyretic action. Anti-inflammatory activity is weak. It is useful for relieving pain in short-lasting conditions like **dysmenorrhea and soft tissue injuries** in a dose of 250–500 mg TDS. It can cause diarrhea, elevation of hepatic enzymes, and hemolytic anemia in rare instances.

Ketorolac is a potent analgesic but poor anti-inflammatory. It is **useful in acute control of postoperative pain for short periods.** It can be used by oral or parenteral routes in a dose of 10–20 mg up to four times a day. It may be used in renal colic, pain of bony metastasis, and migraine. It is used topically as eye drops in inflammatory conditions of the eye like iridocyclitis. Sometimes, it is **combined with opioids** to decrease their dose and adverse effects. In addition to GI adverse effects, it can potentially cause headache, dizziness, somnolence, pain at injection site and hepatic toxicity.

B. Analgesic, Antipyretic, But Weak Anti-inflammatory Drugs

Paracetamol
Paracetamol (PCM) is a de-ethylated active metabolite of phenacetin.

It shows **additive analgesic action with aspirin and other NSAIDs.** Many fixed-drug combinations of paracetamol (PCM) with other NSAIDs are available as over-the-counter drugs.

It has **prompt antipyretic effect** due to good CNS penetration and greater affinity for central cyclooxygenase enzyme than peripheral. Thus, it inhibits prostaglandin synthesis in CNS in response to pyrogens and lowers the temperature setup point in thermoregulatory centre.

Its **anti-inflammatory action is weak**, because COX inhibition by paracetamol is poor in the presence of peroxides (generated at the site of inflammation).

Its **tolerability is much higher** than other drugs of the group. Unlike aspirin, it has no effect on respiration, acid–base balance, cardiovascular system and platelets.

Paracetamol poisoning
This is common in small children, who are unable to metabolise paracetamol properly. Large doses > 150 mg/kg or > 10 g in adults can be fatal. The patient presents with abdominal pain, nausea, vomiting, tenderness in hepatic area due to centrilobular hepatic necrosis; jaundice, renal tubular necrosis, hypoglycemia and death may occur.

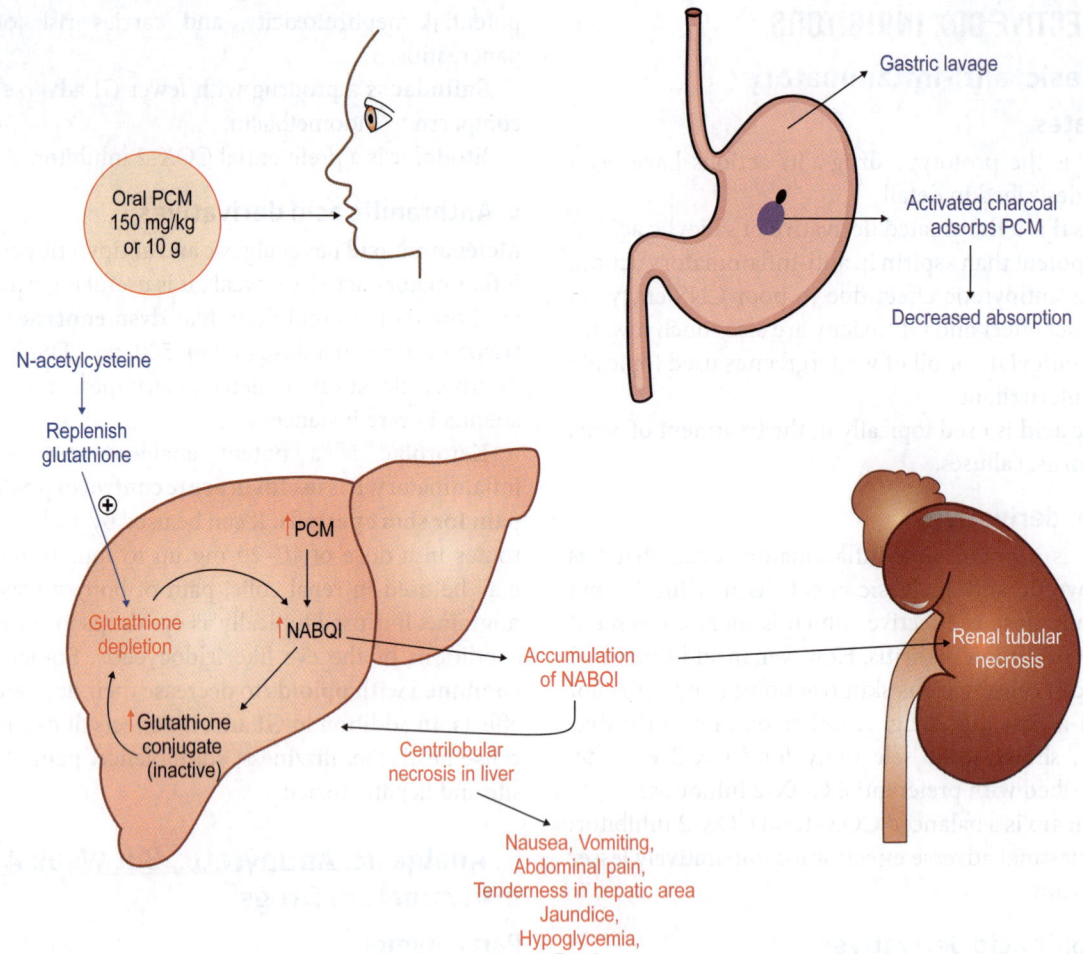

Fig. 23.6 PCM poisoning and treatment

Treatment (Fig. 23.6)
- Gastric lavage is carried out to remove any unabsorbed drug.
- Activated charcoal can help by decreasing the absorption of PCM.
- The specific antidote in paracetamol poisoning is N-acetyl cysteine. A highly reactive metabolite of paracetamol is N-acetyl-p-benzoquinone imine (NABQI). It is further metabolised by glutathione conjugation. In cases of paracetamol poisoning, glutathione depletion results due to its excessive utilisation in conjugating NABQI. This, in turn, leads to accumulation of NABQI, which binds covalently with proteins in hepatocytes and renal tubular cells, causing their necrosis. The risk of toxicity is more in alcoholics, as alcohol induces microsomal enzyme resulting in more formation of NABQI.

N-acetylcysteine replenishes the glutathione stores and prevents cellular necrosis. Its dose is 75 mg/kg every 4–6 hours, for 2–3 days by oral route or I/V infusion of 150 mg/kg in 200 mL of 5% glucose over 15 minutes, followed by the same dose over 20 hours. If treatment with N-acetylcysteine is started later than 16 hours after poisoning, it is not very effective. Patients who fail to respond to N-acetylcysteine may develop fulminant hepatic failure, requiring emergency liver transplantation to save life.

Clinical problem-based questions

18. Which of the following statements about paracetamol is FALSE?
    a. It has good penetration across blood–brain barrier
    b. It causes good COX inhibition in the presence of peroxides at the site of inflammation
    c. N-acetylcysteine is the antidote for PCM poisoning
    d. It does not affect acid–base balance

19. Which of the following NSAIDs is preferred for acute control of post-operative pain?
    a. Diclofenac   b. Ketorolac
    c. Mefenamic acid d. Etoricoxib

20. A 2-year-old child was brought to the emergency department with severe vomiting and abdominal pain. Examination revealed right hypochondrial tenderness and mild jaundice. Random blood sugar was 88 mg/dL, and serum bilirubin was elevated at

2.8 mg/dL. The mother reported a recent episode of high-grade fever with flu-like symptoms the previous week, for which hospital admission was advised but declined. Syrup paracetamol was prescribed (to be given only when the child had fever), but the parents, regardless, administered doses at every 3–4 hour intervals. The child suddenly developed the above symptoms. He was treated with N-acetylcysteine 75 mg/kg every 6 hours, and his condition gradually improved.

  i. Which of the following is the probable cause of the patient's symptoms?
     a. Viral influenza
     b. Paracetamol poisoning
     c. Viral hepatitis
     d. Hypoglycemia
  ii. Explain the pharmacological basis for improvement of this case with N-acetylcysteine.
  iii. What could be the risk of prescribing aspirin instead of PCM in this case?

21. COX-1 is the constitutive and COX-2 the inducible isoform of enzyme. Some NSAIDs have greater affinity for COX-2 than COX-1.
  i. What is the advantage of selective COX-2 inhibitors over non-selective inhibitors?
     a. Lesser risk of bleeding tendency
     b. Lesser risk of cardiovascular events
     c. Lesser risk of peptic ulceration
     d. Better anti-inflammatory effect
  ii. Name selective COX-2 inhibitors and mention their disadvantages.

22. Match the drug with its common therapeutic indication.
    a. Indomethacin   1. Post-operative pain
    b. Mefenamic acid 2. Reserve drug for severe arthritis
    c. Ketorolac   3. Rheumatoid arthritis
    d. Naproxen   4. dysmenorrhea

SERRATIOPEPTIDASE

Serrapeptase is a serine protease obtained from bacteria in the digestive tract of silkworms. Serratiopeptidase is also commercially synthesised. It is a **proteolytic enzyme** having analgesic, anti-inflammatory, fibrinolytic and mucolytic actions.

Mechanism of action

Serine protease binds to COX and **suppresses the release of inflammatory mediators**. It also has affinity for molecules like interleukins and prostaglandins, and degrades them, resulting in anti-inflammatory and analgesic actions. It **interferes with the increase in capillary permeability** in response to histamine and bradykinin. Being a proteolytic enzyme, it **hydrolyses histamine, bradykinin, serotonin**, etc. It also disintegrates abnormal proteins present in exudates; the breakdown products are absorbed into blood or lymph. It **improves microcirculation** at the site of **injury** and improves tissue repair and wound healing.

Serratiopeptidase **prevents the formation of biofilm** and facilitates penetration of antimicrobial agents through preformed biofilms via **dispersion effect**. This effect is useful in various infectious diseases.

It possesses **mucolytic property** that helps to reduce viscosity of tracheobronchial secretions, making it easier to cough out the secretions. During the COVID-19 pandemic, a combination of vitamin D and serratiopeptidase provided good symptomatic relief due to the latter's mucolytic action.

Serine proteases exert **fibrinolytic action, causing clot lysis**. Hence, serratiopeptidase should be stopped two weeks prior to elective surgery. Drug–drug interactions may occur with anticoagulants, antiplatelet and fibrinolytic drugs.

Therapeutic uses

Serratiopeptidase is useful in osteoarthritis, rheumatoid arthritis, painful musculoskeletal conditions, inflammatory bowel disease, ulcerative colitis, sinusitis and other upper respiratory tract infections, chronic obstructive pulmonary disease (COPD), breast engorgement, fibrocystic breast disease and after oral surgery. Adult dose is 5–10 mg, thrice a day, given by oral route, half an hour prior to or 2 hours after meals. It is given as an **enteric-coated tablet**, as it is sensitive to degraded by gastric acid.

ADRs

Serratiopeptidase may cause anorexia, nausea, muscular / joint pain, and allergic reactions such as rashes, erythema and dermatitis. Rarely, Stevens–Johnson syndrome may occur. Bleeding tendencies may be seen due to fibrinolytic action.

> **Summary**
> - Chemically diverse drugs possess analgesic, antipyretic and anti-inflammatory properties to varying extent. The prototype drug is aspirin. Others are derivatives of oxicam, propionic acid, indole, arylacetic acid, pyrazalone and anthranilic acid.
> - Paracetamol and nefopam have analgesic and antipyretic effect, but poor anti-inflammatory action.
> - Major mechanism of action is cyclooxygenase (COX) inhibition, resulting in reduced prostaglandin synthesis.
> - Different members have different affinity for isoenzymes 1 (constitutive) and 2 of COX. NSAIDs may be non-selective, preferential inhibitors of COX-2, or have high selectivity for COX-2.

- Inhibition of PG synthesis is responsible for many useful effects of NSAIDs such as analgesic, anti-inflammatory, antipyretic, anti-aggregatory (with low-dose aspirin) effects and closure of ductus arteriosus.
- At the same time, reduced PG synthesis can cause peptic ulceration, delayed labour, premature closure of ductus arteriosus and Na^+/H_2O retention.
- Diversion of arachidonic acid to the lipoxygenase pathway causing excess LT synthesis may precipitate an attack of bronchial asthma and anaphylactoid reactions.
- Aspirin has dose-dependent effect on urate excretion and respiration.
- Important indications for the use of NSAIDs include fever of any origin, inflammation at any site and mild to moderate pains of musculoskeletal disorders due to any cause.
- Anti-inflammatory dose of aspirin is high (3–6 g/day), whereas for anti-aggregatory effect in post stroke, post-MI patients, aspirin must be used in low dose (75–325 mg). This is because of the more prominent and longer-lasting effect of aspirin on TxA_2 synthesis.
- Aspirin is also useful in newborns with patent ductus arteriosus and familial colonic polyposis.
- Sulfasalazine is used in lower GI inflammatory conditions like ulcerative colitis.
- ADRs of NSAIDs include gastrointestinal side effects, bleeding tendencies, bronchospasm, hypersensitivity reactions, hypertension, edema and central side effects.
- Given in pregnancy, it may delay or prolong labour and cause premature closure of ductus arteriosus.
- In children with viral infection, aspirin can cause Reye's syndrome.
- Acute salicylate poisoning is characterised by hyperventilation, acidotic breathing, vomiting, dehydration, hyperpyrexia and convulsions. It is managed by supportive treatment and forced alkaline diuresis.
- NSAIDs are contraindicated in peptic ulcer, bleeding tendencies, liver disease, history of hypersensitivity, asthma, CHF, pregnant women and children with viral influenza.
- Paracetamol, with good CNS penetration and more affinity for central COX enzyme, is useful as an antipyretic. But it has poor anti-inflammatory property.
- PCM is better tolerated than other NSAIDs, but PCM poisoning is seen in young children, causing abdominal pain, nausea, vomiting, centrilobular hepatic necrosis, and renal tubular necrosis. It needs supportive treatment and N-acetylcysteine that replenishes glutathione and aids in conjugation and elimination of NABQI (N-acetyl-p-benzoquinone imine, a reactive metabolite of PCM).
- Coxibs have more than 50-fold selectivity for COX-2. The advantage of COX-2 selectivity is lesser risk of GI adverse effects like peptic ulcer, but these drugs increase the risk of cardiovascular events like stroke or MI by inhibiting prostacyclin synthesis.
- Serratiopeptidase, a serine protease, has anti-inflammatory, analgesic, antibiofilm, mucolytic and fibrinolytic actions. It is used in osteoarthritis, rheumatoid arthritis, painful musculoskeletal conditions, inflammatory bowel disease, ulcerative colitis, sinusitis and other upper respiratory tract infections, chronic obstructive pulmonary disease (COPD), breast engorgement, fibrocystic breast disease, and after oral surgery. ADRs include anorexia, nausea, muscular /joint pain, and allergic reactions such as rashes, erythema, and dermatitis.

Questions for practice

1. Classify NSAIDs. Enumerate therapeutic uses and adverse effects of aspirin.
2. Comment on the role of
   a. Aspirin in full term pregnant patient.
   b. Aspirin in infants born with patent ductus arteriosus.
   c. Aspirin in primary and secondary prophylaxis of myocardial infarction.
3. Explain why
   a. Alkalinisation of urine is done in aspirin toxicity.
   b. Aspirin overdose can cause both acidosis and alkalosis.
   c. Aspirin should be avoided in children with viral fever.
4. Write short notes on
   a. Acute salicylate poisoning
   b. Paracetamol poisoning
   c. Selective COX-2 Inhibitors

Hints for problem-based questions and MCQs

1. c. Acetylsalicylic acid
2. d. acetaminophen
3. b. Fixed drug eruptions
4. d. > 5 g/day
5. a. Depletion of hepatic glycogen stores
6. a. Anti-aggregatory
7. a–4; b–3; c–1; d–2 (refer to Flowchart 23.1, page 312).
8. i. Refer to Table 23.1, page 313.
   ii. Anti-inflammatory dose of aspirin is 4-6 g/day.
9. Refer to Fig 23.3, page 316.
10. i. Naproxen is a propionic acid derivative that has potent anti-inflammatory action. Its gastric irritant effect is much less than aspirin, so it is preferred for use in osteoarthritis.
    ii. Because of its potential to cause Na^+/H_2O retention (refer to Table 23.1, page 313).
11. i. In post-stroke patients, aspirin is used as a prophylactic agent to prevent the recurrence, because of its anti-aggregatory effect.

ii. For anti-aggregatory effect, aspirin is used in a low dose of 75–162 mg/day (the usual dose is 81 mg) because at a higher dose the beneficial effect may be lost due to prostacyclin PGI_2 synthesis inhibition.

12. i. Acute myocardial infarction
    ii. Refer to page 314
    iii. For anti-aggregatory effect the dose of aspirin is very low. At this dose aspirin is well tolerated, as gastric irritant or other ADRs are mild. Moreover, only aspirin is an irreversible inhibitor of COX, the rest of all NSAIDs are reversible inhibitors. Thus, inhibitory effect of aspirin on platelet TxA_2 synthesis is longer lasting than other NSAIDs.

13. i. Aspirin is rarely used nowadays for the analgesic, antipyretic or anti-inflammatory actions. Other NSAIDs are preferred because of their better tolerability. All NSAIDs have almost equal efficacy, and the choice depends on their relative gastric mucosal damaging effect. Preferential COX-2 inhibitors like diclofenac, aceclofenac, nimesulide and lornoxicam have much better gastric tolerability than non-selective COX inhibitors and are more frequently prescribed.
    ii. Aspirin is still preferred for anti-aggregatory effect in post-MI, post-stroke, transient ischemic attacks. In acute rheumatic fever also, aspirin causes dramatic relief of most of the symptoms and is the preferred drug. Aspirin may have a role in providing symptom relief in familial colonic polyposis and prevention of colonic carcinoma. Topical application of salicylic acid is useful in treating acne, corns, calluses and warts.

14. i. Peptic ulcer
    ii. Refer to page 318.

15. i. Due to blockade of cyclooxygenase pathway by NSAIDs, arachidonic acid is diverted to the lipoxygenase pathway. This results in production of excess leukotrienes. Thus, NSAIDs have a risk of precipitating asthma in susceptible individuals.
    ii. NSAIDs should be avoided in asthma patients as far as possible and they should be warned to always inform the prescriber about their history of asthma.
    iii. In asthma patients selective COX-2 inhibitors are somewhat safer than non-selective drugs.

16. i. The symptoms are due to gastric mucosal damage caused by chronic use of NSAIDs.
    Mucosal damage in GIT occurs even at analgesic doses (0.3–0.6 g, 6–8 hourly) of aspirin. The extent of mucosal damage caused by other NSAIDs varies. The ulcerogenic potential of NSAIDs is due to their ability to suppress prostaglandin (PGE_2, PGI_2) synthesis and knock down ulcer-protective effect of PG. Ion trapping of acidic drugs contributes to mucosal damage.
    ii. Misoprostol, a prostaglandin analogue, when co-administered with NSAIDs, counteracts their GI toxic effects.

17. Aspirin exerts anti-aggregatory effect by causing irreversible COX inhibition in platelets, causing reduced synthesis of TxA_2 and inhibition of platelet aggregation. This can increase blood loss during surgery. So, to avoid risk of excess blood loss during surgery, aspirin should be stopped a week prior to surgery.

18. b. It causes good COX inhibition in the presence of peroxides at the site of inflammation is a wrong statement.

19. b. Ketorolac

20. i. b Paracetamol poisoning
    ii. In cases of paracetamol poisoning, glutathione depletion results due to its excessive utilisation in conjugating NABQI → accumulation of NABQI → bind covalently with proteins in hepatocytes and renal tubular cells, causing their necrosis. N-acetylcysteine replenishes the glutathione stores and prevents cellular necrosis.
    iii. Aspirin used in this child with viral influenza may cause Reye's syndrome.

21. i. c. Lesser risk of peptic ulceration.
    ii. **Selective COX-2 inhibitors** include celecoxib, etoricoxib, parecoxib and valdecoxib. Although the incidence of ulcers is less than most other NSAIDs, but as COX-2 inhibition decreases prostacyclin (anti-aggregatory PG) synthesis, the risk of cardiovascular events like MI or stroke is increased. It can also cause abdominal pain or diarrhea as adverse effects. Parecoxib is a prodrug for valdecoxib and is suitable for parenteral use. It can cause severe injection-site skin reactions.

22. a–2; b–4; c–1; d–3.

CONCEPT MAP - NSAIDs

Mechanism of Action
- Cyclooxygenase inhibition
  ↓
  Decreased PG synthesis
  Irreversible inhibition by Aspirin only
- Divert arachidonic acid to LOX pathway
  ↓
  Increased LT synthesis
- Varying selectivity of drugs for COX-1 & COX-2

Consequences of Reduced PG Synthesis

Beneficial Effects	Harmful Effects
• Analgesic	• Gastric mucosal damage
• Anti-inflammatory	• Na^+ / H_2O retention
• Anti-pyretic	• Delay in onset or prolongation of labour
• Anti-aggregatory	
• Closure of ductus arteriosus	

Important Drugs

Non-selective:
Aspirin, Ibuprofen, Mefenamic acid, Indomethacin, Ketorolac, Lornoxicam

Preferential COX-2 Inhibitor:
Meloxicam, Aceclofenac, Diclofenac, Etodolac, Nimesulide

Selective COX-2 Inhibitors:
Celecoxib, Etoricoxib, Parecoxib

Therapeutic Uses & DOC
- Aches/pains of musculoskeletal origin like headache, toothache, back ache, myalgia, arthralgia, neuralgia: Preferential COX-2 inhibitors
- Dysmenorrhoea: Mefenamic acid
- Mild-to-moderate migraine
- Post operative pain: Ketorolac
- Acute rheumatic fever, Rheumatoid arthritis, Acute gout, Osteoarthritis, Ankylosing spondylitis, Bursitis, Tendonitis: Naproxen
- Fever of any origin: Paracetamol
- Post stroke, Post MI, TIA, Prevention of eclampsia in patients at more risk (after 12 weeks of pregnancy): Aspirin low dose.
- Patent ductus arteriosus: Aspirin, Indomethacin
- Acne, corns, calluses & warts: Topical salicylic acid
- Familial colonic polyposis: Aspirin
- Prevention of carcinoma colon: Aspirin
- Ulcerative colitis: Sulfasalazine, Olsalazine

ADRs

Central: Tinnitus, ataxia, dizziness, mental confusion hallucinations, depression, psychosis

GIT: Nausea, vomiting, dyspepsia, epigastric pain/tenderness, gastric erosions, ulcerations, occult blood loss in stools, abdominal cramps, diarrhea.

Cardiovascular: Hypertension, CHF, rarely MI, harmful in edema, cirrhosis, azotemia, nephritis may occur

Hepatic: Raised serum transaminases, Reye's syndrome or hepatic encephalopathy in children with aspirin, Fulminant hepatic necrosis with nimesulide.

Hypersensitivity as rashes, urticaria, rhinorrhea or fixed drug eruptions. Rarely, serious angioedema, asthma and anaphylactoid reactions

Pregnancy: Premature closure of ductus arteriosus, delayed or prolonged labour, low birth weight baby,

Acute Salicylate Poisoning
Characterised by acidotic breathing, hyperventilation, vomiting, dehydration, petechial hemorrhages, hyperpyrexia, delirium, hallucinations, convulsions, coma, death.
Fatal dose: 15-30 g
Treatment: Supportive, External cooling, Gastric lavage, Blood transfusion or vitamin K, Forced alkaline diuresis, Hemodialysis.

PCM Poisoning
Abdominal pain, nausea, vomiting, tenderness in hepatic area due to centrilobular hepatic necrosis, jaundice may occur, renal tubular necrosis, hypoglycemia and death.
Fatal dose: > 150 mg/kg or > 10 g in adults
Treatment: Supportive, gastric lavage, activated charcoal, N-acetyl cysteine

SECTION 4 Autacoids and Related Drugs

24 Drugs for Gout

PH 2.8 Devise management plan for a case of gout.

Learning objectives

A student of MBBS phase II should be able to:
- Explain pathophysiology of gout.
- Enumerate drugs used in the treatment of gout.
- Describe the mechanism of action of drugs used in acute exacerbation of gout and chronic gout.
- Explain the adverse effects and contraindications of drugs used in gout.
- Describe the management of acute and chronic gout.

PATHOGENESIS OF GOUT

Gout is a metabolic disorder characterised by **recurrent, abrupt, self-limiting episodes of acute arthritis.** The attacks usually occur at night or early morning, and involves one or few joints. The most commonly affected joints are the metatarsophalangeal joint, ankle, heel, wrist and elbow. Fever and generalised malaise may also occur in acute attacks. Chronic **hyperuricemia** always accompanies gouty arthritis. Because uric acid is a product of purine metabolism, hyperuricemia may be aggravated by high intake of proteins. (Gout is often called the 'disease of kings' as rich foods having high protein content may worsen the condition). Hyperuricemia may be primary or secondary.

- **Primary** hyperuricemia occurs due to overproduction of uric acid or reduced excretion of uric acid.
- **Secondary** hyperuricemia occurs due to:
  - other **diseases** like leukemia, lymphoma, polycythemia, diabetic ketoacidosis, psoriasis, and lead poisoning
  - **drugs** like thiazides, furosemide, ethacrynic acid, ethanol, ethambutol, and pyrazinamide

When levels of serum uric acid are high, it precipitates and gets deposited in joints, cartilages, subcutaneous tissues, kidneys, etc.

In joints, phagocytosis of monosodium urate (MSU) crystals, initially by synoviocytes, leads to release of chemotactic factors such as PG, IL-1 and lysosomal enzymes (Fig. 24.1). Polymorphonuclear leukocytes and macrophages migrate into the joint spaces, phagocytose MSU crystals and release a glycoprotein that favours lactic acid production. Lactic acid lowers local pH, favouring more precipitation of MSU and release of lysosomal enzymes, which damage cartilage and articulating surfaces of the bone, resulting in joint immobility.

- Formation of subcutaneous tophi of MSU crystals may occur in the eyelids, pinna of external ear, nose, peri-articular areas, especially near the great toe and wrist.
- Deposition of urate crystals in kidney may cause renal urate stones. Interstitial nephritis can also occur.

MANAGEMENT OF GOUT

Diagnosis

The diagnosis of gout is based upon the presence of hyperuricemia (serum uric acid levels > 7 mg/dL), positive family history, monoarticular or polyarticular disease, presence of tophi, radiological finding of small punched out erosions in periarticular bone, demonstration of MSU crystals in synovial fluid under polarised light, and superadded osteoarthritis changes.

Treatment

Acute gout is managed with drugs such as NSAIDs and colchicine. Among the NSAIDs, piroxicam, naproxen, and indomethacin are preferred, while aspirin and tolmetin are usually avoided.

In patients not responding to NSAIDs, colchicine is tried. Glucocorticoids are reserve drugs for patients not responding to other drugs.

Once the acute attack is controlled, care is taken to avoid precipitating factors.

- Purine-rich foods such as peas, lentils, red meat, and alcohol are omitted from the diet.
- Weight loss is beneficial, especially in obese patients.
- Uric acid synthesis inhibitor, allopurinol, is used as first-choice drug. Febuxostat is an alternative.

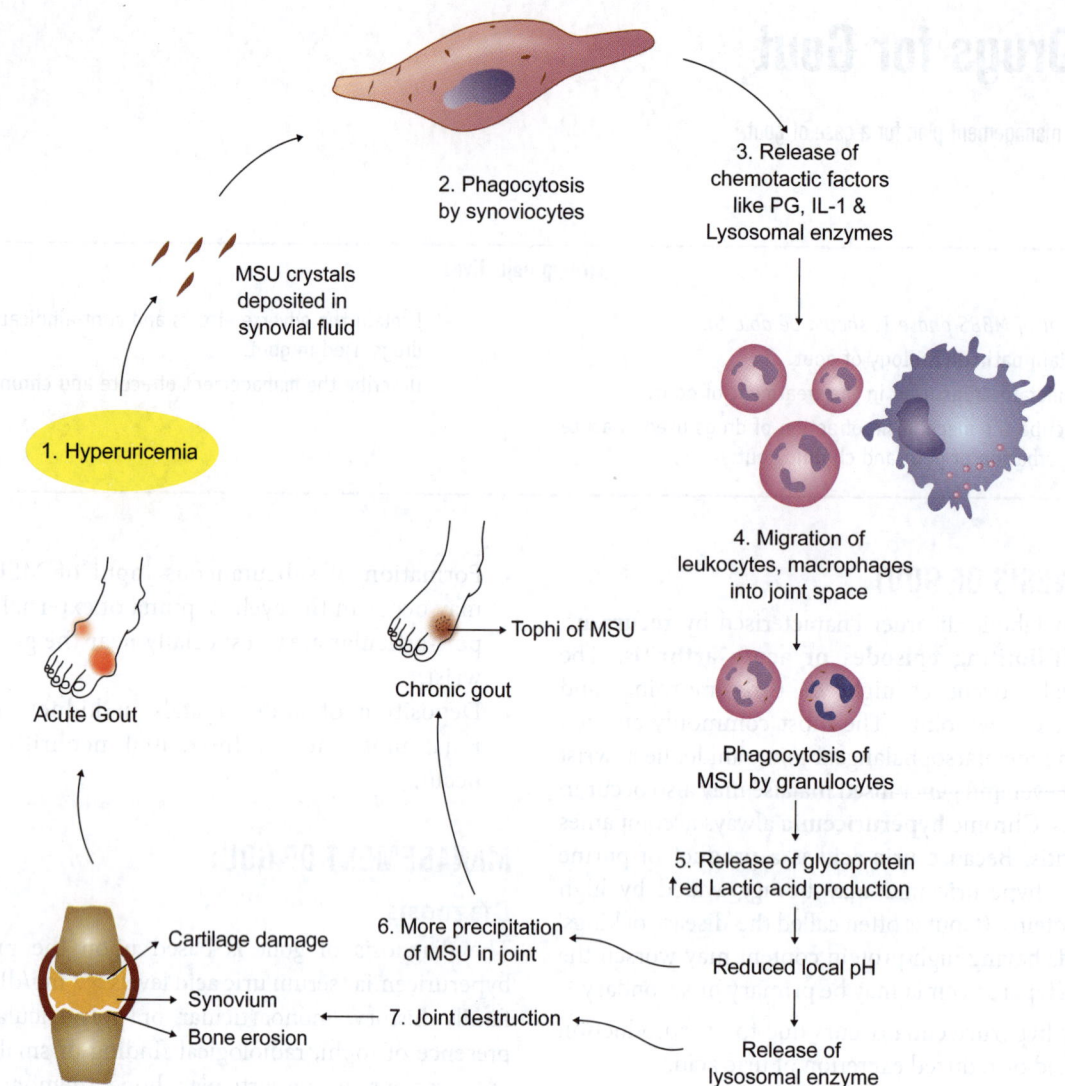

Fig. 24.1 Pathogenesis of gout

- Uricosuric drugs are used if uric acid production is normal, but its excretion is impaired. However, uricosuric drugs are contraindicated in patients with renal failure and urate calculi.

CLASSIFICATION OF DRUGS FOR GOUT

The treatment of an acute attack of gout is different from chronic control of urate levels. Drugs used for chronic gout should not be used during acute attack. In acute gout, NSAIDs, colchicine, glucocorticoids and interleukin inhibitors are useful, whereas in chronic gout, xanthine oxidase inhibitors, uricosuric drugs and mammalian uricase enzyme are useful (Flowchart 24.1).

MECHANISMS OF ACTION OF ANTIGOUT DRUGS

1. Uric acid is an end product of purine metabolism. Hypoxanthine derived from purines is metabolised by enzyme xanthine oxidase to form xanthine and then uric acid. Thus, xanthine oxidase enzyme is an important target for drug action to check uric acid synthesis. For example, **allopurinol and febuxostat act by inhibiting enzyme xanthine oxidase**, and inhibit synthesis of uric acid.

2. In normal individuals, uric acid is freely filtered by glomeruli and then undergoes tubular reabsorption as well as tubular secretion. The organic acid secretory system of the proximal convoluted tubule (PCT) causes the movement of uric acid from the tubular lumen to interstitial fluid. **Uricosuric drugs** like sulfinpyrazone, probenecid, fenofibrate and losartan inhibit the organic acid secretory site OATP (organic anion transporting polypeptides), so that more uric acid stays in the lumen, and is passed out in urine. Thus, these drugs **increase the urinary excretion of uric acid** and are therefore useful in gout.

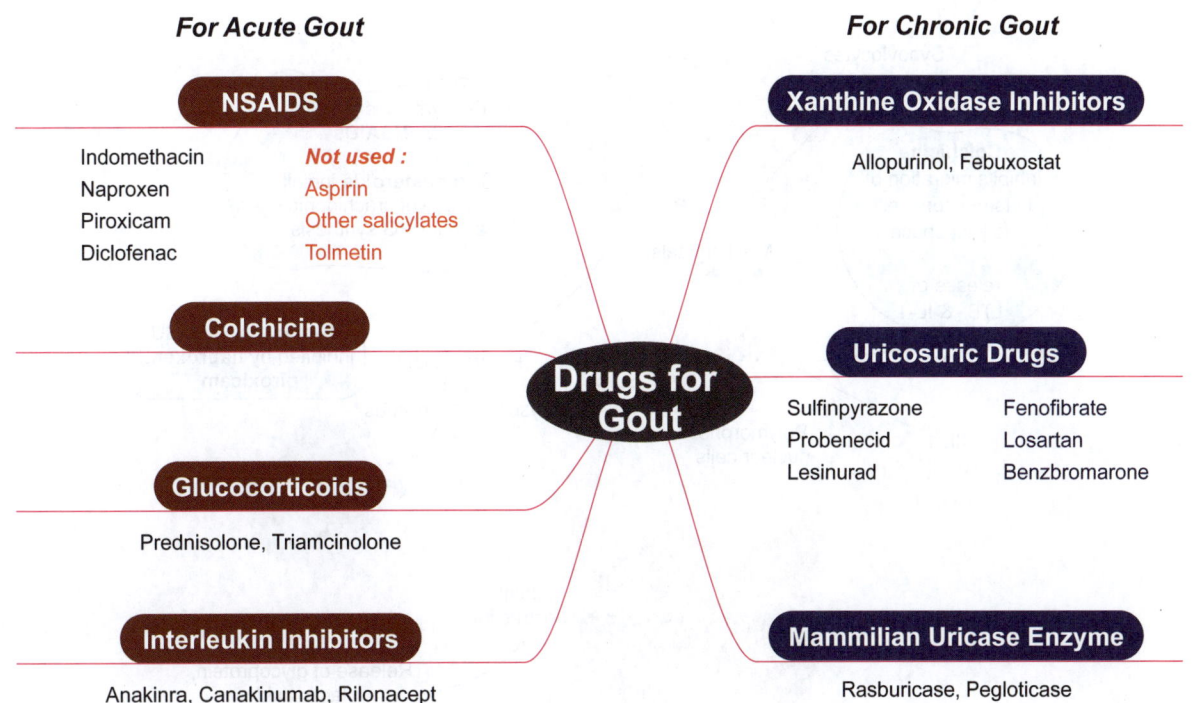

Flowchart 24.1 Drugs for gout

3. **Benzbromarone** has both the above actions, i.e., it causes inhibition of uric acid synthesis by non-competitive inhibition of xanthine oxidase, and also increases uric acid excretion.
4. **NSAIDs** interfere with the process by inhibiting prostaglandin synthesis and **exert anti-inflammatory and analgesic effects**.
5. **Corticosteroids** are useful because of their **non-specific anti-inflammatory** action.
6. **Colchicine** inhibits tubulin polymerisation, migration of leukocytes to the site of inflammation and phagocytosis of urate crystals. Formation of IL-1β and LTB$_4$ is also inhibited.
7. **Interleukin-1 inhibitors** like anakinra, canakinumab and rilonacept are promising drugs for gout as they also oppose IL-1 secretion and actions.

An enzyme called uricase or urate oxidase, present in most birds and mammals, converts uric acid to allantoin that is more soluble and easily excreted by kidneys. However, this enzyme is absent in human beings. **Pegloticase, a recombinant mammalian uricase enzyme** covalently bound to polyethylene glycol, is a new drug that enhances uric acid metabolism and lowers urate levels.

DRUG TREATMENT OF ACUTE GOUT
1. NSAIDs

NSAIDs inhibit enzyme cyclooxygenase, thereby decreasing prostaglandin synthesis and exerting **anti-inflammatory and analgesic** action. In addition, some NSAIDs like **naproxen and piroxicam also inhibit phagocytosis of urate crystals**. This adds to their anti-inflammatory action in acute gout (Fig. 24.2).

Indomethacin 50 mg TDS is the drug of choice. It is commonly given in the beginning of treatment of acute gout. Once the symptoms start improving, the dose can be reduced to 25 mg TDS, and continued for a week or so. Low doses can be continued for a few weeks till the effect of urate lowering drugs becomes manifest.

Other NSAIDs like diclofenac, piroxicam, and naproxen with prominent anti-inflammatory action are also useful. The salicylates (aspirin and tolmetin) are not used in gout patients because **aspirin has a dose-dependent effect on uric acid excretion**. A dose < 2 g/day causes uric acid retention. There is no significant effect on urate excretion with doses between 2–5 g; however, doses > 5 g/day are uricosuric. Although the **response to NSAIDs is slower than to colchicine, these are still preferred as they are better tolerated**.

2. Colchicine

Colchicine was the primary drug for acute gout for many years. It is an alkaloid obtained from plant *Colchicum autumnale*. It possesses **no analgesic or anti-inflammatory activity but still dramatically relieves the symptoms of acute gout**.

Mechanism of action
Colchicine binds to the fibrillar protein, 'tubulin', and prevents its polymerisation to form microtubules, resulting

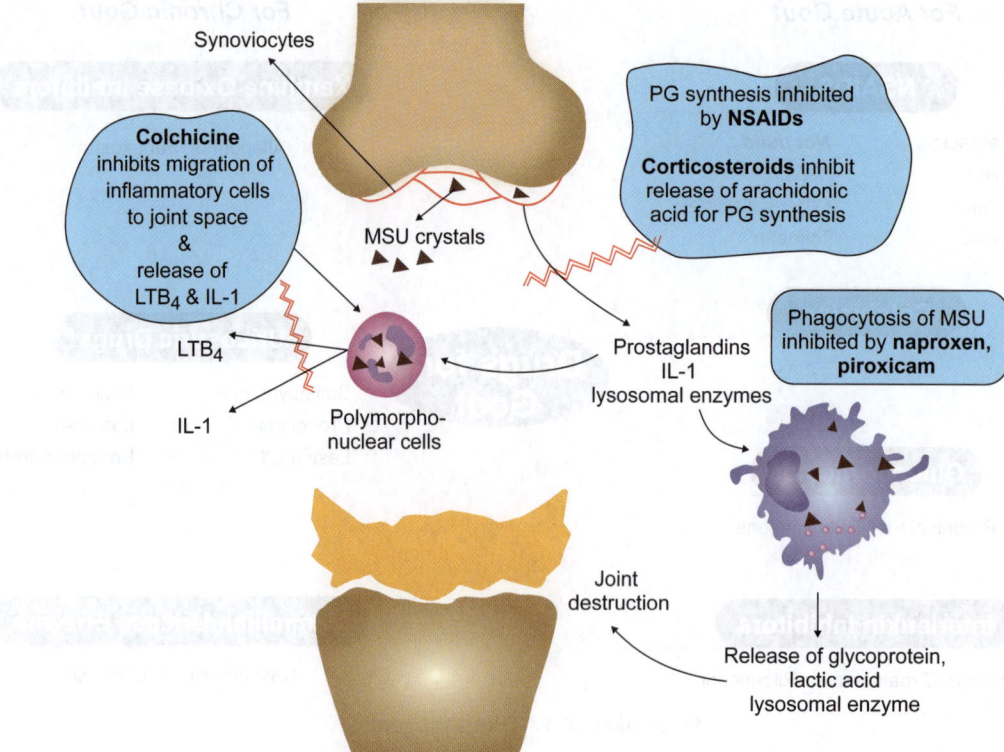

Fig. 24.2 Mechanism of action of drugs in acute gout

in inhibition of leukocytic migration and subsequent phagocytosis. It also inhibits release of chemotactic factors (IL-1 and LTB_4) from neutrophils (Fig. 24.2). Thus, the **vicious cycle of inflammation is interrupted.** During mitosis, colchicine binds to microtubules in the mitotic spindle and causes metaphase arrest Colchicine also increases gut motility.

Therapeutic uses

1. For terminating an **acute attack of gout,** colchicine 1.2 mg, followed by single dose of 0.6 mg, oral, is effective. Intravenous use is associated with serious adverse effects, and has been discontinued.
2. It is used in a low dose of 0.6 mg for **prophylaxis** of gout.
3. It may have some beneficial effects in acute Mediterranean fever, amyloidosis, sarcoid arthritis and hepatic cirrhosis.

ADRs

Though it is very effective in acute gout as well as prophylaxis, it is **not preferred because of its high toxicity**. Dose-related adverse effects include nausea, vomiting, abdominal cramps, diarrhea and intestinal bleeding.

In overdose, colchicine causes:
- Hepatic necrosis
- Disseminated intravascular coagulation
- Acute renal failure
- Convulsions

In rare cases, it can cause bone marrow suppression, hair loss, peripheral neuritis, myopathy and death due to respiratory paralysis.

3. Glucocorticoids

Corticosteroids are very effective in the treatment of acute gout, because of their non-specific anti-inflammatory action. Glucocorticoids inhibit the release of arachidonic acid for prostaglandin synthesis. They produce a **quick response** like colchicine, but because of **too many systemic adverse effects**, steroids are used only as **reserve drug** for patients who do not respond or have some contraindication to the use of NSAIDs.

Prednisolone oral, 30–50 mg/day, for one or two days is advised. Doses are **tapered down** over a week or so. In patients with involvement of one joint or a few joints, **intra-articular** injection of triamcinolone acetonide 10 mg for small joints and 30–40 mg for large joints can be used if patient does not tolerate NSAIDs or colchicine.

4. Interleukin Inhibitors

Anakinra, canakinumab and **rilonacept** target the IL-1 pathway and are **useful in patients who do not respond or develop serious adverse effects to traditional drugs** like NSAIDs/colchicine. Canakinumab is a monoclonal antibody against IL-1β that provides quick, sustained pain relief on **subcutaneous administration**.

These drugs are being studied for their utility in the flare up of gout and at the onset of urate-lowering therapy with synthesis inhibitors or uricosuric drugs.

DRUG TREATMENT OF CHRONIC GOUT

All patients with hyperuricemia may not develop gout, but all patients suffering from gout always have hyperuricemia. The precipitation of monosodium urate crystals is the first step that triggers a series of events resulting in the damage to articular cartilage and joints, causing pain and distress to the patient. Thus, treatment of chronic gout aims at lowering serum uric acid levels by either inhibiting its synthesis or enhancing its renal excretion.

1. Uric Acid Synthesis Inhibitors
a. Allopurinol
Mechanism of action

Allopurinol is a hypoxanthine analogue which causes competitive **inhibition of enzyme xanthine oxidase**. Its active metabolite (alloxanthine) causes non-competitive inhibition of xanthine oxidase (Fig. 24.3).

During uric acid synthesis, xanthine oxidase catalyses the conversion of hypoxanthine to xanthine and then to uric acid. Thus, when the enzyme activity is inhibited, levels of uric acid fall but those of hypoxanthine and xanthine rise somewhat. These two substrates (hypoxanthine and xanthine) are more soluble than uric acid and are hence easily excreted by the kidney. Moreover, raised hypoxanthine causes feedback **inhibition of de novo purine synthesis**.

Uses

1. Allopurinol is the **drug of first choice for chronic gout**, between acute attacks; it prolongs the inter-critical period. The initial dose is 50–100 mg/day; thereafter, the dose is titrated upwards and up to 800 mg/day may be used to achieve serum uric acid levels below 6 mg/dL. However, it **should not be given during an acute attack**. During the initial months of treatment with allopurinol (febuxostat and uricosuric drugs), the levels of urate fluctuate. This may cause intermittent solubilisation and recrystallisation. Thus, an acute attack may be precipitated with allopurinol. Moreover, uric acid inhibits the release of cytokines. This inhibitory effect is knocked out by allopurinol as it reduces uric acid levels. Thus, joint inflammation may get aggravated. So, **NSAIDs/colchicine should be given along with allopurinol at the beginning of therapy**, and discontinued when levels of uric acid fall below 6 mg/dL.
2. Allopurinol is useful in other conditions with hyperuricemia such as Lesch–Nyhan syndrome, tumour lysis syndrome and in patients with organ transplantation.
3. It is used as an adjuvant to sodium stibogluconate in Kala-azar.

ADRs

- It **may precipitate acute gout** that can be prevented by combining NSAIDs at the beginning of therapy.
- **Gastrointestinal** adverse effects such as nausea, vomiting, and diarrhea are frequent.
- **Allergic** maculopapular rash can occur in up to 3% of patients on allopurinol therapy. Some cases of exfoliative dermatitis are also seen. HLA-B*5801 is strongly linked with allopurinol hypersensitivity.
- Rare adverse effects are necrotising vasculitis, peripheral neuritis, myelosuppression, aplastic anemia and cataract.
- Allopurinol also inhibits the enzyme orotidylate decarboxylase that is involved in the final step of pyrimidine biosynthesis, i.e., formation of uridine monophosphate from orotic acid. Thus, it can cause orotic aciduria.

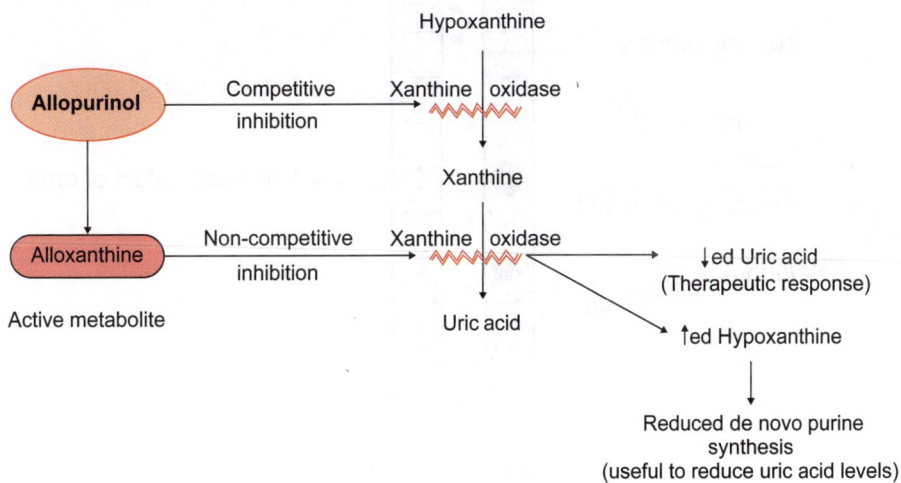

Fig. 24.3 Mechanism of action of allopurinol

Interactions, cautions and contraindications

1. When given to patients on chemotherapeutic purines like azathioprine and 6-mercaptopurine (6-MP), allopurinol inhibits their metabolism, thereby increasing chances of their toxicity. Thus, the **doses of 6-MP and azathioprine should be reduced by 75%.**
2. Allopurinol also inhibits the metabolism of the oral anticoagulant, warfarin, and the thioxanthene derivative, theophylline, and potentiates their effects.
3. Probenecid shortens the half-life of alloxanthine, the active metabolite of allopurinol. However, allopurinol prolongs the half-life of probenecid by decreasing its metabolism.
4. The safety of allopurinol use during pregnancy, lactation and in pediatric age groups is not yet established.
5. In patients with impaired renal and hepatic functions, allopurinol should be used with caution; dose reduction is indicated in renal failure.
6. Allopurinol and ampicillin used together may cause drug rashes in up to 20% of patients.

Contraindications to the use of allopurinol are **acute gout** and **hypersensitivity** to the drug.

b. Febuxostat

Febuxostat is a non-purine drug. It also decreases synthesis of uric acid by inhibition of xanthine oxidase. It reduces uric acid in both over-producers and under-excretors. It is **used in chronic gout as an alternative to allopurinol,** under the cover of NSAIDs or colchicine to prevent flaring up of acute symptoms. The dose is 40–80 mg per day, up to a maximum of 120 mg/day.

It is well tolerated by patients with allopurinol intolerance. The commonly observed adverse effects are nausea, vomiting, diarrhea and headache. Liver damage can occur, so liver function should be monitored. However, in renal failure, dose reduction or adjustment is not required for febuxostat. Hypersensitivity reactions occur rarely, but warrant discontinuation of the drug.

2. Uricosuric Drugs

Drugs which increase urinary excretion of uric acid are called uricosuric drugs. **Sulfinpyrazone** and **probenecid** are useful in chronic gout as they decrease the body's urate pool by increasing urinary excretion of uric acid. **Lesinurad** is a new uricosuric drug, which acts by

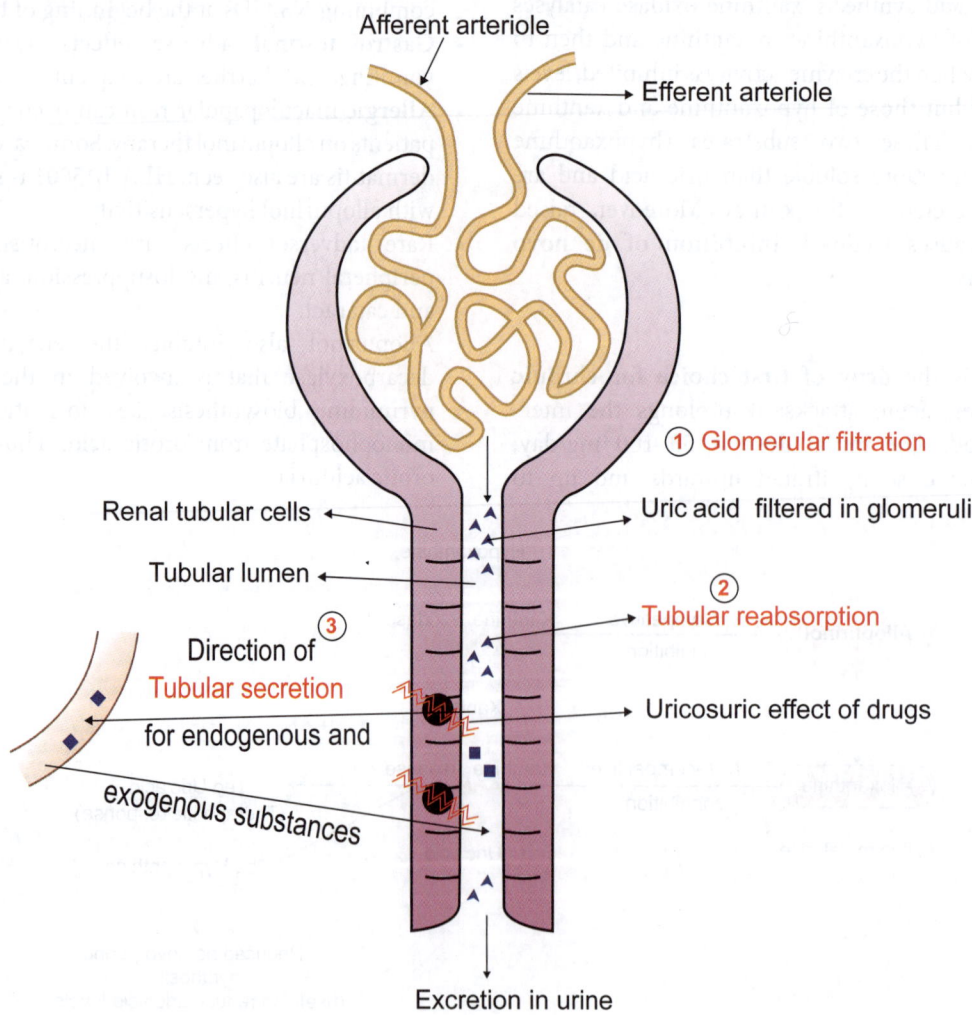

Fig. 24.4 Mechanism of action of uricosuric drug

selective inhibition of uric acid transporter. **Losartan** also possesses uricosuric effect. However, neither of these drugs is effective in renal failure.

Mechanism of action
These drugs act at anion transport sites of the renal tubule and inhibit net reabsorption of uric acid in the PCT (Fig. 24.4). So, urinary excretion of uric acid is increased, resulting in a fall in the body urate pool; however, plasma concentration may not be affected much. The urate deposits from tophi get reabsorbed and bone remineralisation occurs. Arthritis also improves. Care should be taken to **maintain high urine volume and pH above 6**, because excretion of large amounts of uric acid leads to a predisposition to formation of renal urate stones.

Therapeutic uses
These are indicated in **chronic gout with tophaceous deposits,** especially when xanthine oxidase inhibitors are contraindicated or are not tolerated.

Probenecid can decrease renal excretion of penicillin and may be combined with penicillin to prolong duration of its action.

Adverse reactions
- Uricosuric drugs can cause **gastrointestinal irritation** in the form of dyspepsia and pose a risk of peptic ulceration. These irritant effects are more common with sulfinpyrazone, so it is not much in use.
- Rarely, uricosuric drugs can cause rashes, aplastic anemia and nephrotic syndrome.

Contraindications
- These drugs should not be used for at least 2–3 weeks after an acute attack of gout, as there is risk of flaring up and worsening of acute gout.
- These drugs should be given only if creatinine clearance is > 50 mL/min, as they are ineffective in renal insufficiency.
- These should be avoided in patients with peptic ulcer disease and renal stones.
- Uricosuric drugs should be avoided if 24-hour urine sample contains > 800 mg of uric acid.

Interactions
- Probenecid decreases urinary excretion of many drugs like penicillins, cephalosporins, sulphonamides, indomethacin and methotrexate.
- Aspirin, pyrazinamide and ethambutol can decrease the uricosuric effect of probenecid.

Benzbromarone, which is structurally related to amiodarone, an antiarrhythmic drug, is the most potent uricosuric drug. It also causes non-competitive inhibition of xanthine oxidase. It is not preferred, however, due to risk of hepatotoxicity.

3. Mammalian Uricase Enzyme
Pegloticase
Humans are devoid of the enzyme urate oxidase (uricase) that **catalyses the conversion of uric acid to a more soluble and easily excretable compound, allantoin** (Fig. 24.5). **Pegloticase** is a recombinant mammalian urate oxidase enzyme that is covalently bound to methoxy polyethylene glycol (mPEG). It is a rapid-acting drug that reduces urate levels within 24–72 hours of administration. mPEG has 2 benefits: it increases the duration of action of the drug (its effect is maintained for up to 21 days) and reduces immune reactions. Its dose is 8 mg by intravenous infusion, repeated after 2 weeks. However, if antibodies develop against pegloticase, the duration of action is reduced because of its enhanced clearance.

Adverse effects
Like other drugs used in chronic gout, pegloticase can also cause acute gout flare-ups at the beginning of therapy. Thus NSAIDs/colchicine cover is needed during the initial 3–6 months of treatment.

- Immune response is common, resulting in reduced half-life and reduced response to pegloticase. Risk of severe infusion reactions and anaphylaxis is also there.
- Other adverse effects include headache, nausea, anemia, muscle spasms, renal stones and methemoglobinemia.
- Rarely, respiratory tract infection, urinary tract infection, edema and diarrhea may occur.
- It is contraindicated in G6PD deficiency because of risk of hemolysis.

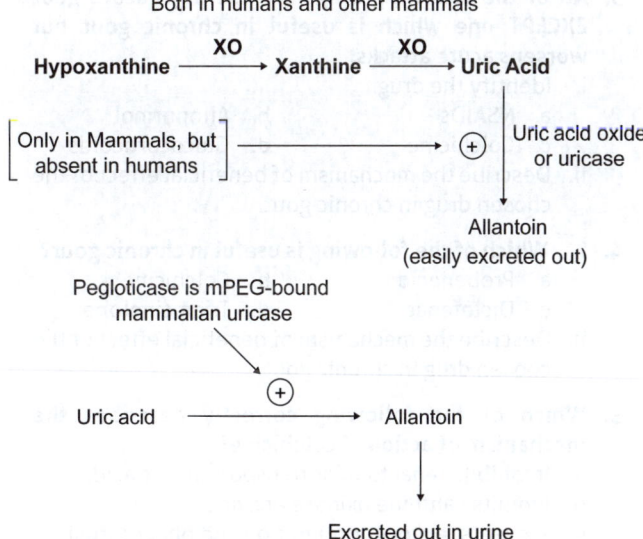

Fig.24.5 Mechanism of action of pegloticase

Rasburicase

Rasburicase is another recombinant uricase analogue used in tumour lysis syndrome.

Uses: Uricase analogues are administered intravenously in chronic gout that does not respond to other drugs.

Clinical problem-based questions and MCQs

1. A 40-year-old woman presented with pain, swelling, and difficulty walking due to inflammation of the right big toe. There was no history of trauma, fever, or injury. Examination revealed the toe to be swollen, warm, and tender. Laboratory tests showed elevated serum uric acid (10.5 mg/dL) and ESR of 30 mm/hr; CBC and other parameters were within normal limits. She mentioned that her mother had similar episodes, which were relieved by allopurinol. The physician explained that allopurinol is not suitable during an acute attack and started her on piroxicam 20 mg twice daily, advising follow-up in 5 days. However, she returned after 2 days with persistent symptoms. She was then prescribed colchicine 0.5 mg four times daily, resulting in symptom relief.
   i. What is this patient suffering from?
   ii. Why does the doctor refuse to prescribe allopurinol to her?
   iii. What is the pharmacological basis of prescribing piroxicam and then colchicine in the next visit?
   iv. What are the possible adverse effects of colchicine?

2. All patients having hyperuricemia may not develop gout, but all patients suffering from gout have hyperuricemia. Therefore, reducing uric acid levels seems to be a useful strategy in treatment of gout. However, none of the uric acid lowering drugs is ever used in acute gout. Justify the statement.

3. All of the following drugs are useful in acute gout EXCEPT one which is useful in chronic gout but worsens acute attacks.
   i. Identify the drug.
      a. NSAIDs   b. Allopurinol
      c. Colchicine   d. Glucocorticoids
   ii. Describe the mechanism of beneficial effect of the chosen drug in chronic gout.

4. i. Which of the following is useful in chronic gout?
      a. Probenecid   b. Colchicine
      c. Diclofenac   d. Triamcinolone
   ii. Describe the mechanism of beneficial effect of the chosen drug in chronic gout.

5. Which of the following correctly describes the mechanism of action of colchicine?
   a. It inhibits renal tubular transport of uric acid.
   b. Inhibits xanthine oxidase enzyme
   c. Prevents leukocytic migration and phagocytosis
   d. Catalyses conversion of uric acid to allantoin

6. Which of the following NSAIDS is not preferred in acute gout and why?
   a. Indomethacin   b. Tolmetin
   c. Diclofenac   d. Piroxicam

7. i. Identify the drug which produces quick response to control acute attack of gout but is kept as a reserve drug?
      a. Prednisolone   b. Piroxicam
      c. Allopurinol   d. Sulfinpyrazone
   ii. Explain the reason for keeping the chosen drug as a reserve drug in acute gout

8. All of the following act by increasing uric acid excretion EXCEPT:
   a. Probenecid   b. Sulfinpyrazone
   c. Febuxostat   d. Lesinurad

9. Which of the following is a noncompetitive inhibitor of xanthine oxidase?
   a. Febuxostat   b. Alloxanthine
   c. Allopurinol   d. Sulfinpyrazone

10. In which of the following conditions is allopurinol contraindicated?
    a. Renal failure   b. Acute gout
    c. Pregnancy   d. All of the above

11. i. Identify the drug that oxidises uric acid to highly soluble products.
       a. Febuxostat   b. Pegloticase
       c. Alloxanthine   d. Colchicine
    ii. Describe the mechanism of action and adverse effects of the chosen drug.

Summary

- Gout is a chronic metabolic disease with recurrent, abrupt, self-limiting episodes of acute arthritis.
- Hyperuricemia is always present in gout → deposition of MSU crystals in synovial fluid results in series of events causing inflammation and subsequent destruction of cartilage and bone.
- **Acute gout** is managed using NSAIDs, colchicine and corticosteroids.
- **NSAIDs** are the drugs of first choice in acute gout because of their anti-inflammatory and analgesic effect. However, aspirin and tolmetin are avoided owing to their dose-dependent effect on urate excretion.
- **Colchicine** prevents tubulin polymerisation → inhibits leukocytic migration and subsequent phagocytosis → interrupts vicious cycle of inflammation.
- Very effective in treatment and prophylaxis of acute gout. Faster acting than NSAIDs, but is not preferred because of high toxicity.

- Dose-related adverse effects of colchicine are nausea, vomiting, diarrhea, abdominal cramps and intestinal bleeding. Overdose can cause convulsions, hepatic necrosis, DIC (disseminated intravascular coagulation), acute renal failure.
- Rarely, bone marrow suppression, hair loss, peripheral neuritis, myopathy and death due to respiratory paralysis occur.
- **Corticosteroids** are very effective but are kept as reserve drugs because of systemic adverse effects. Intra-articular injection of triamcinolone is preferred over oral steroids.
- **Chronic gout** is managed by decreasing synthesis or increasing excretion of uric acid. Allopurinol, uricosuric drugs and pegloticase are useful. However, they may precipitate acute attack through fluctuations in urate levels. So, at the initiation of the therapy, NSAIDs or corticoids are combined.
- **Allopurinol** acts by inhibition of xanthine oxidase. → Uric acid synthesis decreases. Raised levels of hypoxanthine, in turn, reduce de novo purine synthesis.
- Allopurinol may precipitate acute gout. Gastrointestinal adverse effects are frequent, allergic maculopapular rash can occur. Rarely, exfoliative dermatitis, necrotising vasculitis, peripheral neuritis, myelosuppression, aplastic anemia and cataract may occur.
- **Febuxostat**, with the same mechanism of action, is an alternative to allopurinol in patients who do not tolerate allopurinol.
- **Uricosuric drugs** include probenecid and sulfinpyrazone. These act at the anion transport sites of renal tubules and inhibit net reabsorption of uric acid in the PCT. So, urinary excretion of uric acid is increased, resulting in fall of body urate pool. The urate deposits from tophi get reabsorbed and bone remineralisation occurs. Arthritis also improves. These are gastric irritants, and may also cause rashes, aplastic anemia and nephrotic syndrome.
- **Pegloticase** favours conversion of uric acid into allantoin, which is easily excreted. ADRs include headache, nausea, anemia, methemoglobinemia, and respiratory/urinary tract infections.

b. Dose of 6-mercaptopurine should be reduced in patients on allopurinol therapy.
c. Drugs reducing synthesis or increasing excretion of uric acid are not used during acute attack of gouty arthritis.
4. Write short notes on:
   a. Febuxostat
   b. Pegloticase
   c. Allopurinol
   d. Uricosuric drugs
   e. Colchicine

Hints for problem-based questions and MCQs

1. i. Acute gout
   ii. Fluctuating urate levels with allopurinol therapy may cause intermittent solubilisation and recrystallisation. Moreover, uric acid inhibits cytokine release and allopurinol cancels this inhibitory effect by reducing uric acid synthesis. Both these actions may worsen acute gout
   iii. Piroxicam is an NSAID that exerts anti-inflammatory action through COX inhibition and also inhibits phagocytosis of urate crystals. In acute gout, therapy is generally started with one of the NSAIDs. However, as the patient reported no relief in her symptoms with piroxicam, in the next visit colchicine was prescribed. While colchicine has no analgesic or anti-inflammatory activity, it dramatically relieves symptoms in acute gout. It acts by binding to the fibrillar protein, 'tubulin', and prevents its polymerisation to form microtubules and inhibits leukocytic migration and subsequent phagocytosis. Thus, the vicious cycle of inflammation is interrupted.
   iv. Refer to page 332
2. Acute attack may be worsened. (See Answer 1. ii)
3. i. b. Allopurinol
   ii. Refer to page 333
4. i. a. Probenecid
   ii. Refer to page 334
5. c. Prevents leukocytic migration and phagocytosis
6. c. Tolmetin, because it has dose-dependent effect on uric acid excretion.
7. i. a. Prednisolone
   ii. It is a glucocorticoid. Its systemic use is associated with several adverse effects. Hence, systemic steroids are used as reserve drug for patients who do not respond or have some contraindication to the use of NSAIDs.
8. c. Febuxostat
9. b. Alloxanthine
10. d. Allopurinol is contraindicated in all of the above conditions, viz. renal failure, acute gout and pregnancy.
11. i. b. Pegloticase
    ii. Refer to page 335

Questions for practice

1. Describe the pharmacotherapy of acute exacerbation in gouty arthritis.
2. Enumerate the drugs for acute and chronic gout.
3. Explain why:
   a. Allopurinol therapy should be started under the cover of NSAIDs.

CONCEPT MAP - DRUGS FOR GOUT

NSAIDs
Drugs of choice
COX inhibition
↓
Decreased PG synthesis
Action slower than Colchicine
Aspirin avoided due to dose-dependent effect on urate excretion
Indomethacin 25-50 mg TDS used.
Diclofenac, Piroxicam, Naproxen also useful.

Colchicine
Prevents tubulin polymerisation → reduced leukocytic migration → Interrupts vicious cycle of inflammation
Quick response,
Dramatic relief in acute gout
Not preferred due to many ADRs, e.g., nausea, vomiting, diarrhea, abdominal cramps, intestinal bleeding
Overdose: Hepatic necrosis, ARF, convulsions, DIC

Corticosteroids
Non specific anti-inflammatory effect
Quick response
Many ADRs with systemic steroids
Reserved for cases not responding to or not tolerating NSAIDs.
Intra-articular Triamcinolone better tolerated than oral Prednisolone.

Interleukin Inhibitors
Anakinra, Canakinumab, Rilonacept
Useful in patients not responding to NSAIDs/Colchicine or develop serious adverse effects

---

Recurrent, Abrupt, Self-limiting → **Acute Gout** → **Gout** → **Chronic Gout** → **Chronic Hyperuricemia**

Clinical Features
- Metatarsophalangeal, Ankle, Heel, Wrist, Elbow commonly affected
- Throbbing, crushing pain, warmth, redness & immobility of joint
- Fever, Malaise
- Subcutaneous Tophi around joints, on eyelids, nose, pinna
- Renal urate stones, Interstitial nephritis

Pathophysiology
- Increased serum uric acid
- Deposition of MSU crystals in synovial fluid
- Phagocytosis of MSU → Inflammation
- Damage to cartilage
- Fusion of articulating ends of bones
- Joints become immobile

PRIMARY
- Overproduction
- Reduced excretion

SECONDARY
Diseases: Leukemia, Lymphoma, DKA, PCV, Psoriasis
Drugs: Thiazides, Furosemide, Pyrazinamide, Ethambutol

Drugs

Decreasing Synthesis
Allopurinol, Febuxostat

Increasing Excretion
Sulfinpyrazone, Probenecid, Lesinurad

Pegloticase

Decreasing Synthesis
MOA*: Xanthine oxidase inhibition
Allopurinol DOC in chronic gout, prolongs inter-critical period
Dose 50–100 mg/day with NSAIDs/Colchicine at start of therapy
ADRs: At initiation of therapy, fluctuating urate levels may cause intermittent solubilisation and recrystallisation, precipitate acute gout, Nausea, vomiting, diarrhea, allergic reactions
Rare: Necrotising vasculitis, Peripheral neuritis, Myelosuppression, Aplastic anemia, Cataract.
Dose of 6-MP, Azathioprine should be reduced by 75% in patients on allopurinol therapy.
Febuxostat: Alternative to Allopurinol Hepatotoxic, no dose reduction in renal failure.

Increasing Excretion
MOA: Inhibit net reabsorption of uric acid acting at anion transport sites in PCT.
Used in chronic gout with tophaceous deposits
High urine volume & pH above 6 should be maintained to prevent urate renal stones.
ADRs: GI irritant action, dyspepsia, peptic ulceration. Rarely: rash, aplastic anemia, nephrotic syndrome

Pegloticase
MOA: Recombinant mammalian uricase enzyme, catalyses conversion of uric acid to a more soluble & easily excretable compound, allantoin.
ADRs: Can precipitate acute gout, headache, nausea, anemia, muscle spasm, renal stones, UTI, infusion reactions, anaphylaxis, etc.

*MOA: Mechanism of action ; DOC: Drug of choice

SECTION 4 Autacoids and Related Drugs

25 Drugs Used in the Treatment of Rheumatoid Arthritis

PH 2.8 Devise management plan for a case of arthritis.

Learning objectives

A student of MBBS phase II should be able to:
- Explain the pathophysiology of rheumatoid arthritis.
- Describe the goals of drug therapy in rheumatoid arthritis.
- Describe the role of NSAIDs and corticosteroids in rheumatoid arthritis.
- Enumerate disease-modifying anti-rheumatic drugs.
- Describe the mechanism of action, ADRs and contraindications of DMARDs.

RHEUMATOID ARTHRITIS

Rheumatoid arthritis is a chronic inflammatory disorder characterised by inflammation of the small peripheral synovial joints, which results in bone and cartilage destruction that compromises mobility and quality of life. If not treated, it slowly progresses to involve proximal joints. In addition, significant systemic effects also occur.

Pathogenesis

The etiopathogenesis of rheumatoid arthritis (RA) is complex and involves the interaction of many genetic and environmental factors. **Formation of autoantibodies against various protein molecules starts many years before the appearance of the clinical disease.** Rheumatoid factor (RF) and anti-citrullinated protein antibodies (ACPA) are positive in asymptomatic patients.

Immune complexes formed by IgM antibodies activate the complement, which, in turn, cause the release of numerous pro-inflammatory chemokines and cytokines (Fig. 25.1). Mediators like TNF-α, interleukins [mainly IL-1, 6, and 12), interferons and growth factors (such as platelet- derived growth factor (PDGF), fibroblast growth factor (FGF) and vascular endothelial growth factor (VEGF)] play a crucial role in synovial inflammatory process.

Joint damage occurs due to the interaction of synoviocytes with various cytokines released by immune cells (like monocytes, macrophages, mast cells, T cells and B cells). Endothelial cells cause extensive angiogenesis and hyperplastic synovium. Release of cytokines into the synovial fluid induces leukocytic migration and inflammatory changes in the synovial membrane, damaging articular cartilage. Bone erosions occur

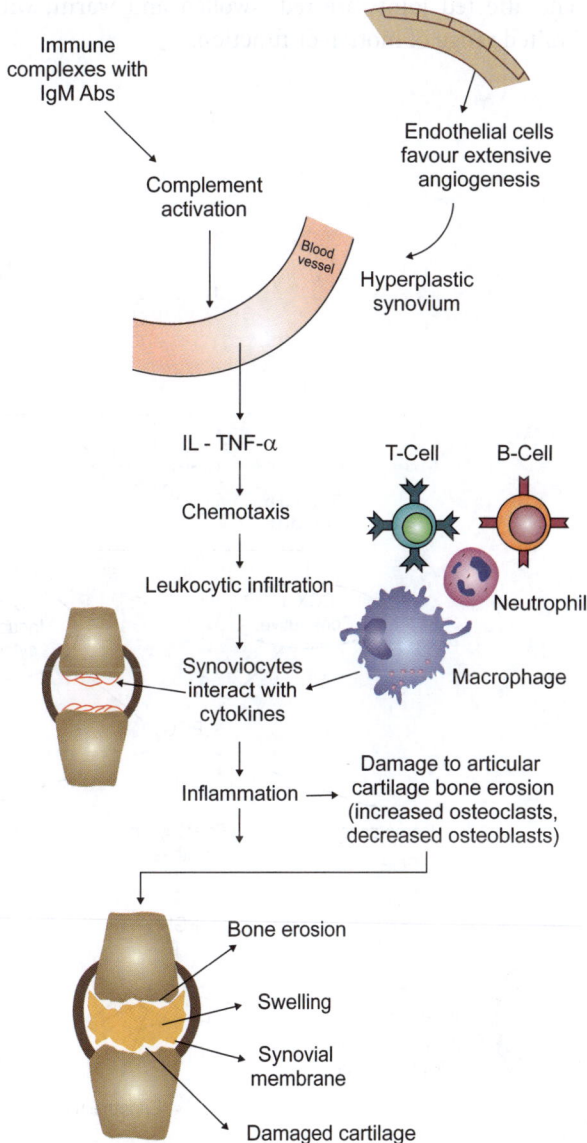

Fig. 25.1 Pathogenesis of rheumatoid arthritis

due to increased osteoclasts and reduced osteoblasts. Subchondral bone destruction follows damage to the articular surface.

Clinical Features

RA has a chronic course characterised by remissions and relapses. Various systemic and articular signs/symptoms occur during periods known as 'relapse or exacerbation'. Between relapses, there are periods of 'remissions' when symptoms clear up completely. While the symptoms of RA can affect several organs in the body, the **joint-related symptoms** include:

- Pain, swelling and stiffness in multiple joints, ultimately leading to deformities and loss of joint function. Joint stiffness is more prominent in the morning upon waking and decreases as day progresses.
- Wrists and small joints of hand and feet are frequently involved.
- The affected joints are red, swollen and warm, with limited range of motion or function.
- Reflexes involving inflamed joints and strength of associated muscles may also be affected.
- No single test can confirm the diagnosis of RA. Levels of rheumatoid factor and anti-citrullinated protein antibodies are raised. ESR and C-reactive protein levels (CRP) are also usually elevated in chronic inflammatory disorders.

Treatment

The treatment of rheumatoid arthritis aims at:
- **Relief of symptoms during relapse**
- **Slowing down or arrest of disease progression**.

For symptom relief, NSAIDs and corticosteroids are used. To slow down disease progression, disease-modifying anti-rheumatic drugs (DMARDs) are used.

1. NSAIDs

NSAIDs exert analgesic, anti-inflammatory action by reducing prostaglandin synthesis through cyclooxygenase inhibition (Fig. 25.2). These are used for **suppressing**

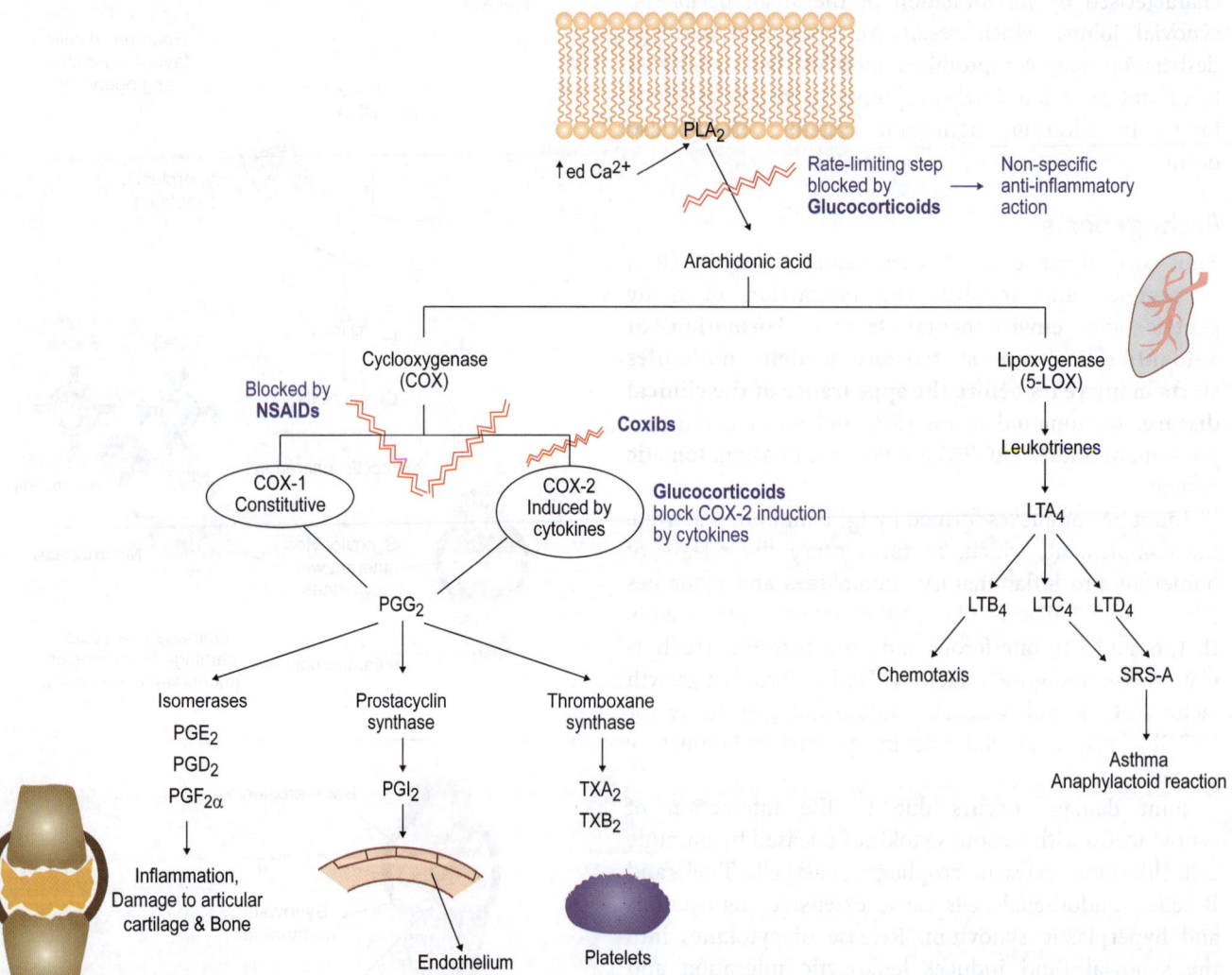

Fig. 25.2 Mechanism of action of drugs relieving symptoms in rheumatoid arthritis

the pain, swelling and morning stiffness of rheumatoid arthritis. They have little effect on the progression of bone and cartilage destruction.

Among NSAIDs, no single drug is superior to all others for every patient, and the choice is largely empirical. High-dose aspirin, indomethacin, naproxen and piroxicam are used to treat exacerbation of rheumatoid arthritis. Initially, the selected drug should be tried for 1–2 weeks; thereafter, it is a matter of trial and observation.

2. Corticosteroids

Prednisone and other glucocorticoids produce **prompt and dramatic symptom relief** in rheumatoid arthritis due to their non-specific anti-inflammatory action. Steroids inhibit phospholipase A2 (the enzyme responsible for liberation of arachidonic acid from membrane lipids). They have recently been shown to selectively inhibit the expression of COX-2 in response to cytokines (Fig. 25.2). They also **slow down the appearance of new bone erosions.**

Corticosteroids are used in rheumatoid arthritis in the following situations:

- They are used **as adjuvants** during periods of exacerbation for an active disease that does not respond or responds only partially to NSAIDs.
- In the presence of serious extra-articular manifestations such as pericarditis or eye involvement
- Corticosteroids are also used as **bridge therapy** with DMARDs, as the effect of DMARDs usually manifests in 2–4 weeks.

When prolonged therapy is required, the dose of prednisolone should not exceed 7.5 mg. Alternate-day therapy is usually not successful in rheumatoid arthritis. **Intra-articular steroids** alleviate painful symptoms and are preferable to increasing the dose of systemic medication. The use of systemic steroids for long durations is associated with **disabling toxic effects** like increased risk of fractures, infections, cataracts, diabetes, hypertension and atherosclerotic heart disease.

3. Disease-modifying antirheumatic drugs (DMARDs)

If NSAIDs alone or along with corticosteroids fail to afford adequate relief, DMARDS are added. **Nowadays, early introduction of DMARDS is favoured.**

DMARDs (Flowchart 25.1) comprise:

- Non-biological agents/drugs
- Biologically derived drugs

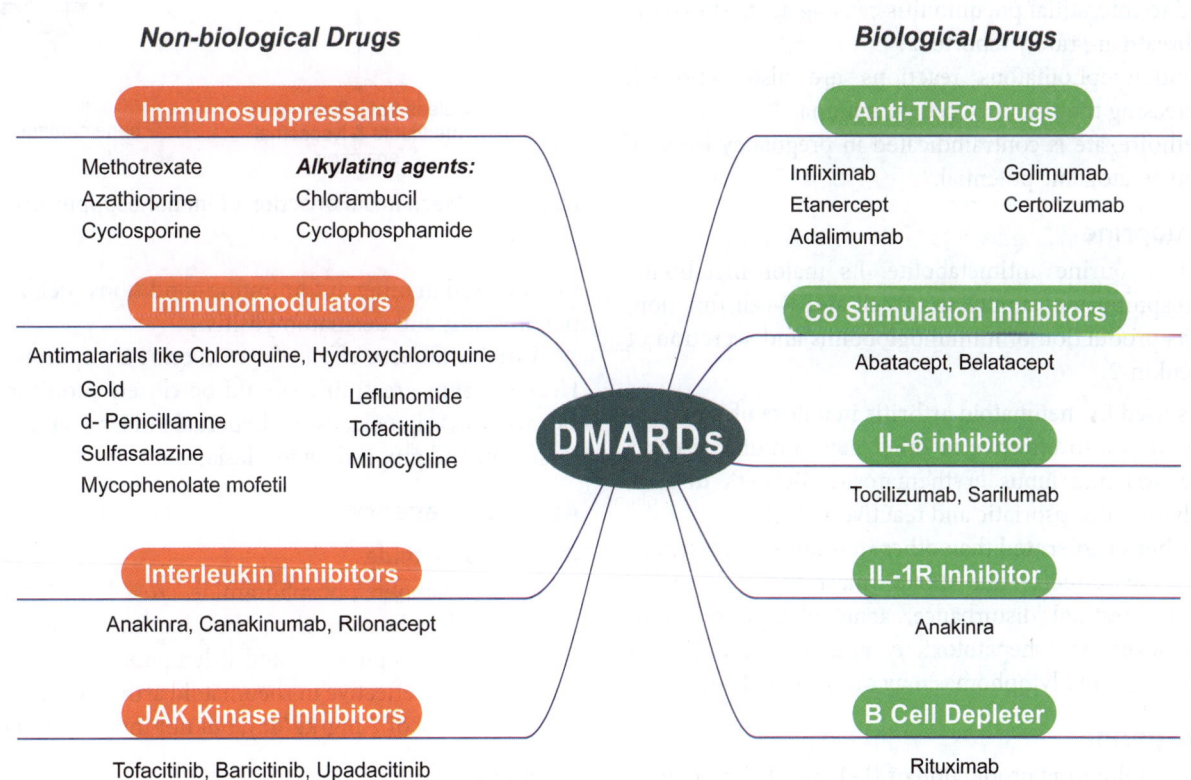

Flowchart 25.1 Classification of disease-modifying antirheumatic drugs (DMARDs)

NON-BIOLOGICAL DMARDs

a. Immunosuppressants

Methotrexate

This is an antimetabolite anticancer drug that also has antirheumatic properties. It works by inhibiting the production of proinflammatory cytokines, suppressing chemotaxis of polymorphonuclear cells, and impairing the function of macrophages and lymphocytes. (Fig. 25.3).

The use of methotrexate in rheumatoid arthritis reduces inflammation and the rate of formation of new bony erosions. It is a DMARD of first choice at doses of 15–25 mg, given orally, once in a week. The dose is much lower than that used for cancer chemotherapy. It is sometimes called the **anchor drug** in rheumatoid arthritis. It is also useful in psoriatic arthritis, ankylosing spondylitis, polymyositis, SLE and vasculitis.

Adverse effects of methotrexate include nausea, mucosal ulcers, pancytopenia and hepatotoxicity, causing fibrosis and cirrhosis. Risk of hepatotoxicity is higher in patients with obesity, diabetes mellitus, heavy alcohol intake, chronic hepatitis and renal dysfunction. So, liver enzymes should be monitored every 3 months in patients receiving methotrexate.

- Methotrexate toxicity can be prevented by leucovorin (folinic acid) 24 hours after each weekly dose of the drug.
- Methotrexate-induced hypersensitivity reactions that lead to interstitial pneumonitis causing acute shortness of breath are rarely reported.
- Pseudolymphomatous reactions are also reported, increasing the risk of B- cell lymphomas.
- Methotrexate is contraindicated in pregnancy because of its teratogenic potential.

Azathioprine

This is a purine antimetabolite. Its major metabolite, 6-mercaptopurine, suppresses T-cell and B-cell function, inhibits production of immunoglobulins and secretion of interleukin-2.

- It is used in rheumatoid arthritis in a dose of 2 mg/kg/day. It is also effective in other autoimmune diseases like systemic lupus erythematosus, Behcet's disease, polymyositis, psoriatic and reactive arthritis.
- It is **better tolerated** than other immunosuppressants.
- **Adverse effects** like bone marrow suppression, gastrointestinal disturbance, acute allergic reactions like fever/rash/ hepatotoxicity and increased risk of infections and lymphomas may occur with its use.

Cyclosporine

It acts by inhibiting production of IL-1 and IL-2 receptors. It also affects T cell and, B cell function. It reduces the rate of appearance of bony erosions in rheumatoid arthritis. It

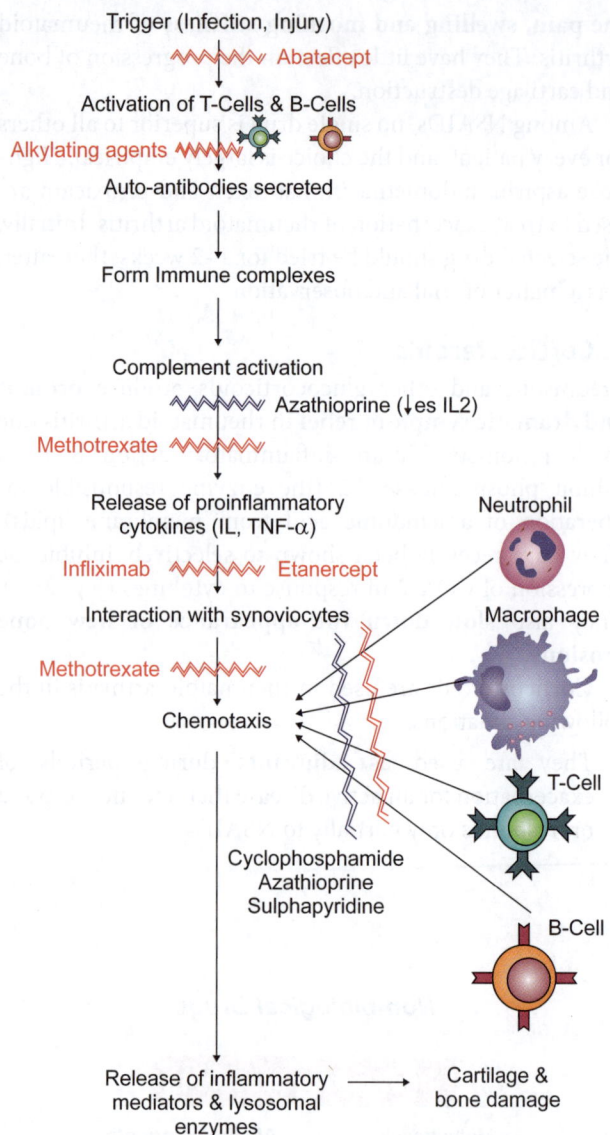

Fig. 25.3 Mechanism of action of immunosuppressants

may be used in other autoimmune conditions such as SLE, polymyositis and dermatomyositis.

A **major adverse** effect of cyclosporine is nephrotoxicity. Hence, serum creatinine should be closely monitored. It can also cause hypertension, hyperkalemia, hepatotoxicity, hirsutism and gingival hyperplasia.

Alkylating agents

Cyclophosphamide

Its active metabolite phosphoramide, cross-links DNA and prevents cell replication. Cyclophosphamide suppresses the function of T-lymphocytes and B-lymphocytes (Fig. 25.3). It appears to be effective in rheumatoid arthritis when given orally in a dose of 2 mg/kg/day, but not intravenously.

Chlorambucil

Chlorambucil, another alkylating agent, and cyclophosphamide are effective as disease-modifying agents in rheumatoid arthritis, systemic lupus erythematosus (SLE), vasculitis and other autoimmune diseases.

Prominent adverse effects of alkylating agents include infertility and bone marrow suppression. Cyclophosphamide can cause hemorrhagic cystitis and carcinoma bladder (rare). Chlorambucil has been associated with a tenfold increased risk of developing leukemia.

b. Immunomodulators

Antimalarials (Chloroquine and Hydroxychloroquine)

Chloroquine and hydroxychloroquine are antimalarial drugs. The exact mechanism of their anti-inflammatory action is not clearly understood, but one or more of the following mechanisms may be responsible.

- Suppression of responsiveness of T-lymphocytes to mitogens
- Decreased leukocyte chemotaxis
- Stabilisation of lysosomal membranes
- Trapping of free radicals

Chloroquine and hydroxychloroquine are often used as **monotherapy in milder non-erosive disease** in a dose not exceeding 5 mg/kg/day for hydroxychloroquine and 200 mg/day for chloroquine. They **improve symptoms and reduce levels of rheumatoid factor,** a marker of disease intensity, after 3–6 months of use, but **they do not decrease the progression of erosive bony lesions.** So, in severe cases, these are used only as **add-on** drugs.

These drugs are also used in Sjogren's syndrome and SLE to reduce serositis, skin manifestations and joint pains. **Adverse effects:** For immunological diseases Sjogren syndrome, and SLE, chloroquine and hydroxychloroquine have to be used for long periods. They have high affinity for melanin-containing tissues and accumulate in them, causing toxicity like retinal damage (bull's eye) and corneal opacity. Hence, biannual or annual ophthalmological monitoring is important. Cumulative toxicity and retinal damage is less common with hydroxychloroquine than chloroquine, so the former is preferred.

Other adverse effects of antimalarials include rashes, graying of hair, irritable bowel syndrome (causing nausea/ vomiting/ abdominal pain), myopathy and neuropathy.

Leflunomide

It is a prodrug which interferes with pyrimidine synthesis by inhibition of enzyme **dihydroorotate dehydrogenase,** resulting in decreased proliferation of B-cells. Thus, formation of autoantibodies by B-cells gets reduced.

(Another dihydroorotate dehydrogenase-inhibiting drug, **teriflunomide,** is useful in relapsing–remitting multiple sclerosis.)

- Leflunomide is **as effective as methotrexate** in rheumatoid arthritis and is used orally. It is a faster-acting alternative to methotrexate. It **can be combined** with methotrexate in patients who do not respond to it alone.
- Common adverse effects include diarrhea, mild alopecia, increase in BP, weight gain, thrombocytopenia and neutropenia.
- It can elevate levels of hepatic enzymes. Elevation of enzymes by more than 3-folds is an indicator to discontinue leflunomide therapy and administer cholestyramine to clear off leflunomide.
- Like methotrexate, it is also contraindicated in pregnancy.

Gold

Gold salts were used extensively in past, but not any longer **because of uncertain efficacy and many toxic effects** like pruritic dermatitis, eosinophilia, pancytopenia, TCP, leukopenia, aplastic anemia, proteinuria and nephrotic syndrome.

d-Penicillamine

The mechanism of its antirheumatic effect is not clearly understood.

- Rh factor titres fall after its administration in a daily dose of 125–250 mg given orally, 1.5 hours after meals.
- It is **reserved for patients with active progressive erosive rheumatoid arthritis who do not respond to other drugs.** Benefits appear within 6 months.
- Nowadays, penicillamine is rarely used because of its adverse effects and interactions with a large number of drugs.
- Used in patients who have not responded to gold therapy.

Sulfasalazine

It consists of sulphapyridine and 5-aminosalicylic acid connected by a diazo bond. It is metabolised by bacteria in the colon to provide constituent moieties. Sulphapyridine is considered as an active moiety for rheumatoid arthritis. Sulfasalazine and its metabolites **reduce release of inflammatory cytokines** like interleukin and TNF-α.

Given in a dose of 2–3 g/day in rheumatoid arthritis, it is more effective than hydroxychloroquine in reducing radiological disease progression. Sulfasalazine is used in patients for whom methotrexate is contraindicated. It is also useful in juvenile arthritis or ankylosing spondylitis.

Adverse effects include nausea, vomiting, rashes, headache, dizziness, pulmonary toxicity, leukopenia and methemoglobinemia.

Minocycline

The mechanism of beneficial effect of minocycline in rheumatoid arthritis is not clear, but it exerts anti-inflammatory action and inhibits collagenase. It is used in mild cases of rheumatoid arthritis in the first year of diagnosis. Dizziness is the most frequent adverse effect encountered.

c. JAK Kinase Inhibitors

Tofacitinib, Baricitinib, and Upadacitinib inhibit JAK kinases, leading to reduced proliferation of lymphocytes and erythrocytes. Tofacitinib is effective orally and checks disease progression in rheumatoid arthritis. It is also useful in psoriatic arthritis and ulcerative colitis.

Adverse effects include GI irritant effects, secondary cancers, opportunistic infections and dyslipidemias.

BIOLOGICAL AGENTS

Biological DMARDs include the following.

a. Anti-TNF α Drugs

These include infliximab, etanercept, and adalimumab.

TNF-α is produced by macrophages and activated T-cells and stimulates the release of other inflammatory cytokines and proteases by activating membrane-bound TNF_1 and TNF_2 receptors. Soluble TNF (sTNF) receptors are the shed portions of TNF-1 and TNF-2 that inhibit the effect of TNF-α. While all inhibitors of TNF-α are administered subcutaneously, infliximab and adalimumab can be administered intravenously as well.

Infliximab: It is a chimeric IgG_1 monoclonal antibody that **binds to TNF-α receptors and slows down the disease progress.** Infliximab is commonly administered with methotrexate as an IV infusion at a dose of 3-10 mg/kg every 8 weeks. This combination therapy is more effective than methotrexate alone in reducing the progression of joint erosions in rheumatoid arthritis.

Etanercept: One molecule of this drug **binds with two molecules of TNF-α.** It is given as subcutaneous injection in a dose of 25 mg twice a week. It is approved for rheumatoid arthritis, juvenile chronic arthritis and psoriatic arthritis.

Adverse effects include injection site reactions such as pain, itching, swelling and redness. There may be increased risk of respiratory infections.

Adalimumab: This is a fully-human IgG_1 anti-TNF monoclonal antibody. It combines with sTNF and down-regulates macrophage and T-cell functions. It is administered as subcutaneous injections on alternate weeks in a dose of 40 mg.

Adverse effects [Mnemonic: **G**o **S**low **O**n **S**lippery **R**oads, i.e., GIT, Secondary carcinoma, Opportunistic infections, Site of injection reaction, Rarely SLE]

- TNF-α inhibitors cause GI ulceration and perforation. Secondary carcinomas like lymphoma and melanoma may occur.
- When infliximab is combined with methotrexate, there is increased risk of upper respiratory tract infections. Latent tuberculosis may get activated. Therefore, patients should be screened for latent TB before starting infliximab therapy. The risk of soft tissue infections, septic arthritis, and opportunist infections increases.
- TNF-α inhibitors can cause erythema, pain, swelling or itching at site of subcutaneous injection.
- Infusion site reactions may also occur with IV infliximab.
- Rarely, infliximab may cause **systemic lupus erythematosus** and demyelinating syndromes; hence, it is contraindicated in patients with multiple sclerosis. Sometimes, it may cause hepatitis, leukopenia, vasculitis, etc.

b. Co-stimulation Inhibitors

These include abatacept and belatacept.

Abatacept

Abatacept acts by inhibiting CD80 and CD86 co-stimulatory molecules on antigen presenting cells (APC), thus inhibiting T-cell activation (refer to Chapter 65, page 848). It reduces clinical signs and symptoms as well as radiographic progression of rheumatoid arthritis. It can be used alone or along with other DMARDs in moderate-to-severe rheumatoid arthritis; however, a combination with another biological agent is usually avoided as two biologic agents together may increase the risk of infection. It is given intravenously at 0, 2 and 4 weeks, and then, monthly. The dose is determined by the bodyweight; it is 500 mg in patients with weight < 60 kg, 750 mg in patients who weigh 60–100 kg and 1000 mg in those above 100 kg. It is given to patients who fail to respond to a combination of methotrexate and TNF-α inhibitors.

ADRs of abatacept include increased risk of upper respiratory tract infections, infusion-related reactions (rare), hypersensitivity reactions such as anaphylaxis and increased risk of lymphomas.

IMMUNOADSORPTION APHERESIS

Immunoadsorption of plasma over columns containing an inert silica matrix and covalently attached, highly purified staphylococcal protein A is designed to remove IgG and immune complexes from plasma. It is done 12-weekly.

Adverse effects include chills, musculoskeletal pain, headache, nausea, GIT symptoms.

DIETARY MANIPULATIONS

Arachidonic acid is an eicosatetraenoic acid metabolised by COX and LOX pathways to yield several mediators of inflammation. If the **diet contains foods like marine fish that are rich in unsaturated fatty acids, e.g., eicosapentaenoic acid,** they will be metabolised in preference to arachidonic acid. The end products of eicosapentaenoic acid are less potent than the end products of arachidonic acid.

It is observed that with eicosapentaenoic acid therapy there is a decrease in both morning stiffness as well as the number of tender joints. There are no adverse effects.

MANAGEMENT PLAN FOR RHEUMATOID ARTHRITIS

The aim of treatment in rheumatoid arthritis is the relief of symptoms, prolonged remission by checking disease progression rate, and prevention of relapse of acute exacerbation.

- NSAIDs are the mainstay of treatment of acute exacerbation of symptoms in rheumatoid arthritis. The choice of NSAID is empirical and no drug has proven superior over the others. Initially, the chosen drug is tried for about two weeks; if it fails to provide adequate symptomatic relief from pain, morning stiffness, etc., an alternative drug is tried. Aspirin, piroxicam, and naproxen are commonly prescribed. Indomethacin is tried as a second choice, if symptoms do not improve.
- Prednisolone (5–7.5 mg/day), is prescribed in patients who do not respond to NSAIDs. Alternate-day therapy is usually not effective in rheumatoid arthritis.
- DMARDs slow down the disease progression and hence prevent relapse of acute symptoms. Methotrexate (15–25 mg, once a week) is the preferred drug for this indication.
- In addition to drug therapy, additional measures such as regular physical activity, dietary manipulation and weight reduction, and psychological counselling of patient are recommended.

Clinical problem-based questions and MCQs

1. **A 40-year-old woman presented with intermittent pain, swelling, and stiffness in the small joints of her hands and feet on and off over the past 3–4 months. The symptoms are more prominent in the morning upon waking and relieved somewhat as the day progresses. The patient claims that she used to take over-the-counter-NSAID diclofenac 75 mg twice daily whenever the symptoms were disturbing. She also reveals that diclofenac initially afforded complete relief, but now, there is partial relief only. On examination, there is swelling, redness and stiffness of metatarsophalangeal and interphalangeal joints in both hands and feet. X-ray of the affected joints shows soft tissue edema and joint abnormalities. ESR and CRP are raised. RA factor is positive.**
   i. What is this patient suffering from?
   ii. What is the role of diclofenac in this case?
   iii. What drug can be used as adjuvant to diclofenac for the short term to control symptoms?
   iv. Name the drugs that can modify the course of the disease in this case.

2. All of the following are disease modifying antirheumatic drugs EXCEPT:
   a. Methotrexate   b. Naproxen
   c. Etanercept   d. Sulfasalazine

3. i. Classify DMARDS.
   ii. Name a DMARD that is a drug of first choice. State the mechanism of its antirheumatic action and dosage.
   iii. List its adverse effects and contraindications of the DMARD of 1st choice and measures to prevent its toxicity.

4. i. Which of the following DMARDs is a TNF-α inhibitor?
   a. Infliximab   b. Sulfasalazine
   c. Leflunomide   d. Cyclosporine
   ii. What are the advantages and disadvantages of combining the chosen TNF-α inhibitor with methotrexate?

5. **DMARDs are used to check disease progression in rheumatoid arthritis. Many diverse drugs can be used as DMARDs.**
   i. Which of the following DMARDs is a prodrug?
   a. Infliximab   b. Sulfasalazine
   c. Leflunomide   d. Cyclosporine
   ii. Describe the mechanism of action of the chosen drug.

Summary

- Rheumatoid arthritis is an **autoimmune disorder** characterised by joint inflammation leading to bone and cartilage destruction. Disease has chronic course with remissions and relapses.
- Involvement of **several small joints and morning stiffness** are characteristic features.
- Drug therapy **aims** at symptom relief and reduction in disease progress rate.
- **NSAIDs** reduce swelling, pain, inflammation and stiffness during acute exacerbation. None of the NSAIDs is superior over others. High-dose aspirin, indomethacin, naproxen and piroxicam are usually used.
- **Corticosteroids** are adjuvants to NSAIDs for symptom control in severe cases with extra-articular manifestations. Daily dose should not exceed 7.5 mg. Alternate day regimens are not effective, but intra-

- articular administration is a better option than high systemic dose. Long-term use is associated with disturbing toxic effects.
- **DMARDs** can be non-biological and biological agents. Non-biological agents are immunosuppressants and immunomodulators.
- Among **immunosuppressants**, methotrexate is the drug of first choice; 15–25 mg is given orally weekly, a dose much lower than the anticancer dose. Important ADRs are nausea, mucosal ulcers, hepatotoxicity and hypersensitivity reactions. Methotrexate toxicity can be checked by leucovorin, given before each weekly dose.
- Other immunosuppressants that may be used as DMARDs include cyclophosphamide, chlorambucil, cyclosporine and azathioprine.
- **Immunomodulators** include chloroquine, hydroxychloroquine, leflunomide, gold, d-penicillamine and sulfasalazine. Anti-malarials, gold and d-penicillamine are not much used because of the many adverse effects associated with their long-term use. Leflunomide may be combined with methotrexate in cases not responding to methotrexate alone. Sulfasalazine has a role in juvenile rheumatoid arthritis.
- Among **biological agents,** anti-TNF-α drug **infliximab** may be used in combination with methotrexate. **Abatacept** can be combined with other DMARDs, but its use with biological agents is associated with increased risk of respiratory infections.

Questions for practice

1. Enumerate DMARDs.
2. Comment on the role of NSAIDs in rheumatoid arthritis.
3. Comment on the role of corticosteroids in rheumatoid arthritis.
4. Write short notes on
   a. Methotrexate as DMARD
   b. Anti-TNF-α as DMARD
5. Explain why
   a. Patients should be screened for latent TB before starting infliximab therapy.
   b. Abatacept is usually not combined with other biological agents.

Hints for problem-based questions and MCQs

1. i. Rheumatoid arthritis
   ii. Symptomatic relief. Refer to page 340
   iii. Prednisone is used as adjuvants to NSAIDs. Refer to page 341
   iv. DMARDs. Refer to Flowchart 25.1, page 341
2. b. Naproxen is the NSAID for symptom control.
3. i. Same as 1.(iv)
   ii. Methotrexate
   iii. Refer to page 342
4. i. a. Infliximab
   ii. Advantage –More reduction in the rate of appearance of new erosions than with methotrexate monotherapy. Disadvantage–Increased risk of upper respiratory tract infections. Latent tuberculosis may get activated. Refer to page 344
5. i. b. Sulfasalazine
   ii. Refer to page 344

Chapter 25 Drugs Used in the Treatment of Rheumatoid Arthritis

CONCEPT MAP - DRUGS FOR RHEUMATOID ARTHRITIS

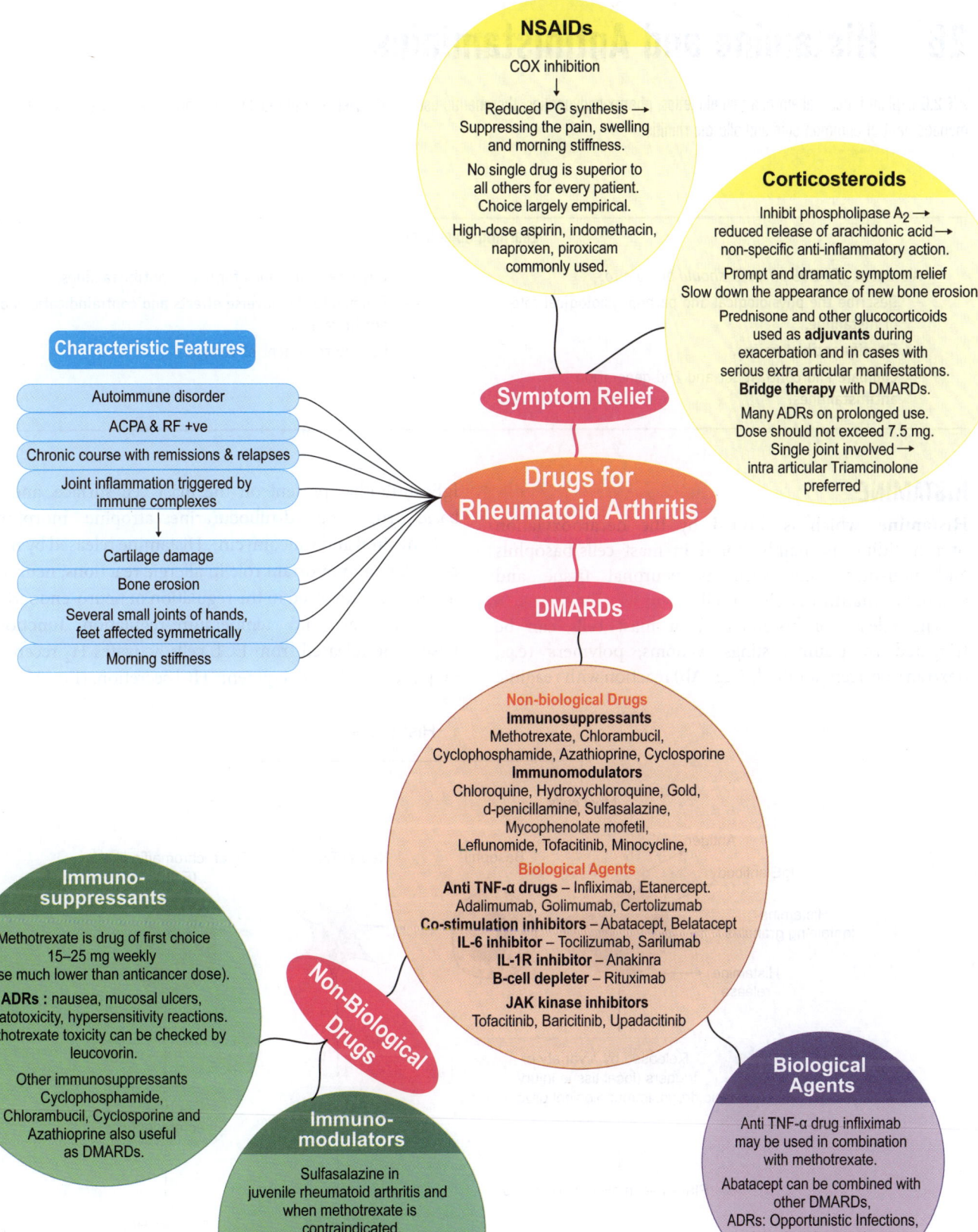

SECTION 4 Autacoids and Related Drugs

26 Histamine and Antihistaminics

PH 2.6 Explain types, salient pharmacokinetics, pharmacodynamics, therapeutic uses, and adverse drug reactions of antihistaminics and explain management of common cold and allergic rhinitis.

Learning objectives

A student of MBBS phase II should be able to:
- Describe the physiological and pathophysiological role of histamine.
- Classify antihistamines.
- Compare and contrast 1st and 2nd generation antihistamines.
- Describe indications for use of antihistamines.
- Enumerate the adverse effects and contraindications of antihistamines.
- Outline treatment of vertigo.

HISTAMINE

Histamine, which is formed by the decarboxylation of L-histidine, is mainly stored in mast cells/basophils and non-mast cells such as neuronal tissue and enterochromaffin-like (ECL) cells.

The release of histamine from mast cells can be triggered by trauma, stings, venoms, polymers (e.g., dextran), antigen–antibody (Ag–Ab) reaction with reaginic IgE antibodies present on the mast cell surface, and by basic drugs (e.g., d-tubocurarine, atropine, morphine, polymyxin B and vancomycin). Histamine released by mast cells plays an important role in allergic reactions; neuronal histamine is involved in the regulation of neuro-endocrine, cardiovascular, and temperature-regulation functions. Histamine released from ECL cells activates H_2 receptors on parietal cells and augments HCl secretion. (Fig. 26.1).

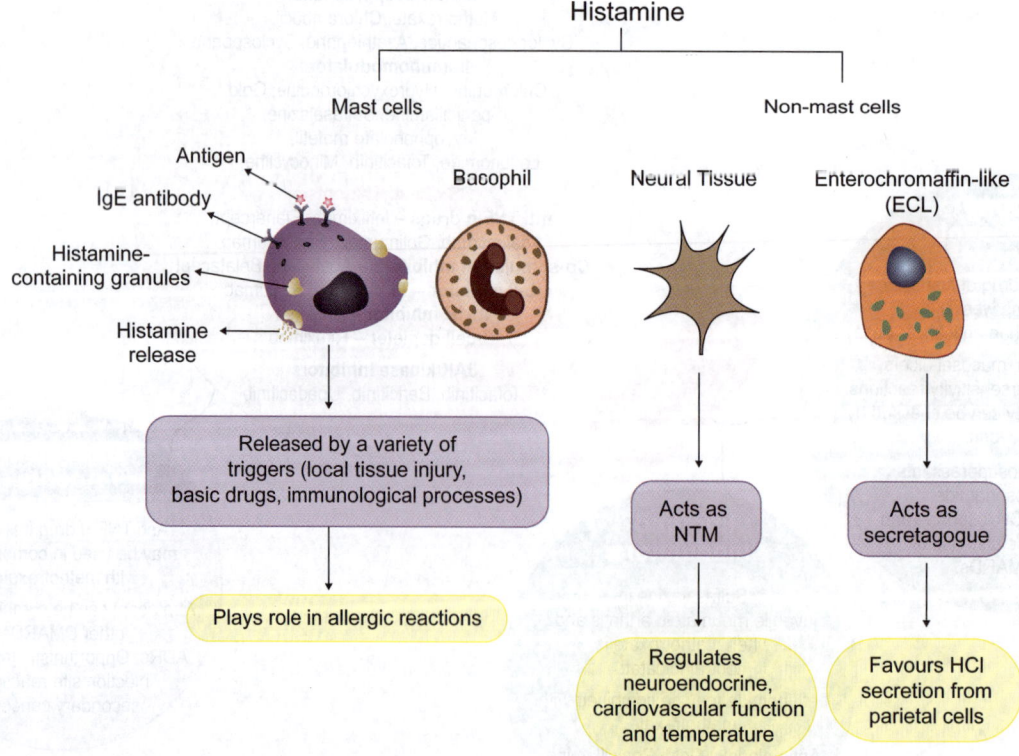

Fig. 26.1 Histamine secretions and functions

Mechanism of Action

Histamine acts through four types of histaminergic receptors, H_1–H_4, all of which are G protein-coupled receptors. Their distribution and major actions are described in Table 26.1.

Pathophysiological Role

a. **Immune reactions:** On exposure to specific antigens, mast cells are sensitised by reaginic IgE antibodies and undergo degranulation, releasing histamine, ATP and other stored mediators. This causes **type I allergic reactions** such as urticaria, hay fever, itching, and anaphylaxis. H_1 receptor-mediated activation of sensory nerve endings causes pain and itching. The most prominent actions of histamine in **immune reactions** are:
   - **Vasodilatation** of smaller blood vessels (capillaries, venules and arterioles) occurs through H1-mediated release of nitric oxide (NO) from the endothelium; this nitric oxide is also called 'endothelium-derived relaxing factor' (EDRF). H1-mediated vasodilatation occurs first, followed by the delayed and persistent vasodilator effects of H2-mediated relaxation of vascular smooth muscles. Vasodilatation results in **flushing**, a sense of **warmth**, **headache, fall in BP, reflex tachycardia** and **increased cardiac output**. However, the larger vessels are constricted through H1-mediated contraction of vascular smooth muscles.
   - **Bronchoconstriction** is mediated by H_1 receptors present on bronchial smooth muscles. The effect is more prominent in bronchial asthma patients with hyper-reactive airways.

b. Histamine is an important **mediator of inflammation** and is released locally upon chemical or mechanical injury to tissues. It causes:
   - Local vasodilatation.
   - Leakage of plasma that is rich in inflammatory mediators such as complement, C-reactive proteins (CRPs) and antibodies.

Table 26.1 *Distribution and actions of histaminergic receptors*

Receptor	Transduction (nature)	Distribution	Actions
H_1	IP_3–DAG → increased Ca^{2+} (**excitatory**)	**Brain** (post-synaptic) on **sensory nerve endings**	Mediate **pain and itching, urticaria, triple response** (red spot, edema and flare) on intradermal injection.
		Midbrain, hypothalamus	**Maintain wakefulness**, suppress appetite
		Ganglia, afferent nerve endings, adrenal medulla	Stimulate ganglia, nerve endings, increase catecholamine release
		Smooth muscles in:	
		- Bronchi	Bronchoconstriction
		- Intestinal muscles	Increased peristalsis → diarrhea
		- Uterine muscles	Contraction → abortion in pregnant women
		- Large blood vessels	Vasoconstriction
		Endothelium in small blood vessels	**EDRF release** → **vasodilatation** of arterioles, relaxation of precapillary sphincters → increased capillary permeability, decrease in SBP and DBP, flushing, warmth and headache → reflex tachycardia.
			Separation of endothelial cells in microcirculation → transudation of fluids → edema
H_2	Activation of adenylyl cyclase → increased cAMP (**excitatory**)	Gastric mucosa	**Increased HCl release** from parietal cells, slight increase in release of pepsin and intrinsic factor (IF)
		Cardiac muscle	Increase in heart rate, contractility
		Smooth muscles of blood vessels	Vasodilatation
H_3	Inhibition of adenylyl cyclase → decrease in cAMP which decreases Ca^{2+} entry through N-type Ca^{2+} channels in nerve endings (**inhibitory**)	Presynaptic in brain, lung, spleen, gastric glands, ileum, myenteric plexus	Reduce release of ACh, histamine and peptide transmitters in brain and peripheral nerves.
			H_3 activation promotes sleepiness.
H_4	Inhibition of adenylyl cyclase → reduced cAMP (**inhibitory**)	Eosinophils, mast cells and basophils	**Chemotaxis** of eosinophils and mast cells in allergic/inflammatory reactions such as rhinitis and asthma

- Chemotaxis of inflammatory cells (e.g., neutrophils, lymphocytes, monocytes, basophils and eosinophils). Intradermal injection of histamine causes a **triple response**, characterised by:
- A red spot due to the dilatation of capillaries upon EDRF release.
- A wheal that is formed as a result of fluid exudation from dilated vessels.
- A flare, or the surrounding redness, caused by axon reflex-mediated arteriolar dilatation.

c. Histamine also plays an important role in the **secretion of gastric acid**, pepsin and IF (intrinsic factor) from gastric parietal cells. This action is mediated through H_2 receptors.

Histamines

Betahistine is a histamine analogue with selective H_1-agonistic effects. It causes vasodilatation of internal ear blood vessels and reduces vertigo in patients suffering from Meniere's disease. It is used orally in a dose of 4–8 mg, four times a day. However, it is contraindicated in patients with asthma as it can worsen bronchoconstriction, and peptic ulcer disease as it increases acid secretion.

The H_3-agonist **pitolisant** is used to reduce daytime sleepiness in narcolepsy.

Other than Meniere's disease and narcolepsy, there are no therapeutic indications for any of the actions of histamine. However, the blockade of histamine actions finds several, diverse uses.

ANTIHISTAMINES

Drugs that block H_1 receptors are called H_1 antihistamines and are extensively used to control allergic reactions. Drugs that block H_2 receptors reduce gastric acid secretion and are used to treat peptic ulcer disease (see Chapter 64). Specific blockers of H_3 and H_4 receptors are not yet available.

Classification of H_1 Antihistamines

H_1 antagonists developed between 1930 and 1980 are called first-generation antihistamines. They are classified based on the intensity of their sedative effect (mild, moderate and highly sedative). H_1 blockers developed after 1980 are classified as second-generation antihistamines (Flowchart 26.1).

Mechanism of Action

These drugs were previously thought to be competitive antagonists, but recent evidence suggests that these are **inverse agonists** at H_1 **receptors.**

H_1 antihistamines bind to and stabilise the inactive state of H_1 receptors, shifting the equilibrium towards the inactive state (refer to the two-state receptor model, page 55), resulting in down-regulation of the constitutive activity of histamine. In addition, different antihistamine drugs possess varying capacities to block muscarinic, α-adrenergic and serotonergic (5-HT_{2A}) receptors.

Pharmacological Actions

- H_1 blockers antagonise most of the actions of histamine, except gastric acid secretion.
- **Central effects** of first-generation H_1 antihistamines vary depending upon their ability to cross the blood–brain barrier. First-generation drugs cause variable degree of **sedation**, with significant inter-individual differences in the intensity of sedative action. In children, however, excitation may occur. Sedative action causes lethargy and reduces cognitive as well as psychomotor performance. Toxic doses can cause **excitation, agitation, convulsions, or coma.** Some H_1 blockers show **antitussive and appetite-stimulating** effects, e.g., cyproheptadine increases appetite by 5-HT_{2A}-blocking action.

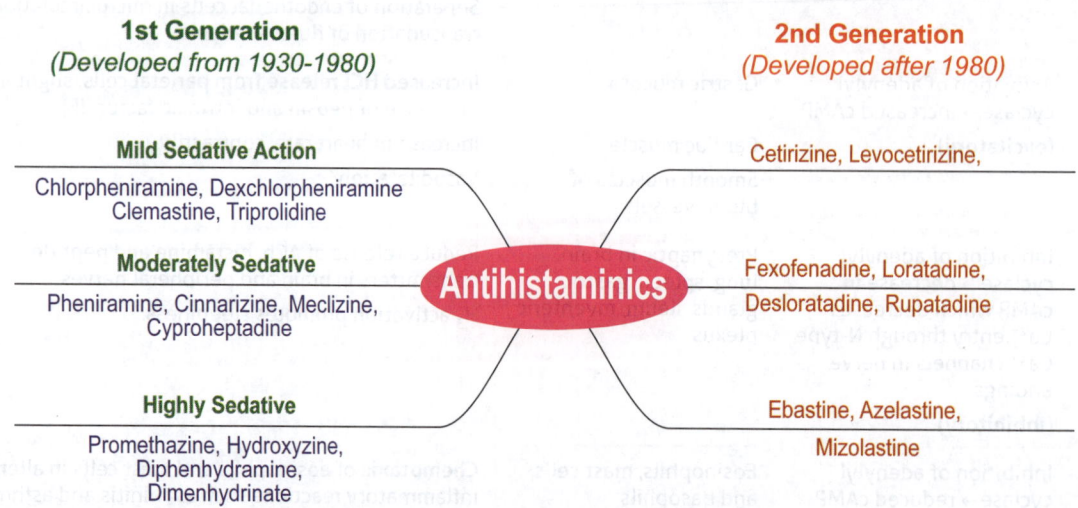

Flowchart 26.1 Classification of antihistamines

Second-generation drugs are free of central sedative as well as excitatory actions.
- **Anticholinergic effects**: Highly sedative first-generation H₁ blockers such as promethazine, diphenhydramine, dimenhydrinate and pheniramine exhibit **antimuscarinic** effects. This contributes to their **antiemetic** effect, which is used to treat morning sickness during pregnancy and motion sickness. They are also effective in reducing symptoms of parkinsonism or extrapyramidal side effects of antipsychotic drugs. The anticholinergic action may cause dryness of mouth, blurring of vision, constipation and urinary retention, especially in elderly males. The antimuscarinic effect is not shown by second-generation drugs.
- **Antiallergic effect**: H₁ blockers control itching, rashes, urticaria, angioedema and prevent type I allergic reactions. However, anaphylactic reaction characterised by fall in BP and bronchoconstriction is not adequately controlled because other mediators such as leukotrienes (C4 and D4) and platelet-activating factor (PAF) also contribute to such reactions. Adrenaline, the physiological antagonist of histamine, can reverse both vasodilatation and bronchoconstriction and is life-saving in anaphylaxis.
- Promethazine has **α-blocking** effects that may cause orthostatic hypotension, dizziness and reflex tachycardia.
- Histamine-induced contraction of intestinal and bronchial smooth muscles is blocked.
- Histamine-induced fall in BP, vasodilatation and triple response is prevented.
- Some H₁ blockers show antitussive and appetite-stimulating effects, e.g., cyproheptadine increases appetite by 5-HT$_{2A}$-blocking action.

Major receptor actions of antihistamines are shown in Fig. 26.2.

Second-Generation Antihistamines
- Second-generation drugs have negligible penetration across the blood–brain barrier. So, they are **devoid of central side effects** such as sedation, lethargy, and decreased concentration.
- Because second-generation drugs **do not possess anticholinergic effects**, they do not cause autonomic adverse effects. However, they are not effective in the treatment of muscular dystonia, parkinsonism and motion sickness.
- Second-generation drugs can **inhibit release or action of mediators** such as cytokines, leukotrienes, PAF from platelets and chemotaxis of eosinophils.
- Azelastine and rupatadine have PAF-antagonistic properties and are useful in allergic rhinitis, hay fever, conjunctivitis, etc.

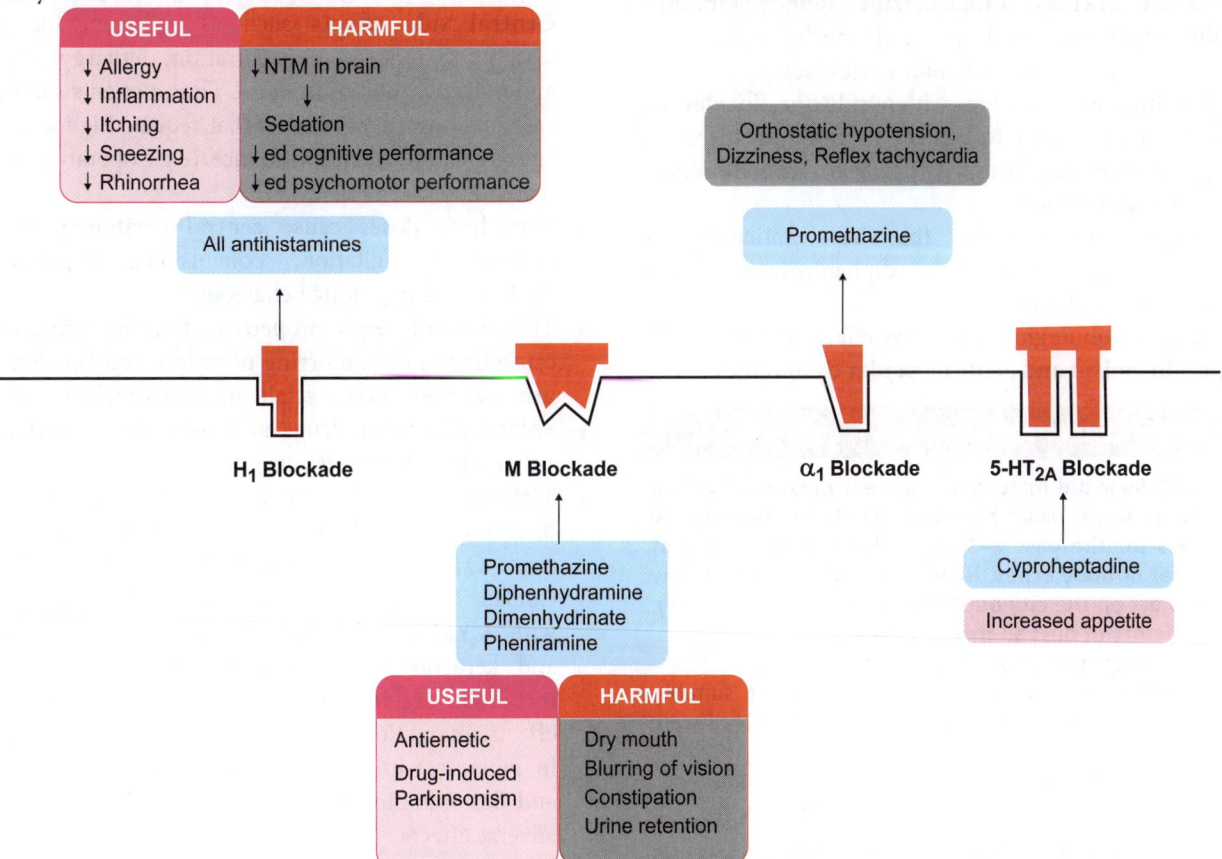

Fig. 26.2 Receptor actions of antihistamines

- Cetirizine is concentrated in the skin and shows better and **longer-lasting effects in the treatment of urticaria, atopic dermatitis and dermographism**.

Therapeutic Uses

- **Type 1 allergic reactions:** H_1 antihistamines are the most frequently used drugs for the prevention and treatment of allergic reactions such as **rashes, urticaria, hay fever, allergic rhinitis, and allergic conjunctivitis**. Second-generation drugs are preferred for these indications because they do not exhibit sedative and autonomic adverse effects. In atopic dermatitis, however, the highly sedative first-generation drug, diphenhydramine, is preferred to reduce the awareness of itching. In angioedema, bronchial asthma and anaphylaxis, the response to antihistamines is not satisfactory, because other mediators are involved. Antihistamines play an adjuvant role to adrenaline in the treatment of these conditions.
- H_1 blockers can effectively treat **insect bites, stings, ivy poisoning** and **drug allergies**.
- **Idiopathic pruritus** responds well to chlorpheniramine, diphenhydramine, or cyproheptadine. In some nonresponsive cases of chronic urticaria, the addition of H_2 blockers may be effective.
- **Motion sickness:** Promethazine, diphenhydramine, dimenhydrinate, cyclizine and meclizine are very effective in prevention of motion sickness.
- **Morning sickness:** Along with pyridoxine, **doxylamine** is extensively used to control morning sickness and hyperemesis gravidarum, though there are a few reports of teratogenic effects.
- **Vertigo:** Antihistamines that have anticholinergic effects (e.g., cinnarizine, diphenhydramine and promethazine) are useful.
- The anticholinergic and sedative effects provide relief in **parkinsonism and acute muscular dystonias**.

Clinical problem-based questions and MCQs

1. A 45-year-old male civil engineer presented with a runny nose, nasal blockage, headache and watery eyes for the past 2–3 days. There is no history of fever or body aches. He was recently allotted a new project on the city outskirts, where it is quite dusty. A history of dust allergy is present.
   i. What is the cause of his symptoms?
   ii. Which of the following drugs is most suitable to relieve his symptoms with minimal adverse effects?
      a. Fexofenadine   b. Diphenhydramine
      c. Pheniramine   d. Promethazine

2. An 8-year-old boy presents with intense itching that worsens at night. Examination showed dry skin with brown-grey patches on ankles, wrists, upper chest, and knees, and lichenification of certain lesions. A diagnosis of atopic dermatitis is made.
   i. Which of the following antihistaminic drugs is the most suitable for this patient?
      a. Doxylamine   b. Levocetirizine
      c. Azelastine   d. Cyproheptadine
   ii. Justify your choice.

3. A 50-year-old male with vertigo, nausea, vomiting and tendency to fall is prescribed betahistine.
   a. Explain the pharmacological basis of use of betahistine.
   b. Enumerate other drugs that may be useful to treat vertigo.

4. All the following antihistamines have anticholinergic property EXCEPT:
   a. Promethazine   b. Fexofenadine
   c. Diphenhydramine   d. Pheniramine

5. Advantages of second-generation antihistamines include:
   a. No sedation
   b. Presence of anticholinergic effects.
   c. Presence of good antitussive effects.
   d. Psychomotor slowing.

Adverse Effects of H_1 Antihistamines

First-generation drugs cause:

- **Central side effects** such as sedation, increased sleepiness, reduced concentration, lethargy, fatigue, and muscular incoordination. Thus, patients should be cautioned against activities that require high attention and psychomotor performance (e.g., operating heavy machinery and vehicles).
- Very high doses cause **central excitatory effects**, restlessness, agitation, convulsions, hypotension, flushing and psychotic behaviour.
- The **anticholinergic** properties of antihistamines may cause dry mouth, blurring of vision, constipation and urinary retention (especially in elderly males).
- Second-generation drugs are mostly free of central and anticholinergic side effects.
- Terfenadine and astemizole (second-generation drugs) have been banned because of their potential to cause QTc prolongation and ventricular arrhythmias (torsade de pointes), especially when combined with CYP3A4-inhibiting drugs (e.g., erythromycin and ketoconazole). While fexofenadine (the active metabolite of terfenadine), is largely free of such adverse effects/interactions, it should be used with caution in patients with prolonged QTc interval. Loratadine and desloratadine are also free of cardiac and central adverse effects.

Levocetirizine, desloratadine and fexofenadine are sometimes considered as third-generation antihistamines.

Therapeutic Uses and ADRs of H_1 Antihistamines

Uses

- **Type 1 allergic reactions**: e.g., rash, urticaria, hay fever, allergic rhinitis, and allergic conjunctivitis. Second-generation drugs are preferred. Cetirizine is a good choice for atopic dermatitis. In the case of sleep disturbance due to itching, highly sedating dimenhydrinate can be used for some time.
- Insect bites, stings, ivy poisoning, or allergic response to drugs.
- **Idiopathic pruritus:** chlorpheniramine, diphenhydramine or cyproheptadine. H_2 blockers may be added if relief is not satisfactory.
- **Motion sickness:** promethazine, diphenhydramine, dimenhydrinate, cyclizine, meclizine.
- **Morning sickness,** hyperemesis gravidarum: doxylamine along with pyridoxine is useful.
- **Vertigo:** Antihistamines that have anticholinergic effects, such as cinnarizine, diphenhydramine, and promethazine are useful. Betahistine is useful in Meniere's disease.
- Parkinsonism and acute muscular dystonia.
- Adjuvant role to adrenaline in **bronchial asthma** and **anaphylaxis**.

ADRs

- Central side effects such as sedation, increased sleepiness, reduced concentration, lethargy, fatigue and muscular incoordination.
- Very high doses cause central excitatory effects, restlessness, agitation, convulsions, hypotension, flushing and psychotic behaviour.
- Anticholinergic adverse effects like dry mouth, blurring of vision, constipation and urinary retention (may occur in elderly males).

VERTIGO

Vertigo is a sensation of movement when it is not actually occurring. Patients usually complain of dizziness, sensation of spinning/rotational motion, nausea and vomiting. It may occur due to a variety of central and peripheral causes, but usually involves vestibular problems.

Drugs for Vertigo

Antihistamines: Cinnarizine, promethazine, diphenhydramine, dimenhydrinate
Histamine analogue: Betahistine
Anticholinergics: Atropine, hyoscine
Neuroleptic: Prochlorperazine
Diuretics: Acetazolamide, thiazides, amiloride
Corticosteroids
Antianxiety/antidepressants: Diazepam, amitriptyline.

Mechanisms of action of antivertigo drugs

Drugs can relieve vertigo by different mechanisms.

- Suppression of central cholinergic pathways or labyrinthine end organ receptors: anticholinergics, antihistaminics with additional anticholinergic effects, phenothiazine with antiemetic action (prochlorperazine) are effective.
- Improving blood flow to the labyrinth: betahistine is used in Meniere's disease.
- Decreasing intralabyrinthine fluid pressure: diuretics
- Decreasing intralabyrinthine edema: corticosteroids
- Modifying perception of vertigo: diazepam, amitriptyline

Cinnarizine has H_1 antihistaminic, antiserotonergic, anticholinergic, sedative and vasodilator actions and is frequently used to treat vertigo. The antivertigo effect may arise from its calcium-channel blocking action, interfering with influx of Ca^{2+} ions from the endolymph to the vestibular sensory cells. Thus, it inhibits vestibular sensory nuclei in the inner ear and suppresses post-rotatory labyrinthine reflexes. It may cause mild GI adverse effects and sedation.

Betahistine is especially useful in Meniere's disease.

Prochlorperazine, a D_2 receptor-blocking neuroleptic drug, is used parenterally in case of severe vertigo associated with vomiting.

Summary

Histamine

- H_1 and H_2 receptors are excitatory, while H_3 and H_4 are inhibitory in nature.
- Released from mast cells, histamine plays an important role in allergic reactions, pain, itching, urticaria, bronchospasm, vasodilatation, hypotension, triple response (through H_1 receptors).
- Neuronal histamine has a role as neurotransmitter (NTM) in temperature, feeding, sleep–wakefulness regulation, cardiovascular and neuroendocrine function regulation (H_1).
- Also plays important role in inflammatory reactions by vasodilatation, leakage of plasma and chemotaxis.
- Regulates gastric acid secretion through H_2 receptors.
- Selective H_1-agonist betahistine is used in Meniere's disease to control vertigo; contraindicated in asthma and peptic ulcer patients.

H_1 Antihistamines

- Classified as first- and second-generation drugs. The first-generation drugs can have mild/moderate/severe sedating effect.

- Act as inverse agonists, down-regulating constitutive activity of histamine.
- Antagonise most actions of histamine except gastric secretion. Sedative effect varies among drugs and from person-to-person. Some drugs have appetite-stimulating and antitussive effects as well.
- Highly sedating H_1 blockers also have anticholinergic and antiemetic effects. Promethazine can cause orthostatic hypotension through $α_1$ blockade.
- Prevent histamine-induced type 1 allergic reactions, vasodilatation, smooth muscle contraction and triple response. However, response in anaphylaxis is partial.
- Release of leukotrienes, cytokines and platelet-activating factor reduced by second-generation drugs. So, these are useful in **allergic rhinitis (azelastine), atopic dermatitis (cetirizine)**.
- Useful in type 1 allergic reactions, idiopathic pruritus, atopic dermatitis, insect bites, stings, ivy poisoning, vertigo, prevention of motion and morning sickness and extrapyramidal adverse effects of antipsychotic drugs.
- Second-generation drugs are not effective in muscular dystonias, parkinsonism and motion sickness as they lack anticholinergic effects.
- Cetirizine is better for urticaria/atopic dermatitis and azelastine for rhinitis.
- Major adverse effects with first-generation drugs are central and anticholinergic. Toxic doses can cause central excitatory response. However, second-generation drugs are free from such adverse effects.

Questions for practice

1. Classify H_1 antihistaminic drugs.
2. Enumerate therapeutic uses and adverse effects of antihistamines.
3. Enumerate differences between first- and second-generation antihistamines.
4. Enumerate antivertigo drugs and describe their mechanisms of action.
5. Explain why:
   a. Promethazine is effective in motion sickness.
   b. Diphenhydramine is used in atopic dermatitis.
   c. Histamine causes triple response.
   d. Betahistine and antihistaminic drugs are useful in vertigo.
   e. Betahistine is contraindicated in patients with peptic ulcer disease.

Hints for problem-based questions and MCQs

1. i. Type I allergic reactions
   ii. a. Fexofenadine is preferred because it does not have sedative and anticholinergic adverse effects.
2. i. b. Cetirizine
   ii. It gets concentrated in the skin and has longer lasting action. Refer to page 352.
3. i. a. Betahistine, a selective H_1-agonist, causes vasodilatation of internal ear blood vessels and increases blood flow to labyrinth.
   ii. Antihistamines that have anticholinergic effects (e.g., cinnarizine, diphenhydramine and promethazine) are useful as they suppress cholinergic pathways in vestibular nuclei. Corticosteroids and antianxiety drugs may also be useful.
4. b. Fexofenadine
5. a. No sedation

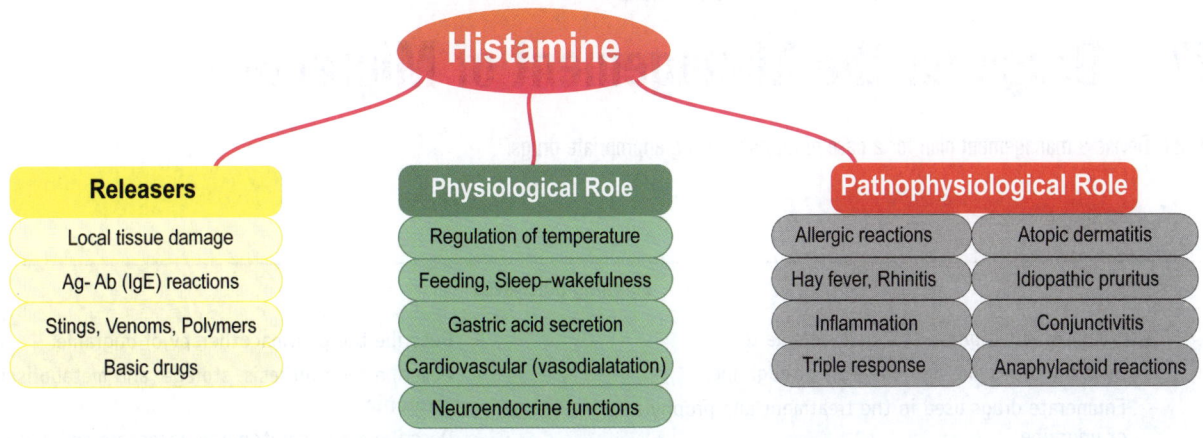

SECTION 4 Autocoids and Related Drugs

27 Drugs for the Management of Migraine

PH 2.8 Devise a management plan for a case of migraine using appropriate drugs.

Learning objectives

A student of MBBS phase II should be able to:
- Describe types and pathogenesis of migraine.
- Enumerate drugs used in the treatment and prophylaxis of migraine.
- Describe mechanism of action and pharmacological actions of drugs used in migraine.
- Describe indications for use, adverse effects, and contraindications of triptans.
- Describe the pharmacotherapy of migraine.
- Describe the synthesis, storage, and metabolism of serotonin.
- Describe major serotonergic receptors and actions mediated through these.
- Describe pathophysiological role and pharmacological actions of serotonin.
- Enumerate drugs that modulate serotonin actions.

Migraine is a neurological syndrome that affects women more commonly than men. The most characteristic feature of migraine is a unilateral throbbing headache that may become severe enough to interfere with routine activity. Treatment aims at relieving the symptoms and preventing further attacks.

TYPES OF MIGRAINE

According to the International Classification of Headache Disorders, migraine can be **episodic** or **chronic**. An acute migraine attack may be precipitated by a variety of **triggers** such as hormonal changes (as during menstruation and use of oral contraceptives), lack of sleep, loud noises, flashing lights, stress and some foods (e.g., aged cheese, red wine, smoked meat, artificial sweeteners, chocolates, alcoholic beverages and dairy products). Trigger factors vary from patient to patient, and can usually be identified by careful maintenance of a pain diary.

a. Migraine is classified as **classical** or **common** based on the presence of an aura.
   - In **classical migraine**, the headache is preceded by an aura. An acute attack of classical migraine is characterised by two phases:
     - The initial **aura phase**, occurring before the headache begins, and usually lasts 5 to 60 minutes. It is caused by **cerebral vessel vasoconstriction** and ischemia that result in visual disturbances and paresthesia (aura), usually unilateral, tingling or numbness, often starting in the fingers or face, and difficulty in speaking or finding words.
     - The **headache phase** is the second phase. Symptoms such as nausea, vomiting, vertigo, and sensitivity to light (photophobia)/sound (phonophobia)/smell (osmophobia) usually accompany the unilateral, pulsatile headache. The symptoms worsen with physical exertion.
   - **Common migraine** → headache manifests without aura in 80% cases.
b. Based on the frequency, duration and severity of symptoms during the attack, migraine can be **mild**, **moderate**, or **severe**.
   - **Mild** cases experience < 1 migraine attack per month; each attack may last up to 8 hours. Pain is of tolerable severity and patient is not incapacitated.
   - **Moderate** cases experience ≥ 1 migraine attacks per month, with each episode lasting 8–24 hours. The pain is more intense, is accompanied by symptoms such as nausea, vomiting and photophobia, and interferes with routine activities.
   - **Severe** cases suffer from > 2–3 attacks of severe throbbing pain per month. Each attack may last for 12–48 hours. Pain is very severe, incapacitating, and accompanied by nausea, vomiting, and vertigo.
   - **Status migrainosus** is when an acute migraine attack lasts longer than 72 hours.

Etiology of Migraine

While the etiology of migraine is not well understood, the following theories have been proposed:

a. **Cerebral ischemia**, due to vasoconstriction or shunting of blood through carotid arteriovenous anastomosis.
b. **Suppression of electrical activity** in cortical neurons is usually implicated in causing migraine.

c. **Disturbance in serotonergic activity** is implicated in the pathophysiology of migraine, as serotonin (5-HT) levels fluctuate across the different phases of a migraine attack. Certain drugs that promote 5-HT release (e.g., reserpine and fenfluramine)—can trigger migraine episodes. Moreover, triptans, which are $5\text{-HT}_{1B/1D}$ receptor agonists, relieve acute migraine symptoms. These 5-HT_1 receptors are inhibitory in nature and their activation reduces the release of 5-HT and other inflammatory neuropeptides. They also cause cranial vessel vasoconstriction, relieving migraine.

The synthesis, storage, release, termination of action of 5-HT, its major receptor actions, pathophysiological role and drugs affecting serotonergic transmission are described later in the chapter (see page 361).

Pathogenesis of Migraine
(Fig 27.1)

1. The **prodromal phase** of migraine is probably due to hypothalamic and thalamic activation, and is characterised by vague symptoms such as irritability, mood swings, food cravings, fatigue, neck stiffness, and photophobia.

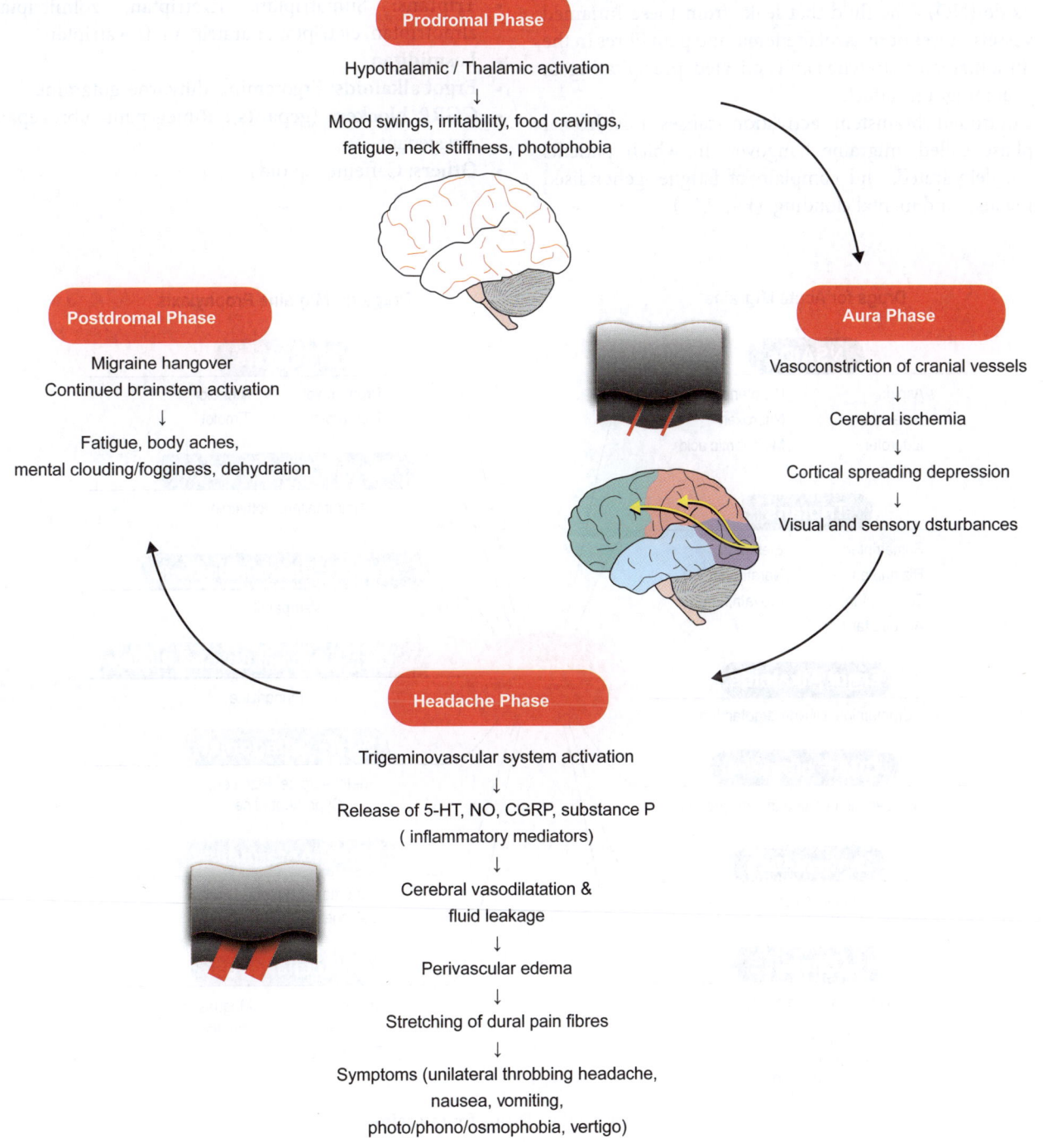

Fig. 27.1 Pathogenesis of migraine

2. **Phase of aura:** Vasoconstriction of cranial vessels in response to 5-HT released from platelets causes cerebral ischemia and is usually the starting point for migraine. The electrical activity in cortical neurons gets suppressed, resulting in visual disturbances and parasthesias. This causes the aura of classical migraine.
3. **Headache phase:** A long phase of cerebral vasodilation that results in pulsatile, throbbing headache, accompanied by nausea, vomiting, photophobia and vertigo follows the aura. **Neurogenic inflammation of vessel** walls, in response to various triggers, causes the release of mediators such as 5-HT, substance P, calcitonin gene-related peptide, (CGRP) and nitric oxide (NO). The fluid that leaks from these inflamed vessels causes perivascular edema, and pain fibres in the dura mater are stretched and activated, precipitating an acute migraine attack.
4. Continued brainstem activation causes postdromal phase called 'migraine hangover', in which patients are dehydrated, and complain of fatigue, generalised malaise, and mental clouding. (Fig. 27.1).

MANAGEMENT OF MIGRAINE

The management of migraine involves both **controlling acute attacks** as well as the prevention of further attacks (Flowchart 27.1).

Drugs that Control Acute Migraine Attacks

Drugs that control acute migraine attacks can be classified as:

- **NSAIDs:** Aspirin, paracetamol, ibuprofen, diclofenac, naproxen, mefenamic acid
- **Antiemetics:** Domperidone, metoclopramide
- **Triptans:** Sumatriptan, rizatriptan, zolmitriptan, almotriptan, eletriptan, naratriptan, frovatriptan
- **Lasmiditan**
- **Ergot alkaloids:** Ergotamine, dihydroergotamine
- **CGRP blockers (gepants):** Rimegepant, ubrogepant, zavegepant
- **Others:** Caffeine, opioids

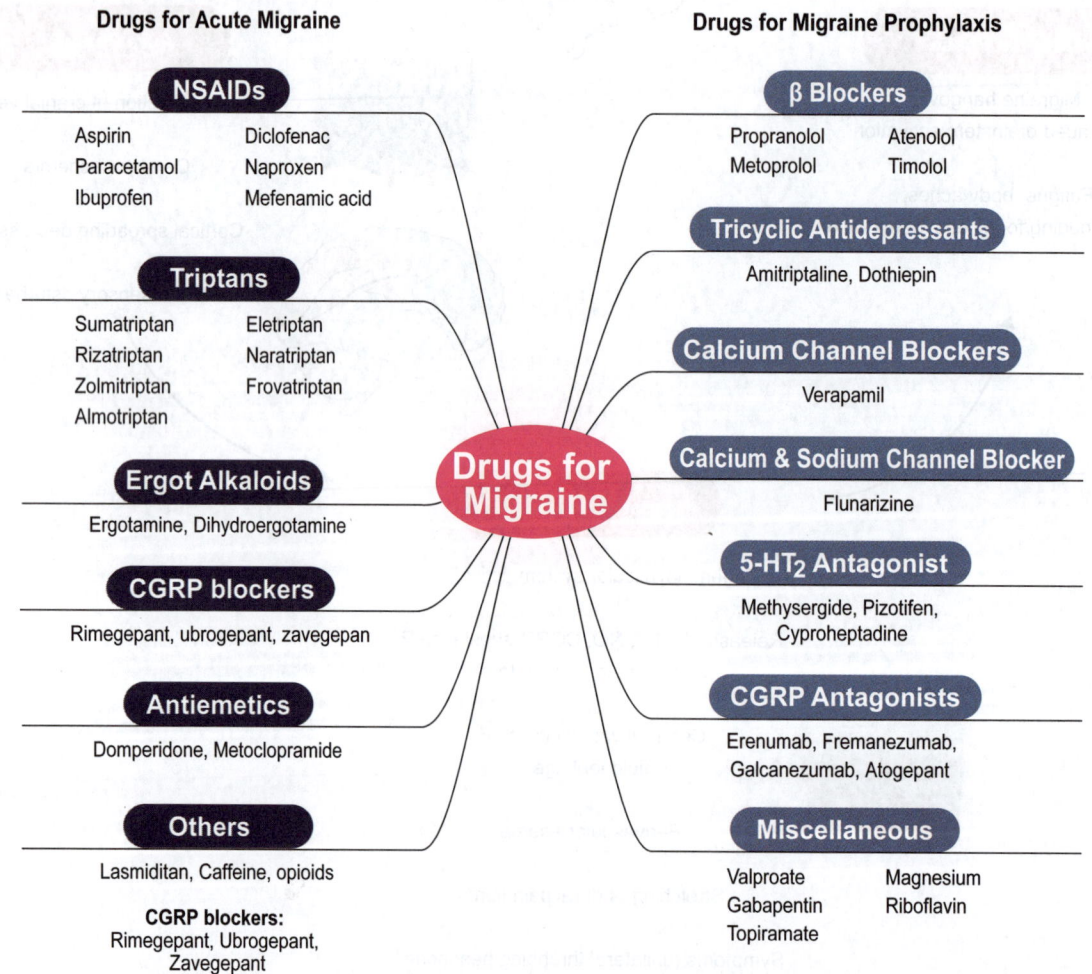

Flowchart 27.1 Drugs for migraine

NSAIDs

NSAIDs are cyclooxygenase inhibitors. They inhibit prostaglandin synthesis and exert analgesic anti-inflammatory action. They relieve headache by their analgesic effect and reduce inflammation surrounding the cranial vessels.

- NSAIDs or their combinations suffice in mild-to-moderate attacks of common migraine without aura.

Commonly prescribed NSAIDs in migraine include paracetamol (0.5–1 g), aspirin (300–600 mg), and ibuprofen (400–800 mg). Some other options are naproxen, diclofenac, and mefenamic acid. In severe refractory cases, opioids may be needed.

Antiemetics

Acute migraine attacks are often accompanied by gastric stasis, which interferes with the absorption of oral drugs.

- Antiemetic drug **metoclopramide** (10 mg, oral or intramuscular) is useful.
- Domperidone (10 mg) is also effective.
- **Diphenhydramine** or **promethazine** may be used for their sedative as well as antiemetic effect.

Antiemetics may be combined with NSAIDs as per the need of individual patients.

Triptans

Triptans include the following drugs: sumatriptan, rizatriptan, frovatriptan, naratriptan, almotriptan, zolmitriptan and eletriptan.

Mechanism of action

These drugs act as **agonists at 5-HT$_{1D/1B}$ receptors**. Sumatriptan can activate other 5-HT$_1$ receptor subtypes also at higher doses, but does not affect 5-HT$_{2-7}$ receptors. The adrenergic, dopaminergic, cholinergic, and GABAergic receptors are not affected.

Pharmacological actions

Sumatriptan promotes the constriction of dilated cranial blood vessels, especially carotid artery arteriovenous shunts. Neurogenic inflammation of dilated cranial vessels and plasma protein extravasation across dural vessels is also suppressed. Triptans can also control the nausea and vomiting associated with migraine attacks.

Pharmacokinetics

The oral bioavailability of sumatriptan is 15%. It gets metabolised quickly by monoamine oxidase isoenzyme A (MAO-A), followed by the excretion of metabolites in urine.

Among the triptans, sumatriptan has the lowest oral bioavailability, plasma protein binding, penetration across the blood–brain barrier, and efficacy. Sumatriptan is safe for use in pregnant women suffering from migraine. It is the only triptan available as a subcutaneous injection as well as nasal spray.

Therapeutic uses

Sumatriptan is the preferred drug for controlling acute migraine attacks that do not respond to analgesic drug combinations.

- Sumatriptan is given orally in a dose of 50–100 mg at the onset of migraine attack; it may be repeated once within 24 hours as per need. About 75% of patients get complete relief from symptoms within 2–3 hours of administration of triptans. Because of the short half-life of sumatriptan, the headache can recur within 24 hours in 20–40% of cases.
- When fast onset of action is required or when the patient is unable to take the drug orally due to migraine-induced vomiting, sumatriptan can be administered by subcutaneous injection (6 mg) or as nasal spray (25 mg).

Rizatriptan exhibits the maximum efficacy among the triptans; it has better oral bioavailability, and is faster-acting and more potent than sumatriptan. It is absorbed rapidly upon oral administration, resulting in fast onset of action. It is the drug of choice for acute attacks (given in a dose of 5–10 mg) and can be repeated once after 2 hours, if needed. Adverse effects include arrhythmias, pain in jaw, and excessive sweating.

Naratriptan and **frovatriptan** have longer half-life than other triptans. Thus, while the pain relief occurs slowly, there is lesser recurrence of headache during the attack. These are valuable in protracted migraine attacks, as seen during the premenstrual or menstrual phase.

ADRs

Triptans cause **mild side effects** such as dizziness, weakness, tightness in chest, heat, and paresthesia of limbs; these are more common after subcutaneous injection.

Serious adverse effects such as bradycardia, coronary vasospasm, and precipitation of myocardial infarction are **rare**. Triptans are preferred over ergots due to their better safety profile and fewer adverse effects.

Contraindications

Triptans are contraindicated in patients with ischemic heart disease, stroke, transient ischemic attack, peripheral vascular disease, hepatic and renal function impairment, and during pregnancy.

Lasmiditan

Lasmiditan, a **5-HT$_{1F}$ agonist**, reduces CGRP release and prevents extravasation of fluid from dural vessels. It can relieve acute migraine symptoms without causing vasoconstriction of cranial vessels. Hence, it is safe for use in migraine patients with co-existent cardiovascular disease.

Its **adverse effects** include sedation, tiredness, numbness and dizziness.

Ergot Alkaloids

These alkaloids are derived from a fungus that grows on millets and rye stored in damp conditions. Consumption of these contaminated grains causes **ergotism**, which is characterised by vasoconstriction, ischemia, gangrene of toes and fingers, hallucinations, dementia and convulsions.

Classification
- **Natural ergot alkaloids:** Ergometrine, ergotamine, ergotoxine
- **Semisynthetic derivatives:**
  - Methylergometrine, dihydroergotamine, dihydroergotoxine
  - Methysergide, lisuride, pergolide, bromocriptine
- **Synthetic derivatives:** Lysergic acid diethylamide (LSD)

Mechanism of action
Ergotamine acts as a $5-HT_{1B/1D}$ receptor agonist → reduced CGRP levels, vasoconstriction → both actions contribute to its antimigraine effect. Vasoconstrictor action is responsible for the ischemic adverse effects of ergots; dihydroergotamine shows a relatively lower vasoconstrictor action.

Pharmacological actions
Ergots have agonistic effects on $5-HT_{1B/1D}$, dopaminergic, and α-receptors.

- **Central actions**
  - **Ergotamine** causes cranial vessel constriction by its agonistic effect on $5-HT_{1B/1D}$ receptors and **relieves migraine pain**. Ergotamine stimulates the chemoreceptor trigger zone (CTZ) and vomiting centre, resulting in **emesis**. Large doses of ergotamine may cause **CNS stimulation, paresthesias, and hallucinations;** LSD, a potent hallucinogen, is a synthetic ergot derivative.
  - **Dihydroergotoxine** increases release of acetylcholine in the cerebral cortex, which may be useful in treating patients with **dementia**.
  - **Bromocriptine** has a relatively selective dopaminergic action; it is a potent agonist at D_2 receptors and partial agonist/antagonist at D_1 receptors. It can quickly relieve symptoms of **Parkinson's disease** but, the dose required is high and poorly tolerated. Bromocriptine reduces prolactin secretion by its D_2-agonistic effect on lactotrophs and causes **suppression of lactation**.
- **Action on blood vessels:** Ergotamine causes **sustained vasoconstriction** due to its slow dissociation from α-adrenergic receptors. This may be responsible for capillary endothelial damage, thrombosis, vascular stasis, and gangrene in cases of chronic ergot exposure. Vasoconstriction is less marked with dihydroergotamine and dihydroergotoxine.

Action on smooth muscles: Methylergometrine acts as a partial agonist at $5-HT_2$ receptors. It causes **myometrial contractions**, especially in full-term pregnant uterus, and contraction of GIT smooth muscles. It is exclusively used for its uterine action and has minimal vasoconstrictor and emetic actions.

Therapeutic uses
- Ergometrine and methylergometrine are useful in controlling **postpartum hemorrhage**.
- Dihydroergotoxine causes some improvement in senile dementia and Alzheimer's disease.
- Ergotamine and dihydroergotamine are effective in relieving **acute migraine attacks**. However, these are not drugs of choice because of the availability of better-tolerated drugs such as triptans.
- Methysergide is useful for **migraine prophylaxis**, but is less efficacious than propranolol.
- Methysergide is effective in the treatment of **carcinoid syndrome**.
- Bromocriptine is useful in **parkinsonism, acromegaly,** and **hyperprolactinemia**, but is not preferred because of its poor tolerability.

Adverse effects
- Most frequent adverse effects of ergots include nausea, vomiting, and diarrhea.
- Hallucinations and paresthesia may occur with larger doses.
- Chronic exposure to ergotamine may cause capillary endothelial damage, thrombosis, vascular stasis, and gangrene due to sustained vasoconstrictor action.
- Ergots should not be used within 24 hours of triptans or other vasoconstrictor drugs, as this may precipitate coronary vasospasm leading to variant angina.

Contraindications
- Pregnancy
- Peripheral vasospastic diseases
- Ischemic heart disease
- Hypertension
- Hepatic/renal function impairment

CGRP blockers (gepants)
Rimegepant, ubrogepant and zavegepant act by blocking receptors of CGRP, resulting in reduced neurogenic inflammation, pain transmission and prevention of cranial artery dilation. All three actions are beneficial in migraine. Thus, gepants relieve migraine pain in about 60% of patients, although they lack vasoconstrictor action. Therefore, gepants are safe for use in patients with ischemic heart disease or cerebrovascular accidents, in whom triptans are contraindicated.

Adverse effects of rimegepant include nausea, dryness of mouth, sedation and hypersensitivity reactions such as rashes, urticaria, angioedema.

Zavegepant is used as nasal spray in patients who are unable to take oral drugs due to nausea and vomiting associated with migraine. However, it may cause nasal discomfort and irritation. Taste disturbances and hypersensitivity reactions are also reported with it.

Caffeine
When used as an **adjuvant to dihydroergotamine (DHE)**, caffeine (100 mg) increases DHE absorption and possesses cranial vasoconstrictor action of its own.

Opioids
Opioid drugs (butorphanol intranasal or pethidine intramuscular) are considered only in resistant cases of migraine, which fail to respond to other drugs.

Drugs for Prophylaxis
The following groups of drugs (Flowchart 27.1) are efficacious in the prevention of acute migraine attacks.
- **β-blockers:** Propranolol, metoprolol, atenolol, timolol
- **Tricyclic antidepressants:** Amitriptyline, dothiepin
- **Calcium channel blockers:** Verapamil
- **Calcium and sodium channel blocker:** Flunarizine
- **5-HT$_2$ antagonists:** Methysergide, pizotifen, cyproheptadine
- **CGRP antagonists:** CGRP antagonists such as erenumab, fremanezumab, and galcanezumab are monoclonal antibodies that block CGRP receptors. They are administered subcutaneously only if >3 prophylactic agents fail to reduce the frequency of migraine attacks. Atogepant is an orally effective CGRP blocker approved for migraine prophylaxis.
- **Miscellaneous:** Valproate, gabapentin, topiramate, magnesium and riboflavin

Cyproheptadine
Mechanism of action
It is a **blocker** of **5-HT$_{2A}$, H$_1$** and **muscarinic receptors**.

Pharmacological actions
Like other antihistaminic drugs, cyproheptadine also has sedative, antiallergic and antipruritic effects; in addition, it can improve appetite.

Therapeutic uses
The 5-HT antagonistic effect of cyproheptadine helps to control **carcinoid tumour symptoms** and relieves dumping symptoms in **post-gastrectomy patients**. It can also relieve fluoxetine-induced orgasmic delay. It is used to treat cold, urticaria, migraine prophylaxis, and serotonin syndrome.

ADRs
Dryness of mouth, confusion because of anticholinergic effects, weight gain, drowsiness and sedation.

Methysergide
Methysergide is another **5-HT$_{2A/2C}$** antagonist used for migraine prophylaxis. Its adverse effects include pulmonary, retroperitoneal, and cardiac fibrosis.

Migraine Prophylaxis
- The first and foremost approach is to **avoid precipitating factors** or situations.
- **Lifestyle modifications** to include a healthy and balanced diet, sufficient sleep, regular food and sleep schedule, regular exercise, yoga/meditation for destressing, and staying well-hydrated are quite effective in reducing migraine frequency.
- The most commonly used drug for migraine prophylaxis is **propranolol** (dose: 40 mg, oral, twice a day). In majority of patients, it decreases the frequency as well as severity of migraine. If the desired response is not obtained, dosage may be increased up to 160 mg, twice a day. The **mechanism** of its migraine prophylactic role **is not clearly understood**.
- For patients who do not respond to the maximum dose of propranolol, **amitriptyline** (dose: 25–50 mg, oral) is tried. It is more suitable for patients suffering from **depression as well as migraine**.
- **Flunarizine**, a **cerebroselective calcium channel blocker**, can also reduce the frequency of migraine attacks and is the **third-choice** drug in migraine prophylaxis after β-blockers and tricyclic antidepressants.
- Many antiepileptic drugs such as valproate, gabapentin, topiramate and verapamil have also shown efficacy in preventing migraine attacks.

Clinical problem-based questions and MCQs

1. A 42-year-old female patient presents with severe headache on the right side of head along with increased sensitivity to light and sound. Past history reveals the occurrence of such episodes a few days before menstruation over the past 3–4 years. The unilateral headache is usually preceded by blurring of vision, flashes of light, lethargy, and nausea. Episode usually lasts for the whole day, > 12 hours, and is severe and incapacitating.
   a. What is the probable diagnosis?
   b. How will you manage this case immediately?
   c. How such attacks can be prevented in future?

2. **Sumatriptan is the preferred drug for acute migraine attacks.**
   i. Identify its correct mechanism of action?
      a. 5-HT$_{1A}$ agonist
      b. 5-HT$_{1A}$ antagonist
      c. 5-HT$_{1D/1B}$ agonist
      d. 5-HT$_{1D/1B}$ antagonist
   ii. What is its dose and route of administration in migraine?
   iii. Enumerate adverse effects and contraindications of sumatriptan.

3. In a 34-year-old female patient with a history of 3 or more severe disabling migraine attacks in a month, a drug is prescribed to reduce the frequency as well as severity of the attacks.
   i. Which of the following drugs is most frequently prescribed for migraine prophylaxis?
      a. Amitriptyline   b. Propranolol
      c. Methysergide   d. Cyproheptadine

ii. What are the dose, duration, and route of administration of the chosen drug?

4. **Explain why:**
   a. Caffeine is combined with ergots in the treatment of migraine.
   b. Triptans are better than ergots for the control of migraine.

SEROTONERGIC TRANSMISSION

(Fig. 27.2)

The steps in the synthesis, storage, release, and termination of serotonin or 5-hydroxytryptamine (5-HT) are broadly similar to those for catecholamines. In serotonergic neuron, tryptophan is first hydroxylated and then decarboxylated to form 5-hydroxytryptamine (5-HT). Upon release, 5-HT acts on its receptors, which are presently grouped into 7 families with a total of 14 receptor subtypes. 5-HT$_1$ receptors are inhibitory in nature, whereas 5-HT$_{2,3,4}$ receptors are excitatory. The clinically relevant receptor subtypes, their actions, and drugs that act on them are listed in Table 27.1.

MAJOR ACTIONS OF 5-HT

5-HT acts as neurotransmitter and local hormone in the gut, causes diarrhea, and has ulcer-protective action.

- **5-HT acts as inhibitory transmitter** in the brain; stimulation of afferent nerve endings causes **tingling, pricking sensation**, and **pain**.
- It plays a role in **temperature regulation, pain perception, appetite, sleep, mood, behaviour**, and **vomiting**. Therefore, drugs affecting central actions of serotonin are useful as antianxiety, antipsychotic, antiemetic drugs, and for migraine relief.

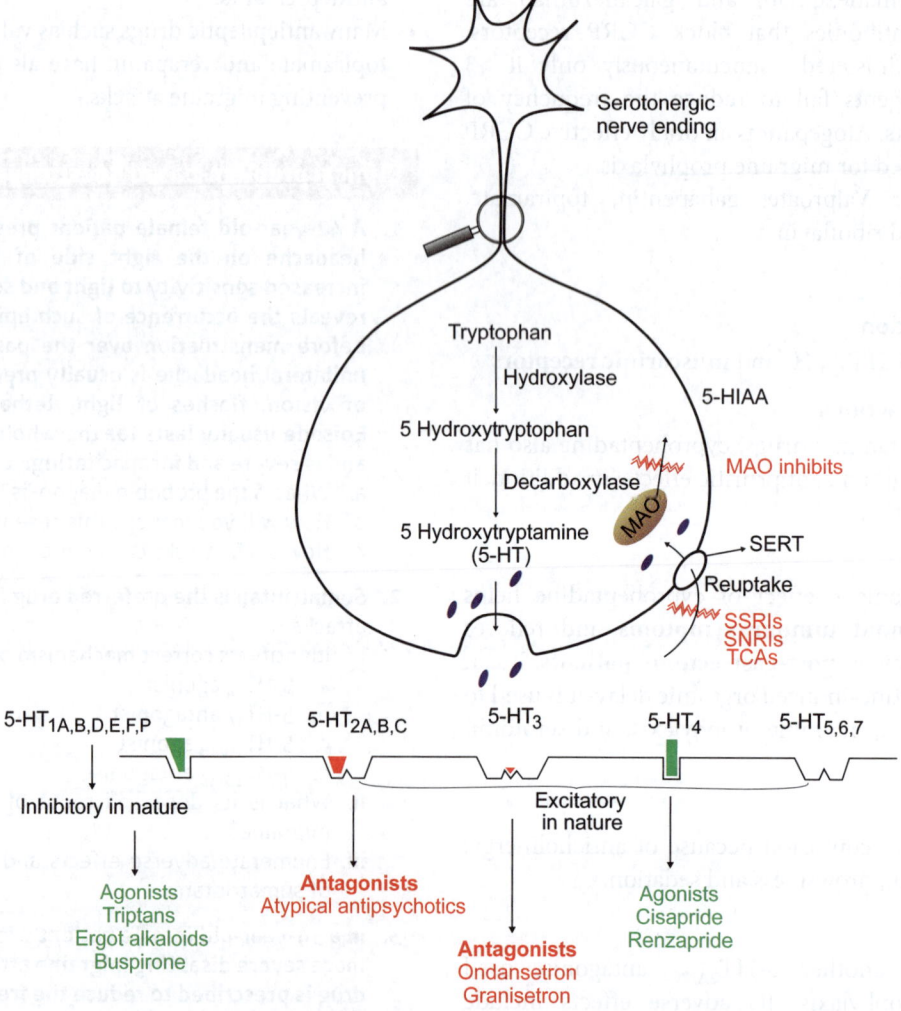

Fig. 27.2 Serotonergic transmission and drugs affecting it
[SERT (serotonin transporter present on platelet membranes and serotonergic nerve endings) causes reuptake of 5-HT, which is then metabolised by MAO-A (monoamine oxidase isoenzyme A) to form 5-HIAA (5-hydroxyindole acetic acid). TCA (tricyclic antidepressants), SSRIs (selective serotonin reuptake inhibitors), SNRIs (serotonin and noradrenaline reuptake inhibitors) and MAO inhibitors interfere with this process.]

Table 27.1 Actions mediated through serotonergic receptor subtypes and the drugs affecting serotonergic transmission

Receptor subtypes	Nature	Major actions	Drugs acting on receptor
5-HT$_1$ → 6 subtypes (5-HT$_{1A,B,D,E,F,P}$)	All 5-HT$_1$ subtypes are G$_i$/G$_o$ protein-coupled (inhibitory)		
5-HT$_{1A}$		Autoreceptors present in the raphe nuclei of brain stem and hippocampus → **Inhibit 5-HT release** from nerve endings.	Antianxiety drugs **buspirone, ipsapirone** and **gepirone** are 5-HT$_{1A}$ partial agonists.
5-HT$_{1D/1B}$		Present in trigeminal nerve and cranial blood vessels. Cause **vasoconstriction** and inhibit inflammatory neuropeptide release from cranial vessel nerve endings. Both these actions are useful in migraine.	**Triptans** are **5-HT$_{1D/1B}$ agonists** that cause cranial vessel vasoconstriction → used for **treatment of migraine.** **Ergot alkaloids** also show agonistic effect at 5-HT$_{1B/1D}$ receptors.
5-HT$_{1F}$		Activation interferes with neural tissue inflammation and interrupts transmission of pain signals to brain.	5-HT$_{1F}$ agonist **lasmiditan** can relieve acute migraine without vasoconstriction of cranial vessels.
5-HT$_{1D}$		Substantia nigra and basal ganglia, where they **regulate dopaminergic function.** Forebrain serotonergic neurons, where they **inhibit 5-HT release.** Sympathetic nerve endings, where they **inhibit catecholamine release.**	Hallucinogenic drug lysergic acid diethyl amide **(LSD)** is a **nonselective agonist** at 5-HT$_{1A}$ and 5-HT$_{2A/2C}$ receptors.
5-HT$_2$ → 3 subtypes (5-HT$_{2A,B,C}$)	G$_q$ protein-coupled receptors → increase in IP$_3$–DAG (excitatory)	Mediates most of the direct postjunctional actions of 5-HT.	5-HT$_2$ agonist **lorcaserin** is an anorectic agent used in obesity management.
5-HT$_{2A}$		Activation causes **vascular and visceral smooth muscle contraction** → Vasoconstriction, intestinal, bronchial and uterine muscle contraction Also causes platelet aggregation Neuronal activation in brain	5-HT$_{2A}$ blockers **ketanserin** and **ritanserin** are used as antihypertensives.
		Neuron **activation**, especially in prefrontal cortex.	5-HT$_{2A/2C}$ blocker or inverse agonists, clozapine, olanzapine, and quetiapine are **atypical antipsychotics** used in resistant cases of schizophrenia. Risperidone is blocker of 5-HT$_{2A}$ and D$_2$ receptors.
			Cyproheptadine has 5-HT$_{2A}$ antagonistic action.
5-HT$_{2B}$		Causes contraction of smooth muscles of gastric fundus in rat.	
5-HT$_{2C}$		Vasodilatation through EDRF release. Regulates CSF formation in choroid plexus.	5-HT$_{2A/2C}$ blockers **methysergide** and **pizotifen** are used in migraine prophylaxis.
5-HT$_3$	Opens up cation channels → Rapid depolarisation (excitatory)	Mediates most of the indirect and reflex effects of 5-HT. Rapid depolarisation of somatic and autonomic nerve endings. Mediates **pain, coronary chemoreflex itching, increased peristaltic activity, nausea, and vomiting.**	Antiemetic drugs **ondansetron, granisetron, palonosetron,** and **ramosetron** are 5-HT$_3$ blockers.

Receptor subtypes	Nature	Major actions	Drugs acting on receptor
$5\text{-}HT_4$	G_s protein-coupled receptor (excitatory)	Augments **peristaltic activity** and **GIT secretions**.	**Cisapride and renzapride** are $5\text{-}HT_4$ agonists.
$5\text{-}HT_{5,6,7}$	Brain	Functions not yet well delineated.	Clozapine shows high affinity for $5\text{-}HT_{6,7}$ receptors, but the effects are not well understood.

- Intravenous 5-HT causes a **triphasic response** on BP, characterised by:
  - An initial sharp fall in BP due to coronary chemoreflex.
  - A brief increase due to vasoconstriction.
  - Prolonged fall due to fluid extravasation.
- **Bronchoconstriction** and **hyperventilation**.
- Weak platelet-aggregating action.
- Vascular effects: 5-HT causes vasoconstriction of both arteries and veins, particularly in pulmonary and renal circulation, whereas it induces vasodilation in the skeletal muscle and coronary vessels. It dilates arterioles and constricts venules, leading to increased capillary pressure and fluid leakage into the surrounding tissues.

Pathophysiological Roles

1. **Nausea and vomiting:** Serotonergic transmission is thought to play role in chemotherapy- and radiotherapy-induced nausea and vomiting (CINV and RINV) by stimulating $5\text{-}HT_3$ receptors in the stomach, small intestine, chemoreceptor trigger zone, and nucleus tractus solitarius. $5\text{-}HT_3$ receptor antagonists like ondansetron, granisetron, palonosetron, and ramosetron are widely used to control chemotherapy-induced nausea and vomiting (CINV).
2. **Schizophrenia:** Serotonergic action through $5\text{-}HT_2$ receptors is implicated in psychotic disorders. $5\text{-}HT_{2A/2C}$ blocker or inverse agonists such as clozapine, olanzapine, quetiapine, and risperidone are atypical antipsychotic drugs used in resistant cases of schizophrenia.
3. **Depression:** Depression is associated with reduced serotonergic and adrenergic transmission in the limbic system. Therefore, selective serotonin reuptake inhibitors (SSRIs) and serotonin and noradrenaline reuptake inhibitors (SNRIs) are used as antidepressants.
4. **Carcinoid syndrome:** Tumours of the enterochromaffin cells of GIT → excessive serotonin release → carcinoid syndrome characterised by diarrhea, dehydration, weakness, hypotension, wheezing, myalgia, arthralgia, and redness and warmth of face and upper chest.
5. **Hypertension:** 5-HT-induced vasoconstriction raises BP in pre-eclampsia. $5\text{-}HT_2$ antagonists ketanserin and ritanserin have mild antihypertensive activity.
6. **Variant angina:** 5-HT and thromboxane A2 released from platelets may cause coronary vasospasm and precipitate variant angina.
7. **Migraine:** Refer to page 357 for the role of 5-HT in migraine.

Among the drugs that act on the serotonergic system (Flowchart 27.2), the triptans, lasmiditan, ergots, cyproheptadine and methysergide are drugs useful in **migraine treatment or prophylaxis**.

Other drugs that modulate serotonergic transmission are discussed in the respective chapters, based on indications for their use.

Clinical problem-based questions and MCQs

5. **A 26-year-old female patient in the second trimester (24 weeks) of pregnancy complains of migraine-like symptoms like unilateral headache, lethargy, nausea, and photophobia. However, the pain is tolerable and not incapacitating. The patient gives history of 2 such attacks since she conceived. Tab paracetamol 500 mg is given by oral route.**
   i. What is role of paracetamol?
   ii. Explain the pharmacological basis for not prescribing the specific antimigraine drug ergotamine.
   iii. Enumerate the adverse effects and contraindications of ergots.
6. Match the drug with correct receptor actions.
   a. Cisapride   1. $5\text{-}HT_{2A}$ antagonist
   b. Ondansetron   2. $5\text{-}HT_4$ agonist
   c. Sumatriptan   3. $5\text{-}HT_3$ antagonist
   d. Risperidone   4. $5\text{-}HT_{1D/1B}$ agonist

Summary

- Migraine can be classical (with aura) or common (without aura).
- Based on the frequency and severity of the attacks, migraine can be mild, moderate, or severe.
- The most characteristic feature of migraine is unilateral throbbing headache.
- Pathophysiology is not well delineated and includes ischemic or neuro-inflammatory theories.
- 5-HT is an inhibitory NTM that plays important pathophysiological roles in many conditions such as migraine, CINV, carcinoid syndrome, and disturbances of mood and behaviour.
- 5-HT itself does not have clinical applications because of its widespread effects that are exerted through 7 types and 14 subtypes of serotonergic receptors.

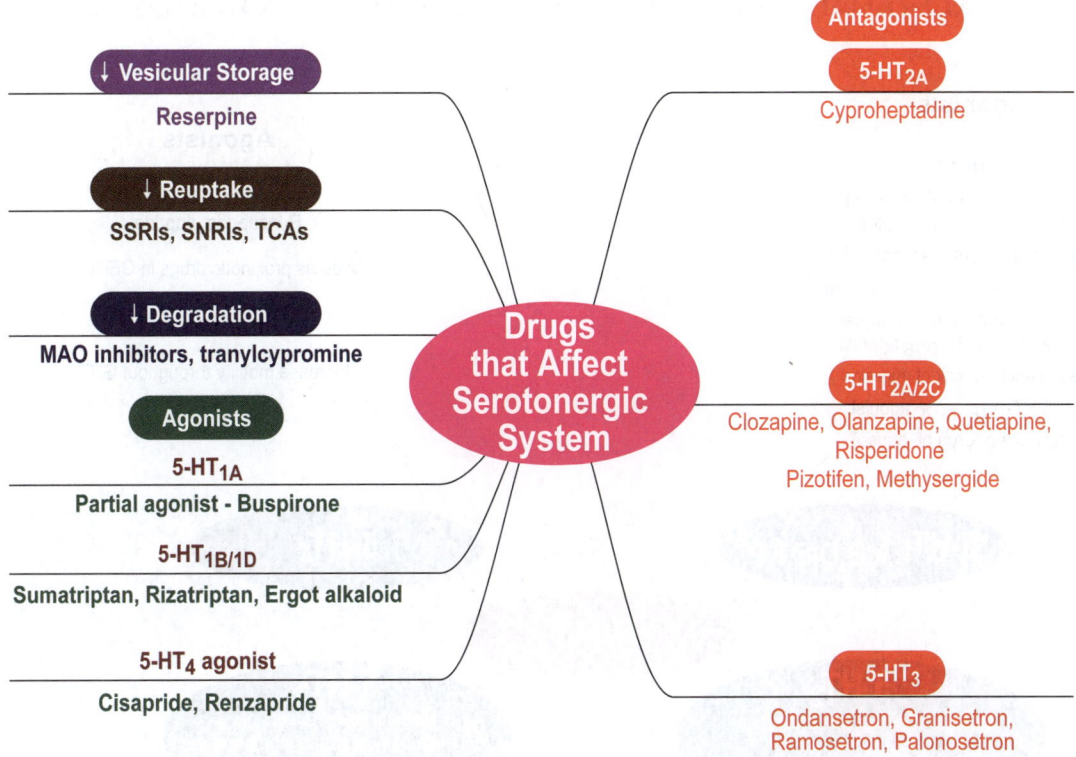

Flowchart 27.2 Drugs that act on the serotonergic system

- Drugs that interfere with its reuptake, agonists, and blockers of specific subtypes of serotonergic receptors are used to treat different clinical conditions such as schizophrenia, depression, migraine, and carcinoid syndrome.
- Mild migraine usually responds to simple analgesics or NSAIDs.
- For moderate migraines, combinations of NSAIDs may be needed. Triptans can also be used if patient does not respond to NSAIDs. Antiemetics may also be prescribed.
- Severe migraine requires triptans (preferred drugs) or ergots along with antiemetics to control acute attacks. Drugs such as propranolol are used for prophylaxis.

Questions for practice

1. Write short notes on:
   a. Triptans
   b. Cyproheptadine
   c. Ergot derivatives
2. Enumerate the drugs used to control acute migraine attacks, based on the severity and frequency of attacks.
3. Enumerate the drugs used for migraine prophylaxis.
4. Comment on the role of the following drugs in the management of migraine.
   a. Sumatriptan
   b. Ergotamine
   c. Propranolol
   d. Flunarizine

Hints for problem-based questions and MCQs

1. a. Severe migraine
   b. Patients with severe migraine should be treated with one of the triptans. Sumatriptan is the most frequently prescribed drug, given in a dose of 50–100 mg orally at the onset of attack. Dose can be repeated once within 24 h, if needed.
   c. Refer to pages 360, 361
2. i. c. 5-HT$_{1D/1B}$ agonist
   ii. Refer to page 359
   iii. Refer to page 359
3. i. b. Propranolol
   ii. Propranolol 40 mg twice daily by oral route should be continued for 6 months at least. Discontinuation may be attempted every 6 monthly, before continuing it further as per need of individual patient.
4. a. Caffeine increases absorption of ergotamine
   b. Refer to page 360
5. a. The patient is pregnant (24 weeks) and has mild migraine with low frequency of attacks (2 attacks since she conceived). Because the severity is also not incapacitating, the patient is given a simple analgesic drug, paracetamol, which is safe in pregnancy.
   b. Specific antimigraine drugs include triptans and ergots. Ergotamine has the potential to cause uterine smooth muscle contractions and is contraindicated in pregnancy. Moreover, simple analgesics are usually prescribed in mild migraine, as seen in this case.
   c. Refer to page 360.
6. a–2; b–3; c–4; d–1.

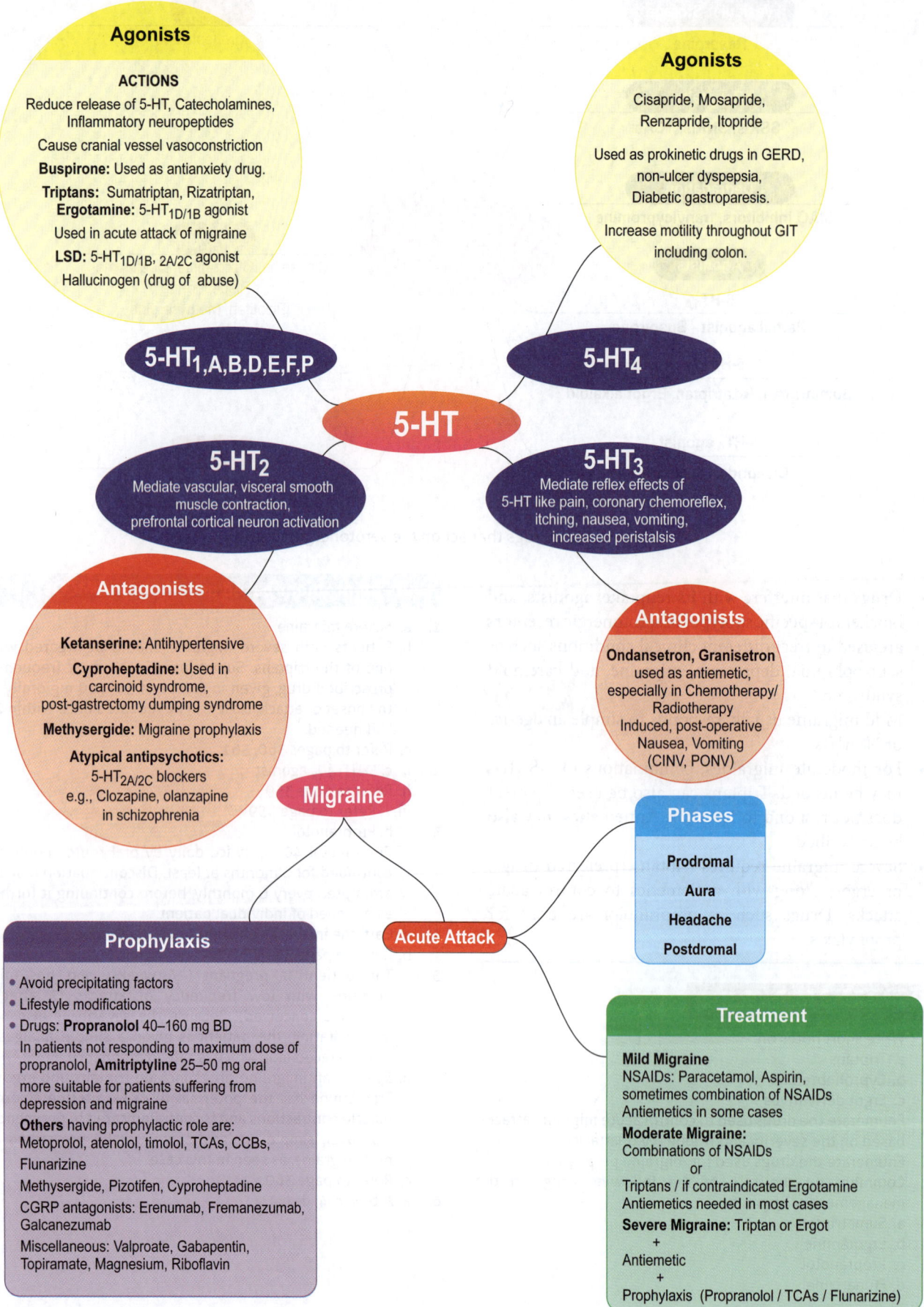

SECTION 5 Drugs Acting on the Respiratory System

28 Drugs Used in Cough and Bronchial Asthma

PH 5.1 Devise management of various stages of bronchial asthma and COPD. Explain salient pharmacokinetics, pharmacodynamics, therapeutic uses, adverse drug reactions of drugs used for the management of bronchial asthma, COPD and rhinitis.

PH 5.2 Explain types, salient pharmacokinetics, pharmacodynamics, therapeutic uses, adverse drug reactions of drugs used for cough management. Describe management of dry & productive cough.

Learning objectives

A student of MBBS phase II should be able to:
- Differentiate between antitussives, expectorants and mucolytics.
- Classify the drug used for cough and describe their mechanism of action.
- Enumerate uses, adverse effects and contraindications of drugs used in treatment of cough.
- Describe management of various types of cough.
- Classify the drugs used for bronchial asthma.
- Describe pharmacological basis for use of various groups of drugs in asthma
- Describe indications, contraindications and ADRs of antiasthma drugs.
- Describe management of bronchial asthma, mentioning doses of drugs.
- Enumerate differences and similarities between bronchial asthma and COPD.
- Describe the differences between COPD and asthma treatment.

COUGH

Coughing is a protective reflex intended to expel any foreign particles or mucus from the respiratory tract. The physiological mechanism of cough production is complex, involving central as well as peripheral mechanisms. Cough occurs when an afferent impulse originating from the cough receptors reaches the cough centre; then an efferent impulse travels from the cough centre to the larynx, lungs, diaphragm and intercostal muscles (Fig. 28.1).

- **Cough receptors** are sensory stretch receptors present in the mucosal cells of the tracheobronchial tree (mechanoreceptors) and lungs (mechanoreceptors and chemoreceptors).
- Impulses from cough receptors travel through afferent fibres in the vagus and glossopharyngeal nerves to the **cough centre**. The cough centre is located in upper part of the dorsal medulla and is different from the respiratory centre. The **cortical cough-modulating centre** is linked to the **medullary cough centre**.
- The cough centre then sends efferent impulses through the parasympathetic and motor nerves to the **larynx, lungs, diaphragm and intercostal muscles**.

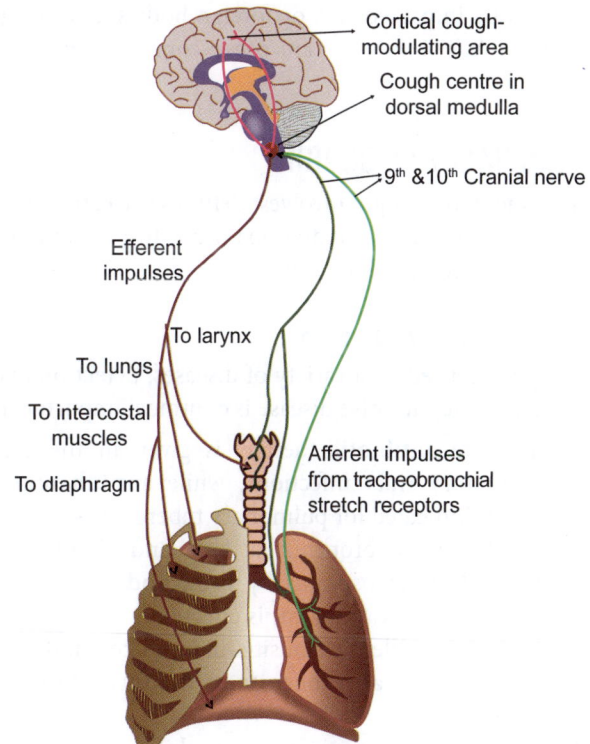

Fig 28.1 The cough reflex pathway

TYPES AND CAUSES OF COUGH

Cough can be of many types; it occurs as a prominent symptom in most respiratory diseases.

1. **Productive cough** or cough with expectoration of sputum occurs in many inflammatory, allergic and irritative diseases of the respiratory tract, e.g., bronchitis, pneumonia, bronchial asthma, tuberculosis,

bronchogenic carcinoma, bronchiectasis, pulmonary edema and infarction.
2. **Nonproductive** or **dry cough** usually occurs following inflammation of the upper respiratory tract, e.g., pharyngitis, laryngitis, tracheitis and early cases of bronchitis.
3. **Whooping cough** is a cough paroxysm followed by a laryngeal spasm that results in an inspiratory whoop. It may occur in pertussis, klebsiella and some viral infections.
4. **Cough associated with change in posture** may occur due to lung abscess, bronchiectasis, bronchopleural fistula, etc. In acute LVF (left ventricular failure) or pulmonary edema, the patient coughs more in the recumbent position.
5. **Nocturnal cough** along with expiratory dyspnea is an important feature of bronchial asthma. However, in chronic obstructive pulmonary disease (COPD), chronic cough occurs intermittently throughout the day.
6. A **sudden and severe paroxysm** of cough may occur in a healthy person due to aspiration of a foreign body.
7. Chronic smoking may diminish mucociliary function and cause **intractable cough**.
8. Bilateral adductor paralysis of vocal cords, gastro-esophageal reflux, pulmonary eosinophilia, postnasal drip caused by sinusitis, stimulation of external auditory meatus by impacted wax or foreign bodies, and drugs such as ACE inhibitors are other common causes of cough.

MANAGEMENT OF COUGH

Management of cough involves definitive treatment of the causative disease, avoiding exposure to precipitating factors, and symptomatic relief.

a. Definitive Treatment

As cough is caused by a variety of diseases, detection and treatment of the causative disease is of utmost importance.
- Appropriate **antibiotic** therapy is given in the case of respiratory tract infections, while **antitubercular** therapy is indicated for pulmonary tuberculosis.
- In cough due to bronchial asthma and COPD, the reversal of bronchospasms by **bronchodilators** (e.g., β_2-agonists and ipratropium) is effective.
- In perennial or allergic sinusitis-induced cough due to postnasal drip, **nasal decongestants** and **antihistaminic** drugs are useful.
- Cough due to pulmonary eosinophilia responds to **diethylcarbamazine** and **inhalational corticoids**.
- Cough associated with GERD responds to acid-lowering **drugs** such as **proton pump inhibitors** and **prokinetic** drugs (e.g., mosapride).
- In ACE inhibitor-induced dry cough, it is important to replace the ACE inhibitors with ARBs.

b. Avoidance of Precipitating Factors

Avoiding smoking, exposure to dust, cow dung and cold weather is advised.

c. Symptomatic Treatment

Cough suppression by antitussive drugs provides only symptomatic relief. Dry or nonproductive cough is usually troublesome and serves no useful purpose; it is commonly treated with cough suppressants or **antitussive drugs**. In contrast, suppression of cough is not useful in productive cough, because coughing helps in expectoration of sputum, and expels harmful substances such as excess respiratory mucus, foreign particles, irritants, exudates and transudates from airways.

However, in patients where the amount of sputum expelled is small in comparison to the effort of coughing, or where coughing can be associated with serious complications (e.g., in hernia, cardiac disease and after ocular surgery), cough suppression is helpful.

Expectorant/mucokinetic and mucolytic drugs assist in the removal of sputum from airways and are beneficial in productive cough.

CLASSIFICATION OF DRUGS USED TO TREAT COUGH

Based on their mechanism of action, antitussive drugs are classified into two types: centrally acting and peripherally acting drugs. These are beneficial only in dry or nonproductive cough, whereas mucokinetic agents/expectorants and mucolytic agents are useful for productive cough (Flowchart 28.1).

A. Centrally Acting Antitussives

1. Opioids

These are the most effective cough suppressants; their antitussive action involves both central and peripheral actions. Central action occurs through increased threshold of the cough centre, while peripheral action decreases the number of cough impulses originating in the respiratory tract. The dose of opioids required for antitussive effect is much lower than their analgesic dose.
- **Codeine**, though qualitatively similar to morphine, is less potent and less efficacious. It has greater selectivity for the cough centre, and is the antitussive agent of choice in mild-to-moderate cough. The dose for cough suppression (10–30 mg) is much lower than its analgesic dose (60 mg), and action lasts for 6 hours. The abuse potential of codeine is lower than that for morphine. However, codeine can cause drowsiness

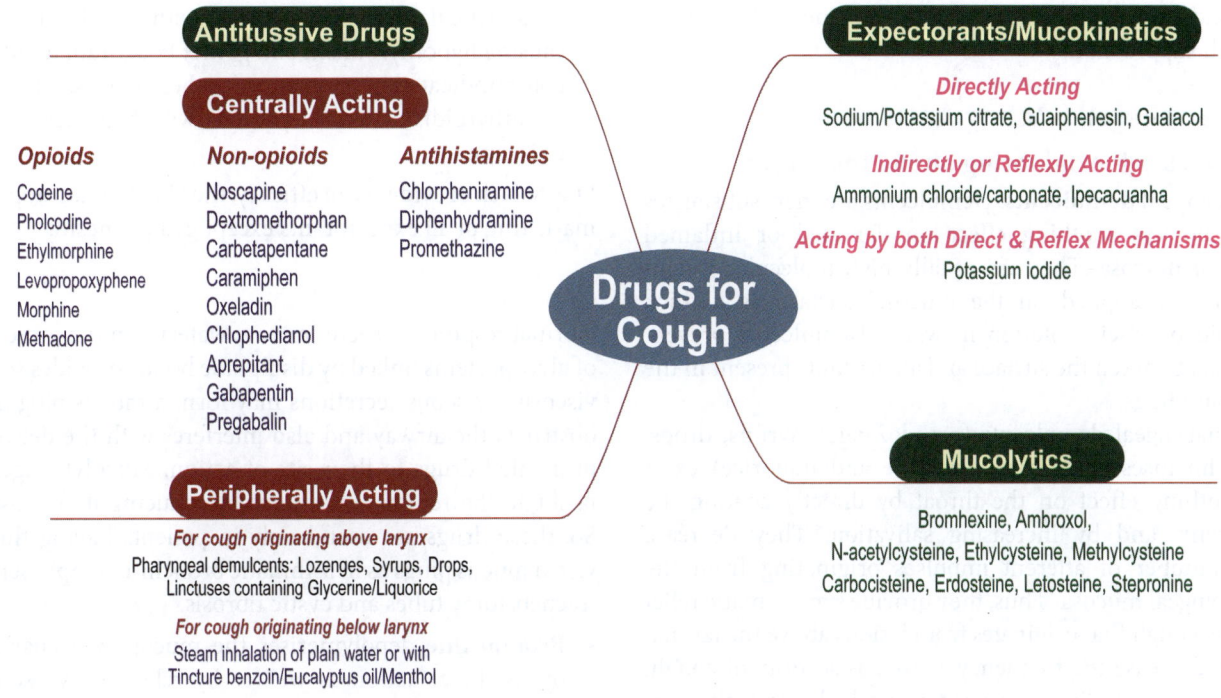

Flowchart 28.1 Classification of antitussive drugs

and constipation. Higher doses of codeine can cause respiratory depression; so, codeine is not used in cough associated with bronchial asthma.
- **Ethylmorphine** is similar to codeine, but causes less constipation.
- **Pholcodine** produces an antitussive effect comparable to that of codeine but with a longer duration of action (~12 hours), allowing for once or twice daily dosing; however, it lacks codeine's analgesic and addictive properties.
- **Levopropoxyphene** is a stereoisomer of the weak opioid agonist dextropropoxyphene. While it lacks the analgesic and addicting effects, it may cause sedation.
- Morphine and methadone are used in severe, intractable cough associated with bronchogenic carcinoma.

2. Non-opioids
- **Noscapine** suppresses cough by its agonistic effect at the sigma opioid receptors. It is used in spasmodic cough in a dose of 15–30 mg. The antitussive action of noscapine is similar to that of codeine, but it has no analgesic, constipating and addicting actions.
Adverse effects of noscapine include nausea and headache, while higher doses may cause histamine release resulting in bronchoconstriction and hypotension. Therefore, it is not used in asthmatic patients.
- **Dextromethorphan**, the d-isomer of methorphan, exerts antitussive effect by central NMDA receptor antagonism, which raises the threshold of cough reflex.

It does not suppress the mucociliary function of the airway mucosa and is used in a dose of 10–20 mg as an **over-the-counter (OTC)** drug for mild cough.
It is as potent as codeine in terms of its antitussive effect, but is free of the addicting, constipating and gastric effects. Its adverse effects include nausea, dizziness, drowsiness, ataxia and hallucination (some illicit use has been reported).
- **Carbetapentane, caramiphen and oxeladin** suppress cough by binding to same site as dextromethorphan. Caramiphen is used in mild cough along with nasal decongestants.
- **Clophedianol** suppresses the cough reflex by direct action on the cough centre in the dorsal medulla. It also possesses local anesthetic, antihistaminic and anticholinergic properties.
- **Aprepitant**, a neurokinin-1 receptor antagonist, has limited use in managing severe cough associated with bronchial carcinoma.
- **Gabapentin** and **pregabalin** play a role in chronic idiopathic cough.

3. Antihistamines
Chlorpheniramine, diphenhydramine and promethazine may afford some relief in cough of allergic origin only, because of their sedative and anticholinergic effects; however, they have poor efficacy in asthma. They have no selectivity for the cough centre and no mucokinetic activity, but reduce mucus secretion by their anticholinergic action.

Second-generation antihistaminics are not effective for cough suppression.

B. Peripherally Acting Antitussives

1. For cough originating above the larynx

Pharyngeal demulcents: Demulcents are inert substances that possess soothing effect on denuded or inflamed skin or mucosa. They are usually high molecular weight substances applied on the mucosal surface as a thick colloid or viscid solution in water. Demulcents prevent contact between the surface and air/irritants present in the surroundings.

Pharyngeal demulcents (e.g., lozenges, syrups, drops, and linctuses containing glycerine and liquorice) exert a soothing effect on the throat by directly coating the pharynx, and by increasing salivation. They decrease the number of afferent impulses originating from the pharyngeal mucosa. Thus, they provide symptomatic relief in dry cough that originates from lesions above the larynx. They decrease the frequency as well as severity of cough. Sometimes, the linctus is used as a vehicle for antitussive drugs.

2. For cough originating below the larynx

Steam inhalation of plain water is very useful for cough originating below the larynx and helps to clear airway secretions. Steam inhalation has no adverse effects and is allowed as and when required. Sometimes, tincture benzoin, eucalyptus oil, menthol, etc., are added to water for steam inhalation. Menthol acts on afferent sensory neurons and produces a cooling sensation on inhalation.

C. Expectorants or Mucokinetics

These drugs act by **increasing the volume** or **decreasing the viscosity** of bronchial secretions; this facilitates the movement/kinesis and removal of such copious, less-viscid secretions. As a result, the cough becomes less tiring and more productive. Hence, expectorants are useful in productive cough.

1. **Sodium and potassium citrate** increase the volume of bronchial secretions and make them thin and loose, so that they can be coughed out easily.
2. **Guaiphenesin** affects the cholinergic innervation of the airway mucous glands and increases bronchial secretion as well as mucociliary action. Plant products such as vasaka and tolu balsam also have similar actions.
3. **Ammonium chloride and carbonate** enhance bronchial secretions, but their taste is unpleasant and nauseating.
4. **Potassium iodide** increases bronchial secretions by its irritant action. However, such irritant action is not desirable when the bronchial mucosa is acutely inflamed. Long-term use of potassium iodide may cause acne flare-ups and interfere with thyroid function causing hypothyroidism and goitre. Potassium iodide is contraindicated in pregnancy (as there is a risk of foetal hypothyroidism) and in patients with hypersensitivity to iodine.

Due to lack of evidence of efficacy, the US FDA has stopped marketing of all expectorants except guaiphenesin.

Mucolytics

Normal respiratory secretions are watery, but the presence of glycoproteins linked by disulphide bonds provides some viscosity. Viscous secretions may form a mucus plug that obstructs the airway and also interferes with the delivery of inhaled drugs to their site of action. Mucolytic agents facilitate the removal of mucus by reducing its viscosity. So, these drugs are useful only in patients having thick, viscid mucus plugs as in asthmatic bronchitis, emphysema, tracheostomy tubes and cystic fibrosis.

- **Bromhexine** depolymerises the mucopolysaccharides by its direct action as well as by releasing lysosomal enzymes. Depolymerisation of the mucopolysaccharides breaks down the network of fibres in tenacious sputum. This makes the bronchial secretions thin and copious. So, bromhexine has both mucolytic and mucokinetic properties. Bromhexine is used in a dose of 8 mg, thrice a day. Adverse effects include rhinorrhea, lacrimation, hypersensitivity reactions and gastric irritation.
- **Ambroxol** is a metabolite of bromhexine with a similar profile of actions, adverse effects and uses (dose: 15–30 mg, three times a day).
- **Acetylcysteine, carbocisteine** and **methylcysteine** have a free –SH group, which breaks the disulphide bonds between glycoproteins and liquefies the viscid sputum.

  Acetylcysteine can be given orally in a dose of 200–600 mg three times a day, or by inhalation of 10–20% nebulised solution. Solution can also be instilled in tracheostomy tubes. Adverse effects include gastrointestinal irritation and rashes.

  Carbocisteine is used orally in a dose of 250–750 mg thrice daily; however, it is contraindicated in peptic ulcer, because of GI irritant action.

  Carbocisteine, erdosteine, letosteine and stepronin liquefy mucus by cleaving disulphide bonds of sialomucins.

The efficacy of mucolytics in cough is doubtful; simple measures such as steam inhalation and proper hydration are more effective in clearing airway secretions. In addition to the above-mentioned antitussive drugs, bronchodilators are used when cough is associated with bronchoconstriction. Prokinetic drugs can relieve cough associated with GERD.

Chapter 28 Drugs Used in Cough and Bronchial Asthma

CONCEPT MAP - COUGH SUPPRESSANT DRUGS

DRUGS FOR COUGH SUPPRESSION

Dry Cough

Uses
- **Codeine:** Drug of choice in mild-to-moderate cough.
- **Noscapine:** in spasmodic cough.
- **Dextromethorphan:** as OTC in mild cough.
- **Morphine, Methadone, Aprepitant:** in severe, intractable cough of bronchial carcinoma.
- **Antihistamines:** in allergic cough
- **Pregabalin, Gabapentin:** in chronic idiopathic cough.

ADRs
- **Codeine:** Constipation, Drowsiness, At high dose, respiratory depression, Contraindicated in asthma.
- **Ethylmorphine** less constipating.
- **Noscapine:** Nausea, Headache, At high dose - Histamine release - contraindicated in asthma.
- **Dextromethorphan:** Nausea, Dizziness, Drowsiness, Ataxia, Hallucinations.

Steam Inhalation
- Useful in clearing airway secretions.
- Inhalation of plain water steam is very useful **for dry cough originating below larynx.**
- Allowed as and when required
- No adverse effects.
- Tincture benzoin, eucalyptus oil, Menthol may be added
- Menthol acts on afferent sensory neurons and produces cooling sensation on inhalation

Centrally Acting
- **Opioids:** Codeine, Pholcodine, Ethylmorphine, Levopropoxyphene, Morphine, Methadone
- **Non-Opioids:** Noscapine, Dextromethorphan Carbetapentane, Caramiphen, Oxeladin, Chlophedianol, Aprepitant, Gabapentin, Pregabalin
- **Antihistamines:** Chlorpheniramine, Diphenhydramine, Promethazine

Peripherally Acting
- **Pharyngeal demulcents:** lozenges, syrups, drops, linctus containing glycerine, liquorice
- **Steam inhalation** of water, Tincture benzoin, Eucalyptus oil, Menthol.

Mechanism of Action
- **Opioids:** Increase the threshold of cough center.
  - Decrease cough impulses originating in respiratory tract.
- **Noscapine:** Sigma receptor agonist
- **Dextromethorphan:** NMDA antagonist Both increase cough centre threshold.

Pharyngeal Demulcents
- **Mechanism:** Coat the pharynx, have soothing effect on throat directly / by increasing salivation. Decrease afferent impulses from pharyngeal mucosa.
- **Use:** Symptomatic relief in **dry cough originating from lesions above larynx.** Decrease frequency as well as severity of cough.

Productive Cough

Mucokinetic/Expectorants
- **Directly acting:** Na/K citrate Guaiphenesin, guaiacol
- **Indirectly or reflexly acting:** Ammonium chloride or carbonate, Ipecacuanha
- **Acting by both direct and reflex mechanisms:** potassium iodide.

Mucolytics
Bromhexine, Ambroxol, Acetylcysteine, Carbocisteine, Methylcysteine.

ADRs
- **Bromhexine:** rhinorrhea, lacrimation, hypersensitivity reaction, gastric irritation.
- **Acetylcysteine, methylcysteine:** gastrointestinal irritation and rashes.

Mechanism
Increase volume of bronchial secretions:
By salt action: Na and K citrate
by irritant action: KI
By reflex action: NH_4Cl, $(NH_4)_2CO_3$
By affecting cholinergic innervations of airway mucous glands: Guaiphenesin
↓
Decreasing viscosity of bronchial secretions
Movement & removal of copious, less viscid secretions is easy.

Uses
Due to lack of evidence of efficacy, US FDA has stopped marketing all expectorants except guaiphenesin.

Mechanism of Action
Bromhexine, Ambroxol: Depolymerisation of mucopolysaccharide
Acetylcysteine, Methylcysteine: Break disulphide bonds
Carbocisteine, Erdosteine, Letosteine, Stepronine liquify mucus and increase secretion of sialomucins
↓
reducing mucosal viscosity
↓
facilitate mucus removal

Uses
Useful **only in patients having thick, viscid mucus plugs** as seen in asthmatic bronchitis, emphysema, tracheostomy tubes cystic fibrosis.

BRONCHIAL ASTHMA AND COPD

Bronchial asthma is an **episodic** disease characterised by recurrent attacks of cough, expiratory dyspnea, wheezing and feeling of tightness in chest. The underlying pathology is **hyper-responsiveness of bronchi** to a variety of stimuli (Fig. 28.2) leading to leukocytic and eosinophilic infiltration, mucus production, and bronchoconstriction. As the disease progresses, pathological remodelling occurs due to hyperplasia of mucosal, vascular and glandular cells resulting in thickening of lamina reticularis. This narrows the airway lumen. Acute asthma attacks are precipitated upon exposure to triggering factors. Antigen–antibody reaction occurs on the surface of mast cells, resulting in degranulation of mast cells and release of mediators such as histamine, leukotrienes, and interleukins. These mediators cause mucosal hyperemia, edema, viscid secretions and bronchoconstriction that are responsible for the characteristic symptoms of asthma.

Status asthmaticus or acute severe asthma is a prolonged, severe form of airway obstruction, which does not respond to routinely used drugs (i.e., inhalational

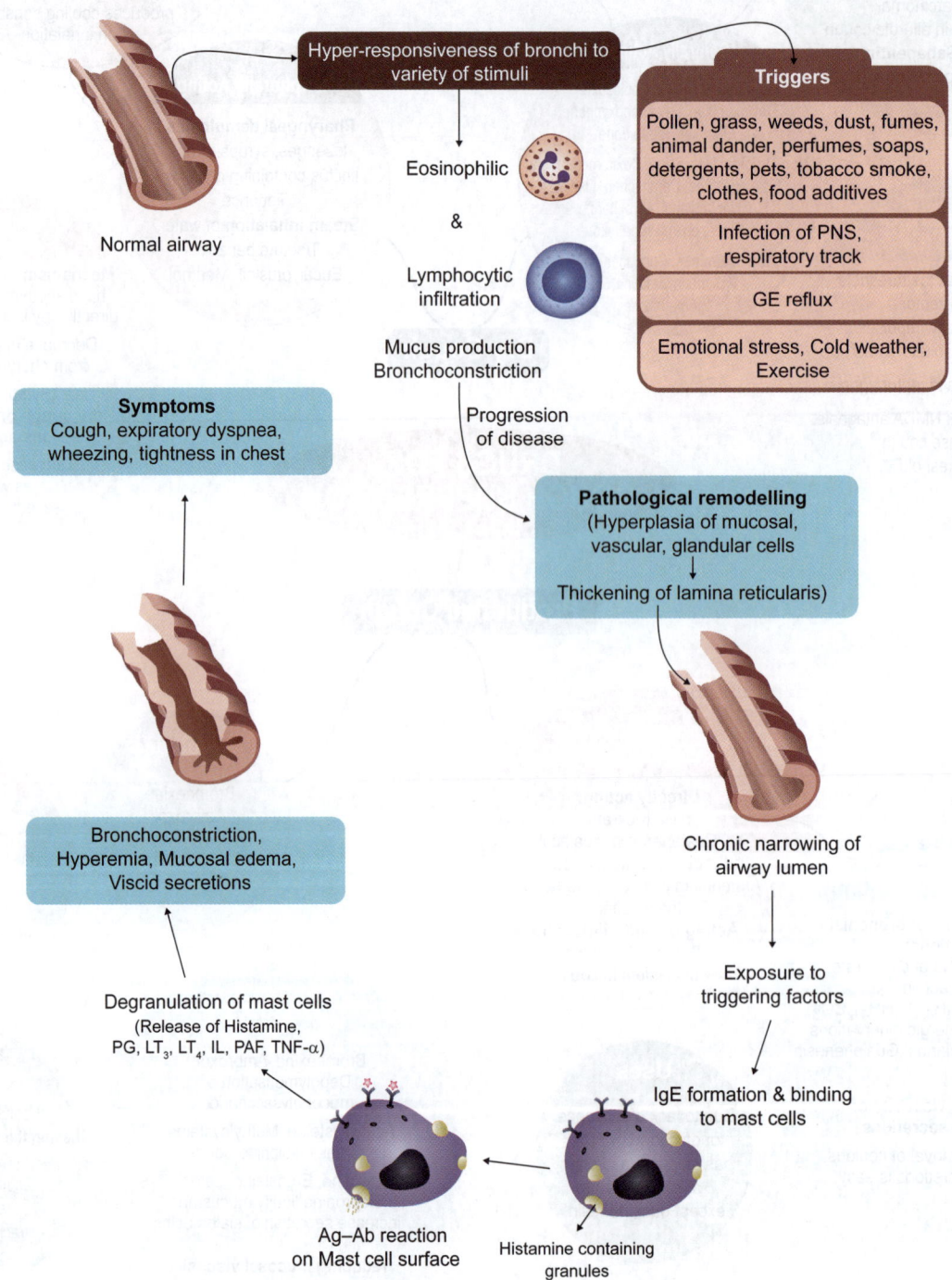

Fig. 28.2 Pathophysiology of bronchial asthma

corticosteroids and bronchodilators), and **may last for > 24 hours**. Patient has cough, wheezing, dyspnea, anxiety along with hypoxia and dehydration. It may lead to respiratory failure and death. Such patients need hospitalisation and intensive treatment.

Chronic obstructive pulmonary disease (COPD) is a progressive disease characterised by **cellular damage** caused by **long-term exposure of lungs to irritants** such as cigarette smoke, tobacco smoke, and toxic chemical fumes. Some **genetic factors** such as $α_1$-antitrypsin (AAT) deficiency are also implicated. While COPD is usually seen in older patients (age > 40 years), bronchial asthma can occur at any age, but is more common in children.

In COPD, chronic obstruction or interference with airflow in the lungs leads to impaired breathing. Symptoms such as chronic cough, dyspnea, excessive mucus and phlegm production, and cyanosis. The symptoms gradually increase in severity, and breathing does not return to normal. While the **symptoms of COPD** are the **same as in asthma**, the latter is episodic and **breathing is normal in between attacks; mucus production** is also **less in asthma** than in COPD.

Treatment strategies are also slightly different in the two conditions. In bronchial asthma, the triggering factors are recognised and avoided. Currently, the mainstay of asthma treatment is **inhalational corticosteroids** and **selective $β_2$-agonists**. The management of COPD involves **quitting smoking, vaccinations to prevent respiratory infections** and **combined bronchodilator therapy**. In general, the prognosis of bronchial asthma is better than that for COPD.

MANAGEMENT OF ASTHMA

It involves reducing the frequency of acute attacks and symptomatic relief during the attack. The strategy of asthma management involves following steps.

- **Prevention of exposure to antigen:** Bronchial asthma is triggered by a variety of allergens and irritants; the detection and avoidance of exposure to these factors is an important part of preventing acute asthmatic attacks. **Hyposensitisation** to the detected antigen also reduces the frequency of asthma attacks.
- Exposure to Ag leads to the production of reaginic antibodies (IgE), which can be neutralised by **monoclonal Abs against IgE (omalizumab)**. Because IgE gets neutralised in circulation, it is not available for Ag–Ab reactions on the mast cell surface.
- If the IgE Abs manage to attach onto the mast cell surface, the Ag–Ab reaction results in mast cell degranulation and release of mediators. This can be controlled by a group of drugs known as **mast cell stabilisers**, e.g., sodium cromoglycate and ketotifen.
- The action of inflammatory mediators released from mast cells can be controlled by **leukotriene antagonists** such as montelukast and zafirlukast. Synthesis of leukotriene (LT) from arachidonic acid can be decreased by the lipoxygenase inhibitor, zileuton.
- Inflammatory response of bronchial mucosa can be controlled by **corticosteroids** that possess non-specific anti-inflammatory action. Inhalational administration of corticosteroids is the first step in the management of asthma. Severe cases may require systemic steroid administration.
- Bronchoconstriction can be reversed by **bronchodilators**, which include anticholinergics, selective $β_2$ agonists, and methylxanthines.
- Treatment of acute **severe asthma/status asthmatics** includes:
  - Humidified oxygen inhalation by nasal catheter/ Venturi mask to control hypoxia.
  - Fluid therapy to make up for excessive insensible fluid loss due to hyperventilation.
  - Sodium bicarbonate to control acidosis.
  - Management of precipitating cause

CLASSIFICATION OF DRUGS USED TO TREAT BRONCHIAL ASTHMA

Drugs useful in the treatment of bronchial asthma include corticosteroids and bronchodilators. Mast cell stabilisers, LT antagonists and monoclonal antibodies also play a significant role (Flowchart 28.2).

I. Corticosteroids

Mechanism of action

Corticosteroids act by binding to intracellular receptors and regulating protein synthesis (refer to page 590). These proteins further regulate the activity of target cells. Corticosteroids are not bronchodilators, but are beneficial in asthma because of their **nonspecific anti-inflammatory action**. They:

- Decrease infiltration of eosinophils, lymphocytes and mast cells into the lungs.
- Inhibit production of cytokines, which are important mediators of the inflammatory process. Thus, corticoids suppress the inflammatory response to the Ag–Ab reactions and other triggers.
- Decrease bronchial hyper-reactivity.
- Steroids cause vasoconstriction of engorged blood vessels in the bronchial mucosa and reduce mucosal edema and airway obstruction.
- Reverse the refractoriness of bronchial smooth muscles to the bronchodilator effect of selective β2-agonists and improve the response.

Thus, steroids provide more **complete and sustained symptomatic relief** (by improving airflow) than other

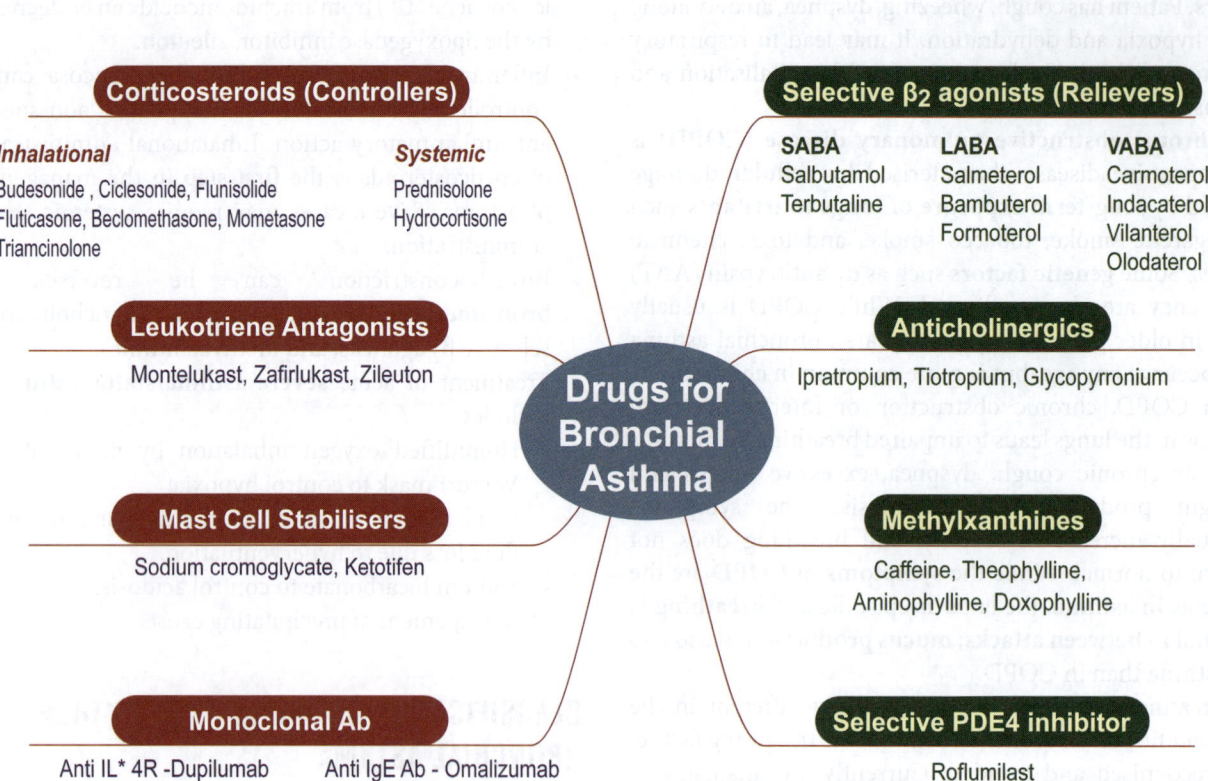

Flowchart 28.2 Classification of drugs for bronchial asthma (IL: interleukin, TSLP: thymic stromal lymphopoietin)

groups of drugs, with increased peak expiratory flow rate (PEFR).

- **They also slow disease progression** by decreasing pathological remodelling.
  Early high-dose ICS reduce the rate of hospital admission during acute asthma exacerbations. After an acute exacerbation, the ICS-formoterol therapy is continued to prevent such relapse episodes, as maintenance-and-reliever-therapy (MART).

Corticosteroids are **not curative** in asthma because the symptoms recur within a few weeks of stopping therapy. These are better labelled as **controllers,** as they provide adequate relief and improve the quality of life of asthma patients.

Role in asthma

Currently, inhalational corticosteroids (ICS) are extensively used in the management of bronchial asthma in children, adults and adolescents. The dose can be low, moderate, or high based on the response. ICS are used in all those patients of **asthma, who need β_2 agonists on a daily basis**. ICS are the **treatment of choice** in persistent bronchial asthma and aspirin/exercise induced asthma.

Drugs such as beclomethasone, fluticasone and budesonide have low systemic bioavailability when administered by the inhalational route. This may be due to poor absorption and/or high presystemic metabolism. Thus, when inhaled, these drugs produce only **local effects** in the airways and the **systemic adverse effects are negligible**. The useful effects in asthma patients, mentioned above along with the lack of systemic adverse effects are largely responsible for making **ICS** along with LABA (e.g., formoterol), as the **first-choice therapy in** regular asthma treatment (MART).

Among inhalational steroids, potency is maximum for fluticasone and least for flunisolide. Beclomethasone and ciclesonide are prodrugs, which are activated by the esterases in bronchial epithelial cells. This further reduces the risk of systemic toxicity; hence these drugs are known as **soft steroids**.

Important adverse effects of ICS are **oropharyngeal candidiasis, sore throat and dysphonia** (hoarseness of voice). To prevent these ADRs, the patient should be instructed to **spit, rinse mouth and gargle with water** after each dose of ICS. The topical antifungal drug nystatin may be used in case of oropharyngeal candidiasis.

Dose of ICS

ICS are available as single drug or in fixed-dose combinations (FDC) with long-acting β_2-agonists (LABA). For fluticasone, which has maximum potency, a low/moderate dose is 100 microgram (mcg) and high dose is 200 mcg, to be applied in different steps of asthma management (as per the GINA guidelines). For budesonide, a low dose is 200–400 mcg, moderate dose is 400–800 mcg, and high dose is > 800 mcg.

Therapy begins with the lowest dose in Step 1 for 4–5 days The **peak effect** occurs about **4–6 days** after **initiating therapy** and persists for few weeks after stopping it. The dose can be increased up to 800 mcg as per the need of individual patient. Increasing the dose further usually has no added benefit. Treatment with inhaled corticoids is continued for **10–12 weeks, and then withdrawn**. If the patient develops asthma symptoms again, treatment is reinstituted.

Systemic corticosteroid therapy is not the preferred method, because of the risk of multiple adverse effects associated with it. It is reserved only for:

- Patients with acute severe asthma may not respond to intensive treatment with bronchodilators (**status asthmaticus**). In these cases, hydrocortisone and methylprednisolone are administered intravenously. The management of status asthmaticus is described in Box 28.1.

> **Box 28.1** Management of status asthmaticus
>
> - Hydrocortisone 100 mg IV, followed by 100–200 mg every 4–8 hours.
> - A short-acting, selective β_2-agonist, such as salbutamol/terbutaline (0.4 mg) is also given, preferably by IM injection. This is because in patients with severe attack, the inhaled drug may not reach smaller airways owing to intense bronchoconstriction and formation of mucus plug by thickened secretions.
> - These patients also need supportive treatment such as controlled-flow humidified oxygen/intubation/mechanical ventilation, fluid therapy, correction of electrolyte/acid–base balance, and management of precipitating factors.
> - IV corticoid therapy usually produces symptomatic relief within 24 hours. Then patient is shifted to oral corticoids only for 5–7 days; these are then stopped abruptly or tapered quickly.

- Systemic corticoids, given orally, are indicated as a last resort in **severe chronic asthma,** where the patient has frequent episodes of increasing severity. Oral prednisolone 20–60 mg is given daily for a few weeks. After adequate control of symptoms, ICS is added and the oral dose is tapered down. Finally, the patient is switched over to ICS. Sudden withdrawal of oral steroid therapy can cause worsening of asthma, myalgias, lassitude, fall in BP and depression. So, the switchover from oral to inhalational corticoids should be carried out with overlapping and very gradually.

Clinical problem-based questions and MCQs

1. For regular treatment of asthma, which of the following routes is preferred for the administration of corticosteroids?
   a. Intravenous
   b. Subcutaneous
   c. Inhalational
   d. Oral

2. Identify inhalational corticosteroid that needs activation in bronchial epithelial cells.
   a. Ciclesonide
   b. Dexamethasone
   c. Fluticasone
   d. Triamcinolone

3. A 42-year-old female patient, a known case of bronchial asthma, presents with cough, wheezing, dyspnea and anxiety, along with hypoxia since the last 24 hours. On examination, the patient is anxious and dehydrated, has laboured breathing and bilateral rhonchi are present. The patient's attendant gives a history of taking regular medicine without relief of symptoms.
   a. What is the diagnosis?
   b. Describe the role of corticosteroids in this patient.

4. Which of the following statements about management of status asthmaticus is NOT correct?
   a. Humidified oxygen is given.
   b. Fluid–electrolyte imbalance is corrected.
   c. Corticosteroids are used by inhalational route.
   d. Short-acting selective β_2-agonists are given by IM injection.

5. Identify the INCORRECT statement about the role of corticosteroids in bronchial asthma.
   a. They reduce the frequency of acute episodes and improve quality of life.
   b. These are labelled as relievers in asthma therapy.
   c. Steroids slow disease progression.
   d. Steroids reverse refractoriness to selective β_2-agonists.

II. Bronchodilators

Three classes of drugs are included in this group.

A. Selective β_2-agonists

These are the **most effective** and **fastest-acting** bronchodilators and are thus useful to relieve acute symptoms. They are better labelled as **relievers**, and have a prominent relaxing effect on bronchiolar smooth muscles (**smaller airways**) as compared to muscarinic blockers that mainly relax larger airways. (Fig. 28.3).

These drugs exert their smooth muscle-relaxing action through G_s protein-coupled β_2 receptors. The binding of the agonist to β_2 receptors activates adenylyl cyclase, which raises cAMP levels. Cyclic AMP inactivates myosin light chain kinase (MLCK) leading to the relaxation of smooth muscles (refer to Table 9.1, page 119). Raised cAMP levels also decrease the release of inflammatory mediators; however, this effect is short-lasting and does not contribute much to the therapeutic effect.

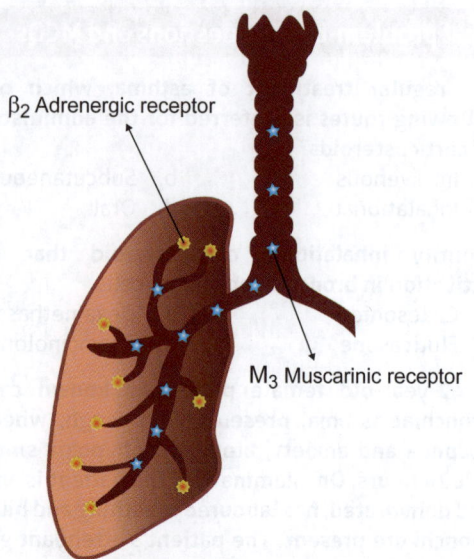

Fig. 28.3 Site of action of β_2 and M_3 receptors on airways

β_2 agonists can be classified into three subtypes, based on their duration of action.

i. Short-acting β_2-agonists (SABAs)

Short-acting β_2-agonists or **SABAs** (e.g., salbutamol and terbutaline) are highly selective for β_2 receptors and achieve adequate bronchodilatation and **relieve asthma exacerbation** within 5 minutes of administration by the inhalational route; the effect lasts for 2–4 hours. Due to such fast onset and brief duration of action, these drugs have been extensively used to **terminate or abort asthma attacks**, but are not suitable for round-the-clock prophylaxis. ICS must always be combined with a SABA.

Dose
Salbutamol is given as 2 puffs (100 mcg per puff) through a metered dose inhaler. Terbutaline is inhaled in a dose of 250 mcg at the beginning of attack to terminate it. Patients who are unable to inhale the drug properly are administered oral salbutamol (2–4 mg) or oral terbutaline (5 mg).

Adverse effects
ADRs are minimal because of the high selectivity. The most common dose-related adverse effect is muscle tremors, while high doses can cause nervousness, palpitation, irritation in throat and ankle edema.

Caution
SABAs **should not be given on regular basis**, because the continuous presence of agonists causes **down-regulation** of the receptors, resulting in **reduced responsiveness** and worsening of bronchial hyper-reactivity. Patients who have frequent asthma episodes and require daily bronchodilator therapy should instead be prescribed inhaled corticoids and long-acting β_2-agonist as maintenance-and-reliever-therapy (MART).

As per the GINA (Global Initiative on Asthma 2019, modified in 2022) guidelines, SABAs, which were prescribed for symptomatic relief for nearly five decades, are not preferred any more. This is because regular usage for even 1–2 weeks is reported to be associated with decreased bronchodilator effect, increased allergic response and increased eosinophils. This may lead to a vicious cycle of allergic response, favouring SABA overuse, more asthma exacerbations and higher mortality.

ii. Long-acting β_2-agonists (LABAs)

Long-acting selective β_2-agonists (LABAs) include bambuterol, salmeterol and formoterol.

- Bambuterol is a prodrug of terbutaline. It is slowly hydrolysed by the pseudocholinesterase enzyme, and releases terbutaline for about 24 hours. Thus, a single evening dose of 10–20 mg by the oral route can be given to patients with nocturnal asthma.
- Salmeterol has a slow onset and longer duration of action than salbutamol. Two puffs (25 mcg per puff) via a metered dose inhaler are prescribed twice a day **for prevention of acute exacerbation**. Similar to salmeterol, formoterol is also long-acting with duration of action (up to 12 hours).
- However, the long-term use of LABAs can cause receptor desensitisation, and worsen the condition. To counter this risk, **long-acting β_2-agonists** are always used in combination with **ICS** as prophylactics in chronic bronchial asthma.
- As per the current GINA guidelines, a low dose of ICS along with formoterol as a reliever is the preferred strategy for asthma control. This combination decreases the risk of exacerbations and provides symptomatic relief similar to that of SABAs.

Salmeterol is as effective as ipratropium in the treatment of COPD; it controls the reversible component of airway obstruction and prevents the closure of airways during exhalation.

iii. VABA

The VABAs (very long-acting β_2-agonists): Indacaterol, vilanterol, and olodaterol are approved for use by the inhalational route in maintenance therapy of COPD.

β_2 agonists are **contraindicated** in patients with hypertension, angina, and those on digoxin therapy.

B. Anticholinergics

This class of drugs includes ipratropium, tiotropium and glycopyrronium.

Mechanism of action

M_3 receptors present on bronchial smooth muscles are excitatory in nature. Activation of these receptors causes bronchoconstriction in response to acetylcholine. Anticholinergic drugs exert bronchodilator effect through

M_3 blockade. Anticholinergics are more effective on **larger airways** that receive **vagal innervations**. Atropine, the prototype anticholinergic drug, causes bronchodilatation, but suppresses the mucociliary function of bronchial epithelium. It also reduces tracheobronchial secretions, which become thick and inspissated to form a mucus plug. These actions make atropine unsuitable for bronchial asthma.

In contrast, anticholinergic drugs such as ipratropium and tiotropium have selective bronchodilator effects, without suppression of secretions and mucociliary clearance. Thus, they are preferred over atropine. Tiotropium and glycopyrronium are longer acting than ipratropium, are called long-acting muscarinic antagonists (LAMA), and are suitable for once-daily administration.

- Anticholinergic drugs have **slow onset of action** and **lower efficacy** in comparison to selective β_2-agonists. Thus, they are more **suitable for regular prophylaxis** rather than during an attack. Current GINA guidelines recommend that **long-acting muscarinic antagonists (LAMA**, e.g., tiotropium and glycopyrronium) should never be used as a monotherapy in asthma and are always used in combination with ICS in step 5 of therapy.
- These may be combined with **selective β_2-agonists** in **severe, refractory asthma** attacks for longer-lasting bronchodilator effect.
- Raised cholinergic tone contributes significantly to airway narrowing in COPD and can be reversed by anticholinergic drugs. Thus, they are **more effective in COPD** than in asthma.
- These drugs improve the functional capacity of COPD patients and reduce the frequency of exacerbations.

C. Phosphodiesterase inhibitors

This group includes methylxanthines such as **theophylline, aminophylline and doxophylline**. Beverages such as tea, coffee and cocoa also contain methylated xanthine alkaloids such as caffeine, theophylline and theobromine.

Mechanism of action

Methylxanthines act by the following three mechanisms.

- **Inhibition of phosphodiesterase (PDE) enzyme**: PDE enzyme inactivates cAMP by converting it to 5′-AMP; hence, its inhibition by theophylline-like drugs raises cAMP levels. In smooth muscles, cAMP inactivates myosin light chain kinase (MLCK) and causes relaxation. This smooth muscle relaxing action leads to bronchodilatation (BD) in bronchial smooth muscles. The BD effect of methylxanthines is not mediated through any receptors; so, they are sometimes called **direct-acting bronchodilators**.

  However, raised cAMP can also cause cardiac stimulation and decreased immune and inflammatory activity of specific cells. The PDE isoform that is most relevant for bronchodilator action is **PDE4**. While selective PDE4 inhibitors such as roflumilast and cilomilast were developed to reduce the adverse effects of methylxanthines, they have not proved useful in clinical trials.

  Phosphodiesterase is also responsible for the conversion of cGMP to 5'-GMP. Thus, PDE inhibitors also raise cGMP levels, resulting in a **vasodilator effect**.

- In contrast to the smooth muscle relaxant effect, methylxanthines also stimulate skeletal and cardiac muscles at high concentrations. This action is mediated through the **release of Ca^{2+}** from the **sarcoplasmic reticulum**, favouring **actin–troponin–tropomyosin interactions.**
- Methylxanthines act as **antagonists at adenosine receptors**

Actions mediated by adenosine

- Smooth muscle contraction leading to bronchoconstriction.
- Depression of cardiac pacemaker activity (cardiac slowing).
- Inhibition of gastric secretions.
- Dilatation of cerebral blood vessels.

Methylxanthines can block these effects of adenosine resulting in:

- Bronchodilatation, highlighting their beneficial effect in airway-obstructive diseases.
- Cardiac stimulant action responsible for their adverse effects.
- Increased gastric acid secretion responsible for gastric irritant effect.
- Constriction of cerebral blood vessels, which is beneficial for migraine.

Actions of methylxanthines

- **Smooth muscles**: The relaxant effect on smooth muscles, especially in the airway, leads to a **slow, sustained bronchodilator** action.
- **Skeletal muscles**: The direct action of calcium release from the sarcoplasmic reticulum and increased ACh secretion leads to an increase in skeletal muscle contractility. Due to this effect, methylxanthines **increase diaphragmatic contractility** and reverse its fatigue. This action is beneficial for COPD patients, along with the bronchodilator action.
- **Mast cells**: Due to increased cAMP levels, methylxanthines **reduce histamine release** from mast cells. The release of other mediators from inflammatory cells is also reduced.
- **Central stimulant**: Caffeine, a methylxanthine present in beverages such as tea and coffee, has a mild central stimulant effect. It increases alertness, reduces fatigue and improves concentration. Higher doses of methylxanthines can cause **anxiety, nervousness, insomnia, medullary stimulation, convulsions and death.**

- **Cardiac action**: Methylxanthines have cardiac stimulant effects because of their adenosine-antagonistic action and direct effect on the sarcoplasmic reticulum of cardiac cells in high doses. Heart rate, contractility and conduction velocity are increased. Thus, ADRs such as **tachycardia, palpitations, increased blood pressure, and rhythm disturbances may occur**.
- Methylxanthines cause contraction of cerebral blood vessels, which is useful in migraine.
- By an unknown mechanism, methylxanthines reduce blood viscosity and improve blood flow. **Podophylline**, a **dimethylxanthine**, is useful in intermittent **claudication** because of this blood thinning effect.
- **Gastric secretions**: Increased gastric acid secretion is responsible for the gastrointestinal adverse effects.
- **Diuretic action**: Increased renal blood flow leading to raised GFR and reduced renal tubular reabsorption are responsible for the mild diuretic action of methylxanthines.

Pharmacokinetics

Theophylline is well absorbed, well distributed, and 50%-bound to plasma proteins. It is metabolised in the liver by demethylation and oxidation. It is important to note that the **metabolism of theophylline becomes saturated** over the therapeutic range, i.e., the metabolism changes from first order to zero order with increasing concentration, increasing the chances of its toxicity. Thus, theophylline has a narrow margin of safety.

Therapeutic uses

- Theophylline is used as a **3rd line drug** in the treatment of **severe bronchial asthma**. The decreased popularity of methylxanthines is attributed to:
  - Low efficacy when compared to selective β_2-agonists and inhalational corticoids
  - Narrow margin of safety
  - Poor tolerability
  - Interindividual variations in response
  - Risk of interactions with several simultaneously used drugs.
- In COPD, theophylline is quite useful in reducing frequency and duration of apnea in premature infants.

Adverse drug reactions

- Theophylline has dose-dependent adverse effects (Fig. 28.4). It has gastric irritant effect upon oral use and causes pain at injection site on parenteral administration. Rectal inflammation occurs with the use of suppositories, while rapid IV administration can cause precordial pain and syncope.
- Headache, nervousness, restlessness, insomnia and dyspepsia are seen in the therapeutic concentration range (5–15 mcg/mL).
- Nausea, vomiting, fall in BP, tachycardia, palpitation and diuresis occur at high concentrations (> 20 mcg/mL).
- Still higher plasma concentrations of theophylline may cause agitation, delirium, flushing, fall in BP, rhythm disturbances, extrasystoles, convulsions, coma, and even death. Figure 28.4 depicts the dose-dependent ADRs of theophylline.
- In addition, there is a high risk of interactions. Enzyme inducers (e.g., phenytoin and rifampicin) and smoking can decrease theophylline efficacy. In contrast, enzyme inhibitors (e.g., ciprofloxacin and erythromycin) and oral contraceptives can precipitate theophylline toxicity.

Thus, theophylline has dose-dependent adverse effects and a narrow safety margin; so, therapeutic drug monitoring is very important.

III. Leukotriene Receptor Antagonists (LTRAs)

Leukotrienes (LT) are synthesised from arachidonic acid by the action of the enzyme lipoxygenase (LOX). These are important mediators causing airway constriction in bronchial asthma. So, drugs interfering with the synthesis/actions of leukotrienes are found to be useful in asthma patients.

- **Zileuton** is an **inhibitor** of the **5-lipoxygenase** enzyme and interferes with leukotriene synthesis. However, it is not used very often because of its hepatotoxic potential.
- **Montelukast** and **zafirlukast** are **competitive antagonists** at the cysteinyl LT receptors and exert the following beneficial effects in bronchial asthma:
  - Bronchodilatation
  - Suppression of airway inflammation
  - Reduced eosinophilic count in sputum

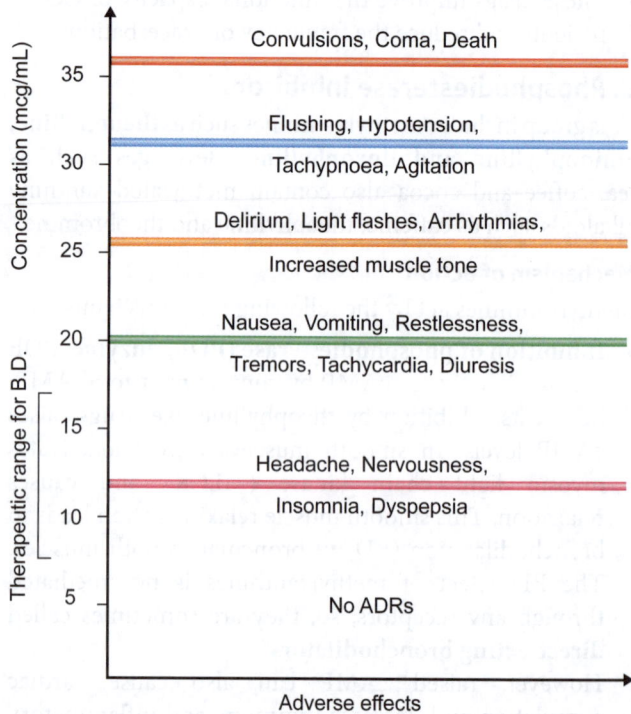

Fig. 28.4 Dose-related adverse effects of theophylline

- LT receptor antagonists are useful alternatives to low-dose ICS in the **prophylaxis of mild-to-moderate asthma** in children at the onset of viral illnesses. In severe cases, these are combined with low dose ICS to reduce the dose of steroids, though they cannot abort an acute attack.

They also provide relief in **NSAID-induced asthma** (NSAIDs act by interfering with the synthesis of prostaglandins from arachidonic acid, by the inhibition of the enzyme cyclo-oxygenase. The excess arachidonic acid is diverted into the lipoxygenase pathway, resulting in the synthesis of excess LTs and precipitating asthma. In such situations, LT antagonists are beneficial as they block the effect of the excess LTs circulating in the blood.

Dose: Montelukast (10 mg); zafirlukast (10–20 mg)

ADRs: LT antagonists are well-tolerated and safe drugs. Minor adverse effects such as headache and rashes may occur. In rare instances, LT antagonists can cause the Churg–Strauss syndrome, characterised by vasculitis and eosinophilia.

IV. Mast Cell Stabilisers

Sodium cromoglycate and ketotifen are useful in asthma because they **prevent the degranulation of mast cells/eosinophils**, and block the release of inflammatory mediators. The mechanism of this mast cell-stabilising action is not well understood, but might involve blockade of chloride channels. Thus, due to decreased release of mediators, chemotaxis (i.e., accumulation of inflammatory cells in the bronchial mucosa), bronchial hyper-responsiveness and bronchoconstriction are prevented.

a. **Sodium cromoglycate** is not absorbed orally because of its poor solubility; it is **used as an aerosol** for long-term prophylaxis in mild-to-moderate asthma to reduce the frequency and severity of acute episodes. It also provides symptomatic relief in allergic rhinitis and allergic conjunctivitis.

   ADRs include headache, dizziness, irritation in throat and cough. In some cases, it may cause rashes, urticaria and joint pain.

b. **Nedocromil** has the same actions as sodium cromoglycate and is used twice daily to decrease frequency and severity of attacks in mild-to-moderate asthma.

c. **Ketotifen** is a H_1-antihistaminic drug that is effective orally; it has a long duration of action (~22 hours). When used for a few (6–12) weeks, it controls the symptoms of asthma, as well as other allergic conditions such as rhinitis, conjunctivitis and atopic dermatitis.

   Adverse effects include sedation, dryness of mouth, dizziness and weight gain.

However, the GINA 2024 guidelines have discontinued the use of sodium cromoglycate and nedocromil via pressurised metered dose inhalers (pMDI) globally, due to low efficacy, despite favourable safety profile.

V. Monoclonal Antibodies

Omalizumab is a humanised monoclonal antibody that **neutralises freely circulating IgE** Abs. Thus, it prevents Ag–Ab reactions on the surface of mast cells and other inflammatory cells. This reduces histamine release from mast cells and prevents asthma attacks. Omalizumab is administered intramuscularly or subcutaneously in a dose of 75 mg (up to 600 mg), every 2 to 4 weeks. Its dose and dosing frequency are determined by serum total IgE levels before starting therapy.

An important limiting factor is its **very high cost**. It, is reserved for use in patients with very severe extrinsic asthma, who do not respond to other drugs. Patients with raised IgE levels, who show positive skin test and need repeated hospitalisation due to severe asthma, also respond well to omalizumab. Other indications for use of omalizumab are chronic spontaneous urticaria and nasal polyposis.

Adverse effects include redness, swelling, pain, burning, bruising and itching at the site of injection, in addition to joint pain, fatigue, headache and nausea.

Recently, **dupilumab** [anti-(interleukin) IL-4 receptor antibody] and **tezepelumab** [anti-thymic stromal lymphopoietin (TSLP) Abs] have also been approved for severe asthma in children older than 6 and 12 years, respectively.

Mepolizumab and reslizumab are anti-IL-5 antibodies. Mepolizumab can be used in children > 6 years, whereas reslizumab should be used only in adults (> 18 years) suffering from severe eosinophilic Type 2 asthma. Anti-IL5 receptor antibody **benralizumab** may be used in patients above 12 years of age, for the same indication.

Clinical problem-based questions and MCQs

6. i. Identify a drug that slowly gets converted into terbutaline, by action of pseudocholinesterase enzyme.
      a. Salmeterol   b. Salbutamol
      b. Bambuterol   d. Formoterol
   ii. Describe mechanism of action of the selected drug and its role in management of bronchial asthma.

7. A 55-year-old bronchial asthma patient gives a history of relief of dyspnea and wheezing upon salbutamol inhalation SOS. During pollen season, however, the patient complains of more frequent attacks and inadequate symptom relief despite daily use of salbutamol therapy.
   i. Explain the cause of inadequate symptom relief with salbutamol in this case.

ii. Which of the following is appropriate in the management of this case?
   a. Increasing the dose of salbutamol.
   b. Switching to longer acting drug, salmeterol.
   c. Switching to ICS-formoterol combination.
   d. Addition of mast cell stabiliser, cromoglycate.
iii. Enumerate the adverse effects of salbutamol.

8. **In current clinical practice, long-acting selective β_2 agonists are combined with ICS for acute asthma exacerbation.**
   i. Name some long-acting selective β_2 agonists.
   ii. Explain the pharmacological basis for combining ICS with LABA for pharmacotherapy of asthma.

9. **The prototype anticholinergic drug atropine causes bronchial smooth muscle relaxation and dilatation, especially of large airways but is still not much used in asthma.**
   i. Explain why atropine does not have a prominent role in the management of asthma despite its bronchodilator action?
   ii. Which anticholinergic drug is better than atropine for the treatment of asthma?
      a. Pirenzepine   b. Tiotropium
      c. Dicyclomine   d. Homatropine
   iii. What is role of the selected drug in asthma and COPD?

10. **Methylxanthines possess which of the following activities?**
    a. Central stimulant
    b. Bronchodilator
    c. Diaphragmatic contraction
    d. All of the above

11. **Methylxanthines are the 3rd line drugs in bronchial asthma in current clinical practice.**
    a. Name some of the methylxanthines.
    b. Describe mechanism of beneficial effect of methylxanthines in asthma and COPD.
    c. Explain why these are not preferred drugs in current practice.
    d. Enumerate the adverse effects of methylxanthines.

12. **A 60-year-old female patient has a history of bronchial asthma that is well controlled with long-acting selective β_2-agonists and ICS used as per need. The patient developed right knee pain due to osteoarthritic changes, for which she took an OTC preparation of diclofenac sodium. Patient reports with cough, expiratory dyspnea and wheezing, which is not responding adequately to her routine drugs.**
    i. What is the cause of asthmatic symptoms in this patient
    ii. Which of the following drugs is most suitable to resolve the symptoms?
       a. Budesonide   b. Zileuton
       c. Zafirlukast   d. Aminophylline
    iii. Justify your choice in this case.
    iv. Enumerate the adverse effects of the selected drug.

13. **Omalizumab is reserved for use in severe extrinsic asthma that does not respond to other drugs.**
    i. Describe mechanism of action of omalizumab
    ii. Why it is reserved for severe, refractory cases only.
    iii. Enumerate adverse effects of omalizumab.

PHARMACOTHERAPY OF ASTHMA

In 1993, WHO established the Global Initiative for Asthma (GINA), which releases an annually updated GINA strategy report. The salient features of the 2019 GINA guidelines (updated in 2023) are:

- **Goals of asthma treatment:**
  - **Symptom control** (few symptoms, no limitation of exercise and no sleep disturbance).
  - **Risk reduction** (maintaining normal lung function and preventing asthma exacerbations, medication adverse effects and asthma deaths).
- **Mild** cases are those that are well controlled by low dose of ICS or as needed only ICS–formoterol.
- **Severe** cases are those that require a high dose of ICS-LABA to prevent it from becoming uncontrollable or those that remain uncontrolled despite optimised treatment with high dose of ICS–LABA.
- Inhalational corticosteroids (ICS) are labelled as **controllers** that target both domains in asthma treatment, i.e., symptom control and future risk reduction.
- Selective β_2-agonists are labelled as **relievers**, and are useful for symptomatic relief, before exercise, or allergen exposure.
- Maintenance therapy is scheduled regularly.
- In GINA 2019, the stepwise therapy of bronchial asthma is instituted. It emphasised the importance of a continuous stepwise process of starting therapy → review of response → assessment → adjustment of treatment.
- The main change in the **2023 update**, was the replacement of short-acting selective β_2-agonists (SABA) with long-acting selective β_2 agonist (LABA: formoterol), because of worsening of asthma symptoms and higher number of exacerbations with SABA.

Treatment Guidelines
Adults and adolescents (> 12 years)

For adults and adolescents (> 12 years) there are **preferred** and **alternative tracks** described in GINA guidelines. The preferred track (see Table 28.1) involves the administration of formoterol (LABA) with low-dose inhalational steroids (ICS) on an 'as needed' basis as **relievers** in all the 5 steps. The **controller** therapy is the same as the reliever in Steps 1 and 2, but the third and fourth steps involve maintenance therapy with low-dose ICS-LABA and medium-dose ICS-LABA respectively. The fifth step of management involves high dose ICS-LABA along with add-on drugs such as long-acting muscarinic antagonist tiotropium with anti-IgE/IL4R/IL5/5R/TSLP Abs.

Table 28.1 Preferred track

Step	Controller	Reliever
1	As needed, only low-dose ICS–formoterol	As needed low-dose ICS–formoterol
2	As needed, only low dose ICS–formoterol	Same as in step 1
3	Low dose maintenance ICS–formoterol	Same as in step 1
4	Medium dose maintenance ICS–formoterol	Same as in step 1
5	High-dose ICS–formoterol, add-on LAMA (tiotropium), with anti-IgE Abs/anti-IL5/5R Ab, anti-IL4R Ab, anti-TSLPs.	Same as in step 1

Alternative track

This track involves the administration of a SABA instead of LABA; ICS are also given as a reliever on an as-needed basis. It is important to ensure the use of ICS whenever SABA is given.

Children (6–11 years)

The updated GINA guidelines for 6-11 year old children involve the administration of low-dose ICS-LABA/SABA as a **reliever** in the first 4 steps listed in Table 28.2. For **controller**, a low-dose ICS is used on an as-needed basis in Step 1, and on a daily-basis in Step 2. Step 3 has either a combination of LABA to low-dose ICS, or a medium dose of ICS given alone. Step 4 involves combining medium-dose ICS with LABA.

Table 28.2 Updated GINA 2022 (6–11 years old)

Step	Controller	Reliever
1	Low dose ICS (as needed)	Low dose ICS–formoterol or SABA
2	Low dose ICS (daily)	
3	Low dose ICS–LABA or Medium dose ICS	Low dose ICS–formoterol or SABA
4	Medium dose ICS–LABA	Low dose ICS–formoterol or SABA

Step 5 involves an **add-on** treatment with
- Long-acting muscarinic antagonist (LAMA), i.e., tiotropium bromide.
- Anti IgE Ab (omalizumab)
- Anti IL5 Ab (mepolizumab in > 6-year-olds)

For children < 5 years of age

For children < 5 years of age, SABA as needed is given as reliever in all the four steps (Table 28.3). For controller, intermittent short course of ICS is given at the onset of viral illness. Leukotriene receptor antagonists are an alternative. In Step 2, low-dose ICS is given on a daily basis. Step 3 involves either a double low-dose ICS or a combination of ICS-LTRA. Step 4 involves specialist care. Step 5 is a high-dose ICS–LABA or an add-on therapy, which could be an anti-IgE Ab (omalizumab).

Table 28.3 Updated GINA 2022 for children < 5 years of age

Steps	Controller	Reliever
1	Intermittent short course ICS at onset of viral illness/LTRA	SABA, as needed
2	Low-dose ICS daily	SABA, as needed
3	Double low-dose ICS/ low-dose ICS+ LTRA	SABA, as needed
4	Continue controller and refer to specialist	SABA, as needed

MANAGEMENT OF STATUS ASTHMATICUS

Status asthmaticus or acute severe asthma is a life threatening condition, requiring emergency hospitalisation and intensive treatment.

- Inhalation of high-flow, **humidified oxygen to control hypoxia** is the first step in management of status asthmaticus. In some cases, intubation and mechanical ventilation may also be required to tide over the crisis.
- IV infusion of normal saline is started to **correct the dehydration and acidosis** associated with hyperventilation and CO_2 retention, respectively. If metabolic acidosis does not respond to this measure, sodium bicarbonate is added to the infusion fluid.
- **Intravenous corticosteroid therapy** with hydrocortisone 100 mg stat IV, followed by IV infusion of 100–200 mg (4–8 hourly) is given. IV dexamethasone with a longer duration of action is also effective for this indication.
- Nebulisation is carried out with **SABA** salbutamol (2.5–5 mg), along with **LAMA** ipratropium bromide (0.5 mg).
- Intramuscular or subcutaneous short-acting β_2-agonists (0.4 mg) are also given because intense bronchoconstriction might prevent inhaled drugs from reaching smaller airways.
- Some patients who are refractory to all the above measures may respond to **IV aminophylline** (250–500 mg) diluted in 5% glucose, administered slowly over 20 minutes.
- If the patient is still not improving, **magnesium sulphate** (2 g) IV infusion in normal saline over 20 minutes may be tried.
- The precipitating cause (e.g., respiratory infection) is treated appropriately.

Clinical problem-based questions and MCQs

14. A 30-year-old woman presented with acute severe expiratory dyspnea. On examination, the patient was dehydrated, exhausted, wheezing and unable to speak in sentences. Her PR was 120 bpm. Bilateral rhonchi were present. She was diagnosed as having acute severe asthma/status asthmaticus. Describe the management of this case.

Summary

- Antitussive drugs are used only in dry cough. In productive cough, expectorants and mucolytic drugs are useful.
- Antitussives can be centrally or peripherally acting.
- **Codeine** is the preferred drug among centrally acting drugs for mild-to-moderate cough. It causes constipation as a major adverse effect. Abuse liability is much less than that for morphine. Codeine is not preferred in asthma due to the risk of respiratory depression at high doses. In severe cough of bronchial cancers, morphine may be used.
- The nonopioid antitussive dextromethorphan is used as an OTC drug.
- Pharyngeal demulcents and steam inhalation are very effective for symptomatic relief by peripheral soothing action on the respiratory tract.
- Mucolytics and expectorants are beneficial only in productive cough. All expectorants other than guaiphenesin are banned by the FDA, due to lack of evidence of their efficacy. Mucolytics such as bromhexine and ambroxol reduce the viscosity of mucus secretions and are effective in conditions involving the formation of mucus plugs (e.g., asthmatic bronchitis, emphysema, tracheostomy tubes and cystic fibrosis).
- **Bronchial asthma** is an episodic disease, characterised by the hyper-responsiveness of airways to various stimuli, pathological remodelling and airway narrowing, resulting in episodes of cough, wheezing and dyspnea.
- Drugs useful in bronchial asthma include corticosteroids, bronchodilators, mast cell stabilisers, leukotriene antagonists and monoclonal antibodies.
- **Corticosteroids** possess nonspecific anti-inflammatory action. Inhalational corticosteroids (ICS) are used for symptom control and future risk reduction, and are called 'controllers'. ICS decrease the frequency of acute attacks and slow down disease progression. Systemic adverse effects are negligible with ICS, especially with the prodrug ciclesonide. Systemic steroids are used intravenously in status asthmaticus and orally in severe chronic asthma.
- **Bronchodilators** include selective agonists at β_2 receptors that activate adenylyl cyclase, resulting in raised cAMP levels. Cyclic AMP inactivates myosin light chain kinase (MLCK) leading to relaxation of smooth muscles. **Short-acting selective β_2-agonists** (salbutamol and terbutaline) relieve symptoms of asthma exacerbation within 5 minutes of administration by the inhalational route, and were extensively used to abort acute attacks. Patients who need frequent (daily) administration of these drugs become refractory to treatment due to receptor down-regulation. So, SABA drugs must always be used in combination with ICS. **Long-acting** drugs such as salmeterol, bambuterol and formoterol are used along with ICS for the prevention of acute bronchial asthma attacks and in COPD; the long-term use of these drugs alone desensitises receptors, worsening the condition. ADRs include muscle tremors, nervousness, palpitation, irritation in throat, and ankle edema.
- **Anticholinergic drugs** or **long-acting muscarinic antagonists (LAMA)** such as ipratropium and tiotropium are given by the inhalational route for regular prophylaxis or combined with selective β_2-agonists in severe refractory type of asthma. Their efficacy is higher in COPD as cholinergic tone is an important contributing factor. Atropine not preferred in asthma because it decreases mucociliary function and tracheobronchial secretions.
- **Methylxanthines** (e.g., theophylline, aminophylline and doxophylline) inhibit PDE4, resulting in bronchodilator and vasodilator action. Through the blockade of adenosine receptors, these cause bronchodilatation, cardiac stimulation, gastric irritation and cerebral vessels constriction. Podophylline reduces blood viscosity and is useful in intermittent claudication. High doses of methylxanthines can cause anxiety, nervousness, insomnia, medullary stimulation, convulsions and even death. They are not preferred because they have many ADRs, low safety margin and risk of drug interactions.
- **LT antagonists (LTRA)** such as montelukast and zafirlukast are used as alternatives to ICS in mild-to-moderate cases and with ICS in severe cases, to reduce the steroid dose. These can relieve NSAID-induced asthma. Adverse effects include headache, rashes, and rarely, the Churg–Strauss syndrome, characterised by vasculitis and eosinophilia.
- **Mast cell stabilisers** such as sodium cromoglycate and ketotifen reduce the frequency and severity of acute attacks. Cromoglycate is used as an aerosol.
- **Omalizumab**, a monoclonal antibody that neutralises circulating IgE, is reserved for severe extrinsic asthma not responding to other drugs. This is due to its high cost, need for parenteral administration and adverse effects (e.g., injection site reactions, fatigue, headache and joint pain).

Questions for practice

1. Classify the drugs used in the management of cough.
2. Comment on the role of the following drugs in management of cough.
   a. Codeine
   b. Dextromethorphan
   c. Prokinetic drugs
   d. Bronchodilators
   e. Mucolytics
3. i. The sale of all mucokinetic drugs EXCEPT one has been stopped by the US FDA. Identify the drug.
      a. Guaiphenesin
      b. Potassium iodide
      c. Ammonium chloride
      d. Sodium citrate
   ii. Describe mechanism of action of the selected drug.
4. Which of the following is responsible for mucolytic action of bromhexine?
   a. Increases bronchial secretions
   b. Breaks disulphide bonds in tenacious sputum
   c. Depolymerises mucopolysaccharides
   d. Affects cholinergic innervations of mucosal glands
5. Which of the following is the site of action of dextromethorphan?
   a. Sigma opioid receptors
   b. Central NMDA receptors
   c. Cough centre in dorsal medulla
   d. Afferent fibres from respiratory mucosa
6. Which of the following cough suppressants is equipotent to codeine, but does not cause constipation?
   a. Noscapine
   b. Bromhexine
   c. Ambroxol
   d. Acetylcysteine
7. Explain why:
   a. Aspirin can precipitate asthma in predisposed individuals.
   b. Ipratropium bromide is more effective in COPD than in bronchial asthma.
   c. Theophylline is useful in asthma.
   d. Beta blockers should be avoided in bronchial asthma.
   e. SABA drugs are always used in combination with ICS.
   f. Use of methylxanthines has declined in asthma treatment.
8. Write short notes on:
   a. Inhaled corticoids
   b. LT antagonists
   c. Mast cell stabilisers
   d. Salmeterol
9. Describe management of
   a. Status asthmaticus or acute severe asthma
   b. Severe, frequent asthma exacerbations
   c. Chronic asthma
10. Describe the stepwise approach in the pharmacotherapy of asthma.

Hints for problem-based questions and MCQs

1. c. Inhalational
2. a. Ciclesonide
3. a. Acute severe asthma or status asthmaticus
   b. Refer to Box 28.1, page 375.
4. c. Corticosteroids are used by inhalational route.
   In status asthmaticus, inhaled drugs may not reach smaller airways owing to intense bronchoconstriction and formation of mucus plug thickened secretions. So, steroids are administered intravenously.
5. b. These are labelled as relievers in asthma therapy
   Steroids are labelled as controllers in asthma therapy, while bronchodilators are relievers.
6. i. c. Bambuterol
   ii. It is a prodrug with slow onset and long duration of action. It is used along with ICS for prevention of acute asthma attacks.
7. i. Daily salbutamol administration, as necessitated by frequent symptoms causes receptor down-regulation and reduced responsiveness.
   ii. c. Addition of inhalational corticosteroid, budesonide is next step to reverse refractoriness to selective β_2-agonists.
   iii. Tremors, nervousness, palpitation, irritation in throat and ankle edema are important adverse effects of selective β_2-agonists.
8. i. Salmeterol, formoterol, bambuterol
   ii. Chronic use of LABA causes receptor desensitisation and worsening of condition.
9. Atropine decreases tracheobronchial secretions and mucociliary function.
   ii. b. Tiotropium has a negligible effect on the mucociliary function and tracheobronchial secretions. So, it is preferred over atropine in bronchial asthma and COPD.
   iii. Anticholinergics (e.g., ipratropium and tiotropium) play a role in step 5 as an add-on drug in the regular prophylaxis of asthma and COPD. Their efficacy is higher in COPD because increased vagal tone is an important factor.
10. d. All of the above
11. i. Theophylline, aminophylline, doxophylline and podophylline.
    ii. PDE4 inhibition → raised cAMP → BD
    Release of calcium from sarcoplasmic reticulum in skeletal muscles, causing diaphragmatic contraction, relieving its fatigue is beneficial in COPD.
    iii. Refer to page 378; less efficacy, more adverse effects, saturable kinetics, higher risk of interaction with other drugs, etc.
    iv. Refer to page 378
12. i. NSAID-induced asthma
    ii. c. Zafirlukast
    iii. NSAIDs divert arachidonic acid to lipoxygenase pathway causing excess LT production that may precipitate asthma symptoms. These can be checked by interfering with synthesis or action of LTs. Zileuton is LOX inhibitor, but not much used due to hepatotoxicity. Zafirlukast is LT antagonist useful to resolve asthma symptoms associated with excess production of LTs.
    iv. Well-tolerated drugs; can cause headache, rashes, etc. The Churg–Strauss syndrome characterised by vasculitis and eosinophilia is a rare adverse effect.
13. i. Neutralises circulating IgE Abs → prevents release of mediators from mast cells and eosinophils.
    ii. Very high cost; needs to be injected; adverse effects
    iii. Refer to page 379
14. Refer to page 381

CONCEPT MAP - DRUGS FOR BRONCHIAL ASTHMA

Classification

Corticosteroids:
Inhalational: Budesonide, Ciclesonide, Flunisolide, Fluticasone, Beclomethasone, Mometasone, Triamcinolone
Systemic: Prednisolone, Hydrocortisone

Bronchodilators:
Selective β₂ agonists: SABA: Salbutamol, Terbutaline
LABA: Salmeterol, Bambuterol, Formoterol
VABA: Carmoterol, Indacaterol, Vilanterol, Olodaterol
Anticholinergics: Ipratropium, Tiotropium, Glycopyrronium
Methylxanthines: Caffeine, Theophylline, Aminophylline, Doxophylline
Selective PDE4 inhibitor: Roflumilast
Leukotriene Antagonists: Montelukast, Zafirlukast, Zileuton
Mast Cell Stabilisers: Sodium cromoglycate, Ketotifen
Monoclonal Abs: Anti-IgE (Omalizumab), Anti-IL4R (Dupilumab), Anti-IL5R (Benralizumab), Anti-IL5 (Mepolizumab, Reslizumab), Anti-TSLP (Tezepelumab)

Corticosteroids

- Non-specific anti-inflammatory action.
- **ICS:** labelled as **'controllers'** for symptom control and future risk reduction.
- Decrease frequency of acute attacks, slow down disease progression.
- Must be combined whenever SABA is used.
- Negligible systemic adverse effects especially with prodrug ciclesonide.
- **Systemic steroids** are used;
- IV in status asthmaticus
- Orally as last resort in chronic severe asthma.

LT Receptor Antagonists (LTRA)

Montelukast, Zafirlukast used as;
- Alternative to ICS in mild-to-moderate cases.
- With ICS in severe cases to reduce steroid doses.
- Relieve NSAID-induced asthma.
- ADRs: Headache, rashes and rarely Churg-Strauss syndrome, characterised by vasculitis and eosinophilia.

Selective β₂ Agonists

- Raise cAMP levels → inactivation of MLCK → smooth muscles relaxation → Bronchodilatation.
- SABA like Salbutamol, terbutaline relieve symptoms within 5 minutes after inhalation. Used as reliever in children only.
- Replaced by Formoterol in GINA 23
- ADRs: Tremors, nervousness, palpitation, irritation in throat and ankle edema. Frequent administration may cause receptor down-regulation → refractoriness.
- LABAs such as Salmetrol, Bambuterol, Formoterol are used for prevention of acute attack of BA and in COPD along with ICS, because use as monotherapy causes desensitisation of receptors and worsening of condition.

Mast Cell Stabilisers

- Sodium cromoglycate, Ketotifen
- Reduce frequency and severity of acute attack.
- Cromoglycate use as pMDI discontinued.

Omalizumab

- Anti-IgE monoclonal antibody, used as 'add-on' drug for severe extrinsic asthma not responding to other drugs,
- ADRs: Injection site reactions, fatigue, headache, joint pain, etc.
- High cost
- Need for parenteral use.

Anticholinergic Drugs

- Ipratropium and long-acting muscarinic antagonists (LAMA) as Tiotropium, glycopyrronium
- Used by inhalational route as 'add-on' drugs in severe refractory type of asthma.
- More efficacious in COPD as cholinergic tone is important contributing factor.
- Atropine decreases mucociliary function and tracheobronchial secretions, hence not preferred in asthma.

Methylxanthines

- Theophylline, Aminophylline, Doxophylline
- PDE4 inhibition → bronchodilatation vasodilatation
- Blockade of adenosine receptors → BD, cardiac stimulation, cerebral vasoconstriction gastric irritant.
- Narrow safety margin, not used much in current clinical practice.
- ADRs: Higher doses cause anxiety, nervousness, insomnia, medullary stimulation, convulsions and death.

SECTION 6 Drugs Acting on the Kidneys

29 Diuretics

PH 4.5 Explain types, salient pharmacokinetics, pharmacodynamics, therapeutic uses, and adverse drug reactions of diuretics, antidiuretics, vasopressin, and analogues.

Learning objectives

A student of MBBS phase II should be able to:
- Classify diuretics.
- Explain the mechanism of action of each class of diuretics.
- Enumerate the indications for use of diuretics.
- Explain the pharmacological basis for each indication of diuretics.
- Comment on therapeutic status of diuretics in different conditions in current clinical practice.
- Enumerate ADRs and contraindications of diuretics.
- Describe renal autacoids.
- Classify and explain therapeutic uses of antidiuretics.
- Enumerate ADRs and contraindications for use of antidiuretics.

DIURETICS

Diuretics are drugs that increase urine output; they are useful in many clinical disorders involving abnormality of fluid volume and electrolyte concentration. Drugs that increase renal sodium excretion are called **natriuretics**, whereas **aquaretics** increase the excretion of solute-free water.

Classification of Diuretics

Diuretics can be classified into low-, medium-, and high-efficacy drugs (Flowchart 29.1). Anti-diuretic hormone

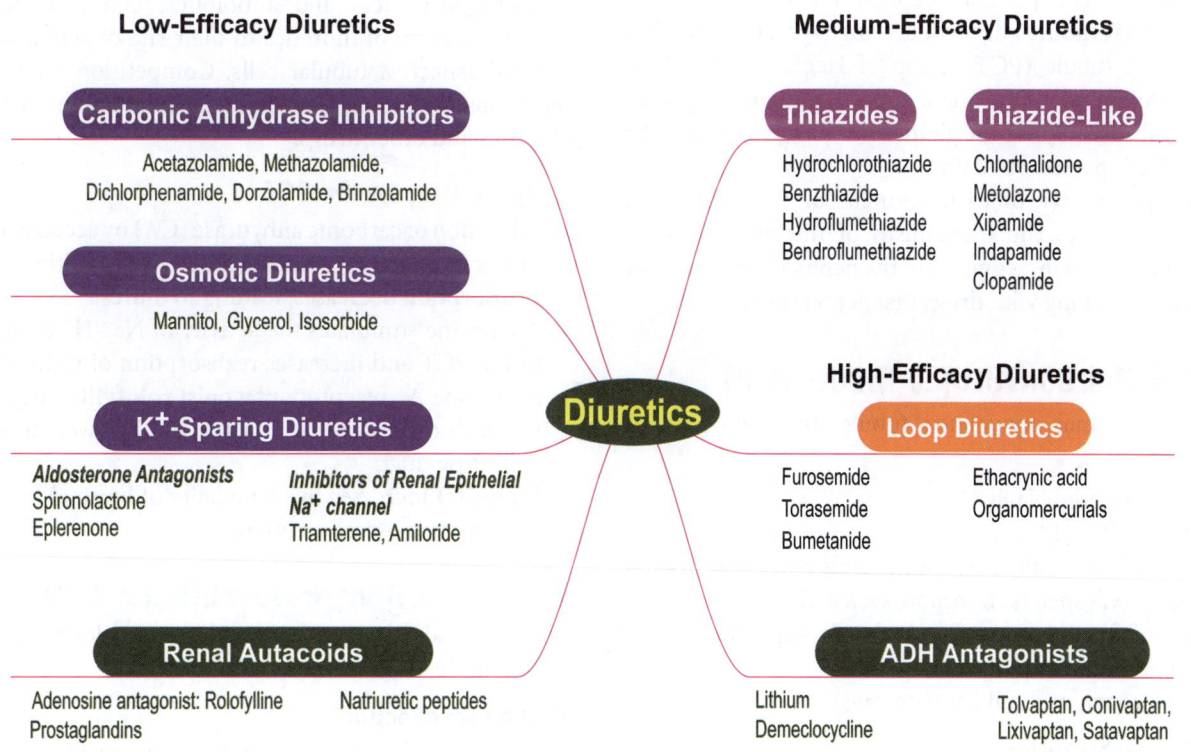

Flowchart 29.1 Classification of diuretics

(ADH) antagonists and renal autacoids also have diuretic effects.

Mechanism of Action

Diuretics act by one of the following mechanisms:

- Inhibition of specific membrane transporters present in renal tubular epithelial cells (thiazides, loop diuretics, triamterene, amiloride).
- Prevention of water reabsorption by osmotic effects (mannitol, glycerol, isosorbide).
- Inhibition of carbonic anhydrase enzyme (acetazolamide).
- Antagonism of hormone effects in renal epithelial cells (spironolactone, eplerenone, vaptans).

Physiology of Urine Formation

The three main functions of kidneys are the excretion of waste products, regulation of fluid–electrolyte balance, and regulation of acid–base balance.

- Renal blood flow is about 20–25% of cardiac output = 1200 mL/min
- Renal plasma flow = 660 mL/min
- Glomerular filtration rate (GFR) = 125 mL/min

The **glomerulus** is a tuft of capillaries projecting into the dilated end of the tubule, i.e., Bowman's capsule. Fluid is driven from the capillaries into the tubular lumen by hydrodynamic forces. The glomerular filtrate contains all the constituents of plasma except plasma proteins.

The **renal tubule** has the following segments: proximal convoluted tubule (PCT), Loop of Henle (LOH), distal convoluted tubule (DCT), and collecting tubule. Together, these reabsorb 99% of the glomerular filtrate and only 1.5 L of urine is passed out daily.

The physiology of each segment of the nephron is closely linked to the mechanism of the diuretic drugs acting on it. Herein, segments of the nephron are described sequentially, along with drugs that act on them.

I. PROXIMAL CONVOLUTED TUBULE (PCT)

In the proximal convoluted tubule, the following are reabsorbed:

- 85% of filtered $NaHCO_3$
- 40% of filtered NaCl
- All the filtered glucose, amino acids and other organic solutes (via specific transport systems).
- 60% of filtered water (passively, through transcellular and paracellular pathways).
- K^+ (through paracellular pathways).

$NaHCO_3$ reabsorption

A Na^+/H^+ exchanger located on the luminal side of the PCT cell (Fig. 29.1) allows the inflow of one Na^+ ion in exchange for the outflow of one H^+ ion. This Na^+ ion is reabsorbed on the basolateral surface by Na^+/K^+-ATPase. In the tubular lumen, H^+ combines with HCO_3^- to form carbonic acid, which then dissociates into H_2O and CO_2; these diffuse inside the cell and recombine to form H_2CO_3. Both these reactions occur under the influence of carbonic anhydrase enzyme. H_2CO_3 then ionises to provide H^+ and HCO_3^- ions; the bicarbonate ions are then reabsorbed into blood by a specific transporter.

NaCl reabsorption

Normally, after the reabsorption of bicarbonate, the luminal fluid in the late PCT resembles a simple NaCl solution. Na^+/H^+ exchange continues, but now the H^+ are not titrated by HCO_3^- ions → luminal pH decreases and activates a poorly defined Cl^-/base exchanger, leading to the reabsorption of NaCl. There is no diuretic available that can prevent NaCl reabsorption in the PCT.

Water reabsorption

Because of the high water permeability of the PCT, water is reabsorbed in direct proportion to salt reabsorption; this increases the concentration of any impermeant solute present in the lumen. So, the osmolality of the luminal fluid increases, which prevents further reabsorption of H_2O. This is the mechanism by which mannitol causes diuresis.

Organic acid secretory systems

The secretory systems located in middle third of the PCT secrete many organic acids such as uric acid, para-aminohippuric acid and antibiotics, and is important for the delivery of diuretics to their site of action on the luminal aspect of tubular cells. Competition for tubular secretions is responsible for many interactions between diuretics and other drugs.

Drugs acting on the PCT

- Inhibition of carbonic anhydrase (CA) by acetazolamide prevents $NaHCO_3$ reabsorption. In addition, H_2O reabsorption decreases, leading to diuresis.
- Adenosine stimulates the activity of Na^+/H^+ exchanger in the PCT and increases reabsorption of sodium. The adenosine A_1-receptor antagonist **rolofylline** decreases the reabsorption of Na^+ in the PCT as well as in the collecting duct.
- **Mannitol** increases the osmolality of luminal fluid and prevents water reabsorption.

1. Carbonic Anhydrase Inhibitors (CAIs)

Acetazolamide, methazolamide, dichlorphenamide, dorzolamide, brinzolamide

Mechanism of action

These drugs decrease bicarbonate reabsorption in the PCT by inhibiting carbonic anhydrase → decrease in H_2O reabsorption → diuresis. Significant HCO_3^- losses result

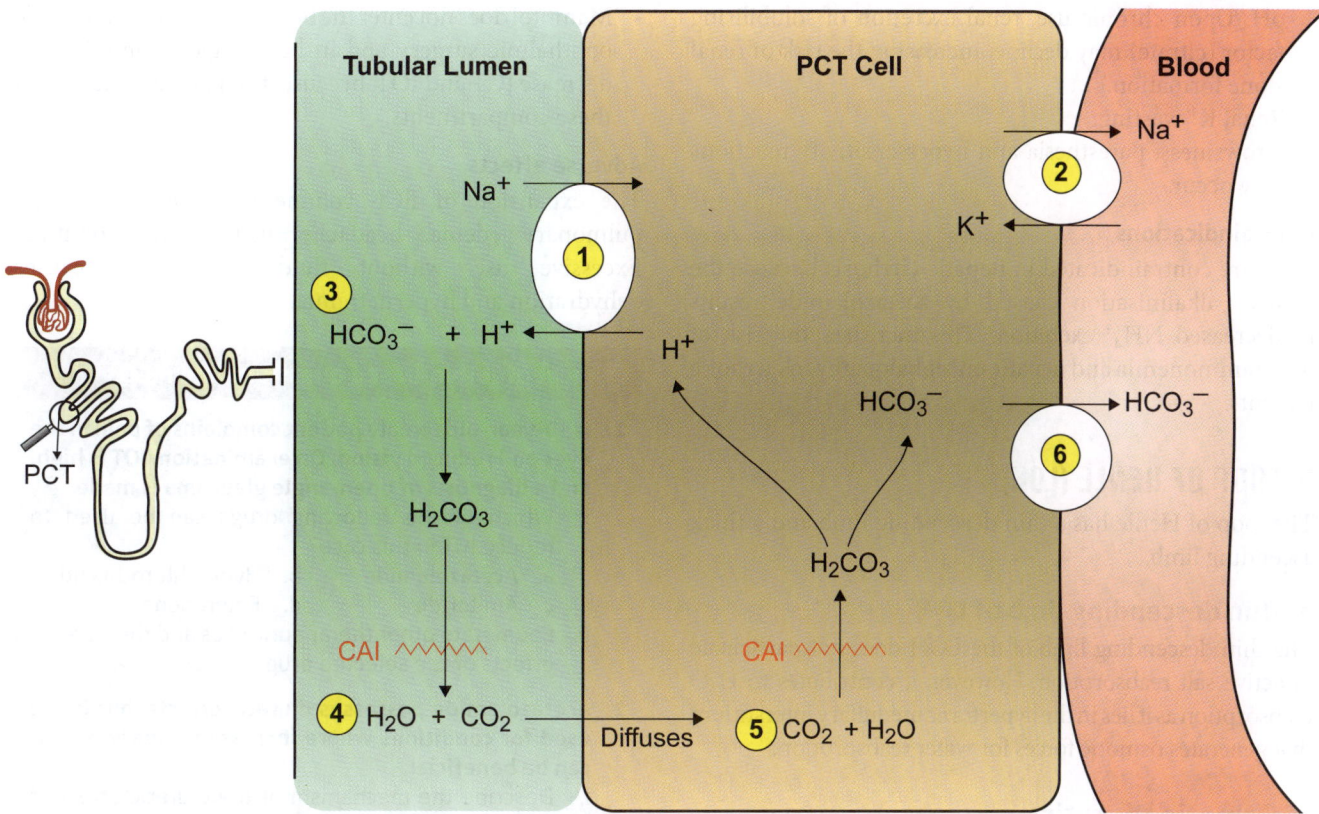

Fig. 29.1 Mechanism of action of carbonic anhydrase inhibitors

① Reabsorption of $NaHCO_3$ occurs by the action of the Na^+/H^+ exchanger located in the luminal membrane of PCT epithelial cells. It allows one Na^+ from the tubular lumen to enter the cell in exchange for a proton from inside the cell.
② Na^+ is transported in exchange for K^+ by Na^+/K^+-ATPase in the basolateral membrane so that the intracellular concentration of Na^+ remains low.
③ H^+ ions secreted into the lumen combine with HCO_3^- ions to form H_2CO_3.
④ Under the action of enzyme carbonic anhydrase (CA), H_2CO_3 forms H_2O and CO_2.
⑤ The CO_2 simply diffuses into the cell, where it recombines with H_2O by the action of CA to form H_2CO_3. This H_2CO_3 spontaneously ionises to H^+ and HCO_3^- so that H^+ is available for exchange with Na^+ on the luminal side.
⑥ HCO_3^- ion is transported across the basolateral membrane by a specific transporter.

in hyperchloremic metabolic acidosis. HCO_3^- depletion → enhanced NaCl reabsorption by the remaining tubule segments in nephron, which decreases the diuretic efficacy over several days.

Therapeutic uses

CAIs are not preferred for diuretic use because of their short-lasting diuretic action. However, they are useful in:

- **Glaucoma**: Carbonic anhydrase plays an important role in the synthesis of aqueous humour. CAIs can reduce the rate of formation of aqueous humour → decrease in intraocular tension (IOT). Brinzolamide and dorzolamide are used topically for this indication.
- **Urinary alkalinisation**: CAIs increase the excretion of HCO_3^- ions in urine. Alkaline urine prevents cystinuria and cystine stones; however, Ca^{2+} precipitates in alkaline urine causing nephrolithiasis.
- **Metabolic alkalosis**: CAIs increase alkali (HCO_3^-) loss from the body; they also help in respiratory alkalosis and obstructive sleep apnea.
- **Acute mountain sickness**: CAIs decrease CSF formation and also lower the pH of CSF. This effect is useful in headache and pseudotumor cerebri.
- CAIs increase CO_2 in central neurons, resulting in **increased GABA release**. This effect can be useful in managing catamenial epilepsy (precipitated by menstruation) and as adjuvants in the treatment of epilepsy.
- In severe **hyperphosphatemia**, CAIs can increase urinary phosphate excretion.

Adverse effects

- Hyperchloremic metabolic acidosis.
- Renal stones caused by **phosphaturia** and **hypercalciuria**: Calcium becomes insoluble in alkaline

pH. Upon chronic use, renal excretion of solubilising factor (citrate) may decline, increasing the risk of renal stone formation.
- Renal K^+ wasting.
- Drowsiness, paresthesia and hypersensitivity reactions may occur.

Contraindications

CAIs are contraindicated in hepatic cirrhosis because the urinary alkalinisation caused by acetazolamide results in decreased NH_4^+ excretion. This increases the risk of hyperammonemia and hepatic encephalopathy in cirrhotic patients.

II. LOOP OF HENLE (LOH)

The loop of Henle has a thin descending limb and a thick ascending limb.

a. Thin descending limb of LOH

The thin descending limb of the LOH does not participate in active salt reabsorption. However, it contributes to H_2O reabsorption as it lies in the hypertonic medullary interstitium that generates osmotic forces for water reabsorption.

2. Osmotic Diuretics

Mannitol, glycerol, isosorbide

Mechanism of action

Osmotic diuretics act on the PCT and thin descending limb of the LOH, which are permeable to water. **Mannitol** is not metabolised and is primarily handled by glomerular filtration without any significant tubular reabsorption or secretion. Because it is poorly absorbed when administered orally, it must be given parenterally.

After glomerular filtration, mannitol stays in tubular lumen → decreases reabsorption of H_2O by interposing a countervailing osmotic force → urine volume and flow rate increase → decrease in contact time between the fluid and the tubular epithelium → decrease in Na^+ reabsorption → **natriuresis**.

However, the natriuresis is of lesser magnitude than aquaresis, resulting in hypernatremia.

Therapeutic uses

Mannitol is used to increase water excretion in preference to Na^+ excretion, as in the following cases:
- When renal hemodynamics are compromised: A decrease in renal blood flow (RBF) → decrease in GFR → nearly complete reabsorption of NaCl and H_2O in the PCT, so that the distal segments of the tubule become dry → cessation of urine flow → acute renal failure. This can be prevented by intravenous mannitol (dose: 1–2 g/kg body weight).
- When large pigment loads are presented to the kidneys as in hemolysis/rhabdomyolysis, mannitol can prevent anuria and maintain urine volume.
- Mannitol does not enter the brain or eye; it is given before ophthalmic surgery and in neurological conditions to decrease ICT and IOT, because it can extract water from these compartments.

Adverse effects

The expansion of ECF volume can complicate CHF, pulmonary edema, headache, nausea and vomiting. Excessive use without fluid replacement causes dehydration and hypernatremia.

> **Clinical problem-based questions and MCQs**
>
> 1. **A 50-year-old female patient complains of pain in the eyes and reduced vision. On examination, IOT is high, and a diagnosis of open-angle glaucoma is made.**
>   i. Which of the following drugs can be used to reduce IOT in this case?
>   a. Acetazolamide   b. Hydrochlorothiazide
>   c. Amiloride   d. Eplerenone
>   ii. Enumerate other therapeutic uses and the adverse effects of the selected drug.
>
> 2. **Acetazolamide possesses diuretic effects, but is not used for conditions where increased urinary output can be beneficial.**
>   i. Describe the mechanism of the diuretic effect of acetazolamide.
>   ii. Explain why it is not used as a diuretic.
>
> 3. i. **Identify the segment of the nephron in which most of the filtered $NaHCO_3$ is reabsorbed.**
>   a. Proximal convoluted tubule
>   b. Loop of Henle
>   c. Distal convoluted tubule
>   d. Collecting tubule
>   ii. Describe the mechanism of $NaHCO_3$ reabsorption in the selected segment.
>   iii. Name the diuretics that act on this segment.
>
> 4. **Mannitol has a natriuretic effect, along with the potential to cause hypernatremia.**
>   i. Describe the mechanism of the natriuretic effect of mannitol.
>   ii. Explain the cause of hypernatremia in spite of its natriuretic effect.
>   iii. Enumerate the therapeutic uses, adverse effects and contraindications of mannitol.
>
> 5. **Which of the following diuretics helps in the excretion of large pigment loads by kidney in hemolysis patients?**
>   a. Acetazolamide   b. Furosemide
>   c. Triamterene   d. Mannitol

b. Thick ascending limb of LOH

In this part of the nephron, nearly 35% of the filtered NaCl is reabsorbed along with Ca^{2+} and Mg^{2+} (through the paracellular space). However, it is extremely impermeable to H_2O, enabling reabsorption of salts but not water. As a result, the fluid in the tubular lumen becomes more dilute, earning this segment the name "diluting segment." **diluting segment**.

NaCl reabsorption in the ascending limb of the LOH occurs via a Na$^+$/K$^+$/2Cl$^-$ cotransporter that is electrically neutral (Fig. 29.2). On the basolateral surface, Na$^+$/K$^+$/ATPase causes Na$^+$ to move out of the cell while a K$^+$ ion moves inside. K$^+$ and Cl$^-$ are cotransported on the basolateral side. This causes accumulation of K$^+$ inside the cell → back diffusion of K$^+$ into the tubular lumen → a lumen positive electrical potential develops, which provides the driving force for the reabsorption of divalent cations, Mg^{2+} and Ca^{2+}, via the paracellular pathway.

3. Loop Diuretics

Furosemide, torsemide, bumetanide

Mechanism of action

Loop diuretics act by selectively blocking the Na$^+$/K$^+$/2Cl$^-$ cotransporter (Fig. 29.2). This inhibits NaCl reabsorption → lumen positive electrical potential does not develop → decrease in paracellular movement of Mg^{2+} and Ca^{2+} → increase in urinary excretion of Mg^{2+} and Ca^{2+}.

Pharmacological actions

- As a consequence of the above actions, loop diuretics decrease NaCl reabsorption in the thick ascending limb of LOH → more solute is delivered to the remaining segments of the nephron, where its osmotic pressure further reduces H$_2$O reabsorption → profuse diuresis → as much as 25% of glomerular filtrate passes out as urine (normally, it is just 1% of the GF).
- Therefore, loop diuretics are the most efficacious diuretics or high ceiling diuretics. In addition they can prevent back diffusion of K$^+$ → increased Mg^{2+} and Ca^{2+} excretion. So, prolonged use can cause significant hypomagnesemia (hypocalcemia does not occur as Ca^{2+} is actively reabsorbed in the next segment, i.e., DCT). However, in patients with hypercalcemia, Ca^{2+} excretion can be greatly enhanced by giving saline infusions along with loop diuretics.
- Loop diuretics also directly affect the blood flow through various vascular beds.
  - Increase RBF and cause redistribution of blood flow within the renal cortex.
  - Relieve pulmonary congestion and decrease the left ventricular filling pressure before measurable increase in urine output occurs.

Pharmacokinetics

- Loop diuretics are orally absorbed and rapid response occurs on intravenous injection.

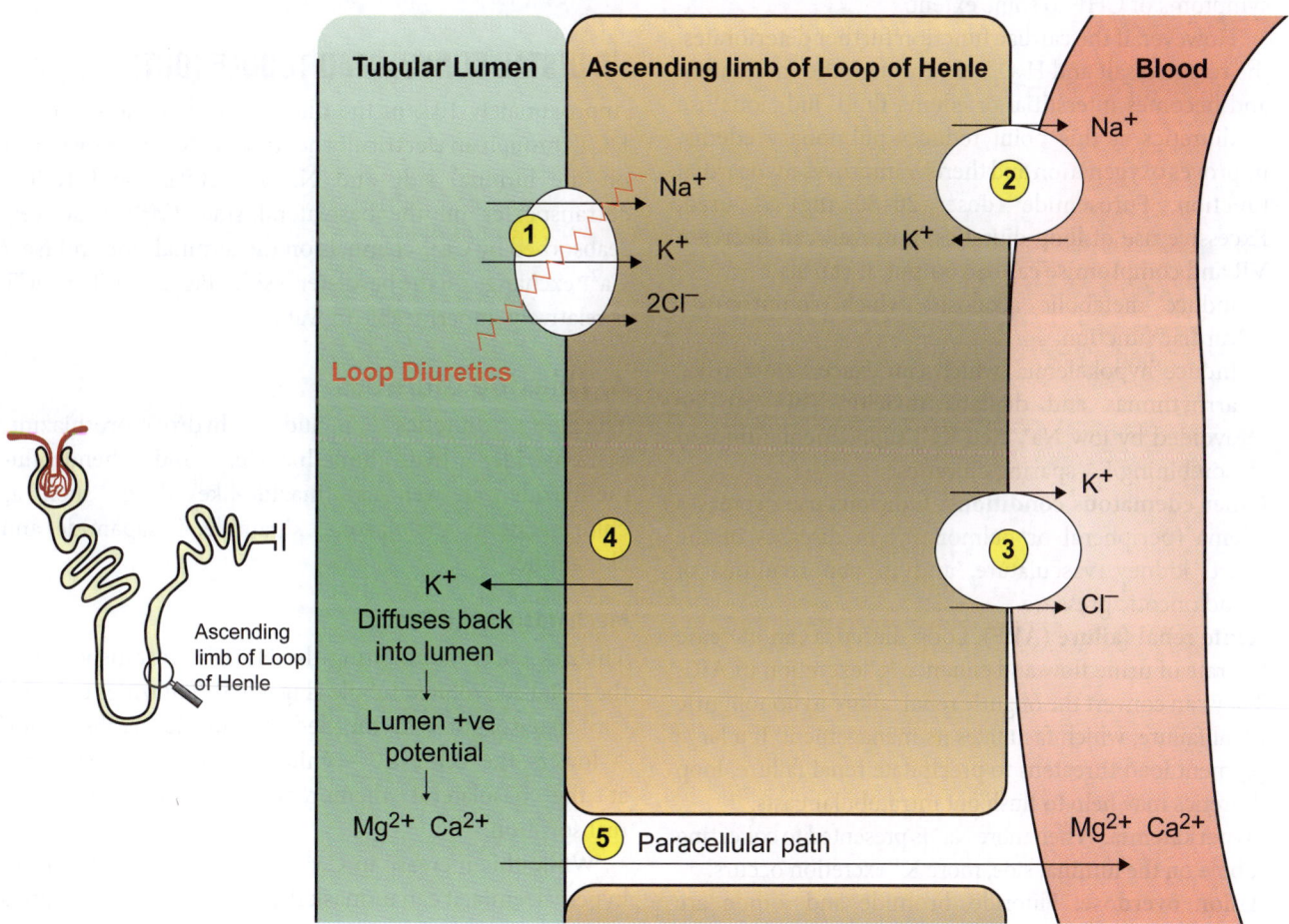

Fig. 29.2 Mechanism of action of loop diuretics

① Na$^+$/K$^+$/2Cl$^-$ cotransporter; ② Na$^+$/K$^+$-ATPase; ③ K$^+$ and Cl$^-$ cotransporter; ④ Back diffusion of K$^+$ into lumen; ⑤ Paracellular reabsorption of divalent cations

- They are strongly plasma protein bound, and so are not filtered in the glomerular filtrate. They reach their site of action on the luminal side by tubular secretion in the middle segment of PCT. Indomethacin and probenecid can inhibit tubular secretion of loop diuretics and decrease their effect.
- Torsemide has an active metabolite, so its duration of action is comparatively longer.

Therapeutic uses

Loop diuretics are used in the following conditions:
- Acute pulmonary edema (CHF)
- Other edematous conditions
- Acute renal failure
- Acute hypercalcemia
- Hyperkalemia
- Anion overdose

Pharmacological basis for use of loop diuretics

- **CHF:** When cardiac contractility and hence cardiac output are reduced by disease, the decrease in RBF leads to compensatory retention of Na^+ and H_2O. This expands the intravascular volume and increases venous return (VR) and preload. Loop diuretics can reduce preload, improve cardiac output (COP) and relieve symptoms of CHF to some extent.

  However, if the cardiac function further deteriorates, the retained salt and H_2O leaks through the vasculature and becomes interstitial or edema fluid. Judicious use of diuretics at this point reduces pulmonary edema, improves oxygenation and thereby improves myocardial function. Furosemide (dose: 20–80 mg) is used. Excessive use of loop diuretics, however, can decrease VR and compromise cardiac output. It can also:
  - induce metabolic alkalosis, which compromises cardiac function.
  - induce hypokalemia, which can exacerbate cardiac arrhythmias and digitalis toxicity. This can be avoided by low Na^+ diet, KCl supplementation and combining K^+-sparing diuretics.
- Other **edematous conditions**: Judicious use decreases edema (peripheral or pulmonary) in diseases of the heart, kidney, vasculature, and in abnormalities of blood oncotic pressure.
- **Acute renal failure (ARF):** Loop diuretics can increase the rate of urine flow and enhance K^+ excretion in ARF. They can convert the oliguric renal failure to nonoliguric renal failure, which facilitates its management. If a large pigment load threatens to precipitate renal failure, loop diuretics may help to flush out intratubular casts.
- **Hyperkalemia:** When more Na^+ is presented to collecting tubule on the luminal side, more K^+ excretion occurs.
- **Anion overdose:** Fluoride, bromide and iodide are reabsorbed in the thick ascending limb of LOH. In the case of toxic ingestion, loop diuretics along with saline infusion are helpful.

ADRs
- **Hypokalemic metabolic alkalosis**: As loop diuretics increase delivery of Na^+ and H_2O to the collecting duct, they enhance K^+ and H^+ secretion.
- **Hypomagnesemia**.
- Severe **dehydration** can occur. If the patient increases water intake in response to thirst caused by dehydration, it can cause **hyponatremia**.
- **Hyperuricemia** and precipitation of gout. Loop diuretics decrease uric acid excretion by inhibiting the voltage-driven drug efflux transporter (NPT4) in the PCT, resulting in hyperuricemia.
- Dose-related ototoxicity and reversible hearing loss, especially in patients with decreased renal function and patients on aminoglycosides.
- Allergic reactions such as skin rash, eosinophilia and interstitial nephritis may occur because of the sulphamoyl moiety.

Contraindications
- Excessive use can be counterproductive in heart failure, renal failure and hepatic cirrhosis.
- Cross-sensitivity can occur in patients who are allergic to sulphonamides.

III. DISTAL CONVOLUTED TUBULE (DCT)

Approximately 10% of the filtered NaCl is reabsorbed in DCT through an electrically neutral Na^+/Cl^- cotransporter on the luminal side and Na^+/K^+-ATPase and K^+/Cl^- cotransporter on the basolateral side. Ca^{2+} is actively reabsorbed by Ca^{2+} channels on the luminal side and Na^+/Ca^{2+} exchange on the basolateral side (Fig. 29.3). The DCT is relatively impermeable to water.

4. Thiazide Diuretics

Thiazide diuretics include hydrochlorothiazide, benzthiazide, hydroflumethiazide, and bendroflumethiazide, as well as 'thiazide-like' drugs such as chlorthalidone, metolazone, xipamide, indapamide and clopamide.

Mechanism of action

Thiazides act by inhibiting the Na^+/Cl^- cotransporter in the distal convoluted tubule (Fig. 29.3). Thiazides enhance Ca^{2+} reabsorption as the decrease in Na^+ reabsorption → lowers the cell Na^+ → enhanced Na^+/Ca^{2+} exchange at the basolateral membrane → increase in Ca^{2+} reabsorption.

While this increase in Ca^{2+} reabsorption rarely causes hypercalcemia, it can unmask the same due to other causes such as hyperparathyroidism, sarcoidosis and carcinomas. However, this effect can be used if patient has renal stones because of hypercalciuria.

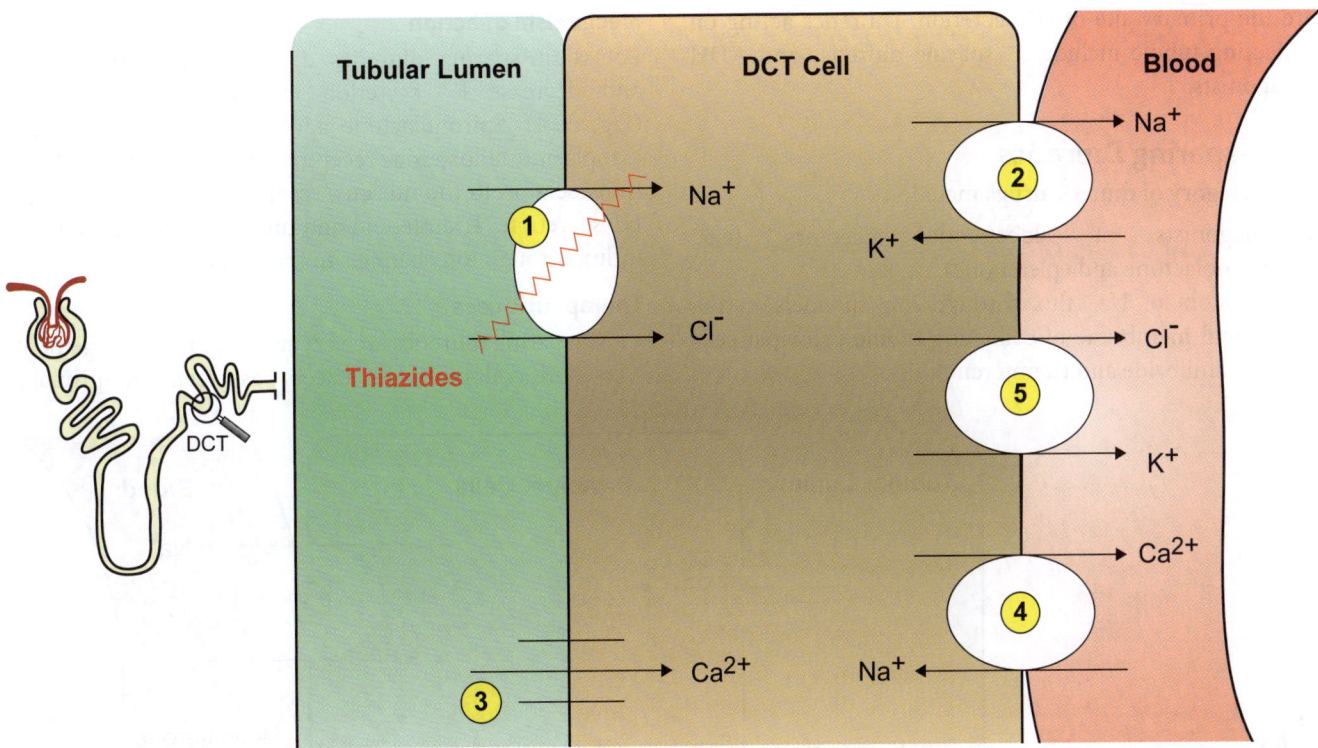

Fig. 29.3 Mechanism of action of thiazides

① NaCl reabsorption in the DCT is carried out by an electrically neutral Na^+/Cl^- cotransporter. ② Na^+ is pumped out at the basolateral surface by Na^+/K^+-ATPase; however, a lumen positive potential does not develop for Ca^{2+}/Mg^{2+} movement (unlike in the LOH). ③ Ca^{2+} is actively reabsorbed via calcium channels on luminal side. ④ Na^+/Ca^{2+} exchangers on the basolateral side. This process is regulated by parathormone. ⑤ Cl^- is reabsorbed on basolateral surface by K^+/Cl^- cotransporter.

Pharmacokinetics

Thiazides are well absorbed orally and secreted in the middle segment of PCT, where they can decrease uric acid secretion → hyperuricemia.

Therapeutic uses

- **Hypertension:** Thiazide diuretics are still among drugs of first choice in mild-to-moderate hypertension (refer to page 422).
- **Congestive heart failure:** Diuretics reduce preload and are useful in symptomatic cases of CHF. Loop diuretics are more useful in this condition; however, thiazides may be combined, if needed.
- **Nephrolithiasis** due to idiopathic hypercalciuria, because thiazides increase calcium reabsorption in the DCT.
- **Nephrogenic diabetes insipidus** (DI). This is paradoxical as a large amount of dilute urine is passed out in DI; thiazides are useful as they cause a state of sustained electrolyte depletion → more complete iso-osmotic reabsorption of the GF in the PCT. So, reduced volume is presented to the diluting segment, resulting in reduced salt reabsorption. Hence, smaller volume of less dilute urine is presented to the CD and passed out. Dose of hydrochlorothiazide for this indication varies from 25–100 mg, given as a single dose.

ADRs

- Hypokalemic metabolic alkalosis
- **Hyponatremia:** hypovolemia leads to elevation of ADH, decreased diluting capacity of the kidney, and increased thirst. It is preventable by decreasing water intake.
- **Hyperlipidemia:** increase in serum cholesterol and LDL
- **Impaired carbohydrate tolerance** as they impair insulin release at high dose.
- **Allergic reactions** include generalised weakness, dermatitis, photosensitivity, fatigue, thrombocytopenia, paresthesia, hemolytic anemia and acute necrotising pancreatitis

Contraindications are same as for loop diuretics.

IV. COLLECTING TUBULE

In the collecting tubule, 2–5% of filtered NaCl is reabsorbed and K^+ secretion occurs under the influence of mineralocorticoids. The principal cells are the major site of $Na^+/K^+/H_2O$ transport. Aldosterone plays important role in sodium reabsorption and K^+, H^+ secretion in collecting tubule. The principal cells have separate channels for Na^+ and K^+ ions on luminal side (Fig. 29.4). The driving force for inflow of sodium is more than that for K^+ secretion, this creates a lumen negative potential that causes reabsorption of Cl^- through paracellular pathway. Water reabsorption occurs under the influence of ADH. The intercalated cells are the primary site of H⁺ secretion. Diuretics acting on collecting tubule include K⁺-sparing diuretics and ADH antagonists.

5. K⁺-sparing Diuretics

This category of diuretic drugs includes:

- Antagonists at aldosterone receptors (e.g., spironolactone and eplerenone).
- Inhibitors of Na⁺ flux through ion channels in the luminal membrane of collecting tubule principal cells (e.g., amiloride and triamterene).

Mechanism of action

Potassium-sparing diuretics decrease Na⁺ reabsorption and decrease K⁺ secretion in the collecting tubule (Fig. 29.4). Spironolactone and eplerenone bind to the cytoplasmic aldosterone receptor complex and prevents its translocation to the nucleus, resulting in reduced K⁺ and H⁺ secretion. Triamterene and amiloride inhibit sodium influx through ion channels in the collecting tubule.

Therapeutic uses

- K⁺-sparing diuretics are very useful in the management of mineralocorticoid excess as seen in primary

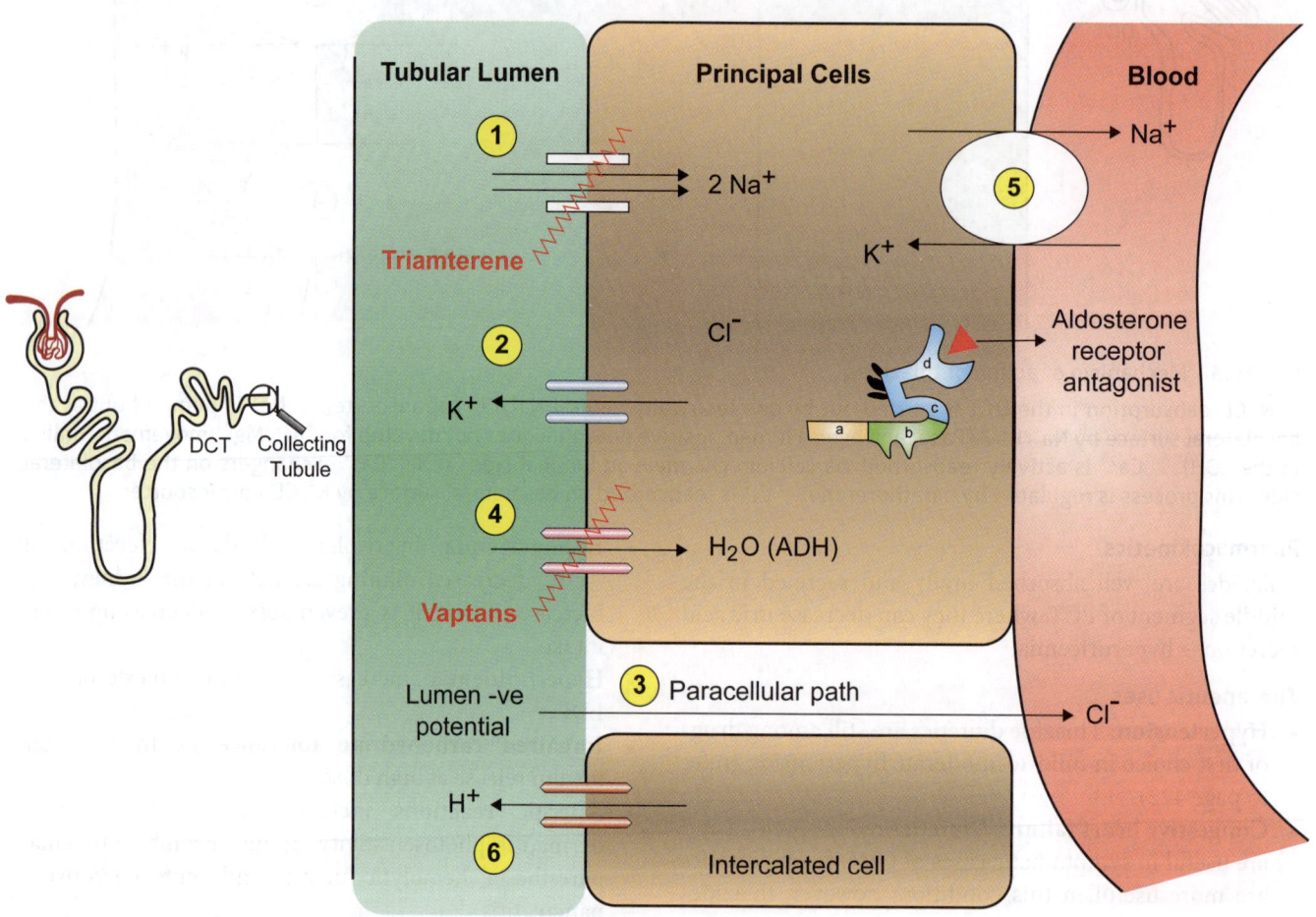

Fig. 29.4 Mechanism of action of potassium-sparing diuretics

① , ② The luminal side of principle cells have separate ion channels for Na⁺ and K⁺; these channels exclude anions.

③ The driving force for Na⁺ entry into the principal cells greatly exceeds that for K⁺ exit; so, Na⁺ reabsorption predominates, leading to the development of a lumen negative electrical potential that drives the transport of Cl⁻ from the lumen to the blood via the paracellular pathway. This also drives K⁺ out of the cell through apical K⁺ channels. Hence, there is an important relationship between Na⁺ delivery to the collecting tubule and the resulting K⁺ secretion.

CAIs, loop diuretics and thiazide diuretics increase Na⁺ delivery to collecting tubule and hence increase K⁺ secretion.

Moreover, diuretics cause volume depletion → increased aldosterone secretion. Aldosterone increases the activity of apical membrane Na⁺/K⁺ channels and basolateral Na⁺/K⁺-ATPase; hence, Na⁺ reabsorption and K⁺ secretion increase.

④ ADH is a key determinant of final urine concentration. While the collecting tubule is impermeable to water in the absence of ADH, its presence increases the membrane permeability to H₂O. Thus, the collecting tubule is the only site of the nephron where H₂O permeability can be regulated and ADH antagonists can be very useful to induce H₂O diuresis.

⑤ Na⁺ reabsorption occurs by Na⁺/K⁺ ATPase on the basolateral membrane.

⑥ Proton (H⁺) secretion occurs from the intercalated cells

hyperaldosteronism (Conn's disease) and ectopic ACTH secretion.
- Secondary hyperaldosteronism, can be caused by CHF, cirrhosis, nephrotic syndrome, and with use of other diuretics due to volume depletion which increases aldosterone secretion. K^+-sparing diuretics are useful in these conditions.
- Spironolactone is drug of choice in cirrhotic edema and resistant hypertension or edema, and for bringing down mortality in patients with a history of MI and chronic CHF.
- The anti-androgenic and anti-progesterone effects of these drugs are useful in PCOD, hirsutism and acne as well.

Amiloride is the drug of choice in Li-induced diabetes insipidus and Liddle syndrome—a condition caused by mutations in epithelial sodium channels that lead to excessive sodium reabsorption, resulting in hypertension and hypokalemia.

ADRs
- Most common adverse toxic effect of potassium sparing diuretics is hyperkalemia which can be mild, moderate, or severe and life-threatening.
- It is more marked in patients with renal disease and patients on drugs that reduce renin or angiotensin II activity, such as β blockers, NSAIDs ACE inhibitors and ARBs (angiotensin receptor blockers). ACE inhibitors and ARBs reduce the amount of aldosterone produced, while spironolactone blocks the action of aldosterone at its receptor. When used together, they have an additive effect.
- Hyperchloremic metabolic acidosis: As these drugs inhibit K^+ as well as H^+ secretion, acidosis occurs.
- The antiandrogenic action of spironolactone causes gynecomastia, impotence and benign prostatic hypertrophy (BPH).
- In women, its antiprogesterone effect may result in menstrual irregularities.
- The poor solubility of triamterene can result in its precipitation in urine, leading to renal stones.

Contraindications
- Oral K^+ supplementation should be discontinued.
- Patients with chronic renal insufficiency are more vulnerable to hyperkalemia.
- Concomitant use of β blockers, NSAIDS, ACE inhibitors and ARBs increases the likelihood of hyperkalemia.

Clinical problem-based questions and MCQs

6. A 60-year-old female patient, a known case of hypertension for the last 20 years, presented with exertional dyspnea and pedal edema. There is no history of fever, chills, cough, wheezing, sputum production, chest pain, etc. On examination HR=74 bpm, RR 24/min, BP = 104/54, and O_2 saturation = 90% on room air. Chest X-ray shows cardiomegaly, prominent interstitial markings suggestive of CHF and small bilateral pleural effusions. Tab furosemide 40 mg (twice daily) is prescribed.
   i. What is the role of furosemide in this patient?
   ii. Describe the mechanism of action of furosemide.
   iii. Enumerate other therapeutic indications and adverse effects of furosemide.

7. A 75-year-old female patient is a known case of CHF on diuretic therapy. Patient presents with history of anorexia, nausea, constipation, muscular weakness and cramping. There is a history of acute exacerbation of CHF (2 weeks earlier) for which the patient was admitted in hospital. At the time of discharge, dose of tab furosemide was doubled (from 40 mg BD to 80 mg BD). On examination, patient is alert and oriented to time, place and person. There is no focal neurologic deficit. HR = 104/min, RR = 24/min, BP = 100/74, audible S1 and S2 sounds. Abdomen is soft and non-distended. Only significant finding in investigations is Serum K^+ levels of 2.1 mEq/L (normal range = 3.5–5.5 mEq/L). Other investigations are within normal range.
   i. What is the possible explanation of the patient's symptoms?
   ii. How should this patient be managed?

8. Identify the condition in which loop diuretics are contraindicated and why.
   a. Acute pulmonary edema
   b. Hepatic cirrhosis
   c. Hypersensitivity to sulphonamide
   d. Acute renal failure

9. i. Which of the following diuretics can precipitate gout?
      a. Mannitol
      b. Loop diuretics
      c. CA inhibitors
      d. Aldosterone antagonists
   ii. Explain why the chosen drug causes hyperuricemia.

10. Identify group of diuretics that may be useful in nephrolithiasis
    a. Loop diuretics   b. Thiazides
    c. CA inhibitors   d. K^+-sparing diuretics
    Justify your choice.

11. Furosemide and hydrochlorothiazide have opposite effects on the excretion of calcium in urine.
    i. Explain the mechanisms of both effects on calcium excretion.
    ii. Mention the clinical implications of these effects.

12. Nephrogenic diabetes insipidus is characterised by the passage of large amounts of dilute urine. Thiazide diuretics are prescribed to reduce urine output; explain the mechanism of this seemingly paradoxical effect.

ADH ANTAGONISTS

These include lithium, demeclocycline and the vaptans such as tolvaptan, conivaptan, lixivaptan and satavaptan.

Mechanism of action

ADH is responsible for water reabsorption in the collecting tubule. **Lithium and demeclocycline** are non-selective drugs that inhibit ADH-mediated cAMP production in the collecting tubule, leading to H_2O diuresis.

Conivaptan, tolvaptan, lixivaptan and satavaptan are ADH receptor antagonists. Vasopressin or ADH exerts its effects through V_1 (V_{1a}, V_{1b}) and V_2 receptors. V_1 receptors are present in CNS and blood vessels, while V_2 receptors are present in the kidney. Drugs like tolvaptan, lixivaptan and satavaptan are selective V_2 antagonists, which inhibit the actions of ADH in the collecting tubule resulting in aquauresis. These drugs are effective orally. Conivaptan can block both V_{1a} and V_2 receptors and is given only intravenously.

Therapeutic uses

- ADH antagonists are tried if H_2O restriction fails to control syndrome of inappropriate ADH secretion (SIADH).
- When ADH is elevated in response to decreased blood volume and volume replacement is not possible (as in CHF or liver disease), H_2O restriction is recommended. If it fails, demeclocycline is given.
- Tolvaptan is approved by FDA for hyponatremia and as adjuvant to standard diuretic treatment in CHF.

Toxicity

- Nephrogenic diabetes insipidus (DI) by Li.
- Renal failure: Both lithium and demeclocycline can cause renal failure.
- Li can cause tremulousness, mental obtundation, cardio-toxicity, thyroid dysfunction and leukocytosis
- Tolvaptan can cause hypotension, abnormal LFT, dry mouth and thirst.
- Demeclocycline should be avoided in liver disease.

Drug–drug interactions of diuretics

- Loop and thiazide diuretics potentiate the effects of all other antihypertensives.
- Hypokalemia caused by diuretics enhances digitalis toxicity.
- Loop diuretics and aminoglycosides are ototoxic.
- Indomethacin and probenecid decrease secretion of diuretics at organic acid secretory sites and decrease their efficacy.
- Potassium-sparing diuretics are useful as adjuvants to loop/thiazide diuretics

RENAL AUTACOIDS

Adenosine, prostaglandin and natriuretic peptides are locally produced in the kidney and have important physiological effects.

a. Adenosine

Adenosine is an unphosphorylated ribonucleoside that acts on A_1, A_{2A}, A_{2B} and A_3 receptors. All 4 receptor types are present in the kidney, but the actions of A_1 receptors are important to understand the diuretic effect of its antagonists.

Receptor	Location	Effect of adenosine
A_1	Preglomerular afferent arteriole	Decrease blood flow to glomerulus and GFR
	PCT, thick ascending limb of LOH, collecting tubules	Increases activity of Na^+/H^+ exchanger in PCT at low concentration but inhibits it at high concentration
		Enhances K^+ secretion in collecting tubule

The diuretic effect of A_1 antagonists such as **rolofylline** is achieved by blocking the stimulant effect of adenosine on the Na^+/H^+ exchanger in the PCT. It also blunts adenosine-mediated K^+ secretion in the collecting tubule. Thus, unlike thiazides and loop diuretics, A_1 antagonists do not cause K^+ wasting and hypokalemia. **Caffeine** and **theophylline** also have nonspecific adenosine receptor blocking effects. However, rolofylline has central toxic effects and newer A_1 blockers are under trial.

b. Prostaglandins

Prostaglandins (PGE_2, PGI_2, PGD_2, $PGF_{2\alpha}$ and TXA_2) are produced by kidney and act on it. Specifically, PGE_2:

- Inhibits the reabsorption of Na^+ in the thick ascending limb of the loop of Henle.
- Blunts ADH-mediated water absorption in the collecting tubule.

These actions contribute to the diuretic action of loop diuretics. NSAIDs blunt loop diuretic response by inhibiting prostaglandin synthesis.

c. Natriuretic Peptides

Natriuretic peptides include atrial natriuretic peptide (ANP), brain natriuretic peptide (BNP), C-type natriuretic peptide (CNP), and urodilatin (which is synthesised in the kidney). All these exert natriuretic effects by different mechanisms.

ANP, BNP and urodilatin have similar actions in the kidney. They:

- Decrease vasomotor tone of glomerular afferent arterioles and increase that of glomerular efferent arterioles, resulting in increased GFR.
- Inhibit Na^+ reabsorption in the PCT.

Both these actions result in natriuretic response. In addition, ANP decreases the release of renin and aldosterone.

- Nesiritide (BNP) and carperitide (ANP) are used clinically in CHF, for their diuretic effect.
- Ularitide is a peptide with the same actions as urodilatin and is under trials for potential clinical use.

CNP has a weaker natriuretic effect, but is a potent vasodilator that has a role in regulating PVR.

Therapeutic uses

The 3 major actions of natriuretic peptides, namely, vasodilation, natriuresis and diuresis, and inhibition of the renin–angiotensin system, appear to be very useful for CHF.

Vasopeptidase inhibitors such as omapatrilat, sampatrilat and fasidotrilat have the dual benefit of increasing natriuretic peptide and decreasing angiotensin II; thus, these drugs show promise for cardiac patients. However, omapatrilat has caused cough, dizziness and angio-edema as side effects, and is not yet approved for clinical use.

Clinical problem-based questions and MCQs

13. Which of the following drugs has the potential to cause renal stones?
    a. Spironolactone   b. Triamterene
    c. Eplerenone   d. Thiazides

14. A 48-year-old male patient, a known case of hypertension, was on hydrochlorothiazide therapy for the last 2 years. After an episode of viral gastroenteritis, the patient presents with anorexia, nausea, extreme weakness, inability to get up from bed and muscular cramps. Investigations revealed that serum potassium was below normal range. Tablet triamterene along with hydrochlorothiazide was prescribed and patient improved satisfactorily at the follow-up examination.
    i. Explain the cause of patient's symptoms.
    ii. Describe the mechanism of action of triamterene.
    iii. Explain the advantage of adding triamterene in this case.

15. Identify the diuretic that is useful in secondary hyperaldosteronism.
    a. Triamterene   b. Spironolactone
    c. Amiloride   d. All of the above

16. Some drugs increase the risk of hyperkalemia when combined with spironolactone and should be used cautiously.
    i. Identify one such drug from the following.
        a. Propranolol   b. Hydrochlorothiazide
        c. Furosemide   d. Acetazolamide
    ii. Explain the pharmacological basis of this drug–drug interaction.

17. i. Identify the vaptan drug which can be given only intravenously.
        a. Lixivaptan   b. Tolvaptan
        c. Conivaptan   d. Satavaptan
    ii. Describe the mechanism of action, uses and adverse effects of vaptans.

ANTIDIURETICS

These drugs inhibit the excretion of water alone, so a better term for them is 'anti-aquaretics'. The chief indication for the use of antidiuretics is **diabetes insipidus**. They can be classified as:

1. **ADH and analogues**: Vasopressin, desmopressin, terlipressin, lypressin
2. **Natriuretics that exert antidiuretic effects**: Thiazides, amiloride
3. **Miscellaneous**: Indomethacin, carbamazepine, chlorpropamide

1. ADH/Vasopressin and Analogues

Antidiuretic hormone (ADH), also known as vasopressin, is a peptide hormone secreted by the posterior lobe of the pituitary gland. Its release is regulated by osmoreceptors and depends on both the extracellular fluid (ECF) volume and the plasma osmolarity. The release of vasopressin is enhanced by prostaglandins, histamine, acetylcholine, neuropeptide Y and angiotensin II.

In contrast, vasopressin secretion is inhibited by GABA, ANP, alcohol, glucocorticoids, phenytoin, etc.

Actions

Vasopressin acts through V_1 (two subtypes: V_{1a} and V_{1b}) and V_2 receptors.

- V_{1a} receptors mediate vasoconstriction and smooth muscle contraction, especially in the uterine muscles. They also increase gluconeogenesis, platelet aggregation and prostaglandin synthesis. Increased PG levels oppose its antidiuretic effect.
- V_{1b} receptors are involved in regulation of body temperature, ACTH release, etc.
- V_2 receptors are responsible for its antidiuretic effect. V_2 activation stimulates adenylyl cyclase → increased cAMP production → insertion of more aqueous channels into the apical membrane of principal cells → increases the water permeability of principal cells → decreased urine volume.

Endothelial V_2 receptors also mediate the vasodilator effect and increase the release of coagulation factor VIII and the von Willebrand factor.

Therapeutic uses

- The deficiency of ADH can result in the passing of a large amount of dilute urine; this condition is called **diabetes insipidus** (DI), which is of two types:
  - Neurogenic DI, arising from the reduced secretion of vasopressin from the pituitary.
  - Nephrogenic DI, which is a result of the reduced response of collecting tubule principal cells to vasopressin.
- Desmopressin, a selective agonist at V_2 receptors is effective in treating neurogenic DI. The dose is individualised and treatment is usually lifelong.

- Lypressin is used to differentiate between the two types of DI.
- In von Willebrand disease: Vasopressin can control bleeding by causing the release of coagulation factors from the vascular endothelium via V_2 receptor activation.
- Vasoconstrictor action through V_1 receptors is used to control bleeding from esophageal varices. Terlipressin is better tolerated than vasopressin for this indication.
- Vasopressin analogues are useful in nocturnal enuresis also.

Adverse drug reactions

Desmopressin has fewer ADRs because of its selectivity for V_2 receptors. The reported ADRs include:

- Headache and flushing, allergic reactions may occur
- Nasal congestion, rhinitis and epistaxis may occur after local application
- Backache in women due to uterine contractions
- Abdominal cramps, belching and nausea
- Fluid retention and hyponatremia

2. Thiazides and Amiloride

While both these drugs are diuretics, they exert an antidiuretic effect in nephrogenic DI. Thiazides can decrease urine volume in neurogenic as well as nephrogenic DI. This **paradoxical** effect is likely because:

- Thiazides reduce the GFR, so less glomerular filtrate is presented to the tubules.
- Thiazides induce sustained electrolyte depletion → more complete reabsorption of glomerular filtrate in the PCT → lower volume of urine presented to the segments of distal nephron → less reabsorption of salt in diluting segment → less dilution of urine

Amiloride is effective in lithium-induced DI. Lithium induces a nephrogenic DI-like state by inhibiting the action of ADH on the distal tubules of the kidney. Because the movement of Li^+ and Na^+ ions in the body is very similar, amiloride can block the entry of Li^+ in the principal cells of the collecting duct, and reverse lithium-induced DI.

3. Miscellaneous

Indomethacin, carbamazepine and chlorpropamide also have antidiuretic effects.

- **Indomethacin** is an NSAID that exerts an antidiuretic effect by inhibiting renal PG synthesis (the diuretic effect of PGs are described under renal autacoids). For this action, it may be used along with thiazides in nephrogenic DI.
- **Carbamazepine** is an antiepileptic drug, which exerts antidiuretic effects in neurogenic DI at high doses, by an unknown mechanism. However, this is of no clinical value as marked adverse effects occur at such high doses.
- **Chlorpropamide** is an antidiabetic drug that sensitises the principal cells of the collecting tubule to the effects of ADH and reduces urine volume in neurogenic DI.

Clinical problem-based questions and MCQs

18. Which of the following is V_2 receptor selective agonist?
    a. Vasopressin   b. Desmopressin
    c. Lypressin   d. None of the above

19. Which of the following is preferred drug in controlling bleeding from esophageal varices?
    a. Vasopressin   b. Desmopressin
    c. Terlipressin   d. Lypressin

20. A 69-year-old male patient, a known case of maniac depressive psychosis (MDP), is on treatment with lithium carbonate (600 mg per day) for the past 4 years. Though his psychiatric symptoms have improved, the patient complains of polyuria, polydipsia and constipation. On examination, the patient has dry skin, urine is colourless instead of pale yellow. The patient was found to have hypotonic polyuria with a 24-hour urine output of 7 L, urine osmolality = 316 mOsm/kg, serum sodium = 151 mmol/L (normal: 136–145 mmol/L), lithium = 0.9 (therapeutic range: 0.8–1.2), calcium= 9.4 mg/dL (normal: 9–10.5 mg/dL), blood urea nitrogen (BUN) = 26 mg/dL (normal: 8–20 mg/dL), and creatinine = 1.1 mg/dL (normal: 0.7–1.3 mg/dL). Upon conducting a desmopressin challenge test, the urine osmolality increased to 485 mOsm/kg (~35% increase from baseline, less than 50% increase indicating partial nephrogenic diabetes insipidus). Patient's symptoms improved with Tab amiloride 5 mg given twice daily.
    i. What is the cause of patient's symptoms?
    ii. Describe the mechanism of reduction of patient's symptoms with amiloride.
    iii. Enumerate the adverse effects of amiloride.

Summary

- **Diuretics** can be classified into low, medium and high efficacy categories.
- **CAIs** act by inhibiting $NaHCO_3$ reabsorption in the PCT, but are not used for diuretic action as diuretic effect decreases with time due to bicarbonate loss.
- Indications for the use of CAIs include open angle glaucoma, acute mountain sickness, metabolic alkalosis and the alkalinisation of urine.
- They cause renal potassium wasting, increased risk of renal stones and metabolic acidosis. These are contraindicated in hepatic cirrhosis.
- **Osmotic diuretics,** e.g., mannitol, act in the PCT and descending loop of Henle. The aquaretic effect > natriuretic effect, resulting in the risk of hypernatremia.
- Used to treat raised ICT or IOT or when renal hemodynamics is compromised
- Expansion of ECF caused by mannitol can be harmful in CHF and pulmonary edema.
- **Loop diuretics,** e.g., furosemide, inhibit NaCl reabsorption from the ascending limb of the loop of

Henle, resulting in brisk diuresis and the loss of K^+, Ca^{2+} and Mg^{2+} ions.
- They are indicated in acute CHF, edematous conditions, hypercalcemia, acute renal failure and hyperkalemia, but should be used judiciously.
- Many ADRs like hypokalemia, hypomagnesemia, hyponatremia, hyperuricemia, ototoxicity and allergic reactions may occur.
- **Thiazides and thiazide-like drugs**, such as hydrochlorothiazide and indapamide, act in the DCT to reduce NaCl reabsorption; however, they increase calcium reabsorption.
- Useful in hypertension, CHF, idiopathic hypercalciuria-induced nephrolithiasis and nephrogenic diabetes insipidus.
- ADRs include hypokalemia, hyponatremia, hyperlipidemia, impaired glucose tolerance and allergic reactions.
- **Potassium-sparing diuretics** antagonise the effect of aldosterone and are weak diuretics that are usually combined with loop or thiazide diuretics to prevent hypokalemia. They are also used in primary and secondary hyperaldosteronism.
- May cause hyperkalemia as an adverse effect, especially when combined with beta blockers, RAAS inhibitors, etc.
- **ADH antagonists** (conivaptan) and **renal autacoids** (adenosine antagonist, prostaglandins and natriuretic peptides) also have diuretic effects.
- ADH and its analogues (vasopressin, desmopressin, terlipressin and lypressin) and other drugs such as indomethacin, carbamazepine and chlorpropamide are used as antidiuretics. Some natriuretics also exert antidiuretic effects, e.g., thiazides and amiloride.
- **ADH analogues** are useful in the management of diabetes insipidus, nocturnal enuresis, von Willebrand disease, and to control bleeding from esophageal varices.

Questions for practice

1. Classify diuretics.
2. Enumerate therapeutic uses and adverse effects of diuretics.
3. Write short notes on:
   a. Osmotic diuretics
   b. Status of diuretics in CHF
   c. Status of diuretics in hypertension
   d. ADH antagonist
4. Explain why
   a. Hypokalemia is caused by furosemide.
   b. Acetazolamide is not used as a diuretic.
   c. Mannitol reduces ICT.
   d. Thiazides reduce urine output in diabetes insipidus.
   e. Spironolactone can cause hyperkalemia when combined with RAAS inhibitors.
5. Classify antidiuretic drugs. Enumerate their therapeutic uses.

Hints for problem-based questions and MCQs

1. i. a. Acetazolamide ii. Refer to page 387.
2. i. Refer to page 386. ii. Refer to page 387.
3. i. a. Proximal convoluted tubule ii. Refer to page 386.
   iii. Carbonic anhydrase inhibitors, mannitol and rolofylline
4. i. Refer to page 388. ii. Refer to page 388.
   iii. Refer to page 388.
5. d. Mannitol
6. i. Reduces preload, improves cardiac output and relieves symptoms. Refer to page 390.
   ii. Refer to page 389. iii. Refer to page 390.
7. i. Hypokalemia induced by high dose furosemide therapy
   ii. Potassium supplementation or addition of K^+-sparing diuretics
8. c. Hypersensitivity to sulphonamides because of cross sensitivity.
9. i. b. Loop diuretics
   ii. Replaces → inhibit. Voltage-driven drug efflux transporter (NPT4) in PCT → uric acid excretion is reduced, leading to hyperuricemia and precipitation of gout.
10. b. Thiazides increase calcium reabsorption. So, in patients having nephrolithiasis associated with idiopathic hypercalciuria, these drugs are useful.
11. i. Furosemide acts in the thick ascending limb of the loop of Henle → reduces NaCl reabsorption, lumen positive electrical potential fails to develop → reduced reabsorption of divalent cations (Ca^{2+} and Mg^{2+}) → increased excretion of these cations.
    In contrast, thiazide diuretics act in the DCT to reduce NaCl reabsorption → reduced cell sodium → increased Na^+/Ca^{2+} exchange on basolateral membrane → increased Ca^{2+} reabsorption from lumen → reduced excretion of calcium.
    ii. Increased calcium excretion by furosemide does not cause hypocalcemia owing to active reabsorption of cations from the DCT. However, loop diuretics can be used along with saline infusion in acute hypercalcemia. Thiazides reduce calcium excretion and are useful in nephrolithiasis associated with idiopathic hypercalciuria. They do not cause hypercalcemia, but may unmask the same due to other causes such as carcinomas, hyperparathyroidism, and sarcoidosis.
12. Refer to page 391. Chronic use of thiazides → sustained electrolyte depletion → more complete iso-osmotic reabsoption of GF in PCT → less volume of tubular fluid is presented to the diluting segment → lesser salt reabsorption in diluting segment. → smaller volume of less dilute urine is passed out.
13. b. Triamterene
14. i. Symptoms due to thiazide induced hypokalemia
    ii. Refer to page 392. Inhibits sodium flux in collecting tubule
    iii. It decreases potassium secretion and thus checks hypokalemia
15. d. All of the above
16. i. a. Propranolol
    ii. Being a β blocker, propranolol reduces renin release → suppresses activity of RAAS → reduced aldosterone secretion → it adds up with aldosterone antagonistic effect of spironolactone
17. i. c. Conivaptan ii. Refer to page 394.
18. b. Desmopressin
19. c. Terlipressin
20. i. Lithium-induced nephrogenic diabetes insipidus
    ii. Amiloride can block the entry of Li^+ in principal cells of collecting tubule and reverse lithium induced DI. Refer to page 396.
    iii. Refer to page 393.

CONCEPT MAP - DIURETICS

DIURETICS

K⁺-Sparing Diuretics
Spironolactone
Triamterene
Amiloride

Mechanism of Action
Aldosterone antagonist or inhibit renal epithelial Na⁺ channel → decrease in NaCl reabsorption and K⁺ secretion.

Uses
In primary hyper-aldosteronism Conn's disease, ectopic ACTH secretion.
Secondary Hyper-aldosteronism in CHF, Cirrhosis, Nephrotic syndrome, Use of other groups of diuretics
Amiloride used in Li-induced DI, Liddle syndrome.
Decrease androgenic activity, so useful in PCOD, Hirsutism and Acne.

ADRs
Hyperkalemia: risk more in patients with renal disease.
Patients taking - β blocker - NSAIDs, ACE inhibitors, ARBs
Hyperchloremic metabolic acidosis
Spironolactone can cause gynecomastia, impotence, benign prostatic hypertrophy (BPH).
Triamterene precipitates in urine → renal stones

Carbonic Anhydrase Inhibitor
Acetazolamide
Brinzolamide
Dorzolamide

Mechanism of Action
Inhibit NaHCO₃ reabsorption in PCT

Uses
Not used as diuretic as HCO₃⁻ loss → enhances NaCl reabsorption in other segments of nephron → limits diuretic effect over few days
Other Uses: Glaucoma
For alkalinisation of urine
Metabolic / respiratory alkalosis
Obstructive sleep apnea
Acute mountain sickness
For catamenial epilepsy.
Severe hyperphosphatemia.
Prevention of cystinuria.

ADRs
Hyperchloremic metabolic acidosis
Renal stones because of phosphaturia, hypercalciuria
Renal K⁺ wasting.
Drowsiness, somnolence, paresthesia, Hypersensitivity reactions
Hyperammonemia → Contraindicated in hepatic cirrhosis.

Thiazides
Hydrochlorothiazide
Benzthiazide
Chlorthalidone
Indapamide
Xipamide
Clopamide

Mechanism of Action
Inhibit Na⁺/Cl⁻ cotransporter → decrease cell Na⁺ → enhance Na⁺/Ca²⁺ exchange on basolateral side → increase Ca²⁺ reabsorption

Uses
Hypertension
Congestive heart failure
Nephrolithiasis due to idiopathic hypercalciuria.
Nephrogenic diabetes insipidus (DI) (paradoxical: chronic use of thiazide → state of electrolyte depletion → more complete, isoosmotic reabsorption of glomerular filtrate in PCT → decreased reabsorption in diluting segment → small volume of less dilute urine passed out.

ADRs
Hypokalemic metabolic alkalosis
Hyponatremia
Hyperlipidemia
Impaired carbohydrate tolerance
Allergic reactions: General dermatitis, Photosensitivity, TCP, Hemolytic anemia, Necrotising pancreatitis
Weakness, Fatigue, Paresthesia

Osmotic Diuretics
Mannitol, Glycerol

Mechanism of Action
Mannitol stays in lumen after glomerular filtration → interposes a countervailing osmotic force → decreases reabsorption of H₂O → aquaresis → increased flow rate → some natriuresis

Uses
When renal hemodynamics are compromised.
When large pigment load is to be excreted.
Raised IOT, ICT

ADRs
Expansion of ECF Volume, Worsening of CHF, pulmonary edema, Headache, Nausea, Vomiting.
Excessive use without fluid replacement causes dehydration, hypernatremia.

Loop Diuretics
Furosemide
Torasemide
Bumetanide

Mechanism of Action
Selectively block Na⁺/K⁺/2Cl cotransporter,
Reduce NaCl reabsorption → more solute delivered to remaining segments → reduce H₂O reabsorption → brisk diuresis

Uses
Acute pulmonary edema (CHF)
Other edematous conditions.
Acute renal failure.
Acute hypercalcemia.
Hyper kalemia
Anion overdose

ADRs
Hypokalemic metabolic alkalosis
Hypomagnesemia.
Severe dehydration → thirst → increased water intake → Hyponatremia.
Hyperuricemia → precipitation of gout.
Ototoxicity → reversible hearing loss
Allergic reactions: skin rash, eosinophilia, interstitial nephritis

SECTION 7 Drugs Acting on CVS

30 Drugs Modulating the Renin–Angiotensin–Aldosterone System (RAAS)

PH 4.6 Explain salient pharmacokinetics, pharmacodynamics, therapeutic uses, and adverse drug reactions of drugs modulating the renin–angiotensin–aldosterone system.

Learning objectives

A student of MBBS phase II should be able to:
- Explain physiology of the renin–angiotensin–aldosterone system.
- Describe regulation of RAAS and pathophysiological role of angiotensin II.
- Enumerate drug classes acting on RAAS.
- Classify ACE inhibitors (ACEIs), angiotensin receptor blockers (ARBs) and direct renin inhibitors.
- Describe the mechanism of action of ACEIs and ARBs.
- Enumerate therapeutic indications of drugs modulating RAAS.
- Describe therapeutic status of drugs modulating RAAS in various clinical conditions.
- Enumerate the adverse effects and contraindications of ACEIs and ARBs.

PHYSIOLOGY OF THE RENIN–ANGIOTENSIN–ALDOSTERONE SYSTEM (RAAS)

Renin is released from the **juxtaglomerular apparatus**, which has three main components:

- **Juxtaglomerular (JG) cells** are epithelial cells located in tunica media of the afferent arteriole as it enters the glomerulus. These cells have secretory granules containing renin.
- **Lacis cells** are present at the junction between the afferent and efferent arterioles. These are agranular cells that contain renin.
- The **macula densa** is a collection of modified tubular epithelial cells, at the origin of the DCT. In this region, the tubule touches the afferent and efferent arterioles of the glomerulus from which it arises. These cells also secrete renin.

TYPES OF RAAS

RAAS exists as tissue/local RAAS and circulating RAAS.

Tissue/Local RAAS

Extrinsic local RAAS: Blood vessels capture angiotensinogen and renin to produce angiotensin II (A-II) at the surface of their walls. A-II then diffuses and acts locally.

Intrinsic local RAAS: Many tissues, especially the heart, brain, kidneys, adrenals and blood vessels, can synthesise all the components of RAAS within their cells as per physiological needs and pathological status.

Prorenin and prorenin receptors (PRR): Prorenin is precursor of renin that can be activated:

- **Enzymatically** by proteases to form renin through an irreversible process.
- **Nonenzymatically** by binding to prorenin receptors (renin also binds to the same receptors). PRRs are abundant in the heart, blood vessels, kidney, brain, eye and liver. Their activation is reversible and leads to active role of prorenin in the local RAAS.

The actions of prorenin in local RAAS are either mediated through angiotensin II or occur directly by the activation of intracellular signalling through mitogen-activated kinase (MAP kinase), plasminogen activator inhibitor-1 (PAI-1), JAK/STAT transcription factor, proto-oncogenes, etc.

Local RAAS plays an important role in cell growth regulation, collagen deposits, inflammation, fibrosis, apoptosis, etc. This can result in **pathological changes** that can cause **end organ damage**, such as hypertensive vascular/ventricular hypertrophy, post-infarction myocardial fibrosis and remodelling in CHF, retinopathy and nephropathy.

Circulating RAAS

It consists of the release of angiotensinogen and its conversion into angiotensin I, II, III and IV (Fig. 30.1).

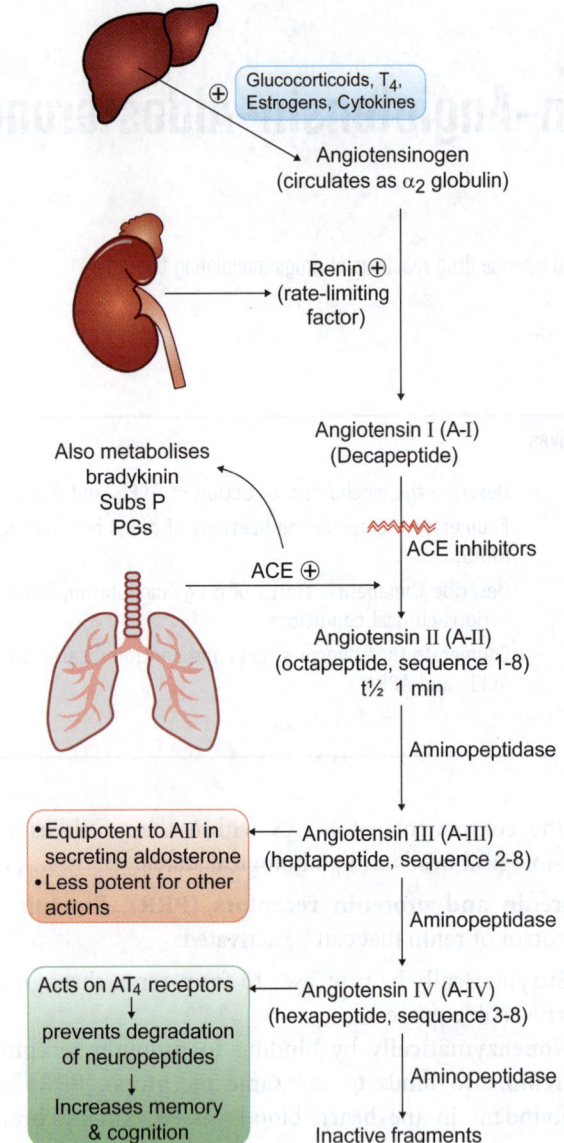

Fig. 30.1 The renin–angiotensin–aldosterone system

Cytokines and some hormones such as thyroxine, corticosteroids, and estrogen favour the release of angiotensinogen from liver. It circulates as α_2 globulin. Renin released from JG cells in the kidneys converts angiotensinogen into angiotensin I (A-I), a decapeptide. A-I is then converted to an octapeptide, angiotensin II (A-II) by the enzyme 'angiotensin converting enzyme' (ACE). This octapeptide A-II causes vasoconstriction, increased aldosterone secretion and cardiac remodelling. ACE has a role in metabolism of bradykinin, prostaglandins and substance P as well. After exerting its action, A-II is metabolised by aminopeptidase to form A-III, A-IV and inactive fragments. A-III is a heptapeptide that has role in aldosterone secretion. A-IV is hexapeptide which may interfere with the degradation of neuropeptides and is known to enhance cognition and memory.

Another carboxypeptidase, angiotensin-converting enzyme 2 (ACE 2), can form a heptapeptide angiotensin (amino acid sequence 1–7) from angiotensin I or angiotensin II. The effects of this heptapeptide are opposite to those of angiotensin II. Thus, it has vasodilator, anti-ischemic, antithrombotic and anti-proliferative actions. ACE 2 is not inhibited by clinically used ACE inhibitors.

Actions of Angiotensin II

There are 2 subtypes of angiotensin II receptors on the surface of target cells, AT_1 and AT_2. Both are G protein-coupled. All the major effects of angiotensin II are mediated through AT_1 receptors, which use different transduction mechanisms in different tissues.

AT_2 receptors are abundant in fetal tissues, than in adults. They are distributed in the adrenal medulla, brain, vascular endothelium and reproductive tissues. The actions mediated through AT_2 receptors are not well delineated. In CHF and myocardial infarction, AT_2 receptors are up-regulated.

Angiotensin III is a weak agonist at AT_1 and AT_2 receptors. Actions of A-II mediated through AT_1 receptors (Fig. 30.2) include:

1. Blood vessels

Angiotensin II causes **vasoconstriction** by the following mechanisms:

- Angiotensin II binds to Gq protein-coupled AT_1 receptors → IP_3–DAG → raised intracellular Ca^{2+} → vascular smooth muscle contraction.
- By increasing adrenaline/noradrenaline release from the adrenal medulla, adrenergic nerve endings and increased central sympathetic outflow.
- By inhibiting the reuptake of noradrenaline.
- By augmenting the responsiveness of vascular smooth muscles to noradrenaline.

Vasoconstriction induced by angiotensin II occurs both in arterioles and venules. Vasoconstriction occurs in all vascular beds, but is less marked in the cerebral, coronary, skeletal and pulmonary vessels. It favours the movement of fluid from vascular to extravascular compartments. However, angiotensin II causes nitric oxide-dependent vasodilatation through AT_2 receptors, which counteracts AT_1-mediated vasoconstriction.

2. Heart

Angiotensin II increases the force of myocardial contractions. The heart rate decreases because of reflex bradycardia (vasoconstriction causes a rise in BP, which decreases heart rate through the baroreceptor reflex). The increased total peripheral resistance due to vasoconstriction causes a fall in cardiac output and increased cardiac workload, although it has little arrhythmogenic activity.

Chronic action of angiotensin II on vascular smooth muscles and myocardium causes:
- Hypertrophy
- Hyperplasia
- Increased intercellular matrix production.

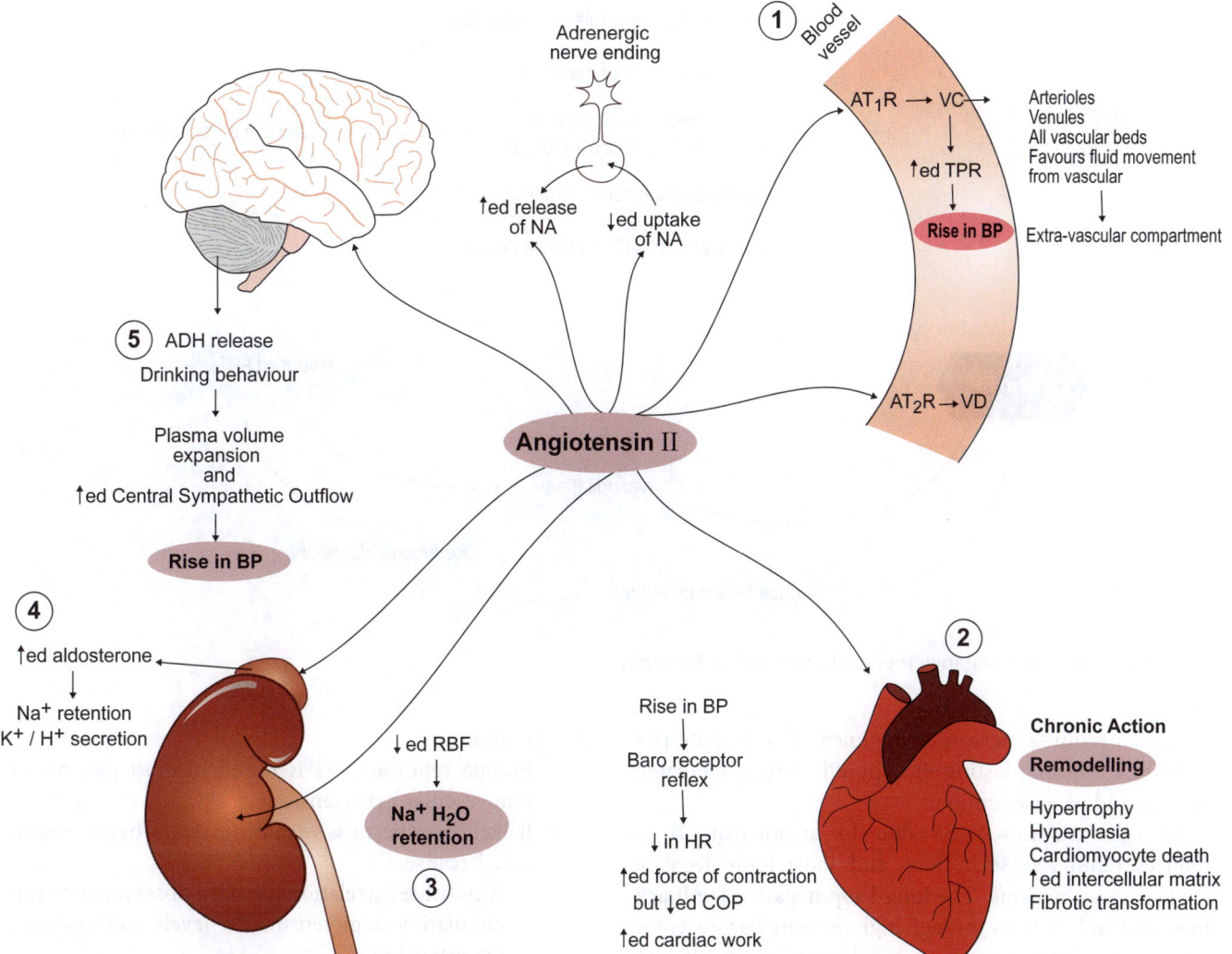

Fig. 30.2 AT$_1$-mediated Actions of angiotensin II

- Remodelling involving abnormal redistribution of muscle mass in heart and blood vessels.
- Increase in vessel wall intimal thickness and ventricular hypertrophy in long-standing hypertension.
- Fibrosis and dilatation of infarcted area and hypertrophy of non-infarcted area in ventricular wall after myocardial infarction (MI).
- Progressive cardiomyocyte death and fibrotic transformation in CHF.

3. Kidney
Angiotensin II increases Na$^+$/H$^+$ exchange in PCT → increased reabsorption of Na$^+$, Cl$^-$ and HCO$_3^-$. Due to vasoconstriction, it decreases RBF → decrease in GFR → intrarenal hemodynamic effects causing Na$^+$/H$_2$O retention.

4. Adrenal cortex
Angiotensin II (along with angiotensin III) increases the synthesis and release of aldosterone from the zona glomerulosa of the adrenal cortex. Aldosterone acts on the kidneys to increase Na$^+$ reabsorption and K$^+$/H$^+$ secretion.

5. CNS
Systemically given angiotensin II gains access to the periventricular areas of the brain

- ADH release induces drinking behaviour and causes plasma volume expansion.
- Increases central sympathetic outflow

Both these actions contribute to rise in BP.

REGULATION OF RAAS ACTIVITY

Decrease in blood volume, BP and Na$^+$ content (due to any reason) leads to renin release by 3 mechanisms:

- **Intrarenal baroreceptor pathway**: Decreased tension in afferent arterioles. → renin release
- **Increased sympathetic outflow**: β$_1$-receptor activation → renin release.
- **Macula densa pathway**: Na$^+$ and Cl$^-$ depletion in tubular fluid → induces COX-2 and nNOS → PGE$_2$ and PGI$_2$ release → renin release.

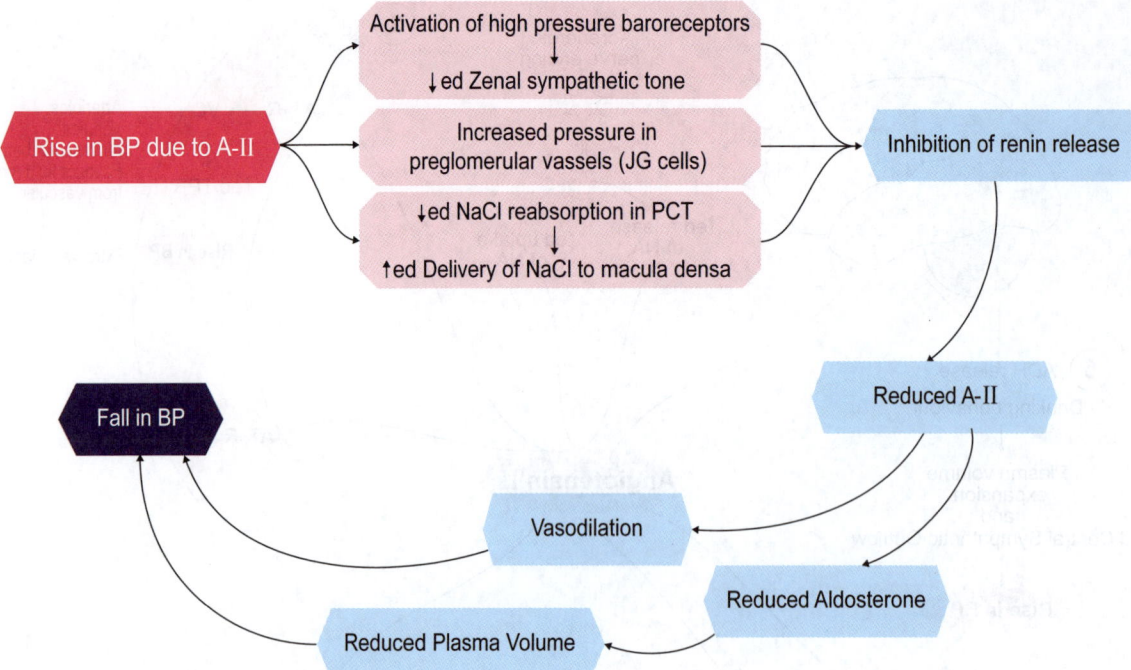

Fig. 30.3 Long-loop negative feedback mechanism for renin

Increased renin → increase in angiotensin II → acute rise in BP by VC → long-lasting effect by aldosterone-mediated sodium and water retention.

In contrast, raised BP due to angiotensin II → reduces renin release by long and short loop negative feedback mechanisms. The **long-loop negative feedback mechanism** functions through high pressure baroreceptor activation, raised pressure in preglomerular vessels and the macula densa pathway. (Fig. 30.3).

The **short-loop negative feedback** mechanism operates within the kidney, where angiotensin II activates AT_1 receptors present on the JG cells and directly inhibits renin release.

Many groups of **drugs** interfere with these regulatory mechanisms:

- ACE inhibitors and ARBs interfere with both short- and long-loop mechanisms → increased renin release.
- Loop diuretics decrease the entry of Na^+ and Cl^- into macula densa cells → increase renin production.
- VDs and diuretics → decrease BP → increased renin release.
- β-blockers and central sympatholytics → decrease renin release.
- NSAIDs, COX-2 inhibitors and nNOS inhibitors → decrease PG production → decrease renin levels.

PATHOPHYSIOLOGICAL ROLE

RAAS plays an important role in:

1. Mineralocorticoid secretion and the homeostasis of electrolyte, blood volume and BP.
2. Hypertension:
   - Plasma renin activity is raised in most patients of renovascular hypertension.
   - It likely has a permissive role in essential hypertension also, because:
     - A positive correlation has been observed between circulating angiotensinogen levels and essential hypertension.
     - ACE inhibitors consistently lower BP in hypertensives, indicating the involvement of RAAS in the pathophysiology of hypertension.
3. Pregnancy-induced hypertension (PIH/pre-eclampsia) probably involves the production of auto-antibodies that activate AT_1 receptors.
4. Angiotensin II is involved in the hypertrophy and remodelling of heart and vascular smooth muscles.
5. RAAS is involved in the development of secondary hyperaldosteronism.

Clinical problem-based questions and MCQs

1. **Identify the RAAS component that possesses vasodilator effect.**
   a. Angiotensin (1–7) b. Aldosterone
   c. Angiotensin II d. Renin

2. **Identify the correct mechanism of angiotensin II-mediated vascular action.**
   a. AT_1 receptor mediated NO release from endothelium
   b. Reduced noradrenaline release from nerve endings

c. Increased noradrenaline uptake
  d. AT_1 receptor-mediated IP_3–DAG pathway
3. **Chronic exposure of tissues to angiotensin II causes:**
   a. Abnormal redistribution of muscle mass
   b. Prevention of apoptosis
   c. Tissue hypoplasia
   d. Decreased intimal thickness in vessel wall
4. **A 60-year-old patient, a known case of hypertension for the last 20 years, shows pathological remodelling. Comment on the changes that occur in heart cells and blood vessels and the role of RAAS in this process.**

DRUGS THAT INHIBIT RAAS

RAAS inhibitors include direct renin inhibitor, angiotensin-converting enzyme inhibitors and angiotensin receptor blockers (Flowchart 30.1). In addition, sympathetic blockers (β blockers and central sympatholytics which decrease renin) and aldosterone antagonists also inhibit RAAS activity. (See Chapters 11 and 29, respectively.)

Angiotensin-Converting Enzyme Inhibitors (ACEIs)

ACE is a dipeptidyl carboxypeptidase, present on the luminal side of vascular endothelium (especially in the lungs).

Actions of angiotensin-converting enzyme

- Its major function is to convert angiotensin I to angiotensin II as blood circulates through the lungs.
- It also functions as kininase II and degrades bradykinin.
- It can split the dipeptidyl segment from substance P and natural stem cell-regulating peptides.

ACE inhibiting drugs include captopril, enalapril, ramipril, lisinopril, fosinopril, and benazepril.

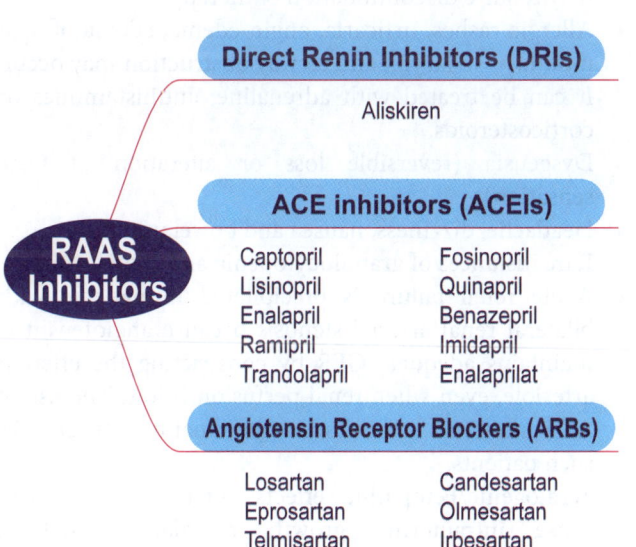

Flowchart 30.1 Classification of RAAS inhibitors

Pharmacodynamics

Mechanism of action

ACE inhibitors act by inhibiting the activity of angiotensin converting enzyme (ACE) leading to:

- Decreased conversion of angiotensin I to angiotensin II. This abolishes the pressor action of angiotensin I, but not that of angiotensin II, because AT receptors are not blocked by these drugs.
- ACE inhibitors reduce angiotensin II levels → feedback increase in renin levels → feedback increase in angiotensin I production. However, because ACE2 is not inhibited by these drugs, angiotensin I is diverted to the ACE2 pathway, forming angiotensin (1–7), a heptapeptide that possesses vasodilator action and possibly contributes to the BP-lowering effect.
- Decrease in degradation of plasma kinins resulting in raised kinin levels. This may contribute to acute vasodepressor action but is not important for long-term hypotensive action.
- Kinins and PGs induced by them lead to cough and angio-edema in susceptible persons.
- Interference in the degradation of substance P.
- Increase in levels of stem cell regulator peptides. This may be partly responsible for their cardio-protective action in CHF.

Effect on BP

ACE inhibitors decrease BP. In the short term, the magnitude of **BP-lowering response** depends upon the **sodium status** and **level of RAAS activity.**

- In normotensive Na^+-replete patients, a modest fall in BP is observed with few initial doses of ACE inhibitors, whereas in Na^+-depleted patients (because of dietary restriction of salt or diuretic use), renin levels are high → more marked fall in BP is observed with ACEIs.
- In CHF also, renin levels are high, leading to a marked fall in BP. In such situations, ACE inhibitors should be started at a much lower dose.
- The fall in BP is more in renovascular, malignant and accelerated hypertension.
- In essential hypertension, RAAS is overactive in 20% of patients, normal in 60% and hypoactive in the remaining 20%. So, RAAS contributes to the maintenance of vascular tone in at least 80% of patients and ACE inhibitors lower the BP.

With long term use of ACE inhibitors, no correlation is seen between plasma renin activity and magnitude of BP lowering effect of ACE inhibitors.

Cardio-renal effects of ACE inhibitors

- ACEIs cause vasodilatation of both arterial and venous vessels, resulting in:
  - Reduced arterial and venous pressure
  - Reduced ventricular preload and afterload

Ventricular preload is determined by the blood volume and venous return, both of which are lowered by ACEIs:

- Less aldosterone activity → less reabsorption of Na^+ and H_2O in principal cells of collecting tubule in kidney → reduction in blood volume.
- Vasodilatation of venous system → reduced venous return.

Ventricular afterload is determined by the total peripheral resistance (TPR).

Vasodilatation of arterial system by ACE inhibitors decreases TPR, and hence the afterload.

- Decrease in blood volume by decreasing aldosterone secretion → reduction of sodium reabsorption and K^+ secretion in the collecting tubule, resulting in natriuresis and diuresis.
- Depress sympathetic activity.
- Inhibit cardiac and vascular hypertrophy and remodelling associated with hypertension, CHF and MI.
- Decrease proteinuria and stabilise renal function by improving intra-renal hemodynamics. This effect is especially useful in diabetic nephropathy.
- ACE inhibitors cause vasodilatation of glomerular efferent arteriole resulting in reduced GFR.; so, they are contraindicated in patients with bilateral renal artery stenosis and renal failure.

Therapeutic uses

1. Hypertension

ACEIs are among the first-line drugs in the treatment of hypertension and are effective in essential, renovascular and malignant hypertension. The **advantages** of ACE inhibitors are as follows:

- ACE inhibitors prevent apoptosis and remodelling in vascular and myocardial tissues. Hence they offer good protective properties against long-term changes and end organ damage.
- Fall in BP caused by ACE inhibitors is not associated with sympathetic stimulation; thus, reflex tachycardia is not a problem, and ACE Inhibitors can be used safely in patients of ischemic heart disease (IHD).
- Even when BP falls substantially, renal blood flow (RBF) is not compromised because of greater dilatation of renal vessels; cerebral and coronary blood flow is also not compromised.
- The basal levels of aldosterone decrease slightly; however, physiologically sufficient secretion occurs under the effect of ACTH and K^+.
- Quality of life (QOL) parameters (e.g., general wellbeing, work, sleep, sex) are minimally affected (unlike beta blockers). There is no risk of hypertensive crisis on withdrawal (unlike clonidine).
- They can be used safely in asthmatics, diabetics, etc. (unlike beta blockers).

2. Congestive heart failure (CHF)

ACE inhibitors assist the failing heart by reducing both the preload and afterload. Long-term use reduces disease progression, morbidity and mortality. In CHF, ACE inhibitors increase stroke volume and cardiac output. They reverse aldosterone-induced sodium retention, edema and reduce remodelling, ventricular hypertrophy and apoptosis. These effects control disease progression.

3. Myocardial infarction (MI)

ACE inhibitors reduce the chances of left ventricular (LV) dysfunction after MI.

4. Diabetic nephropathy

ACEIs decrease proteinuria, stabilise renal function by improving intra-renal hemodynamics, and prevent diabetic nephropathy.

5. Scleroderma crisis

A dramatic improvement is seen in scleroderma renal crisis, characterised by a marked rise in BP and deterioration of renal function.

Adverse Drug Reactions (ADRs)

- Hypotension, especially at initiation of therapy in patients with Na^+ depletion, CHF, MI, etc.
- Hyperkalemia in patients with impaired renal function, or those taking K^+ supplements, K^+-sparing diuretics, NSAIDS, β-blockers, etc.
- Persistent brassy cough (unrelated to dose) is a common adverse effect with ACE inhibitors. It is caused due to inhibition of degradation of bradykinin and substance P. This is a common and disturbing adverse effect and may require discontinuation of therapy.
- Allergic rashes, urticaria, angio-edema, edema of lips/mouth/nose/larynx and airway obstruction may occur. It can be treated with adrenaline, antihistaminics or corticosteroids.
- Dysgeusia (reversible loss or alteration of taste sensation).
- Headache, dizziness, nausea and bowel upset.
- Rare instances of granulocytopenia and proteinuria.
- Acute renal failure is precipitated in patients with bilateral renal arterial stenosis because angiotensin II maintains adequate GFR by constricting the efferent arteriole, even when renal perfusion is low. The use of ACE inhibitors can induce acute renal insufficiency in such patients.
- Teratogenic/Fetopathic effects: ACE inhibitors can cause intrauterine growth retardation (IUGR), hypoplasia of organs and fetal death, when used in the later half of pregnancy. If used in first trimester, the risk of malformations is high.

Drug interactions

ACE inhibitors interact with the following drugs:

- K^+-sparing diuretics or K^+ supplements: Risk of dangerous hyperkalemia because ACE inhibitors decrease aldosterone → decreased Na^+ reabsorption → decreased K^+ secretion.
- Indomethacin attenuates the hypotensive action of ACE inhibitors by causing salt and H_2O retention
- Diuretics cause Na^+ depletion → increased plasma renin activity (PRA). Because ACE inhibitors cause a marked fall in BP at the initiation of therapy in such patients, so, treatment should be started with low doses.
- ACEIs decrease lithium clearance and hence increase chances of Li toxicity.

Individual ACEI drugs

Captopril, the first ACEI to be marketed, **does not need activation** in the body. **Enalapril** is a **prodrug** that is transformed to its active form, enalaprilat, in the liver. **Lisinopril**, a lysine derivative of enalaprilat, is also an **active drug**. All ACE inhibitors are prodrugs (except captopril and lisinopril) and need to be converted into the active metabolites by hepatic esterases.

Captopril, with a $t_{1/2}$ of 8–12 hours, is prescribed twice a day, while enalapril is given once daily despite having a $t_{1/2} < 24$ hours. All other ACEIs have $t_{1/2} > 24$ hours and are given OD. The ACEIs are predominantly eliminated by the kidneys, except fosinopril, which is eliminated by the liver as well as kidneys.

Clinical problem-based questions and MCQs

5. i. Initiation of therapy with ACE inhibitors causes a more marked fall in BP in some patients as compared to others. In such patients, the doses should be kept low at onset of therapy. Such a marked hypotensive response to ACE inhibitors can occur in all of the following subsets of patients, EXCEPT:
    a. Malignant hypertension
    b. Sodium-replete individuals
    c. Patients suffering from CHF
    d. Patients on diuretic therapy
   i. Name drugs that have ACE-inhibiting action.
   ii. Explain the mechanism of hypotensive effect of ACE inhibitors.
   iii. Describe the cardio-renal effects of ACE inhibitors.

6. Describe the advantages of ACE inhibitors over other antihypertensive drugs.

7. Which of the following does not affect RAAS?
    a. Aliskiren   b. Losartan
    c. Prazosin   d. Clonidine

8. A 45-year-old man, a known case of rheumatic heart disease with severe mitral stenosis and severe tricuspid regurgitation, underwent cardiac surgery for mitral valve replacement and tricuspid valve commissurotomy. The postoperative period was uneventful. On discharge, the patient was put on oral therapy with furosemide 40 mg BD, spironolactone 25 mg BD, ecosprin 150 mg, and ramipril 5 mg OD.

   20 days after being discharged from the hospital, patient presented in emergency with extreme weakness, loose stools and vomiting. Patient's wife revealed that he had mild diarrhea since last 3 days and was consuming 3–4 bananas and coconut water, as these are considered good for diarrhea. On examination, PR was 40/min, feeble, irregular. Skin was cold clammy, peripheral pulses not palpable. BP= 80/ not recordable. ECG showed HR = 34/min, wide QRS complexes, and tented T wave. Serum electrolytes were disturbed: serum K^+ = 7.9 mEq/L (normal: 3.5–5.5 mEq/L), and serum Na^+ = 129 mEq/L (normal: 135–145 mEq/L). Patient had hyperkalemia and hyponatremia.
   i. What are the causes of hyperkalemia in this case?
   ii. Which of the following combinations carries a risk of causing hyperkalemia?
       a. Combination of loop and thiazide diuretics
       b. Combination of ACE inhibitor and potassium-sparing diuretic
       c. Combination of potassium supplements with loop diuretics
       d. Combination of ARBs with loop diuretics

9. A 36-year-old woman presented in gynecology OPD with amenorrhea for 6 weeks and retching and vomiting in the morning. Urine test for pregnancy is positive. On antenatal check-up, BP is 150/94 and the doctor decides to put her on antihypertensive drug therapy. Can Tab ramipril 5 mg be prescribed for this patient? Explain the pharmacological basis for your answer.

10. i. Identify the condition in which ramipril is contraindicated.
    a. Malignant hypertension
    b. Scleroderma crisis
    c. Bilateral renal arterial stenosis
    d. Grade III congestive heart failure
   ii. Describe the pharmacological basis for contraindicating ramipril in the chosen condition.

Angiotensin Receptor Blockers/Antagonists (ARBs/ARAs)

The **drugs** in this category include losartan, olmesartan, telmisartan, candesartan, valsartan, irbesartan, and eprosartan.

Mechanism of action

These drugs are specific, competitive antagonists at AT_1 receptors. Different ARBs have different affinities for AT_1 receptors; candesartan exhibits the maximum affinity and losartan the minimum. The affinity of candesartan > irbesartan > telmisartan = valsartan > losartan = eprosartan (CIT = VL = E).

Losartan, which is a competitive antagonist and inverse agonist at AT_1 receptors, is 10000 times more selective for AT_1 than AT_2 receptors. It does not block any other receptor or ion channel except thromboxane A_2 receptors; thus, some platelet anti-aggregatory effect is seen.

Pharmacological actions

Similar to ACE inhibitors, ARBs also block all the overt actions of angiotensin II, i.e., vasoconstriction, sympathetic stimulation, aldosterone release, central actions, renal actions, and growth-promoting actions on heart and blood vessels. In addition, losartan blocks the action of thromboxane A_2, exerts uricosuric action, and reduces insulin resistance. Telmisartan also decreases insulin resistance.

Differences between ARBs and ACEIs

1. Because ARBs do not inhibit the breakdown of bradykinin and substance P, the cough is not frequent. Angio-edema is also less troublesome or rare. Consequently, ARBs are given to patients who do not tolerate ACE inhibitors because of the cough.
2. ARBs inhibit actions of angiotensin II more completely. Because angiotensin II is generated in several tissues (heart, kidney, etc.) by mechanisms other than ACE activity, this synthesis of angiotensin II is not inhibited by ACE inhibitors. However, ARBs block AT_1 receptors and prevent the actions of angiotensin II formed by any mechanism.
3. Short-loop feedback inhibition of renin release by angiotensin II through AT_1 receptors is blocked by ARBs, leading to increased plasma renin activity (PRA) and angiotensin II levels. Angiotensin II, thus formed can act on unblocked AT_2 receptors, contributing to vasodilator activity; however, the clinical relevance of these actions is not very clear.

Therapeutic uses

The therapeutic uses of ARBs are the same as ACEIs.

- **Hypertension**: ARBs are sometimes preferred over ACE inhibitors because they have fewer adverse effects (cough, angio-edema, rash and dysgeusia). However, the superiority of one group over the other is not established.
- Losartan is useful in **portal hypertension**.
- **CHF**: ARBs provide symptomatic as well as long-term benefits.
- **MI** and **diabetic nephropathy**

Adverse effects

While ARBs are well-tolerated drugs, they can cause hypotension; first dose hypotension is uncommon, though. Mild headache, dizziness and GIT adverse effects may occur. Fetopathic potential is same as that for ACEIs.

Alopecia, agranulocytosis and vasculitis are adverse effects of these drugs. Olmesartan can cause sprue-like syndrome, resulting in abdominal pain and weight loss. Hyperkalemia, cough, dysgeusia and angio-edema are infrequent or not seen.

Direct Renin Inhibitors
Aliskiren

Aliskiren is an orally effective, nonpeptide drug that acts by competitively blocking the catalytic site of renin → angiotensin I is not formed → fall in angiotensin II levels. Its anti-hypertensive effect is significantly stronger than ACEIs and ARBs, although the tolerability is the same.

The adverse effects include diarrhea, headache, dizziness and hyperkalemia. Aliskiren is contraindicated in pregnancy. A major drawback is reactive renin secretion and decreased effectiveness, with continued use.

Clinical problem-based questions and MCQs

11. Which of the following is a prodrug?
    a. Captopril   b. Enalapril
    c. Lisinopril   d. All the above

12. Identify drug having minimum antagonistic activity at AT_1 receptors.
    a. Losartan   b. Olmesartan
    c. Telmisartan d. Candesartan

13. Which of the following is NOT an adverse effect of telmisartan?
    a. Teratogenicity   b. Hypotension
    c. Dizziness   d. Dysgeusia

14. ACE inhibitors and ARBs can reduce BP by their RAAS-inhibitory action. Compare the two groups as antihypertensives.

15. i. Identify the RAAS inhibitor whose effectiveness decreases with continued use.
    a. Telmisartan   b. Enalapril
    c. Aliskiren   d. All of the above.
    ii. Describe the cause of reduced efficacy of this drug.

Summary

- The **RAAS** exists as tissue and circulating RAAS.
- Tissue RAAS is involved in cell growth regulation, collagen deposition, inflammation, fibrosis, apoptosis, and is also responsible for the pathological remodelling of tissues.
- In contrast, the circulating RAAS is concerned with mineralocorticoid secretion, BP homeostasis, secondary hyperaldosteronism has a permissive role in renovascular/essential hypertension/pregnancy-induced hypertension.

- Decrease in blood volume, BP and Na$^+$ content leads to renin release that is regulated by the long- and short-loop feedback mechanisms. Drugs such as ACEIs, ARBs, vasodilators, diuretics and NSAIDs interfere with these regulatory mechanisms
- Angiotensin II-mediated vasoconstriction occurs in arterioles, venules and all vascular beds, but is less marked in cerebral, coronary, skeletal and pulmonary vessels. It favours the movement of fluid from vascular to extravascular compartments.
- **ACE inhibitors** include drugs like captopril, enalapril, perindopril, lisinopril and fosinopril.
- The BP-lowering effect is mediated through the reduced formation of angiotensin II, preventing its vasoconstrictor action; excessive angiotensin 1 is diverted to the ACE 2 pathway resulting in the formation of vasodilator angiotensin heptapeptide (1–7).
- In the short term, the magnitude of BP lowering is greater in sodium-depleted patients with raised renin levels, CHF, and malignant/renovascular/accelerated hypertension.
- ACEIs are first-line antihypertensive drugs as they do not cause reflex tachycardia and maintain renal/cerebral and coronary perfusion even while lowering BP. These are safe in diabetics and asthmatic patients, do not have withdrawal reactions, and the QOL is only minimally impaired.
- ACEIs are useful in all grades of CHF, MI, diabetic nephropathy and scleroderma crisis.
- ADRs include dizziness, hypotension (especially at the initiation of therapy), risk of hyperkalemia (especially when combined with K$^+$ supplements/K$^+$-sparing diuretics/β-blockers/NSAIDs or in patients with renal function impairment), rashes, urticaria and angio-edema. Persistent dry cough may occur owing to raised levels of kinins and substance P.
- These drugs may precipitate ARF in bilateral renal artery stenosis. ACE inhibitors have fetopathic effects and are contraindicated in pregnant women.
- **ARBs** include losartan, telmisartan and olmesartan. These are selective, competitive AT$_1$ receptor antagonists and block all the overt actions of angiotensin II more completely than ACEIs.
- They block short-loop feedback inhibition, resulting in raised PRA and angiotensin II, which acts on AT$_2$ receptors → vasodilatation.
- Therapeutic indications for ARBs are same as for ACE inhibitors.
- ARBs are better tolerated than ACEIs as cough angio-edema is less frequent and less troublesome. Hyperkalemia and dysgeusia are not seen. They can cause hypotension, mild headache, dizziness and GI adverse effects.
- **Aliskiren** is a direct renin inhibitor that blocks the active site of renin competitively → fall in levels of angiotensin I and II. Antihypertensive effect is more prominent than ACEI and ARBs, but with continued use its effectiveness decreases owing to reactive renin secretion. ADRs such as diarrhea, hyperkalemia, headache and dizziness may occur.

Questions for practice

1. Classify drugs affecting renin–angiotensin–aldosterone system.
2. Enumerate therapeutic uses and adverse effects of ACE inhibitors.
3. What are differences between ACE inhibitors and ARBs.
4. Write short notes on:
   a. Feedback mechanisms controlling plasma renin activity (PRA)
   b. Pathophysiological role of RAAS in hypertension
   c. Status of ACE inhibitors in treatment of hypertension and CHF
   d. Direct renin inhibitors

Hints for problem-based questions and MCQs

1. a. Angiotensin (1–7)
2. d. AT$_1$ receptor-mediated IP$_3$–DAG pathway
3. a. Abnormal redistribution of muscle mass
4. Refer to page 400, 401
5. i. b. Sodium replete individuals
   ii. Refer to page Flowchart 30.1, page 403
   iii. Refer to page 403
   iv. Refer to page 403
6. Refer to page 404
7. c. Prazosin Aliskiren is DRI. Losartan blocks AT$_1$ receptors and clonidine reduces plasma renin activity on initiation of therapy and also inhibits aldosterone production.
8. i. A combination of K$^+$-sparing diuretic, ACE inhibitor, and intake of K$^+$-rich foods is responsible for hyperkalemia
   ii. b. Combination of ACE inhibitor and potassium sparing diuretic
9. Ramipril is an ACE inhibitor, not safe in pregnancy
10. i. c. Bilateral renal arterial stenosis
    ii. Risk of precipitation of ARF. Refer to page 404
11. b. Enalapril (All ACE inhibitors except captopril and lisinopril are prodrugs.)
12. a. Losartan has minimum AT$_1$ blocking effect
13. d. Dysgeusia occurs with ACE inhibitors, but not with ARBs.
14. Refer to page 406
15. i. c. Aliskiren
    ii. Refer to page 406.

CONCEPT MAP - RAAS INHIBITORS

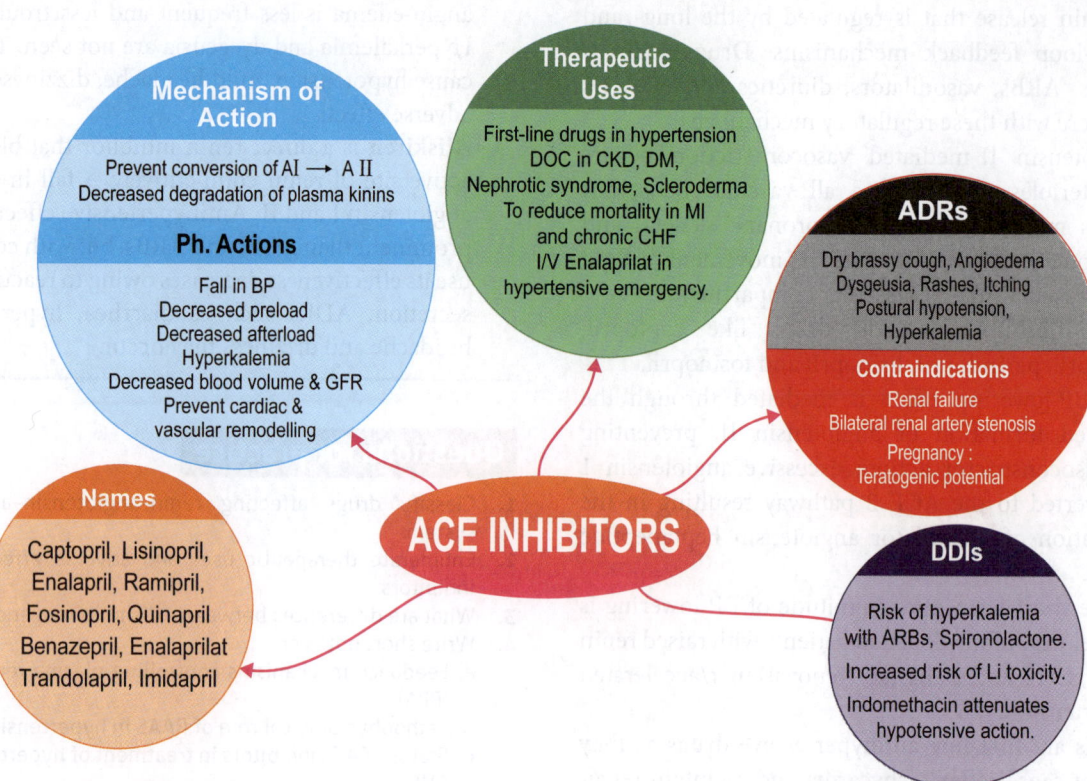

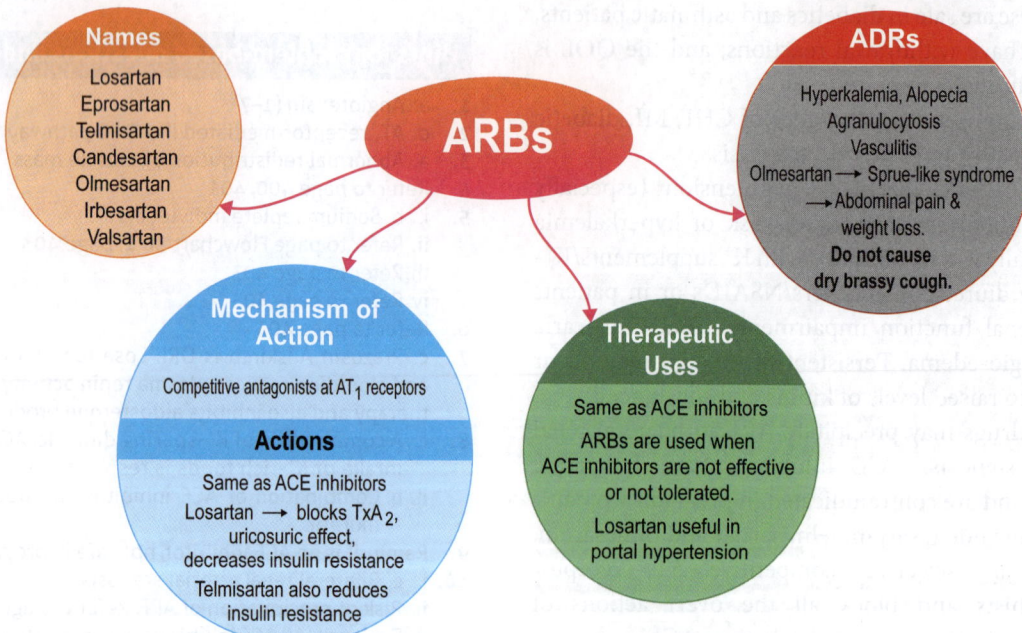

SECTION 7 Drugs Acting on CVS

31 Calcium Channel Blockers

Learning objectives

A student of MBBS phase II should be able to:
- Explain actions mediated through different types of calcium channels.
- Classify calcium channel blockers (CCBs) and describe their mechanism of action.
- Describe the direct and reflex actions of dihydropyridines and non-dihydropyridines.
- Enumerate the therapeutic uses and adverse effects of CCBs.
- Describe the role and status of CCBs in different cardiovascular diseases.

TYPES OF Ca^{2+} CHANNELS

Excitable tissues contain three types of Ca^{2+} channels:

- **Voltage-sensitive channels** that are activated when the membrane potential falls below –40 mV.
- **Receptor-operated calcium channels**: e.g., ryanodine receptors that cause Ca^{2+} release from the sarcoplasmic reticulum. Adrenaline can also trigger calcium influx through these receptors, independent of depolarisation.
- **Leak channels** are stretch-sensitive channels that allow calcium influx in response to mechanical stretching.

Voltage-sensitive Ca^{2+} channels are further classified into:

- **L-type calcium channels** which have long-lasting current and are the most widely distributed (Table 31.1). These channels mediate smooth muscle contraction, impulse generation in the SA node, atrio-ventricular conduction, and release of hormones and neurotransmitters. Drugs that block L-type calcium channels are called calcium channel blockers (CCBs) and are useful in numerous cardiovascular conditions.
- **T-type calcium channels** which have transient current, also play a role in pacemaker activity, AV conduction and hormone/neurotransmitter release. These channels, however, are not present in smooth muscles. T-type CCBs include ethosuximide (used in absence seizures) and flunarizine (anti-vertigo drug).
- **N-type calcium channels**, which are neuronal receptors, are involved in neurotransmitter release, and are blocked by ω-conotoxin.

CLASSIFICATION OF CCBs

CCBs are classified based upon their chemical nature as into DHPs and non-DHPs. The DHPs are further classified into four generations based on their half-lives (Flowchart 31.1).

Table 31.1 Properties of voltage-sensitive calcium channels

	L type (Long-lasting current)	T type (Transient current)	N Type (Neuronal)
Channel kinetics	High threshold → slow activation and inactivation rates	Low threshold → fast inactivation rate	Medium threshold → Medium inactivation rate
Distribution and action	Smooth muscles → excitation–contraction coupling SA node, AV node → impulse generation and conduction Endocrines → hormone release Neurons → NTM release	— SA node, AV node → pacemaker action, AV conduction Endocrines → hormone release Neurons → NTM release	— — Present only in neurons, involved in NTM release
Blocked by	CCBs, DHPs, Non-DHPs	Ethosuximide, flunarizine	ω-Conotoxin

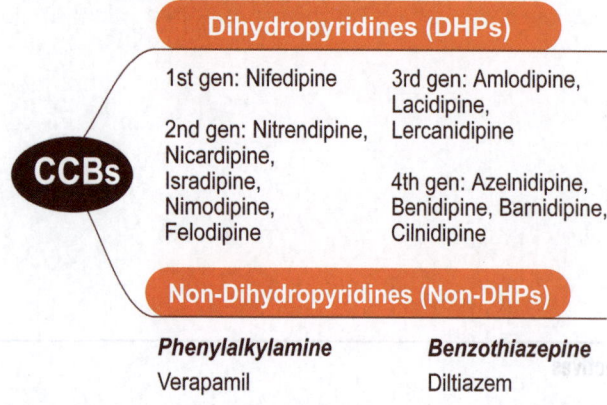

Flowchart 31.1 Classification of calcium channel blockers

MECHANISM OF ACTION

L-type Ca^{2+} channels have $α_1$, $α_2$, $β$, $γ$, and $δ$ subunits. CCBs act by binding to receptors present on the $α_1$-subunit. The binding sites of DHPs are different from those of verapamil and diltiazem.

Blockade of Ca^{2+} channels occurs from the inner side of the membrane. Drugs bind more effectively to the active and inactive states → **decrease in frequency of channel opening** in response to depolarisation → decrease in transmembrane Ca^{2+} current, resulting in smooth muscle relaxation (Fig. 31.1, Box 31.1).

In addition to the effect on the frequency of channel opening, **verapamil** and **diltiazem** delay the recovery of the **inactive** (IA) state of the channel to **resting** (R) state. This effect is not seen with DHPs.

T-type and N-type Ca^{2+} channels are less sensitive to CCBs, as a result of which neurons and secretory glands are not much affected by these drugs.

However, among the 4th generation DHPs, cilnidipine blocks both L- and N-type calcium channels, resulting in reduced sympathetic outflow. Benidipine blocks all three types, i.e., L-, T- and N-type calcium channels and exerts renal protective effect.

PHARMACOLOGICAL ACTIONS OF CCBs

CCBs predominantly affect smooth muscles and cardiac muscles. Skeletal muscles, which depend on intracellular pools of calcium for excitation–contraction coupling, are not much affected by CCBs.

Smooth Muscles

CCBs have a relaxant effect on smooth muscles by the mechanism described in Fig. 31.1 and Box 31.1.

a. Vascular smooth muscle relaxation

- **Arterioles** are markedly **relaxed** → decrease in total peripheral resistance (TPR) → fall in BP → reflex sympathetic stimulation → reflex tachycardia.
- Vasodilatation and reduced peripheral vascular resistance by CCBs is responsible for their beneficial

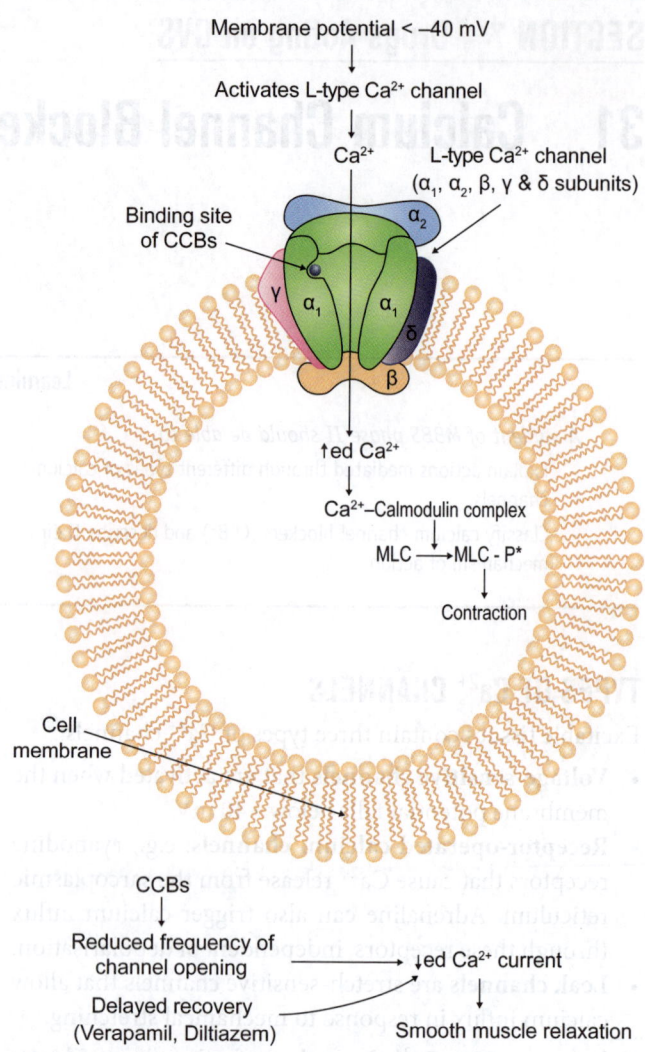

Fig. 31.1 Mechanism of action of CCBs

effect in angina of effort. Coronary artery tone is reduced in patients with variant/vasospastic angina.
- **Arteriolar dilatation > venous dilatation with CCBs**, i.e., CCBs have a mild effect on veins. Thus, there is little vasodilator effect on capacitance vessels, indicating that orthostatic hypotension is not a problem with use of CCBs.

The vascular smooth muscle relaxant effect is strongest with DHPs followed by verapamil and diltiazem (**DHPs > verapamil > diltiazem**). The predominant relaxant action of DHPs may be attributed to:

- Release of NO from endothelium by DHPs → vasodilatation. This may also contribute to anti-atherosclerotic action of DHPs.
- Inhibition of phosphodiesterase → increased cAMP → relaxant action → vasodilatation.
- Greater selectivity of DHPs for L-type calcium channels in smooth muscles.
- Second-generation DHPs like nitrendipine, nicardipine, isradipine, nimodipine and felodipine are more selective for vascular smooth muscles and longer acting than nifedipine. Nimodipine and nicardipine have high affinity

Box 31.1 Mechanism of smooth muscle relaxing action of CCBs

Inward Ca^{2+} movement through voltage-gated Ca^{2+} channels

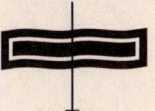
Blocked by CCBs, which decrease intracellular Ca^{2+} availability, resulting in smooth muscle relaxation)

↓

Smooth muscle membrane depolarisation
↓
Ca^{2+} ions trigger further release of Ca^{2+} from intracellular stores
↓
Calcium–calmodulin complex is formed
↓
Phosphorylation of myosin light chain
↓
Excitation–contraction coupling
↓
Contraction of smooth muscles

Arteriolar dilatation > Venous dilatation

On vascular smooth muscles, the **effect of DHPs > Verapamil > Diltiazem**

---

for cerebral blood vessels and appear to reduce morbidity after subarachnoid hemorrhage. They prevent cerebral vasospasm associated with stroke and are reported to reduce cerebral damage after thrombo-embolic episodes.

b. Extravascular smooth muscles

Extravascular smooth muscles (e.g., bronchial, intestinal, biliary, uterine, and vesical) are also relaxed by CCBs.

Cardiac Muscles

The two types of cardiac action potential (fast- and slow-channel AP) and role of the ions involved are described in Box 31.2.

Box 31.2 Cardiac action potential

The ionic movements during various phases of cardiac action potential in different cardiac fibres and the differences between the two action potentials are enumerated below and shown in Figs. 31.2 a,b.

	Fast-channel action potential	Slow-channel action potential
Fibres showing AP	Atria, Ventricles	SA node, AV node, Purkinje fibres
Resting membrane potential	–90 mV	–60 mV
Threshold potential	–60 mV	–40 mV
Ion movement in Phase 0	Na^+ influx	Ca^{2+} influx
Phase 1,2,3	Clearly delineated	Indistinguishable
Phase 4	Potential stable	Potential decays → diastolic depolarisation → automaticity

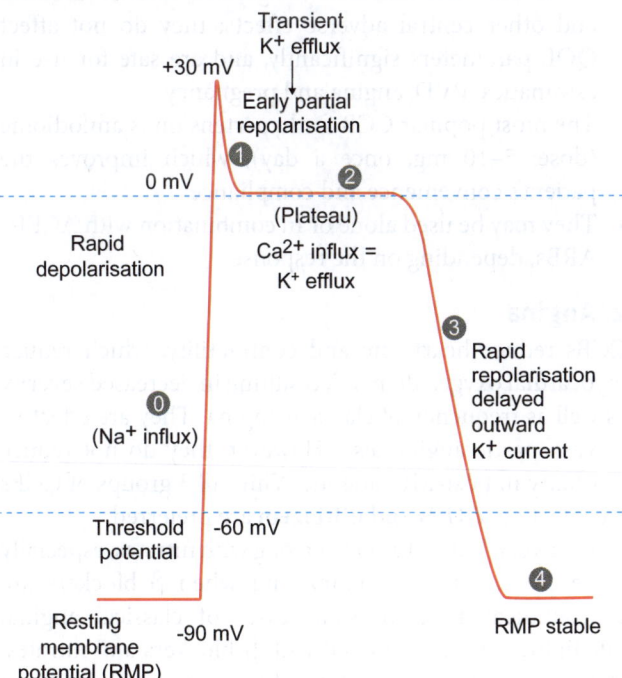

Fig. 31.2(a) Fast-channel action potential in atrial and ventricular fibres

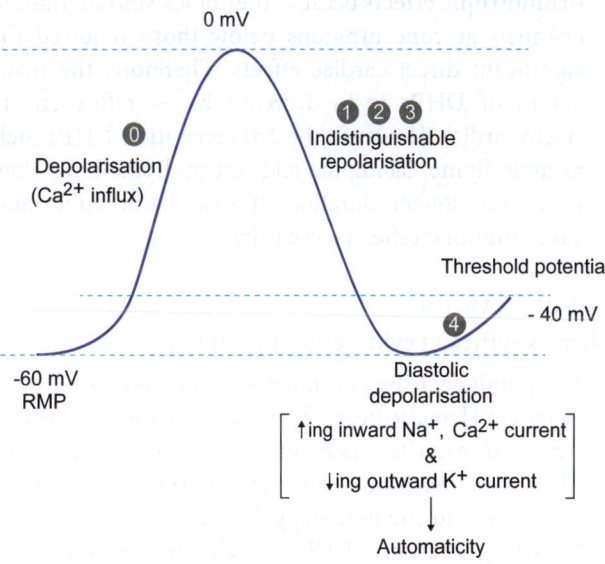

Fig. 31.2(b) Slow-channel action potential in SA nodes, AV nodes, and Purkinje fibres

- In **fast-channel action potential of atrial and ventricular fibres** (Fig. 31.2a), Na$^+$ influx causes 'rapid depolarisation' (Phase 0), and transient K$^+$ efflux causes 'early partial repolarisation' (Phase 1). In Phase 2, the membrane potential plateaus, because Ca^{2+} influx balances the K$^+$ efflux. Ca^{2+} ions moving in during this phase of AP → release more Ca^{2+} from the sarcoplasmic reticulum → excitation–contraction coupling. Rapid repolarisation in Phase 3 occurs due to delayed outward K$^+$ current. Membrane potential remains stable in phase 4. CCBs interfere with calcium influx and exert a **negative inotropic action** → reduced contractility → reduced myocardial O$_2$ demand.
- In **slow-channel action potential of the SA node and AV node**, Phase 0 depolarisation depends on the Ca^{2+} current (Fig. 31.2b). Phases 1, 2, and 3 are indistinguishable and involve K$^+$ efflux. In Phase 4, diastolic depolarisation occurs due to increasing inward Na$^+$, Ca^{2+} currents, and decreasing outward K$^+$ current. Automaticity, i.e., pacemaker activity and conductivity of these cells appears to depend on the rate of recovery of Ca^{2+} channels. As a result, CCBs, especially verapamil and diltiazem, which delay the channel recovery from the **inactive** (IA) to the **resting** (R) state, have **negative chronotropic and negative dromotropic** effects. In other words, they decrease the rate of impulse generation and conduction → bradycardia. The effect of CCBs on the cardiac action potential is shown in Fig. 31.3. Calcium channel blockers reduce the rate of Phase 0 and the maximum potential attained. The slope of repolarisation is also slowed, resulting in increased action potential duration (APD) and effective refractory period (ERP).
- Diltiazem causes less depression of contractility than verapamil.
- **DHPs do not have negative chronotropic and dromotropic effects** because they block smooth muscle channels at concentrations below those required for significant direct cardiac effects. Therefore, the main action of DHPs is to decrease BP → reflex effects (tachycardia). However, the 3rd generation DHPs such as amlodipine, lacidipine and lercanidipine have slow onset and longer duration of vasodilator effect and cause minimal reflex tachycardia.

Other Actions
There is sufficient evidence to suggest that:
- Verapamil decreases insulin release in high doses.
- Verapamil has also beens shown to block P-glycoprotein, which transports many drugs out of cancer cells. Therefore, verapamil can reverse the resistance of cancer cells to chemotherapy drugs.
- Fourth-generation DHPs such as azelnidipine, benidipine, barnidipine and cilnidpine possess

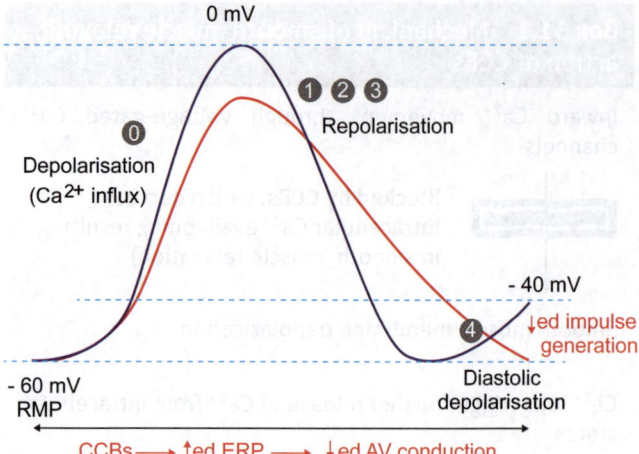

Fig. 31.3 The effect of verapamil and diltiazem on slow-channel action potential

additional organ-protective effects, especially renal-protective action.

THERAPEUTIC USES OF CCBs

1. Hypertension
CCBs are **among the first-line drugs** for the treatment of hypertension. While all 3 groups of CCBs lower BP, **DHPs** are preferred for this indication. The **advantages** of CCBs in treating hypertension include:
- They are specifically indicated for elderly patients with low plasma renin activity and in patients of African descent.
- CCBs are well-tolerated drugs and free of sedative and other central adverse effects; they do not affect QOL parameters significantly, and are safe for use in asthmatics, PVD, angina and pregnancy.
- The most popular CCB for hypertension is amlodipine (dose: 5–10 mg, once a day), which improves the patient's convenience and compliance.
- They may be used alone or in combination with ACEIs/ARBs, depending on the response.

2. Angina
CCBs reduce heart rate and contractility, which reduce myocardial oxygen demand, resulting in decreased severity as well as frequency of classical angina. They are effective in vasospastic angina also. However, they do not reduce mortality in post-MI patients. While all 3 groups of CCBs are effective, **DHPs and diltiazem** are preferred.

CCBs can be used alone or along with nitrates, especially in severe vasospastic angina and when β blockers are contraindicated. In resistant cases of classical angina, nifedipine can be combined with β-blockers and nitrates. However, such a combination of verapamil and diltiazem with β blockers poses the risk of AV blocks and should not be used.

3. Arrhythmia

Verapamil and diltiazem have antiarrhythmic action as they slow down the sinus rate and AV conduction.

- **Verapamil** is a **first-choice drug** to control ventricular rate in atrial flutter and fibrillation in an oral dose of 40–120 mg, though it may be administered intravenously in case of emergency.
- Paroxysmal supraventricular tachycardia (**PSVT**) attacks can be terminated by a 5 mg IV injection over a few minutes.
- Verapamil may be used orally for prophylaxis of PSVT also.
- Diltiazem is a good alternative to verapamil in these conditions, as it causes less marked bradycardia and less suppression of cardiac contractility.

4. Other uses

CCBs also find use in hypertrophic cardiomyopathy, migraine, and Raynaud's syndrome. Nifedipine has some efficacy in preterm labour as well.

Adverse Drug Reactions (ADRs)

Minor adverse effects include flushing, headache, dizziness, nausea, constipation, hypotension and peripheral ankle edema.

Serious adverse effects are:

- **Cardiac depression:** Cardiac adverse effects are more commonly seen with verapamil and diltiazem than with DHPs. They include bradycardia, atrio-ventricular block, heart failure and cardiac arrest.
- **Short-acting DHPs** may **aggravate myocardial** ischemia by reflex tachycardia and fall in mean arterial pressure, which has been reported to increase mortality. However, slow- and long-acting DHP preparations do not pose this risk. Clevidipine, an ultrashort-acting 3rd generation DHP with a half-life of 1 minute, is used by IV infusion in critical care settings. Verapamil (40–160 mg thrice daily, orally) and diltiazem are also free of such effects.
- Patients receiving β-blockers are more sensitive to the depressant effects of verapamil. It can accentuate conduction defects, sinus depression, and precipitate CHF in patients with pre-existing disease, leading to cardiac arrest. However, β-blockers can be combined with nifedipine to check the reflex tachycardia caused by it. Although both verapamil and nifedipine are CCBs, **β-blockers can be combined with nifedipine, but not with verapamil**. This is because verapamil exhibits prominent cardio-depressant action that adds to the similar action of β-blockers. In contrast, nifedipine and other DHPs have prominent vascular action causing vasodilatation and fall in BP, which results in reflex sympathetic stimulation and tachycardia. β-blockers may be added to check the tachycardia caused by DHPs.
- Urinary voiding difficulty in elderly can be exacerbated by DHPs, because of smooth muscle relaxation.
- Gastro-esophageal reflux may be worsened by DHPs because of lower esophageal sphincter (LES) relaxation.

Contraindications

Verapamil and diltiazem are contraindicated in sick sinus syndrome, AV blocks, and digitalis-induced arrhythmias, because of the negative chronotropic and dromotropic effect. CCBs are not used in ventricular tachyarrhythmias as they have poor efficacy and IV use is reported to precipitate ventricular fibrillation in some cases.

Clinical problem based-questions and MCQs

1. i. Identify the calcium channel blocker with the most prominent vasodilator effect.
   a. Verapamil   b. Diltiazem
   c. Nifedipine   d. All have equal effect.
   ii. Describe the pharmacological basis for your choice

2. i. Which of the following correctly describes the antihypertensive role of CCBs?
   a. There is a risk of first-dose hypotension.
   b. Dihydropyridines are preferred over verapamil.
   c. CCBs are preferred hypertension in white persons.
   d. CCBs are preferred in young individuals.

3. i. DHPs have a prominent effect on:
   a. Capacitance vessels
   b. Resistance vessels
   c. Sino-atrial node
   d. Atrio-ventricular node
   ii. What are the clinical implications of the chosen prominent effect?

4. Provide the pharmacological basis for these cautions in the use of CCBs.
   i. Short acting DHPs are not safe in a hypertensive emergency.
   ii. Verapamil should not be combined with β-blockers in patients with resistant angina.

5. Identify the CCB that has greater selectivity for cerebral blood vessels.
   a. Nifedipine   b. Amlodipine
   c. Nimodipine   d. Benidipine

Summary

- L-type calcium channels have high threshold, slow rate of activation and inactivation and long-lasting current; they are mainly distributed in the heart (in the SA and AV nodes) and smooth muscles.
- CCBs include DHPs [divided into 4 generations, e.g., nifedipine (1st), nitrendipine, nicardipine (2nd), amlodipine (3rd), and cilnidipine (4th generation)], and non-DHPs such as verapamil and diltiazem.

- CCBs bind to the active and inactive state of L-type calcium channels, resulting in reduced frequency of channel opening. In addition, non-DHPs delay the recovery of channels from the inactive state to the resting state.
- The two major actions of CCBs are smooth muscle relaxation and cardio-depressant action.
- Vascular smooth muscle relaxation resulting in arteriolar dilatation (more than venous dilatation) is more with DHPs than verapamil and diltiazem; this is because DHPs possess NO-releasing and PDE-inhibiting action in addition to calcium channel blockade, which contributes to vasodilatation.
- Vasodilatation → fall in TPR → fall in BP → reflex tachycardia.
- DHPs are among the first-choice antihypertensive drugs, particularly for elderly individuals with low renin activity and patients of African descent. Orthostatic hypotension is not a problem owing to weak venodilator effect.
- Verapamil and diltiazem exhibit negative inotropic effect in atrial and ventricular fibres. In the SA node and AV node, they reduce the rate of impulse generation and conduction respectively. Oxygen demand is reduced. These are useful in PSVT and atrial flutter/fibrillation to control the ventricular rate.
- CCBs are used in hypertension, angina, and arrhythmias such as PSVT/atrial flutter/fibrillation, hypertrophic cardiomyopathy, migraine and preterm labour.
- DHP-induced reflex tachycardia can be checked by combining with β-blockers, but a combination of non-DHPs, especially verapamil, with β-blockers has the risk of causing AV blocks and is therefore contraindicated.
- ADRs include minor symptoms such as headache, dizziness, flushing, nausea, constipation, and ankle edema. CCBs can worsen GERD and difficulty in voiding in elderly patients The cardio-depressant effect may cause bradycardia, AV blocks, heart failure and cardiac arrest.
- Immediate-release DHPs carry the risk of precipitating MI in hypertensive patients and are banned.
- CCBs are contraindicated in ventricular tachycardia (because of poor efficacy and risk of ventricular fibrillation), AV blocks, sick sinus syndrome and digitalis-induced arrhythmias (because they have negative chronotropic and dromotropic effects).

Questions for practice

1. Classify calcium channel blockers.
2. Differentiate between the cardiovascular effects of DHPs and phenylalkylamines.
3. Enumerate the therapeutic uses and adverse effects of CCBs.
4. Explain why:
   a. Short-acting preparations of DHPs should not be used in angina.
   b. The combination of verapamil and diltiazem with β-blockers should be avoided.

Hints for problem-based questions and MCQs

1. i. c. Nifedipine
   ii. On vascular smooth muscles, the effect of DHPs > verapamil > diltiazem.
2. i. b. Dihydropyridines are preferred over verapamil
3. i. b. Resistance vessels
   ii. Relaxation of resistance vessels (arterioles) reduces TPR and is useful in hypertension and angina.
4. i. Can aggravate myocardial ischemia due to fall in mean arterial pressure and reflex tachycardia. Refer to page 413.
   ii. Patients receiving beta blockers are more sensitive to the cardio-depressant effect of verapamil, leading to risk of sinus depression, accentuation of conduction defects, risk of AV blocks, CHF precipitation, and cardiac arrest in patients with preexisting disease. Refer to page 413.
5. c. Nimodipine

CONCEPT MAP - CALCIUM CHANNEL BLOCKERS

Classification

Dihydropyridines (DHPs)
Nifedipine, Nitrendipine
Nicardipine, Nimodipine, Felodipine
Benidipine, Cilnidipine,
Amlodipine, Lacidipine, Lercanidipine

Non-Dihydropyridines (Non-DHPs)
Phenylalkylamine : Verapamil
Benzothiazepine : Diltiazem

Mechanism of Action

- CCBs bind to active & inactive state of L-type calcium channels
  ↓
  Reduced frequency of channel opening.
  Decreased I/C Ca^{2+}
  Decreased excitation–contraction coupling
  ↓
  Smooth muscle relaxation
- Verapamil, diltiazem also delay recovery of channel from inactive state to resting state.
- DHPs possess NO-releasing and PDE inhibiting action
  ↓
  Smooth muscle relaxation

DDIs

β blockers : DHP-induced reflex tachycardia can be checked.

Combination of Non-DHPs especially Verapamil with β blockers has risk of causing AV block and is therefore contraindicated.

CALCIUM CHANNEL BLOCKERS

Actions

DHPs

Blood vessels : Vasodilatation → fall in TPR → fall in BP → reflex tachycardia

Arteriolar dilatation > venous dilatation. → orthostatic hypotension

Verapamil & diltiazem

Negative inotropic effect

Reduced rate of impulse generation & conduction.

Reduced oxygen demand

ADRs

Minor : Headache, Dizziness, Flushing, Nausea, Constipation, Ankle edema.

Cardiac : Bradycardia, AV blocks, Heart failure and Cardiac arrest.

Risk of precipitating MI in hypertensives with immediate-release DHPs - and are banned

Contraindications

Ventricular tachycardia, AV blocks, Sick sinus syndrome and Digitalis-induced arrhythmias.

Therapeutic Uses

Hypertension in elderly, Low renin activity & African descents DHPs are among first choice drugs.
Hypertrophic cardiomyopathy
PSVT, atrial flutter / fibrillation to control ventricular rate.
Angina
Migraine
Preterm labour

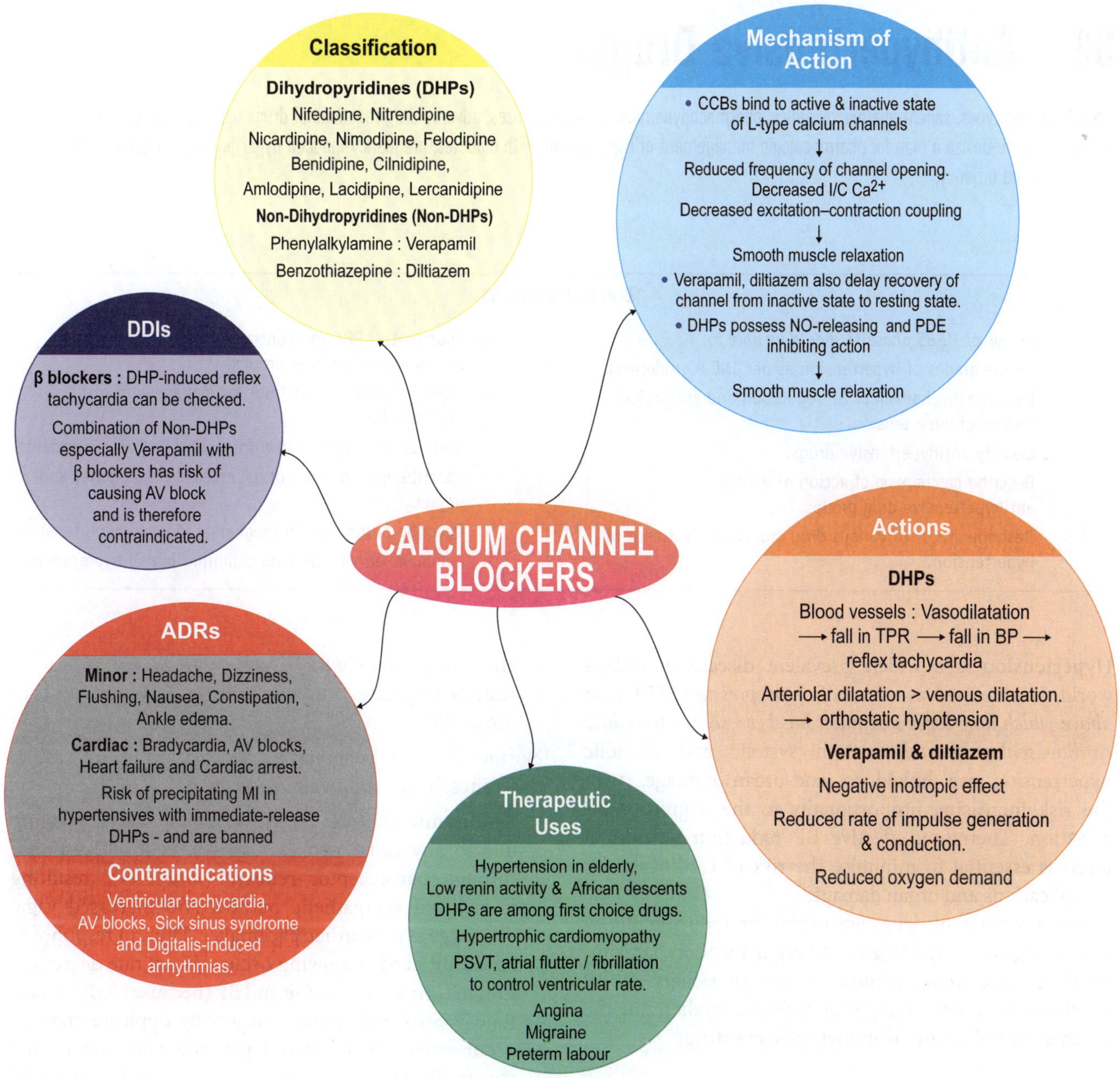

SECTION 7 Drugs Acting on CVS

32 Antihypertensive Drugs

PH 4.7 Explain types, salient pharmacokinetics, pharmacodynamics, therapeutic uses, adverse drug reactions of drugs used for the management of hypertension. Devise a plan for pharmacologic management of hypertension with diabetes, pregnancy-induced hypertension, and hypertensive emergency and urgency.

Learning objectives

A student of MBBS phase II should be able to:
- Define grades of hypertension as per JNC 8 guidelines.
- Describe mechanism of BP regulation and etiological factors of hypertension.
- Classify antihypertensive drugs.
- Describe mechanism of action of various antihypertensive drug groups.
- Describe status of various drug groups in treatment of hypertension.
- Enumerate ADRs and contraindications of various antihypertensive drug groups.
- Describe current guidelines for management of hypertension.
- Describe antihypertensive drugs used in diabetic patients.
- Describe management of hypertensive emergency and urgency.
- Describe drugs used in pregnancy-induced hypertension.
- Comment on various drug combinations in hypertension.

Hypertension is a widely prevalent disease in today's world. It is defined as a *level of blood pressure (BP) at or above which long-term treatment has been shown to reduce cardiovascular mortality*. Both systolic and diastolic hypertension are linked to end-organ damage, with the risk increasing proportionally to the degree of BP elevation. Therefore, effective BP reduction to normal levels is essential to minimise the risk of cardiovascular complications and organ damage.

Many groups of drugs are useful for reducing BP by interfering with physiological BP regulatory mechanisms. Thus, a basic understanding of the physiology of BP regulation is of utmost importance for comprehending the mechanisms of action of antihypertensive drugs.

PHYSIOLOGICAL REGULATION OF BLOOD PRESSURE

Arterial BP is directly proportional to the product of cardiac output (COP) and peripheral vascular resistance (PVR). COP is the amount of blood pumped out by the heart per minute, and PVR is the resistance to the passage of blood through pre-capillary arterioles.

BP = COP × PVR

BP is maintained by the regulation of these two parameters, i.e., COP and PVR, at the following anatomic sites:
- Arterioles (resistance vessels – regulate PVR)
- Postcapillary venules (capacitance vessels regulate venous return and, in turn, COP)
- Heart (regulates COP)
- Kidney (regulates intravascular fluid volume and, in turn, COP)

Normal BP is maintained by coordination of function at these sites, by the following mechanisms:

- **Autonomic control**: Increased mean arterial pressure due to any cause evokes negative feedback response through baroreceptor reflexes (Fig. 32.1), resulting in reduced sympathetic outflow and increased vagal discharge at the cardiac pacemaker. Thus, in response to raised BP, cardiac slowing occurs. Heart rate decreases; this, in turn, reduces COP and BP (because COP = Heart Rate × Stroke Volume). Diagonally opposite changes occur when mean arterial pressure falls due to any reason. Postural baro-reflex helps in rapid adjustment of BP during posture change.
- **Humoral mechanism** including **RAAS**: Reduced BP, due to any reason, induces renin release; this activates RAAS (Fig. 32.2). The vasoconstrictor effect of angiotensin II raises PVR, and aldosterone-induced Na^+/H_2O retention increases intravascular volume. Thus, BP rises towards normal.
- **Local control**: Release of vasoactive substances from the vascular endothelium regulates vascular resistance. Endothelin 1 causes vasoconstriction, while nitric oxide (NO) causes vasodilatation.

These mechanisms are responsible for maintaining BP in normotensive as well as hypertensive individuals. The only difference is that the baroreceptors and renal blood volume

Chapter 32 Antihypertensive Drugs 417

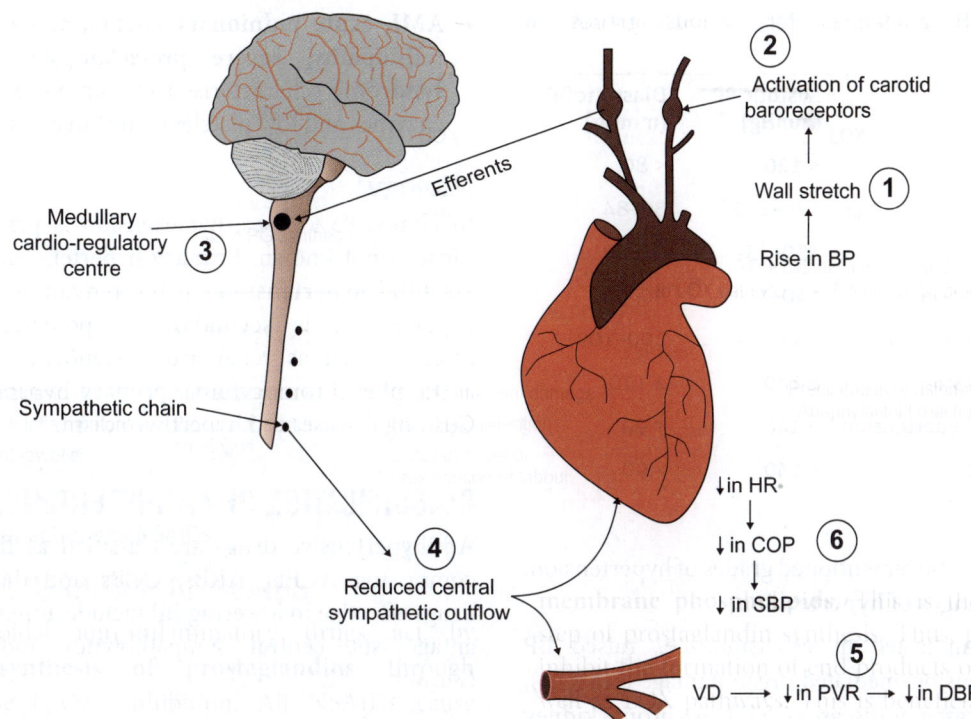

Fig. 32.1 Baroreceptor reflex: Autonomic regulation of BP
Rapid adjustment
① Vessel wall stretch due to internal pressure (arterial pressure) → ② Activation of carotid baroreceptors → ③ Inhibition of tonically active central sympathetic neurons that arise from vasomotor area of the medulla oblongata → ④ Reduced central sympathetic outflow → ⑤ Decreased PVR and COP → ⑥ BP restored to normal.
In contrast, fall in BP → reduced baroreceptor activity → increased sympathetic outflow → raised PVR and COP → BP restored to normal.

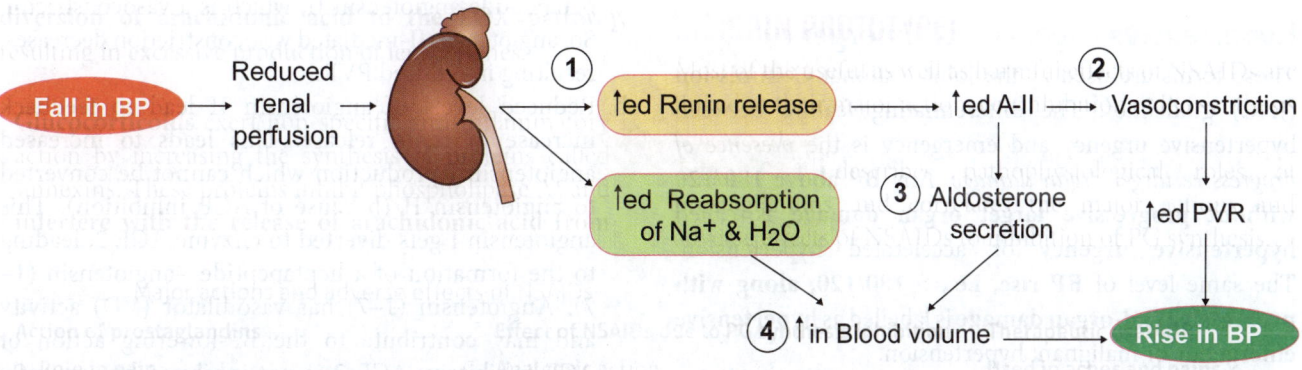

Fig. 32.2 Humoral regulation of BP
Fall in BP → ① Renin release → RAAS activation → ② A-II-induced vasoconstriction → raised PVR. ③ Aldosterone-induced Na⁺/H₂O retention → ④ Increased intravascular volume → BP normalised.

and blood pressure control systems are "set" at higher BP levels in hypertensives compared to normotensives.

Antihypertensive drugs exert their BP-lowering effect by interfering with these normal regulatory mechanisms.

DIAGNOSIS OF HYPERTENSION

Diagnosis is based on repeated, reproducible measurements of elevated BP and not on symptoms reported by the patient. Hypertension usually remains asymptomatic till end-organ damage occurs or is imminent. According to the most recent (2023) guidelines of the European Society of Hypertension (ESH), endorsed by the International Society of Hypertension (ISH), it is recommended to measure BP 3 times, with a gap of 1 min between the three readings. The average of the last two readings is then calculated. There are 3 grades of hypertension. Table 32.1 depicts ESH guidelines for various grades of hypertension.

Table 32.1 ESH guidelines for various grades of hypertension

Category	Systolic BP (mmHg)	Diastolic BP (mmHg)
Optimal	< 120	< 80
Normal	120–129	80–84
High-Normal	130–139	85–89
Grade 1 Hypertension	140–159	90–99
Grade 2 Hypertension	160–179	100–109
Grade 3 Hypertension	≥ 180	≥ 110
Isolated systolic hypertension	> 140	< 90
Isolated diastolic hypertension	< 140	> 90

In addition to the abovementioned grades of hypertension, there are three **stages of hypertension**.

Stage 1: Uncomplicated hypertension, i.e., raised BP **without** hypertension-mediated organ damage (HMOD), diabetes, cardiovascular disease (CVD), or chronic kidney disease (CKD) more severe than stage 3.

Stage 2: HMOD, diabetes, or CKD more severe than stage 3 is present.

Stage 3: CVD or CKD stage 4 or 5 is present.

The **API** (Association of Physicians of India) guidelines 2019 also categorises BP as Grades 1–3 as per ESH guidelines.

Hypertensive Urgency and Emergency

These terms are used in the Joint National Commission (JNC) guidelines. The differentiating feature between hypertensive urgency and emergency is the *presence of progressive target organ damage*. Any **BP above 180/120 without progressive target organ damage** is called **hypertensive urgency** or accelerated hypertension. The same level of **BP rise, i.e., > 180/120, along with progressive end-organ damage** is labelled as **hypertensive emergency** or malignant hypertension.

Hypertensive emergencies include the following conditions:

- Hypertension with **vascular damage,** involving progressive inflammation and necrosis of arterioles. Such lesions in the kidney activate RAAS, causing further increase in BP.
- Hypertensive **encephalopathy**, which is characterised by mental confusion, apprehension, headache, vomiting and neurological deficit. It should be treated aggressively; otherwise, it may progress to convulsions, stupor, coma and death within 48 hours.
- Hypertension with **hemodynamic complications** like heart failure, dissecting aortic aneurysm, and stroke also constitute hypertensive emergencies.

- **AMI, acute pulmonary edema, acute renal failure, retinopathy, severe pre-eclampsia, and HELLP syndrome** (characterised by hemolysis, elevated liver enzymes and low platelet count) may also occur.

Etiology

In almost 95% cases, hypertension is **primary**, i.e., the cause is not known. Primary hypertension is also called **essential hypertension**. In the remaining (~ 5%) cases, hypertension is **secondary** to potentially rectifiable diseases such as renal artery stenosis, co-arctation of aorta, pheochromocytoma, primary hyperaldosteronism, Cushing disease, and hyperthyroidism.

CLASSIFICATION OF ANTIHYPERTENSIVE DRUGS

Antihypertensive drugs are classified as first-line drugs comprising ACEIs, ARBs, CCBs and diuretics. Other drugs effective in lowering BP include adrenergic receptor antagonists, central sympatholytics and vasodilators (Flowchart 32.1).

I. ACE Inhibitors

Mechanism of BP-lowering action

ACE inhibitors (ACEIs) lower BP (Fig. 32.3) by decreasing the peripheral vascular resistance (PVR) through the following mechanisms:

a. ACE inhibitors decrease the formation of the octapeptide angiotensin II, which is a vasoconstrictor. So, angiotensin II-mediated vasoconstriction decreases, resulting in reduced PVR.
b. Reduced levels of angiotensin II lead to feedback increase in renin release. This leads to increased angiotensin I production which cannot be converted to angiotensin II (because of ACE inhibition). This angiotensin I gets diverted to enzyme ACE 2, leading to the formation of a heptapeptide—angiotensin (1–7). Angiotensin (1–7) has vasodilator (VD) activity and may contribute to the BP-lowering action of ACE inhibitors. ACE 2 is not inhibited by currently available ACE inhibitor drugs.
c. ACEIs inhibit the breakdown of bradykinin, increasing its levels. Bradykinin is a potent VD and works at least in part by stimulating the release of NO and PGI_2. The bradykinin-receptor antagonist icatibant blunts the BP-lowering effect of captopril.
d. Reduced A-II decreases aldosterone release → reduction in Na^+ reabsorption, which causes reduction in fluid volume and BP.

In short term, the degree of response to ACE inhibitors varies with renin activity and Na^+ levels. ACE inhibitors cause only a modest fall in BP in normotensive, Na^+-replete individuals; however, when renin levels are high (as seen in renovascular hypertension), the fall in BP is

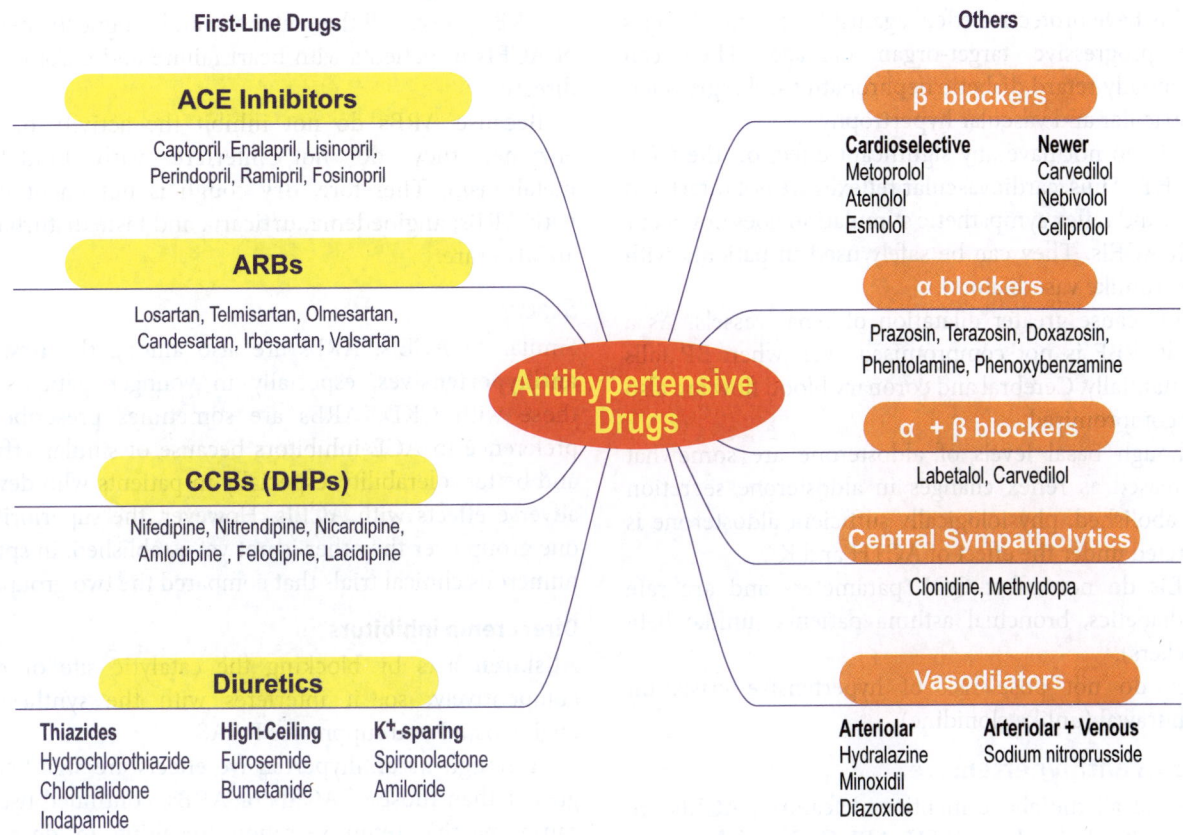

Flowchart 32.1 Classification of antihypertensive drugs

marked. Such a marked fall in BP is also seen in patients with Na$^+$ depletion (due to salt-restricted diet or use of diuretics), malignant/accelerated hypertension, and CHF. In such situations, therapy should be initiated with small doses. However, after long-term use, there is no correlation between plasma renin activity and magnitude of fall in BP with ACE inhibitors.

Advantages

- Dilatation of the arterioles caused by ACEIs, increases the compliance of larger arteries, which lowers total peripheral resistance (TPR) and hence BP. However, there is little dilatation of capacitance vessels. Thus, postural hyertension is not a problem while using ACEIs (unlike α-blockers).

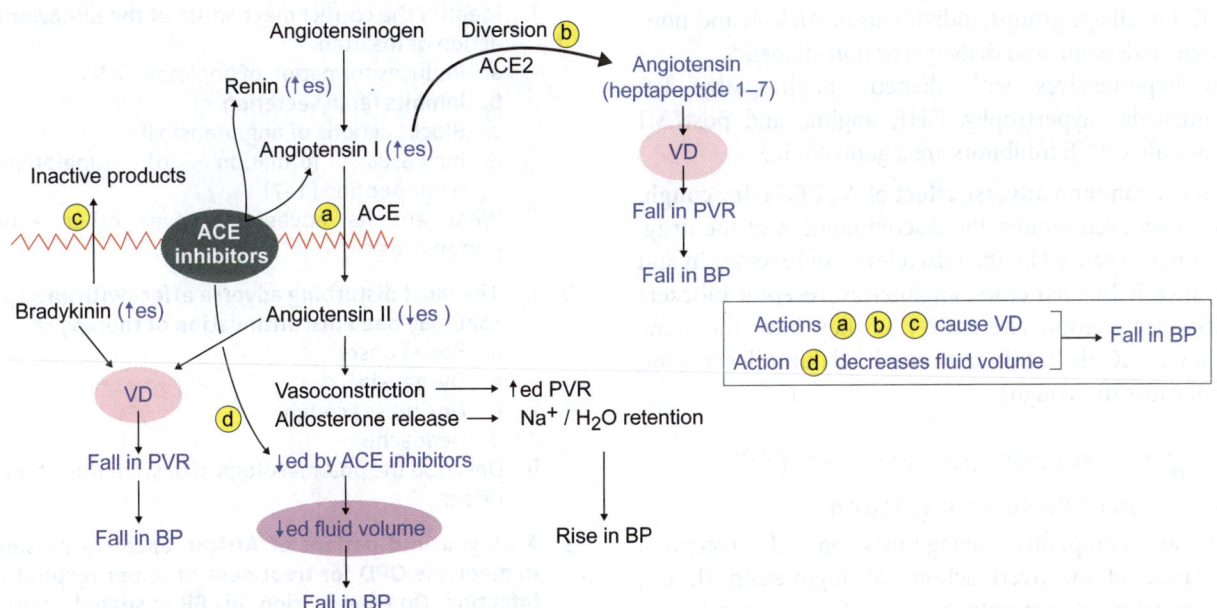

Fig. 32.3 Mechanism of BP-lowering action of ACE inhibitors

- ACEIs have protective effect against long-term changes and progressive target-organ damage. They can potentially retard diabetic nephropathy and regress left ventricular and vascular hypertrophy.
- ACEIs do not have any significant effect on the COP and HR. Thus, cardiovascular reflexes are not interfered with, and reflex sympathetic stimulation does not occur with ACEIs. They can be safely used in patients with IHD (unlike vasodilators).
- ACEIs cause greater dilatation of renal vessels. As a result, RBF is not compromised even when BP falls substantially. Cerebral and coronary blood flow are also not compromised.
- Although basal levels of aldosterone are somewhat decreased as reflex changes in aldosterone secretion are abolished, physiologically sufficient aldosterone is secreted under the effect of ACTH and K^+.
- ACEIs do not affect QOL parameters and are safe in diabetics, bronchial asthma patients (unlike beta blockers).
- They do not pose risk of hypertensive crisis on withdrawal (unlike clonidine).

Status as antihypertensive

Because of all the above mentioned features, ACEIs are among the **1st choice drugs (ESH, API, JNC guidelines)** for all grades of essential as well as renovascular hypertension. These are preferred in patients < 60 years of age, as they appear to be more effective in younger patients than elderly.

- ACEIs are the most suitable drugs in patients of hypertension with chronic kidney disease (CKD). JNC guidelines recommend initiating pharmacotherapy with ACEIs in **hypertensives with CKD**, irrespective of their age and race. In other words, pharmacological treatment with ACEIs is begun in hypertensives with CKD of all age groups, individuals of African and non-African descent, and diabetics or non-diabetics.
- In hypertensives with diabetic nephropathy, left ventricular hypertrophy, CHF, angina, and post MI cases also, ACE inhibitors are a good choice.

The most common **adverse effect of ACEIs is dry cough**, which may even require the discontinuation of the drug. Dry cough is caused by the raised levels of bradykinin and substance P. In such cases, angiotensin receptor blockers (ARBs) are a good alternative, as they have the same efficacy as ACEIs but do not raise bradykinin levels (and do not cause dry cough).

II. Angiotensin Receptor Blockers (ARBs)

Mechanism of BP-lowering action

ARBs are competitive antagonists on AT_1 receptors and block all the overt actions of angiotensin II, i.e., vasoconstriction, sympathetic stimulation, aldosterone release, central actions, renal actions and growth-promoting actions on the heart and blood vessels.

ARBs possess all the metabolic and prognostic benefits of ACEIs in patients with heart failure and chronic renal disease.

Because ARBs do not inhibit the activity of ACE enzyme, they do not interfere with bradykinin metabolism. Therefore, dry cough is not encountered with ARBs; angioedema, urticaria and taste disturbances are also rare.

Status

Similar to ACEIs, ARBs are also among the **first-line antihypertensives**, especially in younger patients and those with CKD. ARBs are sometimes prescribed in preference to ACE inhibitors because of similar efficacy and better tolerability, especially in patients who develop adverse effects with ACEIs. However, the superiority of one group over the other is not yet established, in spite of numerous clinical trials that compared the two groups.

Direct renin inhibitors

Aliskiren acts by blocking the catalytic site of renin competitively; so, it interferes with the synthesis of angiotensin I and suppresses RAAS.

Although its antihypertensive effects are significantly greater than those of ACEIs or ARBs, continued use can cause reactive renin secretion, resulting in decreased effectiveness.

RAAS-inhibiting drugs are contraindicated in pregnancy, hyperkalemia (K^+ > 5.5 mmol/L), bilateral renal artery stenosis and past history of severe angio-neurotic edema.

Clinical problem-based questions and MCQs

1. **A patient with Grade 2 hypertension is prescribed losartan 50 mg daily.**
   i. Identify the correct mechanism of the BP lowering action of losartan.
      a. Reduces formation of angiotensin II
      b. Inhibits renin secretion
      c. Blocks actions of angiotensin II
      d. Increases formation of angiotensin heptapeptide (1–7)
   ii. What are its advantages over other antihypertensives?

2. i. **The most disturbing adverse effect with enalapril that may need discontinuation of therapy is**
      a. Bowel upset
      b. Dysgeusia
      c. Dry, brassy cough
      d. Headache
   ii. Describe the pharmacological basis of this adverse effect.

3. **A 45-year-old patient of African ancestry presents in medicine OPD for treatment of upper respiratory infection. On examination, his BP in seated position was 146/94. The patient was prescribed treatment for URTI and called for follow-up after 2 days. On**

follow-up examination, his BP was 146/92. Patient was advised to sit in a chair with back supported, feet flat on ground, and relax for 3–5 minutes. BP was measured again, twice at a gap of 2–3 minutes. Average of last two readings was 146/92.
  i. Can this patient be labelled as hypertensive?
  ii. If yes, what is the grade of hypertension?
  iii. How this patient should be managed?
  iv. What are the first-line drugs for him?

4. Identify the coexistent condition (a compelling indication) in a young hypertensive that favours use of ACE inhibitors as first-line drugs.
  a. Chronic kidney disease
  b. Chronic obstructive pulmonary disease
  c. Bilateral renal artery stenosis
  d. Hyperkalemia

III. Calcium Channel Blockers (CCBs)

Mechanism of BP-lowering action

CCBs include dihydropyridines (nifedipine, nitrendipine, nicardipine, amlodipine, felodipine, lacidipine, clevidipine, etc.) and non-dihydropyridines (diltiazem and verapamil). They lower BP by decreasing the PVR via the following mechanisms:

- In cardiac and smooth muscles, voltage-gated L-type calcium channels maintain normal resting tone and contractile response. Binding of CCBs to the channel decreases the frequency of channel opening in response to depolarisation, resulting in a marked decrease in calcium current and long-lasting relaxing effect. Vascular smooth muscles are most sensitive to the relaxing effect of CCBs. Among blood vessels, arterioles are more sensitive to the relaxing effect of CCBs than veins. Thus, they decrease peripheral vascular resistance (afterload) and BP. Vasodilator effect of DHPs > verapamil > diltiazem.
- In cardiac muscle, CCBs decrease heart rate and contractility in a dose-dependent manner; cardiac output is not significantly compromised as direct effects on the heart are modified by reflex response to fall in BP.
- In addition to the calcium channel blocking effect, verapamil and diltiazem have a nonspecific anti-adrenergic effect, and block K⁺ channels also. This contributes to their anti-arrhythmic action.

Differences among CCBs

- Among CCBs, the dihydropyridines (**DHPs**) have more effect on **vascular smooth muscles than on the heart**. So, the fall in PVR and BP results in reflex tachycardia.
- In contrast, verapamil has less vasodilator than cardiac effects. The direct cardio-depressant effect is partially countered by reflex effects that are induced by its vasodilator effects; however, verapamil still causes decrease in heart rate, atrio-ventricular conduction and contractility.
- This difference in extent of effect of different CCBs on heart and blood vessels explains why β blockers like **propranolol can be combined with DHPs but not with verapamil**. Propranolol can lower the heart rate that is raised by the reflex effects of DHPs. However, the combined use of propranolol and verapamil (both cardio-depressants) can cause sinus depression, atrio-ventricular blocks and even asystole. Diltiazem should also be avoided in patients with sick sinus or conduction defects. Its combination with β blockers should preferably be avoided or limited to low doses.
- There are **no contraindications** to the use of DHPs. However, in patients with tachyarrhythmias, Class III or IV heart failure, and severe leg edema, CCBs should be used very cautiously. Short-acting preparations of DHPs are reported to worsen angina and increase mortality in post-MI cases; so, short-acting nifedipine preparations are not recommended. Long-acting DHPs, such as amlodipine, are preferred as these provide smooth control of BP. Cilnidipine is useful in hypertension with tachycardia as it reduces sympathetic outflow by blocking N-type calcium channels. Clevidipine is an ultrashort-acting DHP used by IV infusion for reducing BP in critical care settings.

  Verapamil and diltiazem are contraindicated in sino-atrial/AV block, severe left ventricular dysfunction with ejection fraction < 40%, and bradycardia when HR is < 60 bpm.

Status

- Calcium channel blockers are still among the **first-line drugs** for the treatment of hypertension (ESH, API, JNC guidelines). They are especially recommended in **elderly individuals (> 60 years), those with low renin activity, in diabetics, post-stroke patients and in individuals of African descent.**
- ESH guidelines recommend starting the treatment of Stage 2 hypertension with a combination of 2 drugs (ACE inhibitor/ARB + CCB, in a fixed dose combination (FDC)).
- Nicardipine has rapid onset and short duration of action; IV infusion is used in hypertensive emergencies like ischemic/hemorrhagic stroke, aortic dissection and pre-eclampsia. CCBs are most useful in patients with cyclosporine-induced hypertension after renal transplant.
- All CCBs can lower BP, but **DHPs** are preferred because the negative dromotropic action of verapamil/diltiazem can worsen CHF and conduction defects.
- CCBs are among the **first-line antihypertensives** because of their efficacy, good tolerability, favourable kinetics and long-term benefits.
  - CCBs have favourable kinetics as the anti-hypertensive effect is quick in onset and a once-daily dose of long-acting drugs is sufficient to provide round-the-clock BP control.
  - CCBs have better tolerability in comparison to other antihypertensive drug groups. CCBs do not

cause fluid retention despite vasodilatation (unlike vasodilators), affect quality of life parameters or plasma lipid profile (unlike β blockers), or disturb electrolyte balance (unlike diuretics). They have no adverse effects on the fetus in utero (unlike ACEIs/ARBs) and can be used in hypertensives having angina, asthma or PVD.
- CCBs have long-term benefits; amlodipine alone or
- with an ACEI is reported to reduce cardiovascular events in high-risk hypertensive patients, reduce albuminuria and slow down disease progression in nephropathy (hypertensive/diabetic). CCBs also have stroke-preventing potential.

IV. Diuretics

Thiazide diuretics such as hydrochlorothiazide, chlorthalidone and indapamide are useful as antihypertensives. Loop diuretics like furosemide and bumetanide also have a role in severe cases having edema/CHF/renal failure. K^+-sparing diuretics are also used to prevent hypokalemia with thiazides/furosemide.

Mechanism of BP-lowering action

- **Thiazide diuretics** reduce ECF volume and COP initially → PVR may increase in response to reduced COP.
- In 6–8 weeks, compensatory mechanisms regain ECF volume and COP, but the fall in BP is maintained. This reduction in BP, developing over a period of few weeks of diuretic use is attributable to a small but persistent Na^+ and volume deficit.
  Decreased Na^+ concentration in vascular smooth muscles, associated with thiazide use causes:
  - Reduced stiffness of vessel walls
  - Reduced responsiveness of vascular smooth muscles to catecholamines and angiotensin II
  - Increased compliance of blood vessels.

Therefore, **total peripheral resistance decreases** in spite of raised plasma renin activity; this results in fall of BP. Dietary salt restriction also has a similar effect on blood vessels.

Sodium depletion theory of antihypertensive effect of thiazides is confirmed by their reduced efficacy in patients who do not observe dietary salt restrictions (diuretics fail to lower total peripheral resistance if sodium levels are high).

- **Loop diuretics** such as furosemide cause brisk diuresis, reduced ECF volume, cardiac output and BP. After brisk diuresis lasting for 4–6 hours, compensatory responses cause increased tubular reabsorption of Na^+. Therefore, the Na^+-depleted state cannot be maintained round-the-clock and **total peripheral resistance is not reduced by loop diuretics**. Moreover, loop diuretics have greater potential to cause adverse effects. Routine use of loop diuretics is still not recommended in uncomplicated hypertension because they are short acting. Nevertheless, they are indicated in hypertensives with coexisting CHF, chronic renal failure, or other edematous conditions, and those receiving vasodilator therapy.

- K^+-**sparing diuretics**, or aldosterone antagonists like spironolactone prevent K^+ loss with thiazides, and also have a role in preventing hypertension-related ventricular and vascular hypertrophy. Current guidelines recommend the use of spironolactone with ACEIs/ARBs, thiazide diuretics and CCBs if the target BP is not achieved. However, when used with ACEIs/ARBs, the risk of hyperkalemia must be considered, and K^+ levels should be carefully monitored.

Status

Diuretics are still among the **first-line drugs** for hypertension. ESH guidelines recommend using **thiazide diuretics in combination with ACEI/ARBs as Step 1**. They are also recommended **in Step 2 as the 3rd agent** if the combination of **ACEIs/ARBs and DHPs fails** to provide adequate response. This combination controls hypertension in up to 90% of patients. Thiazide diuretics are especially **preferred in elderly individuals**.

Diuretics continue to be the **first-line drugs** because of:

- their efficacy in all grades of hypertension, alone or with other groups of drugs
- convenient once-daily dose regimen
- lack of postural hypotension
- no tolerance to their effect
- low cost.

However, the **disadvantages** of diuretics include risk of hypokalemia, hypomagnesemia, impaired glucose tolerance, and dyslipidemia. Thiazides are contraindicated in hyponatremia and chronic kidney disease due to obstructive uropathy and hypersensitivity to sulphonamides. Diuretics should be cautiously used in gout, metastatic cancer, hypokalemia, hypercalcemia, impaired glucose tolerance and pregnancy.

Clinical problem-based questions and MCQs

5. i. A 68-year-old male patient visits medicine OPD for a routine medical check-up. BP= 146/92. Patient is diagnosed as moderate essential hypertension. No other abnormality is detected on examination and investigations. Which of the following is the preferred diuretic for this case?
   a. Chlorthalidone b. Furosemide
   c. Eplerenone   d. Benzthiazide
   ii. Describe the mechanism of BP-lowering action of the selected drug.
   iii. Explain the pharmacological basis for your choice of drug.
   iv. Comment on the status of the selected drug in the management of hypertension in current clinical practice.

6. Loop diuretics are called high-ceiling diuretics and produce brisk diuresis, but are not preferred for the routine treatment of uncomplicated hypertension.
   i. Explain the pharmacological basis for the above statement.
   ii. Enumerate the conditions where loop diuretics are prescribed as antihypertensive.
7. Aldosterone antagonists offer several benefits in hypertensives. Comment on their role in the management of hypertension.
8. Identify the CCB used as IV infusion in hypertensive emergencies.
   a. Amlodipine   b. Short-acting nifedipine
   c. Nicardipine   d. Felodipine
9. i. Which of the following is the preferred drug class for cyclosporine-induced hypertension?
      a. Selective α_1-blockers
      b. Calcium channel blockers
      c. Vasodilators   d. Diuretics
   ii. Describe the mechanism of hypotensive effect of the selected drug class.
   iii. Comment on the status of the selected drug class in the treatment of hypertension.

V. β blockers

Mechanism of BP-lowering action

Propranolol is a nonselective β-blocker (Fig. 32.4) that blocks all subtypes of β-receptors. Metoprolol, atenolol, acebutolol, esmolol are cardioselectve β blockers. Drugs such as carvedilol, nebivolol have additional vasodilator action.

1. β_1 blockade → cardiac-depressant action → reduction in COP → reduction in SBP.
2. Decreased renin release in response to catecholamines → RAAS-activity suppressed → contributes to lowering of BP.
3. In addition, β blockers reduce secretion of noradrenaline from sympathetic nerve endings, and also reduce central sympathetic outflow. These actions contribute to their BP-lowering action.
4. β_2 blockade → vascular β_2-receptors mediate smooth muscle relaxation and vasodilatation. Initially, β_2 blockers prevent this vasodilatation → rise in PVR → rise in DBP.

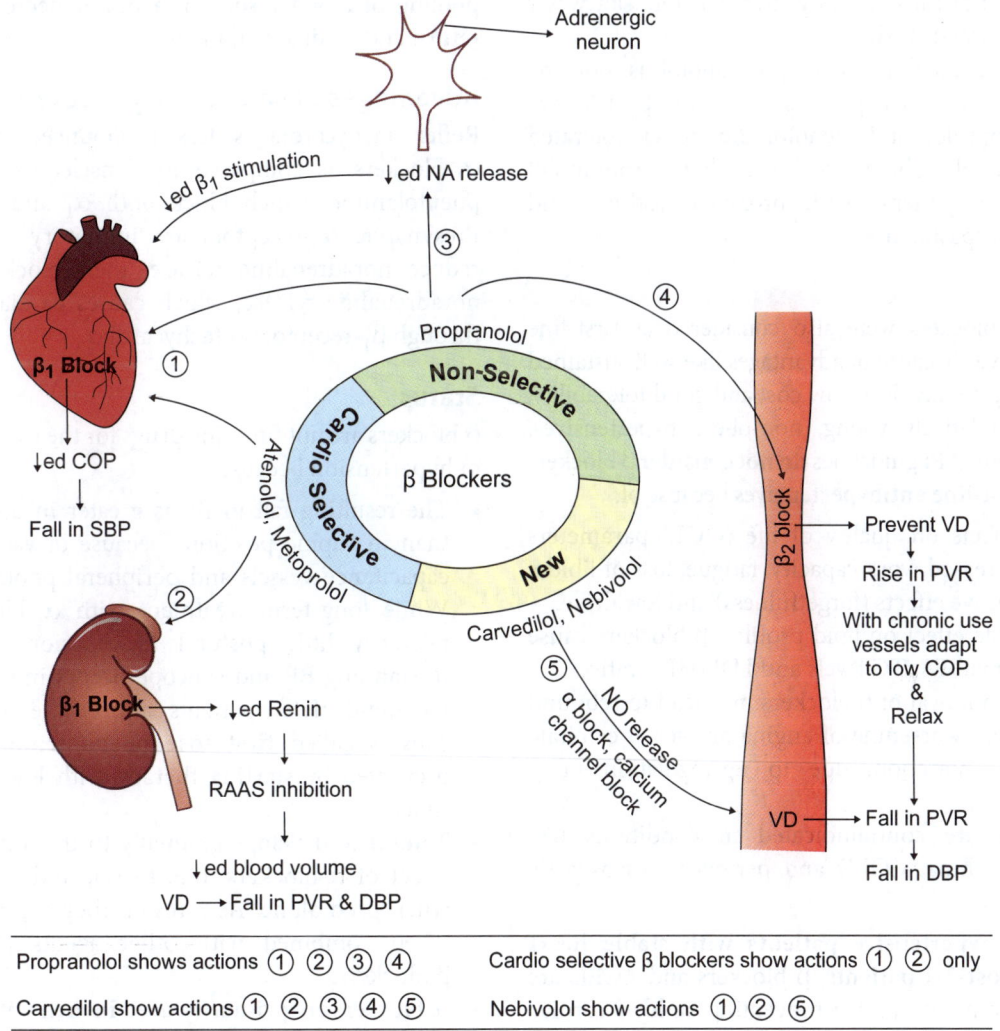

Fig. 32.4 Mechanism of BP-lowering action of β-blockers

Thus, on initiating therapy with β blockers SBP falls but DBP rises. Upon continued use of β blockers, the COP remains low but gradually blood vessels adapt to this chronically reduced COP and relax. Therefore, with continued use of β blockers, the peripheral resistance falls resulting in fall in DBP.

Cardioselective β blockers like atenolol and metoprolol are as potent as propranolol in blocking $β_1$ receptors, resulting in reduced cardiac output and systolic blood pressure. They also reduce renin release, resulting in reduced DBP. However, their $β_2$ receptor blocking effect is negligible; thus, $β_2$ mediated vasodilatation is not blocked by metoprolol and atenolol. Metoprolol is safer than propranolol in hypertensive patients with bronchial asthma and peripheral vasospastic disease.

5. New β blockers have additional mechanisms for vasodilatation, such as $α_1$ blockade (labetalol and carvedilol), NO release (nebivolol and celiprolol), and calcium channel blockade (carvedilol) that contribute to their BP-lowering action.

The hypotensive response to β blockers develops in 1–3 weeks, and then it is well maintained with a single daily dose. They do not cause postural hypotension, salt water retention or bowel disturbance.

In current clinical practice, propranolol is not the preferred β blocker for hypertension. Cardio/$β_1$ selective blockers metoprolol and atenolol are better tolerated than propranolol. These are safer than propranolol in hypertensive patients with bronchial asthma and peripheral vasospastic disease.

Status

Previously, β blockers were also considered as first-line antihypertensives because of advantages like well sustained effect with single daily dose, low cost and good tolerability, especially in relatively young, non-obese hypertensives. However, current API guidelines **do not consider** β blockers **among the first-line antihypertensives** because of:

- Adverse effects on quality of life (QOL) parameters such as decreased work capacity, fatigue, loss of libido, subtle cognitive effects (forgetfulness) and low drive.
- Unfavourable effect on lipid profile—β blockers cause rise in plasma FFA, TG levels and LDL/HDL ratio.
- Sudden withdrawal of β blockers may lead to rebound hypertension, worsening of angina or even precipitate myocardial infarction, due to up-regulation of β receptors
- β blockers are contraindicated in conditions like bronchial asthma, COPD and peripheral vasospastic diseases.

However, in **hypertensive patients with stable heart failure and post-MI patients,** β blockers and ACEIs are the most effective drugs for preventing sudden cardiac death. ESH 2023 guidelines recommend the use of β blockers (metoprolol/bisoprolol/carvedilol/nebivolol) **as monotherapy** or **combination therapy** at any step.

Esmolol has rapid onset and short duration of action, and its effect can be easily titrated by regulating the rate of infusion. Thus, it can be used as 0.5 mg/kg bolus IV injection, followed by IV infusion at the rate of 50–200 mcg/kg/min **in hypertensive emergencies,** such as aortic dissection, where cardiac work and contractility needs to be reduced.

VI. α blockers

Phentolamine and phenoxybenzamine are non-selective alpha blockers. Prazosin, terazosin and doxazosin are selective $α_1$-blockers.

Mechanism of BP-lowering action

By their $α_1$-blocking action, these drugs cause the vasodilatation of both arterioles (resistance vessels) and venules (capacitance vessels); however, the effect on resistance vessels is predominant. Therefore, α blockers cause a significant reduction of the total peripheral resistance that is responsible for their BP-lowering effect. However, dilatation of capacitance vessels and peripheral pooling of blood results in a minor decrease in venous return and cardiac output also.

Advantages of selective $α_1$-blockers

Reflex tachycardia is less pronounced with selective $α_1$-blockers as compared to nonselective blockers like phentolamine, which block both $α_1$ and $α_2$ receptors. Presynaptic $α_2$-receptors are inhibitory in nature and reduce noradrenaline release; their blockade increases noradrenaline release, which causes cardiac stimulation through $β_1$-receptors → tachycardia.

Status

α blockers are not first-line drugs for the routine treatment of hypertension because:

- The resulting fall in BP is greater in upright posture than in supine position (because of vasodilatation of capacitance vessels and peripheral pooling of blood). While long-term treatment with $α_1$-blockers causes relatively little postural hypotension, excessive fall in standing BP and syncope occurs in some salt- and volume-depleted patients shortly after the first dose. This is called **first-dose phenomenon** and can be prevented by starting therapy with low doses at bed time.
- **Tolerance** develops gradually to the antihypertensive effect of α-blockers, due to salt and H_2O retention, when used alone. As a result, they are more effective when combined with other agents like diuretics/β blockers.
- α-blockers are **primarily used in men with concurrent hypertension and benign prostatic hyperplasia**

(BPH), because of their beneficial effect in men with BPH and bladder obstruction symptoms.
- ESH 2023 guidelines recommend adding α-blockers (or spironolactone or β blockers or a centrally acting agent) in **resistant hypertension with CKD**, if a combination of the three first-line drugs (ACEI/ARBs, DHP and thiazide diuretic) fails to adequately control BP.
- The nonselective α-blockers (e.g., phentolamine and phenoxybenzamine) are used in diagnosis and treatment of **pheochromocytoma**, respectively.
- In **emergency** situations like clonidine withdrawal and cheese reaction phentolamine is useful.

VII. α+β Blockers
a. Labetalol
Labetalol is a combined $α_1$, $β_1$, and $β_2$ blocker that reduces BP mainly by decreasing total peripheral resistance. It is faster-acting than pure β blockers. Due to its rapid onset of action, labetalol is administered intravenously in **emergency situations** involving catecholamine excess to quickly reduce blood pressure. Such situations include pheochromocytoma, cheese reaction, clonidine withdrawal syndrome, and eclampsia. It is considered **safe for use during pregnancy**.

Oral labetalol is given in a dose of 100–200 mg, twice a day. It has the adverse effects of both α- and β blockers.

b. Carvedilol
It possesses weak $α_1$-blocking, nonselective β blocking, calcium channel blocking, and antioxidant/free radical scavenging properties. It reduces mortality in patients with heart failure and is particularly useful in patients with both **heart failure and hypertension** because of its cardio-protective action. Treatment is started with a dose of 6.25 mg (twice a day) and can be gradually increased up to 25 mg, twice a day.

VIII. Central Sympatholytics
a. Clonidine
Mechanism of antihypertensive action

Clonidine is a selective agonist at $α_{2A}$ receptors present in the brainstem (especially pre-junctionally) and vasomotor centre in the medulla (post-junctional). $α_2$ receptors are inhibitory in nature.

Clonidine causes → fall in central sympathetic outflow → reduced release of noradrenaline → fall in BP and bradycardia.

Clonidine shows the **therapeutic window phenomenon**, i.e., optimum hypotensive action occurs at plasma concentrations of 0.2–2 ng/mL. This may be attributed to activation of $α_{2B}$ receptors (excitatory in nature) that are present post-junctionally in vascular smooth muscles at concentrations > 2 ng/mL. A transient increase in BP occurs through $α_{2B}$ receptor-mediated VC.

With chronic use, the decreased COP contributes more to the fall in BP than the decreased TPR. Clonidine also inhibits noradrenaline (NA) release from peripheral adrenergic nerve endings by stimulating inhibitory pre-synaptic $α_2$ receptors; however, this effect is not significant at therapeutic doses.

Adverse effects

Clonidine can cause sedation, mental depression, sleep disturbances, dry mouth/nose/eyes, constipation, bradycardia, impotence, and salt and H_2O retention. **Clonidine withdrawal syndrome:** If the dose of clonidine is missed for 1–2 days, withdrawal syndrome results, characterised by tachycardia, restlessness, anxiety, headache, nausea, vomiting, excessive rise in BP, and sweating. Such catastrophic symptoms occur because:

- Clonidine interferes only with the release of catecholamines, not their synthesis. Thus, if a dose is missed, the inhibitory effect on catecholamine release is removed suddenly, resulting in the release of large quantities of stored catecholamines.
- During clonidine therapy, there is chronic reduction of sympathetic tone. So, in the chronic absence of agonists, the receptors become supersensitive. On the sudden withdrawal of clonidine, these supersensitive receptors respond more to the released catecholamines.

Clonidine withdrawal symptoms are controlled by potent vasodilators (sodium nitroprusside), a combination of α- and β blockers (phentolamine + propranolol or labetalol), or by reinstituting clonidine therapy.

Status

Due to its frequent side effects, risk of rebound hypertension upon abrupt withdrawal, and the need for careful dose adjustment, clonidine is considered a third- or fourth-line drug for managing hypertension. Other indications for its use are:

- To suppress sympathetic overactivity associated with opioid withdrawal and reduce craving.
- Clonidine decreases craving in alcohol withdrawal and smoking cessation also.
- Attenuates vasomotor symptoms of menopausal syndrome.
- Controls diarrhea associated with diabetic neuropathy.

Interactions

TCAs and chlorpromazine block α-receptors and abolish the antihypertensive action of clonidine.

b. Methyldopa
Methyldopa is an α-methyl analogue of dihydroxyphenylalanine (DOPA). In the brain, α-methyldopa → leads to formation of α-methylnoradrenaline that acts on central $α_2$-receptors → decreased central sympathetic outflow.

In comparison to clonidine, it causes greater decrease in total peripheral resistance than in COP or HR. Thus, it appears to act on a different population of neurons in the vasomotor centre.

Major adverse effects are sedation, persistent mental lassitude, impaired concentration, depression, vertigo, nightmares, etc.

Status

The only indication for its use is **pregnancy-induced hypertension (PIH)**, because it has a prolonged record of safety, both for the mother and fetus. It is given orally in a dose of 0.25–0.5 g, twice a day, but may be given up to four times daily as required.

Clinical problem-based questions and MCQs

10. **β Blockers were previously regarded as first-line antihypertensive agents but not so in current guidelines such as JNC 8.**
    i. Describe the mechanism of BP-lowering action of β blockers.
    ii. Cite reasons for fall in status of β blockers as antihypertensives.
    iii. In which of the following comorbid conditions are β blockers still used? (or) Identify compelling indications for the use of β blockers as antihypertensives.
       a. Stable heart failure
       b. Chronic kidney disease
       c. Pregnancy-induced hypertension
       d. COPD.
    iv. Which β blocker is most preferred in this comorbid condition
       a. Propranolol   b. Sotalol
       c. Timolol   d. Carvedilol

11. **Identify the β-blocker safe for use in pregnancy-induced hypertension.**
    a. Carvedilol   b. Timolol
    c. Labetalol   d. Atenolol

12. **Which of the following β blockers has a role in hypertensive emergency?**
    a. Carvedilol   b. Timolol
    c. Labetalol   d. Esmolol

13. **Enumerate the indications for use of α-blockers in hypertension.**

14. i. Clonidine is an adrenergic agonist, but lowers BP. Describe the mechanism of BP-lowering action of clonidine.
    ii. Why is clonidine not a preferred antihypertensive?
    iii. What are the indications for use of clonidine?
    iv. Name the most catastrophic adverse effect of clonidine and state its management.

15. i. Identify the antihypertensive drug that is safe in pregnancy.
       a. Clonidine   b. Methyldopa
       c. Esmolol   d. Prazosin

    ii. Describe the mechanism of BP-lowering action of the selected drug.
    iii. Enumerate the adverse effects of the drug selected.

IX. Vasodilators

These include:
- **Arteriolar dilators**, such as hydralazine, dihydralazine, minoxidil and diazoxide.
- **Arteriolar + venous dilators** like sodium nitroprusside.

Mechanism of BP-lowering action

All vasodilators (Fig. 32.5) relax arteriolar smooth muscles → decreased systemic vascular resistance → decreased BP.

The fall in BP elicits compensatory responses mediated via baroreceptors → sympathetic stimulation, sodium/water retention and RAAS activation. As a result, tolerance to their antihypertensive effect develops quickly—a phenomenon known as **tachyphylaxis**.

a. Hydralazine

- Hydralazine **dilates only the arterioles**, and not the veins. BP is lowered by the reduction of TPR (fall in diastolic BP > fall in systolic BP).
- The mechanism of its vasodilator action probably involves the generation of **nitric oxide (NO), reduced Ca^{2+} influx and K^+-channel opening**.
- An important drawback of hydralazine is the compensatory response elicited by the fall in BP that leads to the quick development of **tolerance** to its antihypertensive effect. These compensatory mechanisms (sympathetic stimulation, RAAS activation and Na^+/H_2O retention) can be checked by the addition of β blockers and diuretics.
- Hydralazine gets metabolised by acetylation. There exists a **genetic polymorphism in the rate of acetylation** reactions. In slow acetylators, larger doses (> 400 mg/day) of hydralazine can cause a syndrome resembling lupus erythematosus, characterised by fever, arthralgia and skin rash; this syndrome is reversible upon discontinuation of the drug.
- Other **adverse effects** include throbbing headache, facial flushing, conjunctival injection or redness, nasal stuffiness, fluid retention, edema, and CHF. In some cases, angina and MI may be precipitated; muscle cramps, paresthesia and tremors can also occur.

Status
- Hydralazine is not very commonly used because of tachyphylaxis due to compensatory mechanisms. It is only used as a **2nd line drug with β blockers and/or diuretics** in patients whose hypertension is not controlled by 1st line drugs.
- It is preferred during PIH, especially pre-eclampsia, because of its long record of safe use in pregnancy.

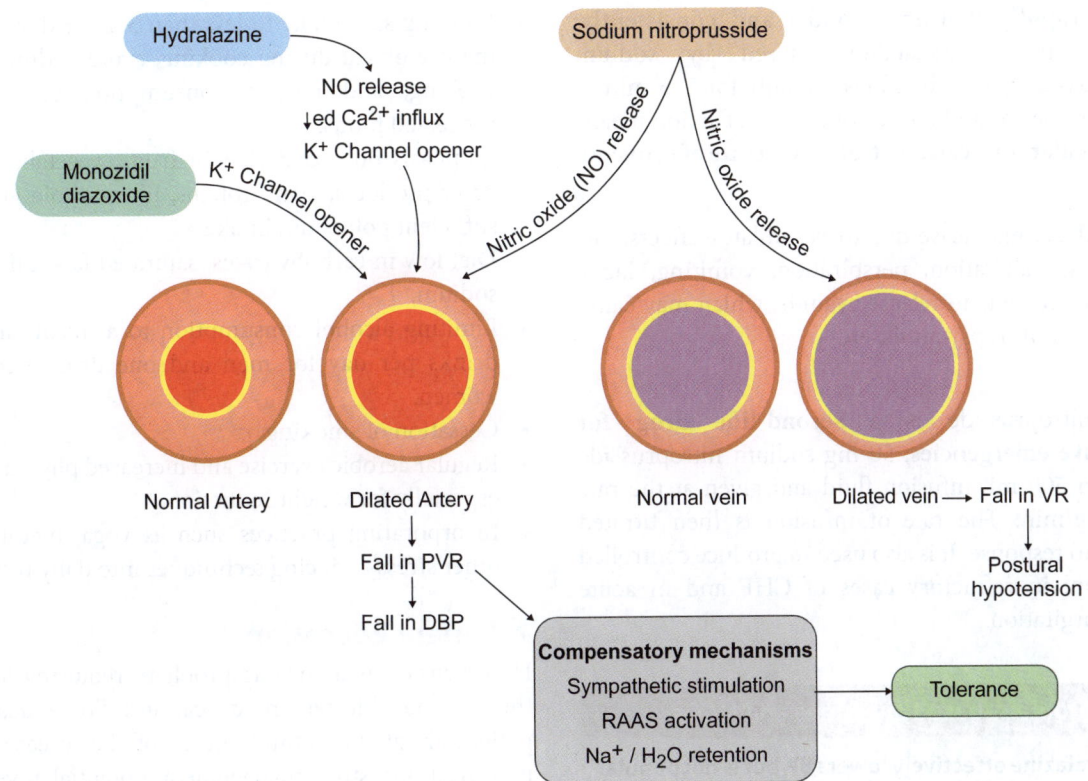

Fig. 32.5 Mechanism of BP-lowering action of vasodilators
PVR : Peripheral vascular resistance; VR : Venous return; DBP : Diastolic blood pressure; NO: Nitric oxide

- It is occasionally used parenterally in hypertensive emergencies.
- Arteriolar dilator action may be useful, when combined with isosorbide dinitrate in CHF, to lower preload and afterload.

Dihydralazine has similar actions and indications as hydralazine

b. Minoxidil

- Minoxidil is also an **arteriolar dilator** that is effective orally. Its active metabolite is minoxidil sulphate → causes **opening of K⁺ channels** in smooth muscles → hyperpolarisation of membrane → relaxation of vascular smooth muscles → vasodilatation (mainly arteriolar dilatation) → reduced TPR and BP (mainly diastolic).
- It also causes reflex sympathetic stimulation and salt/water retention as compensatory mechanisms.
- It increases hair growth by directly stimulating hair follicles and enhancing microcirculation in the vicinity of hair follicles owing to its vasodilator action.
- The only indication for its use is topical application for stimulation of hair growth in **male pattern baldness**. Topical application may cause local irritation, itching, and burning sensations.
- **Adverse effects** include marked tachycardia, palpitation, angina, edema, headache, sweating and hypertrichosis. Because it has a greater risk of precipitating angina and CHF than hydralazine, it is not in use as an oral antihypertensive.

c. Diazoxide

Diazoxide acts as a **K⁺ channel opener**, preventing the contraction of vascular smooth muscles. It causes a rapid fall in vascular resistance and mean BP, along with tachycardia and increase in COP. Diazoxide is a parenterally administered arteriolar dilator, occasionally used in the treatment of **hypertensive emergency** by rapid IV injection.

d. Sodium nitroprusside

Mechanism of VD effect

Endothelial cells and RBCs split nitroprusside both enzymatically and non-enzymatically to generate nitric oxide (NO), which relaxes vascular smooth muscles. The enzymes involved are different from enzymes producing NO from GTN; therefore, tolerance does not develop to its vasodilator action (unlike nitrates).

- It **relaxes arterioles and capacitance vessels**, reducing TPR as well as COP. Reduction in the afterload and preload improves ventricular function in heart failure.
- Myocardial work decreases due to reduced preload and afterload, but it may accentuate ischemia due to the coronary steal phenomenon (refer to page 461).

- It **acts rapidly (within seconds) and consistently**. Because the vasodilatation caused by sodium nitroprusside is very brief, lasting only for 2–5 min, it has to be used as an IV infusion; the brief action means that **vascular tone can be titrated with rate of infusion**.

ADRs
Adverse effects may arise due to vasodilator effects, i.e., nervousness, palpitation, perspiration, vomiting, lactic acidosis, etc. It splits to release cyanide, which may cause toxicity, rise in ICT, psychosis, etc.

Status
Sodium nitroprusside is a **second-line drug for hypertensive emergencies**; 50 mg sodium nitroprusside is added to 500 mL infusion fluid and given at the rate of 0.02 mg/min. The rate of infusion is then titrated according to response. It is also used to produce controlled hypotension, in refractory cases of CHF and in acute mitral regurgitation.

Clinical problem-based questions and MCQs

16. Hydralazine effectively lowers BP, but is not popular for the routine treatment of hypertension.
    i. Explain the mechanism of BP-lowering by hydralazine. Why is it not preferred in clinical practice?
    ii. Enumerate the drugs combined with hydralazine and the pharmacological basis for these combinations.
    iii. Enumerate the adverse drug reactions of hydralazine.
17. i. Which of the following is used topically?
    a. Nitroprusside   b. Hydralazine
    c. Dihydralazine   d. Minoxidil
    ii. What is the indication for topical use of the selected drug and the mechanism of its beneficial effect?
18. Why is sodium nitroprusside used in hypertensive emergencies?

MANAGEMENT OF HYPERTENSION

The **aims** of management of hypertension are:
- Gradual reduction of BP to obtain optimum BP within 3 months and to maintain the same over time.
- Prevention, reversal or delay in the progress of complications.

The management of hypertension includes non-pharmacological measures and drug therapy.

1. Non-pharmacological Measures
Non-pharmacological measures form an essential component of hypertension management at all stages. Lifestyle interventions include:

- Limiting salt intake to less than 5 g per day: minimise the use of salt during cooking, avoid adding salt after cooking, and restrict consumption of canned or processed foods.
- Emphasis on a diet rich in fruits, vegetables, low-fat dairy products, lean proteins, fiber, whole grains, and sufficient potassium intake.
- Diet low in carbohydrates, saturated fats, caffeine, and sodium.
- Limiting alcohol consumption to a maximum of two drinks per day for men and one drink per day for women.
- Cessation of smoking
- Regular aerobic exercise and increased physical activity, especially for weight reduction.
- Incorporating practices such as yoga, meditation, or other stress-reducing techniques into daily routines.

2. Patient Education
Hypertension is a chronic problem, requiring long-term therapy and lifestyle modifications. So, educating the patient about the natural course of the disease, lifestyle modifications, stress management, potential adverse drug effects, importance of compliance with treatment regimen, and regular follow-up go a long way towards achieving treatment goals. All the information should be conveyed to patients in their own language, using simple non-technical terms and in an empathetic manner. The patient's queries should be addressed properly to enable them to participate in their own treatment.

3. Pharmacotherapy
Drug therapy is the mainstay of hypertension management. In addition to BP, the patient's age, presence/absence/severity of target organ damage, presence/absence of cardiovascular risk factors, renal function, and the presence of other diseases must be considered while prescribing for a hypertensive patient. Guidelines recommend that:

- The reduction in BP should be gradual, with low doses of drugs at the beginning of therapy.
- After the BP is controlled, efforts should be made to step down therapy to decrease dose and number of drugs.
- Use of long-acting drugs allows once daily (OD) administration, which improves patient compliance and also ensures smooth, sustained control of BP.
- The current ESH guidelines (2023) recommend starting therapy with a combination of two drugs, given in a fixed-dose combination (FDC) preparation.

a. The 'high-normal' group
Patients with SBP = 130–139 or DBP = 85–89 require treatment only if there is:

- A positive family history of hypertension.

- Patient has diabetes or hypertension-mediated organ damage (HMOD).

b. For Stage 1 patients

These are patients with Grade I (BP 140–159/90–99) or Grade II hypertension (BP 160–179/100–109) who have no symptoms, no HMOD, and no CVD.

If the BP is < **150/95**, patients are advised to:

- Initiate lifestyle modification
- Have home BP monitoring (HBPM) or ambulatory BP monitoring (ABPM), if possible.
- Have at least one additional office visit within 4 weeks.

If BP is not restored to optimum level within 3 months, drug treatment is started.

If BP is > **150/95**, drug treatment is initiated immediately. Therapy is initiated with dual combination for most patients.

As per ESH 2023 (Fig. 32.6):

- **Step 1**: Dual combination of ACE inhibitors/ARBs along with CCBs/thiazide diuretic. It controls BP in up to 60% of patients.
- **Step 2** is a triple combination of ACE inhibitors/ARBs along with a CCB and thiazide diuretic. It controls BP in up to 90% of patients.
- **Step 3** involves addition of further drugs in cases of resistant hypertension not responding to the triple combination.

In patients having Stage 1–3 chronic kidney disease with a GFR > 30 mL/min/1.73 m^2, spironolactone/β-blocker/α-blocker/centrally acting agent is added to three drugs prescribed in **Step 2**.

However, in patients with CKD Stage 4–5 and GFR < 30 mL/min/1.73 m^2, chlorthalidone is the preferred agent. β- or α-blocker or a centrally acting agent may be considered.

Among resistant cases, up to 95% patients respond to such a combined therapy. The remaining patients, who fail to respond, should be referred for specialist consultation.

Monotherapy is considered only in patients with low risk hypertension with BP < 150/95, high normal BP (130–139/85–89), very high risk of CVD, advanced age, and those who are frail.

Choice of drug

The choice of drug depends on the age, concomitant risk factors, presence of other comorbidities, socio-economic factors, drug availability and the physician's past experience. For example:

- In individuals of **non-African descent**, any one among ACEIs/ARBs, CCBs, and thiazide diuretics can be chosen as the first-line drug.
- In **individuals of African descent**, therapy is initiated with either thiazide diuretics or CCBs.
- Among CCBs, amlodipine is the most frequently used drug. It has antihypertensive and anti-anginal effects and is free of metabolic adverse effects. It is recommended for elderly patients, in cases of isolated systolic hypertension and coexistent diabetes or angina.
- **Younger individuals** usually exhibit high renin activity; so, ACEI/ARBs are preferred. Older patients have low-renin hypertension—CCBs or diuretics are preferred.
- In patients with **CKD, diabetes mellitus and previous history of MI**, treatment is initiated with ACEIs/ARBs. ACE inhibitors decrease the onset and rate of progression of renal disease in patients with microalbuminuria and early CKD. However, these are contraindicated in pregnancy, bilateral renal artery stenosis and hyperkalemia.
- In hypertension with **CHF, high risk of coronary artery disease and stroke**, diuretics are preferred over other groups. Currently, low-dose thiazide therapy is recommended (12.5 mg hydrochlorothiazide) as it

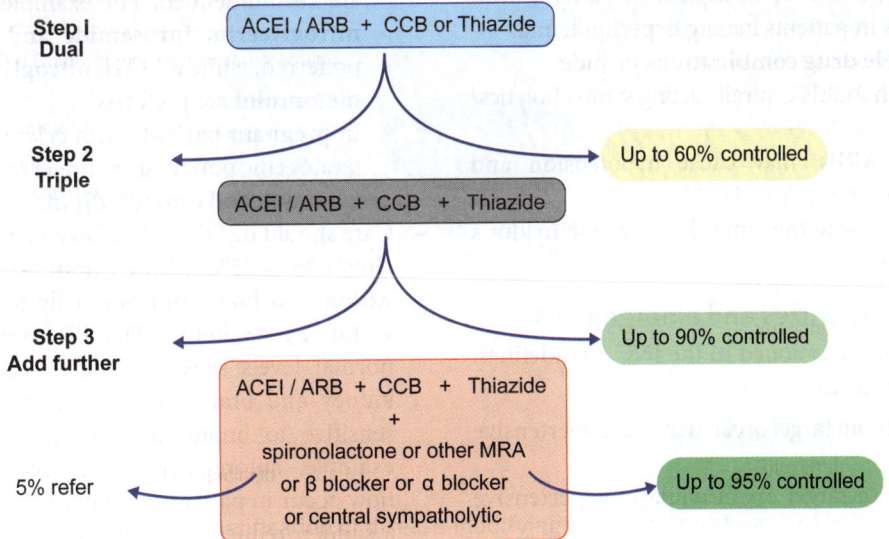

Fig. 32.6 BP control strategy as per ESH 2023 guidelines

has fewer metabolic adverse effects; chlorthalidone is preferred over hydrochlorothiazide.
- In **post-MI and stable heart failure**, β blockers are still preferred over other drug groups.
- If a **pregnant woman** develops hypertension or a hypertensive woman becomes pregnant, the drug chosen for treatment should be safe for fetus. Labetalol, methyldopa, hydralazine and nifedipine are safe in pregnancy; labetalol and methyldopa are most frequently prescribed. Nifedipine, if given, should be stopped near labour as it can relax uterine muscles and delay progress of labour.

> **Patient factors in choice of antihypertensives**
> 1. *Based on race*
>   Individuals of non-African descent: ACEIs/ARBs, CCBs, thiazide diuretics
>   Individuals of African descent: Thiazide diuretics or CCBs
> 2. *Based on age*
>   Elderly: CCBs or thiazides
>   Younger: ACE I/ARBs
> 3. *Based on comorbid conditions*
>   Chronic kidney disease: ACEIs/ARBs
>   DM and other metabolic risk factors: ACEIs/ARBs, CCBs
>   Isolated systolic hypertension: CCBs, thiazides
>   CHF: ACEIs/ARBs, thiazides
>   Angina: CCBs
>   Stable heart failure and post-MI: β blockers, especially carvedilol
>   Post MI: ACEIs/ARBs, β blockers

- **Useful drug combination in hypertension** include:
  - Drugs that have different mechanisms of action are combined, such as ACEIs with diuretics or CCBs.
  - In refractory cases, when 3 drugs are needed, ACEIs/ARBs can be combined with CCBs and thiazide diuretics.
  - Other comorbidities may require a combination of drugs, e.g., low dose of aspirin in patients with stroke, statins in patients having hyperlipidemia.
- Some **undesirable drug combinations** include:
  - β blockers with ACEIs/centrally acting sympatholytics/verapamil.
  - ACEIs with ARBs: may cause hypotension and hyperkalemia.
  - 2 drugs belonging to the same class, e.g., methyldopa with clonidine.

c. Hypertensive urgencies and emergencies

These entities are not mentioned in the JNC 8 guidelines. As per the JNC 7 guidelines:

- BP ≥ 180/120 without target organ damage: hypertensive urgency
- BP ≥ 180/120 with target organ damage: hypertensive emergency

These situations often occur in inadequately treated and noncompliant patients. Patient is usually symptomatic and may present with headache, epistaxis, dyspnea, and anxiety.

- In **hypertensive urgency**, there is no target organ damage; it is sometimes called **severe uncomplicated hypertension**. There is no need of aggressive intravenous therapy; **reinstitution or adjustment of oral medication dose** usually suffices. However, the patient should be **followed-up more frequently** (within one or few days) to see the response and modify the dose and drug as required.
- In **hypertensive emergency**, target organ damage has already occurred. It may be in the form of encephalopathy, seizures, stroke, acute myocardial infarction, acute pulmonary edema, acute aortic dissection, retinopathy, eclampsia, acute renal failure, HELLP syndrome (hemolysis, elevated liver enzymes, low platelets), etc.
- Patient is managed in ICU with **continuous monitoring** of arterial BP, fluid input/output and total body fluid volume.
- **IV drug therapy** is indicated, depending upon the type of organ damage being targeted.
  - In patients with **neurological damage,** drugs like **nicardipine and labetalol** are preferred as these do not raise ICT. Nicardipine is given as 5 mg/hour intravenous infusion. Rate can be increased, guided by the response, up to a maximum of 15 mg/hour.
  - In patients with renal damage, drugs which are not excreted by the renal route and do not have nephrotoxic effects are recommended. For instance, in **scleroderma crisis, ACEIs/ARBs** are useful; in **acute kidney injury, nicardipine and labetalol** are useful.
  - In patients with **cardiac complications,** drugs which do not have the potential to cause or worsen ischemia are recommended. For example, in CHF patients, **nitroglycerin, furosemide and nitroprusside** are preferred, while in AMI, **nitroglycerin, esmolol and metoprolol** are preferred.
  - In **pregnant patients** with eclampsia, drugs without teratogenic potential are preferred, e.g., **hydralazine, labetalol, and oral nifedipine**.
- Care should be taken to **reduce mean arterial pressure slowly by ≤ 25%** within 1 hour, to reach 160/100–110 within 2–6 hour, and gradually to the normal range within 24–48 hours. The BP should be reduced to normal levels slowly, because organs such as heart, kidney and brain contain a microcirculation that is sensitive to broad fluctuations in systemic BP. For example, autoregulatory changes in cerebral blood flow occur in patients with chronically raised BP. Thus, a sudden reduction of BP to normal levels carries the

risk of impaired cerebral perfusion and brain injury. Therefore, BP should be reduced to the normal range over a few hours to prevent organ malperfusion and malfunctioning.
- Acute aortic syndrome is the only exception to above rule, in which case BP should be immediately lowered to normal range.

Clinical problem-based questions and MCQs

19. A 37-year-old patient with low risk Stage I hypertension (BP < 150/95) was advised non-pharmacological measures along with tab Ramipril 5 mg once a day. On follow-up after one month, his BP was still not below 140/90. The physician added another BP-lowering drug to his prescription and called him for follow-up after 10 days.
    i. What are the various non-pharmacological measures?
    ii. What is the mechanism of BP-lowering action of Ramipril?
    iii. What other groups of drugs could have been prescribed to this patient as the second drug on the follow-up visit. Explain the rationale for combining these drug groups.
    iv. What drugs cannot be combined with ramipril?

20. Which of the following is the most preferred drug for patients with hypertensive emergency having neurological damage
    a. Losartan   b. Nitroprusside
    c. Furosemide   d. Nicardipine

21. Identify the condition in which BP should be quickly reduced to normal range
    a. Acute aortic syndrome
    b. Congestive heart failure
    c. Acute MI
    d. Acute renal failure

Summary

- Antihypertensives include RAAS inhibitors, CCBs, diuretics, sympatholytics, and vasodilators.
- ACEI/ARBs, CCBs and thiazide diuretics are among the first-line drugs as per ESH 2023 and API guidelines.
- **ACEIs** inhibit angiotensin II synthesis → reduced vasoconstriction, reduced aldosterone secretion and increased bradykinin and diversion of A-I to ACE 2 pathway → fall in BP.
- ACEIs can be combined with the other two first-line drugs, i.e., CCBs and diuretics, but not with ARBs, as both groups have the same mechanism of action and carry risk of hypotension and hyperkalemia.
- **ARBs** have same actions as ACEIs but do not raise bradykinin levels. These share all the short-term and long-term benefits of ACEIs, and are better tolerated. Thus, they are used in patients who develop intolerable cough with ACEIs.
- ACEIs/ARBs are preferred agents for young, non-African-descent hypertensives and those with comorbid conditions like CKD, DM, metabolic syndromes, heart failure and those with high risk of CAD.
- **CCBs** cause arteriolar dilatation > venous dilatation by blocking voltage-gated L-type calcium channels in vascular smooth muscles → fall in PVR, but no risk of orthostatic hypotension.
- CCBs are preferred in older adults and individuals of African ancestry, particularly in cases of isolated systolic hypertension accompanied by angina. Amlodipine is most frequently used drug, and short-acting nifedipine preparations should be avoided.
- DHPs are preferred over non-DHPs. Reflex tachycardia caused by DHPs can be checked with β blockers, but verapamil should not be combined with propranolol as it increases the risk of AV blocks and cardiac arrest.
- **Diuretics:** In mild-to-moderate, uncomplicated hypertension, especially in patients with edema, CHF, etc., low-dose thiazide therapy is recommended. They produce slowly developing sodium depletion that reduces PVR and BP. K^+-sparing diuretics may be used as add-on drugs in resistant cases. Furosemide does not lower PVR and is used only in patients with severe hypertension, fluid retention, edema and CHF.
- **β blockers** have lost their place among the first-line drugs, because of their adverse effects on the heart, lipid profile and QOL parameters. However, newer drugs like carvedilol are suitable for hypertension associated with stable heart failure, because of its cardio-protective action.
- α_1-**selective blockers** like prazosin and terazosin are added in resistant hypertension if three first-line drugs fail to control BP adequately. Phentolamine has a role in severe emergencies like pheochromocytoma and clonidine withdrawal syndrome.
- **Arteriodilators** like hydralazine and dihydralazine reduce TPR and are useful for short-term treatment of severe hypertension. Tolerance to their action develops quickly because of compensatory mechanisms.
- Another arteriodilator, minoxidil, is used topically in male type baldness.
- **Hypertensive emergencies** are managed by close monitoring; IV drugs like nifedipine, nicardipine, esmolol, labetalol, hydralazine and sodium nitroprusside are preferred.
- Labetalol, hydralazine and methyldopa are safe for use in pregnancy-induced hypertension.

Questions for practice

1. Classify antihypertensive drugs.
2. Comment on the status of the following drugs in hypertension.
   a. β blockers
   b. Thiazide, loop and K⁺-sparing diuretics
   c. Methyldopa
   d. Nicardipine
3. Explain why:
   a. Hydrochlorothiazide is preferred to furosemide in the treatment of hypertension.
   b. Clonidine should not be stopped suddenly.
   c. Clonidine withdrawal responds to phentolamine therapy.
   d. Although both verapamil and nifedipine are CCBs, verapamil cannot be combined with propranolol in the treatment of cardiac conditions, but nifedipine can be combined.
   e. BP should be reduced slowly in hypertensive emergencies.
4. a. Enumerate the drugs that are safe for use in pregnancy-induced hypertension and describe their mechanism of action.
   b. What are hypertensive urgencies and emergencies? Describe their management.

Hints for problem-based questions and MCQs

1. i. c. Blocks actions of angiotensin II
   ii. Refer to page 419, 420 (no cough/angioedema/dysgeusia, long-term survival benefits present, no effect on lipid profile, QOL parameters, no postural hypotension, no withdrawal crisis, safe in diabetes, asthma, IHD)
2. i. c. Dry brassy cough
   ii. Enalapril interferes with bradykinin degradation. Refer to page 420.
3. i. Yes, patient can be labelled hypertensive, as minimum 3 readings are recommended, before diagnosing patient.
   ii. Grade 1 hypertension
   iii. Counselling about lifestyle modifications and pharmacotherapy
   iv. ACE inhibitors
4. a. Chronic kidney disease: ACE inhibitors are contraindicated in bilateral renal artery stenosis and can worsen hyperkalemia. ACEIs cause dry cough, which can be disturbing to a patient of COPD.
5. i. a. Chlorthalidone
   ii. Thiazides lower BP by slowly developing a small and persistent sodium depletion → fall in TPR. Refer to page 422.
   iii. Loop diuretics do not lower TPR; K⁺-sparing are add-on drugs in cases where thiazides do not give adequate response. Among thiazides, hydrochlorothiazide, chlorthalidone and indapamide are equi-efficacious, while others like benzthiazide have lower efficacy as antihypertensives.
   iv. Among the first-line drugs as per JNC 8. Refer to page 422.
6. i. Refer to page 422.
   ii. Refer to page 422.
7. Prevent hypertension-related ventricular and vascular hypertrophy. Also prevent thiazide-induced hypokalemia. Refer page 422.
8. c. Nicardipine
9. i. b. Calcium channel blockers
   ii. Refer to page 421.
   iii. Among the first-line drugs as per JNC 8 (refer to page 421)
10. i. Refer to page 423.
    ii. Refer to page 424.
    iii. a. Stable heart failure
    iv. d. Carvedilol
11. c. Labetalol
12. d. Esmolol because of rapid onset and short duration of action.
13. Selective α₁-blockers in hypertensive men with BPH; phentolamine in emergency situations and pheochromocytoma.
14. i. Clonidine is an agonist at α₂ receptors (inhibitory). So, it lowers NE release leading to fall in BP. Fall in COP contributes more to fall in BP than fall in TPR.
    ii. Clonidine is not preferred because of its many adverse effects, clonidine withdrawal syndrome, and therapeutic window phenomenon.
    iii. Refer to page 425.
    iv. Clonidine withdrawal syndrome, managed by sodium nitroprusside and phentolamine.
15. i. b. Methyldopa
    ii. Methyl dopa → methyl NA → decreases central sympathetic outflow → fall in TPR → fall in BP
    iii Refer to page 426.
16. i. Arteriolar dilatation by NO release, reduced calcium influx, potassium channel opening → fall in PVR. Refer to page 426.
    ii. Hydralazine is combined with β blockers and diuretics to check the compensatory mechanisms and prevent rapid development of tolerance.
    iii. Headache, facial flushing, conjunctival infection. nasal stuffiness fluid retention, edema, CHF, angina.
17. i. d. Minoxidil
    ii. Male pattern baldness due to increase in micro-circulation in the vicinity of hair follicle.
18. Refer to page -- Due to rapid, consistent and titrable vasodilator action on both resistance and capacitance vessels
19. i. Refer to page 428.
    ii. By ACE inhibition.
    iii. CCBs (DHPs) or thiazide diuretics (hydrochlorothiazide/chlorthalidone/indapamide) may be combined
    iv. ARBs and beta blockers should not be combined with ACE inhibitors.
20. d. Nicardipine is preferred as it does not raise ICT.
21. a. Acute aortic syndrome.

CONCEPT MAP - ANTIHYPERTENSIVE DRUGS

CCBs
Nifedipine, Amlodipine

Action: Block L type Ca^{2+} channel
VD (DHPs > Verapamil): arteriolar > venous → fall in TPR, BP & reflex tachycardia, but no risk of orthostatic hypotension.

Cardiodepressant effect (Verapamil > Diltiazem > DHPs).

Uses: Hypertension especially in elderly, individuals of African descent with angina, arrhythmia (PSVT, AF, Af)

ADRs: Headache, flushing, constipation, ankle edema

DHPs can be combined with β blockers but not verapamil → risk of severe AV block & cardiac arrest

ACEIs / ARBs
Ramipril, Enalapril, Lisinopril, Losartan, Telmisartan, Olmesartan

Action: Prevent angiotensin II synthesis/action → fall in BP, blood volume, preload, afterload

Useful in hypertension, CHF (all grades), scleroderma crisis, diabetic nephropathy.

Preferred in young hypertensives with CKD, DM, CHF, high risk of CAD

ADRs: ACEIs cause cough, dysgeusia, angioedema, hypotension, hyperkalemia

ARBs better tolerated

Diuretics
Thiazides inhibit reabsorption of NaCl in DCT → diuresis. Over few weeks → persistent sodium depletion → reduced TPR → fall in BP.

Used in low dose in mild-to-moderate uncomplicated hypertension, as metabolic and electrolyte related ADRs are less frequent with low dose.

Loop diuretics cause brisk diuresis, useful in severe cases with fluid retention, edema, CHF

K^+-sparing diuretics used as add-on drugs

FIRST-LINE DRUGS

ANTIHYPERTENSIVE DRUGS

OTHERS

Central Sympatholytics
Clonidine
Selective α_2 agonist → reduce NA levels, not preferred because of ADRs & withdrawal reaction

Methyldopa: Safe in pregnancy

α Blockers
Selective α_1 blockers: Prazosin, Terazosin in mild-to-moderate cases
&
Phentolamine in Hypertensive emergency

Vasodilators
Arteriolar: Hydralazine reduces TPR, useful in hypertensive emergencies, safe in pregnancy.
Minoxidil used topically for alopecia

Arteriolar + Venodilator:
Nitroprusside → quick, brief action, titrable with rate of infusion, used in hypertensive emergencies

β blockers
β blockers have lost their status as first-line drugs owing to ADRs.

But still- in hypertension with stable heart failure & post-MI cases new β blockers Carvedilol, Nebivolol used

Esmolol with quick onset and brief action used IV in hypertensive emergencies as aortic dissection, where cardiac work and contractility needs reduction.

ESH 2023
Stage 1, grade 1 with BP < 150 / 95: Lifestyle modification, monitoring
Stage 1, grade 1, 2 with BP > 150/95: Drug treatment
Stage 2, grade 1, 2, 3: drug treatment

General strategy for lowering BP

Step 1: Dual combination: ACEIs/ARBs + CCBs or Thiazide
Step 2: Triple combination: ACEIs/ARBs + CCB + Thiazide
Step 3: Add further drugs: ACEIs/ARBs + CCB + Thiazide
+
Spironolactone or β blocker or α blocker or central sympatholytics.

Do not combine: ACEI with ARBs, β blockers with verapamil, 2 drugs of same class.

Safe in pregnancy: Labetalol, Methyldopa, Hydralazine, Nifedipine

SECTION 7   Drugs Acting on CVS

33 Drug Therapy of Congestive Heart Failure (CHF)

PH 4.9 Explain salient pharmacokinetics, pharmacodynamics, therapeutic uses, adverse drug reactions of drugs used for the management of heart failure. Devise a management plan for heart failure patients and describe the strategies to prevent long-term complications of heart failure.

Learning objectives

A student of MBBS phase II should be able to:
- Classify drugs used for congestive heart failure (CHF).
- Explain the mechanism of action of various drugs, based on pathophysiology of CHF.
- Enumerate adverse effects of drugs used in CHF.
- Comment on the status of various drugs in treatment of CHF.
- Enumerate contraindications of drugs used in CHF.

The function of the heart is to pump blood and ensure adequate blood supply to all tissues and organs. The heart begins beating during intrauterine life and continues to function tirelessly till the last breath. Oxygenated blood from the lungs flows to the left atrium, left ventricle, and then to all the tissues/organs; this oxygen is utilised by tissues for their metabolic needs. Thereafter, the deoxygenated blood is returned via the superior and inferior vena cava to the right atrium, right ventricle, and then to the lungs, where it gets oxygenated again; this cycle keeps on repeating. An impairment in the pumping ability of the heart reduces blood supply to tissues and also results in back pressure changes.

TYPES OF HEART FAILURE

a. Left (LHF)/right heart failure (RHF)
b. Systolic/diastolic dysfunction
c. High output/low output failure

a. **LHF:** The left ventricle fails to pump adequately → a part of blood is retained in it. So, it is unable to accept blood from left atrium and in turn from lungs → leading to **pulmonary congestion and edema.**
RHF: The right ventricle fails to pump adequately into the lungs → a part of the blood is retained in it → so, the right ventricle is unable to accept blood from peripheral veins. Thus, RHF is characterised by **peripheral edema and jugular venous distension.**
Usually, left and right heart failure do not occur as separate entities. LHF leads to RHF over time and vice versa.

b. Left ventricular failure can occur as **systolic or diastolic dysfunction.**

Systolic dysfunction is the inability of the heart to pump efficiently. It is characterised by low ejection fraction (fraction of blood present in the ventricle at the end of diastole that is pumped out during systole, i.e., ratio of stroke volume to end diastolic volume).
Diastolic dysfunction is noncompliance of the left ventricle. It receives less blood from the atria during diastole and hence pumps out less, even though the ejection fraction is normal.

c. **Low-output versus high-output failure:**
Of the two types, low-output failure is more common. Here, the metabolic demands of the body are within normal limits, but the heart is unable to meet them. It can have multiple causes such as myocardial infarction (MI), hypertension (HT) and angina.
High-output failure occurs in conditions like anemia, hyperthyroidism and arterio-venous shunts. The metabolic demands of the body are so high that even the increased cardiac output (COP) is insufficient to meet them. It is treated by correcting the underlying cause.

Grades of CHF

According to the New York Heart Association (NYHA), there are 4 classes of heart failure:

- **Class I:** Asymptomatic, no limitation in routine physical activity.
- **Class II:** Mild symptoms, slight limitation during routine physical activity.
- **Class III:** Moderately severe symptoms causing marked limitation in activity, even with less than routine activity.
- **Class IV:** Severe symptoms even during rest.

PATHOPHYSIOLOGY OF CONGESTIVE HEART FAILURE (CHF)

Congestive heart failure, or CHF, is a condition in which:

- The **heart is not able to pump a sufficient amount of blood** to meet the metabolic demands of the body. This leads to symptoms such as fatigue and reduced exercise tolerance.
- As heart is pumping out less → after systole, there is some residual blood in the ventricles each time → so, the heart also receives less blood → this leads to **back pressure changes,** i.e., an edematous state because of congestion and fluid retention. Congestion in the RHF causes peripheral edema, hepatomegaly, anorexia, nausea, vomiting, etc. In LHF, congestion causes pulmonary edema, dyspnea, orthopnea, cyanosis, bilateral crepitations, etc.
- **Compensatory mechanisms** (Fig. 33.1) are activated because the proper functioning of the heart is crucial for tissue oxygenation, function and survival. Activation of the RAAS, sympathetic stimulation, more complete reabsorption in kidney, and myocardial hypertrophy and remodelling are the main compensatory responses to reduced cardiac output. To some extent, the compensatory mechanisms succeed in restoring cardiac output. This stage is called **compensated heart failure.** In the long run, however, these mechanisms increase the work load by:
  - increasing preload (due to sodium and water retention)
  - increasing afterload (due to vasoconstriction)
  - increasing the O_2 demand of the heart (due to increased force of contraction and heart rate owing to sympathetic stimulation).
  - Myocardial hypertrophy → decreased diastolic filling.
  - Remodelling causes ventricular dilatation and changes in the geometry of ventricles.

All these changes further decrease the contractility of heart, leading to **decompensated heart failure**.

Cardiac Performance

Cardiac performance is a function of 4 primary factors—heart rate (HR), contractility, preload, and afterload.

a. **Heart rate** (HR):
   COP = Heart Rate × Stroke Volume.
   In CHF, the intrinsic contractility is low → reduced stroke volume. So, an **increase in heart rate is the first compensatory mechanism.**

b. **Force of contraction or contractility**: Intrinsic **contractility of the heart is decreased in low-output failure** because of:
   - Decreased velocity of muscle shortening
   - Decreased rate of development of intraventricular pressure (dP/dt)
   - This results in reduced SV and hence, COP.

   The force of contraction can be increased by positive inotropic drugs.

c. **Preload:** Preload is synonymous with venous return (VR) and is usually **increased in CHF** because of increased venous tone and increased blood volume. In the left ventricular function curve (Fig. 33.2), a measure

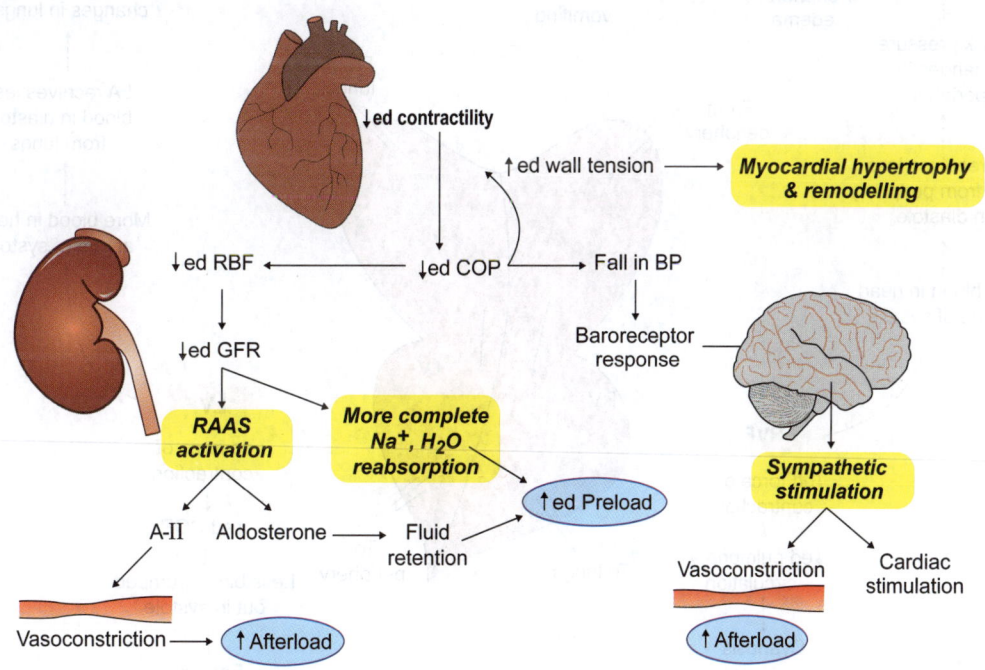

Fig. 33.1 Compensatory mechanisms in CHF

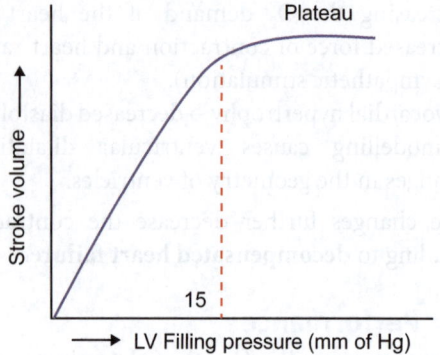

Fig. 33.2 Left ventricular function curve

of LV function (e.g., stroke volume (SV)) is plotted as a function of LV filling pressure. The curve follows Frank–Starling relation up to 15 mm of Hg filling pressure, i.e., as the filling pressure increases, SV also increases, but beyond 15 mm of Hg filling pressure, the cardiac performance plateaus, and SV does not rise any further. Thus, increased preload can increase SV up to a certain limit only; it is counterproductive beyond that point.

As a result, preload needs to be reduced; this reduction is achieved by venodilators, salt restriction, and diuretics.

d. **Afterload**: It is the resistance against which the heart must pump blood; it is represented by aortic impedance and systemic vascular resistance. In CHF, reduced cardiac output elicits compensatory mechanisms:
- Reflex sympathetic stimulation
- Activation of RAAS → formation of angiotensin II
- Endothelin → vasoconstrictor peptide

These result in vasoconstriction and **raised total peripheral resistance → raised afterload**. It can be decreased by using vasodilator (VD) drugs that decrease arteriolar tone.

Pathophysiology of CHF and causes of sign/symptoms are summarised in Flowchart 33.1.

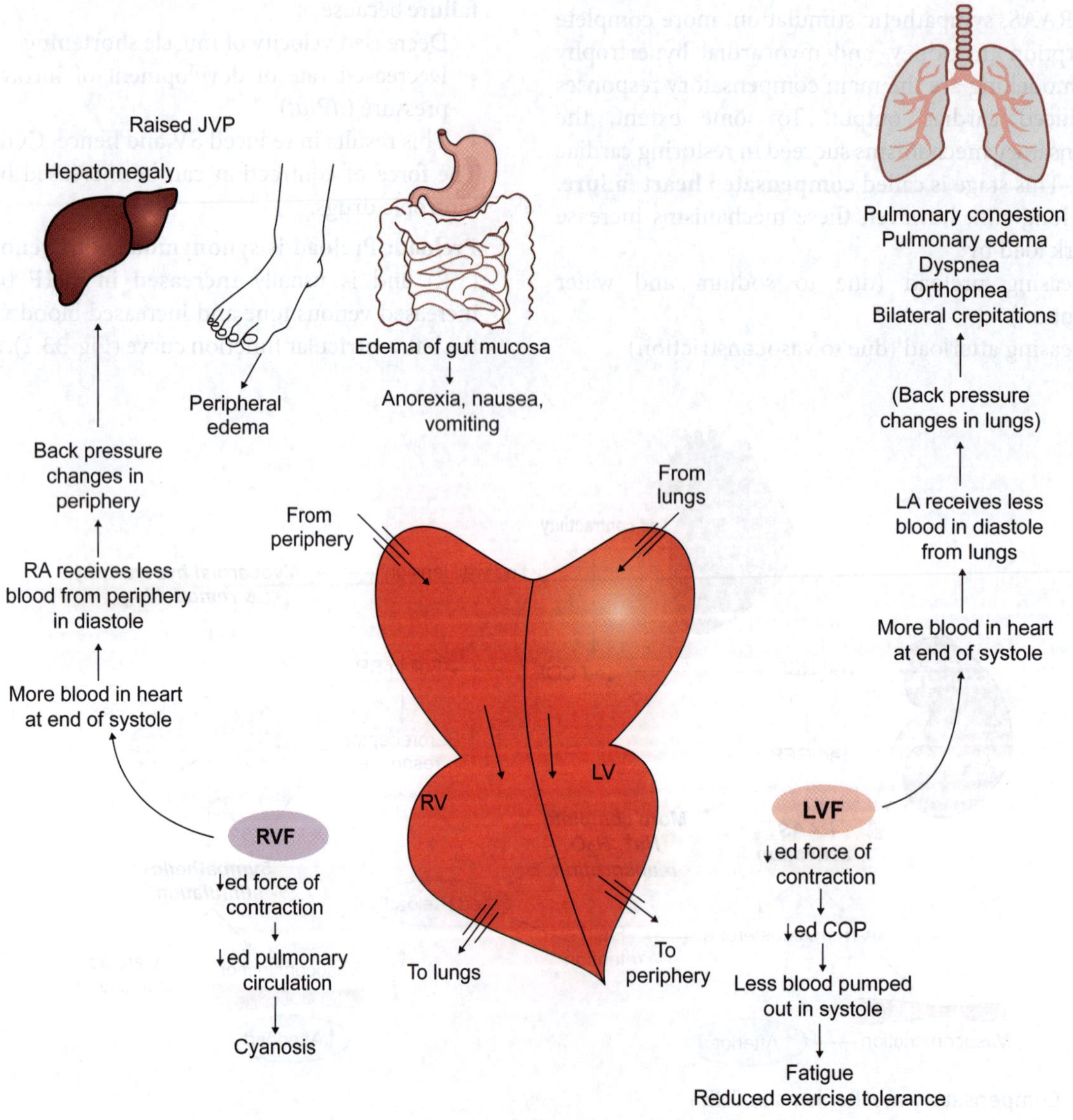

Flowchart 33.1 Pathophysiology of CHF

Thus, the main defect in heart failure is reduced heart contractility. Drugs that are beneficial in CHF act by either increasing cardiac contractility or reducing preload/afterload, resulting in improved cardiac output. An understanding of the physiological control of cardiac contractility is important for understanding the mechanism of action of these drugs.

Control of Normal Cardiac Contractility

The vigour of contraction of heart muscle is determined by several processes that lead to the interaction of calcium with the actin–troponin–tropomyosin system and movement of actin and myosin filaments, in the cardiac sarcomere. The cardiac muscle sarcomere is shown in Fig. 33.3, along with the sites of action of several drugs that alter contractility.

Site 1

Na^+/K^+-ATPase: The sodium pump causes the efflux of 3 Na^+ for influx of 2 K^+. Because it removes intracellular sodium, it is the major determinant of sodium concentration in the cell.

The sodium influx through voltage-gated channels occurring as a normal part of almost all cardiac action potentials is another determinant of intracellular Na^+ concentration.

Drugs acting at site 1: This site appears to be the **primary target of cardiac glycosides**.

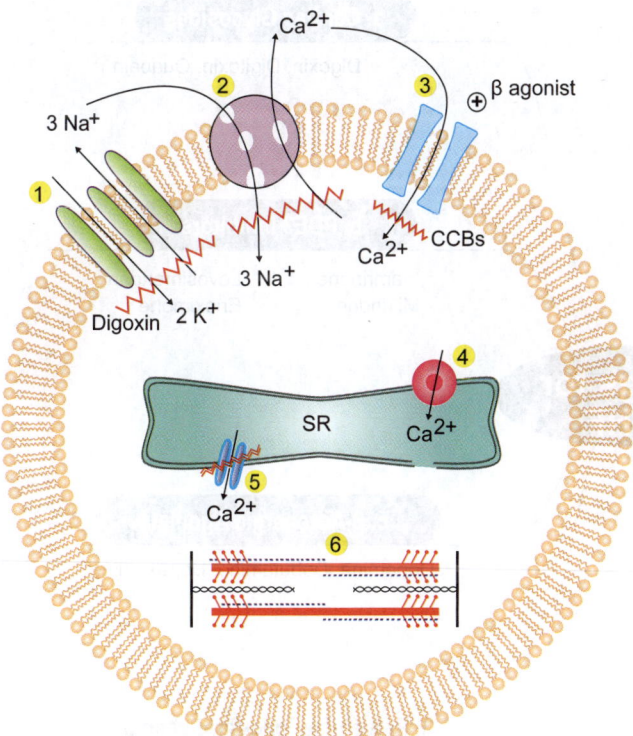

Fig. 33.3 Control of normal cardiac contractility and site of action of various drugs in CHF

Site 2

Na^+/Ca^{2+} exchanger: This antiporter uses the Na^+ gradient to move Ca^{2+} against its concentration gradient, from the cytoplasm to extracellular space. It transports 3 Na^+ ions into the cell in exchange for 1 Ca^{2+} ion moving out of the cell. This exchanger is strongly dependent on the intracellular concentration of both ions, especially Na^+, for its function.

Drugs: Cardiac glycosides such as digoxin inhibit Na^+/K^+-ATPase. When Na^+/K^+-ATPase is inhibited, Na^+ does not move out → intracellular Na^+ remains high. So, there is no need for the Na^+/Ca^{2+} exchangers to bring Na^+ into the cell → thus, the activity of the Na^+/Ca^{2+} exchanger also decreases. Hence, intracellular Ca^{2+} concentration remains high, which increases the force of contraction.

Site 3

L-type Ca^{2+} channel: The amount of trigger Ca^{2+} that enters the cell depends upon the availability of voltage-gated calcium channels and the duration of their opening.

Drugs: β agonists (sympathomimetics) increase the Ca^{2+} influx through these channels. In contrast, calcium channel blockers (CCBs) decrease Ca^{2+} influx → decreased trigger Ca^{2+} → decreased contractility.

Site 4

This is the **calcium transporter that pumps calcium into the sarcoplasmic reticulum** (SR). It maintains free cytoplasmic calcium at low levels. The amount of Ca sequestrated in the sarcoplasmic reticulum (SR) is determined in part by the amount of calcium accessible to this transporter; this, in turn, depends on the balance of:

- Ca^{2+} influx (through voltage-gated Ca^{2+} channels), and
- Ca^{2+} efflux (through Na^+/Ca^{2+} exchanger)

Therefore, the drugs affecting Ca^{2+} influx and efflux affect the amount of calcium present in the SR.

Site 5

This is a **calcium channel in the sarcoplasmic reticular (SR) membrane** that is triggered to release stored calcium. A small rise in free cytoplasmic calcium, brought about by calcium influx during the action potential (AP), triggers the opening of this calcium channel in membrane of SR and a large amount of ions are rapidly released in the vicinity of the actin–troponin–tropomyosin complex. The amount released is proportional to the amount stored in the SR and the amount of trigger calcium that enters the cell through the cell membrane.

Ryanodine interferes with release of calcium from the SR through these channels and is a potent negative inotropic agent.

Site 6

This is the **actin–troponin–tropomyosin complex** at which activator calcium brings about the contractile interaction of actin and myosin.

MANAGEMENT OF CHF

Management of CHF involves:

- Identification and treatment of **risk factors** like hypertension, infective diseases, diabetes mellitus, obesity, arrhythmias and IHD.
- **Nonpharmacological measures** such as salt restriction, weight reduction, and adherence to prescribed drugs.
- **Drug therapy:** Classification of drugs useful in CHF are shown in Flowchart 33.2.

The aim of drug therapy in CHF is:

A. Symptomatic relief and restoration of cardiac performance, achieved by:
  1. Drugs without positive inotropic action (RAAS inhibitors, diuretics, beta blockers, vasodilators, ADH antagonists, etc.)
  2. Drugs with positive inotropic action (cardiac glycosides, PDE3 inhibitors, and beta adrenergic agonists)

B. Reversing or preventing long-term changes: This can be achieved by ACEIs/ARBs, β blockers, aldosterone antagonists and neprilysin inhibitors.

1. DRUGS WITHOUT POSITIVE INOTROPIC ACTION

a. RAAS Inhibitors (ACEIs/ARBs)

Mechanism of beneficial effect in CHF

ACE inhibitors act by the following mechanisms (Flowchart 33.3).

a. ACEIs cause vasodilation by interfering with A-II formation and bradykinin inactivation, resulting in reduced preload and afterload, which improve cardiac function and control symptoms of CHF.
b. ACEIs reduce salt and water reabsorption in PCT → natriuresis → reduced plasma volume, and the reduced aldosterone secretion contribute to the reduction in cardiac preload
c. In addition, ACE inhibitors **prevent pathological remodelling** of the heart and blood vessels. These drugs prevent hypertrophy of the myocardium, apoptosis, fibrosis and intercellular matrix changes.

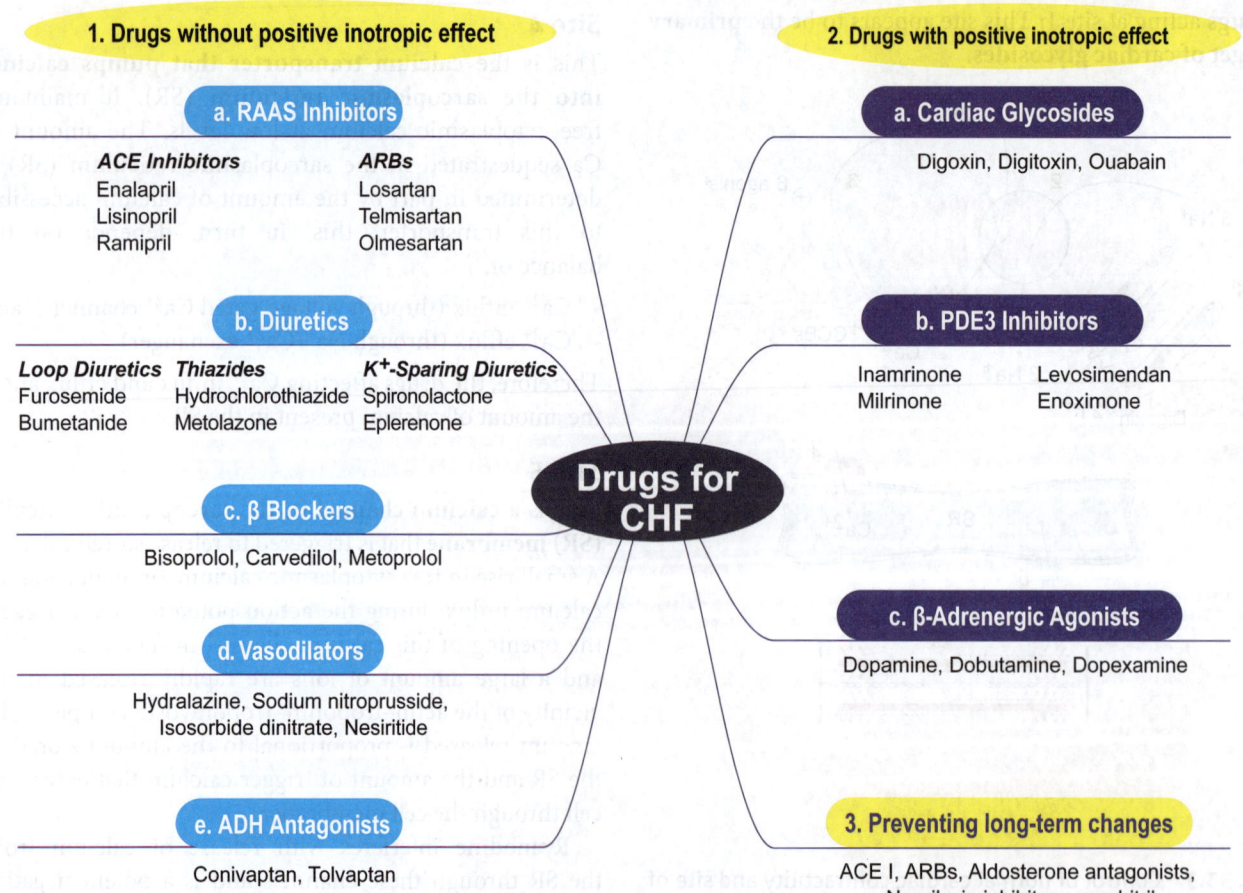

Flowchart 33.2 Drugs used in CHF

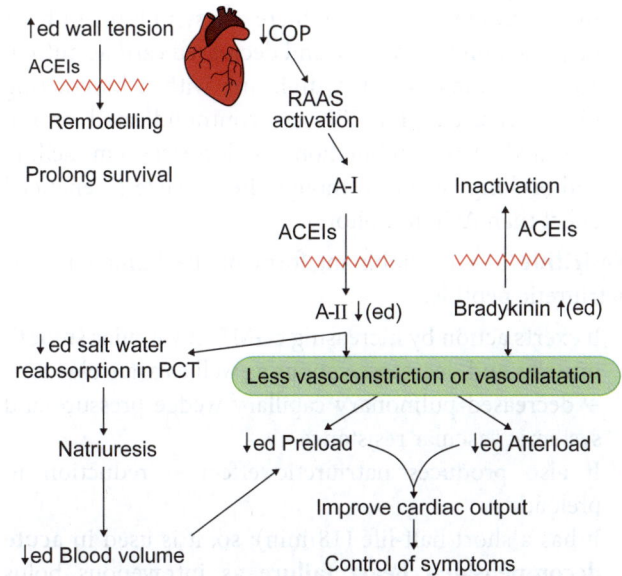

Flowchart 33.3 ACE inhibitors in CHF

They also prolong survival and **decrease mortality** due to arrhythmia, myocardial infarction and stroke.

Status: Angiotensin-converting enzyme inhibitors (ACEIs) are the **drugs of first choice** in the pharmacological management of heart failure. They are **useful in all grades of CHF** (NYHA I–IV), unless contraindicated.

Dosage

Enalapril (2.5 mg BD), lisinopril (2.5–5 mg OD), and ramipril (2.5 mg OD) are commonly used ACE inhibitors.

Angiotensin II is not the only stimulus for aldosterone secretion (there are others, such as ACTH); so, the inhibition of aldosterone secretion by ACE inhibitors is not complete. Moreover, after chronic use, aldosterone levels start returning to normal. This phenomenon is called **aldosterone escape**. Therefore **combining spironolactone (an aldosterone antagonist) with ACE inhibitors** (which decrease aldosterone secretion) is more beneficial than ACEIs alone. This combination further reduces mortality, and maintains beneficial effects on long-term survival; however, the risk of hyperkalemia must be kept in mind, and K⁺ levels should be carefully monitored in patients receiving combination of ACEIs and spironolactone.

Angiotensin receptor blockers **(ARBs) have similar beneficial effects**. While the consensus opinion is to try ACE inhibitors first, if the patient develops troubling cough/angioedema with ACEIs, then ARBs are a better substitute.

b. Diuretics

Mechanism of beneficial effect in CHF

i. Loop diuretics cause rapid or brisk diuresis → decrease in extracellular fluid (ECF) volume → decrease in venous return → **decrease in preload** on right ventricle → decrease in edema and related symptoms → reduced cardiac size → improved pump efficiency.

The brisk diuresis induced by furosemide reduces ECF volume, preload and cardiac size, resulting in improved pump efficiency and symptom relief. So, although **loop diuretics do not influence the primary disease process, these are still widely used** in the management of almost all cases of **symptomatic CHF**, where they relieve symptoms by mobilising edema fluid.

The loss of K^+, H^+, Ca^{2+} and Mg^{2+} ions that occurs with loop diuretics increases the risk of arrhythmias and digitalis toxicity (if combined). To prevent hypokalemia, loop diuretics are combined with K^+-**sparing diuretics**.

ii. Spironolactone is useful in CHF because:

- It enhances diuresis by Na^+ and H_2O excretion.
- It decreases K^+ excretion, which prevents/corrects the hypokalemia caused by loop diuretics.
- It prevents pathological remodelling of the heart by decreasing myocardial and vascular fibrosis and improves survival. There is evidence for the existence of aldosterone receptors on cardiac myocytes, which explains the usefulness of spironolactone in prevention of cardiac remodelling. It should be used in low doses of 12.5–25 mg/day only.
- It also restores the diuretic response to loop diuretics when refractoriness develops upon their chronic use.
- However, there is a risk of hyperkalemia, and K^+ levels must be monitored, especially when spironolactone is combined with RAAS inhibitors.
- Gynecomastia may occur as an adverse effect in males after long-term use.

iii. Thiazides are less frequently used in CHF. In patients with mild CHF, the combination of thiazides and spironolactone may be sufficient. However, in severe CHF, thiazides can be combined with loop diuretics, when resistance to loop diuretics develops after long-term use.

c. β blockers

As a general rule, **β blockers are contraindicated in the decompensated CHF**, because in heart failure, there is decrease in cardiac contractility and cardiac output (COP). Cardiac output is the product of heart rate and stroke volume (COP = SV × HR), Thus an increased heart rate (HR) would be necessary to maintain adequate COP in case of reduced stroke volume, due to CHF. So, β blockers which decrease heart rate and cardiac contractility can produce acute cardiac decompensation in CHF patients.

However, some β blockers like bisoprolol, carvedilol and metoprolol **improve ventricular function and** prolong survival in patients of mild-to-moderate CHF (NYHA Classes II and III) who are undergoing treatment with ACE inhibitors, diuretics, digoxin, etc.

Mechanism of beneficial effect of β blockers in CHF

In CHF there is myocardial stress and hypoxia → increase in circulating noradrenaline (NA) levels. Increased NA levels are associated with damaging effects such as:

- Cardiac hypertrophy, remodelling, apoptosis
- Peripheral vasoconstriction → Increased afterload and preload
- Down-regulation of $β_1$-receptor
- Up-regulation of $β_2$-receptors (as a self-protective mechanism)

These damaging effects can be blocked by β **blockers**. Combined α+β blocker, **carvedilol, is preferred** over selective $β_1$ blockers (e.g., metoprolol and bisoprolol). **Carvedilol** has $α_1$, $β_1$ and $β_2$ blocking effects. It also inhibits free radical-induced lipid peroxidation, and prevents cardiac and vascular mitogenesis.

The maximum utility of β blockers is in **mild-to-moderate dilated cardiomyopathy with systolic dysfunction**. However, these drugs are contraindicated in acute decompensated and severe heart failure (NYHA Class IV) and their benefits are not documented for asymptomatic heart failure (NYHA Class I).

d. Vasodilators

Vasodilators can be classified as:

- Arteriolar dilators: hydralazine
- Venous dilators: nitroglycerin, long-acting nitrates
- Mixed (arteriolar + venous) dilators: sodium nitroprusside

Mechanism of beneficial effect in CHF

Vasodilators reduce both preload and afterload.

- Dilatation of veins → reduction in venous return → decreased preload.
- Arteriolar dilation → reduction in total peripheral resistance → decreased afterload.
- Vasodilators also prevent remodelling.

Vasodilators are used in **acute heart failure for a short duration to tide over the crisis**. The choice of vasodilator depends on patients symptoms:

- In CHF with dyspnea, venodilators are preferred because they may decrease the filling pressure and ultimately pulmonary congestion.
- In CHF patients with low left ventricular output, arteriolar dilators may be useful for increasing COP.

- In severe, chronic failure, there are symptoms of both increased filling pressure and decreased cardiac output. So, a combination of hydralazine with a long-acting nitrate is used (if ACEIs are contraindicated or not tolerated). This combination also decreases remodelling and prolongs survival (though they have less beneficial effect than ACE inhibitors).

Nesiritide is a recombinant form of the human B-type natriuretic peptide.

- It exerts action by increasing cGMP in vascular smooth muscles and decreases venous as well as arteriolar tone → decreased pulmonary capillary wedge pressure and systemic vascular resistance.
- It also produces natriuretic effect → reduction in preload.
- It has a short half-life (18 min); so, it is used in **acute decompensated heart failure** as intravenous bolus dose (2 mcg/kg) followed by continuous intravenous infusion.
- Its most common adverse effect is hypotension.

Neprilysin inhibitor: Sacubitril

Neprilysin or **neutral endopeptidase inhibitor—sacubitril**—is a prodrug, which is converted by esterases into its active form **sacubitrilat**. It acts by inhibiting neutral endopeptidases, resulting in **reduced degradation of atrial natriuretic peptide (ANP) and brain natriuretic peptide (BNP)**. ANP and BNP cause vasodilatation, diuresis and natriuresis. It is approved for use with ARBs (valsartan) to decrease acute cardiac decompensation and mortality in **advanced cases of heart failure**.

e. ADH Antagonists

Vasopressin or antidiuretic hormone (ADH) is released in case of:

- Increased plasma osmolality
- Decreased arterial pressure
- Decreased cardiac filling

V_1 receptors exert vasoconstrictor action; V_2 receptors have antidiuretic effect.

Conivaptan is a mixed V_1 and V_2 receptor-blocker that is approved for a small set of patients of **acute CHF with hyponatremia**. It is administered by the intravenous route. Tolvaptan is an oral V_2-blocker.

Although they are **useful in acute situations**, they do not seem to decrease mortality and their long-term benefits seem doubtful.

The mechanism and site of action of various drug groups effective in CHF that do not possess positive inotropic action are summarised in Flowchart 33.4.

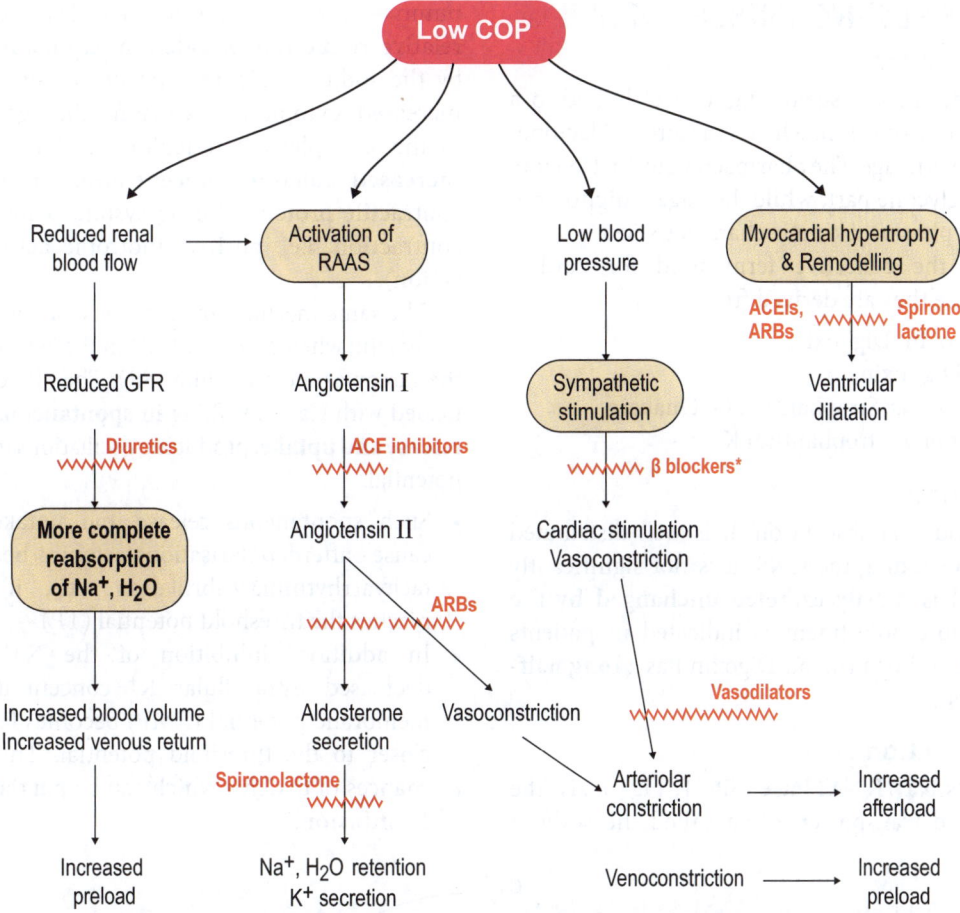

Flowchart 33.4 Sites of action of drugs in CHF (*β blockers are used only in carefully selected cases of CHF with dilated cardiomyopathy)

Clinical problem-based questions and MCQs

1. Low-output CHF occurs due to reduced contractility of the heart, but many drugs without positive inotropic effect are useful in its treatment.
   i. Enumerate such drugs.
   ii. Which of these groups of drugs is the first choice in CHF? Explain the mechanism of action of the chosen drug.

2. A 76-year-old female patient presents with shortness of breath on routine activity, excessive fatigue, weakness, and swelling over face and feet. On examination, PR = 114 beats per minute, BP= 120/78, bilateral pitting edema, hepatomegaly and abdominal distension is present. JVP is raised. On chest auscultation, bilateral basal crepitations are present. Hb is 8.5 g/dL. Chest X-ray shows cardiomegaly. Echocardiography reveals reduced ejection fraction (40%).
   i. What is the probable diagnosis
   ii. Explain the cause of the increased pulse rate, reduced ejection fraction, hepatomegaly and crepitations, based on the pathophysiology of the disease she is suffering from.
   iii. All the following drugs can be useful in this patient except:
   a. Furosemide b. Spironolactone
   c. β-agonists d. CCBs
   Justify your answer.

3. i. Identify most suitable drug from the following to tide over the crisis in a 68-year-old patient suffering from acute CHF with severe dyspnea.
   a. Nitrates b. Hydralazine
   c. Carvedilol d. Nesiritide
   ii. Describe mechanism of beneficial effect of the chosen drug.

4. i. Which of the following β blockers is most suitable in a 46-year-old patient diagnosed with moderate systolic dysfunction with dilated cardiomyopathy?
   a. Atenolol b. Pindolol
   c. Carvedilol d. Propranolol
   ii. Describe the mechanism of beneficial effect of β blockers in this case.
   iii. Justify your choice of drug.

5. A 56-year-old female patient, a known case of CHF on diuretic therapy, developed hyperkalemia on addition of enalapril (2.5 mg, once daily). Identify the diuretic this patient was using.
   a. Indapamide b. Furosemide
   c. Chlorthalidone d. Eplerenone

2. DRUGS WITH POSITIVE INOTROPIC ACTION

a. Cardiac Glycosides

Cardiac glycosides have a sugar (digitoxose) linked to a non-sugar (aglycone or genin, which is a steroidal lactone) moiety by an ether linkage. The pharmacological actions are because of the aglycone part, while the sugar (digitoxose) part governs the pharmacokinetic characteristics.

'Digitalis' is the collective term used for cardiac glycosides because they are derived from:

- *D. lanata*: Digoxin, Digitoxin
- *D. purpurea*: Digitoxin
- *Strophanthus gratus*: Strophanthin G, Ouabain
- *Strophantus kombe*: Strophanthin K

Pharmacokinetics

Digoxin has good oral absorption. It is well distributed in body fluids, including the CNS. It is not significantly metabolised and is **mostly excreted unchanged by the kidney**. Thus, dose adjustment is indicated in patients with renal function impairment. Digoxin has a **long half-life** (36–40 hours).

Mechanism of action

Digoxin **inhibits Na^+/K^+-ATPase** (Site 1, Fig. 33.4), the membrane bound transporter, often called the sodium pump → increased intracellular Na^+ concentration → relative **reduction of calcium expulsion** from the cell by the sodium–calcium exchanger (Site 2, Fig. 33.4) → increased cytoplasmic calcium that gets sequestrated in the sarcoplasmic reticulum (SR) for later release → **increased calcium concentration** in the vicinity of contractile proteins during systole → increased force of contraction, i.e., positive inotropic action (therapeutic action).

The same mechanism is responsible for the toxic effects of digoxin; when excessive Ca^{2+} in the cytosol is taken up by the sarcoplasmic reticulum (SR). The SR gets progressively loaded with Ca^{2+}, resulting in **spontaneous cycles of Ca^{2+} release and uptake**, producing oscillations in the membrane potential.

- Such spontaneous release and uptake of Ca^{2+} can cause afterdepolarisations/ectopic beats/ bigeminy/tachyarrhythmias/fibrillation, etc., if the potential reaches the threshold potential (TP).
- In addition, inhibition of the Na^+ pump causes decreased intracellular K^+ concentration → resting membrane potential (RMP) becomes less negative and closer to the threshold potential. This increases the chances of toxicity, which can be **partially reversed by K^+ infusion**.

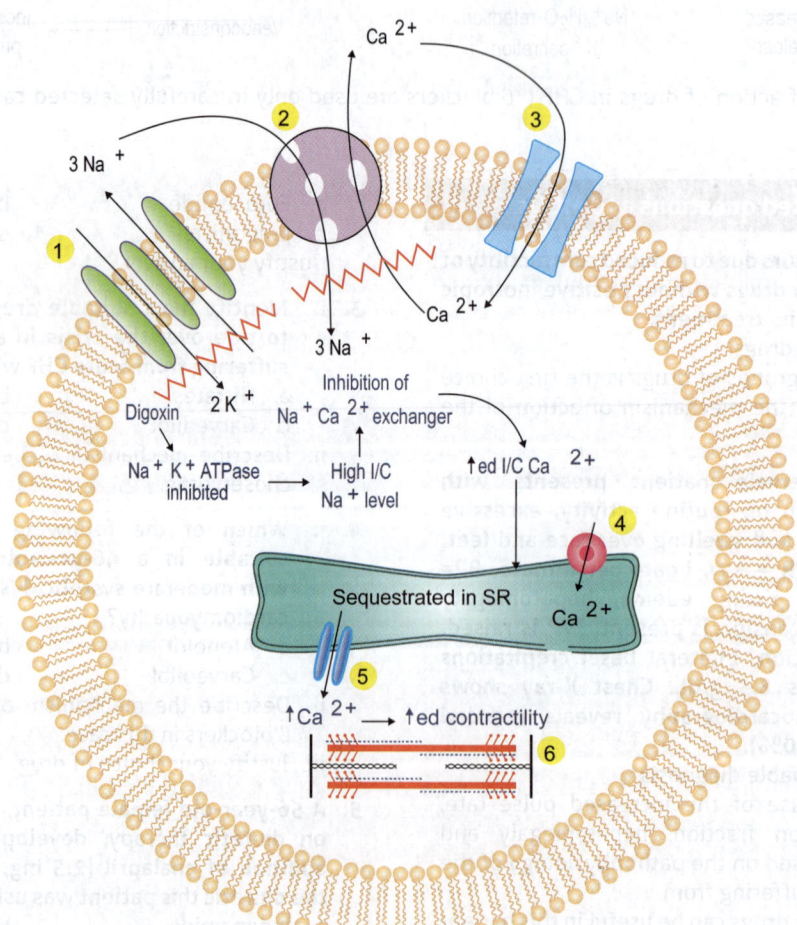

Fig. 33.4 Mechanism of action of digoxin

Because the **therapeutic as well as toxic effects of digoxin occur through same mechanism**, i.e., myocardial sarcoplasmic Ca^{2+} loading, its margin of safety is low.

Pharmacological actions

Heart

Digoxin has direct mechanical and electrical effects as well as autonomic effects on heart.

Direct effects

Mechanical effects

- The failing heart is very sensitive to the positive inotropic action of digoxin that occurs due to Ca^{2+} overloading by the inhibition of the sodium pump. The **velocity of tension development increases → systole shortens and diastole is prolonged.** Thus, the heart contracts more forcefully → more complete emptying of heart during systole → increase in stroke volume and COP → decrease in end-diastolic size.
- The force of contraction increases in normal heart also but it is not translated into increased COP.

Electrical effects

- The **resting membrane potential** (RMP) becomes **less negative** because of the decreased intracellular K^+ due to Na^+/K^+-ATPase inhibition (Fig. 33.5).
- **Phase 0:** Slow rate of Phase 0 because of the less negative RMP.
- **Action potential duration** (APD): The brief early prolongation of APD is followed by a protracted period of shortening. This is because the increased intracellular Ca^{2+} causes increase in K^+ conductance. This results in **shortening of the APD**, especially the plateau phase. The effective refractory period is reduced due to the shortening of APD. This contributes to the arrhythmogenic potential of digoxin.
- **Automaticity**: The slope of Phase 4 depolarisation increases in ectopic pacemakers (because of Ca^{2+} overload) → **increased automaticity.**
- Decreases in automaticity of SA node (vagal effect).

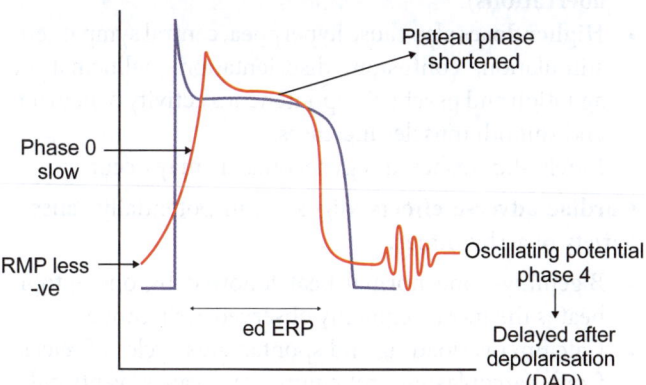

Fig. 33.5 *Effect of digoxin on cardiac action potential*

Thus, arrhythmias like delayed afterdepolarisations (DADs), ectopic beats, bigeminy (one normal beat followed by one ectopic beat), ventricular tachycardia and ventricular fibrillations can occur.

Autonomic effects

At **therapeutic doses,** the cardio-selective, parasympathomimetic effects of digoxin predominate. It is because of the:

- Sensitisation of baroreceptors
- Central vagal stimulation
- Facilitation of muscarinic transmission in myocardial cells.

Cholinergic innervation is greater in the atria than in the Purkinje fibres and ventricular fibres. So, parasympathomimetic actions affect atrial and AV nodal functions more than Purkinje or ventricular functions.

The **vagal cardiac effects** of digoxin include:

- SA node: decrease in automaticity of SA node → decrease in heart rate.
- Atrial muscle: decrease in refractory period → risk of arrhythmias.
- AV node: decrease conduction velocity and increase in refractory period.
- Purkinje system and ventricular muscle: slight decrease in refractory period.
- ECG: PR interval increases (because of slow AV conduction)
- QT interval decreases (because of shortening of systole)

Some of these vagal effects are useful in treatment of certain arrhythmias.

1. **HR decreases** because in CHF patients, a positive inotropic effect translates into increased COP → improved circulation abolishes sympathetic overactivity and restores vagal tone.

   Digitalis has vagal effects at therapeutic doses. It is likely that there is direct antiadrenergic action beyond the receptor level on the SA and AV nodes.

   However, the automaticity of non-pacemaker tissue is increased due to calcium overloading and spontaneous release from sarcoplasmic reticulum, resulting in oscillations in potential.

2. **Contractility increases** due to the positive inotropic action which occurs due to Ca^{2+} overloading upon inhibition of the sodium pump. The velocity of tension development increases → systole shortens and diastole prolongs. Thus, heart contracts more forcefully.

3. **Excitability:**
   - increases at low dose (due to decrease in gap between the resting membrane and threshold potentials).
   - decreases at high dose (as Na^+ channels are inactivated if the RMP is between -75 to -55 mV)

At toxic doses, digoxin increases the sympathetic outflow, and catecholamines sensitise the myocardium and exaggerate all the toxic effects of digoxin. The cardiac effects at toxic dosages include:

- SA node: decreased rate
- Atrial muscle: decreased refractory period and arrhythmias
- AV node: decreased conduction velocity and arrhythmias
- Purkinje system, ventricular muscles: extrasystoles, tachycardia and fibrillation
- ECG shows: tachycardia, fibrillation and cardiac arrest at extremely high dosage.

Blood vessels

Because of the cardiac action of digoxin, cardiac output increases in CHF patients. This abolishes sympathetic overactivity, resulting in reduced PVR and diastolic BP.

- The mild, direct vasoconstrictor action raises the PVR. Thus, **in normal individuals, there is no prominent effect on the BP.** However, in CHF patients, systolic BP increases (because of increase in COP) and diastolic BP decreases (because of reduced PVR). Thus, pulse pressure (PP) increases.
- Nevertheless, hypertension and coronary insufficiency are not contraindications for digoxin use.

The cardiovascular effects of digoxin on the heart are summarised in Box 33.1.

Box 33.1   Summary: Cardiovascular effects of digoxin

1. Automaticity:
   - Increased in non-pacemaker cells; this is because of increased intracellular Ca^{2+} in myocytes, resulting in various arrhythmias.
   - Decreased in SA node; because of vagal stimulation → decreased heart rate.
2. Contractility: increased, i.e., positive inotropic action
3. Conduction: decreased because of vagal effect
4. Excitability: Increased at low dose, but suppressed at high dose.

Digoxin
↓
Positive inotropic action
↓
Increased cardiac output → improved symptoms.
↓
Abolishes sympathetic overactivity → decrease PVR and restores vagal tone
↓
Vagal effects → Decreased heart rate → decreased conduction

5. **Blood vessels**: Direct effect → mild vasoconstrictor effect → increased PVR
   Negligible effect on BP in normal persons.
   In CHF patients:
   - Increase in cardiac output → increased systolic BP
   - Decrease in PVR → decreased diastolic BP
   - Pulse pressure increases.

Kidneys

In CHF patients, improved circulation → increased renal blood flow (RBF) → **diuresis**. Consequently, the retained salt and H_2O are excreted gradually. This diuretic effect is not seen in normal persons or patients with edema due to other reasons.

CNS

There are no apparent central effects at normal therapeutic doses. However, high doses stimulate the chemoreceptor trigger zone (CTZ), resulting in nausea and vomiting.

Status in CHF

Digoxin is a drug with a narrow margin of safety; so, it is considered for use in CHF patients only **after exhausting other safer options**. If ACE inhibitors and diuretics are unable to control the symptoms adequately, digoxin is used. While it relieves symptoms and reduces rate of hospitalisation, any beneficial effect on reducing mortality is not documented. It is also useful in **CHF patients with atrial fibrillation/flutter** to control ventricular rate.

Adverse effects

Digoxin has a low margin of safety; about one-fourth of patients on digoxin therapy develop adverse toxic effects. The ADRs of digoxin include **cardiac** and **extracardiac** effects. Of these, the extracardiac effects usually **occur before** cardiac adverse effects. Thus, the appearance of extracardiac toxic effects, especially visual halos around objects, indicate that digoxin therapy should be stopped.

Extracardiac adverse effects include:

- **GIT:** Anorexia, nausea, vomiting, and diarrhea occur because of vasoconstriction of mesenteric blood vessels, gastric irritant action and stimulation of chemoreceptor trigger zones. These symptoms indicate that dose reduction is required.
- Patient may complain of **generalised malaise, fatigue, headache, and visual disturbances (reduced visual acuity, blurring of vision, photophobia, yellow vision, spots in the visual field and colour perception aberrations)**.
- **Higher doses** also cause hyperpnea, central sympathetic stimulation, confusion, disorientation, hallucination, agitation and psychosis, spontaneous activity of neurons and smooth muscles increases.
- Rarely skin rashes and gynecomastia may occur.

Cardiac adverse effects: digoxin can potentially cause a variety of arrhythmias.

- Bigeminy—one normal beat followed by one ectopic beat is the most frequently observed arrhythmia.
- Calcium overloading and spontaneous cycles of release from sarcoplasmic reticulum can cause ventricular extrasystoles, ventricular tachycardia and fibrillation. Atrial extrasystoles, flutter and fibrillation may also occur.

- Partial-to-complete atrio-ventricular block due to reduced AV conduction is also common.
- Vagal action may cause severe bradycardia

Treatment of digoxin toxicity
- **Withdrawal** of digoxin therapy upon the appearance of visual or other extracardiac adverse effects usually suffices; however, if cardiac rhythm disturbances appear, they should be managed appropriately.
- **K⁺ supplementation** with oral or IV KCl is given to patients on digoxin and diuretic therapy. In diuretic-induced hypokalemic state, there is increased binding of digoxin to sodium pump, resulting in a higher risk of toxic reactions. K⁺ levels are closely monitored and restored to normal by KCl therapy. However, utmost care should be taken to avoid hyperkalemia as it may precipitate AV blocks (see Box 33.2).
- **Lignocaine IV** is drug of choice for ventricular arrhythmias and **propranolol** is useful for supraventricular arrhythmias.
- AV blocks and bradyarrhythmias are treated with **atropine** 0.6–1.2 mg given intramuscularly. In severe cases, cardiac pacing may be needed.
- **Digibind** is a Fab fragment of digoxin specific antibody, useful in severe digoxin toxicity.

> **Box 33.2   Interaction of digoxin with K⁺, Ca²⁺ and Mg²⁺**
>
> K⁺ and digitalis inhibit each other from binding to Na⁺/K⁺-ATPase. So, in hyperkalemia, the enzyme inhibiting action of digoxin is reduced. In hypokalemia, the inhibitory action of digoxin on the Na⁺/K⁺-ATPase enzyme is enhanced.
> Secondly, abnormal cardiac automaticity is inhibited by hyperkalemia. Thus, moderately increased K⁺ concentration reduces the toxic effects of digoxin, whereas hypokalemia is a risk factor for digoxin toxicity.
> Similarly, hypomagnesemia is also a risk factor for digoxin toxicity.
> Ca²⁺ also facilitates the toxic effects of cardiac glycosides by overloading intracellular Ca²⁺ stores.
> Thus, hypercalcemia, hypokalemia and hypomagnesemia may precipitate digoxin toxicity; monitoring of serum K⁺, Mg²⁺ and Ca²⁺ levels, along with ECG monitoring is required during digoxin therapy.

Drug Interactions of digoxin
Loop diuretics, thiazides, corticosteroids → decrease in serum K⁺ levels → increased toxicity of digoxin

Ca²⁺, succinylcholine, catecholamines → digoxin toxicity

Amiodarone, quinidine, verapamil, erythromycin and tetracycline can displace digoxin from the plasma protein binding site → digoxin toxicity.

Antacids, sucralfate and neomycin can decrease digoxin effect by reducing its absorption.

Enzyme inducers like phenobarbitone and phenytoin can also decrease the digoxin effect by increasing its metabolism.

Contraindications
- Hypokalemia
- Children < 10 years of age, and elderly patients with hepatic or renal impairment
- Hypothyroidism: as it slows down drug elimination
- Hyperthyroidism: as it increases the chances of digoxin-induced arrhythmias
- Partial AV block may worsen to complete AV block
- Ventricular tachycardia and Wolff–Parkinson–White (WPW) syndrome: increased risk of ventricular fibrillation.
- Grossly damaged myocardium because of the risk of arrhythmias

b. Phosphodiesterase 3 Inhibitors
Inamrinone, milrinone, levosimendan and enoximone are some phosphodiesterase inhibitors.

Mechanism of action
These bipyridine derivatives are non-glycoside, non-sympathomimetic, inotropic drugs. They act by **inhibiting the phosphodiesterase isoenzyme 3** that is located in myocytes and vascular smooth muscles. These drugs raise cAMP levels by suppressing its degradation.

- In the myocardium, cAMP causes increased contractility by activating the protein kinase, which in turn phophorylates slow Ca²⁺ channels. This results in increased Ca²⁺ inflow and positive inotropic effect.
- In vascular smooth muscles, cAMP has a relaxant effect, causing vasodilation.

Both these effects (**positive inotropic and vasodilator**) are beneficial in CHF. These drugs are administered as intravenous infusions.

ADRs
Inamrinone causes nausea, vomiting, dose-dependent thrombocytopenia, arrhythmias and raised liver enzymes, and is not in use

Milrinone is safer than inamrinone but can also cause arrhythmias. Headache and tremors are minor adverse effects.

Levosimendan: In addition to inhibition of phosphodiesterase isoenzyme 3, it sensitises the contractile mechanism of cardiac myocytes to Ca²⁺ and has some vasodilator effect too.

Enoximone is a congener of inamrinone that is used intravenously in acute heart failure.
- It is better tolerated than inamrinone.
- It improves quality of life and physical mobility in patients (because of the central stimulatory effect of raised cAMP).

Status of phosphodiesterase 3 inhibitors
Their value in management of CHF is limited to patients with **symptoms of low COP who fail to respond to**

intravenous diuretics. Milrinone may help in maintenance of patients awaiting cardiac transplant.

c. β-Adrenergic Agonists

$β_1$ agonism leads to raised cAMP levels → activates protein kinase → increases Ca^{2+} flow into cell → increase in force of contraction by the phosphorylation of slow Ca^{2+} channels.

i. Dobutamine

Dobutamine is the most commonly used inotropic agent after digoxin. It is a $β_1$-**selective** agonist and has a prominent positive inotropic action when compared to its chronotropic effect. It does not cause significant changes in the peripheral vascular resistance (PVR) or blood pressure (BP). Dobutamine has a half-life ($t_{1/2}$) of just 2 minutes; so, it is given by **intravenous infusion for short-term treatment** of acute heart failure.

Disadvantage of dobutamine is an increase in O_2 demand that **may precipitate angina**.

Increased AV condition → can be harmful and cause **arrhythmias**. So, caution should be observed in administering dobutamine to patients with atrial fibrillation. Tolerance may develop on repeated use.

ii. Dopamine

Intravenous infusion of **low dose (2–5 mcg/kg/min)** of dopamine → acts on D_1 receptors in kidney → increased renal blood flow (RBF) → increased glomerular filtration rate (GFR) → increased urine output. This action reduces preload and is beneficial in CHF.

At the **therapeutic dose** (5–10 mcg/kg/min), in addition to D_1 receptors, dopamine stimulates $β_1$ receptors also → increased COP. However, the TPR is unchanged because of renal and splanchnic vasodilator action through D_1 receptors

High doses (**>10 mcg/kg/min**) of dopamine activate $α_1$ receptors also → vasoconstriction (VC) → increased TPR and pulmonary pressure, which may nullify its beneficial effects in heart failure. Consequently, **dopamine (low dose)** is used in treatment of **low-output failure with compromised renal function** (as it causes increase in COP and renal VD); BP, HR and urinary output should be closely monitored.

Clinical problem-based questions and MCQs

6. **Milrinone acts by**
   a. Inhibiting Na^+ ion efflux
   b. Inhibiting Na^+/K^+-ATPase
   c. Raising intracellular cAMP levels
   d. Opening K^+ channels

7. **Sacubitril causes**
   a. Increased ANP levels
   b. Vasodilatation
   c. Inhibition of neutral endopeptidase
   d. All of the above

8. **Digoxin has a narrow margin of safety because of its:**
   a. Vagal stimulant action
   b. Ca^{2+} overloading action
   c. Zero order kinetics
   d. Slow metabolism

9. **All the following have long-term benefits in CHF, except:**
   a. Eplerenone
   b. Lisinopril
   c. Carvedilol
   d. Milrinone

10. A 50-year-old male patient, a known case of CHF, developed atrial fibrillation. He was prescribed a drug for controlling ventricular rate. Patient complained of headache, nausea, reduced visual acuity, blurring of vision, photophobia and yellow vision.
    i. Which of the following may be the offending drug?
       a. Enalapril
       b. Digoxin
       c. Adenosine
       d. Propranolol
    ii. What should be the next immediate action in this patient?

STATUS OF DRUGS IN TREATMENT OF CHF

1. ACE inhibitors are drugs of first choice in all grades (NYHA Classes I–IV) of CHF as they provide symptomatic relief as well as long-term survival benefits.
2. Diuretics:
   - Loop diuretics do not influence the primary disease process, but afford symptomatic relief by mobilising edema fluid; they are still widely used in the management of almost all cases of symptomatic CHF.
   - Spironolactone is combined with loop diuretics to prevent hypokalemia and restore responsiveness in refractory cases after long-term use of loop diuretics. It is combined in low doses with ACE inhibitors to maintain disease-modifying benefits upon long-term use. It also further reduces mortality. However, potassium levels are to be monitored as there is a risk of hyperkalemia. In mild cases of CHF, combination of thiazide diuretic with spironolactone may provide adequate relief.
   - Thiazides are not frequently used in CHF, except in mild cases, along with spironolactone.
3. β Blockers like bisoprolol, carvedilol and metoprolol improve ventricular function and prolong survival in patients of mild-to-moderate CHF (NYHA Classes II and III) being treated with ACE inhibitors, diuretics, digoxin, etc. β blockers are most useful in mild-to-moderate dilated cardiomyopathy with systolic dysfunction. However, they are contraindicated in acute decompensated heart failure.

4. Vasodilators are used in acute heart failure for a short duration to tide over crises.
5. Vasopressin receptor antagonists are used in acute CHF with hyponatremia, but they do not seem to provide any long-term benefits.
6. Digoxin is used if ACEIs and diuretics do not control symptoms adequately. It relieves symptoms, reduces the rate of hospitalisation, and is useful in CHF with atrial fibrillation.
7. Phosphodiesterase 3 inhibitors have a limited role in CHF, in symptomatic patients who fail to respond to diuretics and those awaiting cardiac transplant.
8. β-agonists: Dobutamine is preferred over dopamine. They are useful in low-output failure with compromised renal function.

Summary

- Cardiac performance is a function of 4 primary factors: preload, afterload, contractility and heart rate (HR).
- CHF can be low-output/high-output failure or left/right heart failure.
- Compensatory mechanisms like RAAS, sympathetic stimulation, more complete sodium and water reabsorption, and myocardial hypertrophy can compensate for reduced cardiac output to some extent only.
- Drugs with positive inotropic action, e.g., digoxin, amrinone and milrinone are useful
- Many drugs effective in CHF do not have positive inotropic action, e.g., ACE inhibitors/angiotensin receptor blockers, vasodilators, diuretics and nesiritide.
- **ACE inhibitors** are the preferred drugs because:
  - These reduce angiotensin II levels → decrease angiotensin-induced vasoconstriction → reduced venous return (preload) and peripheral vascular resistance (afterload).
  - In addition, reduced aldosterone levels also decrease salt/water retention → reduced preload.
  - Also reduce cardiac remodelling yielding long-term benefits.
- **Spironolactone** combined in low doses with ACE inhibitors maintains the disease-modifying benefits with long-term use. It also provides added benefit by further reducing mortality. However, potassium levels are monitored as there is a risk of hyperkalemia.
- **ARBs** have the same beneficial effects as ACE inhibitors.
- **Loop diuretics** provide symptomatic relief in CHF by mobilising edema fluid.
  - Widely used in the management of almost all cases of symptomatic CHF.
  - **Spironolactone** can be combined with loop diuretics to prevent hypokalemia and restore responsiveness in refractory cases after long-term use of loop diuretics.
- **Venodilators** like nitrates are valuable for short-term use to tide over crises in acute CHF with predominant dyspnea.
- **Arteriodilators** are more useful in acute CHF with low left ventricular output.
- **β Blockers** like bisoprolol, carvedilol and metoprolol improve the ventricular function and prolong survival in patients of mild-to-moderate CHF (NYHA Classes II and III) being treated with ACE inhibitors, diuretics, digoxin, etc.
  - Maximum benefit in dilated cardiomyopathy with systolic dysfunction.
  - Carvedilol is preferred over other drugs as it has $α_1$, $β_1$ and $β_2$ blocking effects, inhibits free radical-induced lipid peroxidation and prevents cardiac and vascular mitogenesis. However, β blockers are contraindicated in acute decompensated heart failure.
- **Cardiac glycosides** such as digoxin inhibit Na^+/K^+-ATPase (the sodium pump) → which indirectly reduces Ca^{2+} expulsion → intracellular Ca^{2+} increases, gets sequestered in SR → released in the vicinity of actin–myosin, leading to positive inotropic effect.
  - It has direct vagal actions.
  - Overloading of SR with Ca^{2+} may cause spontaneous cycles of its release, resulting in various arrhythmias.
  - Risk of digoxin toxicity increases during diuretic therapy due to hypokalemia.
  - Extracardiac adverse effects on the GIT and visual disturbances are indications for the discontinuation of digoxin as these precede cardiac toxic effects.
- Phosphodiesterase inhibitors like **inamrinone and milrinone** act by inhibiting phosphodiesterase isoenzyme 3 located in myocytes and vascular smooth muscles → raise cAMP levels → positive inotropic and vasodilator effects.
  - Inamrinone is rarely used currently because of its adverse effects.
  - **Enoximone**, a congener of inamrinone, is used intravenously in acute heart failure. It is better tolerated than inamrinone and improves quality of life and physical mobility because of the central stimulatory effects of raised cAMP.
- β-agonist **dopamine** (low-dose IV infusion) can be used in CHF patients with compromised renal function as it maintains renal blood flow. However, BP and PR are to be closely monitored.

- **Dobutamine** is effective but can cause arrhythmias. Angina and tolerance develop on repeated use.
- **Sacubitril** inhibits neprilysin, which is a neutral endopeptidase → reduced degradation of atrial natriuretic peptide and brain natriuretic peptide → vasodilatation, diuresis and natriuresis.
  - Approved for use along with ARBs (valsartan) to decrease acute cardiac decompensation and mortality in advanced cases of heart failure.

Questions for practice

1. Classify drugs used in treatment of CHF.
2. Comment on the role and status of following drugs in treatment of CHF.
   a. Valsartan
   b. Vasodilators
   c. Aldosterone antagonists
   d. Inamrinone
   e. Carvedilol
3. Explain why:
   a. CHF is result of reduced contractility of the heart, but many drugs without positive inotropic effect are useful in its treatment.
   b. Combined use of diuretics and digoxin poses a greater risk of arrhythmias.
   c. Diuretics are given to almost all cases of symptomatic heart failure.
   d. Dobutamine has positive inotropic effect, but is not used in the long-term management of CHF.
4. Describe mechanism of beneficial effect of following drugs in CHF.
   a. Hydralazine
   b. Spironolactone
   c. Sacubitril
5. a. Describe the mechanism of action of digoxin.
   b. Describe the effects of digoxin on the heart, cardiac action potential and ECG.
   c. Enumerate arrhythmias that may be caused in digoxin toxicity and describe the management of digoxin toxicity
   d. Enumerate the ADRs of digoxin.

Hints for problem-based questions and MCQs

1. i. Refer to Flowchart 33.2, page 438.
   ii. ACE inhibitors are the drugs of choice. They reduce venous return (preload) and peripheral vascular resistance (afterload), salt/water retention and cardiac remodelling, and give long-term beneficial effects. (Refer to Flowchart 33.3, page 439)
2. i. Congestive heart failure, low output RHF
   ii. Refer to page 435 (Pathophysiology of CHF)
   iii. d. CCBs are not useful in CHF as they have negative inotropic action.
3. i. a. Nitrates
   ii. Nitrates are venodilators; they reduce venous return resulting in reduced preload or filling pressure. Hence, they are suitable for short-term use to tide over crises in acute CHF with prominent dyspnea.
4. i. c. Carvedilol
   ii. Refer to page 440.
   iii. Refer to page 440.
5. d. Eplerenone is a potassium-sparing diuretic and can cause hyperkalemia when combined with enalapril or other ACE inhibitors.
6. c. By raising cAMP levels due to inhibition of PDE3
7. d. All of the above
8. b. Calcium overloading of SR causes arrhythmias due to spontaneous cycles of Ca^{2+} release from SR
9. d. Milrinone has no long-term benefit in CHF
10. i. b. Digoxin is the offending drug as patient shows extracardiac features of digoxin toxicity
    ii. Digoxin should be stopped immediately. K^+ supplementation also decreases chances of cardiac toxic effects of digoxin.

Chapter 33 Drug Therapy of Congestive Heart Failure (CHF)

CONCEPT MAP–DRUGS FOR CHF

Characteristic Features
Reduced contractility ↓ Low cardiac output, Increased Preload, Increased afterload, Increased HR

Compensatory Mechanisms
RAAS activation, Salt water retention, Sympathetic stimulation, Myocardial hypertrophy & remodeling

Types
- Left heart failure/Right heart failure
- Systolic/Diastolic dysfunction
- Compensated / Decompensated
- Low-output / High-output failure

High-output failure due to beriberi, anemia, hyperthyroidism. Treatment of cause is important for management

Digoxin
$Na^+ K^+$-ATPase inhibitor → ↑ed calcium in SR → ↑ed contractility.
Narrow margin of safety. Used only when ACEI, diuretics fail.
ADRs: Can cause variety of arrhythmias.
Extracardiac (visual) adverse effects warrant dose reduction/stopping.

Inamrinone, Milrinone, Enoximone
- Inhibit PDE3 → raise cAMP levels → ↑ed contractility → +ve inotropic & VD action.
- Used only if symptoms not relieved with IV diuretics
- Enoximone used IV in acute cardiac failure, improves mobility & QOL, better tolerated than inamrinone.

Dopamine Dobutamine
Dopamine low dose IV infusion maintains RBF → Used in acute CHF with compromised renal function.
Dobutamine: Selective β_1 agonist, +ve inotropic action, but risk of arrhythmias and angina. Tolerance develops on repeated use.

DRUGS FOR CHF
CHF — Drugs with +ve inotropic effect — Drugs without +ve inotropic effect

ACE inhibitors/ARBs
- First-line drugs in all grades of CHF.
- Reduce A-II, aldosterone levels → reduced preload, afterload. ↓ Improve symptoms
- Decrease remodelling → reduce mortality & prolong survival.
- Addition of spironolactone maintains long-term beneficial effect.
- K^+ levels need close monitoring due to risk of hyperkalemia with this combination.

Loop Diuretics
- Widely used in all symptomatic cases.
- Mobilise edema fluid, improve pump efficiency, improve symptoms
- Addition of spironolactone prevents hypokalemia and reverses refractoriness

Sacubitril
Inhibits Neprilysin → Raise ANP & BNP levels → VD, diuresis, natriuresis.
Approved for use with ARBs in advanced cases of heart failure to decrease acute decompensation.

β blockers
- Block damaging effects of raised NE.
- Bisoprolol, Carvedilol, Metoprolol → improve ventricular function & prolong survival.
- Carvedilol useful in grade II–III cases especially dilated CMP with systolic dysfunction.
- β blockers are contraindicated in acute decompensated heart failure.

ADH Antagonist Conivaptan
Used only in acute CHF with hyponatremia

Vasodilators
- **Venodilators** reduce preload. Used for short term to tide over the crisis in acute CHF with predominant dyspnoea
- **Arteriodilators** reduce afterload, more useful in acute left ventricular dysfunction.

SECTION 7   **Drugs Acting on CVS**

34   Drugs for Ischemic Heart Disease

PH 4.8 Describe types, salient pharmacokinetics, pharmacodynamics, therapeutic uses, adverse drug reactions of drugs used for the management of ischemic heart disease (stable, unstable angina and myocardial infarction) and devise a management plan for a patient of acute myocardial infarction.

Learning objectives

A student of MBBS phase II should be able to:
- Describe the blood supply of heart.
- Describe etiology and pathophysiology of various types of angina.
- Classify antianginal drugs and describe their mechanisms of action.
- Enumerate therapeutic uses mentioning doses of antianginal drugs.
- Enumerate adverse effects and contraindications of antianginal drugs
- Describe pathophysiology and clinical features of MI.
- Describe management of Non-ST-Elevation MI (NSTEMI) and STEMI.
- Explain the rationale for use of various drugs in MI.

Ischemic heart disease (IHD) is also known as *coronary heart disease* or *atherosclerotic coronary artery disease* (CAD). The imbalance between demand and supply of blood (oxygen) to cardiac muscle is responsible for causing angina that can further progress to unstable angina and myocardial infarction.

ARTERIAL SUPPLY OF HEART

The heart receives its arterial blood supply from the left and right coronary arteries, which originate from the ascending aorta. Both the coronaries and their branches lie in the subepicardial tissue and give rise to collateral branches that form plexuses in the subendocardial region. Blood is supplied to the cardiac walls through these vessels, mainly during diastole.

- **Right coronary artery** gives rise to atrial branches, anterior ventricular branches (including the right marginal artery), posterior interventricular artery and right conus artery to supply the following regions of the heart:
  - Right atrium, SA node, AV node and part of left atrium.
  - Most of the right ventricle, except some parts that adjoin the anterior interventricular groove (Fig. 34.1).
  - Some parts of the diaphragmatic surface of the left ventricle.
  - The posterior 1/3rd of the interventricular septum.
  - AV bundle and some parts of the left bundle branch.

- **Left coronary artery** gives rise to the anterior interventricular or anterior descending branch and the circumflex branch. The circumflex artery gives the left marginal artery. The left coronary artery and its branches supply:
  - Most of the left atrium
  - Most of the left ventricle
  - Some parts of the right ventricle adjoining the anterior interventricular groove
  - The anterior 2/3rd of the interventricular septum (Fig. 34.1)

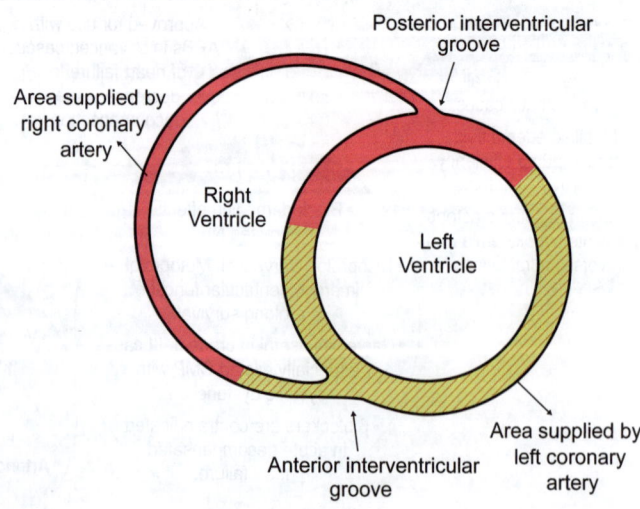

Fig. 34.1 Areas of ventricular walls supplied by the right and left coronary arteries

- Some parts of the AV bundle, right and left bundle branches.

Thus, three major vessels supplying heart are the left anterior descending (LAD) or anterior interventricular artery, posterior interventricular artery and right marginal artery.

ETIOLOGY OF ISCHEMIC HEART DISEASE

The most common etiological factor for angina is **atherosclerosis of large coronary arteries**, which results in narrowing of the lumen (Fig. 34.2a), causing a **fixed** coronary obstruction and reduced blood flow. The blood supplied through these narrow vessels may suffice during rest or normal activity, but fails to meet the increased O_2 demand during exercise, stress, etc. Such patients develop **effort/classical/stable angina**. They experience symptoms during activity/stress that is relieved by rest and antianginal drugs.

In some patients, however, **the atheromatous plaque ruptures**, favouring **platelet deposition** and further narrowing of the coronary artery lumen (Fig. 34.2b). Such patients develop **unstable angina**, characterised by more frequent and more severe attacks that may occur even during rest. Patients of unstable angina should be treated aggressively as they are prone to acute attacks of **myocardial infarction**, which occurs due to complete occlusion of the artery by the platelet plug (Fig. 34.2c).

Sometimes, **localised reversible coronary vasospasm** is responsible for disturbing the O_2 demand-to-supply ratio of the myocardium (Fig. 34.2d). This results in a rare type of angina called **variant/vasospastic/Prinzmetal angina**. In these patients, unpredictable recurrent coronary vasospasm and angina symptoms can occur at any time, even during rest or sleep.

Some of the other causes of cardiac ischemia include;

- Reduced capacity of coronary resistance vessels to dilate (microvascular angina).

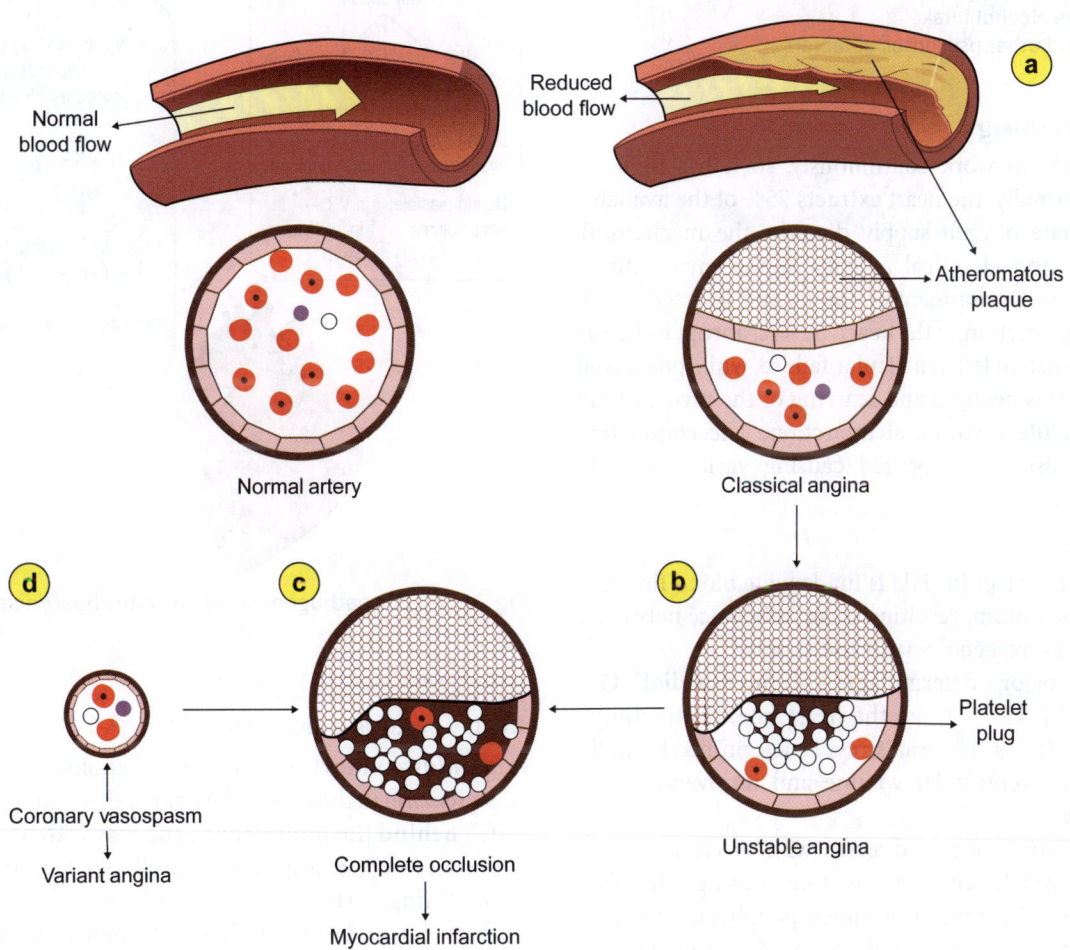

Fig. 34.2 Etiopathogenesis of ischemic heart disease
  a. Atherosclerosis → fixed narrowing of vessel lumen → stable/classical angina.
  b. Rupture of atherosclerotic plaque → formation of platelet plug → unstable angina.
  c. Complete occlusion → myocardial infarction.
  d. Coronary vasospasm → variant angina.

- Aortic stenosis, which causes increased oxygen demand secondary to left ventricular hypertrophy, as well as reduced coronary blood flow.
- Reduced oxygen carrying capacity of blood, as in severe anemia.

Important risk factors for coronary artery disease are enumerated in Box 34.1.

> **Box 34.1** Risk factors for CAD (angina, MI)
>
> **Nonmodifiable risk factors** include:
> - A positive family history in first-degree relatives, especially with onset at young age
> - Males are comparatively at higher risk of developing CAD than females
>
> **Modifiable risk factors are:**
> - Abnormalities in the lipid profile (e.g., hypercholesterolemia, increased LDL and decreased HDL)
> - Diabetes mellitus
> - Hypertension
> - Physical inactivity
> - Abdominal obesity
> - Cigarette smoking
> - Excessive alcohol intake
> - Stress and other psychosocial factors

Pathophysiology

The heart has to work continuously, so it has high O_2 demand. Normally, the heart extracts 75% of the available O_2. Inadequate oxygen supply disturbs the mechanical, biochemical and electrical activity of the myocardium. This results in development of angina and interferes with the pumping function of the heart. Severe, abrupt ischemia can cause transient left ventricular failure, while prolonged ischemia causes necrosis and scarring of the myocardium leading to acute myocardial infarction. The conducting tissue may also get atrophied causing various rhythm disturbances.

- The basic defect in IHD is inadequate blood flow to the myocardium, resulting in an imbalance between the heart's oxygen demand and supply.
- Three major determinants of **myocardial O_2 demand** (Fig. 34.3) are the heart rate, contractility and wall stress. The wall stress is determined by wall thickness, ventricular volume and intraventricular pressure.
  Wall stress varies directly with arteriolar tone during systole and venous tone during diastole. The arteriolar tone determines peripheral vascular resistance, i.e., afterload and arterial BP. During systole, the intraventricular pressure must be greater than the aortic pressure for blood to be pumped forward from the left ventricle to the aorta. Thus, as the arterial (aortic) BP increases, the intraventricular pressure also increases; this, in turn, increases the wall stress.

However, during diastole, wall stress varies directly with the venous return to the heart (preload), which depends on venous tone. With increased venous tone, more blood is returned from the veins to the heart. Thus, increased diastolic filling of heart results in increased ventricular volume and wall stress)
- On the other hand, **myocardial O_2 supply** (Fig. 34.3) depends on the coronary blood flow. Coronary flow is negligible during systole. During diastole, coronary flow varies directly with the duration of the diastolic phase and aortic diastolic pressure, and inversely with coronary vascular resistance. Damage to the endothelium of coronary vessels reduces their ability to dilate; hence, coronary vascular resistance increases.

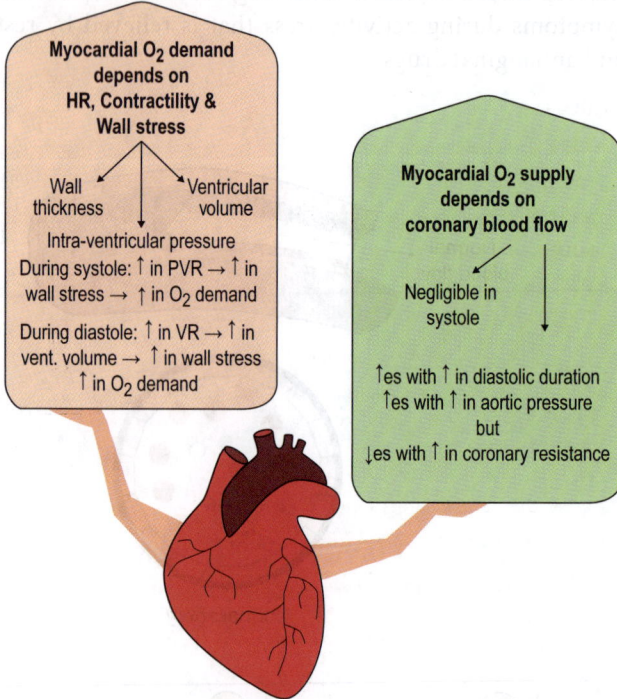

Fig. 34.3 Etiopathogenesis of ischemic heart disease

Clinical Features of IHD

Angina pectoris is characterised by:
- **Pain/discomfort** or sensation of **choking/ tightness / squeezing** in the chest. The pain or discomfort is usually felt **behind the midsternum** and may **radiate** to the left shoulder, upper arm (up to the elbow), forearm, and 4th or 5th finger. However, it can radiate to any dermatome from C8 to T4, right shoulder, right arm, lower jaw, back or neck. In some patients, there may not be any pain, resulting in **ambulatory/silent** CAD.
- Anginal symptoms usually **last for short durations and subside completely**. Angina precipitated by exertion is relieved within a few minutes (< 3 minutes) of rest, whereas that precipitated by a heavy meal or stressful outburst may

take 15–20 minutes to subside. Symptoms **lasting longer than 30 minutes indicate more severe ischemia, such as acute coronary syndrome or myocardial infarction,** and need emergency hospitalisation and treatment.

- Resting ECG is normal in most of the patients. Exercise ECG or treadmill test (TMT) with successively increasing speed and elevation every 3 minutes, indicates ischemic changes in the form of **ST segment depression /elevation.**
- Treadmill test should not be attempted in patients having rest angina, as they are at higher risk of infarction during the test.
- **Echocardiography** provides indirect evidence of coronary branch blockage.
- Coronary angiography and contrast CT angiography are carried out to confirm the diagnosis and determine the extent of blockage of coronaries.

Management of IHD

Treatment of ischemic heart disease involves following strategies:

- **Risk factor modification** is a very important part of management of CAD. It includes smoking cessation, weight reduction, and regular exercise. Alcohol intake should be stopped or moderated to less than 1 drink per day in women and 2 drinks per day in men. Co-morbidities that may cause or contribute to angina, such as obesity, diabetes, hypertension, hyperthyroidism, anemia and aortic valve disease, should be identified and aggressively treated.
- **Adaptation of activity** to a **level below the ischemic threshold** is very helpful in decreasing the frequency of angina episodes. Reducing the speed at which given tasks are performed and reducing energy requirements in the morning/after meals/in cold weather may help to decrease the frequency of angina attacks. A regular program of isotonic exercises within ischemic threshold is also quite beneficial.
- **Symptomatic treatment** of angina is based on **correcting the imbalance between myocardial O_2 demand and supply,** either by decreasing the demand or increasing the supply. Another recent strategy is to enable efficient utilisation of substrates by the heart, e.g., by pFOX inhibitors.
  - Most of the drugs used in classical angina (nitrates, calcium channel blockers, β blockers) decrease the O_2 demand by decreasing HR, contractility and wall stress. ACEIs/ARBs reduce wall stress by decreasing the afterload and preload. Nitrates also cause favourable redistribution of coronary flow to the ischemic site.
  - In variant angina, vasodilator drugs reverse coronary vasospasm and increase myocardial O_2 delivery.
  - In acute coronary syndrome or unstable angina, both decreasing the demand and increasing the supply of O_2 are attempted.
- **Treatment of the underlying cause,** i.e., atherosclerosis: Administration of lipid-lowering drugs can modify the course of the atherosclerotic disease process and improve the long-term outcome. HMG-CoA reductase inhibitors or statins lower LDL, raise HDL, and improve patient outcomes.
- **Revascularisation** by percutaneous coronary intervention **(PCI) or stenting** and **coronary artery bypass grafting** are indicated in patients with:
  - Intolerable symptoms.
  - Left coronary stenosis > 50%, even without symptoms.
  - Triple vessel disease with ejection fraction < 50%.
  - Post-myocardial infarction patients with continued angina.
- **Planned rehabilitation** programmes offer repeated reassurance and support to patients for controlling risk factors and improving exercise tolerance.

DRUGS FOR IHD

Drug groups such as nitrates, β blockers, CCBs, K^+-channel openers, and ACEIs have a role in the management of IHD (Flowchart 34.1). Nitrates can be short-acting and useful for control of acute attacks or long-acting for

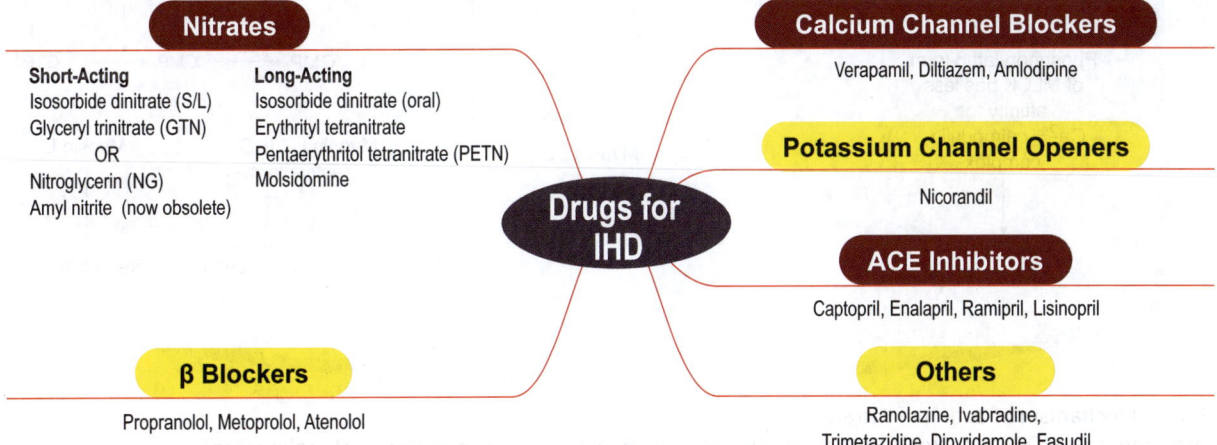

Flowchart 34.1 Classification of drugs for IHD

chronic maintenance therapy. In addition, drugs such as ranolazine, ivabradine, trimetazidine, dipyridamole and fasudil have beneficial effects in IHD.

1. Nitrates

Mechanism of action

The mechanism of action of all nitrates is the same, whether they are used for controlling acute attacks or for maintenance therapy of angina.

- GTN and PETN are activated by the enzymatic action of aldehyde dehydrogenase isoform 2 (and possibly isoform 3) to release nitric oxide (NO). Different enzymes may be responsible for NO release from isosorbide dinitrate and mononitrate.
- Once formed, NO (which is complexed with cysteine) activates guanylyl cyclase, resulting in the production of cyclic GMP from GTP (Fig. 34.4).
- Cyclic GMP causes inactivation of myosin light chain (LC) by dephosphorylation and the smooth muscles relax.
- In addition, other mechanisms such as reduced calcium entry, synthesis of PGE_2 and PGI_2, and membrane hyperpolarisation may also contribute to the smooth muscle relaxant action of nitrates.

- Hypotensive doses of nitrates evoke reflex sympathetic stimulation. The β_2-agonistic action generates cAMP that causes phosphorylation of myosin LC kinase, which decreases its affinity for Ca–calmodulin, resulting in vascular smooth muscle relaxation (this mechanism may not be involved in the primary nitrate response).

Tolerance develops rapidly to the action of nitrates. It may be due to:
- Decrease in tissue –SH groups (cysteine).
- Increased generation of oxygen free radicals.
- Less availability of calcitonin gene-related peptide (CGRP) which is a potent vasodilator.
- Compensatory mechanism: vasodilatation → hypotension → reflex sympathetic stimulation → tachycardia and Na^+/H_2O retention.

Molsidomine has the same mechanism of action as nitrates; however, no tolerance develops to its action.

Organ system effects

The major action of nitrates is to relax all types of smooth muscles; however, they have no effect on cardiac and skeletal muscles.

1. **CVS**
   a. **Blood vessels**: Nitrates relax the vascular smooth muscles from large arteries to large veins. The degree

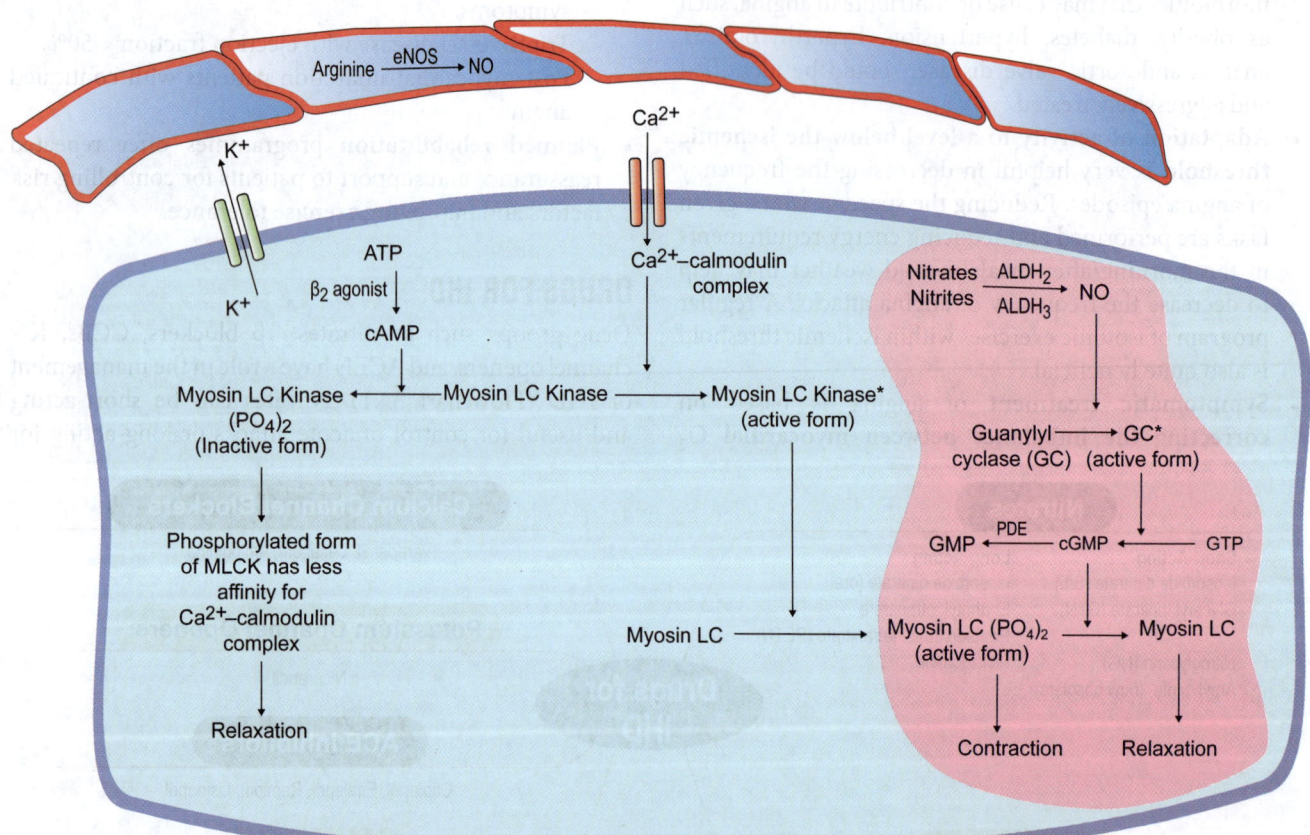

Fig. 34.4 Mechanism of action of nitrates.
[Nitrates generate NO → activate GC → form cGMP → inactivate myosin LC → smooth muscle relaxation]

of relaxation depends upon the capacity of different vessels to release NO from the drug.
- The veins are most sensitive to the **vasodilator** effect of nitrates and venodilatation occurs at the lowest concentrations. Arteries dilate at slightly higher concentrations, whereas arterioles and precapillary sphincters are the least affected → vasodilator effect of nitrates on veins > arteries > arterioles and precapillary sphincters.
- The **marked venodilatation** induced by nitrates results in decreased venous return (preload) to the heart → reduced end-diastolic volume, which reduces wall stress (a major determinant of myocardial O_2 demand) (Fig. 34.5). However, pooling of blood in the peripheral veins causes orthostatic hypotension and syncope.
- Hypotension caused by nitrates evokes reflex responses resulting in tachycardia and salt/water retention. Tachycardia increases myocardial O_2 demand; salt and H_2O retention also increases O_2 demand by increasing blood volume, which in turn increases preload and wall stress. These effects contribute to the **development of tolerance** to nitrates.
- The coronaries supply the layers of heart through large epicardial vessels that lie in the subepicardial layer of connective and adipose tissue. Many conducting vessels arising from these epicardial vessels pass through the myocardium to form the subendocardial arteriolar plexus (resistance vessels, Fig. 34.6).
- Dilation of the large epicardial coronary arteries can increase total coronary blood flow in normal subjects; however, there is no evidence of increased total coronary blood flow in patients with atherosclerotic coronary artery obstruction. However, the graded effect of nitrates (more on the conducting vessels than resistance vessels) causes **favourable redistribution of coronary flow** from the normal to ischemic myocardium; this may contribute to the beneficial effect of nitrates in angina.
- Ischemia (anoxia) itself induces vasodilatation of subendocardial resistance vessels in the ischemic zone (Fig. 34.6 a, b). Nitrates dilate the larger epicardial arteries more than the resistance vessels. Thus, resistance vessels in the non-ischemic areas are not dilated much (Fig. 34.6 b). Dilated epicardial vessels conduct more blood to the ischemic zone, resulting in favourable redistribution. Cardiovascular effects of nitrates are summarised in Box 34.2 and Fig. 34.7.
- Temporal and meningeal artery pulsations may result in throbbing headache as an adverse effect.

b. Relaxation of smooth muscles of GIT, biliary tract, bronchi, and genitourinary tract occurs, but is of no clinical utility due to brief duration of action.

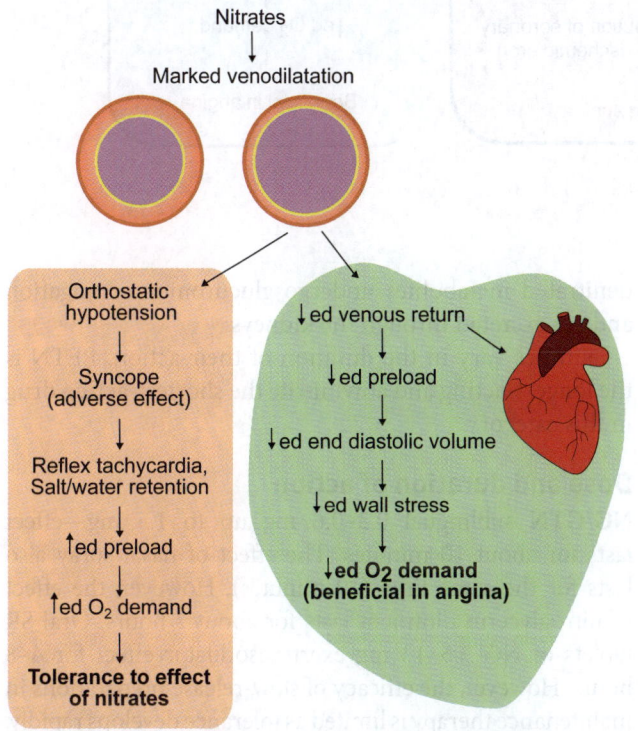

Fig. 34.5 Consequences of nitrate-induced venodilatation

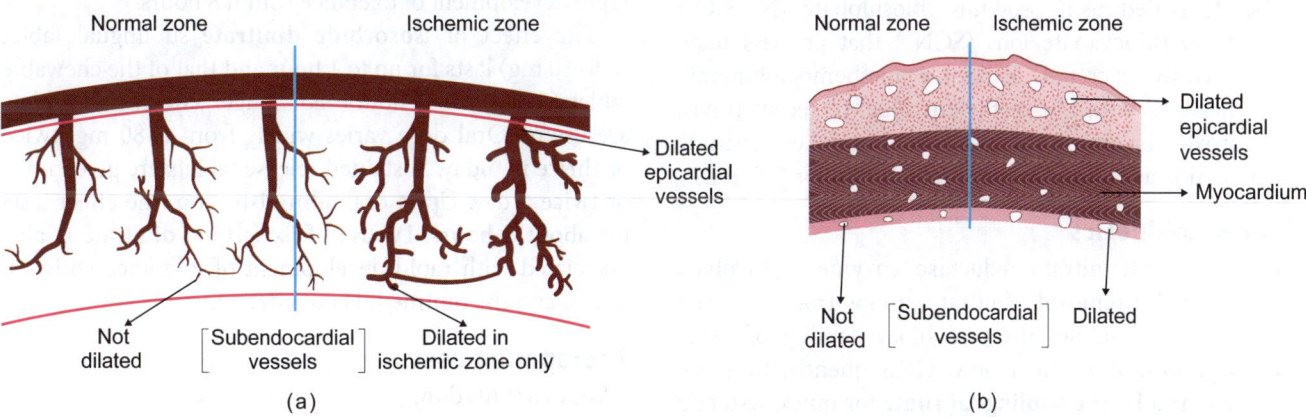

Fig. 34.6 Graded effect of nitrates. Effect of nitrates on larger epicardial arteries > subendocardial arterioles → Favourable redistribution of blood from normal to ischemic zone.

Box 34.2 Cardiovascular effects of nitrates

Nitrates have a graded vasodilator effect on different vessels. Venodilatation > arterial dilatation > arteriolar dilatation. The usefulness of each effect in angina is shown in Fig. 34.7.

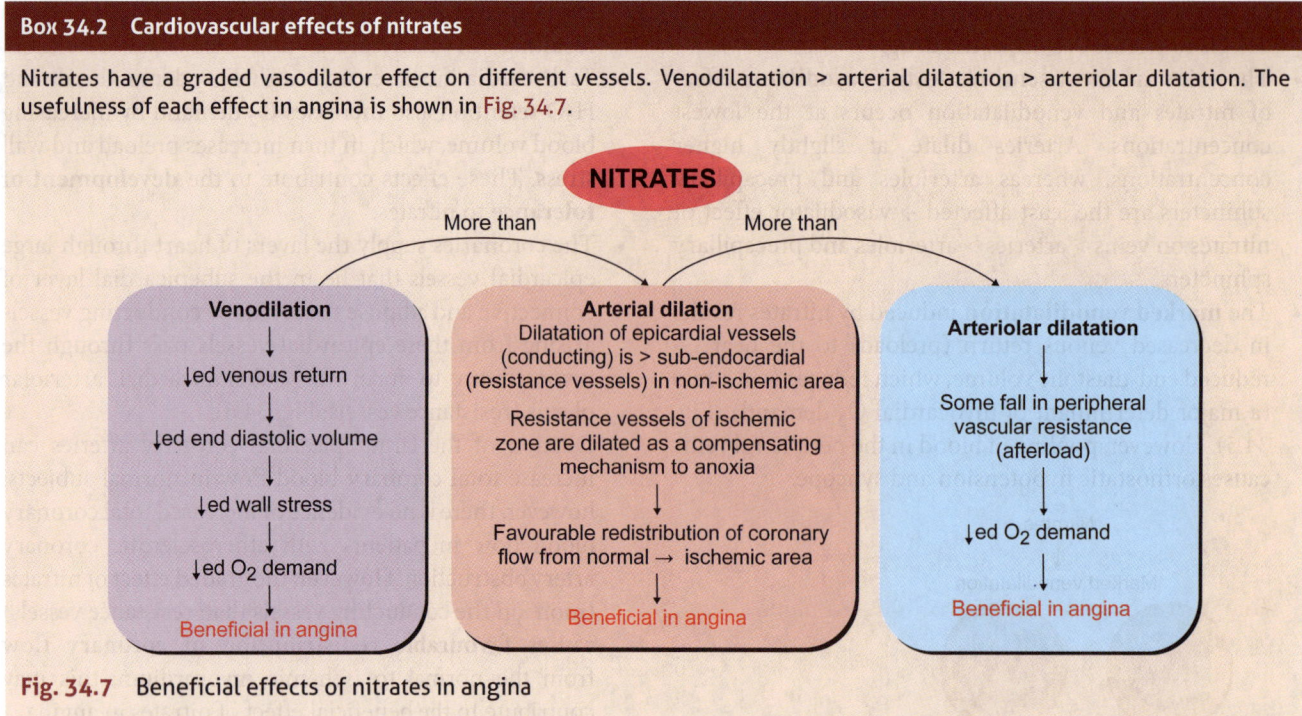

Fig. 34.7 Beneficial effects of nitrates in angina

2. **Antiaggregatory effect** is seen because of increased cGMP in the platelets. While this may contribute to beneficial effect of nitrates in unstable angina, there is no evidence of its benefit in acute myocardial infarction.
3. Nitrite (not nitrate) ions react with Hb to form methemoglobin, which has very low O_2-carrying capacity. Inadvertent exposure to high concentrations of nitrite ion causes pseudo-cyanosis and tissue anoxia and can be fatal. Fortunately, even large doses of nitrates (when used therapeutically) do not yield nitrite ion concentrations sufficient to cause clinically significant **methemoglobinemia.**

However, sodium nitrite ($NaNO_2$) administration is **useful in cyanide poisoning.** Nitrite ions convert Hb into methemoglobin, which has very high affinity for cyanide ions. The resulting cyan methemoglobin can be detoxified using sodium thiosulphate ($Na_2S_2O_3$) to form thiocyanate ions (SCN^-) that are less toxic and easily excreted. Excessive methemoglobinemia is managed with I/V methylene blue. In recent times, hydroxocobalamine is used in cases of cyanide poisoning as it also has very high affinity for CN^- ions.

Pharmacokinetics

Hepatic organic nitrate reductase enzyme is involved in the stepwise removal of nitrate groups from the drug and inactivates it. So, the oral bioavailability of GTN and isosorbide dinitrate is low. Consequently, they are **administered by the sublingual route** for quick systemic absorption and better bioavailability, as this route bypasses the liver. For longer lasting effect, oral, transdermal, and buccal routes and slow-release preparations are used. The denitrated metabolites undergo glucuronide conjugation and are excreted through the kidneys.

Nitrates vary in the duration of their action. PETN is the longest-acting and amylnitrite the shortest-acting drug in this category.

Dose and duration of action

NG/GTN sublingual 0.3–0.6 mg up to 1.5 mg—effect lasts for about 10 minutes. The effect of nasal spray also lasts for the same time (10 minutes). However, the effect of nitroglycerin ointment lasts for about 7 hours. Oral SR tablets of NG 2.5–13 mg exert vasodilator effect for 4–8 hours. However, the efficacy of slow-release preparations in maintenance therapy is limited as tolerance develops rapidly. Transdermal patches are effective for longer durations (8–12 hours). IV use of NG (5–200 mcg/minute) is associated with rapid development of tolerance within 8 hours.

The effect of **isosorbide dinitrate** sublingual tablet (2.5–10 mg) lasts for up to 1 hour and that of the chewable tablet (5 mg) for 2 hours. For longer effect, oral tablets are useful. Oral dose varies widely from 5–80 mg, twice or thrice in a day. Sustained release tablets are given once or twice a day. Upon oral administration, the effect lasts for about 8 hours. IV use of isosorbide dinitrate is also associated with rapid development of tolerance within 8 hours, and the ointment is not effective.

Therapeutic uses

Nitrates are used in:

- **Stable angina pectoris**: Nitrates reduce myocardial oxygen demand and cause redistribution of coronary flow from the non-ischemic to ischemic zone.

- **Unstable angina** and acute coronary syndrome: Nitrates improve oxygen demand:supply ratio of the myocardium and also have antiaggregatory effects.
- In **variant angina**, nitrates help by reversing coronary spasms and improving O_2 supply to the myocardium.
- **Acute myocardial infarction**.
- **CHF**: Nitrates help by decreasing both preload and afterload.
- In **portal hypertension**, nitrates decrease the hepatic venous pressure gradient; in combination with vasopressin, they can control acute variceal bleeding.

Adverse drug reactions

1. Orthostatic hypotension
2. Throbbing headache, pallor, weakness, dizziness (syncopal attack)
3. Tachycardia
4. Facial flushing
5. **Tolerance/Tachyphylaxis**: There is rapid development of tolerance on continued exposure. Tolerance to the action of nitrates develops quickly, due to the decreased capacity to release NO (**true vascular tolerance**) and compensatory mechanisms (**pseudotolerance**). Therapeutically, development of tolerance can be prevented by providing nitrate-free interval for at least 8 hours daily, usually at night, when the O_2 demand of heart is lower. SH donors such as N-acetylcysteine and L-methionine, antioxidants, statins, ACEIs and ARBs, carvedilol and hydralazine are also used to prevent development of tolerance to nitrates.
6. Prolonged therapy causes endothelial dysfunction. PETN does not have side effects like tolerance and endothelial dysfunction.
7. **Occupational exposure** to high levels nitrate occurs in the explosives manufacturing industry. Such severe contamination with volatile organic nitrates results in the development of tolerance in workers. When the exposure to nitrates is discontinued over the weekend, the tolerance also disappears. Workers experience symptoms like headache and dizziness on Monday morning; these settle down in a day or so, once tolerance develops again. Such recurrence of symptoms every Monday (or first day of the work week) is called the **Monday disease**.
8. Occupational exposure can cause **dependence** also; however, therapeutic exposure even to high doses of nitrates do not have this adverse effect.

Contraindications of nitrates

1. Nitrates should not be combined with phosphodiesterase-5 inhibitors, such as sildenafil, tardenafil and vardenafil, because of the risk of severe hypotension.
2. In patients with increased intracranial tension.
3. Transdermal NG patches may get ignited during external defibrillator electroshock, so it should be removed before defibrillation.

Clinical problem-based questions and MCQs

1. i. Identify the preferred route of administration of GTN during anginal attack.
   a. Oral
   b. Sublingual
   c. Intravenous
   d. Transdermal
   ii. Justify your choice.

2. i. A 60-year-old man was walking to his home. He experienced sudden presternal pain radiating to his left shoulder. The pain disappeared after he rested for a few minutes. A decision is made to treat him with nitroglycerin. Identify the correct action of NG for relief of angina symptoms.
   a. Decreasing oxygen demand
   b. Increasing O_2 supply.
   c. Increasing aortic impedance
   d. Decreasing venous capacitance
   ii. Describe the mechanism of beneficial effect of nitrates in angina.

3. Identify the vessels on which the effect of nitrates is most prominent.
   a. Veins
   b. Large arteries
   c. Capillaries
   d. Arterioles

4. Identify the drug effective for treatment as well as prophylaxis of angina pectoris.
   a. Pentoxifylline
   b. Diltiazem
   c. Dipyridamole
   d. Isosorbide dinitrate

5. Identify the correct mechanism of beneficial effect of NG in variant angina.
   a. Increased O_2 supply
   b. Decreased ventricular contractility
   c. Decreased cardiac automaticity
   d. Reduction of afterload

6. A 56-year-old worker in an explosive manufacturing factory complains of headache and dizziness for the first two days of the week, i.e., Monday and Tuesday. Symptoms are relieved from Wednesday onwards without any treatment. This is repeated every week. No abnormal findings are detected on GPE.
   i. What is this patient suffering from?
   ii. Identify most likely cause of relief of symptoms without any treatment in this case.
   a. Tolerance to nitrates
   b. Resistance to nitrates
   c. Dependence on nitrates
   d. Withdrawal from nitrates

7. Nitrates are the mainstay of angina treatment; however, they show the phenomenon of tachyphylaxis.
   i. What is tachyphylaxis? Describe the mechanisms for tachyphylaxis to the effect of nitrates.
   ii. Describe the measures to prevent tachyphylaxis while using nitrates over a long term.

8. Sodium nitrite administration followed by sodium thiosulphate and methylene blue is used for the management of cyanide poisoning. Describe the pharmacological basis for this particular sequence of drugs.

2. β Blockers in Angina

β-blockers include propranolol, metoprolol and atenolol.

- β-blockers (except a few like carvedilol and nebivolol) do not possess vasodilator effects, but are useful in angina. The beneficial effect of β blockers in angina involves **decreased myocardial O_2 demand at rest and during exercise** secondary to decrease in HR, contractility and BP (Fig. 34.8).
- In addition, the decrease in HR leads to an **increase in diastolic perfusion time** that may increase coronary perfusion. However, an increase in end-diastolic volume may be counterproductive, and can be balanced by combining with nitrates.
- β-blockers improve exercise tolerance, relieve the symptoms and improve patient outcome in stable angina.
- Long-term therapy with β-blockers may be useful in silent ischemia by **reducing the frequency and duration of ischemic episodes.**
- β-blockers are used in acute myocardial infarction for **myocardial salvage and secondary prophylaxis.** For myocardial salvage, β-blockers (given intravenously within 4–6 hours of acute myocardial infarction and subsequently by oral route) are helpful in decreasing infarct size and preventing rhythm disturbances. However, patients should be carefully selected; β blockers should not be given to patients who are:
  - **in shock**
  - **have HR < 50**
  - **have > first degree AV block.**

For secondary prophylaxis → long-term (minimum 2 years) treatment with β-blockers decreases the mortality by 20% because they prevent reinfarction and ventricular fibrillation during subsequent attacks. β-blockers are the only antianginal drugs that may reduce mortality in post-MI cases (Fig. 34.8).

- However, β-blockers are **contraindicated in vasospastic angina** because they can worsen coronary vasospasms.
- Other contraindications to the use of β-blockers include bronchial asthma, severe bradycardia, AV blocks and severe LVF.

3. Calcium Channel Blockers (CCBs) in Angina

Verapamil, diltiazem and amlodipine are some examples of CCBs used in angina.

Mechanism of action

Smooth muscles need transmembrane calcium influx to maintain normal resting tone and contractile response. Voltage-gated L-type calcium channels in heart and smooth muscles contain α_1 (pore forming), α_2, β, γ and δ subunits. Drug-binding sites are present on the α_1 subunit (refer to Fig. 31.1). Drugs act on the channel from the inner side of the membrane and have greater affinity for open and inactive channels (like Na^+ channel blockade by local anesthetics). Binding of CCBs to the channel **decreases frequency of opening** in response to depolarisation. This results in a marked decrease in the calcium current, which causes long-lasting relaxing effect in smooth muscles.

Role of CCBs in angina

- The beneficial cardiovascular effects of CCBs in angina are summarised in Fig. 34.9.
- Vascular smooth muscles are the most sensitive to CCBs, though bronchiolar, gastrointestinal and uterine muscles also relax. **Arterioles are more sensitive to the relaxing effect of CCBs than veins** (unlike nitrates, which have a stronger relaxing effect on veins). Thus, they decrease peripheral vascular resistance (afterload) and BP.
- The lower the peripheral vascular resistance (PVR) → lower is the required intraventricular pressure to push the blood into aorta → wall stress is also lower, and

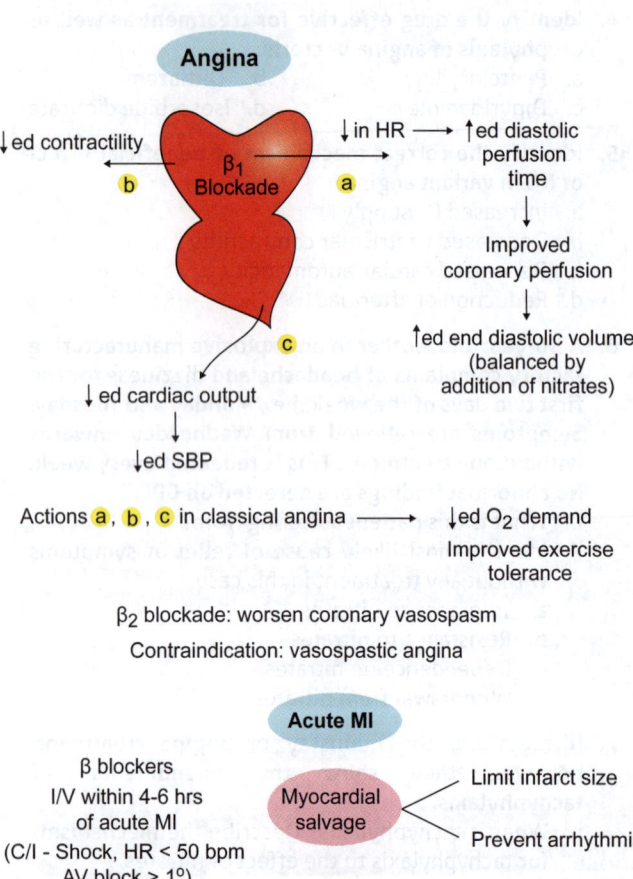

Fig. 34.8 Role of β-blockers in IHD

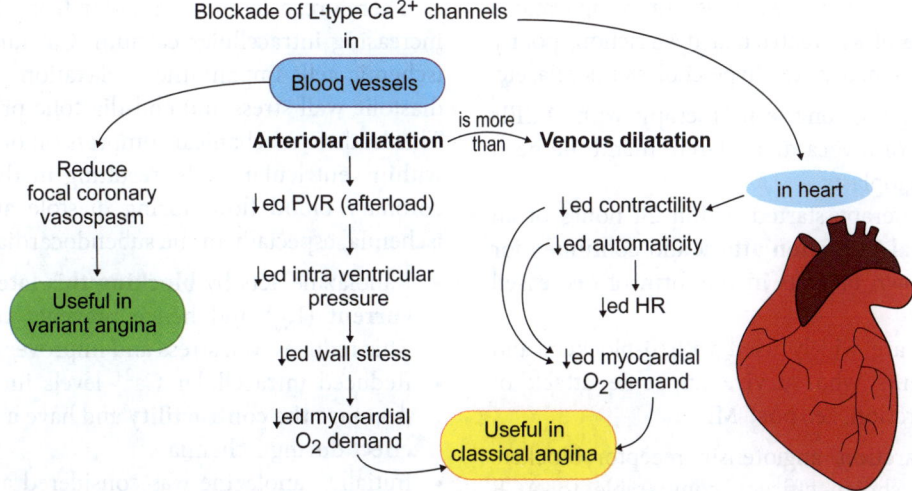

Fig. 34.9 Role of CCBs in IHD

hence **myocardial O$_2$ demand decreases**. Thus, the CCBs are useful in angina of effort.
- In cardiac muscle, CCBs decrease contractility in a dose-dependent manner. CCBs decrease oxygen demand by **reduction of cardiac mechanical function**. They also reduce automaticity, leading to a decrease in HR. This effect causes further decrease in O$_2$ demand and makes them useful in angina of effort.
- In addition, verapamil and diltiazem have **nonspecific antiadrenergic effects** that may contribute to their vasodilator action. There are **variations** in the effect of different CCBs.
  - Dihydropyridines (DHPs) have greater effect on vascular smooth muscles than cardiac effects. Different DHPs may vary in their effect on different vascular beds because of the differences in the structure of α$_1$ subunits.
  - Verapamil has greater cardiac effects than vascular effects, because it blocks K$^+$ channels also in vascular smooth muscles that limit its vasodilator effect.
- In patients with variant or vasospastic angina, CCBs **reduce focal coronary artery vasospasm** that improves coronary flow. Thus, CCBs are useful in prophylaxis of this type of angina.
- However, in patients of **unstable angina**, CCBs are not first-line drugs. These may be used only as add-on therapy in cases having prominent coronary vasospasm. The **immediate-release preparations of rapid- and short-acting CCBs** (nifedipine/nimodipine/nicardipine) are **contraindicated** because a quick and sharp fall in BP caused by such preparations may compromise organ (cerebral and myocardial) perfusion. This can result in catastrophic outcomes like cerebrovascular accidents, acute MI, conduction defects and may be fatal.

4. K$^+$-channel Openers in Angina

Minoxidil and diazoxide are K$^+$-channel openers that are useful in severe hypertension and hypertensive emergencies.

Another K$^+$-channel opener, nicorandil, has a dual mechanism of action:
- It activates ATP-sensitive K$^+$-channels (K$_{ATP}$) in membranes of smooth muscles, resulting in membrane-hyperpolarisation and relaxation.
- Nitrate-like NO-releasing action, resulting in cGMP production that causes dephosphorylation of myosin light chains, leading to smooth muscle relaxation.

Role of nicorandil in angina
- Nicorandil causes **arterial as well as venous dilatation** leading to reduction in both preload and afterload. Coronary flow is increased.
- While its cardiac effects are not significant, it has **cardioprotective** action due to the activation of cardiac mitochondrial K$_{ATP}$ channels. This results in brief periods of ischemia and reperfusion. This **ischemic preconditioning** exerts a cardioprotective action during total vascular occlusion.
- It reduces frequency of angina attacks and improves exercise tolerance in stable as well as variant angina; however, its long term effects are less well-established. Thus, it is used as a **2nd line antianginal drug** along with other drugs for resistant angina.

Pharmacokinetics
Nicorandil is well-absorbed orally, completely metabolised by the liver, and excreted in urine.

Adverse effects include flushing, palpitation, weakness, headache, dizziness, nausea, vomiting and painful aphthous ulcers in the mouth.

Tolerance does not occur to the vasodilator effect of nicorandil, but it can interact with PDE5 inhibitors, e.g., sildenafil (in a manner similar to nitrates).

5. ACEIs in IHD

Although ACE inhibitors do not have direct antianginal effect, they provide maximum benefit to patients suffering from **chronic IHD** with increased risk of complications due to the presence of left ventricular dysfunction, poorly controlled hypertension, diabetes, hypercholesterolemia, etc.

- In **unstable angina**, long-term therapy with ACEIs reduces the risk of myocardial infarction and the need for coronary angioplasty.
- ACE inhibitor therapy started within 24 hours of an **acute myocardial infarction attack** and continued for 6 weeks has shown benefits in the form of decreased mortality.
- ACE inhibitors are widely used with β-blockers and statins in patients who survive an acute attack of myocardial infarction, i.e., **post-MI**.

In myocardial infarction, angiotensin receptor blockers (ARBs) have also shown efficacy comparable to ACE inhibitors.

6. Ranolazine
Mechanism of action

In the ischemic myocardium, a late inward sodium current (I_{Na}) contributes to an increase in intracellular sodium that promotes reverse mode sodium–calcium exchange (The sodium–calcium exchanger works in two modes. In the forward mode, one Ca^{2+} is eliminated for influx of 3 Na^+ to accomplish diastolic relaxation (refer to Fig. 33.6). In its reverse mode, 2 Ca^{2+} move into the cell in exchange for the elimination of 3 Na^+ (Fig. 34.10). The direction of transport depends on the membrane potential and intracellular sodium and calcium concentrations).

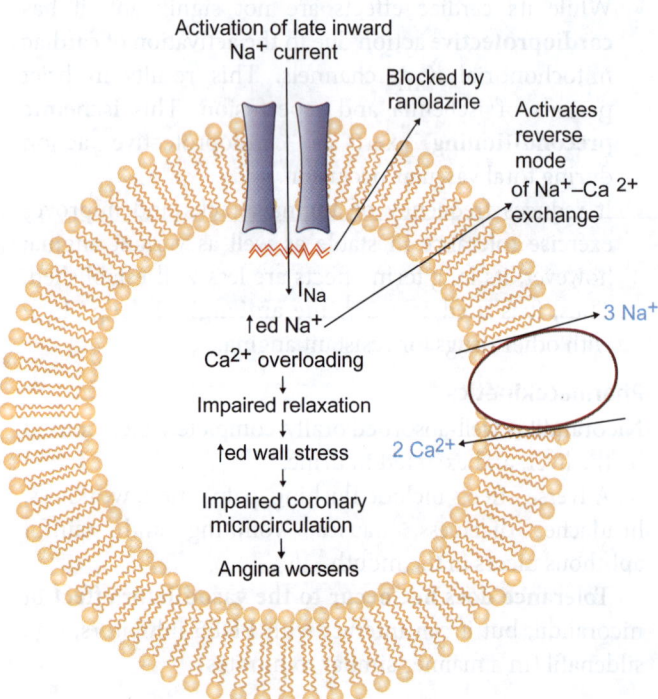

Fig. 34.10 Ionic movements in an ischemic cell and mechanism of action of ranolazine

Therefore, calcium elimination from the cell is reduced, increasing intracellular calcium. Calcium overloading of ischemic cells impairs their relaxation. Thus, ventricular diastolic wall stress and end-diastolic pressure are raised. This leads to mechanical compression of microcirculation within ventricular walls, resulting in the impairment of coronary blood flow during diastole and worsening of ischemia, especially in the subendocardial region.

- Ranolazine acts by **blocking this late inward sodium current** (I_{Na}) and hence prevents calcium overload. This reduces wall stress and improves coronary flow.
- Reduced intracellular Ca^{2+} levels in the myocardium **decrease the contractility** and have **a cardioprotective effect** during ischemia.
- Initially, ranolazine was considered a partial inhibitor of the fatty acid oxidation pathway (pFOX inhibitor) in the ischemic myocardium by inhibition of enzyme LC 3-KAT (long chain 3-ketoacyl-CoA thiolase). However, this action is not seen at therapeutically attained concentrations of ranolazine.
- Ranolazine has no effect on the HR and BP, but improves exercise duration in angina patients and decreases frequency of angina attacks. Thus, it is **effective in chronic stable angina, but does not reduce mortality in acute coronary syndrome**.
- It can be **safely** used with **sildenafil**.

ADRs

The adverse effects include headache, dizziness, postural hypotension, weakness, constipation, and dyspepsia; it may also prolong QT interval.

Contraindications: Ranolazine should not be combined with drugs that can prolong the QT interval, such as quinidine, procainamide, and sotalol. It is also contraindicated in liver and kidney disease.

7. Ivabradine

Ivabradine inhibits **hyperpolarisation-activated sodium channels in the SA node** (called funny current, I_f), resulting in reduced heart rate and hence reduced myocardial O_2 demand. No other hemodynamic effects are seen. Decrease in HR leads to prolongation of diastole to allow more time for coronary perfusion. Thus, ivabradine improves exercise tolerance and decreases frequency of angina attacks. Its **antianginal efficacy is the same as β-blockers and CCBs**.

Ivabradine is **used in stable angina when β-blockers are contraindicated**. Other uses include sinus tachycardia and Grades II–IV heart failure due to systolic dysfunction.

The most important ADRs of ivabradine are visual disturbances, extrasystoles, prolonged PR interval, headache and dizziness.

Contraindications to use of ivabradine are HR < 60, sick sinus syndrome and atrial fibrillation.

8. Trimetazidine

It has no effect on myocardial O_2 demand at rest or during exercise, but still decreases angina frequency and increases exercise tolerance. It acts by inhibiting the mitochondrial LC 3-KAT enzyme involved in fatty acid metabolism in ischemic myocardium, i.e., it is a **pFOX inhibitor**. Thus, **glucose oxidation is promoted instead of fatty acid oxidation**. For generating the same amount of ATP, glucose oxidation consumes lesser oxygen than fatty acid oxidation. This decreases the O_2 demand of the ischemic myocardium.

Trimetazidine is used as **add-on** drug to conventional treatment in angina and post-MI patients.

ADRs are mild gastric irritation, fatigue, dizziness and muscle cramps.

9. Dipyridamole

Adenosine is a local mediator causing auto regulation of coronary flow in response to ischemia. Dipyridamole acts by **preventing uptake and degradation of adenosine**. It is not useful as an antianginal drug, because it diverts blood to the non-ischemic zone by dilating small autoregulatory vessels in this zone. Vessels in the ischemic area are already dilated as a compensatory mechanism to anoxia; these cannot dilate further under the drug's effect (**coronary steal phenomenon**). Dipyridamole is, however, useful as an adjuvant antiplatelet drug (refer to page 518).

10. Fasudil

Rho-kinases prevent the dephosphorylation of myosin LCs and hence inhibit vascular relaxation. Excess activity of Rho-kinases is implicated in coronary vasospasm and pulmonary hypertension.

By exerting an **inhibitory effect on smooth muscle Rho-kinases**, fasudil reduces coronary vasospasm in experimental animals. Fasudil has also shown improvement of performance of CAD patients in stress tests in clinical trials.

Clinical problem-based questions and MCQs

9. A 50-year-old male patient diagnosed with acute myocardial infarction is given metoprolol 6 hours after an ischemic episode.
   i. Describe pharmacological basis for use of metoprolol in this case.
   ii. What conditions must have been excluded before prescribing metoprolol to this patient?
10. A 56-year-old female patient suffering from stable angina is prescribed a combination of atenolol and nitrates.
    i. Describe the mechanism of beneficial action of atenolol in stable angina.
    ii. Describe the rationale for combining nitrates with atenolol in this case.
11. CCBs have an important role in the management of angina of effort as well as vasospastic angina. However, immediate-release, short-acting CCBs are contraindicated in unstable angina.
    i. Describe mechanism of beneficial effect of CCBs in
        a. Angina of effort
        b. Vasospastic angina
    ii. Explain why short-acting CCBs are contraindicated in unstable angina
12. i. Identify the drug contraindicated in vasospastic angina.
        a. GTN   b. Atenolol
        c. Nifedipine   d. Diltiazem
    ii. Describe the pharmacological basis for your answer.
13. i. Which of the following drugs is contraindicated in unstable angina?
        a. GTN   b. Atenolol
        c. Nifedipine   d. Diltiazem
    ii. Describe the pharmacological basis for your answer.
14. i. Identify the mechanism of vasodilator effect of nicorandil.
        a. β-blocker
        b. Reduces inward Na current
        c. Calcium channel blocker
        d. Potassium channel opener
    ii. Describe mechanism of beneficial effect of nicorandil in angina
15. Match the following antianginal drugs with their mechanism of action.

a.	Trimetazidine	1.	Inhibits hyperpolarisation-activated sodium channels
b.	Ivabradine	2.	Inhibits smooth muscle Rho-kinases
c.	Ranolazine	3.	Promotes glucose oxidation over FA oxidation
d.	Fasudil	4.	Inhibits ischemia-induced inward sodium current

16. The antianginal effect of propranolol may be attributed to:
    a. Block exercise-induced tachycardia
    b. Dilatation of constricted coronary vessels
    c. Increased cardiac force
    d. Increased resting heart rate
17. Propranolol is contraindicated in a patient of angina pectoris who is already receiving:
    a. Nifedipine   b. Aspirin
    c. Verapamil   d. Isosorbide mononitrate
18. Coronary steal phenomenon is caused by:
    a. Dipyridamole   b. Diltiazem
    c. Propranolol   d. Verapamil

MANAGEMENT OF ACUTE CORONARY SYNDROMES

Acute coronary syndromes can be graded as:
- **Unstable Angina** (UA)
  - Vascular obstruction is incomplete.
  - Myocardial necrosis is not present.
  - Markers of ischemia (myoglobin, CK–MB, troponin I) are not seen
  - ST segment is not elevated
- **Non-ST-Elevation MI** (NSTEMI)
  - Vascular obstruction is incomplete
  - Partial thickness of ventricular wall is involved
  - Small area of necrosis is present
  - Biochemical markers appear
  - ST segment is not elevated
- **ST Elevation MI** (STEMI)
  - Vascular obstruction is complete
  - Full thickness of ventricular wall is involved
  - Large area of necrosis is present
  - Biochemical markers are prominently raised
  - ST segment is elevated

Treatment of Unstable Angina (UA) and Non-ST-elevation MI (NSTEMI)

- Patients with UA and NSTEMI are advised **bed rest**.
- **Constant monitoring of ECG** is done for ST elevation and any rhythm disturbances. If the patient does not show any recurrence of ischemia for 12–24 hours, ambulation is permitted.
- **Anti-ischemic treatment**: NG is given by S/L route (0.3–0.6 mg), repeated after 5 minutes if pain is not relieved. Three such doses can be given. If ischemic pain is still not controlled, I/V NG (5–10 mcg/min) is administered every 3–5 min till symptoms resolve or systolic BP falls to < 100 mm of Hg.
- Oral β-blockers, to achieve HR 50–60 bpm, are the mainstay of anti-ischemic therapy. If the symptoms persist after administering the full dose of nitrates and β-blockers, CCBs with prominent cardiac action (verapamil or diltiazem) are used.
- ACEIs and statins are indicated for secondary prevention.
- Antithrombotic therapy with low dose aspirin (75–325 mg) and clopidogrel reduces chances of MI, stroke and cardiovascular mortality. Prasugrel and ticagrelor are the other alternative drugs for antithrombotic therapy.
- Anticoagulant therapy can be provided with unfractionated heparin (UFH), low molecular weight heparin/enoxaparin (LMWH) or fondaparinux.

Major adverse effect of all antithrombotic and anticoagulant drugs is excessive bleeding, which can be checked by carefully adjusting the dose for weight and existing renal function.

Management of STEMI

Myocardial infarction involves ischemic necrosis of some part of the myocardium due to sudden obstruction of a branch of the coronary artery. 25% of patients of myocardial infarction die before they can get medical help. Those who are hospitalised need continuous monitoring of hemodynamic parameters, biochemical markers and ECG to guide selection of drugs and dosages. Important steps of management of acute MI include:

1. **Emergency management** involves recognition and treatment of rhythm disturbances and pump failure, resuscitative manoeuvres (defibrillation and advanced cardiac life support), and reperfusion therapy.
   - Fibrinolytics (alteplase/tenecteplase) are indicated in STEMI or high-risk non-STEMI within 1–2 hours of MI onset to reperfuse the infarcted area.
   - PCI stenting is the preferred revasculation procedure.
2. **Supportive treatment:** This involves maintenance of oxygenation by O_2 inhalation and assisted respiration if needed.
   - Maintenance of tissue perfusion by slow IV infusion of 5% dextrose or normal saline. Extra care should be taken to avoid volume overloading which will be counterproductive.
   - Correction of acidosis by intravenous sodium bicarbonate infusion.
3. **Control of acute symptoms** like pain and anxiety by GTN (up to 3 doses can be given). If the patient develops acute left ventricular failure or acute pulmonary edema, parenteral opioid administration is indicated. Morphine is useful as it shifts the blood away from the pulmonary to the systemic circulation and also relieves the associated anxiety. Pentazocine and pethidine cause tachycardia and may worsen the patient's condition.
4. **β blockers** are given intravenously or orally within 4–6 hours of an acute attack, if there is no contraindication to their use (i.e., patient is not in cardiac failure or shock, HR > 50, and AV block not > 1st degree). Such early use of β-blockers aid myocardial salvage to limit the infarct size and also decreases the risk of dangerous arrhythmias and mortality during acute MI.
5. **Management of coexistent arrhythmias:** Intravenous lignocaine, procainamide or amiodarone is used to treat tachyarrhythmias occurring during acute MI. Atropine and electrical pacing are useful for treatment of bradyarrhythmias and heart blocks.
6. **Maintenance of pumping function of heart:** Useful drugs are
   - Loop diuretics: Furosemide
   - Vasodilators: GTN slow IV infusion, esmolol or labetolol may be added
7. **Inotropic drugs** (dopamine/dobutamine) may be needed to tide over the crisis.
8. **Secondary prophylaxis** aims to prevent reinfarction. Important measures include:
   - Long-term usage of oral β-blockers reduces the risk of reinfarction. They also prevent ventricular fibrillation during subsequent attacks.

- Hyperlipidemia control by use of unsaturated fats and statins reduce the risk of cardiovascular events.
- **Prevention of thrombosis:**
  - Antiaggregatory drugs like low-dose aspirin (162–325 mg chewable tab), clopidogrel or ticagrelor.
  - Anticoagulants (heparins initially, followed later by oral anticoagulants) are given to prevent deep vein thrombosis (DVT), and check coronary thrombus extension. However, their benefits are uncertain.
- **Prevention of remodelling and CHF development:** ACEIs/ARBs are started as soon as the patient is stable. They have proven efficacy and long-term survival benefits.

Clinical problem-based questions and MCQs

19. Which of the following drugs is used for control of acute symptoms in MI?
    a. Morphine   b. Butorphanol
    c. Cocaine   d. Pethidine

20. A 56-year-old male patient is brought to emergency with severe presternal pain radiating to root of neck and left shoulder. Patient is sweating profusely. On examination BP is 90/50, ECG shows a raised ST segment and biochemical markers (CK–MB and troponin 1) are raised.
    i. Comment on the role of β-blockers in this case.
    ii. Comment on role of nitrates in this case.
    iii. Which drug is not useful in this case?
       a. GTN   b. Alteplase
       c. Phentolamine d. Dopamine

Summary

- The three major blood vessels supplying the heart are the left anterior descending (LAD) or anterior interventricular artery, posterior interventricular artery and right marginal artery.
- Imbalance between myocardial oxygen demand and supply causes IHD.
- HR, contractility and wall stress determine myocardial oxygen demand. Wall stress depends on ventricular volume, intraventricular pressure and wall thickness.
- Myocardial oxygen supply depends on diastolic duration (as coronary flow is negligible during systole), aortic diastolic pressure and coronary vascular resistance.
- Chronic stable angina/exertional angina, unstable angina (UA), non-ST-elevation myocardial infarction (NSTEMI) and ST-elevation myocardial infarction (STEMI) represent the same disease process with increasing severity.
- Severe, prolonged ischemia results in necrosis and fibrous replacement (scarring) of the myocardium, which interferes with the pumping function of the heart → atrophy of conducting tissue → arrhythmias.
- Treatment of IHD involves risk factor modification, symptom control with antianginal drugs, correction of underlying cause with antiplatelet/fibrinolytic/hypolipidemic drugs and rehabilitation.
- Drugs useful in IHD include nitrates, β-blockers, calcium channel blockers, potassium channel openers, ACE inhibitors/ARBs and miscellaneous drugs (ranolazine, ivabradine, trimetazidine, dipyridamole, fasudil, etc.)
- **Nitrates** are the mainstay of angina treatment. They act by releasing NO → cGMP production → dephosphorylation of myosin light chain → smooth muscle relaxation.
  - Venodilatation > arterial > arteriolar dilatation.
  - Reduce oxygen demand and cause redistribution of coronary blood flow from non-ischemic to ischemic zones.
- Nitrite ion can cause methemoglobinemia that may be useful in cyanide poisoning.
- Nitrates are used in stable angina, unstable angina, myocardial infarction, congestive heart failure and portal hypertension.
- It is important to provide an 8-hour nitrate-free interval for preventing tolerance.
- ADRs of nitrates include throbbing headache, dizziness, facial flushing, orthostatic hypotension, syncopal attack and tachycardia. Occupational exposure to high concentration of nitrates can cause development of tolerance (Monday disease) and even dependence.
- **β-blockers** in angina reduce myocardial oxygen demand by reducing HR, contractility and BP. Increased duration of diastole → more time for coronary perfusion → improved perfusion.
- β-blockers are used in acute MI for myocardial salvage to reduce the infarct size and prevent arrhythmias. However, they are given only to patients who are not in shock, have HR > 50 and AV block not > 1st degree. They are also useful for secondary prophylaxis to prevent reinfarction and arrhythmias during subsequent attacks.
- Contraindications to the use of β-blockers include vasospastic or variant angina, bronchial asthma, COPD, bradycardia, AV blocks and severe LVF.
- In angina, **CCBs** cause vascular smooth muscle relaxation by decreasing the frequency of channel opening → reduced intracellular calcium.
- Arterioles are more sensitive to the VD effect of CCBs; reduced wall stress → reduced myocardial oxygen demand → useful in classical angina.
- Cardiac effects of CCBs reduce myocardial oxygen demand → useful in classical angina.

- CCBs can reverse coronary vasospasm → useful in variant angina.
- Immediate-release, short-acting CCBs are contraindicated as they can impair organ perfusion resulting in catastrophic outcomes.
- **Nicorandil** activates K_{ATP} channels in smooth muscles → hyperpolarisation → smooth muscle relaxation → **arterial as well as venodilatation** → reduced preload and afterload
  - It is a second-line drug in resistant cases.
  - Ischemic pre-conditioning of myocardium through K_{ATP} channel activation is cardioprotective.
- **Ranolazine** acts by reducing the late I_{Na} → reduced activity of reverse Na^+/Ca^{2+} exchanger → reduced intracellular calcium → reduced contractility → cardioprotective effect in angina. Ranolazine improves exercise tolerance in angina and decreases frequency of angina attacks.
  - It is used in chronic stable angina, but has no utility in acute coronary syndromes.
- **Ivabradine** decreases HR by inhibiting hyperpolarisation-activated sodium channels (I_f) in SA node → prolonged diastolic duration allows better coronary perfusion → used in stable angina if β-blockers are contraindicated, sinus tachycardia and Grades II–IV heart failure due to systolic dysfunction.

  Contraindications are sick sinus syndrome, AF and severe bradycardia with HR < 60.
- **Trimetazidine** favours use of glucose for ATP generation instead of fatty acids. Improves exercise tolerance and reduces frequency of angina episodes. It is used as an add-on drug in angina and post-MI patients.
- **Management of acute coronary syndromes**: They are graded as unstable angina, non-ST-elevation MI (NSTEMI) and ST elevation MI (STEMI), based on severity of ischemia. Patients need hospitalisation and close monitoring of ECG for ST elevation and rhythm disturbances. Treatment of acute myocardial infarction (STEMI) involves O_2 inhalation or assisted respiration, maintenance of tissue perfusion with caution to prevent volume overloading, control of pain and anxiety with nitrates/opioids, maintenance of pump function of heart, prevention and treatment of rhythm disturbances, antiaggregatory drugs and hypolipidemic drugs.

Questions for practice

1. Classify antianginal drugs. What is the rationale for the use of nitrates in angina?
2. Describe the mechanism of action, clinical uses and adverse drug reactions of nitrates.
3. Explain the pharmacological basis for use of:
   a. β-blockers in angina
   b. β-blockers in myocardial infarction
   c. CCBs in angina
   d. Ranolazine in angina
4. Explain why:
   a. Nitroglycerin is given sublingually in acute attack of angina.
   b. β-blockers are contraindicated in Prinzmetal angina.
   c. ACE inhibitors are used in IHD.
5. Write short notes on:
   a. Nicorandil
   b. Ranolazine
   c. Ivabradine

Hints for problem-based questions and MCQs

1. i. b. Sublingual route
   ii. Quick absorption, better bioavailability.
2. i. a. Decreasing O_2 demand
   ii. Refer to pages 455, 457.
3. i. a. Veins
4. d. Isosorbide dinitrate
5. a. Variant angina involves coronary vasospasm. Its reversal increases O_2 supply.
6. i. Monday disease (refer to page 457)
   ii. a. Tolerance to nitrates
7. i. Tachyphylaxis is the rapid development of tolerance to the effects of drugs. Tolerance to nitrates occurs because of reduced capacity to release NO, compensatory mechanisms, reduced SH groups. reduced CGRP, and generation of free radicals. Refer to pages 455, 457.
   ii. Provide an 8-hour nitrate-free interval each night, when oxygen demand is low; SH donors, antioxidants, other drugs such as ACEIs and carvedilol.
8. Sodium nitrite converts Hb to methemoglobin, which forms cyanmethemoglobin. Sodium thiosulphate forms thiocyanate → readly excreted. Methylene blue is given to manage excess metHb. Refer to page 456.
9. i. Limit infarct size and prevent arrhythmia.
   ii. Patient not in shock, HR not < 50, not > first degree AV block.
10. i. Atenolol acts by reducing O_2 demand, resulting in prevention of reinfarction. It also prevents arrhythmias during subsequent attacks.
    ii. Increase in end-diastolic volume caused by atenolol is countered by nitrates. Refer to page 458.
11. i a. Refer to page 458.
    i b. Refer to page 459.
    ii. Refer to page 459.
12. i. b. Atenolol
    ii. Can worsen coronary vasospasm.
13. i. c. Nifedipine
    ii. Refer to page 459.
14. i. d. Potassium channel opener
    ii. Vasodilator and cardioprotective effect by activating K_{ATP} channels → preconditioning of myocardium.
15. a–3; b–1; c–4; d–2.
16. a. Block exercise induced tachycardia
17. c. Verapamil
18. a. Dipyridamole
19. a. Morphine.
20. i. Limit infarct size and prevent arrhythmia
    ii. Relieve acute symptoms
    iii. c. Phentolamine

Chapter 34 Drugs for Ischemic Heart Disease

CONCEPT MAP - DRUGS FOR IHD

DRUGS FOR IHD

NITRATES

Uses
- Stable angina
- Unstable angina
- MI
- CHF
- Portal hypertension

ADRs
- Throbbing headache, Dizziness, Facial flushing, Orthostatic hypotension, Syncope, Tachycardia.
- With occupational exposure 'Monday disease', Dependence

Mechanism of Antianginal Effect
- Release NO → ↑cGMP → inactivates MLC → vasodilatation
- VD of veins > large arteries > arterioles
- VD veins → Reduced preload, end diastolic volume, wall stress → reduced O_2 demand
- VD arteries → redistribution from non-ischemic to ischemic area

Classification

- **Short Acting:** Isosorbide dinitrate (S/L), Glyceryl trinitrate (GTN) OR Nitroglycerin (NG), Amyl Nitrite (now obsolete)
- **Long Acting:** Isosorbide dinitrate (oral), Erythrityl tetranitrate, Pentaerythritol tetranitrate (PETN), Molsidomine
- **β Blockers:** Propranolol, Metoprolol, Atenolol
- **CCBs:** Verapamil, Diltiazem, Amlodipine
- **KCO:** Nicorandil
- **ACE Inhibitors:** Captopril, Enalapril, Ramipril, Lisinopril
- **Others:** Ranolazine, Ivabradine, Trimetazidine, Dipyridamole, Fasudil

Others

- **Nicorandil:** Potassium channel opener → VD
- **Ranolazine:** reduces late I_{Na} in ischemic cells
- **Ivabradine:** reduces I_f in SA node → ↓ed HR
- **Trimetazidine:** pFOX inhibitor
- **Fasudil:** Rho kinase inhibitor

β Blockers

Mechanism of Antianginal Effect
- Reduce HR, contractility, BP → reduced myocardial O_2 demand
- With decrease in HR → diastolic duration ↑es → coronary perfusion improves

Uses
- AMI : For myocardial salvage to reduce infarct size and prevent arrhythmias.
- For secondary prophylaxis to prevent reinfarction and arrhythmias during any subsequent attack.
- With nitrates for stable and unstable angina

Contraindications
- In AMI cases with shock, HR < 50 bpm and > first degree AV block.
- In vasospastic angina

CCBs

Mechanism of Antianginal Effect
- Antianginal action: Vascular smooth muscle relaxation → vasodilatation.
- Arteriolar VD → reduced PVR → reduced wall stress → reduced myocardial O_2 demand.
- Reverse coronary spasm in variant angina.

Contraindications
- Immediate release, nifedipine contraindicated in unstable angina as they cause tachycardia & accentuate angina
- Verapamil not to be given in sick sinus syndrome & with β blockers.

Uses
- Classical angina if Nitrates + β blockers fail.
- Vasospastic angina

Acute Coronary Syndromes

UA & NSTEMI
Bed rest → ambulation after 12–24 hours.
NG : 0.3–0.6 mg, 3 doses, 5 minutes apart
β blockers (target HR 50–60 bpm)
Verapamil/diltiazem added in resistant cases

STEMI
O_2 inhalation, IV infusion
GTN up to 3 doses
IV morphine in acute LVF, IV $NaHCO_3$
Management of arrhythmias
For pump function: furosemide/ vasodilators/Inotropics
Fibrinolytics/PCI
Secondary prophylaxis: ACE inhibitor, Aspirin/clopidogrel
UFH/LMWH/Fondaparinux

SECTION 7 Drugs Acting on CVS

35 Drugs for Peripheral Vascular Disease (PVD) and Management of Shock

PH 4.8 Describe types, salient pharmacokinetics, pharmacodynamics, therapeutic uses, and adverse drug reactions of drugs used for the management of peripheral vascular disease.
PH 2.3 Explain the rationale and demonstrate the emergency use of various sympathetic and parasympathetic drug agonists/antagonists (like noradrenaline/adrenaline/dopamine/dobutamine, atropine) in case-based scenarios (see also Chapters 2 and 71).

Learning objectives

A student of MBBS phase II should be able to:
- Enumerate drugs used for peripheral vascular diseases.
- Describe the management of peripheral vascular diseases.
- Define shock.
- Describe different types of shock.
- Describe stepwise approach to diagnose type of shock.
- Describe the general principles in management of shock.
- Explain role of drugs in management of different types of shock.
- Classify plasma volume expanders and discuss their mechanism of action.
- Explain the indications for use of plasma volume expanders and enumerate their ADRs and contraindications.

PERIPHERAL VASCULAR DISEASE (PVD)

Peripheral vascular disease (PVD) is a broad term for diseases of all blood vessels, i.e., arteries, veins and lymphatics. However, diseases of the peripheral arteries, called peripheral arterial diseases (PAD), commonly affecting lower limb arteries, are more frequently encountered; the two terms (PVD and PAD) are often used interchangeably.

Types of PAD

PAD is mainly of two types—organic and functional.
 Organic PAD is characterised by **structural changes in the blood vessels** such as formation of atheromatous plaques, inflammation and tissue necrosis, as seen in, arteriosclerosis, intermittent claudication and thromboangiitis obliterans (Buerger's disease). The formation of atherosclerotic plaques initiates a series of changes that result in the formation of platelet plugs and thrombi. Such atheromas and thrombi obstruct the flow of blood through medium and large arteries and cause ischemia of peripheral skeletal muscles, especially in the lower limbs.
 Functional PAD is characterised by the **exaggerated response of blood vessels** to emotional stress and temperature changes **leading to episodic spasms of vessels**. It is also called peripheral vasospastic disease or Raynaud's disease/phenomenon, characterised by symmetrical vasospasm of digital arteries, arterioles and cutaneous arterio-venous shunts, precipitated by extreme cold or emotional stress, resulting in tissue ischemia.

Risk Factors

Important risk factors for developing PVD include:
- Age > 50 years.
- Gender: more common in male than female patients.
- Positive family history of atherosclerotic disease.
- Obesity, cigarette smoking, sedentary life style, etc.
- Hyperlipidemia, especially raised LDL and triglyceride levels; low HDL is also an important risk factor for development of atherosclerosis.
- Diabetes mellitus, chronic renal failure and hypertension.

In PVD, the **effect of risk factors is additive**. Thus, persons with > 1 risk factor are more likely to suffer from more severe types of PVD.

Etiopathogenesis

- Atherosclerosis causes narrowing of blood vessels. Thromboembolic phenomenon may follow, causing

complete obstruction and catastrophic outcomes due to tissue necrosis.
- Vasculitis associated with injury to blood vessels, surgery and clotting disorders may also cause tissue ischemia and necrosis.
- Exposure to cold environment or stress can cause vasoconstriction, leading to tissue ischemia, as seen in Raynaud's disease.

Clinical Features and Diagnosis

While nearly 50% patients with PVD or PAD are asymptomatic, others may present with the following signs/symptoms:

- **Intermittent claudication** is characterised by cramping pain in legs or arms upon exercise that is relieved with rest. The most common site for pain in intermittent claudication is the calf muscles. The pain slowly increases while walking and the patient needs to stop; once they rest, the pain quickly disappears.
  - In severe cases with critically reduced blood supply, pain in legs and feet occurs even during rest. Such pain is more disturbing at night.
  - Weakness and atrophy of calf muscles.
  - Cold legs or feet.
- In **Raynaud's disease**, patients complain of numbness of fingertips, toes, nose, and ears. The colour of overlying skin may change to pale and then blue. Touch sensation may be reduced. There may be throbbing pain in fingers/toes in severe cases.
  - The colour of skin over the feet may change upon changing the position of feet. When elevated, the skin is pale, but when dropped, in dependent position, the skin is dusky red.
  - Poor wound healing due to reduced blood supply.
  - In the late stages, ulcers, cyanosis and gangrene may occur in toes.
  - On examination, peripheral pulses are weak or absent.

Investigations

- Doppler ultrasound calculates the ankle brachial index (ABI), which is the ankle blood pressure divided by the brachial blood pressure.
  - ABI 0.9–1.3 is normal.
  - ABI < 0.9 indicates peripheral arterial disease in legs.
  - ABI < 0.5 indicates severe disease.
- Duplex ultrasound detects the exact site and degree of narrowing or obstruction. Angiography using X-rays, CT scans and MRI is useful to get an exact view of the location and extent of obstruction; this helps in surgical correction

Management

The goal of treatment in PVD is to:
- Improve exercise tolerance and increase the distance at which onset of claudication occurs.
- Achieve symptomatic relief.
- Prevent severe complications like ulcers, gangrene, stroke and limb amputation.

These goals are achieved by:

a. **Lifestyle modification** including:
   - Dietary modifications.
   - Physical therapy, increased activity and exercise for weight reduction. Further, regular supervised exercise is reported to improve oxygenation of muscles, formation of collateral vessels and reduce symptoms.
   - Smoking cessation.

b. **Risk reduction**: Diseases like DM, hypertension and dyslipidemia should be adequately treated, as these are important risk factors.

c. **Pharmacotherapy**: Drug treatment primarily **aims** at:
   - Reversing or controlling the atheromatous process with lipid-lowering drugs or prevention of clotting in the region of atheromatous plaque by antiplatelet drugs, fibrinolytics, and anticoagulants.
   - Improving blood flow through partially obstructed vessels by reducing blood viscosity and increasing erythrocyte flexibility: pentoxifylline, cilostazol, and naftidrofuryl oxalate are used.
   - Conventional vasodilators are not very beneficial in PVD. Blood vessels distal to the obstruction become dilated as a compensatory mechanism. Vasodilators can cause the **steal phenomenon**, i.e., vasodilatation of other arteries diverts blood away from the ischemic to non-ischemic areas.
   - **Drugs** useful in the treatment of PVDs include:
     1. Phosphodiesterase inhibitors: Pentoxifylline and cilostazol are used exclusively in PVD.
     2. 5-HT$_2$ blocker: Naftidrofuryl oxalate
     3. Antiplatelet, fibrinolytic or anti-coagulant drugs
     4. Lipid-lowering drugs: Statins
     5. Vasodilators: Cyclandelate, xanthinol nicotinate, α-blockers (Thymoxamine, tolazoline)

d. **Surgical interventions are needed** in severe cases. These include:
   - Percutaneous transluminal angioplasty (**PTA**) involves the insertion of a thin catheter from the groin artery. The catheter is advanced till the occluded area, and a balloon on its tip is inflated to enlarge the narrow artery.
   - Insertion of **stent** (a cylindrical wire mesh) via PTA into the narrowed region of the artery.

- Surgical treatment for PAD includes **bypass vascular surgery** and **endarterectomy**.

DRUGS USED IN PVD

1. Pentoxifylline

Mechanism of action

- Pentoxifylline is a methyl xanthine derivative that causes phosphodiesterase inhibition → it increases erythrocytic ATP and cyclic nucleotide levels → increased flexibility of RBCs. This is called **rheology modifying** effect.
- Pentoxifylline also decreases erythrocyte and platelet aggregation and plasma fibrinogen concentration. It also stimulates fibrinolysis. All these effects contribute towards **reducing blood viscosity** so that blood can flow easily through vessels partially obstructed by atheromatous plaques. Thus, blood flow to the ischemic area increases, and there is **no steal phenomenon**. The effect on cutaneous blood flow is greater than in skeletal muscles.

Uses

Pentoxifylline is used exclusively in PVD affecting the legs. It is also useful in venous leg ulcers secondary to trauma or varicose veins. It is given orally in a dose of 400 mg, twice a day.

ADRs

It can cause gastric irritant effects like nausea, vomiting, dyspepsia, abdominal pain and distension.

2. Cilostazol

Cilostazol is another phosphodiesterase 3 inhibitor that facilitates blood flow through partially obstructed vessels and also causes vasodilatation. It is useful to prevent claudication in the legs in PVD. The dosage is 100 mg orally, twice daily.

3. Naftidrofuryl Oxalate

Naftidrofuryl oxalate has multiple effects in PVD. It is a 5-HT$_2$ receptor blocker → reduces 5-HT-induced vasoconstriction and platelet aggregation. Similar to pentoxifylline, it also reduces plasma fibrinogen and improves flexibility of erythrocytes. This results in reduced blood viscosity and increased blood flow to the ischemic area.

- It has greater effect on the cutaneous flow, making it useful in healing of venous leg ulcers. Dose is 100–200 mg, twice or thrice a day, for a minimum period of 3 months.
- It is also useful in cerebral vascular disorders that cause confusion and mental deterioration, especially in the elderly.

- **ADRs**: It can cause headache, dizziness, agitation, insomnia, epigastric pain, esophagitis, diarrhea, renal stones, rashes, hepatitis and hepatic failure.
- **Contraindications**: It is contraindicated in patients < 18 years of age, hyperoxaluria, and nephrolithiasis. It should be used cautiously in pregnancy and lactation. Dose should be reduced in case of renal function impairment.

3. Others

Vasodilators like cyclandelate, xanthinol nicotinate and α-blockers (thymoxamine and tolazoline) are sometimes used in PVD. However, their efficacy is uncertain as they may cause greater vasodilatation in normal tissue than in diseased areas. Adverse effects like hypotension, headache, flushing and reflex tachycardia may occur.

Glyceryl trinitrate (GTN) may be tried in resistant cases.

Selective β$_2$-agonist **isoxsuprine** and calcium channel blockers (like **nifedipine and amlodipine**) may be useful in some mild cases.

Antiplatelet, **fibrinolytic** and **hypolipidemic** drugs are important **adjuvants** in treatment of PVD (Chapters 38, 39).

Clinical problem-based questions and MCQs

1. A 46-year-old patient complained of severe pain in their calf muscles on walking about 200 metres. Pain is severe enough to require stopping the activity and rest. Pain is relieved upon resting. Patient is a chain smoker since last 10 years and suffering from moderate hypertension.
   a. What is this patient probably suffering from?
   b. How the diagnosis can be confirmed?
   c. How this patient can be managed?

2. i. What is 'steal phenomenon' in PVD?
   ii. Which of the following drugs does NOT cause 'steal phenomenon' in PVD?
      a. Cyclandelate
      b. Xanthinol nicotinate
      c. Pentoxifylline
      d. Thymoxamine
   iii. Describe the mechanism of beneficial action of the selected drug in PVD.
   iv. Explain the pharmacological basis for lack of steal phenomenon of the selected drug.

3. i. Identify the drug that has a role in the management of venous leg ulcers.
      a. Naftidrofuryl oxalate
      b. Amiodarone
      c. Lignocaine
      d. Dobutamine
   ii. Describe the mechanism of beneficial effect of the selected drug.

CONCEPT MAP – DRUGS FOR PVD

Etiology
- Atherosclerosis → narrowing of vessel lumen
- Thromboembolic phenomenon → complete obstruction → tissue necrosis
- Episodic spasm of vessels due to exposure to cold or stress

Risk Factors
Males > 50 years, Obesity, Hyperlipidemia, DM, Smoking, Positive family history

Clinical Features
Cramping pain in legs/arms, worsens on walking, relieved with rest
Calf muscle atrophy
Numbness
Ulcers
Cyanosis
Weak peripheral pulses

Management
Lifestyle modification, Risk reduction, Physical therapy, Exercise training, Surgical (Percutaneous transluminal angioplasty, stenting/ vascular bypass surgery / endarterectomy)

Drugs
Phosphodiesterase inhibitors: Pentoxifylline, Cilostazol.
5-HT_2 blocker: Naftidrofuryl oxalate
Vasodilators: Cyclandelate, Xanthinol nicotinate
α blockers: Thymoxamine, Tolazoline
Adjuvants: Antiplatelet, fibrinolytic or anti-coagulants, Lipid-lowering drugs

Types
Organic
Arteriosclerosis, Intermittent claudication, Buerger's disease
Functional
Peripheral vasospastic disease or Raynaud's disease

DRUGS FOR PVD

Vasodilators
Cyclandelate, Xanthinol nicotinate, α blockers like thymoxamine, tolazoline
Uncertain efficacy in PVD as they may cause more vasodilation in normal tissue than in diseased area → steal phenomenon
Uses: GTN tried in resistant cases. Isoxsuprine (Selective $β_2$ agonist), Nifedipine, Amlodipine (CCBs) may be useful in some mild cases
ADRs: Hypotension, headache, flushing, reflex tachycardia

Naftidrofuryl Oxalate
Mechanism: 5-HT_2 receptor blocker → Reduction of 5-HT induced VC and platelet aggregation
Reduces plasma fibrinogen, improves flexibility of erythrocytes, reduced blood viscosity and increased blood flow to ischemic area.
Effect is more on cutaneous flow.
Uses: Useful in healing of venous leg ulcers, cerebral vascular disorders causing confusion and mental deterioration, especially in the elderly.
ADRs: Headache, dizziness, agitation, insomnia, epigastric pain, esophagitis, diarrhea, renal stones, rashes, hepatitis and hepatic failure

PDE3 Inhibitors
Pentoxifylline
Mechanism: Causes PDE inhibition → raised ATP and cyclic nucleotide levels → rheology modifying effect (increased-flexibility of RBCs).
Antiaggregatory, antiplatelet and fibrinolytic effect.
Reduced viscosity of blood
No steal phenomenon
Uses: PVD of legs, venous ulcers.
ADRs: Nausea, vomiting, dyspepsia, abdominal pain, distension.

Cilostazol
Same as pentoxifylline, also causes VD

SHOCK

Shock is a syndrome of reduced tissue perfusion due to any cause. A state of shock can occur as a manifestation of a variety of conditions such as severe hypersensitivity to drugs/food/insect bites, massive blood/fluid loss, sepsis, heart failure, and nerve injury. If left untreated, it rapidly progresses from the stage of tissue hypoperfusion to multi-organ damage and death, in about 40–60% cases.

Reduced tissue perfusion → reduced supply of oxygen to organs → oxygen demand–supply imbalance → cellular dysfunction → structural/functional changes in microvasculature → multi-organ failure → fatal outcome.

DIAGNOSIS OF SHOCK

The indicators of tissue hypoperfusion are:
- **Altered mentation**.
- **Hypotension**: Systolic BP < 90 mm of Hg or mean arterial pressure < 65 mm of Hg.
- **Tachypnea**: Respiratory rate > 20 per minute.
- **Tachycardia**: Heart rate > 100 bpm.
- **Oliguria**: Urine output < 0.5 mL/kg/h.
- **Lactic acidosis:** Due to excess formation of lactic acid in anaerobic metabolism, serum lactate > 4 mmol/L.

The presence of any four indicators is required to make a diagnosis of shock.

TYPES OF SHOCK

Broadly speaking, tissue hypoperfusion can occur due to less volume of available blood, less volume of blood pumped out by heart (low cardiac output), or low capacity of blood vessels to transport blood to tissues.

- **Less volume of fluid** in intravascular compartments (hypovolemia) can be:
  - Absolute: due to blood/plasma/fluid loss, as in **hypovolemic** shock.
  - Relative: due to abnormal distribution of fluid in different compartments (**distributive** shock).
- **Less amount of blood is pumped** out of the heart because of:
  - Diseased heart, as in **cardiogenic** shock
- An obstruction to blood flow in heart or great vessels, leads to **obstructive** shock.

Box 35.1 Analogy

To water plants, we need water, a pump to create pressure for the water to flow, and pipes to transport this water. The plants cannot be watered properly if:
- If there is less/no water available
- If the pump is not functioning properly
- If the pipe lumens are very narrow or compressed from outside.
- If pipes are leaky

Now, considering the heart as the pump, blood vessels as pipes, intravascular fluid as water, and tissues as plants, it is obvious that tissue hypoperfusion may occur due to:
- Less intravascular volume—hypovolemic shock.
- Abnormal pump function—cardiogenic shock.
- Intense vasoconstriction or compression of vessels—obstructive shock.
- Fluid is abnormally redistributed due to increased capillary permeability—distributive shock.

Thus, depending upon the underlying pathophysiological process, shock can be of four types: hypovolemic, distributive, cardiogenic and obstructive.

Hypovolemic Shock

Hypovolemic shock can occur due to:
- Loss of **blood**, as in internal hemorrhage (e.g., ulcer perforation and post-traumatic) or external hemorrhage (traumatic).
- Loss of **plasma**, as in burns.
- Loss of **fluid/electrolytes**, as in diarrhea, dehydration and heat stroke.

Patient has history of blood/fluid loss, cold, clammy skin, low central venous pressure However, lung crepitations are absent.

Distributive Shock

Distributive shock occurs due to endothelial dysfunction resulting in excessive capillary leakage, i.e., excessive movement of fluid to extravascular compartments. This causes relative hypovolemia. Such abnormal redistribution of fluids is seen in:

- **Septic** shock: It is commonly caused by gram-negative septicemia. The endotoxins produced by pathogenic bacteria cause excessive vasodilatation, resulting in fall in BP and shock. Septic shock is called 'warm shock' as the patient has warm extremities. Patient has a history of fever; infections and necrotic tissue may be present.
- **Neurogenic** shock: It is associated with spinal injuries due to trauma or as a complication of spinal anesthesia. The sympathetic tone is reduced and reflex vagal stimulation causes vasodilatation, hypotension, bradycardia, syncope and warm extremities.
- **Anaphylactic shock** occurs due to severe Type 1 hypersensitivity reaction to bee stings, other insect bites, and some foods or drugs. It involves an Ag–Ab reaction-mediated release of mediators (mainly histamine) that causes bronchoconstriction, vasodilatation, and warm extremities.

In the early phase of distributive shock, extremities are warm, central venous pressure (CVP) is low and pulse pressure wide. However, in the late phase, extremities are cold and patient is refractory to fluid therapy.

Cardiogenic Shock

Cardiogenic shock occurs following a fall in cardiac output due to a variety of cardiac diseases such as AMI or IHD, and atrial fibrillation, or other arrhythmias, valvular dysfunction, cardiomyopathy, etc. Patient has cold clammy skin, jugular venous pressure (JVP) is raised and pulse pressure is narrow; history is suggestive of previous cardiac diseases, and bilateral lung crepitations are present.

Obstructive Shock

Obstructive shock involves obstruction to flow of blood in heart or great vessels resulting in reduced cardiac output as seen in tension pneumothorax. Patient may have history of trauma leading to hemothorax or pneumothorax. JVP is high, but there are no lung crepitations.

These salient features of different types of shock enable the diagnosis of type and cause of shock to decide on the specific treatment. Features like temperature of extremities, pulse pressure, jugular venous pressure (JVP), lung crepitations in lungs help in differentiating different types of shock.

STEPWISE DIAGNOSIS OF TYPE OF SHOCK

1. **History**
   - History of (H/O) trauma, diarrhea, vomiting, hemorrhage, burns, or electrocution indicates hypovolemic shock.
   - H/O trauma along with weak heart sounds indicates obstructive shock, as in tension pneumothorax
   - H/O trauma to spinal cord or spinal/epidural anesthesia indicates neurogenic shock.
   - H/O previous cardiac disease or chest pain indicates cardiogenic shock.
   - H/O fever, infection, or lab investigations indicating infection are suggestive of septic shock.
   - H/O bee sting or food/drug intake points towards anaphylactic shock.
2. **Temperature of extremities** and **pulse pressure (PP):**
   - The pulse pressure (PP) is the difference between systolic and diastolic BP. A value of 25–60 mm of Hg is considered normal.
   - Warm extremities and wide PP (> 60 mm of Hg) indicate distributive shock (septic, neurogenic and anaphylactic shock). Pulse pressure is wide in these conditions due to hyperdynamic circulation (Fig. 35.1 a, c).
   - Cold, clammy skin with narrow PP (< 25 mm of Hg) indicates low cardiac output state, as seen in obstructive, hypovolemic, and cardiogenic shocks (Fig. 35.1 a, c).

3. **Jugular venous pressure** and **lung crepitations:**
   Jugular venous pressure (JVP) is assessed by keeping the patient inclined at 45° and observing pulsations of the jugular vein between the sternal and clavicular head of the sternocleidomastoid muscle (Fig. 35.1 b). The vertical distance of highest level of pulsation of jugular vein from the sternal angle is measured, and 5 cm is added to it (because the right atrium lies 5 cm below the sternal angle). Normal value of JVP is 6–8 cm of H_2O. A JVP value that is < 5 cm of H_2O is considered low and > 9 cm of H_2O is labelled as raised (Fig. 35.1 d).
   - Low JVP and no crepitations indicate hypovolemic shock.
   - Raised JVP and no crepitations indicate obstructive shock.
   - Raised JVP with bilateral lung crepitations indicate cardiogenic shock.

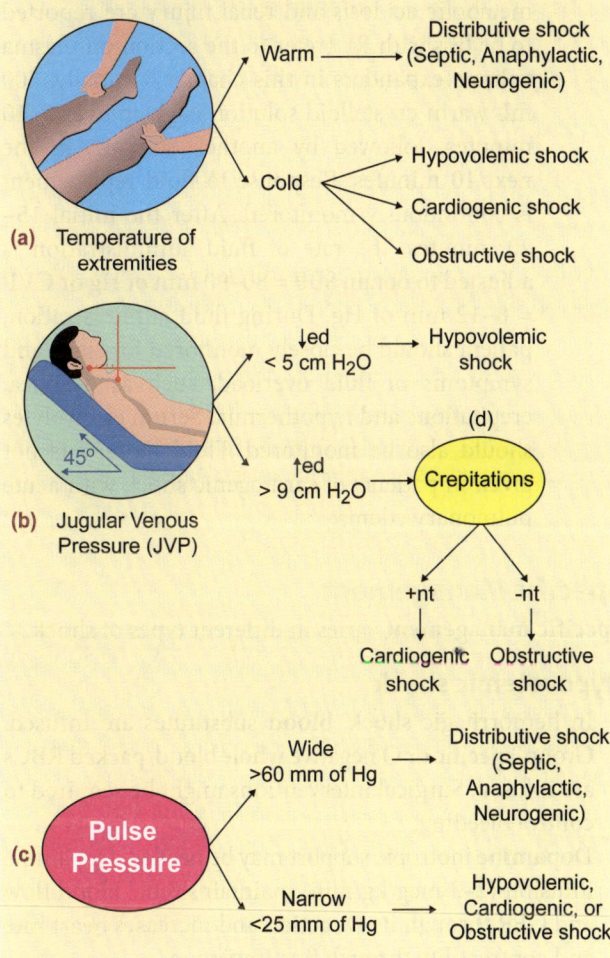

Fig. 35.1 (a–d) Diagnostic plan for type of shock

MANAGEMENT OF SHOCK

The aim of treating a patient in shock is to restore tissue perfusion with general supportive measures, followed by specific management of each type of shock.

General Supportive Treatment

General supportive treatment is given in all types of shock to stabilise the patient.

- Maintain **ABC**, i.e., **A**irway, **B**reathing and **C**irculation
  - Maintain patency of airways
  - Maintain adequate breathing by high flow oxygen to maintain $SpO_2 > 94\%$.
  - Maintain adequate circulation with **fluid resuscitation**.
    - IV line or central venous line is secured at the earliest with a wide bore needle of 14–16 G to infuse fluid rapidly.
    - Crystalloids (e.g., ringer lactate (**RL**) and normal saline (**NS**)) are preferred over colloids (e.g., albumin and hetastarch) in hypovolemic shock, because colloids have higher incidence of adverse effects and are costlier. Among crystalloids, RL is preferred over NS as chances of hyperchloremic metabolic acidosis and renal injury are reported to be less with RL (refer to the section on plasma volume expanders in this chapter). Initially, 500 mL warm crystalloid solution is given over 5–10 minutes, followed by another 500 mL in the next 10 minutes. Response to fluid replacement is continuously monitored. After the initial 15–20 minutes, the rate of fluid administration is adjusted to obtain SBP = 80–90 mm of Hg or CVP = 8–12 mm of Hg. During fluid administration, patient should be closely monitored for signs and symptoms of fluid overload, such as dyspnea, crepitations and hypothermia. Serum electrolytes should also be monitored. Fluid therapy is not given in patients of cardiogenic shock with acute pulmonary edema.

Specific Management

Specific management varies in different types of shock.

Hypovolemic shock

- In hemorrhagic shock, **blood** substitutes are infused. Group-specific or O negative whole blood/packed RBCs are infused. Surgical interventions might be required to control bleeding.
- **Dopamine** inotropic support may be needed. Dopamine infusion (2–3 mcg/kg/min) maintains renal blood flow and GFR through its D_1 action and increases heart rate and contractility through β_1 stimulation.
- Vasopressors are usually not indicated because intense reflex vasoconstriction occurs as a compensatory mechanism in case of fluid loss from body. Rather, the α_1-blocker phenoxybenzamine can help by shifting blood from the pulmonary to systemic circulation and from the extravascular to intravascular compartments.

Cardiogenic shock

- **Dopamine or dobutamine** treatment for positive inotropic effect is given after fluid therapy.
  Dobutamine is a selective β_1-agonist, given as an IV infusion (2.5 mcg/kg/min). It increases contractility and cardiac output. Reflex sympathetic tone decreases; PVR and afterload also decrease. Low-dose dopamine infusion (2–3 mcg/kg/min) is an alternative. In refractory cases, noradrenaline (2–4 mcg/min) is sometimes effective. Maximum dose of noradrenaline is 15 mcg/min, because further increase does not provide any extra benefit.
- Patients with ST elevation MI (STEMI) may need invasive interventions (see Chapter 34).
- Rhythm disturbances, if any, are treated appropriately.

Distributive shock

Distributive shock can be neurogenic, septic or anaphylactic, each of which is managed differently.

Neurogenic shock

- After fluid therapy, hemorrhage is ruled out. **Noradrenaline** or pure α-agonist **phenylephrine** can be given to increase vascular resistance and maintain arterial pressure.

Septic shock

After the patient's vitals are maintained with fluid therapy:
- Samples are collected for culture/sensitivity testing and empirical **antibiotic** therapy is instituted with combinations of ticarcillin/clavulanic acid and meropenem. Later on, antibiotics are changed based on the culture reports
- A recombinant form of human-activated protein C preparation—**drotrecogin alfa**—is approved by the FDA for reducing mortality in severe septic shock with multiple organ failure. It has anti-inflammatory, anticoagulant. and fibrinolytic actions.
- **Vasopressin** causes peripheral vasoconstriction, reduces NO synthesis and augments the effect of catecholamines on blood vessels. So, it can raise blood pressure in severe septic shock.
- **Corticosteroids** suppress the formation of NO and prostaglandins. They also reduce mortality in septic shock.

Anaphylactic shock

Adrenaline is a physiological antagonist of histamine and can reverse bronchoconstriction and vasodilatation caused by histamine. Adrenaline 1:1000, given intramuscularly in a dose of 0.3–0.5 mL, is lifesaving. **Corticosteroids** and H_1 **antihistamines** are also useful as adjuvants to adrenaline.

Obstructive shock

Treatment is cause-specific, e.g., in case of tension pneumothorax, immediate decompression by inserting a large bore needle of 14–16 gauge into the 2nd intercostal space is a lifesaving measure. In case of pericardial tamponade, fluid from the pericardial sac is drained using a needle.

Quick recognition and prompt treatment are the keys to success in shock management. General management to maintain vitals should be immediately instituted. At the same time, efforts to elicit the history pointing towards cause of shock and relevant investigations should be ordered, so that specific treatment can be started at the earliest.

PLASMA VOLUME EXPANDERS

Distribution of Total Body Water (TBW)

- Water makes up **60 % of the total body weight**. Thus, the total body water (TBW) in an average adult weighing ~70 kg is about 42 L.
- The TBW is distributed in **intra- and extracellular** compartments in a ratio of 2:1 (Fig. 35.2).
- The extracellular fluid (ECF; 14 L out of 42 L) is further divided between **extravascular and intravascular** compartments in approximately 3:1 ratio. So, out of 14 L of ECF, ~3 L is intravascular (plasma, circulating inside blood vessels) and the rest (11 L) is extravascular (interstitial fluid)
- **Plasma** is a clear, straw coloured fluid. **Blood** contains plasma with different blood cells suspended in it. So, blood is a colloid, fluid connective tissue. It keeps on circulating through the body to provide oxygen to all the tissues. Plasma devoid of clotting factors is called **serum.**

A variety of clinical conditions (burns, trauma, surgical blood loss and medical conditions involving loss of blood or plasma from the body) may cause hypovolemic shock

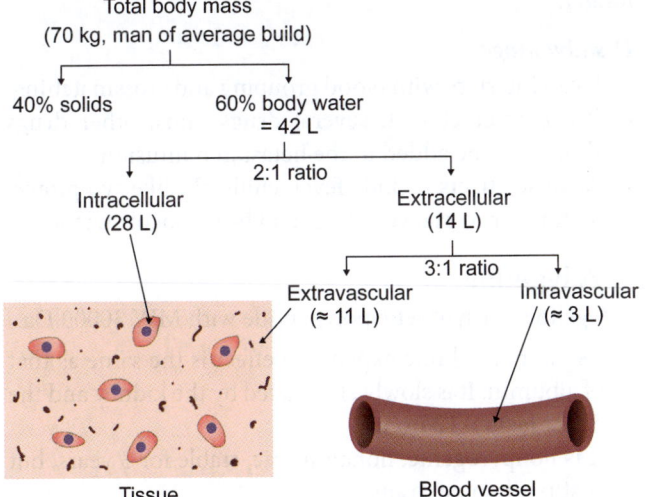

Fig. 35.2 Distribution of total body water

and require replacement therapy. While the ideal option is to replace whatever is lost, blood transfusion needs prior grouping and crossmatching. Moreover, human blood or plasma infusion has availability problems and carries the risk of transmitting infections such as HIV, HBV, and HCV.

Plasma volume expanders (PVEs) are substances with high molecular weight (MW) that are infused intravenously. These exert **oncotic osmotic pressure** (osmotic pressure is pressure exerted by solutes dissolved in water across a selectively permeable membrane. The part of osmotic pressure which is created by larger colloidal solute components is called oncotic pressure). Due to osmotic pressure, **water is drawn from the interstitial fluid** and the volume of fluid in the intravascular compartment increases. However, these **do not have oxygen carrying capacity.** Moreover, volume replacement with synthetic colloids., other than fresh blood can cause dilution of the cellular and homeostatic protein components, which may result in coagulopathies.

Properties of an ideal PVE

Following are properties desired in an ideal PVE

- It should be **iso-oncotic** with plasma, i.e., the oncotic pressure exerted by the PVE should be comparable to that exerted by plasma.
- It should get **distributed only in the intravascular** compartments and not leak out of vessels.
- It should not have any other pharmacological actions or organ system effects, i.e., PVE should be pharmacodynamically **inert**.
- It should be **nonpyrogenic** (no potential to cause fever) and **nonantigenic** (no potential to cause Ag–Ab reactions in the body) or **nonallergenic**.
- It should not interfere with blood grouping and crossmatching.
- It should have the **appropriate viscosity** for intravascular administration.
- It should be **stable** during storage, easily sterilisable and not expensive.

CLASSIFICATION

Chemically, PVEs can be classified into colloids and crystalloids (Flowchart 35.1).

A. Colloidal PVEs

1. Human albumin

After human plasma, human albumin is the most suitable agent for correcting hypovolemia. It is a nonglycosylated, hydrophilic protein with MW = 69000 Da. 100 mL of 20% human albumin solution exerts the same oncotic pressure as 400 mL of fresh frozen plasma.

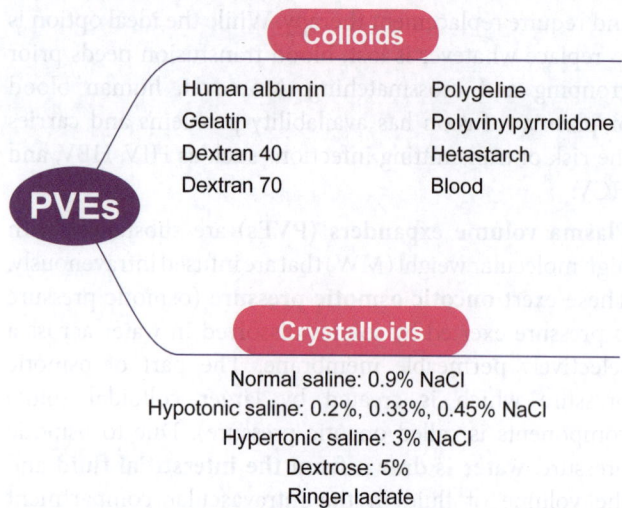

Flowchart 35.1 Classification of plasma volume expanders

Advantages
- Unlike blood or plasma, it can be used without blood grouping and crossmatching
- There is no risk of transmitting HIV or hepatitis viruses as it is heat-treated during preparation.
- There is no interference with coagulation although it may cause hemodilution.
- On repeat administration, risk of sensitisation is not there.

Disadvantages
- Sometimes febrile reactions occur.
- High cost is the most important disadvantage with human albumin. It is very costly as it is prepared from pooled human plasma.

Indications
- It is used as an **isotonic (4–5%) solution** in hypovolemia, shock, and burns to increase intravascular volume.
- **Hypertonic solution 20–25%** of human albumin is used in acute liver failure, hypoproteinemia and dialysis to maintain the balance of fluid distribution between various compartments.

2. Dextrans
These are branched polysaccharides. Two commonly used dextran preparations are dextran70 and dextran 40, which are named after their average molecular weight.
- For dextran 70, average molecular weight is 70000 Da.
- For dextran 40, average molecular weight is 40000 Da.

Pharmacodynamics of dextrans is largely dependent on their molecular weight.

a. Dextran 70
Dextran 70 is the most frequently used colloid, because it has most of the properties of an **ideal PVE**. Dextrans are iso-oncotic with plasma, stable for about 10 years, non-pyrogenic, largely non-antigenic, pharmacologically inert, and have appropriate viscosity and low cost.

It is slowly excreted by glomerular filtration (GF) and the plasma volume expanding action lasts for about 24 hours. Dextran 70 is used as a 6% solution, which is hypertonic and draws fluid into intravascular compartment from other tissues. Therefore, **concurrent administration of additional fluids is important**, especially in patients with poor hydration status.

Disadvantages
- Dextran 70 can decrease levels of clotting factors (factor VIII and vWF); thus, it can decrease coagulation, resulting in **prolonged bleeding time**. Because of this, it is contraindicated in conditions where coagulation is already poor, such as thrombocytopenia, hypofibrogenemia, afibrogenemia and bleeding tendencies.
- It interferes with RBC rouleaux formation. So, samples for blood grouping and crossmatching should be taken before starting dextran administration.
- There is some risk of **anaphylactoid reactions** like itching, urticaria, fall in BP, wheezing and bronchoconstriction.
- Risk of electrolyte disturbance.

b. Dextran 40
It is **faster and shorter acting** than dextran 70, and is used as a 10% solution. It may improve microcirculation by reducing blood viscosity and coating RBCs. It is rapidly excreted by glomerular filtration. As a result, **urine flow rate should be sufficient for its excretion**; otherwise it may cause tubular obstruction.

3. Hydroxyethyl starch or hetastarch
It is an ethoxylated amylopectin; the molecular weight of particles ranges from 10000–10 lakhs Da, with an average MW of 4.5 lakhs Da. The oncotic pressure exerted by 6% hydroxyethyl starch is almost the same as that exerted by human albumin. Its action lasts for 24 hours or longer.

Disadvantage
- It can interfere with blood grouping and crossmatching.
- It can interact with several drugs; thus, other drugs should not be added to the hetastarch infusion.
- Adverse effects include fever, chills, flu-like symptoms, itching, urticaria, vomiting, and bronchoconstriction.

4. Polygeline
Polygeline is a synthetic polypeptide with MW 30000 Da.
- Its plasma-volume expanding effect is the same as that of albumin. It is slowly eliminated by the kidney and the **effect lasts > 12 hours.**
- It is nonpyrogenic, nonantigenic, stable for 3 years, but costlier than dextrans.
- It is used for PVE and priming of heart–lung and dialysis machines.

5. Gelatins

Gelatins (MW = 30000–35000 Da) are iso-oncotic, stable for 3–5 years and do not interfere with blood grouping/crossmatching; blood coagulation and renal function is maintained.

Adverse effects can occur as local cutaneous reactions, fall in BP and histamine release. Gelatins can cause a hypercoagulable state, but impair platelet function.

6. Polyvinylpyrrolidone (PVP)

PVP is not commonly used as a PVE; however, it is used in shampoos, toothpastes, hair gels, sprays, etc. In pharmaceutics, it is used as a binding agent. PVP complexed to iodine is a very frequently used disinfectant called povidone–iodine.

B. Crystalloids

In contrast to colloids, crystalloids are electrolyte solutions with smaller molecules that **diffuse freely in the extracellular fluid**. 75–80% of administered crystalloid solutions is distributed in the interstitial space. Thus, **these expand interstitial fluid volume rather than plasma volume**, e.g.:

- Isotonic saline (0.9% NaCl) has a solute concentration which is the same as in plasma. It does not move inside cells; thus, ECF volume increases, especially intravascular volume.
- Hypotonic solutions, such as 0.2, 0.33, and 0.45% NaCl, have lower solute concentrations than ICF. So, these hydrate the cells.
- Hypertonic solutions, such as 3% NaCl and D5NS, draw water out of the ICF and increase ECF; these are used as volume expanders.

Indications and contraindications of crystalloids:

Normal saline (**NS**) and ringer lactate (**RL**) are the first-line crystalloids for **fluid resuscitation**.

- NS is administered in fluid volume deficit as seen in severe diarrhea, vomiting, dehydration, hemorrhage, shock, diabetic ketoacidosis, and along with blood products. There is a **risk of hyperchloremic metabolic acidosis** with NS given at a rate of 30 mL/kg/hour.
- In ringer lactate, K^+ and Ca^{2+} concentrations are the same as in plasma, but Na^+ concentration is kept low for electrical neutrality. It is used to replace fluid loss from GIT as in diarrhea/vomiting and in burns and trauma. The risk of metabolic acidosis is eliminated with large volume infusions of ringer lactate solution. However, it is **contraindicated for use as a diluent for blood transfusions**. It is also contraindicated in lactic acidosis and in patients with liver disease.

- **Dextrose 5%** is also isotonic, but becomes hypotonic after dextrose metabolism. Being small molecules, they can move freely and **expand both intracellular and extracellular compartments**. It is used in hypernatremia (as it has no electrolyte) and hypoglycemia, but is contraindicated in patients with renal failure, cerebral edema, with blood and for fluid resuscitation.

CONTRAINDICATIONS TO PVE

PVE use is contraindicated in:

- Severe anemia, as these cause further hemodilution
- Cardiac failure
- Liver disease
- Pulmonary edema
- Renal insufficiency

Clinical problem-based questions and MCQs

4. A 36-year-old female patient presents with history of persistent diarrhea and vomiting since last 2 days. On examination, the patient is drowsy, extremities are cold, peripheral pulses are feeble, HR = 124 bpm, RR = 24/min and BP = 86/60. Chest is clear, heart sounds are normal and JVP is not raised. Capillary refill time is prolonged. There is no history of chest pain, trauma, insect bite or drug intake.
   i. What are the indicators of shock in this patient?
   ii. What is the type of shock in this case, and how do you rule out other types of shock.
   iii. Describe the management of this patient.

5. A 38-year-old woman, gravid 4, presents in emergency after home-conducted vaginal delivery, with profuse vaginal bleeding. On examination patient is pale, anxious and confused. Extremities are cold and clammy. BP = 84/50, HR = 120 bpm and RR = 24/min, prolonged capillary refill time. On chest auscultation, there are no crepitations and heart sounds are normal. JVP is not raised.
   i. What parameters indicate that patient is in shock?
   ii. What type of shock is this patient suffering from?
   iii. Describe the management of this patient.

6. A 10-year-old boy was injured in a fall from his cycle. Although the injuries were mild abrasions only, injection TT was given. Suddenly, the patient developed severe itching and redness at the site of injection, followed by rashes all over the body, urticaria, swelling of lips, wheezing and difficulty in breathing. On examination, patient had warm extremities, there was a bilateral wheeze (but no crepitations), PR = 124 bpm and BP = 110/68 (wide PP).
   i. What is the type and cause of shock in this case?
   ii. Which of the following drugs is lifesaving in this patient?
       a. H_1 antihistamines
       b. Prednisolone

       c. Adrenaline
       d. Dobutamine
    iii. Explain pharmacological basis for use of chosen drug in (ii).
7. Describe cause and management of septic shock in detail.
8. Which of these is NOT an indication for use of hypertonic human albumin?
    a. Burns   b. Acute liver failure
    b. Dialysis   d. Hypoproteinemia
9. i. Enumerate the properties of an ideal plasma volume expander.
    ii. Which of the following has most of the properties of an ideal PVE?
       a. Dextrose 5%   b. Dextran 70
       b. Ringer lactate   d. Normal saline
    iii. Enumerate the disadvantages of the selected PVE.
10. Why are colloids preferred over crystalloids for volume expansion?
11. Which of the following conditions is an indication for use of plasma expanders?
    a. Severe anemia
    b. Trauma
    c. Pulmonary edema
    d. Congestive heart failure

Summary

- **Plasma volume expanders** include colloids and crystalloids. Colloids are preferred for volume expansion as these are more effective and longer acting than crystalloids.
- An ideal PVE should be iso-oncotic with plasma, stable, non-pyrogenic, largely non-antigenic, pharmacologically inert, and have appropriate viscosity and low cost. Dextran 70 has most of the properties of an ideal PVE.
- Colloids include human albumin, gelatin, dextran 70/40, polygeline, hetastarch and blood. Isotonic solution of albumin (4–5%) is preferred in hypovolemia, shock and burns to increase intravascular volume, while a hypertonic solution 20–25% of human albumin is used in acute liver failure, hypoproteinemia and dialysis to maintain the balance of fluid distribution between various compartments.
- Crystalloids include normal saline, dextrose and ringer lactate. NS and ringer lactate are first-line crystalloids for fluid resuscitation.
- Dextrose 5% is used in hypernatremia and hypoglycemia, but is contraindicated in renal failure, cerebral edema and with blood in fluids resuscitation.
- Contraindications to the use of PVEs include severe anemia, cardiac failure, liver disease, pulmonary edema and renal insufficiency.

Hints for problem-based questions and MCQs

1. a. Intermittent claudication
   b. ABI < 0.9, duplex ultrasound to detect the exact site and degree of narrowing. Angiography using X-rays, CT scans and MRI to get an exact view of the location and extent of obstruction. Refer to page 467.
   c. Management is with lifestyle modification, risk reduction, pharmacotherapy and surgical methods (refer to page 467).
2. i. Vasodilatation in normal region, diverting blood from ischemic to normal region is called 'steal phenomenon'.
   ii. c. Pentoxifylline
   iii. **Rheology-modifying** action and reduced viscosity of blood (refer to page 468).
   iv. Due to increased flexibility of RBCs, reduced viscosity of blood, it blood can flow easily through vessels obstructed partially by atheromatous plaques. Thus, blood flow to ischemic area is increased, i.e., no steal phenomenon.
3. i. a. Naftidrofuryl oxalate
   ii. 5-HT_2 receptor blocking action leading to reduction of 5-HT induced vasoconstriction and platelet aggregation.
4. i. Low BP, tachycardia, tachypnea, altered mentation
   ii. Hypovolemic shock.
       History rules out cardiogenic, obstructive and anaphylactic shock.
       JVP is not raised; this rules out cardiogenic and obstructive shock
       Cold extremities rule out distributive shock.
   iii. Refer to page 472.
5. i. Low BP, tachycardia, tachypnea and confused state of mind
   ii. Hypovolemic (hemorrhagic) shock
   iii. Refer to page 472.
6. i. Anaphylactic shock, due to hypersensitivity to injection TT
   ii. c. Adrenaline
   iii. Adrenaline is a physiological antagonist of histamine
7. Refer to pages 470, 472.
8. a. Burns, in which isotonic albumin is used to increase intravascular volume.
9. i. Refer to page 473.
   ii. b. Dextran 70.
   iii. Refer to page 474.
10. Colloids have larger molecules that have better retention in the intravascular compartment; so they are better than crystalloids. Thus, these are **more effective** in increasing oncotic osmotic pressure and restoring plasma volume. Moreover, duration of action of colloids is **longer** than crystalloids. Overall, **colloids are preferred over crystalloids for volume expansion**.
11. b. Trauma.

Chapter 35 Drugs for Peripheral Vascular Disease (PVD) and Management of Shock

CONCEPT MAP - MANAGEMENT OF SHOCK

Shock
Reduced tissue perfusion due to any cause → Multiorgan failure → Fatal outcome

Diagnosis
Presence of any 4 features: Hypotension, Tachycardia, Tachypnea, Oliguria, Altered mentation, Serum lactic acid > 4 mmol/L

Hypovolemic Shock
Causes: Hemorrhage, Burns, Diarrhea, Dehydration

Diagnosis: Suggestive history, Cold clammy skin, Narrow pulse Pressure (PP), Low JVP, No Crepitations.

Treatment: General supportive: Maintain airways, breathing, circulation.
Hemorrhagic shock: Whole blood/packed RBCs.
Dopamine 2–3 mcg/kg/min
Phenoxybenzamine may be useful
No role of vasopressors.

Cardiogenic Shock
Causes: Acute MI or IHD, Atrial fibrillation, Valvular diseases, Cardiomyopathy → decreased cardiac output

Diagnosis: H/S/O cardiac disease, Cold clammy skin, Narrow PP, JVP raised, Crepitations present

Treatment: Supportive
Dopamine 2–3 mcg/kg/min or Dobutamine 2.5 mcg/kg/min or Noradrenaline 2–4 mcg/kg/min (maximum 15 mcg/kg/min)
Correction of coronary obstruction by PCTA, stenting, bypass surgery
Correction of valvular defect
Appropriate drugs for arrhythmias.

Obstructive Shock
Causes: Trauma → Cardiac tamponade
Tension pneumothorax → fall in cardiac output

Diagnosis: H/O trauma, Cold clammy skin, JVP raised, weak heart sounds, No crepitations

Treatment: Supportive treatment
Decompression of pneumothorax by putting needle in 2nd intercostal space,
Drainage of fluid from pericardial space in cardiac tamponade

Septic Shock
Cause: Gram –ve septicemia, endotoxin induced VD

Diagnosis: History of severe infection, Warm extremities, Wide PP due to hyperdynamic circulation

Treatment: Supportive, Empirical AMAs, Culture/sensitivity testing → Appropriate antimicrobial therapy

Distributive Shock
Warm extremities, cause can be septic/anaphylactic/neurogenic

Anaphylctic Shock
Cause: Type 1 hypersensitivity reaction to bee sting, insect bite, drugs, food

Diagnosis: Suggestive history, Warm extremities, Wide PP

Treatment: Adrenaline 1:1000, in a dose of 0.3–0.5 mL, Steroids, H_1 blockers

Neurogenic Shock
Cause: Spinal cord injury above T6 level, interrupting sympathetic system, parasympathetic preserved.

Diagnosis: H/O trauma, Profound hypotension, Bradycardia, Decreased contractility and cardiac output

Treatment: Fluid resuscitation.
Vasopressors if symptoms persist: Phenylephrine, dopamine, NA
Atropine for bradycardia

SECTION 7   Drugs Acting on CVS

36   Antiarrhythmic Drugs

PH 4.10 Explain salient pharmacokinetics, pharmacodynamics, therapeutic uses, adverse drug reactions of drugs used for cardiac arrhythmias. Devise a plan to manage a patient with supraventricular, ventricular arrhythmias, cardiac arrest and fibrillations.

Learning objectives

A student of MBBS phase II should be able to:
- Describe normal electrophysiology of fast channel and slow channel cardiac action potential.
- Define cardiac arrhythmias and describe different types and mechanisms of arrhythmias.
- Classify antiarrhythmic drugs and explain their mechanisms of action.
- Explain uses of drugs in different types of arrhythmias, mentioning doses.
- Enumerate the adverse effects of and contraindications to antiarrhythmic drugs.
- Devise a management plan for supraventricular/ventricular arrhythmia/cardiac arrest/ fibrillation.

ARRHYTHMIAS

A normal heart:
- Beats at a rate of **60–100 beats per minute** (bpm).
- Beats with an impulse which originates from the **sino-atrial (SA node)**.
- Follows a **normal conduction path**, i.e., atrioventricular (AV) node, bundle of His, right and left bundle branches, Purkinje fibres (PF).
- Has a **normal velocity of conduction**, such that there is a delay of about 0.1 seconds at the AV node to provide time for atrial contraction to pump blood into the relaxed ventricles; the impulse then spreads to all parts of the ventricles in < 0.1 seconds to cause synchronous contraction of all ventricular muscles that is hemodynamically effective.

Any deviation from this description is called arrhythmia.

> Any abnormality in site of origin of impulse, its rate, regularity and conduction is called an arrhythmia or dysrhythmia.

Causes of arrhythmias

Rhythm disturbances in the heart can occur due to myocardial ischemia, anoxia, injury, stretching, electrolyte disturbances (especially hypokalemia), pH disturbances, drugs and neurogenic factors.

NORMAL ELECTROPHYSIOLOGY OF HEART

Knowledge of the normal electrophysiology of cardiac action potential is important to understand the mechanisms of occurrence of various arrhythmias and actions of antiarrhythmic drugs

There are **2 types** of action potentials in cardiac tissues:
- **Fast channel action potential**, which is shown by myocardial contractile tissue—atrial and ventricular fibres.
- **Slow channel action potential**, which is shown by pacemaker/conducting tissue—SA node, AV node, and the His–Purkinje system.

The **transmembrane potential** of cardiac cells is determined by the **concentration of Na^+, K^+ and Ca^{2+} ions** on either side of the membrane. They cannot diffuse freely across the membrane, but move through specific ion channels according to their electrochemical gradient at specific times during the action potential (AP).

Fast Channel Action Potential

Fast channel action potential (AP) is shown by atrial and ventricular tissue. The distribution of Na^+ and K^+ ions at the **resting membrane potential** (RMP) of –90 mV is shown in Fig. 36.1.

At this stage, the distribution of Na^+ ions is such that there is a substantial concentration gradient—the Na^+ concentration is 140 mmol/L outside and only 10–15 mmol/L inside the cell. An electrical gradient (0 mV outside, –90 mV inside the cell) along with a concentration gradient can drive Na^+ into cell. However, Na^+ does not enter the cell at rest because the Na^+ channels are closed.

The situation is different for K^+ in the resting cardiac cell. At RMP, the concentration gradient of K^+ (4 mmol/L outside, 140 mmol/L inside) tries to drive K^+ out of the cell; however, the electrical gradient (0 mV outside, –90 mV inside) tries to drive K^+ in. Hence, although certain K^+ channels (called inward rectifier channels) are open in the

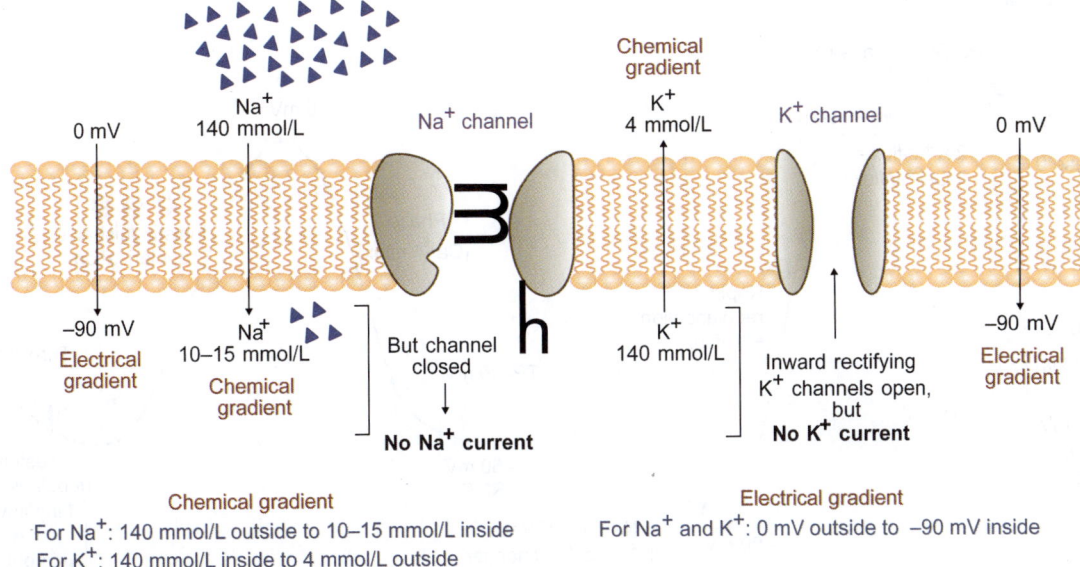

Fig. 36.1 Ionic concentrations at RMP in atrial and ventricular fibres

resting phase, little current flows through them because of this balance between the electrical and concentration gradients of K$^+$.

There are **5 phases in the fast channel AP**, i.e., Phases 0, 1, 2, 3, and 4 (Fig. 36.2a).

Rapid depolarisation (Phase 0): When the RMP (−90 mV) reaches the **threshold potential** (TP; −60 to −70 mV) the m gates of the Na$^+$ channels open [called the **active (A) state** of the channel] and permeability increases markedly. **Quick Na$^+$ influx** occurs (because of concentration and electrical gradient) → thus, the membrane potential shoots up rapidly to +30 mV.

The opening of m gates at the TP is promptly followed by closing of h gates [called **inactive (IA)** state of the Na$^+$ channel] over a potential range of −75 to −55 mV.

Early/partial repolarisation (Phase 1): This phase of partial repolarisation occurs because of the inactivation of the Na$^+$ current and transient **voltage-sensitive K$^+$ efflux**. K$^+$ efflux occurs because the membrane potential (MP) is +30 mV at the end of Phase 0 (that is, the potential is positive inside) and K$^+$ concentration is lower outside the cell. So, the electrical gradient drives the K$^+$ out, and the membrane potential (MP) rapidly returns towards isoelectric (0 mV) potential.

Plateau (Phase 2): The plateau phase occurs because of a balance between **inward Ca^{2+}** and **outward K$^+$ flow**. The Ca^{2+} channels (L type) are activated and inactivated in the same manner as Na$^+$ channels, albeit at a more positive potential and with slower dynamics. So, 2 K$^+$ ions move out for one Ca^{2+} ion and the membrane potential stabilises, forming a plateau.

Rapid repolarisation (Phase 3): In this phase, the Ca^{2+} channels close but a delayed outwardly rectifying K$^+$ current is activated. It is augmented by:

- Another K$^+$ current activated by the high intracellular Ca^{2+} concentration during the plateau phase.
- Sometimes, other K$^+$ currents are activated by acetylcholine and arachidonic acid.

Thus, the membrane potential (MP) becomes negative again (−90 mV) because of the **outward K$^+$ flow**. Now, although the membrane resumes its negativity, ions have changed their position when compared to the resting stage, i.e., more Na$^+$ ions are inside the cell (moved in during Phase 0) and more K$^+$ ions are outside (moved out during Phases 1, 2 and 3). The ions are again distributed by the **Na$^+$/K$^+$ ATPase** or **sodium pump** to restore intra- and extracellular ion concentrations of Na$^+$ and K$^+$ ions to their pre-excitation levels.

In Phase 4, the RMP is stable because of the activity of the **Na$^+$/K$^+$ pump, outward K$^+$ flow** and **Na$^+$/Ca^{2+} exchanger**.

Slow Channel Action Potential

Slow channel AP is seen in the SA nodes, AV nodes and His–Purkinje system. It differs from the fast channel AP in the following aspects (Fig. 36.2b).

1. The **RMP is around −60 mV**, at which most of the Na$^+$ channels are in the 'inactive' IA stage (m gate open, h gates closed). Because Na$^+$ channels are in the IA state, Ca^{2+} influx is largely responsible for the upstroke in Phase 0. Upstroke velocity is reduced and overshoot is less. At the **end of Phase 0, potential becomes isoelectric** (0 mV), in comparison to +30 mV in the fast channel action potential.
2. **Phases 1, 2 and 3 are indistinguishable and are due to K$^+$ efflux**
3. **Phase 4** shows **diastolic depolarisation** that is responsible for automaticity. Automaticity is the ability of a cell to alter its RMP (−60 mV) towards threshold

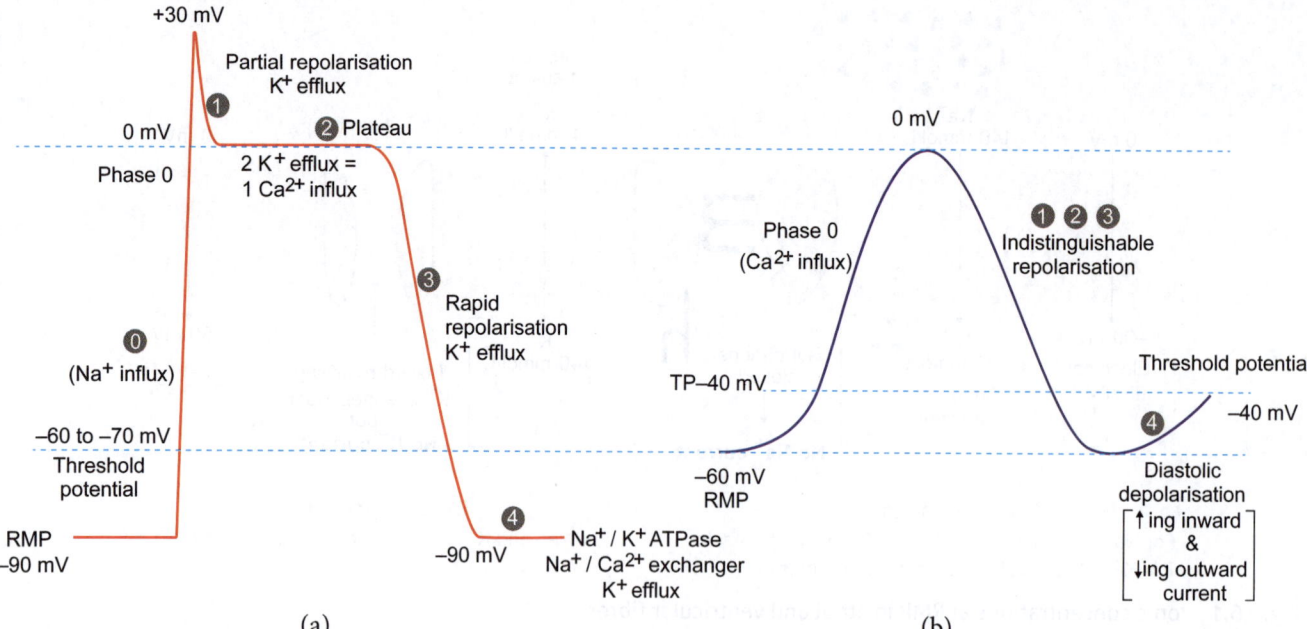

Fig. 36.2 (a) Fast channel action potential in atrial and ventricular fibres (b) Slow channel action potential in SA nodes, AV nodes and Purkinje fibres

potential TP (−40 mV), without the influence of any stimulus. This is because of **increasing inward currents**, which are:

- Background conductance due to Na^+.
- Increased inward Ca^{2+} current, because Ca^{2+} channel inactivation wears off during diastole.
- Activation of T-type Ca^{2+} channel during late diastole.
- **Decreasing outward currents**, because the delayed outward rectifier K^+ current is turned off by negative membrane potential early in diastole.

These two factors lead to the movement of RMP towards TP, causing diastolic depolarisation, which gives a **slope to Phase 4** in nodal tissue. The rate of diastolic depolarisation determines the slope of Phase 4, which is maximum in the SA node. Thus, the SA node sets the pace for the whole heart.

- Other automatic fibres act as latent pacemakers, i.e., they possess the ability to provide automaticity when the SA node is not functioning properly. In a normal heart, these latent pacemakers are excited at the pace set by the SA node.
- Thus, during Phase 4, the MP is stable in atrial and ventricular fibres, but decays in nodal tissues, leading to their automaticity.
- The Na^+/K^+ ATPase pump and Na^+/Ca^{2+} exchanger also act in this phase to return the ion concentrations to pre-excitation levels, so that the tissue is ready to respond to next impulse.

Refractory period

Once depolarisation starts, the myocardial cell remains refractory (does not respond to the next stimulis). This refractory period includes the:

- **Absolute** refractory period (ARP): From Phase 0 till mid-Phase 3, the cell does not respond to any stimuli.
- **Relative** refractory period (RRP): From mid-Phase 3 to the end of Phase 3, the cell can respond to strong stimuli as the Na^+ channels are recovering from the inactive (IA) to resting (R) state.
- **Effective** refractory period (ERP) is the total of the ARP and RRP; it represents the minimum interval between 2 successive propagated responses.

MECHANISMS OF ARRHYTHMIAS

Arrhythmias occur due to:

I. **Disturbed generation of impulse** that may result in:
  a. Increased automaticity
  b. Decreased automaticity
  c. Triggered automaticity.

II. **Disturbed conduction of impulse** that can manifest as conduction blocks and re-entry phenomenon.

I. Disturbed Generation of Impulse

a. Increased automaticity

Increased automaticity (Fig. 36.3a) can occur because of:

- **Increased slope of diastolic depolarisation** or **Phase 4** depolarisation as seen with acidosis, β-agonists, positive chronotropic drugs, etc. [A mnemonic for the causes of increased slope of Phase 4 is **A-B-C**, i.e., **A**cidosis, **B**eta agonists and **C**hronotropic drugs.]
- Partial depolarisation of the membrane or RMP becomes less negative, i.e., gap between **RMP and threshold potential** reduces as seen in ischemia, anoxia, injury, and stretching of cardiac muscles.

The increased automaticity caused by these two mechanisms results in tachyarrhythmias.

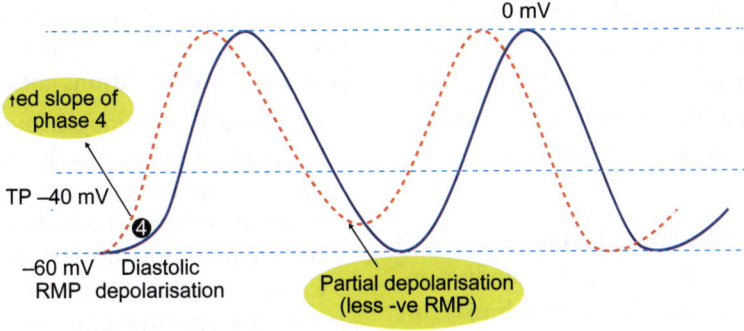

Fig. 36.3 (a) Mechanism of increased automaticity

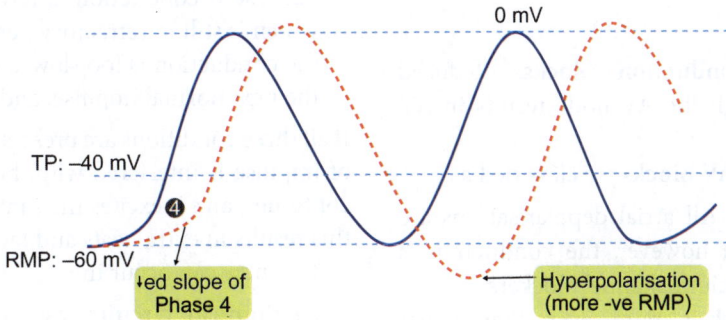

Fig. 36.3 (b) Mechanism of decreased automaticity

b. Decreased automaticity

In contrast, decreased automaticity is the result of a decrease in the slope of Phase 4 depolarisation (by β-blockers and calcium channel blockers) and hyperpolarisation or more negative RMP (by vagal stimulation); reduced automaticity results in bradyarrhythmias (Fig. 36.3b).

c. Triggered automaticity

A normal action potential is essential for initiation of triggered automaticity, which includes:

- **Early afterdepolarisations (EADs)** interrupt Phase 3 of the action potential (Fig. 36.4). They occur when the action potential duration (APD) and hence QT interval is prolonged, as in bradycardia, hypokalemia, hypomagnesemia, hypocalcemia, and by drugs like terfenadine, astemizole, cisapride, potassium channel blockers (Class III antiarrhythmics) and Class IA antiarrhythmics (such as quinidine). EADs are the starting point for a self-sustaining tachyarrhythmia called torsade de pointes (TDP).

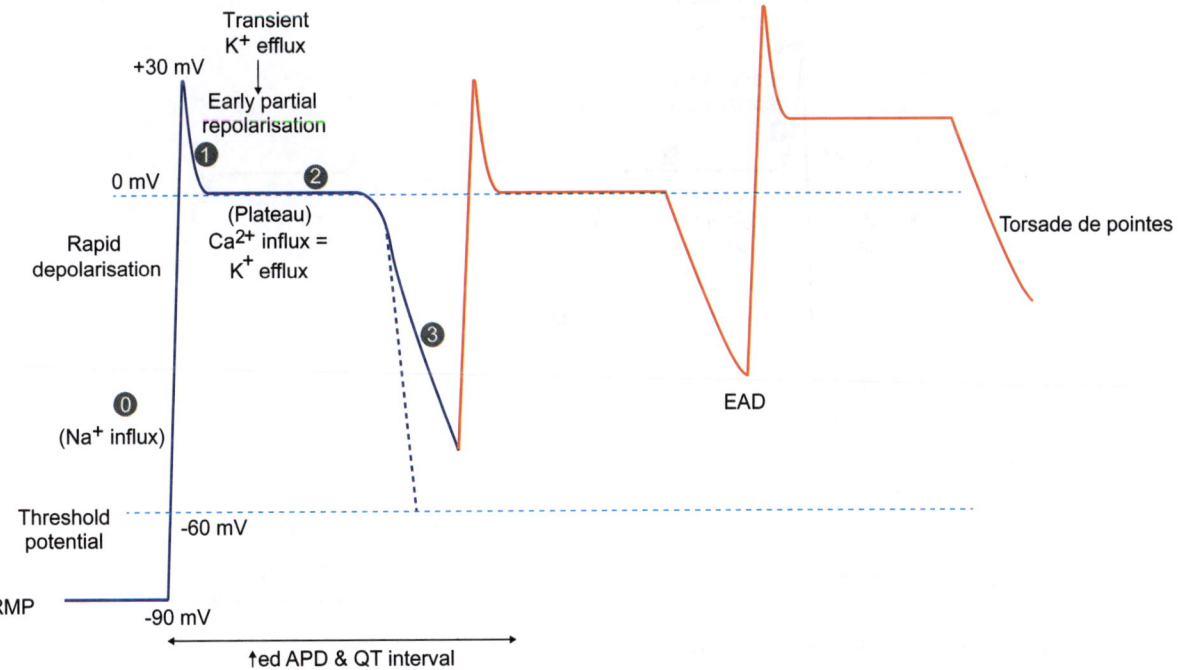

Fig. 36.4 Mechanism of early afterdepolarisation (EAD)

- **Delayed afterdepolarisations** (DADs) interrupt Phase 4; the RMP oscillates and causes an extra beat if the threshold potential is reached (Fig. 36.5). It occurs because of cation overloading secondary to ischemia, injury, increased catecholamines, digoxin, etc.

II. Disturbed Conduction of Impulse

Defects in conduction velocity and conduction pathways may result in various bradyarrhythmias or tachyarrhythmias.

a. Bradyarrhythmias

Bradyarrhythmias or conduction blocks: Reduced conduction velocity through the AV node results in **AV blocks**.

Based on their severity, **AV blocks** are classified as:

- **First degree AV block**: All atrial depolarisations are conducted to ventricles; however, the conduction is slow, e.g., β-blockers, calcium channel blockers.
- **Second degree AV block** is more severe than a first degree block. Here, some atrial depolarisations (P waves) are not transmitted to the ventricles.
- **Third degree AV block**: P waves are not conducted to the ventricles; these start beating at their own rate (atria and ventricles beat at their own rates, called AV dissociation).

b. Tachyarrhythmias

Tachyarrhythmias caused by conduction defects occur due to a phenomenon known as re-entry.

One impulse re-enters and excites areas of the heart more than once (Fig. 36.6). Re-entry occurs only if the following **three conditions coexist**:

1. An obstacle to homogeneous conduction, which may be a scarred non-excitable area of the myocardium, so that the impulse starts moving around the obstacle.
2. A unidirectional conduction block, i.e., anterograde conduction of impulse is stopped but not the retrograde.
3. Conduction time around the obstacle should be greater than the effective refractory period (ERP). In other words, conduction should be reduced to a critical extent, because if conduction is too fast, it reaches the tissue which is still in refractory period. On the other hand, if the conduction is too slow, an impulse will collide with the next normal impulse, and is lost or dies out.

If all three conditions are present, anterograde propagation of impulse is interfered with, but retrograde propagation continues, and it excites the same areas of the heart again; this results in extra beats and tachyarrhythmias.

Re-entry can occur in:

- **Anatomical circuits**, as seen in **Wolff–Parkinson–White** (WPW) syndrome. In a normal heart, the AV node is the only pathway for conduction of impulses between the atria and ventricles. In WPW syndrome, there exists an abnormal connection between the atria and ventricles, called the *bundle of Kent*. It is further attached to the bundle of His via a piece of myocardium that has moderate conduction velocity.

  When a patient has a sinus rhythm, re-entry does not occur through the bundle of Kent. However, when an ectopic focus develops near the bundle of Kent (such as due to smoking, alcohol consumption, caffeine intake,

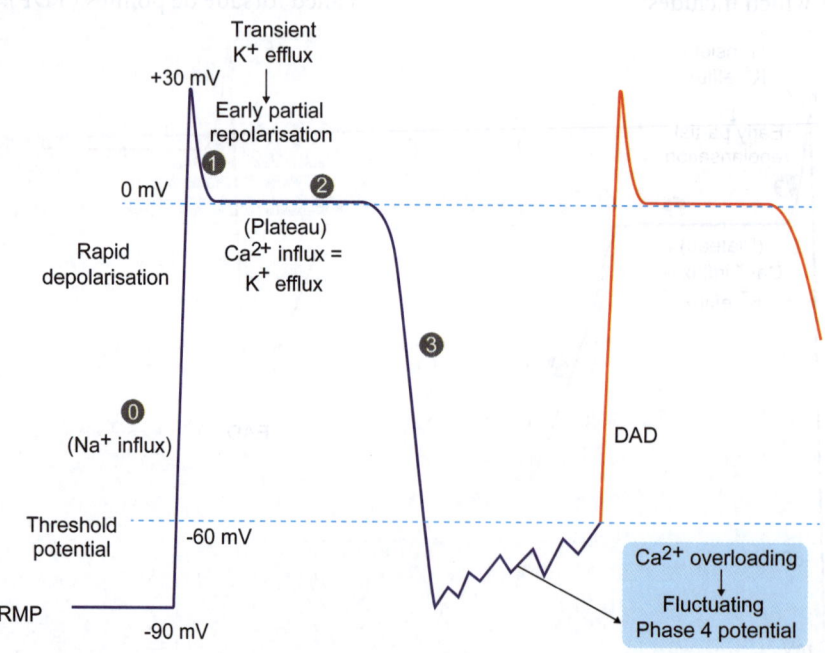

Fig. 36.5 Mechanism of delayed afterdepolarisation (DAD)

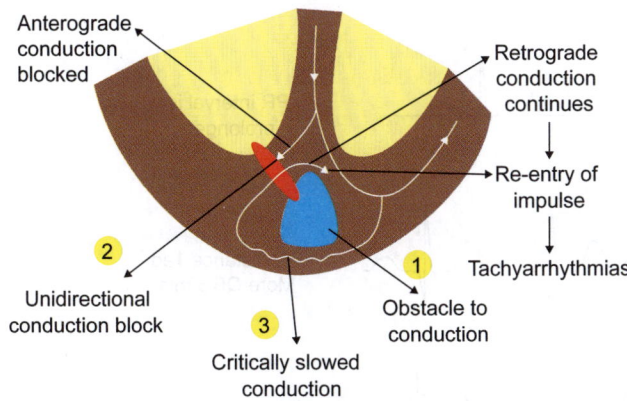

Fig. 36.6 The re-entry phenomenon

stress, excess catecholamines), the abnormal impulse enters bundle of Kent and a re-entry circuit is formed with the AV node via the connecting myocardial tissue. As the rate of conduction through the bundle of Kent is greater than in the AV node, the PR interval decreases and the Q wave is missing
- **Functional circuits** may be formed in atrial, AV nodal or ventricular tissues or two pathways having varying conduction velocity may be present within the AV node, resulting in re-entry and tachyarrhythmias.

Thus, re-entry can be the underlying mechanism for paroxysmal supraventricular tachycardia (PSVT), atrial flutter (AF), atrial fibrillation (Af), atrio-ventricular reciprocal tachycardia, ventricular extrasystole (VES), ventricular tachycardia (VT), ventricular flutter (VF), ventricular fibrillation (Vf), etc.

TYPES OF ARRHYTHMIAS

Arrhythmias can be categorised depending on the rate and site of impulse generation.

a. Depending upon the **rate**, arrhythmias can be tachyarrhythmias or bradyarrhythmias. Normal heart rate is 60–100 beats per minutes (bpm).

Bradyarrhythmias	Tachyarrhythmias
Bradycardia	Tachycardia: 100–250 bpm
Mild: 40–60 bpm	Flutter: 250–350 bpm
Moderate: 20–40 bpm	Fibrillation: > 350 bpm
Severe: < 20 bpm	

b. Depending upon the **site of origin** of abnormal rhythm:
   - SA node: Sinus arrhythmias
   - Within the atrium: Atrial arrhythmias
   - AV node/junctional tissue: Junctional arrhythmias
   - Within the ventricles: Ventricular arrhythmias.

Sinus, atrial and junctional arrhythmias are also known as supraventricular arrhythmias, as these originate above the ventricular area.

ECG CHANGES

Supraventricular Arrhythmias

These include sinus, atrial and junctional arrhythmias.

Sinus and atrial arrhythmias

a. In a normal ECG, the P wave represents atrial depolarisation, QRS complex indicates ventricular depolarisation, and PR interval indicates AV conduction. The **ECG changes** seen in sinus and atrial arrhythmias are shown in Fig. 36.7.
b. Sinus tachycardia: ECG pattern is normal, but there are more QRS complexes per minute (or) RR distance decreases.
c. Sinus bradycardia: ECG pattern is normal, but there are fewer QRS complexes per minute (or) RR distance increases.
d. Sick sinus syndrome: Occasionally, sinus tachycardia occurs, while at other times sinus bradycardia is seen. The number of QRS complexes per minute and RR distance in the ECG is variable.
e. Atrial tachycardia: P waves are well formed, but each P wave is not followed by a QRS complex.
f. Atrial flutter: P waves are not well formed and a **sawtooth** pattern called flutter (F) waves is seen. The atrial rate is high and fewer QRS complexes are seen.
g. Atrial fibrillation: Atrial electrical activity is not well defined. P wave occurs as a small fluctuation called fibrillation (f) waves. QRS complexes occur occasionally.

Junctional Arrhythmias

These occur as varying degrees of AV blocks (Fig. 36.8).

a. In **first degree AV blocks**, all P waves are followed by QRS complexes, but the PR interval is prolonged.
b. **Second degree AV blocks** present as the following subtypes:
   - Mobitz type I: The PR interval increases progressively till one atrial beat is not transmitted to the ventricles, i.e., one beat is missed.
   - Mobitz type II: The PR interval is stable but somewhere a beat is missed.
   - **2:1 block:** One atrial depolarisation is transmitted to the ventricles but the next one is missed. Two P waves are followed by one QRS complex.
c. In **third degree AV blocks**, there is no relation or pattern between the P waves and QRS complexes. In WPW syndrome, as the rate of conduction through the bundle of Kent is greater than in the AV node, the PR interval decreases and Q waves are missing.

Ventricular Arrhythmias

The **ECG changes** seen in ventricular arrhythmias are shown in Fig. 36.9.

a. In ventricular premature beats (VPBs), there is a wider-than-normal QRS complex in an otherwise normal ECG.

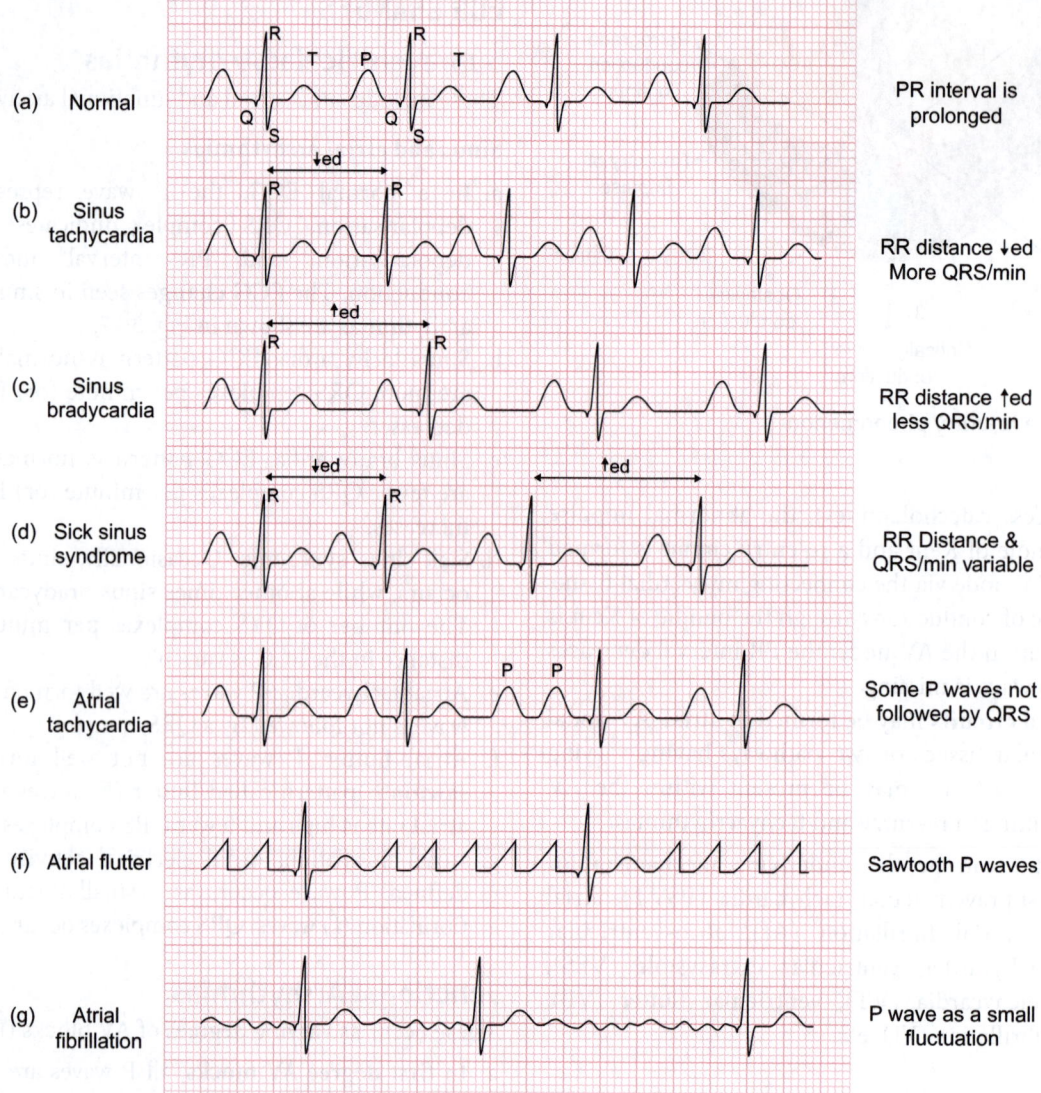

Fig. 36.7 ECG changes in sinus and atrial arrhythmias

b. In ventricular tachycardia, a series of wider QRS complexes or VPBs are seen.
c. Ventricular flutters (VF) occur as a curved line in ECG.
d. Ventricular fibrillation (Vf): Hardly any electrical activity is seen.

MANAGEMENT OF ARRHYTHMIAS

Rhythm disturbances in the heart cannot be left untreated; whether too fast, too slow, or asynchronous, the cardiac output decreases. Moreover, some rhythm disturbances carry the risk of precipitating more severe, life-threatening arrhythmias, e.g., premature ventricular depolarisation can lead to ventricular fibrillation.

Arrhythmias can be managed by **drugs** as well as **non-pharmacological measures** such as pacemakers, cardioversion, catheter ablation, and surgical treatment. However, antiarrhythmic drugs can have adverse reactions and can themselves precipitate arrhythmias. So, in general, treatment of asymptomatic or minimally symptomatic arrhythmias should be avoided. After successful control of arrhythmia, the patient is counseled for lifestyle modifications such as healthy diet, regular exercise, weight reduction, reduced alcohol intake, smoking cessation, adequate sleep, stress management and adequate control of BP and LDL cholesterol levels.

CLASSIFICATION OF ANTIARRHYTHMIC DRUGS

Antiarrhythmic drugs are classified into **4 types**, based on their major mechanism of action (Flowchart 36.1).

Class I drugs, the Na channel blockers (NaCBs), are further divided into **three subgroups** based on their effect on **potassium channels** and the **kinetics of their binding and dissociation from sodium channels**. Class II drugs are β blockers, while potassium channel blockers (KCBs) and calcium channel blockers (CCBs) form classes III and IV, respectively. In addition, adenosine. ATP and magnesium also possess anti-arrhythmic actions.

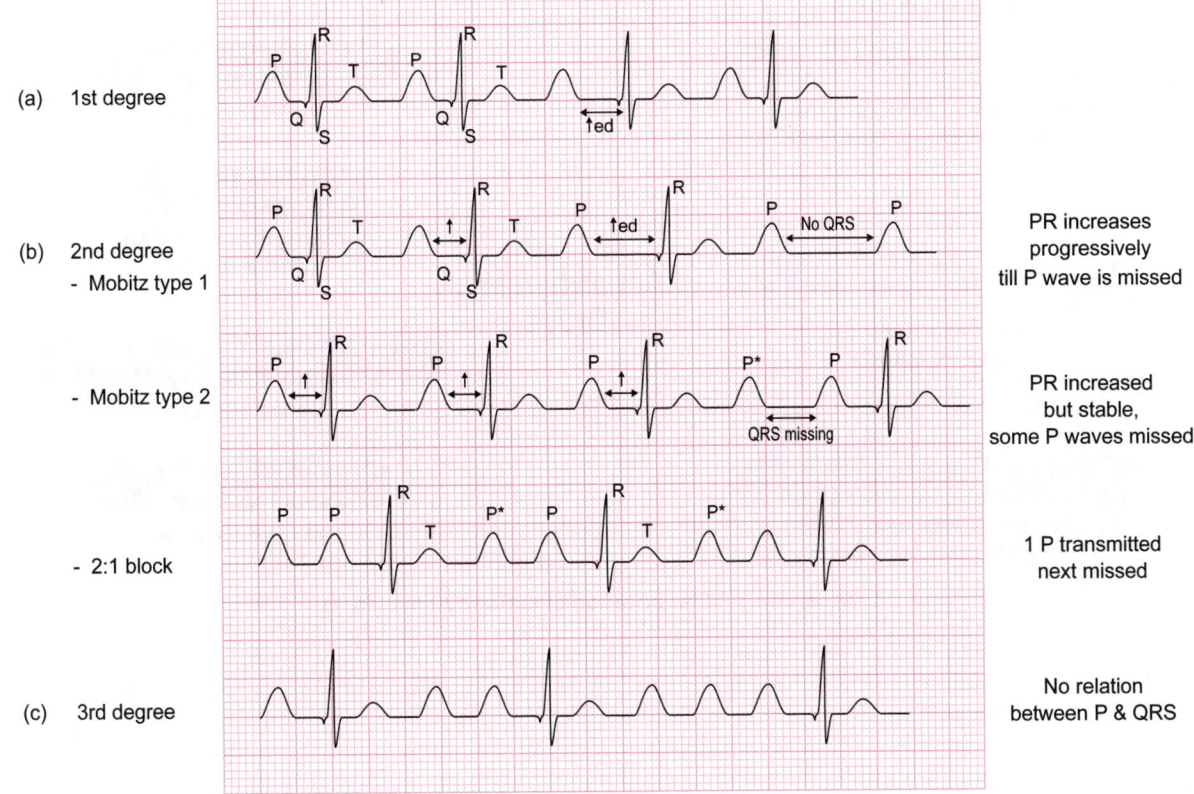

Fig. 36.8 ECG changes in AV blocks

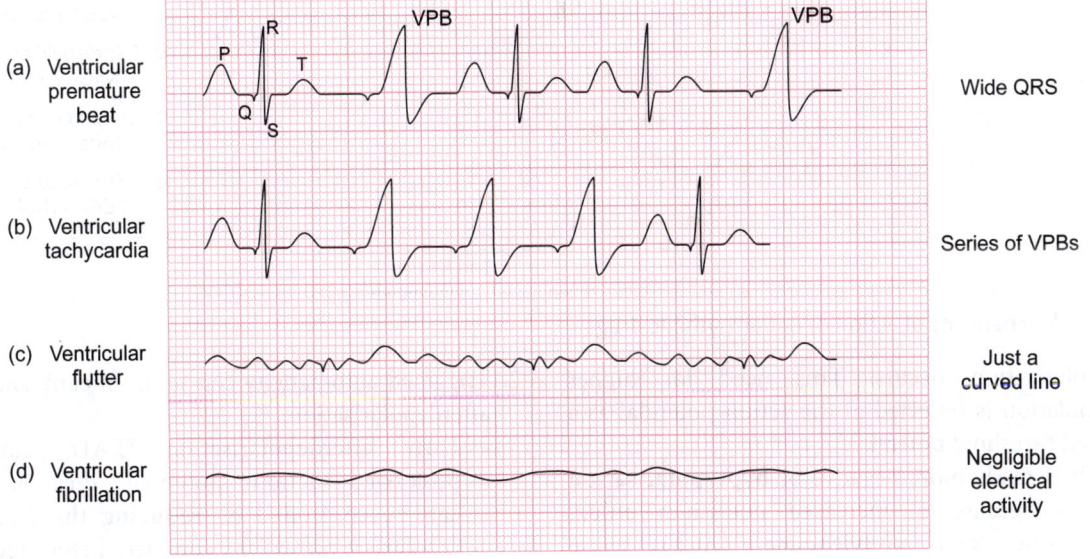

Fig. 36.9 ECG changes in ventricular arrhythmias

MECHANISM OF ANTIARRHYTHMIC ACTION OF DRUGS

Antiarrhythmic drugs alter the electrophysiological properties of heart cells by their effect on sodium/potassium/calcium channels that determine the cardiac action potential.

1. If tachyarrhythmia occurs due to **increased spontaneous automaticity**, drugs can **reduce automaticity** by the following mechanisms (Fig. 36.10).

   a. The slope of diastolic depolarisation or **Phase 4 depolarisation is reduced** by NaCBs (Class I), β-blockers (Class II), CCBs (Class IV), adenosine, and vagal stimulation/digoxin. This is because of reduced cation influx into the cell.

   b. **Threshold potential (TP) is raised** or made less negative, because some channels are blocked by NaCBs (Class I) and CCBs (Class IV) drugs. Therefore, stronger stimulus is required, so that even the partially blocked channels open and

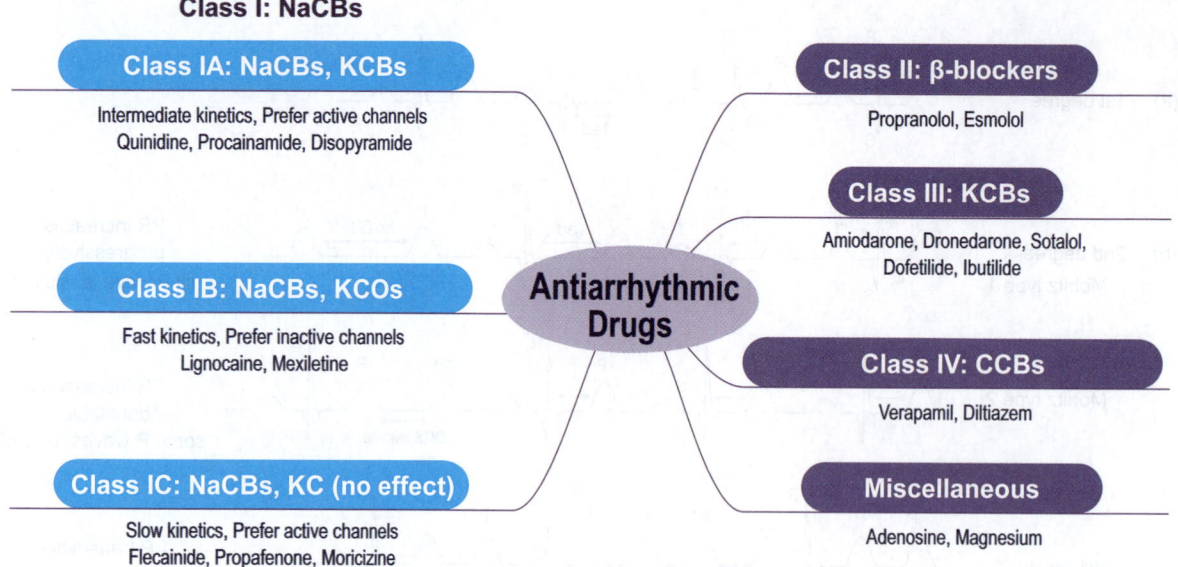

Flowchart 36.1 Classification of antiarrhythmic drugs

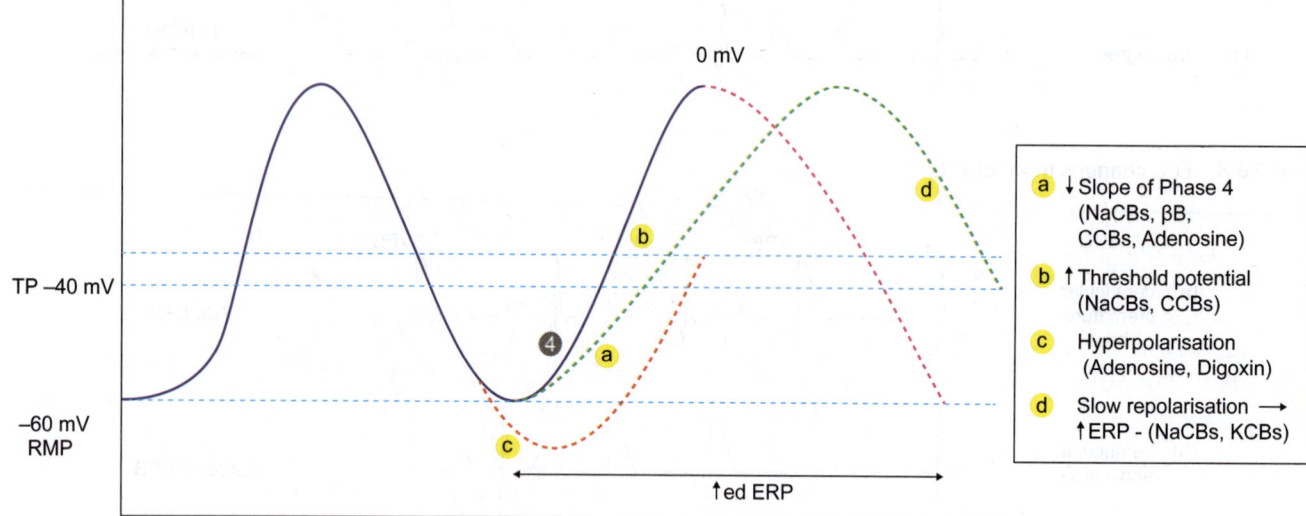

Fig. 36.10 Mechanisms of action of antiarrhythmic drugs

depolarisation occurs. This need for higher stimulation is reflected in the action potential as a raised threshold potential.

c. RMP is made more negative or **hyperpolarisation** occurs because of increased potassium efflux. Adenosine and acetylcholine (ACh) cause hyperpolarisation. However, ACh itself is not used as a drug. The vagotonic effect of digoxin or reflex vagal stimulation (by Valsalva manoeuvre, splashing cold water on face, and hyperflexion of neck by bending the head between knees) can also bring about hyperpolarisation. These electrophysiological changes decrease the automaticity, as more time is needed for the RMP to reach the threshold potential.

d. In the Purkinje fibres, raised automaticity can be reduced by potassium channel blockers as they delay repolarisation and **prolong the effective refractory period**.

2. Triggered automaticity can result in early and delayed afterdepolarisation.
   - Early afterdepolarisation (EAD) caused by prolonged action potential duration (APD) can be controlled by **reducing the APD.** Thus, repolarisation will be complete before recovery of most of the sodium channels from the inactive to resting stages. APD can be reduced by pacing and isoproterenol. Magnesium is also useful in EAD as it interferes with the recovery of sodium channels by an unknown mechanism.
   - Delayed afterdepolarisation (DAD) is a result of cation overloading, e.g., calcium overloading caused by digoxin toxicity. These can be controlled by CCBs (Class III, which check calcium entry into the cell) and NaCBs (Class I, which raise the threshold potential), so that oscillations of the potential in

Phase 4 fail to reach the threshold and the extra beat is prevented.

3. **Conduction defects:** In AV blocks, atropine and isoproterenol are useful as they **increase AV conduction**.
   - Re-entry can be controlled by **increasing the ERP**, so that the unidirectional block is converted to a bidirectional block. In fast response tissues, the ERP can be increased by NaCBs (Class I, which delay the recovery of sodium channels) and KCBs (Class III, which delay repolarisation).
   - In the case of anatomical re-entry as seen in WPW syndrome, the re-entrant circuit is broken by **further decreasing AV conduction** using CCBs, β-blockers, digoxin, etc. If the re-entry circuit is in the AV node, CCBs (Class IV) can be used to further decrease the conduction in AV node. Adenosine is effective but usually not preferred because of its very short duration of action (just 10 seconds) and in WPW syndrome, tachyarrhythmia can recur because of the presence of an anatomical defect. These mechanisms of action of anti-arrhythmic drugs are summarised in Table 36.1.

Table 36.1	Mechanism of action of antiarrhythmic drugs
Reduced automaticity	a. Decreasing slope of Phase 4 depolarisation: NaCBs, β-blockers, CCBs, adenosine, vagal stimulation b. Raised threshold potential: NaCBs, CCBs c. Hyperpolarisation or RMP more negative: adenosine, ACh (reflex vagal stimulation)
Reducing APD	d. Pacing, isoproterenol, magnesium
Increasing ERP	e. NaCBs, KCBs
Decreasing AV conduction	f. Adenosine, β-blockers, CCBs, digoxin

PHARMACOLOGICAL ACTIONS OF ANTIARRHYTHMIC DRUGS

Class IA Antiarrhythmics

This class of drugs includes quinidine, procainamide and disopyramide.

Pharmacological actions

Class IA drugs have sodium channel blocking effect with intermediate kinetics of binding and dissociation; they preferentially block active channels. These drugs **delay the recovery of sodium channels from inactive to resting state**. They also have potassium channel blocking action.

NaCB action leads to slowing of Phase 0 depolarisation in fast channel action potentials → prolongation of QRS complex in ECG (Fig. 36.11a).

- Decrease in slope of Phase 4 or diastolic depolarisation → reduced automaticity (Fig. 36.11b).
- Increase in threshold potential (TP made less negative) → reduced automaticity (Fig. 36.11b).
- KCB action leads to → slowing down of repolarisation or Phase 3 → prolonged APD → prolongation of QT interval in ECG. Prolonged QT interval is associated with risk of torsade de pointes (TDP) arrhythmia, which leads to syncope (Fig. 36.12).

Status: Class IA drugs are **not used frequently** because of the adverse effects associated with their use.

1. Quinidine

Quinidine is **rarely used** because of its adverse effects.
- Gastrointestinal effects: nausea, vomiting, diarrhea and abdominal pain.
- Cinchonism: headache, delirium, tinnitus, and hearing and visual impairment.
- Allergic reactions: fever, rash, angio-neurotic edema, hepatitis, thrombocytopenia, hemolytic anemia.

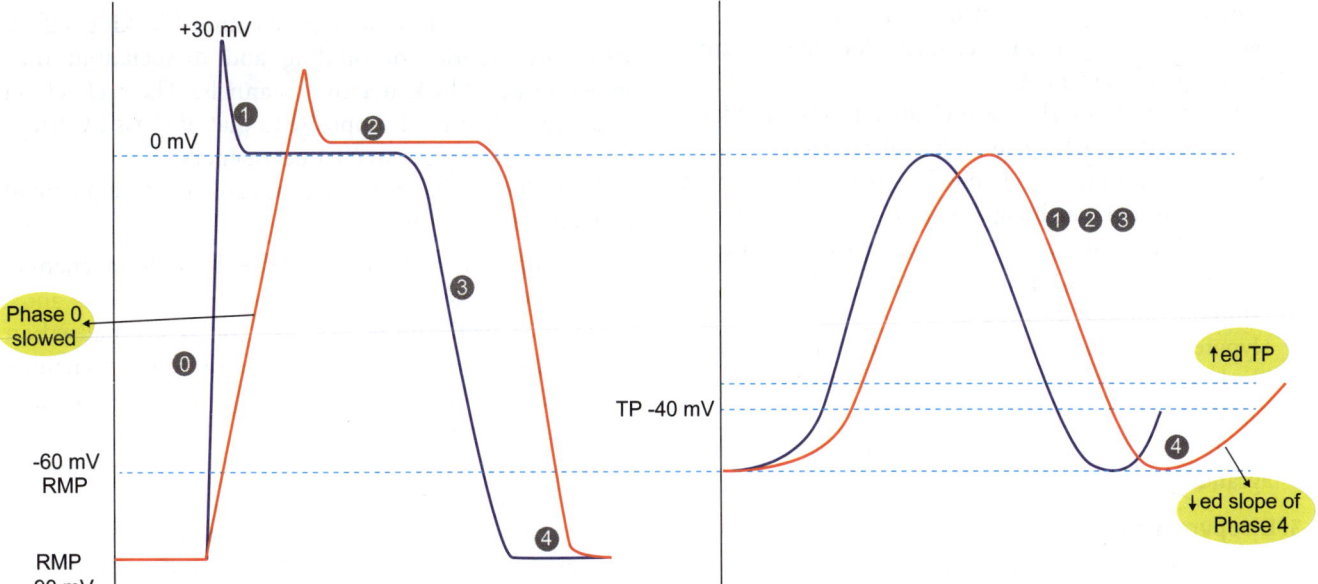

Fig. 36.11 (a, b) Effect of sodium channel blockade on cardiac action potential

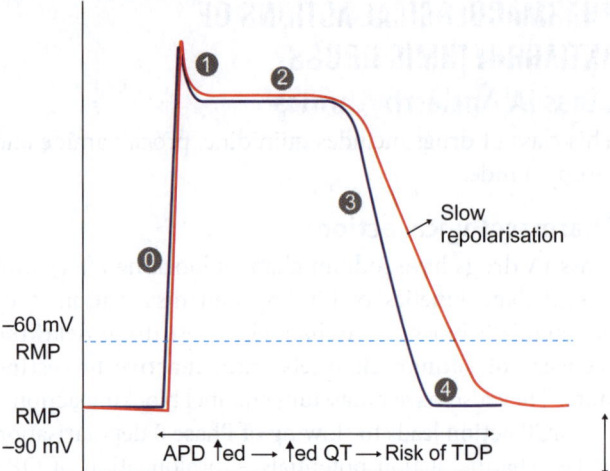

Fig. 36.12 Effect of K+-channel blockade on cardiac action potential

- Torsade de pointes (TDP) can be precipitated because of prolongation of QT interval
- Quinidine can cause severe hypotension by its α-blocking action
- Hypoglycemia can occur.
- Quinidine decreases renal as well as biliary clearance of digoxin and precipitates digoxin toxicity.

2. Procainamide

- Procainamide is used as the **2nd or 3rd choice** drug in tachyarrhythmias, if lignocaine or amiodarone are not tolerated or are contraindicated.
- It is metabolised by acetylation to form N-acetyl procainamide (NAPA), which is then excreted in urine. Therefore, dose reduction is indicated in patients with renal function impairment.
- There is genetic polymorphism in the rate of acetylation of procainamide to form NAPA, which possesses potassium channel blocking effects. Thus, in rapid acetylators, a large amount of NAPA is formed. This causes excessive potassium channel blockade, resulting in precipitation of TDP.

  In contrast, in slow acetylators, procainamide is metabolised slowly, and lupus-like reactions may occur on chronic use. Lupus-like reactions manifest as rash, myalgia, arthralgia, pleuritis and pericarditis. Antinuclear antibodies (ANAs) are present in almost 60–70% patients on procainamide therapy; once the symptoms appear, the drug should be discontinued.
- Hypotension can occur because of the ganglion-blocking effect of procainamide, but is less severe than that caused by quinidine.
- The most dangerous adverse effect of procainamide is agranulocytosis.

3. Disopyramide

Disopyramide is also rarely used because of its adverse effects.

- Anticholinergic adverse effects like dryness of mouth, blurring of vision, constipation, and urinary retention.
- Prolonged QT interval leading to torsade de pointes (TDP).
- Negative inotropic effect that can precipitate or worsen congestive heart failure.

Clinical problem-based questions and MCQs

1. **Torsade de pointes (TDP) can be precipitated by Class IA antiarrhythmic drugs. What is the mechanism of causation of TDP?**
   a. Delayed recovery of sodium channels
   b. Blockade of potassium channels
   c. Blockade of alpha receptors
   d. Vagal stimulation

2. **The risk of TDP with procainamide increases in:**
   a. Slow acetylators   b. Rapid acetylators
   c. Sick sinus syndrome   d. WPW syndrome

3. **Which of the following is not an electrophysiological effect of quinidine?**
   a. Decreases APD
   b. Decreases slope of diastolic depolarisation
   c. Increases threshold potential
   d. Prolongs QT interval

4. **Enumerate Class IA antiarrhythmic drugs. Explain why:**
   i. Quinidine is rarely used in clinical practice.
   ii. Disopyramide worsens CHF.
   iii. Procainamide can cause lupus-like reaction in some patients.

Class IB Antiarrhythmics

Lignocaine and mexiletine are examples of Class IB drugs.

Pharmacological actions

Class IB drugs have sodium channel blocking effect, with fast kinetics of binding and dissociation; they preferentially block inactive channels. Their effect on potassium channels is opposite to that of Class IA drugs, i.e., these are potassium channel openers.

The effects of lignocaine on the cardiac action potential includes (Fig. 36.13):

- Slowing down of Phase 0, due to sodium channel blockade (NaCB).
- RMP is made more negative (or is normalised in partially depolarised cells) due to sodium channel blocking (NaCB) and potassium channel opening (KCO) actions.
- Action potential duration (APD) is reduced due to KCO action, causing quick repolarisation.
- Effective refractory period (ERP) is reduced.
- Class IB drugs (lignocaine and mexiletine) **preferentially bind to the inactive state of sodium**

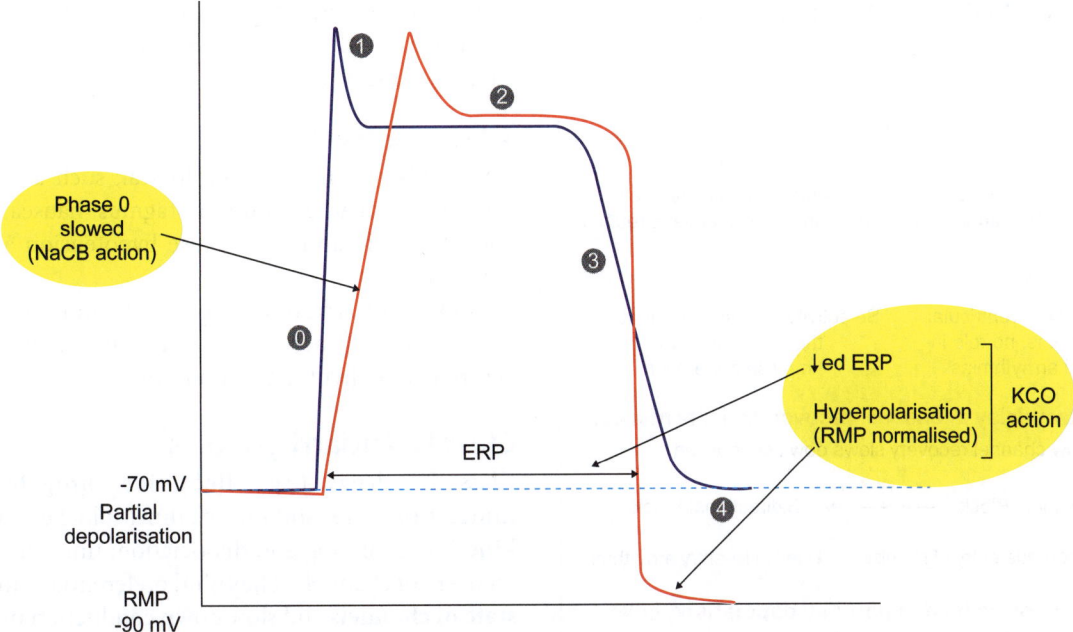

Fig. 36.13 Effect of lignocaine on the action potential in partially depolarised cells

channels. Therefore, lignocaine has a greater effect on myocytes, where more sodium channels remain in the inactive state for longer durations (e.g., in **cells with long APD** and **partially depolarised** cells).

- Ventricular and Purkinje fibres have longer APDs compared to atrial cells, and are more strongly affected by lignocaine, because they have more sodium channels in the inactive state. Therefore, **lignocaine is used only in ventricular arrhythmias** and has practically no value in atrial arrhythmias.
- Partially depolarised cells are those affected by ischemia, anoxia, injury and stretching. These are commonly the focus for starting ectopic beats. Thus, the greater propensity of lignocaine to bind to the inactive state of sodium channels confers it selectivity. In this manner, lignocaine exerts greater action on partially depolarised cells, which serve as foci of abnormal impulse generation.
- Lignocaine does not cause any delay in channel recovery in normal cells because of its **fast kinetics** of binding and dissociation with channels. However, in ischemic or injured cells, the kinetics of lignocaine binding/dissociation is comparatively slow. Therefore, lignocaine selectively delays channel recovery and causes blockade of conduction in such injured/ischemic cells. It can change a unidirectional block to a bidirectional block.
- The **potassium channel opening** effect of lignocaine → shortening of APD and some decrease in the effective refractory period; so, there is no risk of TDP. Sodium channel blocking and potassium channel opening effects help to make the RMP more negative. Thus, the RMP is normalised in partially depolarised cells (Fig. 36.13) and conduction improves. In this manner, lignocaine can abolish one-way blocks.
- Lignocaine decreases the automaticity of ectopic foci but has no effect on the SA node. It has no effect on conduction in the AV node but selectively alters conduction of partially depolarised fibres. It may abolish a one-way block or convert it to a two-way block. Thus, lignocaine is useful to control ventricular re-entrant arrhythmias.
- Lignocaine has no autonomic actions.
- Its arrhythmogenic potential, i.e., risk of causing arrhythmias, is minimal because it has no effect on SA nodal automaticity, AV nodal conduction and the QT interval. It is the least cardiotoxic of the antiarrhythmic drugs.
- Lignocaine is very useful in ventricular tachycardia, ventricular re-entrant arrhythmias and digoxin-induced ventricular tachycardia. The salient features of lignocaine action are summarised in Flowchart 36.2.

Pharmacokinetics

Lignocaine has a short half-life (10–20 min) because of its rapid redistribution. It is metabolised in the liver; its metabolism depends on hepatic blood flow. Therefore, it should be used cautiously in conditions like congestive heart failure, where hepatic blood flow is reduced. Lignocaine is administered as an intravenous bolus injection (50–100 mg followed by 20–40 mg every 10–20 minutes) or as a 1–3 mcg/min infusion. It has quick and easily titrable action. Therefore, it is

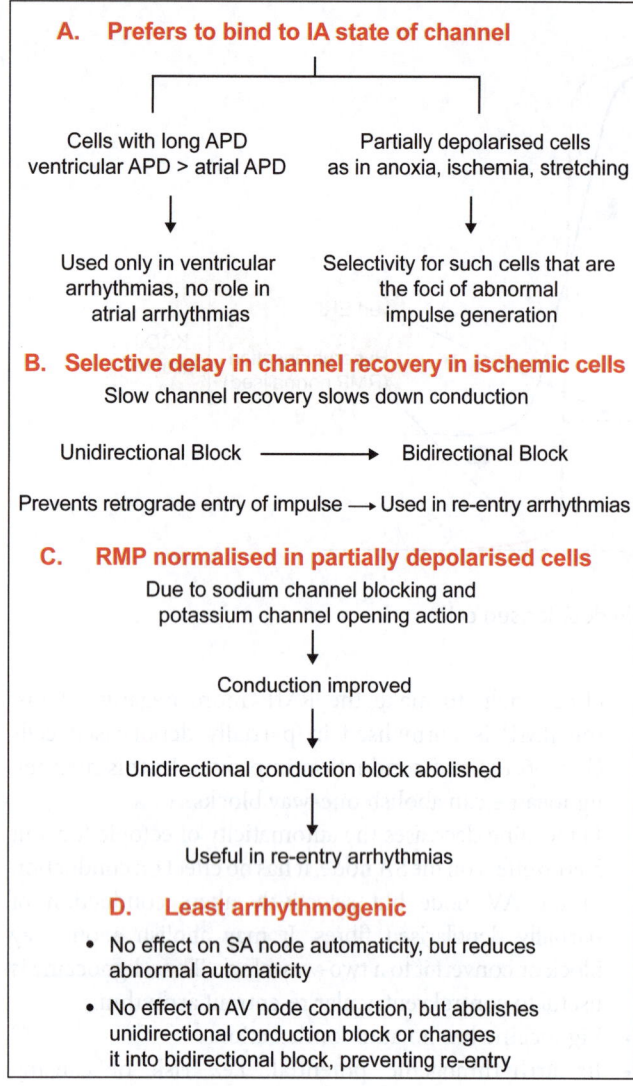

Flowchart 36.2 Lignocaine as an antiarrhythmic drug

suitable for emergency conditions such as arrhythmias associated with acute myocardial infarction (AMI), cardiac surgery, etc.

Adverse effects

The ADRs are mainly neurological, such as paresthesia, drowsiness, disorientation, nystagmus, nausea, twitching, and fits. Toxic doses can cause hypotension and cardiac depression.

Mexiletine is an oral congener of lignocaine. It is rarely used as the efficacy of the oral drug in prophylaxis of ventricular arrhythmias is doubtful.

Class IC Antiarrhythmics

Class IC drugs (e.g., **flecainide, propafenone and moricizine**) are sodium channel blockers with **slow kinetics** of binding and dissociation; thus, they delay the recovery of channels. They bind preferentially to the **active state of channels** and slow down conduction markedly. In the ECG, the PR interval is prolonged and QRS complexes are wide. However, they do not have a noticeable effect on potassium channels. Thus, **QT prolongation is not seen**.

- Propafenone can be useful in WPW syndrome as it converts one-way blocks into two-way blocks.
- Propafenone may be useful to control ventricular rate in supraventricular arrhythmias.
- It is also useful in the prophylaxis of PSVT.
- In addition to Class I effects, it causes β blockade, which could result in bronchospasm and precipitate CHF.
- In patients with ischemic heart disease, it can precipitate life-threatening arrhythmias. So, it is not commonly used.

A comparison of the characteristics of the three categories of Class I antiarrhythmics is presented in Table 36.2.

Table 36.2 Characteristics of Class I antiarrhythmic drugs (sodium channel blockers)

	Characteristic	IA	IB	IC
1	Kinetics at Na channel	Intermediate	Fast in normal cells Slow in partially depolarised cells	Slow
2	Preferred state of Na channel for binding	Active	Inactive	Active
3	Effect on Na channel recovery from IA to R state	Delayed	Selectively delayed in partially depolarised cells only	Delayed
4	Effect on potassium channels	Blocked	Opened	No effect
5	Effect on APD/QT interval	Prolonged	Shortened	No effect
6	Risk of torsade de pointes	Present	No risk	No risk
7	Current status	Not used because of many ADRs	Lignocaine used in ventricular arrhythmias	Useful in WPW and controlling ventricular rate in PSVT, but not used commonly.

> **Clinical problem-based questions and MCQs**
>
> 5. A 50-year-old male patient, a known case of unstable angina, lands in emergency with severe precordial pain radiating to the left shoulder and arm, cold sweating, anxiety and palpitation. ECG shows T wave inversion and ventricular tachycardia. Patient is diagnosed as having AMI with VT. Injection lignocaine 50 mg bolus IV, followed by IV infusion 1–3 mcg/minute is given.
>   i. Describe the pharmacological basis for preferring lignocaine in this emergency situation.
>   ii. Describe the mechanism of action and cardiac effects of lignocaine.
>   iii. Lignocaine is said to have the least arrhythmogenic potential among antiarrhythmic drugs. Explain.
>   iv. Lignocaine is not effective in SVT. Explain.
>
> 6. Explain the re-entry phenomenon seen in WPW syndrome. Why is propafenone effective in this case, though not used frequently?
>
> 7. Which of the following drugs decreases conduction through the AV node?
>   a. Lignocaine   b. Mexiletine
>   c. Propafenone   d. All of the above

Class II Antiarrhythmics (β-blockers)

Class II antiarrhythmics (β-blockers) such as propranolol and esmolol are useful in the treatment of sinus tachycardia, atrial tachycardia and junctional tachycardia, especially when these are induced by sympathetic overactivity as in emotional stress, exercise, during halothane anesthesia, and pheochromocytoma.

- In PSVT, Class IV drugs, i.e., CCBs and adenosine are more effective than β-blockers.
- In cases of atrial flutter and fibrillation, propranolol controls the ventricular rate by causing AV blockade.
- In WPW syndrome, propranolol can be combined with Class IA and IC drugs.
- Propranolol prophylaxis can reduce mortality in AMI due to sudden arrhythmias.

Esmolol is a short-acting β-blocker with rapid onset of action. It is used intravenously to control the ventricular rate in atrial flutter and fibrillation. It is used to terminate supraventricular tachycardia associated with anesthetic use.

Class III Antiarrhythmics

Class III antiarrhythmics drugs are potassium channel blockers (KCBs) such as amiodarone, dronedarone, sotalol, vernakalant, ibutilide and dofetilide. These drugs block potassium channels → prolonged repolarisation → increased APD → increased QT interval.

The blockade of potassium channels is '**reverse use dependent**', i.e., the drugs prefer to bind to channels in the resting state. Therefore, the risk of TDP is greater in patients with slow heart rate, which is when the channels remain in resting state for longer.

However, the potential to cause torsade de pointes varies from drug to drug. Sotalol has a greater risk of causing TDP when compared to amiodarone.

1. Amiodarone

It has a **wide spectrum** of antiarrhythmic effects, including NaCB, β-blocker, KCB, CCB, α-blocker and vasodilator activity. Therefore, it is effective in atrial fibrillation as well as recurrent ventricular arrhythmias. Because of its **long half-life** of 40–50 days, a loading dose is required. The effects of this drug persist for a long time after discontinuation.

The adverse **effects** of amiodarone (Fig. 36.14) include:

- **Photosensitiv**ity reactions
- **O**ptic neuritis
- An iodine-containing compound, amiodarone interferes with **th**yroid function and can cause hypo- or hyperthyroidism.
- **Peripher**al neuropathy
- **My**ocardial damage
- **Pulmonary** fibrosis
- **Liver** damage, causing hepatic enzymes to be raised
- Slate blue **skin** discoloration
- **Corneal** deposits

[Mnemonic: **Photosensitivity of the periphery** of **my lung**, **liver**, **skin** and **cornea**]

2. Dronedarone

Its mechanism of action is similar to amiodarone. Important differences from amiodarone include:

- It lacks iodine therefore, does not cause thyroid dysfunction as an adverse effect.

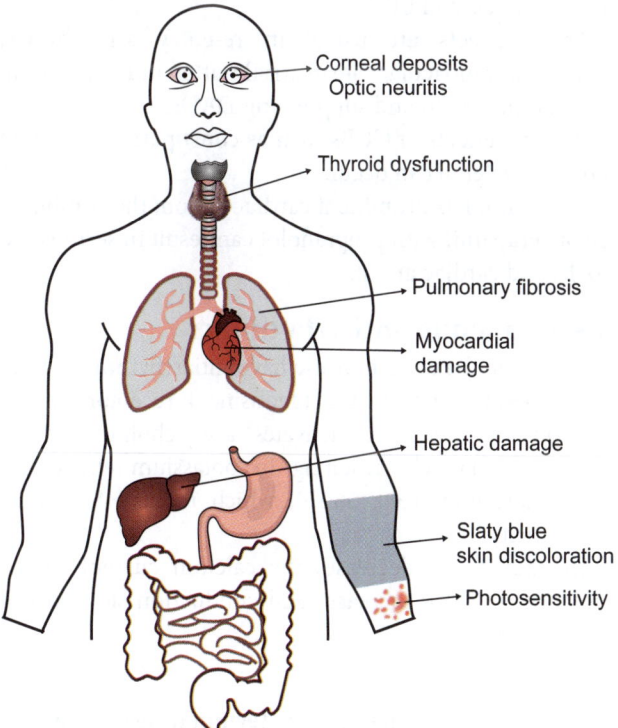

Fig. 36.14 Adverse effects of amiodarone

- Its half-life is shorter (24 hours).
- Dronedarone is less effective than amiodarone and is used only for supraventricular arrhythmias, whereas amiodarone is used in ventricular as well as supraventricular arrhythmias (see Fig. 36.17).
- Dronedarone is less toxic than amiodarone. Its adverse effects include gastrointestinal symptoms, weakness, cough, bradycardia and skin reactions. The risk of TDPs is lower; thyroid dysfunction or pulmonary fibrosis do not occur.

3. Sotalol
Sotalol possesses both β-blocking and potassium channel blocking actions. It has a greater risk of causing TDP than amiodarone. Sotalol is approved for the treatment of supraventricular and ventricular arrhythmias in pediatric populations.

4. Dofetilide and ibutilide
Dofetilide and ibutilide are pure potassium channel blockers and carry the risk of causing TDP. They are used for maintaining atrial flutter and fibrillation converts in the sinus rhythm.

Class IV Antiarrhythmics (Calcium Channel Blockers)
Class IV drugs (e.g., verapamil and diltiazem) exert antiarrhythmic effect by blocking L-type calcium channels in the active and inactive states.

SA node: The direct action of calcium channel blockers decreases the automaticity of the SA node, but hypotensive action can cause some reflex tachycardia.

AV node: CCBs decrease conduction through the AV node → increase in ERP.

These effects are useful in re-entry arrhythmias, controlling ventricular rate in atrial flutter and fibrillation, terminating PSVT, and suppressing DADs.

Adverse effects of CCBs such as constipation, lassitude and pedal edema can occur.

Verapamil has prominent cardiac action; the combined use of verapamil with propranolol can result in serious AV blocks and cardiac arrest.

Miscellaneous Antiarrhythmics
Adenosine and magnesium also have antiarrhythmic action.

Adenosine binds to the adenosine 1 receptors in the SA and AV nodes. It activates acetylcholine-sensitive potassium channels, resulting in potassium efflux and hyperpolarisation (Fig. 36.15), which reduces SA nodal automaticity.

In addition, it decreases the calcium current in the AV node; so, ERP increases and conduction slows down (Fig. 36.16).

Uses
Adenosine is better than CCBs in **terminating acute attack of PSVT**. It is also useful in the diagnosis of AV node-

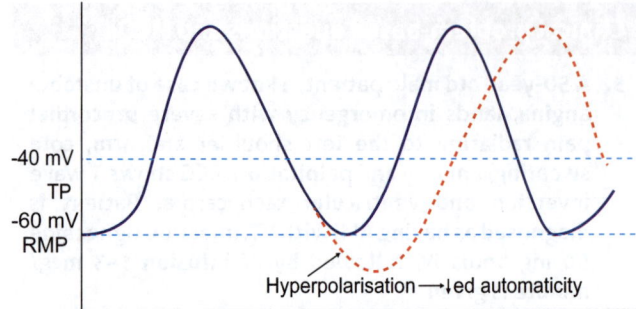

Fig. 36.15 Effect of adenosine on the cardiac AP in the SA node

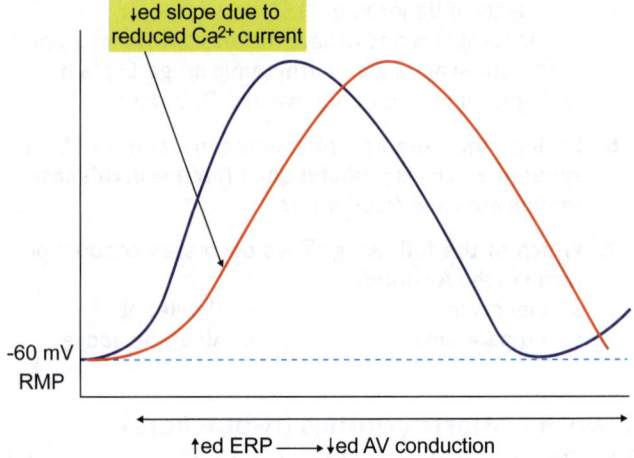

Fig. 36.16 Effect of adenosine on the cardiac AP in the AV node

dependent tachycardia. Adenosine produces controlled hypotension during surgery and is also useful for brief coronary vasodilation.

Pharmacokinetics
Adenosine is rapidly taken up by endothelial cells and RBCs and metabolised to 5-AMP and inosine. It has to be injected as a bolus injection into a large vein for noticeable effect. Because the **half-life of adenosine is very short** (just 10 seconds), adverse effects like chest pain, dyspnea, hypotension, flushing and even cardiac arrest are transient. However, it is of no value in prophylaxis of recurrent arrhythmias because of its very short duration of action.

DRUG THERAPY OF VARIOUS ARRHYTHMIAS
Tachyarrhythmias
Diagnosis is based on symptoms and investigations. Symptoms of patients suffering from tachyarrythmias are similar, irrespective of their site of origin. Patients usually complain of a feeling of rapid thumping/fluttering/pounding/racing heartbeat that is associated with uneasiness, lightheadedness, dizziness, anxiety, profuse sweating, syncope, tachypnea, etc. Chest pain or tightness may also occur. In paroxysmal arrhythmias, the onset of such symptoms is very abrupt. The symptoms also disappear abruptly upon termination of a paroxysmal attack.

Diagnosis of type of arrhythmia

ECG shows characteristic features of rhythm disturbances. The electrocardiogram is recorded for a full day or longer, using a Holter monitor. Patients who have normal ECGs, but complain of symptoms suggestive of arrhythmias, are advised to wear a portable ECG device called an 'event recorder' and press the button to record the ECG upon onset of symptoms. The 'event recorder' may be implanted under the skin in the chest area in patients with infrequent arrhythmias.

Some other tests (e.g., stress test with treadmill, tilt table test, and electrophysiological mapping) are also helpful in detecting arrhythmias.

Drug treatment

It depends on the type of arrhythmia, as described below:

Sinus tachycardia

β-blockers and CCBs are the drugs of first choice. They are useful as they decrease the automaticity in the SA node. When the use of β-blockers and CCBs is contraindicated, ivabradine—a purely bradycardiac drug—is useful.

PSVT

Reflex vagal stimulation can terminate a PSVT attack. The vagus can be stimulated by the Valsalva manoeuvre, splashing of ice cold water on face, hyperflexion of neck (bending head between knees) and carotid sinus massage with the patient in a recumbent position (only one side at a time).

- Adenosine, given as a rapid intravenous injection (6–12 mg), can quickly terminate an acute attack of PSVT.
- β-blockers: Short-acting β-blocker esmolol is useful in PSVT for terminating acute illness.
- CCBs (verapamil and diltiazem) may be effective.
- Dronedarone, a KCB drug, may be useful.
- Digoxin can also slow down AV conduction by its vagotonic action.

In patients who do not respond to drug treatment, DC shock may be required.

- In SVT due to WPW syndrome, radio frequency ablation of the bundle of Kent, the abnormal conducting pathway, is effective in controlling tachyarrhythmia.
- In serious life-threatening arrhythmias such as incessant SVT, atrial flutter, and atrial fibrillation, catheter ablation is attempted when medicines fail to correct the rhythm disturbance.

Ventricular tachycardia

The occurrence of three or more ventricular ectopic beats in succession is called ventricular tachycardia (VT). It occurs due to pre-existing cardiac diseases (such as IHD, myocarditis, and cardiomyopathies), electrolyte disturbances, digoxin toxicity, etc. Symptoms are similar to SVT and diagnosis is based on ECG changes. The management of VT is more aggressive, as it can progress to ventricular fibrillation, and the patient may go into shock. Mortality rate is high.

- In uncomplicated cases of VT, ventricular re-entrant arrhythmia and digoxin-induced arrhythmia, lignocaine is the drug of choice. It is given as a 2% solution by IV bolus injection in a dose of 50–100 mg. If cardiac rhythm is not normalised, 20–40 mg dose of lignocaine can be repeated every 10–20 minutes, up to a maximum total dose of 250 mg. For maintenance therapy, lignocaine 1 g in 500 mL of 5% glucose is infused at a rate of 2–4 mg/min. The maintenance dose is tapered off in 48–72 hours.
- In patients with recurring arrhythmia, other useful drugs are procainamide, disopyramide, amiodarone and beta-blockers (after lignocaine therapy).
- If the patient is in shock, a synchronised DC shock (100–150 Joules) is given immediately. Drugs like dopamine may be required (refer to page 472).
- A grave complication of VT with fatal outcomes is ventricular fibrillation (Vf). It needs immediate defibrillation with a DC shock of 300–400 Joules. Implantable Cardioverter Defibrillators (ICDs) are devices that detect VT/Vf, and automatically deliver a DC shock of appropriate strength.
- There is a chance of recovery of brain function if cardiac rhythm is restored within three minutes of onset of Vf. Life support measures, e.g., mouth-to-mouth respiration and external cardiac massage are provided till patient reaches the specialised cardiac centre.

Drugs for Supraventricular and Ventricular Arrhythmias

SVT only: Adenosine, CCBs, digoxin, dronedarone

VT only: lignocaine, mexiletine

For SVT and VT: Amiodarone, β-blockers (propranolol, esmolol andsotalol), Class IA drugs (quinidine, procainamide and disopyramide) and Class IC drugs (flecainide, propafenone and moricizine) (Fig. 36.17).

AV blocks

The definitive treatment of AV blocks is pacing by implanting a cardiac pacemaker. Drugs are used in the short term for acute control. If the AV block caused by vagal overactivity as seen in digoxin toxicity and AMI, atropine is given intravenously in a dose of 0.6–1.2 mg. Sympathomimetics such as adrenaline and isoprenaline are also used sometimes.

Cardiac arrest

Cardiac arrest occurs most commonly as a complication of VF and asystole. Irreversible brain damage occurs if it is not corrected within 3–4 minutes. Cardiac arrest can be managed by teamwork only. If the pulse is not palpable and no cardiac activity is seen, resuscitation should be started. Important steps of cardiac resuscitation include the following:

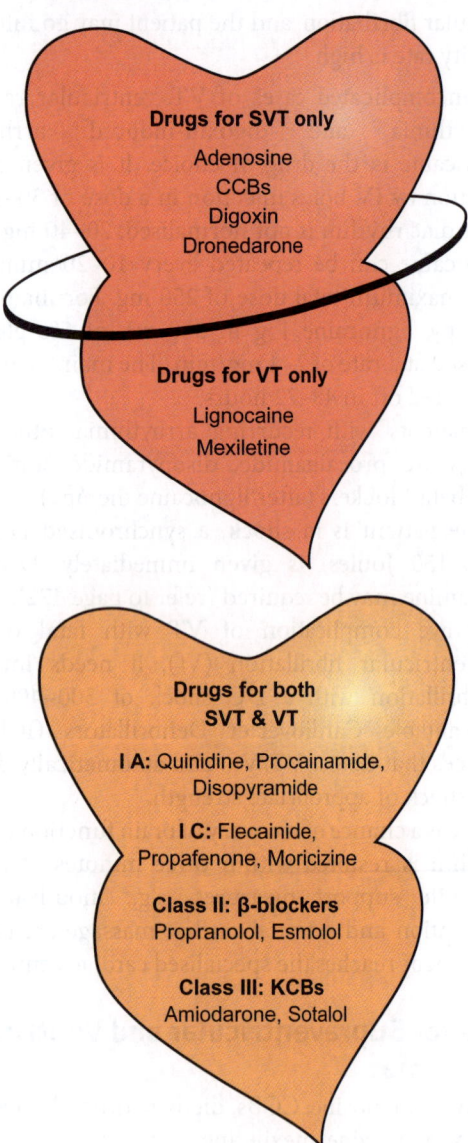

Fig. 36.17 Drugs for SVT and VT

- **Clearing airways**: chin is moved up to prevent the tongue falling back and secretions from air passages are removed by suction.
- Simultaneously, **artificial ventilation** is started by mouth-to-mouth breathing/ Ambu bag/ tracheal intubation, depending upon the facility that is available immediately.
- **External cardiac massage** by pressing firmly over sternum at a rate of 50–60 times per minute. It is continued till SBP reaches 70–80 mm of Hg.
- **IV line** is secured with 5% glucose to facilitate administration of medicines.
- Intracardiac injection of **adrenaline** 0.5 mg, into the right ventricle, through the 3rd or 4th left intercostal space or intravenously for ventricular asystole; adrenaline may convert asystole into VF, which is then managed with DC shock.

- Sodium bicarbonate 100 mmol is given IV to correct metabolic acidosis.
- In patients not responding to cardiac massage and adrenaline injection, repeat dose of adrenaline and sodium bicarbonate is tried.
- If the patient still does not respond, 20 mL of 5% solution of calcium chloride is injected IV.

Resuscitation is discontinued after 1 hour, if the patient fails to respond to these measures.

Clinical problem-based questions and MCQs

8. A 76-year-old female patient presents with palpitation, anxiety and sweating. Pulse is feeble, HR = 280, ECG shows sawtooth appearance of P wave. Patient is diagnosed with atrial flutter. Which of the following drugs is most suitable to control ventricular rate in this patient?
   a. Esmolol   b. Propranolol
   c. Lignocaine   d. Quinidine
   Justify your choice.

9. i. Identify the drug that has a wide spectrum of antiarrhythmic activity
      a. Lignocaine   b. Verapamil
      c. Amiodarone   d. Adenosine
   ii. Enumerate the adverse effects of the chosen drug.

10. Explain why:
    i. Propranolol and verapamil are useful to control ventricular rate in atrial tachyarrhythmias, but their combined use is hazardous.
    ii. Adenosine is preferred over CCBs in PSVT.

11. Describe the emergency management of ventricular fibrillation.

12. Describe resuscitation measures for patients with cardiac arrest.

Summary

- Arrhythmias arise from a disturbance in the site or rate of generation of cardiac impulse and rate or route of conduction. They can be tachy- or bradyarrhythmias, supraventricular or ventricular arrhythmias and re-entrant arrhythmias.
- Antiarrhythmic drugs are of **4 classes**.
- Class I drugs are NaCBs. Based on the kinetics of binding and effect on potassium channels these are further grouped into three subtypes.
  - **Class IA drugs** (quinidine, procainamide and disopyramide) are not used much because of their adverse effects.
  - Among **Class IB** drugs, lignocaine is very useful for ventricular arrhythmias, especially in

Chapter 36 Antiarrhythmic Drugs

emergency situations; however, it has no role in supraventricular arrhythmias.
- **Class IC drugs** (flecainide and propafenone) slow down conduction; they are also not much in use.
- **Class II** drugs include β-blockers like propranolol and esmolol. Esmolol is a short-acting drug with rapid onset of action. It is used intravenously to control the ventricular rate in atrial flutters and fibrillations. It is used to terminate supraventricular tachycardia associated with anesthetic use.
- **Class III** drugs are potassium channel blockers like amiodarone, dronedarone and sotalol. They cause reverse use dependent blockade.
- **Amiodarone** has a very long half-life and several adverse effects. It can prolong APD, QT interval and increase the risk of precipitating TDP, especially in patients with slow HR.
- **Class IV** drugs are CCBs that exert antiarrhythmic effect by blocking L-type calcium channels in the active and inactive states. They decrease the automaticity of SA node, (but hypotensive action can cause some reflex tachycardia), decrease conduction through AV node, and increase ERP.
- These effects are useful in re-entry arrhythmias, controlling ventricular rate in atrial flutters and fibrillations, terminating PSVT and suppressing delayed afterdepolarisations (DADs).
- **Adenosine** is a miscellaneous antiarrhythmic drug that activates acetylcholine-sensitive potassium channels causing hyperpolarisation. It decreases calcium current in the AV node, SA nodal automaticity and AV node conduction, and is better than CCBs in terminating acute PSVT attacks. It has very short duration of action so its adverse effects are transient.

Questions for practice

1. Classify antiarrhythmic drugs.
2. Describe the mechanism of action of antiarrhythmic drugs.
3. Explain why:
   a. Class I A antiarrhythmics are not used frequently.
   b. Lignocaine is used in ventricular arrhythmias.
   c. Esmolol is used in atrial flutters and fibrillations.
   d. Among patients receiving Class III antiarrhythmics, risk of TDP is greater in patients with slow heart rate.
   e. Combined use of propranolol and verapamil can be hazardous in cardiac patients.
   f. All arrhythmias do not need drug treatment.
4. Describe the drug therapy of:
   a. Sinus tachycardia
   b. Paroxysmal supraventricular tachycardia
   c. AV blocks
5. Write short notes on:
   a. Amiodarone
   b. Adenosine

Hints for problem-based questions and MCQs

1. b. Blockade of potassium channels prolongs QT interval which can precipitate self-sustaining TDP.
2. b. Rapid acetylators, because N-acetyl procainamide (formed by acetylation of procainamide) has excessive potassium channel blocking effect, resulting in prolongation of QT interval and precipitation of TDP.
3. a. Decreases APD. Quinidine is a Class IA drug that has NaCB as well as KCB action. Because of the KCB action, repolarisation slows down and APD increases.
4. i. Rarely used because of many adverse effects. Refer to page 487.
   ii. Because of its negative inotropic effect.
   iii. Procainamide is metabolised by acetylation. In slow acetylators, it may cause a lupus-like reaction. Refer to page 488
5. i. Lignocaine has quick and easily titrable action. Therefore, it is suitable for emergency conditions such as arrhythmias associated with acute myocardial infarction (AMI), cardiac surgery, etc. In this case of AMI with VT, lignocaine is highly effective because ischemia causes the partial depolarisation of myocardial cells. Lignocaine has a greater propensity to bind to IA sodium channels, so it selectively exerts action on partially depolarised cells (as they have more Na channels in IA form), which serve as the foci of abnormal impulse generation.
   ii. Sodium channel block with higher affinity for IA state of channel.
   Fast kinetics of channel association and dissociation.
   Potassium channel opening action.
   (Refer to pages 488, 489.)
   iii. Its affinity for the IA state of channel, which is seen in partially depolarised (injured/ischemic) cells, results in selective action. Refer to page 489.
   iv. Lignocaine binds preferentially to the inactive state of sodium channels For instance, ventricular and Purkinje fibres have longer APDs than atrial cells and are affected more by lignocaine. Hence, lignocaine is not effective in SVT. Refer to page 489.
6. Propafenone can be useful in WPW syndrome as it delays conduction and converts one-way block to two-way block. However, it is not used because of the risk of bronchial asthma, CHF, and arrhythmia. Refer to pages 482, 490.
7. c. Propafenone markedly reduces conduction.
8. a. Esmolol is a short-acting β-blocker with a rapid onset of action. It is used intravenously to control the ventricular rate in atrial flutters and fibrillations. Propranolol is useful but esmolol is preferred. Lignocaine has no role in supraventricular tachycardias. Quinidine is not used because of its numerous adverse effects.
9. i. c. Amiodarone
   ii. Refer to page 491.
10. i. The combined use of verapamil with propranolol can result in serious AV blocks and cardiac arrest.
    ii. Adenosine acts by binding to adenosine 1 receptors in the SA and AV nodes, resulting in activation of acetylcholine-sensitive potassium channels. This results in hyperpolarisation, reduced SA node automaticity AV conduction. In addition it decreases calcium current in AV node.
    Adenosine is better than CCBs in terminating an acute attack of PSVT. Moreover ADRs are transient because of its very short duration of action.
11. Refer to page 493.
12. Refer to page 494.

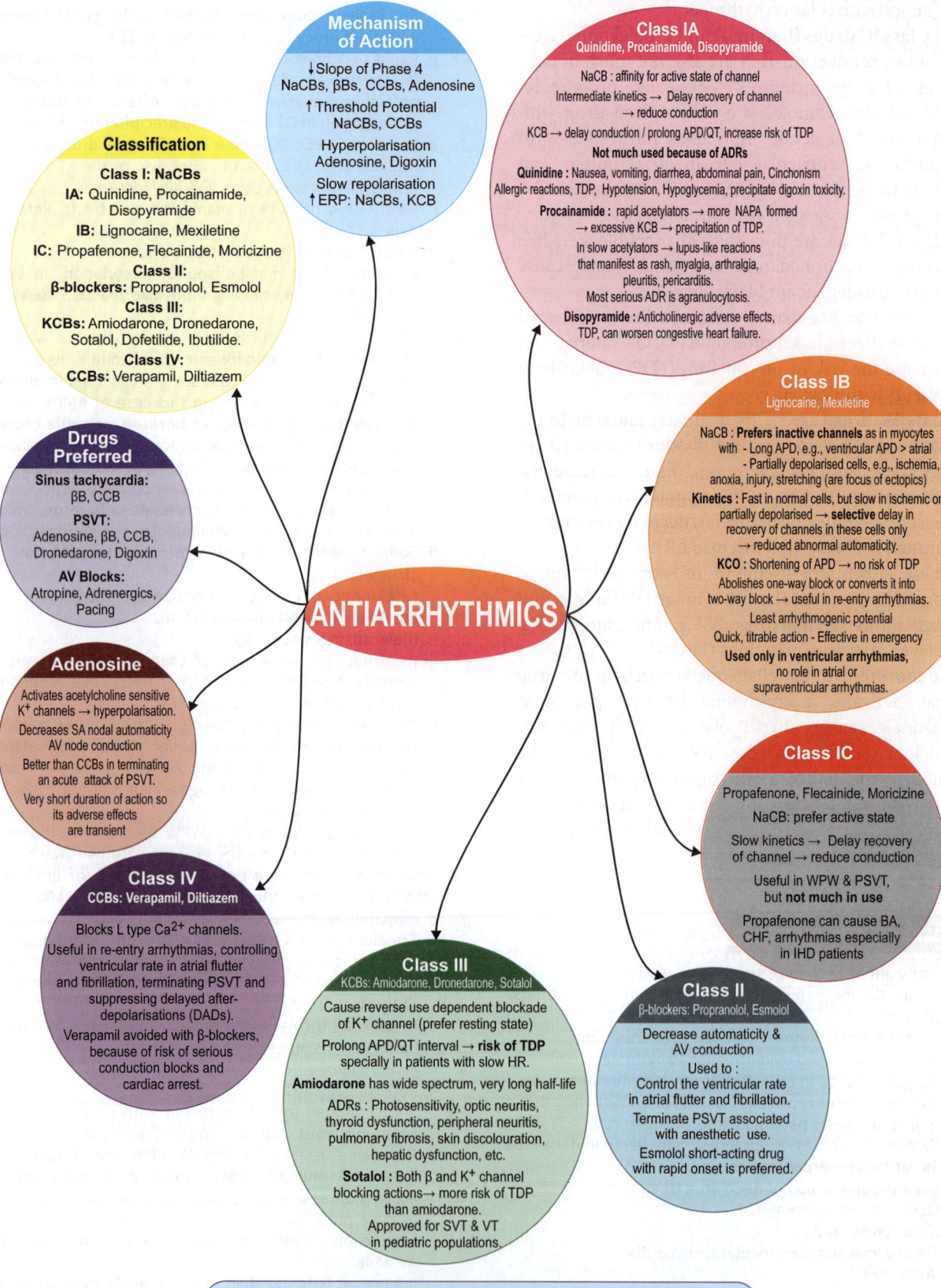

SECTION 8   Drugs Affecting Blood

37   Coagulants and Anticoagulants

PH 4.2 Explain types, salient pharmacokinetics, pharmacodynamics, therapeutic uses, adverse drug reactions of drugs acting on coagulation system (coagulants/anticoagulants) and devise a plan to monitor therapy and management of adverse effects.

Learning objectives

A student of MBBS phase II should be able to:
- Describe the steps of the coagulation process and its regulation.
- Classify coagulants and describe their mechanisms of action.
- Enumerate therapeutic uses, adverse effects and contraindications of coagulants.
- Classify anticoagulants and describe their mechanisms of action.
- Enumerate therapeutic uses of anticoagulants mentioning doses.
- Enumerate adverse effects and contraindications of anticoagulants.
- Describe the monitoring of anticoagulant therapy and management of adverse effects of anticoagulants.
- Comment on the advantages of LMWH over UFHs.
- Describe factors which can potentiate or decrease anticoagulant effect of warfarin.

PROCESS OF COAGULATION

Under normal circumstances, circulating platelets and clotting factors do not adhere to the vascular endothelium. However, when the **vascular endothelium is injured**, primary and secondary hemostasis follow, which involve the formation of a **platelet plug** and **fibrin clot**, respectively.

Formation of Platelet Plug (Primary Hemostasis)

An injury to the vascular endothelium (Fig. 37.1) exposes subendothelial matrix proteins like collagen and von Willebrand factor (vWF) that bind to GP_{1a} and GP_{1b} receptors on the platelet surface, respectively, resulting in platelet adherence and activation. The activated platelets secrete thromboxane A_2 (TxA_2), adenosine diphosphate (ADP) and 5-hydroxytryptamine (5-HT), which induce platelet aggregation. At the same time, conformational changes occur in the $GP_{IIb/IIIa}$ receptors of activated platelets, which favour binding to fibrinogen, cross-linking of adjacent platelets, and formation of a platelet plug.

Formation of Fibrin Clot (Secondary Hemostasis)

As the platelet plug is formed, the coagulation cascade is activated simultaneously. Factor VII forms an activated complex (Fig. 37.2) with tissue factors (TF), TF–VII_a, which catalyses the activation of factor IX to IX_a. This is followed by the activation of factor X, factor II (prothrombin to form thrombin), and then I to I_a (fibrinogen to fibrin), which

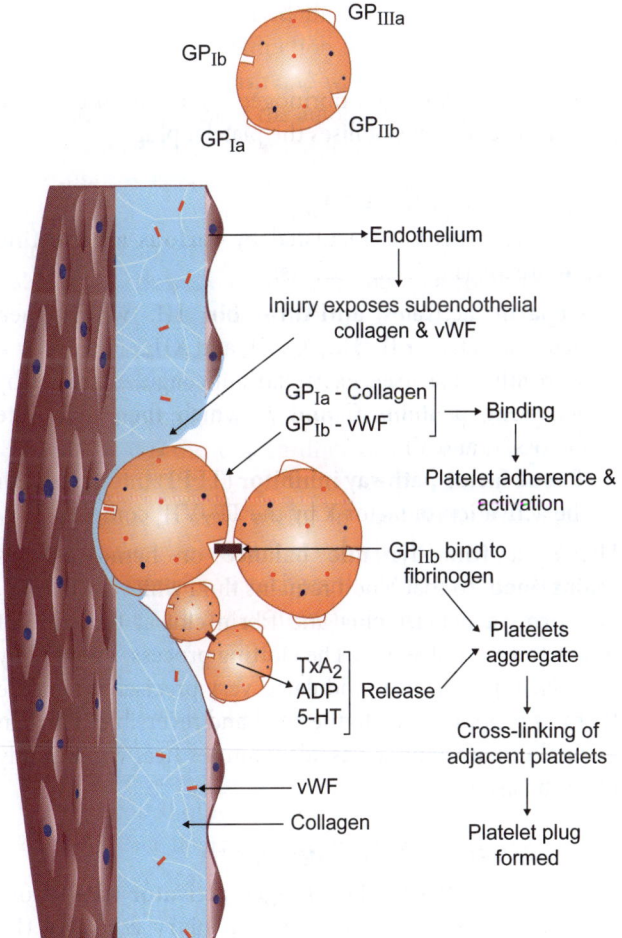

Fig. 37.1 Formation of platelet plug

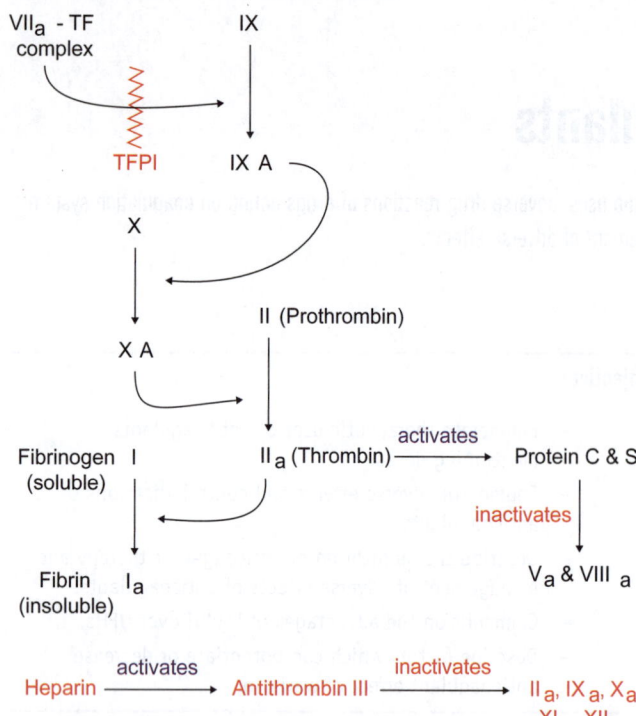

Fig. 37.2 Mechanism of clotting and its regulation

forms a fibrin clot from fibrinogen. Fibrin is an essential part of the clot as it stabilises the platelet plug.

Regulation of Clotting

The above process is regulated by **various anticlotting mechanisms** (Fig. 37.2) such as:

- **Heparin** activates **anti-thrombin III**, which then inactivates factor II_a, IX_a, X_a, XI_a and XII_a.
- **Thrombin IIa** itself exerts an anticoagulant effect by activating **proteins C and S**, which then inactivate factors V_a and VIII_a.
- **Tissue factor pathway inhibitor (TFPI)** interferes with the activation of factor X by the TF–VII_a complex.

Hence, a **fine dynamic balance or hemostasis is maintained**, so that blood remains fluid while circulating, but forms a platelet plug and fibrin clot at the time of injury to arrest bleeding. The clotting process, initiated by vascular injury is also modulated very precisely to ensure that it is proportionate to the need and reversible. Thus, in normal circumstances, vascular injuries heal without any thrombosis.

Fibrinolysis (Fibrin Digestion)

The release of **tissue plasminogen activator (tPA)** from endothelial cells in response to an injury **activates the fibrinolytic system** and limits extension of the thrombus (Fig. 37.3). Tissue plasminogen activator (tPA), as its name indicates, catalyses the activation of plasminogen, (the inactive precursor), to form plasmin. Plasmin then binds to exposed lysines on the fibrin clot and degrades fibrin and fibrinogen, and thus, **clot-specific fibrinolysis** occurs. However, such clot specificity of fibrinolytic activity is **lost at pharmacological levels of tPA**, leading to a systemic fibrinolytic state and risk of bleeding.

Negative regulators of fibrinolysis are:

- **Plasminogen activator inhibitor (PAI),** synthesised and released from endothelial cells in response to injury. It inhibits tPA, and prevents the activation of plasminogen to plasmin.
- α_2-**antiplasmin** circulating in the plasma can rapidly inactivate free plasmin that is not clot-bound.

DISTURBANCES OF HEMOSTATIC MECHANISMS

Breakdown or disturbance of the hemostatic mechanism can cause:

- Suboptimal coagulability resulting in **bleeding disorders.**
- Excessive coagulability resulting in **thrombo-embolic disorders**.

Such an imbalance of hemostatic regulation may occur due to hereditary or acquired defects of the coagulation cascade or may be secondary to infective and malignant diseases. Important disorders of coagulation include:

I. Disseminated intravascular coagulation (DIC)
II. Bleeding disorders
III. Thrombo-embolic disorders

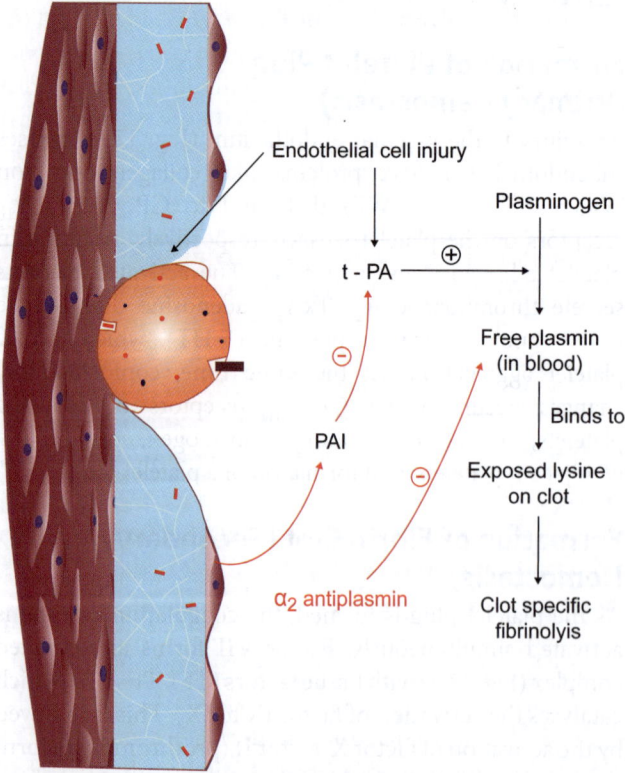

Fig. 37.3 Fibrinolysis and its regulation

I. Disseminated Intravascular Coagulation (DIC)

Pathological activation of coagulation and fibrinolytic systems in patients with massive tissue injury, advanced carcinoma, sepsis and obstetric emergencies, leads to disseminated intravascular coagulation (DIC). It is characterised by **generalised intravascular clotting as well as bleeding**. For treating DIC, the causative disease process should be controlled quickly; otherwise, it may have a fatal outcome.

II. Bleeding Disorders

Formation of the platelet plug (primary hemostasis) and fibrin clot (secondary hemostasis) are two important parts of blood clotting. Defects of either of these two functions present as excessive bleeding.

However, in **defects of formation of platelet plug** (e.g., in platelet function defect and von Willebrand disease) the **bleeding usually occurs from surface sites** like the skin and gums, and excessive menstrual loss. Also, there is an **inciting event** such as an injury or menstruation.

In contrast, in **defects of the coagulation cascade** (e.g., hemophilia and Christmas disease), bleeding usually occurs in **deeper tissues** such as muscles, joints, and retroperitoneal bleeding. Such bleeding usually occurs unpredictably, **without an apparent inciting event.**

Bleeding disorders are managed with fresh whole blood, fresh frozen plasma and coagulants. **Fresh whole blood and fresh frozen plasma** are the most suitable treatment for deficiency of any factor, because these can **provide all** the **factors** and **act almost immediately.**

COAGULANTS

The coagulants used in clinical practice include vitamin K, plasma fractions, fibrinolysis inhibitors, and some local agents called styptics (Flowchart 37.1).

a. Vitamin K

Vitamin K is a fat-soluble vitamin which exists in **two natural forms:**

- Vitamin K_1 (phytonadione) found mainly in green leafy vegetables, cheese.
- Vitamin K_2 (menaquinone) synthesised by bacteria colonised in human intestines.

Synthetic compound is called vitamin K_3 (menadione).

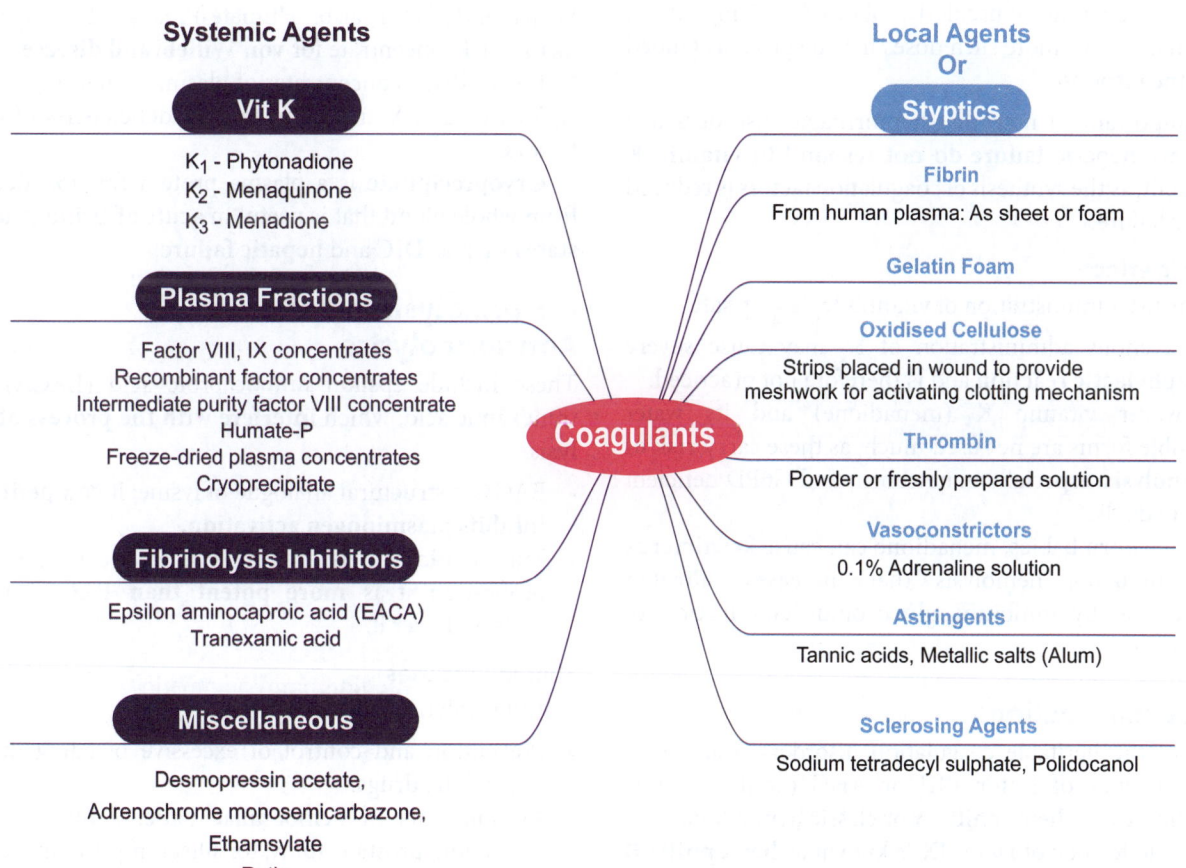

Flowchart 37.1 Coagulants used in clinical practice

Mechanism of action

The vitamin K-dependent γ-carboxylation of glutamate residues of factors II, VII, IX and X in the liver is essential for their participation in coagulation cascade (Fig. 37.4). Vitamin K changes from its hydroquinone to the epoxide form in this reaction.

Therapeutic uses

- **Deficiency of vitamin K**, secondary to malabsorption, liver disease, uremia, obstructive jaundice and prolonged antimicrobial therapy.
  - Vitamin K deficiency manifests as excessive bleeding tendency. Bleeding commonly occurs from the urinary tract, GIT, nose and as subcutaneous ecchymosis. Usually, hematuria is the first feature of vitamin K deficiency.
  - Oral or parenteral **vitamin K_1, 10 mg/day**, is indicated in treatment of bleeding tendencies due to such conditions.
- **Neonates**, especially **premature babies**, have low levels of clotting factors. So, vitamin K_1 (1 mg) is routinely injected intramuscularly routinely, in all newborns, to prevent hemorrhagic disease.
- **Overdose of anticoagulant medications**: Hypoprothrombinemia and bleeding due to overdose of oral anticoagulants is treated with vitamin K_1 10 mg, injected intramuscularly, followed by 5 mg after 4 hours. One or more such doses may be given as guided by the response.

It is important to note that hemorrhagic disorders due to **severe hepatic failure do not respond to vitamin K** treatment, as the synthesis of coagulation factors is reduced in liver failure.

Adverse effects

Oral or IM administration of vitamin K_1 is very safe.

- Intravenous administration of K_1 may cause **severe anaphylactic reaction** and is therefore not practiced.
- However vitamin K_3 (menadione) and its water soluble forms are not used much, as these carry **risk of hemolysis**, especially in newborns and G6PD deficient individuals.
- In newborn babies, menadione can cause **kernicterus** by inducing hemolysis that increases bilirubin load and by inhibiting glucuronide conjugation of bilirubin.

b. Plasma Fractions

Most of the heritable coagulation disorders result from the deficiency of factor VIII or AHG (antihemophilic globulin), called **hemophilia A** or classic hemophilia.

The deficiency of factor IX is known as **hemophilia B** or Christmas disease.

Bleeding tendencies associated with these conditions are treated with concentrated plasma fractions. Factor

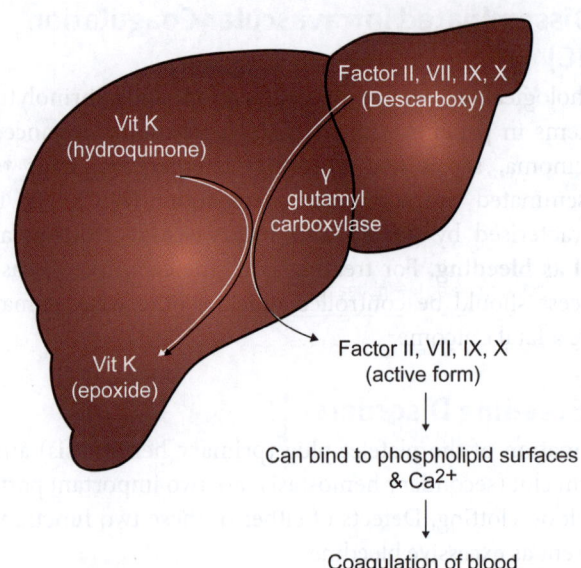

Fig. 37.4 Role of Vitamin K in coagulation

concentrates, which are plasma derived or recombinant (high purity concentrates), constitute the standard treatment for hemophilia.

Intermediate purity factor VIII concentrates have von Willebrand factor also. Humate-P is a FDA-approved factor VIII concentrate for **von Willebrand disease.**

Freeze-dried concentrates of plasma containing factors II, VII, IX and X are useful to treat deficiencies of these factors.

Cryoprecipitate is a plasma protein fraction derived from whole blood that is useful in **acute afibrinogenemia states** such as **DIC** and **hepatic failure**.

c. Fibrinolysis Inhibitors or Antifibrinolytics

These include epsilon-aminocaproic acid (EACA) and tranexamic acid, which **interfere with the process of clot lysis**.

- EACA is structural analogue of lysine; it **competitively inhibits plasminogen activation.**
- Tranexamic acid is an EACA analogue with similar properties; it is **more potent than EACA** and is preferred over it.

Therapeutic uses

Antifibrinolytic drugs are used in:

- Prevention and control of excessive bleeding due to fibrinolytic drugs.
- As adjuvants in hemophiliac patients during tooth extraction, prostatectomy, tonsillectomy, trauma, etc.
- Prevention of re-bleed from peptic ulcers, aneurysms, epistaxis, bleeding from bladder due to radiation/drug-induced cystitis, etc.

- Useful in menorrhagia associated with intrauterine contraceptive devices.

The dosage of tranexamic acid is 1–1.5 g, three times a day, orally. For severe bleeding, 0.5–1 g is given thrice a day by slow intravenous infusion.

Adverse effects of tranexamic acid include nausea, GI upset, nasal stuffiness, myopathy, hypotension and intravascular thrombosis.

d. Styptics or Local Hemostatics

Styptics are agents that help to stop bleeding from an approachable site upon local application. These include:

- **Strips of absorbable materials** such as fibrin, gelatin foam, and oxidised cellulose provide a meshwork that can activate clotting process.
- **Thrombin** is applied as a dry power or freshly prepared solution; it can stop surface bleeding in hemophiliacs.
- Cotton gauze soaked in **vasoconstrictors** such as adrenaline 0.1% solution can be packed in a bleeding tooth socket or nasal cavity in epistaxis.
- Bleeding from gums can be checked by **astringents** like tannic acid and alum.
- **Sclerosing agents** like sodium tetradecyl sulphate and polidocanol are used as local injections to treat varicose veins and hemorrhoids. As these are irritants, they cause local inflammation and fibrosis, which checks the bleeding from these sites.

e. Miscellaneous

- **Desmopressin acetate** can increase the release of factor VIII and von Willebrand factor from the endothelium. It is effective in patients of mild hemophilia A and von Willebrand disease during preparation for minor surgical procedures; it is administered intranasally.
- **Adrenochrome monosemicarbazone** reduces capillary fragility and prevents microvessel bleeding. It is used to **control the oozing of blood** from raw surfaces, wounds, epistaxis, hematuria, etc.
- **Ethamsylate and rutin** were used to prevent and treat capillary bleeding as seen in epistaxis, after tooth extraction, abortion, menorrhagia, and hematuria; however, their efficacy is uncertain.

Clinical problem-based questions and MCQs

1. A 27-year-old primigravida presented with labour pains at 32 weeks of gestation. On examination, cervix was soft, fully effaced, 5 cm dilated. Uterine contractions were good, fetal heart rate was normal and regular. After normal vaginal delivery (NVD) was conducted, injection vitamin K_1 (1 mg) was given intramuscularly to the baby.
   i. Describe the pharmacological basis for injecting vitamin K_1.
   ii. Can vitamin K_3 be used instead of vitamin K_1 in this setting? Justify.
   iii. What are the other indications for use of vitamin K_1?

2. A 49-year-old patient with severe alcoholic liver disease and hepatic failure develops subcutaneous ecchymosis and hematuria. Vitamin K_1 (10 mg) is injected, but there is no improvement in bleeding symptoms.
   i. Explain the cause of bleeding and non-responsiveness to vitamin K therapy in this patient.
   ii. Identify the suitable drug in this case.
      a. Vasoconstrictors   b. Vitamin K_3
      c. Cryoprecipitate   d. Ethamsylate

3. All of the following can occur as adverse effects of Vitamin K, EXCEPT:
   a. Hemolysis   b. GI disturbance
   c. Kernicterus   d. Anaphylaxis

4. A 51-year-old female patient presents with polymenorrhea and menorrhagia. Examination reveals pallor and PR = 90/min. Investigations showed Hb = 8.0 mg/dL. USG abdomen shows multiple small fibromyomas of uterus. Patient is advised surgical treatment at a time convenient to her. Iron 60 mg oral (daily for 15 days) and tranexamic acid (1 g, three times daily, till uterine bleeding stops) are prescribed.
   i. Describe the pharmacological basis for prescribing tranexamic acid.
   ii. What are other indications for use and adverse effects of tranexamic acid?

5. Identify the most suitable agent for controlling surface bleeding in hemophiliacs.
   a. Tetradecyl sulphate   b. Polidocanol
   c. Adrenaline   d. Thrombin

CONCEPT MAP – COAGULANTS

Plasma Fractions

Deficiency of factor VIII: hemophilia A or classic hemophilia.
Deficiency of factor IX: hemophilia B or Christmas disease.

Factor concentrates are high purity concentrates: Plasma derived or recombinant
Intermediate purity factor VIII concentrates that also contain von Willebrand factor.
Humate-P is factor VIII concentrate for von Willebrand disease.
Freeze-dried concentrates of plasma containing factor II, VII, IX and X
Cryoprecipitate is a plasma protein fraction, derived from whole blood useful in acute afibrinogenemia states like DIC, and hepatic failure.

Vitamin K

K_1 (Phytonadione), K_2 (Menaquinone), K_3 (Menadione)

Mechanism
Vit K plays crucial role in γ carboxylation of factors II, VII, IX, X

Uses
- Deficiency of vitamin K, secondary to malabsorption, liver disease, uremia, obstructive jaundice and prolonged antimicrobial therapy.
- To prevent hemorrhagic disease in neonates, especially premature, vitamin K_1 1 mg is given IM.
- Overdose of anticoagulants: IM vit K_1 10 mg, followed by 5 mg after 4 hours.

Adverse effects
Oral or IM vitamin K_1 is very safe.
- Risk of severe anaphylactic reaction on IV use.
- Risk of hemolysis, kernicterus with water-soluble vitamin K_3 especially in newborns and G6PD deficiency.

Antifibrinolytics

Epsilon-aminocaproic acid (EACA) competitively inhibits plasminogen activation.
Tranexamic acid more potent EACA analogue, with similar properties. Preferred over EACA.

Therapeutic Uses
Prevention and control of excess bleeding due to fibrinolytic drugs.
As adjuvants in hemophiliac patients undergoing tooth extraction, prostatectomy, tonsillectomy, trauma.
For preventing re-bleed from peptic ulcers, aneurysms, epistaxis, bleeding from bladder due to radiation or drug-induced cystitis.
Menorrhagia associated with intra-uterine contraceptive devices.

Adverse effects
Nausea, GI upset, nasal stuffiness, myopathy, hypotension and intravascular thrombosis

COAGULANTS

Styptics or Local Hemostatics

Used to stop bleeding from an approachable site on local application.

Strips of absorbable materials like fibrin, gelatin foam, oxidised cellulose provide a meshwork that activates clotting process.
Thrombin dry powder or freshly prepared solution used in hemophiliacs to stop surface bleeding
Vasoconstrictors like adrenaline 0.1% solution soaked cotton gauze can be packed in bleeding tooth socket or nasal cavity in epistaxis.
Astringents like tannic acid for bleeding from gums.
Sclerosing agents like sodium tetradecyl sulphate, polidocanol are used as local injections in varicose veins, hemorrhoids to check bleeding from these sites due to local irritant action.

Miscellaneous

Desmopressin acetate
Increases release of factor VIII and vWF from endothelium.
Used in mild hemophilia & von Willebrand disease by intranasal route for preparation of minor surgical procedures.

Adrenochrome monosemicarbazone
Prevents microvessel bleeding by reducing capillary fragility.
Used to control oozing of blood from raw surfaces, wounds, epistaxis, hematuria etc.

Ethamsylate, Rutin were used to prevent and treat capillary bleeding as in epistaxis, after tooth extraction, abortion, menorrhagia, and hematuria, but their efficacy is uncertain.

III. Thrombo-Embolic Disorders

A fine dynamic balance between various clotting and anticlotting mechanisms ensures that blood remains fluid and circulates through blood vessels, endlessly, throughout life. However, whenever there is an injury, blood loss is checked by formation of a platelet plug and fibrin clot. Disturbances in this balance may result in bleeding or thrombotic disorders.

Thrombosis is the pathological formation of a platelet plug within the vasculature, in absence of bleeding. Breaking away of the thrombus results in the formation of **emboli** that may be carried with the circulation, get lodged in distant organs and are usually associated with disastrous outcomes.

Risk factors for thrombo-embolic disorders

Virchow's triad is a triad of factors that predisposes an individual to the development of thrombi. These are:
- Injury to vascular endothelium, e.g., by the rupture of atheromatous plaque.
- Altered blood flow, as seen in leg veins of patients with prolonged immobilisation, atrial flutter.
- Hypercoagulability of blood, as seen in patients on oral contraceptive pills (OCPs) or during late pregnancy.

Conditions that predispose an individual to venous thrombosis include:
- **Inherited disorders** with qualitative or quantitative deficiency of the physiological anticoagulant system (e.g., antithrombin III, protein C, protein S), or elevated levels of clotting factors or their cofactors.
- **Acquired factors**: The risk of venous thrombosis is higher in patients with atrial fibrillation, mechanical heart valves, prolonged immobilisation due to any cause, pregnancy or OCP use, and malignant diseases. Another important risk factor for deep vein thrombosis is antiphospholipid antibody syndrome (APS) or APLA syndrome.

Types of thrombi

Based on vessels involved, thrombosis can be mainly classified into arterial and venous thrombosis.

Arterial thrombi mainly consist of platelets and leukocytes in a fibrin mesh; these are called **white thrombi**. They interrupt blood flow resulting in **ischemia or infarction of tissues distal to the thrombus,** such as stroke, angina, and MI.

In contrast, **venous thrombi** have a small **white head and jelly-like red tail**. While the composition of the white head is the same as an arterial thrombus, the red tail contains blood cells trapped in the diffuse fibrin meshwork. A part of the thrombus can breakdown (embolus) and reach distant sites with catastrophic results (Fig. 37.5).

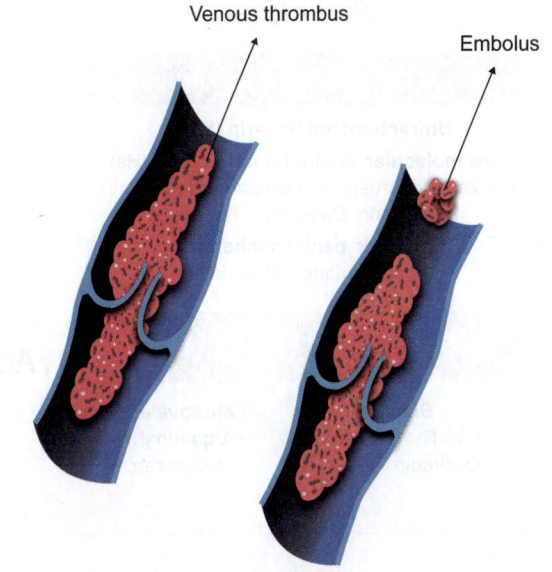

Fig. 37.5 Venous thrombo-embolism

The **three main groups of drugs** useful in diseases associated with excessive clotting of blood within vessels are:
1. Antiplatelet drugs
2. Fibrinolytic drugs
3. Anticoagulant drugs

Platelet activation is considered to be an essential step in arterial thrombosis. Therefore, **drugs that inhibit** platelet aggregation, such as aspirin, clopidogrel and ticlopidine, are the mainstay of treatment in conditions secondary to arterial thrombosis.

Fibrinolytic drugs like streptokinase, anistreplase, and alteplase are useful **in acute situations** associated with thrombo-embolism such as pulmonary embolism, superior vena cava syndrome, and ascending thrombophlebitis of ileofemoral vein.

As venous thrombi are associated with the hypercoagulable state and are fibrin rich, the mainstay of treatment in deep vein thrombosis and thrombo-embolic diseases is **anticoagulant drugs** such as heparin (unfractionated/LMWH) and warfarin.

ANTICOAGULANTS

Anticoagulants are classified based on their mechanism of action and route of administration as shown in Flowchart 37.2. Based on their mechanism of action, anticoagulant drugs can be indirect thrombin inhibitors (IDTIs), direct thrombin inhibitors (DTIs), direct factor X_a inhibitors, and vitamin K antagonists. All the IDTIs are administered parenterally, whereas all vitamin K

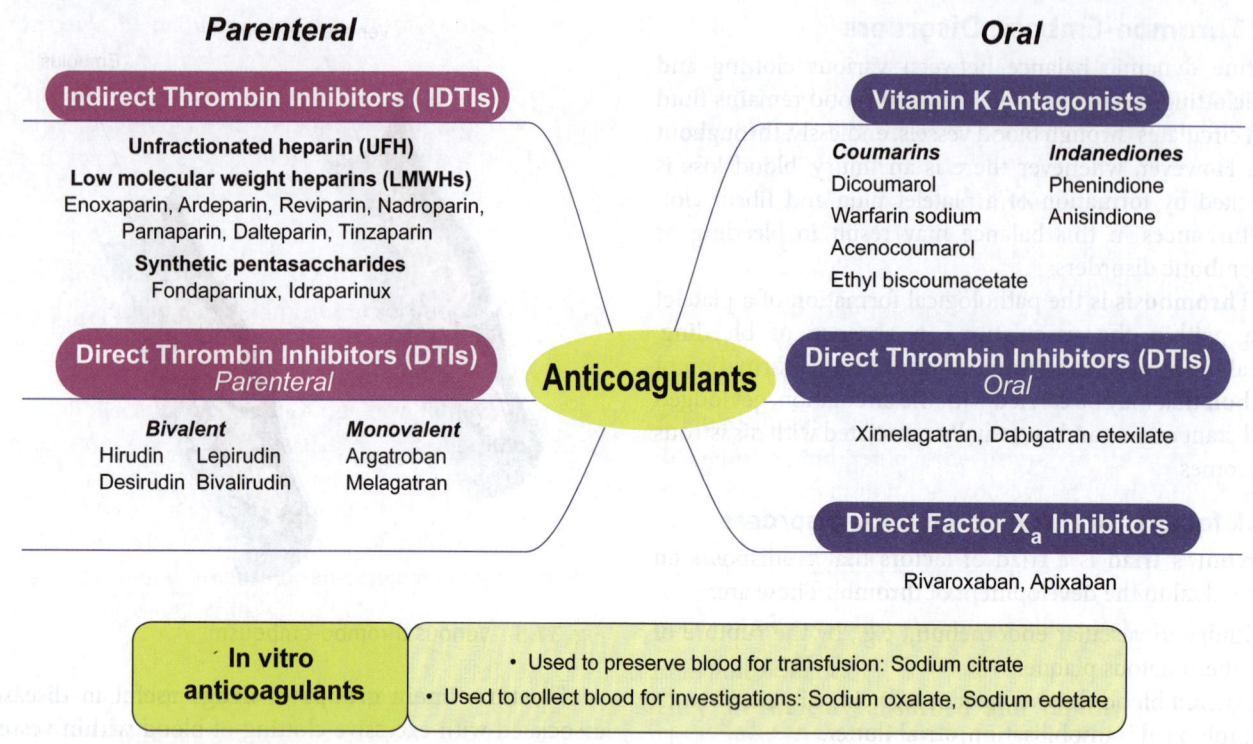

Flowchart 37.2 Classification of anticoagulant drugs

antagonists and direct X_a inhibitors are given orally. DTIs are used both orally and parenterally.

INDIRECT THROMBIN INHIBITORS (IDTIS)

These include unfractionated heparin (UFH), low molecular-weight heparins (LMWHs) and synthetic pentasaccharides such as fondaparinux and idraparinux.

a. Heparin

Mechanism of anticoagulant action: Heparin exerts its anticoagulant action indirectly through antithrombin III (AT_{III}). AT_{III} is a suicide inhibitor of protease clotting factors, because it is itself a substrate for these factors. AT_{III} forms **stable equimolar complexes with clotting factors** (II_a, X_a and IX_a) and interferes with coagulation; however, the rate of this reaction is very slow.

Heparin **enhances the rate** of this reaction **1000-fold**. A specific pentasaccharide sequence present in heparin molecules causes a conformational change in AT_{III}, and increases its interaction with clotting factors, leading to inactivation of factors II_a, X_a, and IX_a. Thus, heparin serves as a **cofactor for the AT_{III}–clotting factors reaction**, and is released intact once the AT_{III}–clotting factor complex is formed. The same effect is produced by UFH, LMWH and fondaparinux.

In addition, unfractionated heparin **provides a scaffold** for the interaction of AT_{III} and factors X_a and II_a (Fig. 37.6). This effect is not shown by LMWHs and fondaparinux.

As a result, UFH inhibits factors X_a, II_a and also IX_a to some extent; LMWHs inhibit factor X_a but have little effect on factor II_a.

b. Low Molecular-Weight Heparins (LMWHs)

These include drugs like enoxaparin, ardeparin, reviparin, nadroparin, parnaparin, dalteparin and tinzaparin.

Mechanism of action: LMWHs induce conformational changes in AT_{III} and catalyse its binding to factor X_a. They also increase binding to factor II_a but have no scaffolding effect as the molecule is smaller than UFH. Thus, the inhibitory effect on thrombin (II_a) is lesser than that of UFH (Fig. 37.7).

Comparison of LMWHs and UFH

Advantages

- LMWHs have little inhibitory effect on factor II_a (thrombin). Therefore, while LMWHs are **equi-efficacious** as UFH, the adverse effects in the form of **bleeding tendencies are less**.
- Because LMWHs have lesser effect on aPTT (activated partial thromboplastin time) and whole blood clotting time than UFH, **laboratory monitoring of aPTT is not required** while prescribing LMWHs (except in patients with renal insufficiency, obesity and in pregnant women).
- The bioavailability of UFH given by subcutaneous route is inconsistent, because heparin is a highly ionised molecule with high molecular weight (10000–

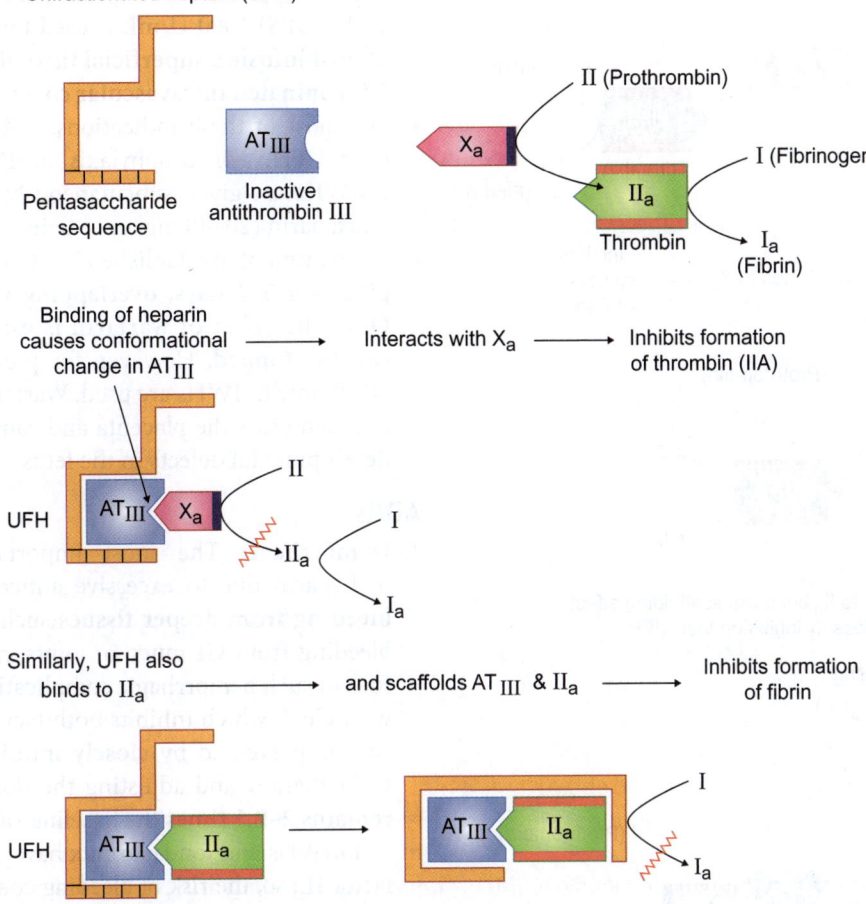

Fig. 37.6 Mechanism of action of unfractionated heparin (UFH)

20000 Da). Its average half-life is 1 hour at dose < 100 U/kg; this increases up to 4 hour at doses > 100 U/kg due to dose-dependent kinetics of elimination. UFH is given 8–12 hourly.

In contrast, LMWHs have molecular weight varying from 3000–7000 Da and their **bioavailability after subcutaneous administration is higher** (100%) when compared to UFH (90%). Their **half-life is longer** (17 hours) in comparison to that of UFH; **once or twice daily dosing** is sufficient. Therefore, LMWHs have better bioavailability and a more convenient dosing regimen than UFH.

- After long-term use, the risk of adverse effects such as **osteoporosis, thrombocytopenia and hemorrhagic complications is lower** for LMWHs than for UFH.

Disadvantages
- LMWHs are not very effective in the prevention of catheter thrombosis. So, in patients with epidural catheters and those selected **for cardiopulmonary bypass surgery, UFH is preferred** over LMWHs.
- LMWHs are not given to patients undergoing concomitant thrombolysis, because of their longer half-life and lack of specific antidote.
- LMWHs are mainly eliminated through the renal route. So, these are **not suitable for patients with severe chronic renal failure,** with creatinine clearance < 30 mL/min. UFH is preferred in these cases.
- UFH is preferred in patients with venous thromboembolism, who are at greater risk of bleeding (such as post-operative cases).

c. Fondaparinux

It is a synthetic drug containing the **specific pentasaccharide of heparin that has a high affinity for binding to AT_{III}** and causes an irreversible conformational change in it. It inactivates factor X_a but has no effect on factor II_a (Fig. 37.7). Its subcutaneous **bioavailability is 100%** and the effect lasts longer (half-life = 17 hour). The risk of **bleeding, thrombocytopenia and osteoporosis is also much lower** than that for UFH and LMWHs.

The dose for prophylaxis of DVT is 2.5 mg (S/C, once daily), while dose for treatment of DVT is larger, i.e., 5–10 mg. However, like LMWHs, fondaparinux is also eliminated unchanged by the renal route; so, it should not be given to patients with renal failure.

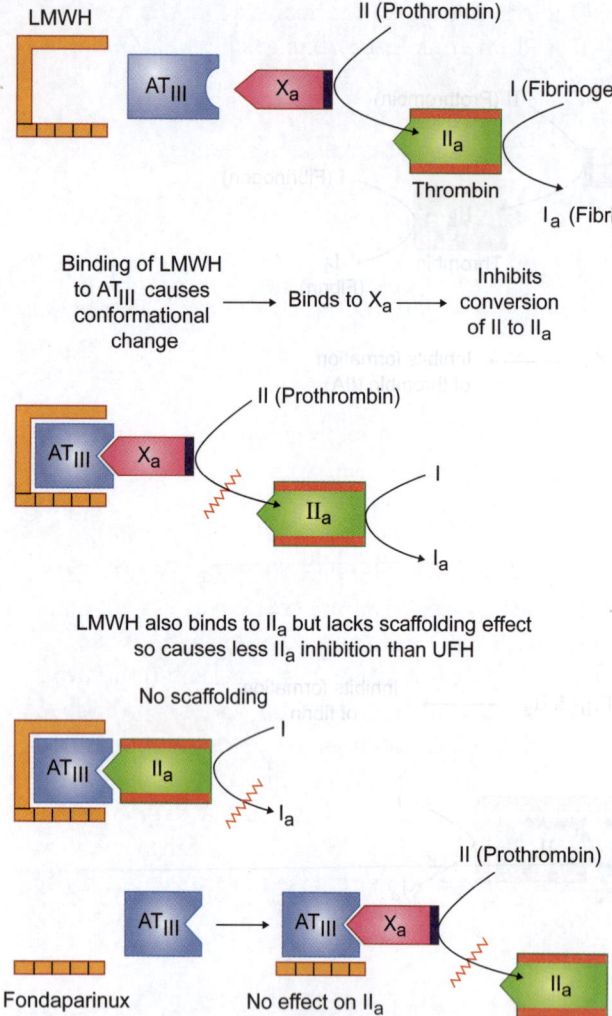

Fig. 37.7 Mechanism of action of low molecular weight heparins (LMWHs) and fondaparinux

Idraparinux is similar to fondaparinux, but it has a longer half-life of 5–6 days.

Therapeutic uses of IDTIs or heparin

- Heparin is the mainstay of **prophylaxis and treatment of deep vein thrombosis** (DVT) and **pulmonary embolism** (PE) in patients with prolonged immobilisation, undergoing surgery or other high-risk patients.
- For patients having unstable angina and myocardial infarction, especially **STEMI and bundle branch block**, the outcome is best when heparin therapy is started within 6 hours of onset of MI.
- Used for maintaining **patency of canulas or shunts in patients on dialysis**.
- A plasma concentration of 0.3–0.7 U/mL of UFH (by anti-X_a units) is sufficient to prevent pulmonary embolism in patients suffering from DVT. It corresponds to an **aPTT value** that is **2–3 times the baseline** value.
- Topical application of quick penetrating solution of UFH (QPS) 1000 U/mL is used for improving healing of **post infusion superficial thrombophlebitis**.
- **Disseminated intravascular coagulation**.
- For most of these indications, LMWHs are preferred over UFH. For prophylaxis of DVT, low doses of LMWHs are given subcutaneously, e.g., subcutaneous enoxaparin (20–40 mg, once daily).
- For treatment of established DVT, initially **LMWHs are given for 5–7 days, overlapping with oral warfarin. Once the effect of warfarin is established, heparins can be stopped**. However, for pregnant women with DVT, only LMWHs are used. Warfarin is not combined as it can cross the placenta and cause hemorrhage and developmental defects in the fetus.

ADRs

1. **Hemorrhage:** The most important adverse effect of heparin due to excessive anticoagulant activity is **bleeding from deeper tissues** such as hematuria, and bleeding from GI mucosa, joints, muscles, and brain. Risk of such hemorrhagic complications is much higher with UFH, which inhibits both factors X_a and II_a. This can be prevented by **closely monitoring** patients on UFH therapy and adjusting the dose such that **aPTT remains 2–2.5 times** the baseline values.

   LMWHs and fondaparinux have negligible effects on factor II_a; so, the risk of bleeding complications is much lower and monitoring of aPTT or clotting time is not required (except in patients with renal insufficiency, obesity and during pregnancy).

2. **Heparin-induced thrombocytopenia** (HIT): The platelet count falls below 1 lakh/μL, usually 5–10 days after starting heparin therapy. Mild transient **thrombocytopenia** is caused by heparin because of platelet aggregation, which can cause serious thrombo-embolic complications. This affects the veins more commonly, but arteries may also be involved. In rare instances, antibodies directed against the platelet–heparin complex are responsible for severe thrombocytopenia.

   - **Management:** For all patients on heparin therapy, the **blood platelets count should be monitored frequently**. If the platelet count is < 1 lakh/μL heparin therapy is replaced by fondaparinux or DTIs. Lepirudin is safe in hepatic failure and argatroban in renal failure. When the platelet count recovers and reaches 1 lakh/μL, DTIs are discontinued; warfarin is started and should be continued for at least 30 days.
   - Danaparoid is also useful in patients with heparin-induced thrombocytopenia (HIT). It consists of heparan sulphate (a low-sulfated glycosaminoglycan) along with dermatan sulphate and chondroitin sulphate.

3. Because heparin is obtained from porcine intestinal mucosa or bovine lung tissue, **hypersensitivity reactions** such as rashes, urticaria, rigors, and anaphylactic reactions may occur.
4. Heparins can cause **reversible alopecia, osteoporosis and raised hepatic enzymes** upon prolonged use.

Contraindications

Heparins are contraindicated in:

- Patients with **bleeding tendencies and active bleeding** such as hemophilia, intracranial hemorrhage, severe hypertension, ulcerative gastrointestinal lesions (bleeding peptic ulcer, hemorrhoids, ulcerative colitis), and threatened abortion.
- Advanced **malignant diseases**, because of the risk of bleeding in necrosed tumour tissue.
- **Active tuberculosis**, as it can cause hemoptysis, i.e., blood in sputum.
- **Alcoholic liver disease** (ALD), cirrhosis, **advanced hepatic or renal failure**, etc.; in these conditions, its elimination is decreased, increasing the risk of hemorrhagic complications.
- Patients with deficient platelet function such as **thrombocytopenia, previous history of HIT, purpura, and patients on antiplatelet drug therapy** (e.g., aspirin and clopidogrel).
- In subacute bacterial endocarditis (**SABE**), heparin use is associated with the risk of embolisation.
- Heparin should be avoided in **postoperative patients**, especially after ocular surgery, neurosurgery or in patients selected for lumbar puncture.
- **Pregnancy:** Although heparin is a large molecule and does not cross the placental barrier, it may cause hemorrhagic complications. It should be **avoided in pregnancy as far as possible**, but may be used if there is an absolute indication.

The effect of heparin can be rapidly antagonised by administering 1 mg of protamine sulphate I/V for every 100 units of heparin. Protamine sulphate is a strongly basic protein obtained from fish sperm. The effect of LMWHs is only partially reversed and fondaparinux is not antagonised by protamine. Adverse effects of protamine are due to its histamine releasing action, leading to vasodilatation, flushing, dyspnea, hypotension, etc.

2. DIRECT THROMBIN INHIBITORS (DTIs)

Direct thrombin inhibitors (DTIs) can be categorised into **parenteral and oral drugs**. The action of these drugs is independent of ATIII activity (unlike heparin). They are classified into bivalent or monovalent types based on how they bind to thrombin (Flowchart 37.2).

Bivalent DTIs

Parenteral DTI drugs, which exert action by binding to both catalytic and substrate recognition sites of thrombin (II_a) are called **bivalent DTIs**, e.g., hirudin, bivalirudin, lepirudin and desirudin.

Hirudin is a polypeptide obtained from leech saliva, while **bivalirudin** is its synthetic analogue. **Lepirudin** and **desirudin** are the recombinant forms of hirudin.

Mechanism of action: Bivalent DTIs bind firmly to both the **substrate recognition and catalytic sites of thrombin** and **inhibit its action directly** (Fig. 37.8) without any role of AT_{III} activity. The activity of **clot-bound as well as circulating thrombin is inhibited** by these drugs.

Lepirudin is **approved by FDA for 'heparin-induced thrombocytopenia'** (HIT) as it does not inhibit platelet function. It is excreted by renal route, and caution should be observed in patients with renal function impairment. Antibodies formed against the lepirudin–thrombin complex may cause **severe anaphylactic reaction** on re-exposure.

Bivalirudin, a synthetic analogue of hirudin, has same mechanism of anticoagulant action, albeit with **quick onset and short duration** of action. It gets metabolised by proteolysis and excreted by the kidney. While it **inhibits thrombin-mediated platelet aggregation**, there is **no risk of thrombocytopenia** (unlike heparins). It is FDA-approved for **STEMI** patients undergoing PCI (percutaneous coronary intervention), **unstable angina and NSTEMI**, when early intervention is needed. Dose is 0.75 mg/kg body weight (IV bolus dose), followed by 1.75 mg/kg/hour infusion for up to 4 hours after PCI. Adverse

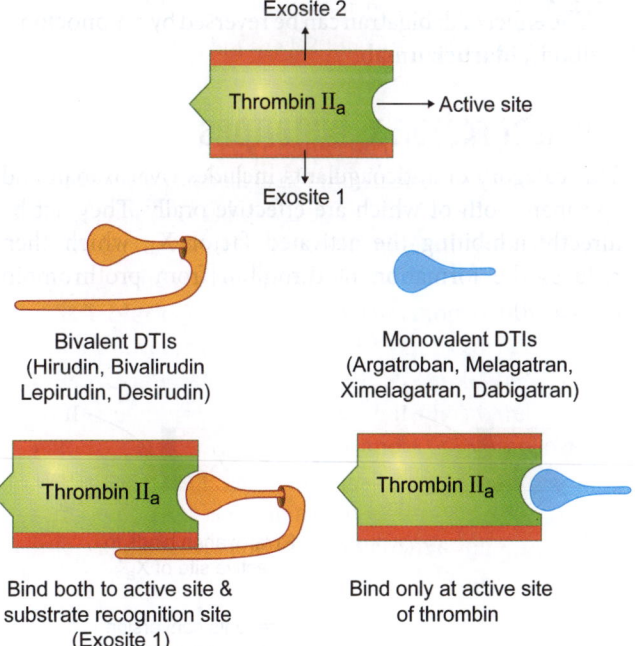

Fig. 37.8 Mechanism of action of direct thrombin inhibitors

effects include risk of bleeding, back ache, headache and hypotension.

Monovalent DTIs

Monovalent DTIs such as argatroban and melagatran inhibit thrombin by binding to its catalytic site alone (Fig. 37.8).

Argatroban has a rapid onset and short duration of action as it is rapidly metabolised and cleared by the liver. It is also **approved by FDA for HIT** patients who require coronary angioplasty and is preferred over lepirudin in patients with renal function impairment. It is given as 350 mg/kg bolus dose followed by 25 mg/kg/min infusion; its effect is monitored by aPPT.

Melagatran is another another monovalent DTI used intravenously.

Oral DTIs

Ximelagatran is a prodrug of melagatran; it is **not used now** because of reports of **hepatotoxicity**.

Dabigatran etexilate is also a **prodrug** which gets hydrolysed to release dabigatran; that has a direct thrombin inhibiting effect by **binding at the catalytic site of thrombin**. Its action starts within 2 hours and lasts for 24 hours. The advantages include oral administration and consistent anticoagulant effect. Moreover, lab monitoring of aPTT is not required. It is approved for the prevention of venous thrombo-embolism after hip/knee replacement and atrial fibrillation in a dose of 110 mg, once a day.

ADRs include the risk of hemorrhagic complications, though it is much lower than for heparin and warfarin. Dyspepsia and other GIT adverse effects may also occur.

The effect of dabigatran can be reversed by a monoclonal antibody, **idarucizumab**.

3. DIRECT FACTOR X_a INHIBITORS

This category of anticoagulants includes rivaroxaban and apixaban, both of which are effective orally. They act by directly inhibiting the activated factor X_a, which then reduces the formation of thrombin from prothrombin (Fig. 37.9).

The anticoagulant action of **rivaroxaban** develops within 3–4 hours of intake, and lasts for 24 hours.

- It is used in **joint replacement (hip/knee) surgery to prevent venous thrombo-embolism (VTE)**: 10 mg, given 6–10 hours before surgery and continued as 10 mg, once daily, for about 2 weeks after knee replacement and 5 weeks after hip replacement surgery.
- It is also used in **atrial fibrillation** for prevention of stroke.
- Treatment of DVT and pulmonary embolism: Dose is 15 mg, twice a day, for 3 weeks and then 20 mg once daily.
- It can be used along with antiplatelet drugs like low-dose aspirin or clopidogrel for **prophylaxis in acute coronary syndrome**.

Adverse effects include nausea, fall in BP, tachycardia, edema and bleeding tendencies; however, routine monitoring of PT or aPTT is not required.

Apixaban is similar to rivaroxaban and has same indications for use; the risk of bleeding is lower with apixaban. It is useful for prophylaxis of VTE after joint replacement (2.5 mg twice daily), prophylaxis of stroke in AF (5 mg twice daily) and treatment of DVT and PE (10 mg twice a day for first 7 days, followed by 5 mg twice a day).

Direct factor X_a inhibitors have an **advantage over warfarin** as:

- They do not have a lag period and the effect appears within 3–4 hours of administration.
- Duration of action is also short (24 hours).
- No need to monitor PT or aPTT.
- Equally efficacious as warfarin.
- Risk of bleeding is much lower than that for warfarin.
- Risk of drug–drug interactions (DDIs) is also lower than that for warfarin.

Clinical problem-based questions and MCQs

6. All of the following are used as in vitro anticoagulants, EXCEPT:
    a. Sodium carbonate
    b. Sodium citrate
    c. Sodium oxalate
    d. Sodium edetate

7. Identify the anticoagulant that has action independent of AT_{III} activity.
    a. Fondaparinux
    b. Argatroban
    c. Nadroparin
    d. Heparin

8. i. In which of the following conditions is heparin contraindicated?
    a. Post-infusion superficial thrombophlebitis.
    b. Disseminated intravascular coagulation.
    c. Patient receiving antiplatelet drugs
    d. Patient receiving oral anticoagulants
   ii. Enumerate all the contraindications for heparin use.

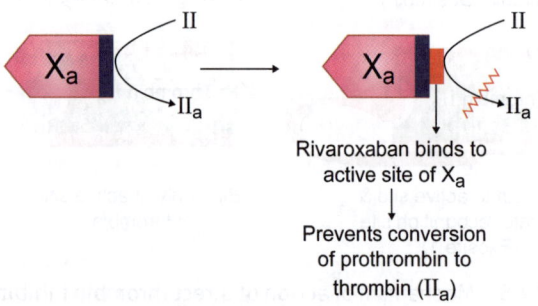

Fig. 37.9 Mechanism of action of rivaroxaban

9. In current clinical practice, LMWHs are preferred over UFH as they have many advantages.
   i. Which of the following is not an advantage of LMWHs?
      a. Better bioavailability after subcutaneous administration
      b. Safety in renal failure
      c. Lower risk of osteoporosis
      d. No need for laboratory monitoring
   ii. Enumerate the advantages and disadvantages of LMWHs.
   iii. Enumerate the therapeutic uses and ADRs of heparins.

10. A DVT patient receiving heparin is being monitored regularly for aPTT and platelet count. At a follow-up visit, aPTT is double the baseline value, but platelet counts are reduced.
    i. Explain the cause of heparin-induced thrombocytopenia (HIT).
    ii. Which of the following drugs is approved for HIT
       a. Low dose aspirin   b. Tranexamic acid
       c. Lepirudin   d. Clopidogrel
    iii. Describe the mechanism of action of the selected drug.

11. Identify the DTI given by oral route
    a. Ximelagatran   b. Lepirudin
    c. Argatroban   d. Melagatran

12. i. Which of the following group of drugs is preferred for prophylaxis of DVT?
       a. Fibrinolytics   b. Antifibrinolytics
       c. Anticoagulants   d. Antiplatelet drugs
    ii. Justify your choice.

13. i. Which of the following drug groups is preferred in treatment of arterial thrombosis and why?
       a. Fibrinolytics   b. Antifibrinolytics
       c. Anticoagulants   d. Antiplatelet drugs
    ii. Justify your choice with the pharmacological reason.

14. i. Identify a drug that causes direct factor X_a inhibition.
       a. Argatroban   b. Apixaban
       c. Ximelagatran   d. Fondaparinux
    ii. Enumerate the advantages of direct factor X_a inhibitors over warfarin.

VITAMIN K ANTAGONISTS

This category consists of warfarin-like drugs, conventionally called coumarins. The drugs in this group include dicoumarol, warfarin sodium, acenocoumarol and ethyl biscoumacetate.

Mechanism of action

Coumarins exert their anticoagulant action by interfering with the **synthesis of vitamin K-dependent clotting factors** in the liver. Hydroquinone is the active form of vitamin K; it acts as a cofactor for the enzyme γ-glutamyl carboxylase, and enables γ carboxylation of the glutamate residues of factors II, VII, IX, and X. Only after γ carboxylation are these factors capable of binding to Ca^{2+} and phospholipid surfaces during coagulation (Fig. 37.10).

During this reaction, the hydroquinone form of vitamin K changes into the epoxide form. Regeneration of the active hydroquinone form of vitamin K requires the catalytic activity of the **vitamin K epoxide reductase (VKOR)** enzyme.

Coumarin anticoagulants act by inhibiting this enzyme, which prevents formation of the active form of vitamin K. Thus, γ carboxylation of glutamate residues of factor II, VII, IX and X is interfered with; warfarin inhibits synthesis of clotting factors within **2–4 hours** of administration.

However, before the anticoagulant effect manifests, the coagulation factors already present in the body must be eliminated. The levels of factor VII fall first, followed by

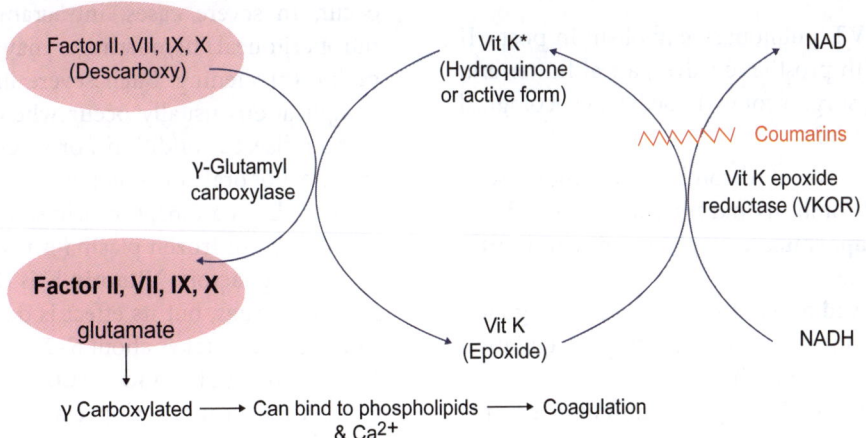

Fig. 37.10 Mechanism of action of coumarins. Coumarins inhibit VKOR → interferes with regeneration of hydroquinone form of vitamin K → interfere with → γ-carboxylation of clotting factors II, VII, IX, and X → anticoagulant effect.

levels of factors IX, X and II. Thus, the **anticoagulant effect of coumarin drugs is delayed** and develops gradually over 1–3 days, implying that the main role of these drugs is in maintenance anticoagulant therapy.

In addition to clotting factors, coumarin anticoagulants **inhibit the** γ carboxylation of anticoagulant **proteins (C and S) and osteocalcin** as well. The half-life of protein C is 8 hours, shorter than that of most clotting factors. Therefore, levels of protein C decline first; this results in a hypercoagulable state and dermal vascular necrosis at the beginning of warfarin therapy. To avoid such early onset adverse effects, indirect-acting thrombin inhibitors (IDTIs) are combined at the beginning of warfarin therapy. Later on, the effects of inhibition of proteins C and S are overshadowed by the inhibition of clotting factors. Inhibition of osteocalcin synthesis may suppress new bone formation.

- **Warfarin** is used as a racemic mixture of dextro and levorotatory enantiomers.
- Warfarin is completely and rapidly absorbed after oral administration and is highly plasma protein bound. Metabolism occurs in the liver by oxidation/side-chain reduction followed by glucuronide conjugation, and excretion occurs via renal route. Its half-life is 36–48 h.
- **Dicoumarol** is not preferred because of its slow unpredictable absorption and frequent gastrointestinal adverse effects.
- **Acenocoumarol** acts **more rapidly** than warfarin.
- **Ethyl biscoumacetate** also has **rapid onset, short-lasting** action. These may be **used to initiate anticoagulant** therapy.

The dosage of coumarin anticoagulants is individualised to achieve the international normalised ratio (INR), which varies from 2–3.5 based on the indication for use.

Therapeutic uses

Coumarin anticoagulants are used for:

- Maintenance treatment in DVT and pulmonary embolism.
- Prophylaxis of DVT, pulmonary embolism in post MI cases, patients with prosthetic valves, atrial flutter and those undergoing surgery for orthopedic, gynecological and cardiac conditions.

In patients at high risk of thrombosis or those with established venous thrombosis, **parenteral anticoagulants like LMWHs/fondaparinux are given concomitantly with warfarin** because:

- Warfarin has **delayed onset** of action; the anticoagulant effect manifests only after the existing coagulation factors are eliminated from the body.
- Warfarin **monotherapy has a procoagulant effect** due to decrease in levels of proteins C and S (which are endogenous anticoagulants). This can be counteracted by combining a parenteral anticoagulant at initiation of warfarin therapy, which is continued for at least 2–5 days after achieving the target INR. Then, warfarin alone is continued for at least 3–6 months, depending on the clinical condition.

Warfarin is usually started at 5–10 mg dose and adjusted as required to obtain 25% of normal prothrombin activity.

Warfarin therapy is monitored by measuring the prothrombin time (PT). Testing for PT involves adding a reagent, thromboplastin (that contains TF, Ca^{2+} and phospholipids), to citrated plasma.

$$\text{International normalised ratio (INR)} = \left(\frac{\text{Patient PT}}{\text{PT of normal pooled sample}}\right)^{ISI}$$

ISI is the International Sensitivity Index that serves to relate the measured PT to the WHO reference standard thromboplastin. For the instruments and reagents in current use, ISI ≈ 1. Thus, the INR is an approximate ratio of the patient's PT to the mean normal PT of pooled sample. For prophylaxis and treatment of thrombotic diseases, INR = 2–3 is recommended. However, in recurrent cases, and patients with MI and prosthetic valves, INR between 3–3.5 is recommended.

During anticoagulant therapy, the prothrombin time–international normalised ratio (PT–INR) should be checked at frequency given below:

- Daily, while it is not in target range or for the first five days.
- Then, 3 times every week for 2 weeks.
- Once the patient is stable, the INR should be monitored every 3–4 weeks.

ADRs

- The most common adverse effect of warfarin is the extension of its pharmacological action to cause **bleeding**. Epistaxis, ecchymosis, hematuria, etc. may occur. In severe cases, intracranial/ gastrointestinal/ retroperitoneal hemorrhage may occur, which can be life threatening. Such severe internal hemorrhagic complications usually occur **when INR exceeds 4**, in certain disease conditions, or when drugs potentiating the effect of oral anticoagulants are coadministered.

  In such situations, warfarin should be stopped; fresh blood or fresh frozen plasma is transfused to replenish the clotting factors. **Vitamin K is the specific antidote** for these drugs, but its effect is delayed as synthesis of clotting factors takes about 6–24 hours.

- **Gastrointestinal and cutaneous side effects:** Coumarins cause alopecia, dermatitis and GI disturbances such as anorexia, nausea and diarrhea.
  - Acenocoumarol may cause oral ulcerations and urticaria.

- Bishydroxycoumarin can also cause GI intolerance.
- Ethyl biscoumacetate can cause bad taste and alopecia.
- Warfarin and acenocoumarol are better tolerated than other coumarins.
- Due to reduced activity of protein C, **cutaneous necrosis** may occur during the first week of treatment with coumarins. In rare cases, frank infarction of fatty tissues, breast, intestines or extremities may occur.
- In rare cases, it may cause **osteoporosis, purple toe syndrome, leukopenia**, etc.
- Warfarin can easily cross the placental barrier resulting in hemorrhagic disorder and impairment of synthesis of proteins that are crucial for the formation of bones and cartilages. **Fetal warfarin syndrome or DiSalvo syndrome** (named after the scientist who first described it in 1966) is characterised by growth retardation, stippled epiphysis and hypoplasia of bones of nose/eye socket/hands, choanal atresia, short neck, laryngeal abnormalities and airway obstruction. Therefore, warfarin is contraindicated during pregnancy.
- However, warfarin can be used safely in lactating women, as it is not secreted in breast milk.

Interactions

Many conditions can enhance/decrease the effect of coumarin anticoagulants. Therefore, therapy should be monitored by repeated PT measurements.

Factors that **enhance** the effect of coumarins:

- Conditions in which **vitamin K supply to liver is reduced** such as malnutrition, debilitating diseases, malabsorption syndrome and prolonged therapy with broad spectrum antibiotics.
- Conditions in which **synthesis of clotting factors is reduced**, e.g., chronic alcoholism and hepatic function impairment.
- Conditions in which **clotting factors are degraded** quickly, e.g., hyperthyroidism.
- Conditions in which the **PPB of drug is reduced**, such as hypoproteinemia.
- Some **drugs** augment the effect of coumarins:
  - Cephalosporins (cefoperazone/ceftriaxone) cause hypoprothrombinemia and have additive effect with coumarins.
  - The antiplatelet action of aspirin may cause GI bleeding in patients on coumarin therapy.
  - Several drugs can displace warfarin from its plasma protein binding site, e.g., sulphonamides, phenytoin, and indomethacin, resulting in its toxic effects.
  - Enzyme inhibitors like erythromycin, chloramphenicol and metronidazole inhibit the hepatic metabolism of warfarin.
  - Tolbutamide and phenytoin also inhibit warfarin metabolism.
  - Absorption of vitamin K is reduced by liquid paraffin.
  - Broad spectrum antimicrobials suppress gut flora and vitamin K synthesis.

Factors that **diminish** the effect of coumarins:

- **Increased plasma protein binding** of coumarins, e.g., in pregnancy, when plasma albumin levels are raised.
- **Increased loss of the protein bound form of drug in urine** occurs in nephrotic syndrome.
- In some patients, coumarins have **low affinity for the VKOR enzyme**. Thus, they show genetic resistance to effect of warfarin.
- **Drugs:**
  - Oral contraceptive pills increase levels of clotting factors and reduce the effect of warfarin.
  - Enzyme inducers like barbiturates, rifampicin, griseofulvin and carbamazepine increase metabolism of warfarin and reduce its effect.

Because of these factors that may enhance or inhibit effect of anticoagulants, **their use requires great caution and continuous monitoring.**

- **Phenindiones** are not much in use, as they carry risk of hepatic and renal damage. These also cause orange discoloration of urine.

Choice among anticoagulants for various clinical conditions:

- Parenteral anticoagulants are suitable for rapid, short-term use and oral drugs for maintenance therapy, e.g., embolism.
- For prophylaxis of DVT and pulmonary embolism in bed-ridden high-risk patients. Anticoagulants are very effective in preventing recurrences by limiting the extension of venous thrombus and embolisation, though they do not dissolve already formed thrombi.
- In most conditions, LMWHs/fondaparinux have several advantages and are preferred over UFH, followed by warfarin. However, in patients with kidney disease, UFH is preferred because its clearance is less affected by renal dysfunction. In patients with heparin-induced thrombocytopenia (HIT), bivalirudin is used. Warfarin or rivaroxaban is used for maintenance therapy.
- In patients with joint (knee/hip) replacement surgery, oral factor X_a inhibitors and DTIs are most frequently used for the prevention of venous thrombo-embolism.
- Oral drugs are also useful in patients of non-valvular AF and transient ischemic attack to prevent stroke. These are also useful with antiplatelet drugs to prevent re-occlusion in STEMI patients.

The differences between heparin and oral anticoagulants (warfarin) are tabulated in Table 37.1.

Table 37.1 Comparison of heparin and oral anticoagulants

Differentiating feature	Heparin	Warfarin
Method of administration	Subcutaneous or intravenous injection	Oral
Mechanism of action	Causes conformational changes in antithrombin III Catalyses inhibition of factors X_a and II_a.	Interferes with vitamin K-dependent γ-carboxylation of factors II, VII, IX and X.
Onset of action	Fast	Delayed for 1–3 days (time needed for elimination of preformed factors)
Use	To initiate anticoagulant therapy	For maintenance anticoagulant therapy
Monitoring of action by	aPTT	PT, INR
Antidote	Protamine	Vitamin K
Safety in pregnancy	Safe	Can cause fetal warfarin (DiSalvo) syndrome
Activity	In vitro and in vivo	only in vivo

Clinical problem-based questions and MCQs

15. A 60-year-old male patient was on bed rest for the last 8 weeks, because of a fractured neck of femur following a fall down the stairs. He developed leg vein thrombosis and was prescribed injection fondaparinux 5 mg via subcutaneous route, once daily, and tablet warfarin 5 mg twice daily. INR is monitored daily.
    i. Describe the pharmacological basis for giving both fondaparinux and warfarin in this patient.
    ii. Explain the mechanism of anticoagulant action of fondaparinux and warfarin with help of suitable diagrams.
    iii. For how long should each drug be continued?
    iv. What is INR? Explain the importance of monitoring INR during anticoagulant therapy.

16. Identify a drug with the potential to enhance the anticoagulant effect of warfarin.
    a. Carbamazepine b. Cefoperazone
    c. Oral contraceptives d. All of the above

17. The recommended INR range for a patient with a prosthetic valve during warfarin therapy is:
    a. 1.5–2 b. 2–2.5
    c. 2.5–3 d. 3–3.5

Summary

- Coagulants are useful in hemorrhagic states. These include vitamin K_1, K_3, fibrinogen, antihemophillic factors, rutin, desmopressin, ethamsylate, and adrenochrome monosemicarbazone.
- Vitamin K_1 is the most frequently used coagulant, in conditions such as dietary deficiency of vitamin K, obstructive jaundice, prolonged therapy with AMAs, hepatic diseases, premature neonates and patients with overdose of anticoagulant drugs.
- Vitamin K_3 (menadione) has delayed onset of action, poor efficacy, and higher toxicity than vitamin K_1. In neonates, menadione can cause dose-dependent hemolysis and kernicterus; so, it cannot be used instead of K_1 in premature babies.
- Local hemostatics or styptics include thrombin, fibrin, oxidised cellulose, gelatin foam and tannic acid. These are used to stop bleeding from an approachable site by local application.
- **Indirect thrombin inhibitors (IDTIs)** are UFH, LMWH and fondaparinux (a pentasaccharide).
- UFH inactivates factor X_a and II_a after binding to AT_{III}. UFH has low bioavailability, so it is used subcutaneously for prevention and intravenously for treatment of DVT.
- LMWHs like enoxaparin, tinzaparin and nadroparin have smaller chains than UFH. These mainly inactivate X_a with negligible effect on II_a. These have equal efficacy, better bioavailability, longer half-life and fewer adverse effects in comparison to UFH.
- ADRs of heparin include alopecia, hypercalcemia, osteoporosis and TCP (HIT). Heparin is contraindicated in alcoholism, TCP, hepatic cirrhosis, hypertension and renal failure.
- Fondaparinux is an active pentasaccharide that has higher bioavailability and longer half-life than LMWHs.
- LMWHs and fondaparinux are preferred over UFH, except in renal failure patients undergoing cardio-pulmonary bypass surgery or concomitant thrombolysis; in these cases, UFH is still the preferred drug.
- Specific antidote for heparin is protamine.
- **Direct thrombin inhibitors (DTIs)** can be oral and parenteral.
- Among the oral DTIs, ximelagatran is not used much due to its hepatotoxic potential. Dabigatran is used for prevention of DVT in patients undergoing knee/hip surgery, but it needs dose reduction in renal failure.
- Parenteral DTIs can be bivalent (hirudin, lepirudin, desirudin and bivalirudin) and monovalent

(melagatran and argatroban). These are used in HIT, DVT (desirudin) and STEMI for PCI (bivalirudin).
- An important ADR of DTIs is bleeding tendency. Consequently, aPTT monitoring is important for all drugs, except argatroban. All DTIs are contraindicated in renal failure, except argatroban, which is metabolised in liver.
- **Direct factor X_a inhibitors** (rivaroxaban and apixaban) have several advantages over warfarin such as equal efficacy, no lag period (effect appears within 3–4 hours of administration), short duration of action, lower risk of adverse effects and drug interactions and no need to monitor PT or aPTT.
- **Warfarin** acts by inhibiting the VKOR enzyme, thus interfering with the activation of vitamin K. There is a lag period of ~5 days for its anticoagulant effect to set in, as some time is needed for elimination of already synthesised clotting factors. Because it also inhibits proteins C and S, prothrombotic effect is seen with monotherapy. So, at initiation of therapy, warfarin is combined with LMWHs or fondaparinux. It is used in antiphospholipid antibody syndrome and prevention of thrombosis in patients with mechanical valves and AF.
- ADRs of warfarin are bleeding, worsening of HIT, alopecia, skin necrosis and purple/blue discolouration of toes/feet. It also has teratogenic potential and is contraindicated in pregnancy. Warfarin therapy is monitored by INR which is the ratio of the patient's PT to the normal PT of a pooled sample.

Questions for practice

1. Write short notes on:
   a. Styptics
   b. Role of plasma fractions in bleeding disorders
2. a. Classify anticoagulants.
   b. Enumerate therapeutic uses of anticoagulants
   c. Enumerate adverse effects and contraindications for use of heparins
3. Explain why:
   a. LMWHs are generally preferred over UFH. In which condition is UFH still used?
   b. Warfarin is contraindicated in pregnancy.
   c. Warfarin toxicity can occur in hyperthyroidism.
   d. Vitamin K_3 is not given in infants.
   e. Parenteral anticoagulants are combined with warfarin at the beginning of therapy.
4. a. Enumerate the factors that can potentiate or inhibit effect of coumarin anticoagulants.
   b. Enumerate the adverse effects of coumarin anticoagulants.
5. Write short notes on:
   a. Direct thrombin inhibitors
   b. Direct factor X_a inhibitors
   c. Heparin-induced thrombocytopenia

Hints for problem-based questions and MCQs

1. i. Delivery was conducted at 32 weeks of gestation. Premature babies have low levels of clotting factors; so, vitamin K was given to prevent hemorrhagic disease.
   ii. Vitamin K_3 should not be used because of the risk of hemolysis and kernicterus.
   iii. Vitamin K deficiency states and overdose of anticoagulants.
2. i. Synthesis of coagulation factors is reduced in liver failure, leading to bleeding disorders. Vitamin K is not effective as it exerts its coagulant action through activation of coagulation factors by gamma carboxylation.
   ii. c. Cryoprecipitate
3. b. GI disturbance
4. i. Tranexamic acid interferes with the process of clot lysis by competitively inhibiting plasminogen activation.
   ii. Other uses include prevention and control of excess bleeding due to fibrinolytic drugs, as adjuvants in hemophiliac patients undergoing tooth extraction, prostatectomy, tonsillectomy, trauma and to prevent re-bleed from peptic ulcers, aneurysms, epistaxis, bleeding from bladder due to radiation or drug-induced cystitis. ADRS are nausea, GI upset, nasal stuffiness, myopathy, hypotension and intravascular thrombosis.
5. d. Thrombin applied as dry power or freshly prepared solution can stop surface bleeding in hemophiliacs. Tetradecyl sulphate and polidocanol are sclerosing agents injected in varicose veins and hemorrhoids. Adrenaline is a vasoconstrictor for control of epistaxis or bleeding from tooth socket.
6. a. Sodium carbonate
7. b. Argatroban is a DTI; all the others are IDTIs acting through AT_{III}.
8. i. c. Patient receiving antiplatelet drugs, because heparin is used in DIC, post-infusion thrombophlebitis and at the beginning of warfarin therapy.
   ii. Refer to page 507.
9. i. b. Safety in renal failure
   ii. Refer to page 504, 505.
   iii. Refer to page 506.
10. i. Heparin-induced TCP occurs due to platelet aggregation or formation of Abs against platelet-heparin complex.
    ii. c. Lepirudin
    iii. Direct thrombin inhibitor, parenteral, bivalent DTI, binds to the substrate binding as well as catalytic sites of thrombin and inhibits it directly.
11. a. Ximelagatran
12. i. c. Anticoagulants.
    ii. Venous thrombi are associated with the hypercoagulable state and are fibrin rich
13. i. d. Antiplatelet drugs
    ii. Arterial thrombus is platelet rich.
14. i. b. Apixaban
    ii. Refer to page 508.
15. i. Effect of warfarin takes some time to manifest, and it causes prothrombotic state at beginning of therapy.
    ii. Refer to page 506, 509.
    iii. Fondaparinux given till 2 days after achieving target INR, and warfarin for 3–6 months depending on condition of patient
    iv. Refer to page 510.
16. b. Cefoperazone has additive effect with warfarin, because it causes hypoprothrombinemia. Carbamazepine and oral contraceptives are enzyme inducers, so reduce warfarin effect.
17. d. 3–3.5

CONCEPT MAP – ANTICOAGULANTS

ADRs
- **Bleeding** from deeper tissues like hematuria, GI bleeding, joints, muscles, brain
- **Heparin-induced thrombocytopenia (HIT):** can be mild, transient due to platelet aggregation or severe life-threatening due to immune reaction. Platelet counts must be monitored. Switch over to Fondaparinux or DTIs.
- **Hypersensitivity:** Rashes, urticaria, rigors, anaphylaxis
- On long-term use reversible alopecia, osteoporosis, raised hepatic enzymes.
- **Antidote:** Protamine

Contraindications
- Active bleeding, bleeding tendency e.g. hemophilia, severe hypertension, intracranial hemorrhage, ulcerative colitis, peptic ulcers, threatened abortion.
- Advanced malignant disease → risk of bleeding from necrosed tumour tissue.
- Active TB → risk of hemoptysis.
- Alcoholic liver disease, H/O heparin induced TCP (HIT), purpura, hepatic/renal failure.
- Ocular/ neurosurgery.
- SABE → risk of embolisation.
- Patients on antiplatelet drug therapy.
- Pregnancy: Avoided till there is a clear indication for use.

Advantages
- Equi-efficacious as UFH, but lesser ADRs (bleeding tendency). Lab monitoring of aPTT not required.
- More bioavailability and longer half-life than UFHs → OD or BD dose sufficient
- Lower risk of long-term complications like TCP, osteoporosis

LMWHs
Enoxaparin, Nadroparin, Reviparin, Dalteparin
Mechanism same as UFH, but **no scaffolding** provided for clotting factors → less inhibitory effect on factor II_a than UFH.

Disadvantages
- Not effective in preventing catheter thrombosis → in cardiopulmonary bypass surgery, UFH preferred.
- Not suitable in patients with renal failure.

Uses
- Prophylaxis & treatment of DVT, Pulmonary embolism
- STEMI and Bundle branch block
- To maintain patency of shunts/cannulas in dialysis patients.
- Disseminated intravascular coagulation
- To improve healing of post infusion superficial thrombophlebitis (Quick penetration solution-QPS of UFH is used topically).

UFH Mechanism
Binds to AT_{III}, causes conformational change, increasing its binding to clotting factors → **inactivates X_a.**
Also provides **scaffolding for II_a**.
UFH prevents conversion of prothrombin to thrombin and that of fibrinogen to fibrin.
Effective in vivo & in vitro

Fondaparinux
Binds only to AT_{III} & inactivates factor X_a only. **No effect on II_a.**
Bioavailability and duration of action longer than LMWHs
Risk of bleeding, TCP, osteoporosis, even less than LMWHs
Useful in HIT

Direct X_a inhibitors
Rivaroxaban, Apixaban directly inhibit factor X_a and prevent thrombin formation
Effective orally
Uses: To prevent thrombosis after joint replacement, atrial fibrillation. Prophylaxis in stroke, acute coronary syndrome, Treatment of DVT, PE.
Advantages over warfarin: No lag period in onset of effect, Short duration of action, Efficacy same as warfarin, Risk of bleeding lower → no need to monitor PT or aPTT, Risk of DDIs less than warfarin
ADRs: nausea, hypotension, tachycardia, edema, bleeding tendency

IDTIs

ANTICOAGULANTS

DTIs
Oral DTIs (Ximelagatran, Dabigatran) & **Monovalent parenteral DTIs** (Argatroban, Melagatran) bind only to active site of thrombin (II_a)
Bivalent parenteral DTIs (Hirudin, Lepirudin, Bivalirudin, Desirudin) bind both to active and substrate recognising (exosite) of thrombin (II_a)
DTIs inhibit circulating as well as clot-bound thrombin and prevent conversion of fibrinogen to fibrin.

Uses
- **Lepirudin** used in HIT, **Argatroban** preferred in HIT patients having renal dysfunction.
- **Bivalirudin** in STEMI patients undergoing intervention, unstable angina, NSTEMI. It inhibits thrombin-mediated platelet aggregation, but has no risk of TCP.
- **Dabigatran** used to prevent venous thrombosis after joint replacement, in atrial fibrillation

ADRs
Bleeding, backache, headache, hypotension
Ximelagatran is hepatotoxic
Dabigatran causes dyspepsia.

Vit K Antagonists
Coumarins (Dicoumarol, Warfarin, Acenocoumarol) interfere with gamma carboxylation of factors II, VII, IX, X.
Anticoagulant effect delayed till preformed factors are eliminated
Also decrease carboxylation of protein C, S and osteocalcin

Uses
Maintenance treatment of DVT, PE
Prophylaxis of DVT, PE in post MI, atrial flutter, prosthetic valve, patients undergoing orthopedic, gynecological, cardiac surgery
Parenteral anticoagulants are given with warfarin for first 5 days or for 2 days after achieving target INR

ADRs
- **Bleeding** like hematuria, epistaxis, ecchymosis, retroperitoneal/intracranial/ GI hemorrhage. Antidote is vitamin K
- Alopecia, dermatitis, anorexia, nausea, diarrhea, bad taste
- Cutaneous necrosis, osteoporosis
- Purple toe syndrome
- **Contraindicated in pregnancy** → can cause fetal warfarin syndrome (growth retardation, hypoplasia of nose, eyeballs, hands)

DDIs
Warfarin effect increased by:
- Reduced vitamin K supply to liver e.g. Malnutrition, malabsorption syndrome, prolonged antimicrobial therapy
- Reduced clotting factor synthesis as in chronic alcoholism, hepatic function impairment
- Hypoproteinemia
- Drugs which displace it from PPB site
- Drugs which can inhibit metabolism

Warfarin action reduced by enzyme inducers, Increased PPB as in pregnancy, nephrotic syndrome
With OCPs → levels of clotting factors increased

SECTION 8 Drugs Affecting Blood

38 Antiplatelet and Fibrinolytic Drugs

PH 4.3 Describe the types, salient pharmacokinetics, pharmacodynamics, therapeutic uses and adverse drug reactions of fibrinolytics.
PH 4.4 Explain the types, salient pharmacokinetics, pharmacodynamics, therapeutic uses, adverse drug reactions of antiplatelets agents.

Learning objectives

A student of MBBS phase II should be able to:
- Classify antiplatelet drugs.
- Describe mechanism of action of antiplatelet drugs.
- Discuss the indications for use of antiplatelet drugs, mentioning their doses.
- Enumerate contraindications to use and adverse effects of antiplatelet drugs.
- Enumerate fibrinolytic/thrombolytic drugs.
- Describe mechanism of action of fibrinolytic drugs.
- Discuss the indications for use of fibrinolytic drugs, mentioning their doses.
- Enumerate contraindications to use and adverse effects of fibrinolytic drugs.

ANTIPLATELET DRUGS

MECHANISM OF PLATELET AGGREGATION

Platelet aggregation and the formation of platelet plug is an important initial step in the process of clot formation. The function of platelets is regulated by many substances **synthesised outside or within the platelets** such as adenosine diphosphate (ADP), thromboxane A_2 (TxA_2), prostacyclin (PGI_2), PGD_2, PGE_2, collagen, thrombin, serotonin, Ca^{2+}, cAMP, and cGMP. These substances act on receptors present on the surface of or inside platelets and serve as important targets for drugs that inhibit platelet action.

Receptors present on the surface or membrane of platelets are:

GP_{Ia} receptors: These have affinity for collagen that is exposed at the site of injury to vessel wall.

GP_{Ib} receptors: These can bind to von Willebrand factor (vWF)

$GP_{IIb/IIIa}$ receptors: These can bind to fibrinogen and other macromolecules.

$P2Y_{12}$, $P2X_1$ and $P2Y_1$ receptors that bind to ADP.

The steps of process of platelet aggregation are described below (Fig. 38.1)

a. Whenever there is an injury to a vessel wall, subendothelial matrix proteins like collagen and vWF get exposed.
b. Platelets adhere to collagen and vWF (at GP_{Ia} and GP_{Ib} receptors, respectively) and get activated.
c. Platelet activation results in the synthesis and secretion of TxA_2, ADP, 5-HT, etc. These agents induce platelet aggregation. However, PGI_2 released from endothelial cells opposes platelet aggregation. Platelet activation also causes conformational changes in $GP_{IIb/IIIa}$ receptors, enabling it to bind to fibrinogen and other macromolecules.
d. In this way, fibrinogen serves to cross-link adjacent platelets and causes platelet aggregation that results in the formation of a platelet plug.

The coagulation cascade is also activated concurrently, resulting in the formation of a fibrin mesh that stabilises the platelet plug.

CLASSIFICATION OF ANTIPLATELET DRUGS

Depending upon their mechanism of action, antiplatelet drugs are classified as drugs that inhibit TxA_2 synthesis, block $P2Y_{12}$ purinergic receptors, and block $GP_{IIb/IIIa}$ receptors (Flowchart 38.1).

1. TxA_2 Synthesis Inhibitors

TxA_2 is a pro-aggregatory substance synthesised in platelets from arachidonic acid, via the action of cyclo-oxygenase 1 (COX1) enzyme.

Aspirin, a TxA_2 synthesis inhibitor, causes:

- Acetylation and **irreversible inhibition** of platelet cyclo-oxygenase I resulting in reduced synthesis of TxA_2.
- Platelets cannot synthesise new COX enzyme (because platelets are non-nucleated). Thus, the inhibiting effect of aspirin on TxA_2 synthesis persists for the lifespan of platelets (8–10 days). Aspirin, in a dose of 75–150 mg per day, causes maximal inhibition of platelet function.
- In addition to COX inhibition, aspirin **decreases the release of ADP** from platelets which may contribute to its anti-aggregatory effect.

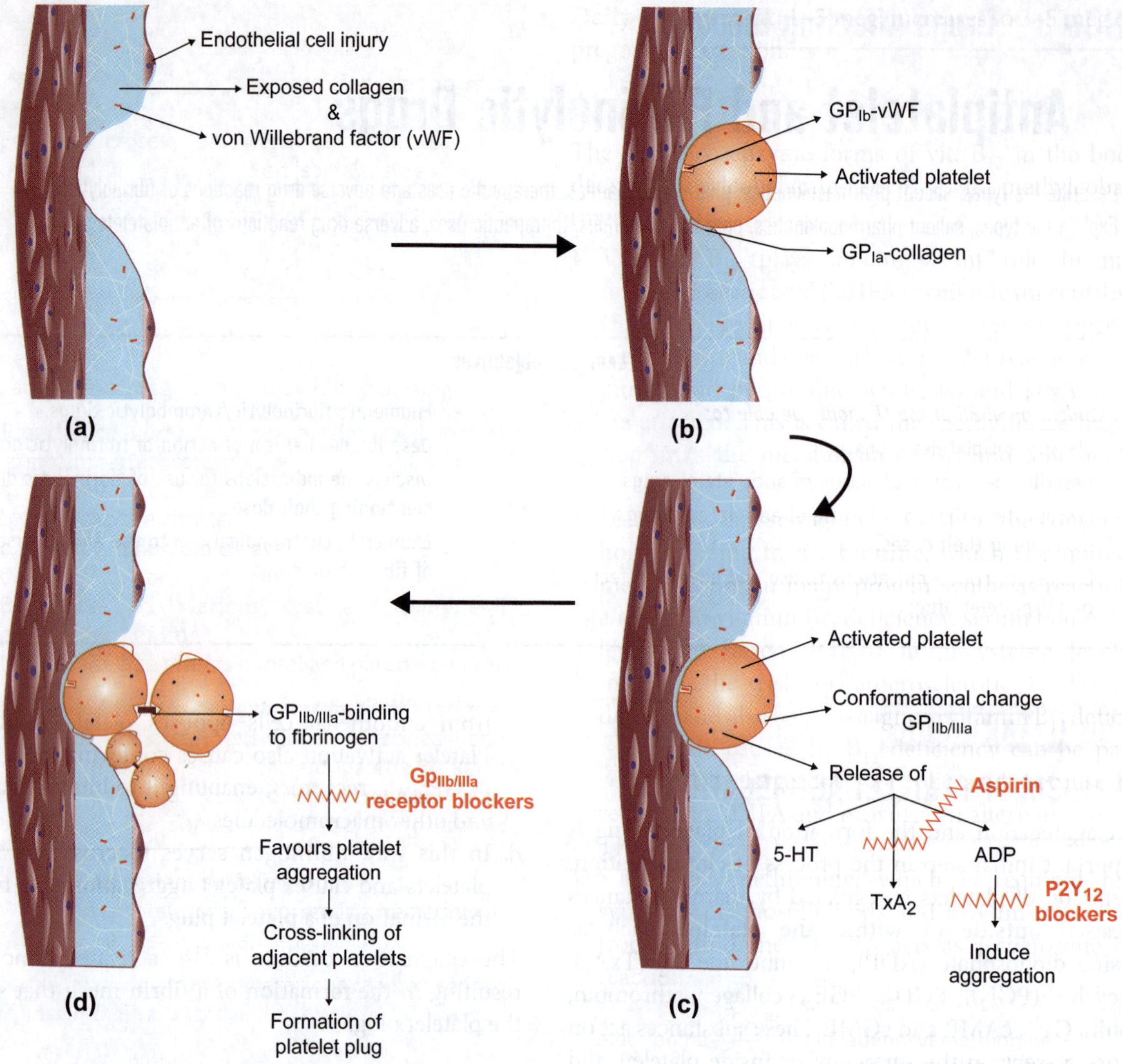

Fig. 38.1 Mechanism of platelet aggregation and site of action of antiplatelet drugs

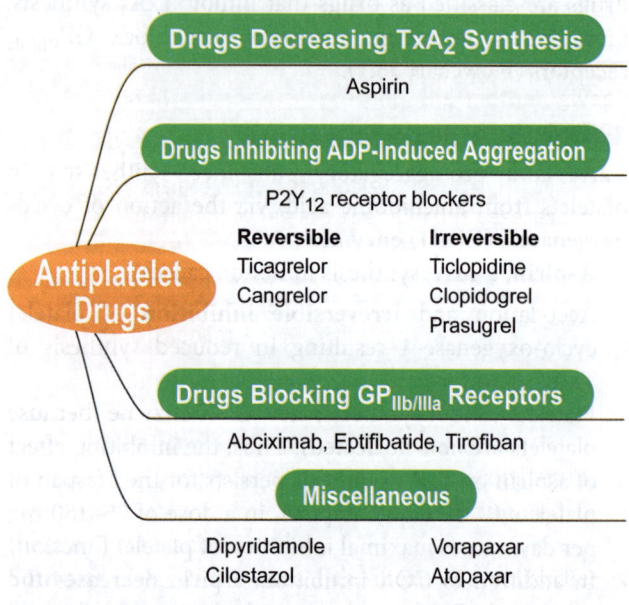

Flowchart 38.1 Classification of antiplatelet drugs

- Aspirin also **decreases the tendency of platelets to stick to each other**; however, it has no effect on the binding of platelets to subendothelial matrix proteins and the survival time of platelets.
- Notably, **the anti-aggregatory effect of aspirin decreases at higher doses** because of the reduced synthesis of PGI_2 from endothelial cells. Therefore, the recommended anti-aggregatory dose of aspirin for long-term prophylaxis is 75–125 mg/day.
- Other NSAIDs are competitive inhibitors of COX; their platelet-inhibiting effect is of shorter duration and not clinically useful.

2. Drugs that inhibit ADP-induced platelet aggregation

$P2Y_{12}$ is a G_i protein-coupled purinergic receptor present on the surface of platelets. The binding of ADP to $P2Y_{12}$ receptors inhibits adenylyl cyclase → reduced cAMP → platelet aggregation. This process is blocked by $P2Y_{12}$

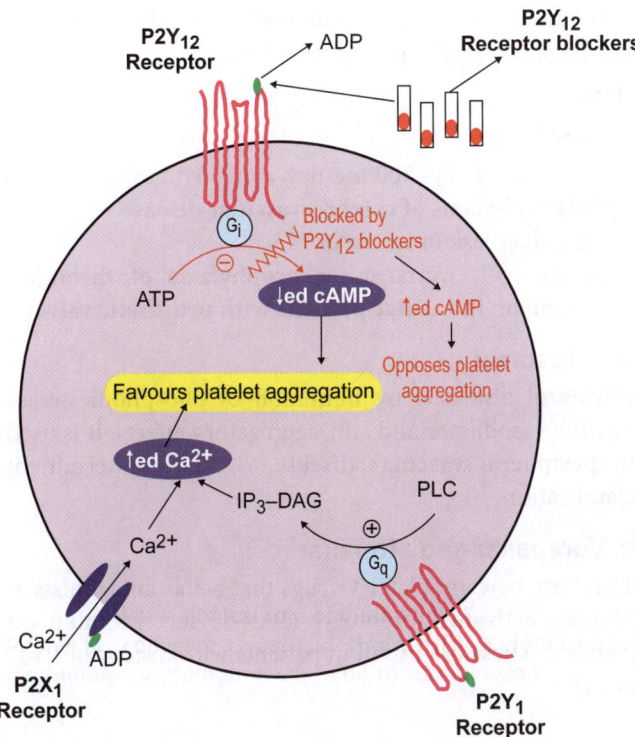

Fig. 38.2 ADP-induced platelet aggregation and mechanism of P2Y$_{12}$ receptor blockers

receptor blockers, resulting in raised cAMP levels that oppose platelet aggregation.

In addition to P2Y$_{12}$ receptors, ADP acts on calcium-channel linked P2X$_1$ receptors and G$_q$-linked P2Y$_1$ receptors. Activation of both these receptors raises intracellular calcium and favours platelet aggregation (Fig. 38.2).

a. Ticlopidine

Ticlopidine is a thienopyridine, which acts by **irreversibly blocking P2Y$_{12}$ purinergic receptors** and inhibits the platelet aggregation induced by ADP.

Ticlopidine has **many adverse effects** such as:

- GI upset: Nausea, diarrhea, dyspepsia
- Hemorrhage
- Hemolysis, jaundice, thrombocytopenic purpura, hemolytic uremic syndrome
- Bone marrow suppression: Neutropenia, leukopenia, TCP, etc.

Other drugs like clopidogrel, prasugrel and ticagrelor are preferred.

b. Clopidogrel

Clopidogrel has the same mechanism of action and efficacy of anti-aggregatory effect as ticlopidine, but is **more potent and better tolerated**.

Clopidogrel is a prodrug which gets activated slowly in the liver by the enzyme CYP2C19 into an active thiol that blocks P2Y$_{12}$ receptors and ADP-induced aggregation.

The anti-aggregatory effect **develops slowly (over a few days) and lasts for the lifespan of the platelets,** because of the irreversible block.

Wide interindividual variation in the antiplatelet effect of clopidogrel is due to the genetic polymorphism of the enzyme (CYP2C19) that activates this prodrug. **Omeprazol decreases the effect of clopidogrel** as it inhibits CYP2C19 and interferes with the generation of active thiol from clopidogrel.

Clopidogrel acts **synergistically with aspirin** to prevent arterial thrombosis and ischemic episodes. Such **dual antiplatelet therapy (DAPT)** is used for:

- **Unstable angina and non-STEMI** for reducing risk of MI, stroke and cardiovascular deaths.
- **Prevention of restenosis** of coronaries after stenting.

Clopidogrel is given as 300 mg loading dose, followed by 75 mg once daily.

Adverse effects

These occur in the form of nausea, epigastric pain, diarrhea, rashes and risk of bleeding. Addition of aspirin to clopidogrel further increases the risk of hemorrhagic complications. However, the risk of bone marrow toxicity and leukopenia is much **lower with clopidogrel than ticlopidine.**

c. Prasugrel

Prasugrel is **more potent, faster and longer-acting than clopidogrel**. It is also a **prodrug** activated by CYP2C19, but activation is fast and not much affected by genetic polymorphism or enzyme inhibitors like omeprazole.

- Owing to the faster onset of action, it is preferred in **acute coronary syndromes and STEMI.**
- Prasugrel is contraindicated in patients with a history of TIA and stroke because the risk of **intracranial hemorrhagic complications** is high.

Ticlopidine, clopidogrel and prasugrel are hit-and-run drugs, i.e., their action lasts longer than their half-life, owing to the irreversible interaction with P2Y$_{12}$ receptors.

d. Ticagrelor

It does not need activation through CYP2C19, and directly inhibits the binding of ADP and P2Y$_{12}$ receptors on the platelet surface.

- Thus, its **onset of action is faster** than previous drugs of the same class; it is unaffected by genetic polymorphism or enzyme inhibitors.
- It has a **more potent and consistent** effect
- Moreover, the effect is **reversible**; therefore, the duration of action is also less, necessitating twice daily administration.
- It is recommended for **all patients of ACS requiring urgent percutaneous intervention.** The recommended dose is 180 mg loading dose, followed by 90 mg twice a day. The treatment may be continued for up to one year.

Adverse effects

These include nausea, dizziness, irregular pulse, shortness of breath, tightness in chest and increased risk of intracranial hemorrhages.

3. Drugs that Block GP$_{IIb/IIIa}$ Receptors

The activation of the GP$_{IIb/IIIa}$ receptor complex serves as a final common pathway in the aggregation of platelets. Absence of these receptors causes a condition called 'Glanzmann thrombasthenia' characterised by excessive bleeding. Thus, the blockade of GP$_{IIb/IIIa}$ receptors, by drugs such as abciximab, eptifibatide and tirofiban, inhibits the binding of fibrinogen to platelets.

a. Abciximab

Abciximab was the first drug in this group.

- It is the **Fab fragment of the monoclonal antibody** against the GP$_{IIb/IIIa}$ receptor complex. It binds to these receptors and inhibits platelet aggregation for 12–24 hours (abciximab has the shortest half-life in this group), but action lasts longer due to maximum affinity for GP$_{IIb/IIIa}$ receptors.
- It is given as 0.25 mg/kg **intravenous** bolus dose, followed by 10 mcg/min IV infusion for 12 hours.
- It is used in **unstable angina, ACS and 10–60 min before PCI** along with aspirin and heparin. With the addition of abciximab, incidence of subsequent restenosis, MI and death is reduced.
- It is also useful in **acute ischemic stroke**.

Adverse effects

The major ADRs of abciximab are the risk of bleeding and thrombocytopenia.

b. Eptifibatide

This cyclic peptide is an analogue of the carboxyl-terminal of the delta chain of fibrinogen.

- It **binds to GP$_{IIb/IIIa}$ receptors in place of fibrinogen** and inhibits platelet aggregation. However, it dissociates from the receptors in a short while and the **effect lasts only for 6–10 hours.**
- Indications for use include unstable angina and just before coronary angioplasty along with aspirin and heparin.
- Similar to abciximab, it can cause bleeding and thrombocytopenia (TCP).

c. Tirofiban

Tirofiban has the same mechanism of action, uses and adverse effects as eptifibatide; however, it is not a peptide.

4. Miscellaneous Antiplatelet Drugs

a. Dipyridamole

Dipyridamole increases levels of cAMP in platelets by:

- Inhibition of phosphodiesterase enzyme
- Inhibiting uptake of adenosine

The raised cAMP level **potentiates the effect of PGI$_2$** resulting in an anti-aggregatory effect.

Uses

It is used:

- In a dose of 150–300 mg/day, along with aspirin 25 mg for **prophylaxis of cerebro-vascular disease**.
- To reduce risk of stroke in TIA.
- Along with warfarin for **prophylaxis of thrombo-embolism in cardiac patients with prosthetic valves.**

b. Cilostazol

Cilostazol also acts by inhibition of phosphodiesterase causing vasodilator and anti-aggregatory effects. It is used in **peripheral vascular disease** to relieve intermittent claudication.

c. Vorapaxar and atopaxar

These are new antiplatelet drugs that act as antagonists at protease-activated receptor-1 (PAR-1) for thrombin on platelets. These are useful in patients with history of PVD or MI.

THERAPEUTIC USES OF ANTIPLATELET DRUGS

As arterial thrombi are platelet-rich, most of the indications for use of antiplatelet drugs **are related to arterial thrombosis**, such as:

- Coronary artery disease (CAD): aspirin, clopidogrel, or both (in **dual antiplatelet therapy**) are used for prevention of reinfarction in post-MI patients.
- In acute coronary syndromes, including conditions such as unstable angina, NSTEMI and STEMI, antiplatelet drugs along with heparin followed by warfarin reduce incidence of restenosis, subsequent MI and death.
- Prevention of stroke: Antiplatelet drugs prevent stroke in patients with TIAs and atrial fibrillations. For these indications, antiplatelet drugs can be used alone or in combination with dipyridamole.
- Antiplatelet drugs, along with warfarin, are used to prevent microthrombi formation on prosthetic heart valves.
- Antiplatelet drugs are used to improve patency of grafts and for hemodialysis.
- In peripheral vascular diseases, for symptomatic improvement of intermittent claudication cilostazol is used.

Clinical problem-based questions and MCQs

1. A 50-year-old patient complains of chest pain radiating to left shoulder whenever he walks for about 10 minutes, which is relieved upon rest. Patient is diagnosed with classical angina pectoris.
    i. Identify the most suitable drug for long-term prevention of myocardial infarction in this case.
        a. Aspirin   b. Prasugrel
        c. Abciximab   d. Ticagrelor

ii. Describe the mechanism of antiplatelet action and dosage of the selected drug.
2. A 60-year-old post-MI patient needs an antiplatelet drug for prevention of ACS and reinfarction. History of transient ischemic attacks is present. Which of the following antiplatelet drugs is contraindicated?
   a. Clopidogrel   b. Prasugrel
   c. Dipyridamole   d. All of the above.
3. i. Which of the following drugs interferes with the binding of platelets to fibrinogen?
   a. Abciximab   b. Ticagrelor
   c. Prasugrel   d. Ticlopidine
   ii. Describe the mechanism of action, uses and adverse effects of the selected drug.
4. i. Identify the CORRECT statement about clopidogrel.
   a. Acts as antagonist at $GP_{IIb/IIIa}$ receptors
   b. Has faster onset of action
   c. Used in dual antiplatelet therapy
   d. Not suitable for patients with stroke
   ii. Why is the efficacy of clopidogrel reduced by omeprazole?
5. i. Which drug is used in intermittent claudication?
   a. Ticagrelor   b. Cilostazol
   c. Dipyridamole   d. Abciximab
   ii. Describe the mechanism of beneficial effect of the selected drug.
6. Which drug has the maximum affinity for $GP_{IIb/IIIa}$ receptors?
   a. Abciximab   b. Eptifibatide
   c. Tirofiban   d. Ticagrelor

FIBRINOLYTIC/THROMBOLYTIC DRUGS

Fibrinolytic or thrombolytic drugs **break (lysis means breakdown) the fibrin meshwork of the already formed thrombi** or clots, reopening the occluded vessels. Plasminogen, plasmin and tissue plasminogen activator (tPA) are important components of the natural fibrinolytic system. All fibrinolytic drugs **activate the natural fibrinolytic system** and can be nonspecific, moderately specific or highly specific for clot (fibrin)-bound plasminogen (Flowchart 38.2).

Classification
1. Streptokinase
The oldest drug of this group, streptokinase, was obtained from β-hemolytic streptococci.
Mechanism of action: tPA binding sites are present on plasminogen molecules. tPA, which is released at the time of endothelial cell injury, converts plasminogen to plasmin. This binds to the exposed lysine on clots, breaks down fibrin, and dissolves the clot (Fig 38.3). However, action of the tPA on circulating plasminogen increases the risk of bleeding. Streptokinase binds to plasminogen and uncovers the tPA binding site, leading to increased formation of plasmin.

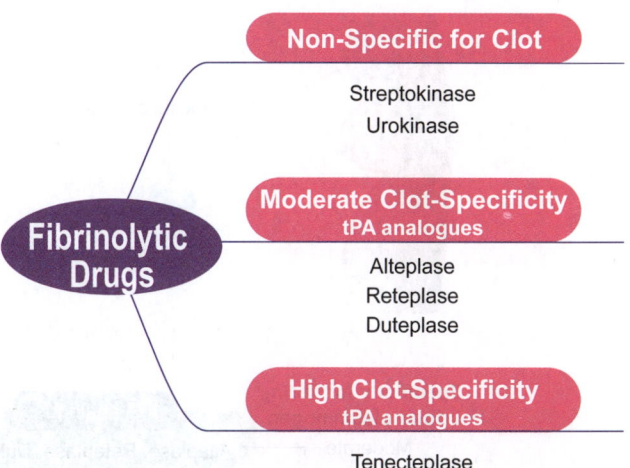

Flowchart 38.2 Classification of fibrinolytic drugs

A major drawback of streptokinase is that it is **not fibrin specific**, i.e., it activates not only the fibrin-bound plasminogen, but also circulating plasminogen. Because circulating fibrinogen is depleted, the **risk of bleeding is greater.** It is not currently preferred for thrombolysis.

Streptokinase can cause transient hypotension due to raised bradykinin levels.

2. Urokinase
Urokinase is also non-clot specific; it is obsolete because of the availability of better-tolerated newer drugs.

3. Alteplase
It is a recombinant tissue plasminogen activator (**rtPA**) produced by recombinant DNA technology that activates plasminogen to form plasmin. It has **moderate specificity** for fibrin-bound plasminogen; so, the risk of bleeding is lower than with streptokinase.

It has a **half-life of just a few minutes**, and is thus administered as a slow intravenous infusion for 90 minutes along with heparin, for myocardial infarction (MI), pulmonary embolism (PE) and ischemic stroke.

ADRs to alteplase include fever, nausea and fall in BP.

Reteplase
Reteplase is **longer-acting than alteplase** with a half-life of 13–16 minutes. Consequently, it can be given as two IV bolus doses of 18 mg given with 30 minutes gap in STEMI and PE cases.

Tenecteplase
Tenecteplase has **greater specificity for fibrin-bound plasminogen**, which decreases the risk of bleeding tendencies. Its **duration of action is longer** than other drugs in this group; so, it is given as a single IV injection over 10 seconds.

Therapeutic Uses of Fibrinolytic Drugs
Fibrinolytic drugs are more **useful for dissolving venous thrombi** than arterial thrombi. Important therapeutic uses of fibrinolytic drugs include:

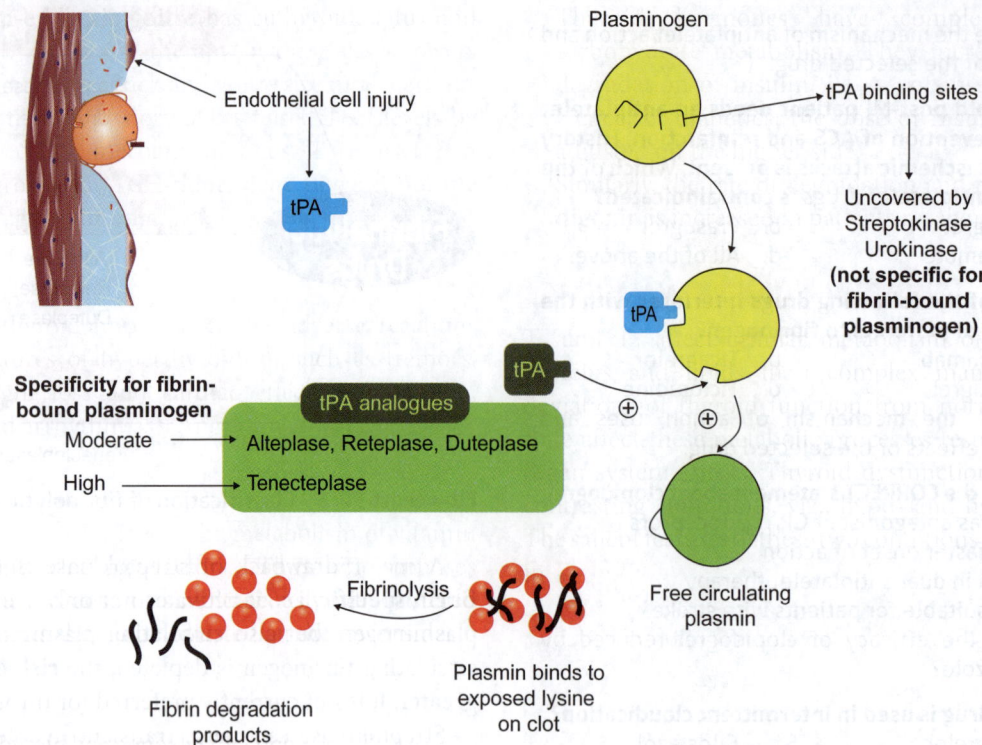

Fig. 38.3 The plasminogen–plasmin system and mechanism of action of fibrinolytic drugs

- In **DVT** of legs, shoulders and pelvis: These drugs reduce pain, swelling, and risk of embolisation, and preserve venous valves.
- For **reperfusion therapy** in STEMI: Fibrinolytics are the alternative first-line approach to PCI and stenting. The efficacy of alteplase, reteplase and tenecteplase in achieving lysis of thrombi and recanalisation of occluded coronaries is similar, but tenecteplase has the advantage of lower risk of bleeding and single IV bolus dose. In acute myocardial infarction, thrombolytics should be used within 12 hours to achieve significant reduction in mortality. Once the vessel is recanalised, its reocclusion is prevented by anticoagulants (heparin) and antiplatelet drugs (aspirin).
- Fibrinolytics are useful to preserve lung function in pulmonary embolism.
- In ischemic stroke: These drugs are useful if given within 3–4 hours of onset, but it is important to rule out the risk of intracranial hemorrhages before giving fibrinolytics.
- These drugs are used in limb artery occlusion, if a surgical thrombectomy is not possible.

ADRs of Fibrinolytic Drugs

Major adverse effect is risk of bleeding, especially intracranial bleeding. These drugs may also cause fall in BP and allergic reactions.

Contraindications of Fibrinolytic Drugs

These drugs are not given in conditions which cause a predisposition to risk of bleeding, such as:

- Peptic ulcer and esophageal varices.
- Any wound/fracture/tooth extraction/major surgery in the preceding 3 weeks.
- Brain tumour, aneurysm, intracranial hemorrhage within the last one year (absolute contraindication), head injury.
- Bleeding disorders.
- Pregnancy.

Clinical problem-based questions and MCQs

7. A 60-year-old patient, a known case of angina, presents with severe, penetrating chest pain radiating to the root of neck and back, with anxiety and cold sweats. ECG shows ST elevation; cardiac enzymes are raised. Patient is diagnosed as STEMI and needs PCI. However, the patient lives in a remote area, with no facility for stenting.
   i. Identify the preferred alternative drug for reperfusion?
      a. Warfarin   b. Tenecteplase
      c. Streptokinase   d. Ticagrelor
   ii. Justify your choice.
   iii. Enumerate the therapeutic uses and contraindications of the selected drug.

8. i. Identify the drug having maximum clot-specific action.
      a. Streptokinase   b. Urokinase
      c. Alteplase   d. Tenecteplase
   ii. What are the clinical implications of the clot-specific action?

9. Reperfusion by use of thrombolytic drugs reduces mortality in AMI if the drug is given within a certain time limit. Identify the appropriate time limit.
   a. 2 hours
   b. 6 hours
   c. 12 hours
   d. 24 hours

10. Which condition is an absolute contraindication for thrombolytic therapy?
    a. History of stroke in past one year
    b. Pregnancy
    c. Tooth extraction
    d. Hypertension

11. Which fibrinolytic drug can be given as a single dose?
    a. Streptokinase
    b. Alteplase
    c. Tenecteplase
    d. Duteplase

Summary

- Aspirin, a non-selective COX inhibitor, is used in a low dose (75–125 mg, daily) for its antiplatelet effect (at higher doses, prostacyclin (PGI_2) synthesis in the endothelium is also inhibited, and the useful antiplatelet effect is lost).
- ADP-mediated platelet aggregation is inhibated by $P2Y_{12}$ receptor blockers such as ticlopidine, clopidogrel, prasugrel and ticagrelor
- Ticlopidine has many adverse effects like GI disturbance, agranulocytosis, TCP and hemolytic uremic syndrome and is not preferred. Clopidogrel is more potent and better tolerated.
- Dual antiplatelet therapy is a combination of aspirin and clopidogrel for secondary prophylaxis of MI and stroke.
- Prasugrel is faster- and longer-acting than clopidogrel, and used in ACS. However, it is contraindicated in TIA, because of high risk of intracranial hemorrhage.
- Ticagrelor is a fast-acting, orally effective drug, with consistent effect that is useful in ACS along with aspirin or clopidogrel.
- Abciximab is a $GP_{IIb/IIIa}$ inhibitor with maximum affinity for receptors and is useful in ACS and stroke.
- **Fibrinolytic drugs**: Streptokinase and urokinase are not clot/fibrin-selective and carry a greater risk of causing bleeding tendencies and are not much in use.
- The fibrin-specific action of recombinant tPAs such as alteplase, reteplase and duteplase is moderate, while that of tenecteplase is maximum. These drugs have a lower risk of causing bleeding.
- These drugs are used in STEMI, ischemic stroke for thrombolysis, and massive pulmonary embolism.
- Contraindications are a history of intracranial hemorrhage in the past one year, pregnancy, head injury, aneurysm, peptic ulcer, esophageal varices, recent surgery, tooth extraction, etc.

Questions for practice

1. Classify antiplatelet drugs.
2. Enumerate the therapeutic uses of antiplatelet drugs.
3. Explain why:
   a. Aspirin is used in low dose for its anti-aggregatory effect.
   b. Clopidogrel and aspirin may be combined for their antiplatelet action.
   c. There are wide interindividual variations in the antiplatelet effect of clopidogrel.
   d. Omeprazole decreases the antiplatelet effect of clopidogrel.
4. Write short notes on:
   a. Ticagrelor
   b. Abciximab
   c. Dipyridamole
5. Enumerate the therapeutic uses and adverse effects of fibrinolytic drugs.
6. Explain why:
   a. Fibrinolytics are the first-line alternative approach to PCI in STEMI.
   b. Risk of hemorrhagic complications is lower with alteplase than streptokinase.
   c. Fibrinolytics are useful in established DVT.
   d. Alteplase therapy is contraindicated in DVT patients having concurrent peptic ulcer disease.

Hints for problem-based questions and MCQs

1. i. a. Aspirin is useful for long-term prophylaxis of MI in angina. The other three are useful in acute coronary syndromes, because of their faster onset of action.
   ii. Irreversible COX inhibition in platelets → reduced TxA_2 synthesis → antiplatelet action → reduced risk of arterial thrombosis. Dose 75–125 mg/day.
2. b. Prasugrel increases the risk of intracranial hemorrhage in TIA patients; so, it is contraindicated.
3. i. a. Abciximab
   ii. $GP_{IIb/IIIa}$ receptor blocker; useful in unstable angina, ACS and before PCI. ADRs are bleeding and TCP.
4. i. c. Clopidogrel is used with aspirin in dual antiplatelet therapy.
   ii. Clopidogrel is a prodrug activated by CYP2C19. Omeprazole interferes with activation of clopidogrel by inhibition of CYP2C19.
5. i. b. Cilostazol
   ii. PDE inhibition → raised cAMP → VD and antiplatelet effect.
6. a. Abciximab has greater affinity for $GP_{IIb/IIIa}$ receptors than eptifibatide and tirofiban. Ticagrelor has no action on these receptors.
7. i. b. Tenecteplase
   ii. Thrombolytics are used for reperfusion. Streptokinase is not fibrin- or clot-specific; so, the risk of bleeding is higher. Tenecteplase has maximum clot-specific action and is the preferred drug. Warfarin is an anticoagulant and ticagrelor is an antiplatelet drug. These have role in secondary prophylaxis in post-MI cases.
   iii. Refer to page 520.
8. i. d. Tenecteplase
   ii. Lower risk of bleeding.
9. c. 12 hours
10. a. History of stroke in past year
11. c. Tenecteplase as single IV injection over 10 minutes, due to a longer half-life than other fibrinolytic drugs.

CONCEPT MAP – ANTIPLATELET AND FIBRINOLYTIC DRUGS

ANTIPLATELET DRUGS

Irreversible (P2Y12 blockers)
Ticlopidine: Many ADRs, not preferred.
Clopidogrel: Prodrug activated by CYP2C19 → DDIs with omeprazole, interindividual variations
Slower-acting, more potent, better tolerated than ticlopidne
Used with aspirin as dual antiplatelet therapy (**DAPT**) for unstable angina & non-STEMI and for prevention of re-stenosis of coronaries after stenting
ADRs: Nausea, epigastric pain, diarrhea, rashes, risk of bleeding.
Prasugrel: More potent, faster & longer acting than clopidogrel → preferred in acute coronary syndromes & STEMI.
Contraindicated in TIA & stroke due to high risk of intracranial hemorrhage

Reversible
Ticagrelor
Faster onset of action than irreversible drugs, more potent
No effect of genetic polymorphism or enzyme inhibitors.
Effect is reversible → shorter duration of action → necessitating BD dose.
Recommended for all patients of ACS requiring urgent percutaneous intervention,
May be continued for up to one year.
ADRs: Nausea, Dizziness, Irregular pulse, Shortness of breath, Tightness in chest
Increased risk of intracranial hemorrhages.

P2Y$_{12}$ Antagonists
Binding of ADP to P2Y$_{12}$ receptors (G$_i$PCR) decreases cAMP & favours aggregation.
Antagonists raise cAMP → oppose aggregation.

TxA$_2$ Synthesis Inhibitors
Aspirin: Irreversible COX inhibition → decreases TxA$_2$ synthesis in platelets for lifespan of platelets (8–10 days)
Also decreases ADP release and sticking of platelets to each other.
Dose: 75–125 mg/day
At higher dose antiplatelet effect is lost due to decreased PGI$_2$ synthesis from endothelial cells.

Gp$_{IIb/IIIa}$ Blockers
Abciximab, Eptifibatide, Tirofiban inhibit the binding of fibrinogen to platelets → inhibit platelet aggregation
Abciximab: Inhibits platelet aggregation for 12–24 h.
Abciximab has shortest half-life in this group, but action lasts longer due to maximum affinity for GP$_{IIb/IIIa}$ receptors.
Uses: Unstable angina, ACS and 10–60 min before PCI along with aspirin and heparin → reduces incidence of subsequent restenosis, MI and death.
Also used in acute ischemic stroke
ADRs: Risk of bleeding, TCP

Miscellaneous
Dipyridamole and Cilostazol are PDE inhibitors that raise cAMP levels, which, in turn, decreases platelet aggregation.
Dipyridamole is useful in prophylaxis of thromboembolic phenomena in patients with TIA, prosthetic valves.
Cilostazol has role in PVD.
Vorapaxar and Atopaxar are protease activated receptor 1 (PAR-1) antagonists, used in patients with H/O MI or PVD.

Classification
TxA$_2$ synthesis inhibitors: Aspirin, other NSAIDs
P2Y$_{12}$ blockers
Irreversible: Ticlopidine, Clopidogrel, Prasugrel
Reversible: Ticagrelor, Cangrelor
GP$_{IIb/IIIa}$ receptor blockers: Abciximab, Eptifibatide, Tirofiban
Miscellaneous: Dipyridamole, Cilostazol, Vorapaxar, Atopaxar

FIBRINOLYTIC DRUGS

Streptokinase Urokinase
Mechanism of action: Exposes tPA binding site on plasminogen.
Activate both circulating & fibrin-bound plasminogen, → Greater risk of bleeding.
Not preferred

tPA Analogues
Moderate clot specificity: Alteplase, Reteplase, Duteplase.
High clot specificity: Tenecteplase.
Alteplase: Has half-life of only few minutes → slow intravenous infusion is used with heparin for MI, PE & stroke.
ADRs fever, nausea, fall in BP.
Reteplase: Has longer half-life → given as two IV bolus doses 30 minutes apart in STEMI & PE cases.
Tenecteplase: More specificity for fibrin-bound plasminogen → Lower risk of bleeding tendencies
Longer duration of action → single IV injection sufficient.

Uses
DVT of legs, shoulders, pelvis
For reperfusion therapy in STEMI.
To preserve lung function in pulmonary embolism.
Ischemic stroke
Limb artery occlusion if surgical thrombectomy cannot be done.

Contraindications
Conditions which predispose to risk of bleeding:
Peptic ulcer, esophageal varices
Any wound/fracture/tooth extraction/major surgery within preceeding 3 weeks
Brain tumours, aneurysm, intracranial hemorrhages within last one year (absolute contraindication),
Head injury
Bleeding disorders
Pregnancy

ADRs
Risk of bleeding especially intracranial bleeding
Fall in BP
Allergic reactions

SECTION 8 Drugs Affecting Blood

39 Hypolipidemic Drugs

PH 4.11 Explain salient pharmacokinetics, pharmacodynamics, therapeutic uses, adverse drug reactions of drugs used for the management of dyslipidemias and enumerate drugs leading to dyslipidemias.

Learning objectives

A student of MBBS phase II should be able to:
- Describe the various types of hyperlipidemias.
- Enumerate the drugs that disturb lipid levels.
- Classify the drugs used for hyperlipidemia.
- Describe the mechanisms of lipid-lowering action of various hypolipidemic drugs.
- Enumerate therapeutic uses of various hypolipidemic drugs and their doses.
- Enumerate ADRs and contraindications for the use of hypolipidemic drugs.

LIPID METABOLISM AND TRANSPORT

Lipids circulate in the body as **lipoproteins (LPs)** that have:

- A hydrophobic core with a variable amount of triglycerides (TGs) and cholesteryl esters (CHEs).
- An outer polar layer made up of phospholipids, apolipoproteins and cholesterol (Fig. 39.1).

There are **6 types** of LPs: Chylomicron, its remnants, very low density lipoproteins (VLDLs), intermediate density lipoproteins (IDLs), low density lipoproteins (LDLs), and high density lipoproteins (HDLs). The diameter of LP molecules increases from chylomicrons to HDL.

When LDL is linked to an (a) protein by a disulphide bond, it forms Lp(a). While LP(a) levels are genetically determined, they are also raised in some inflammatory conditions. Lp(a) is present in atheromatous plaques and raised Lp(a) levels may be associated with risk of coronary artery disease.

Lipid metabolism and transport in the body is described in Fig. 39.2.

1. Plant-based foods do not contain cholesterol. The TG content in the diet (100 g) is much higher than the cholesterol content (1 g).
2. Dietary lipids are absorbed from the intestine with the help of bile acids.
3. Dietary lipids exist in circulation as chylomicrons having TG >> CHE.
4. Endothelium-bound lipoprotein lipase enzyme (LPL) releases fatty acids (FAs) from chylomicrons, which are used by peripheral tissues as a source of energy or stored as TG in adipose tissue.
5. Chylomicron remnants, which are rich in CHE, are formed.
6. They are taken up by hepatocytes. CHE is de-esterified to release free cholesterol that is excreted in bile, incorporated in VLDL, or stored as TG (if in excess).
7. TGs are also formed by the liver from excess dietary carbohydrates.
8. TG-rich lipoprotein (VLDL) is released by the liver into circulation.
9. LPL releases FAs from TGs in VLDLs, forming IDLs that have CHE > TG.
10. IDLs keep on losing TG to form LDLs that have CHE >> TG.
11. LDL is internalised by receptor-mediated endocytosis and digested in liver and other tissues such as renal cells, muscles, lymphocytes and adrenal cortex.

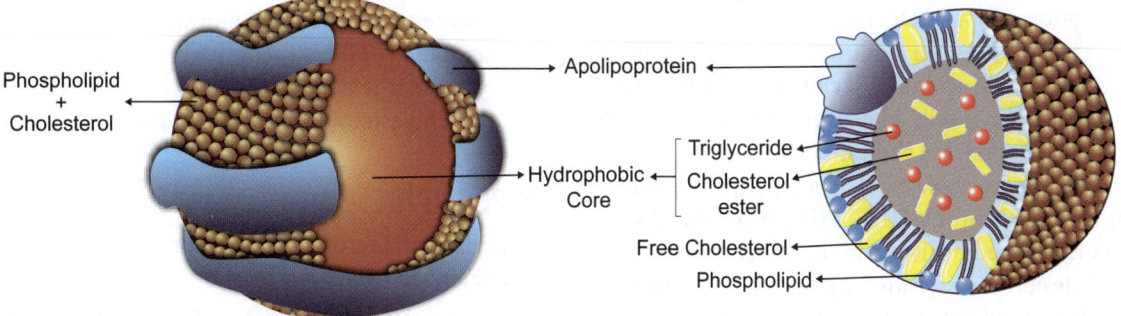

Fig. 39.1 Structure of lipoproteins

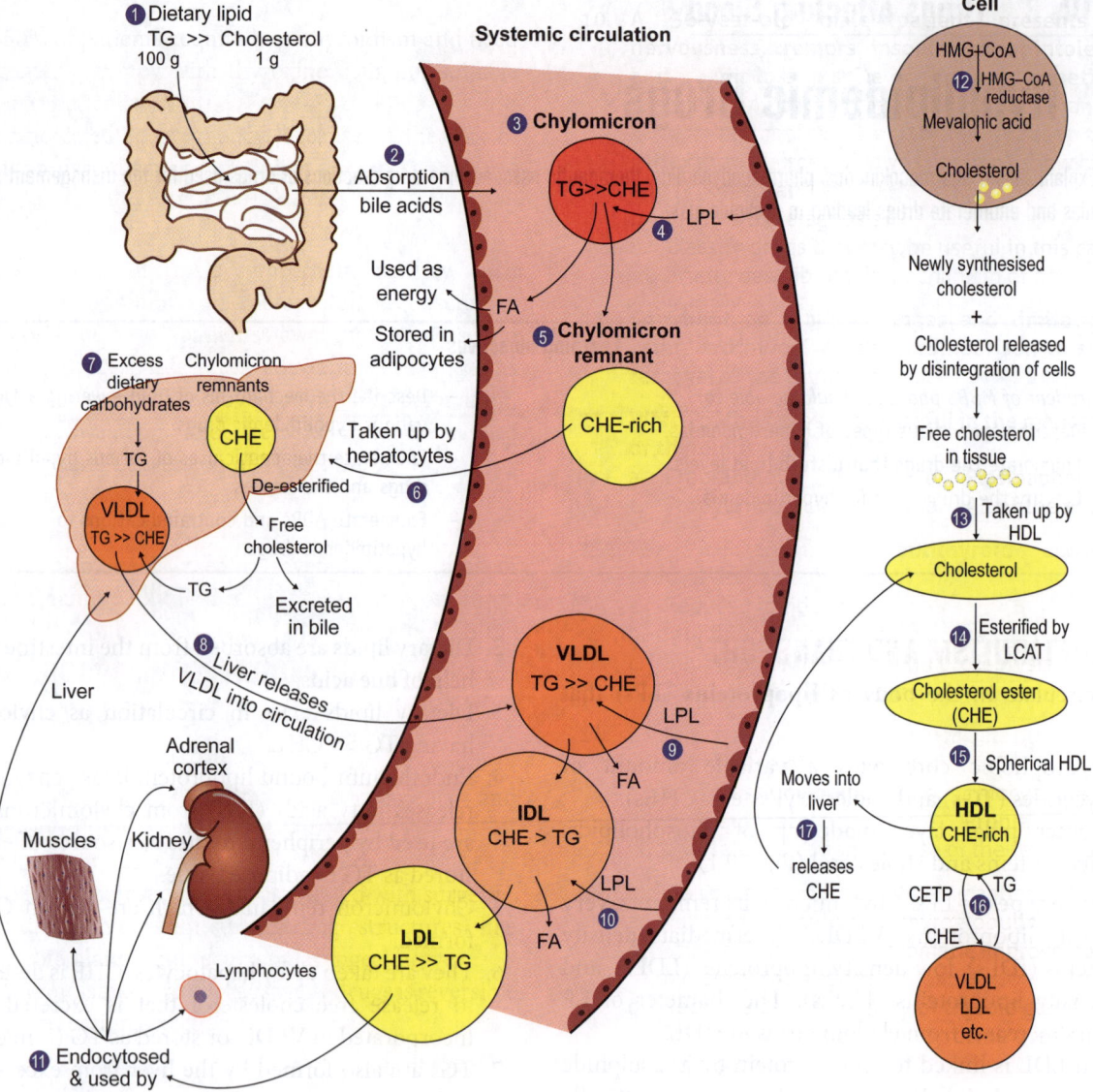

Fig. 39.2 Lipid metabolism and transport

Cholesterol released by de-esterification of CHE of LDL is utilised in body functions like the formation of membranes and steroidal hormone synthesis.

12. Cholesterol is also synthesised in cells by the reduction of HMG-CoA to mevalonic acid by action of the enzyme HMG-CoA reductase. The cholesterol content of the cell regulates both processes (LDL endocytosis and new cholesterol synthesis) by regulating the transcription of the LDL receptors and HMG-CoA reductase enzymes. In addition, liver cells convert cholesterol to bile acids and secrete it in the bile. Later on, disintegrating cells like liver parenchymal cells, and phagocytes release cholesterol.
13. This free excess cholesterol from peripheral tissues is rapidly taken up by HDL. HDL is a thin, discoid molecule secreted by liver and intestinal cells.
14. Free cholesterol is esterified by the LCAT enzyme to form cholesteryl esters (CHEs) in the hydrophobic core of HDL.
15. With the accumulation of CHE in its core, the HDL molecule becomes spherical.
16. The CHEs from spherical HDL molecules is then transferred to other lipoproteins (such as VLDL and LDL) in exchange for TG with help of cholesterol ester transport protein (CETP). Thus, the removal of excess cholesterol from peripheral tissues by HDL continues.
17. The HDL laden with CHEs moves into the liver and releases its CHE, following which the molecule is re-circulated. HDL is considered as 'good cholesterol', because it is the only lipoprotein that removes excess free cholesterol from peripheral tissues.

HYPERLIPIDEMIA

Hyperlipidemia or hyperlipoproteinemia (H↑LP) is characterised by:

- Plasma cholesterol levels > 200 mg/dL and TG > 150 mg/dL.

- Excess TGs (also called hyperlipemia) are stored in the adipose tissue and cause complications like obesity, diabetes, ketosis and other obesity-related problems.
- Raised LDL (> 500 mg/dL) is associated with the risk of acute pancreatitis.
- Increased levels of VLDLs and LDLs (prebeta-and beta-LPs) favour atheromatous deposition. Thus, they are considered as unfavourable or bad lipids.

In contrast, HDL or alpha LPs help in the removal of free cholesterol from peripheral tissues and have a protective role against atherogenesis; these are considered as good or favourable lipids.

Classification of Hyperlipidemia

I. Based on the cause

Hyperlipidemias (H↑LP) can be primary (1°) or secondary (2°).

a. Primary hyperlipidemia

Primary hyperlipidemia occurs due to single or multiple gene defects (called monogenic or polygenic, respectively). Dietary factors, lack of physical activity, and smoking contribute to the causation of hyperlipidemia.

b. Secondary hyperlipidemia

Secondary hyperlipidemia occurs because of other diseases or drugs.

- Diseases like DM, hypothyroidism, acromegaly, hypopituitarism, biliary obstruction, nephrotic syndrome, and pancreatitis.
- Chronic alcoholism and drugs like OCPs, β-blockers, and corticosteroids are commonly associated with hyperlipidemias.

Other drugs which may cause dyslipidemias are enumerated in Box 39.1.

> **Box 39.1 Drugs that cause dyslipidemia**
>
> 1. Drugs that increase both LDL and TG
>   - Corticosteroids, diuretics (loop and thiazides), estrogen, protease inhibitors, cyclosporine, tacrolimus, retinoids.
> 2. Drugs that increase only LDL:
>   - Amiodarone, anabolic steroids, anticonvulsant drugs (e.g., valproate, carbamazepine, gabapentin), direct-acting antiviral drugs against HCV, danazol, growth hormone.
> 3. Drugs that increase TG only:
>   - β blockers (especially non-selective blockers that lack ISA, e.g., propranolol, nadolol, timolol, etc.), antipsychotics (clozapine, olanzapine, quetiapine), tamoxifen.
> 4. Drugs that lower HDL levels:
>   - Anabolic steroids, β blockers, clozapine/olanzapine/quetiapine, danazol.

Metabolic syndrome, also called **syndrome X** or **Reaven syndrome**, is characterised by abdominal obesity, hypertension, impaired glucose tolerance, coronary artery disease and dyslipidemias. Marked lipoprotein abnormalities are present such as hypertriglyceridemia (H↑TG), fall in serum HDL levels, and LDL molecules that are smaller, denser and more atherogenic.

II. Frederickson classification

The classification has six types of hyperlipidemias: Types I, IIa, IIb, III, IV and V, of which **Types IIb and IV** are the most common.

a. Type I H↑LP

This is a rare type of hyperlipidemia involving familial deficiency of the LPL enzyme. Because the LPL enzyme is responsible for hydrolysis of TGs in the chylomicron core, its deficiency raises **chylomicron levels** in the plasma. Thus, both TG and CHE levels are raised.

b. Type II H↑LP

In this type of H↑LP, taking up and digestion of LDL by peripheral tissues is faulty due to gene-mediated receptor defects. It is characterised by **raised levels of LDL and cholesterol** and is further classified as: **Type IIa** (due to genetic causes; rare) and **Type IIb** (due to multiple causes; very common).

c. Type III H↑LP

Type III H↑LP is a rare genetic disorder called familial dysbetalipoproteinemia in which **IDL and chylomicron remnant levels are raised**. Plasma levels of both cholesterol and TG are slightly raised.

d. Type IV H↑LP

Type IV H↑LP is hypertriglyceridemia (H↑TG) involving **raised VLDL and TG** levels. However, cholesterol levels are normal.

e. Type V H↑LP

Type V H↑LP is familial combined hyperlipidemia in which levels of both **VLDL and LDL are raised**. Therefore, both cholesterol and TG levels in plasma increase.

III. Based on the lipid (cholesterol or TG)

Hyperlipidemias can be grouped into 3 groups (I, II and III), based on which lipid level is raised.

a. Group I

It is characterised by:

- Increase in cholesterol levels, up to 260–500 mg/dL.
- Increase in LDL or beta-lipoprotein levels.
- Normal triglycerides and clear serum.
- Defect in receptor-mediated endocytosis of LDL.

It is an autosomal dominant inherited disorder in 5% patients, and is aggravated in the majority by environmental factors. Raised LDL cholesterol is associated with increased risk of premature ischemic heart disease, painless tendon and tuberous xanthomas, xanthelasma (yellowish plaques near medial aspect of eyelids) and premature corneal arcus.

HMG-CoA reductase inhibitors, niacin and ezetimibe may be used in this condition.

b. Group II
The category is characterised by:
- Increase in triglyceride levels and cloudy serum.
- Increase in VLDL or prebeta-lipoproteins
- Cholesterol, however, is normal or moderately raised

This type of hyperlipidemia is associated with obesity, diabetes mellitus, gout, and increased risk of ischemic heart disease. If TG levels exceed 700 mg/dL, the LPL clearance mechanism becomes saturated, leading to a risk of acute pancreatitis.

c. Group III
This is a rare familial hyperlipidemia due to the deficiency of LPL enzyme, resulting in raised chylomicron levels even after 10 hours of fasting. Both TG and CHE levels are raised.

TG levels may reach 2000–3000 mg/dL; acute pancreatitis may occur, as well as eruptive xanthomas, hypersplenism, enlargement of liver and spleen, with presence of foam cells.

- VLDL may be moderately elevated.
- Marked restriction of dietary fat intake to < 15 g/day can effectively reduce TG levels. Niacin/ fibrates may reduce VLDL.

d. Others
Rarely, **HDL deficiency** may occur due to Tangier disease and LCAT deficiency. HDL levels may fall below 35–45 mg/dL, causing premature atherosclerotic changes. In some cases, it coexists with hypertriglyceridemia (H↑TG). Niacin may be useful.

MANAGEMENT OF HYPERLIPIDEMIA

Hyperlipidemia can be managed by various non-pharmacological and pharmacological measures.

Non-pharmacological Measures

Non-pharmacological measures such as dietary restrictions, aerobic exercises, weight reduction, restriction of alcohol, and smoking cessation are useful. Dietary restrictions are the initial measures to control hyperlipidemias.

- Total fat, excess calories and alcohol tend to raise TG levels, whereas saturated and trans fats increase LDL levels.
- Alcohol increases hepatic secretion of VLDL leading to H↑TG
- Excess caloric intake also increases synthesis and secretion of VLDL.

Thus, calorie restriction, weight reduction and alcohol avoidance are advised to reduce VLDL and LDL.

In patients with hyperlipidemias:
- Calories from fats should be 20–25% of the total daily calorie intake.
- Saturated fat should be < 8%.
- Total daily fat intake should be 10–20 g/day and cholesterol intake should be < 200 mg/day.
- Complex carbohydrates, fibre and cis-monounsaturated fats should predominate.
- Intake of omega-3 fatty acids, such as in fish oil, can markedly reduce TG levels.
- Fat-soluble vitamins are useful in primary chylomicronemia.
- In patients with homocysteinemia (homocysteine is proatherogenic), protein intake is restricted.
- Vitamin B and folic acid supplements are given.

Pharmacological Measures

Pharmacological measures or lipid-lowering drugs are used if normal lipid levels are not achieved by non-pharmacological measures alone.

CLASSIFICATION OF HYPOLIPIDEMIC DRUGS

These drugs are classified on basis of their mechanisms of action. Lipid levels can be lowered by:
- Decreasing the synthesis of TGs and cholesterol
- Increasing degradation
- Reducing absorption.

Drugs can lower lipid levels by interfering with biosynthesis (of TGs and cholesterol), decreasing intestinal sterol absorption, decreasing enterohepatic circulation, increasing hydrolysis of TGs and inhibiting CETP (Flowchart 39.1).

First-line hypolipidemic drugs include statins, bile acid binding resins and ezetimibe, whereas fibrates and niacin are considered as second-line drugs.

1. Statins: Drugs That Inhibit Cholesterol Synthesis

Atorvastatin, rosuvastatin, lovastatin, pravastatin, pitavastatin, and simvastatin belong to this class.

Mechanism of action

The fundamental lipid, **cholesterol**, is synthesised from acetyl-CoA in three stages.

Stage 1: The key building block of cholesterol, i.e., isopentenyl pyrophosphate is synthesised from acetyl-CoA, in the cytosol.

The formation of mevalonate from HMG-CoA, catalysed by the action of enzyme HMG-CoA reductase, is an irreversible step. It is the rate-limiting step in cholesterol biosynthesis (Fig. 39.3).

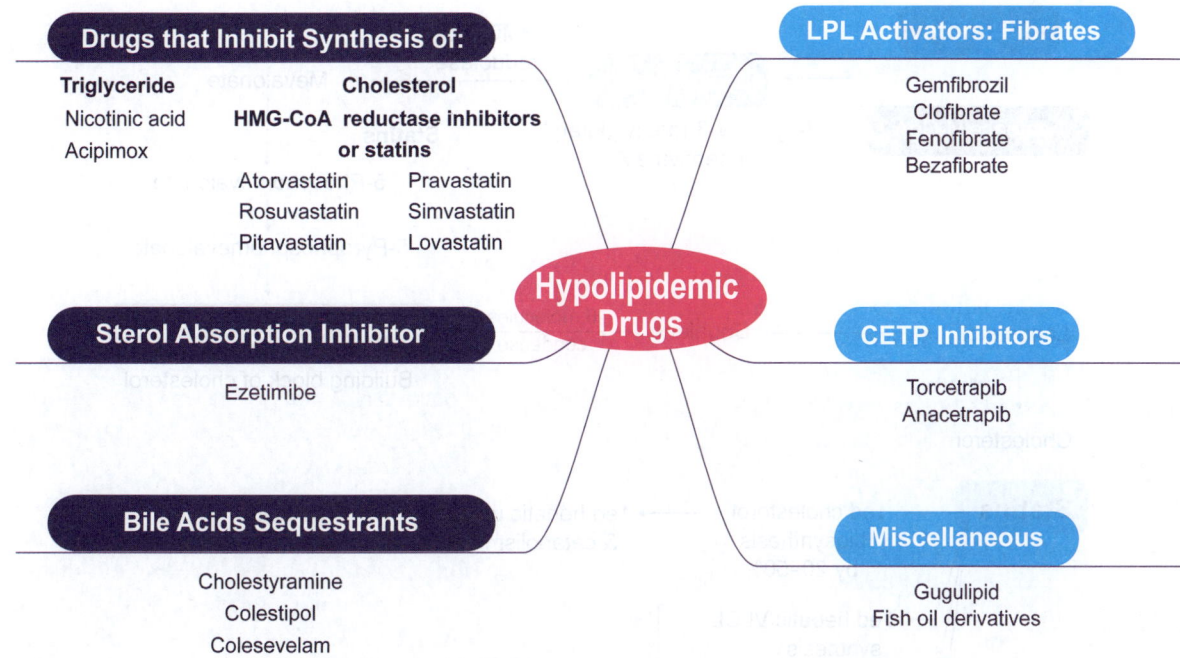

Flowchart 39.1 Classification of hypolipidemic drugs

Stage 2: Six molecules of isopentenyl pyrophosphate undergo condensation to form squalene.

Stage 3: The cyclisation of squalene yields a tetracyclic compound, which rearranges to forms lanosterol. Next, lanosterol is converted to cholesterol through a complex process

- Statins interfere with cholesterol biosynthesis by the **partial inhibition of enzyme HMG-CoA reductase**. Thus, cholesterol synthesis is reduced by 20–50%.
- Reduced biosynthesis of cholesterol induces increased expression of high affinity LDL receptors on hepatic cells which in turn **increase the hepatic uptake and catabolism of LDL**. Finally, after 1–2 weeks of therapy, **LDL cholesterol levels fall** in a dose-dependent manner.
  Different statins differ in potency and efficacy of LDL cholesterol-lowering effect. Lovastatin, pravastatin and simvastatin have low-to-moderate efficacy, whereas **rosuvastatin and atorvastatin have high efficacy**; pitavastatin is the most potent drug among statins.
- In addition, statins also reduce hepatic VLDL synthesis and increase its removal from plasma → **reduced VLDL levels** → 10–30% fall in plasma triglycerides.
- Some **rise in HDL cholesterol** is reported, especially with rosuvastatin.

Other mechanisms contributing to the anti-atherosclerotic action of statins include:

- Increased nitric oxide (NO) production and improvement of endothelial function.
- Reduced LDL oxidation.

In addition, statins also possess anti-inflammatory, anti-proliferative and anti-oxidant properties. These pleiotropic effects of statins lower the risk of stroke and MI.

Therapeutic uses

- Statins can be used alone or in combination with other lipid-lowering drugs to reduce LDL levels in patients having **moderate-to-severe hypercholesterolemia** with raised LDL cholesterol and total cholesterol, **with or without hypertriglyceridemia** (Type IIa, IIb, and V). Atorvastatin is the most commonly used statin. At a dose of 80 mg/dL, it decreases LDL cholesterol by 55–60%. It also reduces raised triglycerides and possesses antioxidant activity.
- In children, use of statins is restricted to **familial hypercholesterolemia** or familial combined hyperlipidemias.
- They are the **drugs of choice for dyslipidemias in diabetics**.
- Statins reduce the incidence of all atherosclerotic cardiovascular diseases such as ACS, unstable angina, stroke and peripheral arterial disease. These are also useful in the **secondary prophylaxis of MI**.
- Statins are used after knee/hip joint replacement surgery to **decrease the risk of venous thrombo-embolism (VTE)**.

The half-life of statins is 1–4 hours, except atorvastatin and rosuvastatin that have long plasma half-lives. **Atorvastatin is given as a single daily dose in the evening**, because the activity of HMG-CoA reductase peaks at midnight. Atorvastatin is given in a dose of 5–20 mg (maximum 40 mg).

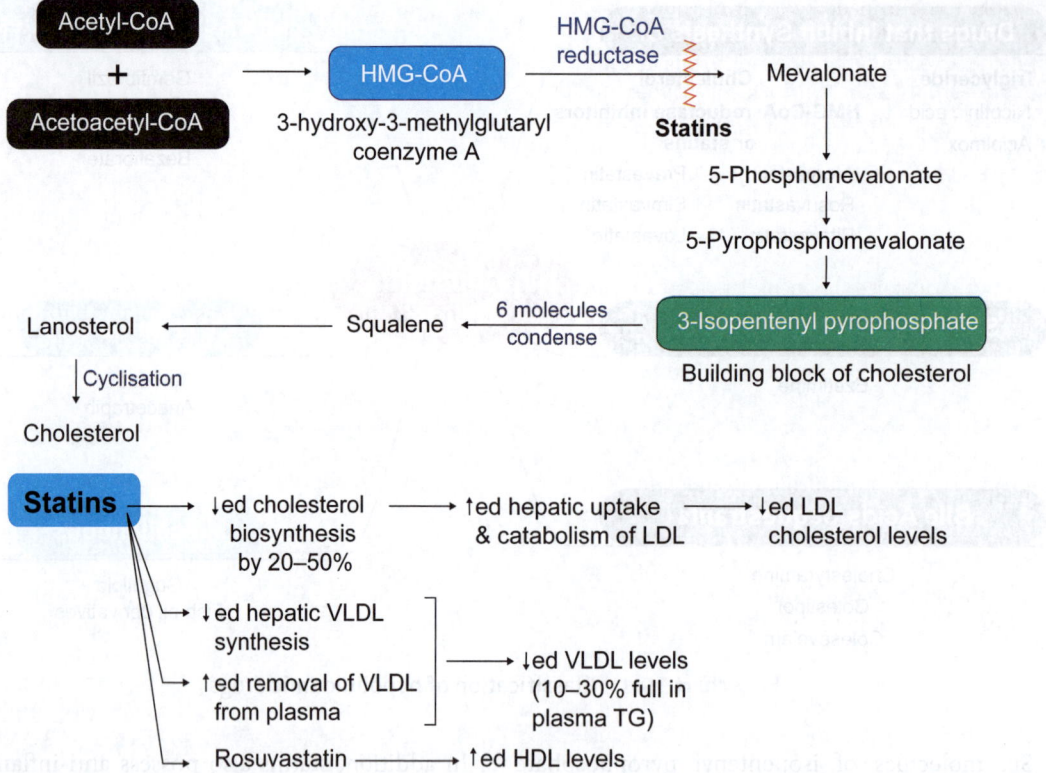

Fig. 39.3 Cholesterol biosynthesis and mechanism of action of statins

Adverse effects

These are well-tolerated drugs and can be continued indefinitely.

- Minor adverse effects like mild headache, muscle aches, and gastrointestinal symptoms may occur.
- Rarely, rashes, sleep disturbance, increased serum transaminase levels and myopathy may occur. CPK levels may rise.

Cautions/contraindications

Risk of liver injury and myopathy with statins is increased by renal insufficiency, old age and when used concurrently with drugs like:

- Nicotinic acid/gemfibrozil, which decrease the hepatic uptake of statin.
- Cytochrome P450 enzyme inhibitors like erythromycin, ketoconazole, and cyclosporine.

Statins should not be used in pregnant/lactating women or those planning pregnancy as data on their safety is not available.

2. Drugs That Inhibit Triglyceride Synthesis

Niacin (nicotinic acid) and acipimox are drugs that belong to this class.

Mechanism of Action

- **Niacin inhibits lipolysis by lipases in fat cells**, resulting in a decreased supply of free fatty acids (FFAs) from fat cells to the liver. Thus, production of TGs and VLDL in the liver decreases (Fig. 39.4). Niacin rapidly reduces VLDL and triglyceride levels by 20–50%.
- Direct **inhibition of TG synthesis in hepatic cells** and **increased clearance of TGs by LPL** may contribute to the TG-lowering effect of niacin.

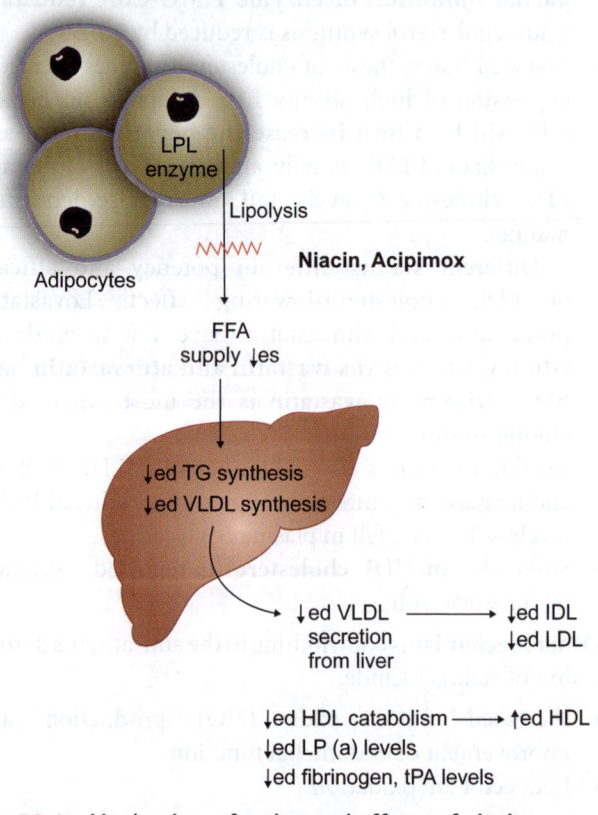

Fig. 39.4 Mechanism of action and effects of niacin

- Reduced secretion of VLDL from liver, in turn decreases levels of IDL and LDL cholesterol by 15–25%. It has no direct effect on cholesterol and bile acid metabolism.
- Niacin also decreases the rate of HDL catabolism; it **significantly raises HDL cholesterol levels** by 20–35%. This effect is achieved at a lower dose (1 g/day)
- Niacin also reduces levels of fibrinogen, tPA and LP(a), which is highly atherogenic. Niacin is the only hypolipidemic drug having LP(a) lowering effect.

Therapeutic uses

Niacin is effective in hypertriglyceridemia, with or without hypercholesterolemia (Type IIb and IV). However, it is used to lower VLDL and raise HDL levels in **high-risk cases only**.

- Niacin is useful to **control pancreatitis** associated with severe hypertriglyceridemia and for reducing the risk of such attacks in the future.
- Niacin may be used with statins or bile acid binding resins in some patients of nephrosis, familial and other hypercholesterolemias, combined hyperlipidemias, and dysbetalipoproteinemia.
- It is not used alone or with other drugs for atherosclerotic cardiovascular disease because of uncertain benefits.

Adverse effects

It is **poorly tolerated** in lipid-lowering doses.

- At the beginning of therapy, every dose of niacin causes a harmless **cutaneous vasodilation**, flushing (especially in the blush area), and a sensation of warmth and itching. This effect is prostaglandin-mediated and can be prevented or decreased by aspirin given half hour before niacin. Tolerance to this reaction develops within a few days.
- Nausea, abdominal pain, dyspepsia, diarrhea, vomiting, and peptic ulceration are common adverse reactions to the full dose. Thus, dose should **not exceed 2 g/day**.
- In some patients, rashes, dryness of skin and mucous membrane, pigmentation, pruritus, acanthosis nigricans (formation of dark, velvety patches in body creases/folds) and maculopathy may occur. If acanthosis nigricans occurs, niacin is contraindicated.
- Most important adverse effect is **serious hepatic damage** causing acute necrosis. Drug should be stopped in such cases. Thus, in all patients receiving niacin, liver function should be monitored regularly.
- Reversible impairment of glucose tolerance may occur in some latent diabetics.
- Hyperuricemia can occur, resulting in precipitation of acute gouty arthritis.
- Atrial arrhythmias, blurring of vision and reversible amblyopia may occur rarely.
- It should not be used in pregnancy, as teratogenic effects have been reported in animal studies.

Acipimox is a derivative of nicotinic acid that has fewer adverse effects; however, its plasma lipid lowering efficacy is also low.

Clinical problem-based questions and MCQs

1. i. Which of the following lipid lowering drugs inhibits cholesterol biosynthesis?
   a. Ezetimibe b. Lovastatin
   c. Colestipol d. Niacin
   ii. Describe the mechanism of action of the selected drug.
   iii. Enumerate the uses and adverse effects of the selected drug.

2. Which of the following is the most potent statin?
   a. Atorvastatin b. Pitavastatin
   c. Rosuvastatin d. Lovastatin

3. Which of the following statins has the most efficacious LDL-lowering action?
   a. Lovastatin b. Rosuvastatin
   c. Pravastatin d. Simvastatin

4. i. Which of the following drugs is most useful in hypertriglyceridemia?
   a. Nicotinic acid b. Ezetimibe
   c. Gemfibrozil d. Rosuvastatin
   ii. Describe mechanism of action and enumerate uses and adverse effects of the selected drug.

5. A 60-year-old male patient had NSTEMI a year ago. He is receiving treatment with ARBs, lisinopril, β-blocker metoprolol and aspirin. On examination, his BMI = 35 kg/m^2 and BP = 140/85. Investigation revealed that his lipid profile is disturbed; total cholesterol = 220 mg/dL, TG = 154 mg/dL, HDL = 39 mg/dL and LDL cholesterol = 156 mg/dL. He is prescribed rosuvastatin 20 mg/day
   i. What is the pharmacological basis for giving rosuvastatin?
   ii. Enumerate the adverse effects of rosuvastatin.

3. Drugs that Increase Lipid Breakdown (Lipolysis)

This category includes fibrates like clofibrate, gemfibrozil, bezafibrate and fenofibrate.

Mechanisms of action of fibrates

Fibrates act through nuclear peroxisome proliferator-activated receptor α (PPAR-α) present in liver, muscle and fat cells (Fig. 39.5). Activation of PPAR-α receptor regulates gene transcription resulting in:

- **Increased LPL synthesis** → VLDL degradation leading to lowering of VLDL secretion by liver and circulating TG levels by 20–50%.
- **Increased LDL receptor expression** in liver → causes increase in uptake and utilisation of LDL → reduces LDL levels by 10–15%.

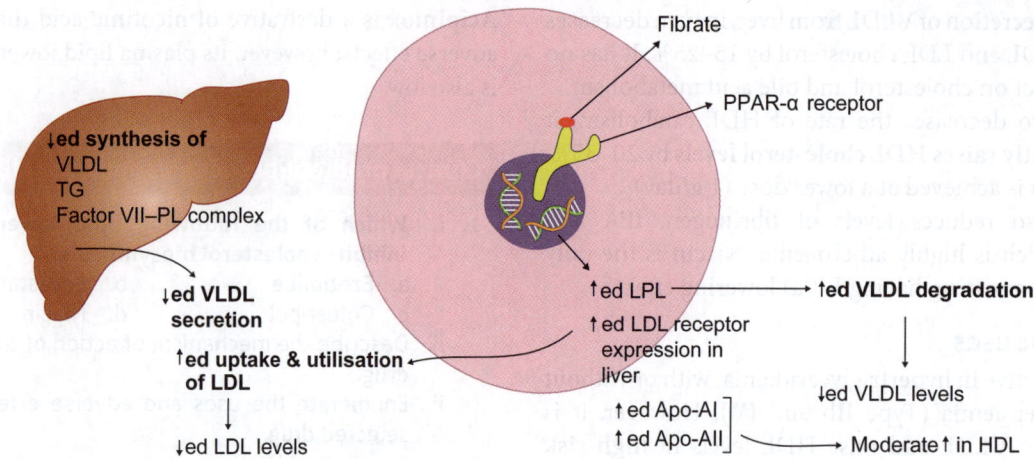

Fig. 39.5 Mechanism of action and effects of fibrates

- Increased fatty acid oxidation in liver and striated muscles.
- Down-regulation of apo-CIII, which is an inhibitor of lipolysis.
- Moderate increase in HDL cholesterol occurs because of increased transport of surface lipids from degraded VLDL to HDL and the increased production of apo-AI and apo-AII.
- In addition, gemfibrozil suppresses hepatic synthesis of TG, factor VII–phospholipid complex and promotes fibrinolysis.

Therapeutic uses

These are useful in hypertriglyceridemias and dysbetalipoproteinemia.

- Hypertriglyceridemia that occurs after use of viral protease inhibitors also responds to fibrates.
  Gemfibrozil (600 mg, twice a day before meals) is a **first-line drug in hypertriglyceridemia** (type III, IV and V) and the **acute pancreatitis** associated with it. Chylomicronemia can be prevented.
- It is also useful in patients with low HDL cholesterol as diabetes type 2 and metabolic syndrome.

Bezafibrate and fenofibrate are second-generation fibrates with greater efficacy in raising HDL and lowering VLDL levels, with fewer adverse effects. These do not increase the risk of rhabdomyolysis when combined with statins.

Saroglitazar acts as an agonist at PPAR-α and γ receptors. It lowers blood glucose (FBS, HbA_{1c}) as well as plasma TG and total cholesterol. It is approved in India only for treatment of **diabetic dyslipidemia and H↑TG not responding to statins**.

However, routine use of fibrates in primary or secondary prophylaxis of atherosclerotic CVD, chronic renal disease or diabetes is not recommended.

Adverse effects

Common ADRs seen with fibrates include:

- Epigastric pain, dyspepsia and diarrhea.
- Headache, blurring of vision, body aches and myalgias.
- Rashes.
- In patients with impaired renal function, fibrates can cause rhabdomyolysis, myoglobulinuria and acute renal failure.
- Risk of myopathy is greater if they are combined with statins. However, such a risk is minimal with second-generation fibrates such as bezafibrate and fenofibrate.
- Fibrates are not used during pregnancy.
- Currently, clofibrate is not used because of high mortality (due to malignancy and post-cholecystectomy complications) associated with its use.

4. Drugs That Decrease Lipid Absorption

Ezetimibe is a new drug that interferes with absorption of dietary and biliary cholesterol from the intestine. It acts by inhibiting the action of cholesterol transporter protein, Niemann-Pick C1-Like 1 (NPC1L1), in the intestinal mucosa → the reduced intestinal absorption of cholesterol, in turn, leads to increased hepatic cholesterol synthesis, which can be blocked by combining statins.

Thus, **ezetimibe and statins have synergistic cholesterol-lowering effect.** Consequently, ezetimibe (10 mg once a day) is mainly used as an adjuvant to statins in primary hypercholesterolemia to achieve good LDL cholesterol-lowering effect with low dose of statins.

ADRs such as reversible liver dysfunction and myositis may occur.

5. Drugs That Decrease Enterohepatic Circulation of Bile Acids

These include bile acid sequestrants or resins like cholestyramine, colestipol and colesevelam.

Mechanism of action

- The liver synthesises bile acids from cholesterol by 7-α-hydroxylation. Bile acids normally undergo enterohepatic circulation (EHC, Fig. 39.6). These drugs

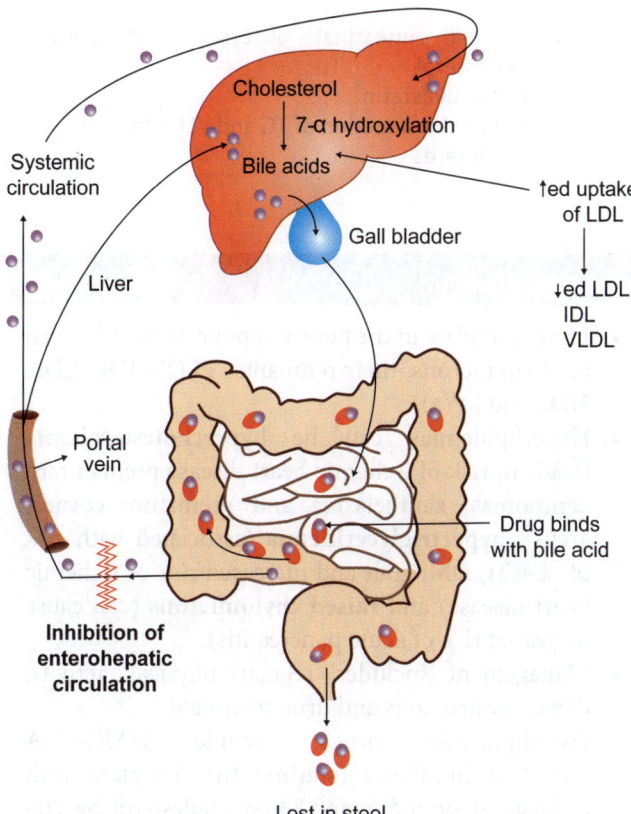

Fig. 39.6 Mechanism of action of cholestyramine
Loss of bile acids in stool → increased conversion of cholesterol to bile acids → Hepatic pool of cholesterol decreases

bind to bile acids in the intestinal lumen and interfere with their enterohepatic circulation. So, excretion of bile acids and cholesterol in the stool is increased up to 10 times the normal amount.
- Indirect effects include increased hepatic metabolism of cholesterol to bile acids via 7-α-hydroxylation → leading to reduction in the hepatic cholesterol pool (Fig. 39.6).
- Up-regulation of LDL receptors on hepatocytes and clearance of LDL (and indirectly that of IDL and VLDL) also increases.

Uses
Bile acid sequestrants are useful in **primary hypercholesterolemia**. These are the drugs of choice for lowering cholesterol levels during pregnancy and lactation and in children.
- Pruritus occurring in patients of cholestasis may be relieved by these drugs.
- They can bind to unabsorbed digoxin and increase its elimination in stool; so, they may be useful in digitalis toxicity.

ADRs
- These drugs are **not preferred** because large doses (up to 20 g/day) are required, the taste is unpleasant, multiple doses may cause GI disturbances, they are inconvenient, and have poor patient acceptability.
- Constipation, bloating sensation and dyspepsia may occur.
- These drugs impair the absorption of fat soluble vitamins and folic acid. Deficiency of vitamin K leads to hypoprothrombinemia.
- They may increase the risk of gallstones, especially in obese patients.
- These interfere with the absorption of many other drugs like digoxin, thiazide diuretics, iron, warfarin, aspirin, and statins. Thus, drug administration should be delayed for 1–2 hours after giving bile acid sequestrants.

6. CETP Inhibitors
Cholesteryl ester transfer protein (CETP) transfers cholesterol from HDL to LDL and VLDL. Torcetrapib and anacetrapib inhibit this transport of CE, significantly increasing HDL and decreasing LDL.

7. Miscellaneous
a. Gugulipid is derived from guggul gum and contains E and Z guggulsterones. It acts by:
- Decreasing cholesterol synthesis.
- Increasing cholesterol excretion.

Thus, it reduces total cholesterol and LDL, causes a modest fall in TG levels, and increases HDL.

ADRs: Loose stools are the main adverse effect; otherwise, it is very well tolerated.

b. Fish oil derivatives contain polyunsaturated fatty acids, omega-3 fatty acids. They have membrane-stabilising and antioxidant properties, and are used for prevention of IHD in high-risk CAD patients with hyperlipidemias.

> ### Clinical problem-based questions and MCQs
> 6. A 20-year-old female patient presents with dull upper abdominal pain that radiates to the back, accompanied by vomiting for the past 24 hours. Pain is relieved slightly on bending forward. On examination, the patient has epigastric tenderness and high-grade fever. Investigations show raised levels of serum amylase and triglycerides.
>   i. Identify the drug of first choice to lower TG levels in this case.
>   a. Atorvastatin   b. Niacin
>   c. Gemfibrozil   d. Acipimox
>   ii. Explain the mechanism of action of the chosen drug.
>   iii. Enumerate the therapeutic uses and adverse effects of the selected drug.

7. Which of the following fibrates may be combined with rosuvastatin if needed?
   a. Gemfibrozil
   b. Clofibrate
   c. Fenofibrate
   d. None of the above

8. Identify the drug used for diabetic dyslipidemia not responding to statins.
   a. Niacin
   b. Ezetimibe
   c. Saroglitazar
   d. Torcetrapib

9. i. Identify the drug that acts synergistically with statins in primary hypercholesterolemia.
      a. Ezetimibe
      b. Saroglitazar
      c. Acipimox
      d. Gemfibrozil
   ii. Describe the mechanism of synergistic action of the selected drug with statins.

10. i. Identify the drug that interferes with enterohepatic circulation of bile acids
       a. Gemfibrozil
       b. Acipimox
       c. Colestipol
       d. Ezetimibe
    ii. Describe mechanism of action, uses and adverse effects of the selected drug.

11. A 45-year-old hypertensive patient on thiazide therapy shows raised cholesterol levels in his routine follow-up examination. The patient is put on cholestyramine therapy but advised to take this drug after 1–2 hours of thiazides. Describe the pharmacological basis of using cholestyramine and advised time gap between the two medications.

12. Fibrates lower lipids by all the following mechanisms, EXCEPT:
    a. Increased degradation of VLDL
    b. Increased LDL uptake and utilisation
    c. Apo-CIII down-regulation
    d. Inhibition of cholesterol transporter protein

13. i. Identify the inhibitor of Niemann-Pick C1-Like 1 protein responsible for intestinal cholesterol absorption.
       a. Anacetrapib
       b. Ezetimibe
       c. Gemfibrozil
       d. Colestipol
    ii. Describe the interaction of the selected drug with statins.

14. i. Identify the dual PPAR-α and γ inhibitor.
       a. Fenofibrate
       b. Saroglitazar
       c. Pitavastatin
       d. Colesevelam
    ii. Describe the effects and uses of the selected drug.

15. Match the lipid-lowering action with the drug that exhibits it.
    a. Reduced enterohepatic circulation of bile acids
       1. Niacin
    b. Inhibition of cholesterol biosynthesis
       2. Ezetimibe
    c. Reduced intestinal absorption of dietary cholesterol
       3. Rosuvastatin
    d. Reduced production of TG and VLDL in liver
       4. Fibrates

Summary

- Lipids circulate in the body as lipoproteins (LP) such as chylomicrons, their remnants, VLDL, IDL, LDL, HDL and LP(a).
- Hyperlipidemias can be **hypercholesterolemia** (leads to risk of ischemic heart disease prematurely, xanthomas, xanthelasma and premature corneal arcus), **hypertriglyceridemia** (associated with risk of obesity, DM, gout and increased risk of ischemic heart disease) and **raised chylomicrons** (can cause increased risk of acute pancreatitis).
- Management includes regular physical activity, dietary restrictions and drug treatment.
- Hypolipidemic drugs include HMG-CoA reductase inhibitors (**statins**) that interfere with cholesterol synthesis and lower cholesterol by 20–50%. Atorvastatin and rosuvastatin are the most efficacious, while pitavastatin is the most potent statin. These are useful in primary and secondary hyperlipidemias with raised cholesterol levels, with or without raised TG. ADRs like GI upset, rashes, sleep disturbances, headache and myalgias are common.
- **Nicotinic acid** inhibits lipolysis by lipases in fat cells, leading to the reduced production of TGs and VLDL in the liver. Niacin rapidly reduces levels of VLDL and triglycerides, and is effective in hypertriglyceridemia and risk of acute pancreatitis; it is not used frequently due to many adverse effects like cutaneous vasodilatation at initiation of therapy, GI upset, severe hepatic damage, and cardiac arrhythmias.
- **Fibrates** activate the PPAR-α receptor, that regulates gene transcription, and results in increased LPL synthesis, LDL receptor expression in liver → causes increased uptake and utilisation of LDL → thus reducing LDL levels. Gemfibrozil is a first-line drug in hypertriglyceridemia, acute pancreatitis associated with H↑TG. It is not combined with statins as it increases the risk of myopathy. However, second-generation drugs (bezafibrate and fenofibrate) can be combined with statins as they do not increase the risk of rhabdomyolysis.

- **Ezetimibe** interferes with intestinal absorption of dietary cholesterol by inhibiting NPC1L1 and synergises with statins for cholesterol-lowering action.
- **Bile acid sequestrants** such as cholestyramine, colestipol and colesevelam lower cholesterol by interfering with their enterohepatic circulation. These are the drugs of choice during pregnancy and lactation and in children with **primary hypercholesterolemia**. However, they are **not preferred** in other patients because of the need of large doses (up to 20 g/day), unpleasant taste, GI disturbances, inconvenient dose schedule and poor patient acceptability.

Questions for practice

1. Classify lipid lowering drugs.
2. Describe mechanism of lipid lowering effect of:
   a. Rosuvastatin
   b. Ezetimibe
   c. Fenofibrate
   d. Niacin
   e. Colestipol
3. Explain why:
   a. Statins are usually given as a single evening dose.
   b. Niacin rapidly reduces TG levels but is not a preferred drug for hypertriglyceridemia.
   c. Gemfibrozil is usually not combined with statins.
   d. Ezetimibe is used as adjuvant to statins.
   e. Bile acid sequestrants are not preferred in treatment of hypercholesterolemia.
4. Enumerate ADRs of:
   a. Nicotinic acid
   b. Bile acid sequestrants
5. Enumerate drugs useful in:
   a. Hypercholesterolemia
   b. Hypertriglyceridemia

Hints for problem-based questions and MCQs

1. i. b. Lovastatin
   ii. HMG-CoA reductase is a rate-limiting enzyme in cholesterol biosynthesis. Its inhibition by statins prevents the conversion of HMG-CoA into mevalonate.
   iii. Statins are used in primary and secondary hyperlipidemias with raised cholesterol, with or without raised triglycerides. ADRs include GIT upset, rashes, sleep disturbances, headache and myalgia.
2. b. Pitavastatin
3. b. Rosuvastatin
4. i. a. Nicotinic acid
   ii. It acts by inhibiting lipolysis in fat cells, leading to reduced production of TG and VLDL in liver. Niacin is useful in hypertriglyceridemia and to reduce the risk of acute pancreatitis. ADRs include initial cutaneous vasodilatation, GI intolerance, severe hepatic damage and cardiac arrhythmias.
5. i. It inhibits cholesterol biosynthesis by HMG-CoA reductase inhibitor action
   ii. Refer to page 528.
6. i. c. Gemfibrozil
   ii. Activation of PPAR-α receptor regulates gene transcription that results in LPL synthesis, LDL receptor expression in liver, and hence reduced LDL levels.
   iii. Used in hypertriglyceridemia and acute pancreatitis. ADRs include increase in risk of rhabdomyolysis
7. c. Fenofibrate can be combined with statins as it does not increase risk of rhabdomyolysis.
8. c. Saroglitazar.
9. i. a. Ezetimibe
   ii. Ezetimibe decreases intestinal absorption of cholesterol, which stimulates hepatic synthesis that can be blocked by adding statins.
10. i. c. Colestipol
    ii. Useful in hypercholesterolemia, but not preferred, because of adverse effects. Refer to page 531.
11. Cholestyramine can interfere with absorption of thiazides.
12. d. Inhibition of cholesterol transport protein.
13. b. Ezetimibe inhibits NPC1L1 and reduces intestinal absorption of cholesterol.
14. i. b. Saroglitazar
    ii. It is used for diabetic dyslipidemia and hypertriglyceridemia not responding to statins.
15. a–4; b–3; c–2; d–1.

CONCEPT MAP – HYPOLIPIDEMIC DRUGS

Classification

Drugs Inhibiting Synthesis of

Triglyceride: Nicotinic acid, Acipimox

Cholesterol: HMG-CoA reductase inhibitors or statins like
Atorvastatin, Rosuvastatin, Pitavastatin
Pravastatin, Simvastatin, Lovastatin

Sterol Absorption Inhibitors: Ezetimibe

Bile Acid Sequestrants:
Cholestyramine, Colestipol, Colesevelam

LPL Activators: Fibrates:
Gemfibrozil, Clofibrate, Fenofibrate, Bezafibrate

CETP Inhibitors:
Torcetrapib, Anacetrapib

Miscellaneous:
Gugulipid, Fish oil derivatives

Statins

Mechanism:
- Inhibit HMG-CoA reductase → decrease cholesterol biosynthesis
- Decrease hepatic VLDL synthesis
- Increase VLDL removal
- Increase hepatic LDL uptake,
- Rosuvastatin raises HDL

Uses:
Drug of choice for dyslipidemia in diabetics
Moderate-to-severe hypercholesterolemia (IIa, IIb, V)
Familial hypercholesterolemia or combined hyperlipidemia
Secondary prophylaxis of MI
Joint replacement to prevent thrombo-embolism

ADRs:
GI upset, rashes, sleep disturbances, headache, myalgias, raised serum transaminases & CPK

Caution:
- Pregnancy, lactation
- With niacin, fibrates, enzyme inhibitors
    ↓
    increased risk of hepatic injury & myopathy

Types of hyperlipidemias

Primary: Monogenic, polygenic
Secondary: to diseases or drugs
Frederickson's types: I, IIa, IIb, III, IV, V
Based on lipid raised:
Group I: Cholesterol raised, TG normal
Group II: TG raised, Cholesterol normal
Group III: Both TG & cholesterol raised.
Tangier's disease, LCAT deficiency : HDL decreased.

HYPOLIPIDEMIC DRUGS

Ezetimibe

Mechanism: Interferes with intestinal absorption of dietary cholesterol by inhibiting cholesterol transport protein in intestinal mucosa, in turn causes increased biosynthesis, that is blocked with statins.

Uses: Used as adjuvant to statins to reduce their dose

ADRs: Reversible liver damage
Myositis

Torcetrapib

Mechanism: Causes CETP inhibition → reduced transfer of CHE from HDL to LDL & VLDL
    ↓
Marked increase in HDL, fall in LDL

Bile acid Sequestrants

Mechanism: Cholesterol forms bile acids which undergo enterohepatic circulation.
Cholestyramine binds to bile acids, reduces their enterohepatic circulation → increased loss of bile acids & cholesterol in stool

In turn hepatic synthesis of bile acids from cholesterol increases → reduced hepatic cholesterol pool
Also increases clearance of LDL, VLDL

Uses: Effective in primary hypercholesterolemia, but not preferred
Pruritus associated with cholestasis
Digoxin toxicity

ADRs: High dose, unpleasant taste → poor patient acceptability
GI intolerance, constipation, bloating, dyspepsia,
Vitamin K deficiency, hypo-prothrombinemia
Increased risk of gallstones

Fibrates

Mechanism:
Activate PPAR-α receptors in liver/muscle/fat cells
    ↓
Increased LPL synthesis
Increased degradation of VLDL
Increased uptake and utilisation of LDL
Moderate increase in HDL cholesterol
Gemfibrozil reduces TG synthesis in liver, promotes fibrinolysis

Uses: Gemfibrozil is DOC in hypertriglyceridemia (after viral PI use)
Dysbetalipoproteinemia
Acute pancreatitis (in type III, IV, V)
Chylomicronemia,
Type 2 DM & metabolic syndrome

ADRs: Epigastric pain, dyspepsia, diarrhea, headache, visual disturbances, rash, myalgia, rhabdomyolysis, ARF
Myopathy (more when combined with statins, niacin)
Not used in pregnancy

2nd generation fibrates:
Bezafibrate, Fenofibrate have more efficacy,
Fewer ADRs, do not increase rhabdomyolysis with statins

Saroglitazar:
PPAR-α and γ agonist → Reduces FBS, HbA1C, TG, Total cholesterol
Used in diabetic dyslipidemias, hypertriglyceridemia unresponsive to statins

Nicotinic Acid, Acipimox

Nicotinic Acid
Mechanism: inhibit lipolysis in adipocytes → decreased supply of FFA to hepatocytes for TG & VLDL synthesis
- Decrease VLDL secretion from liver → fall in IDL, LDL
- Decrease rate of HDL catabolism → rise in HDL levels

Uses: Hypertriglyceridemia with or without hypercholesterolemia (type IIb, IV)
To control and prevent pancreatitis
No benefit in atherosclerotic cardiovascular disease

ADRs: Poorly tolerated
PG-mediated cutaneous vasodilatation → warmth, itching, prevented with aspirin pretreatment
GI intolerance, rashes, dry skin, pigmentation, pruritus, acanthosis nigricans
Acute hepatic necrosis (liver function to be monitored)
Hyperuricemia, glucose intolerance, arrhythmias
Blurring of vision, amblyopia
Teratogenic

Acipimox: Niacin derivative, less efficacious, better tolerated

SECTION 8 Drugs Affecting Blood

40 Hematinics

PH 4.1 Explain types, salient pharmacokinetics, pharmacodynamics, therapeutic uses, adverse drug reactions of drugs used for different anemias and thrombocytopenia.

Learning objectives

A student of MBBS phase II should be able to:
- Enumerate the causes of anemia.
- Describe the process of absorption, transport, storage and utilisation of iron.
- Enumerate iron preparations.
- Enumerate indications for use and adverse effects of oral and parenteral iron preparations.
- Calculate total iron dose for a patient with iron deficiency anemia.
- Describe the features and management of acute and chronic iron poisoning.
- Describe the physiological role of vitamin B_{12}.
- Describe features and management of vitamin B_{12} deficiency.
- Describe physiological role of folic acid.
- Describe features and management of folic acid deficiency.
- Enumerate colony stimulating factors (CSFs).
- Describe mechanism of action of CSFs.
- Enumerate indications, adverse effects of and contraindications to CSFs.
- Comment on use of CSFs in cancer chemotherapy.

Hematopoiesis is the process of formation of undifferentiated stem cells in the bone marrow, which then differentiate to form erythrocytes, leukocytes and platelets. Adequate functioning of the hematopoietic machinery essentially requires three nutrients—**iron, folic acid and vitamin B_{12}**—called **hematinics**. The proliferation and differentiation of hematopoietic cells is regulated by **hematopoietic growth factors**. Therefore, inadequate supply of these hematinics or growth factors manifests as a deficiency of functioning blood cells.

- Deficiency of erythrocytes results in reduced oxygen carrying capacity of blood and is called **anemia**. This is the most frequently encountered hematological disorder.
- Deficiency of leukocytes, called **leukopenia or neutropenia,** weakens the body's defence against infection.
- Deficiency of platelets is called **thrombocytopenia** and causes defective clot formation, leading to bleeding disorders.

ANEMIA

A variety of factors involving imbalance between the rate of production and destruction of RBCs can cause **anemia**. **Common causes** of anemia include:
- **Impaired formation** of RBCs because of:
  - **Deficiency of essential nutrients,** i.e., iron, vitamin B_{12} and folic acid. Iron deficiency causes microcytic, hypochromic anemia, whereas deficiency of vitamin B_{12} and folic acid causes megaloblastic anemia. These are easily treated by supplementing the deficient nutrients.
  - **Bone marrow suppression** may occur due to several diseases or drugs. This results in deficiency of all types of blood cells, leading to aplastic anemia, leukopenia and thrombocytopenia. Such anemias are difficult to treat and need correction of the underlying cause.
  - **Erythropoietin deficiency** may occur in chronic kidney disease resulting in anemia that requires treatment with erythropoietin stimulating agents (ESA).
- **Increased destruction of RBCs** due to a variety of diseases (inherited blood disorders such as sickle cell anemia, infections, autoimmune or malignant diseases and hypersplenism) or drugs causes hemolytic anemias. Here, treatment of the cause is important.
- **Acute or chronic blood loss** causes anemia

Anemic patients present with pallor, easy fatigability, dyspnea on exertion, generalised malaise, dizziness, etc.

HEMATINICS FOR MANAGEMENT OF ANEMIA

Hematinics are nutrients that are essential for hematopoiesis. Nutritional deficiency anemias are easily preventable and treatable using iron, vitamins B_{12} and folic acid.

I. IRON

Iron acts as a cofactor for several hemoproteins/heme proteins and non-heme proteins.

- Hemoproteins are hemoglobin (Hb), myoglobin, catalase, peroxidase and cytochromal enzymes. These are involved in O_2 binding and transport, electron transport and mitochondrial respiration.
- Non-heme proteins play a crucial role in cell proliferation, differentiation, gene regulation, drug metabolism and steroid synthesis.

Total Body Iron

The total body iron in adults is 50–60 mg/kg body weight, i.e., 3500–4000 mg in an adult weighing 70 kg.

- Hemoglobin contains 65% of the total body iron.
- Myoglobin and other heme-containing enzymes contain 10%.
- Iron is stored only in the ferric (Fe^{3+}) form, in combination with a large protein called apoferritin.

    Apoferritin + Fe^{3+} → Ferritin → Aggregates to form hemosiderin.

    The most important storage sites are the reticuloendothelial cells (RE) that contain approximately 12% of the total body iron. Ferritin content in hepatocytes varies from 5–25%, depending upon the iron status.

- Bone marrow cells have 3–4% of the total body iron.

Daily iron requirement: 0.5–1 mg iron is required daily in men and 1–2 mg in women to make up for the daily loss. However, pregnant women require about 3.5 mg iron daily in the last 2 trimesters for the expansion of RBCs, transfer to the fetus, and to compensate for loss during delivery. Infants require about 60 mcg/kg body weight and children, 25 mcg/kg body weight iron daily.

Dietary sources of iron include:

Rich sources—Liver, egg yolk, dry beans, dry fruits, yeast, etc.
Medium sources—Meat, chicken, fish, banana, spinach, apple, etc.

Iron absorption

The average daily diet has 10–20 mg of iron, which is absorbed all over the intestine but mainly in the upper part of the duodenum. Iron constantly changes between various oxidation states during the process of absorption. Among them, the divalent (ferrous, Fe^{2+}) and trivalent (ferric, Fe^{3+}) states are the most common. Dietary iron is present in 2 forms (Fig. 40.1):

- Heme form—It is the smaller fraction of dietary iron that is better absorbed (up to 35%). The heme form is absorbed from the intestinal lumen to enterocytes via the 'heme carrier protein 1' (HCP-1); this process is largely unaffected by the presence of other foods.
- Inorganic form—It is present in the ferric form (Fe^{3+}) and is reduced to the ferrous (Fe^{2+}) form and absorbed

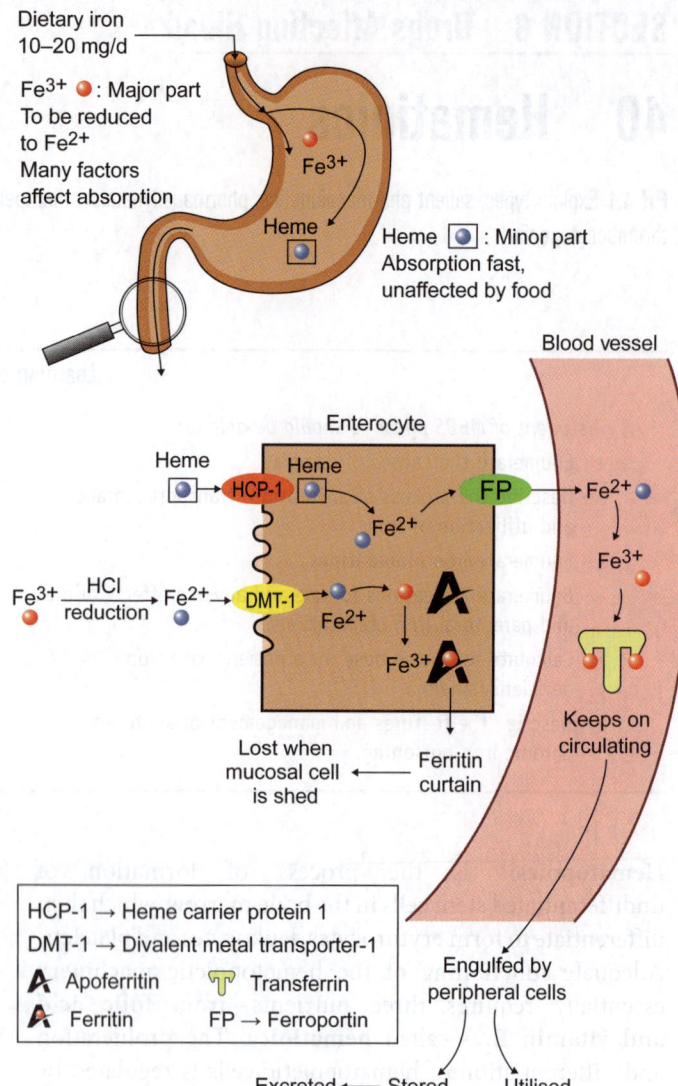

Fig. 40.1 Iron absorption

via 'divalent metal transporter 1' (DMT-1) into enterocytes. The extent of absorption is just 5%, and is affected by several factors.

Once iron enters a mucosal cell, it is either transported into the plasma [as Fe^{2+} via ferroportin (FP)] or stored as ferritin.

- The iron that stays back inside mucosal cells is oxidised to Fe^{3+} ($Fe^{2+} \rightarrow Fe^{3+}$). The Fe^{3+} form combines with apoferritin to form **ferritin**, which is the **stored form of iron in mucosal cells** and lost when the cells are shed (lifespan = 2–4 days). This is the **ferritin curtain,** which blocks the entry of excess iron into the plasma; however, this mucosal block can be overcome by a gross excess of iron.
- In the plasma, Fe^{2+} is oxidised to Fe^{3+} → Fe^{3+} binds to **transferrin** and keeps on circulating. The total iron content in the plasma = 3 mg; it is recycled 10 times/day, indicating that the daily turnover of iron is 30 mg.

Transferrin can get attached to specific membrane-bound receptors (Fig. 40.2) → Fe^{3+}–transferrin complex is engulfed and iron is released intracellularly.

In this manner, iron is either used for erythropoiesis or stored. Iron is **stored in reticulo-endothelial cells in the liver, spleen, bone marrow, myocytes and hepatocytes.** In iron deficiency, the number of transferrin receptors in erythropoietic cells increases.

Normally, the balance between these 2 processes is governed by the iron status of the body, e.g., a larger percentage of iron moves into the plasma during a state of iron deficiency. So, in iron deficiency, either the formation of ferritin is less or it dissociates soon and transcription of apoferritin does not occur (the reverse occurs in iron overload).

Iron derived from the destruction of old RBCs, from iron stores, and from intestinal absorption forms a common pool available for erythropoiesis and to replenish iron stores.

Iron excretion: On a daily basis, 0.5–1 mg iron is lost in the form of:
- Exfoliated gastrointestinal mucosal cells, some RBCs, and bile lost in feces.
- Desquamation of skin
- Small amount excreted in sweat and urine also contribute to iron loss.
- During menstruation, additional iron loss is 0.5–1 mg/day.

Therapeutic Uses of Iron
- Treatment of iron deficiency anemia.
- Prophylaxis of iron deficiency anemia in menstruation, pregnancy, infants, menorrhagia, blood loss, chronic illness, etc.
- Megaloblastic anemia: Stimulation of erythropoiesis after correction of vitamin B_{12} and folic acid deficiencies may unmask iron deficiency; accordingly, iron should be administered.
- Ferric chloride is used as an astringent in throat pain.

Iron Preparations and Doses
Important preparations of iron (oral and parenteral) are shown in Flowchart 40.1.

Oral iron preparations
Dissociable ferrous salts are better absorbed than ferric salts. These are cheaper and have high iron content.

Carbonyl iron is a very finely powdered form of high purity iron. It has better gastrointestinal tolerability than other preparations.

The combination of iron and folic acid containing hematinics with vitamin B complex and zinc is **not recommended**. Sustained release (SR) preparations of iron are also irrational because most of iron absorption occurs in upper intestines, whereas these preparations release major part of their iron in the lower intestines, which is excreted in the feces.

Dose: Total **200 mg** elemental iron (child: 3–5 mg/kg) given daily in 3 divided doses yields maximal hematopoietic response. Prophylactic dose = **30 mg** daily.

Though iron absorption is better when taken on an empty stomach, it is usually given as **small doses between meals** because of gastric irritant effects.

Adverse effects of oral iron
- Epigastric pain, nausea, and vomiting.
- Heartburn
- Constipation due to astringent action or diarrhea due to irritant action of iron may occur. Such gastric irritant effects are related to total quantity of elemental iron administered.
- Metallic taste.
- Teeth-staining is more likely with liquid iron preparations.

Parenteral iron preparations
Parenteral iron preparations are indicated in the following conditions:
- Oral iron is not tolerated (intolerable bowel upset).

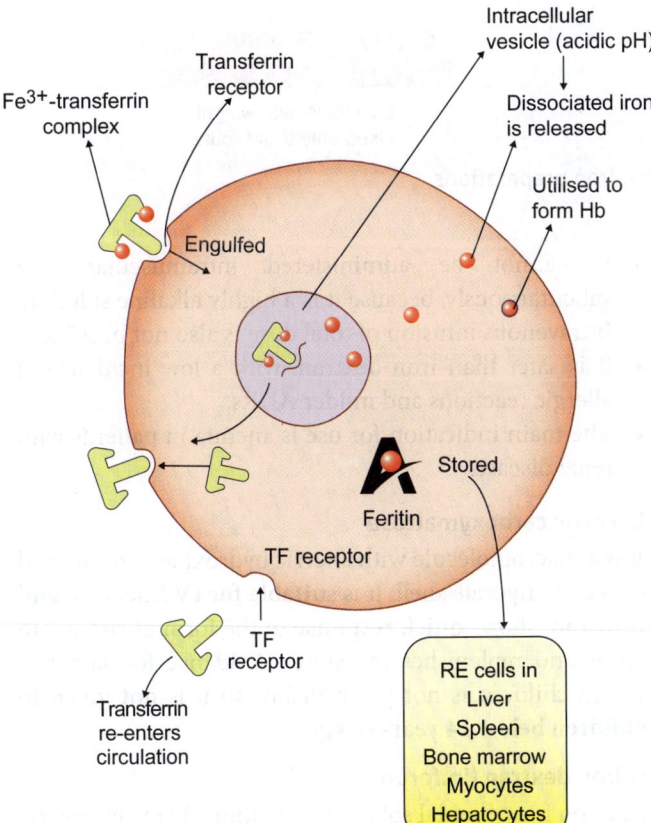

Fig. 40.2 Transport, storage and utilisation of iron in an erythropoietic cell

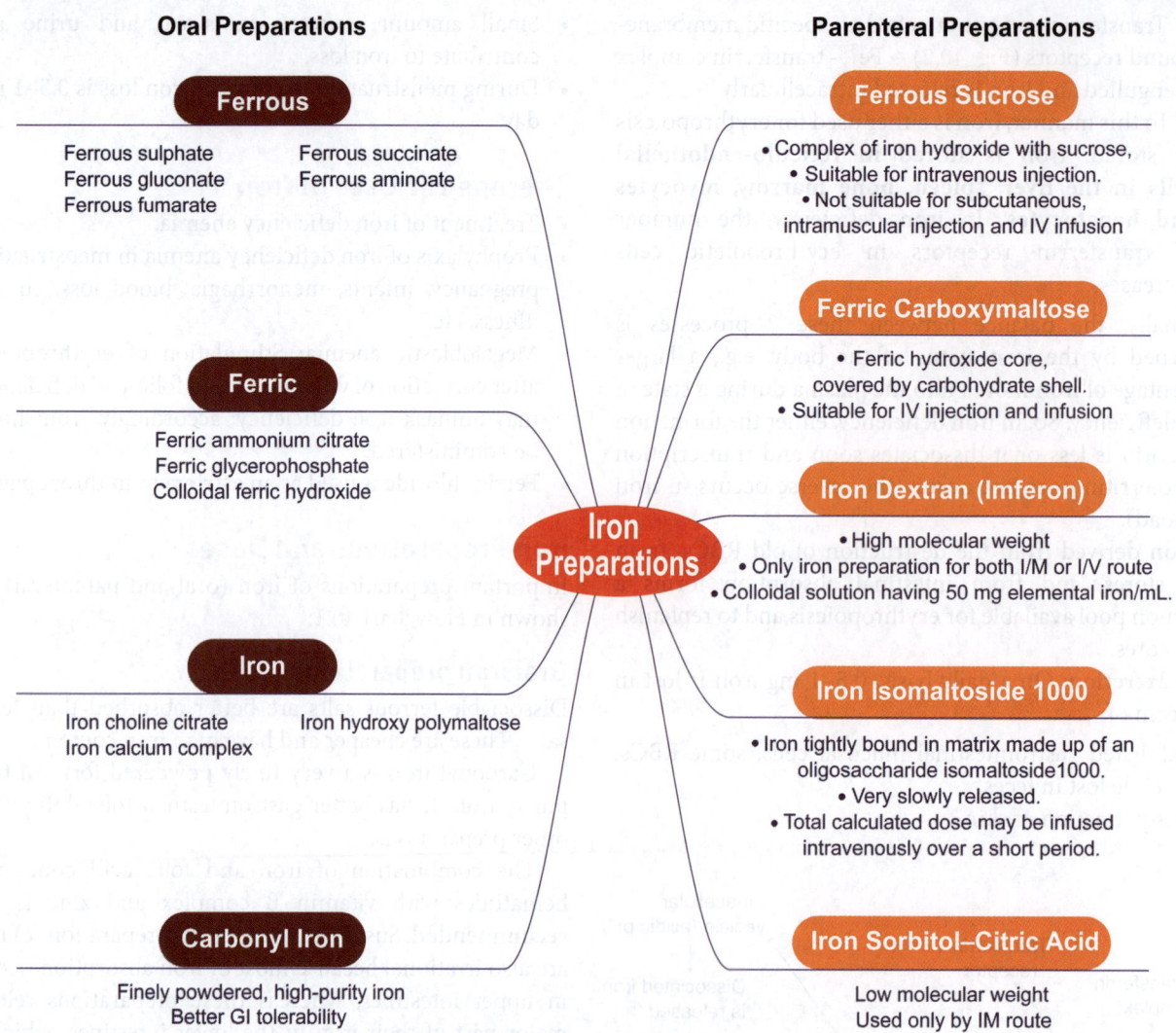

Flowchart 40.1 Different iron preparations

- Oral iron is not absorbed (malabsorption, inflammatory bowel disease (IBD), and chronic inflammation).
- Noncompliance to oral iron therapy.
- Severe deficiency with chronic bleeding.
- Along with erythropoietin (oral iron may not be absorbed at a rate sufficient to meet the demands of induced rapid erythropoiesis).

Total dose of iron required = 4.4 × Body Weight (kg) × Hb Deficit (g/dL)

Important features of parenteral iron preparations are described below:

a. Ferrous sucrose

Ferrous sucrose is a complex of iron hydroxide with sucrose, suitable for intravenous injection in a dose of 200 mg in 5 minutes, daily or weekly, till the total calculated dose is given. It is taken up by the reticulo-endothelial cells, where it dissociates and makes the iron available. It is not suitable for subcutaneous and intramuscular injections or for intravenous infusion.

- It cannot be administered intramuscularly or subcutaneously, because it is a highly alkaline solution. Intravenous infusion of total dose is also not possible.
- It is safer than iron dextran, with a low incidence of allergic reactions and milder ADRs.
- The main indication for use is anemia in patients with renal disease.

b. Ferric carboxymaltose

It is a macromolecule with a ferric hydroxide core covered by a carbohydrate shell. It is **suitable for IV injection and infusion**, shows **quick response** in the form of rise in Hb levels and replenishes the stores. Evidence for safety of use in children is not yet available, so it is **not given to children below 14 years of age.**

c. Iron dextran (Imferon)

Imferon is a colloidal solution containing 50 mg elemental iron/mL.

- High molecular weight

- It is the only iron preparation that can be used by both I/M or I/V routes.
  - **Intramuscular** administration: It is administered deeply in gluteal region by the Z-track technique (to avoid skin staining). Because 10–30% local binding occurs, the actual dose administered is 25% more than the calculated dose. After I/M use, absorption occurs through the lymphatics. The injection **causes local pain** that may last for many weeks.
  - **Intravenous** administration: After a test dose of 0.5 mL, iron dextran is given as 2 mL intravenous injection over 5–10 minutes daily. For total dose infusion (TDI), the total calculated dose is diluted in 500 mL glucose/saline and infused over 6–8 hours under observation. If the patient complains of symptoms like **giddiness, paresthesia, and chest constriction**, the infusion is stopped.
- It is taken up by macrophages and slowly made available for erythropoiesis.

d. Iron isomaltoside 1000

It is most recent parenteral iron preparation where iron is tightly bound in a matrix made up of an oligosaccharide, isomaltoside 1000. After IV injection, it is taken up by reticulo-endothelial cells. Because the iron is tightly bound to the matrix, it is released very slowly. Doses as large as 1–2 g can be given intravenously over 15–30 minutes. Thus, it is more convenient and economical, because **total calculated dose may be infused intravenously over a short period**.

- It has low potential to cause immune reactions.
- ADRs are milder.

e. Iron sorbitol–citric acid

The iron sorbitol–citric acid complex has low molecular weight. It is meant only for intramuscular use and there is no local binding of the drug. From the site of IM injection, it is directly absorbed into the systemic circulation and is available for heme synthesis; it binds to transferrin with high affinity and may saturate it.

Important differences between iron dextran and iron sorbitol–citric acid are listed in Table 40.1.

ADRs of parenteral iron

Local ADRs: Pain at I/M injection site, skin pigmentation, sterile abscess (especially in old debilitated patients).

Systemic ADRs: Fever, headache, joint pain, flushing, palpitation, chest pain, dyspnea, lymphadenopathy. Metallic taste is more frequently seen with IV use than IM use.

Acute Iron Poisoning

Acute iron poisoning occurs mostly in infants and children after consuming 10–20 tablets. Patients present with vomiting, abdominal pain, hematemesis, diarrhea, dehydration, lethargy, cyanosis, acidosis, convulsions, shock, cardiovascular collapse, and death.

Treatment is:

- Supportive: Fluid–electrolyte balance, respiratory support, correction of acidosis, diazepam for convulsions, etc.
- Induce vomiting or gastric lavage with $NaHCO_3$.
- Milk and egg yolk are given because they can form complexes with iron and decrease further absorption.
- Desferrioxamine is a chelating agent, given intramuscularly in a dose of 0.5–1 g, and can be repeated after 4–12 hours as required.
- Calcium edetate may be an alternative, but BAL is contraindicated as a chelating agent, because the iron–BAL chelate is also toxic.

Chronic iron toxicity or overload may occur in an inherited disorder known as **hemochromatosis**, which is characterised by excessive iron absorption, and in patients receiving repeated blood transfusions, e.g., for thalassemia major. Excessive deposition of iron in the heart, liver, pancreas and other organs may cause organ failure and death. It is treated using iron chelating agents like desferrioxamine and deferasirox and by intermittent phlebotomy (where a unit of blood is removed weekly).

Table 40.1 Comparison of iron dextran and iron sorbitol–citric acid

Property	Iron dextran	Iron sorbitol–citric acid
Molecular weight	High	Low
Route of administration	IV or IM route	Only by IM route
Local binding	10–30% binding to the local tissue upon IM injection	No local binding at site of IM injection
Absorption after IM administration	Through lymphatic system	Directly into systemic circulation
Availability for heme synthesis	First taken up by macrophages and then slowly made available for heme synthesis	Directly available for heme synthesis
Affinity for transferrin	Low, does not bind to transferrin	High, may saturate transferrin

Clinical problem-based questions and MCQs

1. Which of the following iron preparations can be used by both IM and IV routes?
   a. Ferrous sucrose
   b. Ferric carboxymaltose
   c. Iron dextran
   d. Iron isomaltoside

2. All of the following occur in iron deficiency anemia EXCEPT:
   a. Content of Hb in erythrocyte decreases
   b. Size of erythrocyte decreases
   c. Number of erythrocytic transferrin receptors decreases
   d. Larger percentage of iron moves into plasma.

3. i. Identify the oral iron preparation with better gastrointestinal tolerability.
      a. Ferrous gluconate
      b. Iron choline citrate.
      c. Ferric ammonium citrate
      d. Carbonyl iron
   ii. Enumerate the various oral and parenteral preparations of iron.
   iii. List the adverse effects of oral and parenteral iron.

4. A 35-year-old female patient presents with fatigue, generalised malaise, exertional dyspnea and dizziness. On examination, patient weighs 60 kg, is pale, finger nails are soft, scooped out (koilonychia). Hb = 6 g/dL, PBF shows microcytic, hypochromic anemia.
   i. What is this patient suffering from?
   ii. What is the total dose of correcting hematinic, if total dose infusion is planned?

5. All of the following iron preparations can be used for total dose infusion, except:
   a. Ferrous sucrose
   b. Iron dextran
   c. Iron carboxymaltose
   d. Iron isomaltoside 1000

6. A 6-year-old boy is brought to emergency with vomiting, diarrhea, dehydration, abdominal pain and convulsions. Patient is lethargic and semiconscious; peripheral cyanosis is present. His mother gives history of intake of about 20 tablets of sugar-coated iron preparation.
   i. What is the likely diagnosis?
   ii. All of the following are useful in this case, except:
      a. Gastric lavage with $NaHCO_3$
      b. BAL
      c. Calcium edetate
      d. Diazepam

II. VITAMIN B_{12}

Vitamin B_{12} (cyanocobalamin or hydroxocobalamin) is synthesised only by microorganisms and acquired from them by plants and animals.
Sources: Liver, kidney, sea fish, meat, egg yolk, cheese, legumes (pulses).

Daily requirement: 1–3 mcg; increases to 3–5 mcg during pregnancy/lactation.

Role of B_{12} in the Body

The active co-enzyme forms of vit. B_{12} in the body are deoxyadenosylcobalamin (DA B_{12}) and methylcobalamin (methyl B_{12}).

1. Vitamin B_{12} plays an important role in **making tetrahydrofolic acid (THFA) available for reutilisation** (Fig. 40.3). In vit. B_{12} deficiency, THFA is trapped in the methyl form and one-carbon transfer reactions (such as purine and pyrimidine synthesis) and DNA synthesis are affected. This is called the **methylfolate trap**. This step links the metabolism of B_{12} and folic acid (Fig. 40.4).

2. Methyl B_{12} is essential (Fig. 40.3) for the conversion of **homocysteine to methionine**, which is required as a methyl donor in many protein synthesis reactions. As a result, in vitamin B_{12} deficiency, serum homocysteine levels are raised. **Raised homocysteine levels** can increase the risk of atherosclerotic cardiovascular disease and also help to diagnose vitamin B_{12} deficiency.

   Anemia caused by B_{12} deficiency can be partially corrected by large doses of folic acid, because it gets reduced to DHFA and provides an alternative source of THFA (Fig. 40.4).

3. S-adenosyl methionine, which is required for the synthesis of phospholipids and myelin, is synthesised from methionine; DA B_{12} acts as a coenzyme in this reaction.

$$\text{Methionine} \xrightarrow{\text{DA } B_{12}} \text{S-adenosyl methionine}$$
(used for myelin, PL synthesis)

Therefore, in B_{12} deficiency, **demyelination and neurological damage** occur. Because THFA has no role in this reaction, the administration of folic acid cannot prevent neurological damage caused by B_{12} deficiency; however, anemia improves. So, if folic acid alone is given in B_{12} deficiency, it stimulates erythropoiesis and **hematological improvement occurs. However, neurological symptoms keep on deteriorating**, as the meagre amount of available B_{12} is diverted to erythropoiesis. Thus, folic acid should not be used alone in B_{12} deficiency anemias.

4. DA B_{12} is required for the **formation of succinyl-CoA** from methylmalonyl-CoA by the action of enzyme methylmalonyl-CoA mutase.

$$\text{Methylmalonyl-CoA} \xrightarrow[\text{DA } B_{12}]{\text{Methylmalonyl-CoA mutase}} \text{Succinyl-CoA}$$

Thus, in vitamin B_{12} deficiency, **serum and urine concentrations of methylmalonyl-CoA** and methylmalonic acid increase; this helps to establish

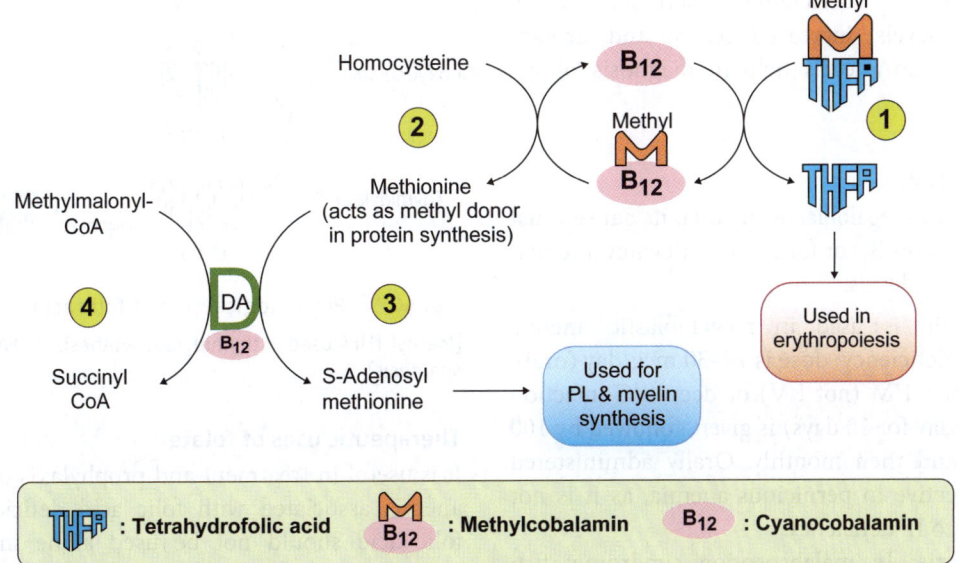

Fig. 40.3 Physiological role of vitamin B_{12}.
Methyl B_{12} converts: 1. Methyl THFA to THFA; 2. Homocysteine to methionine. DA B12 converts: 3. Methionine to S-adenosyl methionine; 4. Methylmalonyl-CoA to succinyl-CoA

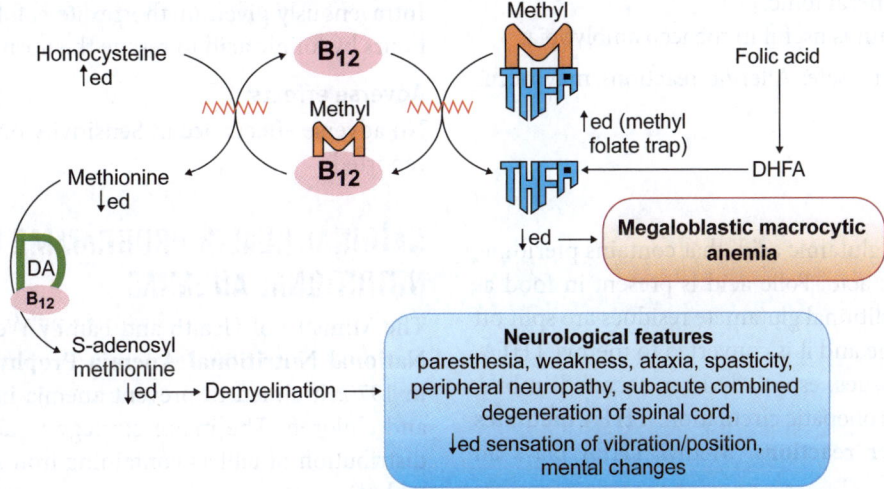

Fig. 40.4 Deficiency of vitamin B_{12}. → Fall in THFA → hematological features. Reduced S-adenosyl methionine → neurological features. Increased serum homocysteine, methylmalonyl-CoA → help in diagnosis of vitamin B_{12} deficiency.

the diagnosis and has been implicated in causation of neurological manifestations of B_{12} deficiency.

- Intrinsic factor (IF) secreted by the stomach helps in the oral absorption of B_{12}.
- Transcobalamin II (TC II) transports B_{12} in the blood.
- It is taken up and stored by liver cells.
- Vitamin B_{12} is not degraded in the body, undergoes enterohepatic circulation, and is excreted in bile.

Deficiency of B_{12}

Deficiency of vitamin B_{12} can occur in pernicious anemia involving defective IF secretion from gastric mucosa, malabsorption syndrome, IBD, diseases of the distal ileum, total/partial gastrectomy and small bowel resection. Patient presents with:

- Megaloblastic, macrocytic anemia, glossitis and GI disturbances,
- Neurological syndromes starting with paresthesia and weakness, progressing to ataxia, spasticity, etc. These may be accompanied by subacute combined degeneration of the spinal cord, peripheral neuritis, decrease in vibration and position senses and mental changes.
- Mild-to-moderate leukopenia and thrombocytopenia may also occur.
- Hypercellular bone marrow with accumulation of megaloblastic erythroid cells and other precursors.

Diagnosis of B_{12} deficiency: increased serum homocysteine levels, increased serum and urinary methylmalonyl CoA levels help in diagnosis of B_{12} deficiency

Therapeutic uses

When a patient has megaloblastic anemia, its **cause must be identified** (vitamin B_{12} or folic acid deficiency anemia) by measuring serum levels.

- Cyanocobalamin is used in megaloblastic anemia caused by B_{12} deficiency; dose is 10–30 mcg/day (oral). In IF deficiency, I/M (not I/V) or deep S/C injection (30–100 mcg/day for 10 days) is given, followed by 100 mcg weekly and then monthly. Orally administered B_{12} is not effective in pernicious anemia, as it is not absorbed due to IF deficiency.
- For **prophylaxis**: In malabsorption syndrome, fish tapeworm infestation, pregnancy, infant, chronic gastritis, etc., dosage is 3–10 mcg/day.
- In neuropathies, cutaneous sarcoid and psychiatric disorders, as a general tonic.
- Hydroxocobalamin is useful in tobacco amblyopia.

Adverse effects: Very safe. Allergic reactions may occur on parenteral use.

III. FOLIC ACID

Folic acid is 'pteroylglutamic acid' that contains pteridine, PABA and glutamic acid. Folic acid is present in food as polyglutamates. Additional glutamate residues are split off in the upper intestine and it is converted to methyl THFA. This is stored in tissues, especially liver, secreted in bile, and undergoes enterohepatic circulation. **THFA mediates one-carbon transfer reactions**. Methyl THFA plays an important role in:

- Conversion of homocysteine to methionine (Fig. 40.3).
- Generation of thymidylate from deoxyuridylate (Fig. 40.5).
- THFA plays a role in the conversion of serine to glycine.

Thus, folic acid is important for purine synthesis and the generation and utilisation of the formate pool.

Deficiency of folic acid can be dietary or because of malabsorption syndrome, biliary fistula, chronic alcoholism, liver disease or increased demand (e.g., pregnancy and hemolysis). Drugs such as methotrexate, trimethoprim and pyrimethamine, which inhibit dihydrofolate reductase, can also cause folic acid deficiency.

Clinical features of deficiency

Megaloblastic anemia, glossitis, diarrhea, steatorrhea, generalised weakness, weight loss and sterility. However, unlike B_{12} deficiency, there are **no neurological symptoms**.

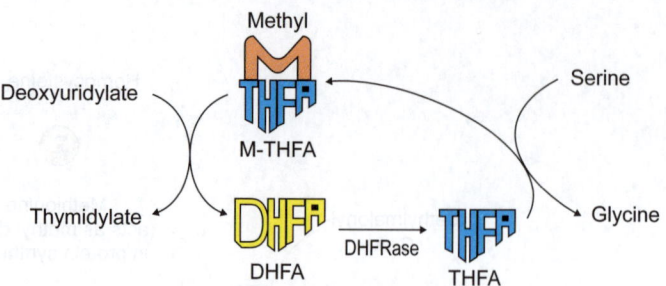

Fig. 40.5 Physiological role of folic acid
[Methyl THFA used in thymidylate synthesis; THFA used in glycine synthesis]

Therapeutic uses of folate

It is useful in treatment and prophylaxis of megaloblastic anemia associated with folic acid deficiency. However, folic acid should not be used alone in patients with B_{12} deficiency anemia, as there is a risk of worsening of neurological features.

Methotrexate toxicity: Folinic acid (5-formyl-THFA) or citrovorum factor rescue prevents methotrexate toxicity. Intravenously given methotrexate is followed within ½–2 hours by folinic acid to rescue the normal cells).

Adverse effects

No adverse effects occur. Sensitivity on injection is rarely reported.

NATIONAL HEALTH PROGRAMME FOR NUTRITIONAL ANEMIAS

The Ministry of Health and Family Welfare launched the **National Nutritional Anemia Prophylaxis Programme** in 1970. It aimed to prevent anemia in pregnant women and children. The major strategy to achieve this was by distribution of tablets containing iron and folic acid (IFA tablets).

In 2013, the **National Iron Plus Initiative** was launched for the supplementation and treatment of anemia in children, adolescents, and pregnant/lactating women through the life cycle approach.

In 2018, the **Anemia Mukt Bharat** strategy was launched by Government of India. It aimed at reducing anemia in vulnerable age groups using the 6×6×6 strategy, in which there are six target beneficiaries, six interventions and six institutional mechanisms to implement the National Iron Plus Initiative.

The **target beneficiaries** of Anemia Mukt Bharat strategy are:

- Children between 6 months to 59 months of age (preschool children).
- Children 5–9 years of age (Classes 1–5 of government/aided schools, and children who did not join school).
- Adolescents between 10–19 years of age.

- Women 20–24 years.
- Pregnant women.
- Lactating women having children up to 6 months of age.

Interventions

Key interventions in the Anemia Mukt Bharat strategy include supplementation with IFA, deworming, IFA fortification of foods in public health programs, intensified behaviour change communication (BCC) for solid body/ smart mind/ delayed cord clamping, using digital methods for anemia testing, and addressing non-nutritional causes of anemia like malaria and hemoglobinopathies.

IFA Supplementation

The age-wise dose regimens of elemental iron and folic acid given under **Anemia Mukt Bharat** are tabulated in Table 40.2.

Outcomes

In spite of enthusiastic planning and timely implementation, the outcomes of programme have been far from satisfactory, due to the following reasons:

- The problem of anemia is poorly perceived by the people.
- The education and training components in this programme were not given adequate importance. As a result, beneficiaries as well as functionaries had poor knowledge of the disease, its complications and the importance of prophylactic supplementation, resulting in poor compliance.
- Outreach to the target population was not adequate.
- Medicines supplied were inadequate and of poor quality.
- The programme was not evaluated properly.

HEMATOPOIETIC GROWTH FACTORS

Hematopoietic growth factors are glycoprotein hormones that regulate the hematopoietic process. These include:

1. Erythropoiesis-stimulating agents (ESAs) which include:
   a. Erythropoietin
   b. Epoietin alfa, darbepoetin alfa, epoetin beta, methoxy PEG-epoetin beta
2. Myeloid growth factors
   a. Granulocyte colony-stimulating factor (G-CSF): Filgrastim, Pegfilgrastim, Lenograstim
   b. Granulocyte-macrophage colony-stimulating factor (GM-CSF): Sargramostim, Molgramostim
3. Megakaryocyte growth factors
   a. Thrombopoietin (TPO) and its recombinant forms (rHuTPO, rHuMGDF)
   b. (IL-11, oprelvekin)
   c. Romiplostim
   d. Eltrombopag

1. Erythropoiesis Stimulating Agents (ESAs)

a. **Erythropoietin** was the first hematopoietic growth factor, initially isolated from the urine of severely anemic patients. It is a glycoprotein that is **mainly produced** by the **kidney**. Formation of erythropoietin increases in response to tissue hypoxia in anemic patients. It acts by binding to 'erythropoietin receptors' present on the surface of red cell progenitors in bone marrow. Erythropoietin receptors are JAK/STAT tyrosine kinase receptors that cause protein phosphorylation and activation of transcription factors, resulting in erythroid proliferation and differentiation. It also induces Hb formation and reticulocyte release from bone marrow into circulation.

Normally, there is an **inverse relationship between Hb and erythropoietin levels.** Most anemic patients (aplastic anemia, myelodysplastic diseases, nutritional deficiency anemias, etc.), have significantly raised erythropoietin levels, except **patients of anemia due to CKD.** This is because the kidneys fail to produce this hematopoietic growth factor in CKD, resulting in poor erythropoiesis and anemia. Thus, anemia of CKD responds best to erythropoietin therapy.

Table 40.2 Age-wise dose regimens of elemental iron and folic acid given under Anemia Mukt Bharat

Beneficiary	Dosage form	Elemental iron (mg)	Folic acid (mcg)	Frequency of administration
Preschool children (6–59 months)	Syrup 50 mL 1 mL contains →	20	100	Biweekly
5–9 year old children	Sugar coated (Pink tablet)	45	400	Weekly
Adolescents	Sugar coated (Blue tablet)	60	500	Weekly
Pregnant, lactating women	Sugar coated (Red tablet)	60	500	180 days in pregnancy, continued for 180 days postpartum.
Women in reproductive age *(WRA)	Sugar coated(Red tablet)	60	500	Weekly

*If women of reproductive age group (WRA) are planning pregnancy, they are advised to stop IFA supplementation and start only folic acid supplementation, to be continued till 12 weeks of pregnancy.

b. **Epoetin alfa and beta** are recombinant human erythropoietins. The half-life of **darbepoetin alfa** is 2–3 times **longer** than that of epoetin alfa and is suitable for once a week administration. **Methoxy polyethylene glycol-epoetin beta** is a longer-acting erythropoietin suitable for fortnightly or monthly administration.

Therapeutic uses of ESAs

- These are routinely used in **anemia due to CKD** along with iron and folate supplementation to support increased erythropoiesis. Dose is 25–100 U/kg, given by subcutaneous or IV route, thrice a week.
- ESAs are also useful in anemias associated with **chronic inflammation**, HIV-infected patients on **zidovudine** therapy, and patients receiving myelosuppressive **anticancer drugs**.
- It may be used to decrease the need for blood transfusion in high-risk patients undergoing elective nonvascular, noncardiac surgeries.

Response to erythropoietin therapy is good if endogenous levels are < 100 IU/L.

ADRs

- **Allergic** reactions are common.
- Transient flu-like symptoms may occur.
- Sudden increase in hematocrit can cause **thrombotic complications** leading to hypertension, increased rate of stroke, MI, worsening of CHF and death.
- Main ADR with epoietin is hypertension and polycythemia.

So, it is recommended to treat anemia due to CKD with ESAs only until Hb = 10–11 g/dL is achieved. In cancer chemotherapy patients also, ESAs should be **given only when Hb falls below 10 g/dL**, with lowest dose needed, so as to avoid blood transfusion.

2. Myeloid Growth Factors

a. Granulocyte colony-stimulating factor (G-CSF)

Filgrastim is a recombinant human granulocyte colony-stimulating factor.

Filgrastim acts through **JAK/STAT tyrosine kinase-linked receptors**, and activates colony forming units of the myeloid series. This results in increased neutrophil count, neutrophil release into circulation from the bone marrow, and phagocytic activity of neutrophils.

Therapeutic uses

Filgastrim is useful in neutropenia due to:

- Myelosuppressive anticancer drugs.
- Acute myeloid leukemia patients receiving chemotherapy
- After stem cell transplantation
- HIV-infected patients on zidovudine therapy
- Also useful in aplastic anemia, myelodysplasia

ADRs: It can cause reactions at the site of subcutaneous injection, fever, bone pains, thrombocytopenia, etc. Rarely, splenomegaly, splenic rupture, and acute respiratory distress may occur.

Pegfilgrastim: It is a complex of filgrastim with polyethylene glycol that has a much longer half-life. Thus, it can be used once in each cycle of chemotherapy.

Lenograstim is a glycosylated rG-CSF with the same efficacy as filgrastim for peripheral mobilisation of blood stem cells in cancer patients. However, in healthy donors, lenograstim is more efficacious than filgrastim for this action.

b. Granulocyte-macrophage CSF (GM-CSF)

Sargramostim is a recombinant human GM-CSF. It stimulates the differentiation of progenitor cells to neutrophils, monocytes, eosinophils, macrophages and myeloid derived dendritic cells. It also stimulates the function of mature macrophages and granulocytes.

- It is used in autologous bone marrow transplantation.
- Used in bone marrow transplant failure to improve survival.

Adverse effects include fever, chills, rashes, breathlessness and bony pains.

Molgramostim is another rGM-CSF useful in patients receiving myelosuppressive drugs/ganciclovir to reduce the severity of neutropenia and for quick myeloid recovery after transplantation.

In addition to ADRs shown by sargramostim, it may cause cardiac rhythm disturbance, pleural or pericardial effusion, hypotension and flushing.

3. Megakaryocyte Growth Factors

a. **Thrombopoietin (TPO)** is a glycoprotein produced by liver cells. TPO levels decrease in hepatic cirrhosis and thrombocytopenia (TCP). Recombinant human thrombopoietin (rHuTPO) and recombinant human megakaryocyte growth and development factor (rHuMGDF) are used in idiopathic thrombocytopenic purpura (ITP).

b. **IL-11** is a protein formed by fibroblasts and stromal cells in the bone marrow. Its recombinant form, **oprelvekin,** is approved for prevention of thrombocytopenia associated with cancer chemotherapy. However, both thrombopoietin and IL-11 are antigenic in nature. So, their use is associated with allergic reactions. They cause formation of auto-antibodies against thrombopoietin in normal human subjects, resulting in thrombocytopenia.

c. **Romiplostim** belongs to a new class called peptibodies, which are biologically active peptides linked to antibody fragments.

d. **Eltrombopag** is a small molecule that acts as agonist at thrombopoietin receptors, useful in the treatment of idiopathic thrombocytopenia. Romiplostim and eltrombopag are free of immunogenic effects.

Clinical problem-based questions and MCQs

7. A 56-year-old patient, a known case of IBD, presents with excessive fatigue, pallor, dizziness, paresthesia and muscular weakness. Hb = 8 g/dL, PBF shows macrocytes. A diagnosis of megaloblastic anemia is made. The physician advises further investigations to confirm the cause, before starting treatment.
    i. Why is the confirmation of cause of megaloblastic anemia important in this case?
    ii. What investigations can be advised here?
    iii. How can this patient be managed?

8. i. Which vitamin deficiency causes paresthesia, ataxia, subacute combined degeneration of spinal cord, peripheral neuritis, and decrease in vibration and position senses?
    ii. Explain the cause of such neurological changes in this vitamin deficiency?

9. All of the following may cause megaloblastic anemia in a patient with subclinical folate deficiency, EXCEPT:
    a. Chloroquine   b. Co-trimoxazole
    c. Chronic alcoholism d. Pyrimethamine

10. Which of the following is used for rescue therapy in methotrexate toxicity?
    a. DHFA   b. 5-formyl-THFA
    c. Methyl THFA   d. Folic acid

11. i. Which of the following is correct indication for use of epoietin?
    a. Pernicious anemia
    b. Anemia associated with chronic renal failure
    c. Hemolytic anemia
    d. Sickle cell anemia
    ii. Describe the mechanism of action of epoietin and pharmacological basis for its use in the selected condition.

12. i. Which of the following is a peptibody?
    a. Romiplostim   b. Filgrastim
    c. Oprelvekin   d. Epoietin
    ii. What is the indication for its use?

Summary

- Dietary intake of **iron** is 10–20 mg per day. It is mainly absorbed in the upper part of intestine. Daily iron turnover is 30 mg. Iron that reaches mucosal cells is either transported into plasma or stored in mucosal cells as ferritin. Excess iron stored as ferritin is lost with the shedding of mucosal cells (ferritin curtain). Plasma iron circulates in the form of a complex with transferrin, which is engulfed by cells. Number of transferrin receptors increases in iron deficiency.
- Iron deficiency causes microcytic, hypochromic anemia
- It is corrected by oral or parenteral iron preparations.
- Oral preparations include ferrous sulphate/gluconate/fumarate, ferric ammonium citrate/glycerophosphate, colloidal ferric hydroxide, iron choline citrate, iron calcium complex, iron hydroxyl polymaltose, and carbonyl iron, used for prophylaxis (30 mg) and treatment (200 mg) of iron deficiency anemia. ADRs like epigastric pain, constipation/diarrhea, heart burn, nausea, vomiting, metallic taste and teeth-staining occur with oral iron.
- Parenteral preparations include iron dextran, iron carboxymaltose, ferrous sucrose and iron isomaltoside. Iron dextran is the only preparation given by IV as well as IM route. TDI can be given via all preparations except ferrous sucrose. Parenteral iron is indicated when oral iron is not tolerated, not absorbed, or there is severe deficiency with chronic bleeding. It is also indicated along with erythropoietin. Dose for TDI is calculated as (4.4 × Body weight × Hb deficit). Adverse effects of parenteral iron include pain, skin pigmentation at I/M injection site, sterile abscess and systemic effects (fever, headache, joint pain, flushing, palpitation, chest pain, dyspnea, lymph adenopathy and metallic taste).
- **Methyl B_{12}** is involved in the conversion of homocysteine to methionine and makes THFA available for reutilisation. **Deoxyadenosyl B_{12}** aids in the conversion of methylmalonyl-CoA to succinyl-CoA and methionine to S-adenosyl methionine that is used for phospholipid and myelin synthesis.
- Deficiency of B_{12} causes raised levels of methylmalonic acid, homocysteine and demyelination of nerves, resulting in neurological damage. Patient develops megaloblastic, macrocytic anemia and neurological symptoms. Large doses of folic acid can reverse hematological but not the neurological changes.
- Dose of B_{12} is 3–10 mcg for prophylaxis and 10–30 mcg for treatment of deficiency. In IF deficiency causing pernicious anemia, oral B_{12} is not effective; 30–100 mcg is given IM or SC, daily, for 10 days and then once a month.
- **Folic acid** plays a role in one-carbon transfer reactions. Methyl THFA helps in the conversion of homocysteine to methionine, deoxyuridylate to thymidylate; THFA helps in conversion of serine to glycine. Folic acid deficiency also causes megaloblastic anemia, but there are no neurological symptoms.
- **Erythropoietin** or its recombinant form, epoietin, is used in anemia caused by chronic renal failure (CKD), chronic inflammation and myelosuppressive drugs and in HIV patients on zidovudine. These

- increase hematocrit and reticulocyte counts. Major ADRs are polycythemia, hypertension, allergic reactions and thrombotic complications. So, ESAs should be used only when Hb is below 10 mg/dL.
- **Filgrastim** is an rG-CSF, useful in leukopenia caused by anticancer drugs and in HIV patients on zidovudine therapy. **Sargramostim** is a GM-CSF used in bone marrow transplantation. Bone pain is common adverse effect
- **Thrombopoietin** or IL-11 and their recombinant forms are used in TCP. However, antigenic properties are a problem. In chronic ITP, peptibodies like **romiplostim**, which are free of antigenic effects, are useful

Questions for practice

1. a. Describe oral and parenteral iron preparations.
   b. Enumerate the adverse effects of iron.
2. Explain why:
   a. Folic acid improves the hematological picture of pernicious anemia.
   b. Folic acid should not be used alone in pernicious anemia.
   c. Vitamin B_{12} deficiency causes both hematological and neurological symptoms.
3. Comment on the role of:
   a. Erythropoietin in CKD.
   b. Filgrastim in patient on anticancer drugs.
   c. Colony-stimulating factors in bone marrow transplantation.

Hints for problem-based questions and MCQs

1. c. Iron dextran
2. c. Number of erythrocytic transferrin receptors decreases.
3. i. d. Carbonyl iron
   ii. Refer to Flowchart 40.1, page 538.
   iii. Refer to page 537, 539
4. i. Iron deficiency anemia
   ii. Total dose of iron required = $4.4 \times 60 \times (12 - 6) = 1584$ mg
   Total calculated dose is diluted in 500 mL glucose/ saline and infused over 6–8 hours under observation.
5. a. Ferrous sucrose
6. i. Acute iron poisoning
   ii. b. BAL has no role in this case as BAL–iron chelate is also toxic.
7. i. Both folic acid and vit. B_{12} deficiency cause megaloblastic anemia. Folic acid and vit. B_{12} metabolism are linked at the step of conversion of homocysteine to methionine. So, large doses of folic acid given in vit. B_{12} deficiency may cause improvement of hematological features. Vit. B_{12} deficiency causes reduced synthesis of S-adenosyl methionine required for synthesis of myelin sheath. Thus, deficiency causes demyelination and neurological findings. Folic acid cannot improve these neurological symptoms, so the cause must be determined.
   ii. In deficiency of vit. B_{12}, levels of homocysteine and methylmalonoic acid are raised. Serum B_{12} levels are low. In folic acid deficiency, serum folic acid levels are low.
   iii. Replacement therapy with vit. B_{12} or folic acid, whichever is the cause of anemia.
8. i. Vitamin B_{12} deficiency
   ii. Due to reduced S-adenosyl methionine, which is required for synthesis of phospholipid and myelin sheath.
9. a. Chloroquine.
10. b. 5-Formyl-THFA
11. i. b. Anemia associated with chronic renal failure
    ii. Epoeitin is an rHuEPO that acts on JAK/STAT TK-linked receptors on the surface of RBC progenitor cells, resulting in activation of transcription factors → erythroid proliferation and differentiation.
12. i. a. Romiplostim
    ii. ITP

CONCEPT MAP – HEMATINICS

HEMATINICS

Iron

Therapeutic Uses
- Treatment of Iron deficiency anemia
- Prophylaxis of iron deficiency anemia in menstruation, pregnancy, infant, menorrhagia, blood loss, chronic illness, etc.
- Megaloblastic anemia: stimulation of erythropoeisis after correction of vitamin B_{12} and folic acid deficiency, may unmask iron deficiency.
- Ferric chloride is used as astringent in throat pain.

Oral Preparations
Ferrous: Ferrous sulphate, gluconate, fumarate, succinate, aminoate
Ferric: Ferric ammonium citrate, glycerophosphate, Colloidal ferric hydroxide
Iron: Iron choline citrate, Iron calcium complex, Iron hydroxyl polymaltose, Carbonyl iron
ADRs: Epigastric pain, Heartburn, nausea, vomiting, metallic taste. Constipation or diarrhea and staining of teeth

Parenteral Preparations
Ferrous Sucrose: Suitable for IV injection. Not suitable for SC/IM inj., IV infusion
Ferric Carboxymaltose: Suitable for IV inj & infusion
Iron Dextran: High molecular weight, Only iron preparation that can be used by both IM or IV route.
Iron Sorbitol Citric Acid: Low molecular weight, Used only by IM route
Iron Isomaltoside 1000: Very slowly released. Total calculated dose may be infused IV over a short period.

Absorption, Transport, Storage
Daily requirement: 0.5–1 mg in men, 1–2 mg in women
Dietary sources: Liver, egg yolk, dry beans, dry fruits, yeast, meat, chicken, fish, banana, spinach, apple 10–20 mg of iron as Fe^{3+} & heme form in daily diet.
Absorption: Mainly from upper part of duodenum
Transport: Circulates bound to transferrin in plasma. Hemoglobin contains 65% of total body iron (50–60 mg/kg body weight),
Storage: Apoferritin Fe^{3+} + Fe → Ferritin → aggregates to form Hemosiderin, is stored in RE cells in liver, spleen, bone marrow, myocytes, hepatocytes.
Excretion: Daily 0.5–1 mg iron is lost as exfoliated gastro intestinal mucosal cells, some RBCs & bile in feces. Some excretion in sweat, urine, desquamation of skin and menstrual blood.

Indications
Oral iron is not tolerated
Oral iron is not absorbed - malabsorption, inflammatory bowel disease (IBD), chronic inflammation
Non-compliance to oral iron.
Severe deficiency with chronic bleeding.
Along with erthropoietin
Total iron required = $4.4 \times$ Body weight (Kg) $\times$ Hb deficit (g/dL).

ADRs
Local: Pain at IM injection site, Skin pigmentation, Sterile abscess
Systemic: Fever, headache, joint pain, flushing, palpitation chest pain, dyspnea, lymphadenopathy, metallic taste are more frequently seen with IV use than IM use.

Vitamin B_{12}

Absorption, Transport, Storage
Cyanocobalamin, hydroxocobalamin
Daily requirement 1–3 mcg,
In pregnancy/lactation = 3–5 mcg
Sources: Liver, kidney, sea fish, meat, egg yolk, cheese, legumes (pulses).
Absorption: IF in stomach helps in oral absorption.
Transport: In blood with transcobalamin II (TC-II)
Storage: In liver cells.
Excretion: It is not degraded in body, gets excreted in bile,
Undergoes enterohepatic circulation

Physiological Role
Conversion of homocysteine to methionine which is required as methyl donor in protein synthesis.
Makes THFA available for reutilisation.
So B_{12} deficiency anemia can be partially corrected by large doses of folic acid that provides alternative source of THFA.
Formation of succinyl-CoA from methylmalonyl-CoA, DA B_{12} acts as coenzyme in synthesis of S-adenosyl methionine from methionine, which is utilised in synthesis of phospholipids & myelin. (no role of folic acid in this reaction)

Deficiency
Raised levels of methylmalonic acid, homocysteine and demyelination of nerves.
Megaloblastic, macrocytic anemia
Glossitis, GI disturbances
Neurological symptoms such as paresthesia and weakness progressing to ataxia, and spasticity
Subacute combined degeneration of spinal cord, peripheral neuritis, decrease in vibration and position senses and mental changes
Large doses of folic acid can reverse hematological changes, but not the neurological ones.
Mild-to-moderate leukopenia and thrombocytopenia may also occur
Hypercellular bone marrow

Therapeutic Uses
Treatment of B_{12} deficiency megaloblastic anemia
IF deficiency: Pernicious anemia (effective only parenterally)
For prophylaxis of B_{12} deficiency: In malabsorption syndrome, fish tapeworm, pregnancy, infants, chronic gastritis, etc.
As general tonic in neuropathies, cutaneous sarcoidosis, psychiatric disorders.
Hydroxocobalamin is used in tobacco amblyopia.
Dose is 3–10 mcg for prophylaxis and 10–30 mcg for treatment of B_{12} deficiency.
In IF deficiency 30–100mcg is given IM or SC, daily for 10 days and then once a month.
ADRs: Very safe.
Allergic reactions may occur on parenteral use.

Folic Acid

Daily Requirement
Daily requirement = < 0.1 mg,
In pregnancy/ lactation 0.8 mg/d
Sources – Liver, egg, meat, milk, green leafy vegetables.

Physiological Role
Conversion of homocysteine to methionine (Methyl THFA)
Deoxyuridylate to thymidylate, Purine synthesis (Methyl THFA)
Serine to glycine (THFA)
Generation & utilisation of formate pool

Deficiency
Can be: Dietary or in malabsorption syndrome, biliary fistula, chronic alcoholism, liver disease, in pregnancy and hemolysis,
Drugs like methotrexate, trimethoprim, pyrimethamine
C/F: Megaloblastic anemia, glossitis, diarrhea, steatorrhea, generalised weakness, weight loss, sterility.
Unlike B_{12} deficiency, there are no neurological symptoms

Uses
Treatment & prophylaxis of megaloblastic anemia
Methotrexate toxicity : folinic acid (5-formyl-THFA) citrovorum factor rescue

SECTION 9 Drugs Affecting the Endocrine System

41 Anterior Pituitary Hormones

PH 7.4 Describe the types, mechanisms of action, adverse effects, indications and contraindications of the drugs which modify the release of anterior pituitary hormones.

Learning objectives

A student of MBBS phase II should be able to:
- Enumerate the anterior pituitary hormones.
- Describe the regulation of secretion of anterior pituitary hormones.
- Enumerate the mechanism of action of growth hormone.
- Describe the therapeutic uses and ADRs of growth hormone, its analogues and antagonists.
- Describe the uses and ADRs of gonadotropins, GnRH analogues and antagonists.
- Describe the mechanism of action, uses and ADRs of drugs used in hyperprolactinemia.

The pituitary gland lies in the sella turcica at the base of the brain, and has anterior and posterior lobes. It is connected to the hypothalamus through a stalk. The function of the pituitary gland is controlled by the hypothalamus (Fig. 41.1).

The **anterior lobe** of the pituitary gland secretes six hormones:

- Thyroid-stimulating hormone (TSH)
- Gonadotropins: Follicle-stimulating hormone (FSH), luteinising hormone (LH)
- Adrenocorticotropic hormone (ACTH)
- Growth hormone (GH)
- Prolactin (PRL)

The **posterior lobe** of the pituitary secretes the following two hormones:

- Oxytocin
- Vasopressin or antidiuretic hormone (ADH)

The secretion of hormones from anterior pituitary is regulated by the hypothalamus and feedback mechanisms. The hypothalamus secretes the following hormones or factors:

a. Thyrotropin-releasing hormone (TRH)
b. Dopamine (prolactin inhibitory hormone, PIH)
c. Gonadotropin-releasing hormone (GnRH)
d. Corticotropin-releasing hormone (CRH)
e. Growth hormone-releasing hormone (GHRH)
f. Somatostatin, which inhibits secretion of the growth hormone

- TRH, GnRH, and CRH secreted from the hypothalamus regulate secretion of TSH, gonadotropins (FSH, LH) and ACTH, respectively, from the anterior pituitary.
- TSH, gonadotropins (FSH, LH) and ACTH increase the secretion of thyroid hormones, sex hormones and cortisol, respectively; these, in turn, exert negative feedback effect on their tropic hormones from the anterior pituitary and hypothalamus (Fig. 41.2).
- GHRH from the hypothalamus increases secretion of growth hormone from the anterior pituitary.
- Somatostatin (SST) has an inhibitory effect on GH secretion.
- GH mediates its actions through insulin-like growth factor-1 (IGF-1), which exerts negative feedback effect on GH secretion.
- The secretion of prolactin (PRL) from the anterior pituitary is inhibited by prolactin inhibitory hormone (PIH; chemically, dopamine) and acts through D_2 receptors. High concentration of thyrotropin-releasing hormone (TRH) can enhance PRL secretion.

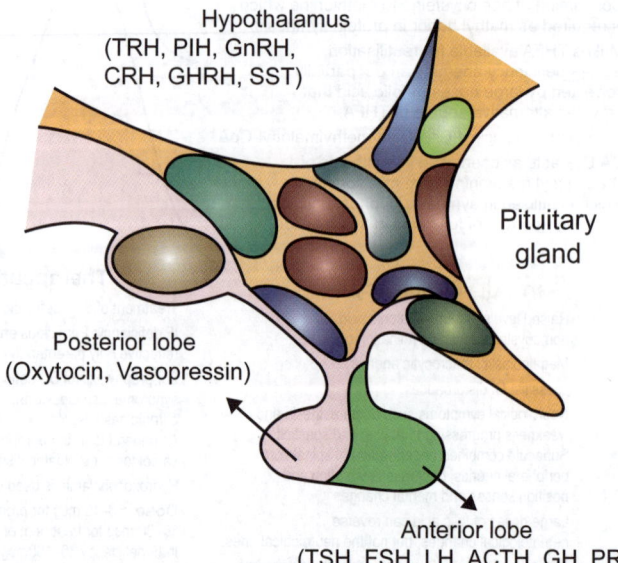

Fig. 41.1 The hypothalamus and pituitary glands and hormones secreted by them

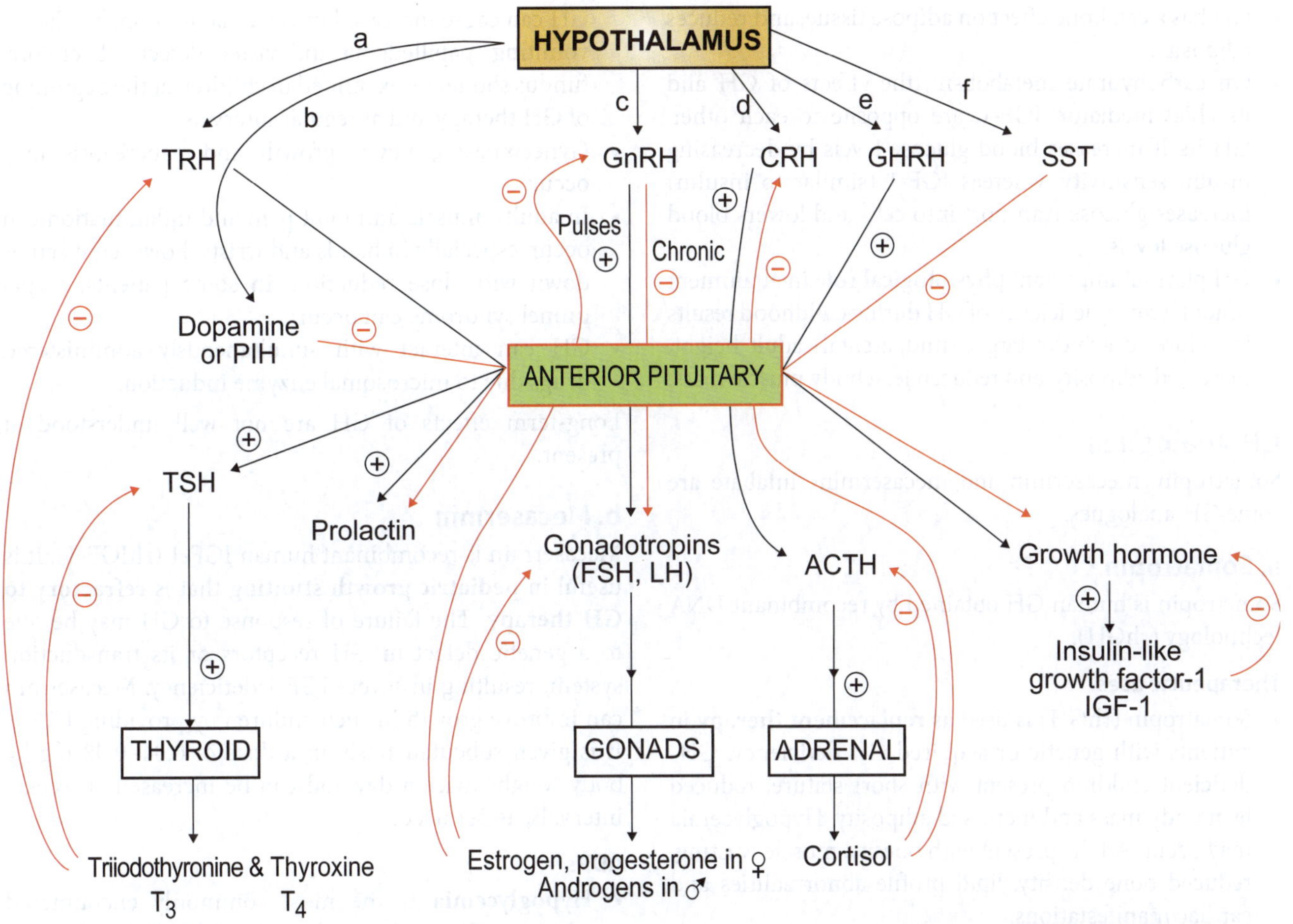

Fig. 41.2 Regulation of anterior pituitary hormones by the hypothalamus and negative feedback mechanisms

All these hypothalamic and anterior pituitary hormones have some diagnostic and/or therapeutic indications. However, in case of diseases involving the thyroid gland, adrenal cortex and gonads, the use of target hormones (thyroxine, corticosteroids and sex hormones, respectively) is more convenient, economical and thus preferred over their regulating hormones from the anterior pituitary and hypothalamus. GH, SST, GnRH, their analogues, and antagonists are used in clinical practice.

1. GROWTH HORMONE (GH)

Growth hormone (GH) is also known as somatotropin.
Mechanism of action: Somatotropin (GH) exerts its action by binding to JAK/STAT cytokine receptors, leading to synthesis of insulin-like growth factor-1 (IGF-1) in the liver, kidney, muscles and bones (Fig. 41.3).

- IGF-1 mediates the growth-promoting action of GH. Longitudinal growth of bones in children occurs before the closure of epiphyses. Muscle mass and lean body mass also increase. GH plays a role in the growth of all the organs of the body, except eye and brain.

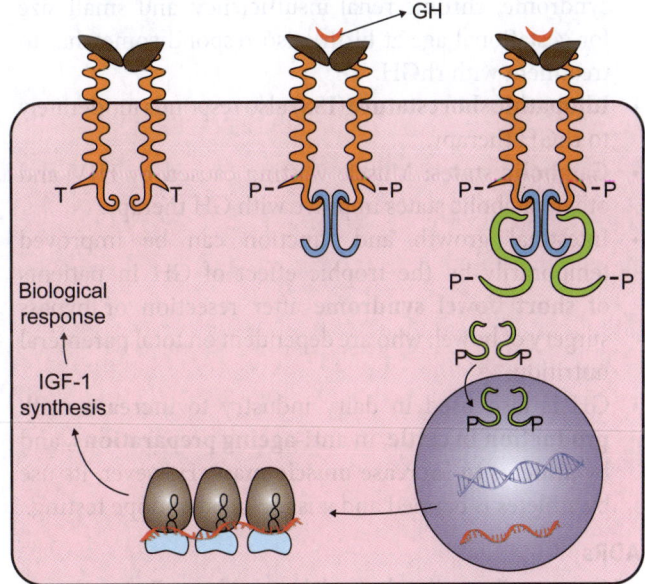

Fig. 41.3 Mechanism of action of GH through JAK/STAT binding receptors

[J → JAK   S → STAT]

- GH has a catabolic effect on adipose tissue, and reduces adiposity.
- On carbohydrate metabolism, the effects of GH and its chief mediator, IGF-1, are opposite to each other. GH itself increases blood glucose levels by decreasing insulin sensitivity, whereas IGF-1 (similar to insulin) increases glucose transport into cells and lowers blood glucose levels.
- GH plays an important **physiological role** in attainment of adult size. A deficiency of GH during childhood results in failure to achieve target (midparental) adult height, increased adiposity, and reduced lean body muscle mass.

GH Analogues

Somatropin, mecasermin and mecasermin rinfabate are some GH analogues.

a. Somatropin

Somatropin is human GH obtained by recombinant DNA technology (rhGH).

Therapeutic uses

- Somatropin (rhGH) is used **as replacement therapy** in patients with genetic or acquired GH deficiency. GH-deficient children present with short stature, reduced lean body mass and increased adiposity. Hypoglycemia may occur. Adults present with obesity, muscle wasting, reduced bone density, lipid profile abnormalities and cardiac manifestations.

Early initiation of therapy can help achieve target adult height in these children and reversal of symptoms in adults.

- **Pediatric growth failure and short stature** due to some other conditions (e.g., Turner syndrome, Prader–Willi syndrome, chronic renal insufficiency, and small size for gestational age at birth) also respond somewhat to treatment with rhGH.
- **Idiopathic short stature** (ISS) also responds moderately to rhGH therapy.
- **Catabolic states:** Muscle wasting caused by HIV and other catabolic states improve with GH therapy.
- Intestinal growth and function can be improved temporarily by the trophic effect of GH in patients of **short bowel syndrome** after resection or bypass surgery of bowel, who are dependent on total parenteral nutrition.
- GH is also used in dairy industry to **increase milk production in cattle**, in **anti-ageing preparations,** and by **athletes to increase muscle mass.** However, its use by athletes is banned and it is included in dope testing.

ADRs

GH is usually well tolerated by children. Rare adverse effects include:

- Slipped epiphysis of femur, hyperglycemia, edema, scoliosis, pseudotumor cerebri and sleep apnea. Rarely, GH can cause increased intracranial tension, headache, vomiting, papilledema and visual defects. Therefore, fundus should be examined in children at the beginning of GH therapy and at regular intervals.
- Gynecomastia, nevus growth and pancreatitis may occur.
- In adults, muscle and joint pain and inflammation can occur, especially in hands and wrists; however, it settles down with dose reduction. In some patients, carpal tunnel syndrome can occur.
- GH can interact with simultaneously administered drugs due to microsomal enzyme induction.

Long-term effects of GH are not well understood at present.

b. Mecasermin

Mecasermin is recombinant human IGF-1 (rhIGF-1). It is useful in **pediatric growth stunting** that is **refractory to GH therapy**. The failure of response to GH may be due to a genetic defect in GH receptors or its transduction system, resulting in severe IGF-1 deficiency. Mecasermin can improve growth in such children by providing IGF-1. It is given subcutaneously in a dose of 0.04–0.08 mg/kg body weight twice a day and can be increased at weekly intervals, as per need.

ADRs

- **Hypoglycemia** is the most commonly encountered adverse effect of mecasermin (rhIGF-1). Because IGF-1 increases glucose uptake like insulin, patients are advised to consume a carbohydrate-rich meal within 20 minutes of its use.
- Liver enzymes may be raised.
- Intracranial tension may be raised.

c. Mecasermin rinfabate

It is a complex of recombinant human IGF-1 (rhIGF-1) and its binding protein-3 (rhIGFBP-3). This complexing of IGF-1 with binding protein decreases its clearance, resulting in **increased half-life**.

2. GH ANTAGONISTS

Excessive release of GH (as in case of pituitary adenoma) results in **acromegaly** in adults and **gigantism** in children. The treatment of pituitary adenoma is primarily surgical, but if GH levels remain high after resection of tumour, GH antagonists are used. These include:

a. **Somatostatin analogues** such as **octreotide and lanreotide** (because somatostatin released from the hypothalamus has an inhibitory effect on GH release).
b. GH-receptor antagonist, **pegvisomant,** prevents the activation of signalling pathways by GH.
c. **Dopamine agonists** can also reduce GH secretion.

a. Somatostatin Analogues

Somatostatin is an important paracrine factor that is secreted by the hypothalamus, GIT and pancreatic δ cells. It has **inhibitory effect on the secretion** of:

- GH, TSH and prolactin from the anterior pituitary.
- Insulin and glucagon from the pancreas.
- All gastrointestinal secretions, including HCl and gastrin. This antisecretory effect of somatostatin may be used in patients with biliary, intestinal or pancreatic fistulae.
- Somatostatin causes **vasoconstriction** of renal, hepatic and splanchnic blood vessels. This effect may be used to control bleeding from esophageal varices and bleeding peptic ulcers.

Somatostatin is mainly metabolised and excreted by the kidneys at a very rapid rate. Its **half-life is very short** (1–3 minutes). Thus, its clinical usefulness is limited, owing to short duration of action and multiple effects. Somatostatin analogues used in clinical practice are octreotide and lanreotide.

Octreotide

Octreotide is **longer-acting** in comparison to somatostatin. It is **more selective** for inhibiting GH release than insulin release. Thus, hyperglycemia is rarely seen with octreotide.

Uses

It is useful for controlling symptoms in many **hormone-releasing tumours** such as acromegaly, carcinoid syndrome, insulinoma, glucagonoma, gastrinoma, and TSH-secreting adenoma.

- Radiolabelled octreotide can help **to localise neuroendocrine tumours** by somatostatin-receptor scintigraphy.
- It is useful in portal hypertension to **control esophageal variceal bleeding**; dose is 50–200 mcg subcutaneously, 3 times daily.
- It is useful in secretory diarrhea.

[Mnemonic: Somatostatin analogues are used in 'SEATS', i.e., Secretory diarrhea, Esophageal varices, Acromegaly, Tumours secreting hormones, Scintigraphy]

ADRs

- Nausea, vomiting, bulky stools, flatulence and abdominal cramps.
- In some patients, continued treatment leads to formation of gallstones.
- Vit. B_{12} deficiency may occur.
- Decrease in heart rate and AV conduction can occur.

Lanreotide

Lanreotide is longer acting than octreotide and is useful for the treatment of acromegaly.

Vapreotide, pasireotide and seglitide are some other somatostatin analogues.

b. Pegvisomant

It is a polyethylene glycol (PEG) derivative of GH with differential affinity of its two binding sites for GH receptors, which results in **blockade of the signal transduction pathway**. It is useful in treatment of acromegaly.

Important adverse effects are the raised hepatic enzymes and lack of inhibitory effect on the secretion of GH, which may result in increased adenoma growth.

Clinical problem-based questions and MCQs

1. An 8-year-old boy is brought to pediatric OPD with complaints of short stature, obesity. On examination, lean body mass is very low and adiposity is high. After appropriate investigations, patient is diagnosed to have growth hormone deficiency.
   i. Identify a suitable drug for this child
      a. Pegvisomant
      b. Octreotide
      c. Somatropin
      d. Somatostatin
   ii. Describe the uses and adverse effects of the selected drug.

2. A 30-year-old male patient with portal hypertension and hematemesis due to bleeding from esophageal varices reports to medicine OPD for treatment.
   i. Choose the most suitable drug for the patient
      a. Somatropin
      b. Somatostatin
      c. Octreotide
      d. Mecasermin
   ii. Describe the mechanism of action of the selected drug.
   iii. Enumerate the therapeutic uses and adverse effects of the chosen drug.

3. Somatostatin inhibits the secretion of:
   a. Growth hormone
   b. Gastrin
   c. Prolactin
   d. All of the above

4. i. Identify a suitable drug for pediatric growth stunting, refractory to GH.
      a. Somatropin
      b. Mecasermin
      c. Lanreotide
      d. Pegvisomant
   ii. Justify your choice with the pharmacological basis.

5. Pegvisomant, a growth hormone antagonist used for the treatment of acromegaly, may increase growth of pituitary adenomas. Explain.

6. Both somatropin and mecasermin are growth hormone analogues. Somatropin causes hyperglycemia, but mecasermin causes hypoglycemia as an adverse effect. Explain the pharmacological basis.

> 7. Differentiate between somatotropin and somatostatin.
> 8. i. Which of the following is a somatostatin analogue?
>   a. Mecasermin   b. Lanreotide
>   c. Pegvisomant   d. Somatropin
>   ii. Enumerate the therapeutic uses and adverse effects of the selected drug.

3. GONADOTROPINS

Follicle-stimulating hormone (FSH) and luteinising hormone (LH) are gonadotropins secreted by the anterior pituitary. These promote secretion of gonadal hormones and gametogenesis. Secretion of both **FSH and LH** is increased by **GnRH/gonadorelin** secreted by the hypothalamus in a pulsatile manner. However, sustained action of GnRH inhibits the release of FSH and LH by desensitising pituitary gonadotrophic cells. **Inhibin** secreted from the gonads inhibits release of FSH only, while dopamine inhibits the release of LH only.

Inadequate secretion of gonadotropin may result in delayed puberty in both sexes, amenorrhea in females and oligozoospermia in males. In contrast, excessive gonadotropin secretion causes precocious puberty, polycystic ovarian disease (PCOD), uterine fibroids, endometriosis and prostatic carcinoma.

Gonadotropins for Medicinal Use

- Menotropin obtained from the urine of menopausal women contains both FSH and LH.
- Urofollitropin contains FSH only.
- Follitropin α and β are recombinant human FSH (rhFSH).
- Lutropin is recombinant human LH (rhLH).
- Human chorionic gonadotropin (hCG) is obtained from the urine of pregnant females.
- Choriogonadotropin is recombinant hCG (rhCG).

Therapeutic uses of gonadotropins

In female infertility, if clomiphene citrate fails to induce ovulation, gonadotropins are tried.

- These are useful to induce ovulation in females with **polycystic ovarian disease.** Dose of menotropins is 75 IU of FSH and LH each, given intramuscularly for 10 days, followed by injection hCG 10000 IU.
- For **controlled ovarian stimulation** in women undergoing **in vitro fertilisation**, menotropins are given along with GnRH agonists or antagonists, so that the endogenous secretion of gonadotropins is suppressed.
- In males with **delayed puberty, oligozoospermia and sterility**, hCG is given biweekly as intramuscular injections to increase testosterone secretion. After a few months of giving hCG, FSH and LH 75 IU each are injected to induce spermatogenesis.

Adverse effects

- The most frequently encountered adverse effect with gonadotropins is **ovarian hyperstimulation syndrome.**
- Abortion and multiple pregnancies may occur.
- Lower abdominal pain, polycystic ovary, ovarian bleeding and even shock may occur during induction of ovulation.
- Use of gonadotropins in children may cause precocious puberty.
- Headache, edema and mood disturbances are also reported.

4. GONADORELIN/ GONADOTROPIN-RELEASING HORMONE (GnRH) AGONISTS

Buserelin, goserelin, nafarelin, triptorelin, histrelin and leuprolide are gonadorelin agonistic drugs. These analogues are much more potent and longer-acting than natural GnRH.

Pharmacological actions

GnRH causes an increase in Gn secretion if given in pulsatile manner. So, with acute use, these drugs increase gonadotropin secretion at initiation of therapy. However, upon continuous use for 1–2 weeks, down-regulation and desensitisation of receptors occurs, leading to reduced gonadotropin secretion. Due to decreased secretion of FSH and LH, gonadal function is suppressed. Levels of estradiol (in females) and testosterone (in males) decrease drastically, as if castration has been carried out. Ovulation and spermatogenesis stops. Gonadal functions remain suppressed as long as the drug is given; it recovers after a few months of stopping the drug.

Therapeutic uses

GnRH analogues are used for reversible pharmacological (**medical**) **oophorectomy** in precocious puberty, endometriosis, pre-menopausal carcinoma breast, uterine fibroid and polycystic ovarian disease. Medical orchidectomy is indicated in precocious puberty in males and prostatic carcinoma. These drugs are used as **nasal sprays or subcutaneous injections.**

Adverse effects include hot flushes, loss of libido, vaginal dryness, osteoporosis and emotional lability as seen in menopausal women.

5. GONADOTROPIN-RELEASING HORMONE (GnRH) ANTAGONISTS

Ganirelix, cetrorelix, degarelix and abarelix are GnRH antagonists.

- They inhibit Gn secretion. There is no stimulation of Gn release at initiation of therapy.

- These are used in females undergoing in vitro fertilisation (IVF) to inhibit LH surges during **controlled ovarian stimulation.**
- Degarelix and abarelix are approved for androgen withdrawal therapy in patients with **advanced carcinoma prostate.**
- **Risk of ovarian hyperstimulation is lower** with these drugs.

6. PROLACTIN

Prolactin is secreted from anterior pituitary, and plays an important role in:

- Growth and development of breast tissue
- Synthesis of lactose and milk proteins during pregnancy
- Milk secretion after delivery.
- During breastfeeding, high levels of prolactin inhibit the release of GnRH. This causes lactational amenorrhea, anovulation and infertility.

Prolactin inhibitory factor (PIF) released from the hypothalamus is dopamine; this inhibits prolactin secretion by acting on D_2 receptors of pituitary lactotrophs. Thus, **dopamine agonists decrease prolactin secretion and antagonists cause hyperprolactinemia.**

Hyperprolactinemia

Dopamine antagonists such as metoclopramide, and antipsychotics (haloperidol chlorpromazine) can cause hyperprolactinemia as an adverse effect. Prolactin secreting tumours or raised thyrotropin-releasing hormone (TRH) in hypothyroid patients can also cause hyperprolactinemia.

It manifests as galactorrhea, amenorrhea and infertility in females and loss of libido in males.

Treatment of hyperprolactinemia involves administration of dopamine agonists like bromocriptine, cabergoline and quinagolide.

a. Bromocriptine

It is a synthetic ergot derivative that acts as a potent dopamine agonist.

Actions

- It acts on D_2 receptors causing decreased prolactin secretion from the pituitary.
- Bromocriptine increases secretion of GH in normal persons, but decreases GH release from pituitary tumours (which cause acromegaly).
- It has anti-parkinsonian effects in CNS.
- The chemoreceptor trigger zone is stimulated, resulting in severe nausea and vomiting.
- Weak α-blocking effect and suppression of postural reflexes by bromocriptine cause hypotension.
- Gastrointestinal motility is reduced.

Therapeutic uses

- Bromocriptine is useful in **hyperprolactinemia**, in an oral dose of 2.5–10 mg daily.
- Bromocriptine is used for **suppression of lactation.**
- In **acromegaly**, it has lower efficacy than somatostatin or octreotide. (For both these indications, cabergoline is now preferred over bromocriptine.)
- It is approved as adjunctive drug in type 2 **diabetes.**
- It is used as an **adjuvant** in **parkinsonism.** Newer D_2 receptor agonists like ropinirole and pramipexole are preferred over bromocriptine for this indication.

[Mnemonic for the therapeutic uses of bromocriptine: 'Highly Sensitive ADP', i.e., Hyperprolactinemia, Suppression of lactation, Acromegaly, Diabetes and Parkinsonism]

ADRs

It has many disturbing, dose-related adverse effects like:

- Nausea, vomiting due to CTZ stimulation, and constipation due to reduced gastrointestinal motility.
- Nasal blockade, postural hypotension and syncope due to α-blocking effect and suppression of postural reflexes.
- Late adverse effects include confusion, behavioural alterations, hallucinations and psychosis. Abnormal movements and livedo reticularis may occur.

b. Cabergoline

Cabergoline is a newer agonist at D_2 receptors in pituitary lactotrophs.

- It has **more potency and longer duration of action** than bromocriptine; so, twice weekly administration is sufficient.
- It is **better tolerated** than bromocriptine, with risk of nausea and vomiting.
- It is effective in patients not responding to bromocriptine.

Because of these advantages, cabergoline has replaced bromocriptine as a **first-line drug in hyperprolactinemia.** Prolactinomas regress in size during therapy with cabergoline. However, the beneficial effect persists till drug is given and symptoms usually recur on stopping the drug. Although teratogenic effects are not reported, it is better to discontinue use of cabergoline once the patient conceives.

c. Quinagolide

It is a non-ergot dopamine agonist with fewer adverse effects than bromocriptine and cabergoline.

Clinical problem-based questions and MCQs

9. A female patient with infertility was not responding to clomiphene. Identify the most suitable gonadotropin to treat such a case.
    a. Lutropin
    b. Menotropin
    c. Follitropin α
    d. Follitropin β

10. Comment on the role of gonadotropin RH agonists in medical oophorectomy.

11. The method of 'controlled ovarian stimulation' is opted in women undergoing 'in vitro fertilisation'. Which of the following drug groups is useful for this indication?
    a. GnRH agonists
    b. GnRH antagonists
    c. Menotropins
    d. All of the above

12. Which of the following is free from the risk of ovarian hyperstimulation?
    a. Nafarelin
    b. Degarelix
    c. Leuprolide
    d. Follitropin

13. Which of the following is a GnRH antagonist?
    a. Nafarelin
    b. Degarelix
    c. Cabergoline
    d. Octreotide

14. A 48-year-old schizophrenic patient on treatment with antipsychotic drugs presents with gynecomastia and galactorrhea.
    i. Which could be the offending antipsychotic drug?
        a. Chlorpromazine
        b. Risperidone
        c. Clozapine
        d. Aripirazole
    ii. Explain how the selected drug causes gynecomastia.

15. A 30-year-old female patient presents with inability to conceive since last 3 years and galactorrhea. She has amenorrhea for last 2 months. Urine for pregnancy test is negative. Serum prolactin levels are raised.
    i. Identify the drug of first choice in this case.
        a. Bromocriptine
        b. Dopamine
        c. Cabergoline
        d. Amantidine
    ii. Describe the mechanism of beneficial effect of the selected drug?
    iii. Why it is preferred over other drugs in this case?

Summary

- Growth hormone (GH), prolactin (PRL), thyroid-stimulating hormone (TSH), gonadotropins (follicle-stimulating hormone FSH, luteinising hormone LH), and adrenocorticotropic hormone (ACTH) are secreted from the anterior pituitary.
- Secretion of these hormones is under hypothalamic control through GHRH, somatostatin, prolactin inhibitory hormone, TRH, GnRH, and CRH; it is also regulated through negative feedback mechanism.
- **GH analogues include** somatropin (recombinant human GH), mecasermin (recombinant human IGF-1) and mecasermin rinfabate (complex of recombinant human IGF-1 and its binding protein-3).
- Somatropin is used for replacement therapy in GH deficiency states, pediatric growth stunting, idiopathic short stature, short bowel syndrome and as anti-ageing preparations.
- Mecasermin is useful in pediatric growth stunting that does not improve with somatropin.
- **Somatostatin** decreases the release of many hormones (GH, TSH, PRL, insulin, glucagon and gastrin), HCl in stomach, and causes vasoconstriction of renal, hepatic and splanchnic blood vessels. However, it is not used therapeutically because of its short half-life (1–3 minutes).
- **Octreotide**, a longer-acting analogue of somatostatin, is useful in many hormone-secreting tumours like acromegaly, insulinoma, glucagonoma, prolactinoma, and carcinoid syndrome, and in portal hypertension to control esophageal variceal bleeding. It causes ADRs like nausea, vomiting, flatulence, bulky stools, and abdominal cramps.
- Pegvisomant blocks signal transduction in response to GH binding to its receptors and may be useful in acromegaly.
- **Gonadotropins** in clinical use include menotropins (containing both FSH and LH), urofollitropin/follitropin α, β (FSH only), lutropin (LH only) and human chorionic gonadotropin (hCG).
- These are useful for ovulation induction in female infertility, in cases not responding to clomiphene and for controlled ovarian stimulation in IVF and oligozoospermia in males.
- Most important ADR is ovarian hyperstimulation syndrome.
- **GnRH agonists** like buserelin and nafarelin increase gonadotropin secretion upon pulsatile administration and decrease secretion on continuous use. These are used as nasal sprays and

subcutaneous injections for medical oophorectomy and orchidectomy. ADRs resemble menopausal symptoms.
- **Prolactin** secretion is inhibited by dopamine (prolactin inhibitory hormone). Dopamine agonists such as bromocriptine and cabergoline are useful in prolactinomas.
- Cabergoline is preferred over bromocriptine as it is more potent, has a longer half-life and is better tolerated. Dopamine antagonists like metoclopramide and antipsychotics, can cause hyperprolactinemia resulting in galactorrhea and gynecomastia as adverse effects.

Questions for practice

1. Describe therapeutic uses and adverse effects of somatropin.
2. Explain why:
   a. Somatostatin is not useful in clinical practice.
   b. Cabergoline is preferred over bromocriptine
   c. GnRH agonists can cause medical oophorectomy.
3. Write short notes on:
   a. Octreotide
   b. Menotropin
   c. Nafarelin

Hints for problem-based questions and MCQs

1. i. c. Somatropin
   ii. Refer to page 550.
2. i. c. Octreotide
   ii. Somatostatin analogue with longer duration of action than SST; causes vasoconstriction of renal/hepatic/splanchnic vessels.
   iii. Refer to page 551.
3. d. All of the above
4. i. b. Mecasermin
   ii. Mecasermin is rhIGF-1; failure to respond to GH may be due to a genetic defect in GH receptors or its transduction pathway resulting in severe IGF-1 deficiency.
5. Because it does not check secretion of GH.
6. GH and its chief mediator IGF-1 have opposite effects on carbohydrate metabolism.
   - GH itself increases the blood glucose levels by decreasing insulin sensitivity
   - Like insulin, IGF-1 increases glucose transport into cells, resulting in lowering of blood glucose
     Somatropin is rhGH and Mecasermin is rhIGF-1. So their effects on blood glucose levels are opposite to each other.
7. Somatotropin is growth hormone, whereas somatostatin inhibits the release of growth hormone. Refer to page 549, 550.
8. i. b. Lanreotide
   ii. Refer to page 551.
9. b. Menotropin, as it contains both FSH and LH.
10. Gonadotropin RH agonists include buserelin, nafarelin, triptorelin, and goserelin. Their continued use suppresses the release of gonadotropins due to down-regulation and desensitisation of receptors. This is useful for getting medical oophorectomy or orchidectomy.
11. d. All of the above. (GnRH agonists when given continuously; GnRH antagonists as well as menotropins are used for **controlled ovarian stimulation**.)
12. b. Degarelix, because it is a GnRH antagonist. Both nafarelin and leuprolide are GnRH agonists, which cause initial ovarian stimulation. Follitropin is FSH, which can cause ovarian hyperstimulation as an adverse effect.
13. b. Degarelix.
14. i. a. Chlorpromazine
    ii. The antipsychotic drug chlorpromazine is a D_2 antagonist. So, it blocks the inhibitory effect of dopamine on pituitary lactotrophs, resulting in hyperprolactinemia. Raised prolactin levels in this patient result in galactorrhea and gynecomastia.
15. i. c. Cabergoline
    ii. D_2 agonist
    iii. More potent, longer acting and better tolerated than bromocriptine. Dopamine and amantidine are not used in hyperprolactinemia.

CONCEPT MAP – ANTERIOR PITUITARY HORMONES

Growth Hormone : Somatotropin
Acts through JAK/STAT binding receptors
Actions: Longitudinal bone growth & epiphyseal closure in children.
Increased muscle & lean body mass, reduced adiposity.
GH increases, but IGF-1 reduces glucose levels
Excess release of GH (as in case of pituitary adenoma) results in 'acromegaly' in adults and 'gigantism' in children
Deficiency: Short stature in children, increased adiposity, abnormal lipid profile, cardiac manifestations, reduced lean body/muscle mass, decreased bone density, hypoglycemia.

Somatropin: rhGH
Therapeutic uses:
- As replacement therapy in patients with genetic or acquired GH deficiency. (Early initiation of therapy beneficial).
- Pediatric growth failure and short stature (due to Turner's syndrome, Prader–Willi syndrome, chronic renal insufficiency, small for gestational age at birth) Idiopathic short stature also responds.
- Muscle wasting of HIV and other catabolic states.
- Short bowel syndrome after resection.
- Used in anti-ageing preparations.
- Used by athletes to build up muscle mass.
- Used in cattle to increase milk production.

ADRs: Usually well tolerated by children
- Rare adverse effects include Slipped epiphysis of femur, hyperglycemia, edema, scoliosis, pseudotumor cerebri, sleep apnea, gynecomastia, nevus growth, and pancreatitis.
- In adults muscle & joint pain, inflammation especially in hands and wrists, carpal tunnel syndrome.
- GH can interact with simultaneously administered drugs due to microsomal enzyme induction.
- Its use in athletes is banned → included in dope testing.

Mecasermin: rhIGF-1
Uses: Useful in pediatric growth stunting, refractory to treatment with GH.
Given subcutaneously in a dose of 0.04–0.08 mg/kg body weight, twice a day and can be increased at weekly interval as per need.
ADRs: Hypoglycemia → patients are advised to have carbohydrate rich meal within 20 minutes of its use.
May raise liver enzymes & Intracranial tension.
Mecasermin rinfabate: It contains a complex of (rhIGF-1) & its binding protein-3 (rhIGFBP-3). Its half-life is longer than mecasermin.

Somatostatin
A paracrine factor present in hypothalamus, GIT and pancreas.
Inhibits secretion of GH, TSH, prolactin, Insulin, glucagon and all gastrointestinal secretions including HCl and gastrin
Uses: May be used in patients with biliary, intestinal or pancreatic fistulae.
Somatostatin causes vasoconstriction of renal, hepatic and splanchnic blood vessels → may be used to control bleeding from esophageal varices and bleeding peptic ulcers.
Limited clinical usefulness due to very short half-life (1–3 minutes only) and multiple effects.

Somatostatin Analogues
Octreotide: Longer acting and more selective for inhibiting GH release than insulin release in comparison to somatostatin. Thus, hyperglycemia is rarely seen with octreotide.
Uses: To control symptoms in hormone releasing tumours like acromegaly, carcinoid, insulinoma, glucagonoma, and gastrinoma.
To localise neuro-endocrine tumours by Somatostatin receptor scintigraphy (radiolabelled Octreotide used)
To control esophageal variceal bleeding in portal hypertension.
ADRs: Nausea, vomiting, bulky stools, flatulence, abdominal cramps. In some patients, continued treatment leads to formation of gallstones.
B_{12} deficiency may occur
Decrease in heart rate and AV conduction can occur
Lanreotide, Longer acting than octreotide, useful in acromegaly

Pegvisomant
Polyethylene glycol (PEG) derivative of GH with differential affinity of its two binding sites for GH receptors → blockade of signal transduction pathway.
Uses: Useful in treatment of acromegaly.
ADRs: raised hepatic enzymes
Lacks inhibitory effect on secretion of GH → increased adenoma growth.

ANTERIOR PITUITARY HORMONES

- GH Analogues
- GH Antagonists
- Growth Hormone
- Gonadotropins
- Prolactin

Gonadotropins
Drugs: Menotropin (FSH+LH), Urofollitropin (only FSH), Follitropin α and β (rhFSH), Lutropin (rhLH), Human chorionic gonadotropin (hCG), Choriogonadotropin (rhCG)
Therapeutic uses: To induce ovulation in infertility, if clomiphene citrate fails in polycystic ovarian disease.
For controlled ovarian stimulation in women undergoing 'in vitro fertilisation'.
Delayed puberty, oligozoospermia and sterility in males.
ADRs: 'Ovarian hyperstimulation syndrome'
Abortion and multiple pregnancies
Lower abdominal pain, polycystic ovary, ovarian bleeding and even shock may occur during induction of ovulation.
Precocious puberty in children
Headache, edema, mood disturbances

GnRH Agonists
Buserelin, Goserelin, Nafarelin, Triptorelin, Histrelin, Leuprolide.
More potent and longer acting than natural GnRH
Cause increase in Gn secretion if given in pulsatile manner.
So, with acute use → increase in gonadotropin secretion.
Continuous use, for 1–2 weeks → down-regulation, desensitisation of receptors → reduced gonadotropin secretion → gonadal function suppressed → drastic fall in estradiol levels in females and testosterone in males.
Therapeutic uses: Used as nasal spray or subcutaneous injections
For reversible pharmacological (medical) oophorectomy in precocious puberty, endometriosis, pre-menopausal carcinoma breast, uterine fibroid, polycystic ovarian disease.
Medical orchidectomy is indicated in precocious puberty in males and prostatic carcinoma.
ADRs: Hot flushes, loss of libido, vaginal dryness, osteoporosis and emotional lability as seen in menopausal women.

GnRH Antagonists
Ganirelix, Cetrorelix, Degarelix, Abarelix
Inhibit Gn secretion, without initial stimulation of Gn release
Used during IVF, to inhibit LH surges during controlled ovarian stimulation. So, risk of ovarian hyperstimulation is less.
Degarelix and Abarelix approved for androgen withdrawal therapy in patients with advanced carcinoma prostate.

Prolactin
Dopamine is prolactin inhibitory hormone (PIH).
Dopamine agonists like bromocriptine and cabergoline are useful in prolactinomas. Cabergoline is preferred due to longer half-life and fewer ADRs.
Dopamine antagonists like metoclopramide and antipsychotics can cause hyperprolactinemia → galactorrhea, gynecomastia as adverse effects.

SECTION 9 Drugs Affecting the Endocrine System

42 Drugs for Thyroid Disorders

PH 7.3 Describe the types, kinetics, dynamics, adverse drug reactions of drugs used in thyroid disorders, and devise a management plan for a case with thyroid disorder.

Learning objectives

A student of MBBS phase II should be able to:
- Describe the synthesis, storage, release of thyroid hormones.
- Describe the physiological role of thyroid hormones.
- Describe the indications for use and ADRs of thyroid hormones.
- Classify antithyroid drugs and describe their mechanisms of action.
- Enumerate therapeutic uses, ADRs and contraindications for use of antithyroid drugs.
- Devise management plan for a case of thyroid disorder.

THYROID HORMONES

The thyroid gland is present anterior to the trachea, between the thyroid cartilage and the suprasternal notch. It consists of two lobes (left and right), joined by an isthmus (Fig. 42.1). The basic functional unit of the thyroid gland is a **follicle**, which consists of a thyroglobulin-rich 'colloid' surrounded by follicular cells. Follicular cells secrete two hormones:

- T_3: Triiodothyronine
- T_4: Thyroxine

Parafollicular cells secrete calcitonin, which regulates Ca^{2+} homeostasis. Thyrotropin or thyroid stimulating hormone (TSH) is released from the anterior pituitary under the influence of thyrotropin releasing hormone (TRH) from the hypothalamus. In contrast, somatostatin (SST) released from the hypothalamus reduces TSH secretion. TSH stimulates all the steps of T_3 and T_4 synthesis and is the most important physiological marker of thyroid function. An endocrine feedback loop exists between the hypothalamus, anterior pituitary and thyroid gland. T_3 and T_4 exert negative feedback effect on TRH and TSH production (Fig. 42.1).

Hence, in patients with **hyperthyroidism, raised T_3 and T_4 levels** exert negative feedback effect and **TSH levels are reduced**.

In contrast, in **hypothyroidism, T_3 and T_4 are reduced**. This reduces their negative feedback effect and **TSH levels are elevated**.

Synthesis, Storage and Release of Thyroid Hormones

Synthesis of T_3 and T_4 in thyroid follicles and their release into the blood stream is a multistep process which can be interrupted by drugs at many sites (Fig. 42.2).

① The critical first step in thyroid hormone synthesis is the **uptake of iodides**. Iodide (I^-) is taken up by the basement membrane of follicular cells via an active transport mechanism using a sodium/iodide symporter (Na^+/I^- symporter or NIS). The **NIS can be competitively inhibited by monovalent anions** such as thiocyanate (SCN^-), perchlorate (ClO_4^-) pertechnetate (TcO_4^-) and nitrates (NO_3^-). So, all these anions exert an antithyroid effect.

② **Organification and coupling:** At the apical membrane of follicular cells, I^- is oxidised by the thyroid peroxidase enzyme (TPO) to form reactive iodine (iodinium ions: I^+, hypoiodus acid: HOI, enzyme-linked hypoiodite: EOI).

③ These reactive iodine species cause iodination of the tyrosine residues present in thyroglobulin, forming mono- and diiodotyrosine (MIT, DIT; organification).

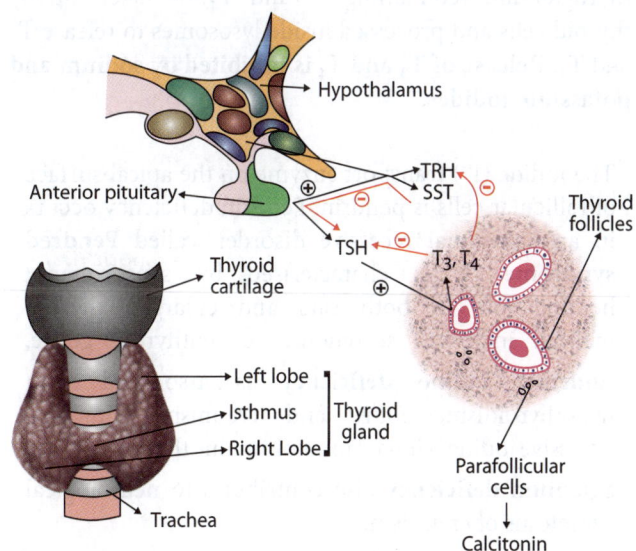

Fig. 42.1 Regulation of thyroid hormone secretion

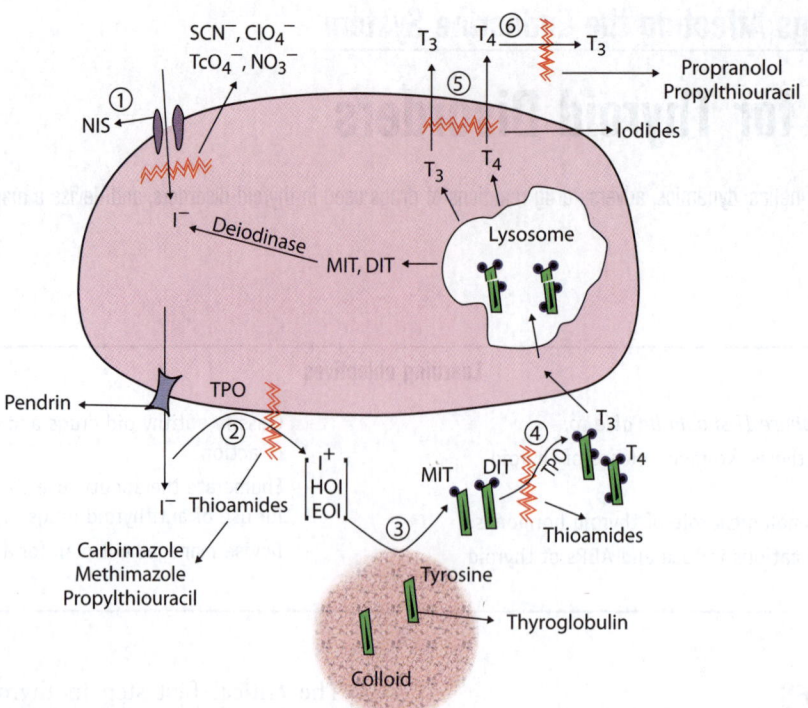

Fig. 42.2 Synthesis and release of thyroid hormones and site of action of antithyroid drugs. [① Iodide uptake; ② Oxidation of iodide to form reactive iodinium ions, hypoiodus acid, and enzyme-linked hypoiodite; ③ Organification; ④ Coupling; ⑤ Storage and release; ⑥ Conversion of T_4 to T_3.]

④ Further coupling of these iodotyrosines forms T_3 and T_4. DIT combines with MIT to form T_3 (3,5,3'-triiodothyronine) and with another DIT to form T_4 (3,5,3',5'-tetraiodothyronine). This coupling reaction is also catalysed by TPO. Unused MIT and DIT are de-**iodinated** by the enzyme called **deiodinase**, and iodine is recycled.

Thioamides such as carbimazole, methimazole and propylthiouracil **inhibit all TPO-catalysed steps** of thyroid hormone synthesis and exert an antithyroid effect.

⑤ **Storage and release**: After organification and coupling, thyroglobulin (containing T_3 and T_4) is taken up by thyroid cells and processed inside lysosomes to release T_3 and T_4. **Release of T_3 and T_4 is inhibited by sodium and potassium iodides.**

> The iodide (I⁻) transport enzyme on the apical surface of follicular cells is pendrin. Pendrin deficiency occurs in an autosomal recessive disorder, called **Pendred syndrome**. It is characterised by sensorineural hearing loss in both ears and enlarged thyroid without increased secretions, i.e., euthyroid goitre.
> **Endemic iodine deficiency** is associated with hypothyroidism, goitre and cretinism. However, excessive iodine is linked to autoimmune thyroid disease.
> **Selenium deficiency** also contributes to neurological symptoms of cretinism.
> These conditions can be prevented by consumption of iodine-rich/fortified foods.

⑥ T_4 is the major circulating hormone. In the liver and kidney, T_4 is converted into T_3 by the action of the enzyme, 5'-deiodinase; T_3 is the active form of thyroid hormone, which is taken up by target tissues and exerts action. This peripheral conversion is inhibited by propylthiouracil and propranolol. However, the pituitary gland takes up T_4 and converts it into T_3 intracellularly.

Pharmacokinetics
Oral absorption
Absorption of orally administered thyroxine (T_4) occurs in the small intestine. Oral bioavailability of T_4 is 70%. However, T_3 is completely absorbed after oral administration. Various intraluminal factors (food, gastric acidity and other drugs) interfere with T_4 absorption. Therefore, thyroxine (T_4) **is always given on an empty stomach**. In severe myxedema coma, the oral absorption of T_4 is seriously impaired; T_4 is given intravenously in this situation.

Plasma protein binding
After secretion from the thyroid gland into the blood stream, or after exogenous administration, T_3 and T_4 circulate while bound to plasma proteins such as thyroxine binding globulin (TBG), thyroxine binding pre-albumin (TBPA) and thyroxine binding albumin (TBA). The extent of binding varies for T_3 and T_4. The protein binding delays hormone clearance and increases the circulating hormone pool. Approximately **0.4% of T_3 and 0.04% of T_4 are present in the free form to exert actions.**

Deficiency of thyroxine binding globulin (TBG) results in reduced total T_3 and T_4. In contrast, elevated TBG levels (as in pregnancy and contraceptive use) raise total T_3 and T_4 levels. However, levels of free T_3 and free T_4 remain normal in both the situations.

Metabolism

T_4 gets converted to T_3 by the process of **de-iodination**. The catalysing enzyme is deiodinase 1 in the liver and kidney, whereas it is deiodinase 2 in the brain, pituitary, skeletal muscles and cardiac muscles. In fetal tissue, deiodinase 3 catalyses the formation of reverse T_3, which is indicative of fetal thyroid function.

Subsequent de-iodination of T_3 and **conjugation with glucuronyl and sulphate** forms inactive metabolites that are excreted in the urine. The half-life of T_4 is longer (7 days) than that of T_3 (24 hours).

Pharmacodynamics

The **mechanism of action** of thyroid hormones resembles that of corticosteroids. Free T_3 and T_4 enter the cell by active transport. T_4 is deiodinated to T_3. T_3 enters the nucleus, binds to intranuclear T_3 thyroid receptor protein (a protein from the c-erb oncogene family), and mediates transcription and protein synthesis. There is a time lag of hours or days between thyroxine administration and clinical response due to this **gene-mediated mechanism** of action. The number of thyroid receptors is larger in more responsive tissues such as liver, kidney, heart, lungs, intestine, skeletal muscles, and pituitary and widespread effects are seen.

Physiological Role

- Thyroid hormones **increase the basal metabolic rate (BMR)** by increased cellular metabolism of carbohydrates, proteins and lipids.
  - Thyroid hormones increase use of glucose by tissues for ATP production. However, increased gluconeogenesis, glycogenolysis and intestinal absorption of glucose result in hyperglycemia and diabetes-like state.
  - T_3 and T_4 enhance synthesis of some proteins. However, they also increase use of proteins as a source of energy, resulting in a net catabolic effect and negative nitrogen balance.
  - Lipolysis increases, resulting in raised levels of FFAs, lowered cholesterol and more conversion of cholesterol into bile acids.
- **Calorigenic effect** is seen because of facilitation of ATP utilisation, which liberates heat and raises body temperature.
- Thyroid hormones **stimulate growth** and development of all tissues, but effect on CNS is most prominent.
- These hormones cause **up-regulation of β-receptors** and **sensitise the heart to catecholamines**. Heart rate, force of contraction and stroke volume are increased, causing hyperdynamic circulation.
- **Other actions**: Thyroid hormones facilitate propulsive activity of gut, urine flow and hemopoiesis.

Therapeutic Uses

- **Hypothyroidism**: Replacement therapy using thyroid hormones is the only treatment available for hypothyroid patients.

T_4 is the preferred preparation for replacement therapy because:
  - Its longer half-life allows only once daily dosing, which is more convenient.
  - Easy monitoring of serum concentrations.
  - More stability.
  - Lack of allergic reactions.
  - Low cost.
  - Lower risk of cardiac adverse effects than T_3.

Moreover, patients should maintain the same brand of T_4 to avoid changes in the bioavailability, i.e., bioinequivalence. The differences between T_3 and T_4 are listed in Table 42.1.

Dose of thyroxine: The average adult dose of thyroxine is 1.7 mcg/kg/day; however, it is given orally as 50–100 mcg (adjusted by age and comorbidity), on empty stomach. Pregnant women with hypothyroidism may need 20% higher doses of thyroxine to meet the demands of fetal brain development. As TBG is raised in pregnancy, free T_4 should be monitored for dose adjustment.

- **Cretinism**: The dose of levothyroxine for 6–12-month-old infants is 10–15 mcg/kg/day. Dose decreases with increasing age. The drug is to be continued throughout life with monitoring and dosage adjustment.
- **Myxedema coma needs intravenous administration of levothyroxine** (as oral absorption is impaired) in a dose of 200–500 mcg, followed by 100 mcg, once a day. Once the patient's condition improves, oral treatment is started.

Table 42.1 Differences between T_3 and T_4

	Levothyroxine (T_4)	Liothyronine (T_3)
Chemical name	3,5,3′,5′-tetraiodothyronine	3,5,3′-triiodothyronine
Potency	Less potent	More potent
Activity	Less active	More active
Onset of action	Slow	Fast
Duration of action	Long acting	Short acting
Use	Suitable for long-term use in hypothyroidism	Suitable for emergency situations, i.e., myxedema coma

- **Simple non-endemic goitre** has euthyroid status and raised TSH. Thyroxine therapy in these cases lowers TSH by negative feedback and goitre size may regress.
- Administration of T_4 normalises raised TSH levels by negative feedback mechanism. Thus, T_4 is useful in checking growth of **TSH-dependent thyroid nodule and papillary carcinoma**.

Adverse drug reactions
Overdose of thyroid hormone causes adverse reactions similar to features of hyperthyroidism such as tremors, diarrhea, weight loss and cardiac effects (tachycardia, palpitation and arrhythmias). Angina may worsen.

Drugs interactions
- Thyroid hormones increase the metabolism of vitamin K-dependent clotting factors. Thus, T_4 opposes coagulation; the dose of simultaneously administered **anticoagulants** should be adjusted on the lower side.
- Thyroid hormones have complex effects on carbohydrate metabolism. They increase the rate of degradation of insulin, i.e., $t_{½}$ of insulin is reduced. Hence, in diabetics, the dose of **insulin** needs to be adjusted on the higher side.
- Similarly, the rate of degradation and required dose of **digoxin** is increased in patients receiving thyroxine.

ABNORMAL THYROID FUNCTIONS
T_3 and T_4 affect cellular metabolism of carbohydrates, proteins and lipids in a complex manner. Therefore, deviations of thyroid function from normal (euthyroid) state affect these metabolic processes resulting in various organ system effects. Thyroid dysfunction occurs as two contrasting conditions, viz., hypo- and hyperthyroidism. The salient features of these two conditions are summarised in Table 42.2.

Table 42.2 Thyroid hormone dysfunction

Parameter	Hypothyroidism	Hyperthyroidism
1. Basic defect	Deficiency of thyroid hormones	Excess of thyroid hormones
2. Etiology	**Impaired synthesis** of thyroid hormones. May be due to: • Iodine deficiency • Drug induced (Li, amiodarone) Destruction of gland due to: • Autoimmune process as in Hashimoto's thyroiditis • Surgical removal • Radioactive iodine (^{131}I) • Secondary to pituitary disease • TSH receptor-blocking antibodies (congenital)	- Graves' disease (**autoimmune** process involving the formation of immunoglobulin that stimulates growth and biosynthetic activity similar to TSH) - Toxic uninodular or multinodular **adenomas** or goitre - **Viral infection** of thyroid gland causing parenchymal destruction and release of stored thyroid hormones
3. Manifestation		
General symptoms	Lethargy, muscular weakness, decreased deep tendon reflexes, facial puffiness, deep hoarse voice	Insomnia, nervousness, tremors, weakness, muscle wasting. Increased deep tendon reflexes, exophthalmos
- Skin/hair	Dry skin, hair loss of outer 1/3rd of eyebrows, low body temperature, cold sensitivity	Warm moist skin, heat intolerance
- Metabolic	Reduced BMR, hypertriglyceridemia, weight gain	Raised BMR, hyperglycemia, negative nitrogen balance, weight loss.
- Cardiac	Bradycardia, risk of low output cardiac failure	Tachycardia, arrhythmias, angina may be precipitated, risk of high output cardiac failure.
- Gastrointestinal	Decreased appetite, constipation, ascites	Increased appetite, diarrhea
- Reproductive	Decreased libido, menorrhagia, infertility, oligospermia, impotence	Menstrual irregularities, amenorrhea, infertility

Parameter	Hypothyroidism	Hyperthyroidism
- Kidneys	Decreased renal blood flow, impairment of water excretion	Increased renal blood flow, mild polyuria.
- Goitre	May or may not be present	May be present in toxic adenomas
4. Investigations	Low level of free thyroxine, raised TSH levels	Raised (total and free) T_3 and T_4 levels, and reduced TSH levels
5. Treatment	Replacement therapy with **oral levothyroxine** given on empty stomach. Average **adult** dose 1.7 mcg/kg/day. Higher dose for **infants**: 10–15 mcg/kg/day for 6–12 months age. Dose decreases as age increases.	**Antithyroid drugs** that reduce synthesis or release of hormones are preferred in young patients having mild disease. In patient > 21 years ^{131}I can be used. **Surgical treatment** (subtotal thyroidectomy) is done for patients with very large gland or multinodular goitre
6. Severe form of disease	**Myxedema coma** is characterised by stuporous condition, progressive muscular weakness, hypoglycemia, hypothermia, hypoventilation, hyponatremia, hypercapnia, water intoxication, shock and death. Management: - Patient may need mechanical or ventilator **support**. - Associated illness should be vigorously treated. - Caution in use of I/V fluids because of fear of water intoxication. - Oral drugs are only partly absorbed; so, therapy is given intravenously. T_3 may be used as its onset of action is faster, but it is not preferred because of higher cardiotoxicity potential. Dose is 20 mcg stat, repeated after 4 hours. - Levothyroxine sodium 500 mcg intravenous stat, followed by 100 mcg daily is used	**Thyroid storm or thyrotoxicosis crisis** is a life-threatening condition characterised by acute exacerbation of all symptoms of thyrotoxicosis. It may be precipitated by acute infection, trauma, surgery, stress and ketoacidosis. Patient develops hyperpyrexia, profuse sweating, diarrhea, tachyarrhythmias, pulmonary edema and cardiac failure. Management: - Involves **supportive therapy** to control heart rate, fever and treatment of precipitating disease. - **Hydrocortisone** 100 mg/IV can protect from shock. - β-blocker **propranolol** (1–4 mg slow I/V or 40–80 mg oral every 4 hours) is effective to control symptoms of sympathetic overactivity. It also prevents peripheral conversion of T_4 to active T_3 form. - Thioamides block new synthesis of hormone. **Propylthiouracil** is faster-acting than carbimazole. It is given orally as 500 mg loading dose, followed by 250 mg 4-hourly maintenance dose. If patient is not fit to take dose orally, rectal route can be tried. - After 1 hour of initiating thioamide therapy, **5 drops of KI** are given **orally**, 6-hourly, to block release of thyroid hormone. - In very severe cases, **plasmapheresis** may be needed.

Clinical problem-based questions and MCQs

1. A 41-year-old female patient presents with lethargy, muscular weakness, dry skin and menorrhagia. On examination, deep tendon reflexes are depressed. Investigations show raised TSH and reduced T_4 levels.
   i. What is the diagnosis?
   ii. Which of the following is drug of choice in this patient?
      a. Carbimazole   b. Liothyronine
      c. Levothyroxine   d. Propylthiouracil
   iii. Justify your choice with the pharmacological basis.

2. Which of the following factors interfere with oral absorption of thyroxine?
   a. Gastric acidity   b. Food
   c. Other drugs   d. All of the above

3. i. In patients using oral contraceptives:
   a. Total (T_3, T_4) levels are raised, but free (fT_3 and fT_4) levels are low.
   b. Total (T_3, T_4) levels are raised, but free (fT_3 and fT_4) levels are normal.
   c. Both total and fT_3 and fT_4 levels are raised.
   d. Both total and fT_3 and fT_4 levels are low.
   ii. Describe the interaction between oral contraceptives and thyroid hormones.

4. In patients suffering from hypothyroidism, T_4 is preferred over T_3 because of its:
   a. Longer half-life
   b. Fewer adverse effects
   c. Lack of allergic reactions
   d. All of the above

5. Which of the following is true about the metabolic effects of T_4?
   a. Inhibits lipolysis.
   b. Facilitates ATP production and utilisation.
   c. Inhibits protein synthesis.
   d. Decreases cellular metabolism of proteins.

6. i. Identify the best parameter for thyroxine dosage adjustment in pregnant females with hypothyroidism.
   a. Free T_3 and T_4
   b. Total (T_3, T_4)
   c. TSH
   d. Both free and total, T_3 and T_4
   ii. Justify your choice with the pharmacological basis.

7. Thyroxine is indicated in all of the following except
   a. Hypothyroidism
   b. Simple non-endemic goitre
   c. Graves' disease
   d. Chronic thyroiditis

8. A 56-year-old female patient is brought to emergency in a stuporous condition, with a history of progressive muscular weakness. On examination, patient has hypothermia (body temperature = 36.2 °C), respiratory rate: 10 per minute (hypoventilation), and tendon reflexes diminished. Investigations show hypoglycemia, hyponatremia, hypercapnia, raised TSH and low (T_3, T_4) levels.
   i. What is the diagnosis?
   ii. Describe the management of this case.

CLASSIFICATION OF ANTITHYROID DRUGS

Based on their mechanism of action, antithyroid drugs are classified (Flowchart 42.1) into drugs which reduce hormone synthesis by inhibiting either iodide trapping or thyroid peroxidase enzyme. Some drugs inhibit release of thyroid hormones, while others relieve symptoms

1. Ionic Inhibitors

Monovalent anions such as SCN^-, ClO_4^-, TcO_4^- and NO_3^- **competitively inhibit NIS** and iodide uptake by the follicular cells. While the synthesis of T_3 and T_4 is inhibited in this manner, these are **not clinically useful** because:

- Competitive inhibition can be overcome by large doses of iodides; so, their effects are unpredictable.
- These ions are very toxic, e.g., potassium perchlorate increases the risk of aplastic anemia.

2. Thioamides

Thioamides include carbimazole, methimazole and propylthiouracil (PTU).

Mechanism of action

Thioamides act by inhibiting thyroid peroxidase (TPO) enzyme. So, they inhibit:

- Oxidation of iodide (I^-) to form reactive iodine species (I^+, HOI, EOI).
- Iodination (organification) of tyrosine residues of thyroglobulin, preventing the formation of iodotyrosines (MIT and DIT).
- Coupling of iodotyrosines, so that T_3 and T_4 are not formed from MIT and DIT.

Hence, thioamides inhibit TPO-catalysed reactions (iodide oxidation, organification and coupling), which leads to lowering of T_3 and T_4 levels slowly and colloid depletion. So, the onset of action of these drugs is delayed for 1–3 weeks, till the hormonal deposits in the gland are used up.

- In addition, propylthiouracil (PTU) prevents peripheral conversion of T_4 to T_3.

However, thioamides have no effect on iodide trapping by the thyroid and release of T_3 and T_4 from the thyroid gland. These drugs do not affect the actions of T_3 and T_4 on target organs.

Pharmacokinetics

Thioamides are **well-absorbed orally**. Carbimazole is a prodrug; it is converted into methimazole in vivo. While the absorption of PTU is faster than that of methimazole, methimazole is 10 times more potent and longer-acting than PTU.

Thioamides are **widely distributed**, with the volume of distribution being equal to the total body water. They accumulate in the thyroid gland and can cross the placental barrier to suppress fetal thyroid function. Methimazole has been rarely associated with an increased risk of congenital malformations. PTU is more strongly bound to plasma proteins than methimazole, and so, less drug crosses the

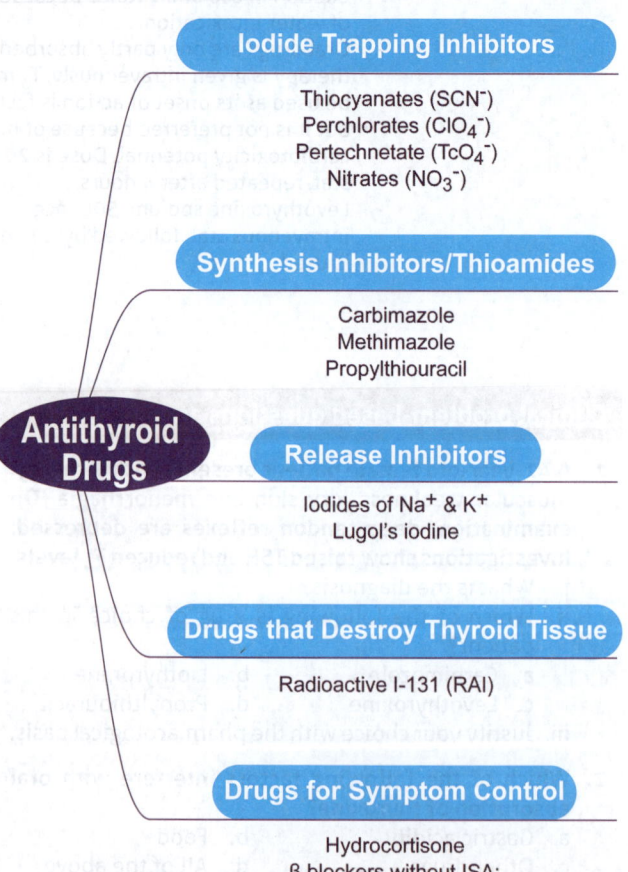

Flowchart 42.1 Classification of antithyroid drugs based on their mechanism of action.

placenta. Consequently, **PTU is preferred in hyperthyroid patients during the 1st trimester of pregnancy.**

Metabolism of thioamides occurs by **conjugation in the liver** and inactive metabolites are excreted in urine. Methimazole ($t^{½} = 6$ hours) is longer acting than PTU ($t^{½} = 1.5$ hours). However, the **duration of antithyroid action is much longer than expected from the half-life,** because of drug concentration in the thyroid gland. The effect of a single dose of PTU lasts for 6–8 hours and methimazole for > 24 hours.

Therapeutic uses
- It is used for the **definitive treatment of hyperthyroid** patients with Graves' disease and toxic goitre. Remission occurs within 1–2 years of treatment. The drug therapy can be then stopped and reinstituted as and when required.
- **Preoperatively:** Thioamides are used to make patients euthyroid before attempting subtotal thyroidectomy.
- In older patients selected for radioactive iodine (RAI) therapy also, thioamides are given first to prevent flaring up of hyperthyroidism by RAI (due to release of stored hormone).

Adverse reactions
Over-dosing can cause **hypothyroidism**, i.e., lowering of T_3 and T_4 levels → increase in TSH and goitre. These adverse effects are reversible on dose reduction. Other common adverse effects are:
- **Gastrointestinal** intolerance (nausea and gastrointestinal distress, altered taste and smell) with methimazole.
- **Allergic reactions** as maculopapular pruritic rash is reported in 4–6% of patients treated with thioamides. Rarely, severe reactions may occur in the form of urticaria, lupus-like reaction, exfoliative dermatitis, polyserositis, cholestatic jaundice and acute arthralgia.
- PTU carries the risk of severe hepatitis, which may even be fatal. Therefore, it is reserved for use in emergency situations such as thyroid storm and in the 1st trimester of pregnancy.
- An infrequent but very serious adverse effect of these drugs is **agranulocytosis.** Risk is greater in patients receiving higher doses and in the elderly. Hence, it is important to monitor patients on thioamide therapy. The reaction is reversible upon stopping the drug.

3. Iodides
Iodides include sodium iodide, potassium iodide and Lugol's solution (5% iodine in 10% KI).

Mechanism of action
- The most important action of sodium and potassium iodides and Lugol's solution is the **inhibition of thyroglobulin proteolysis** and **hormone release.** As a consequence, the symptoms improve rapidly within 2–7 days of starting therapy. This is sometimes called the **thyroid-constipating action** of iodides.
- Excess iodide **inhibits its own uptake** by the gland and also **the iodination of tyrosine residues** of colloidal thyroglobulin, leading to reduced synthesis.
- Preoperative use of, iodides **reduces the size, fragility and vascularity** of the thyroid gland.

However, after 2–8 weeks of iodide therapy, **thyroid escape** occurs, and hyperthyroidism appears with greater severity, because of the iodine stored in the gland. So, iodides should never be used alone. **Thioamide therapy is initiated** to achieve euthyroid state before initiating iodide therapy, because iodides may delay the onset of thioamide action.

Uses
Lugol's solution is given **preoperatively** for 10 days in an oral dose of 5–10 drops daily, to make the thyroid gland firm, less vascular and smaller. Propranolol may be added for symptom control, if needed.
- In thyroid storm or **thyrotoxic crisis,** iodides inhibit the release of T_3 and T_4
- Iodine is also used as an **antiseptic** (tincture iodine and povidone–iodine) and in iodised salt for **prophylaxis of endemic goitre.**

Adverse reactions
- **Acute reactions** such as swelling of lips and eyelids, angioedema of larynx, fever and joint pain may occur.
- Overdose may cause **iodism** in the form of acneiform eruptions, mucous membrane ulcerations, rhinorrhea, swelling in salivary glands, headache, rashes, bleeding disorders, and even anaphylactic reactions.
- In pregnancy, fetal goitre and hypothyroidism may occur.

4. Radioactive Iodine (RAI) I-131
The sodium salt of **I-131** dissolved in H_2O gets concentrated in the thyroidal colloid upon oral use. It emits β-particles that can penetrate up to 400–2000 µm and **damage follicular cells from within**, without damaging surrounding tissues. Dose is 4–5 millicuries (mCi), orally, for Graves' disease and multinodular goitre. Although response develops gradually and takes 3 months to attain its peak effect, the cure is permanent.

Therapeutic uses
Radioactive I is used in hyperthyroidism due to Grave's disease and toxic goitre. It is the treatment of choice for patients > 35 years of age.
- It is used in patients where surgery is contraindicated.
- It is useful in palliative treatment of medullary carcinoma of thyroid.

ADRs

- Over 50% of patients acquire hypothyroidism and need replacement therapy with thyroxine; it is not suitable for young patients.
- Contraindicated in pregnancy, because of the risk of fetal hypothyroidism and cretinism.

5. β-Blockers

β-blockers without intrinsic sympathetic activity, such as propranolol, esmolol and metoprolol, are useful in thyrotoxicosis and in patients awaiting response to **I-131**. These drugs cause rapid alleviation of symptoms associated with sympathetic overactivity like palpitation, nervousness, sweating, and tremors. β-blockers also prevent peripheral conversion of T_4 to T_3.

6. Corticosteroids

Methyl prednisolone is used intravenously in cases of Graves' ophthalmopathy. RAI can aggravate this condition.

COMPARISON OF ANTITHYROID DRUGS, SURGERY AND I-131

Advantages of antithyroid drugs:

- Easy administration, simple, convenient and inexpensive therapy.
- There is no surgical scar.
- Patient is not exposed to risks associated with surgery.
- No risk of injury to surrounding structures like parathyroid glands and recurrent laryngeal nerve.
- Hypothyroidism due to overdosage of drugs is reversible on dose reduction, except for RAI.
- Antithyroid drugs can be used even in children and young adults.

Disadvantages of antithyroid drugs:

- Prolonged treatment is needed because relapse rate is after discontinuation.
- Risk of toxicity to fetus in pregnancy, as the drugs can cross the placental barrier and cause fetal hypothyroidism and cretinism. Propylthiouracil is comparatively safer than other antithyroid drugs for pregnant patients.
- Compliance is poor in less educated patients.
- Agranulocytosis caused by thioamides (though rare) can be life-threatening.
- With radioactive iodine, the onset of action is delayed by about 2 weeks, and peak response is achieved after 3 months of therapy.

Clinical problem-based questions and MCQs

9. Which of the following causes competitive inhibition of the sodium-iodide symporter (NIS)?
   a. Thiocyanate b. Carbimazole
   c. Propylthiouracil d. Radioactive iodine

10. A 36-year-old male patient presents with nervousness, tremors, insomnia, heat intolerance, and weight loss in spite of increased appetite. On examination, patient has exophthalmos and skin is warm and moist. HR = 120/minute, deep tendon reflexes are increased. Investigations show high fT_3 and fT_4 levels and low TSH.
    i. What is the diagnosis?
    ii. Classify drugs that may be useful in this case.
    iii. Briefly describe their mechanism of action.

11. Comment on the advantages and limitations of using antithyroid drugs in comparison to surgical removal of the thyroid gland.

12. Which of the following is useful in the management of thyroid storm?
    a. Propranolol b. Plasmapheresis
    c. Propylthiouracil d. All of the above.

13. The mechanism of antithyroid action of propylthiouracil involves:
    a. Reduced iodide trapping
    b. Inhibition of thyroid peroxidase
    c. Inhibition of thyroglobulin proteolysis
    d. Destruction of thyroid tissue

14. i. Which of the following drugs acts by decreasing the release of thyroid hormones?
    a. Potassium iodide b. Thiocyanate
    c. Methimazole d. Propranolol
    ii. What are indications for use of the selected drug?

15. Iodides cause all of the following actions, EXCEPT:
    a. Increase proteolysis of thyroglobulin.
    b. Bring about rapid symptomatic improvement in a hyperthyroid patient.
    c. Reduce size and fragility of thyroid gland.
    d. Reduce iodination of tyrosine residues of thyroglobulin.

16. A 50-year-old male patient, known case of hyperthyroidism on carbimazole therapy, develops acute respiratory tract infection. Patient presents with hyperpyrexia, profuse sweating, diarrhea and palpitation. On examination HR = 110 bpm. Features of pulmonary edema and cardiac failure are positive. TSH is very low and fT_3 and fT_4 are markedly raised. Patient is diagnosed with thyrotoxic crisis.
    i. Describe the management of this case.
    ii. Comment on the role of various drugs in this case.

17. Iodides are known to cause a phenomenon called 'thyroid escape'. Describe the cause of this phenomenon and measures to prevent it.

18. A 25-year-old pregnant woman presents with anxiety, heat intolerance and palpitation. On examination, patient is 8-weeks pregnant. Skin is warm and moist. HR is increased, tendon reflexes are increased. On investigation T_3 and T_4 levels are raised and TSH is low. She is diagnosed with hyperthyroidism.
    i. Identify the drug of choice in this case.
    a. Radioactive iodine b. Propylthiouracil
    c. Methimazole d. Propranolol

ii. Justify your choice with the pharmacological basis.
19. Identify the life-threatening adverse effect of carbimazole.
    a. Thrombo-embolism   b. Pulmonary edema
    c. Agranulocytosis   d. Anaphylactic shock
20. Identify the drug that prevents peripheral conversion of thyroxine to T_3.
    a. Methimazole   b. Potassium iodide
    c. Propylthiouracil   d. Thiocyanates

MANAGEMENT PLAN FOR THYROID DISEASES

The management of thyroid disorders needs a comprehensive holistic approach. For a patient with history suggestive of thyroid dysfunction (refer Table 42.2), a variety of approaches are initiated, as described below.

Initial Assessment

A medical specialist or endocrinologist determines the type and severity of thyroid disorder. Clinical examination can show many classical features, such as;

- Weight gain, dry/coarse/sparse hair, scanty eyebrows, thick/dry/lustreless skin, macroglossia, non-pitting edema, periorbital edema in hypothyroidism.
- Soft, moist skin, lid lag, stare, reduced blinking, unilateral/bilateral exophthalmos, tremors, tachycardia in hyperthyroidism.

Investigations

Baseline investigations include free T_3, T_4, and TSH levels. Thyroid antibody test may also be needed.

- In **hypothyroidism**: T_3, T_4 levels are reduced, and TSH is raised above the reference range.
- In **hyperthyroidism**: T_3, T_4 levels are raised, while TSH levels are below reference range.
- Goitre may or may not be present in both hypothyroidism and hyperthyroidism.

Further investigations, such as TRH stimulation test, free needle aspiration cytology (FNAC) from thyroid swelling, ultrasound/CT scan/ MRI, thyroid auto-antibodies test and thyroid scintiscanning, may be done as needed for confirmation of diagnosis.

Treatment

Thyroid diseases are managed by pharmacotherapy and non-pharmacological measures.

Hypothyroidism

Hypothyroid patients require replacement therapy with levothyroxine.

- Adult dose of thyroxine is 1.7 mcg/kg/day. It is usually given orally, on an empty stomach, as a tablet containing 50–100 mcg thyroxine.
- Patient should be informed about need for lifelong therapy with thyroid hormones, and the need to take thyroxine ½–1 hour before meals.
- Patient should be instructed regarding proper storage of thyroxine tablets in a cool, dark, dry place.
- In hypothyroidism, fluctuations in thyroid function are common and the disease is slowly progressive. Thus, periodic follow up and dose adjustment is needed, according to the response. Adherence to drug therapy should be ensured before changing dose.
- **Non-pharmacological measures**: In addition to replacement therapy with thyroxine, patients should be instructed about iodine intake, overall nutrition, regular physical activity and weight reduction.

Myxedema coma

Myxedema coma is a medical emergency and requires hospitalisation.

- Gradual warming up of patient, maintenance of airways, ventilation, and circulation is of prime importance.
- Triiodothyronine is given intravenously. Dose is 20 mcg stat, repeated after 4 hours; however, it is not preferred because of its cardiotoxicity.
- Levothyroxine sodium 500 mcg as a stat dose, followed by 100 mcg daily.
- If parenteral preparations of triiodothyronine/ levothyroxine are not available or intravenous line is not accessible, thyroxine 100 mcg may be given through a nasogastric tube. Dose is repeated 3–4 times a day.
- Injection hydrocortisone 100 mg, intravenous 3–4 times a day is used to prevent hypoadrenal crisis, and helps in recovery from shock. Injection dexamethasone 2 mg, intravenous 6-hourly may be used as an alternative.
- Treatment of concurrent infections and diseases that precipitate myxedema coma is important.

Hyperthyroidism

- Patients with hyperthyroidism should be offered various available treatment modalities/options, i.e., drugs, radioactive iodine, surgery, etc. Pros and cons of each modality should be discussed with the patient for shared decision making. Antithyroid drugs are the first line of management. Treatment is started with low dose and modified based on response.
- Carbimazole is most frequently used drug, given orally in a dose of 10–15 mg, every 6 hours. The effect of the drug manifests in 2–3 weeks. So, dose adjustment should be done at this stage. The dose, once stabilised, is maintained for 18–24 months. As the condition of the patient improves, tapering down of the dose is attempted to maintain treatment with a lower dose or to discontinue the drug. If symptoms of hyperthyroidism reappear, treatment is re-instituted.

- Propylthiouracil is preferred in pregnant women with hyperthyroidism.
- Thioamides have potential adverse effects such as leukopenia, thrombocytopenia and agranulocytosis. Patients should be counselled about the risks and advised to get periodic blood counts to detect any adverse events at the earliest.
- Surgical treatment is offered in patients showing the pressure effects of a large goitre, inadequate response, intolerable adverse effects, or poor compliance with drugs. Two weeks prior to surgery, potassium iodide 60–100 mg per day is given to decrease the size and vascularity of the thyroid gland.
- Patient may develop features of hypothyroidism after subtotal thyroidectomy. They should be informed about the symptoms of hypothyroidism and advised to seek medical help if such symptoms appear. These patients may need thyroxine supplementation therapy for rest of their lives.
- Patients with small to moderate goitres who are poor operative risks or develop repeated thyrotoxicosis are given I-131 (4–5 millicurie); the same dose may be repeated after 3–6 months. These patients may also develop hypothyroidism, many years after radioactive I-131 therapy.

Thyrotoxic crisis

Thyrotoxic crisis is also considered a medical emergency, and hospitalisation is required.

- Glucose saline intravenous infusion with 100 mg hydrocortisone is given every 4–6 hours to combat shock.
- Diazepam (5–10 mg) intravenous to quieten the patient.
- Propranolol (1–4 mg) stat intravenous over 5 minutes is useful to control tachycardia and other symptoms of sympathetic stimulation. Once the condition improves, oral propranolol is given.
- Sodium iodide (300–600 mg) is given intravenously, every 8 hours, till the crisis condition is controlled.
- An alternative to sodium iodide is propylthiouracil—500 mg loading dose, followed by 250 mg 4-hourly maintenance dose by oral/rectal route or through nasogastric tube. After 1 hour of initiating thioamide therapy, **5 drops of KI** are given **orally**, every 6 hours, to block the release of thyroid hormone. Carbimazole (15–20 mg) may be given through nasogastric tube.
- Sodium ipodate (500 mg/day oral), an iodine containing radio-contrast dye, can restore T_3 levels to the normal range in 2–3 days. After 14 days, sodium ipodate and propranolol should be withdrawn

Medical Applications and Devices

Monitoring devices such as fitness trackers and smart watches are useful to monitor heart rate and blood pressure. Weight changes should be tracked on a digital scale. Mobile health applications to track iodine intake, sleep trackers, medical alert devices are quite frequently advised in current clinical practice.

Patient Education

Increasing awareness about course of disease, need for long-term therapy, periodic investigations especially during dose adjustment, periodic follow up, importance of compliance to drug therapy is of utmost importance in successful management of thyroid disorders. Regular communication with health team, follow up by mobile health monitoring applications, telemedicine, and patient support groups for emotional and mental support can significantly improve the outcomes.

IODINE DEFICIENCY

Iodine is one of the essential micronutrients; 100-150 mcg is required daily for normal growth and development in humans.

Burden and Spectrum of Iodine Deficiency Diseases

Nutritional deficiency of iodine causes a spectrum of diseases called iodine deficiency disorders (IDD). IDDs affect people of all ages, both genders and different socio-economic groups in all the continents, resulting in huge burden of disease.

- Deficiency of iodine during pregnancy can cause abortions, stillbirth, congenital defects like squint, deaf-mutism, and mental retardation.
- Neonates may develop goitre and hypothyroidism.
- Perinatal and infant mortality increases.
- Children born to hypothyroid mothers may develop cretinism, dwarfism, spastic diplegia and psychomotor defects.
- In children and adolescents, conditions like goitre, juvenile hypothyroidism, growth retardation and impaired mental function may develop.
- Adults may suffer from goitre, hypothyroidism and impairment of mental function.

Goitre (IDD) is diagnosed by inspection and palpation of the neck. The disease is graded as:

- **Grade 0**: No visible swelling or palpable mass in neck, i.e., no goitre.
- **Grade 1**: No swelling is visible in neck in normal position. However, a mass consistent with enlarged thyroid is palpable in neck, it moves upwards while swallowing.
- **Grade 2**: A swelling is visible when the neck is in normal position. On palpation, a mass consistent with thyroid enlargement is present.

Severity of public health problem

Severity of disease burden and public health problem is labelled as mild, moderate or severe, based on population having goitre grade higher than zero and median urine iodine excretion (UIE) as shown in table below.

	Mild	Moderate	Severe
Goitre grade > 0 (%)	5–19.9	20–29.9	≥ 30
Median urine iodine excretion (UIE; mcg/L)	50–99	20–49	< 20

IDDs can be prevented by a very simple measure, i.e., intake of iodised salt. Thus, the Central Govt. started the National Goitre Control Programme (NGCP) in 1962 (renamed as **National Iodine Deficiency Disorder Control Programme (NIDDCP)** in 1992), keeping in mind the broad range of diseases caused by iodine deficiency.

The goal of the NIDDCP is to reduce the prevalence below 5% and ensure 100% consumption of iodised salt at the household level. This was envisaged to be achieved by surveys, supply of iodised salt, health education and publicity activities etc.

State IDD cells create demand of iodised salt, coordinate with food and civil supplies department to ensure adequate distribution, monitor consumption and check iodine levels in salt with wholesalers and retailers. These cells also conduct surveys, trainings, information dissemination, communication and public awareness activities.

Indicators in NIDDCP

Manufacturing and sale of uniodised salt is banned in India with effect from May 2006. Adequate iodine content in salt is 15 parts per million (ppm). The iodine content of salt is measured in the laboratory by iodometric titrations.

More than 90% households should be consuming adequately iodised salt (containing 15 ppm iodine) in an amount > 150 mcg/day. However, iodised salt intake from 150–1000 mcg is considered safe, as any excess iodine is easily excreted by kidneys in urine. Thus, adequate supply should ensure 150 mcg iodised salt/person/day.

Median urinary iodine excretion (UIE) should be 100–199 mcg/L in general population and 150–249 mcg/L in pregnant women.

Across the world, 21 October is observed as Global IDD Prevention Day.

Summary

- Thyroid gland secretes triiodothyronine (T_3), thyroxine (T_4) and calcitonin.
- Secretion of T_3 and T_4 is regulated by thyrotropin or thyroid-stimulating hormone (TSH), which is regulated through TRH and SST from the hypothalamus. TSH secretion is increased by TRH and reduced by SST. T_3 and T_4 exert negative feedback effect on TRH and TSH secretion.
- Synthesis of thyroid hormones: iodide trapping is transport of iodide into the thyroid gland by sodium/iodide symporter (NIS) → oxidation at the apical cell membrane of thyroid follicular cells catalysed by thyroid peroxidase (TPO) to form I^+, HOI and EOI → which iodise tyrosine residues within thyroglobulin molecules forming monoiodotyrosine (MIT) and diiodotyrosine (DIT) called **organification** → **coupling** of two molecules of DIT or one molecule of MIT with one molecule of DIT results in the formation of L-thyroxine (T_4) or triiodothyronine (T_3), respectively.
- Synthesis is inhibited by **monovalent anions** like thiocyanate (SCN^-), perchlorate (ClO_4^-), pertechnetate (TcO_4^-) and nitrates (NO_3^-), which interfere with iodide trapping and TPO inhibitors like **thioamides**.
- T_3 and T_4 are stored, bound to thyroglobulin, in the thyroid colloid → endocytosis of thyroglobulin by follicular cells and proteolysis by lysosomal enzymes results in the release of T_3 and T_4 into circulation. This release is inhibited by **iodides of sodium and potassium**.
- T_3 is the active form of the thyroid hormone. T_4 is converted into T_3 in the periphery. This conversion is inhibited by **propranolol and propylthiouracil**.
- **Hypothyroidism**, typically manifests as bradycardia, cold intolerance, constipation, fatigue, menorrhagia, and weight gain. Replacement therapy with levothyroxine (1.7 mcg/kg body weight) is the treatment of choice for hypothyroidism. Severe form of hypothyroidism causes myxedema coma. It is managed by supportive treatment and intravenous **levothyroxine in a loading dose of 300–400 mcg** to occupy vacant binding sites followed by maintenance dose 50–100 mcg/day. Other uses of thyroxine are for non-toxic goitre, thyroid nodule and papillary carcinoma of thyroid.
- **Thyroxine is preferred over T_3** because of its longer half-life, greater stability, low cost, lack of allergic reactions, lower risk of cardiac adverse effects than T_3, and easy monitoring of serum concentrations.
- **Hyperthyroidism** occurs in Graves' disease (autoimmune), toxic nodular goitre and toxic adenoma. Patients present with weight loss, heat intolerance, diarrhea, fine tremors, and muscle weakness.
- **Antithyroid drugs include thiocyanates and perchlorates**, which inhibit iodide trapping by the sodium/iodide symporter. However, these are not

used much because of toxicity and unpredictable effect.
- **Thioamides** such as carbimazole, methimazole and propylthiouracil inhibit TPO → inhibition of hormone synthesis. Thus, the onset of effect is delayed. Propylthiouracil also inhibits the peripheral conversion of T_4 to T_3. So, it is useful in thyrotoxic crisis, where fast onset of action is required. Propylthiouracil is more plasma protein-bound; hence, less of it crosses the placenta, resulting in fewer adverse effects on the fetus. Consequently, propylthiouracil is preferred for the management of hyperthyroidism in the first trimester of pregnancy. Adverse effects of thioamides include skin rash, gastrointestinal intolerance, and rarely, agranulocytosis.
- **Iodides** of Na and K inhibit hormone release and are the fastest-acting thyroid inhibitors. However, they are not used for long term because peak effect is seen in 10–15 days, following which, **thyroid escape** occurs. The adverse effects of iodides include rashes, inflammation of mucous membranes, acneiform eruptions, and petechial hemorrhages.
- **Radioactive iodine** (^{131}I) given in a dose of 3–6 microcurie (orally) gets concentrated inside the thyroid follicles β particles → β particles penetrate the thyroid tissue and cause its destruction from within. However, it may cause hypothyroidism and is not suitable for young patients.
- **Beta-blockers**: Propranolol helps in controlling symptoms arising from sympathetic overactivity in thyrotoxicosis. These also prevent the peripheral conversion of T_4 to T_3.
- **Thyroid storm or thyrotoxic crisis** is a severe form of hyperthyroidism, which is managed by supportive measures, hydrocortisone, propranolol, propylthiouracil and iodides.

Questions for practice

1. Enumerate the therapeutic uses and adverse effects of thyroxine.
2. Explain why:
   a. T_4 is preferred over T_3 for replacement therapy in hypothyroidism.
   b. Free T_3 and T_4 are monitored in pregnant females with hypothyroidism.
   c. Loading dose of thyroid hormones is given in myxedema coma.
   d. Dose of anticoagulants needs adjustment in patients on thyroxine therapy.
3. Classify antithyroid drugs.
4. Enumerate therapeutic uses and adverse effects of thioamides.
5. Explain why:
   a. Propranolol is used in the management of thyrotoxic crises.
   b. Carbimazole has delayed onset of antithyroid effect.
   c. Propylthiouracil is preferred over methimazole in pregnant women with hyperthyroidism.
   d. Thioamide therapy is initiated before iodides.
6. Describe the management of:
   a. Thyrotoxic crisis
   b. Myxedema coma

Hints for problem-based questions and MCQs

1. i. Hypothyroidism
   ii. c. Levothyroxine
   iii. Levothyroxine is used as replacement therapy and preferred over T_3 (refer to page 559). Carbimazole and propylthiouracil are antithyroid drugs useful in hyperthyroidism.
2. d. All the above factors (food, gastric acidity and other drugs) interfere with the absorption of thyroxine. So, it should be given empty stomach.
3. i. b. Total T_3 and T_4 levels are raised, but fT_3 and fT_4 levels are normal
   ii. Raised levels of thyroxine binding globulin in pregnancy and OCP use raises total T_3 and T_4, although fT_3 and fT_4 remain normal.
4. d. All of the above. Refer to page 559.
5. b. Thyroxine facilitates ATP production and utilisation.
6. i. a. Free T_3 and T_4, because increased TBG in pregnancy increases plasma protein binding and levels of total T_3 and T_4.
   ii. Refer to pages 558, 559.
7. c. Graves' disease
8. i. Myxedema coma
   ii. Refer to page 561.
9. a. Thiocyanates
10. i. Hyperthyroidism
    ii. Refer to page 562.
    iii. Refer to pages 562, 563.
11. Refer to page 564.
12. d. All of the above.
13. b. Inhibition of thyroid peroxidase.
14. i. a. Potassium iodide.
    ii. Pre-operatively before thyroidectomy and in thyrotoxic crisis.
15. a. Increase proteolysis of thyroglobulin. Iodides decrease proteolysis of thyroglobulin and reduce release of thyroid hormones.
16. i. Supportive, hydrocortisone, propranolol, PTU, KI, plasmapheresis
    ii. Refer to page 561.
17. More severe form of hyperthyroidism after 2–8 weeks of iodides therapy.
18. i. b. Propylthiouracil,
    ii. PTU is highly bound to plasma proteins when compared to other thioamides. So, chances of the drug crossing the placental barrier and causing fetal adverse effects are lower and it is preferred in the first trimester of pregnancy.
19. c. Agranulocytosis
20. c. Propylthiouracil

CONCEPT MAP – THYROID AND ANTITHYROID DRUGS

Thyroid Hormones T_3, T_4

Physiological Role
- Growth & development
- Increased BMR, Calorigenesis.
- Increased metabolism of carbohydrates, proteins and lipids, Hyperglycemia, Negative nitrogen balance, Low cholesterol

Uses
- Replacement therapy in:
  - Hypothyroidism
  - Cretinism
  - Myxedema coma
- To reduce TSH in simple endemic nontoxic goiter, Papillary carcinoma
- T_4 is preferred over T_3 because of long half-life, more stability, low cost, less ADRs & easy monitoring

ADRs
Resemble features of hyperthyroidism like tachycardia, palpitation, tremors, weight loss, heat intolerance, hyperglycemia, hyperpyrexia

ANTITHYROID DRUGS

Classification
- **Iodide Trapping Ionic Inhibitors**
  Thiocyanates (SCN^-), Perchlorates (ClO_4^-), Pertechnetate (TcO_4^-), Nitrates (NO_3^-)
- **Hormone synthesis inhibitors**
  Carbimazole, Methimazole, Propylthiouracil
- **Drugs that Inhibit Hormone Release**
  Iodides of Na & K, Lugol's solution
- **Drugs that Destroy Thyroid Tissues**
  Radioactive iodine^{131} (RAI)
- **Drugs for Symptom Control**
  β-blockers without ISA like Propranolol, Metoprolol, Esmolol
  Hydrocortisone

Monovalent Anions
SCN^-, ClO_4^-, TcO_4^- and NO_3^-
Inhibit iodide trapping by blocking Na^+ iodide symporter (NIS)
Not much in use due to unpredictable effect and toxicity.

Thioamides
Carbimazole, Methimazole and Propylthiouracil (PTU).
Mechanism: Act by inhibiting thyroid peroxidase (TPO) → inhibition of hormone synthesis → delayed onset of effect.
Ph/K: Well absorbed orally, well distributed, can cross placenta, but PTU is more plasma protein bound → less of it crosses placenta, → fewer adverse effects on fetus → preferred in managing hyperthyroidism in first trimester of pregnancy.
PTU also inhibits peripheral conversion of T_4 to T_3 → fast onset → useful in thyrotoxicosis
ADRs: Include skin rash, gastrointestinal intolerance, rarely agranulocytosis may occur.

β Blockers
Symptomatic relief
Prevent peripheral conversion of T_4 to T_3
Used in thyrotoxicosis

Radioactive Iodine
I^{131} gets concentrated inside the thyroid follicles → emits β particles → β particles penetrate the thyroid tissue and cause its destruction from within.
ADRs: Hypothyroidism, mutagenic, carcinogenic potential, not suitable for young patients

Iodides of Na^+ & K^+
Mechanism: Inhibit hormone release → fastest acting
Uses: Used in thyrotoxic crisis
Not used for long term, because peak effect is seen in 10–15 days, later on 'thyroid escape' occurs.
ADRs: Rashes, inflammation of mucous membranes, acneiform eruptions, petechial hemorrhages

---

Antithyroid Drugs versus Subtotal Thyroidectomy

Advantages: No scar, no risk of damage to surrounding structures, no surgery/anesthesia related risks, hypothyroidism caused is reversible on dose reduction.

Disadvantages: Prolonged treatment needed, poor compliance especially in less educated, risk of agranulocytosis, risk of adverse effects in fetus when used in pregnancy.

SECTION 9 Drugs Affecting the Endocrinal Action

43 Insulin and Antidiabetic Drugs

PH 7.1 Describe the types, kinetics, dynamics and adverse drug reactions of drugs used in diabetes mellitus and devise management for an obese and non-obese diabetic patient, and also comment on prevention of complication of diabetes.

Learning objectives

A student of MBBS phase II should be able to:
- Describe the mechanism and regulation of insulin secretion.
- Describe the mechanism of action of insulin.
- Explain the metabolic effects of insulin.
- Classify insulin preparations.
- Describe therapeutic uses of insulin mentioning doses.
- Enumerate adverse effects and contraindications for use of insulin.
- Classify oral antidiabetic drugs and describe their mechanisms of action.
- Enumerate adverse effects of and contraindications to oral antidiabetic drugs.
- Explain management of obese and non-obese diabetic patient.
- Explain management of diabetic ketoacidosis.
- Describe measures to prevent complication of diabetes.

DIABETES MELLITUS

Diabetes mellitus (DM) is a metabolic disorder characterised by hyperglycemia, glycosuria, hyperlipidemia, negative nitrogen balance, and occasionally, ketonemia.

In DM, carbohydrate metabolism is reduced, while that of lipids and proteins is increased. Virtually all forms of diabetes are either due to decreased circulating levels of insulin, i.e., **insulin deficiency** or decreased tissue responsiveness to insulin, i.e., **insulin resistance**. Polyuria, polydipsia and polyphagia are the **clinical hallmarks** of DM.

According to the American Diabetes Association (ADA), **diagnostic criteria** for DM are:

- Fasting plasma glucose level > 126 mg/dL or 7 mmol/L on more than one occasion.
- Random plasma glucose > 200 mg/dL or venous blood glucose > 11.1 mmol/L.

Types of Diabetes

Type I: Insulin-dependent diabetes mellitus (IDDM).

Type II: Non-insulin-dependent diabetes mellitus (NIDDM).

Type III: Hyperglycemia secondary to other diseases (e.g., chronic pancreatitis) or drugs (e.g., glucocorticoids, thiazides, diazoxide and growth hormone)

Type IV: Gestational DM occurs in 4–5% pregnancies as placental hormones promote insulin resistance. It is observed in $2^{nd}/3^{rd}$ trimester of pregnancy and resolves in the postpartum period.

Differences in the cause, patient characteristics, severity, pathogenesis and treatment of Type I and Type II DM are listed in Table 43.1.

Complications

1. **Ketoacidosis** is more common in uncontrolled Type I DM. In the absence of insulin, glucose cannot enter the skeletal muscles and body cells → so, cells use fatty acids for ATP generation → accelerated fat breakdown leads to production of ketone bodies, i.e., acetyl-CoA, acetoacetic acid, and β-hydroxybutyric acid. The acetoacetic acid is converted to acetone in the liver; which is exhaled out through the lungs, giving a fruity odour to breath. Glycosuria, renal excretion of nitrogenous substances and ketone bodies, promote osmotic diuresis → dehydration → polydipsia. The metabolic products of fatty acid breakdown (acetone, acetoacetic acid and β-hydroxybutyric acid) lead to decreased blood pH, i.e., metabolic acidosis called diabetic ketoacidosis, which can lead to coma/death.
2. **Hyperosmolar coma**, characterised by severe hyperglycemia and dehydration, is more common in Type II DM.
3. **Microvascular complications** of diabetes occur over many years. Diabetic retinopathy and nephropathy are caused by sorbitol accumulation, leading to thickening of the basement membrane of capillary endothelium. Neuropathy is the result of demyelination of axons.
4. **Macrovascular complications** like atherosclerosis and diabetic dyslipidemia (increased LDL and TG) may occur.

Table 43.1 Comparison of Type I and Type II diabetes mellitus

	Type I (IDDM)	Type II (NIDDM)
Patient characteristics	Usually juvenile, sometimes non-obese adults or elderly	Usually obese adults, sometimes adolescents
Cause	Immune-mediated β-cell destruction, insulin is absent, glucagon increased	Deficiency of insulin or resistance to action of insulin.
Pathogenesis	- Genetic predisposition (HLA-DR3 and DR4 are more prone) - Auto-aggression - β cells do not respond to any insulinogenic stimulus	Insulin levels are subnormal or relatively inadequate because of tissue insensitivity. - β-cell response to glucose is deficient.
Severity	More severe form, commonly associated with ketosis if not treated	Less severe form
Treatment	Only insulin, dietary restrictions, exercise	Dietary restriction, weight reduction, oral antidiabetic drugs, sometimes insulin may be required.

5. **Cataract** occurs because of deposition of sorbitol in the lens.

Glycosylated Hb: Blood glucose may vary on a day-to-day basis. Glycosylated Hb, called HbA1c, is a better measure of glycemic control over the lifespan of red blood cells (120 days). Hb is glycosylated at its valine amino acid terminal, at a rate directly proportional to glucose concentration. The goal of treatment in DM is to maintain HbA1c below 7%. HbA1c > 8% indicates poor glycemic control.

INSULIN

Insulin is a peptide hormone made up of 2 chains, A and B, containing a total of 51 amino acids.

The basal secretion of insulin is 1 unit/hour. It is stimulated by various chemical, hormonal and neural stimuli.

Chemical stimuli:
- Glucose
- Amino acids, mainly arginine and leucine
- Fatty acids
- Food: Meal-induced insulin bursts are larger and last for 2–3 hours

Hormonal stimuli:
- Glucagon increases insulin release
- Somatostatin decreases insulin release

Neural stimuli:
- Muscarinic and β_2 activation increases insulin release
- α_2 activation decreases insulin release

PHYSIOLOGY OF INSULIN SECRETION AND ACTION

In a resting cell, insulin release is minimal as ATP levels are low and K^+ diffuses out through ATP-regulated K^+ channels (Fig. 43.1). This maintains the intracellular potential at a negative level, i.e., the membrane is fully polarised.

The most important insulinogenic stimulus is glucose. Glucose levels > 70 mg/dL stimulate insulin synthesis and release through a series of regulatory steps (Flowchart 43.1).

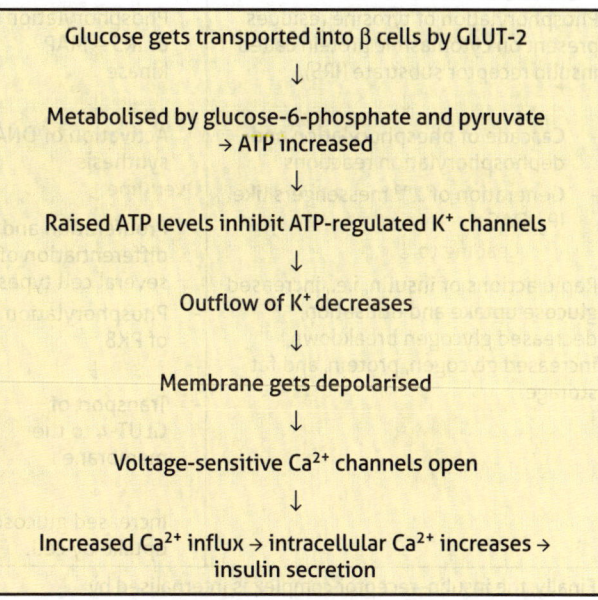

Flowchart 43.1 Insulin secretion

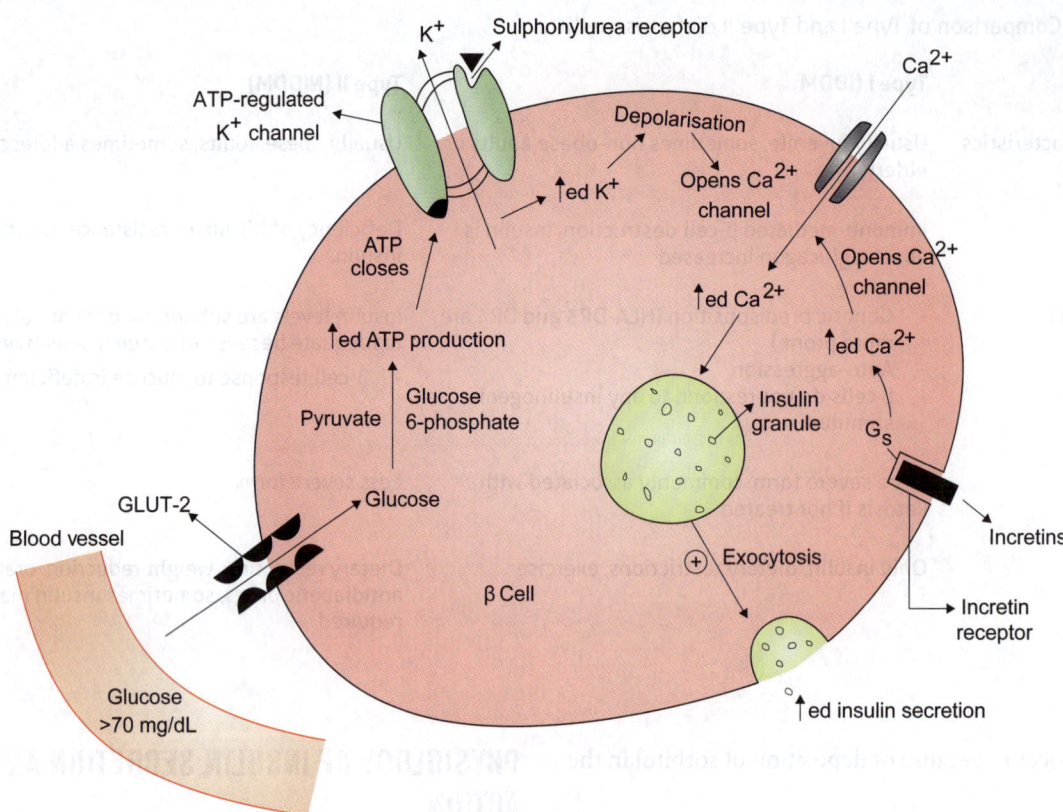

Fig. 43.1 Mechanism of insulin secretion from pancreatic β-cells and effect of glucose, incretins and sulphonylureas on insulin secretion.

MECHANISM OF ACTION OF INSULIN

An insulin receptor has 2 extracellular α-subunits and 2 membrane-spanning β-subunits linked by disulphide bonds (Fig. 43.2). Binding of insulin to α-subunit stimulates tyrosine kinase activity in the β-subunit. This leads to autophosphorylation of adjacent β-subunits, and a series of reactions depicted in Flowchart 43.2 and Fig. 43.2.

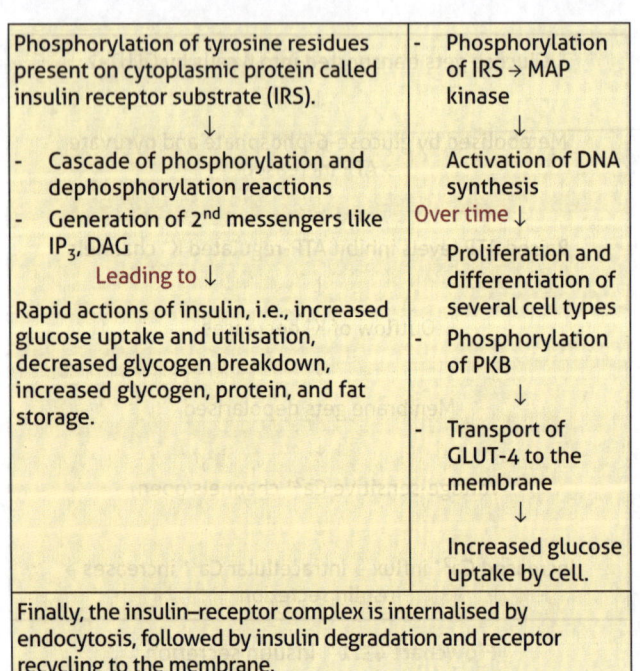

| Phosphorylation of tyrosine residues present on cytoplasmic protein called insulin receptor substrate (IRS).
 ↓
 - Cascade of phosphorylation and dephosphorylation reactions
 - Generation of 2nd messengers like IP$_3$, DAG
 Leading to ↓
 Rapid actions of insulin, i.e., increased glucose uptake and utilisation, decreased glycogen breakdown, increased glycogen, protein, and fat storage. | - Phosphorylation of IRS → MAP kinase
 ↓
 Activation of DNA synthesis
 Over time ↓
 Proliferation and differentiation of several cell types
 - Phosphorylation of PKB
 ↓
 - Transport of GLUT-4 to the membrane
 ↓
 Increased glucose uptake by cell. |

Finally, the insulin–receptor complex is internalised by endocytosis, followed by insulin degradation and receptor recycling to the membrane.

Flowchart 43.2 Mechanism of action of insulin

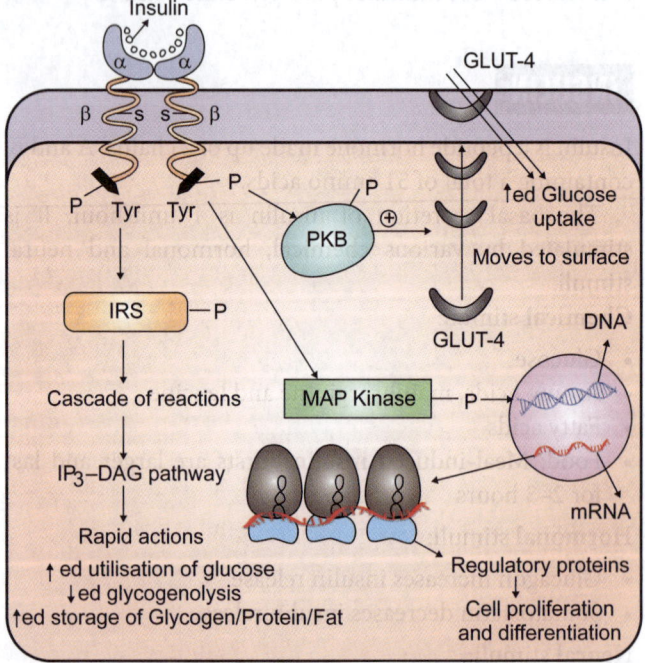

Fig. 43.2 Mechanism of action of insulin

[MAP Kinase; Mitogen-activated protein kinase; IRS: Insulin Receptor Substrate; GLUT-4: Glucose Transporter-4] PKB - Protein Kinase B

Effect of Insulin on Metabolism

Carbohydrates
- Translocation of GLUT-4 to cell surface → increased uptake of glucose.
- Increased glucose utilisation by activation of glucokinase.
- Increased glycogen synthesis by activation of glycogen synthase.
- Decreased glycogenolysis by inhibition of phosphorylase.
- Decreased gluconeogenesis by inhibition of PEP carboxykinase.

Proteins
- Decreased protein breakdown in liver.
- Increased protein synthesis and amino acid uptake in muscles. So, insulin produces a positive nitrogen balance.

Fats
- Increased lipogenesis in liver
- Increased synthesis and storage of FA and TG in fat cells and decreased lipolysis
- Stimulates vascular endothelial lipoprotein lipase (LPL) → increased clearance of VLDL and chylomicrons.

PHARMACOLOGY OF INSULIN

Pharmacokinetics
- Insulin cannot be used orally because it is a peptide in nature.
- It is injected subcutaneously or intravenously. Upon subcutaneous administration, the rate of absorption varies depending upon the site of injection. The most common site for subcutaneous administration is the abdomen, as it provides the most reliable and fastest absorption. However, insulin glargine has the same rate of absorption from all the sites.
- Half of the dose undergoes first-pass metabolism in the liver.
- Metabolism occurs inside cell after internalisation of insulin–receptor complex.

Insulin Preparations
Source: Human insulin differs from bovine insulin by 3 amino acids, and from porcine insulin by just 1 amino acid. Thus, porcine insulin is less immunogenic than bovine insulin (which carries a risk of 'mad cow disease' as well). These insulins are purified by gel filtration and ion-exchange chromatography to obtain single peak and monocomponent insulins.
- Human insulin is prepared using recombinant DNA technique by inserting the human proinsulin gene into *E. coli*/yeast. With growth and multiplication of *E. coli*/yeast → human proinsulin is synthesised, which is then extracted and processed to form human insulin for therapeutic use.
- Some insulins are **modified** by genetic engineering to make analogues with better pharmacokinetic properties, e.g., insulin glargine, lispro, aspart and glulisine.

CLASSIFICATION

According to their **duration of action**, insulin preparations are classified as ultrashort-acting, short-acting, intermediate-acting and long-acting insulins (Flowchart 43.3).

1. Ultrashort-acting (Rapid/Fast-acting)
Insulin **lispro**, insulin **aspart** and insulin **glulisine** are human-modified analogues that are absorbed rapidly from subcutaneous tissues. Thus, their **action starts within 15–30 minutes and lasts for 3–4 hours**.
- They are monomers, which promotes their rapid absorption.
- They are soluble insulins, dispensed as a clear solution at neutral pH.
- They are useful to control immediate post-meal hyperglycemia.
- These are **usually combined** with a long-acting preparation to maintain baseline levels of insulin between two meals.

2. Short-acting Insulins
These include regular and semilente insulins.

a. Regular insulin
Regular insulin is a soluble human insulin preparation produced using recombinant DNA technology. It exists in crystalline form. Zinc ions are added to regular insulin to enhance its stability; in solution, it exists as hexamer. However, in the interstitial fluid, it breaks into dimers and monomers that are quickly absorbed. Action starts **within 1 hour and lasts for 4–8 hours**. Regular insulin is the drug of choice for control of post-meal hyperglycemia; it is the **only insulin preparation that can be used intravenously** in conditions such as ketoacidosis and hyperkalemia. It can be mixed with all the insulins except long-acting analogues.

b. Semilente insulin
Semilente insulin is amorphous with smaller particles; it is a short-acting preparation, with onset of action in 1–2 hours and duration of action of 8–12 hours.

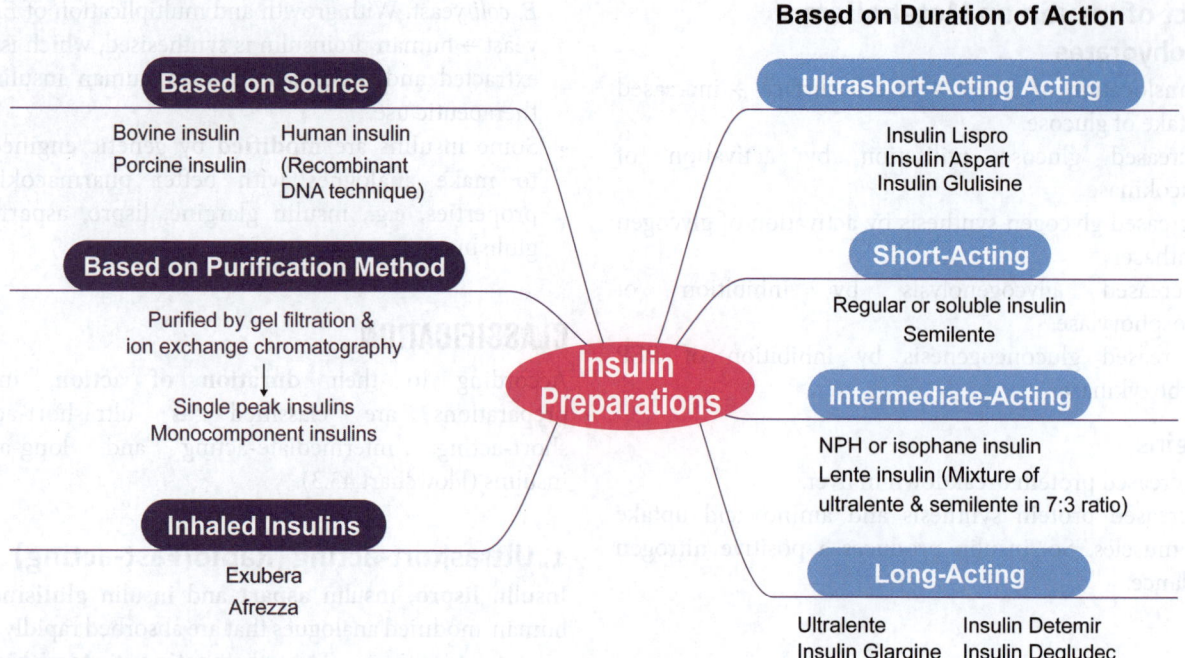

Flowchart 43.3 Classification of insulin preparations

3. Intermediate-acting Insulins
These include NPH and lente insulin.

a. NPH or isophane insulin
This preparation has neutral pH, is **conjugated with protamine** (an arginine-rich protein obtained from fish sperm) and was developed by Hans Christian Hagedorn. Consequently, it is called NPH (Neutral-Protamine-Hagedorn) insulin. NPH insulin is a **cloudy suspension** (all other insulins are clear solutions), having insulin conjugated with protamine. Isophane insulin is NPH insulin that has 6 molecules of insulin per molecule of protamine. It has a slower onset of action, i.e., about 2 hours; this is because upon subcutaneous injection, proteolytic enzymes in tissues slowly degrade protamine resulting in sustained absorption of insulin. The duration of action is also longer (16–20 hours).

b. Lente insulin
Lente insulin is a 7:3 mixture of ultralente and semilente insulins and is intermediate acting. Lente insulin **must be shaken prior to administration**; it is used subcutaneously twice or thrice daily (not intravenous) to control DM, but not for diabetic ketoacidosis.

4. Long-acting Insulins
Ultralente, insulin glargine, insulin detemir and insulin degludec are some long-acting insulin preparations.

a. Ultralente insulin
It is an insulin–Zn suspension with large crystalline particles and is insoluble in H_2O. It is long-acting, with onset of action in **4–6 hours** and duration of action of **20–36 hours**.

b. Insulin glargine
This is a long-acting insulin analogue, which is **soluble at pH 4**. At the physiological pH of 7.4, it is less soluble and more stable. Thus, it forms a microfine precipitate in subcutaneous tissue from which insulin is released in a slow, sustained manner (with **no troughs or peaks in levels**). Consequently, the plasma concentration–time curve obtained with insulin glargine is smooth and peakless (Fig. 43.3). Insulin glargine **cannot be mixed with any other form of insulin** for injection, because it forms white precipitates when mixed with any other insulin. It remains in solution form for injection only at pH 4.

c. Insulin detemir
Insulin detemir has a fatty acid side chain, which increases its binding to albumin. It is then **slowly released from albumin** for slow, sustained absorption. This preparation also should **not be mixed with any other insulin preparation**.

d. Insulin degludec
This insulin preparation also has a fatty acid side chain which allows the formation of a subcutaneous depot of **multihexamers** for slow, sustained release. The duration of action of these preparations is 24 hours. These are used **once or twice daily**, subcutaneously, for maintenance treatment in diabetes.

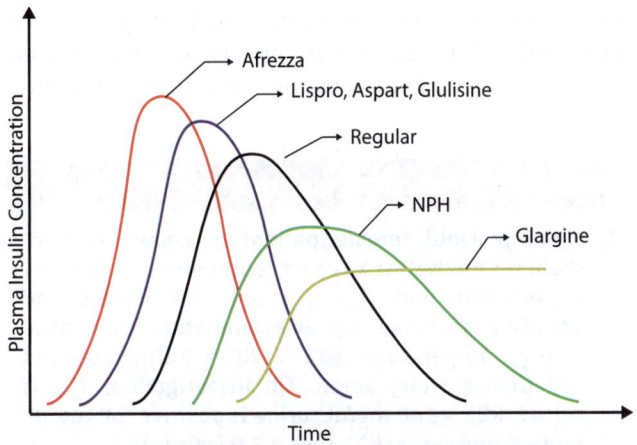

Fig. 43.3 The plasma insulin concentration–time curve for different insulin preparations

5. Inhaled Insulins

Currently, two FDA-approved inhaled insulin preparations—Exubera and Afrezza—are available. **Afrezza** is the **fastest-acting** insulin with the **shortest duration of action**. They are inhaled at meal time, **immediately before food**, to control the rapid rise in blood glucose levels.

Afrezza is available as cartridges of different colours, wherein the blue, green, and yellow cartridges contain 4, 8, and 12 units, respectively. Inhaled insulins can cause pharyngitis, pulmonary fibrosis and lung cancer. These are **contraindicated in patients with bronchial asthma, chronic obstructive pulmonary disease and in smokers.**

Inhaled insulin, regular insulin and NPH insulin are insulin preparations, while the rest are insulin analogues.

NEW INSULIN DELIVERY DEVICES

To improve the ease and accuracy of insulin administration for tight glycemic control, several delivery devices have been innovated. They include:

- **Insulin syringes** are prefilled, disposable syringes containing specific types or mixtures of regular and modified insulins. These syringes avoid the need to carry vials, etc.
- **Pen devices** are fountain pen-like syringes with a cartridge that contains insulin. Dose is set by a dial and injected subcutaneously by pushing the plunger. It is also convenient and there is no need to carry vials, syringes, etc.
- **Insulin pumps** are portable infusion devices, connected to a subcutaneous cannula for providing **CSII (continuous subcutaneous insulin infusion)**. The pump can be programmed to deliver insulin at a low basal rate (1 unit/hour) and pre-meal bolus doses (4–15 times the basal rate) for controlling postprandial hyperglycemia. Only regular insulin or fast-acting insulin analogues are used in insulin pumps.
- **Implantable pumps** are percutaneous, refillable reservoirs with insulin delivery regulated through electromechanical mechanisms.
- **Jet injections** deliver insulin subcutaneously without the use of needles.
- **External artificial pancreas** is a microprocessor-controlled device connected through an intravenous line. It measures blood glucose and infuses the appropriate amount of insulin in a continuous feedback manner.
- **Other** routes such as oral, rectal, intraperitoneal and intranasal are being evaluated for insulin administration.

THERAPEUTIC USES

Insulin is used for the control of hyperglycemia in the following situations.

1. All cases of Type I DM
2. Type II DM
   - Not controlled by diet, exercise and oral drugs
   - When oral drugs are not tolerated
   - To tide over stressful conditions like surgery, trauma, infection, and pregnancy.

> Intensive insulin therapy is a complex regimen of 2–4 injections of various preparations to achieve round-the-clock tight glycemic control. It markedly reduces the occurrence and rate of progression of microvascular complications of DM, but has higher incidence of severe hypoglycemic episodes. Hence, intensive insulin therapy is best avoided in children and the elderly.

3. **Nonketotic, hyperosmolar coma:** Insulin, fast I/V fluid infusion, and heparin are administered.
4. **Diabetic ketoacidosis** is precipitated by stressful conditions. It is characterised by dehydration, hyperventilation, acidosis and impaired consciousness. The **treatment** involves:
- **Intravenous fluids:**
   - Normal saline 1 L/hour followed by 0.5 L/ 4 hour.
   - Half-normal saline is given when the blood pressure and pulse rate stabilise.
   - 5% glucose in normal saline is given when blood glucose reduces to 300 mg/dL.
- **Insulin:** *Regular insulin*
   Dose
   - 0.1–0.2 U/kg IV bolus injection, followed by
   - 2–3 U/Kg/h IV infusion, till blood glucose levels reach 300 mg/dL
   - 2–3U/h IV infusion

Adrenaline can increase insulin release by β2-receptor stimulation.

Thus, it helps in diabetic ketoacidosis with hyperkalemia to shift K^+ back into the cells.
- **KCl:** 10–20 mEq/hour is added to intravenous fluids after 4 hours of treatment. This is because ketosis subsides on starting insulin therapy and potassium is driven intracellulary, leading to dangerous hypokalemia.
- **NaHCO$_3$:** It is not required routinely, but if pH is < 7.1, 50 mEq of NaHCO$_3$ is administered in intravenous fluids.
- Supportive treatment, phosphates, and antibiotics are also required in some cases.

ADVERSE REACTIONS

- **Hypoglycemia** is the most frequent and most serious adverse effect of insulin. It can occur because of a larger dose of insulin, a delayed/missed meal, or unusual physical exertion.
  There are 2 types of symptoms in hypoglycemia:
  - Symptoms associated with autonomic regulatory hyperactivity such as anxiety, sweating, tremors and palpitation.
  - Symptoms due to neuroglycopenia (lack of glucose and essential nutrients to brain) such as headache, hunger, dizziness, weakness, fatigue, and muscular incoordination.

  In patients taking regular insulin, hypoglycemia can develop rapidly leading to autonomic regulatory symptoms, whereas in elderly patients developing hypoglycemia due to long-acting insulin preparations, neuroglycopenic symptoms are predominant.
  In order to manage hypoglycemia:
  - Glucose solution is given **orally** if patient is conscious. However, if patient is unconscious → 25–50 mL of 50% glucose is given intravenously.
  - If intravenous line is not accessible, glucagon (1 mg, intramuscular or subcutaneous) is given. Patient regains consciousness in about 15 minutes, and then, glucose solution can be administered, orally.
- **Allergic reactions** such as urticaria and angioedema can be seen with bovine and porcine insulins, but are rare with human insulin.
- **Lipodystrophy** at the site of subcutaneous injection; this is not much of a problem with newer preparations and can be managed by changing the injection site.
- Transient dependent **edema** may occur at the beginning of insulin therapy.
- **Insulin resistance** is said to have developed if the daily insulin requirement is > 100 U/day. It can develop:
  - **Acutely**, because of stress, surgery, inflammation, trauma due to release of steroids, and other hormones that oppose insulin action.
  - **Chronically**, because of development of high Ab titre against insulins.

Insulin resistance may also occur in pregnancy, OCP use, acromegaly, Cushing syndrome, pheochromocytoma, hypertensives, etc. The treatment is to switch over to purer preparations.

Clinical problem-based questions and MCQs

1. A 43-year-old female patient, a known case of diabetes for the last 25 years, is brought to emergency department with fever, cough, drowsiness and vomiting since one day. On examination, her tongue is dry, temperature: 102 °F, RR = 26/minute, and breath has fruity smell. On investigation, TLC is raised, RBS = 540 mg/dL, urine is positive for ketone bodies, and serum K^+ levels = 5.9 (raised).
   i. What is this patient likely suffering from?
   ii. Describe the management of this patient.
   iii. Which of the following can control raised K^+ levels in this patient?
   a. Glucagon   b. Atropine
   c. Adrenaline d. All of the above

2. Identify the insulin preparation used in diabetic ketoacidosis.
   a. Lente insulin   b. NPH insulin
   c. Regular insulin d. Semilente insulin

3. A 10-year-old school boy, a known case of IDDM, receiving 8 units of insulin twice daily, is brought to hospital emergency in unconscious state. On examination, his PR was 130 bpm. There is history of participation in a sports activity (400 m relay race) during school time, in which he was absolutely fine and performed well. After a while, he developed weakness, tremors, sweating, muscular incoordination, and then became unconscious on way to hospital.
   i. What is probable diagnosis?
   ii. What is the immediate treatment?

4. Identify the diabetic complication that needs heparin injection for immediate management.
   a. Diabetic nephropathy
   b. Diabetic ketoacidosis
   c. Hypoglycemic coma
   d. Hyperosmolar coma

5. Identify the insulin preparation with a smooth, peakless insulin concentration–time curve.
   a. Insulin glulisine   b. Regular insulin
   c. Isophane insulin   d. Insulin glargine

6. In an insulin preparation, protamine is complexed to insulin in a ratio of 1:6.
   i. Identify the insulin preparation containing protamine
   a. Isophane insulin   b. Lente insulin
   c. Regular insulin   d. Insulin aspart
   ii. What is role of protamine in this preparation?

7. Which of the following devices delivers insulin subcutaneously without need for injection prick?
   a. Pen device   b. Insulin syringes
   c. Jet injector   d. Insulin pump

ANTIDIABETIC DRUGS

This category of drugs was called oral hypoglycemic drugs because most of them are administered orally to lower blood glucose levels. However, the GLP-1 analogues are given subcutaneously, and the word *oral* has been dropped. Moreover, some of these drugs are euglycemics, i.e., they reduce raised blood glucose to normal levels, but do not cause hypoglycemia. So, the term 'hypoglycemic' is also not suitable. This class is now called 'antidiabetic drugs'.

CLASSIFICATION

Based on their mechanism of action, antidiabetic drugs are classified (Flowchart 43.4) into those that increase insulin secretion (sulphonylureas, meglitinides and incretin mimetics), drugs that have peripheral actions similar to insulin (biguanides and thiazolidinediones), drugs that decrease intestinal absorption of glucose (α-glucosidase inhibitors) and those that reduce renal tubular reabsorption (SGLT-2 inhibitors). In addition, D_2-agonist bromocriptine, amylin mimetic pramlintide, bile acid sequestrant colesevelam, and dual PPAR agonist drugs also also lower blood glucose levels.

A. Drugs That Enhance Insulin Secretion

I. Drugs which bind to sulphonylurea receptors

1. Sulphonylureas

First-generation sulphonylureas (SU) include chlorpropamide and tolbutamide; of these, only tolbutamide is infrequently used. Chlorpropamide is not much in use because it is long-acting and can cause prolonged hypoglycemia (especially in the elderly). ADRs like hyponatremia, cholestatic jaundice and disulfiram reaction with alcohol (due to aldehyde dehydrogenase inhibition) may be caused by chlorpropamide.

Currently, second-generation **sulphonylureas** are preferred; these include glibenclamide, glipizide, gliclazide and glimepiride.

Mechanism of action

The major action of sulphonylureas is to **increase insulin release** (refer to Fig. 43.1). They bind to a high-affinity SU receptor associated with ATP-regulated K^+ channel (K_{ATP}) on pancreatic β-cells and inhibit the efflux of K^+ ions → membrane depolarisation → Ca^{2+} influx → release of preformed insulin. Thus, SU are effective only in patients who have at least 30% functioning pancreatic β-cells. In addition, they also:

- Suppress glucagon levels.

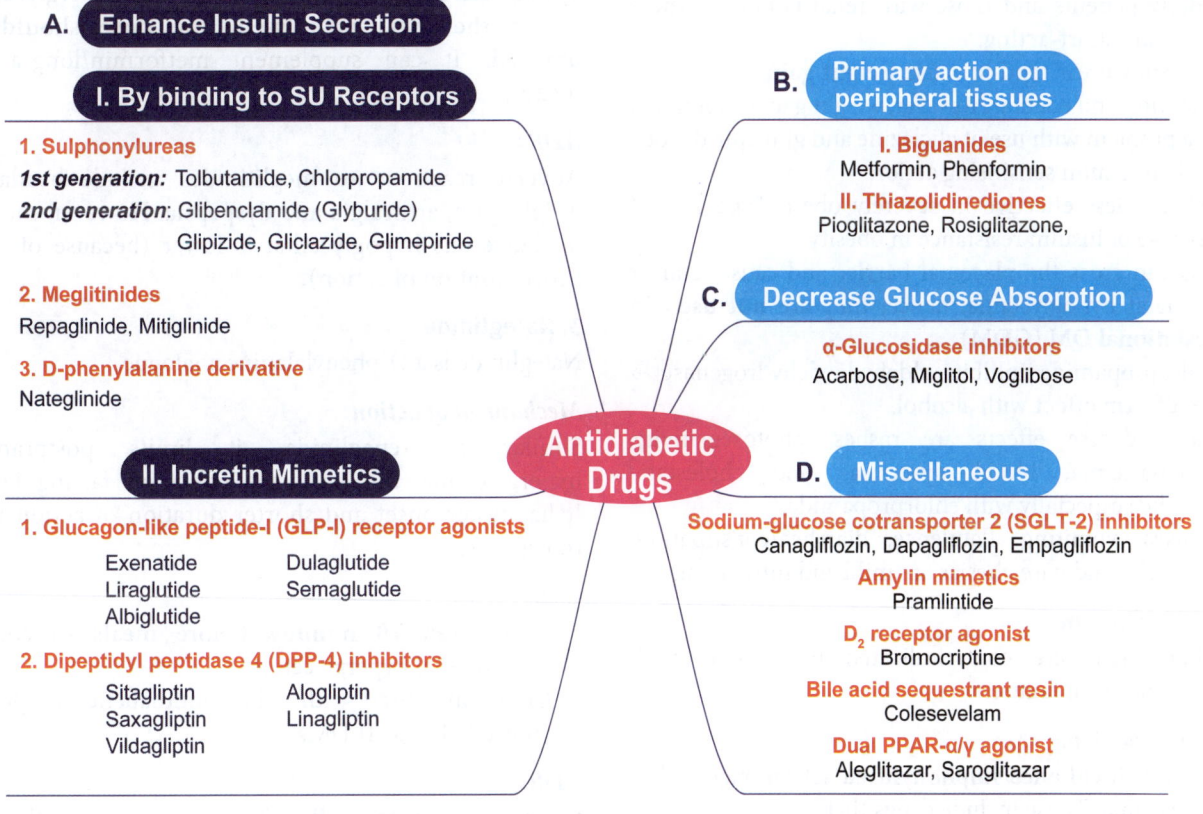

Flowchart 43.4 Classification of antidiabetic drugs

- Increase the number of insulin receptors on target cells, especially the liver.
- Glipizide, gliclazide and glimepiride increase sensitivity of peripheral tissues to insulin.
- Gliclazide possesses antiplatelet action also.
- Second-generation drugs have more potency than the first-generation drugs.

Pharmacokinetics

- Well-absorbed orally (glipizide absorption is delayed by food).
- 90–98% plasma protein bound.
- Metabolised in liver, and excreted by kidney.
- Duration of action varies. Among the first-generation drugs, tolbutamide is shortest-acting while chlorpropamide has long duration of action. Among 2nd-generation SUs, the effect of glibenclamide lasts for > 24 hours, because of an active metabolite that is sequestrated in β cells.

ADRs

Second-generation drugs have fewer ADRs than first-generation drugs.

- The most important ADR is **hypoglycemia** (drugs that increase insulin secretion cause hypoglycemia as an adverse effect). Severe hypoglycemia can cause coma, especially in elderly patients who are on long-acting drugs. Tolbutamide and glipizide are safe for use in elderly patients and those with renal failure, as these drugs are short-acting.
- Sulphonylureas tend to cause **weight gain** due to fluid retention and edema. However, weight gain is not much of a problem with use of gliclazide and glimepiride, due to their insulin sensitising action.
- SUs are less effective in severely obese Type II DM because of insulin resistance in obesity
- SUs can cross the placental barrier and cause fetal or neonatal hypoglycemia; hence, they are **not used in gestational DM (GDM)**.
- Chlorpropamide inhibits aldehyde dehydrogenase → **disulfiram effect** with alcohol.
- Rare adverse effects are rashes, photosensitivity, hyponatremia, blood dyscrasias and cholestatic jaundice especially with chlorpropamide.
- Nausea, vomiting, flatulence, diarrhea/constipation, headache and paresthesias are mild and infrequent.

Contraindications

Sulphonylureas are contraindicated in patients with hepatic and renal failure.

Drug interactions

Drugs which **enhance sulphonylurea action** may lead to hypoglycemia. These include drugs that:

- Displace sulphonylureas from plasma protein binding sites: sulphonamides, salicylates, phenylbutazone, sulfinpyrazone.
- Inhibit metabolism/excretion: sulphonamides, ketoconazole, warfarin, chloramphenicol
- Synergise with pharmacodynamic action: propranolol, salicylates, antihypertensives (sympatholytics), lithium, theophylline.

Drugs which **decrease sulphonylurea action** and vitiate diabetic control include:

- Enzyme inducers: phenobarbitone, phenytoin, chronic alcoholism, rifampicin.
- Drugs that oppose action of SU, i.e., insulin release or action: thiazides, corticosteroids, furosemide, OCPs.

2. Meglitinides

Repaglinide and mitiglinide belong to this class. Their mechanism of action is the same as that of sulphonylureas. They are K_{ATP} channel blockers with **quick but short-lasting insulin secreting action**. The onset of insulin-secreting action is fast, but the effect is short lasting. Repaglinide normalises mealtime glucose excursions.

Pharmacokinetics

They are **quickly absorbed and rapidly metabolised**. These pharmacokinetic features provide them fast onset and short-duration of action, respectively.

Uses

Repaglinide is used in selected Type II DM patients with **pronounced postprandial hyperglycemia**. It is given before each meal to control postprandial hyperglycemia. So, if **the meal is missed, the dose should be omitted**. It can supplement metformin/long-acting insulin.

ADRs

Adverse reactions to meglitinides include headache, weight gain, arthralgia and dyspepsia. However, the risk of dangerous hypoglycemia is lower (because of their short duration of action).

3. Nateglinide

Nateglinide is a D-phenylalanine analogue.

Mechanism of action

Similar to repaglinide, it limits postprandial hyperglycemia, but has little effect on fasting levels. It has faster onset and shorter duration of action than repaglinide.

Uses

- It is given **10 minutes before meals** to control postprandial hyperglycemia.
- Commonly used with other antidiabetics in poorly controlled Type II DM.

ADRs

Dizziness, nausea, flu-like symptoms, arthralgia and weight gain can occur; however, episodes of hypoglycemia are less frequent because of shorter duration of action.

Caution

Meglitinides and nateglinide should be avoided in case of liver failure. Dose should be reduced in patients with hepatic and renal disease.

II. Drugs which mimic or prolong incretin effect

Oral glucose load provokes a higher insulin response than equivalent intravenous glucose load, because oral glucose leads to the release of gut hormones called 'incretins' [glucagon-like peptide-I (**GLP-I**) and glucose-dependent insulinotropic peptide (**GIP**)]. These incretins amplify glucose-induced insulin secretion. **GLP-I receptors** are present on:

- α cells → decrease glucagon release.
- β cells → **increase insulin release in response to glucose** (i.e., insulin release is more pronounced when glucose levels are high, but less so when glucose levels are normal. So, **lower risk of hypoglycemia than with sulphonylureas**).
- GIT mucosa → delays gastric emptying → slows the rate of nutrient absorption (may lead to decreased appetite and **weight loss**).
- Hypothalamus → probably decrease appetite (induce weight loss).
- The incretin system appears to promote β-cell health; failure of incretins is implicated in the progression of Type II DM. So, GLP-I-based therapy can be useful to **decrease the disease progression rate** in Type II DM.

After exerting its action, **GLP-I** is **rapidly metabolised by dipeptidyl peptidase 4** (DPP-4) and endopeptidases ($t_{½}$ is just 1–2 minutes). So, DPP-4 inhibitors → interfere with the degradation of GLP-1 → mimic incretin effects and enhance the effects of GLP-I receptor agonists.

1. GLP-I receptor agonists

These include exenatide, liraglutide, albiglutide, dulaglutide and semaglutide.

Exenatide is a long-acting analogue that is resistant to DPP-4 degradation because of glycine substitution. Due to its peptide nature, it is is not effective by oral route, and is given subcutaneously (5–10 mcg, BD). It acts on GLP-I receptors and causes:

- Increased insulin secretion in response to glucose
- Decreased glucagon secretion.
- Delayed gastric emptying.
- Decreased appetite and causes **weight loss**
- In Type II DM, exenatide decreases postprandial glucose, fasting blood glucose, HbA1c and causes weight loss. It is approved for use as adjunctive therapy in patients with suboptimal glycemic control with metformin used alone or with sulphonylureas.

Liraglutide can be used as subcutaneous injection, given **once daily**.

Albiglutide and **dulaglutide** have a long $t_{½}$ of 5 days; so, they are used **once a week** as a subcutaneous injection.

Semaglutide is also given as an injection, **once a week**. It is the **first GLP-I agonist** that is effective by oral route also. However, oral semaglutide should be taken daily, on empty stomach as the first thing in the morning, preceding the first meal and other oral medications by at least 30 minutes with only 4 oz. plain water. If the patient fails to strictly follow these instructions, efficacy is reported to decrease.

Semaglutide and liraglutide can be used for obesity as they decrease appetite and weight. **Semaglutide is the drug of choice for obesity**.

ADRs

- GLP-I agonists have low risk of causing hypoglycemia when used alone, because they increase insulin secretion only in response to raised glucose levels.

Anorexia, nausea and vomiting are seen in approximately 50% patients, but decrease with passage of time.

- All these drugs increase the **risk of pancreatitis**. So, patients are counselled to seek immediate medical care in case of unexplained, severe, persistent abdominal pain.
- Cases of **renal impairment** have been reported.
- Exenatide and liraglutide stimulate **parafollicular tumours in rodents**; however, its relevance in humans is not known at present. Nevertheless, they should not be used in patients with past/family history of medullary thyroid cancer or multiple endocrine neoplasia (MEN) syndrome Type II.

2. Dipeptidyl peptidase 4 (DPP-4) inhibitors

Sitagliptin, vildagliptin, saxagliptin, alogliptin and linagliptin are DPP-4 inhibitors.

Mechanism of action

The first drug introduced in this category, sitagliptin, is a **competitive and selective inhibitor of DPP-4** → interferes with degradation of GLP-1 and GIP → so, it increases postprandial insulin release and decreases glucagon secretion → lowers mealtime as well as fasting blood glucose in Type II DM, also decreases HbA1c.

- No effect on gastric emptying time or appetite is noted. So, it is **body weight neutral.**
- Lower risk of hypoglycemia, when used alone.
- It is used as **adjuvant** to other drugs in Type II DM that is not controlled by metformin and/or SU/thiazolidinediones, etc.
- One advantage over GLP-1 agonists is that these drugs are **effective orally**.
- Sitagliptin is mainly excreted unchanged by the kidney with $t_{½}$ = 12 hours → so **dose should be adjusted in case of renal disease.**

Vildagliptin binds covalently to **DPP-4** and **inhibits it for a longer duration**. Its duration of action is 12–24 hours despite a short $t_{1/2}$ of 2–4 hours. Thus, it is given **once or twice daily**. It is metabolised in the liver and excreted by the kidney; so, dose should be reduced in hepatic and renal disease. **Hepatotoxicity** has been reported with vidagliptin.

Saxagliptin also binds covalently and has **duration of action of 24 hours,** despite a $t_{1/2}$ of 2–4 hours.

Alogliptin and linagliptin are newly approved members of this class.

ADRs
- Nausea, diarrhea and allergic reactions (rashes/edema).
- **Nasopharyngitis** may occur because DPP-4 degrades substance P also; cough occurs in some patients.

B. Drugs That Lower Glucose by Acting on Peripheral Tissues
I. Biguanides

Metformin and phenformin are prominent examples of this class of drugs. While phenformin is not used because of the high risk of lactic acidosis, **metformin is the most useful drug in DM.**

Mechanism of action
Metformin reduces blood glucose levels by following mechanisms (Fig. 43.4):

1. **Slowing of glucose absorption** from GIT → more glucose available to enterocytes for conversion into lactates.
2. It stimulates AMP-activated protein kinase (AMPK) → inhibition of hepatic gluconeogenesis → **decreased hepatic glucose output.** Reduced ability of glucagon to generate cAMP in hepatocytes may also contribute to this action.
3. Renal gluconeogenesis is also reduced.
4. **Increased uptake and utilisation** of glucose by skeletal muscles, which decreases insulin resistance.
5. Promotes **binding of insulin to its receptors,** reducing insulin resistance.

Advantages over sulphonylureas
- Metformin does not increase insulin release; so, it is not dependent on functional β-cells for its action (unlike SU) and does not lower glucose levels in normal persons. In other words, metformin is **euglycemic, not hypoglycemic.**
- It does **not** cause **weight gain**, and can be given to obese patients with diabetes.
- It has **favourable effect on lipids**—it lowers LDL, VLDL and elevates HDL.
- **Decreases risk of** micro-as well as macrovascular complications

Pharmacokinetics
- Orally effective
- No plasma protein binding
- No metabolism
- Excreted unchanged by the kidney
- Its $t_{1/2}$ is 2–3 hours, and duration of action is 6–10 hours.

Uses
- It is often the drug of **first choice** in **obese Type II patients with diabetes** because it causes anorexia, preventing weight gain. It also decreases insulin resistance.

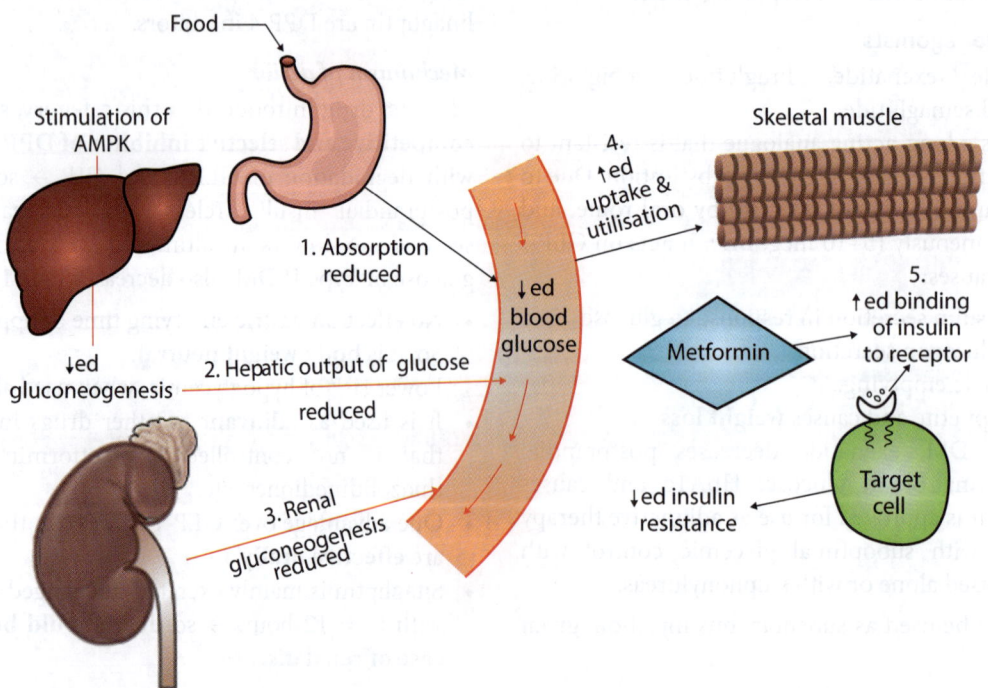

Fig. 43.4 Mechanism of action of metformin

- Can be given alone or in combination with sulphonylureas, thiazolidinediones and meglitinides to treat **insulin resistance syndrome**.
- It has been used to treat hirsutism in patients with **polycystic ovarian disease** (PCOD) and may enhance fertility in such women by increasing insulin sensitivity and decreasing androgen levels.
- Metformin is reported to be useful in **fatty liver** in nonalcoholic patients.

ADRs
- **Gastrointestinal** effects like anorexia, nausea, vomiting, flatulence, diarrhea and metallic taste.
- **Decreased B_{12} absorption** leading to megaloblastic anemia is common with metformin. So, B_{12} supplements should be given to patients on metformin therapy.
- **Lactic acidosis** is a rare side effect which occurs because more glucose remains unabsorbed in intestines and is converted by anaerobic glycolysis into lactic acid by enterotrophs. Lactates normally get utilised in gluconeogenesis, which is inhibited by biguanides. Risk of lactic acidosis is higher in elderly individuals, chronic alcoholics, in patients with renal/hepatic/heart failure and severe pulmonary disease.

II. Thiazolidinediones

Rosiglitazone and **pioglitazone** belong to this category; of these, only pioglitazone is in use currently.

Mechanism of action
They are **selective agonists** for nuclear **peroxisome proliferator-activated receptor gamma** (PPAR-γ) expressed mainly in fat cells, but also in muscles → activation of this receptor leads to transcription of several insulin-responsive genes resulting in **increased expression and translocation** of GLUT-4 to the cell surface → increased entry of glucose into muscle and fat cells. Thus, **insulin resistance is reversed**.
- Also suppresses hepatic gluconeogenesis.
- Lowers blood glucose and HbA1c without increasing insulin levels.
- Sensitises adipose tissue to insulin action → adipocyte turnover and differentiation is accelerated.
- Lowers triglycerides and raises HDL levels, without much change in LDL levels.
- Thiazolidinediones stimulate epithelial sodium channels (ENaC), resulting in **sodium and water retention**.

Uses
Pioglitazone is used as an adjuvant drug in Type II DM, but not in Type I.

ADRs
- Thiazolidinediones can cause **plasma volume expansion** → edema, weight gain, headache, myalgia, mild anemia and may precipitate or worsen CHF.
- Rosiglitazone is banned in India because of the unacceptable increase in risk of CHF, MI, stroke and death.
- Hepatic dysfunction may occur.
- These drugs can also cause osteoporosis and increase **risk of bone fractures, especially in women.**

Thiazolidinediones are **contraindicated** in liver disease and CHF.

C. Drugs that Decrease Glucose Absorption

α-Glucosidase inhibitors

Acarbose, miglitol and voglibose belong to this category.
Acarbose is a complex oligosaccharide that inhibits α-glucosidase reversibly. This is the final enzyme for digestion of carbohydrates in the brush border of small intestine mucosa. Inhibition of α-glucosidase slows down digestion and absorption of polysaccharides. In addition, GLP-1 release is increased → significant increase in insulin levels. Postprandial hyperglycemia is reduced. HbA1c also reduces upon chronic use.

Acarbose is antihyperglycemic but not hypoglycemic and is used as an **adjuvant** to diet restriction in **obese Type II DM**. It is also useful in postprandial hyperglycemia, and is **taken after taking a few bites** of a meal.

ADRs
It is not a well-tolerated drug. Unabsorbed polysaccharides get fermented and cause gastro-intestinal adverse effects such as flatulence, abdominal discomfort and loose stools (osmotic diarrhea).

D. Miscellaneous

1. Sodium-glucose cotransporter 2 (SGLT-2) inhibitors

These include canagliflozin, dapagliflozin and empagliflozin. SGLT-2 inhibitors are a new therapeutic approach in the treatment of Type II DM. These drugs have their site of action in kidneys.

Canagliflozin is a reversible, selective inhibitor of sodium-glucose cotransporter-2. Thus, it decreases reabsorption of glucose in the kidney, resulting in **increased excretion of glucose in urine**, lowering plasma glucose level. It is effective orally, and is used as a **third-line drug** in the management of Type II DM.

ADRs
- Increased glucose excretion in urine causes polyuria, hypotension, and increased risk of genital thrush, UTI and vaginal infections.
- It can also increase LDL levels
- Constipation.
- Risk of hypoglycemia is greater if SGLT-2 inhibitors are combined with sulphonylureas.
- Canagliflozin can cause osteoporosis and **increased risk of bone fractures, especially in elderly patients**; there is no predilection for any sex.

- Dapagliflozin increases risk of breast and bladder cancer.

Contraindications

These are contraindicated in patients with renal function impairment and Type I DM (may increase risk of diabetic ketoacidosis). Another contraindication is in patients receiving diuretic therapy.

2. Amylin mimetics

Pramlintide

Amylin is a hormone secreted by β-cells, in same manner as insulin, after a meal. Amylin improves glycemic control by:

- Modulating the gastric emptying rate—it **slows down the absorption** of food.
- Preventing postprandial rise in glucagon levels. Thus, glucose production by the liver is reduced.
- **Increase in sensation of satiety**, which reduces calorie intake, resulting in weight loss.

Diabetic patients are deficient in amylin.

Pramlintide is an amylin-mimetic drug that can be **used as adjuvant in Type I and II diabetes patients** in whom adequate glycemic control is not achieved with preprandial insulin therapy. Pramlintide is administered subcutaneously as it is peptide in nature.

ADRs

Adverse effects include nausea, vomiting, abdominal pain, headache, fatigue, weight loss and risk of hypoglycemia on combining with insulin.

3. D2 agonists

Bromocriptine has a modest effect in improving insulin sensitivity. It can be used as adjuvant in Type II DM, in addition to diet and exercise. It can also be combined with metformin and/or sulphonylureas.

4. Bile acid sequestrant

Colesevelam is a bile acid sequestrant that decreases hepatic glucose output, blood glucose and HbA1c. It can also be used as adjuvant with metformin/ SUs/insulin.

5. Dual PPAR-α/γ agonist

Dual PPAR agonists at alpha and gamma receptors such as aliglitazar and saroglitazar reduce levels of LDL, TG, blood glucose, HbA1c and raise HDL levels. These are approved for diabetic dyslipidemia (in a dose of 4 mg, once a day) that is not controlled using statins alone.

Effect of antidiabetic drugs on weight

Weight **gain**: Sulphonylureas, thiazolidinediones
Weight **loss**: GLP-1 analogues, pramlintide
Weight **neutral**: Metformin, DPP-4 inhibitors

Clinical problem-based questions and MCQs

8. i. Identify the antidiabetic drug that needs at least 30% functional β-cells to exert its hypoglycemic effect.
   a. Metformin b. Glipizide
   c. Voglibose d. Dapagliflozin
   ii. Describe the mechanism of action of the chosen drug with a suitable diagram.
   iii. Enumerate the adverse effects of the chosen drug.

9. Which antidiabetic drug has quick, short-lasting effect of controlling postprandial hyperglycemia?
   a. Glibenclamide b. Chlorpropamide
   c. Repaglinide   d. Pioglitazone

10. A 46-year-old male presents with increased frequency of micturition, especially during night, dryness of mouth, and weight loss in spite of increased appetite. No abnormality is detected on examination. On investigation, FBS = 186 mg/dL, HbA1c = 7.9%. Patient is prescribed Tab metformin 500 mg, twice daily.
    i. Name the group to which metformin belongs.
    ii. Describe the mechanism of beneficial effect of metformin in this case.
    iii. What are the advantages of metformin over sulphonylureas?
    iv. Enumerate the therapeutic uses and adverse effects of metformin.

11. Which of the following is the first-choice antidiabetic drug in obese diabetics?
    a. Glipizide   b. Exenatide
    c. Metformin   d. Vildagliptin

12. Identify the antidiabetic drug that is contraindicated in CHF
    a. Chlorpropamide b. Metformin
    c. Pioglitazone   d. Exenatide

13. Identify the oral hypoglycemic drug that increases the risk of bone fractures in women.
    a. Voglibose   b. Rosiglitazone
    c. Liraglutide d. Canagliflozin

14. Match the antidiabetic drug with its mechanism of action.
    a. Chlorpropamide   1. DPP-4 inhibitor
    b. Sitagliptin   2. Closure of K_{ATP} channel
    c. Pioglitazone   3. Incretin mimetic
    d. Albiglutide   4. Increased GLUT-4 expression

15. GLP-1 analogues have lower risk of hypoglycemia than sulphonylureas. Explain.

16. A 75-year-old male patient, a known case of Type II DM on oral hypoglycemic drug therapy, missed his lunch while travelling. He presents in medicine OPD with excessive fatigue, muscular weakness, palpitation and slurring of speech. On examination, patient is anxious and sweating profusely. PR is 136 bpm; RBS = 40 mg/dL.
    i. What is the diagnosis for this case?

ii. Which group of antidiabetic drugs is more prone to cause such symptoms?
iii. Describe the management of this case.
iv. How should this patient be counseled to avoid such symptoms in future?

MANAGEMENT PLAN FOR DIABETES MELLITUS

Diagnosis

Classical symptoms of diabetes, i.e., polyuria, polydipsia and polyphagia help in making clinical diagnosis of diabetes. However, a large number of cases are asymptomatic; so, a high degree of suspicion and biochemical tests are important for confirmation of diagnosis. American Diabetes Association (ADA), defines plasma glucose value of 100 mg/dL as normal. A value between 100–126 mg/dL is labelled impaired fasting plasma glucose or prediabetic.

- Diagnostic criteria for DM are fasting plasma glucose level > 126 mg/dL or 7 mmol/L on more than one occasion. The fasting state is defined as no calorie intake for the last 8 hours.
- Random or postprandial plasma glucose > 200 mg/dL or venous blood glucose > 11.1 mmol/L.
- During oral glucose tolerance test, a glucose load containing equivalent of 75 g anhydrous glucose dissolved in water is given orally. A plasma glucose value of 200 mg/dL, 2 hours after the glucose load, is diagnostic of diabetes.

Treatment

Aim of treatment in diabetes is to maintain normal blood glucose levels (euglycemia) round the clock, relieve the symptoms (if any) and prevent complications. The treatment strategy for diabetes involves both nonpharmacological and pharmacological approaches.

Nonpharmacological measures

Nutrition/Dietary therapy

This is the first step in management of Type II diabetes, along with exercise. Nutrition therapy should be advised and the response is evaluated after 4–8 weeks.

- Nutritional advice should be given after appropriate assessment of the caloric needs of each patient based on their occupation, activities, etc.
- The desirable body weight of the patient is calculated by subtracting 100 from their height in cm.

    Ideal body weight (kg) = Height (cm) – 100

- The recommended caloric requirement/kg of ideal body weight varies from 20–45 calories/kg, based on weight and level of activity (Table 43.2). Calorie requirement is 35 calories/kg in a patient with normal body weight and moderate activity.

Table 43.2 Recommended caloric requirement/kg of ideal body weight

Activity level	Optimum calories/kg of ideal body weight		
	Obese	Normal	Underweight
Sedentary	20	30	35
Moderate	25	35	40
Heavy	30	40	45

- The total number of calculated calories is then divided into three main meals and two mini meals or snacks. 60% of the calories should be derived from carbohydrates and 20% each from proteins and fats.
  - **Carbohydrates**: Intake of complex carbohydrates and fibre in the form of foods such as pulses, legumes and vegetables is favoured over refined carbohydrates.
  - **Fats**: Equal intake of saturated, mono- and polyunsaturated fats is recommended. Dietary cholesterol intake should be kept < 300 mg/day.
  - **Protein** intake from vegetarian (lentils and cereals) and non-vegetarian (lean meat and fish) sources is recommended. However, in diabetic nephropathy and renal failure, dietary protein is restricted.
  - Daily intake of salt should not exceed 6 g.
  - Alcohol intake should be altogether avoided or restricted to a maximum 20–40 mL/day
- While explaining dietary therapy, it is important to counsel patient that it is only diet modification, not reduction. In initial stages, patients or relatives should be encouraged to ask questions about methods of weighing the quantity and calculating the calories in common food articles used in that particular country/region/state.
- The socioeconomic status, cultural habits and education level of the patient must be kept in mind while prescribing diets for chronic diseases like diabetes.

Exercise

Regular exercise is an important component of diabetes management and provides many benefits such as improved insulin sensitivity, decreased blood glucose, reduced triglycerides/LDL and raised HDL. Aerobic exercise also causes cardiovascular conditioning, reduces weight, provides a feeling of well-being and improves quality of life. Aerobic exercises such as brisk walking, cycling and swimming are reported to provide maximum benefit. The practice of Yoga has also been reported to reduce blood glucose, HbA1c levels and prevent long-term complications.

However, the exercise program should be carefully planned and supervised. Unsupervised exercise routine may be counterproductive in uncontrolled diabetes and may precipitate cardio-vascular events or worsen long-term diabetic complications.

Approximately 50% of patients achieve the euglycemic stage with non-pharmacological measures alone. However, drug therapy is indicated for the remaining patients.

Pharmacological measures

1. **In Type I diabetes**, insulin replacement therapy is the mainstay of treatment. Insulin injections are given subcutaneously in the anterior abdominal wall, arms or lateral aspect of thighs.
   - Intensive insulin therapy involves 3–4 injections of insulin per day or continuous subcutaneous insulin infusion (CSII) to maintain tight, round-the-clock glycemic control.
   - Metformin is combined with insulin to improve insulin sensitivity, resulting in insulin dose reduction
2. **Type II DM** : Antidiabetic drugs are used only in Type II DM.
   - Metformin is the most frequently prescribed first-choice drug in obese Type II diabetics; it is given in a dose of 500–2500 mg, based on the severity of the disease. Vitamin B_{12} supplementation should be given to patients on metformin therapy
   - In some patients, sulphonylureas may be combined with metformin to allow adequate control of blood glucose with oral medication only. However, sulphonylureas are less effective in obese diabetics, as obesity leads to insulin resistance and SUs exert their action through insulin. Moreover, SUs have a tendency to cause fluid retention, edema and weight gain; thus, they are not preferred for use in obese diabetics.
   - GLP-1 analogues are approved for use as adjunctive therapy in patients with suboptimal glycemic control with metformin used alone or with sulphonylureas.
   - DDP-4 inhibitors are also used as adjuvant to other drugs in Type II DM not controlled by metformin and/or SU/thiazolidinediones, etc.
   - Acarbose is used as adjuvant to diet restriction in obese Type II DM.
   - In patients with pronounced post-prandial hyperglycemia, drugs having fast onset and short duration of action (such as repaglinide and nateglinide) are given 10–15 minutes before meals. Acarbose is taken after consuming a few bites of a meal and is also useful in postprandial hyperglycemia,
   - Type II diabetics may need short-term insulin therapy to tide over the crisis in stressful situations such as diabetic ketoacidosis, hyperosmolar nonketotic coma, lactic acidosis, infections and pregnancy.

Monitoring of diabetes control

The best indicator to periodically monitor diabetic control after institution of various nonpharmacological and/or pharmacological measures is by measuring plasma glucose levels in both fasting and postprandial states. While FBS levels should be checked as frequently as possible in Type I diabetes, they should be checked at an interval of about 4–6 weeks in Type II diabetes. Target fasting and postprandial blood glucose levels for good control of diabetes are 90–130 and < 180 mg/dL, respectively. In addition, diabetic control can be checked with:

- Estimation of HbA1c every 3 months. A level of < 7% indicates good diabetic control.
- Renal function test should be carried out every 3–6 months.
- Lipid profile, urine microalbumins, ECG, chest X-ray and ophthalmic examination should be carried out annually.

Patient education and counselling

DM is a chronic disease requiring lifelong dietary modification and drug therapy or insulin therapy.

Prevention of Complications

Diabetes is a chronic disease associated with numerous acute and chronic complications.

- Acute complications such as diabetic ketoacidosis, hyperosmolar nonketotic coma, drug/insulin-induced hypoglycemia, lactic acidosis, and intercurrent infections need intensive treatment, as described earlier.
- Long-term complications can involve almost every organ and system in body, such as IHD, nephropathy, retinopathy, neuropathy, and skin/respiratory/bones/joints infections. For prevention of various chronic complications, the following measures are suggested:
  - Strict diabetic control using insulin, while also being extra cautious to prevent hypoglycemia, is important to retard the rate of progress of various microvascular complications.
  - Smoking cessation, correction of dyslipidemia, and control of BP are useful.
  - Retinal check-up using fluorescein angiography should be carried out every three years to detect and manage retinal changes at an early stage.
  - Panretinal photocoagulation with laser diminishes retinal oxygen demand and reduces neovascularisation.
  - Early detection of microalbuminuria by periodic monitoring, dietary protein restriction, ACE inhibitors, and angiotensin receptor blockers can slow down the rate of progression of diabetic nephropathy. Lisinopril (2.5–20 mg), ramipril (1.25–5 mg), losartan (25–100 mg), etc., are effective in retarding the progress of renal lesions.
  - Prophylactic use of antiplatelet drugs in patients at high risk of cerebrovascular disease.
  - Neuropathy can result in many other complications. Analgesics and antidepressants may have a role in reducing pain, insomnia and other psychological

symptoms associated with neuropathy. Electrical stimulation at site of pain with a cutaneous nerve stimulator may also be helpful.
- A diabetic foot needs meticulous care. To prevent it, diabetics should avoid walking barefoot or wearing tight/hard footwear. They should also avoid use of hot water bottles, heating pads etc.

Summary

- DM is a chronic metabolic disorder arising from insulin deficiency or insulin resistance.
- Type I is IDDM managed only by insulin, a peptide hormone from pancreatic β-cells.
- Numerous chemical, hormonal and neural stimuli regulate insulin secretion.
- Plasma glucose is taken up by β-cells and raises ATP levels, which reduce K^+ outflow → membrane depolarisation that in turn opens Ca^{2+} channels → increase Ca^{2+} influx, causing insulin secretion.
- **Insulin** acts through tyrosine kinase receptors causing rapid actions such as increased uptake/utilisation of glucose; transport of GLUT-4 to the surface; decreased glycogen breakdown; increased store of glycogen, protein, fat.
- Insulin lispro, insulin aspart and insulin glulisine are ultrashort-acting preparations. Regular or soluble insulin is short-acting and the most commonly used preparation; it is the only insulin that can be given by IV route. It can be mixed with all other preparations, except longer-acting insulins such as degludec and detemir. Isophane and lente are intermediate-acting insulins.
- Numerous novel delivery devices (syringes, pen devices, jet injectors, pumps, implants and external artificial pancreas) and alternative routes (nasal, oral, inhalational and intraperitoneal) are being developed to improve ease of administration.
- Insulin is used in Type I DM, uncontrolled Type II and diabetic complications such as ketoacidosis and hyperosmolar coma.
- Hypoglycemia, lipodystrophy at injection site, allergic reactions and dependent edema may occur as adverse effects of insulin.
- **Oral hypoglycemic drugs** such as sulphonylureas (glibenclamide, chlorpropamide, tolbutamide, etc.) and meglitinides (rapeglinide) act on sulphonylurea receptors → reduce K^+ outflow → resulting in increased insulin secretion.
- Due to this, sulphonylurea can cause hypoglycemia as an ADR. Weight gain is another important drawback. Hypoglycemia risk is lower with meglitinides due to fast action and short duration of effect
- **Incretin mimetics** include GLP-1 analogues (exenatide and liraglutide) and DPP-4 inhibitors (sitagliptin and vildagliptin)
- **GLP-1 analogues** such as **exenatide** need subcutaneous administration. These increase insulin and reduce glucagon secretion. Weight loss occurs due to the hypothalamic and gastrointestinal effect. They are used as adjuvants to metformin or sulphonylureas. Semaglutide is orally effective in obesity.
- **DPP-4 inhibitors** (e.g., sitagliptin and vildagliptin) are also used as adjuvants, but these are body weight neutral.
- Pancreatitis may occur with incretin mimetic drugs.
- **Metformin** is a biguanide that inhibits gluconeogenesis, increases uptake and utilisation of glucose by peripheral tissues, reduces GI absorption of glucose, and can reverse insulin resistance. It is the drug of choice in obese Type II diabetics, and also useful in PCOD.
- Metformin is preferred over sulphonylureas because it does not cause hypoglycemia and weight gain, causes favourable changes in lipid profile, and decreases risk of complications. However, lactic acidosis is an important adverse effect.
- **Pioglitazone** is an agonist at nuclear peroxisome proliferator-activated receptors that increases the expression of GLUT-4 and can reverse insulin resistance. However, it can cause volume expansion and is contraindicated in CHF.
- **Acarbose and voglibose** are α-glucosidase inhibitors that interfere with the digestion and absorption of polysaccharides; however, these are not well tolerated as they cause flatulence, abdominal discomfort and loose stools.
- Drugs like **canagliflozin** reduce renal tubular reabsorption of glucose and Pramlintide has amylin-mimetic action. These drugs also reduces circulating glucose levels and are useful as adjuvants in DM.

Questions for practice

1. a. Classify insulin preparations
   b. Describe the characteristic features of various insulin preparations.
   c. Describe the novel insulin delivery systems.
2. Describe the metabolic effects of insulin.
3. Enumerate the therapeutic uses and adverse effects of insulin.
4. Classify oral hypoglycemic drugs. Describe the mechanism of action, therapeutic uses and adverse effects of biguanides.
5. Write short notes on:
   a. Vildagliptin

b. GLP-1 analogues
c. SGLT-2 inhibitors
d. Pramlintide
e. Glipizide
6. What is the advantage of sitagliptin over exenatide?

Hints for problem-based questions and MCQs

1. i. Diabetic ketoacidosis
   ii. Patients of diabetic ketoacidosis are managed with intravenous fluid replacement with NS, half NS and 5% dextrose in NS. Regular insulin given by IV route, adrenaline to shift potassium ions into the cells. KCl is added in IV fluids after 4 hours of insulin treatment to prevent hypokalemia. NaHCO$_3$ is needed if patient has PH< 7.1. Refer to page 575 for details.
   iii. c. Adrenaline can increase insulin release by β_2 stimulation, which drives K$^+$ into the cell and controls hyperkalemia.
2. c. Regular insulin
3. i. Hypoglycemia
   ii. Intravenous glucose (refer to page 576.)
4. d. Hyperosmolar coma
5. d. Insulin glargine.
6. i. a. Isophane insulin
   ii. Protamine allows slow, sustained absorption
7. c. Jet injector
8. i. b. Glipizide
   ii. Glipizide is a SU, it binds to SU receptors on ATP regulated K channels on pancreatic beta cells, and inhibits the efflux of potassium ions → membrane depolarization → influx of calcium ions → release of preformed insulin. Refer to Fig. 43.1, page 572.
   iii. Refer to page 578.
9. c. Repaglinide
10. i. Metformin is a biguanide
    ii. Metformin slows down absorption of glucose from GIT, inhibits hepatic and renal gluconeogenesis, increases uptake and utilisation of glucose by skeletal muscles and reduces insulin resistance. All these actions result in lowering of blood glucose levels.
    iii. Advantages of metformin over SUs include: no risk of hypoglycaemia, no weight gain, favourable effect on lipids and reduced risk of microvascular as well as macrovascular complications.
    iv. Metformin is drug of choice for obese type II diabetics. Also useful in insulin resistance syndrome, PCOD, and non-alcoholic fatty liver disease. ADRs include GI symptoms as anorexia, nausea, vomiting, metallic taste. B$_{12}$ deficiency resulting in megaloblastic anemia and lactic acidosis may occur.
11. c. Metformin (Glipizide, a sulphonylurea drug, causes weight gain, exenatide causes weight loss, but it needs subcutaneous administration, while vildagliptin is body weight neutral.)
12. c. Pioglitazone, as it can cause volume expansion resulting in worsening of CHF.
13. b. Rosiglitazone. Canagliflozin also increases osteoporosis and risk of fractures in elderly, but there is no sex predilection.
14. a–2; b–1; c–4; d–3.
15. They increase insulin secretion only in response to glucose.
16. i. Hypoglycemia, as patient has missed a meal, symptoms are also suggestive of hypoglycemia and RBS is less than normal.
    ii. Sulphonylureas, especially long-acting drugs, have high risk of causing hypoglycemia in elderly individuals.
    iii. Patient is conscious, oral glucose is given.
    iv. Patient should be counselled about importance of regular meals, correct use of drug, and warning symptoms of hypoglycemia. They should be advised to always keep something sugary (containing simple carbohydrates) with them.

CONCEPT MAP – INSULIN AND ANTIDIABETIC DRUGS

DIABETES MELLITUS
Cause: Insulin deficiency / resistance
Types:
Type 1- IDDM Type 2- NIDDM
Type 3- Secondary Type 4-Gestational
Management: Lifestyle modification, Insulin replacement, Antidiabetic drugs

Insulin
Mechanism: Acts through tyrosine kinase receptors, that phosphorylate IRS causing rapid and slow effects
Rapid actions: Increased glucose uptake & utilisation, Reduced gluconeogenesis, Glycogen deposition, Positive nitrogen balance, Lipogenesis

Preparations
Ultra-short acting: Insulin Lispro, Aspart, Glulysine
Short-acting: Regular insulin (preferred, can be mixed with all except long-acting preparations)
Intermediate-acting: Isophane, Lente (mixture of semilente & ultralente)
Long-acting: Glargine, Detemir, Degludec

New Delivery Devices
Syringes, Pen devices, Jet injectors, Pumps, Implants, External artificial pancreas
Uses: Type 1 DM, Type 2 DM not controlled with drugs, Diabetic ketoacidosis, Hyperosmolar coma
ADRs: Hypoglycemia, lipodystrophy at injection site, allergic reactions and dependent edema

DRUGS FOR DIABETES MELLITUS

Hypoglycemic Drugs (Increase Insulin Secretion)

Sulphonylurea
Tolbutamide, Chlorpropamide, Glibenclamide, Glipizide, Gliclazide.
Mechanism: Act on sulphonylurea receptors → reduce K⁺ outflow → membrane depolarises → calcium influx → raised intracellular calcium → increased insulin secretion.
Also increase tissue sensitivity to insulin.
ADRs: Hypoglycemia - risk more in elderly patients, on long-acting drugs.
Fluid retention & edema → weight gain.
Less effective in severely obese Type 2 DM because of insulin resistance in obesity
Cross placental barrier → fetal or neonatal hypoglycemia → not used in gestational DM (GDM).
Chlorpropamide inhibits aldehyde dehydrogenase → disulfiram effect with alcohol.
Mild, infrequent ADRs: Nausea, vomiting, flatulence, diarrhea or constipation, headache, paresthesias.
Rarely rashes, photosensitivity, blood dyscrasias & cholestatic jaundice.
Contraindications: sulphonylureas are contraindicated in patients with hepatic and renal failure.

Meglitinides
Repaglinide: Mechanism same as SU, but quick onset and short duration of action reduces risk of hypoglycemia.
Mainly used for control of postprandial hyperglycemia
ADRs: Headache, Weight gain, Arthralgia, Dyspepsia

Incretin Mimetics
Uses: Useful as adjunctive therapy in patients with suboptimal glycemic control with Metformin used alone or with Sulphonylurea.
GLP-1 analogues (Exenatide, Liraglutide), increase insulin secretion in response to glucose → low risk of causing hypoglycemia, when used alone.
Decrease glucagon secretion
Delay gastric emptying
Decrease appetite and cause weight loss
Need subcutaneous administration.
ADRs: Anorexia, nausea, vomiting → decrease with passage of time.
May cause renal impairment
Should not be used in patients with past or family history of medullary thyroid cancer multiple endocrine neoplasia (MEN) syndrome Type 2, due to reports of parafollicular tumours in rodents.
DPP-4 inhibitors: e.g., Sitagliptin, Vildagliptin interfere with breakdown of incretins. Actions same as GLP-1 analogues but are body weight neutral and effective orally.
ADRs: Nausea, diarrhea and allergic reactions like rashes/edema
All incretin mimetic drugs increase the risk of pancreatitis. Patients counselled to seek immediate medical care in case of unexplained, severe persistent abdominal pain.

Euglycemic Drugs (Do not Increase Insulin Secretion)

Metformin
Mechanism: Inhibits gluconeogenesis
Inhibits glycogenolysis,
Increases uptake & utilisation of glucose by peripheral tissues
Reduces GI absorption of glucose
Reverses insulin resistance.
Uses: It is drug of choice in obese Type 2 diabetics, It is preferred over sulphonylurea because it does not cause hypoglycemia and weight gain, causes favourable changes in lipid profile and reduces risk of micro - as well as macrovascular complications
Insulin resistance syndrome
PCOD
ADRs: Anorexia, nausea, vomiting, flatulence, diarrhea, metallic taste
Decreased B₁₂ absorption
Lactic acidosis: Higher risk in elderly individuals, chronic alcoholics, renal/ hepatic/ heart failure and severe pulmonary disease.

Pioglitazone
Mechanism: Nuclear peroxisome proliferator receptors agonist → increases expression of GLUT-4 → reverses insulin resistance.
ADRs: Potential to expand volume → contraindicated in CHF.

Acarbose, Voglibose
Mechanism: α-glucosidase inhibitors that interfere with digestion and absorption of polysaccharides,
May be used as adjuvants
ADRs: Flatulence abdominal discomfort, loose stools.

Miscellaneous
Canagliflozin
SGLT-2 inhibitor that reduces renal tubular reabsorption of glucose
Pramlintide
Amylin mimetic action,
Reduce circulating glucose levels and are useful as adjuvants in DM.

SECTION 9 Drugs Affecting Endocrine System

44 Corticosteroids

PH 7.5 Explain the types, kinetics, dynamics, adverse effects, indications and contraindications of corticosteroids and communicate to patient the appropriate use of corticosteroids.

Learning objectives

A student of MBBS phase II should be able to:
- Name hormones secreted from the adrenal cortex and their regulation.
- Classify corticosteroids used as drugs.
- Describe mechanism of action of corticosteroids.
- Describe pharmacological actions of glucocorticoids and mineralocorticoids.
- Enumerate therapeutic uses of corticosteroids mentioning doses.
- Describe pharmacological basis for uses of corticosteroids in specific clinical conditions.
- Describe adverse drug reactions of corticosteroids and general principles to minimise ADRs.
- Enumerate cautions and contraindications of corticosteroids.
- Monitor a patient receiving corticosteroids.
- Communicate the appropriate use of corticosteroids to the patient.

The adrenal cortex secretes steroidal hormones under the influence of corticotropin or adreno-corticotropic hormone (ACTH) secreted by the anterior pituitary. The secretion of ACTH is controlled by the corticotropin-releasing hormone (CRH) released from the hypothalamus. Cortisol secreted from the adrenal cortex exerts negative feedback effect on both CRH as well as ACTH. This constitutes the **hypothalamic–pituitary–adrenal axis** (Fig. 44.1).

The adrenal cortex consists of the following three zones, each of which secretes different hormones (Fig. 44.1).

- **Zona glomerulosa**, which secretes mineralocorticoids such as **aldosterone** (0.125 mg per day).
- **Zona fasciculata**, which secretes glucocorticoids such as **hydrocortisone or cortisol** (10 mg per day, half of which is secreted during few morning hours).
- **Zona reticularis** secretes **dehydroepiandrosterone**, which then changes into androstenedione and testosterone.
- The adrenal medulla secretes **adrenaline**, a catecholamine.

CLASSIFICATION OF CORTICOSTEROIDS

I. Based on Their Major Actions

Corticosteroids are classified as glucocorticoids and mineralocorticoids. Glucocorticoids are further classified based on the duration of their action into short-, intermediate- and long-acting drugs, with duration of action < 12, 12–36, and > 36 hours, respectively. (Flowchart 44.1).

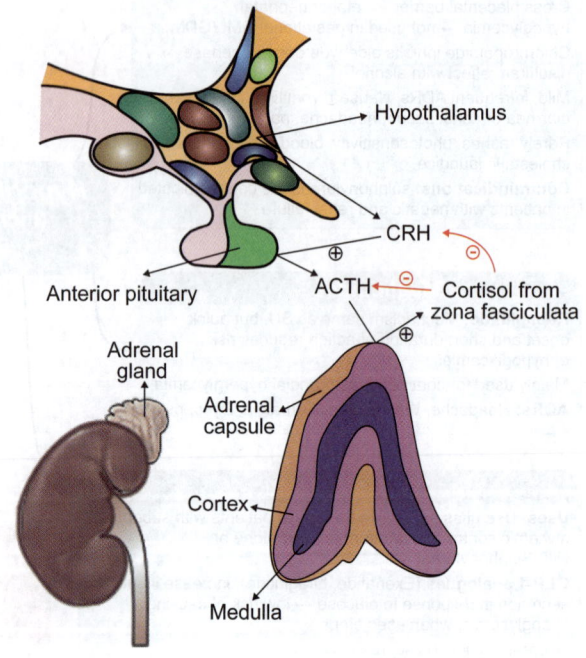

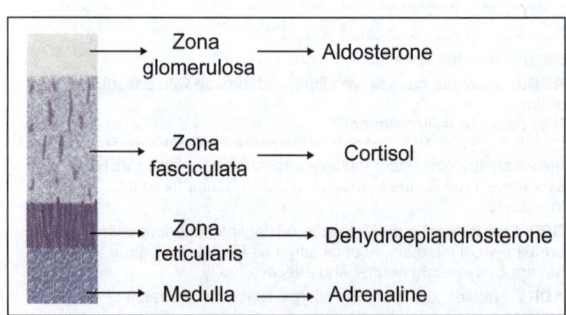

Fig. 44.1 The hypothalamic–pituitary–adrenal axis

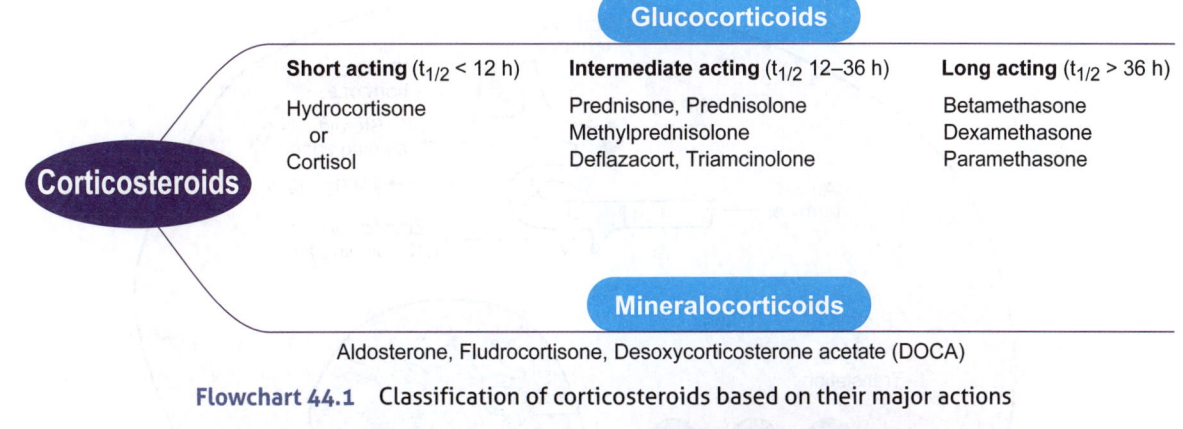

Flowchart 44.1 Classification of corticosteroids based on their major actions

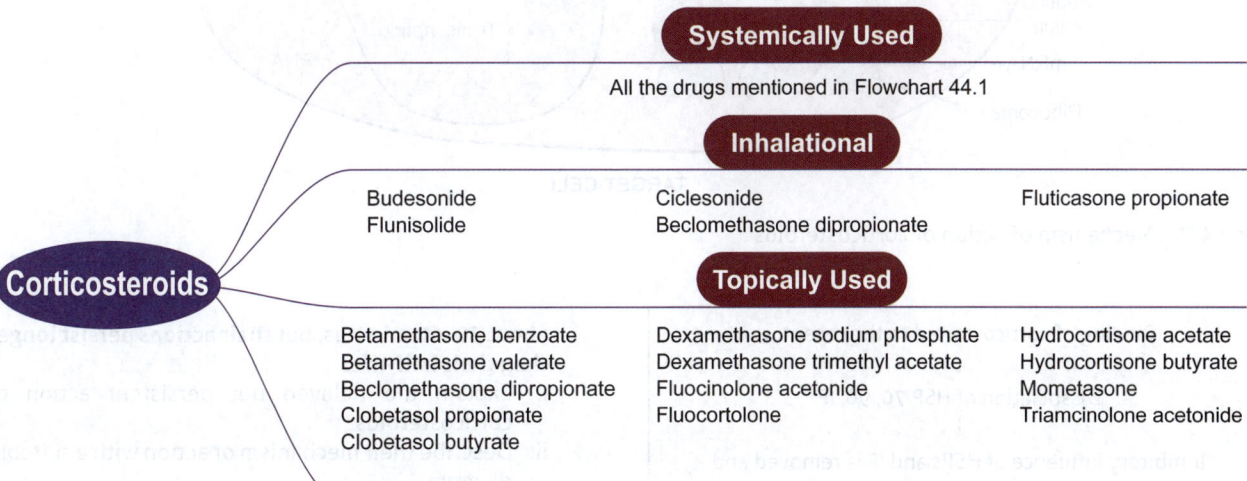

Flowchart 44.2 Classification of corticosteroids based on the route of administration

II. Based on the Route of Administration

Corticosteroids can be divided as systemically used, inhalational and topically used drugs (Flowchart 44.2).

- All natural and synthetic corticosteroids (except DOCA) are effective by the **oral** route.
- Water soluble esters, e.g., hydrocortisone hemisuccinate and dexamethasone sodium phosphate can be given **intravenously and intramuscularly**. These achieve high concentration in tissue fluids quickly and are rapidly acting, suitable for emergency conditions.
- Insoluble esters e.g., hydrocortisone acetate and triamcinolone acetonide cannot be administered intravenously, but are slowly absorbed after intramuscular injection. They are useful in conditions where prolonged effect is required.
- Triamcinolone can be given as **intra-articular** injections also.
- Some corticosteroids used by **inhalational** route for quick action and reduced systemic adverse effects, e.g., budesonide, fluticasone propionate.
- Some corticosteroids, e.g., fluocinolone acetonide, clobetasol propionate and fluocortolone are applied **topically** in various dermatological conditions.

MECHANISM OF ACTION

Corticosteroids bind with high affinity to **cytoplasmic receptors** that are present in almost all cells. Because of the wide distribution of receptors, corticosteroids have far-reaching actions in the body, resulting in a long list of therapeutic uses as well as adverse effects.

Glucocorticoid receptors (GR) have the following **4 functional domains** (Fig. 44.2).

a. **Amino (NH_2) terminal** has a role in activating gene-specific transcription.
b. **DNA binding domain** has 2 zinc fingers that wrap around the DNA helix. It controls transcriptional activation.
c. **Hinge domain or dimerisation region** overlaps the steroid binding domain and plays a role in nuclear localisation, transcription and dimer formation.
d. **Steroid binding domain** attaches 3 other proteins called Heat Shock Protein 90 (HSP 90), HSP 70 and called Heat Shock Protein 90 (HSP 90), HSP 70 and immunophilin (IP). It is located near the carboxy terminal. It binds with steroidal hormones and also has a role in nuclear localisation and dimer formation.

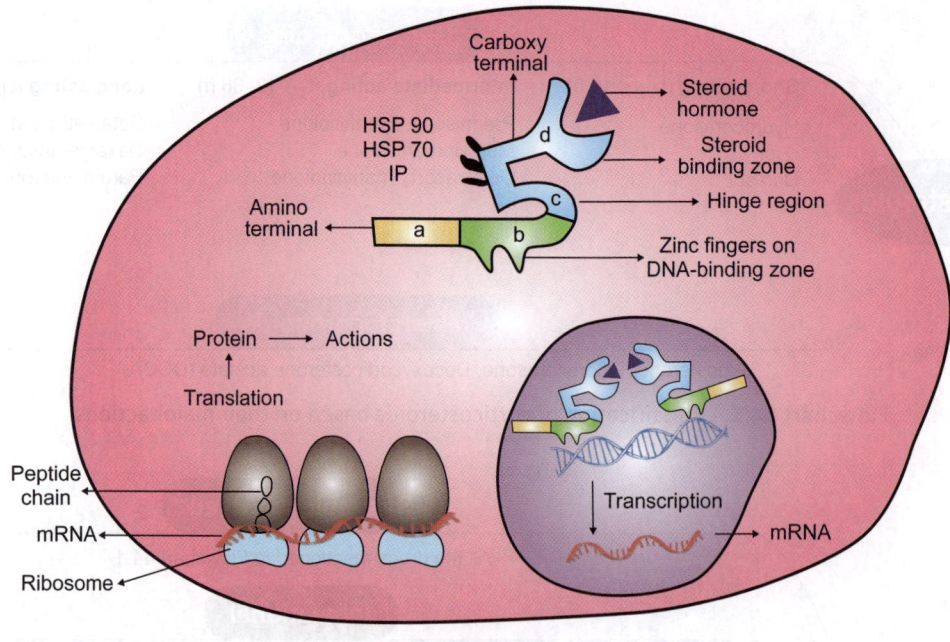

Fig. 44.2 Mechanism of action of corticosteroids

Binding of corticosteroid to the receptor
↓
Dissociation of HSP 70, 90, IP
↓
Inhibitory influence of HSPs and IP is removed and dimerisation region is exposed
↓
Dimerisation of steroid hormone-occupied receptor to form a homodimer
↓
The homodimer then translocates to the nucleus
↓
Here, the 'DNA binding domain' interacts with specific DNA sequences called 'glucocorticoid response elements (GREs)'
↓
Altered expression of genes, i.e., promotion/suppression of their transcription, producing specific mRNA → directed to ribosomes → specific protein synthesis. This, in turn, modifies cell function.

All these steps take some time, delaying the actions of corticosteroids for about 30–60 minutes. However, once these specific regulatory proteins are synthesised, their effect persists for a time longer than the half-life of steroidal hormones. Nevertheless, negative feedback effect of corticosteroids to decrease ACTH release from the pituitary is quick in onset, because it does not involve a gene expression-related mechanism.

Clinical problem-based questions and MCQs

1. Corticosteroids are useful in a variety of clinical indications. The onset of their action is delayed by about 30–60 minutes, but their actions persist longer than their half-life.
   i. Explain the delayed but persistent action of corticosteroids.
   ii. Describe their mechanism of action with a suitable diagram.

2. Identify the correct transduction pathway for metabolic effects of glucocorticoids.
   a. IP_3–DAG pathway
   b. cAMP pathway
   c. Gene expression alteration
   d. Ionic exchange pathway

3. Which part of the corticosteroid receptor possesses zinc fingers?
   a. DNA binding domain
   b. Steroid binding domain
   c. Dimerisation region
   d. Heat shock protein region

4. Identify the inhalational corticoid.
   a. Hydrocortisone   b. Triamcinolone
   c. Budesonide   d. Deflazacort

5. Which of these is a long-acting steroid?
   a. Hydrocortisone   b. Deflazacort
   c. Prednisolone   d. Dexamethasone

6. Which of the following has maximum glucocorticoid activity?
   a. Hydrocortisone   b. Prednisolone
   c. Dexamethasone   d. Fludrocortisone

7. Identify the corticosteroid that has selective mineralocorticoid activity.
   a. Desoxycorticosterone acetate

b. Triamcinolone
   c. Deflazacort
   d. Methylprednisolone
8. Inhalational corticosteroid therapy is preferred over systemic therapy in bronchial asthma. Which of the following steroids is suitable for administration by the inhalational route?
   a. Betamethasone benzoate
   b. Fluticasone propionate
   c. Clobetasol propionate
   d. Dexamethasone sodium phosphate

GLUCOCORTICOIDS

The glucocorticoids include hydrocortisone, prednisone, prednisolone, methylprednisolone, deflazacort, triamcinolone, betamethasone, dexamethasone, and paramethasone. Their actions are markedly different from those of mineralocorticoids.

- Hydrocortisone exhibits both glucocorticoid and mineralocorticoid activity to the same extent (1:1).
- Methylprednisolone, triamcinolone, betamethasone, dexamethasone and paramethasone have selective glucocorticoid activity, i.e., no mineralocorticoid activity. Dexamethasone has maximum glucocorticoid activity—30 times the activity of hydrocortisone.

Pharmacological Actions

1. Metabolic actions

The metabolic effects of glucocorticoids appear to play a **role in maintaining blood glucose during starvation,** so that nutrient supply to brain continues.

i. Carbohydrate metabolism

a. Glucocorticoids cause translocation of glucose transporters from the cell surface to deeper sites → decreased uptake and peripheral utilisation of glucose (its effect is opposite to that of insulin).
b. Hepatic gluconeogenic enzymes are induced, resulting in increased glucose production from amino acids.
c. Increased blood glucose due to both the above actions leads to increased insulin secretion as well as hepatic glycogen synthesis and deposition.

Hence, glucocorticoids increase insulin levels but cause resistance to insulin and a DM-like state.

ii. Protein metabolism

Glucocorticoids cause protein breakdown and amino acid mobilisation from peripheral tissues, resulting **in muscle wasting, loss of bone osteoid and thinning of skin.** The amino acids released upon protein breakdown reach the liver and are used for gluconeogenesis. Thus, corticoids cause negative nitrogen balance.

iii. Fat metabolism

> Glucocorticoids have a **permissive role*** in lipolytic response to catecholamines, growth hormone, glucagon, thyroxine, etc.
> ↓
> These hormones act by increasing cAMP concentration inside the cell.
> ↓
> Raised cAMP activates cAMP-dependent kinase. Synthesis of this kinase requires the presence of glucocorticoids
> (*Permissive role of glucocorticoids → their presence facilitates other hormones to exert their action.)
> ↓
> In turn, cAMP-activated kinase activates lipase.
> ↓
> Lipolytic response, i.e., enhanced triglyceride breakdown.

However, this **lipolytic response to glucocorticoids is differential**, i.e., fat depots in different body parts respond differently. This differential lipolytic response occurs because one action of glucocorticoids favours lipolysis, while other actions oppose it in adipose tissues.

Inhibits lipolysis	Favours lipolysis
Glucocorticoids increase insulin levels ↓ Insulin inhibits lipolysis in adipose tissue. This effect is especially predominant in truncal adipocytes ↓ Long-term use of glucocorticoids causes fat deposition over face, neck, shoulders ↓	GH, glucagon, thyroxine and catecholamines have lipolytic action (and) Glucocorticoids have permissive role in this action. The lipolytic effect is prominently seen in peripheral adipose tissue. ↓ With long-term use of corticosteroids, fat is lost from subcutaneous tissue over extremities ↓

These two effects lead to **redistribution of body fat** → thin extremities, moon facies, fish mouth and buffalo hump, seen in a state of corticoid excess called **Cushing syndrome.**

iv. Calcium metabolism

Glucocorticoids tend to cause **negative calcium balance** due to:

- Decrease in intestinal absorption of Ca^{2+}.
- Increased renal excretion of Ca^{2+}.
- Loss of calcium from bone indirectly due to loss of osteoid **predisposes to osteoporosis.** Spongy bones (vertebrae and ribs) are more sensitive.

2. CVS

Glucocorticoids:

- maintain the tone of arterioles and have a permissive role in the pressor action of adrenaline and angiotensin.

- maintain myocardial contractility.
- restrict capillary permeability.
- Na^+/H_2O retention and K^+ loss may occur as some mineralocorticoid activity is seen at non-physiological doses of glucocorticoids.

Thus, glucocorticoids have a **permissive role in hypertension** and should be used cautiously in hypertensives. On the other hand, acute adrenal insufficiency causes arteriolar dilatation, increased capillary permeability, hypovolemia, reduced cardiac output, and cardio vascular collapse.

3. Skeletal muscles

Muscular weakness occurs both in hypo- and hypercorticism.

In hypocorticism, deficiency of corticosteroids causes hypodynamic circulation leading to diminished work capacity and weakness. In hypercorticism, however, excessive mineralocorticoid action causes hypokalemia leading to muscular weakness. Excessive glucocorticoid action causes **muscle wasting, myopathy and weakness**.

4. CNS

Mild **euphoria** is fairly common with pharmacological doses of corticosteroids. This is a direct effect on the brain, independent of relief of symptoms of the disease for which corticoids were used. In some cases, it may progress to **increased motor activity, insomnia, anxiety or depression**. High doses of glucocorticoids **lower the seizure threshold**. So, these should be used cautiously in psychosis and epilepsy.

5. Negative feedback effect: HPAA suppression

Both endogenous and exogenous corticosteroids have a **negative feedback effect on CRH and ACTH** secretion. Exogenous glucocorticoid administration depresses the secretion of CRH and ACTH; this, in turn, inhibits the secretion of endogenous glucocorticoids and causes atrophy of the adrenal cortex. With prolonged glucocorticoid therapy, the hypothalamic–pituitary–adrenal axis (HPAA) is suppressed and may take many months to return to normal levels. Thus, sudden withdrawal of corticosteroids after prolonged systemic administration may cause symptoms like fatigue, weakness, anorexia, weight loss, nausea, vomiting, abdominal pain and diarrhea. Though these symptoms resemble the symptoms of many other medical problems, the recent history of stopping steroid intake suggests HPAA suppression. Therefore, corticosteroids should never be stopped abruptly and **should be slowly tapered off** over weeks or months.

6. Stomach

Glucocorticoids increase the secretion of gastric acid and pepsin, and may aggravate peptic ulcers.

7. Blood and lymphoid tissue

Glucocorticoids increase the number of RBCs, platelets, and neutrophils in circulation, but decrease the number of lymphocytes, eosinophils and basophils. They enhance the rate of destruction of lymphoid cells. T cells are more sensitive to this **lympholytic action** than B cells. Moreover, the lytic response is more marked in malignant lymphatic cells than in normal lymphoid tissue. This action forms the basis for use of steroids in lymphomas.

8. Anti-inflammatory action

Glucocorticoids have a **nonspecific anti-inflammatory effect** that covers all stages and components of inflammation. Moreover, the effect is exerted irrespective of the type of injury or insult, i.e., inflammations caused by invading pathogenic organisms, chemical stimuli, physical stimuli, hypersensitivity reactions, autoimmune reactions, etc. respond to corticosteroid therapy.

a. **Effect on inflammatory cells**

Corticosteroids:
- decrease the egress of neutrophils and macrophages from blood vessels
- decrease the activity of neutrophils, macrophages, fibroblasts, and T helper cells.
- decrease the clonal proliferation of T cells.
- decrease fibroblast function. Thus, production of collagen and glycosaminoglycans is reduced. While this action suppresses chronic inflammation, healing and repair also slow down.
- decrease the function of osteoblasts, but increase the activity of osteoclasts, thus favouring osteoporotic tendency.

b. **Effect on inflammatory mediators**
- Decrease production of prostaglandins and leukotrienes due to inhibition of phospholipase A_2.
- Decrease production of cytokines, interleukins (IL-1, 2, 3, 4, 5, 6, and 8), tumour necrosis factor (TNF-α), cell adhesion factors, and GM-CSF owing to decreased transcription of their genes.
- Decrease concentration of complement in plasma.
- Decrease generation of induced nitric oxide (NO).
- Decrease histamine release from mast cells.
- Decrease formation of IgG.

Thus, the anti-inflammatory effect of corticosteroids includes:
- Reduction of capillary permeability, local exudation, cellular infiltration, and phagocytic activity
- Reduction of late responses like capillary proliferation, collagen deposition, fibroblastic activity and scar formation.

However, it is important to note that corticosteroids only have a palliative role, and do not correct the cause of inflammation. So, while they suppress the inflammation and symptoms related to it, the underlying disease process continues to progress.

9. Immunosuppressive effect

Glucocorticoids suppress the body's immune response and all types of hypersensitivity and allergic phenomena. The immune suppression is because of the reduced recruitment of leukocytes at the site of contact with the antigen as well as reduced inflammatory response to immunological insults. The effect is more pronounced on cell-mediated immune responses, because **T lymphocytes (involved in CMI) are more sensitive to corticosteroids than B lymphocytes**. This effect is useful in **graft rejections and delayed hypersensitivity reactions**. However, impairment of antibody production and complement function is usually not seen at therapeutic doses.

At high concentrations, glucocorticoids can interfere with practically every step of immune response, making the patient immunosuppressed and **more prone to infections**.

The important actions of corticosteroids are summarised in Flowchart 44.3.

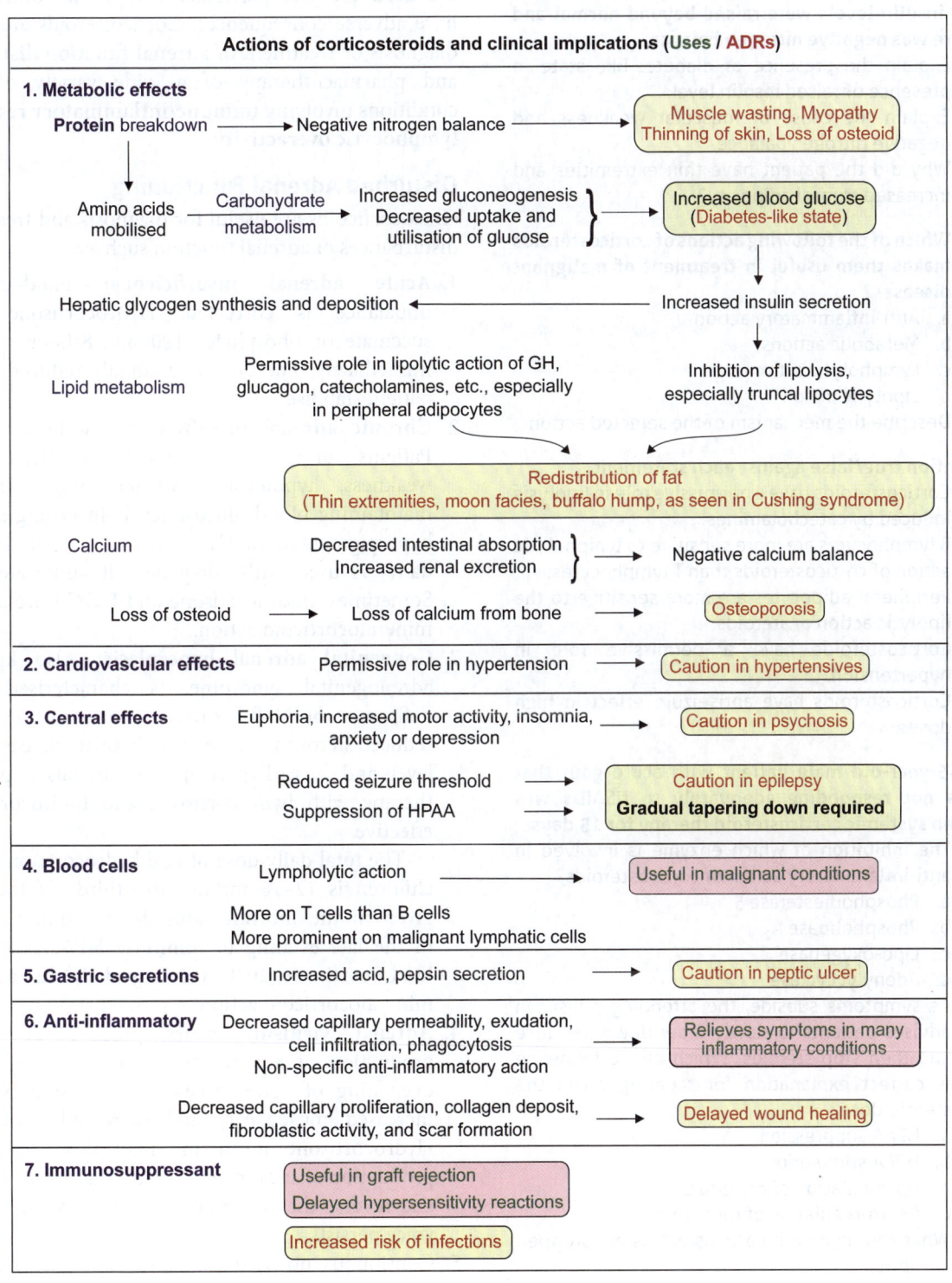

Flowchart 44.3 Major actions of corticosteroids

Clinical problem-based questions and MCQs

9. A 45-year-old male patient suffering from acute gouty arthritis, not responding to NSAIDs, is on corticosteroid therapy for about five months. He complained of nocturnal polyuria, polydipsia and polyphagia. On examination, patient had muscular weakness and thinning of skin, thin extremities, increased truncal adipocity (buffalo hump and moon facies). On investigating, FBS = 140 mg/dL, but insulin levels were raised beyond normal and there was negative nitrogen balance.
   i. Explain the presence of diabetes-like state in presence of raised insulin levels.
   ii. Explain the cause of muscular weakness and negative nitrogen balance.
   iii. Why did the patient have thin extremities and increased truncal adiposity?

10. i. Which of the following actions of corticosteroids makes them useful in treatment of malignant diseases?
    a. Anti-inflammatory action
    b. Metabolic actions
    c. Lympholytic action
    d. Lipolytic action
    ii. Describe the mechanism of the selected action.

11. Mention true/false against each statement.
    a. Corticosteroids have a permissive role in lipolysis induced by catecholamines.
    b. B lymphocytes are more sensitive to lympholytic action of corticosteroids than T lymphocytes.
    c. Peripheral adipocytes are more sensitive to the lipolytic action of steroids.
    d. Corticosteroids have a permissive role in hypertension.
    e. Corticosteroids have antiseizure effect in high doses.

12. A 55-year-old male patient with acute gout that was not responding adequately to NSAIDs was given systemic corticosteroid therapy for 15 days.
    i. The inhibition of which enzyme is involved in anti-inflammatory action of corticosteroids?
       a. Phosphodiesterase 5
       b. Phospholipase A_2
       c. Lipo-oxygenase
       d. Adenylyl cyclase
    ii. As symptoms subside, the attending physician advises patients to slowly taper down the dose and then stop steroids. Which of the following is correct explanation for tapering down the steroid dose?
       a. HPAA suppression.
       b. HPAA stimulation.
       c. Up-regulation of receptors.
       d. Down-regulation of receptors.
    iii. What can happen if corticosteroids are stopped abruptly?

13. Corticosteroids are used for symptomatic relief in many inflammatory conditions. Describe their mechanism of anti-inflammatory action.

Therapeutic Uses of Glucocorticoids

Owing to the wide distribution of their receptors, glucocorticoids have widespread effects and many indications for use (see Box 44.1). However, when they are used for one particular action, the other actions have adverse consequences. Corticosteroids are used for diagnosis or treatment of **adrenal function disturbances** and pharmacotherapy of a wide variety of clinical conditions involving **immune/inflammatory response or lymphocytic overactivity**.

Disturbed Adrenal Functioning

Glucocorticoids are useful for diagnosis and treatment in disturbances of adrenal function such as:

1. **Acute adrenal insufficiency:** Fluid–electrolyte imbalance is corrected. Hydrocortisone sodium succinate or phosphate (100 mg, 8-hourly) is given immediately. The dose is gradually reduced once the patient stabilises.

2. **Chronic adrenal insufficiency** (Addison's disease): Patients of chronic adrenal insufficiency have weakness, hypotension, weight loss, difficulty in maintaining blood glucose levels in fasting state, and hyperpigmentation. Hydrocortisone (oral, 20–30 mg daily) is used with adequate salt and water intake. Sometimes, fludrocortisone and DOCA are added for mineralocorticoid action.

3. **Congenital adrenal hyperplasia:** Also known as adrenogenital syndrome, is characterised by the deficiency of 21-β-hydroxylase enzyme, resulting in reduced steroid secretion; this, in turn, increases ACTH levels and causes hypertrophy of adrenals. Replacement therapy with hydrocortisone and fludrocortisone is effective.

    The total daily dose of oral hydrocortisone in these children is 12–18 mg/m^2; two-thirds of the dose is given in the morning and the remaining one-third in the late evening to minimise HPAA suppression. Fludrocortisone (0.05–0.2 mg daily) is added for mineralocorticoid action.

4. **Adrenal virilism** occurs because of excessive production of adrenal androgens resulting in acne, deepening of voice, excessive facial and body hair, increased muscularity and increased sexual drive. Hydrocortisone given in small doses can reduce production of androgens in cases of adrenal hyperplasia and reverse the symptoms; however, the deepening of voice persists.

5. Continuous intravenous infusion of hydrocortisone (up to 300 mg) is given during surgical removal of **ACTH-**

secreting pituitary adenomas. Slowly, the dose is reduced to normal replacement levels.
6. Diagnostic use of glucocorticoids: **Dexamethasone suppression test** helps in distinguishing patients having ACTH-secreting pituitary adenoma (Cushing disease) from other causes of Cushing syndrome, such as ectopic ACTH syndrome or steroid-producing tumours of adrenal cortex

Pharmacotherapy

Glucocorticoids are also used empirically in a variety of conditions that do not involve adrenal disturbance. While their use is mostly palliative, it can be life-saving in some situations owing to their anti-inflammatory, antiallergic or immunosuppressive and lympholytic action

a. Therapeutic uses based on anti-inflammatory action

7. **Arthritis**: Glucocorticoids are useful in various types of arthritis like **rheumatoid arthritis, osteoarthritis,** and **gout** during periods of exacerbation, because of their anti-inflammatory action. In conditions like **bursitis and tenosynovitis** also, steroids relieve symptoms.
8. **Eye conditions** such as conjunctivitis, iritis, iridocyclitis, choroiditis, retinitis, optic neuritis and uveitis are relieved using glucocorticoids.
9. **Gastrointestinal diseases**: Patients suffering from diseases like irritable bowel syndrome, nontropical sprue, and subacute hepatitis experience symptomatic relief.
10. **Dermatological conditions**: Steroids are very frequently used topically or systemically in various dermatological conditions such as atopic dermatitis, pemphigus, seborrheic dermatitis, lichen simplex chronicus, xerosis, eczema, and mycosis fungoides.
11. **Bronchial asthma:** Corticosteroids are useful in bronchial asthma because of their nonspecific anti-inflammatory and antiallergic actions. Inhalational corticosteroids (ICS) are indicated along with β_2-agonists in chronic asthma. In cases of acute severe attack of asthma or status asthmaticus, intravenous administration is indicated
12. They are used in other **lung diseases** such as aspiration pneumonia, pulmonary edema, prevention of respiratory distress in infants, and to accelerate recovery in acute respiratory distress syndrome (ARDS), and sarcoidosis.
13. Mountain sickness, neurological conditions such as cerebral edema, multiple sclerosis, and neurocysticercosis.
14. Dexamethasone is used to prevent **nausea and vomiting** associated with cancer chemotherapy [chemotherapy-induced nausea and vomiting (CINV)] and general anesthesia.

b. Therapeutic uses based on antiallergic/immunosuppressive actions

15. **Allergic reactions**: Glucocorticoids effectively suppress severe allergic reactions such as anaphylaxis, angioedema, urticaria, serum sickness, drug reactions, bee stings, and allergic rhinitis.
16. **Autoimmune diseases**: Glucocorticoids are useful in autoimmune diseases because of their immunosuppressant action. They are effective in conditions like **hemolytic anemia, thrombocytopenia, rheumatic fever, chronic active hepatitis, and myasthenia gravis.**
17. Collagen diseases like systemic lupus erythematosus (SLE), nephrotic syndrome, dermatomyositis, polymyositis, giant cell arteritis, and temporal arteritis.
18. Prevention of **transplant rejection**: Methylprednisolone pulse therapy (1 g, IV infusion) at 6–8 weeks intervals is preferred. Pulse therapy provides good results with minimal suppression of the pituitary–adrenal axis.
19. Thyroid conditions like malignant exopthalmos and subacute thyroiditis.
20. Hematological conditions like leukemia, multiple myeloma, acquired hemolytic anemia, and idiopathic thrombocytopenic purpura.

c. Uses based on lympholytic action

21. Corticosteroids are used in **cancer chemotherapy** along with other anticancer drugs for acute lymphoid leukemia, Hodgkin and non-Hodgkin lymphoma, carcinoma breast, etc.

d. Other uses

22. Hypercalcemia
23. **Premature births**: Corticosteroids are used to **accelerate lung maturity** in premature delivery.
24. Betamethasone and dexamethasone are devoid of mineralocorticoid action, and are useful in reducing **cerebral edema associated with TB or malignant diseases.**
25. Glucocorticoids are useful to **tide over crises in acute conditions like lepra reactions, tubercular meningitis, and septicemia.** Glucocorticoids are used for a short time, under the cover of specific antitubercular drugs or antibiotics.

Box 44.1 Therapeutic uses of corticosteroids

Corticosteroids are used in many clinical conditions [Mnemonic: Alphabets from A–V, excluding J, K, and Q]
A. **Arthritis** (rheumatoid/gout/osteoarthritis, bursitis, tenosynovitis), **Allergic reactions** (anaphylaxis, angioedema, urticaria, serum sickness, drug reactions, bee stings, allergic rhinitis), **Autoimmune disorders** (chronic active hepatitis, myasthenia gravis)
B. **Bronchial asthma**

C. **C**ollagen disorders (systemic lupus erythematosus (SLE), nephrotic syndrome, dermatomyositis, polymyositis, giant cell arteritis, temporal arteritis), **C**erebral edema due to tubercular or malignant diseases
D. **D**ermatological conditions (atopic dermatitis, pemphigus, seborrheic dermatitis, lichen simplex chronicus, xerosis, eczema, mycosis fungoides)
E. **E**xopthalmos (malignant type)
F. **F**ungoides: a type of non-Hodgkin lymphoma
G. **G**astrointestinal conditions (irritable bowel syndrome, nontropical sprue, subacute hepatitis)
H. **H**ypercalcemia, **H**emolytic anemia
I. **I**diopathic TCP
J. —
K. —
L. **L**epra reaction
M. **M**ountain sickness, **M**ultiple sclerosis, **M**ultiple myeloma
N. **N**eoplastic conditions (lymphomas, leukemias), **N**eurocysticercosis
O. **O**phthalmic conditions (conjunctivitis, iritis, iridocyclitis, choroiditis, retinitis, optic neuritis, uveitis)
P. **P**ulmonary conditions (aspiration pneumonia, pulmonary edema, prevention of respiratory distress syndrome), **P**remature labour
Q. —
R. **R**heumatic fever, **R**espiratory distress syndrome, **R**eplacement therapy (acute/chronic adrenal insufficiency, congenital adrenal hyperplasia, removal of ACTH-secreting pituitary adenomas)
S. **S**ubacute thyroiditis, **S**epticemia
T. **T**ransplant rejection, **T**ubercular meningitis
U. **U**rticaria
V. **V**omiting associated with cancer chemotherapy and general anesthesia

Clinical problem-based questions and MCQs

14. Corticosteroids receptors are very widely distributed, so corticosteroids have clinical utility in a variety of clinical conditions, as well as many adverse effects.
    i. Enumerate the therapeutic uses of corticosteroids
    ii. Enumerate the pharmacological basis for use of corticosteroids in:
        a. Congenital adrenal hyperplasia
        b. Malignant conditions

15. A 45-year-old male patient with diabetic nephropathy had undergone renal transplant. Post-operatively, methylprednisolone pulse therapy is given (1 g, intravenous infusion, every 6 weeks).
    i. Describe the pharmacological basis for use of methylprednisolone in this case.
    ii. What is the advantage of pulse therapy?

16. Corticosteroids are used in all of the following conditions, EXCEPT:
    a. Subacute thyroiditis   b. Peptic ulcer
    c. Multiple sclerosis   d. Cerebral edema

17. While corticosteroids cause dramatic improvement in many clinical conditions, their use is associated with numerous adverse effects. In order to minimise adverse effects of corticosteroids, some general principles are adopted. Which of the following statements is correct to ensure safe use of steroids?
    a. Long-acting steroids are preferred.
    b. Multiple daily doses are safer than single dose.
    c. Alternate day therapy is preferred.
    d. Maximum tolerated dose should be given.

Adverse Effects of Corticosteroids

Corticosteroids can cause many adverse effects.
[Mnemonic: Most of the ADRs can be derived from the alphabets of word **CORTICOSTEROID**: **C**ushing syndrome, **O**steoporosis, **R**etention of salt and water, **T**B may worsen or latent TB may be activated, **I**nfections occur more commonly or may worsen, **C**ataract, **O**edema, **S**uppression of HPAA, **T**opical use in eye can cause glaucoma, **E**pilepsy may worsen, **R**enal failure may worsen, **I**mpaired healing, **D**iabetes may occur as these cause hyperglycemia]

1. **Cushing syndrome**: Most of the patients receiving steroids in a dose of 100 mg daily, for more than 2 weeks develop **iatrogenic Cushing syndrome** (Fig. 44.3) characterised by:

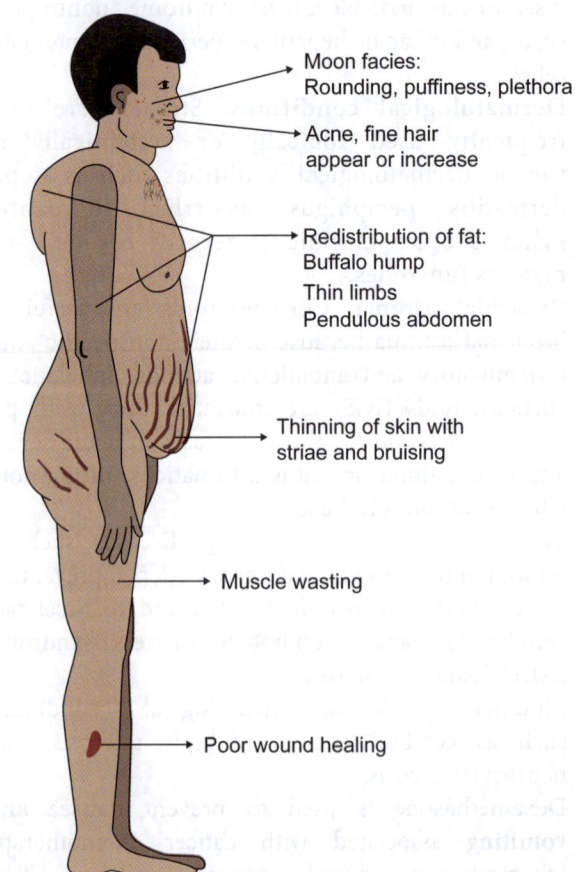

Fig. 44.3 Cushing syndrome

- Face: Rounding, puffiness and plethora appear (called 'moon facies'.)
- Fat is redistributed from extremities to trunk, back of neck, supraclavicular area (buffalo hump) and face.
- Growth of fine hair on thighs, trunk and face.
- Acne appear or increase.
- Insomnia
- Increased appetite, weight gain, visceral fat deposition.
- Muscle wasting, thinning of skin with striae and bruising
- Hyperglycemia: Eventually diabetes may occur
- Osteoporosis and aseptic necrosis of hip can occur
- Impaired wound healing

Patients using corticosteroids should be given high protein diet and increased K^+; anabolic steroids can be used when required.

2. **Hypothalamic–pituitary–adrenal axis suppression**: Administration of steroids for more than a few days causes adrenal suppression. Additional dose is then required during stressful conditions. It takes 2–3 months for the pituitary to become responsive again. **If the dose is reduced rapidly, symptoms of the disease (for which steroids were given) will appear again** with greater intensity. **Anorexia, nausea, vomiting, headache, lethargy, weight loss, fever, myalgia, arthralgia, postural hypotension**, etc. may also occur. To avoid such adverse effects, the dose should be slowly tapered down and stopped gradually over 2–12 months.

3. Other adverse effects include:
   - Benign intracranial hypertension
   - Psychosis can occur with large doses
   - Posterior subcapsular cataract develops with long-term therapy.
   - Increased IOT and glaucoma may be induced
   - Development of peptic ulcers and their complications may occur.
   - Nausea, dizziness, and (in some patients) weight loss occurs with triamcinolone and methyl prednisolone. It is treated with reduction of dose, drug change, increased K^+ and protein intake
   - Growth retardation in children with doses ≥ 45 mg/m² per day.
   - Clinical findings of bacterial and mycotic infections may be masked by corticosteroids. Patients must be watched carefully, especially when large doses are being used.
   - Myopathy of unknown origin is more frequently seen with triamcinolone.
   - Cortisone and hydrocortisone cause sodium and fluid retention and K^+ loss due to mineralocorticoid action at high doses. In patients with normal cardiovascular and renal function, it leads to hypokalemic and hypochloremic alkalosis, and eventually, to a rise in BP. However, in patients with heart disease, even little sodium retention can precipitate CHF. In hypoproteinemia and renal or liver diseases, such fluid retention causes development of edema. It is managed with salt restriction and judicious K^+ supplementation.

Cautions
Patients receiving corticosteroids on a long-term basis should be monitored for the development of hyperglycemia, glycosuria, sodium retention, edema, hypertension, hypokalemia, peptic ulcer, osteoporosis, and hidden infections.

Contraindications
- Peptic ulcer
- Heart disease
- Hypertension with CHF
- Infections
- Psychosis
- Diabetes
- Osteoporosis
- Glaucoma
- Herpes simplex infections

General Principles of Corticosteroid Therapy
Corticosteroids can cause **dramatic improvement but equally dramatic ADRs**. Therefore, the following general principles should be followed while using corticosteroids for any therapeutic indication.

1. **Single dose** is usually not harmful; even **short courses** are not harmful in the absence of contraindications. However, if long-term use is required for a particular condition, after exhausting all less harmful options, care should be taken to minimise the adverse consequences.
2. Corticosteroids **having medium-to-intermediate duration of action** such as prednisone and prednisolone should be preferred over longer-acting drugs, as these cause less suppression of the HPAA.
3. The **dose should be the minimum** dose at which the useful effect is obtained. However, dose should be increased during stressful conditions such as infection, injury, and surgery.
4. **Alternate day therapy** should be preferred over daily use, wherever possible.
5. Once steroids have been used for > 2–3 weeks, they should not be abruptly discontinued. Dose should be **tapered down very slowly** over 2–12 months, so that hypothalamic–pituitary axis recovers from the suppressing effect of exogenous steroids. Quick dose reduction may worsen the condition for which steroids were used. Patient may also develop symptoms suggesting glucocorticoid deficiency like anorexia, nausea, vomiting, headache, lethargy, fever, arthralgia, myalgia, postural hypotension, and weight loss.

6. Larger portion of dose should be **given in morning**. This minimises HPAA suppression.
7. During **stress**: Dose of steroids should be increased.

Clinical problem-based questions and MCQs

18. Identify the condition in which corticosteroids are contraindicated and explain why.
    a. Hypertension
    b. Bronchial asthma
    c. Rheumatoid arthritis
    d. Pulmonary edema

19. While corticosteroids are known to cause dramatic improvement in many diseases, they can produce equally dramatic adverse effects.
    i. Enumerate adverse effects of corticosteroids.
    ii. Describe the general principles of corticosteroid use to minimise their adverse effects.

20. Identify the glucocorticoid that is totally devoid of mineralocorticoid action and may be used to reduce cerebral edema due to tubercular meningitis.
    a. Prednisolone
    b. Prednisone
    c. Hydrocortisone
    d. Methylprednisolone

21. A patient of bronchial asthma is prescribed an inhalational corticosteroid. Identify the drug.
    a. Betamethasone
    b. Beclomethasone
    c. Triamcinolone
    d. Dexamethasone

22. Corticosteroids are contraindicated in all of the following conditions EXCEPT:
    a. Diabetes mellitus
    b. Angioedema
    c. Hypertension
    d. Epilepsy

Monitoring Steroid Therapy

Corticosteroids can be compared to a double-edged sword; while they possess numerous and varied therapeutic applications, their use is also associated with several adverse consequences. So, in clinical practice, corticosteroids should be prescribed and used very carefully to obtain optimum treatment outcomes, with minimal adverse effects.

- **Before prescribing** corticosteroids for any therapeutic indication, patient history should be elicited and physical examination should be conducted to rule out the presence of contraindications or conditions that may be worsened by steroids such as diabetes, hypertension, CHF, dyslipidemias, psychiatric illnesses, and osteoporosis.
- **Baseline measurements** of height, weight, nutritional status, puberty (especially in children/ adolescents), blood pressure, bone mineral density, lipid profile, fasting blood sugar, and ophthalmological examination should be conducted before starting steroid therapy.
- **Follow-up**: At each follow-up visit:
  - Fluid–electrolyte levels should be monitored.
  - To detect HPAA suppression with corticosteroids, early morning cortisol should be measured. Low-dose ACTH testing may be beneficial. If HPAA suppression is detected, daily physiological dose is given and stress doses are added as per need of individual patient.
  - In patients on long-term steroid therapy, bone mineral density should be measured at one-year intervals and the patient should be screened for fragility fractures. If adverse effects on bones are not detected, the frequency of repeat BMD testing is reduced to every 2–3 years.
  - Patient should be evaluated for any joint pain and range of joint mobility.
  - Concurrently used medications should be evaluated because many drugs like anticoagulants, antidiabetics, and NSAIDs interact with steroids and need dosage adjustment.
  - In case of children, any live or live-attenuated vaccination should be delayed for about three months after discontinuation of steroid therapy; this is because the patient becomes more prone to infections while receiving steroid therapy.

Communication with patient

Proper, on-going communication with patient in their preferred language, taking care to clarify their doubts about dose/route/duration/time of administration, etc., goes a long way toward optimising benefits of corticosteroid therapy and minimising the risks. The dialogue with patient starts before starting therapy and is continued throughout the course of treatment till slow, gradual tapering down of dose to stop the treatment. This whole process may take weeks, months or even longer. Healthcare professionals should be committed to provide all necessary information and repeat it as many times as needed, till patient is confident about correct use of medication.

- All members of the healthcare team should be enabled to communicate with patients in an empathetic manner, and to highlight the importance of strictly **adhering to corticosteroid prescription and follow-up schedule**. Patients are educated to take the dose as advised, at a specific time, with specified frequency, and for appropriate duration.
- Patients should not continue treatment for a period longer than prescribed. They must come for follow-up examination as and when called by physician to decide to continue or taper down the dose; this is based on improvement of symptoms of disease for which steroids were prescribed, and evaluation for presence of any adverse effects.

- Patient should be educated about the risk of potential adverse effects and **measures that can prevent/minimise the adverse effects.** All risks and benefits should be explained to patient to involve them in the decision-making process to ensure optimum treatment outcomes.
- Patients on long-term therapy should be advised to carry **treatment card/tag** that may be applied to patient's treatment charts for notifying other team members about corticosteroid use.
- Oral dose should be preferably **taken with food** to reduce the gastric irritant effect, and **in the morning**, to prevent HPAA suppression.
- If a patient on once-daily dosage misses a dose, they should take it as soon as they remember on the same day; however, if they remember it on the next day, the **dose should not be doubled**.
- Patients with history of gastric ulcers or receiving NSAIDs concurrently, should be given **proton pump inhibitors** to reduce the risk of ulcer or its complications.
- Patients are advised **low calorie, high protein diet** that is **potassium-rich and low in sodium**.
- **Alcohol consumption/cigarette smoking** should be minimised or stopped completely.
- Medicine should be **stored** in an airtight container at room temperature, away from direct light, heat and moisture.

MINERALOCORTICOIDS

These include aldosterone, desoxycorticosterone acetate (DOCA), and fludrocortisone.

Aldosterone

Aldosterone is synthesised mainly in the zona glomerulosa of the adrenal cortex; its secretion is influenced by ACTH and angiotensin.

Mechanism of action

Aldosterone acts by binding to mineralocorticoid receptors in the cytoplasm of target cells, especially principal cells of the collecting tubules of the kidney. It affects gene transcription and increases the activity of both apical membrane channels and basolateral Na^+/K^+ ATPase, resulting in the increase in both Na^+ reabsorption and K^+ secretion.

Actions

- Aldosterone has maximum mineralocorticoid activity (about 3000 times the activity of hydrocortisone). It promotes reabsorption of sodium from tubular fluid in collecting tubules. Sodium reabsorption is loosely coupled to the secretion of K^+ and H^+.
- Increased sodium reabsorption in the sweat and salivary glands, gastrointestinal mucosa and across cell membrane in general.

Excess aldosterone (as seen in patients with overdose of synthetic mineralocorticoids or tumours) causes increased plasma volume, hypertension, hypokalemia and metabolic alkalosis. Thus, aldosterone antagonists (e.g., spironolactone) are used adjuvantly to diuretics in various cardiovascular conditions.

Desoxycorticosterone Acetate

Desoxycorticosterone acetate (DOCA) is a precursor of aldosterone. DOCA has selective mineralocorticoid activity (i.e., no glucocorticoid activity). When injected I/V, it has a half-life of 70 min. Its secretion is primarily under ACTH control and increases markedly in adrenal carcinoma and congenital adrenal hyperplasia.

Fludrocortisone

This is the most widely used mineralocorticoid. It has both gluco- and mineralocorticoid activity It is used in the treatment of adrenocortical insufficiency, in a dose of 0.1 mg, 2–7 times a week; it has potent salt-retaining effect. However, these doses are too small to have any anti-inflammatory action.

Summary

- Corticosteroids can be glucocorticoids or mineralocorticoids. Glucocorticoids can be short-, intermediate- and long-acting.
- Their mechanism of action involves gene regulation after binding to a widely distributed cytoplasmic receptor.
- They have nonspecific, anti-inflammatory, immunosuppressive, antiallergic and lympholytic actions.
- Corticosteroids are used clinically in a variety of conditions; however, they also have frequent and dramatic adverse effects.
- So, corticosteroids should be used very carefully, only when indicated, for the shortest possible duration, and as single early morning dose or alternate-day therapy. Care should be taken to taper down the dose slowly, after use for 2 or more weeks.
- Important therapeutic uses include replacement therapy in deficiency disorders and as pharmacotherapy in many clinical conditions, owing to their anti-inflammatory and immunosuppressant actions. These are used for replacement therapy in acute/chronic adrenal insufficiency and congenital adrenal hyperplasia.

- Pharmacotherapy with corticosteroids is empirical, palliative and life-saving in clinical conditions such as rheumatoid arthritis, osteoarthritis, gout, acute rheumatic fever, collagen diseases (SLE, nephrotic syndrome, dermatomyositis), severe allergic reactions (anaphylaxis, urticaria, angioedema, serum sickness), bronchial asthma, autoimmune disorders (hemolytic anemia, TCP, myasthenia gravis, chronic active hepatitis), ocular conditions (conjunctivitis, iritis, retinitis, keratitis, optic neuritis), aspiration pneumonia, pulmonary edema, dermatological conditions (atopic dermatitis, pemphigus, seborrheic dermatitis, xerosis), subacute thyroiditis, mountain sickness, IBS, nontropical sprue, and transplant rejection.
- Corticosteroids can cause variety of adverse effects due to suppression of the HPAA, metabolic actions and other effects. HPAA suppression causes anorexia, nausea, vomiting, headache, lethargy, weight loss, fever, myalgia and postural hypotension. Upon stopping therapy, symptoms of the disease for which steroids were used initially reappear with increased severity. Metabolic adverse effects include Cushing syndrome characterised by moon facies, buffalo hump, muscle wasting, thinning of skin, weight gain, hyperglycemia, osteoporosis, impaired wound healing etc. Other ADRs include peptic ulcer, myopathy, psychotic behaviour, glaucoma, hypertension, fluid retention, posterior subcapsular cataract and growth retardation in children.
- Corticosteroids are contraindicated in epilepsy, diabetes, psychosis, peptic ulcer, hypertension, congestive heart failure, herpes simplex keratitis, renal failure and osteoporosis.

Questions for practice

1. Classify corticosteroids on the basis of their duration of action.
2. Enumerate the therapeutic uses and adverse effects of corticosteroids.
3. Explain why:
   a. Corticosteroids should be given as single morning dose.
   b. Dose of corticosteroids should be slowly tapered down.
   c. Corticosteroids are contraindicated in diabetic patients.
   d. Corticosteroids are used in lymphomas along with other anticancer drugs.

Hints for problem-based questions and MCQs

1. i. Delayed and persistent action of corticosteroids is because of their mechanism of action through altered expression of genes, which involves many steps. Refer to page 590.
   ii. Refer to Fig. 44.2, page 590
2. c. Gene expression alteration.
3. a. DNA binding domain possesses zinc fingers
4. c. Budesonide is given by inhalational route
5. d. Dexamethasone has long duration of action >36 hours
6. c. Dexamethasone has maximum glucocorticoid activity (30 times that of hydrocortisone).
7. a. Desoxycorticosterone acetate
8. b. Fluticasone dipropionate.
9. i. Decreased uptake and peripheral utilisation of glucose, increased glucose production from amino acids → increased blood glucose → increased insulin secretion and hepatic glycogen synthesis and deposition. Refer to page 591.
   ii. Due to catabolic effect on proteins. Refer to page 591.
   iii. Due to redistribution of fat because of differential lipolytic response. Refer to page 591.
10. i. c. Lympholytic action
    ii. Steroids enhance the rate of destruction of lymphoid cells; malignant cells are affected more than normal lymphoid tissue. Refer to page 592.
11. a. T; b. F; c. T; d. T; e. F.
12. i. b. Phospholipase A2
    ii. a. HPAA suppression
    iii. HPAA suppression --> fatigue, weakness, anorexia, weight loss, nausea, vomiting, abdominal pain and diarrhea.
13. Nonspecific anti-inflammatory action due to PLA2 inhibition → reduced PG, LT, IL, cytokines production:
    - Reduced capillary permeability, exudation, cell infiltration, and phagocytosis.
    - Decreased late responses such as cell proliferation, collagen deposition, and fibroblastic scar formation. Refer to page 592.
14. i. Refer to page 595, 596.
    ii. a. Replacement therapy with corticosteroids decreases ACTH levels and checks adrenal hypertrophy. Refer to page 594.
    iii. b. Due to lympholytic action, steroids are useful in lymphomas
15. i. Because of immunosuppressant action
    ii. Pulse therapy provides good results with minimal HPAA suppression
16. b. Peptic ulcer
17. c. Alternate-day therapy is preferred (to minimise suppression of HPAA).
18. a. Corticosteroids are contraindicated in hypertension as they have a permissive effect on the pressor action of adrenaline and angiotensin and maintain the tone of arterioles.
19. i. Corticosteroids can cause variety of adverse effects due to suppression of HPAA, metabolic and other actions. Refer to page 596.
    ii. General principles include single morning dose, minimal dose, drugs with medium-to-intermediate duration of action, short courses and alternate-day therapy are preferred as far as possible. Dose can be increased during stressful conditions. Withdrawal should be very gradual by slowly tapering down doses. Refer to page 597.
20. d. Methylprednisolone has no mineralocorticoid activity.
21. b. Beclomethasone is an inhalational steroid.
22. b. Angioedema

CONCEPT MAP - CORTICOSTEROIDS

Mechanism of Action

Bind to a **cytoplasmic receptor** present in all the cells → dimerisation of steroid hormone occupied receptor → homodimer translocates to nucleus → interacts with glucocorticoid response elements (GREs) → promotes/ suppresses their transcription → **specific protein synthesis** → modification of cell function. Onset of actions delayed for 30–60 minutes, but last longer than their half-life

Classification

Based on Major Actions

Glucocorticoids

Short acting: Have a half-life < 12 hours
Hydrocortisone or cortisol

Intermediate acting: Half-life is 12–36 hours
Prednisone, Prednisolone, Methylprednisolone, Deflazacort, Triamcinolone

Long acting: Half-life is > 36 hours
Betamethasone, Dexamethasone, Paramethasone

Mineralocorticoids
Aldosterone, Fludrocortisone, Desoxycorticosterone acetate (DOCA)

Major Actions

- **Metabolic effects:**
  Increase insulin levels but cause resistance to insulin and DM like state.
  Cause protein breakdown and amino acid mobilisation from peripheral tissues,
  Negative nitrogen balance → causes muscle wasting, myopathy and weakness
  Permissive role in lipolytic response to other hormones. However, lipolytic response to glucocorticoids is differential
- Non-specific anti-inflammatory, immunosuppressive, antiallergic and lympholytic actions
- Permissive role in hypertension
- Negative calcium balance → predisposes to osteoporosis.

CORTICOSTEROIDS

Contraindications

Epilepsy, Diabetes, Psychosis, Peptic ulcer, Hypertension, Congestive heart failure, Herpes simplex keratitis, Renal failure, Osteoporosis.

ADRs

HPAA suppression → anorexia, nausea, vomiting, headache, lethargy, weight loss, fever, myalgia, postural hypotension.
Upon stopping therapy, symptoms of the disease for which steroids were used reappear with increased severity.
Metabolic adverse effects include Cushing syndrome characterised by moon facies, buffalo hump, muscle wasting, thinning of skin, weight gain, hyperglycemia, osteoporosis, impaired wound healing, etc.
Other ADRs include peptic ulcer, myopathy, psychotic behaviour, glaucoma, hypertension, fluid retention, posterior subcapsular cataract, growth retardation in children.

Therapeutic Uses

For replacement therapy in acute/ chronic adrenal insufficiency, Congenital adrenal hyperplasia

Pharmacotherapy
- Arthritis (RA, OA, gout), Autoimmune disorders Acute rheumatic fever, Severe allergic reactions
- Pulmonary conditions: Bronchial asthma, Aspiration pneumonia, Pulmonary edema
- Collagen disorders
- Dermatological conditions (atopic dermatitis, pemphigus, seborrheic dermatitis)
- Ocular conditions (conjunctivitis, iritis, retinitis, keratitis, optic neuritis)
- Subacute thyroiditis, mountain sickness, IBS, Nontropical sprue, Transplant rejection, etc.

General Principles of Corticosteroid Therapy

- Single dose, short courses, with minimum dose of drugs having medium-to-intermediate duration of action should be preferred
- Alternate-day therapy preferred over daily use, with larger portion of dose given in morning.
- Once steroids have been used for > 2-3 weeks, they should not be abruptly discontinued. Dose should be tapered down very slowly over 2-12 months,

SECTION 9 Drugs Affecting the Endocrine System

45 Female Sex Hormones and Antagonists

PH 7.7 Explain the types, kinetics, dynamics, adverse effects, indications and contraindications of drugs which modify the female reproductive functions.

Learning objectives

A student of MBBS phase II should be able to:
- Describe the secretion, regulation and physiological role of estrogen and progesterone.
- Classify drugs used as female sex hormones and their analogues (estrogens and progestins).
- Describe the mechanism of action of estrogens, progestins and drugs opposing their action.
- Describe the pharmacological actions of estrogen, antiestrogens, SERMs, SERDs, aromatase inhibitors, and antiprogestins.
- Enumerate therapeutic uses and adverse effects of estrogen, progestins, and drugs opposing their actions.

The ovary has gametogenic as well as hormonal functions. In humans, the ovary is relatively quiescent during childhood. A cyclic function called the **menstrual cycle** begins at puberty, under the influence of gonadotropins (FSH, LH) secreted by the anterior pituitary. The onset of the menstrual cycle is called **menarche**. After approximately 30–40 years, this cyclic function ceases and menstrual bleeding stops; this is called **menopause**.

PHYSIOLOGY OF SECRETION AND REGULATION OF FEMALE SEX HORMONES

Hormonal Changes at Puberty

The age of puberty in girls is about 12–13 years. The hormonal changes that occur at this age are shown in Fig. 45.1. Gonadotropin releasing hormone (GnRH) secreted from the hypothalamus in a pulsatile manner (frequency of one discharge per hour), induces the release of gonadotropins (FSH, LH) from the anterior pituitary. These, in turn, stimulate estrogen secretion from the ovaries, resulting in pubertal changes.

Physiology of the Menstrual Cycle

The onset of menstruation at puberty is called menarche. While the first few menstrual cycles may be anovulatory, normal ovulatory function is established later. **Estrogen and progesterone** are the main female sex hormones that regulate the menstrual cycle. Estrogen causes proliferative changes in the endometrium, whereas progesterone causes secretory changes in the estrogen-primed endometrium (Fig. 45.2).

Estrogen secretion varies from 10–100 mcg/day. Estrogen secretion begins during the follicular phase, then rises gradually and continues after ovulation, till 2 days before menstruation. **Progesterone is secreted** (10–20 mg/day) by the corpus luteum during the luteal phase. Levels fall sharply a few days before menstruation. (Fig. 45.2) These cyclic changes in estrogen/progesterone levels continue throughout the reproductive years.

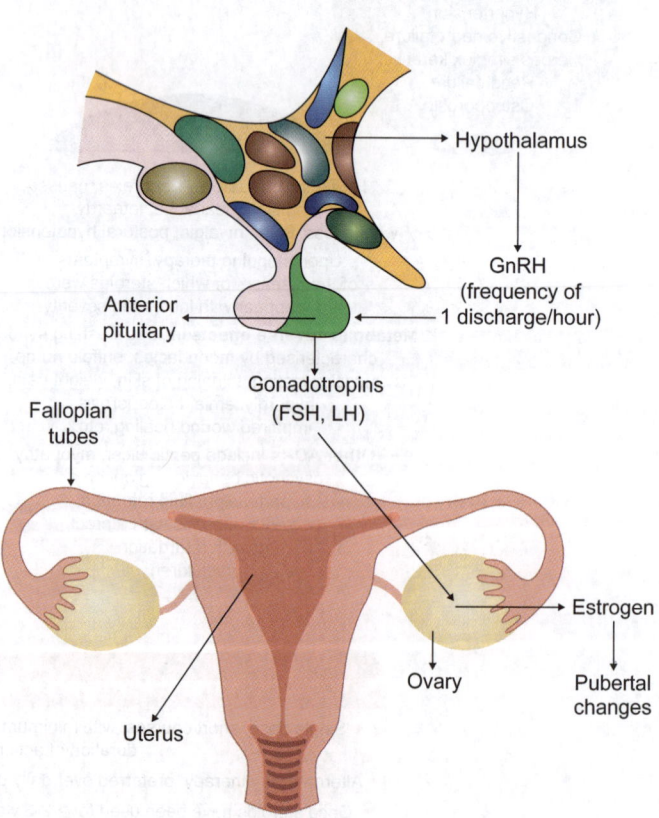

Fig. 45.1 Hormonal changes at puberty in females

FSH secreted from the anterior pituitary is responsible for maturation of the Graafian follicles in the ovary. Graafian follicles contain granulosa cells immediately surrounding the oocyte and theca cells forming supporting wall for the follicle (Fig. 45.3). As the follicle matures, a follicular cavity containing liquor folliculi develops. Estrogen is secreted by the **theca interna** of the dominant Graafian follicle.

Estrogen exerts a negative feedback effect on FSH and also conditions the pituitary to secrete LH, resulting in series of changes that are responsible for the menstrual cycle (Fig. 45.4).

During early pregnancy, human chorionic gonadotropin (HCG) secreted by the blastocyst sustains the corpus luteum. From the 2nd trimester of pregnancy till term, the placenta secretes large amounts of estrogen and progesterone; however, after delivery, the hormone levels decrease sharply.

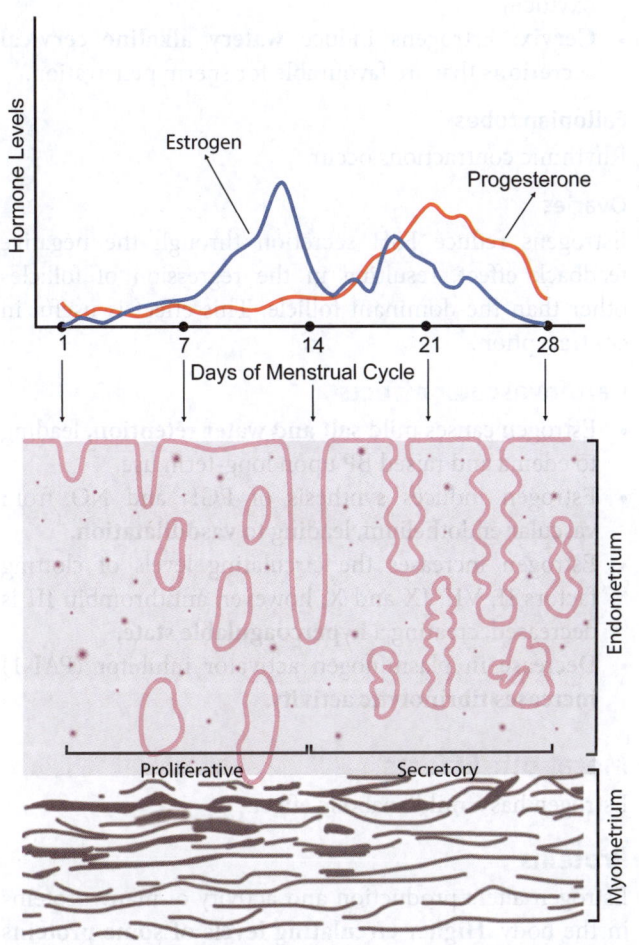

Fig. 45.2 Cyclic hormonal and endometrial changes during an ovulatory menstrual cycle

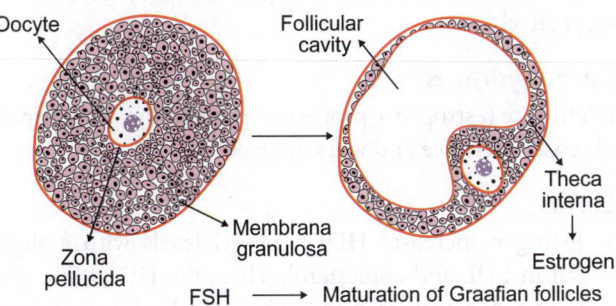

Fig. 45.3 Maturation of a Graafian follicle

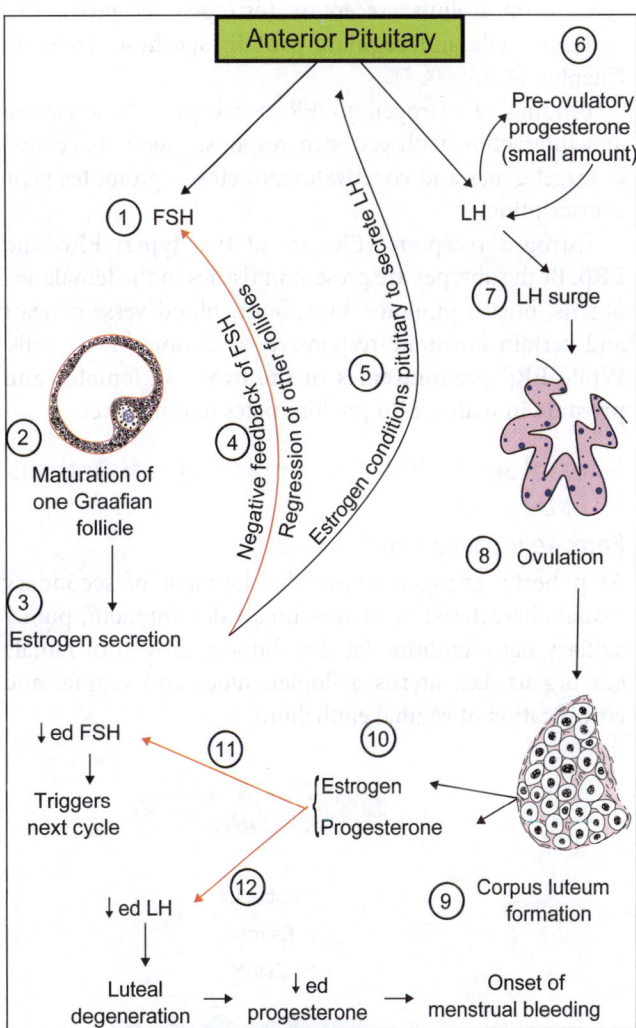

Fig. 45.4 Regulation of gonadotropins and ovarian hormones

① Anterior pituitary secretes FSH in response to GnRH → ② Maturation of Graafian follicles in the ovary → ③ Mature Graafian follicle secretes estrogen → ④ Negative feedback of FSH → Regression of other follicles and ⑤ high levels of estrogens condition pituitary to release LH in response to GnRH → ⑥ Release of small amount of progesterone in pre-ovulatory period → ⑦ Positive feedback causes LH surge → ⑧ Ovulation and ⑨ Formation of corpus luteum → ⑩ Secretes both estrogens and progesterone ⑪ Negative feedback → Reduced FSH (that triggers next cycle) and ⑫ Reduced LH → Luteal degeneration → Reduced progesterone → Menstrual bleeding

ESTROGENS

Classification
Based on their **source**, estrogens are classified as natural and synthetic estrogens. Synthetic estrogens are further categorised into **steroidal and nonsteroidal** estrogens, based on their **chemical structure** (Flowchart 45.1).

Mechanism of Action
Estrogens (like other steroidal hormones) act through specific intracellular receptors (estrogen receptors, ER) in target cells and **regulate protein synthesis** (refer to Chapter 44, Fig. 44.2).

Binding of estrogen to ER → receptor dimerisation and interaction with estrogen response elements (EREs) of target genes and coactivator proteins → promotes gene transcription.

Estrogen receptors (ER) are of **two types: ERα** and **ERβ**. Both subtypes are present in tissues in the female sex organs, breast, pituitary, liver, bone, blood vessels, heart and certain hormone-responsive carcinoma breast cells. While **ERβ predominates in the ovary in females and prostate in males**, ERα predominates in other sites.

Physiological Role/Pharmacological Actions of Estrogens

Female maturation
At puberty, estrogen causes development of secondary sexual characteristics such as breast development, pubic/axillary hair, feminine fat distribution, growth of female sex organs, i.e., uterus, fallopian tubes and vagina, and cornification of vaginal epithelium.

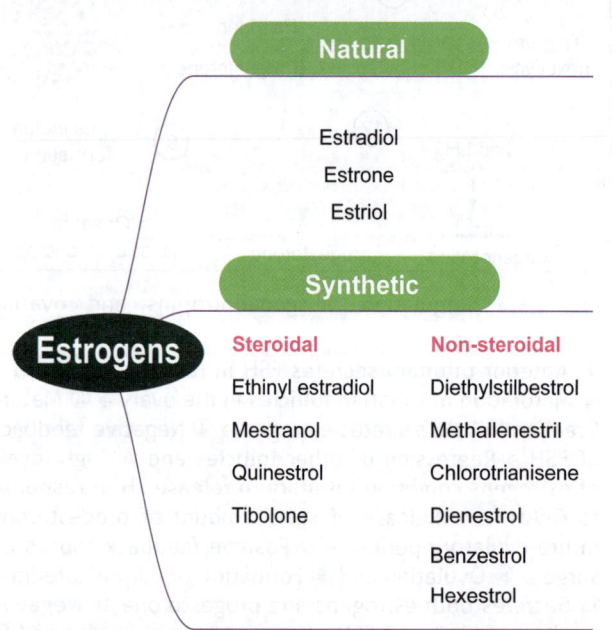

Flowchart 45.1 Classification of estrogens based on the source

Female sex organs
Uterus
- **Endometrium**: Estrogen causes **proliferative changes** in the pre-ovulatory phase of the menstrual cycle. Progestins then bring about secretory changes in the estrogen-primed endometrium (Fig. 45.2). However, continuous administration of estrogens without progesterone causes **endometrial hypertrophy** and delays menstruation.
- **Myometrium**: Estrogens cause **rhythmic contractions** and increase the sensitivity of the myometrium to oxytocin.
- **Cervix**: Estrogens induce **watery alkaline cervical secretions** that are favourable for sperm penetration.

Fallopian tubes
Rhythmic contractions occur.

Ovaries
Estrogens reduce FSH secretion through the negative feedback effect, resulting in the regression of follicles other than the dominant follicle. This effect is useful in contraception.

Cardiovascular effects
- Estrogen causes mild **salt and water retention,** leading to edema and raised BP upon long-term use.
- Estrogen induces synthesis of PGI_2 and NO from vascular endothelium, leading to **vasodilatation.**
- Estrogen increases the circulating levels of clotting factors II, VII, IX and X; however, antithrombin III is decreased, creating a **hypercoagulable state.**
- Decrease in plasminogen activator inhibitor (PAI-1) **increases fibrinolytic activity.**

Metabolic Effects
Estrogen has a mild anabolic effect.

Proteins
Estrogen alters production and activity of many proteins in the body. **Higher circulating levels of some proteins** such as corticosteroid binding globulin (CBG), thyroxine binding globulin (TBG), sex hormone binding globulin (SHBG) and transferrin may lead to increased levels of corticosteroids, thyroxine, estrogen/testosterone, and iron, respectively.

Carbohydrates
High-dose (estrogen + progestin) preparations can **impair glucose tolerance** and worsen diabetes.

Lipids
- Estrogen increases HDL and TG levels with a slight fall in LDL and cholesterol. Thus, the HDL:LDL ratio is raised, which is responsible for the **lower risk of atherosclerosis in premenopausal women.** This

protective effect is lost when estrogen levels fall to 2–10 mcg/day after menopause.
- Estrogen increases cholesterol secretion, but reduces that of bile salt. This **increases risk of cholelithiasis** (gall bladder stone formation) in females. **Four Fs** are commonly linked with increased risk of cholelithiasis, i.e., **F**at, **F**ertile, **F**emale and **F**orty.

Bones
- Estrogen helps to **maintain bone mass**, as it reduces the rate of bone resorption by:
  - Decreasing maturation and activity of osteoclasts and inhibiting osteoclast pit formation.
  - Increasing expression of bone matrix proteins (osteonectin, osteocalcin, collagen, etc.).
  - Maintaining positive calcium balance

  Therefore, estrogen deficiency in post-menopausal women is associated with reduced bone density, osteoporosis and spontaneous fractures.
- Estrogenic action **favours epiphyseal fusion** in both genders.

Pharmacokinetics
- **Absorption**: Natural estrogens (estradiol, estrone, and estriol) are orally inactive due to rapid hepatic metabolism. However, synthetic estrogens (such as ethinyl estradiol, dinestrol, mestranol, quinestrol, and diethylstilbestrol) are well-absorbed orally. Estradiol, ethinyl estradiol and estriol are absorbed through intact skin and are useful as transdermal patches/ gels/cremes etc. Estradiol esters (estradiol valerate/ cypionate/ enanthate) are absorbed slowly from intramuscular injection sites, resulting in prolonged action.
- **Distribution**: Estrogen is strongly bound to sex hormone binding globulin (SHBG); a small amount binds to albumin also.
- **Termination of action**: Estradiol is converted in the liver (and other tissues) to estrone and then to estriol. These are further metabolised by glucuronide and sulphate conjugation. Inactive conjugates are excreted in urine. Some excretion in bile and enterohepatic circulation also occurs.

THERAPEUTIC USES OF ESTROGENS

1. Contraceptive
Estrogen in combination with progesterone is used as **contraceptive** (Chapter 46).

2. Hormone replacement therapy (HRT)
Estrogen is used for **hormone replacement therapy** in the following conditions:
a. **Primary hypogonadism:** It is a state of estrogen deficiency due to primary failure of development of ovaries. Small doses of ethinyl estradiol (5–10 mcg) are given on days 1–21 of each month in this condition. Treatment in primary hypogonadism is usually started at 11–13 years of age in order to:
  - Obtain development of secondary sex characteristics and regular menstruation.
  - Stimulate optimal growth.
  - Prevent osteoporosis.
  - Avoid psychological consequences of delayed puberty.

  When growth is completed, chronic therapy consists mainly of the administration of both estrogen and progesterone.

b. **Post-menopausal hormone replacement therapy**
  At around 45 years of age, ovarian function ceases, resulting in the loss of menstrual periods and variable symptoms such as:
  - Vasomotor symptoms such as hot flushes /flashes (feeling of sudden warmth), inappropriate sweating, faintness, aches and pains.
  - Genital atrophy: Vaginal dryness, vulval shrinkage, vaginitis, recurrent urinary tract infection.
  - Accelerated bone loss, especially in vertebral, hip, and wrist joints.
  - Lipid profile changes, atherosclerotic cardiovascular disease.
  - Psychological disturbances, such as irritability, depression, and loss of self-confidence.

  Optimal management of post-menopausal syndrome requires careful assessment of the patient's symptoms, consideration of her age and risk for CVS disease, osteoporosis, HRT is not routinely prescribed to all post-menopausal women. The need for HRT and dosage are decided on individual basis.
  - If the patient has vasomotor symptoms (such as hot flashes) as the dominant feature within 10 years of menopause, therapy is required with the **lowest** dose of estrogen and for limited period of time.
  - In patients with low risk of osteoporosis, symptoms such as mild atrophic vaginitis are easily managed with **topical preparations** like vaginal creams.
  - Osteoporosis after menopause depends on the amount of bone present in the beginning, vitamin D and calcium intake, and on the degree of physical activity. Estrogen in the smallest dose consistent with symptomatic relief is given for the first 21–25 days of each month, along with calcium supplements (1500 mg/day). In patients with early menopause, it is advisable to continue HRT till the age of natural menopause in order to check bone loss and osteoporosis.
  - HRT decreases the risk of coronary artery disease (CAD) only in the early post-menopausal period; however, risk of MI and stroke may be increased in elderly females. In addition, it improves physical and mental well-being.

Disadvantages of HRT

HRT **increases risk of some diseases** such as carcinoma breast, carcinoma endometrium, gallstones, and may cause worsening of migraine. However, HRT does not check cognitive decline; rather, it increases the risk of dementia. This risk may be reduced somewhat by the following measures:

- Prescribing HRT only when necessary.
- Addition of progestin to estrogen for the last 10-12 days decreases risk of carcinoma endometrium; however, menopausal symptoms may return in the estrogen-off period.
- Using transdermal estrogen patches (Box 45.1).

3. Other uses

a. **Senile vaginitis:** Topical preparations are preferred over oral drugs to prevent and treat atrophic vaginitis in elderly women.
b. **Intractable dysmenorrhea:** Estrogen along with progestins is used to suppress ovulation in these patients.
c. **Dysfunctional uterine bleeding:** Cyclic progestin is better for this indication. Estrogen has an adjuvant role only.
d. **Lactation suppression**: High dose of estrogen is required to suppress lactation; bromocriptine is preferred for this indication.
e. **Acne and hirsutism** associated with increased androgen secretion may improve with estrogens.
f. **Carcinoma prostate** is an androgen-dependent tumour. Estrogen has a palliative role in this case.

> **Box 45.1 Transdermal estrogen patch**
>
> **Size**
> These patches are available in 3 sizes:
> - **5 cm²**: Delivers 0.025 mg of estradiol in 24 hours.
> - **10 cm²**: Double the size of the 5 cm² patch and delivers double the amount (0.05 mg) of estradiol in 24 hours.
> - **20 cm²**: Four times the size of the 5 cm² patch; delivers 0.1 mg of estradiol in 24 hours.
>
> A single patch is effective for 3–4 days. Cyclic therapy with this patch (3 weeks on, 1 week off) along with oral progestin for last 10–12 days is advised.
>
> **Advantages**
> - Ease of administration → more compliance by patient.
> - Comparable efficacy → beneficial effects in improvement of menopausal symptoms with the transdermal patch are comparable to those of oral estrogen therapy. Vaginal epithelium and bone density also improve with transdermal patches.
> - Better tolerability → systemic side effects of transdermal patch are the same as oral estrogen, but milder
>
> High hepatic delivery avoided → plasma levels of CBG, TBG, angiotensinogen, and clotting factors are not increased. Therefore, risk of thrombo-embolic phenomenon may not be increased.
>
> **Disadvantage**
> Improvement in lipid profile is less favourable with transdermal patch as compared to oral use of estrogen.

Adverse Effects

1. Nausea and breast tenderness are common side effects. These can be minimised by using the smallest effective dose.
2. Hyperpigmentation.
3. **In pregnancy** (especially in the 1st trimester), stilbestrol increases the risk of carcinoma vagina and cervix in female offspring (during childhood or early adulthood), and genital abnormalities in male offspring.
4. **In post-menopausal women**, estrogen replacement therapy is associated with:
   - Increased risk of carcinoma endometrium, leading to post-menopausal bleeding. However, addition of progestin prevents this risk.
   - Increased risk of carcinoma breast with prolonged therapy (low doses are probably safer).
   - Increased risk of benign hepatoma, gallstones, worsening of migraine, and endometriosis.
   - Increased incidence of thrombo-embolic phenomenon
5. **In males**, when used for carcinoma prostate, estrogen may cause suppression of libido, gynecomastia, and feminisation
6. **In children**, early fusion of epiphyses may result in reduced adult height.

Contraindications

Estrogens are contraindicated in the case of:

- Hormone-dependent malignancies (carcinoma breast, uterus)
- Severe liver disease
- Thrombo-embolic disease
- Migraine
- Epilepsy
- Heavy smokers

TIBOLONE

- It is a synthetic steroid that possesses estrogenic + progestational + weak androgenic activity
- It is useful for menopausal symptoms (dose: 2.5 mg, daily); addition of progestin is not required.
- It improves vasomotor, psychological, vaginal atrophy, cardiovascular and osteoporotic symptoms.
- However, it is **not popular** because of **ADRs** like growth of facial hair, weight gain, and vaginal spotting.

> **Clinical problem-based questions and MCQs**
>
> 1. Identify the CORRECT statement about the effect of estrogens on lipid levels.
>   a. Decreases HDL   b. Decreases triglycerides
>   c. Decreases LDL   d. Increases cholesterol

2. i The advantages of transdermal patches of estradiol over oral estrogen include all of the following EXCEPT:
   a. More compliance
   b. Comparable effect on bone density
   c. Favourable changes in lipid profile
   d. Lower risk of thrombo-embolic phenomenon
   ii. Enumerate the therapeutic uses, ADRs and contraindications of estrogens.
3. A 54-year-old post-menopausal female patient presents with complaints of hot flushes, chilly sensations, and aches and pains. On investigation, there are osteoporotic changes and bone density is reduced.
   i. Describe role of HRT for management of this case.
   ii. Enumerate risks associated with such treatment.
4. Drug 'A' possesses estrogenic, progestational and weak androgenic activity. Identify A.
   a. Tibolone   b. Stilbestrol
   c. Ethinyl estradiol d. Estrone
5. Identify the nonsteroidal estrogen among the following.
   a. Mestranol   b. Quinestrol
   c. Ethinyl estradiol d. Dienestrol
6. Which of the following statements about cyclic hormonal changes in the menstrual cycle is correct?
   a. LH surge results in luteal degeneration.
   b. Progesterone causes secretory changes in the estrogen-primed endometrium.
   c. Sudden rise in progesterone causes menstrual bleeding.
   d. Corpus luteum secretes only progesterone.

DRUGS OPPOSING ESTROGEN ACTIONS

Drugs that oppose the actions of estrogen can be classified as partial agonists, selective estrogen receptor modulators and down-regulators, and aromatase inhibitors (Flowchart 45.2).

1. Partial Agonist
Clomiphene citrate

Mechanism of action
Clomiphene is a partial agonist at estrogen receptors. Thus, it blocks the action of the full agonists, i.e., estrogens.

Clomiphene **blocks negative feedback effect of estrogen** on the pituitary → increased release of gonadotropins → maturation of Graafian follicles and ovulation (if ovaries are responsive to gonadotropins).

Therapeutic uses
- Clomiphene is used for **ovulation induction** in patients suffering from infertility due to ovulatory disturbances. It is effective orally, given in a dose of 50 mg for 5 days, starting from the 5th day of the menstrual cycle and is

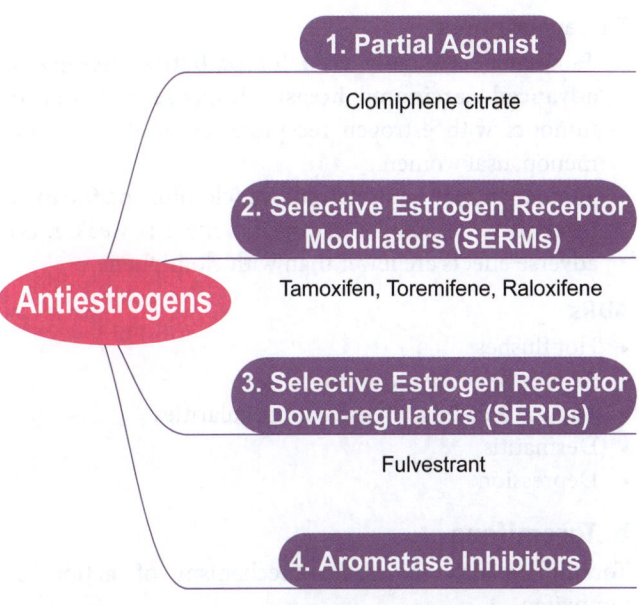

Flowchart 45.2 Classification of antiestrogens (drugs that oppose estrogen actions)

repeated every month. If the patient fails to conceive, the dose can be doubled. Concurrent use of gonadotropins increases the success rate.
- Clomiphene is useful in **oligozoospermia** in men. The dose for this indication is 25 mg, orally (for 25 days in a month, then stopped for 6 days). It can be given in this manner for up to 6 months.

Adverse effects
Clomiphene, a partial agonist, blocks the peripheral actions of estrogen, resulting in **hot flushes**.
- Several ova mature simultaneously, resulting in **multiple pregnancy** (such as twins or triplets).
- Polycystic ovaries
- Allergic dermatitis may occur.

2. Selective Estrogen Receptor Modulators (SERMs)
These drugs oppose estrogen action selectively in some tissues, but exert weak estrogenic effect in other tissues. Therefore, they are known as selective estrogen receptor modulators, e.g., tamoxifen, toremifene and raloxifene.

a. Tamoxifen citrate
It has antiestrogen and partial agonistic effects:
- Antiestrogen effects cause inhibition of human carcinoma breast cells and hot flushes.
- Partial agonist effects lower gonadotropins and prolactin (PRL) levels in post-menopausal women, stimulate endometrial proliferation, and improve bone density.

Therapeutic uses
- Tamoxifen is mainly used for **palliative therapy of advanced carcinoma breast.** Response is better in tumours with estrogen receptors, especially in post-menopausal women.
- Tamoxifen may be preferred over clomiphene **for male infertility**, because its estrogenic effect is weaker. So, adverse effects are fewer than with clomiphene.

ADRs
- Hot flushes
- Anorexia, nausea, vomiting
- Vaginal bleeding, menstrual irregularities
- Dermatitis
- Depression

b. Toremifene
Toremifene has the same mechanism of action as tamoxifen.
- Its antiestrogenic effect is useful in **carcinoma breast.**
- Estrogenic effect is useful **in post-menopausal women** to prevent expected loss of lumbar spine bone density and to decrease the risk of atherosclerosis by causing plasma lipid changes.

It has the same ADRs as tamoxifen. It also increases the risk of carcinoma endometrium.

c. Raloxifene
- It has partial agonistic action at estrogen receptors in bone, CVS and lipid metabolism. So, it improves bone density and lipid profile in post-menopausal women.
- Raloxifene is reported to decrease the risk of ER-positive carcinoma breast.
- It does not cause endometrial proliferation, so there is **no increase in risk of carcinoma endometrium** in post-menopausal women receiving raloxifene.
- It is useful as a second-line drug for prevention of post-menopausal osteoporosis.
- Drawback with raloxifene therapy is adverse effects like hot flushes, occasional vaginal bleeding and increased risk of thrombo-embolism.

3. Selective Estrogen Receptor Down regulators (SERDs)

Fulvestrant, a selective estrogen receptor down regulator (SERD), is a pure estrogen antagonist and causes **down-regulation of estrogen receptors (ER)**. It acts by preventing the dimerisation of estrogen receptors, resulting in reduced effect of estrogen on protein synthesis and causes fast degradation of receptors.

It is used in **advanced ER+ve carcinoma breast resistant to tamoxifen.** Fulvestrant 250–500 mg is given intramuscularly at monthly intervals.

ADRs of fulvestrant include hot flashes, headache, aches/pains, nausea, asthenia, and injection-site reactions.

4. Aromatase Inhibitors

These include letrozole, anastrozole and exemestane. Aromatase is an enzyme that catalyses the final step of estrogen synthesis from androstenedione and testosterone.

Locally produced estrogen plays a role in the growth of carcinoma breast.

Mechanism of action
Inhibition of aromatase **interferes with the production of estrogen** from androstenedione and testosterone. In post-menopausal women, estrogen deprivation is almost complete.

Therapeutic uses
Newer aromatase inhibitors like letrozole, anastrozole and exemestane are widely used in treatment of **carcinoma breast, especially in post-menopausal women.** However, these drugs are not as effective in pre-menopausal patients, as some estrogen secretion continues from the ovary.

- Aromatase inhibitors are very useful as adjuvants after surgical removal of carcinoma breast in early stage of disease. These are especially useful in post-menopausal women having ER-positive carcinoma breast.
- In palliative treatment of advanced metastatic carcinoma breast, aromatase inhibitors are currently **preferred over tamoxifen** as they have higher response rates, longer survival and lower treatment failure rates. Another advantage of letrozole over tamoxifen is the lack of risk of thrombo-embolism and carcinoma endometrium.
- Letrozole is also useful in carcinoma breast that does not respond to tamoxifen.

Adverse effects
- Aromatase inhibitors may cause dyspepsia, nausea, diarrhea, hot flushes, and vaginal atrophic changes.
- Accelerated bone loss, arthritis and risk of fractures are associated with prolonged use of letrozole.
- However, unlike tamoxifen, the risk of endometrial carcinoma and thrombo-embolism does not increase.

Clinical problem-based questions and MCQs

7. Drugs having agonistic/partial agonistic/antagonistic effects on estrogen receptors are useful in varied clinical conditions.
   i. Identify a drug that has partial agonistic effect on ER
      a. Letrozole   b. Mestranol
      c. Exemestane   d. Clomiphene
   ii. Describe the usefulness of the selected drug in clinical practice, along with its adverse effects.

8. i. A 65-year-old post-menopausal woman, diagnosed with carcinoma breast stage 1 undergoes surgical treatment (mastectomy). The tumour is ER+ve. Which of the following

is the most suitable drug for the prevention of recurrence in this case?
   a. Letrozole   b. Methallenstril
   c. Tamoxifen   d. Clomiphene
   ii. Justify your choice with the pharmacological basis.

9. i. Identify a drug that has pure estrogen antagonistic action.
   a. Clomiphene   b. Letrozole
   c. Fulvestrant   d. Tamoxifen
   ii. Describe the mechanism of action, uses and adverse effects of the selected drug.

10. i. Drug 'X' is useful for infertility, but increases the risk of PCOD. Identify X.
    a. Anastrozole   b. Ethinyl estradiol
    c. Clomiphene   d. Raloxifene
    ii. Describe the mechanism of action of the selected drug.
    iii. Describe dose and duration of administration of the selected drug in male and female infertility.

11. i. Identify the correct mechanism of action of anastrozole.
    a. Prevents dimerisation of estrogen receptors
    b. Causes down-regulation of estrogen receptors
    c. Prevents conversion of androstenedione into estrogen
    d. Favours formation of progestin from cholesterol
    ii. Describe its therapeutic uses and adverse effects.

PROGESTINS

CLASSIFICATION

Progestins are categorised into **natural and synthetic progestins**. Natural progestin, or **progesterone,** is a steroid with 21 carbons. It is synthesised in the ovaries, testes, and adrenals from circulating cholesterol. The daily secretion in the second half of the menstrual cycle is 10–20 mg by the corpus luteum. In pregnancy, large amounts of progesterone are secreted by the placenta.

Synthetic progestins are further classified based on their chemical structure (Flowchart 45.3).

- **21-carbon progesterone derivatives**, which are pure progestins with low antiovulatory effect.
- **19-nortestosterone derivatives** that are further divided into estranes and gonanes.
  - **Estranes** have progestational, weak estrogenic and androgenic activity. Antiovulatory effect is prominent.
  - **Gonanes** have an ethyl substitution at C13. These are more potent antiovulatory drugs than estranes.

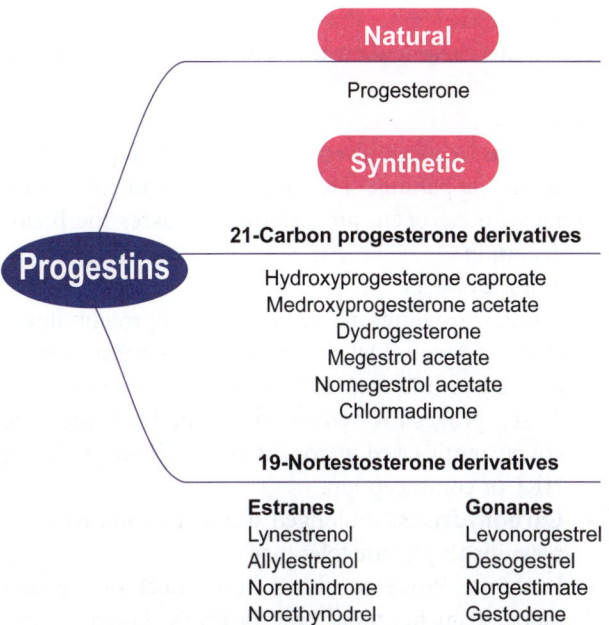

Flowchart 45.3 Classification of progestins

However, their androgenic activity is weaker than that of estranes.

Natural Progestins: Progesterone

Mechanism of action

- Progestin receptors are present in the female genital tract, breast, CNS and pituitary.
- Progestins exert their action by binding to specific receptors present in target cells → the progesterone–receptor complex dimerises, moves into nucleus → binds to progesterone response elements (PRE) on target genes and regulates DNA-mediated RNA transcription and protein synthesis.

Pharmacological actions

1. **Pituitary**

Progesterone is a weak inhibitor of gonadotropin (Gn) secretion. When progesterone is given during the follicular phase, it suppresses the LH surge and prevents ovulation; this effect is useful in contraception.

2. **Uterus**
   - **Endometrium:** Progestins bring about secretory changes in the estrogen-primed endometrium, leading to normal menstruation. However, continued action of progestins, as during pregnancy, causes decidual changes in the endometrium.
   - **Myometrium**: Progestins decrease the sensitivity of the myometrium to oxytocin.
   - **Cervix**: Under the influence of progestins, cervical secretions become thick, scanty, cellular and hostile to sperm penetration. This effect of progesterone is used in contraception.

3. **Vagina**
   Progestins cause leukocytic infiltration of the cornified vaginal epithelium.
4. **Breast**
   Progestins cause alveolo-lobular development of secretory apparatus, i.e., acini development. Thus, along with estrogen, progesterone prepares the breast for lactation.
5. **Metabolic effects**
   - **Lipids**: Progesterone stimulates lipoprotein lipase (LPL) → favours fat deposition. 19-Nortestosterone derivatives increase LDL and lower serum HDL → so, progestins reduce the beneficial effect of concurrently used estrogens on the lipid profile in HRT or contraception.
   - **Carbohydrates**: Prolonged use as in contraception may impair glucose tolerance.
   - **Proteins**: Progestins have little effect on protein metabolism, but they lower the levels of many amino acids in the plasma. Urinary nitrogen excretion increases.
6. **Kidney**
   Progesterone competes with aldosterone for receptors in the renal tubule → decrease Na^+ reabsorption → increased aldosterone secretion by adrenal cortex (as seen during pregnancy).
7. **CNS**
   High doses of progesterone have a CNS-depressant effect → hypnotic effect.
   - Hypothalamic temperature centre is reset at a higher level. This causes a 0.5 °C rise in the basal body temperature (BBT) during the luteal phase. This effect of progesterone is used to detect ovulation.
   - Progesterone increases ventilatory response to CO_2. Thus, there is a measurable reduction in alveolar and arterial pCO_2 during the luteal phase of menstrual cycle and pregnancy.

Synthetic Progestins

- **21-carbon progesterone derivatives** include hydroxyprogesterone caproate, medroxyprogesterone acetate, megestrol, nomegestrol and dydrogesterone. These are pure progestins (except chlormadinone) with weak antiovulatory effect; they are **mainly used in HRT** as adjuvants to estrogen. They inhibit Na^+ reabsorption induced by aldosterone. **Nomegestrol** possesses antiandrogenic effects. It has strong effect on the endometrium, but comparatively less effect on ovulation suppression.
- **19-nortestosterone derivatives** such as estranes (lynestrenol, allylestrenol, norethindrone, etc.) and gonanes (levonorgestrel, desogestrel, norgestimate, etc.) produce decidual changes in the endometrium during pregnancy.
  - These are potent gonadotropin (Gn) secretion inhibitors; thus, they have potent antiovulatory effect and are **useful in contraception**.
  - Minimal estrogenic and androgenic activity may be present. However, gonanes (desogestrel, norgestimate and gestodene) have no androgenic effect and are used in contraception along with estrogen. An advantage is that the beneficial effect of estrogen on the lipid profile is not neutralised. Moreover, the potent antiovulatory effect allows for reducing dose of ethinyl estradiol, thus reducing estrogenic adverse effects.

Therapeutic uses

1. **Contraception**: Progestins are used alone or along with estrogens for hormonal contraception. 19-nortestosterone derivatives, especially gonanes such as levonorgestrel, desogestrel, norgestimate and gestodene that have weak androgenic but potent antiovulatory effect, are preferred.
2. **HRT**: In non-hysterectomised post-menopausal women, estrogen given for first 21–25 days of a month with progestin combined with it in last 10–14 days counteracts the increased risk of carcinoma endometrium. 21-carbon progesterone derivatives (pure progestins) or gonanes that lack androgenic activity are preferred, because they do not counteract the beneficial effect of estrogen on the lipid profile.
3. **Dysfunctional uterine bleeding** (DUB): Initially, large doses are given to arrest bleeding; later on, cyclic treatment is given with estrogen to regularise menstrual flow.
4. **Endometriosis**: Progesterone may be used, but danazol is preferred.
5. **Pre-menstrual syndrome (PMS)**: Severe cases require combined estrogen and progesterone therapy to suppress ovulation.
6. For **palliative care** in carcinoma endometrium, high doses are needed.
7. **Threatened/habitual abortion**: Not very beneficial.
8. **Diagnostic use:** In amenorrhea, if progesterone administration is followed by withdrawal bleeding → it shows that the endometrium has been stimulated by estrogen.

Adverse effects

- Headache, breast engorgement, increase in body temperature, esophageal reflux and mood swings.
- Progestins with androgenic effects lower HDL levels.
- Progestins may precipitate diabetes in predisposed individuals upon long-term use.
- BP may increase in some patients.
- Combined estrogen and progestin HRT may increase risk of carcinoma breast.

ANTIPROGESTINS

1. Mifepristone

Mechanism of action

Mifepristone strongly binds to progesterone receptors, resulting in inhibition of progesterone activity. However, in the absence of progesterone, as in post-menopausal women, mifepristone exerts a partial agonistic effect.

Pharmacological actions

The effect of mifepristone on the uterus depends on the phase of the menstrual cycle:

- Follicular phase: Mifepristone exerts an antiovulatory effect.
- Luteal phase: It prevents secretory changes in the endometrium.
- Midluteal phase: Mifepristone causes luteolysis by an unknown mechanism, resulting in decreased progesterone secretion and cervical softening.
- Later in the cycle: It blocks progesterone support to the endometrium → induces menstruation. It also blocks the inhibitory effect of progesterone on prostaglandin (PG) release. Thus, PG is released, resulting in uterine contractions.
- If implantation has occurred, mifepristone blocks decidualisation → dislodges the conceptus.
- However, in menopausal women (in the absence of progesterone), it exerts a partial agonistic effect and causes predecidual changes.
- It also binds to and acts as antagonist at glucocorticoid receptors; thus, high dose is useful in Cushing syndrome.

Therapeutic uses

1. As a **contraceptive**: Mifepristone, given as a single 600 mg dose within 72 hours of unprotected coitus, prevents implantation and is effective as an emergency postcoital contraceptive.
   If given within 10 days of expected day of menses, it can dislodge the conceptus, if any, in about 90% cases.
2. To **terminate early pregnancy** (up to 7 weeks): Mifepristone in a dose of 400–600 mg (daily, for 4 days) or 800 mg (daily, for 2 days) can successfully terminate pregnancy in > 85% users.
   A single 600 mg dose of mifepristone is combined with PGE_1 analogue, oral misoprostol, or vaginal pessary of gemeprost, for termination of early pregnancy. This combination successfully terminates pregnancy in about 95% cases.
3. Mifepristone is useful for **induction of labour** in cases of intrauterine fetal death (IUFD) or abnormal fetuses. It promotes labour by blocking the relaxant effect of progesterone on the pregnant uterus.
4. Mifepristone, given in a dose of 600 mg (24 hours prior to induction of labour or surgical abortion), causes **cervical softening and ripening** that facilitates labour.
5. High dose of mifepristone is beneficial in Cushing syndrome.
6. It may be useful in endometriosis, tumours having progesterone or glucocorticoid receptors (such as carcinoma breast, meningioma, and uterine fibroids).

Adverse effects

- Nausea, vomiting and diarrhea.
- Abdominal or pelvic pain.
- Some patients have severe vaginal bleeding that may require some other intervention.

2. Gestrinone

- It acts as a partial agonist at progesterone receptor or selective progesterone receptor modulator (SPRM). It also possesses weak agonistic effect at androgen receptor.
- Gestrinone activates progesterone and androgen receptors in the pituitary, resulting in weak antigonadotropin activity.
- In the endometrium, gestrinone has antiestrogenic activity. Therefore, it is approved for use in **endometriosis**; it is better tolerated than danazol.
- It causes shrinkage of **uterine fibroids** and reduces menstrual blood loss in **menorrhagia**.
- ADRs include acne, hirsutism, breast hypoplasia, hair loss, and weight gain.

3. Ulipristal

It is also a selective progesterone receptor modulator (SPRM) that:

- It suppresses LH surge, resulting in suppression of ovulation. Ulipristal also has some direct suppressant effect on Graafian follicle rupture.
- It prevents secretory changes in the endometrium and interferes with implantation.

Uses

Ulipristal 30 mg is approved for use as an emergency postcoital contraceptive, and is as effective as levonorgestrel 1.5 mg when taken within 120 hours of unprotected coitus. Thus, ulipristal increases the window period for effectiveness of postcoital contraceptives from 72 hours (with mifepristone) to 120 hours.

ADRs

It may cause ADRs like headache, nausea, vomiting, abdominal pain and delayed menstruation.

Clinical problem-based questions and MCQs

12. A 28-year-old female patient, with 2 living children, comes to the gynec OPD for contraceptive advice. She decides to use oral contraceptive pills.
    i. Identify the most suitable progestin for combining with estrogen in this case.
        a. Megestrol acetate   b. Lynestrenol
        c. Allylestreno   d. Levonorgestrel
    ii. Justify your choice along with the pharmacological basis.
    iii. Enumerate the therapeutic uses and adverse effects of progestins.

13. Identify the correct statement about the central effects of progestins.
    a. Reduced ventilator response to CO_2
    b. Fall in basal body temperature (BBT)
    c. Hypnotic effect
    d. Causes LH surge

14. Comment on the role of the combination of mifepristone and misoprostol in termination of early pregnancy.

15. i. Identify the drug that is better than danazol for endometriosis.
        a. Mifepristone   b. Ulipristal
        c. Gestrinone   d. d.Gestodene
    ii. Describe the pharmacological basis for use of the selected drug in endometriosis.

Summary

- Estrogen and progesterone are the two main female sex hormones; both are steroidal in nature and exert their action by binding to intracellular receptors and regulating protein synthesis.
- **Estrogen** causes pubertal changes at 12–13 years of age and proliferative changes in the endometrium. Bone resorption is reduced, HDL raised, LDL lowered, and blood coagulability enhanced.
- Estrogen is mainly used clinically for HRT in primary hypogonadism, postmenopausal symptoms, and for oral contraception. For these indications, combination with progesterone is beneficial. Other indications for use are senile vaginitis, dysfunctional uterine bleeding and palliation of carcinoma prostate.
- ADRs of estrogen include postmenopausal bleeding, breast tenderness, hyperpigmentation, migraine, increased risk of thrombo-embolic phenomena/ carcinoma endometrium and breast/ hepatoma/gall stones.
- **Antiestrogens** include the partial agonist clomiphene citrate, which is useful for the induction of ovulation in infertility and for oligozoospermia in males.
- **SERMs:** Tamoxifen is used for the palliation of carcinoma breast, especially ER+ve cases. Toremifene and raloxifene are useful for the prevention of postmenopausal osteoporosis.
- **SERD**: Fulvestrant has pure estrogen antagonistic actions and is useful in tamoxifen-resistant carcinoma breast.
- **Aromatase inhibitors**: Letrozole and anastrozole inhibit peripheral estrogen synthesis and are effective in carcinoma breast palliation in postmenopausal women.
- **Progestins** can be natural (progesterone) or synthetic. Synthetic progestins can be either 21-C progesterone derivatives or 19-nortestosterone derivatives. The latter are further classified into estranes and gonanes.
- Progesterone causes secretory changes in the estrogen-primed endometrium, makes cervical secretions hostile for sperm penetration (thick / scanty), and promotes alveolo-lobular development in the breast. HDL is lowered and carbohydrate tolerance is impaired. Central effects are sedation, raised BBT, suppression of LH surge and antiovulatory effect.
- Mainly used with estrogens in a cyclic manner for HRT and oral contraception. Beneficial effects are seen in DUB, PMS, and endometriosis.
- ADRs to progestins include headache, engorgement of breast, and lowering HDL; it may also precipitate DM and hypertension.
- **21-C progesterone derivatives** (medroxy-/ hydroxylprogesterone acetate, megestrol) have poor antiovulatory effect; they are mainly useful with estrogen in HRT.
- In contrast, **19-nortestosterone derivatives** have good antiovulatory effect. Gonanes are preferred for use in OCPs as they have poor androgenic effect; so, the beneficial effect of estrogens on lipids is not lost.
- **Antiprogestins**: Mifepristone prevents actions of progesterone by strongly binding with progesterone receptors. It is useful for emergency postcoital contraception, termination of early pregnancy (combined with PGE_1 analogue misoprostol), cervical priming, and induction of labour in IUFD. However, major drawbacks are nausea, vomiting, diarrhea, abdominal pain and severe vaginal bleeding.
- **Ulipristal,** a selective progesterone receptor modulator, is also useful as a postcoital emergency contraceptive with a longer window period of up to 120 h.
- **Gestrinone**, another SPRM, is better than danazol in endometriosis.

Questions for practice

1. Classify estrogens and progesterone. Comment on their combination in:
   a. Hormone replacement therapy
   b. Oral contraception
2. Explain why:
   a. Estrogen and progesterone are given in cyclic manner for long-term uses.
   b. Letrozole is not very effective in carcinoma breast in premenopausal women.
   c. Clomiphene is useful in infertility.
   d. Tamoxifen is used in carcinoma breast.
   e. Levonorgestrel is preferred over estranes for use as oral contraceptives.
   f. Mifepristone and misoprostol are combined for termination of early pregnancy.
3. Write short notes on:
   a. SERMs
   b. Aromatase inhibitors
   c. Mifepristone

Hints for problem-based questions and MCQs

1. c. Decreases LDL and cholesterol. However, HDL and TG are raised with estrogen
2. i. c. Favourable changes in lipid profile
   ii Uses: Contraceptive, HRT, senile vaginitis, DUB, dysmenorrhea, to suppress lactation, acne, hirsutism, carcinoma prostate. ADRs: Nausea, breast tenderness, hyperpigmentation, increased risk of carcinoma endometrium/ breast, benign hepatoma, gallstones, worsening of migraine, endometriosis. Contraindications: Carcinoma breast/ uterus, severe liver disease, thromboembolism, migraine, epilepsy, etc.
3. i. The patient is a post-menopausal woman with vasomotor symptoms and osteoporotic changes. For these symptoms, treatment is with lowest dose of estrogen consistent with symptom relief, for the first 21–25 days of each month and continued for limited period of time. Progestin can be added for the last 10–12 days.
   ii. Refer to page 606.
4. a. Tibolone
5. d. Dinesterol is nonsteroidal.
6. b. Progesterone causes secretory changes in estrogen-primed endometrium
7. i. d. Clomiphene
   ii. Used in infertility. ADRs include hot flashes, multiple pregnancy, polycystic ovary and allergic dermatitis.
8. i. a. Letrozole
   ii. Letrozole is an aromatase inhibitor that prevents estrogen synthesis completely in postmenopausal patients. However, the response is less in premenopausal patients as secretion continues from the ovary. Letrozole is preferred over tamoxifen in postmenopausal women with ER+ve carcinoma breast. Methallenestril is nonsteroidal estrogen which may aggravate growth of carcinoma breast. Clomiphene is a partial agonist of estrogen with a role in infertility, but not in carcinoma breast.
9. i. c. Fulvestrant
   ii. Prevents dimerisation of estrogen receptors, causing down-regulation of ER. It is used in advanced ER+ve carcinoma breast, not responding to tamoxifen. ADRs include headache, nausea, asthenia, aches, hot flashes, injection site reactions.
10. i. c. Clomiphene
    ii. Partial agonist at ER; blocks negative feedback effect of estrogen on pituitary resulting in increased gonadotropin secretion, maturation of Graafian follicles, and ovulation.
    iii. In females, 50 mg for 5 days starting from the 5th day of menstrual cycle, and in males, 25 mg for 25 days followed by a gap of 6 days (treatment continued for 6 months).
11. i. c. Prevents conversion of androstenedione into estrogen
    ii. Aromatase inhibitors are useful in post-menopausal carcinoma breast, palliative treatment of advanced carcinoma breast, not responding to tamoxifen, Adverse effects include dysplasia, nausea, diarrhea, hot flashes, accelerated bone loss, arthritis, vaginal atrophy, etc.
12. i. d. Levonorgestrel
    ii. Levonorgestrel is a 19-norethindrone derivative with strong antiovulatory action. It is a gonane with ethyl group at position 13; so, androgenic activity is poor.
    iii. Refer to page 611.
13. c. Hypnotic effect. Progestins increase ventilator response to CO_2, raise BBT and prevent LH surge.
14. Refer to page 611
15. i. c. Gestrinone
    ii. Refer to page 611.

CONCEPT MAP – ESTROGENS AND ANTIESTROGENS

ESTROGENS

Therapeutic Uses
- Hormone replacement therapy (HRT) in primary hypogonadism and post-menopausal syndrome.
- Oral contraception.
- Senile vaginitis, dysmenorrhea, Dysfunctional uterine bleeding
- Acne, Hirsutism, Palliation of carcinoma prostate

Actions
- Pubertal changes in females at age of 12–13 years,
- Proliferative changes in endometrium.
- Rhythmic contractions of myometrium and fallopian tubes & increased sensitivity of myometrium to oxytocin
- Watery alkaline cervical secretions
- Estrogens reduce FSH secretion and suppress development & rupture of Graafian follicles.
- Reduced bone resorption
- HDL raised, LDL lowered
- Increased blood coagulability.
- Mild salt and water retention,
- Vasodilatation
- Increased circulating levels of CBG, TBG, SHBG & Transferrin

ADRs
- Post-menopausal bleeding, breast tenderness, hyperpigmentation, migraine
- Increased risk of thrombo-embolic phenomenon / carcinoma endometrium / breast / hepatoma / gallstones
- **Teratogenic:** Stilbestrol increases risk of carcinoma vagina and cervix in female offspring and genital abnormalities in male offspring.
- Suppression of libido, gynecomastia, feminisation in males.
- Fusion of epiphyses and reduced adult height in children

Classification
Based on Source
Natural Estrogens: Estradiol, Estrone, Estriol
Synthetic Estrogens:
Steroidal: Ethinyl estradiol, Mestranol, Quinestrol, Tibolone
Non steroidal: Diethylstilbestrol, Methallenestril, Chlorotrianisene, Dienestrol, Benzestrol, Hexestrol

Contraindications
- Hormone dependent malignancies (carcinoma breast, uterus)
- Severe liver disease
- Thrombo-embolic disease
- Migraine
- Epilepsy
- Heavy smokers

ANTIESTROGENS

SERMs
Tamoxifen, Raloxifene, Toremifene

These drugs oppose estrogen action selectively in some tissues → inhibition of human carcinoma breast cells and hot flushes

In some other tissues exert weak estrogenic effect → reducing Gn & PRL levels in post-menopausal women, endometrial proliferation and improved bone density.

Uses: Palliation of carcinoma breast especially ER+ve cases.
Prevention of post menopausal osteoporosis
Tamoxifen may be preferred over clomiphene for male infertility, due to fewer estrogenic adverse effects.

ADRs: Hot flushes, anorexia, nausea, vomiting, vaginal bleeding, menstrual irregularities, dermatitis, depression

SERD
Fulvestrant causes down-regulation of estrogen receptors (ER). It acts by preventing dimerisation of estrogen receptor, resulting in reduced effect of estrogen on protein synthesis and fast receptor degradation.

Fulvestrant has pure estrogen antagonistic actions and is useful in tamoxifen-resistant carcinoma breast.

Aromatase Inhibitors
Letrozole and anastrozole interfere with production of estrogen from androstenedione & testosterone → almost complete estrogen deprivation in post-menopausal women

Uses: As adjuvants after surgical removal of carcinoma breast in early stage of disease, especially in ER +ve tumours in post menopausal women.

Preferred over tamoxifen in palliative treatment of advanced metastatic carcinoma breast as these have higher response rate, longer survival, lower treatment failure rates & no risk of thrombo-embolism and carcinoma endometrium

ADRs: Dyspepsia, nausea, diarrhea, hot flushes, vaginal atrophic changes. Prolonged use may cause accelerated bone loss, arthritis and risk of fractures

CONCEPT MAP – PROGESTINS AND ANTIPROGESTINS

Actions
Secretory changes in estrogen-primed endometrium
Thick /scanty cervical secretions, hostile for sperm penetration
Alveolo-lobular development in breast.
HDL is lowered, carbohydrate tolerance impaired.
Central effects: Sedation, raised basal body temperature (BBT), suppression of LH surge and anti-ovulatory effect.

Classification
Natural: Progesterone
Synthetic:
21-Carbon progesterone derivatives
Hydroxyprogesterone caproate
Medroxyprogesterone acetate
Dydrogesterone, Megestrol acetate, Nomegestrol acetate, Chlormadinone
19-Nortestosterone derivatives
Estranes: Lynestrenol, Allylestrenol, Norethindrone, Norethynodrel
Gonanes: Levonorgestrel, Desogestrel, Norgestimate, Gestodene

Uses
With estrogens in a cyclic manner for:
Hormone replacement therapy (HRT)
Oral contraception
Dysfunctional uterine bleeding (DUB)
Premenstrual syndrome (PMS)
Endometriosis

ADRs
Headache, Engorgement of breast, Lowering HDL, May precipitate DM and hypertension.

Progestins

Antiprogestins

Mifepristone
Prevents actions of progesterone by strongly binding with progesterone receptors.
Uses: For emergency post-coital contraception
Termination of early pregnancy (combined with PGE_1 analogue misoprostol),
Cervical priming
Induction of labour in IUD.
ADRs: Nausea, vomiting, diarrhea, abdominal pain and severe vaginal bleeding

Gestrinone
Selective progesterone receptor modulator (SPRM) with weak androgenic effect
Activates progesterone and androgen receptors in pituitary, resulting in weak anti-gonadotropin activity
Antiestrogenic activity in endometrium
↓
Reduces menstrual blood loss in menorrhagia, Shrinkage of fibroids
Useful in endometriosis
ADRs: Acne, hirsutism, breast hypoplasia, hair loss, weight gain, etc.

Ulipristal
A selective progesterone receptor modulator that is useful as post-coital emergency contraceptive with longer window period of up to 120 hours.

SECTION 9 Drugs Affecting the Endocrine System

46 Hormonal Contraceptives

PH 7.7 Explain the types, kinetics, dynamics, adverse effects, indications and contraindications of drugs which modify the female reproductive functions including contraceptives. Explain the important instructions for use of female and male contraceptives.
PH 10.14 Communicate with the patient regarding optimal use of a drug therapy using empathy and professionalism, e.g., oral contraceptives.

Learning objectives

A student of MBBS phase II should be able to:
- Enumerate contraceptive preparations.
- Describe the mechanism of action of contraceptive preparations.
- Describe uses of contraceptives, mentioning doses.
- Describe adverse effects and contraindications to use of contraceptives.
- Communicate correct method of use of contraceptives to female/male subjects.

Contraceptives are drugs used for suppressing fertility in a reversible manner for the purpose of family planning. Contraception methods for males and females are different and are hence described separately.

FEMALE CONTRACEPTION

Hormonal contraceptives can be used in following ways:
- Oral intake of hormonal pills (most frequently used method of female contraception)
- Intramuscular injection of depot preparations every 2–3 months
- Hormonal implants
- Hormone-impregnated intrauterine devices

Important contraceptives are shown in Flowchart 46.1.

1. Oral Contraceptives

The most frequently used method of female contraception is the daily oral intake of hormonal pills called oral contraceptive pills (OCPs). These pills are of 4 types: combined pills, phased pills, progesterone-only pills and post-coital pills.

a. Combined pills

Combined pills contain a combination of estrogen and progestins.
- The estrogen used in all the preparations is ethinyl estradiol (EE)
- Progestins used include norgestrel (NG), levonorgestrel (LN) and desogestrel (DG)

Preparations
- **EE with NG**
  - EE 50 mcg + NG 0.5 mg
  - EE 30 mcg + NG 0.3 mg
- **EE with LN**
  - EE 50 mcg + LN 0.25 mg
  - EE 30 mcg + LN 0.15 mg
  - EE 20 mcg + LN 0.10 mg
- **EE with DG**
  - EE 30 mcg + DG 0.15 mg
  - EE 20 mcg + DG 0.15 mg
- For the majority of women, pills containing EE 30 mcg suffice.
  - Pills containing larger doses (50 mcg) are indicated in obese patients and in those having breakthrough bleeding with lower doses of EE.
  - Lower dose (20 mcg) is indicated in patients > 40 years of age and those who have cardiovascular risk factors.

b. Phased pills

The content of estrogen and progestins is varied in accordance with the phase of the menstrual cycle, so that the steroidal hormone content is reduced. Such phased pills are indicated in women > 35 years of age and those with other risk factors.

In current practice, triphasic pills are usually preferred. The estrogen in most preparations is ethinyl estradiol (EE), which is kept constant at 35 mcg or may be slightly varied (30–40–30 mcg). The progestins may be levonorgestrel (LN) or norethindrone enanthate (NEE) in varying doses as described below.

- **Triquilar**
  - 6 pills containing EE 30 mcg + LN 50 mcg
  - 5 pills containing EE 40 mcg + LN 75 mcg
  - 10 pills containing EE 30 mcg + LN 125 mcg

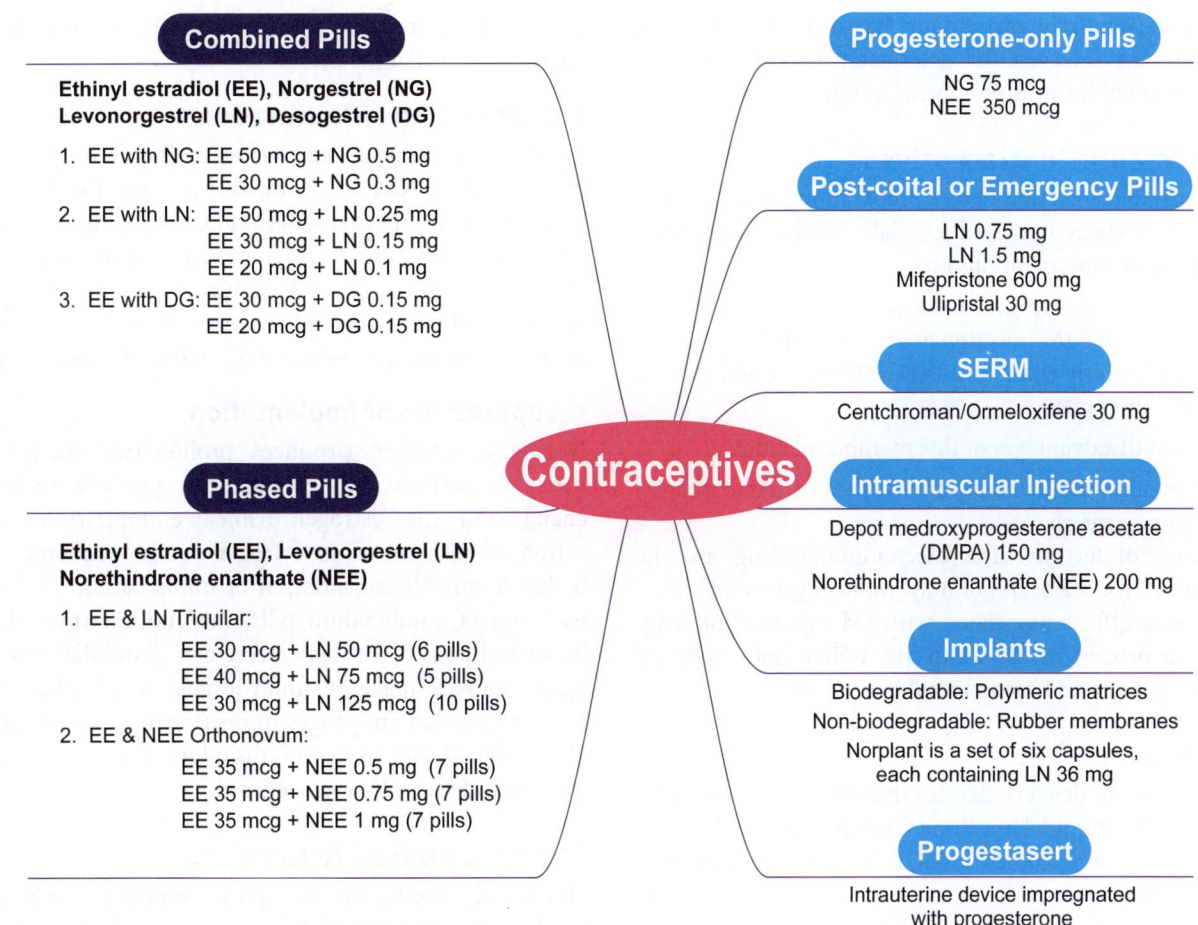

Flowchart 46.1 Classification of hormonal contraceptives

- Orthonovum
  - 7 pills containing EE 35 mcg + NEE 0.5 mg
  - 7 pills containing EE 35 mcg + NEE 0.75 mg
  - 7 pills containing EE 35 mcg + NEE 1 mg

c. Progestin-only pills

The adverse effects of combined or phased pills are mostly attributed to the estrogen component. These can be prevented by use of pills containing only progestins, such as norgestrel 75 mcg or norethindrone 350 mcg. Such progestin-only pills or mini pills are taken continuously daily, without any gap.

Progestin-only pills are indicated in women for whom the use of estrogens is contraindicated. With continuous use of progestins, the menstrual cycle becomes anovulatory. However, ovulation occurs in up to 30% users. In these subjects, the changes in cervical mucus (thick, scanty) and inhibition of implantation are responsible for the contraceptive effect. These pills are not frequently used, because they have lower efficacy than combined pills and the menstrual cycle becomes irregular.

d. Post-coital contraceptive pills

These pills are used for emergency contraception after unprotected coitus, such as in rape victims and in case of condom rupture.

The Yuzpe method that was used previously involved administration of two combined pills (each pill containing EE 50 mcg and LN 0.25 mg) within 72 hours of unprotected coitus and repeated after 12 hours.

Various pills used in current practice are:

1. Levonorgestrel 0.75 mg alone, within 48 hours of unprotected coitus, and repeated after 12 hours.
   (OR) Levonorgestrel 1.5 mg, single dose, within 72 hours of unprotected coitus. Such LN-containing pills are more effective and better tolerated than the Yuzpe method.
2. The antiprogestin mifepristone (600 mg, single dose) has high success rate and fewer adverse effects.
3. Selective progesterone receptor modulator (SPRM), ulipristal (30 mg, single dose within 120 hours of coitus), is as effective and well tolerated as the levonorgestrel method.

For all the above-mentioned regimens, the failure rate and adverse drug effects are greater than those for combined pills used regularly on a daily basis. Therefore, these methods are reserved for emergency use and are not recommended for routine contraception.

2. Injectable Contraceptives

Intramuscular injection of oily preparations at 2–3 month intervals obviates the need for daily intake. Commonly used injectable preparations are:

1. Depot medroxyprogesterone acetate (DMPA; 150 mg) given by deep IM injection every 3 months.
2. Norethindrone enanthate (NEE; 200 mg) given IM at 2 month intervals.

Important disadvantages of this method include:

- Menstrual irregularities (amenorrhea or menorrhagia) occur commonly.
- Return of fertility after discontinuing drug may be delayed (for > 2 years) or may not be regained at all.
- Adverse effects associated with IM injection of long-acting progestins are headache, weight gain, reduced bone density and menopausal symptoms.

3. Implants

These are drug delivery devices that are implanted under the skin. The steroidal hormone is released slowly from the implant, over a period of about 1–5 years. There are two types of implants:

- Biodegradable: These are polymeric matrices, which need not be removed from body and undergo degradation by themselves.
- Nonbiodegradable: These are rubber membranes that must be removed on expiry, e.g., norplant, a set of six capsules each containing 36 mg of levonorgestrel implanted subcutaneously.

4. Intrauterine Devices

Copper T (Cu T) is the most frequently used intrauterine device for contraception. Progestasert is an intrauterine device impregnated with progesterone for exerting local action on the endometrium; however, it has low efficacy.

Mechanism of Contraceptive Action of Hormonal Pills

Combined pills containing estrogen and progestins exert their contraceptive effect via the suppression of ovulation, fertilisation and implantation.

a. Suppression of ovulation

Selective inhibition of pituitary function by negative feedback mechanism leads to reduced secretion of gonadotropins. Estrogen mainly reduces the secretion of FSH, while progestin reduces the number of secretory pulses of LH per unit time. The midcycle LH surge is prevented by the synergistic action of both estrogen and progestins, resulting in the inhibition of ovulation. In contrast, progestin-only pills may not suppress ovulation in about one-third of the cycles.

b. Suppression of fertilisation

Changes in cervical mucus are mainly brought about by progestins. Cervical mucus becomes thick, scanty and hostile to sperm penetration. Thus, the progestin component of hormonal contraceptives decreases the chances of fertilisation of the ovum. Moreover, changes in motility and secretions of the uterine tube, brought about by progestins further reduce the likelihood of conception.

c. Suppression of implantation

Normally, estrogen produces proliferative changes in the endometrium, while progestins produce secretory changes in the 'estrogen-primed endometrium'. This action of progestins on estrogen-primed endometrium makes it suitable for nidation or implantation. However, with use of combination pills, the endometrium shows hyperproliferative or hypersecretory glandular atrophy. Such changes make it unfavourable for implantation. Mifepristone, an antiprogestin present in post-coital pills, blocks decidualisation and dislodges the blastocyst, if implantation has already occurred.

Pharmacological Actions

Hormonal contraceptive pills suppress ovulation, fertilisation and implantation as mentioned above. Other actions include effects on breasts, CNS, and the endocrine glands.

- Estrogen component of OCPs stimulates breast growth. Breast enlargement occurs in most OCP users.
- Central effects are not prominent, but the progestin component raises the basal body temperature and may cause depression.
- Prolonged use of OCPs causes increased rennin activity and increased aldosterone secretion. Levels of thyroxine, sex hormones and corticosteroid-binding globulins (TBG, SHBG, CBG) are also raised.

Therapeutic Uses

Contraception

Oral contraceptives are the most commonly used method of family planning due to their effectiveness, convenience, and affordability.

Instructions for use

1. Both the combined and phased pills are given daily for 21 days, starting from the 5th day of the cycle (day 1 being the beginning of menstrual bleeding). Patient is advised to take one pill daily in a row, followed by a gap of 7 days. In most preparations, a placebo or some other nutritional supplement tablets without any hormonal content are given for these 7 days. Withdrawal bleeding occurs within this gap in hormone administration. This

practice of giving inert tablets for the duration of the gap improves patient compliance and reduces the risk of patient forgetting to restart pills after the gap period.
2. Patient should be counselled properly, in a language easily understood by her, to use the pills as per instructions given on the pack. In most of the packs of combined or sequential pills, arrowed lines indicate from where to start taking pills and how to proceed. These arrows and pills to be taken on each day should be explained and demonstrated to patients for effective use. Patients should be given opportunities to ask questions and clarify their doubts about the correct use of OCPs.
3. If patient starts taking the pill on any other day of menstrual cycle (other than day 5), she should use some additional birth control method for at least 7 days for better protection.
4. Patient is advised to take the pill around same time every day (to reduce chances of missing the dose). Alarms, calendar reminders or birth control app may be beneficial in remembering the daily dose. In case of progestin-only pills, patient is advised to take the pill during the same 3-hour window, every day, for better efficacy.
5. If the patient misses one pill, she can take two pills the next day; but if more than 2 pills are missed, the patient is advised to stop OCPs and use some other method of contraception for that cycle. OCPs can then be restarted from day 5 of the next cycle.

Non-contraceptive uses

6. In addition to their use as contraceptives, these drugs have beneficial effects in benign breast disease, fibroid uterus, ovarian cysts, endometriosis, malignancy of ovaries/ endometrium/colon, premenstrual tension syndrome and osteoporosis.

Adverse Drug Reactions
Mild ADRs

- Nausea, vomiting
- Breast tenderness
- Mild headache/migraine may be triggered
- Amenorrhea
- Edema
- Rarely, breast discomfort and abdominal distension may occur with progestin-only pills
- Breakthrough bleeding can occur with progestin-only pills. It can be reduced by using phased pills.

Late ADRs
Some ADRs that can occur upon continued use of OCPs for prolonged period are mentioned below.

Moderately severe ADRs
- The progestin component can cause:
  - **Acne** is a problem with progestins that have androgenic effect, but addition of estrogen causes improvement.
  - Progestins having androgenic effect can also cause **hirsutism**. Norgestrel and desogestrel are preferred for their low androgenic activity.
  - **Weight gain, mood swings and depression** on prolonged use.
- The estrogen component can cause **pigmentation** of nose, cheeks, forehead resembling chloasma of pregnancy and increased incidence of **gallstones**; cholangitis and cholestatic jaundice may be seen.
- Both estrogen and progestin components contribute to rise in BP secondary to increased renin and aldosterone activity. However, the risk of **hypertension** is lower with currently used low-dose preparations.

Serious ADRs
- Increased risk of **thrombo-embolic phenomena** such as DVT and pulmonary embolism is because of the estrogen component of OCPs.
- In hypertensives, smokers, and elderly women, the risk of cerebrovascular accidents, **CVA**, and **stroke** is higher.
- Risk of **myocardial infarction** is higher in women with hypertension, history of smoking, pre-eclampsia, hyperlipidemias, and diabetes.
- Estrogens have a beneficial effect on the lipid profile as it raises the HDL:LDL ratio; however, this is countered by the progestin component. Triglyceride levels are slightly raised.
- **Risk of malignancies**: OCPs reduce the risk of ovarian carcinoma due to prolonged suppression of gonadotropin secretion. The risk of **vaginal, cervical, and breast cancer** is increased only in predisposed individuals, e.g., the risk of cervical carcinoma is increased in women with human papilloma virus infection who are on OCPs. The risk of benign **hepatic adenoma** is also somewhat increased in OCP users.

Cautions
OCPs should be used cautiously or avoided if possible in smokers, obese women, those > 35 years of age, and in women with uterine fibroids, mild hypertension, gall bladder disease, migraine, and epilepsy, etc.

Contraindications of OCPs
- History of thrombo-embolism, stroke, and MI
- Suspected hormone-responsive malignancy of genitals or breast
- Liver disease
- Hyperlipidemia
- Moderate/severe hypertension

Drug–drug interactions
- Enzyme inducers such as rifampicin, phenytoin, and carbamazepine can cause contraceptive failure.
- Antimicrobial agents such as tetracyclines and ampicillin suppress intestinal microbial flora and

interfere with enterohepatic circulation of OCPs, causing their failure.

Centchroman/Ormeloxifene

It is a nonsteroidal selective estrogen receptor modulator (SERM) that has prominent antiestrogenic effect on the uterus and breast.

- Endocrine function of the pituitary–ovarian axis remains unaffected.
- Menstrual cycle is not disturbed, as hormone levels are not altered.
- It exerts contraceptive effect by causing embryo–uterus asynchrony. It accelerates transport of the embryo through the tubes, whereas decidual changes in the endometrium are delayed due to down-regulation of endometrial estrogen receptors and suppression of endometrial proliferation. Thus, when the embryo reaches the uterine cavity, the endometrium is not favourable for implantation.
- Because of its long half-life, it is administered twice weekly, in a dose of 30 mg for 12 weeks, and then weekly. The drug is continued till contraception is required.
- Its antiestrogenic effect on the uterus is useful in dysfunctional uterine bleeding (DUB) as well. Dosage in DUB is 60 mg, twice weekly for 12 weeks, and then weekly for 12 more weeks.
- Adverse effects include headache, nausea, fluid retention, increase in BP, and weight gain.

MALE CONTRACEPTION

In contrast to the availability of a variety of effective contraceptives for women, none of the drugs investigated for use as male contraceptives are satisfactory. Challenges in male contraception include:

- Poor compliance with treatment, as men themselves do not get pregnant.
- Low efficacy of drugs in suppressing spermatogenesis, as millions of sperms are released per ejaculation in comparison to a single ovum released per menstrual cycle in females. Thus, failure rate is high as complete azoospermia may not be achievable.
- Adverse effects of drugs used for suppression of spermatogenesis such as impotence and loss of libido are not acceptable to most couples.

Drug groups studied for male contraception include estrogens, progestins, androgens, antiandrogens, gonadotropin-releasing hormone analogues and cytotoxic drugs; however, none of them show satisfactory efficacy, tolerability and acceptability.

Gossypol

Gossypol is an orally effective drug obtained from cotton seeds.

- It appears to have a direct toxic effect on seminiferous tubules, and suppresses spermatogenesis and motility of sperms in 99.9% users.
- Testosterone levels are not reduced; thus, loss of libido and impotence are not a problem with this drug.
- The most disturbing adverse effect is hypokalemia, which causes muscular weakness and even paralysis. Diarrhea, edema, and neurological symptoms may also occur. Currently, it is not much in use.

In the absence of safe and effective hormonal method of contraception for men, coitus interruptus, barrier methods using condoms with/without spermicidal creams, and vasectomy are more useful options.

INSTRUCTIONS FOR EFFECTIVE USE

- Use of barrier contraceptives should be promoted as it decreases chances of pregnancy, reduces transmission of sexually transmitted infectious diseases, and has no hormonal adverse effects. Condoms should be used as per instructions given on the pack, not to be reused or used beyond expiry date. It should be unrolled and worn properly, leaving space at the tip for the ejaculate. It should be removed carefully after use and disposed of. A lubricant or spermicidal cream may facilitate condom use. The protection against pregnancy is also better when condoms are combined with spermicidal creams.
- Vasectomy is a permanent birth control method for men who have completed their family. It takes about 3 months for a vasectomy to become fully protective. Thus, patients are advised to continue using alternative contraceptive methods during this time.

Clinical problem-based questions and MCQs

1. **A 29-year-old female patient with two live children was using combination pills containing EE and LN for contraception for the last 3 years. Two months back, patient developed cough with expectoration and was diagnosed with pulmonary TB. First-line anti-tubercular drug regimen was prescribed and patient responded well. Patient presents to gynec OPD with amenorrhea for 20 days and tests positive for pregnancy**
   i. What is the cause of her present symptoms?
   ii. Identify the drug that might have interacted with contraceptives and describe the mechanism of its interaction.
   iii. Enumerate other drugs that can cause similar interactions with contraceptives.

2. i. **Levonorgestrel and ethinyl estradiol pills have contraceptive as well as non-contraceptive uses. Which of the following is a non-contraceptive use?**
   a. Premenstrual syndrome
   b. Post-coital pill

c. Carcinoma breast
d. Hepatic adenoma
ii. Enumerate other non-contraceptive indications for levonorgestrel.

3. A 39-year-old female patient visits the OBG outpatient department for contraceptive advice. Careful history reveals that she is a smoker with H/O angina attack 3 years back and is on regular treatment for the same. Which of the following methods of contraception is contraindicated in this case?
   a. Intrauterine device
   b. Levonorgestrel
   c. Combined contraceptive pill
   d. Condoms

4. i. Identify the progestin used in emergency contraception.
   a. Micronised progesterone
   b. Depot medroxyprogesterone acetate
   c. Levonorgestrel
   d. Desogestrel
   ii. Name two other drugs used for the same indication.

5. Identify an adverse effect of progesterone-only pills.
   a. Hypertension
   b. Chloasma
   c. Cholestatic jaundice
   d. Breakthrough bleeding

6. i. Identify the drug that exerts contraceptive effect through embryo–uterus asynchrony.
   a. Levonorgestrel
   b. Ethinyl estradiol
   c. Ormeloxifene
   d. Mifepristone
   ii. What is the dose and frequency of administration of the selected drug?

7. All of the following are means of male contraception, EXCEPT:
   a. Centchroman
   b. Gossypol
   c. Coitus interruptus
   d. Barrier methods

8. OCPs increase the risk of all the following malignancies, EXCEPT:
   a. Endometrium
   b. Breast
   c. Ovaries
   d. Vagina

Summary

- Contraceptives are drugs used for the reversible suppression of fertility.
- **Female contraception**: Combined oral contraceptive pills (OCPs) are the most frequently used method for female contraception. They are started from day 5 of the menstrual cycle and given daily for 21 days, followed by a gap of 7 days during which placebos or other nutritional supplement tablets without any hormonal content are given. Withdrawal bleeding occurs within these 7 days.
- OCPs contain a combination of an estrogen (ethinyl estradiol, EE) with one of the progesterones [norgestrel (NG), levonorgestrel (LN), desogestrel (DG)].
- The dose of EE in different preparations of **combined pills** varies from 20–50 mcg. The dose is kept low (20 mcg) in patients > 40 years of age and those who have cardiovascular risk factors. However, obese patients or those who have breakthrough bleeding with low dose EE pills, require higher dose of EE, i.e., 50 mcg. The dose of progestins also varies as 0.3 and 0.5 mg for NG, 0.1, 0.15, and 0.25 mg for LN and 0.15 mg for DG.
- **Phased pills** have a variable amount of estrogen and progesterone in accordance with the phase of menstrual cycle, to reduce the content of steroidal hormones. These are indicated in women > 35 years of age or having other risk factors. EE is kept constant at 35 mcg or varied slightly (30–40–30 mcg). The progestin (levonorgestrel, LN) is varied as 50 mcg for the first 6 days, 75 mcg for next 5 days, and 125 mcg for the next 10 days.
- **Progesterone-only pills** containing norgestrel (NG, 75 mcg) or norethindrone (NEE, 350 mcg) taken continuously daily, without any gap, are indicated in women who have contraindications to the use of estrogens.
- **Post-coital or emergency contraceptive pills** are used for after unprotected coitus (e.g., in rape victims or condom rupture). Such pills have LN 0.75 mg or LN 1.5 mg and are given within 48 or 72 hours of unprotected coitus and repeated after 12 hours. A single dose of an antiprogestin such as mifepristone (600 mg) or ulipristal (30 mg) is also useful.
- **Centchroman or ormeloxifene** exerts its contraceptive effect by causing embryo–uterus asynchrony, without altering hormone levels and the menstrual cycle. Dose is 30 mg twice weekly for 12 weeks and then weekly, continued till contraception is required. ADRs like headache, nausea, retention of fluid, increase in BP, and weight gain may occur.
- **Intramuscular injection** of oily preparations such as DMPA 150 mg or NEE 200 mg at 2–3 month intervals obviates the need for daily intake, but may cause menstrual irregularities, headache, weight gain, reduced bone density and menopausal symptoms. Recovery of fertility after discontinuing use may be delayed.

- **Implants** are biodegradable or nonbiodegradable devices that are placed under the skin, which release the hormone slowly, for 1–5 years.
- **Progestasert** is an intrauterine device impregnated with progesterone.
- Hormonal contraceptive pills suppress ovulation (by reducing Gn secretion), fertilisation (by making cervical mucus thick, scanty and hostile to sperm penetration) and implantation (by making the endometrium unfavourable for implantation).
- **Mild ADRs** are nausea, vomiting, breast discomfort/tenderness, headache/migraine, amenorrhea, edema and abdominal distension.
- **Moderately severe late ADRs** caused by the progesterone component include acne, hirsutism, weight gain, hypertriglyceridemia, mood swings, and depression; those caused by the estrogen component include pigmentation, increased incidence of gallstones, cholangitis, cholestatic jaundice and hypertension.
- **Serious adverse effects** of contraceptives include thrombo-embolic phenomena like DVT/pulmonary embolism, increased risk of myocardial infarction/CVA or stroke, and vaginal/cervical/breast cancer/benign hepatic adenoma.
- OCPs are **contraindicated** in thrombo-embolism, stroke, MI, suspected hormone-responsive malignancy of genitals or breast, liver disease, hyperlipidemia and moderate/severe hypertension.
- If possible, OCPs are avoided in smokers, obese women, when age > 35 years, uterine fibroids, mild hypertension, gall bladder disease and migraine.
- **Male contraception:** Many hormonal and cytotoxic drugs have been investigated but found unsatisfactory. Gossypol suppresses spermatogenesis and motility of sperms without affecting libido and testosterone levels. However, it is not in use because of ADRs like hypokalemia, diarrhea, edema and neurological symptoms.

Questions for practice

1. Enumerate the therapeutic uses and adverse effects of:
   a. Progestins
   b. Mifepristone
2. Describe the various oral contraceptive preparations used for contraception in females.
3. Enumerate the adverse effects and contraindications for use of OCPs.
4. Describe the challenges in male contraception.

Hints for problem-based questions & MCQs

1. a. Contraceptive failure
   b. Enzyme inducing action of rifampicin
   c. Phenobarbitone, carbamazepine, griseofulvin etc.
2. i. a. Premenstrual syndrome is a non-contraceptive indication for the use of levonorgestrel. Post-coital pill is a contraceptive use. It has no role in carcinoma breast and prostate.
   ii. Benign breast disease, uterine fibroids, ovarian cyst, endometriosis, osteoporosis, malignancy of ovary/endometrium/colon, etc.
3. c. Combined contraceptive pill is contraindicated in angina and MI and should be avoided in patients > 35 years of age.
4. i. c. Levonorgestrel
   ii. Mifepristone, Ulipristal
5. d. Breakthrough bleeding
6. i. c. Ormeloxifene
   ii. 30 mg, twice weekly for 12 weeks or as long as contraception is desired.
7. a. Centchroman
8. c. Ovaries

CONCEPT MAP – HORMONAL CONTRACEPTIVES

Mechanism of Action

Estrogen, progesterone pills

Suppression of ovulation:
Reduced secretion of gonadotropins.
Estrogen reduces FSH secretion,
Progestin reduces number of secretory pulses of LH per unit time.
Both prevent midcycle LH surge → inhibition of ovulation.

Suppression of fertilisation: Progestins make cervical mucus thick, scanty and hostile to sperm penetration. Changes in motility and secretions in uterine tube → decreased chances of fertilisation of ovum.

Suppression of implantation: Endometrium shows glandular atrophy, hyperproliferative or hypersecretory, making it unfavourable for implantation.

Mifepristone blocks decidualisation and dislodges the blastocyst, if implantation has already occurred

Centchroman causes embryo–uterus asynchrony as it accelerates the transport of embryo through tubes, but delays decidual changes in endometrium.

Combined Pills

Contain estrogen (ethinyl estradiol: EE) & progesterone (Norgestrel NG/Levonorgestrel LN/Desogestrel DG).

Dose of EE in different preparations of combined pills varies from 20–50 mcg.

Dose is kept low 20 mcg in patients > 40 years of age or those who have cardiovascular risk factors.

Higher dose EE 50 mcg given in obese patients, or those who have breakthrough bleeding with low dose EE pills

Dose of progestins varies as 0.3, 0.5 mg for NG,
0.1, 0.15, 0.25 mg for LN
0.15 mg for DG.

How to use:
Combined pills are started from day 5 of menstrual cycle, given daily for 21 days, followed by a gap of 7 days in which placebos or other nutritional supplements without any hormonal content are given. Withdrawal bleeding occurs within these 7 days.

Classification

Oral contraceptives
Combination pills
Phased pills
Progesterone-only pills
Post-coital pills
Centchroman

Injectable contraceptives
DMPA
NEE

Implants
Biodegradable
Non-biodegradable
Norplant

Intrauterine device
Progestasert

CONTRACEPTIVES

Phased Pills

Have variable amount of estrogen and progesterone in accordance with the phase of menstrual cycle, **to reduce content of steroidal hormones.**

Indicated in **women > 35 years** of age or those who have other risk factors.

Dose of EE is kept constant at 35 mcg or varied slightly (30-40-30 mcg).

Dose of Progestins: Levonorgestrel (LN) is varied as: 50 mcg for first 6 days,
75 mcg for next 5 days &
125 mcg for next 10 days

Dose of NEE is varied as 0.5 mg, 0.75 mg and 1 mg for 7 days each

Method of administration is same as combined pill

Progesterone-Only Pills

Contain only progestins like norgestrel (NG) 75 mcg or norethindrone (NEE) 350 mcg.

Indicated in women who have some condition contraindicating use of estrogens

Given continuously daily, without any gap.

With continuous use of progestins, menstrual cycle becomes anovulatory (but in up to 30% users ovulation occurs). In these subjects, changes in cervical mucus (thick, scanty) and inhibition of implantation are responsible for contraceptive effect.

Disadvantage: Low efficacy than combined pills.
The menstrual cycle becomes irregular

Injectable Contraceptives

Depot medroxyprogesterone acetate (DMPA) 150 mg given by deep IM injection at 3 month intervals
Norethindrone enanthate (NEE) 200 mg given IM at 2 month intervals.
Disadvantages: Menstrual irregularities
Delayed return of fertility after discontinuing drug

Centchroman

Contains ormeloxifene
Exerts contraceptive effect by causing embryo-uterus asynchrony without altering hormone levels and menstrual cycle.
Dose is 30 mg twice weekly for 12 weeks and then weekly, continued till contraception is required.
ADRs like headache, nausea, retention of fluid, increase in BP, weight gain may occur

Post-coital Pills

Used for emergency contraception after unprotected coitus.
Yuzpe method: Administration of two combined pills (each containing EE 50 mcg and LN 0.25 mg) within 72 hours of unprotected coitus and repeated after 12 hours.
Levonorgestrel 0.75 mg alone within 48 hours of unprotected coitus and repeated after 12 hours
Levonorgestrel 1.5 mg single dose within 72 hours of unprotected coitus.
Such LN containing pills are more effective and better tolerated than Yuzpe method.
Antiprogestin, mifepristone 600 mg single dose has high success rate and fewer ADRs.
SPRM ulipristal 30 mg single dose within 120 hours of coitus is as effective and well tolerated as levonorgestrel method
Disadvantage: Not recommended for routine contraception, as failure rate and adverse drug effects are more than combined pills.

ADRs of Hormonal Contraceptives

Mild: Nausea, vomiting, breast discomfort/tenderness, headache/migraine, amenorrhea, edema and abdominal distension.
Moderately severe late ADRs: Due to progesterone: acne, hirsutism, weight gain, hypertriglyceridemia, mood swings, depression
Due to estrogen: Pigmentation, increased incidence of gallstones, cholangitis, cholestatic jaundice and hypertension.
Serious late adverse effects: Thrombo-embolic phenomena like DVT/pulmonary embolism,
Increased risk of myocardial infarction/CVA or stroke,
Vaginal/cervical/breast cancer/benign hepatic adenoma
Contraindication: Thrombo-embolism, stroke, MI, suspected hormone responsive malignancy of genitals or breast, liver disease, hyperlipidemia and moderate/severe hypertension
Avoided in smokers, obese women, > 35 years of age, uterine fibroids, mild hypertension, gall bladder disease and migraine.

SECTION 9 Drugs Affecting the Endocrine System

47 Drugs Acting on the Uterus

PH 7.8 Explain the types, kinetics, dynamics, adverse effects, indications and contraindications of uterine relaxants and stimulants.

Learning objectives

A student of MBBS phase II should be able to:
- Enumerate drugs that stimulate the uterus.
- Describe the mechanism of action and pharmacological actions of uterine stimulants.
- Describe the salient pharmacokinetic features of uterine stimulants.
- Enumerate the therapeutic uses and adverse effects of uterine stimulants.
- Enumerate uterine relaxants.
- Describe the mechanism of action and indications for use of uterine relaxants.
- Enumerate the adverse effects and contraindications for use of uterine relaxants.

The uterus consists of uterine muscles called the **myometrium**, which are covered on the inner side by the **endometrium**. The endometrium is mainly acted upon by the female sex hormones—estrogen, progestins, and their antagonists. The myometrium is supplied by sympathetic and parasympathetic nerves; as a result, uterine contractility is affected by many autonomic drugs. In addition, some drugs possess direct action on the myometrium and cause uterine contraction or relaxation.

Drugs that act on the uterine myometrium are broadly classified into **uterine stimulants** and **relaxants**.

UTERINE STIMULANTS

Uterine stimulant drugs are also called ecbolics, oxytocics, and abortifacients; these include oxytocin, its analogues, ergot alkaloids and prostaglandins (Flowchart 47.1).

Oxytocin and its Analogues
Oxytocin synthesis and release
Oxytocin is an octapeptide hormone mainly synthesised by the paraventricular nuclei of the hypothalamus; it is transported along axons to be stored in the neurohypophysis. A small quantity of oxytocin is synthesised in the supraoptic hypothalamic nuclei, corpus luteum in the ovary, uterus and fetal membranes as well.

Oxytocin is released from the posterior pituitary in a pulsatile manner, in response to various stimuli such as persistent distension of the cervix and vagina, coitus, suckling, pain, and apprehension. Stimuli for ADH release (water deprivation, hypertonic saline, etc.), also cause some release of oxytocin. On the other hand, relaxin (released by the ovaries) and alcohol reduce oxytocin secretion.

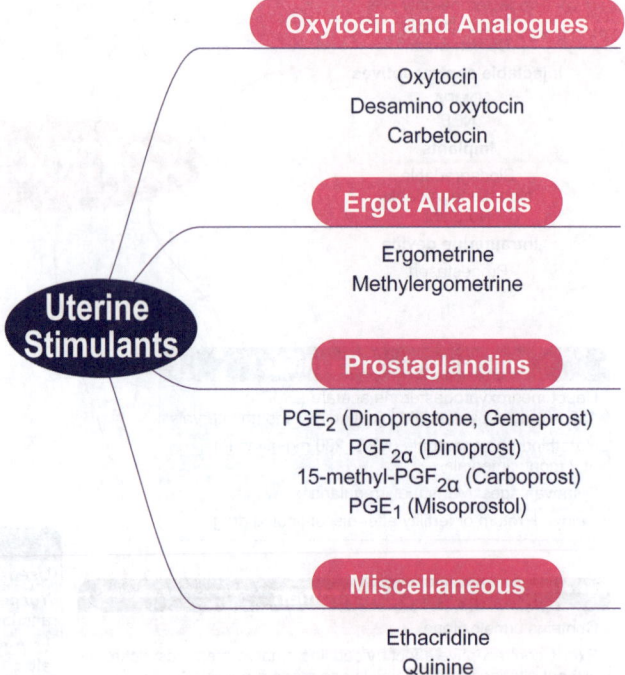

Flowchart 47.1 Classification of uterine stimulants

Mechanism of action
Oxytocin acts through G protein-coupled receptors present on smooth muscles in the myometrium and myoepithelial cells in the breast. Binding of agonists to oxytocin receptors causes membrane depolarisation and Ca^{2+} influx, as well as calcium release from intracellular stores. Raised intracellular calcium leads to smooth muscle contraction. Oxytocin also increases prostaglandin synthesis and release from the endometrium. These prostaglandins contribute to its uterine stimulant action to some extent.

Pharmacological actions

1. Uterine smooth muscles

Oxytocin causes sustained uterine contraction. It **increases the force and frequency of uterine contractions**. The fundus and body of the uterus contract, but the **lower segment is not much affected** or even relaxes at full-term pregnancy. With low dose of oxytocin, the **uterine muscles relax completely between the contractions**; however, at higher doses, the basal tone increases.

The sensitivity of the uterus to oxytocin action is affected by the female sex hormones. Estrogen increases and progesterone decreases myometrial sensitivity to oxytocin. Thus, sensitivity of the uterus to the action of oxytocin is low in the non-pregnant state and during early pregnancy. High progesterone levels and the accompanying low oxytocin sensitivity help to maintain pregnancy. However, at term, progesterone decreases and estrogen increases. So, the sensitivity of the pregnant uterus to oxytocin sharply increases near term, and then falls quickly during puerperium. Consequently, oxytocin is not used as an abortifacient. While oxytocin is not necessarily required for initiation of labour, it has a facilitatory role in labour. PGs and platelet-activating factor (PAF) complement the action of oxytocin during labour.

2. Breast

The **milk ejection reflex** initiated by suckling is mediated through oxytocin. Suckling stimulates oxytocin release from the neurohypophysis; oxytocin causes contraction of myoepithelial cells surrounding the mammary alveoli, resulting in milk ejection or let-down reflex.

3. Other actions

Other actions of oxytocin are not seen at doses used in obstetric practice. However, larger doses can cause vasodilatation, leading to a brief fall in BP, flushing and reflex tachycardia. Large doses of oxytocin given with lots of IV fluids can cause ADH-like action and pulmonary edema.

Pharmacokinetics

Oxytocin is a peptide hormone, susceptible to proteolytic enzymes. Therefore, it is not effective orally. Upon parenteral administration, oxytocin is quickly metabolised in the liver and excreted by the kidney. The pregnant uterus and placenta can secrete oxytocinase enzyme that contributes to oxytocin metabolism. Owing to rapid inactivation, oxytocin has a short half-life of 5–10 minutes. So, when given as IV infusion, its effect can be easily controlled and quickly terminated.

Therapeutic uses

1. Oxytocin is used as drug of first choice for **induction of labour** in:
   - Postmaturity [condition in which pregnancy continues beyond two weeks after the expected date of delivery (EDOD)]
   - Conditions requiring early delivery, e.g., pre-eclampsia, Rh incompatibility, maternal diabetes, and placental insufficiency.

   Oxytocin is used by IV infusion. 1 IU is equivalent to 2 mcg of pure hormone. 5 IU (10 mcg of oxytocin) dissolved in 500 mL saline and infused intravenously at a rate of 0.2–2 mL/min, till sufficiently strong contractions are achieved. The oxytocin drip is then discontinued, because exceedingly strong contractions can cause many complications.

2. Oxytocin is useful for **augmenting dysfunctional labour** in cases of uterine inertia—by IV infusion in the same dose as for induction. However, if labour is progressing normally, oxytocin cannot hasten the process and should not be used.

   In both these indications for using oxytocin, all contraindications to its use must be ruled out before starting oxytocin drip. It is important to confirm fetal presentation, lung maturity, and rule out fetal distress, placenta previa, cephalopelvic disproportion and uterine scars from any previous surgery.

   Oxytocin is the drug of choice for both these indications, i.e., induction and augmentation of labour and is preferred over PG and ergometrine, because:
   - Oxytocin has a consistent effect on the strength of uterine smooth muscle contractions.
   - At low doses, oxytocin causes relaxation between contractions, because of which fetal oxygenation is not affected.
   - At term, oxytocin increases the force and frequency of contractions only in the fundus and body of the uterus, whereas the lower segment of the uterus is relaxed. This action favours fetal descent through the birth canal and childbirth.

3. **Postpartum hemorrhage**: In hypertensive patients, where ergometrine is contraindicated, oxytocin is used for the treatment of atonic postpartum hemorrhage (PPH). Dose for the control of PPH is higher. 10 IU given intramuscularly or dissolved in 500 mL saline and infused at a rate of 10 mL/min after the delivery of the placenta.

4. In **breast engorgement after delivery**, due to impaired milk ejection, oxytocin can be used as a nasal spray, in a dose of one puff about 2–3 minutes before feeding baby. However, oxytocin is not effective if milk secretion is deficient.

Adverse effects

Oxytocin has almost no adverse effects at recommended doses and rates.
- However, injudicious use during labour can result in excessively strong uterine contractions that force the presenting part through an incompletely dilated cervix, resulting in maternal and fetal soft tissue injuries.

Catastrophic outcomes like uterine rupture, fetal asphyxia, fetal death, and maternal death may occur.
- Water intoxication may occur if high doses are given with excess IV fluids, especially in patients with toxemia of pregnancy and renal insufficiency. This occurs due to the ADH-like action, and leads to symptoms such as headache, drowsiness and convulsions.

Contraindications

Induction/augmentation of labour with oxytocin is contraindicated in:
- Prematurity
- Fetal distress
- Cephalopelvic disproportion
- Abnormal presentation
- Presence of uterine scars
- With sympathomimetic drugs

Desamino oxytocin

It has the same actions, indications and contraindications as oxytocin; however, its effect is less consistent.

It is used as a buccal formulation (tablets) of 50 IU, repeated every 30 minutes up to a maximum of 10 tablets.

For breast engorgement and uterine inertia, the dose is 25–50 IU.

For promoting uterine involution during puerperium, 25–50 IU is given 5 times a day and continued for 7 days.

Carbetocin

Carbetocin is a newer, long-acting oxytocin analogue with a half-life of 90–100 minutes. It is useful for preventing PPH due to uterine atony after LSCS, in a dose of 100 mcg by IM or slow IV injection, given only once. If uterine atony persists, other uterine stimulants should be considered, because sufficient safety data about repeated doses of carbetocin is not yet available.

2. Ergot Alkaloids

Among the ergot alkaloids obtained from *Claviceps purpurea*, **ergometrine/ergonovine** and **methylergometrine** have significant effects on uterine muscles.

Mechanism of action

Ergot alkaloids act on several receptors (α-adrenoceptors, 5-HT_2 receptors, and dopamine receptors) as agonists, partial agonists, and antagonists. The uterine stimulant action is probably associated with their agonistic or partial agonistic action at 5-HT_2 and α-adrenoceptors).

Pharmacological actions

Uterus

Ergometrine and methylergometrine **increase the force, frequency and duration of uterine contractions**. At very low doses, phasic contractions occur with relaxation in between; however, at higher doses, basal tone is raised and contracture occurs. Moreover, unlike oxytocin, the stimulant action of ergometrine **contracts the lower uterine segment also**.

Therefore, it is not used before delivery for induction or augmentation of labour, because contractions of the lower segment interfere with fetal descent. The sensitivity of the uterus to ergometrine is much higher at full-term than in early pregnancy and in the nonpregnant state.

Blood vessels

The vasoconstrictor action of ergometrine is much weaker than that of ergotamine and is not significant at therapeutic doses; however, high doses can cause vasoconstriction and rise in BP.

CNS

Central effects do not occur at the usual dose. However, higher doses may cause complex actions on various receptors.

GIT

High doses increase peristaltic activity in the gut.

Methylergometrine

The methyl derivative of ergometrine is 1.5 times more potent than ergometrine in uterine stimulant action. However, its actions on blood vessels, CNS and GIT are negligible. As a result, methylergometrine is preferred over ergometrine for obstetric indications.

Therapeutic uses

- Methylergometrine is used for prevention and control of PPH. It can decrease blood loss during parturition, but is not used in all cases. It is given in a dose of 0.2–0.3 mg IM at delivery of anterior shoulder to prevent PPH in grand multipara, uterine atony, etc.

  Methylergometrine is preferred over oxytocin for the control of PPH, because it causes sustained contractions that result in the compression of perforated uterine arteries that stops bleeding. However, in severe PPH 0.5 mg methylergometrine can be combined with 5 mg oxytocin.
- Methylergometrine is useful to prevent uterine atony after LSCS or instrumental delivery.
- It is used orally for uterine involution in a dose of 0.125 mg, three times daily, for 7 days in multipara, where slow involution is expected. If the uterus is active and firm, its involution occurs rapidly in puerperium. Because ergots cannot hasten normal involution further, they are not indicated routinely in all cases.

Adverse effects

Usual doses are well tolerated. Sometimes, ergometrine may cause headache, nausea, vomiting, and rise in BP. High doses given for many days may stop milk secretion as it decreases prolactin secretion.

Contraindications

Ergometrine and methylergometrine should not be used in hypertension, toxemia of pregnancy, sepsis, liver and kidney diseases, and before the third stage of labour in pregnancy.

3. Prostaglandins

Mechanism of action

Prostaglandins exert their actions through prostanoid receptors, which are Gq-linked GPCRs in uterine muscles. Binding of prostaglandins to these receptors results in activation of PLC and generation of IP_3 and DAG; these, in turn, raise the intracellular calcium ion concentration resulting in smooth muscle contraction. Prostaglandins can cause contraction of the pregnant as well as nonpregnant uterus; the sensitivity of a pregnant uterus is greater and keeps increasing as the pregnancy advances. This effect is more prominent with $PGF_{2\alpha}$. Prostaglandins **increase the basal tone and amplitude of uterine contractions**. At term, they cause cervical softening and dilation by breaking down the collagen fibres in cervix, and make it more compliant for delivery. PGE_2 has more prominent effect on cervical ripening. Prostaglandins are thought to be responsible for initiation and progression of labour.

Increased prostaglandin synthesis by the endometrium is implicated in the causation of dysmenorrhea. Prostaglandin-induced uncoordinated uterine contractions can compress blood vessels, causing uterine ischemia and pain. So, prostaglandin synthesis inhibitors, i.e., NSAIDs, are very effective in dysmenorrhea.

Therapeutic uses

- Prostaglandins are mainly used as **abortifacients** because of their uterine stimulant action.
  - For medical termination of pregnancy (MTP) up to 49 days (7 weeks) of gestation, **mifepristone** (an antiprogestin) is given as a single dose of 600 mg, orally. It is followed after 2 days with a single 400 mcg dose of misoprostol, a prostaglandin E_1 analogue. Increased uterine contractions cause expulsion of the conceptus; this method is preferred over suction evacuation. Sometimes, low dose of methotrexate (due to its toxic effect on trophoblastic tissue) is used along with misoprostol intravaginal (4 tablets of 200 mcg each) to induce abortion in first few weeks of gestation. However, adverse effects of misoprostol such as nausea, vomiting, diarrhea, vaginal bleeding, and uterine cramps may occur.
  - In first trimester abortions, suction of the products of conception through the cervix (transcervical suction evacuation) is the procedure of choice. However, to reduce the cervical resistance to dilatation, an intravaginal pessary containing 1 mg PGE_2 (gemeprost) is inserted 3 hours before attempting cervical dilatation. This minimises the risk of cervical trauma during the procedure.
  - In late abortions, such as midterm abortions, missed abortion, and molar pregnancy, prostaglandins can be used to convert an oxytocin-resistant uterus to an oxytocin-sensitive uterus. A single extra-amniotic injection of PGE_2, followed by an oxytocin drip or a single intra-amniotic injection of $PGF_{2\alpha}$ with hypertonic saline solution is effective. Pretreatment with mifepristone can increase the efficacy of prostaglandins as abortifacients.
- For cervical priming: PGE_2 cervical gel containing 0.5 mg in 2.5 mL prefilled syringe is administered in the cervical canal or vagina. It makes the cervix soft and compliant. At such low doses, uterine contractions are not induced. After 12 hours of cervical priming, oxytocin IV infusion is started, to induce labour.
- Prostaglandins do not have any advantage over oxytocin for induction or augmentation of labour. However, they may be used for induction in patients with toxemia of pregnancy and renal failure, because unlike oxytocin, prostaglandins do not cause fluid retention. They are preferably given by the intravaginal route
- In PPH, due to uterine atony that does not respond to methylergometrine or oxytocin, an important alternative is 15-methyl-$PGF_{2\alpha}$ (carboprost), given intramuscularly in a dose of 0.25 mg. The dose can be repeated after 30–120 minutes if adequate response is not achieved

ADRs

Prostaglandins frequently cause adverse effects such as nausea, vomiting, watery diarrhea, uterine cramps, vaginal bleeding, flushing, shivering, fall in BP, tachycardia, fever, malaise, and chest pain.

However, the adverse effects of prostaglandins are negligible upon intravaginal administration.

Other Uterine Stimulants

Other uterine stimulants such as ethacridine and quinine are rarely used in current obstetric practice. Ethacridine (150 mL of 50 mg/50 mL solution injected slowly in the extra-amniotic space) is an alternative method for MTP in the 2nd trimester. The uterine stimulant action of quinine is unpredictable and not suitable for clinical use.

Clinical problem-based questions and MCQs

1. A 36-year-old woman presents with postmaturity (gestation period of 42 weeks). Fetal heart sounds are normal. There is no cephalopelvic disproportion or any other contraindication to normal delivery. On examination, cervix is undilated and uneffaced.
    i. Which of the following drugs is used for cervical priming?
    a. PGE_2
    b. Methylergometrine
    c. Ergometrine
    d. Oxytocin

ii. Which of the following is most suitable for induction of labour?
   a. PGE$_2$ b. Methylergometrine
   c. Ergometrine d. Oxytocin
iii. Justify your choices with the pharmacological basis.

2. A 39-year-old multipara presents in a shock-like state with excessive vaginal bleeding after home-conducted normal vaginal delivery. Abdominal examination revealed that uterus is atonic and relaxed.
   i. Identify the first-choice uterine stimulant in this case.
      a. PGE$_2$ b. Methylergometrine
      c. Ergometrine d. Oxytocin
   ii. Give pharmacological basis to justify your choice.

UTERINE RELAXANTS (TOCOLYTICS)

These drugs are used to decrease uterine contractility

CLASSIFICATION OF TOCOLYTICS

The classification of tocolytic drugs is shown in Flowchart 47.2.

Mechanism of tocolytic action: As is evident from the classification, drugs can bring about uterine smooth muscle relaxation by varied mechanisms such as β$_2$-agonism, calcium channel blockade/competing with calcium for influx through calcium channels, oxytocin antagonism, and reduced PG synthesis.

Indications for use of tocolytics: Tocolytics are clinically useful to suppress premature labour. If premature onset of labour occurs, attempts are made to delay or postpone it, in an effort to buy time for:
- The fetus to mature.
- Starting glucocorticoid therapy for fetal lung maturation.
- Shifting the mother to a centre that has proper facilities for the care of a premature baby.

However, if the patient has severe toxemia, antepartum hemorrhage, intrauterine infection, or ruptured membranes, then delaying labour can be counterproductive. So, in these conditions, the use of tocolytics is contraindicated. Moreover, attempts to delay labour are unlikely to succeed if cervical dilatation is already > 4 cm and the lower segment is taken up or effaced.

Other conditions that may benefit from the use of uterine relaxants include threatened abortion and dysmenorrhea.

1. Selective β$_2$-agonists

Ritodrine is a selective β$_2$-agonist with prominent relaxant effect on the uterus. It is approved for suppression of premature labour and for delaying delivery in acute fetal distress. Ritodrine is given as IV infusion in a dose of 50 mcg/min. Dose can be increased after every 10 minutes, till uterine contractions are controlled or maternal pulse rate becomes 120/min. It can be given as intramuscular injection, 10 mg, every 4–6 hours, for 12–48 hours and then orally to keep uterine contractions suppressed.

Salbutamol and **terbutaline**, given as 5–20 mcg/min IV infusion are alternatives to ritodrine.

Isoxsuprine is given by oral or IM route in uncomplicated premature labour and threatened abortion. Oral therapy is started with dose of 20 mg, 6-hourly, and then reduced to 10 mg, three times a day.

ADRs

These drugs may cause cardiovascular and metabolic adverse effects, increasing maternal morbidity.
CVS: Hypotension, tachycardia, arrhythmias, pulmonary edema.
Metabolic: Hyperglycemia, hyperinsulinemia, hypokalemia
Central side effects: Anxiety, restlessness and headache may occur.
Neonate may develop hypoglycemia, pulmonary edema and ileus.

Contraindications

If the mother is diabetic, has heart disease, or is receiving β-blockers/steroids, selective β$_2$-agonists are contraindicated.

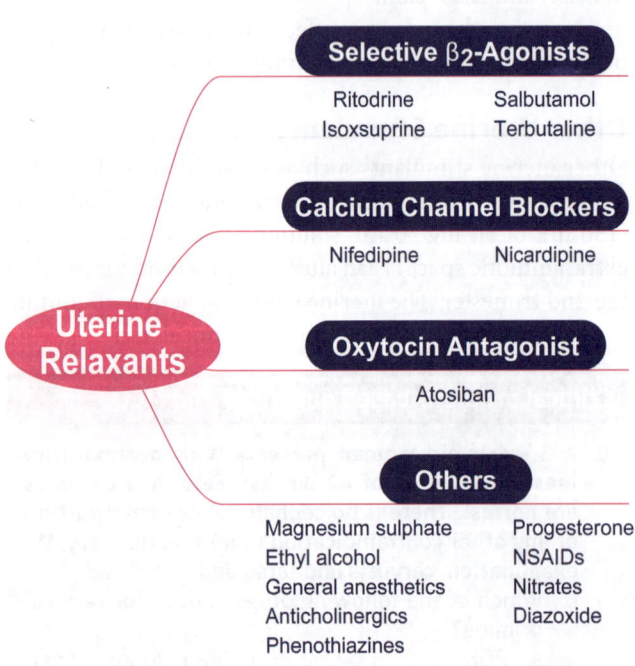

Flowchart 47.2 Classification of uterine relaxants

It is recommended that treatment with ritodrine in acute fetal distress should not be continued beyond 48 hours as fetal outcome does not improve, and there is a risk of adverse effects for the mother.

2. Calcium Channel Blockers

Influx of Ca^{2+} ions plays an important role in uterine contractions. Therefore, Ca^{2+} channel blockers can oppose the contractions and reduce myometrial tone. Dihydropyridines such as nifedipine and nicardipine have prominent smooth muscle relaxant action and can postpone labour if used early. Nifedipine given orally in a dose of 10 mg can be repeated after every 20–30 minutes and then given 6-hourly; this is as effective as selective $β_2$-agonists, with the added advantage of fewer adverse effects. CCBs can cause hypotension, tachycardia, and risk of reduced placental perfusion causing fetal hypoxia.

3. Oxytocin Antagonists

Atosiban is more effective than selective $β_2$-agonists and equally effective as nifedipine in acute treatment of premature labour at 24–33 weeks of gestation. IV infusion of atosiban suppresses premature uterine contractions and postpones preterm delivery. Cardiovascular and metabolic adverse effects are less than seen with selective $β_2$-agonists. ADRs include nausea, vomiting, hyperglycemia, and vasodilatation.

Other Uterine Relaxants

- NSAIDs can also cause uterine relaxation and delay labour, but are not used for this indication; this is because of their unpredictable efficacy, risk of intrauterine closure of ductus arteriosus, and risk of oligohydramnios. However, they are useful in dysmenorrhea, because PGs produced locally in the uterus are largely responsible for it.
- Halothane is used as a general anesthetic when an internal or external version is attempted to correct the fetal presentation/lie, because it has good uterine relaxant action.
- Magnesium sulphate competes with Ca^{2+} ions for passage through voltage-sensitive and ligand-gated Ca^{2+} channels. However, it may increase perinatal mortality, and is not recommended for delaying premature labour.
- Ethyl alcohol given IV can stop labour, but is not useful for this indication as there is risk of marked maternal CNS depression and fetal hypoxia.
- Progesterone decreases the sensitivity of the uterus to oxytocin. It is used in threatened and habitual abortion; however, its efficiency in the absence of progesterone deficiency remains uncertain.
- Nitrites, diazoxide, phenothiazines, etc., also have uterine relaxant action, but their efficacy is so low that they cannot be depended on to delay labour or relieve dysmenorrhea.

Clinical problem-based questions and MCQs

3. A 26-year-old primigravida at 23 weeks of pregnancy presents with pain in abdomen and mild bleeding per vagina. She is diagnosed with threatened abortion. Tab isoxsuprine is prescribed.
    i. Which group does isoxsuprine belong to?
        a. Prostaglandin analogue
        b. Ergot derivative
        c. Selective $β_2$-agonist
        d. Anticholinergic
    ii. Explain the pharmacological basis for administration of isoxsuprine.
    iii. Enumerate the adverse effects of isoxsuprine.

4. Which of the following drugs is not useful in preterm labour, although it can relax uterine muscles?
    a. Ritodrine   b. Nicardipine
    c. Isoxsuprine   d. Magnesium sulphate

5. Which of the following drugs is not a uterine relaxant?
    a. Dinoprost   b. Magnesium sulphate
    c. Ethyl alcohol   d. Nicardipine

Summary

- Drugs causing stimulation or suppression of uterine contractions are useful in varied clinical conditions.
- **Uterine stimulants** include the posterior pituitary hormone oxytocin, its derivatives (desamino oxytocin and carbetocin), ergometrine, methylergometrine, PGE_2, $PGF_{2α}$, 15-methyl-$PGF_{2α}$ and misoprostol.
- Their therapeutic indications are determined by the differences in sensitivity of the pregnant and nonpregnant uterus to different drugs, effect of these drugs on the basal tone of uterine muscles and on the lower uterine segment.
- Oxytocin given by slow IV infusion is the drug of choice for induction and augmentation of labour; it allows relaxation of the uterus between contractions and relaxes the lower part of the uterus, which is favourable during parturition.
- In contrast, methylergometrine is contraindicated before the third stage of labour as it can increase basal tone and contracts lower segment also. However, due to sustained contractions, it is preferred over other drugs for control of PPH in grand multiparas and uterine atony. In severe PPH, however, oxytocin and methylergometrine can be combined.

- Prostaglandins are mainly useful as abortifacients. In first trimester abortions, before 7 weeks of gestation, mifepristone followed by misoprostol is an effective alternative to suction evacuation. If suction evacuation is to be carried out, an intravaginal PGE_2 pessary (gemeprost) increases cervical compliance to dilatation. Cervical priming is useful before inducing labour with oxytocin.
- **Uterine relaxants or tocolytics** include selective β_2-agonists (ritodrine and isoxsuprine), calcium channel blockers (nifedipine and nicardipine), and the oxytocin antagonist atosiban.
- These are indicated in suppression or postponement of preterm labour to allow time for fetal maturation, glucocorticoid therapy for fetal lung maturity and referral of patient to a centre that can care for premature neonates.
- Ritodrine is useful in acute treatment of premature labour for up to 48 hours. Isoxsuprine is useful in threatened abortion. These are associated with many cardiovascular and metabolic adverse effects.
- So, nifedipine, which is equally efficacious and has fewer adverse effects, is a better choice.
- Atosiban is a new drug, a better-tolerated alternative for acute management of preterm labour for up to 48 hours.
- Many other drugs like ethyl alcohol, magnesium sulphate, NSAIDs, progesterone, and diazoxide have a tocolytic effect; however, these are not therapeutically useful in preterm labour.

Questions for practice

1. Explain why:
   a. Oxytocin is the drug of first choice for induction of labour.
   b. Methylergometrine is not useful for induction of labour
   c. Postpartum hemorrhage is prevented by administration of methylergometrine at delivery of anterior shoulder.
   d. Oxytocin is not effective as abortifacient.
2. Enumerate tocolytic drugs and the indications for their use.

Hints for problem-based questions and MCQs

1. i. a. PGE_2
   ii. d. Oxytocin
   iii. Prostaglandins make the cervix soft and compliant; so, they are used for cervical priming. Oxytocin is the first-choice drug for inducing labour as it relaxes the uterus between contractions and does not cause contractions of the lower part of the uterus. This favours fetal descent into the birth canal and childbirth.
2. i. b. Methylergometrine
   ii. As ergots cause sustained contraction of the uterine myometrium and rise in basal tone, the perforated blood vessels get compressed; this is useful in control of PPH. Methylergometrine is more potent than ergometrine for uterine action, whereas other actions are negligible. So, for obstetric indications methylergometrine is preferred over ergometrine.
3. i. c. Selective β_2-agonist
   ii. Selective β_2-agonists have uterine relaxant effect. Because the patient is diagnosed with threatened abortion, uterine relaxants can relax the muscles and help in continuation of pregnancy till fetal maturity for a favourable outcome.
   iii. Selective β_2-agonists can cause hypotension, tachycardia, arrhythmias, hyperglycemia, hyperinsulinemia, hypokalemia and central side effects such as anxiety, restlessness and headache.
4. d. Magnesium sulphate may increase perinatal mortality.
5. a. Dinoprost

CONCEPT MAP – DRUGS ACTING ON THE UTERUS

Drugs that Act on the Uterus

Uterine Stimulants

Oxytocin and Analogues

Mechanism: Acts through G_q-linked receptors & ↑es endometrial PG synthesis.

Action: ↑es force and frequency of uterine contractions.
Fundus and body of uterus contract, but lower segment relaxes
Contracts myoepithelial cells in mammary alveoli → milk ejection
Larger doses → VD → brief fall in BP, flushing and reflex tachycardia.
→ cause ADH-like action & pulmonary edema

Uses: DOC for inducing labour in prematurity, pre-eclampsia, maternal DM, Rh incompatibility, placental insufficiency.
To augment dysfunctional labour in uterine inertia,
Atonic PPH in hypertensive patients
Breast engorgement after delivery.
Oxytocin is **preferred over PG & ergometrine for induction & augmentation** of labour because of consistent effect on uterine contraction, short half-life, relaxation between contractions which maintains fetal oxygenation & relaxation of lower segment that favours fetal descent.

ADRs: No adverse effects at recommended doses and rate.
However, injudicious use may cause maternal and fetal soft tissue injuries, uterine rupture, fetal asphyxia, fetal death, maternal death.

Contraindications: Prematurity, Fetal distress, Cephalopelvic disproportion, Abnormal presentation, Presence of uterine scars & along with sympathomimetic drugs

Desamino oxytocin: Same as oxytocin, but effect is less consistent

Carbetocin: Long-acting analogue, $t_{1/2}$: 90–100 minutes, useful in preventing atonic PPH after LSCS, given IV, only once.

Ergometrine

Mechanism: Agonistic or partial agonistic action at $5-HT_2$ and α-receptors → uterine stimulant action

Actions: Increase the force, frequency and duration of uterine contractions. At higher dose, basal tone is raised and contracture occurs. Sustained contraction results in compression of perforating uterine arteries that stops bleeding → **preferred over oxytocin in PPH**.

Unlike oxytocin ergometrine contracts the lower uterine segment also → can interfere with fetal descent → **never used before delivery**.

High dose causes VC & increases peristaltic activity

Methylergometrine is more potent, so preferred over ergometrine.

Uses: Prevention of PPH in grand multipara, uterine atony, in dose of 0.2–0.3 mg IM at delivery of anterior shoulder.
To control severe, atonic PPH, dose is 0.5 mg, can be combined with 5 mg oxytocin.
To prevent uterine atony after LSCS or instrumental delivery.
Used orally for uterine involution in multipara

ADRs: Nausea, vomiting, rise in BP, decreased milk secretion with high doses

Contraindications: Hypertension, toxemia of pregnancy, sepsis, liver, kidney diseases and before third stage of labour

Prostaglandins

PGE_2, $PGF_{2α}$:
- Cause contraction of pregnant as well as nonpregnant uterus, increase basal tone as well as amplitude of uterine contractions.
- At term they soften the cervix and make it more compliant for delivery.
- Role in initiation and progression of labour

Uses: Mainly used as **abortifacients**
- MTP: up to 7 weeks of gestation, mifepristone 600 mg single dose orally, is followed after 2 days by misoprostol (PG analogue) 400 mg single dose.
- PGE_2 1 mg intravaginal pessary inserted 3 hours before attempting cervical dilatation in first trimester abortions.
- In late abortions such as midterm abortions, missed abortion, and molar pregnancy, PG converts oxytocin-resistant uterus to oxytocin-sensitive.
- For cervical priming, PGE_2 cervical gel administered in cervical canal or vagina to make cervix soft and compliant, before inducing labour with oxytocin.
- PG may be used for induction of labour in patients with toxemia of pregnancy and renal failure, as they do not cause fluid retention.
- Atonic PPH, not responding to methylergometrine or oxytocin, 15-methyl-$PGF_{2α}$ (carboprost) 0.25 mg is given IM

ADRs: Nausea, vomiting, watery diarrhea, uterine cramps, vaginal bleeding, flushing, shivering, fall in BP, tachycardia, fever, malaise, chest pain etc.
- ADRs are negligible after intravaginal administration

Uterine Relaxants

Selective β₂-Agonists

Uses: Ritodrine approved for suppression of premature labour, for delaying delivery in acute fetal distress by IV infusion 50 mcg/minute, can be increased after every 10 minutes till uterine contractions are controlled or maternal PR becomes 120/minute.
Salbutamol & terbutaline may be used as alternatives as 5–20 mcg/minute IV infusion

ADRs: Hypotension, tachycardia, arrhythmias, pulmonary edema.
Hyperglycemia, hyperinsulinemia, hypokalemia
Central side effects like anxiety, restlessness and headache may occur.
Neonate may develop hypoglycemia, pulmonary edema and ileus
Ritodrine use in acute fetal distress should not exceed 48 hours as fetal outcome is not improved and there is risk of adverse effects in mother.

Uses & Contraindications

Uses: Used to suppress premature labour in an effort to buy time for fetus to mature, for starting lung maturation glucocorticoid therapy & for shifting mother to a higher centre.
Threatened abortion
Dysmenorrhea

Contraindications: When delaying labour can be counterproductive e.g. severe toxemia, antepartum hemorrhage (APH), intrauterine infection, ruptured membranes
When cervical dilatation is already > 4 cm and lower segment is taken up or effaced.

CCBs

Nifedipine and Nicardipine → smooth muscle relaxing action → can postpone labour.
As effective as selective β₂-agonists with fewer adverse effects.

ADRs: Hypotension, tachycardia and risk of fetal hypoxia.

Atosiban

Oxytocin antagonist is as effective as nifedipine & more effective than selective β₂-agonists in acute treatment of premature labour

ADRs: Nausea, vomiting, hyperglycemia, vasodilatation

SECTION 9 Drugs Affecting the Endocrine System

48 Male Sex Hormones and Their Analogues

PH 7.6 Describe the types, kinetics, dynamics, adverse effects, indications and contraindications of androgens

---

Learning objectives

A student of MBBS phase II should be able to:
- Enumerate drugs used as male sex hormones and their analogues.
- Describe therapeutic uses, adverse effects of and contraindications to male sex hormones and their analogues.
- Enumerate drugs used as anabolic steroids.
- Enumerate therapeutic uses and adverse effects of anabolic steroids.
- Enumerate drugs having antiandrogenic action, their uses and adverse effects.

MALE SEX HORMONES (ANDROGENS)

The testes perform gametogenic as well as endocrinal functions, namely, spermatogenesis and testosterone secretion, respectively.

- Sperm production (gametogenic function) occurs in the seminiferous tubules of the testes. It is controlled by **follicle stimulating hormone (FSH)** from the anterior pituitary and requires high local testosterone concentration.
- The endocrinal function of the testes is testosterone production from the interstitial or Leydig cells that are scattered between seminiferous tubules. Testosterone secretion is stimulated by **luteinising hormone (LH)** from the anterior pituitary. In normal adult males, 8 mg testosterone is produced daily. 95% of total testosterone production occurs in Leydig cells and 5% in adrenals. After puberty, the normal plasma testosterone level in males is 0.6 mcg/dL. In females, testosterone is derived from the adrenals, ovaries and peripheral conversion of other hormones and levels are low (0.03mcg/dL). The regulatory control of testosterone secretion is depicted in Fig. 48.1.
- In addition to testosterone, the testes also secrete small amounts of dihydrotestosterone, androstenedione and dehydroepiandrosterone (DHEA).
- Negative feedback inhibition of gonadotropin secretion is driven by testosterone, its active metabolite dihydrotestosterone, estradiol, and inhibin, whereas activin stimulates FSH secretion. Both inhibin and activin are secreted by Sertoli cells.

CLASSIFICATION

Androgens can be natural or synthetic, as shown in Flowchart 48.1.

Mechanism of Action

Like other steroidal hormones, testosterone also crosses the cell membrane and binds with cytoplasmic androgen receptors. The hormone–receptor complex is transported to the nucleus and regulates transcription, resulting in growth, differentiation, and synthesis of several enzymes and functional proteins.

Physiological Role/Pharmacological Actions

Androgens have androgenic and anabolic functions.

Androgenic role

1. Testosterone brings about pubertal changes in males which include:
   - Growth of prostate and seminal vesicles, and penile and scrotal growth.
   - Appearance of pubic hair, axillary hair, moustache, beard, body hair, and male pattern of its distribution.

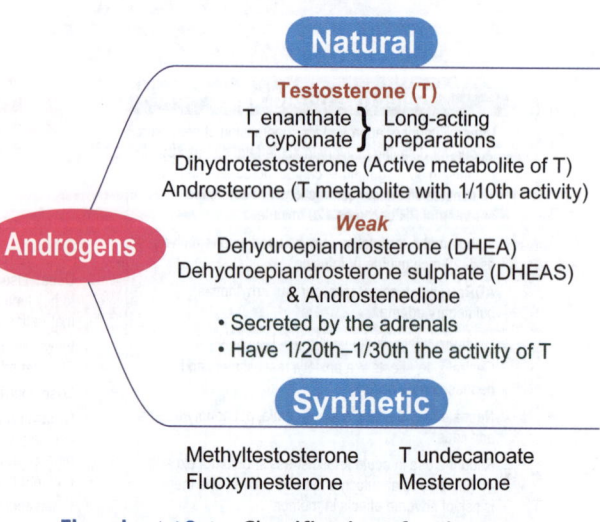

Flowchart 48.1 Classification of androgens

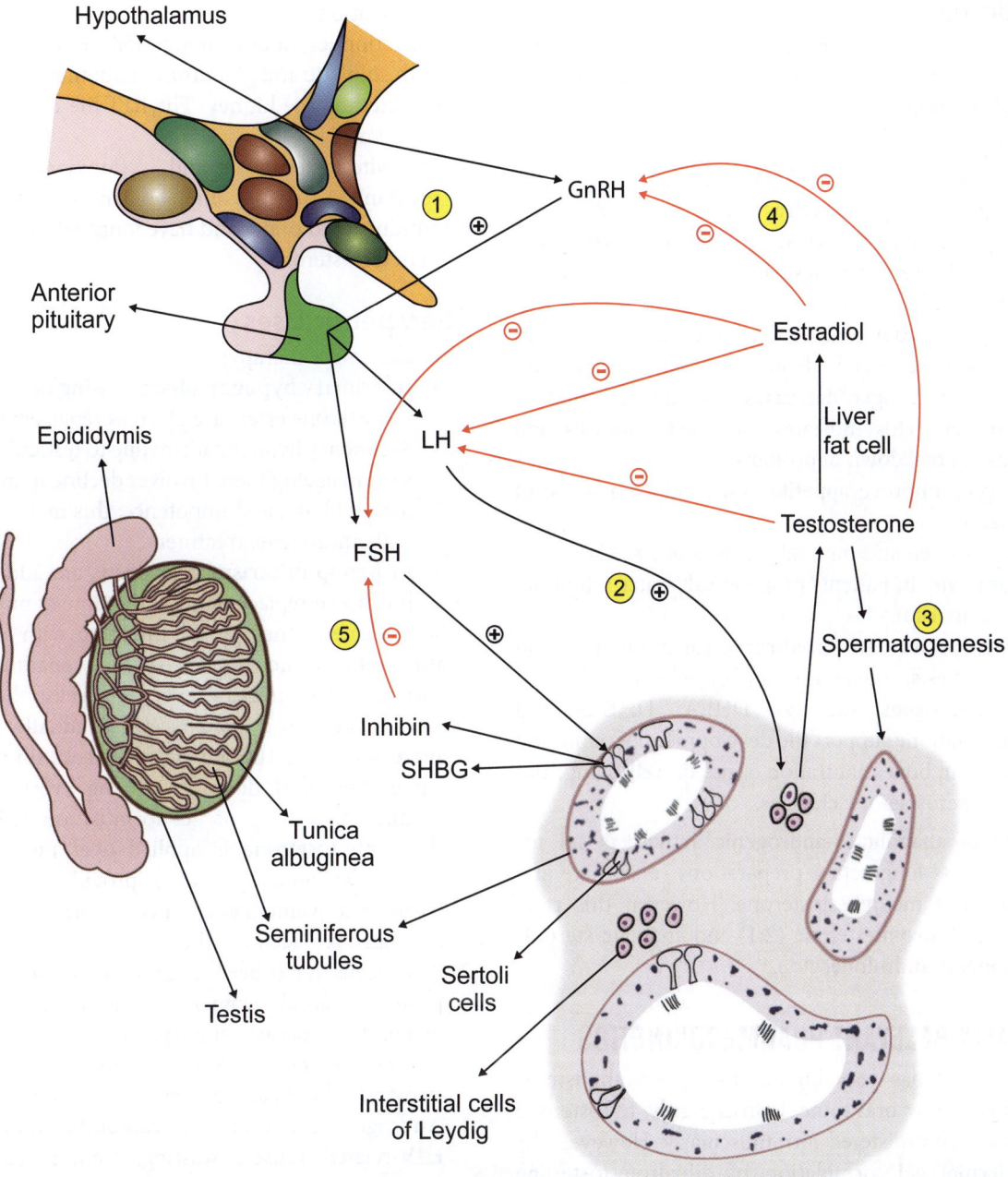

Fig. 48.1 Testosterone secretion and regulation
① GnRH from the hypothalamus causes secretion of Gn (FSH, LH) from the anterior pituitary; ② LH stimulates testosterone production from interstitial cells of Leydig; ③ High testosterone and FSH stimulate spermatogenesis in seminiferous tubules; ④ Negative feedback effect is exerted on GnRH and Gn secretion by testosterone and estradiol (formed from testosterone in fat and liver cells); ⑤ Inhibin secreted from Sertoli cells decreases FSH.

- Thickening and darkening of skin, increased greasiness of skin, especially on the face due to increased activity of sebaceous glands that predisposes to acne.
- Loss of subcutaneous fat, so that veins look prominent.
- Growth of larynx and thickening of vocal cords causing low-pitched voice or hoarsening of voice.
- Behavioural changes such as increased vigour and aggressiveness.

2. Androgens stimulate and maintain sexual function in males.
3. Testosterone is needed in high concentration for normal spermatogenesis and maturation of spermatozoa.
4. Fetal testes produce large amount of testosterone that is needed for the development of male phenotype.
5. Large doses of testosterone in adult males can cause negative feedback inhibition of gonadotropin secretion from the anterior pituitary, resulting in some atrophy of interstitial tissue and testicular tubules.

Anabolic role

Androgens also have an anabolic role; however, the ratio of androgenic-to-anabolic activity varies and determines their clinical utility.

1. Androgens are responsible for the pubertal growth spurt in boys and to a small extent in girls.
2. Bones grow in length as well as thickness. However, after puberty, the epiphyses close and linear growth stops. Estradiol derived from testosterone causes epiphyseal closure in males.
3. Androgens favour muscle building, especially with regular exercise. Lean body mass increases, and urinary excretion of nitrogen decreases, especially in children and women. This indicates increased synthesis and decreased breakdown of proteins.
4. Androgens improve appetite and produce a sense of well-being.
5. Water, nitrogen and minerals such as Na, K, Ca, P, and S accumulate. In patients prone to salt water retention, edema can occur.
6. Testosterone increases erythropoietin production and heme synthesis, accelerating erythropoiesis.
7. Weak androgens such as DHEA, DHEAS and androstenedione support the development of pubic and axillary hair, bone maturation, sense of well-being, and reduce atherosclerotic changes.

The ratio of anabolic-to-androgenic activity is 1:1 for testosterone, its long-acting preparations (enanthate and cypionate) and methyltestosterone. However, this ratio is higher for fluoxymesterone (2:1) and anabolic steroids (nandrolone, oxandrolone, etc.).

CLINICALLY RELEVANT PHARMACOKINETICS

- Testosterone has very high first-pass metabolism → not effective by oral route. Consequently, testosterone esters are administered intramuscularly. However, the transdermal gel formulation of dihydrotestosterone bypasses hepatic first-pass metabolism.
- Testosterone is 98% bound to plasma proteins; 65% is bound to a specific globulin [**sex hormone-binding globulin** (SHBG)] and 33% is bound to albumin. The actions are exerted by 2% free testosterone, which crosses cell membranes to bind with cytoplasmic receptors.
- In tissues such as skin, prostate, seminal vesicles, and epididymis, testosterone is converted into 5α-testosterone by the enzyme 5α-reductase, which brings about the actions.
- In some tissues such as the liver, adipose tissue, hypothalamus and Sertoli cells of seminiferous tubules, testosterone is converted to estradiol by the enzyme P450 aromatase.
- Inactivation of testosterone in the liver involves reduction of double bond, followed by conjugation with sulphate and glucuronic acid; these conjugates are excreted by the kidney. The half-life of testosterone is 10–20 min.
- Methyltestosterone and fluoxymesterone are resistant to first-pass metabolism. Therefore, they are administered orally and have longer duration of action than testosterone.

Therapeutic Uses

1. Replacement therapy:
   - In primary **hypogonadism** causing delayed puberty, testosterone esters are given as replacement therapy.
   - Secondary hypogonadism due to testicular failure, as seen in ageing men, involves decline in muscle mass, loss of libido, and impotence; this may also improve with androgenic treatment.
   - In **hypopituitarism**, androgens are added to other hormonal replacements at the time of puberty.

   Replacement therapy is initiated with long-acting preparations such as testosterone enanthate 50 mg intramuscular, initially every 4 weeks, then every 3 weeks and then every 2 weeks. Gradually, the dose is increased up to 100 mg every 2 weeks till maturation. Then, the adult dose of 200 mg every 2 weeks is continued. 5–10 g of gel formulation (25 mg/g) of dihydrotestosterone is applied over nonscrotal skin, once a day. Such application provides uniform blood levels, is convenient and hence the preferred method of androgen replacement therapy.

2. Androgens have been used in **carcinoma breast** in postmenopausal women, along with estrogens in postpartum **breast engorgement**, and in hormone replacement therapy **(HRT)** for postmenopausal women to increase libido and prevent endometrial bleeding.

3. Androgens are useful in **catabolic conditions** like HIV-related muscle wasting, trauma, surgery, and chronic debilitating diseases to make up for protein loss. However, for these indications, anabolic steroids with high anabolic-to-androgenic activity ratios are preferred over testosterone.

4. Methyltestosterone and stanozolol are useful in **hereditary angioneurotic edema**, because of their stimulant action on complement (C1) esterase inhibitor synthesis.

Adverse drug reactions

1. **In males:**
   - Painful and sustained penile erection occurs in the beginning of therapy, which subsides after sometime.
   - Acne, erythrocytosis, and behavioural changes like aggressiveness, psychological dependence and psychosis may occur.

- Moderate doses for a few weeks may cause reduced testicular size, oligozoospermia, and azoospermia due to negative feedback effect on Gn secretion. Upon stopping therapy, these changes take some time to reverse.
- In elderly males, androgens can cause prostatic hyperplasia and urinary retention.
2. **In females**: Most adverse effects are due to masculinising actions. More than 200–300 mg testosterone per month can cause acne, hirsutism, clitoral enlargement, hoarseness of voice and menstrual irregularities. Administration in pregnant women can cause virilisation of female fetus.
3. **In children**: Administration of androgens for more than few weeks in children causes precocious puberty, early epiphyseal closure, and short stature.
4. In patients with cardiac or renal disease, large doses can cause salt water retention and edema.
5. In patients with liver disease, more testosterone is peripherally converted to estradiol, which can cause gynecomastia and breast pain.
6. Methyltestosterone can cause fall in HDL and rise in LDL levels, reversible cholestatic jaundice and increased risk for hepatic carcinoma.

Contraindications

Androgens are contraindicated in carcinoma prostate, male breast carcinoma, liver disease, kidney disease and pregnancy.

They should be avoided in infants, young children and patients with CHF, migraine and epilepsy.

ANABOLIC STEROIDS

These are compounds that have anabolic-to-androgenic activity ratio greater than 1 (Flowchart 48.2).

Mechanism of Action

The mechanism of action is the same as that of testosterone, i.e., through gene-linked intracellular receptors. However, their anabolic actions are more pronounced in comparison to androgenic actions, i.e., anabolic-to-androgenic activity ratio is greater than 1 (2.5–4:1 for nandrolone and 3–13:1 for oxandrolone).

Therapeutic Uses

1. Anabolic steroids are mainly useful in catabolic states such as during **convalescence** as in:
   - Acute illness
   - Severe trauma
   - After major surgery, etc., to reduce nitrogen loss over short period of time. These drugs improve appetite and produce a sense of well-being.
2. These are useful to counteract glucocorticoid-induced osteoporosis and catabolism. They improve **osteoporosis** secondary to prolonged immobilisation, especially in elderly males. However, bisphosphonates are preferred over anabolic steroids for this condition.
3. These drugs can **reduce frequency of dialysis** in renal failure cases by reducing urea production. However, the benefits are transient in chronic renal failure.
4. Anabolic steroids can be used carefully in **children with suboptimal growth**. They may cause a brief growth spurt. Use for longer than 6 months is not recommended, as they may cause early epiphyseal closure. Somatropin is more suitable for this indication.
5. They can be given for 2–3 months in malignancy-associated and aplastic **anemias**; however, there are reports of development of hepatocellular carcinoma in patients of aplastic anemia these drugs. Therefore, erythropoietin and colony-stimulating factors are a better option than anabolic steroids to induce erythropoiesis.
6. Anabolic steroids are **misused** for improving physical ability and performance in athletes. Therefore, athletes are tested for these drugs in **dope tests**.

Dose

Nandrolone decanoate: 25–100 mg, intramuscularly, every 3 weeks
Oxymetholone: 5–10 mg, once daily, orally
Methandienone: 2–5 mg, OD or BD, orally
Stanozolol: 2–6 mg, orally

Adverse effects and **contraindications** are the same as those for androgens. There is a risk of cholestatic jaundice with stanozolol and oxymetholone.

ANTIANDROGENS

Antiandrogen drugs are shown in Flowchart 48.3.

Danazol

Danazol is an orally active drug that has mild androgenic, anabolic, progestational and glucocorticoid activity.

- It suppresses gonadotropin secretion from the pituitary in both males and females, resulting in inhibition of testicular/ovarian function. Amenorrhea and endometrial atrophy occurs after use for few weeks.
- Danazol inhibits steroidogenic enzymes also, resulting in direct suppression of gonadal function.

Anabolic Steroids: Nandrolone decanoate, Oxymetholone, Oxandrolone, Methandienone, Stanozolol

Flowchart 48.2 Anabolic steroids

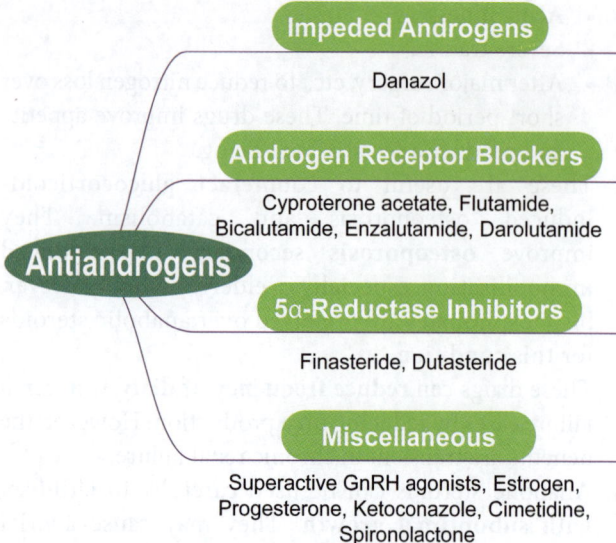

Flowchart 48.3 Antiandrogen drugs

- Danazol binds to androgenic receptors, moves into the nucleus and causes synthesis of some androgen-specific RNA. Therefore, it is called an impeded androgen.

Therapeutic uses
In females
1. **Endometriosis**: Danazol is one of the most effective drugs. It causes marked improvement and promptly relieves dysmenorrhea. Other symptoms like pain, dyspareunia and bleeding respond slowly. Prolonged or permanent relief of symptoms is achieved in more than 50% patients with 3–6 months of danazol therapy. However, androgenic adverse effects are a disturbing feature.
2. **Menorrhagia**: A daily dose of 200 mg of danazol reduces menstrual blood loss. It is continued for 3 months and then stopped. Menstrual blood flow remains low even after discontinuation of danazol. However, oral progestin is preferred for this indication.
3. **Fibrocystic breast disease**: Danazol causes remarkable symptomatic improvement, causing reduced pain, engorgement and nodularity after 3–6 months of use.
4. **Infertility**: Ovulation resumes after withdrawal of danazol after use for 3 months, causing rebound fertility.

In males
5. It has a role in gynecomastia and precocious puberty in boys.

In both genders
6. Like methyltestosterone and stanozolol, danazol has a prophylactic role in hereditary angioneurotic edema. The beneficial effect is mediated through increased synthesis of complement esterase inhibitors.

Adverse effects
Danazol can cause complete amenorrhea with higher dose.
- Androgenic adverse effects like acne, hirsutism, deepening of voice, weight gain, and edema can occur, and are more disturbing in females.
- It can cause hot flushes and night sweats in females and loss of libido in males.
- Other ADRs include GI upset and muscle cramps; hepatic enzymes are elevated.

Cyproterone Acetate
Cyproterone acetate inhibits LH release from the anterior pituitary, leading to reduced testosterone levels. It is beneficial in precocious puberty in boys and for acne/hirsutism in females. However, it is hepatotoxic, and not commonly used in clinical practice.

Flutamide
Flutamide is a nonsteroidal drug that acts as antagonist on androgen receptors. An active metabolite of flutamide is 2-hydroxyflutamide, which blocks androgenic action on accessory sex organs and the pituitary. Flutamide blocks the negative feedback effect of androgens on the pituitary, resulting in raised LH and testosterone levels that may partially overcome its direct antiandrogenic effect. Thus, flutamide is not used as monotherapy. It is always used along with GnRH agonists for **'combined androgen blockade' (CAB)** therapy, or after castration in metastatic carcinoma prostate to check LH and testosterone secretion.

Therapeutic uses
It is used for palliative therapy of carcinoma prostate after castration, or in combination with GnRH agonists. This is known as **combined androgen blockade** (CAB).

In female hirsutism, flutamide may be used along with OCPs.

Adverse effects
Flutamide can cause gynecomastia, breast tenderness and liver damage.

Bicalutamide
It is more potent and longer-acting than flutamide and is suitable for once-a-day administration in metastatic carcinoma prostate. It is also less hepatotoxic than flutamide. Other ADRs are edema, hot flushes and diarrhea.

5α-Reductase Inhibitors
Finasteride and dutasteride are included in this class of drugs

Mechanism of action
Testosterone is converted into its more active form, **dihydrotestosterone (DHT)**, in many tissues such as the

prostate gland and hair follicles. This reaction is catalysed by the enzyme 5α-reductase. Finasteride acts by inhibiting 5α-reductase isoenzyme 2, which is prominent in the male urogenital tract. This results in a lowering of circulating and prostatic DHT levels. LH and testosterone levels remain the same.

Therapeutic uses

- Because of interference with the activation of testosterone, finasteride decreases the size of the prostate gland and improves peak urine flow rate in **benign prostatic hypertrophy (BPH)**. Finasteride, given orally in a dose of 5 mg, once daily, improves the static component of BHP; these effects are seen only after the drug has been used for 6 months and are maintained up to 3 years. Withdrawal of the drug causes regrowth of prostate. It is combined with the uroselective α-blocker **tamsulosin** for this indication. Tamsulosin improves the dynamic component and produces quick symptomatic relief. It also reduces risk of development of carcinoma prostate.
- Finasteride is also useful in male pattern baldness to prevent further hair loss and promote hair growth.

ADRs: It is well-tolerated, but may cause decreased libido, impotence, gynecomastia, and allergic reactions like rashes, swelling of lips, etc.

Dutasteride is similar to finasteride, but it inhibits both isoenzymes 1 and 2 of 5α-reductase in hair follicles and the male urogenital tract, respectively.

Other drugs with antiandrogenic effects

- Estrogen reduces gonadotropin secretion by the negative feedback effect, which then reduces testosterone levels. This effect of estrogen is useful in 'gender affirming hormone therapy', to increase feminine characteristics and suppress masculine features in transgender females.
- Superactive GnRH agonists such as leuprolide, nafarelin, and triptorelin inhibit gonadotropin secretion by desensitisation and down-regulation of GnRH receptors. These are useful in central precocious puberty, both in girls and boys, and are given till 11 and 12 years of age, respectively.
- High doses of ketoconazole interfere with testosterone production by inhibiting the steroidogenic CYP450 enzyme. However, it is not used as an antiandrogen due to toxic effects at high dose.
- Cimetidine displaces dihydrotestosterone from androgen receptors, whereas spironolactone and progesterone have weak antagonistic effect on androgen receptors. However, the antiandrogen effect of these drugs is not clinically useful and manifests as their adverse effects, e.g., impotence, erectile dysfunction, loss of libido and oligospermia.

Clinical problem-based questions and MCQs

1. A 76-year-old male patient presents with difficulty in micturition, hesitancy, urgency, frequency, thinning of stream, and dribbling of urine. Per rectal examination shows prostatic enlargement. PSA is not raised. Patient is prescribed finasteride 5 mg once daily and tamsulosin 0.4 mg, once daily.
    i. What is the probable diagnosis?
        a. Prostate carcinoma
        b. Urinary tract infection
        c. Benign prostatic hypertrophy
        d. Cystitis
    ii. Describe the pharmacological basis for combining finasteride and tamsulosin in this patient.
    iii. Describe the mechanism of action, uses and adverse effects of finasteride.

2. A 53-year-old man complaining of loss of libido, lack of energy, and reduced muscle strength and mass, is on testosterone gel therapy for the last 4 months. What is the likely adverse effect?
    a. Hypotension   b. Stomatitis
    c. Virilisation   d. Breast pain

3. An 82-year-old patient is diagnosed with metastatic carcinoma prostate.
    i. Which of the following drugs are useful in palliative treatment?
        a. Bicalutamide   b. Leuprolide
        c. Both a and b   d. None of the above
    ii. Justify your choice with the pharmacological basis.

4. An 80-year-male patient of carcinoma prostate is administered injection leuprolide IM every month. What is the mechanism of beneficial effect of leuprolide in this case?
    a. It is a GnRH analogue that decreases LH production from the anterior pituitary.
    b. It antagonises the action of gonadotropins on the testes.
    c. It prevents the activation of testosterone.
    d. It induces testosterone inactivation.

5. A 34-year-old female patient complains of chronic pelvic pain and is diagnosed with endometriosis of the uterus, bladder and pelvic wall.
    i. Identify the drug used for symptom control
        a. Finasteride   b. Leuprolide
        c. Danazol   d. Stanozolol
    ii. Justify your choice with the pharmacological basis
    iii. Identify the correct mechanism of action of the selected drug.
        a. Inhibition of aromatase
        b. Androgen receptor blockade
        c. Decreased level of FSH
        d. Inhibition of 5α-reductase

6. Identify the drug useful in precocious puberty in boys.
    a. Stanozolol   b. Methyltestosterone
    c. Mesterolone   d. Cyproterone

7. i. To which of the following pharmacological classes does stanozolol belong?
   a. Anabolic steroid b. Corticosteroid
   c. Impeded androgen d. Antiandrogen
   ii. Name three other drugs in the selected drug class.
   iii. Enumerate the therapeutic uses and adverse effects of these drugs.

8. A 13-year-old athlete wanted to improve his athletic performance, for which he took fortnightly intramuscular injections of nandrolone decanoate 50 mg. What is the most likely consequence if he continues the medication for a year?
   a. Hepatotoxicity   b. Testicular hyperplasia
   c. Psychiatric symptoms d. Epiphyseal closure

9. Which of the following is contraindicated in carcinoma prostate?
   a. Flutamide   b. Mesterolone
   c. Leuprolide   d. All of the above

Summary

- **Testosterone** is an **androgen** secreted by the interstitial cells of Leydig in the testes. Its secretion is influenced by GnRH from the hypothalamus and LH from the pituitary.
- Androgens such as testosterone, methyltestosterone, fluoxymesterone and mesterolone are useful in primary and secondary hypogonadism, idiopathic infertility in males, AIDS-related muscle wasting and hereditary angioneurotic edema.
- ADRs associated with androgens are oligozoospermia, testicular atrophy, edema, cholestatic jaundice, gynecomastia and breast pain in males and acne, hirsutism and menstrual irregularities in females.
- **Anabolic steroids** like nandrolone, methandienone, stanozolol and oxymetholone have more anabolic activity than androgenic activity. These are useful in catabolic states, osteoporosis, refractory anemias and renal insufficiency. Because they improve athletic performance, they are included in dope testing.
- ADRs of anabolic steroids include reduced testicular function, growth stunting due to epiphyseal closure in long bones, gynecomastia, breast pain and virilisation in children. Stanozolol can cause abnormal lipid levels and jaundice.
- Danazol is an **impeded androgen** useful in endometriosis, fibrocystic breast disease, and menorrhagia. It has androgenic adverse effects such as acne, hirsutism, weight gain, edema, and loss of libido in men.
- **Antiandrogens** include androgen receptor antagonists (flutamide and bicalutamide) and 5α-reductase inhibitors (finasteride and dutasteride), which prevent activation of testosterone to DHT.
- Flutamide prevents negative feedback effect of androgens → increased LH levels, which counteracts its direct antiandrogenic effects. So, it is combined with GnRH analogues given continuously to check rise in LH levels. This combination is useful in metastatic carcinoma prostate for palliation as CAB.
- Finasteride checks prostate growth in BPH and improves the static component after about 6 months of use. It is combined with tamsulosin for improving the dynamic component in BPH.

Questions for practice

1. Enumerate the therapeutic uses and adverse effects of:
   a. Methyltestosterone
   b. Anabolic steroids
   c. Antiandrogens
2. Explain why:
   a. Finasteride improves the symptoms of BPH.
   b. Danazol is useful in endometriosis.
   c. Flutamide–leuprolide combination is used in carcinoma prostate.

Hints for problem-based questions and MCQs

1. i. c. Benign prostatic hypertrophy (PSA is not raised, which rules out carcinoma prostate. Symptoms mentioned are not suggestive of UTI or cystitis).
   ii. Finasteride for the static and tamsulosin for the dynamic component. Refer to page 637.
   iii. Finasteride is a 5α-reductase inhibitor that interferes with the conversion of testosterone to DHT. It is useful in BPH and male type baldness. **ADRs**: reduced libido, impotence, gynecomastia and allergic reactions.
2. d. Breast pain and gynecomastia are important adverse effects of testosterone in adults. BP is somewhat raised, and virilisation occurs in the female fetus when androgens are given in pregnancy; stomatitis does not occur with testosterone therapy.
3. i. c. Both (a) and (b). Both bicalutamide and leuprolide are used in combination for metastatic prostate cancer.
   ii. Bicalutamide is an androgen receptor blocker, which increases LH secretion by blocking negative feedback effect of androgen. This can be checked by the GnRH analogue leuprolide; this is called 'combined androgen blockade' therapy (CAB).
4. a. Leuprolide is GnRH analogue that decreases LH production from the anterior pituitary on continued use. This effect reduces the growth of carcinoma prostate.
5. i. c. Danazol
   ii. Danazol decreases gonadotropin secretion from pituitary, inhibiting ovarian function in females.
   iii. Danazol decreases FSH levels.
6. d. Cyproterone has antiandrogenic effects, which makes it beneficial in boys with precocious puberty.
7. i. a. Anabolic steroids
   ii. Nandrolone, methandienone, oxymetholone
   iii. Refer to page 635.
8. d. Premature closure of epiphysis of long bones causes reduced adult height with use of anabolic steroids.
9. b. Mesterolone is contraindicated as androgens increase growth of prostate.

CONCEPT MAP – ANDROGENS & ANTIANDROGENS

ANDROGENS

Actions
- Have androgenic and anabolic actions.
- **Androgenic actions:**
- Needed for development of male phenotype
- Bring about pubertal changes
- Stimulate and maintain sexual function in males
- High concentration is required for normal spermatogenesis and maturation of spermatozoa.
- Large dose in adult males can inhibit Gn secretion → some atrophy of interstitial tissue & testicular tubules.
- **Anabolic actions:**
- Increase length & thickness of bones, favour muscle building, improve appetite and produce a sense of well-being, cause accumulation of water, nitrogen and minerals (Na, K, Ca, P, S) and accelerate erythropoiesis.

Classification
- **Natural androgens:**
- Testosterone (T), T enanthate, T cypionate
- Dihydrotestosterone (DHT), Androsterone
- **Weak androgens:**
- Dehydroepiandrosterone (DHEA)
- Dehydroepiandrosterone sulphate (DHEAS) & androstenedione
- **Synthetic androgens:**
- Methyltestosterone, Fluoxymesterone
- T undecanoate, Mesterolone

Therapeutic Uses
- Replacement therapy
  - in primary & secondary hypogonadism
  - in hypopituitarism, along with other hormonal replacements.
- In breast carcinoma in postmenopausal women,
- Along with estrogens in postpartum breast engorgement and hormone replacement therapy (HRT)
- In catabolic conditions like HIV-related muscle wasting, trauma, surgery, chronic debilitating diseases
- Methyltestosterone, & stanozolol are useful in hereditary angioneurotic edema

ADRs
- **In males:**
- Painful, sustained penile erection, acne, erythrocytosis, behavioural changes.
- Moderate doses may cause reduced testicular size, oligozoospermia, azoospermia → reverse after stopping the therapy.
- Prostatic hyperplasia and urinary retention in elderly
- **In females:**
- Acne, hirsutism, clitoral enlargement, hoarseness of voice and menstrual irregularities.
- **In children:**
- Precocious puberty, early epiphyseal closure and short stature
- **Other ADRs:** Salt water retention, edema, fall in HDL, rise in LDL levels, reversible cholestatic jaundice and increased risk for hepatic carcinoma.

Anabolic Steroids
- Nandrolone decanoate, Oxymetholone, Oxandrolone, Methandienone, Stanozolol have anabolic-to-androgenic activity ratio >1
- **Uses:** In catabolic states like acute illness, severe trauma, major operation
- To counteract glucocorticoid-induced osteoporosis and osteoporosis secondary to immobilisation in elderly males → Bisphosphonates are preferred.
- To cause brief growth spurt in children with suboptimal growth → not to be used for > 6 months.
- To reduce urea production & frequency of dialysis in renal failure cases
- To induce erythropoiesis in malignancy-associated and aplastic anemias → erythropoietin and CSF are better.
- Are misused for improving physical ability and performance in athletes. Therefore, these drugs are tested in 'dope test'

ANTIANDROGENS

5α-reductase Inhibitors
- Finasteride: inhibits 5α-reductase isoenzyme 2 (more prominent in male urogenital tract.) → inhibits activation of testosterone to form DHT.
- **Uses:** BPH: It decreases size of prostate gland and improves peak urine flow rate in BPH, improves static component, given 5 mg orally once daily, effects seen only after 6 months of drug use and are maintained for up to 3 years.
- Also useful in male pattern baldness
- **ADRs:** Decreased libido, impotence, gynecomastia and allergic reactions
- Dutasteride inhibits both isoenzyme 1 and 2 of 5α-reductase enzyme in hair follicles and male urogenital tract, respectively.

Danazol
- Mild androgenic, anabolic, progestational and glucocorticoid activity.
- Suppresses Gn secretion → inhibition of testicular/ovarian function
- Amenorrhea and endometrial atrophy occurs after few weeks of use
- Labelled as impeded androgen as it causes synthesis of some androgen-specific RNA.
- **Therapeutic uses:**
- **In females:** Menorrhagia, endometriosis, fibrocystic breast disease and infertility
- **In males:** Gynecomastia and precocious puberty in boys
- **In both sexes:** Prophylactic role in hereditary angioneurotic edema, mediated through increased synthesis of 'complement esterase inhibitor'
- **ADRs:** complete amenorrhea, acne, hirsutism, deepening of voice, weight gain, edema, hot flushes, night sweats are more disturbing in females.
- Loss of libido in males.
- GI upset, muscle cramps, hepatic enzymes are elevated.

Flutamide
- Blocks negative feedback effect of androgens on pituitary → raised LH and testosterone levels → partially overcome direct antiandrogenic effect.
- So not used as monotherapy, but with GnRH agonists as 'combined androgen blockade' (CAB), for palliative therapy of carcinoma prostate
- Along with OCPs, in female hirsutism.
- **ADRs:** Gynecomastia, breast tenderness and liver damage.
- **Bicalutamide:** Is more potent and longer acting than flutamide, less hepatotoxic.
- ADRs are edema, hot flushes and diarrhea.

SECTION 9   Drugs Affecting the Endocrine System

49 Drugs for Infertility and Erectile Dysfunction

PH 7.6 Describe the types, kinetics, dynamics, adverse effects, indications and contraindications of drugs used in erectile dysfunction.
PH 7.9 Describe drugs used for treatment of infertility.

Learning objectives

A student of MBBS phase II should be able to:
- Enumerate drugs used in the treatment of infertility in males and females.
- Describe the mechanism of action of drugs used in treatment of infertility.
- Mention doses of drugs used for inducing ovulation/spermatogenesis.
- Describe the ADRs of drugs used in the treatment of infertility.
- Enumerate drugs used in erectile dysfunction.
- Describe the mechanism of action and indications for use of drugs for erectile dysfunction.
- Describe adverse drug reactions and contraindications of drugs used in erectile dysfunction.

Infertility is defined as the failure of a couple to conceive even after 12 months of having regular, unprotected sexual intercourse. **Primary** infertility is the failure to conceive for the first time, whereas in **secondary** infertility, patient has conceived at least once in the past, irrespective of the outcome of that pregnancy.

Causes of **male infertility** include reduced sperm count (oligozoospermia), absence of sperms (azoospermia), abnormalities of shape and motility of sperms, and ejaculatory problems. Important causes of **female infertility** include diseases of the uterus, e.g., structural defects, fibroids, endometriosis, polycystic ovary disease (PCOD), anovulatory cycles, tubal blockade due to inflammatory adhesions or pressure by any mass in close vicinity, and hormonal disturbances.

Treatment of infertility is challenging and varies from patient to patient, based on the underlying cause. Moreover, in some cases, the cause of infertility may not be clearly identified.

- Some causes require **surgical treatment**, e.g., structural deformities of the uterus, tubal blockade, and fibroids. Surgical removal of adhesions, scars and cysts may result in restoration of fertility when these are the underlying cause.
- However, some causes of infertility, such as anovulation, endometriosis, polycystic ovarian disease (PCOD) and hormonal disturbances can be managed by drug treatment.

DRUGS USED IN INFERTILITY

Hormonal disturbances are managed with appropriate drugs. For example, infertility associated with thyroid dysfunction, insulin resistance, etc., is managed by correcting the hormonal derangements. Drugs that induce ovulation/spermatogenesis and drugs for endometriosis and PCOD are described herein.

1. Drugs That Induce Oogenesis and Spermatogenesis

Anovulation in females can be caused by hypogonadism and hormonal disturbances (e.g., hyperprolactinemia, estrogen-to-progesterone imbalance), while in males, **oligozoospermia** is usually associated with hypogonadism. Drugs that induce oogenesis and spermatogenesis, such as clomiphene citrate, rHCG, and menotropin can be used in both genders. Mesterolone is used only in males, while bromocriptine, cabergoline, nafarelin and triptorelin have a role in female infertility only.

Drugs useful in both genders

a. **Clomiphene citrate**, an antagonist at estrogen receptors (ERα and ERβ), blocks the negative feedback effect of estrogen on the pituitary, resulting in increased secretion of gonadotropins. This induces ovulation in females and spermatogenesis in males. Thus, clomiphene can be used in both male and female infertility.

Dosage: In males, dose is 25 mg per day, given for 25 days in a month, followed by a gap of 5 days; such a regimen may be continued for 3–6 months. In females, however, the dose is higher, but it is given only for 5 days in each cycle. Clomiphene 50 mg is given orally starting from 5th day of the menstrual cycle, for 5 days. This regimen is repeated for 2 or 3 cycles. If desired results are not obtained, dose may be increased up to a maximum of 200 mg/day. It can be tried for 6 menstrual cycles.

ADRs: Important adverse effects of clomiphene include hot flashes, hyperstimulation of ovary causing multiple pregnancy, polycystic ovaries, vertigo, and allergic dermatitis.

Menotropin or chorionic gonadotropin given with clomiphene for the last two days of its use is reported to increase chances of ovulation in infertile females with anovulatory cycles.

b. **Recombinant human chorionic gonadotropin (rHCG)** and menotropin are used in cases of male and female infertility that fail to respond to clomiphene treatment.
Dosage: In men with hypogonadism and oligozoospermia, first, HCG 1000–2000 IU (intramuscular, 2–3 times in a week) is continued for 3–4 months; HCG stimulates secretion of testosterone. This is followed by menotropin (75 IU of FSH and LH each) given IM, three times a week, to stimulate spermatogenesis. This is continued for about 4–6 months.

In women who have PCOD or anovulatory cycles not responding to clomiphene therapy, menotropin (75 IU each of FSH and LH) is first given intramuscularly daily for 10 days, followed by HCG 5000–10000 IU. In about 3/4th of cases, ovulation occurs within 48 hours of HCG injection.
Adverse effects of gonadotropins include headache, edema, mood changes, hyperstimulation of ovary and allergic reactions

Drugs used in males only

c. **Mesterolone**, an anabolic androgenic steroid, is a dihydrotestosterone derivative. It is preferred over testosterone for idiopathic male infertility as it induces spermatogenesis, but does not cross the blood–brain barrier well. Consequently, feedback inhibition of gonadotropin secretion is less, and its effect on FSH and LH levels is minimal.

Drugs used in females only

d. **Bromocriptine and cabergoline** are D_2 receptor agonists. These inhibit the release of prolactin from pituitary lactotrophs and can be used to induce ovulation in patients with hyperprolactinemia.
ADRs: Bromocriptine frequently causes adverse effects like nausea, vomiting, marked postural hypotension, nasal blockade, behavioural and psychological symptoms. Therefore, cabergoline, which has greater selectivity for pituitary lactotrophs, longer duration of action, and fewer adverse effects is preferred over bromocriptine.
Dose: Cabergoline 0.25 mg (oral, twice a week) lowers the raised prolactin levels to normal range in 2–4 weeks; fertility returns within a year in most cases.

e. **Gonadotropin-releasing hormone agonists (e.g., nafarelin and triptorelin)** can increase gonadotropin (FSH, LH) secretion and induce ovulation, when used in a pulsatile manner. However, to mimic pulsatile physiological secretion, their schedule of administration needs to be very accurate and is complicated. Any error in administration time or frequency can reduce gonadotropin secretion and is counterproductive. So, these are not currently preferred for treatment of infertility.

f. **Aromatase inhibitors** such as letrozole can also induce ovulation. However, they are not preferred for this indication as they can cause adverse effects resembling post-menopausal symptoms.

2. Drugs for Endometriosis

Endometriosis is a chronic problem, characterised by presence of endometrial cells outside the uterus, at ectopic sites in the pelvic or abdominal cavity. These ectopic endometrial cells respond to estrogen and progesterone. Patients commonly complain of abnormalities of menstrual cycle, such as menorrhagia, dysuria, dysmenorrhea, and dyspareunia (i.e., excessive menstrual blood loss, pain during urination, menstruation, and intercourse, respectively). Infertility is common among women with endometriosis. Drugs used in endometriosis include:

a. **Nonsteroidal anti-inflammatory agents** like naproxen and mefenamic acid are commonly employed for pain relief.
b. **Oral contraceptive pills** containing both estrogen and progesterone are given for at least 3 months. This is the preferred method for controlling symptoms of endometriosis.
c. **Continuous administration of progesterone** converts ovulatory cycles to anovulatory cycles and inhibits gonadotropin release, which, in turn, reduces estrogenic activity. Thus, proliferation of ectopic endometrial cells is controlled and symptoms are relieved. Long-term treatment with progesterone for up to 6 months causes regression of the ectopic endometrium and improves fertility. Progesterone is usually well-tolerated. The progesterone-only pill, progestasert, is used frequently.
d. **Gestrinone** is a new progesterone antagonist that is reported to be very effective in endometriosis. It has the same actions and effectiveness as danazol in endometriosis, with fewer adverse effects. It can cause acne, seborrhea, hirsutism, loss of hair, weight gain, etc. as adverse effects.
e. **Gonadotropin-releasing hormone agonists:** Nafarelin 200 mcg given as a nasal spray (twice daily, for maximum 6 months) is also effective in the treatment of endometriosis. Others like triptorelin, goserelin, and leuprolide are also effective. These drugs create a state of medical menopause. Thus, their adverse effects (hot flashes, osteoporosis, decreased libido, depressive symptoms, etc.) resemble menopausal symptoms.

f. **Danazol**, a derivative of ethisterone, has affinity for SHBG and CBG. It binds to androgens, progesterone and glucocorticoid receptors, but not to estrogen receptors. Dehydrogenase and hydroxylase, enzymes involved in steroid synthesis, are inhibited, but not aromatase (which is responsible for estrogen synthesis). Its metabolite, ethisterone, possesses progestational and weak androgenic activity.

Mechanism of action: Danazol inhibits the secretion of gonadotropins from the anterior pituitary, resulting in the suppression of gonadal (testes and ovaries) function. When danazol is continued for a few weeks, endometrial atrophy occurs. This effect of danazol is useful in endometriosis.

Dose: It is given as a single daily dose of 600 mg for first month, then reduced to 400 mg for next 2 months, followed by 200 mg for up to 6 months. Dysmenorrhea associated with endometriosis is quickly relieved; however, other symptoms are controlled gradually with continued use.

ADRs of danazol include weight gain, edema, muscular cramps, hot flashes, decrease in breast size, hirsutism, amenorrhea, and acne. Hepatic damage may occur in patients with liver dysfunction. Even though danazol is effective in controlling symptoms of endometriosis, it is not preferred currently because of frequent and disturbing adverse effects.

g. **Aromatase inhibitors like letrozole and anastrozole** interfere with the final step of estrogen synthesis from testosterone and androstenedione. These may be used in nonresponsive cases of endometriosis, but are not preferred as they carry the risk of causing osteoporosis and menopausal symptoms.

3. Drugs for Polycystic Ovary Disease

Polycystic ovary disease (PCOD) or syndrome (PCOS) is a common endocrinal disorder in females of reproductive age. It runs in families and a variety of genetic and environmental factors are implicated in its causation. Patients of PCOD commonly present with obesity, insulin resistance, hirsutism, anovulation, irregular menstruation, and infertility. Treatment varies depending on the patient's need to conceive and presence of comorbid conditions.

In addition to **lifestyle modifications** such as regular exercise, healthy eating (high protein/low carbohydrate diet) and sleeping patterns, and maintaining good hydration, several drugs are employed for the treatment of PCOD.

- **Insulin-sensitising agents,** notably **metformin**, improves menstrual irregularities, anovulation, hirsutism, obesity, and insulin resistance.
- The **ovulation-inducing agent** clomiphene may be used. Metformin and clomiphene may be used in combination.
- **Rosiglitazone and pioglitazone** can also decrease insulin resistance and hirsutism.
- Topical **eflornithine** reduces growth of unwanted facial hair by irreversible inhibition of ornithine decarboxylase in the skin. It may cause rashes, redness and burning sensation as adverse effects.
- In **PCOD** patients who have already completed their family, **oral contraceptives** may be used. The aldosterone antagonist **spironolactone** can decrease hirsutism. Antiandrogens like **flutamide** and **finasteride** may control acne and hirsutism.

Clinical problem-based questions and MCQs

1. A 36-year-old female patient presents with inability to conceive after 4 years of marriage and regular, unprotected intercourse. Patient gives history of scanty menstruation since menarche and frequent menstrual irregularities. On examination, the patient is overweight for her age and height, BMI is 31 kg/m^2, has thick hair on face, and acne on chin and neck; scalp hair is thin. Skin over nape of neck is thick and dark-pigmented. Patient is anxious and wants to have quick conception. USG shows multiple cysts in both ovaries.
   i. What is the probable diagnosis?
   ii. Enumerate various drugs that may be used in this disease.
   iii. Which of the following antidiabetic drugs is used in such cases?
      a. Glibenclamide   b. Lente insulin
      c. Metformin   d. Acarbose

2. Infertility can be due to oligozoospermia in males and anovulation in females.
   i. Identify the drug that can be used to augment gametogenesis in both sexes.
      a. Mesterolone   b. Cabergoline
      c. Clomiphene   d. Nafarelin
   ii. Describe the mechanism of action of the selected drug in inducing spermatogenesis in males and ovulation in females.
   iii. Mention doses and duration of treatment in both cases.

3. A 36-year-old woman, married for the last 12 years, presents with secondary infertility. Menstrual cycles are regular and painless. No other abnormality is detected in general physical and gynecological examination. The attending gynecologist decides to induce ovulation with drugs.
   i. Which is most suitable drug for this patient?
   ii. Describe the mechanism of beneficial effect and dosage schedule of chosen drug.
   iii. Enumerate the adverse effects of the drug used.

4. A 42-year-old woman, a known case of type 2 DM, presents with galactorrhea, oligomenorrhea, and hirsutism. On examination, patient is obese, BP is 160/100, and changes related to diabetic retinopathy are present. On investigation, her prolactin levels are found to be abnormally raised. Pituitary MRI shows

a microadenoma. Patient was prescribed cabergoline (0.25 mg, twice a week) and called for follow-up after 2 months.
 i. What is the probable diagnosis?
 ii. What is the pharmacological basis of using cabergoline?
 iii. What are advantages of cabergoline over other drugs suitable for this case?
 iv. Which of the following drugs may be useful in this case?
   a. Menotropin b. Clomiphene
   c. Danazol d. Bromocriptine

5. Endometriosis is an important cause of infertility in females. Endometrial tissue is present at ectopic sites in the pelvic and abdominal cavity.
 i. Which of the following drugs is useful in the treatment of endometriosis?
   a. Mesterolone b. Clomiphene
   c. Danazol d. Tamoxifen
 ii. Describe the mechanism of beneficial effect and adverse effects of the chosen drug in endometriosis.
 iii. Enumerate all the drugs that may have a role in the management of endometriosis.

6. Which of the following is useful in male infertility?
   a. Mestranol b. Gestodene
   c. Tamoxifen d. Mifepristone

7. Which of the following is used for induction of ovulation?
   a. Letrozole b. Clomiphene
   c. Exemestane d. Mifepristone

ERECTILE DYSFUNCTION

Erectile dysfunction (ED) is the inability to achieve or maintain penile erection for satisfactory coitus. Normal penile erection involves vasodilatation of cavernosal vessels and filling of cavernosal sinusoids with blood.

Sexual arousal due to any cause results in release of nitric oxide from the endothelium of penile blood vessels. NO increases cGMP levels, leading to inactivation of myosin light chain kinase and relaxation of smooth muscles (Refer to Fig. 34.4, page 454). In the penis, smooth muscles of arteries, arterioles, and cavernosal sinusoids are relaxed and these vessels are filled with blood, resulting in penile erection. cGMP is then inactivated by phosphodiesterase 5 (PDE5) to form 5GMP. PDE5 is selectively present in penile smooth muscles.

ED can have a variety of causes like cardiovascular disease, diabetes mellitus, psychological causes, alcoholism, substance abuse, hypogonadism, and may be drug induced. Common drugs that have the potential to cause erectile dysfunction include antipsychotic drugs (phenothiazines), TCAs, SSRIs, levodopa, phenytoin, carbamazepine, thiazide diuretics, and β-blockers.

Management

The management of erectile dysfunction involves:

- **Psychosexual counselling** has a very important role as psychological causes are responsible for about 15% cases of ED. Alcoholics and drug addicts also benefit from counselling.
- **Discontinuation of the offending drug** may reverse the problem in about one-fourth of ED cases.

DRUG TREATMENT OF ED

Drugs for ED can be given by oral, intracavernosal, intramuscular, and transurethral routes.

- **Oral drugs**
  - Phosphodiesterase 5 (PDE5) inhibitors: Sildenafil, vardenafil, tadalafil, udenafil, and avanafil.
  - Others: Yohimbine, trazodone, apomorphine, and bromocriptine are rarely used.
- **Intracavernosal injections**
  - PIPE therapy, i.e., papaverine/phentolamine-induced penile erection
  - Alprostadil (PGE$_1$)
  - Thymoxamine
  - Aviptadil
- **Transurethral pellets**
  - Alprostadil pellet used as **medicated urethral system for erection** (MUSE).
- **IM injections**
  - Testosterone

A. Oral Drugs for ED

1. PDE5 inhibitors

Sildenafil, vardenafil, tadalafil, udenafil, and avanafil are orally administered PDE5 inhibitors. They are the **first-line drugs** for ED in current clinical practice because of the convenience of oral administration and good efficacy.

Mechanism of action

The PDE5 enzyme, selectively present in penile smooth muscles, is responsible for the inactivation of cGMP. Drugs like sildenafil inhibit this enzyme and interfere with the conversion of cGMP to 5GMP. Thus, the smooth muscle relaxing effect of cGMP lasts longer. Vasodilatation of cavernosal vessels and filling of cavernosal sinusoids with blood results in good penile erection.

Sildenafil is 70 times more selective for PDE5 than other isoforms PDE1, 2, 3, and 4. However, higher doses can cause PDE6 inhibition in eyes, resulting in difficulty to distinguish between green and blue colours.

PDE5 inhibitors are not effective if erectile disorder is associated with loss of libido or neurogenic causes (such as spinal cord injury). These drugs have no aphrodisiac action (i.e., they do not increase sexual pleasure and satisfaction).

Oral bioavailability of sildenafil is 40% and its effect lasts for about 4 hours.

Uses

- **Male erectile dysfunction (MED)**: Sildenafil is used in a dose of 25–50 mg, given orally, an hour before intercourse. It may be repeated in case of inadequate response; however, the total dose in 24 hours should not exceed 100 mg.
- **Pulmonary hypertension**: NO plays an important role in regulating the tone of pulmonary vasculature. NO-induced vasodilatation of pulmonary blood vessels is augmented by PDE5 inhibitors, especially sildenafil. Thus, it is useful in pulmonary hypertension in neonates with congenital heart disease.

Adverse effects

- Due to vasodilatation: Headache, nasal stuffiness, facial flushing, hypotension, dizziness.
- Reduced tone at lower esophageal sphincter causes dyspepsia and gastro-esophageal reflux.
- In some patients with leukemia, sickle cell anemia, etc., it may cause prolonged/persistent/painful penile erection called priapism, which may be reversed by α-agonists.
- PDE6 inhibition in eye causes problems in blue–green discrimination.
- In patients of nonarteritic anterior ischemic optic neuropathy (NAION) or retinitis pigmentosa, these drugs may cause sudden loss of vision.

Contraindications

In patients of angina and MI on nitrate therapy, the vasodilator effect of nitrates is potentiated. Profound vasodilatation and tachycardia in such patients has caused some sudden deaths. So, PDE5 inhibitors are contraindicated in patients with IHD on nitrate therapy. If it is used, there should be a gap of at least 24 hours between administration of nitrates and sildenafil.

- Because sildenafil is metabolised by CYP3A4, it should not be used in patients receiving enzyme inhibitors like ketoconazole, verapamil, and cimetidine.
- Peptic ulcer, liver dysfunction, impaired renal function, NAION and retinitis pigmentosa are other contraindications for using these drugs.

Tadalafil is more potent and longer-acting than sildenafil. The required gap after nitrate usage is therefore longer, i.e., 3 days. It is used in erectile dysfunction (ED) in patients of prostatic hypertrophy. Backache and myalgias may occur with its use.

Vardenafil is similar to sildenafil. However, its onset of action is in 30 minutes and so can be used 30 minutes before intercourse. It has potential to prolong the QT interval.

Udenafil also has rapid onset and long duration.

Avanafil is the fastest-acting; action starts within 15–30 minutes and lasts for 36 hours. As a result, it is called the **weekend pill**.

2. Other oral drugs for ED

Yohimbine

It is an α_2-selective blocker that increases noradrenaline release. It was traditionally used in South Africa as an aphrodisiac and dietary supplement. It is proposed to be useful for erectile dysfunction as it increases blood flow and nerve impulses to the penis. It is useful orally, alone or in combination with sildenafil, in a dose of 5–15 mg. However, it can cause ADRs like tachycardia, hypertension, tremors, insomnia, headache, anxiety, nausea, and diarrhea.

Trazodone

Trazodone is a sedative, antidepressant drug. It is used empirically in erectile dysfunction. The response to trazodone is reported to be higher in younger subjects, in psychogenic ED, and when the duration of ED is <12 months. The efficacy of trazodone in ED is greater at higher doses of 150–200 mg/day. Important ADRs include dryness of mouth, sedation, fatigue and dizziness.

Apomorphine

It is a dopaminergic agonist with greater affinity for D_2 receptors in the paraventricular nucleus in hypothalamus. Activation of these receptors is known to generate erectogenic signals. It is effective in ED in a dose of 2–3 mg, sublingually. Important ADRs are nausea, vomiting and vasovagal syncope.

Bromocriptine

Bromocriptine is another orally effective dopaminergic drug reported to improve frequency and quality of erections in males on maintenance hemodialysis, provided their serum testosterone values are within normal range. However, its use is associated with frequent adverse effects like nausea, vomiting, nasal blockade, hypotension, and syncope. Long-term use may cause behavioural and psychotic symptoms.

B. Drugs Given as Intracavernosal Injections

1. Alprostadil (PGE1)

Alprostadil is a PGE_1 analogue. It can be given as an intracavernosal injection with a fine needle. Penile erection after alprostadil injection in the cavernosum lasts for 1–2 hours. It causes less local pain than papaverine injections. Risk of priapism and fibrosis is also lower when compared to PIPE therapy. Therefore, alprostadil is a **second-line drug** for patients in whom sildenafil is contraindicated or gives no response.

2. PIPE therapy

Papaverine/phentolamine-induced penile erection (PIPE) therapy: Papaverine is an opium alkaloid with prominent antispasmodic action. The exact mechanism of its action is not well understood, but it probably acts by inhibiting PDE enzyme, raising levels of cAMP and cGMP and smooth muscle relaxation. It is a selective inhibitor of PDE10A subtype, which is present in the brain striatum. Inhibition of this enzyme subtype is demonstrated to cause motor and cognitive deficits in mice. Papaverine is used to reverse visceral spasms of the gastrointestinal tract, bile ducts, and ureter, e.g., acute mesenteric ischemia. Papaverine is also useful in subarachnoid hemorrhage and coronary artery bypass surgery (CABS), due to its cerebral and coronary vasodilator actions, respectively.

Injection of papaverine into the penile cavernosal tissue exerts direct smooth muscle relaxant action, resulting in filling of corpus cavernosal sinusoids with blood, achieving penile erection. Papaverine may be used alone in a dose of 3–15 mg or along with α-blocker phentolamine (0.5–1 mg) for this indication.

ADRs of papaverine commonly include constipation, tachycardia, somnolence, vertigo and increased levels of alkaline phosphatase and serum transaminase. Intracavernosal PIPE therapy may cause pain and priapism, which is reversible with α-agonist phenylephrine. Local tissue damage, hematoma and infection can occur. Chronic, repeated use may cause penile fibrosis and permanent damage. It is used only in patients who do not respond to first-line (oral PDE5 inhibitors) and second-line (alprostadil) therapy.

3. Thymoxamine

Thymoxamine or moxisylyte is the only $α_1$ adrenergic receptor antagonist useful for ocular indications. It is useful in ED due to its vasodilator action.

4. Aviptadil

Aviptadil is an analogue of vasoactive intestinal peptide (VIP) that causes visceral smooth muscle relaxation; it can be used alone or with phentolamine by the intracavernosal route in ED.

C. Drugs Given as Transurethral Pellet

Alprostadil pellet can be used as a **medicated urethral system for erection** (MUSE). It is inserted through the urethra with a plunger (after passing urine), in a dose of 250–1000 mcg per application. The first application should be carried out under supervision, as there is a risk of hypotension, vasovagal shock, bleeding and priapism. Urethral burning may also occur.

D. Drugs Given by IM Route

Testosterone intramuscular injection is useful to improve ED only in patients with testosterone deficiency. However, nowadays, dihydrotestosterone (25 mg/g) gel formulation, once a day application over nonscrotal skin is preferred.

Clinical problem-based questions and MCQs

8. A young man visits psychiatry OPD for treatment of impotence. On careful history and examination, patient is diagnosed to have psychogenic erectile dysfunction. It is decided to start oral drug therapy along with psychosexual counseling. Name all the drugs which can be given orally in ED.

9. Which of the following drugs cannot be given orally to treat erectile dysfunction?
    a. Sildenafil   b. Bromocriptine
    c. Alprostadil   d. Trazodone
    i. By which routes can the selected drug be used in this case?
    ii. Enumerate the adverse effects of the selected drug.

10. i. Name the orally effective first-line drugs for a patient complaining of erectile dysfunction.
    ii. Describe the mechanism of action, adverse effects and contraindications for use of these drugs.

11. i. Identify the PDE5 inhibitor that is called the weekend pill.
    a. Udenafil   b. Avanafil
    c. Sildenafil   d. Vardenafil
    ii. Why it is called the weekend pill?

12. Match each drug to its mechanism that makes it useful in ED
    a. Alprostadil   (1) D_2 receptor agonist
    b. Avanafil   (2) PGE_1 analogue
    c. Apomorphine   (3) $α_2$ blockade
    d. Yohimbine   (4) PDE5 inhibition

Summary

- **Infertility** is the inability to conceive in spite of regular, unprotected coitus for 12 months.
- Treatment is challenging and depends upon the underlying cause.
- Most commonly, **clomiphene** is used to induce ovulation. It is useful in males also to treat oligozoospermia. It can cause hot flushes, hyperstimulation of ovary causing multiple pregnancy, polycystic ovaries, vertigo, allergic dermatitis, etc., as adverse effects.
- In patients unresponsive to clomiphene, **rHCG** and menotropin can be tried. Headache, edema, mood changes, hyperstimulation of ovary, and allergic reactions can occur as adverse effects of gonadotropins.
- **Menotropin or chorionic gonadotropin** can be given with clomiphene for the last two days of its use to increase chances of ovulation in infertile females with anovulatory cycles.

- Patients with infertility due to PCOD are given **metformin** alone or in combination with clomiphene.
- Endometriosis is also an important cause of infertility and responds to treatment with **OCPs, progesterone alone for continuous use, danazol**, NSAIDs, etc.
- In patients with hyperprolactinemia due to drugs or pituitary adenoma, cabergoline, a dopaminergic agonist, is used. It is preferred over bromocriptine as it is better tolerated, is more selective for pituitary lactotrophs, and has longer duration of action.
- **Erectile dysfunction** in males can be due to variety of causes. Psychosexual counselling has an important place in the management of this condition.
- Orally used **PDE5 inhibitors** like **sildenafil** are first-line drugs for ED. However, these can potentiate the effect of nitrates and are contraindicated in IHD patients on nitrate therapy. Many other oral drugs are also tried and used empirically (trazodone, apomorphine, yohimbine, etc.).
- In patients unresponsive to to first-line PDE5 inhibitors, **alprostadil, a PGE$_1$ analogue** is given via intracavernosal injections or transurethral pellets. PIPE therapy with local injection **of papaverine** (an opium alkaloid with prominent smooth muscle relaxing action) and α-blocker **phentolamine** into cavernosal sinusoids is useful, but is associated with many adverse effects (pain at injection site, fibrosis, risk of priapism).
- IM **testosterone** is effective only in patients with deficiency of this hormone as the underlying cause of erection problem. However, topical gel formulation of DHT is preferred.

Questions for practice

1. Enumerate the drugs that have a role in the treatment of:
   a. Endometriosis
   b. PCOD
2. Comment on the role of the following drugs in the treatment of infertility in males and females.
   a. Clomiphene
   b. GnRH analogues
   c. rHCG
   d. Menotropin
3. Describe the mechanism of action, adverse effects and contraindications for the use of sildenafil.
4. Explain why:
   a. Sildenafil is a first-line drug in the management of MED.
   b. Sildenafil is contraindicated in patients with ischemic heart disease on nitrate therapy.
   c. PIPE therapy is rarely used now-a-days.
   d. First administration by MUSE should be under supervision.

Hints for problem-based questions and MCQs

1. i. This is a case of polycystic ovarian disease or syndrome
   ii. Insulin-sensitising drugs (metformin, rosiglitazone), ovulation-inducing drug (clomiphene), aldosterone antagonist (spironolactone), antiandrogens (flutamide, finasteride) and OCPs may have a role in treatment of this condition. In this specific case, however, because the patient presents with infertility, clomiphene and metformin will be preferred.
   iii. c. Metformin, as it improves insulin sensitivity.
2. i. c. Clomiphene can be used in both male and female infertility.
   ii. Blocks estrogen receptors → prevents negative feedback effect of estrogen on pituitary → increased gonadotropin secretion → induces ovulation/spermatogenesis.
   iii. Refer to page 640.
3. i. Clomiphene
   ii. Refer to page 640.
   iii. Refer to page 640.
4. i. Patient has microadenoma of pituitary with hyperprolactinemia
   ii. Cabergoline acts as a D$_2$ agonist at pituitary lactotrophs and decreases prolactin secretion. Cabergoline 0.25 mg, given orally, twice a week, lowers raised prolactin levels to the normal range in 2–4 weeks.
   iii. Refer to page 641.
   iv. d. Bromocriptine
5. i. c. Danazol
   ii. Danazol inhibits the secretion of gonadotropins from the anterior pituitary resulting in suppression of gonadal (testis and ovaries) function. When danazol is continued for a few weeks, endometrial atrophy occurs. This effect of danazol is useful in endometriosis.
   ADRs of danazol: refer to page 642.
   iii. NSAIDs, oral combined contraceptive pill, progesterone-only pill, danazol, gestrinone, and nafarelin may have beneficial effect in endometriosis.
6. a. Mestranol
7. b. Clomiphene
8. PDE5 inhibitors (sildenafil, vardenafil, tadalafil), yohimbine, trazodone, apomorphine, bromocriptine
9. i. c. Alprostadil
   ii. It can be used as intracavernosal injection or transurethral pellet
   iii. Adverse effects of alprostadil: pain at injection site, priapism, fibrosis
10. i. First-line drugs in ED, effective by oral route are PDE5 inhibitors like sildenafil, vardenafil, and tadalafil.
    ii. Sildenafil causes selective PDE5 inhibition, resulting in decreased metabolism of cGMP. So, vasodilator effect of cGMP in cavernosal vessels and sinusoids lasts longer, achieving adequate penile erection.
    ADRs of PDE5 inhibitors: refer to page 644.
    Contraindications: refer to page 644
11. i. b. Avanafil
    ii. It is called the weekend pill because of its fast onset (within 15 min) and long duration (up to 36 hours) of action.
12. a–2; b–4; c–1; d–3.

CONCEPT MAP – DRUGS FOR INFERTILITY

In both Males & Females

Clomiphene citrate: ERα & ERβ antagonist → blocks negative feedback effect of estrogen on pituitary, resulting in increased Gn secretion → induces ovulation/spermatogenesis.

Dose: In males is 25 mg/day, for 25 days in a month → gap of 5 days, regimen continued for 3–6 months.

In females 50 mg/day for 5 days starting from 5th day of menstrual cycle → repeated for 2 or 3 cycles. Maximum dose 200 mg, for maximum 6 months.

rHCG, Menotropin: Used in male and female infertility unresponsive to clomiphene treatment.

In Males Only

Mesterolone: DHT derivative → induces spermatogenesis → preferred over testosterone for idiopathic male infertility
Does not cross blood–brain barrier → less feedback inhibition of Gn secretion.

In Females Only

Bromocriptine and Cabergoline: D_2 agonists → inhibit release of PRL from pituitary lactotrophs → used to induce ovulation in patients with hyperprolactinemia.
Cabergoline preferred over bromocriptine due to greater selectivity for pituitary lactotrophs, longer duration of action and fewer adverse effects.
Nafarelin, Triptorelin: GnRH agonists increase Gn (FSH, LH) secretion and induce ovulation, when used in a pulsatile manner → their schedule of administration needs to be very accurate and is complicated → not preferred.
Letrozole: Aromatase inhibitor → induce ovulation
Can cause adverse effects resembling post menopausal symptoms → not much used for infertility.

Drugs that Induce Ovulation/Spermatogenesis

Treatment

Varies based on cause
Surgical treatment for structural deformities of uterus, adhesions, tubal blockade, fibroids
Drugs for anovulation, endometriosis, PCOD and hormonal disturbances

Types & Causes

Primary, Secondary
Causes of male infertility
Oligozoospermia, azoospermia, abnormal shape /motility of sperms and ejaculatory problems
Causes of female infertility
Structural defects, fibroids, endometriosis, PCOD, anovulatory cycles, tubal blockade

Drugs for Endometriosis

Endometriosis is characterised by presence of endometrial cells outside uterus at ectopic sites in pelvic or abdominal cavity.
NSAIDs are used for symptom relief.
OCPs for at least 3 months, preferred for controlling symptoms
Long-term treatment with **Progesterone** only, for up to 6 months → regression of ectopic endometrium and improves fertility.
Danazol: Inhibits Gn secretion → suppression of gonadal function. Causes endometrial atrophy after few weeks of use. Effective but not preferred due to frequent ADRs like weight gain, edema, muscular cramps, hot flushes, decrease in size of breast, hirsutism, amenorrhea, acne & hepatic damage.
Gestrinone, a progesterone antagonist, is as effective as danazol with fewer adverse effects.
Nafarelin, a GnRH agonist, given as nasal spray for maximum 6 months is effective.
Letrozole, Anastrozole may be used in non-responsive cases of endometriosis, but not preferred as they carry risk of causing osteoporosis and menopausal symptoms.

DRUGS FOR INFERTILITY

Management of Erectile Dysfunction

Psychosexual counseling
Discontinuation of offending drugs like phenothiazines, TCAs, SSRIs, levodopa, phenytoin, carbamazepine, thiazide diuretics, and β blockers may reverse the problem
Drug for ED include drugs used by oral, intracavernosal, intramuscular, transurethral routes.

Drugs for Erectile Dysfunction

Drugs for PCOD

Insulin-sensitising agents, notably **metformin**, improve menstrual irregularities, anovulation, hirsutism, obesity and insulin resistance. **Rosiglitazone, pioglitazone** can also decrease insulin resistance and hirsutism.
Ovulation-inducing agent clomiphene may be used. Metformin and clomiphene may be used in combination.
Topical eflornithine reduces growth of unwanted facial hair by irreversible inhibition of ornithine decarboxylase in skin. It may cause rashes, redness and burning sensation
Oral contraceptives may be used in patients who have already completed their family.
Spironolactone, aldosterone antagonist can decrease hirsutism.
Antiandrogens like flutamide, finasteride may control acne and hirsutism.
In case of infertility associated with hormonal disturbances like thyroid dysfunction, insulin resistance etc., treatment of cause improves the fertility also.

Oral Drugs

Phosphodiesterase 5 inhibitors (PDE5 inhibitors): Sildenafil, Vardenafil, Tadalafil, Udenafil, Avanafil
Others: Yohimbine, Trazodone, Apomorphine, Bromocriptine
Intracavernosal injections:
PIPE therapy, i.e., papaverine/phentolamine-induced penile erection: Alprostadil (PGE_1), Thymoxamine, Aviptadil
IM injection: Testosterone
Transurethral pellet: Alprostadil

PDE5 Inhibitors

Sildenafil, Vardenafil, Tadalafil, Udenafil, Avanafil
Prolong VD effect of cGMP → therapeutic response
ADRs: Headache, nasal stuffiness, facial flushing, hypotension, dizziness.
Dyspepsia, and gastro-esophageal reflux.
Problems in blue–green discrimination, may cause sudden loss of vision.
In some patients with leukemia, sickle cell anemia etc., it may cause prolonged/persistent painful penile erection called priapism (which may be reversed by α agonists).
Contraindications: IHD patients on nitrate therapy. If used, there should be a gap of atleast 24 hours between administration of nitrates and sildenafil.

SECTION 9 Drugs Affecting the Endocrine System

50 Drugs for Osteoporosis

PH 7.2 Describe the types, kinetics, dynamics, therapeutic uses, and adverse drug reactions of drugs used in osteoporosis. Devise management plans for a female and male patient with osteoporosis.

Learning objectives

A student of MBBS phase II should be able to:
- Enlist drugs that have a role in the treatment of osteoporosis.
- Describe the mechanism of action of various drugs used in osteoporosis.
- Enumerate uses, ADRs and contraindications of drugs used in osteoporosis.
- Devise management plans for a female and male patients with osteoporosis.

The human skeleton contains two types of bones: 80% is cortical bone, which is the dense outer part, while the remaining 20% is trabecular bone, which forms the inner meshwork. Cortical bone is mainly present in the shaft of long bones of limbs, while trabecular bone is predominantly present in the epiphyses of long bones, iliac crest and vertebrae. A gradual increase in bone mass occurs until the early thirties, but thereafter, with increase in age, bone mass decreases slowly.

Remodelling of bones is the continuous lifelong process of bone resorption and renewal. The process of bone remodelling involves a balanced activity of bone resorption by osteoclasts and new bone formation by osteoblasts. Millions of small remodelling units are active on the surface of bone trabeculae and Haversian canals. The process of bone remodelling is depicted in Fig. 50.1.

- Osteoclasts (bone resorbing cells) are derived from monocytes. Osteoclast precursor cells have receptors for activation of nuclear factor κB (RANK) on their surface.
- The specific ligand for these receptors (called RANKL) is secreted by activated osteoblasts.
- Binding of RANKL to its receptors (RANK) activates the formation of mature, multinucleated osteoclasts, which have a ruffled surface and possess bone lysing effect.
- Mature osteoclasts release acid and proteolytic acid hydrolases, which help in digging 'resorption pits' on the bone surface.
- Once the resorption pit is formed, bone marrow stem cells form pre-osteoblasts that migrate to the base of the pit and get converted to mature osteoblasts. These osteoblasts lay down osteoid or new bone that gets mineralised. Thus, bone resorption is always followed by laying down of bone. The whole cycle takes about 4–6 months.
- Osteoblasts secrete osteoprotegerin (OPG), which binds with RANKL and prevent their binding to RANK, resulting in reduction in osteoclastic activity.

Thus, osteoclastic activity is regulated by osteoblasts through the secretion of two proteins, namely RANKL (which increases osteoclastic activity) and OPG (which decreases osteoclastic activity). This finely balanced remodelling process can be affected by various lifestyle factors, hormones, and drugs, e.g., parathormone and calcitriol induce RANKL production from osteoblasts, thereby favouring bone resorption, but calcitonin directly inhibits bone resorption.

OSTEOPOROSIS

Osteoporosis is a metabolic disorder characterised by an imbalance between bone resorption and bone formation during the remodelling process. Bone deficit occurring over several years results in osteopenia (reduced bone mass), decreased bone density, disturbance of micro-architecture, bone pains, vertebral collapse, loss of height and fractures upon minimal trauma or without trauma (spontaneous fractures). Trabecular bone, being more metabolically active than cortical bone, is more prone to metabolic disturbances and osteoporotic changes. Therefore, sites with predominantly trabecular bone (e.g., vertebrae, wrists and hips) show more frequent spontaneous fractures. The diagnosis of osteoporosis is confirmed by DEXA (dual-energy X-ray absorptiometry), which assesses the decrease in bone mass density (BMD).

Risk Factors for Osteoporosis

The important risk factors include:
- Lack of estrogen in post-menopausal period
- Inadequate dietary intake of calcium and vitamin D
- Increasing age

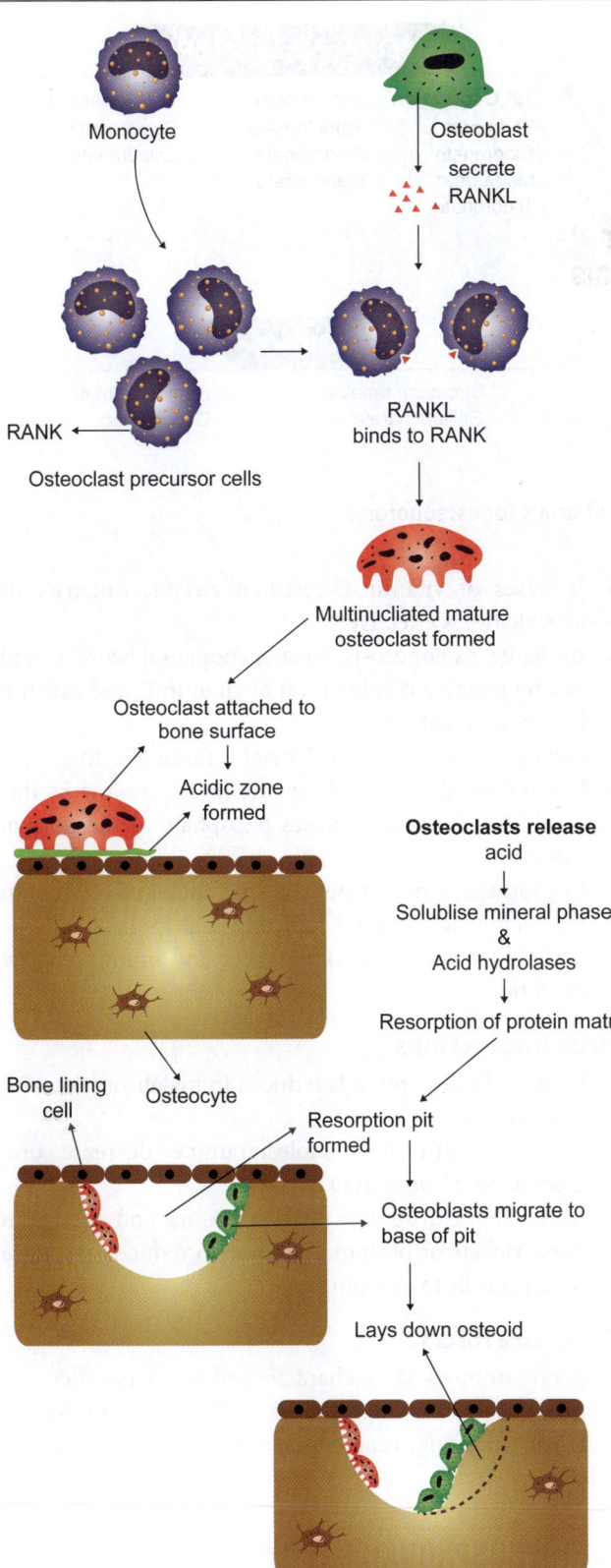

Fig. 50.1 Process of bone remodelling

- Lifestyle factors such as lack of physical activity, smoking, alcoholism and excessive caffeine intake
- Diseases like vitamin D deficiency, malnutrition, scurvy, rheumatoid arthritis, hyperparathyroidism, leukemias, and gastrointestinal, hepatic and renal diseases
- Drugs like corticosteroids, thyroxine and phenobarbitone

DRUGS USED IN OSTEOPOROSIS

Drugs that may be beneficial in osteoporosis are shown in Flowchart 50.1. These include dietary supplements (calcium, vitamin D), bisphosphonates, and hormonal drugs.

A. DIETARY SUPPLEMENTS

1. Calcium

Calcium is stored in bones as crystalline hydroxyapatite deposited on bone matrix osteoid. Calcium alone or in combination with vitamin D_3 has only an adjuvant role in the treatment of osteoporosis with bisphosphonates or hormone replacement therapy. The aim of calcium intake is to ensure that its levels are adequate for supporting bone mineralisation. Reportedly, calcium and D_3 supplements given without other drugs do not decrease the risk of fractures in patients on an adequate diet. Also, the beneficial effect of calcium, if any, is limited to cortical bones and in subjects having inadequate dietary intake.

Calcium preparations used for oral supplementation include calcium carbonate, calcium citrate, calcium gluconate, calcium lactate and calcium dibasic phosphate. The dose of calcium varies with age.

- For children up to the age of 10, the dose is 0.8–1.2 g/day.
- For pregnant, lactating, and post-menopausal women without HRT, the dose is 1.5 g/day.
- For post-menopausal women on HRT, the dose is 1.0 g/day.

Phytates, phosphates, oxalates and tetracyclines form complexes with calcium in the intestine and interfere with its absorption. Other drugs like glucocorticoids and phenytoin also decrease calcium absorption.

Other uses of calcium

Calcium gluconate is injected intravenously for immediate treatment of tetany, dermatoses, paresthesias and weakness. Oral calcium carbonate is used as an antacid.

Adverse effects

Oral calcium is usually well tolerated. Sometimes, constipation and abdominal bloating may occur.

2. Vitamin D

Vitamin D exists in three forms: D_1, D_2 and D_3.
- Vitamin D_1 is obtained from food.
- Vitamin D_2 is present in irradiated food, yeast, fungi, bread, milk, etc.
- Vitamin D_3 is synthesised in skin under the influence of UV light.

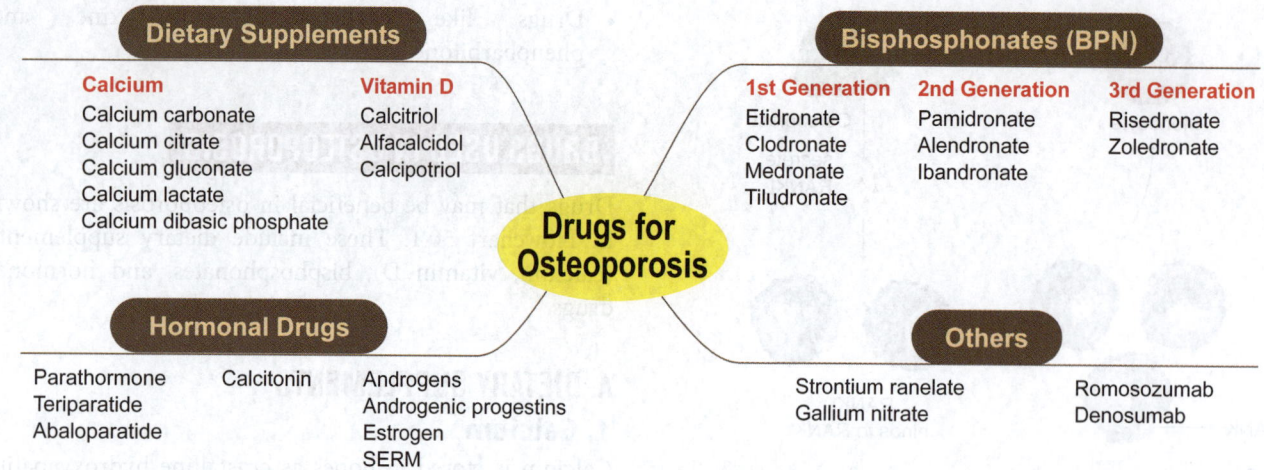

Flowchart 50.1 Classification of drugs for osteoporosis

Vitamin D gets activated by sequential hydroxylation at position 25 in the liver and then at position 1 in the kidneys to form 1,25-dihydroxy calcitriol, the active form of vitamin D. Final hydroxylation at position 1 is the rate-limiting step. It is induced by calcium, parathormone, estrogens, and prolactin, and inhibited by calcitriol in a feedback manner.

Actions

The active form of vitamin D (1,25-dihydroxy calcitriol):

- Increases intestinal absorption of calcium and phosphate.
- Increases bone resorption by inducing RANKL secretion from osteoblasts, which, in turn, increases recruitment and differentiation of osteoclast precursor cells in remodelling units (Fig. 50.1). Subsequent to resorption, vitamin D also promotes laying down of new osteoid and mineralisation.
- Increases renal tubular reabsorption of calcium and phosphate in PCT.

These three actions raise plasma calcium levels. Therefore, vitamin D deficiency is characterised by hypocalcemia, which induces parathormone (PTH) secretion. PTH, in turn, causes calcium mobilisation from bones. Thus, mineralisation in newly formed bone is affected, causing rickets in children and osteomalacia in adults.

Other tissues like immune cells, epidermal cells, neuronal cells, skeletal muscles and some malignant cells also possess vitamin D receptors and are affected by vitamin D.

Therapeutic uses

- Vitamin D is used as a nutritional supplement for prophylaxis and treatment of vitamin D deficiency. The dose for prophylaxis is 400 IU per day and for treatment, it is 3000–4000 IU per day. A convenient alternative is to give 3–6 lakh IU orally or intramuscularly, once in 2–6 months.
- In cases of vitamin-D-resistant rickets, calcitriol or alfacalcidol is effective.
- In senile osteoporosis, post-menopausal women and elderly males, a combination of vitamin D and calcium has an adjuvant role.
- Hypoparathyroidism – calcitriol is more effective.
- Fanconi syndrome – phosphate levels are low in this condition. Vitamin D raises phosphate to the normal value.
- In psoriasis, a non-hypercalcemic analogue of vitamin D, calcipotriol, is used topically. Calcipotriol may be useful systemically in skin cancer and immunological conditions.

Drug interactions

- Vitamin D absorption is reduced in malabsorption and steatorrhea.
- Liquid paraffin and cholestyramine decrease oral absorption of vitamin D.
- Antiepileptic drugs like phenobarbitone and phenytoin cause rickets or osteomalacia due to reduced response of target cells to vitamin D.

Adverse effects

Hypervitaminosis D is characterised by hypercalcemia, fatigue, weakness, sluggishness, polyuria, albuminuria, diarrhea, vomiting, renal stones and ectopic deposits of calcium.

B. BISPHOSPHONATES (BPN)

These include three generations of drugs based on the chronology of their development, route of administration, potency, etc. The 1st-generation drugs (etidronate, clodronate, medronate, tiludronate) are not used much. Among the 2nd-generation drugs, alendronate is orally effective, whereas pamidronate is given intravenously. Similarly, of the 3rd-generation drugs, risedronate is a highly potent drug used orally, while zoledronate is given parenterally.

Bisphosphonates are pyrophosphates that have strong affinity for calcium phosphate. As a result, their action is selective for calcified tissues.

Mechanism of Action

- A protein matrix and solid mineral phase consisting of crystalline hydroxyapatite are the two main components of bone structure (Fig. 50.2). The osteoclasts secrete acid and acid hydrolases at their ruffled border. So, a clear acidic zone is formed in the resorption pit. In this acidic zone, the mineral phase gets solubilised and calcium ions are released from the bone surface. Then, acid hydrolases secreted by osteoclasts cause resorption of the protein matrix. BPNs first get localised in this acidic zone under osteoclasts because of their high affinity for calcium, and are then internalised in osteoclasts by the process of endocytosis. This accelerates apoptosis of osteoclasts and disrupts the cytoskeleton from the ruffled border of osteoclasts.
- BPNs also inhibit differentiation of osteoclast precursors through suppression of IL-6.
- Potent BPNs like alendronate and pamidronate interfere with the mevalonate pathway for isoprenoid lipid synthesis. This interferes with cytoskeletal organisation and reduces the membrane ruffling of osteoclasts. Thus, BPNs interfere with the bone resorption process.

Therapeutic Uses

- BPNs are the first-line drugs for the prevention and treatment of age-related, post-menopausal, steroid-induced and idiopathic osteoporosis. Alendronate is equally effective as HRT and SERM (selective estrogen receptor modulators) in conserving BMD and is better tolerated. Alendronate is given orally on an empty stomach, in a dose of 5–10 mg, once daily, with a full glass of water, to be swallowed without chewing. The patient should be advised not to lie down or eat food for 30 minutes after taking BPNs orally. This caution is aimed at preventing exposure of the esophageal mucosa to the drug, which may result in esophagitis, ulcers, etc.
- In Paget's disease of bone, BPNs can reduce bony pains, relieve secondary symptoms, and prevent further bone loss. Long-term remission is induced. Calcitonin combined with BPNs gives better results.
- In cancerous diseases with osteolytic bony metastasis, the third-generation BPN, pamidronate, given intravenously in a dose of 30–90 mg over 4–12 hours, once daily to once in 2 months, is effective in reducing bone pain, controlling hypercalcemia of malignancy, and arresting further osteolytic lesions.

ADRs

- Orally used BPNs cause gastric irritation, metallic taste, retrosternal pain and flatulence.
- Intravenous use is associated with thrombophlebitis of veins, bone pains, fever, leukopenia, flu-like symptoms, nausea, vomiting, dizziness, etc.
- Headache, pyrexia
- Hypersensitivity reactions
- Bone pains
- Osteomalacia may occur with continuous therapy as they interfere with bone mineralisation.

Adverse effects can be minimised by giving the drug once a week, in a dose of 35–70 mg.

Interactions

- Many substances like tea, coffee, fruit juice, mineral water, iron and calcium form complexes with BPNs and decrease their absorption.
- When NSAIDs are administered concurrently with BPNs, the gastric irritant effect of NSAIDs is augmented.

The first BPN to be used clinically, **etidronate**, carries the risk of causing osteomalacia as it inhibits bone mineralisation. Therefore, for prevention and treatment of osteoporosis in both genders, it has been largely replaced by other drugs like **alendronate** and **risedronate**. Alendronate is an orally-effective second-generation drug.

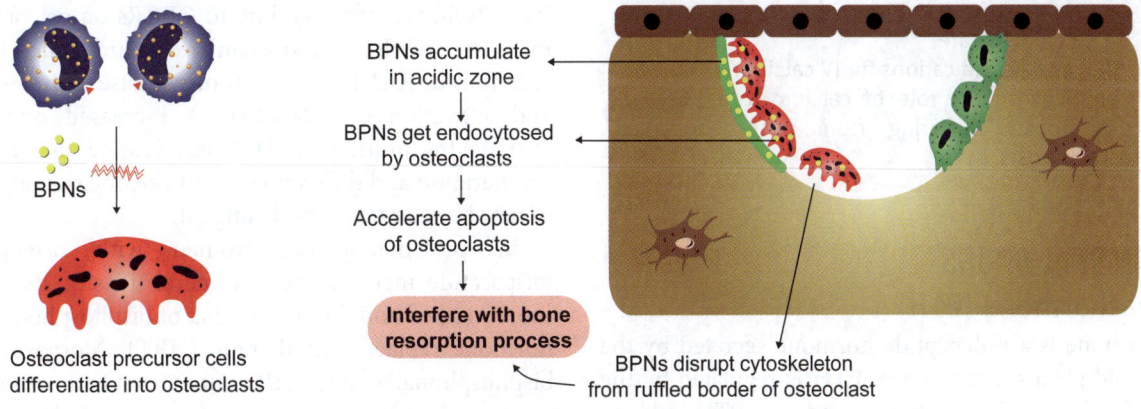

Fig. 50.2 Mechanism of action of bisphosphonates (BPNs)

Pamidronate is a second-generation BPN with intermediate potency, used intravenously in Paget's disease, osteolytic metastasis and hypercalcemia associated with malignant diseases. Risedronate is a third-generation drug with high potency, given orally in a daily dose of 5 mg. Zoledronate is a third-generation parenteral drug. It has higher efficacy, faster action and causes less venous irritation than pamidronate. So, zoledronate is the drug of first choice in hypercalcemia of malignancy. It can arrest osteolytic metastasis in multiple myeloma, carcinoma breast, carcinoma prostate, etc.

> **Clinical problem-based questions and MCQs**
>
> 1. **A 76-year-old male, a diagnosed case of carcinoma prostate, presents with severe bone pains. Investigations show osteolytic bony lesions. The patient is given zoledronate by intravenous administration.**
>   i. What is the pharmacological basis for administration of zoledronate in this case?
>   ii. Which of the following bone cells is the target site of zoledronate?
>   a. Osteoclast
>   b. Osteoblast
>   c. Stem cell
>   d. Osteocyte
>   iii. Why is zoledronate preferred over pamidronate for this indication?
>
> 2. i. In which of the following conditions is vitamin D indicated?
>   a. Hyperparathyroidism
>   b. Osteomalacia
>   c. Hypercalcemia
>   d. Hyperphosphatemia
>   ii. Describe the pharmacological basis for use of vitamin D in the selected clinical condition.
>   iii. What is the dose of vitamin D in selected clinical condition?
>
> 3. i. Identify the calcium preparation that is administered intravenously.
>   a. Calcium carbonate
>   b. Calcium citrate
>   c. Calcium gluconate
>   d. Calcium lactate
>   ii. What are the indications for IV calcium?
>   iii. Comment on the role of calcium in a 56-year-old woman suffering from post-menopausal osteoporosis.

C. HORMONAL DRUGS

(i) Parathormone (PTH)

Parathormone is a polypeptide hormone secreted by the parathyroid glands. Secretion of PTH is regulated by the levels of calcium. Hypocalcemia induces PTH release; hypercalcemia inhibits it.

Mechanism of action

PTH acts through G protein-coupled receptors (GPCRs), increases cAMP and intracellular calcium concentration.

- In bones, the target cell for PTH is the osteoblast. It induces RANKL secretion, which, in turn, increases osteoclastic differentiation and activity. **A high concentration of PTH, when present continuously, causes increased resorption** of calcium from bones. Because resorption is followed by the laying down of new bone, this process is also activated by intermittent administration of low-dose PTH. Thus, intermittent presence of PTH favours new bone formation.
- PTH also increases calcium reabsorption from the DCT in the kidney and provides moment-to-moment regulation of calcium excretion. However, in cases of hyperparathyroidism, the effect of raised plasma calcium levels is of overriding importance and calcium excretion in urine increases.
  [Because of these two effects, it is said that in hyperparathyroidism, bones are resorbed and passed out in urine.]
- PTH increases intestinal absorption of calcium indirectly by increasing the activation of 25-hydroxy vitamin D through hydroxylation at position 1.

All the above actions increase calcium levels, but **PTH is not used therapeutically** because:

- It cannot be given orally, so administration is inconvenient.
- It is costlier than vitamin D.

Thus, vitamin D therapy, which is useful in hypocalcemia, is preferred over PTH therapy as it is cheaper and orally effective.

(ii) Teriparatide

Teriparatide is a recombinant preparation containing an amino acid sequence similar to the first 34 residues at the amino terminal of PTH.

Actions of teriparatide

The actions of teriparatide in bone resemble those of PTH itself, i.e., after binding to GPCRs on osteoblasts, it increases cAMP and intracellular calcium, which induces secretion of RANKL. This, in turn, causes differentiation and activation of osteoclasts → increased number of remodelling units. Like PTH, teriparatide also enhances proliferation and differentiation of osteoblastic deposition of new bone in the remodelling pit.

In post-menopausal women with osteoporosis, teriparatide increases bone mineral density. Its effect is more marked and faster than that of bisphosphonates and hormone replacement therapy (HRT). Moreover, while bisphosphonates and HRT only decrease resorption, teriparatide increases new bone formation. It decreases the risk of vertebral and non-vertebral compression fractures.

So, it is used in severe post-menopausal osteoporosis and glucocorticoid-induced osteoporosis.

Dose: Because teriparatide is a peptide, it cannot be used orally. It is administered once daily as a 20 mcg subcutaneous injection. It has a half-life of just an hour, and after a single subcutaneous injection, the action lasts for 2–3 hours. So, with single daily administration, its intermittent presence leads to predominantly bone-forming action.

ADRs
Headache, nausea, dizziness and leg cramps may occur. It should not be continued for more than 2 years. Moreover, daily subcutaneous injection is inconvenient for the patient. So, teriparatide is reserved only for post-menopausal women with severe osteoporosis.

(iii) Abaloparatide
Abaloparatide resembles teriparatide and is useful in women who have severe, resistant-type of post-menopausal osteoporosis associated with high risk of fractures.

(iv) Calcitonin
This is a polypeptide hormone secreted from parafollicular 'C' cells of the thyroid gland. Its secretion is induced by hypercalcemia and inhibited by hypocalcemia.

Actions of calcitonin
The actions of calcitonin are just the opposite of those of parathormone.
- In the bone, it decreases the ruffled surface of osteoclasts. Hence, their bone lysing effect decreases. Thus, calcitonin is a potent inhibitor of bone resorption. It causes hypocalcemia, which lasts for about 8 hours.
- Calcitonin decreases the reabsorption of calcium and phosphate in the PCT by direct action; however, it causes hypocalcemia. Also, glomerular filtration is markedly reduced and in spite of decreased reabsorption, the net excretion of calcium in urine is actually reduced.

Therapeutic uses
In post-menopausal osteoporosis, calcitonin 100 IU is given by subcutaneous or intramuscular injection, once daily, together with calcium and vitamin D supplementation. It is also available for use as nasal spray in a dose of 200 IU per day. It is usually indicated in women after > 5 years of menopause and in conditions where HRT with estrogens is contraindicated.

Other uses of calcitonin include:
- Hypercalcemic states like hyperparathyroidism and hypervitaminosis D
- Osteolytic bony metastasis
- Paget's disease of bone – It is the second-line drug after bisphosphonates.

ADRs of calcitonin include urticaria, swelling of hands, nausea and abdominal cramps. Use as nasal spray may cause headache, rhinitis, ulceration and epistaxis.

(v) Androgens
Testosterone has a useful positive effect on bone mineralisation and muscle mass, and hence may be useful in elderly men. Androgens in small amounts are added to HRT in post-menopausal women. However, the cardiovascular and metabolic adverse effects of androgens are a limitation of such use in aged individuals.

(vi) Estrogen
Estrogen opposes the process of bone resorption by:
- Inhibiting formation of osteoclastic pits.
- Inducing formation of bone matrix proteins like osteocalcin and osteonectin.
- Maintaining positive calcium balance by promoting activation of vitamin D.

Thus, estrogen has an important role in maintaining bone mass and is used as HRT in post-menopausal women to prevent bone loss. However, because of the metabolic and cardiovascular adverse effects, estrogen should be used in very small doses and not continued beyond 5 years. Progestin combined with estrogen in HRT can lower the risk of adverse metabolic and cardiovascular consequences.

(vii) Selective Estrogen Receptor Modulators (SERMs)
SERMs include drugs like **raloxifene** and **ormeloxifene**. Raloxifene has partial agonistic action at estrogen receptors in bone, cardiovascular system and adipose tissue, and antagonistic action in the breast and endometrium. It decreases bone loss and improves BMD, especially in the lumbar vertebrae. However, its efficacy in preventing fractures is lower than that of bisphosphonates. So, raloxifene is used as a second-line drug after BPNs to reduce the risk of spine fractures in post-menopausal osteoporosis.

(viii) Other Drugs
Other drugs that have a role in osteoporosis include:

Strontium ranelate: It inhibits osteoclast differentiation, but increases their apoptosis. Thus, bone resorption is reduced. In addition, bone formation is stimulated. However, owing to its serious cardiovascular adverse effects, its use is restricted to preventing vertebral and hip fractures only in cases of severe osteoporosis in patients who are very prone to fractures and cannot tolerate other drugs like BPNs.

Denosumab: It is a monoclonal antibody against RANKL and hence, interferes with differentiation of osteoclast precursors. Its inhibitory effect on bone resorption is equivalent to third-generation BPNs and is useful for limiting bone metastasis associated with prostate and breast cancers.

Romosozumab is a monoclonal antibody that opposes the actions of sclerostin. Sclerostin acts by interfering with the proliferation of osteoblasts but increases osteoclast action through increased RANKL secretion. Romosozumab is useful in post-menopausal women at high risk of fractures.

Gallium nitrate inhibits ATP-dependent proton pumps on ruffled surfaces of osteoclasts and decreases bone resorption. However, it is nephrotoxic and its use is therefore restricted to severe resistant cases of malignancy-related hypercalcemia only.

MANAGEMENT PLAN FOR OSTEOPOROSIS

Diagnosis

Clinical features: Osteoporosis usually causes no symptoms till a fracture occurs. '**Fragility fractures**' that occur after falling from standing height or even lower are typically seen in osteoporosis. Symptoms associated with the fracture are pain, local tenderness and deformity.

Assessment and Evaluation

The guidelines (2020) issued by the American Association of Endocrinologists recommend that all women aged ≥ 50 years should be evaluated for risk of osteoporosis.

Initial evaluation involves detailed history, physical examination and clinical assessment using a 'fracture risk assessment tool'.

Bone mineral density

Indications for measurement of bone mineral density (BMD) include:

- Females > 65 years of age and males > 70 years of age
- Early onset menopause.
- Post-menopausal women with osteopenia/history of fracture without major trauma/ family history of osteoporotic fractures/need long-term glucocorticoid therapy for some other medical condition.
- Secondary osteoporosis (such patients need laboratory tests to measure levels of serum 25-hydroxyvitamin D, calcium, creatinine, and thyroid-stimulating hormone).
- Heavy smoking/alcoholism.

For those who have normal bone mineral density on initial screening, intervals of at least four years appear safe for re-screening.

Aim of management in osteoporosis

The aim is to maintain healthy BMD and bone mass, maximise the patient's ability to carry out routine daily activities, prevent falls/fractures, provide relief for symptoms and prevent disability if fractures occur.

Treatment

The treatment of osteoporosis involves **non-pharmacological** and **pharmacological measures.**

Non-pharmacological measures

These involve various lifestyle modifications.

- A **calcium-rich diet** is advocated, especially during childhood, to ensure adequate bone mass and density. Milk, cheese and yogurt are rich sources of calcium.
- **Vitamin-D-rich diet** including foods such as fortified dairy products, egg yolk, saltwater fish and supplements in elderly to maintain optimum levels.
- Regular **exercise**, including muscle strength training and increasing weight bearing exercises, which help in maintaining bone mass.
- **Minimise caffeine intake** and abstain from **cigarette smoking and alcohol consumption.**

Pharmacological measures

No treatment can fully reverse osteoporotic changes. Treatment can only prevent osteoporosis or decrease the rate of progression.

- Treatment is tailored to the individual patient, with risks and benefits discussed in detail to involve them in decision-making.
- Patients who need corticosteroids for some other medical condition should be given minimum effective dose of steroids, and attempt should be made to taper down and withdraw corticosteroids as early as possible.
- **Bisphosphonates** are the mainstay of treatment in osteoporosis in men and post-menopausal women. Alendronate is given orally in a dose of 70 mg per week. The patient should swallow the drug with a large glass of water 30 minutes before breakfast, while sitting in upright position, and should not lie down for the next 30 minutes.
- The therapy is **continued for 5 years**. At end of 5 years oral or 3 years IV BPN therapy, the patient is reassessed. If the risk of fracture is no longer high, a '**drug holiday' for 2–3 years** may be attempted. During this time, bone turnover and BMD are monitored, and therapy is reinstituted as and when needed. However, in patients having high risk of hip/vertebral fractures or compression, **BPNs may be continued for 5 more years**, with periodic evaluations.
- Patients who do not tolerate BPNs or do not respond to BPNs need other alternative drugs such as raloxifene, teriparatide and denosumab
- Secondary osteoporosis needs treatment of the primary condition that is responsible for precipitating bone loss and fractures.

- If fracture occurs, the patient needs **local measures** such as moist hot packs, transcutaneous electrical nerve stimulation (TENS) and oral analgesics to control the symptoms. Orthotics, i.e., custom-molded shoe inserts or ankle braces are used to reduce flexion force and pressure on the fracture site, and prevent worsening of kyphosis.
- Painful vertebral compression fractures may need **vertebroplasty**, i.e., injection of methyl methacrylate into vertebral body under local anesthesia (methyl methacrylate is an organic liquid widely used in medicine and dental practice for making prosthetic devices).
- **Kyphoplasty**, involving the insertion of a needle into the affected vertebral body and inflation and filling of a balloon with methyl methacrylate, may be a useful alternative to vertebroplasty.
- **Surgical management** of fractures may be needed in some cases.

Clinical problem-based questions and MCQs

4. i. Parathormone increases renal tubular reabsorption of calcium, but in a 45-year-old male, a known case of hyperparathyroidism, urinary excretion of calcium is increased. Explain the clinical finding.
   ii. Describe the effect of parathormone in bone remodelling.
5. i. Which of the following is a first-line drug for post-menopausal osteoporosis?
      a. Alendronate
      b. Teriparatide
      c. Raloxifene
      d. Testosterone
   ii. Justify your choice.

Summary

- Osteoporosis is a metabolic disease caused by the imbalance in osteoclastic and osteoblastic activity, resulting in disturbance of bone remodelling.
- Post-menopausal women, elderly individuals of both genders, patients suffering from diseases such as vitamin D deficiency, malnutrition, scurvy, rheumatoid arthritis, hyperparathyroidism, leukemias, and gastrointestinal, hepatic and renal diseases, and those taking drugs like corticosteroids, thyroxine and phenobarbitone are more prone to osteoporosis.
- Many dietary supplements and drugs have a role in the prevention and treatment of osteoporosis.
- Calcium and vitamin D have only an adjuvant role in patients receiving HRT or bisphosphonates.
- Vitamin D increases bone resorption, intestinal absorption of calcium and renal tubular reabsorption of calcium. All three actions cause hypercalcemia.
- Thus, vitamin D deficiency causes hypocalcemia → increased PTH secretion, that mobilises calcium from bones. This affects mineralisation in newly formed bones, resulting in rickets and osteomalacia.
- Bisphosphonates (BPNs) reduce bone resorption by increasing osteoclast apoptosis, cytoskeletal disruption and decreasing ruffling of osteoclasts; they are first-line drugs for osteoporosis. Other indications for their use include Paget's disease, osteolytic bony metastasis and hypercalcemia of malignancy. Care should be taken to swallow oral BPNs without chewing, on an empty stomach, and along with a full glass of water; this precaution decreases their esophageal irritant action. High-potency BPNs like pamidronate and zoledronate are useful in bone metastasis and hypercalcemia associated with malignancy.
- Parathormone (PTH) causes activation of 25-hydroxy vitamin D, thus indirectly increasing intestinal calcium absorption. It also increases calcium reabsorption in the DCT. PTH increases calcium resorption from bones when used continuously, but its intermittent presence increases bone formation All these actions result in hypercalcemia, which in turn causes increased excretion of calcium in urine in hyperparathyroidism.
- However, in spite of this role, PTH is not used in osteoporosis because it has to be injected subcutaneously daily, which is inconvenient for the patient.
- Calcitonin decreases bone resorption, causing hypocalcemia. It reduces calcium reabsorption also in renal tubules; however, calcium excretion is reduced because of hypocalcemia.
- Bisphosphonates and HRT only decrease bone resorption, whereas teriparatide, containing the first 34 amino acids of PTH, increases new bone formation. It decreases the risk of vertebral and non-vertebral compression fractures.
- HRT, SERMs, and androgens also have a role in post-menopausal women. However, because of risk of associated metabolic and cardiovascular adverse effects, these are not the first choice of treatment.

Questions for practice

1. Comment on the role of following drugs in post-menopausal osteoporosis.
   a. Bisphosphonates
   b. Teriparatide
   c. Raloxifene
2. Explain why:
   a. Alendronate is the first-choice drug in osteoporosis.
   b. Parathormone is not used in osteoporosis.
   c. Teriparatide is used only in severe cases.

Hints for problem-based questions and MCQs

1. i. Zoledronate is a third-generation bisphosphonate. BPNs get localised in the acidic zone under osteoclasts because of their high affinity for calcium and are then internalised in osteoclasts by the process of endocytosis. This accelerates apoptosis of osteoclasts and disrupts the cytoskeleton from the ruffled border of osteoclasts, resulting in inhibition of bone resorption. In this case, with osteolytic bony lesions, zoledronate can effectively reduce bone pain, control hypercalcemia of malignancy and arrest further osteolytic lesions.
   ii. a. Osteoclast is the target cell of zoledronate, like other BPNs.
   iii. Zoledronate has higher efficacy, faster action and causes less venous irritation compared to pamidronate.

2. i. b. Osteomalacia is caused in adults because of vitamin D deficiency. It is also useful in hypoparathyroidism, but not in hyperparathyroidism. Hypocalcemia is a feature of vitamin D deficiency; thus, vitamin D has no role in hypercalcemia. Vitamin D is also used in Fanconi syndrome, in which phosphate levels are low; thus, it has no role in hyperphosphatemia
   ii. Vitamin D increases bone resorption, intestinal absorption and renal tubular reabsorption of calcium. All three actions raise plasma calcium levels. Thus, deficiency of vitamin D is characterised by hypocalcemia that induces parathormone secretion. PTH, in turn, causes calcium mobilisation from bones. Thus, mineralisation in newly formed bone is affected, causing rickets in children and osteomalacia in adults. So, osteomalacia responds if vitamin D levels are restored to normal.
   iii. Dose of vitamin D in treatment of osteomalacia is 3000–4000 IU per day. A convenient alternative is to give 3–6 lakh IU orally or intramuscularly, once in 2–6 months.

3. i. c. Calcium gluconate
   ii. Calcium gluconate is used as intravenous injection for immediate treatment of tetany, dermatoses, paresthesias and weakness.
   iii. In the treatment of osteoporosis, calcium alone or in combination with vitamin D_3 has only an adjuvant role while treating osteoporosis with bisphosphonates or hormone replacement therapy. The aim is to ensure that calcium levels are adequate to support bone mineralisation.

4. i. PTH increases calcium reabsorption from DCT in the kidney and provides moment-to-moment regulation of calcium excretion. However, in cases of hyperparathyroidism, the effect of raised plasma calcium levels is of overriding importance and calcium excretion in urine increases as glomerular filtration increases.
   ii. Target cell for PTH in bones is the osteoblast. It induces RANKL secretion, which, in turn, increases osteoclastic differentiation and activity. When high concentration of PTH is present continuously, it causes increased resorption of calcium from bone. Since resorption is followed by laying down of new bone, it also gets activated by intermittent administration of low dose of PTH.

5. i. Alendronate a second-generation bisphosphonate, effective orally is the first-choice drug in post-menopausal osteoporosis.
   ii. Teriparatide has to be given subcutaneously; so, it is used as reserve drug in severe osteoporosis and in patients with high risk of fractures. Raloxifene, a selective estrogen receptor modulator has lower efficacy than alendronate.
   Testosterone can cause disturbing metabolic and cardiovascular adverse effects, especially in aged individuals.

CONCEPT MAP – DRUGS FOR OSTEOPOROSIS

Calcium
Given to ensure calcium levels adequate to support bone mineralisation.
Adjuvant role to BPNs/hormonal drugs
Dose varies with age
up to 10 years: 0.8–1.2 g per day,
For pregnant and lactating women, post-menopausal women without HRT, 1.5 g/day
For post-menopausal women on HRT 1.0 g/day

Management
Lifestyle modifications:
Measures like Calcium, Vitamin D rich diet, Regular exercise, stopping cigarette smoking/ alcohol & caffeine intake.
Drug treatment:
Dietary supplements: Calcium, vitamin D
Bisphosphonates (BPNs)
1st-generation BPNs (least potent)
Etidronate, Clodronate, Medronate, Tiludronate
2nd-generation BPNs (intermediate potency)
Pamidronate, Alendronate, Ibandronate
3rd-generation BPNs (most potent)
Risedronate, Zoledronate.
Hormonal drugs: Parathormone, Teriparatide, Abaloparatide, Calcitonin, Androgens, Androgenic progestins, Estrogen, SERM
Others: Strontium ranelate, Denosumab, Romosozumab, Gallium nitrate, etc.

Vitamin D
Active form is 1,25-dihydroxy calcitriol
Actions: Raises plasma calcium levels by:
- Increasing intestinal absorption of Ca & P
- Increasing bone resorption by inducing RANKL secretion from osteoblasts
- Increasing renal tubular reabsorption of Ca & P in PCT
Uses: Adjuvant role in senile osteoporosis
- Prophylaxis and treatment of vitamin D deficiency, Hypoparathyroidism, Fanconi syndrome.
- Calcipotriol is used in psoriasis, skin cancers & immunological conditions.
ADRs: Hypervitaminosis D characterised by hypercalcemia, fatigue, weakness, sluggishness, polyuria, albuminuria, diarrhea, vomiting, renal stones and ectopic deposits of calcium

Nutritional Supplements

DRUGS FOR OSTEOPOROSIS

Osteoporosis
Metabolic disorder characterised by imbalance of bone remodelling, osteopenia, decreased bone density, disturbed micro-architecture, bone pains, vertebral collapse & spontaneous fractures

Hormonal Drugs

Parathormone
Actions: Induces RANKL secretion from osteoblast, which, in turn, increases osteoclastic differentiation and activity → increased resorption of calcium from bone.
Increases calcium reabsorption from DCT in kidney.
Indirectly increases intestinal absorption of calcium, by favouring activation of vitamin D
Not used because of high cost & inconvenience of administration (not effective orally)

Teriparatide
Actions: Same as PTH, also enhances proliferation and differentiation of osteoblastic deposition of new bone in remodeling pit.
Uses: Used in severe post-menopausal osteoporosis & glucocorticoid-induced osteoporosis as 20 mcg SC injection once daily. In post-menopausal women, increases bone density, reduces risk of fractures & effect is more marked and faster than BPNs & HRT.
ADRs: headache, nausea, dizziness, leg cramps may occur.
It should not be continued for more than 2 years.

Calcitonin
Mechanism: Decreases the ruffled surface of osteoclasts and hence their bone lysing effect → hypocalcemia
Also decreases the reabsorption of calcium and phosphate in PCT, but net calcium excretion decreases due to hypocalcemic action.
Uses: In women after > 5 years of menopause and where HRT with estrogens is contraindicated.
Hypercalcemic states like hyperparathyroidism, hypervitaminosis D, Osteolytic bony metastasis
2nd line drug in Paget disease of bone
ADRs: Urticaria, swelling of hands, nausea, abdominal cramps.
After nasal spray, headache, rhinitis, ulceration and epistaxis may occur

Bisphosphonates (BPNs)
Mechanism: Interfere with differentiation of osteoclast precursor cells.
First, they get localised in the acidic zone under osteoclasts, then endocytosed by osteoclasts → accelerate apoptosis of osteoclasts, disrupt cytoskeleton from ruffled border of osteoclasts → interfere with bone resorption process.
Uses: First-line drugs for prevention and treatment of age-related, post-menopausal, steroid-induced and idiopathic osteoporosis.
Also used in Paget disease of bones, osteolytic bony metastasis
ADRs: *Oral:* Gastric irritation, metallic taste, retrosternal pain, flatulence.
IV: Thrombophlebitis of vein, bony pains, fever, leukopenia, flu-like symptoms, nausea, vomiting, dizziness, etc.
May also cause headache, pyrexia, hypersensitivity reactions & bone pains.
Caution: Oral BPNs to be taken with full glass of water, without chewing, on empty stomach. Patient advised not to lie down or take food for 30 minutes to prevent exposure of esophageal mucosa to drug that may result in esophagitis, ulcers, etc.

SECTION 10 Chemotherapeutic Drugs

51 General Principles of Chemotherapy

PH 8.1 Discuss general principles of chemotherapy with emphasis on antimicrobial resistance.
PH 8.2 Discuss rational use of antimicrobials and describe the antibiotic stewardship program (ASP) of your institute.

Learning objectives

A student of MBBS phase II should be able to:
- Define common terms used in chemotherapy.
- Classify antimicrobial agents based on their chemical structure, mechanism of action, spectrum of action, etc.
- Describe problems associated with rampant and irrational use of AMAs like drug resistance and superinfection.
- Describe the general principles of antimicrobial use, mentioning factors to be considered while selecting AMA, prophylactic use of AMAs and combined use of AMAs.
- Enumerate causes of failure of antimicrobial therapy.
- Describe the components of antibiotic stewardship program (ASP).
- Describe the AWaRe classification as a tool for ASP.

INTRODUCTION

In the early 20th century, **Paul Ehrlich**, known as the **father of chemotherapy**, pioneered the use of drugs with known chemical structures to selectively target microbes while sparing host cells. Notably, he used 'arsenicals' to treat diseases like syphilis and sleeping sickness. As the chemical structure of most of the other drugs used was not known at that time, Ehrlich coined the term **'chemotherapy' for drugs of known chemical structure**. This was followed by the advent of many drugs having selective toxic effect on microbes, like sulphapyridine in 1938, penicillin in 1941, and streptomycin in 1944. Soon after, tetracycline, chloramphenicol, erythromycin, many cephalosporins, and fluoroquinolones were developed for use as antimicrobial agents. The new agents included ketolides, glycopeptides, and oxazolidinones. However, in the recent past, research has focussed on developing semisynthetic derivatives of older antibiotics with desirable pharmacokinetic properties and different antimicrobial spectra.

Definitions

1. **Chemotherapy:** It is the **treatment of systemic infections** with specific drugs, which are natural or synthetic **chemicals**, that possess **selective suppressing effect** on the infecting microorganism but do not affect the host cells significantly.
2. **Selective toxicity:** It is the ability of chemicals to **selectively suppress foreign cells without causing any significant damage to the host cells.** Such selectivity arises from the **affinity of the drug for microbial cell constituents** such as cell wall, specific cellular enzymes and microbial nucleic acids, which are not of any relevance to the host cell. Macromolecules of the host cells are not affected by these drugs.
3. **Antibiotics, chemotherapeutic agents, antimicrobial agents (AMA):** These three terms are commonly used interchangeably, though they differ slightly. **Antibiotics are chemicals produced by microorganisms that have the capacity to inhibit or kill other microorganisms, when used in very low concentrations**. However, substances produced by higher organisms (antibodies produced by humans) as well as substances produced by microbes but needed in higher concentrations to inhibit/kill other microbes (e.g., hydrogen peroxide and ethanol) are excluded from this terminology. The term **'chemotherapeutic agents' includes only synthetic drugs possessing anti-infective activity**. **'Antimicrobial agents' (AMAs)** is a broad term that includes drugs of **natural origin** (i.e., antibiotics) as well as **synthetic drugs** (i.e., chemotherapeutic agents that possess anti-infective activity). AMAs include antibacterial, antiviral, antifungal, antiprotozoal and anthelmintic agents.
4. **Chemotherapeutic index:** This index provides an insight into the safety margin of an AMA. It is defined as the **ratio of lethal dose (LD) 0.1** and **curing dose (CD) 99.9**. Here, LD 0.1 is the dose of the AMA that kills all experimental animals except 0.1% and CD 99.9 is the dose of AMA that cures 99.9% of the experimental animals (i.e., cures all animals except 0.1%).
5. **Minimum inhibitory concentration (MIC):** This is the **lowest concentration of an AMA** (determined by serial dilutions of the drug) that **inhibits multiplication** and

prevents visible growth of a susceptible bacterium in culture plates. It reflects the **activity per mg** or the **potency** of the AMA.

6. **Minimum bactericidal concentration (MBC):** This is the **concentration of the AMA that kills 99.9% of the susceptible bacteria.** To determine the MBC of an AMA, subculturing is done from culture tubes having no visible growth. **If the difference between the MBC and MIC is small,** the drug is labelled as **bactericidal (killing bacteria); a larger difference between the two** indicates that the drug is **bacteriostatic (inhibits multiplication).**

7. **Post-antibiotic effect (PAE):** After exposure to an AMA, when the organism is placed again in an antibiotic-free medium, it resumes multiplication after some time lag. This **lag period in resuming growth by the microorganism after a brief exposure to AMA** is called PAE. Drugs such as fluoroquinolones, aminoglycosides and β-lactams have long PAE. [Mnemonic: FAB]

CLASSIFICATION OF AMAs

AMAs can be classified in many ways, based on their source, chemical nature, types of organisms they affect, mechanism, spectrum, and type of action.

1. Based on the source
AMAs can be obtained from natural sources, such as:
- Fungi, e.g., penicillin, cephalosporins, griseofulvin
- Bacteria, e.g., bacitracin, colistin, polymyxin B
- Actinomycetes, e.g., aminoglycosides, macrolides, tetracyclines, and chloramphenicol.

However, most AMAs used in current clinical practice are synthesised chemically, e.g., fluoroquinolones, cephalosporins and lincosamides.

2. Based on types of organisms affected
AMAs can be grouped as antibacterial, antiviral, antifungal, antiamoebic, antimalarial, antitubercular, anthelminthic, etc.

3. Based on chemical nature and major mechanism of action
The classes of AMAs based on chemical nature and major mechanism of action are shown in Flowchart 51.1.

4. Based on spectrum of action
AMAs can be divided into broad-spectrum or narrow-spectrum drugs.
- Broad-spectrum AMAs: tetracyclines, chloramphenicol
- Narrow-spectrum: benzylpenicillin, streptomycin, erythromycin, etc.

5. Based on concentration or time-dependent effect
- Certain AMAs show a concentration-dependent effect, e.g., aminoglycosides and fluoroquinolones. In these drugs, the clinical response depends on the peak AMA concentration achieved at the site of infection in relation to MIC. Such drugs have a long post-antibiotic effect.

Based on Chemical Nature
- Sulphonamides, Diaminopyrimidines, Quinolones, Fluoroquinolones
- β-lactams: Penicillins, Cephalosporins, Monobactams, Carbapenems
- Tetracyclines, Chloramphenicol, Aminoglycosides, Macrolides
- Lincosamides, Glycopeptides, Polypeptides, Oxazolidinones
- **Miscellaneous**: Mupirocin, Fusidic acid, Spectinomycin, Daptomycin, Quinupristin/Dalfopristin

Antimicrobial Agents (AMAs)

Based on Mechanism of Action
- **Drugs that inhibit protein synthesis**: Macrolides, Tetracyclines, Chloramphenicol, Aminoglycosides, Lincosamides, Oxazolidinones
- **Drugs that inhibit cell wall synthesis**: β-lactams, Glycopeptides, Bacitracin
- **Drugs that inhibit DNA gyrase**: Quinolones, Fluoroquinolones.
- **Drugs that inhibit intermediary metabolism**: Sulphonamides, Diaminopyrimidines, Metronidazole, para-aminosalicylic acid
- **Drugs that increase membrane permeability**: Colistin, Bacitracin, Polymyxin B, Aminoglycosides

Flowchart 51.1 Classification of AMAs based on chemical nature and major mechanism of action

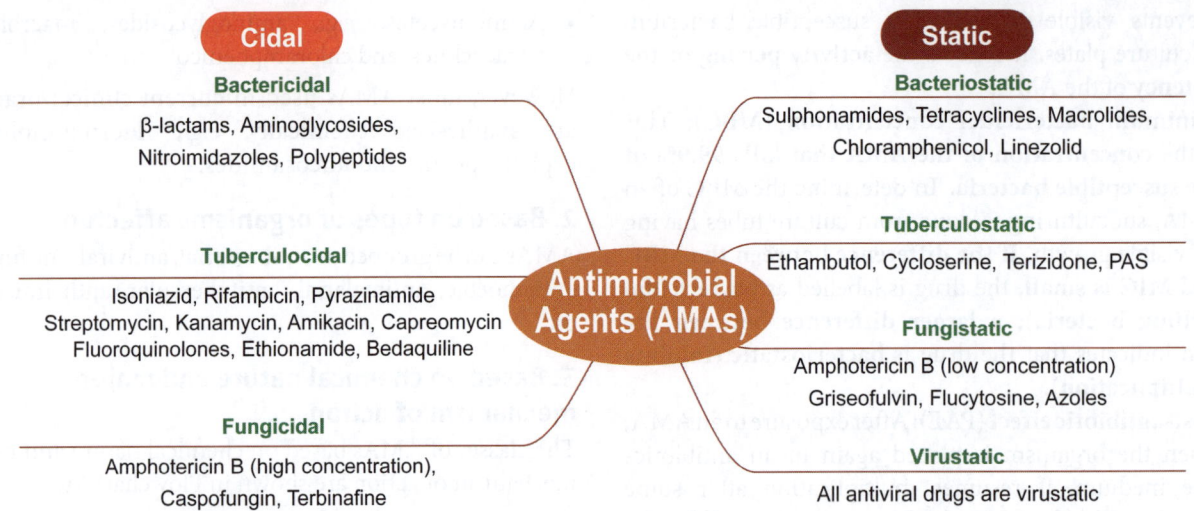

Flowchart 51.2 Classification of antimicrobial agents based on type of action

- Certain other AMAs such as β-lactams and macrolides show time-dependent effects. Their concentration should be kept above the MIC for maximum time between doses to ensure clinical efficacy.

6. Based on the type of action

AMAs can be classified as 'cidal' (which kill microorganisms) or 'static' (which inhibit growth of microbes) (Flowchart 51.2).

However, such classification of AMAs into static or cidal is arbitrary and less used nowadays, as some static drugs can be cidal at high concentrations. For example, sulphonamides, nitrofurantoin and erythromycin show bactericidal effect in urine, where they attain high concentrations. Moreover, the effect of cidal drugs is more pronounced against rapidly multiplying organisms. Static drugs slow the rate of multiplication of microorganisms and thus protect them from the killing effect of cidal drugs. Such mutual antagonism of AMAs having static and cidal effects must be kept in mind while choosing antimicrobial combinations.

Clinical problem-based questions and MCQs

1. **Differentiate between the following terms.**
   i. Antibiotic and antimicrobial agents
   ii. Bacteriostatic and bactericidal drugs
   iii. MIC and MBC

2. **Identify the antimicrobial agent that inhibits bacterial protein synthesis.**
   a. Penicillins   b. Monobactams
   c. Macrolides   d. Quinolones

3. **Which of the following antimicrobial groups has long post-antibiotic effect?**
   a. Penicillins   b. Monobactams
   c. Macrolides   d. Fluoroquinolones

4. **Identify the bactericidal drugs from the following:**
   a. Carbapenems   b. Tetracyclines
   c. Sulphonamides   d. Macrolides

5. **Penicillin G is a:**
   a. Broad-spectrum cidal drug
   b. Broad-spectrum static drug
   c. Narrow-spectrum cidal drug
   d. Narrow-spectrum static drug

6. **Some AMAs exert their antibacterial effect by inhibiting intermediary metabolism. Identify the group.**
   a. Diaminopyrimidines   b. Fluoroquinolones
   c. Monobactams   d. Chloramphenicol

PROBLEMS ASSOCIATED WITH USE OF AMAs

In current clinical practice, antimicrobial agents are amongst the most frequently prescribed drugs. Very often, these are used without rational justification. Such rampant overuse of AMAs is associated with a variety of problems including adverse toxic effects, hypersensitivity reactions (type B ADRs), nutritional deficiencies, superinfection, and drug resistance.

1. Adverse Effects of AMAs

Every drug has the potential to cause some adverse effects, and AMAs are not an exception.

- Some AMAs may cause **local irritant effect at the site of administration,** resulting in gastric irritant effects on oral use or pain at the site of IM injection. Sometimes, a sterile abscess may be formed. Inflammation of the injected vein may occur, causing thrombophlebitis. Chloramphenicol, tetracycline and erythromycin, for example, show such local irritant actions.

- **Organ specific systemic toxicity** is associated with use of aminoglycosides, tetracyclines, chloramphenicol, vancomycin, amphotericin B, etc.
- Unpredictable adverse effects, not related to dose, e.g., **hypersensitivity reactions** (rashes, itching, urticaria), angioedema, bone marrow suppression, blood dyscrasias, and even anaphylaxis are frequently associated with the use of penicillins, sulphonamides and cephalosporins. They may, however, occur with any agent.

2. Nutritional Deficiency

Prolonged use of AMAs can alter the normal intestinal flora and cause deficiency of vitamin B complex and vitamin K. Malabsorption syndrome and steatorrhea may occur.

3. Masking of Chronic Infection

Masking of chronic infections may occur with short-term use of an AMA for some trivial concurrent infection. For example, short-term use of streptomycin for trivial respiratory infection may mask tuberculosis, which manifests later in a more severe form.

4. Superinfection

Superinfection is the occurrence of a new infection while receiving antimicrobial therapy for an infectious disease.

The normal flora of the body competes with pathogens for nutrients and also secretes substances like bacteriocins, which suppress the growth of pathogenic bacteria (Fig. 51.1). **Prolonged use of broad-spectrum AMAs like tetracyclines, ampicillin, and chloramphenicol suppresses or alters normal bacterial flora and predisposing the body to infection by organisms of low pathogenicity** (e.g., Candida). This mostly occurs in immunocompromised individuals with impaired host defence mechanisms, as seen in patients of AIDS, agranulocytosis, diabetes mellitus, or those receiving corticosteroids or immunosuppressant therapy.

Common sites for superinfection are the ones harbouring normal commensals like oropharynx, gastrointestinal tract, genitourinary tract, respiratory tract and skin.

Examples of superinfections and drugs useful in managing these:

1. Thrush, vulvovaginitis, and monilial diarrhea caused by Candida are managed using antifungal drugs (clotrimazole, nystatin, etc).
2. Enteritis caused by resistant strains of *Staphylococcus* responds to cloxacillin.
3. The use of AMAs like clindamycin, tetracyclines, aminoglycosides and ampicillin is associated with pseudomembranous enterocolitis, especially after colorectal surgery. In this condition, an enterotoxin released by *Clostridium difficile* damages the gut mucosa and plaques are formed. This condition is managed with metronidazole and vancomycin.
4. UTIs and enteritis caused by *Proteus* and *Pseudomonas* respond to cephalosporins and penicillins, respectively.

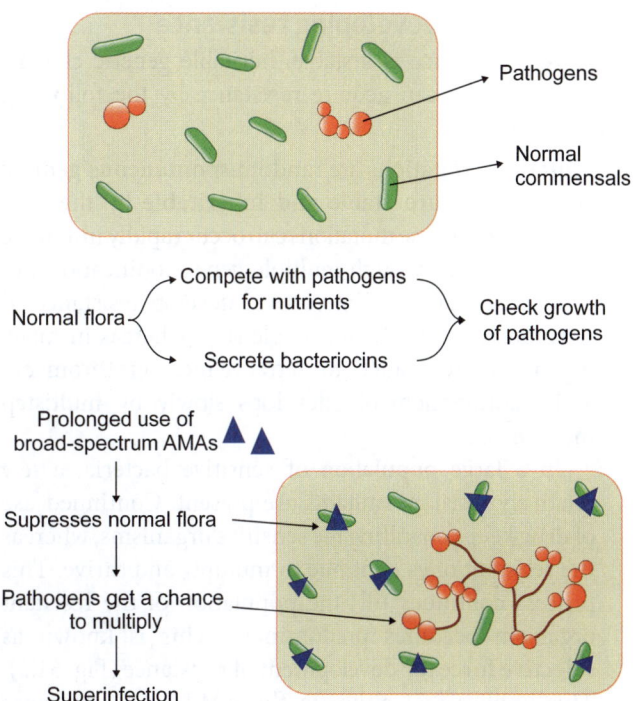

Fig. 51.1 Superinfection

While managing superinfections, in addition to the use of organism-specific drugs, it is important to discontinue the offending drug that caused the superinfection. Superinfections can be prevented by the rational use of antibiotics, e.g., avoiding antibiotics for trivial infections, using them only when necessary, in appropriate doses for appropriate durations, and selecting narrow-spectrum drugs.

5. Antimicrobial Drug Resistance

This is the major medical problem associated with antimicrobial use. Resistance refers to the **unresponsiveness of a microorganism to an AMA.**

Microbial resistance to drugs can be natural or acquired.

a. **Natural resistance** is not much of a hazard. It is a characteristic of an entire species or particular strains within a species. This type of resistance to AMAs occurs because the organism lacks a metabolic pathway or target site specific for that drug. However, alternative drugs are available and the infection can be easily managed.

b. **Acquired resistance** is a major clinical problem. Here, the organism, which was initially sensitive to the drug, develops resistance to the drug upon its use over a period of time.

Mechanism of developing resistance

Acquired resistance is a stable, heritable genetic change. Microorganisms can acquire resistance by the following mechanisms:

1. **Mutation**: Mutations are random **spontaneous genetic changes that are stable and inheritable** by the next generations. These mutations can occur rapidly in a single step or slowly through multiple gene modifications, in a stepwise manner. Enterococci develop resistance to streptomycin rapidly in a single step, whereas in many organisms, resistance to tetracyclines, erythromycin and chloramphenicol develops slowly by multistep mutations.

   In a large population of sensitive bacteria, a few relatively resistant mutants are present. Continued use of drug keeps on killing the sensitive organisms, whereas the resistant ones continue to multiply and thrive. This process continues till the population of the resistant organism becomes predominant. This is known as **selective force** for development of resistance (Fig. 51.2). This implies that although the AMA does not cause the mutation, it is acting as a force that selectively kills sensitive organisms and favours the growth of resistant strains.

2. **Adaptation**: Microorganisms have the potential to synthesise **drug-destroying enzymes** or possess such enzymes in low concentrations. Upon exposure to antimicrobial agents (AMAs), the microorganisms can be induced to synthesise these enzymes in larger quantities. This adaptation enables them to break down the drug molecules more effectively. For example, exposure to semisynthetic penicillins induces synthesis of penicillinase in certain strains of *Staphylococcus*.

3. **Transfer of the gene coding for resistance 'R factor' from resistant to susceptible organisms**: R factor, the genetic material coding for resistance, may be associated with chromosomal or plasmid DNA. This gets transferred from resistant strains to sensitive strains by any of the following processes: **conjugation, transduction, or transformation** (Fig. 51.3).

   In conjugation, the 'R factor' is transferred from cell to cell by direct contact **through a bridge or sex pilus**. The presence of resistance transfer factor (RTF) is also mandatory for this process. Transduction involves transfer of an 'R factor' carrying plasmid **through the agency of a bacteriophage.** In transformation, the resistant strain releases R factor-carrying **DNA into medium**; this free DNA may be imbibed by another sensitive organism.

The response of resistant organisms to an AMA is suboptimal due to following reasons:

- **Increased destruction of drug by enzymes** released by resistant organisms, e.g., β-lactamases released

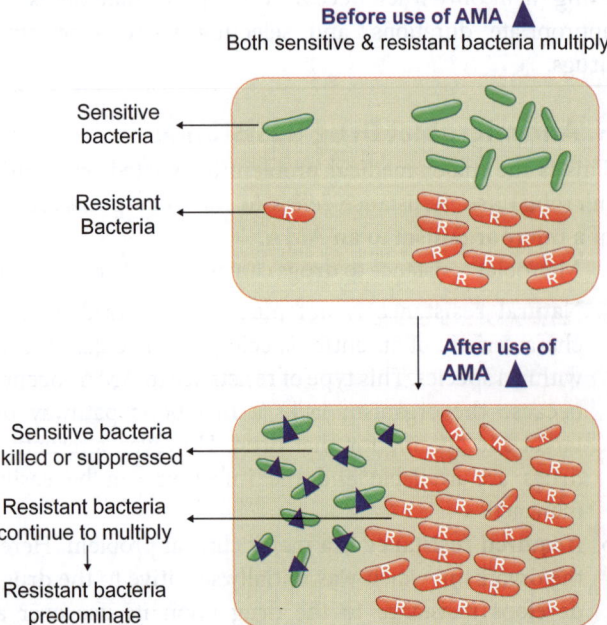

Fig. 51.2 Selective force for development of resistance

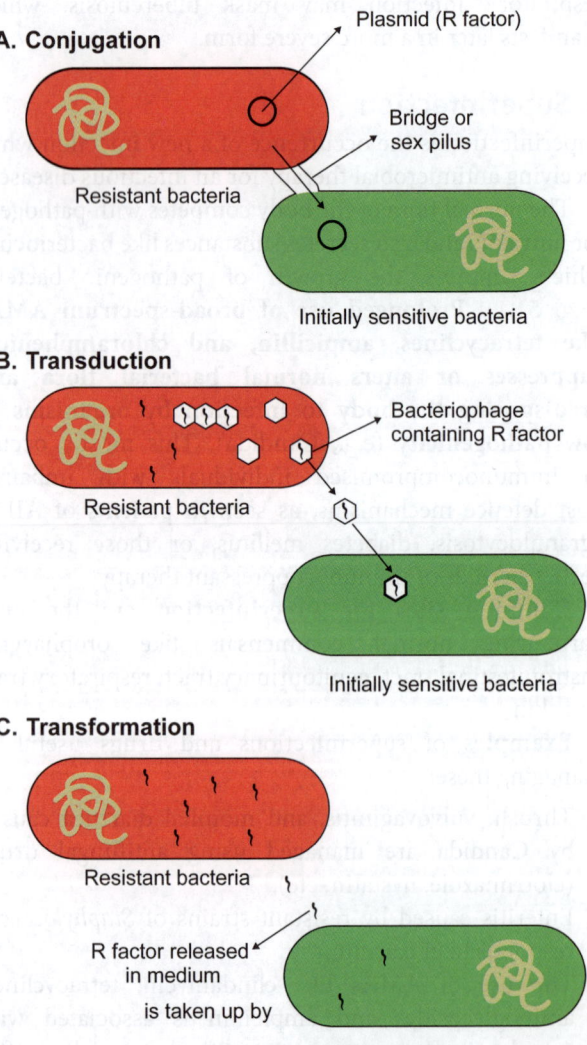

Fig. 51.3 Mechanism of transfer of resistance

by staphylococci destroy penicillins; acetylating/phosphorylating enzymes released by gram-negative bacilli can inactivate aminoglycosides.
- **Change in permeability of the bacteria** so that the drug is not transported into it, e.g., resistance to polymyxins and tetracyclines.
- The target site of the drug may be altered to **lose or have reduced affinity** for the drug, e.g., 30S ribosomal subunit is altered, resulting in resistance to aminoglycosides; tetrahydropteroic acid synthase of resistant bacteria has less affinity for sulphonamides.
- **Cross-resistance**: Organisms that have become resistant to a particular drug after exposure to it are sometimes found to be resistant to another drug, even without exposure to this drug.

Cross-resistance commonly occurs between chemically related drugs, e.g., resistance to one of the sulphonamides confers resistance to all other sulphonamides. This is called **complete cross-resistance**. Tetracyclines also show complete cross-resistance.

Partial cross-resistance is seen among aminoglycosides. e.g., resistance to gentamicin causes resistance to streptomycin/neomycin, but the reverse is not true. Partial cross-resistance may occur between chemically unrelated drugs—for example, tetracyclines and chloramphenicol, or erythromycin and lincomycin.

Prevention of Development of Resistance

Development of resistance by an increasing number of organisms to existing drugs causes failure of therapy, necessitating repeated determination of drug sensitivity pattern, revision of therapy, and introduction of newer drugs. Therefore, some general principles must be followed while prescribing AMAs to prevent resistance.

- **AMAs should be used only when necessary.** In case of minor viral infections, colds, etc., antimicrobials should not be given.
- When antimicrobials are needed, **specific narrow-spectrum drugs should be preferred over broad-spectrum drugs**. Only when a specific drug is unsuitable or unavailable should broad-spectrum drugs be used.
- The **dose and duration of treatment with AMAs should be adequate**. Infections caused by organisms that are notorious for developing resistance, such as staphylococci and proteus, should be treated intensively.
- Antimicrobial therapy should not be unduly prolonged. When prolonged therapy is required, such as in tuberculosis, **combination of antimicrobials should be used to prevent selective force** and development of resistance.

Clinical problem-based questions and MCQs

7. A 10-year-old boy is diagnosed with meningococcal meningitis. There is a history of allergic reaction to cephalosporins. Chloramphenicol succinate is given as IV injection. Next day, the patient develops edema in the arm where the injection was administered, along with pain, warmth and, bluish discolouration at the site of injection.
   i. What is the cause of his symptoms?
   ii. Name two other antimicrobial drugs that can cause a similar reaction.

8. Identify the antimicrobial drugs that have low therapeutic index.
   a. Penicillins   b. Erythromycin
   c. Aminoglycosides   d. Cephalosporins

9. Penicillins are notorious for causing hypersensitivity reactions. Identify the manifestation of hypersensitivity.
   a. Paresthesia   b. Blood dyscrasia
   c. Thrombophlebitis   d. Renal damage

10. A 55-year-old female patient suffering from otitis media is put on oral ampicillin 60 mg/kg body weight /day for 7 days. On the third day, the patient complains of diarrhea.
    i. What is the cause of diarrhea?
    ii. Describe the phenomenon involved in detail.

11. A 35-year-old male with gonorrhea fails to respond to penicillin treatment. On microbiological investigation, organisms are seen to be resistant to drug.
    i. Describe drug resistance.
    ii. Explain the various mechanisms responsible for development of resistant strains.
    iii. Describe measures to prevent emergence of resistant strains.

GENERAL PRINCIPLES OF ANTIMICROBIAL THERAPY

Introduction of antimicrobial agents is one of the biggest advances in the treatment of infectious diseases. The appropriate AMA, given in adequate dose for adequate duration, provides dramatic relief and cures many infective diseases. However, inappropriate selection and rampant, irrational use of AMAs has resulted in numerous problems. Among them, the development of resistance by organisms is the most important and requires immediate attention and remedial actions.

Some general principles should be followed while treating infectious diseases with AMAs.

1. **Make precise diagnosis**: For treating infectious diseases properly, first of all, a precise and correct diagnosis should be made. As far as possible, the **site** where the infection has occurred, **the infecting organism, and its sensitivity to various drugs** should be determined before prescribing AMAs. Ideally, biological samples (blood, urine, sputum, etc.) should be collected

for culture sensitivity testing before giving empiric antibiotics.
2. **Ascertain the necessity of antimicrobial use**: Acute infections generally require antimicrobial chemotherapy. However, some acute infections may be managed by symptomatic treatment, e.g., gastroenteritis. For chronic infections like abscess and empyema, it is important to drain the abscess, remove tissue barriers, and remove any obstructions from the respiratory tract or urinary tract (urinary catheters, IV cannula, etc). **Surgery to break down tissue barriers should be done under chemotherapeutic cover** to prevent flaring up or dissemination of the infection.
3. **Select the best antimicrobial drug**: It is important to choose the AMA after **considering various factors** related to the patient, drug, infecting organism, and infection site. It is always best to **use a specific AMA**, i.e., the organism responsible must be covered in the spectrum of the chosen drug. Local sensitivity patterns and culture/sensitivity reports help in selecting the appropriate antibiotic. Patient's history should be carefully elicited to **rule out any allergic reactions** to the chosen drug. It should be ensured that the patient's **drug-metabolising hepatic system and drug-excreting renal system are functioning normally** and can handle the drug. The site of infection must also be considered and drugs that **can reach the site of infection** should be chosen. To improve compliance, it is also important to consider the **affordability and ease of use** of the antimicrobial regimen for the patient. Use of broad-spectrum drugs should be avoided as far as possible, as indiscriminate use of such drugs for common infections increases selection pressure and favours development of resistance.
4. **Appropriate dose, route and duration**: Once the drug is chosen, the appropriate dose and route of administration for the patient should be decided. Treatment should be **continued till an apparent cure** is achieved. Most acute infections resolve within 5–10 days of antimicrobial therapy. Cure is microbiologically confirmed in some cases.
5. **Monitoring effectiveness of therapy**: Once antibiotic therapy is started, response should be evaluated at an early stage to ensure suitability of treatment. **'Streamlining, sequential use, stepping down, switching' actions** should be carried out as required.
   a. **Streamlining** refers to replacing the intravenous broad-spectrum antibiotic with a narrow-spectrum drug, which specifically targets the offending organism as confirmed by culture–sensitivity reports.
   b. **Sequential** change relates to changing the IV formulation of an antibiotic to its oral formulation, ensuring no loss of potency.
   c. **Switching** involves changing the IV antibiotic to an oral formulation of another antibiotic, but without any loss of potency.
   d. **Stepping down** is the change of IV antibiotic to an oral agent of same or different class of similar antibiotics, with reduction in potency
6. **Indications for combining AMAs**: Antimicrobial combinations are required in some situations. The use of fixed-drug combination (FDC) preparations improves patient compliance in such cases. These include:
   a. In chronic infections requiring **prolonged therapy,** such as tuberculosis and infective endocarditis, to prevent development of resistant strains. For example, isoniazid, rifampicin, pyrazinamide and ethambutol are used together in the intensive phase of tuberculosis treatment.
   b. In known **mixed infections,** e.g., peritonitis after gut perforation, antimicrobials can be combined to broaden the spectrum of activity.
   c. When it is **difficult to predict the causative organism** but necessary to start treatment before microbiological confirmation by culture/sensitivity tests, e.g., septicemia in neutropenic patients and severe community-acquired pneumonia.
   d. Sometimes, drugs are combined **for their synergistic action.** For example, a combination of gentamicin and penicillin is used in enterococcal SABE, as penicillin acts on the cell wall and increases permeability of the organism to aminoglycosides. Cotrimoxazole, which is a combination of sulphamethoxazole and trimethoprim, causes sequential blockade of folic acid synthesis and reduction. It exerts cidal action, even though each component is bacteriostatic when used alone.
   e. **To decrease dose of one component** to reduce adverse effects, e.g., combined use of flucytosine and amphotericin B for cryptococcal meningitis.
   f. Topical antimicrobial combinations are used **to cover a broad range** of gram-positive and negative organisms, e.g., a combination of neomycin, polymyxin B and bacitracin is available for topical use on the skin and eye.

However, combinations of static and cidal drugs should be avoided, as antagonism may occur (cidal drugs act on fast-multiplying organisms and static drugs reduce the rate of their multiplication). For example, the combination of penicillin with tetracycline/chloramphenicol in pneumococcal meningitis and the combination of nalidixic acid and nitrofurantoin in E. coli infection are less efficacious than the cidal drug used alone.

In the absence of the above-mentioned indications, casual use of antimicrobial combinations increases the risk of superinfections, adverse effects, toxicity, cost of treatment, and favours the emergence of resistant organisms.

Prophylactic Use of Antimicrobial Agents

This involves the use of antimicrobial agents for preventing infection or for suppressing a contracted infection from becoming manifest.

Prophylactic use of antimicrobial drugs is justified in the following situations:

a. **Against specific organisms:**
   - Benzathine penicillin against rheumatic fever
   - Isoniazid for 6 months, for children exposed to open cases of tuberculosis
   - Azithromycin against *Mycobacterium avium* complex (MAC)
   - Post-exposure prophylaxis for HIV with tenofovir and emtricitabine
   - Rifampicin for prevention of meningococcal meningitis Ampicillin for prevention of gonorrhea, immediately after exposure
   - Malaria prophylaxis with mefloquine for travellers to endemic areas
   - Cholera prophylaxis with tetracycline

b. **When** the **patient is at a high risk for infection** such as in patients with indwelling catheters, abnormalities of urinary tract, COPD, valvular defects, and immune-compromised status due to some disease or drugs.

c. **Surgeries where the procedure lasts for > 2 hours** or a **prosthesis is inserted**; surgeries involving **perforation and spillage** of secretions from the GI/biliary/respiratory/urinary tract; **opening of pus-containing sites, penetrating injuries,** etc., need antimicrobial prophylaxis. However, care should be taken not to unduly prolong the duration of AMA use. Adequate antibiotic activity at the time of closure of the wound and a few hours beyond is sufficient to prevent surgical site infections (SSIs).

Antimicrobial prophylaxis is not at all required in babies born after prolonged labour, in women after normal vaginal delivery, in mild upper respiratory viral infections, in routine clean, elective surgeries, and unconscious patient on respirator. Use of AMAs in these conditions unnecessarily exposes the patient to adverse effects and increases the risk of development of drug resistance.

Failure of Antimicrobial Therapy

The effectiveness of antimicrobial agents is judged by clinical improvement of the patient and eradication of the infecting organism from biological samples. However, failure to respond to antimicrobials is frequently encountered in clinical practice. Important causes of failure of antimicrobial therapy include:

a. **Noncompliance by patient:** The patient may not be taking drug in prescribed dose or for adequate duration. This may be due to high cost of drugs, adverse effects of drugs, symptom relief occurring before biological cure, and inability of the patient to understand the concerns for drug resistance.

b. **Wrong selection** of drug, dose, and route of administration for a particular case: The selected drug should be effective against the offending pathogen and must be given in a dosage form by a route which achieves adequate concentration at the site of infection.

c. If there are **tissue barriers** that interfere with the movement of drug to infective site, they should be removed surgically under the cover of antimicrobials.

d. **Duration of treatment** may be inadequate.

e. The response of patients with **compromised immune functions** (e.g., those on corticosteroid and anticancer drugs, HIV positive patients, diabetics) is poor, especially to static drugs.

f. The presence of dormant or resistant organisms may cause treatment failure.

ANTIBIOTIC STEWARDSHIP PROGRAM (ASP)

Antimicrobials are the most **overused, misused** and **abused** of all therapeutic drugs.

- **Overuse** refers to prescription of AMAs for conditions where they are not indicated (e.g., non-infective diarrheas, minor viral infection of the upper respiratory tract, prophylaxis in clean/elective surgery) or extending antimicrobial therapy beyond a time when there is no further clinical benefit, e.g., in surgical prophylaxis, antimicrobials are continued for many days postoperatively).

- **Misuse** is the use of antibiotics reserved for serious nosocomial infections in patients having trivial community-acquired infections; not prescribing or changing the antimicrobial in accordance with the culture sensitivity report is also misuse.

- **Abuse** involves prescribing an AMA or a particular brand in preference to other more effective or less costly options for financial or other benefits.

Irrational use of antibiotics is a **hazard** to individual patients as well as the community. Patients are exposed to adverse effects, toxic effects, extra cost and prolonged hospital stay if parenteral drugs are prescribed without actual need. The total healthcare costs also escalate. In addition, inappropriate use of AMAs favours development of resistant strains that are difficult to treat. As a result, the entire community is at greater risk of exposure to resistant infections.

The term '**stewardship**' means supervising or taking care of something. This term was used in the context of antimicrobial use for the first time in 1996, with the purpose of **monitoring and optimising antibiotic use to check rapid development of antimicrobial resistance**

(AMR). A global action plan on AMR was adopted by WHO in 2015. In India, a National Action Plan (NAP) for AMR was released in April 2017. The Indian Council for Medical Research (ICMR) released recent stewardship guidelines in November 2018.

Definition

Antibiotic stewardship is defined as the "optimal selection of antimicrobial drug, its dose and duration of treatment to ensure best clinical outcomes for patient with minimum adverse toxic effects and minimum impact on antimicrobial resistance subsequently".

Goals of ASP

1. To reduce the development of antimicrobial resistance (AMR) among organisms
2. To promote rational use of AMAs
3. To prevent antimicrobial overuse, misuse and abuse

Governance of ASP: The ASP is to be run by a **stewardship team** (ASP team) established in each hospital. The constitution of the team may vary based on the priorities and needs of the individual hospital. However, it is recommended that the team should include **an infectious disease physician, a microbiologist, a pharmacist and an administrator.**

Activities of ASP

Important activities of antibiotic stewardship program include the following.

- **Identifying current problems** specific to a hospital with regard to pathogens and their sensitivity patterns
- Networking and **sharing AMR data** with healthcare providers in the same hospital as well as other hospitals at the regional and national levels.
- **Designing antibiotic order forms** for the hospital: These facilitate consideration of various factors before prescribing antimicrobial drugs to ensure that the drug, dose and duration selected are appropriate.
- **Formulating treatment algorithms** as a pocketbook guide, mentioning appropriate antibiotics for different infections, trend of sensitivity or resistance in that particular hospital, doses as per body weight, low-cost alternative options, indications/options for empiric and prophylactic antibiotic use.
- **Pre-prescription intervention** to identify **restricted AMAs,** for which permission from ASP team is mandated before prescribing and supplying to patients. Carbapenems, linezolid, glycopeptides, some higher-generation cephalosporins and clindamycin are the commonly restricted antimicrobials. This restriction favours the use of antimicrobial drugs only for specific indications, and prevents the development of resistance against these drugs.
- **Post-prescription intervention** allows the ASP team to **review an antibiotic order** and advise the treating doctor accordingly. This intervention facilitates the use of specific drugs for a case and its **de-escalation,** such as changing from combination therapy to monotherapy, from broad-spectrum empiric drug to specific drug as guided by the microbiological report, or discontinuation of antimicrobial therapy.
- **Optimising the dose, route of administration and duration** of the antimicrobial therapy by educating healthcare providers about the various pharmacokinetic and pharmacodynamic properties of drugs.

AWaRe Classification

A WHO expert committee on the 'Selection and Use of Essential Medicines' developed the AWaRe classification of antibiotics in 2017. It is a tool to support ASP activities at the local, national and global levels and optimise antibiotic use. In this classification, antibiotics are classified as **Access**, **Watch** and **Reserve** groups, based on their impact on antimicrobial resistance. The list was updated in 2019 to include 170 commonly used antimicrobial drugs.

Access: Antimicrobial agents that possess activity against a wide range of commonly encountered susceptible organisms and have lower resistance potential than the other two groups (watch and reserve) fall in this category. These drugs are often recommended as the first- or second-choice drugs for empiric treatment. It is recommended that 60% of the total antibiotic consumption at country level should be from the Access group.

There are 48 drugs in this category. Notable examples are:

- Benzylpenicillin or penicillin G, benzathine penicillin G, procaine penicillin G, phenoxymethyl penicillin
- Ampicillin, amoxicillin, amoxicillin + clavulanic acid, cloxacillin
- Cephalexin, cefazolin, cotrimoxazole
- Doxycycline, gentamicin, metronidazole, chloramphenicol, nitrofurantoin.

Watch: Antibiotic classes that have higher potential for development of resistance are included in this group. These are the key targets of ASP and monitoring. These drugs are recommended for use in specific infectious diseases as an essential first or second-choice empiric option. There are 110 drugs in this category, e.g., quinolones, fluoroquinolones, third-generation cephalosporins, macrolides, glycopeptides, and carbapenems.

Reserve: These are last resort antibiotics that are reserved for treatment of suspected/confirmed infections by multidrug-resistant organisms. These drugs should be accessible, but their use should be limited to highly specific cases where no suitable alternative is available. There are 22 drugs in this group: fourth- and fifth-generation cephalosporins, oxazolidinones, aztreonam, tigecycline, polymyxin, fosfomycin, daptomycin, etc.

Clinical problem-based questions and MCQs

12. Prescription of antibiotics reserved for serious nosocomial infections in a patient with trivial community-acquired infection is considered as:
    a. Overuse
    b. Misuse
    b. Abuse
    c. Prophylaxis
13. Continued administration of AMAs in the postoperative period to prevent SSIs constitutes:
    a. Overuse
    b. Misuse
    c. Abuse
    d. Prophylactic use
14. Identify the drug that belongs to the 'watch' category:
    a. Amoxicillin
    b. Cephalexin
    c. Aztreonam
    d. Moxifloxacin
15. As per the AWaRe classification, to which category does tigecycline belong?
    a. Access
    b. Watch
    c. Reserve
    d. None of the above

Summary

- Chemotherapy is the use of drugs of known chemical structure for the inhibition of growth or killing of infecting microorganisms without significantly affecting the host cells.
- Antibiotics are obtained from microorganisms and have an inhibitory effect on microorganisms when used in low concentration. Synthetic drugs with such effect are called chemotherapeutic agents. Antimicrobial agents (AMAs) is a broad term that includes both antibiotics and chemotherapeutic agents.
- AMAs are classified based on their source (natural/synthetic), mechanism of action (inhibition of cell wall synthesis/protein synthesis/nucleic acid synthesis/DNA gyrase enzyme/folate synthase enzyme/DHFRase enzyme), extent of action (cidal/static drugs), chemical nature (β-lactams/sulphonamides/diaminopyrimidines/fluoroquinolones/aminoglycosides/tetracyclines/macrolides/glycopeptides, etc.)
- Chemotherapeutic index reflects the margin of safety of an AMA. It is the ratio of the lethal dose (LD) 0.1 and curing dose (CD) 99.9.
- Minimum inhibitory concentration (MIC) is the lowest concentration of an AMA that inhibits multiplication and prevents visible growth of a susceptible bacterium in culture plates and reflects the activity per mg or the potency of an AMA.
- Minimum bactericidal concentration (MBC) is the concentration of an AMA that kills 99.9% of susceptible bacteria. A small difference between MBC and MIC indicates bactericidal action, while a larger difference indicates bacteriostatic action.
- Problems associated with the use of antimicrobial agents include organ-specific toxicities (e.g., aminoglycosides and vancomycin are nephrotoxic; pyrazinamide is hepatotoxic), nutritional deficiencies, masking of chronic infection, superinfection and development of drug resistance.
- Superinfection is the occurrence of a new infection by an organism of low pathogenicity during prolonged AMA use, e.g., thrush, enteritis, pseudomembranous enterocolitis, and UTIs.
- Resistance to AMAs can be natural or acquired. Acquired resistance can occur due to mutation or transfer of the R factor from resistant to sensitive organisms via conjugation (through sex pilus/bridge), transduction (through bacteriophage) and transformation (through medium). Resistant bacteria develop drug-destroying enzymes and have reduced affinity for concentrating or binding to the drug. Cross-resistance (total or partial) may occur among drugs that share chemical structure or mechanism of action.
- To prevent the development of drug resistance among microorganisms, antibiotics should be used only when necessary, in adequate dose, and for an appropriate duration. Specific, narrow-spectrum drugs are preferable over broad-spectrum drugs, and drug combinations are used if prolonged therapy is needed, e.g., for tuberculosis and leprosy.
- Antibiotic stewardship (ASP) is defined as the optimal selection of antimicrobial drug, its dose, and duration of treatment to ensure the best clinical outcomes for the patient with minimum adverse toxic effects and minimum impact on antimicrobial resistance.
- ASP aims to prevent development of antimicrobial resistance and ensure rational use of AMAs, while avoiding overuse, abuse and misuse.
- Important activities under ASP include identifying problems regarding the sensitivity of pathogens in the hospital, sharing these with the treating doctors, preparing treatment algorithms, controlling prescription of restricted antibiotics, monitoring of antibiotic orders to ensure de-escalation as needed, and ensuring appropriate dose, route and duration of antimicrobial therapy.
- AWaRe classification: WHO has divided antibiotics into access, watch and reserve groups and provided extensive lists to support ASP activities and rational use of antibiotics.

Questions for practice

1. Enumerate the various problems associated with the use of AMAs.
2. Comment on the mechanisms responsible for the development of drug resistance and suggest measures to prevent the same.
3. Enumerate situations where antimicrobial prophylaxis is useful.
4. Comment on the possible causes of failure of antimicrobial therapy.
5. Explain why:
   i Superinfections are frequently reported with antimicrobial therapy.
   ii Organisms that have acquired resistance to one of the penicillins fail to respond to other penicillins also.
   iii Antimicrobial combinations are preferred over single drug use when prolonged therapy is required.
   iv Combination of static and cidal drugs may produce antagonistic effects.
6. Describe the goals and activities of antibiotic stewardship program.

Hints for problem-based questions and MCQs

1. i. Antibiotics are chemicals produced by microorganisms that have the capacity to inhibit or kill other microorganisms when used in very low concentrations, whereas the term 'antimicrobial agents (AMAs)' is a broad term including drugs of natural origin, i.e., antibiotics, as well as synthetic drugs, i.e., chemotherapeutic agents that possess anti-infective activity.
   ii. Drugs which inhibit the multiplication of bacteria are static drugs, whereas drugs that kill bacterial cells are bactericidal. For example, tetracycline, sulphonamides and macrolides are bacteriostatic; penicillin and aminoglycosides are cidal.
   iii. MIC is the lowest concentration of an AMA that prevents visible growth of susceptible organisms in culture plates. MBC is the concentration of the AMA that kills 99.9% of susceptible organisms.
2. c. Macrolides (Refer to Flowchart 51.1, page 659)
3. d. Fluoroquinolones, as they have a concentration-dependent effect.
4. a. Carbapenems are ß-lactam drugs with cidal effect (refer to Flowchart 51.2, page 660).
5. c. Narrow-spectrum cidal drug (refer to page 660)
6. a. Diaminopyrimidines (Refer to Flowchart 51.1, page 659)
7. i. The patient has developed thrombophlebitis of the injected vein due to the irritant nature of chloramphenicol.
   ii. Erythromycin, tetracyclines are also irritant in nature.
8. iii. Aminoglycosides have low therapeutic index as they show toxic effects on kidney and the 8th cranial nerve. (Refer to page 661)
9. b. Blood dyscrasia (refer to page 661)
10. i. Diarrhea associated with use of ampicillin is a result of alteration of intestinal bacterial flora and superinfection.
    ii. Superinfection is the appearance of a new infection while receiving antimicrobial therapy for an infectious disease. Refer to page 661.
11. i. Resistance refers to the unresponsiveness of a microorganism to AMAs. Refer to page 661.
    ii. Resistance develops due to mutation, adaptation or transfer of the 'R factor' from the resistant bacteria to sensitive bacteria by conjugation, transduction or transformation (refer to page 662.)
    iii. Refer to page 663.
12. b. Misuse
13. a. Overuse
14. d. Moxifloxacin
15. c. Reserve

CONCEPT MAP – GENERAL PRINCIPLES OF CHEMOTHERAPY

Terms

Chemotherapy: It is treatment of systemic infections with specific drugs that are natural or synthetic chemicals and possess selective suppressive effect on the infecting microorganism but do not affect host cells significantly

Minimum inhibitory concentration (MIC): It is the lowest concentration of an AMA that inhibits multiplication and reflects the activity per mg or potency of the AMA

Minimum bactericidal concentration (MBC): It is the concentration of AMA that kills 99.9% of susceptible bacteria

Post-antibiotic effect (PAE): The lag period in resuming growth by microorganisms after brief exposure to AMA is called PAE. Drugs like fluoroquinolones, aminoglycosides and β-lactams have long PAE.

Classification

Based on chemical nature:
Sulphonamides, Diaminopyrimidines
Quinolones, Fluoroquinolones

β-lactams: Penicillins, Cephalosporins, Monobactams, Carbapenems

Tetracyclines, Chloramphenicol, Aminoglycosides, Macrolides

Lincosamides, Glycopeptides, Polypeptides, Oxazolidinones

Miscellaneous: Mupirocin, Fusidic acid, Spectinomycin, Daptomycin, Quinupristin/Dalfopristin

Mechanism of Action

Inhibition of protein synthesis: Macrolides, tetracyclines, chloramphenicol, aminoglycosides, lincosamides, oxazolidinones

Inhibition of cell wall synthesis: β-lactams, glycopeptides, bacitracin

Inhibition of DNA gyrase: Quinolones and fluoroquinolones.

Inhibition of intermediary metabolism: Sulphonamides, diaminopyrimidines, metronidazole, para aminosalicylic acid

Increase in membrane permeability: Colistin, bacitracin, polymyxin B, aminoglycosides.

CHEMOTHERAPY

ADRs

Local irritant effect at the site of administration: Gastric irritant effect, pain at site of IM injection, sterile abscess, inflammation of injected vein causing thrombophlebitis.

Organ-specific systemic toxicity with aminoglycosides, tetracyclines, chloramphenicol, vancomycin, amphotericin B, etc.

Allergic reactions such as rashes, itching, urticaria, angioedema, bone marrow suppression and even anaphylaxis, mainly with penicillins, sulphonamides, cephalosporins.

Nutritional deficiency: Deficiency of vitamin B complex and vitamin K. Malabsorption syndrome and steatorrhea with prolonged use of AMAs that alter normal intestinal flora.

Masking of chronic infection with short-term use of an AMA for some trivial concurrent infection.

Superinfection, Antimicrobial drug resistance

Superinfection

Definition: Prolonged use of broad-spectrum AMAs like tetracyclines, ampicillin, and chloramphenicol suppresses or alters normal bacterial flora and predisposes one to infection by organisms of low pathogenicity like Candida. Mostly affects individuals with impaired host defence mechanisms.

Common sites are those that harbouring normal commensals like oropharynx, GIT, genitourinary tract, respiratory tract and skin.

Examples: Thrush, vulvovaginitis, monilial diarrhea caused by Candida are managed with antifungal drugs like clotrimazole and nystatin.

Enteritis caused by resistant strains of *Staphylococcus* responds to cloxacillin.

Use of AMAs like clindamycin, tetracyclines, aminoglycosides and ampicillin is associated with pseudomembranous enterocolitis, especially after colorectal surgery. In this condition, an enterotoxin released by *Clostridium difficile* damages gut mucosa and plaques are formed. This condition is managed with metronidazole, vancomycin.

UTIs and enteritis caused by *Proteus* and *Pseudomonas* respond to cephalosporins and penicillins, respectively.

Drug Resistance

It is the unresponsiveness of a microorganism to an AMA.

Types: Natural resistance occurs due to lack of metabolic pathway or target site specific for a drug in that organism.

Acquired resistance develops after the use of AMA over a period of time in organisms that were initially sensitive to the drug.

Mechanism of developing resistance: Microorganisms can acquire resistance by the following mechanisms;

Mutation: Mutations are random, spontaneous genetic changes that are stable and inheritable.

Adaptation: Microorganisms have the potential to synthesise drug-destroying enzymes, change in permeability of bacteria.

Transfer of gene coding for resistance 'R factor' from resistant to susceptible organisms by conjugation, transduction, transformation

Cross-resistance: Organisms that have become resistant to a particular drug after exposure to it are sometimes found to be resistant to another drug even without exposure to that drug.

Prevention of resistance: AMAs should be used only when necessary.

Specific narrow-spectrum drugs are preferred over broad-spectrum drugs.

Dose and duration of treatment with AMAs should be adequate.

Antimicrobial therapy should not be unduly prolonged. When prolonged therapy is required, say, as in tuberculosis, combination of antimicrobials should be used to prevent 'selective force' and development of resistance.

General Principles of Antimicrobial Therapy

- A precise, correct diagnosis should be made. The site of infection, infecting organism and its sensitivity to various drugs should be determined, before prescribing AMAs.
- Necessity of antimicrobial use should be ascertained. Acute infections generally require antimicrobial chemotherapy. For chronic infections, removal of tissue barriers/obstruction, if any, in respiratory or urinary tract is important and is usually done under antibiotic cover.
- Choose the best AMA after evaluating various factors related to patient/drug/infecting organism/infection site.
- Dose, route and duration should be appropriate.
- Whenever prolonged therapy with AMAs is required, antimicrobial combinations are used.

SECTION 10 Chemotherapeutic Drugs

52 Antimicrobial Agents (AMAs)

PH 8.3 Explain the kinetics, dynamics, adverse effects, indications of the following antibacterial drugs: Sulphonamides, Quinolones, Beta lactams, Macrolides, Tetracyclines, Aminoglycosides, and newer antibacterial drugs.

Learning objectives

A student of MBBS phase II should be able to:
- Classify different chemical groups of AMAs.
- Describe the mechanism of action of important groups of AMAs.
- Describe the mechanisms of development of resistance by organisms against different AMAs.
- Enumerate therapeutic uses and adverse effects of important groups of AMAs.

CLASSIFICATION OF AMAs

AMAs are classified based on different characteristics, such as:

- Concentration-/time-dependent killing
- Chemical nature
- Mechanism of action

Concentration-/Time-dependent Killing

Cidal drugs can be of 2 types:

a. **Drugs with concentration-dependent killing effect:** The cidal effect of these drugs is greater when the **ratio of peak concentration to MIC is higher**. Therefore, a better response is obtained upon administering a large single-dose of these drugs, e.g., fluoroquinolones and aminoglycosides.

b. **Drugs with time-dependent killing effect:** The cidal effect of these drugs is greater when the **drug concentration remains above MIC for a long period of time**. Therefore, a better response is obtained on administering multiple daily doses of these drugs, such as beta lactams and vancomycin.

It is interesting to note that the inhibitory effect of an AMA persists even after its concentration falls below the MIC. This is known as **post-antibiotic effect (PAE)**. Most drugs have long PAE against gram-positive organisms. Some drugs have long PAE against gram-negative organisms also. For example, chloramphenicol, aminoglycosides, tetracyclines, quinolones, tigecycline, rifampicin, and carbapenems [Mnemonic: Can A Tiger Question The Royal Cat] have a long PAE for gram-negative organisms also.

Based on Chemical Nature

- **Sulphonamides:** Short-acting, intermediate-acting, long-acting and special purpose sulphonamides
- **Diaminopyrimidines:** Trimethoprim and pyrimethamine (**cotrimoxazole** is a fixed-dose combination (FDC) of trimethoprim and sulphamethoxazole)
- **Quinolones and fluoroquinolones (FQs)**, which are divided into two generations based on the chronology of their development.
- **β-lactams:** These include penicillins, cephalosporins, monobactams, and carbapenems
  - **Penicillins:** Naturally obtained penicillin, semisynthetic penicillins such as acid-resistant, penicillinase-resistant, and extended-spectrum penicillins. Extended-spectrum penicillins include aminopenicillins, carboxypenicillins, and ureidopenicillins.
  - **Cephalosporins** are grouped into five generations, based on their chronology of development.
  - **Monobactams:** Aztreonam
  - **Carbapenems:** Imipenem, meropenem, faropenem, doripenem, ertapenem
- **Tetracyclines:** Tetracycline, oxytetracycline, demeclocycline, doxycycline, minocycline, tigecycline
- **Chloramphenicol**
- **Aminoglycosides** are systemic and topical
- **Macrolides:** Erythromycin, clarithromycin, azithromycin, roxithromycin, telithromycin, spiramycin
- **Others:** These include lincosamides, glycopeptides, polypeptides, oxazolidinones and miscellaneous drugs such as mupirocin, fusidic acid, spectinomycin, daptomycin, and quinupristin/dalfopristin.

Based on Mechanism of Action

AMAs can act by the following major mechanisms:

A. Interfering with folic acid metabolism: sulphonamides, diaminopyrimidines, dapsone
B. DNA gyrase inhibitors: quinolones, FQs

C. Cell wall synthesis inhibitors: β-lactams, glycopeptides, bacitracin, cycloserine
D. Protein synthesis inhibitors: Tetracyclines, chloramphenicol, aminoglycosides, macrolides, ketolides, oxazolidinones, lincosamides, streptogramins, etc.

The salient features of important antimicrobial agents are described below.

SALIANT FEATURES OF INDIVIDUAL ANTIMICROBIAL GROUPS

A. ANTIFOLATE ANTIMICROBIALS

These include sulphonamides, diaminopyrimidines and cotrimoxazole.

1. Sulphonamides

Classification

Depending upon their duration of action, sulphonamides can be short-acting, intermediate-acting or long-acting, as shown in Flowchart 52.1. In addition, there are some special-purpose sulphonamides such as sulfacetamide sodium, sulfasalazine, silver sulfadiazine and mafenide.

Mechanism of action

Sulphonamides are structural analogues of para-aminobenzoic acid (PABA). These drugs exert bacteriostatic action by interfering with conversion of PABA into folic acid by competitive inhibition of the folate synthase enzyme. Pus present at site of infection is rich in PABA, which can displace sulphonamides from the binding site on folate synthase enzyme. Therefore, sulphonamides are not effective in the presence of pus.

Pharmacokinetics

Sulphonamides are well absorbed from the gastrointestinal tract and widely distributed in body fluids. They also cross the blood–brain barrier and placental barrier. They are metabolised in the liver by acetylation and excreted by the kidney through glomerular filtration. The metabolites of sulphonamides have poor solubility in acidic urine; hence, they may get precipitated and cause crystalluria.

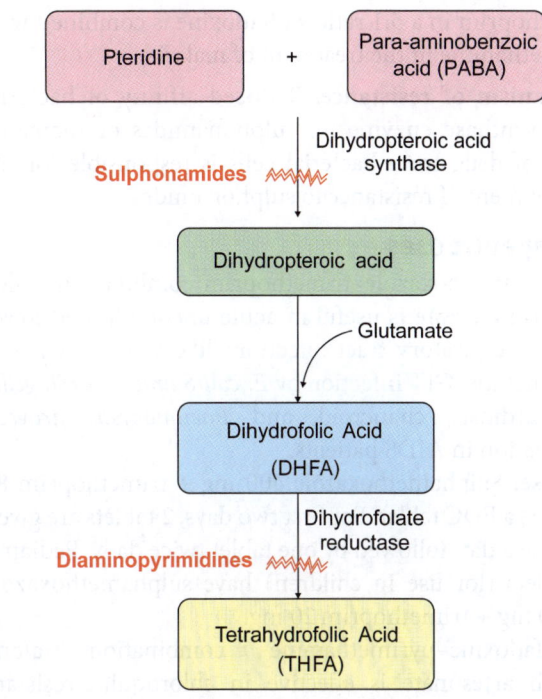

Fig. 52.1 Sequential block by cotrimoxazole

2. Diaminopyrimidines

Diaminopyrimidines (trimethoprim and pyrimethamine) inhibit the conversion of dihydrofolate (DHF) into tetrahydrofolate (THF) by competitive inhibition of dihydrofolate reductase enzyme.

3. Combination of Sulphonamides and Diaminopyrimidines

These combinations cause sequential blockade of synthesis and activation of folic acid in the bacterial cell, resulting in bactericidal effect (Fig. 52.1). One such combination is cotrimoxazole, which contains sulphamethoxazole and

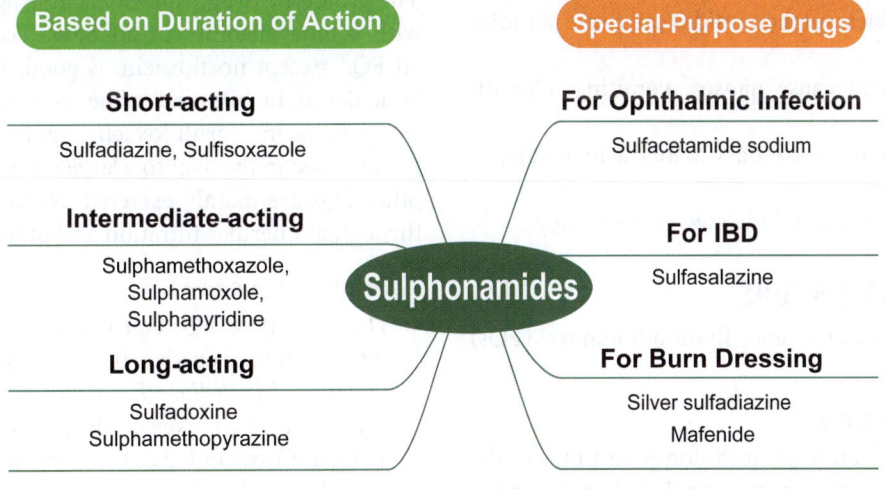

Flowchart 52.1 Classification of sulphonamides

trimethoprim in a 5:1 ratio. Sulfadoxine is combined with pyrimethamine in the treatment of malaria.

Mechanism of resistance: Reduced affinity of bacterial folate synthase enzyme for sulphonamides or increased efflux of drug from bacterial cells is responsible for the development of resistance to sulphonamides.

Therapeutic uses

- Sulphamethoxazole–trimethoprim combination called **cotrimoxazole** is useful in acute uncomplicated lower UTI, respiratory tract infections like acute or chronic bronchitis, GIT infection by *E. coli/Salmonella/Shigella*, nocardiosis, chancroid, and *Pneumocystis jirovecii* infection in AIDS patients.
- **Dose:** Sulphamethoxazole 400 mg + trimethoprim 80 mg is a FDC tablet. For first two days, 2 tablets are given twice a day, followed by one tablet twice daily. Pediatric tablets (for use in children) have sulphamethoxazole 100 mg + trimethoprim 20 mg.
- Sulfadoxine–pyrimethamine combination along with artesunate is effective in chloroquine-resistant falciparum malaria.
- Sulfadiazine–pyrimethamine is the preferred drug for toxoplasmosis.
- Sulfasalazine is used in rheumatoid arthritis, inflammatory bowel disease (IBD), and ulcerative colitis.
- Local sulphonamides: Sulfacetamide sodium eye drops are used for ophthalmic infections, especially trachoma, and silver sulfadiazine and mafenide for the dressing of burns to prevent secondary infection.

Adverse drug reactions

- Sulphonamides may cause crystalluria, hematuria and urinary tract obstruction. To prevent these adverse effects, excess fluid intake and urinary alkalinisation is advised.
- Hypersensitivity reactions like rashes, itching, drug fever, exfoliative dermatitis and Stevens–Johnson syndrome may occur.
- Sulphonamides can cause hemolysis in patients with G6PD deficiency.
- In premature babies, sulphonamides can cause jaundice and kernicterus.
- Cotrimoxazole can cause nausea, vomiting, glossitis and stomatitis.
- Megaloblastic anemia secondary to folic acid deficiency may occur.
- Sulphonamides are contraindicated in pregnancy.

B. DNA GYRASE INHIBITORS

These include quinolones and fluoroquinolones (FQs) (Flowchart 52.2).

Mechanism of Action

The mechanism of action of quinolones and FQs is the same. These drugs exert bactericidal action in gram-

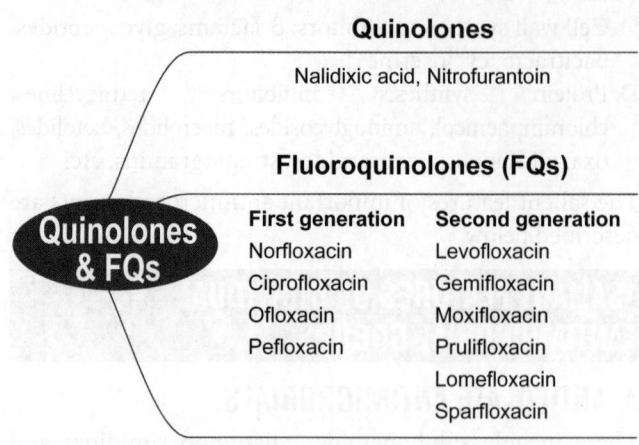

Flowchart 52.2 Classification of quinolones and FQs

negative bacteria through **inhibition of DNA gyrase enzyme.** When the two strands of double-helical DNA are separated for replication, excessive positive supercoiling/overwinding occurs in front of the 'separation point'. This overwinding is undone (corrected) by the DNA gyrase enzyme, which has two 'A' and two 'B' subunits. The 'A' subunit has nicking and resealing functions, while the 'B' subunit introduces a negative supercoil in (unwinds) the DNA strands. FQs bind to subunit 'A' and inhibit the nicking and resealing action of DNA gyrase enzyme, resulting in excessive coiling of DNA, and cell death (Fig. 52.2).

In gram-positive bacteria, inhibition of topoisomerase IV enzyme occurs, interfering with the separation of DNA strands for replication.

Mechanism of resistance

Resistance occurs due to a chromosomal mutation resulting in reduced affinity of DNA gyrase/topoisomerase IV for FQs. Decreased entry of drug into organisms or increased efflux may also contribute to development of resistance to FQs.

Pharmacokinetics

The prototype drug, ciprofloxacin, is well absorbed orally, with a bioavailability of 60–80%. Tissue penetration of all FQs, except norfloxacin, is good. High concentration is achieved in bile and urine as well. Few drugs, such as pefloxacin, prulifloxacin and moxifloxacin, are metabolised in the liver to a large extent (> 70%), while the other FQs are mainly excreted unchanged by the kidney through glomerular filtration and tubular secretion.

Therapeutic uses

- The prototype FQ, ciprofloxacin, is effective against aerobic gram-negative bacteria (*Salmonella, Shigella, Proteus, Klebsiella, E. coli, N. gonorrhoeae, H. influenzae*, etc.). Newer drugs such as moxifloxacin and gemifloxacin have some activity against anaerobes as well.

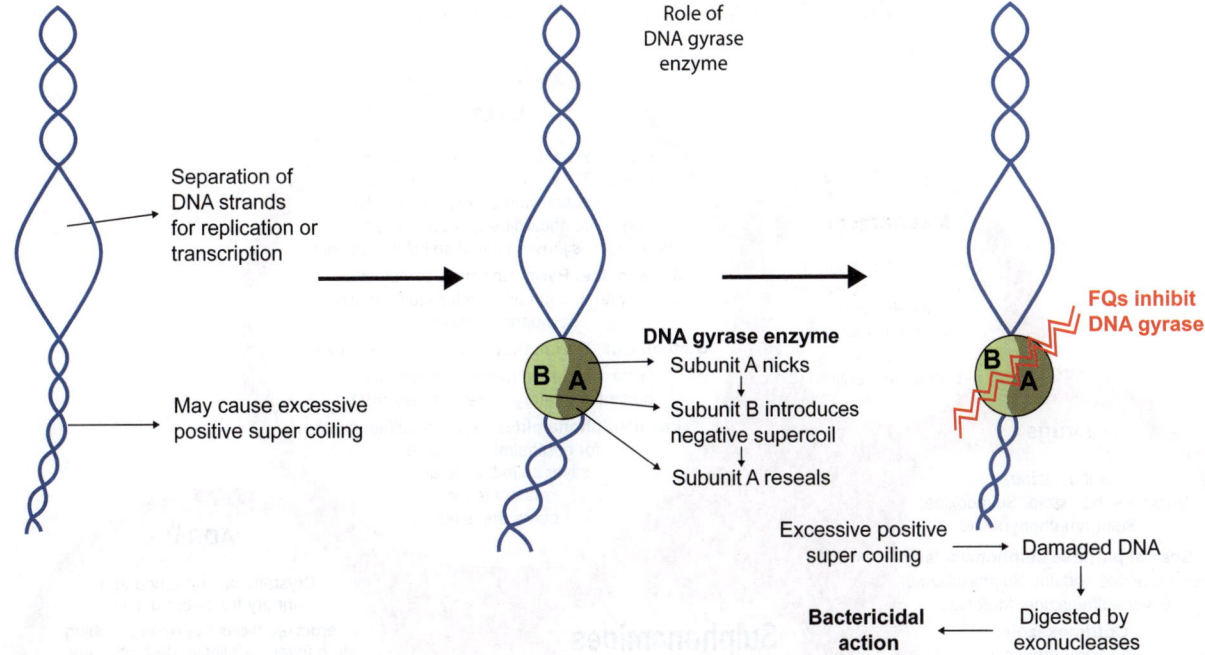

Fig. 52.2 Mechanism of action of FQs

- FQs are better than cotrimoxazole for UTI, prostatitis, bacterial diarrhea, etc. They are the **drugs of choice for uncomplicated lower UTI** caused by E. coli. Norfloxacin (400 mg), ciprofloxacin (250–750 mg), ofloxacin (200–400 mg) are typically administered twice daily by the oral route. Levofloxacin (500 mg) and moxifloxacin (400 mg) are given once daily.
- These are also used in **amoxicillin-resistant cases of UTI** in patients with prostatitis and indwelling catheters. Infections caused by *Pseudomonas* **also respond** to ciprofloxacin.
- Ofloxacin is an alternative drug for **urethritis caused by** *Chlamydia*.
- For **chronic UTIs**, norfloxacin is given for 8–12 weeks.
- Pefloxacin, moxifloxacin and trovafloxacin are FQs that are safe in renal failure.
- **Other indications** for use of ciprofloxacin include bacterial gastroenteritis, enteric fever, typhoid carrier state, infections of the skin, soft tissues and bones, wound infections, community-acquired pneumonia, bronchitis, conjunctivitis, STDs, and prophylaxis in immunocompromised patients.
- In serious infections caused by gram-negative bacteria, like septicemia, ciprofloxacin can be used along with third-generation cephalosporins or aminoglycosides.
- In MDR tuberculosis, FQs are used along with other drugs.

Adverse effects

FQs have mild adverse effects.

- Anorexia, nausea, bad taste in mouth, and even vomiting may occur.
- Central adverse effects like headache, dizziness, confusion, anxiety, insomnia, restlessness and impaired concentration can occur.
- Chances of tendonitis and rupture of tendons are higher in elderly patients and those receiving corticosteroids.
- These may cause cartilage damage in children.
- Moxifloxacin can cause QT prolongation, resulting in risk of arrhythmias.
- Sparfloxacin causes photosensitivity.
- Hypersensitivity reactions are usually mild, such as rashes, urticaria, and pruritus.
- FQs are also contraindicated in pregnancy.

Drug interactions

- Antacids can decrease absorption of FQs.
- Ciprofloxacin can cause enzyme inhibition, and hence there is a risk of toxicity of drugs like warfarin and theophylline.

Clinical problem-based questions and MCQs

1. **A patient with 50% burns is admitted in the burns unit. In addition to fluid therapy, burn dressing using AMAs is advised to prevent secondary infection of burnt skin.**
   i. Identify the most suitable drug from the following for burn dressing.
      a. Sulfacetamide   b. Sulphamethoxazole
      c. Silver sulfadiazine d. Sulfadoxine
   ii. Describe the mechanism of action of the drug selected.

2. i Which of the following shows synergism with sulphonamides?
      a. Diaminopyrimidines   b. Nalidixic acid
      c. Fluoroquinolones   d. Tetracyclines

CONCEPT MAP – SULPHONAMIDES AND FQS

AMAs

Sulphonamides

Mechanism
Sequential blockade of formation and activation of folic acid by cotrimoxazole
↓
bactericidal action

Drugs
Sulfadiazine, Sulphamethoxazole, Sulfadoxine, Sulphamethopyrazine
Special purpose sulphonamides: Sulfacetamide sodium, Sulphasalazine, Silver sulfadiazine, Mafenide
Cotrimoxazole: Sulphamethoxazole and trimethoprim in 5:1 ratio.

Uses
Cotrimoxazole: Acute uncomplicated lower UTI, acute or chronic bronchitis, GIT infection with *E.coli*, *Salmonella*, *Shigella*, nocardiosis, chancroid and *Pneumocystis jirovecii* infection in AIDS patients.
Sulfadoxine: Pyrimethamine combination along with artesunate in chloroquine resistant falciparum malaria.
Sulfadiazine: Pyrimethamine for toxoplasmosis.
Sulfasalazine in rheumatoid arthritis and inflammatory bowel disease (IBD).
Local sulphonamides: Sodium sulfacetamide for ophthalmic infections, silver sulfadiazine and mafenide for burns dressing.

ADRs
Crystalluria, hematuria and urinary tract obstruction.
Allergic reactions like rashes, itching, drug fever, exfoliative dermatitis and Stevens–Johnson syndrome.
Hemolysis in patients with G6PD deficiency.
Jaundice and kernicterus in premature babies
Nausea, vomiting, glossitis, stomatitis
Contraindicated in pregnancy.

Quinolones & Fluoroquinolones

Drugs
Quinolones: Nalidixic acid, nitrofurantoin
Fluoroquinolones:
1st generation: Norfloxacin, Ciprofloxacin, Ofloxacin and Pefloxacin
2nd generation: Gemifloxacin, Levofloxacin, Moxifloxacin, Prulifloxacin, Lomefloxacin & Sparfloxacin

Mechanism
Inhibition of DNA gyrase enzyme → interfere with nicking & resealing of DNA strands → excessive supercoiling of DNA strands → damaged DNA → digested by exonucleases → **bactericidal** action.

Uses
- **UTI:** Lower uncomplicated UTI caused by *E. coli*, amoxicillin-resistant cases, patients with prostatitis and indwelling catheters, *Pseudomonas* infections, urethritis caused by Chlamydia, chronic UTIs,
- Bacterial gastroenteritis, enteric fever, typhoid carrier state, infections of skin, wounds, soft tissues, bones,
- Community-acquired pneumonia, bronchitis, conjunctivitis, prophylaxis in immunocompromised patients and in STDs.
- Gram-negative septicemia: Ciprofloxacin along with third-generation cephalosporins or aminoglycosides.
- MDR tuberculosis along with other anti-TB drugs.

ADRs
Anorexia, nausea, vomiting, bad taste in mouth.
Headache, dizziness, confusion, anxiety, insomnia, restlessness, impaired concentration.
Tendonitis and rupture of tendons (in elderly and patients on corticosteroids).
Cartilage damage in children.
QT prolongation with Moxifloxacin → risk of arrhythmias.
Photosensitivity with Sparfloxacin.
Mild hypersensitivity reactions: rash, urticaria, pruritus, etc.
Contraindicated in pregnancy.

ii. Describe the mechanism of synergistic action of the selected group of AMAs with sulphonamides.
iii. Name the synergistic combination of the selected drug with sulphonamides and enumerate its therapeutic uses.

3. A 56-year-old male patient is diagnosed with inflammatory bowel disease. Identify the drug used in IBD.
   a. Tetracycline   b. Sulfasalazine
   c. Gemifloxacin   d. Clarithromycin

4. Ciprofloxacin exerts bactericidal effect against gram-negative organisms. Identify the correct mechanism of its action.
   a. Inhibits reduction of dihydrofolate reductase
   b. Inhibits cell wall synthesis
   c. Inhibits protein synthesis
   d. Inhibits nicking and resealing of DNA chain

5. i Which of the following is the drug of choice for lower UTI caused by *E. coli*?
   a. Norfloxacin
   b. Methenamine
   c. Nitrofurantoin
   d. Cotrimoxazole
   ii. Describe the mechanism of action, therapeutic uses and adverse effects of the selected drug.

6. Dose adjustment for FQs is needed in patients with renal failure. Which of the following FQs is safe in renal failure with low creatinine clearance?
   a. Pefloxacin   b. Norfloxacin
   c. Sparfloxacin   d. Ciprofloxacin

7. Identify the FQ that causes: (i) Photosensitivity, (ii) QT prolongation.
   a. Moxifloxacin   b. Norfloxacin
   c. Sparfloxacin   d. Ciprofloxacin

C. CELL WALL SYNTHESIS INHIBITORS

These include:
- β-lactams (penicillins, cephalosporins, carbapenems, monobactams)
- Glycopeptides: Vancomycin, teicoplanin, oritavancin, telavancin, dalbavancin
- Fosfomycin
- Bacitracin
- Cycloserine

β-Lactam Antimicrobials

These include penicillins, cephalosporins, carbapenems and monobactams as shown in Flowchart 52.3.

a. Penicillins

Crystalline Penicillin
- Penicillin G
- Procaine Penicillin G
- Benzathine Penicillin G

Acid-Resistant
- Phenoxymethylpenicillin or penicillin V

Penicillinase-Resistant Drugs
- Cloxacillin, Dicloxacillin, Methicillin

Extended-Spectrum Drugs

Carboxypenicillin	Aminopenicillin	Ureidopenicillin
Carbenicillin	Ampicillin	Piperacillin
Ticarcillin	Bacampicillin	Mezlocillin
	Amoxicillin	

b. Cephalosporins

First Generation

Oral	Parenteral
Cephalexin	Cefazolin
Cefadroxil	

Second Generation

Oral	Parenteral
Cefaclor	Cefuroxime
Cefuroxime axetil	Cefoxitin

Third Generation

Oral	Parenteral	
Cefixime	Ceftriaxone	Cefotaxime
Cefpodoxime proxetil	Cefoperazone	Ceftazidime
Cefdinir	Ceftizoxime	

Fourth Generation
- Cefepime, Cefpirome

Fifth Generation
- Ceftaroline, Ceftobiprole

d. Carbapenems
- Imipenem, Faropenem, Ertapenem
- Meropenem, Doripenem

c. Monobactams
- Aztreonam

Flowchart 52.3 Classification of β-lactam AMAs

Mechanism of action

β-lactam AMAs act by inhibition of cell wall synthesis. These drugs inhibit transpeptidases, thereby disturbing cross-linking of the peptidoglycan layer and the closeknit structure of the bacterial cell wall (Fig. 52.3). Under the influence of β-lactam AMAs, cell-wall-deficient (CWD) bacteria are formed, which swell up due to hypertonicity of intracellular contents and burst, resulting in bactericidal action. In case of rapidly multiplying organisms, cell wall synthesis also occurs at a rapid rate. Hence, the bactericidal effect of drugs is more pronounced.

a. Penicillins

Penicillins are divided into two categories: natural (penicillin G and its repository forms) and semisynthetic (Flowchart 52.3). Semisynthetic penicillins include penicillin V (acid-resistant), penicillinase-resistant drugs (cloxacillin, diclocacillin, methicillin), and extended-spectrum drugs (carboxy/amino/ureidopenicillins).

- Carboxypenicillins: carbenicillin, ticarcillin
- Aminopenicillins: ampicillin, bacampicillin, amoxicillin
- Ureidopenicillins: piperacillin, mezlocillin

Mechanism of development of resistance

- Some bacteria produce enzyme penicillinase, which opens up the β-lactam ring and inactivates the drug, e.g., staphylococci, gonococci, *B. subtilis*, *E. coli*, and *H. influenzae*.
- Some penicillins, e.g., methicillin, cloxacillin and dicloxacillin, however, have a side chain that partially protects their β-lactam ring from penicillinase enzyme. These drugs are useful in penicillin-resistant *Staphylococcus aureus* infections, but are not capable of protecting the β-lactam ring from penicillinase produced by gram-negative bacteria. Hence, they are not useful in penicillinase-producing *E. coli* infections.
- Resistance to methicillin in *S. aureus* (MRSA) develops due to an altered 'penicillin-binding site' to which the drug cannot bind effectively.
- In some gram-negative bacteria, decreased entry of the drug into the organism is responsible for development of resistance.

Pharmacokinetics

Crystalline penicillin G is acid-labile, i.e., it is destroyed by gastric acid. Consequently, it is not effective orally and is given by IM or IV route every 4–6 hours. However, phenoxymethyl penicillin (penicillin V) is resistant to gastric acid and can be used orally. Repository forms, i.e., procaine penicillin G and benzathine penicillin G are given by deep intramuscular injection. While penicillin G is widely distributed in body cavities such as pleural and synovial cavities, it fails to cross the blood–brain barrier. Penicillins are mainly excreted unchanged by kidneys via tubular secretion. Probenecid increases the duration of action of penicillin by competing at tubular secretory sites.

Therapeutic uses

- **Penicillin G** is useful in **s**treptococcal infections (rheumatic fever, subacute bacterial endocarditis, otitis media, pharyngitis), **a**ctinomycosis, **l**eptospirosis, **s**yphilis and **a**nthrax infections [Mnemonic: **SALSA**]. It is also effective in meningitis, pneumonia, gonorrhea, etc. Dosage in pneumonia is 0.5–5 million units, intravenously, every 6 hours. In meningitis, the dosage is 12–24 million units, by IV route.
- **Cloxacillin**, dicloxacillin and methicillin are useful in penicillinase-producing **staphylococcal** infections. Among these penicillinase-resistant drugs, cloxacillin is effective orally, given in a dose of 250-500 mg every 6 hours. Methicillin is acid-labile, and is therefore administered as injection. However, use of methicillin has declined due to development of MRSA strains.
- **Ampicillin** is partly excreted in the bile and shows enterohepatic circulation; it is the drug of choice in patients with listeria, meningitis and UTI due to *E. faecalis*. Dose varies from 0.5–2 g every 6 hours.
- **Amoxicillin** is preferred over ampicillin for **bronchitis, UTIs, SABE** and **gonorrhea** because of its better oral absorption, more convenient dosing and lower incidence of diarrhea. Dose varies from 0.25–1 g, three times a day.
- Amoxicillin is also used in most triple-drug regimens for **eradication of *H. pylori*** in peptic ulceration.
- Amoxicillin can be used along with metronidazole for acute necrotising **ulcerative gingivitis** and with gentamicin for septicemia and mixed infections.
- Single dose of amoxicillin 3 g with clavulanic acid 500 mg and probenecid 1 g is curative for gonorrhea caused by penicillinase producing *Neisseria gonorrhoeae* (**PPNG**).
- **Ticarcillin** is useful in infections caused by ***Pseudomonas* and *Proteus***. It can be combined with gentamicin and clavulanic acid. Dose is 3 g IM or IV, every 6 hours.
- **Piperacillin** is also effective against *Pseudomonas, Klebsiella, Enterobacteriaceae* and bacteroides. It is used in **serious gram-negative infections in immunocompromised** patients. Dose of piperacillin is 100–150 mg/kg daily, in 3 divided doses, by IM/IV route.

ADRs

- Hypersensitivity reactions are seen in up to 10% of patients treated with penicillin G. These can occur as rashes, itching, fever, urticaria, angioneurotic edema, anaphylaxis, serum sickness, exfoliative dermatitis, etc.

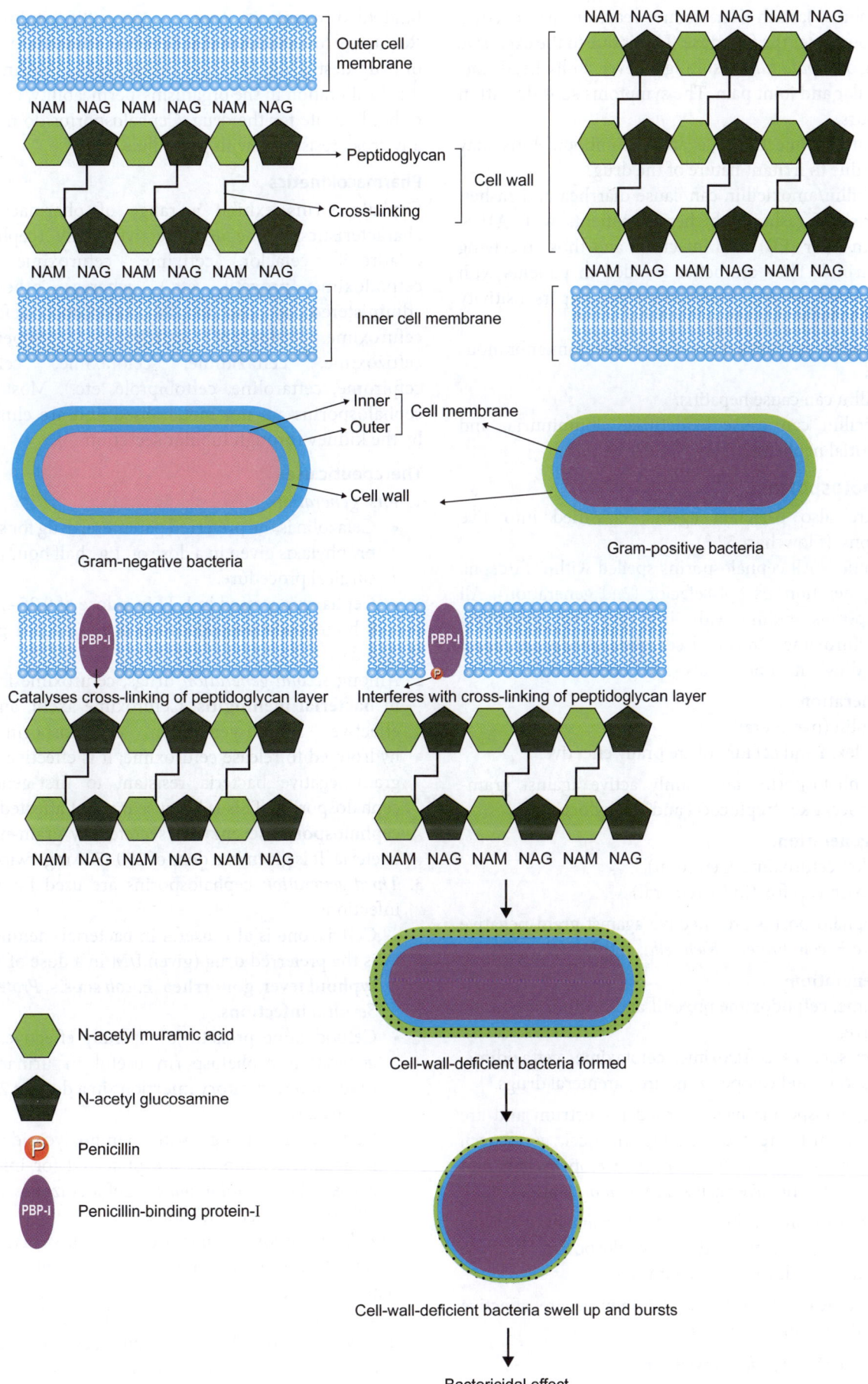

Fig. 52.3 Mechanism of action of penicillin

- In syphilis, Jarisch–Herxheimer reaction may occur a few hours after the first dose. This is due to the excessive killing of *T. pallidum*, resulting in fever, chills, headache, muscular and joint pain. The symptoms subside within 48 hours.
- Pain at the injection site and thrombophlebitis may occur due to irritant nature of the drug.
- Ampicillin/amoxicillin can cause diarrhea and rashes. The risk of rashes is higher in patients with AIDS, Epstein–Barr (EB) viral infection, and those receiving allopurinol. They are better avoided in patients with history of severe immediate-type hypersensitivity reactions with penicillins.
- Ampicillin can sometimes cause pseudomembranous colitis.
- Oxacillin can cause hepatitis.
- Methicillin can cause hematuria, albuminuria, and interstitial nephritis.

b. Cephalosporins

These are also β-lactam agents, classified into five generations. (Flowchart 52.3)

[Mnemonic – All cephalosporins spelled with cefa/cepha are 1st generation, except cefaclor (2nd generation). All cephalosporins ending with 'ime' are 3rd generation except cefuroxime (2nd) and cefepime (4th generation). Those ending with 'one' are also 3rd generation.]

First generation:
- Cefazolin (parenteral)
- Cephalexin and cefadroxil are orally effective.

These cephalosporins are mainly active against gram-positive cocci like streptococci and staphylococci.

Second generation:
- Cefaclor, cefuroxime axetil (oral)
- Cefuroxime, cefoxitin (parenteral)

These cephalosporins are effective against gram-negative bacilli like *E. coli*, *Proteus*, *Klebsiella*, and *H. influenzae*.

Third generation:
- Cefixime, cefpodoxime proxetil and cefdinir are orally effective.
- Others such as ceftizoxime, cefotaxime, ceftazidime, ceftriaxone, and cefoperazone are parenteral drugs.

These cephalosporins have a broader spectrum and are effective against streptococci, staphylococci, gonococci, *Enterobacteriaceae* and bacteroides. Cefoperazone and ceftazidime are effective against *Pseudomonas* also.

Fourth generation: Cefepime and cefpirome have actions similar to the 3rd generation cephalosporins, but are resistant to breakdown by β-lactamases.

Fifth generation: Ceftaroline, ceftobiprole are effective against MRSA and *Pseudomonas*.

Mechanism of action and resistance

Similar to penicillins, cephalosporins also exert bactericidal effect by inhibiting cell wall synthesis, although they bind to different site (not the 'penicillin-binding site'). Resistance to cephalosporins develops due to the evolution of drug-destroying enzymes called 'cephalosporinases' or due to alteration in the organisms' permeability, or affinity of binding site for the drug. Cephalosporins do not show any cross-resistance with penicillins.

Pharmacokinetics

Cephalosporins exhibit a range of pharmacokinetic characteristics. Some are effective orally (cephalexin, cefadroxil, cefaclor, cefixime, cefuroxime axetil, cefpodoxime proxetil, etc.), whereas others are administered by IM or IV injections (ceftazolin, cefuroxime, cefoxitin, ceftriaxone, cefoperazone, ceftizoxime, ceftazidime, cefotaxime, cefepime, cefpirome, ceftaroline, ceftobiprole, etc.). Most of the cephalosporins are not metabolised and are eliminated by the kidney through tubular secretion.

Therapeutic uses

1. *First generation:*
   - Cefazolin is the preferred parenteral drug for surgical prophylaxis given in a dose of 1 g, half hour prior to surgical procedure.
   - Cephalexin is used in UTI in a dose of 0.25–1 g, 6 to 8 hourly, whereas cefadroxil is given 0.5–1 g, twice a day.
2. Among *second-generation* drugs, cefuroxime is useful in **bacterial meningitis**. Cefuroxime axetil, an orally effective second-generation cephalosporin, gets hydrolysed to release cefuroxime; it is effective against gram-negative bacteria resistant to first-generation cephalosporins. This is because it is not affected by the **cephalosporinase enzyme** secreted by gram-negative bacteria. It is given in a dose of 250–500 mg, twice a day.
3. *Third-generation* cephalosporins are used for serious infections.
   - Ceftriaxone is also useful in bacterial meningitis. It is the preferred drug (given I/M in a dose of 1 g) for **typhoid fever, gonorrhea,** *E. coli* **sepsis,** *Proteus* **and** *Serratia* **infections**.
   - Cefpodoxime proxetil is an orally effective, third-generation cephalosporin useful in urinary, soft tissue and respiratory infections in a dose of 200 mg, twice daily.
   - Ceftazidime along with aminoglycosides and ß-lactamase inhibitors are preferred for infections caused by *Pseudomonas*. Cefoperazone is also effective for such infections.
4. *Fourth-generation* cephalosporins are useful in infections caused by organisms resistant to third-generation drugs.
5. *Fifth-generation:* Ceftaroline and ceftobiprole are reserved for MRSA and hospital-acquired bacterial infections resistant to penicillins.
6. Other indications for the use of cephalosporins as a group include **penicillin-resistant gonorrhea, typhoid**

fever, and mixed aerobic–anaerobic infections in patients undergoing obstetric/colorectal surgery/ suffering from cancers.
7. Higher-generation cephalosporins are extensively used in current clinical practice in serious gram-negative septicemia, hospital-acquired respiratory infections in ICU patients, and in meningitis.

Adverse reactions
These are well tolerated drugs.
- Oral cephalosporins may cause diarrhea due to their irritant effect or due to changes in gut flora.
- Incidence of hypersensitivity reactions is less than with penicillins. Rashes are more frequent; angioedema, asthma, urticaria and even anaphylaxis may occur.
- Injectable drugs cause pain at the site of injection and thrombophlebitis.
- Ceftriaxone may cause biliary sludging syndrome and gall stones.
- In rare cases, ceftazidime may cause neutropenia and thrombocytopenia (TCP). Cefoperazone and ceftriaxone can cause hypoprothrombinemia and bleeding, especially in patients with renal failure or malignant disease.
- Some cephalosporins like cefoperazone and cefamandole can inhibit aldehyde dehydrogenase enzyme, resulting in disulfiram reaction. Hence, patients taking these drugs should be cautioned against the use of alcohol.

c. Monobactams
Aztreonam is a narrow-spectrum β-lactam AMA with the same mechanism of action as penicillins and cephalosporins, i.e., it inhibits cell wall synthesis. It is effective against β-lactamase-producing gram-negative bacilli including *Pseudomonas* and *H. influenzae*. Aztreonam is not effective against gram-positive cocci and anaerobes. It has no cross-sensitivity with penicillins or cephalosporins (except ceftazidime). Thus, aztreonam can be used in hospital-acquired infections of the GI, biliary and genitourinary tract in patients who show hypersensitivity reactions to penicillins or cephalosporins.

Adverse effects include rashes and raised serum aminotransferases.

d. Carbapenems
These include imipenem, meropenem, faropenem, doripenem and ertapenem.

Imipenem is a broad-spectrum β-lactam AMA active against gram-positive cocci (including penicillinase-producing staphylococci), gram-negative bacilli, *Pseudomonas,* enterobacteriacae, *Listeria* and anaerobes like *Claustridium difficile* and *B. fragilis*.

- Imipenem is resistant to hydrolysis by most of the β-lactamases. Therefore, it is effective against extended-spectrum β-lactamase (ESBL)-producing organisms.
- Imipenem gets rapidly hydrolysed by the enzyme dehydropeptidase 1 present on the brush border of renal tubular epithelial cells. Therefore, it is always combined with the reversible dehydropeptidase 1 inhibiting drug, cilastin. A combination of imipenem and cilastin (in equal ratio; 250 or 500 mg of each) is used in serious hospital-acquired infections of urinary tract, respiratory tract, skin, soft tissues, abdominal and pelvic cavity, especially in immunocompromised patients. The dose is 500 mg, intravenously, every 6 hours.
- ADRs include rashes, vomiting and diarrhea. Seizures may be precipitated at higher doses.

Meropenem is the most active carbapenem against *Pseudomonas*. It is kept as a reserve drug in serious septicemia, diabetic foot, abdominal and pelvic sepsis caused by organisms resistant to cephalosporins.

Doripenem has the same uses as meropenem, but is effective against resistant *Pseudomonas*.

Faropenem is orally effective, whereas imipenem and meropenem are injectables.

Ertapenem has poor activity against *Pseudomonas*, but is highly effective against *E. coli, H. influenzae, Klebsiella pneumoniae, Moraxella, Proteus*, etc. It is useful in resistant skin and soft tissue infections, diabetic foot, complicated UTIs, and for prophylaxis in colorectal surgery. It is given as a 1 g IV infusion once daily.

Cilastin need not be combined with meropenem, doripenem, faropenem and ertapenem, as these are not metabolised by dehydropeptidase 1 enzyme.

β-Lactamase Inhibitors
β-lactamase the enzyme produced by resistant bacteria, causes opening of the β-lactam ring and inactivates β-lactam AMAs. β-lactamase inhibitors include clavulanic acid, sulbactam, tazobactam and avibactam.

- Clavulanic acid has a β-lactam ring, but no antimicrobial action of its own. When used along with penicillins in infections caused by organisms that produce β-lactamase, clavulanic acid acts as a 'suicide inhibitor', i.e., it binds to the β-lactamase enzyme and gets inactivated; this saves the β-lactam ring of penicillin from attack of β-lactamase enzyme.
- A combination of clavulanic acid and amoxicillin, called co-amoxiclav, is useful in empirical therapy of hospital-acquired infections of the respiratory, urinary and biliary tracts, skin and soft tissue infections, and abdominal and pelvic sepsis.
- Sulbactam has poor oral absorption; so, it is commonly used parenterally with ampicillin for mixed aerobic–anaerobic infections of the abdominal cavity, pelvic cavity and surgical sites. It is also effective in

penicillinase-producing *N. gonorrhoea* (PPNG). ADRs like pain at the injection site, thrombophlebitis, rashes and diarrhea may occur.

- Tazobactam is combined with piperacillin for severe respiratory, urinary tract, and pelvic infections and peritonitis caused by β-lactamase-producing bacilli. The combination is however not active against piperacillin-resistant *Pseudomonas* and *Enterobacteriaceae*.
- Avibactam is combined with ceftazidime in complicated urinary tract infections like pyelonephritis and intra-abdominal sepsis.

Other AMAs that Inhibit Cell Wall Synthesis

1. Glycopeptides

Vancomycin is a narrow-spectrum drug active against penicillin-resistant pneumococci, methicillin-resistant *Staphylococcus aureus* (MRSA), *Clostridium difficile* and *Corynebacterium jeikeium*. It is administered **only by IV route** for serious infections in patients who have penicillin hypersensitivity, MRSA and *Corynebacterium jeikeium* infections. Dose is 150 mg, infused over 1 hour, every 6 hours. Oral vancomycin is useful in pseudomembranous colitis caused by *C. difficile* and staphylococcal enterocolitis. It is given in a dose of 125–500 mg, 6-hourly.

- Rapid IV injection of vancomycin induces histamine release, resulting in diffuse flushing called 'red man syndrome'.
- It also causes chills, ototoxicity, nephrotoxicity. Because vancomycin is nephrotoxic and is excreted unchanged by the kidneys, dose should be reduced in renal dysfunction.

Teicoplanin is as effective as vancomycin against MRSA and enterococci. Even vancomycin-resistant enterococci (VRE) and vancomycin-intermediate *Staphylococcus aureus* (VISA) respond to teicoplanin. It has a longer half-life than vancomycin, and is free of adverse effects like nephrotoxicity and red man syndrome.

Oritavancin and **telavancin** are useful in MRSA and complicated skin and soft tissue infections.

Dalbavancin is effective against MRSA as well as VRSA (methicillin/vancomycin-resistant *Staphylococcus aureus*).

2. Fosfomycin

Fosfomycin inhibits enol pyruvate transferase and interferes with cell wall synthesis. It is the preferred drug for uncomplicated UTIs. Diarrhea is a common ADR associated with fosfomycin use.

3. Bacitracin

Bacitracin is effective only against gram-positive organisms. It is used only topically, as it is too toxic for systemic use.

4. Cycloserine

Cycloserine is used as a second-line drug in tuberculosis. It can cause tremors, seizures and neuropsychiatric symptoms as adverse effects.

Clinical problem-based questions and MCQs

8. All the following drugs are effective against *Pseudomonas*, EXCEPT:
   a. Azlocillin
   b. Ticarcillin
   c. Cefoperazone
   d. Ertapenem

9. Which of the following is a 4th-generation cephalosporin?
   a. Cefepime
   b. Cefotaxime
   c. Cefoperazone
   d. Cefadroxil

10. Which of the carbapenems is orally effective?
    a. Imipenem
    b. Meropenem
    c. Farropenem
    d. Ertapenem

11. i In which of the following conditions is vancomycin given orally?
    a. MRSA
    b. ESB-producing organisms
    c. Pseudomembranous colitis
    d. All of the above
    ii. Describe the mechanism of action, uses and adverse effects of vancomycin.

12. i Identify the correct single-dose therapy for PPNG.
    a. Amoxicillin, probenecid and clavulanic acid
    b. Amoxicillin, sulbactam
    c. Imipenem, cilastin
    d. Meropenem, tazobactam, probenecid
    ii. Describe the mechanism of action and dose of each component drug used in single-dose therapy of PPNG.

13. i Which of the following possesses β-lactamase inhibitory action?
    a. Tazobactam
    b. Piperacillin
    c. Cefoperazone
    d. All of the above
    ii. Describe clinical utility of β-lactamase inhibitors.

14. Imipenem is always combined with cilastin for treatment of infections caused by ESBL-producing organisms. Explain why.

15. i Identify the AMA effective against vancomycin-resistant *Staphylococcus aureus* (VRSA) infection.
    a. Dalbavancin
    b. Tazobactum
    c. Fosfomycin
    d. Faropenem
    ii. Describe the mechanism of action of the selected drug VRSA.

CONCEPT MAP – β-LACTAM DRUGS

β-Lactams

Penicillins

Classification
- Penicillin G, Penicillin V
- **Penicillinase-resistant drugs:** Cloxacillin, Dicloxacillin, Methicillin
- **Extended-spectrum drugs:**
  - *Carboxypenicillins*: Carbenicillin, Ticarcillin
  - *Aminopenicillins*: Ampicillin, Bacampicillin, Amoxicillin
  - *Ureidopenicillins*: Piperacillin, Mezlocillin

Uses
- **Penicillin G** in streptococcal infections (rheumatic fever, SABE, otitis media, pharyngitis), actinomycosis, leptospirosis, syphilis, anthrax, meningitis, pneumonia, gonorrhea.
- **Ampicillin** drug of choice in listeria, meningitis and UTI due to *E. faecalis*.
- **Amoxicillin** in bronchitis, UTIs, SABE, gonorrhea, *H. pylori* in peptic ulceration
- Amoxicillin with metronidazole for acute necrotising ulcerative gingivitis and with gentamicin for septicemia and mixed infections.
- Single dose of amoxicillin with clavulanic acid and probenecid for PPNG.
- **Ticarcillin** in *Pseudomonas* and *Proteus* infections
- **Piperacillin** in serious gram-negative infections with *Pseudomonas, Klebsiella, Enterobacteriaceae* and bacteroides in immunocompromised patients.

ADRs
- Hypersensitivity reactions as rashes, itching, fever, urticaria, angioneurotic edema, anaphylaxis, serum sickness, exfoliative dermatitis.
- Pain at injection site, thrombophlebitis.
- Ampicillin/amoxicillin can cause diarrhea, rashes, pseudomembranous enterocolitis.
- Hepatitis with oxacillin and interstitial nephritis with methicillin

Carbapenems

Imipenem, Meropenem, Faropenem, Doripenem, Ertapenem.

Imipenem is broad-spectrum AMA, effective against extended-spectrum β-lactamases (ESBL) producing organisms.

Always combined with reversible dehydropeptidase 1 inhibiting drug, cilastin, in serious HAIs of urinary tract, respiratory tract, skin, soft tissues, abdominal and pelvic cavity, especially in immunocompromised patients.

Meropenem is a reserve drug in serious septicemia, diabetic foot, abdominal and pelvic sepsis caused by cephalosporin-resistant organisms.

Cilastin need not be combined with meropenem, doripenem, faropenem and ertapenem, as these are not metabolised by dehydropeptidase 1 enzyme

ADRs include rashes, vomiting, diarrhea, seizures.

Mechanism of Action

Inhibit transpeptidases → cross-linking & close-knit structure of bacterial cell wall is disturbed → **inhibit cell wall synthesis** → cell-wall-deficient (CWD) bacteria formed → swell up due to hypertonicity of intracellular contents and burst → **bactericidal** action.

Monobactams

Effective against β-lactamase-producing gram-negative bacilli including *Pseudomonas* and *H. influenzae* → used in HAIs of GI, biliary and genitourinary tract in patients showing hypersensitivity reactions with penicillins or cephlosporins.

Adverse effects:
Rashes and raised serum aminotransferases.

Cephalosporins

Classification
- **1st Generation:** Cefazolin (parenteral) Cephalexin & Cefadroxil (oral)
- **2nd Generation:** Cefaclor, Cefuroxime axetil (oral) Cefuroxime, cefoxitin (parenteral)
- **3rd Generation:** Cefixime, Cefpodoxime proxetil, Cefdinir (oral) Ceftriaxone, Cefoperazone, Ceftizoxime, Cefotaxime, Ceftazidime (parenteral)
- **4th Generation:** Cefepime, Cefpirome
- **5th Generation:** Ceftaroline, Ceftobiprole

Uses
- **1st Generation:** Cefazolin for surgical prophylaxis. Cephalexin, Cefadroxil in UTI
- **2nd Generation:** Cefuroxime in bacterial meningitis & gram-negative bacteria resistant to first-generation drugs.
- **3rd Generation:** Ceftriaxone in bacterial meningitis, typhoid fever, gonorrhea, *E. coli* sepsis, *Proteus* and *Serratia* infections.
  Cefpodoxime in urinary, soft tissue and respiratory infections.
  Ceftazidime with aminoglycosides for *Pseudomonas* infections.
- **4th Generation:** For infections caused by organisms resistant to 3rd generation drugs.
- **5th Generation:** Reserved for MRSA and penicillin-resistant HAIs.

ADRs
- Diarrhea, pain at site of injection & thrombophlebitis.
- Hypersensitivity reactions less than with penicillins. Rashes, angioedema, asthma, urticaria & even anaphylaxis may occur.
- Biliary sludging syndrome & gall stones with Ceftriaxone.
- Neutropenia with Ceftazidime.
- Disulfiram reaction with Cefoperazone, Moxalactam, Cefamandole

D. PROTEIN SYNTHESIS INHIBITORS

These include:
- Broad-spectrum drugs like tetracyclines, chloramphenicol, and pleuromutilin
- Moderate-spectrum drugs like macrolides and aminoglycosides
- Narrow-spectrum drugs like lincosamides, linezolid, and streptogramins

a. Broad-Spectrum Drugs

1. Tetracyclines

These include tetracycline, oxytetracycline, chlortetracycline, methacycline, demeclocycline, doxycycline, minocycline and a tetracycline analogue, tigecycline.

Mechanism of action

Bacterial protein synthesis occurs at 30S and 50S ribosomal subunits. The acceptor site (A) accepts new tRNA carrying amino acids, while the peptidyl (P) site stores accumulated amino acids and the ejector (E) site ejects the tRNA (Fig. 52.4a). When a new tRNA molecule carrying an amino acid attaches at A site (Fig. 52.4b), the stored amino acids (peptide chain) are transferred from the A site to P site by the action of peptidyl transferase enzyme. This process is known as transpeptidation (Fig. 52.4c).

- The tRNA at P site has already performed its function, so it is ejected out (Fig. 52.4d).
- The tRNA with amino acid translocates from A site to P site.
- New tRNA with next an amino acid attaches at A site (Fig. 52.4e).

This cycle is repeated till a polypeptide chain is formed.

This process is interrupted by various drugs is repeated to the 30S or 50S subunits of ribosomes. Tetracyclines **bind to the 30S subunit, interfering with binding of tRNA at the acceptor site and exert bacteristatic effect**. These **broad-spectrum** drugs are effective against gram-positive and gram-negative bacteria excluding *Proteus*, *Pseudomonas* and *Providencia*. Tetracyclines are not active against anaerobic organisms. **Several initially sensitive organisms have also developed resistance**. Resistance develops mainly due to excessive efflux of drug from the microbial cell. However, enzymatic inactivation of the drug molecule and reduced binding of the drug to 30S ribosomal subunit is also responsible for tetracycline resistance in some cases.

Pharmacokinetics

Oral absorption of tetracycline and oxytetracycline is partial (60–80%). Tetracyclines can potentially form complexes with calcium and other metals, thus absorption is reduced by food, milk, iron, antacids, etc. To prevent this, there should be a time interval between administration of food/milk/antacids and tetracyclines. Doxycycline and minocycline are absorbed more completely and are not much affected by food.

Tetracyclines are widely distributed and achieve high concentration in teeth, bones, liver and spleen. Excretion is largely through the kidneys, except for doxycycline, which is metabolised in the liver.

Therapeutic uses

Tetracyclines have **few indications** for use in current clinical practice. These are administered orally or

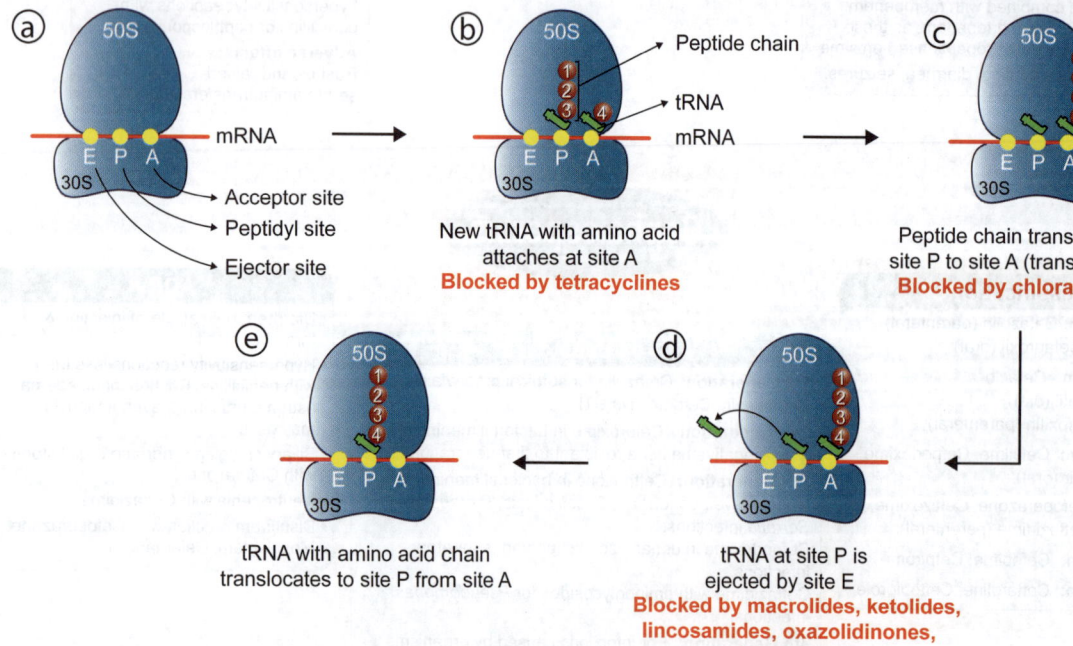

Fig. 52.4 Inhibition of bacterial protein synthesis by drugs

intravenously, but never intramuscularly, as they cause pain and inflammation at the injection site.
- Doxycycline is useful in chlamydial non-specific urethritis, LGV, granuloma inguinale and endocervicitis. Dose of doxycycline is 100 mg, once or twice daily for 1–3 weeks.
- Tetracyclines are useful in mycoplasma pneumonia, cholera, brucellosis, plague, typhus and Rocky Mountain spotted fever.
- Minocycline is used in acne, nocardiosis and leprosy.
- Demeclocycline is used in ' Syndrome of inappropriate ADH' (SIADH) because of its ADH antagonistic action.
- *Newer tetracyclines*: Sarecycline is useful in acne, eravacycline in severe abdominal infection and omadacycline in pneumonias and skin infections.

[Mnemonic for uses of tetracyclines: '**AC M**anufactured **B**y **LG C**ompany **R**uns **S**moothly', i.e., Atypical pneumonia, cholera, meningococcal carrier state, brucellosis, lymphogranuloma venereum, granuloma inguinale, chlamydial infections, rickettsial infections, SIADH]

- **Tigecycline**, a synthetic analogue of minocycline, is effective against tetracycline-resistant organisms. It is not effective orally and is always given intravenously. It is effective against gram-positive, negative organisms as well as anaerobes. However, tigecycline is reserved for serious infections caused by resistant organisms like MRSA, VRSA, carbapenem-resistant gram-negative infections like *E. coli, Klebsiella, Acinetobacter* and *Enterobacter*. Tigecycline is given as an intravenous infusion of 100 mg, followed by 50 mg every 12 hours, infused over 30–60 minutes. The treatment is continued for 1-2 weeks.

ADRs
The most common adverse effects after oral use of tetracyclines are nausea, vomiting, and esophagitis. Tetracyclines can form unabsorbable complexes with calcium, and food decreases their absorption. So, these should always be taken on empty stomach along with a full glass of water; the patient is advised not to lie down for at least half an hour afterwards.

- These have the potential to get deposited on bones and teeth, causing abnormal growths on bones and yellow staining of teeth. Moreover, there is a risk of hepatotoxicity in pregnant women, and hence are not given during pregnancy and also to children.
- Demeclocycline causes diabetes-insipidus-like situation due to ADH antagonistic action.
- Minocycline is vestibulotoxic.
- Minocycline, doxycycline and tigecycline are nephrotoxic.
- Tetracyclines can also cause anti-anabolic effects, pseudotumor cerebri and photosensitivity reactions like sunburn on exposed areas of skin.

- Outdated/expired tetracycline preparations may cause Fanconi syndrome, characterised by nausea, vomiting, altered sensorium, acidosis, and excretion of glucose/ proteins/ amino acids in urine.

2. Chloramphenicol
Chloramphenicol binds to the **50S ribosomal subunit** and interferes with peptide bond formation between the newly added amino acid and nascent peptide chain to exert bacteristatic action. It blocks the step following the one blocked by tetracyclines (Fig. 52.4c).

Pharmacokinetics
Oral absorption of chloramphenicol is fast and complete; it is partly bound to plasma proteins and well distributed. Chloramphenicol easily enters serous body cavities; it also crosses the blood–brain barrier as well as the placental barrier. Metabolism occurs through glucuronide conjugation and inactive metabolites are excreted in urine. Therefore, dose reduction is indicated in patients with hepatic cirrhosis and newborns who have lower ability to inactivate chloramphenicol.

The most significant disadvantage of chloramphenicol is its potential to inhibit protein synthesis in mammalian cells at high doses, which can lead to bone marrow suppression. This leads to agranulocytosis, aplastic anemia, thrombocytopenia and pancytopenia. In rare cases, chloramphenicol can cause idiosyncratic myelosuppression that is not dose-related, which can be severe and even fatal. High doses of chloramphenicol administered to premature infants can cause 'grey baby syndrome', characterised by ashen-grey cyanosis, abdominal distension, irregular respiration, hypothermia and cardiovascular collapse. Hence, it is not a preferred drug and used only in case of resistant infections caused by organisms like *H. influenzae*, meningococci, pneumococci and *Rickettsia*. For most of the other indications, it has been superseded by other better tolerated drugs. Dose of chloramphenicol should not exceed 2–3 g and the duration of therapy not exceed 2 weeks. Repeated courses should be avoided and blood counts should be closely monitored in patients receiving chloramphenicol.

3. Pleuromutilins
Retapamulin acts by inhibiting protein synthesis by binding to the 50S ribosomal subunit. These drugs interfere with the correct positioning of tRNA and peptide bond formation. It is effective against gram-positive, fastidious gram-negative organisms, mycoplasma, chlamydia, legionella, etc.

Pleuromutilins **do not show cross-resistance with other AMAs** and have **extremely low resistance rates.** It is approved only for topical use in impetigo (a highly contagious bacterial skin infection).

ADRs associated with topical use is irritation at the site of application.

Lefamulin is a new drug effective against pneumococcus, *Klebsiella*, *Chlamydia* and *Mycoplasma*. It is administered by the oral or intravenous route in community-acquired pneumonia. Systemic use causes many adverse effects such as nausea, vomiting, diarrhea, headache, insomnia, hypokalemia, QT prolongation and raised liver enzymes.

b. Moderate-Spectrum Drugs
These include aminoglycosides and macrolides.

1. Aminoglycosides
These include drugs obtained from streptomyces (with suffix mycin), such as streptomycin, neomycin, tobramycin and paromomycin. Some are obtained from micromonospora (the suffix used is micin); e.g., gentamicin, amikacin, and netilmicin.

Mechanism of action

Aminoglycosides get transported into bacterial cell via a multistep process involving:
- Diffusion across the outer coat through porin channels in gram-negative bacteria.
- Movement across cytoplasmic membrane by carrier-mediated transport linked to electron transport chain. Because drug transport into bacterial cells is oxygen-dependent, anaerobic bacteria fail to transport aminoglycosides into the bacterial cell. Therefore, aminoglycosides are not effective against anaerobes.

Streptomycin binds to 30S, while other aminoglycosides bind to **30S, 50S, and the interface of 30S–50S subunits**. They freeze the initiation of protein synthesis by **preventing the formation of polysomes and cause misreading of the mRNA code**, which results in the incorporation of wrong amino acids in the peptide chain. Secondarily, this causes changes in the integrity of bacterial cell membrane, leading to a *bactericidal effect* (in contrast to the bacteriostatic effect of other protein synthesis inhibitors like tetracyclines, chloramphenicol and macrolides).

Mechanism of resistance

Resistance to aminoglycosides develops due to synthesis of enzymes that inactivate the drug by acetylation/phosphorylation/adenylation. Amikacin and netilmicin are not inactivated by resistant bacteria. In some resistant bacteria, decreased binding of the drug to ribosomes and reduced transport of the drug across membranes may be responsible for conferring resistance to drug action.

Pharmacokinetics

Aminoglycosides, being polar in nature, are not absorbed orally. So, these are **always used by the parenteral (intramuscular/intravenous) route** for systemic effect. However, **neomycin is used orally** for its local effect in the gut.

Aminoglycosides are not metabolised in the body. These are excreted unchanged by the kidney through glomerular filtration. Tubular secretion or reabsorption is not significant. Therefore, dose reduction is indicated in elderly individuals, newborns, and patients with impaired renal function.

Therapeutic uses

1. **Gentamicin**
   - It is useful in the prevention and treatment of respiratory infections in immunocompromised patients (on corticosteroid/anticancer drug therapy or those with HIV infection) and critically ill patients (like those in ICU, or on ventilator).
   - Gentamicin combined with tetracyclines is the drug of choice for plague and tularemia.
   - Gentamicin along with ampicillin is used for subacute bacterial endocarditis.
   - Gentamicin is used in combination with third-generation cephalosporins or piperacillin to treat serious infections caused by *Proteus*, *Pseudomonas* and *Klebsiella*. Aminoglycosides are combined with cephalosporins for meningitis and other serious gram-negative infections. The dose of gentamicin for systemic infections is 3–5 mg/kg body weight, in patients with normal creatinine clearance (CLCr). Dose is appropriately reduced if CLCr falls below 70 mL/minute.
   - In patients with burns, it may be used topically.
2. **Streptomycin, amikacin, capreomycin and kanamycin** have a role in the management of drug-resistant tuberculosis (Refer to Chapter 54).
3. **Tobramycin** is effective in some gentamicin-resistant infections caused by *Proteus* and *Pseudomonas*.
4. **Amikacin** is used as a reserve drug for empirical treatment of hospital acquired gram-negative infections in a daily dose of 15 mg/kg body weight.
5. **Neomycin** is used orally in a dose of 250–1000 mg every 6 hours for bowel preparation before surgery and in the management of hepatic encephalopathy. It reduces ammonia (NH_3) production by suppressing intestinal bacterial flora, thereby improving the clinical status of patients with hepatic encephalopathy. However, lactulose is preferred.
6. Neomycin is frequently used topically along with polymyxin and bacitracin for burns, ulcers, and ear and eye infections.
7. **Framycetin** is also very toxic, and its use is restricted to topical application in skin, eye and ear infections.
8. **Paromomycin** is effective against protozoa such as *Entamoeba histolytica*, *Giardia lamblia*, *Leishmania*, and *Trichomonas*. It is used orally for intestinal amoebiasis and parenterally in visceral leishmaniasis.

ADRs

Characteristic toxic effects associated with use of aminoglycosides include ototoxicity, nephrotoxicity and neuromuscular blockade.

- Kanamycin, amikacin and neomycin cause maximum hearing loss [Mnemonic: KAN, the Hindi word for ear]. Streptomycin possesses maximal vestibular toxicity, while netilmicin is the least ototoxic aminoglycoside. These should not be combined with other ototoxic drugs like furosemide, vancomycin and minocycline.
- Nephrotoxicity is maximum with neomycin [Mnemonic: Nn for Nephrotoxicity → neomycin] and minimum with streptomycin. Hence, aminoglycosides should be avoided in renal dysfunction and elderly individuals, and should not be combined with other nephrotoxic drugs like amphotericin B, vancomycin, and cyclosporin.
- All aminoglycosides have the potential to reduce release of acetylcholine from motor nerve endings and accentuate muscular weakness in myasthenia gravis. However, this effect is negligible upon IM or IV injections, and manifests only when streptomycin was instilled into the peritoneal/ pleural cavity during the operation.
- Aminoglycosides are contraindicated in pregnant women, as there is a risk of fetal ototoxicity.

2. Macrolides

These include erythromycin, clarithromycin, azithromycin and telithromycin.

Mechanism of action

Macrolides bind to 50S ribosomal subunit and interfere with the translocation of peptide chain from the A site to P site (Fig. 52.4 d, e), resulting in **inhibition of protein synthesis** and bacteriostatic effect in susceptible bacteria. Many initially sensitive organisms have developed resistance to erythromycin by **acquiring the ability to pump out the drug.** Some organisms produce enzymes that inactivate drugs. In some organisms, resistance occurs due to reduced affinity of the ribosomal binding site for the drug.

Macrolides are effective against gram-positive bacteria (like *Streptococcus, Corynebacterium*), gram-negative organisms (*Mycobacterium, Campylobacter, Bordetella pertussis*) and atypical bacteria like *Mycoplasma, Legionella* and *Chlamydia*.

Pharmacokinetics

Because erythromycin is susceptible to hydrolysis by gastric acid, it is administered as an enteric-coated preparation. Oral absorption is incomplete and delayed by food. It is widely distributed in body cavities, but cannot cross the blood–brain barrier. It is partly metabolised and excreted in bile. Renal excretion is negligible; thus, dose adjustment is not required in patients with renal dysfunction.

Uses

- **Erythromycin** is the drug of choice in diphtheria and pertussis. It is also used in prophylaxis of rheumatic fever in patients showing hypersensitivity to penicillins. The dose of erythromycin is 250–500 mg, every 6 hours.
- **Clarithromycin** is effective in mycobacterium tuberculi, lepri, mycobacterium avium complex (MAC) and kansasii infections.
- Clarithromycin (250 mg, twice daily) is part of the triple-drug regimen for *H. pylori* eradication in patients with peptic ulcer.
- **Azithromycin**, an azalide congener of the prototype macrolide erythromycin, has better tolerability and a more extended spectrum than erythromycin. It is used as the drug of first choice in urethritis caused by *Chlamydia trachomatis* and penicillinase-producing *Neisseria gonorrhoeae* (PPNG). However, it shows cross-resistance with erythromycin.
- Other indications for use of azithromycin include otitis media, tonsillitis, pharyngitis, sinusitis, acute bronchitis, typhoid and community-acquired pneumonia. Dose of azithromyin is 500 mg, once a day.
- Azithromycin is the drug of choice in pregnant women and children who have cholera infection.

ADRs

- Erythromycin can cause diarrhea, cholestatic jaundice, hypertrophic pyloric stenosis and prolongation of QT interval, predisposing patients to rhythm disturbances.
- Azithromycin is well tolerated with mild adverse effects such as mild gastrointestinal upsets, abdominal cramps, headache and dizziness.

3. Ketolides

Telithromycin and solithromycin are ketolides that have the same mechanism of action as macrolides. **Telithromycin** has higher affinity for the 50S ribosomal subunit and is useful in macrolide-resistant infections. Telithromycin is effective in community-acquired pneumonia. ADRs include hepatotoxicity and neuromuscular blockade. Hence, it may worsen myasthenia gravis.

c. Narrow Spectrum Drugs

These include lincosamides, oxazolidinones and streptogramins.

1. Lincosamides

Clindamycin binds to the 50S subunit and interferes with translocation of the peptide chain from the P to A site (Fig. 52.4d), resulting in inhibition of protein synthesis and bacteriostatic action.

Uses

They are used topically in bacterial vaginosis and acne.
- It is the drug of choice for **toxic shock syndrome**, as it inhibits synthesis of toxins by staphylococci and streptococci. Vancomycin is combined with clindamycin for these infections.
- Other indications for use include **osteomyelitis, nocardiosis and gas gangrene.**
- Clindamycin is drug of choice for *Prevotella* infection of oral cavity, lungs and pleural cavity.
- It has role in infections caused by *Pneumocystis, Toxoplasma* and malarial parasite.

ADRs

- Clindamycin can cause severe allergic reactions such as Stevens–Johnson syndrome.
- It causes thrombophlebitis of the injected vein due to its irritant nature.
- The most important adverse effect of clindamycin is **pseudomembranous enterocolitis**.
- Neuromuscular blockade and worsening of myasthenia gravis may be caused.

2. Oxazolidinones

These include linezolid, tedizolid and sutezolid.

They have the same mechanism of action as clindamycin. **Linezolid** is effective against staphylococci, enterococci and mycobacteria. However, because of its potential to cause myelosuppression, it is reserved for infections caused by vancomycin-resistant bacteria. i.e., MRSA, VRSA, VRE, MDR and XDR tuberculosis. Linezolid has very good oral bioavailability (100%) and is given orally, twice daily.

Tedizolid has lower potential to cause bone marrow suppression than linezolid. It is useful in MRSA and VRSA. **Sutezolid** is used for drug-resistant tuberculosis.

3. Streptogramins

Streptogramins include dalfopristin and quinupristin. They interfere with translocation and protein synthesis after binding to the 50S ribosomal subunit. The binding of quinupristin to the erythromycin-binding site at 50S ribosomal subunit is facilitated by dalfopristin. Hence, these two are always combined in a 3:7 ratio for bactericidal effect against MRSA and VRSA. They can cause injection site reactions as an important adverse effect.

Clinical problem-based questions and MCQs

16. i. Which of the following is effective against anaerobic organisms?
    a. Doxycycline
    b. Tigecycline
    c. Ticarcillin
    d. Amoxicillin
    ii. Describe the mechanism of action and uses of the selected drug.

17. i. Which tetracycline is useful in SIADH?
    a. Minocycline
    b. Demeclocycline
    c. Tigecycline
    d. Doxycycline
    ii. Explain the pharmacological basis for the use of the selected drug in SIADH.

18. Match the drug with typical adverse effect.
    a. Chloramphenicol   1. Pseudomembranous enterocolitis
    b. Tetracyclines   2. Grey baby syndrome
    c. Vancomycin   3. Nephrotoxicity
    d. Neomycin   4. Fanconi syndrome
    e. Clindamycin   5. Red man syndrome

19. All of the following AMAs are too toxic for systemic use, EXCEPT:
    a. Netilmicin
    b. Framycetin
    c. Bacitracin
    d. Mupirocin

20. Name the antimicrobial agent effective in toxic shock syndrome. Describe its mechanism of action, other uses and adverse effects.

21. i. Identify the drug that is effective against vancomycin-resistant enterococcal infection.
    a. Clindamycin
    b. Meropenem
    c. Linezolid
    d. Azithromycin
    ii. Describe mechanism of action and adverse effects of the selected drug.

22. A patient diagnosed with vancomycin-resistant staphylococcal infection is prescribed a combination of quinupristin and dalfopristin. Describe the mechanism of action of these drugs and explain the pharmacological basis for combining the two in VRSA.

23. A 35-year-old patient is diagnosed with toxic shock syndrome.
    i. Identify the most suitable drug:
    a. Vancomycin
    b. Clindamycin
    c. Linezolid
    d. Tigecycline
    ii. Describe the mechanism of action and adverse effects of the selected drug.

24. i. What is post-antibiotic effect?
    ii. Which of the following shows long PAE against gram-negative bacteria?
    a. Aminoglycosides
    b. Sulphonamides
    c. Macrolides
    d. Vancomycin

25. Identify an AMA that is effective against VRSA:
    a. Linezolid
    b. Piperacillin
    c. Methicillin
    d. All are effective

Drugs effective against *Pseudomonas* and MRSA/VRSA are enumerated in Box 52.1 and Box 52.2, respectively.

Box 52.1   AMAs effective against *Pseudomonas*

1. **Penicillins** – Carbenicillin, Ticarcillin, Azlocillin, Mezlocillin, Piperacillin.
2. **Cephalosporins** – Ceftazidime, Cefoperazone, Ceftolazone, Moxalactam, Cefepime, Cefpirome
3. **Monobactams** – Aztreonam
4. **Carbapenems** – Imipenem, Meropenem, Doripenem
5. **Fluoroquinolones** – Ciprofloxacin, Levofloxacin
6. **Aminoglycosides** – Gentamicin
7. **Polypeptides** like Colistin, Polymyxin B

> **Box 52.2** Drugs against methicillin, vancomycin-resistant *S. aureus* (MRSA, VRSA)
>
> **MRSA:**
> - **Glycopeptides** – Vancomycin, Teicoplanin, Oritavancin, Telavancin, Dalbavancin
> - **Fifth-generation cephalosporins** – Ceftaroline, Ceftobiprole
> - **Oxazolidinones** – Linezolid, Tedizolid
> - **Rifampicin**
> - **Tigecycline**
> - **Streptogramins** – Quinupristin + Dalfopristin
>
> **VRSA:**
> - Dalbavancin
> - Tigecycline
> - Linezolid, Tedizolid
> - Quinupristin, Dalfopristin

Some AMAs possess organ toxic effects. Drugs having nephrotoxic and hepatotoxic potential are listed in Box 52.3.

> **Box 52.3** AMAs with organ toxicity on liver, kidney
>
> **Nephrotoxic drugs**
> - Aminoglycosides
> - Amphotericin B
> - Vancomycin
> - Cephalothin
> - Cephaloridine
> - Nitrofurantoin
> - Nalidixic acid
> - Tetracyclines (with the exception of doxycycline)
> - Ethambutol
>
> **Hepatotoxic drugs**
> - Isoniazid, Rifampicin, Pyrazinamide
> - Erythromycin
> - Tetracyclines
> - Pefloxacin
> - Chloramphenicol
> - Clindamycin

Summary

- AMAs are classified based on mechanism of their action.
- Drugs that **interfere with folate synthesis** are sulphonamides and diaminopyrimidines. These cause sequential blockade of folic acid synthesis and reduction of DHFA to THFA. Thus, combinations of sulphamethoxazole and trimethoprim (cotrimoxazole) exert bactericidal action. Main indications for its use are cystitis, prostatitis, nocardiosis, pneumocystis infection, skin and soft tissue infections. ADRs include crystalline urine. Hence, excess fluid intake and frequent voiding is advised.
- Sulfadoxine combined with pyrimethamine and artesunate, is useful in drug-resistant malaria infection.
- Sulfacetamide, silver sulfadiazine and mafenide are topically used sulphonamides.
- Quinolones and FQs **inhibit DNA gyrase enzyme**. Ciprofloxacin is the drug of choice in meningococcal meningitis, typhoid, anthrax, plague, and *Pseudomonas* infections. Norfloxacin is preferred in UTI, prostatitis and traveller's diarrhea. Adverse effects are gastrointestinal symptoms, tendon rupture, cartilage damage, QT prolongation, photosensitivity, etc.
- **Cell wall synthesis inhibitors** include β-lactams such as penicillins, cephalosporins, monobactams and carbapenems. **Penicillin G** is useful in streptococcal infections (rheumatic fever, sub-acute bacterial endocarditis, otitis media, pharyngitis), actinomycosis, leptospirosis, syphilis, anthrax infections [Mnemonic: Salsa]. The extended-spectrum penicillin, amoxicillin, is used in UTI, RTI, SABE, gonorrhea, and *H. pylori* infection. Combination therapy of amoxicillin with clavulanic acid and probenecid is used in PPNG. The most important adverse effects of penicillins are the hypersensitivity reactions. Cloxacillin, dicloxacillin and methicillin are resistant to penicillinase enzyme. Carbenicillin, ticarcillin, azlocillin, mezlocillin and piperacillin are penicillins effective against *Pseudomonas*.
- **Cephalosporins** are divided into five generations. These are useful in surgical prophylaxis, UTI, RTI, bacterial meningitis, typhoid fever and soft tissue infections. Ceftazidime, cefoperazone and ceftolazone are effective against *Pseudomonas*. Higher generation drugs are reserved for hospital-acquired infections caused by MRSA and penicillin-resistant organisms. ADRs include gastrointestinal irritant symptoms, pain at the injection site, thrombophlebitis, hypersensitivity reactions, biliary sludging syndrome and gall stones. Cefoperazone and cefamandole can inhibit aldehyde dehydrogenase enzyme, resulting in disulfiram reaction.
- **Aztreonam** has no cross-resistance with penicillins or cephalosporins. It is useful in hospital-acquired infections of GI, biliary and genitourinary tract in patients showing hypersensitivity reactions with penicillins or cephalosporins.
- **Imipenem** is always used along with cilastin to prevent its degradation by dehydropeptidase 1 enzyme in the renal brush border. It is used in hospital-acquired infections of the urinary tract, respiratory tract, skin, soft tissues, abdominal and pelvic cavity, especially in immunocompromised patients. It has the potential to precipitate seizures.
- **Protein synthesis inhibitors** include broad-spectrum drugs like tetracyclines, chloramphenicol and pleuromutilins. Aminoglycosides and macrolides are moderate-spectrum drugs. Clindamycin,

oxazolidinones and streptogramins are narrow-spectrum drugs.
- **Tetracyclines** are never given by the intramuscular route. These should be taken orally before meals with water to avoid formation of complexes with calcium in food and milk. Patients are advised not to lie down for some time after taking the medicine to avoid esophagitis. They are useful in **A**typical pneumonia, **c**holera, **m**eningococcal carrier state, **b**rucellosis, **l**ymphogranuloma venereum, **g**ranuloma inguinale, **c**hlamydial infections, **r**ickettsial infections, **S**IADH [Mnemonic for uses of tetracyclines: Ac manufactured by LG company runs smoothly.]
- Important ADRs include photosensitivity, GI symptoms, hepatotoxicity, nephrotoxicity, deposition in bones and teeth, and pseudotumor cerebri; outdated drugs cause Fanconi syndrome. These are contraindicated in pregnancy and children.
- **Chloramphenicol** has the potential to cause bone marrow suppression and grey baby syndrome. So, it is not preferred, except in cases of resistant pneumococci, meningococcal, rickettsial and *H. influenzae* infections.
- **Aminoglycosides** cause freezing of chain initiation, misreading of mRNA code and structural damage to cell membrane, resulting in cidal effect. These require parenteral administration for systemic effect. Gentamicin is useful in serious respiratory infections in critically ill, immunocompromised patients, plague, tularemia, and with other drugs in SABE, meningitis, *Proteus*, *Pseudomonas* and *Klebsiella* infections. Streptomycin, capreomycin, kanamycin and amikacin have roles in resistant TB. Major adverse effects are hepatotoxicity, nephrotoxicity and neuromuscular blockade.
- **Macrolides** interfere with translocation of peptide chain after binding to the 50S subunit. Clarithromycin and azithromycin are used in *H. pylori* infections and urethritis caused by *Chlamydia trachomatis* and penicillinase-producing *Neisseria gonorrhoeae* (PPNG), respectively. ADRs like diarrhea, cholestatic jaundice, hypertrophic pyloric stenosis and prolongation of QT interval, predisposing one to rhythm disturbances, abdominal cramps, headache and dizziness may occur.
- Other protein-synthesis inhibitors include clindamycin, linezolid, and quinupristin + dalfopristin. These are reserved for methicillin- and vancomycin-resistant staphylococcal infections.

Questions for practice

1. Comment on the combined use of:
   a. Sulphamethoxazole and trimethoprim
   b. Sulfadoxine and pyrimethamine
   c. Probenecid and penicillin
   d. Cephalosporin and alcohol
   e. Amoxicillin and clavulanic acid
   f. Tetracyclines and milk
   g. Imipenem and cilastin
2. Enumerate adverse effects of:
   a. Cephalosporins
   b. Fluoroquinolones
   c. Aminoglycosides
3. Enumerate:
   a. Anti-*Pseudomonas* drugs
   b. Drugs for MRSA
   c. Drugs fo VRSA

Hints for problem-based questions and MCQs

1. i. c. Silver sulfadiazine
   ii. Inhibits folate synthase enzyme
2. i. a. Diaminopyrimidines
   ii. Sequential blockade of folate synthase and DHF reductase enzyme.
   iii. Cotrimoxazole. Refer to page 672.
3. b. Sulfasalazine
4. d. Inhibits nicking and resealing of DNA chain.
5. i. a. Norfloxacin
   ii. Refer to page 672, 673.
6. a. Pefloxacin is safe (moxifloxacin and trovafloxacin are also safe in renal failure).
7. i. c. Sparfloxacin
   ii. a. Moxifloxacin
8. d. Ertapenem
9. a. Cefepime
10. c. Faropenem
11. i. c. Pseudomembranous colitis
    ii. Refer to page 680.
12. i. a. Amoxicillin, clavulanic acid, probenecid
    ii. Amoxicillin is a cell wall synthesis inhibitor; clavulanic acid is a β-lactamase inhibitor; probenecid interferes with tubular secretion of amoxicillin, increasing its duration of action. Doses are 3 g, 0.5 g and 1 g, respectively.
13. i. a. Tazobactam
    ii. Refer to pages 679, 680.
14. Cilastin inhibits dehydropeptidase 1 and prevents hydrolysis of imipenem. Refer to page 679
15. i. a. Dalbavancin
    ii. Cell wall synthesis inhibitor
16. i. b. Tigecycline
    ii. Tigecycline causes protein synthesis inhibition, is useful in MRSA, VRSA, carbapenem-resistant gram-negative infections. (Refer to page 683.)
17. i. b. Demeclocycline
    ii. Useful in SIADH because of its ADH antagonistic action.
18. a–2; b–4; c–5; d–3; e–1.
19. a. Netilmicin
20. Clindamycin. Refer to page 685.
21. i. c. Linezolid
    ii. Refer to page 686.
22. Dalfopristin facilitates binding of quinupristin to the 50S ribosomal subunit (refer to page 686).
23. i. b. Clindamycin
    ii. Refer to page 685.
24. i. Refer to page 670.
    ii. a. Aminoglycosides
25. a. Linezolid

CONCEPT MAP – BACTERIAL PROTEIN SYNTHESIS INHIBITORS

Tetracyclines (Broad-Spectrum Drugs)

Uses
Atypical pneumonia, Cholera, Meningococcal carrier state, Brucellosis, Lymphogranuloma venereum, Granuloma inguinale, Chlamydial infections, Rickettsial infections, SIADH.
Used orally or intravenously, but never intramuscularly

Mechanism
Tetracyclines bind to 30S subunit, interfere with binding of tRNA at acceptor site → **bacteriostatic** effect
Resistance due to excessive efflux of drug from microbial cells, enzymatic inactivation of drug molecule and reduced binding of drug to 30S.

Drugs
Tetracycline, Oxytetracycline, Chlortetracycline, Methacycline, Demeclocycline, Doxycycline, Minocycline

ADRs
Nausea, vomiting, esophagitis
Can form unabsorbable complexes with calcium and food.
Get deposited on bone and teeth → abnormal growths on bones and yellow staining of teeth.
Risk of hepatotoxicity in pregnant women.
Demeclocycline → diabetes insipidus
Minocycline → vestibulotoxic.
Minocycline, doxycycline and tigecycline are nephrotoxic
Tetracyclines can also cause anti-anabolic effects, pseudotumor cerebri and photosensitivity reactions like sunburn on exposed areas of skin.
Outdated/expired tetracycline preparations → Fanconi syndrome.

Chloramphenicol (Broad-Spectrum Drugs)

Mechanism
Binds to 50S ribosomal subunit → interferes with peptide bond formation between newly added amino acid and nascent peptide chain → **bacteriostatic** effect

Uses
Used only in case of resistant infections caused by organisms like *H. influenzae*, meningococci, pneumococci and Rickettsia. Dose not > 2–3 gm and duration of therapy not > 2 weeks.

ADRs
At high dose, bone marrow suppression → agranulocytosis, aplastic anemia, thrombocytopenia and pancytopenia.
Rarely, idiosyncratic myelosuppression, not dose-related, more severe and can be fatal.
In premature infants, 'grey baby syndrome' characterised by ashen grey cyanosis, abdominal distension, irregular respiration, hypothermia and cardiovascular collapse.

Pleuromutilins (Broad-Spectrum Drugs)
No cross-resistance with other AMAs, extremely low resistance rates.
Approved only for topical use in impetigo
ADRs: Irritation at site of application

Aminoglycosides (Moderate-Spectrum Drugs)

Drugs
Streptomycin, Neomycin, Tobramycin, Paromomycin, Gentamicin, Amikacin, Netilmicin

Mechanism
Bind to 30S–50S interface → freeze initiation of protein synthesis, misreading of mRNA code → incorporation of wrong amino acids → changes in integrity of cell membrane → **bactericidal** effect

Uses
Gentamicin for prevention and treatment of respiratory infections in immuno-compromised patients.
Gentamicin + tetracyclines for plague and tularemia.
Gentamicin + ampicillin/vancomycin for SABE
Gentamicin + 3rd generation cephalosporins or piperacillin for serious infections caused by *Proteus, Pseudomonas, Klebsiella*
Streptomycin, Amikacin, Capreomycin and Kanamycin as 2nd-line antitubercular drugs
Neomycin oral for preparation of bowel before surgery, hepatic coma

ADRs
Ototoxicity - hearing loss and vestibular toxicity.
Nephrotoxicity
Neuromuscular blockade.
Contraindicated in pregnancy.

Macrolides (Moderate-Spectrum Drugs)

Drugs
Erythromycin, Clarithromycin, Azithromycin, Telithromycin

Mechanism
Bind to 50S ribosomal subunit → interfere with translocation of peptide chain → **bacteristatic** effect
Resistance due to drug efflux, inactivating enzymes and reduced affinity for 50S binding site.

Uses
Erythromycin is the DOC in diphtheria, pertussis
Clarithromycin is effective in *H. pylori, Mycobacterium tuberculi/lepri/avium/kansasii* infections.
Azithromycin is the DOC in urethritis caused by *Chlamydia trachomatis* and PPNG, cholera infection in pregnant women/children, otitis media, tonsillitis, pharyngitis, sinusitis. acute bronchitis typhoid and community-acquired pneumonia.

ADRs
Diarrhea, cholestatic jaundice, hypertrophic pyloric stenosis and prolongation of QT interval predisposing to rhythm disturbances.

SECTION 10 Chemotherapeutic Drugs

53 Drugs Used in UTIs and STDs

PH 8.4 Devise a pharmacotherapeutic plan for UTI and STDs and explain to patient the instructions and adherence to treatment.

Learning objectives

A student of MBBS phase II should be able to:
- Describe the general principles of management of UTIs.
- Enumerate drugs used in UTIs.
- Describe the mechanism of action of drugs of choice in UTIs.
- Enumerate therapeutic uses and adverse effects of the drugs of choice in UTIs.
- Enumerate alternative drugs in UTI.
- Describe chemoprophylaxis of UTI.
- Describe the management of UTI in pregnancy.
- Describe the management of UTI in patients with impaired renal function.
- Describe common STDs and the drugs used to manage them.

URINARY TRACT INFECTIONS (UTIs)

Types of UTIs

Urinary tract infections (UTIs) commonly affect the lower urinary tract, causing **urethritis, cystitis, cystourethritis, vulvovaginitis**, and **prostatitis** (Fig. 53.1). Patients typically present with the following symptoms:

- Increased frequency of micturition
- Dysuria, i.e., lower abdominal /suprapubic pain, burning sensation while passing urine
- Pus in urine (pyuria)
- Urine may appear blood-stained (hematuria)

Normally, acute lower UTIs are self-limiting or respond to **treatment** with:

- urinary antiseptics.
- antimicrobial agents (AMAs) given for 3–5 days.

However, in patients with indwelling catheters, obstruction to the flow of urine, and dryness/atrophy and bacterial colonisation of the vagina (as seen in post-menopausal women), the infection may become chronic and recurrence is common.

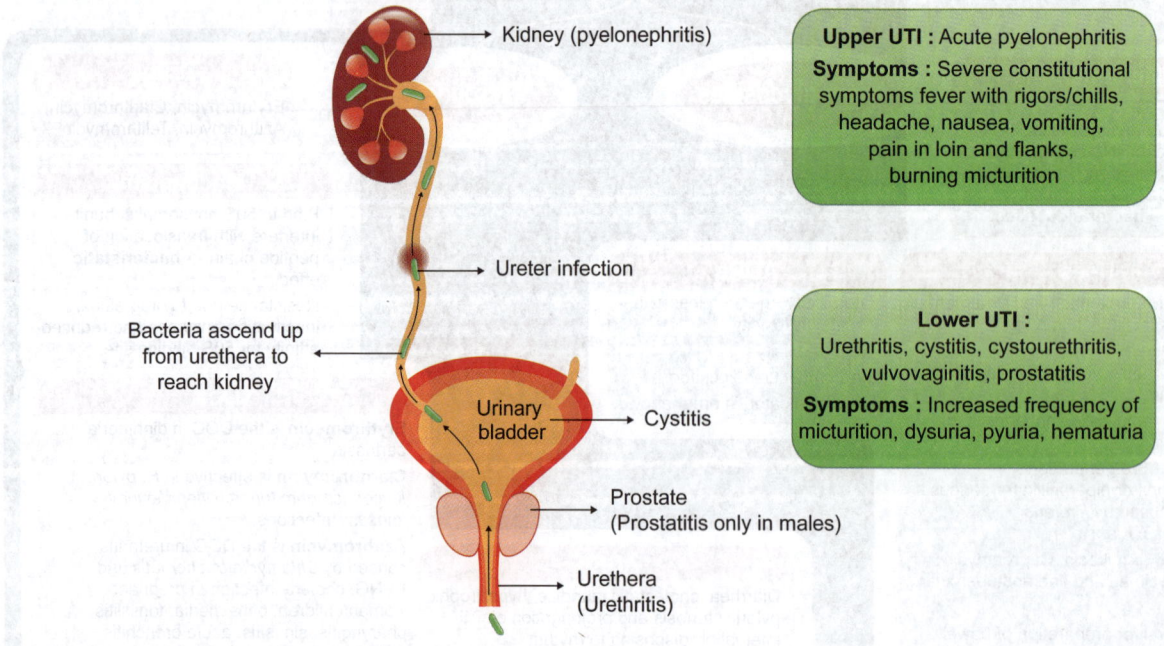

Fig. 53.1 Sites of urinary tract infections

In severe, untreated, or incompletely treated cases, infection may spread upwards in the urinary tract, causing upper UTI. In **acute pyelonephritis,** the patient presents with severe constitutional symptoms such as:

- Fever with rigors/chills.
- Headache, nausea and vomiting.
- Pain in the loins and flanks, burning micturition are also reported.

Severe, complicated pyelonephritis may result in **renal failure and gram-negative septicemia**. So, upper UTIs must be **treated aggressively.** Administration of a specific antimicrobial agent, based on culture and sensitivity reports, is usually required for a longer duration, often up to two weeks.

Diagnosis of UTI

UTI is confirmed by urine analysis. Urine may be turbid, foul-smelling, or blood-stained. The pH of urine is acidic in *E. coli* and *Klebsiella* infections, while it is alkaline in *Proteus* infections. Pus cells and pus cell casts are present. Culture sensitivity confirms the causative organism and AMAs to which it is sensitive. The sample for culture sensitivity testing should be obtained prior to initiation of empirical antibiotic therapy.

Organisms Responsible for UTIs

Most UTIs are caused by gram-negative bacteria, with *Escherichia coli* being responsible for a majority of the uncomplicated lower UTIs. The common source of coliform infections is the rectum. Other organisms that cause UTIs include *Proteus, Klebsiella, Pseudomonas, Enterobacteriaceae,* enterococci, *Chlamydia,* and *Gardnerella vaginalis*. These organisms (other than *E. coli*) are mostly responsible for UTIs in patients with structural or functional obstruction to the flow of urine, indwelling urinary catheters, or immunocompromised status (such as the use of immunosuppressive drugs or AIDS). Mixed infections with more than one organism may also occur in such patients.

MANAGEMENT OF UTIs

Many acute lower UTIs are self-limiting and respond to **increased fluid intake and high urine flow rate**. Treatment of UTI includes symptomatic relief, urinary antiseptics, antimicrobial therapy, and sometimes, change in urinary pH.

1. Drugs for Symptomatic Relief

a. **Anticholinergic drugs with vesicoselective action**, such as flavoxate, oxybutynin, tolterodine, darifenacin and solifenacin, are useful. These have a relaxant action on the ureter and urinary bladder, exerted through the blockade of muscarinic cholinergic receptors (mainly M_3 subtype). **Flavoxate** is the most commonly used drug in this group. It relieves dysuria, frequency and urgency in UTI. It is given orally in a dose of 200 mg three times a day.

Anticholinergic antispasmodic drug **valethamate** is useful in relieving urinary colic, e.g., in UTI associated with renal calculi. These drugs can cause **atropinic adverse effects** such as dryness of mouth, skin, eyes, blurring of vision, urinary retention (especially in elderly males), and constipation.

b. **Drotaverine,** a phosphodiesterase 4 inhibitor that causes smooth muscle relaxation, is also useful in renal colic. It is free of atropinic adverse effects, but may cause headache, dizziness, flushing and fall in BP.

c. **Phenazopyridine** is a dye that has urinary analgesic action. It relieves symptoms associated with cystitis. Dose is 200–400 mg, three times a day. Nausea, vomiting and epigastric pain are frequent adverse effects.

2. Urinary Antiseptics

These are AMAs that attain effective antibacterial concentration only in the urinary tract, at their orally tolerated doses. They are concentrated in the renal tubules and are **indicated only in UTIs**. Although these drugs are administered orally, they exert antibacterial effect only in the urinary tract (acting as a local therapy), and are hence called 'urinary antiseptics'. The drugs in this category include nitrofurantoin, nalidixic acid and methenamine.

a. Nitrofurantoin

The mechanism of action of nitrofurantoin involves enzymatic reduction by susceptible bacteria to generate reactive intermediates that damage bacterial DNA. Action is mainly **bacteriostatic**; however, the higher concentrations achieved in acidic urine **may be bactericidal.** Nitrofurantoin is active against gram-negative bacteria, but due to emergence of resistant strains and adverse effects, it is not used much nowadays. It is useful only for the treatment of **uncomplicated lower UTI caused by *E. coli*.** Nitrofurantoin does not show cross-resistance with any other antimicrobial drug. It can be used for **prophylaxis** of UTI in patients with catheterisation and women with recurrent UTIs, in a dose of 100 mg at bedtime.

Adverse effects of nitrofurantoin include gastrointestinal intolerance like nausea, vomiting, epigastric pain and tenderness, fever, chills and leukopenia. In patients with G6PD deficiency, hemolysis may occur. Long-term use may cause neurological complications, liver damage, pulmonary fibrosis, etc.

b. Methenamine

Methenamine is hexamethylene tetramine which decomposes slowly in acidic urine to release formaldehyde that inhibits all the bacteria. Methenamine does not have any antimicrobial effect in the blood or any other tissues, as it is activated only in acidic pH (< 5.5). So, **urine must be acidified** using mandelic or ascorbic acid to exploit the antibacterial effect of methenamine. Adequate concentration of formaldehyde in urine is ensured by modulating fluid intake to keep daily urine output at 1–1.5 litres. Methenamine is effective in chronic resistant UTI, in a dose of 1 g three times a day; however, the development of many resistant strains has limited its usage.

Adverse effects of methenamine include:

- Gastritis due to release of formaldehyde in acidic pH of stomach. This is prevented by use of enteric-coated tablets.
- It may cause central adverse effects, dizziness, lightheadedness, fainting, etc.
- High dose can cause chemical cystitis and hematuria.
- Serious allergic reactions can occur.

c. Nalidixic acid

It was the **first quinolone** introduced in clinical practice. Its mechanism of action involves bactericidal action through **inhibition of bacterial DNA gyrase** enzyme. DNA gyrase has two subunits, A and B. Subunit A of DNA gyrase carries out nicking and resealing of DNA, while subunit B introduces a negative supercoil. DNA gyrase acts by preventing excessive positive supercoiling of DNA strands during strand separation prior to replication or transcription. Quinolones bind to subunit A of DNA gyrase and inhibit the nicking and resealing function, resulting in excessive supercoiling of DNA; this leads to DNA damage and cell death (refer to Fig. 52.2).

Nalidixic acid is mainly **effective against gram-negative organisms** like *E. coli, Klebsiella, Proteus, Shigella,* and *Enterobacter,* but not against *Pseudomonas.* With the usual oral dose, it attains therapeutic concentration only in the urine and gut lumen. Hence, it was used for urinary infections and infective diarrheas in a dose of 500–1000 mg, three or four times a day. However, nowadays, it is rarely used, as **fluorinated quinolones (FQs) provide better efficacy and tolerability.**

Adverse effects associated with the use of nalidixic acid include gastrointestinal intolerance, rashes, headache, drowsiness, visual problems, vertigo and even convulsions in children.

> **Clinical problem-based questions and MCQs**
>
> 1. A 65-year-old post-menopausal woman presents with a history suggestive of chronic, recurrent, resistant urinary tract infection.
>   i. Identify the most suitable urinary antiseptic for this case.
>   a. Methenamine   b. Formaldehyde
>   c. Nalidixic acid   d. Nitrofurantoin
>   ii. Describe the mechanism of action and adverse effects of the chosen drug.
>
> 2. i. Which of the following is a non-anticholinergic antispasmodic used in renal colic?
>   a. Solifenacin   b. Drotaverine
>   c. Oxybutynin   d. Flavoxate
>   ii. Describe the mechanism of action and adverse effects of the chosen drug.
>
> 3. Which drug requires acidic pH of urine as a mandatory condition for its urinary antiseptic action?
>   a. Methenamine   b. Nalidixic acid
>   c. Nitrofurantoin   d. All of above
>
> 4. Match the drug with its mechanism of action.
>   a. Nalidixic acid   1. PDE4 inhibition
>   b. Nitrofurantoin   2. DNA gyrase inhibition
>   c. Methenamine   3. M_3 receptor blockade
>   d. Flavoxate   4. Formaldehyde release in acidic urine
>   e. Drotaverine   5. Reduction to form reactive intermediates that damage DNA

3. Antimicrobial Therapy

It is the mainstay of the management of UTI. Most UTIs respond well to antimicrobial therapy.

The **choice of AMA** depends on the suspected organisms and bacteriological investigations, i.e., culture sensitivity report of midstream urine. **Empirical treatment** is usually given for *E. coli* infection and initial treatment of other infections. Efficacy of the drug against the causative organism, safety, patient characteristics and cost of drug are important factors for consideration while selecting AMAs for empirical treatment. In general, **low-cost drugs with lower risk of serious adverse effects are preferred.** If the patient responds adequately to the empirical AMA, the course is continued to completion (3–5 days for uncomplicated lower UTIs). However, if the clinical response is inadequate, the AMA is changed as per the culture sensitivity report. Commonly used AMAs in UTIs are listed below.

a. Cotrimoxazole

Cotrimoxazole is effective against many urinary pathogens. It is a fixed-dose combination of sulphamethoxazole and trimethoprim in a ratio of 5:1.

Mechanism of action: Sulphamethoxazole, one of the sulphonamides, is a PABA analogue that acts by **interfering with bacterial folate synthesis** (refer to Fig. 52.1). Trimethoprim is a diaminopyrimidine that **inhibits bacterial DHFRase** and prevents conversion of dihydrofolate into tetrahydrofolate. Although the individual components of cotrimoxazole are bacteriostatic, their combination causes **sequential blockade of the steps in bacterial THFA synthesis,** resulting in bactericidal action against many organisms.

Resistance develops due to plasmid-mediated mutation resulting in DHFRase that has low affinity for trimethoprim. Most of the originally sensitive bacterial strains have developed resistance to it.

Therapeutic uses: Cotrimoxazole, a combination of sulphamethoxazole and trimethoprim, is used to treat **acute uncomplicated UTIs** like acute cystitis and chronic recurrent prostatitis. Trimethoprim gets concentrated effectively in the acidic environment of the prostate.

Dosage: 800 mg sulphamethoxazole + 160 mg trimethoprim, taken twice daily for 3–10 days.

Other uses include bacterial diarrhea, dysentery, chronic bronchitis, otitis media, facio-maxillary infections, pneumonia in AIDS patients caused by *Pneumocystis jirovecii*. However, its utility in severe systemic infections has decreased due to development of resistant strains.

ADRs: Headache, rashes, nausea, vomiting, glossitis, stomatitis, and megaloblastic anemia secondary to folate deficiency may occur.

The dose should be reduced in patients with renal dysfunction, as it may cause uremia. In rare cases, blood dyscrasias and bone marrow suppression may occur, especially in elderly individuals.

b. Fluoroquinolones

The **mechanism of action** of FQs is the same as that of nalidixic acid. These exert bactericidal action by **inhibiting DNA gyrase enzyme**.

Therapeutic uses

- Norfloxacin 400 mg or ciprofloxacin 500 mg or ofloxacin 200–400 mg given twice daily, orally, are the **drugs of choice for lower uncomplicated UTI** caused by *E. coli*.
- These are also used in cases of **amoxicillin-resistant UTI** in patients with prostatitis and indwelling catheters. Cure rates are higher than with cotrimoxazole. Infections caused by *Pseudomonas* also respond to ciprofloxacin.
- Ofloxacin is alternative drug for **urethritis** caused by *Chlamydia*.
- For chronic UTIs, norfloxacin is given for 8–12 weeks.

c. Amoxycillin + clavulanic acid

Amoxycillin is an extended-spectrum penicillin, while clavulanic acid is a penicillinase inhibitor.

Mechanism of action: Like all β-lactam AMAs, amoxicillin is a bactericidal drug that acts by inhibiting bacterial cell wall synthesis. **Resistance** to penicillins develop due to the **production of enzyme penicillinase by bacteria.** This enzyme **opens up the β-lactam ring and inactivates the drug.** Bacteria such as staphylococci, gonococci, *B. subtilis*, *E. coli*, and *H. influenzae* commonly produce the penicillinase enzyme, which breaks down penicillin. As a result, urinary tract infections (UTIs) caused by penicillinase-producing *E. coli* are often resistant to most penicillin antibiotics.

Clavulanic acid, sulbactam and tazobactam are inhibitors of enzyme penicillinase or β-lactamase. These have a β-lactam ring but negligible antimicrobial action. **Clavulanic acid is a progressive inhibitor of β-lactamase enzyme**. Initially, it binds to β-lactamase enzyme reversibly and then by a covalent bond. Clavulanic acid when combined with a penicillin or β-lactam AMA acts as a **'suicide inhibitor'**. Clavulanic acid contains a β-lactam ring. It binds to the active site of β-lactamase enzyme and inhibits it irreversibly, saving the β-lactam ring of the concurrently administered penicillin. Clavulanic acid permeates through the outer layers of the cell wall in gram-negative bacteria and protects penicillins from attack by penicillinase enzyme in the periplasm. Therefore, combinations of these β-lactamase inhibitors with β-lactam antibiotics, e.g., amoxicillin (250/500 mg) + clavulanic acid (125 mg), re-establishes antimicrobial activity in resistant organisms like staphylococci, *E. coli*, *Proteus*, and *Klebsiella*.

d. Cephalosporins

Like penicillins, cephalosporins also have a β-lactam ring and the same mechanism of action, i.e., inhibition of cell wall synthesis. However, cephalosporins and penicillins bind to different sites. This explains the differences in their spectrum of action and lack of cross-resistance with penicillins. **Resistance** occurs due to production of β-lactamases called cephalosporinases, which specifically destroy cephalosporins. Cephalexin (250–1000 mg, 6–8 hourly), cefadroxil (500–1000 mg, twice a day), and cefuroxime axetil (250–500 mg, twice daily) are among the drugs of choice for the management of UTIs. Cefpodoxime proxetil (200 mg, twice daily) can be used as an alternative drug.

e. Macrolides

These include erythromycin, clarithromycin, azithromycin and telithromycin that act by **inhibiting protein synthesis** in susceptible bacteria. Resistance occurs due to pumping out of the drug from bacterial cells, release of drug-inactivating enzymes by bacteria, and reduced affinity of the drug for ribosomal binding sites.

With a wider spectrum of activity and better tolerability, **azithromycin is the drug of first choice in urethritis** caused by *Chlamydia trachomatis* and penicillinase-producing *Neisseria gonorrhoeae* (PPNG). However, it shows cross-resistance with erythromycin. It also causes mild gastrointestinal upset, abdominal cramps, headache and dizziness as adverse effects.

f. Fosfomycin

It is a phosphonic antibiotic that acts by **inhibiting the initial step of cell wall synthesis involving enzyme phosphoenolpyruvate synthetase in both gram-positive and gram-negative bacteria.** There is no cross-resistance with other drugs. It is effective in the treatment of **lower UTIs, cystitis and prostate infections**. However, it should be kept as a **reserve drug** to delay the development of resistance to its action. **ADRs** include headache, nausea and vaginal fungal infections.

> *Duration of antimicrobial therapy*
> **In uncomplicated infections** of the lower urinary tract, single-dose therapies have been successful. To ensure eradication of organisms, a **3–5 days** regimen is usually advocated. However, upper UTI needs aggressive antimicrobial therapy for **up to 2 weeks**.

4. Changes in urinary pH

Some AMAs are **more effective in acidic urine**, e.g., nitrofurantoin, methenamine, tetracyclines, methicillin and cloxacillin. In contrast, cotrimoxazole, aminoglycosides, cephalosporins and FQs are **more effective in alkaline pH**.

However, alteration of pH by giving acidifying or alkalinising agents is not usually required, except in the case of methenamine (which can act only in acidic urine). In patients who exhibit inadequate response to antimicrobial therapy, measuring the pH of urine and applying corrective measures may be helpful.

Certain urease-positive organisms like *Proteus* convert urea to NH_3. In such cases, it becomes impossible to acidify urine. So, drugs that are active in an alkaline pH should be prescribed.

UTI in pregnancy

Urinary tract infections are a common occurrence during pregnancy. Infection of the lower urinary tract predisposes to pyelonephritis and poses risk to the fetus as well. Hence, **prophylaxis and early treatment** are advised.

For prevention of recurrent UTIs, pregnant women are **screened for bacteriuria** during antenatal visits, even if there are no symptoms suggestive of UTI. If UTI is diagnosed, it should be treated promptly. **Amoxicillin (alone or with β-lactamase inhibitor), cephalexin, cefadroxil** and **cefuroxime axetil** are safe for use in pregnant women. Empirical therapy is given with any of these drugs after obtaining a sample for culture sensitivity testing. **Fosfomycin and macrolide** antibiotics are also safe. Macrolides are useful in chlamydial or gonococcal urethritis.

Follow-up of patient is important to prevent recurrent infection and associated complications.

UTI in renal impairment

It is difficult to treat urinary infections in patients with impaired renal function. Most **antimicrobial agents fail to attain adequate concentration in urine** and thus become less efficacious. Many **drugs, otherwise effective in UTIs, are not safe** in renal dysfunction, e.g., methenamine, nalidixic acid, nitrofurantoin, cephalosporins, and tetracyclines. In such patients, **culture sensitivity testing** should be done to choose the appropriate antimicrobial agent. Follow-up culture testing is required to confirm eradication of the infection.

> **Instructions to patients with UTI**
> - Patients must strictly follow the prescribed treatment and follow-up schedules. Incomplete treatment can lead to the development of drug-resistant bacterial strains.
> - Drink at least 8–10 glasses of water daily to ensure frequent urination, which helps to flush out bacteria from the urinary tract.
> - Use the correct method of wiping from 'front-to-back', after defecation. This prevents migration of coliform bacteria from the anal region to the vagina, and reduces the risk of ascending urinary infections.

Clinical problem-based questions and MCQs

5. Match the antimicrobial agent to the correct mechanism of its action.
   - a. Cefuroxime
   - b. Amoxicillin
   - c. Trimethoprim
   - d. Ofloxacin

   1. DNA gyrase inhibition
   2. DHFRase inhibition
   3. Cell wall synthesis inhibition
   4. β-lactamase inhibition

6. A 30-year-old patient complained of generalised aches and pains, pain in the iliac region while passing urine, and burning micturition for the past two days. There has been no such symptoms earlier. Urine analysis shows turbid, foul-smelling urine with numerous pus cells.
   i. What other investigation is indicated?
   ii. Describe the pharmacotherapy of this patient.
   iii. Describe the duration of treatment required and conditions in which change of therapy may be needed.

7. A 45-year-old patient suffering from UTI was given amoxicillin in combination with clavulanic acid. Describe the mechanism of action of both drugs and justify their combination.

8. Which of the following AMAs has the risk of causing tendon rupture in elderly individuals?
   a. Amoxicillin   b. Ciprofloxacin
   c. Clavulanic acid d. Cefuroxime

9. Identify an AMA safe for use in a pregnant woman suffering from acute UTI.
   a. Gentamicin   b. Amoxicillin
   c. Ofloxacin   d. Cotrimoxazole

10. Which of the following AMAs acts by inhibiting bacterial protein synthesis?
    a. Ciprofloxacin   b. Fosfomycin
    c. Cefadroxil   d. Azithromycin

TREATMENT OF SEXUALLY TRANSMITTED DISEASES

Sexually transmitted diseases encountered commonly in clinical practice are gonorrhea, syphilis, granuloma inguinale, chancroid, urethritis, endocervicitis, lymphogranuloma venereum, vaginitis, and genital herpes. The important features of these diseases are described below.

Gonorrhea

Gonorrhea is caused by *Neisseria gonorrhoeae* or gonococcus. Females with gonococcal infection are generally asymptomatic but develop infertility or complications during pregnancy. Their neonates may acquire eye infection (ophthalmia neonatorum) during passage through the birth canal. Men suffering from gonorrhea usually present with dysuria, penile discharge and testicular pain.

Gonococcal infection responds well to penicillins, though many strains have developed resistance due to penicillinase production. Extended spectrum penicillins like amoxicillin, given in a dose of 3–3.5 g orally, is the drug of first choice. Probenecid competes with penicillins at tubular acid secretory sites in the kidney and prolongs their duration of action. Thus, probenecid 1 g is combined with amoxicillin.

Resistant strains are labelled as penicillinase-producing *N. gonorrhoeae* (PPNG). They are managed with cephalosporins such as ceftriaxone 1 g or cefuroxime 1.5 g, given intramuscularly, in combination with probenecid 1 g given orally. Azithromycin given orally as a 1 g-single-dose is also effective against PPNG.

In patients hypersensitive to or not tolerating penicillins, cephalosporins/doxycycline/erythromycin are good alternatives.

Syphilis

Syphilis is a highly contagious disease caused by *Treponema pallidum*. Infection is transmitted by sexual activity, direct contact and from mother to fetus via the placenta during pregnancy. Syphilis occurs as early syphilis (comprising primary, secondary, and latent stages) and late/tertiary syphilis.

- In **primary syphilis**, firm, round, painless sores called chancres are formed on the genitals, anus, lips, mouth, etc.
- In **secondary syphilis**, rashes appear on the trunk, palms of hands or soles. The rashes are usually non-itchy, reddish-brown in colour and have a rough surface.
- **Latent or hidden syphilis** is the asymptomatic stage and may last for many years. If left untreated, it progresses to the next stage.
- **Tertiary or late syphilis** involves spread of infection to distant organs like the brain, eyes, ears, heart, and blood vessels. Infection in the brain, called 'neurosyphilis', causes symptoms such as severe headache, myalgia, difficulty in concentrating, confusion, dementia and paralysis. Ocular infection may cause pain, redness in eye, visual disturbances and even blindness. Otosyphilis may cause tinnitus, hearing loss, dizziness and vertigo.

Congenital syphilis spreads from an infected mother to the unborn baby via the placenta, and may cause abortion, stillbirth and increased risk of neonatal mortality.

Patients with early syphilis, i.e., primary, secondary and latent syphilis of less than one year duration respond well to penicillins. Benzathine penicillin G 2.4 million units (MU), given intramuscularly as 1–3 weekly injections, is the treatment of choice in such cases. In late/tertiary syphilis, it is given as weekly injections for 4 weeks. Procaine penicillin, given in a dose of 1.2 MU daily by intramuscular injection, for 10 days in early syphilis and 20 days in late syphilis is an alternative to weekly benzathine penicillin.

In patients with a history of hypersensitivity to penicillins, ceftriaxone 1 g daily is given intramuscularly for 7 days. Doxycycline or erythromycin used orally are other effective alternative drugs.

Granuloma inguinale or donovanosis

This infection is caused by *Calymmatobacterium granulomatis* (also known as *Klebsiella granulomatis*). The characteristic lesions are slowly-progressing ulcers in the genital or perineal regions. There is no pain or regional lymphadenopathy. The infection disseminates to the pelvis, abdominal organs, bones, mouth and skin. Highly vascular, subcutaneous granulomas of beefy red colour may form.

Granuloma inguinale responds well to oral treatment with doxycycline 100 mg, twice a day, for 3 weeks. Oral azithromycin 500 mg once daily, for one week, is a good alternative. It has the advantage of once-daily dose and shorter duration of treatment.

Chancroid

Chancroid is caused by *Hemophilus ducreyi* infection and presents as a soft ulcer on the genitals. The ulcer may be accompanied by pain, redness and pus formation, but unlike syphilis, the edges of the ulcer are not hard.

H. ducreyi responds well to single-dose therapy of intramuscular ceftriaxone 0.25 g, or azithromycin 1 g given orally. Ciprofloxacin 500 mg BD for 3 days is an important alternative treatment. Doxycycline is also effective.

Chlamydia trachomatis infection

Chlamydia trachomatis **infection** can cause nonspecific urethritis, endocervicitis and lymphogranuloma venereum (LGV). *Chlamydia* infection can occur in both sexes. Female patients present with lower abdominal pain/discomfort, vaginal discharge, dysuria, dyspareunia and bleeding between menstrual periods. Newborns of mothers with chlamydial infection may have eye infection, and pneumonitis.

Male patients usually present with dysuria, penile discharge and pain/discomfort in testicles. In lymphogranuloma venereum (LGV), fever, severe inflammation in urogenital and anorectal region, genital ulcers and lymphadenopathy may occur. Patients usually complain of constipation/diarrhea and painful defecation.

Patients usually respond well to antimicrobial therapy. Macrolides (erythromycin, azithromycin), doxycycline and levofloxacin are effective against *Chlamydia trachomatis*. **Urethritis and endocervicitis** respond well to a single-dose therapy of azithromycin 1 g given orally. However, for LGV, azithromycin 1g, oral, is given once a week, for 3 weeks.

Doxycycline is an important alternative, used as 100 mg twice daily for 1–3 weeks.

Trichomonas vaginitis

Trichomonas vaginitis is a protozoal disease caused by *Trichomonas vaginalis*. Female patients usually present with vaginal discharge, itching and pelvic pain. Dysuria and dyspareunia may also occur. However, males infected with *Trichomonas vaginalis* are usually asymptomatic.

The treatment of choice is a single dose of metronidazole 2 g. For patients who cannot tolerate this high dose, metronidazole 400 mg, three times daily (TDS), for 7 days, is an alternative regimen. Tinidazole is also effective, given as a single dose of 2 g or 600 mg daily for 7 days.

Additionally, clotrimazole 100 mg intravaginally at night, after urination, for 6–12 days, is helpful.

Instructions to patients with STDs
- Sexual partners should be identified, tested, and treated to prevent reinfection and further transmission.
- Address the psychological trauma and social stigma associated with STDs through counselling and support.
- Educate patients on safe sexual practices and the importance of regular follow-up examinations, particularly for high-risk groups such as sex workers.
- Advise patients to abstain from sexual activity until they test negative for infection.
- Promote consistent and correct use of condoms to prevent the spread of infections.
- Recommend available vaccines (e.g., HPV, Hepatitis B) to protect against certain sexually transmitted diseases.

Clinical problem-based questions and MCQs

11. A 30-year-old male patient complains of testicular pain and penile discharge. Culture sensitivity shows gram-negative, bean-shaped diplococci. Phenotypic sensitivity testing shows greater zone of inhibition in cefoperazone–sulbactam culture plates, confirming PPNG infection.
    i. What is the diagnosis?
    ii. Which of the following drugs is effective orally in this case?
        a. Ciprofloxacin   b. Metronidazole
        c. Azithromycin   d. Amoxicillin

12. Which of the following is most common mechanism of acquired resistance to penicillins in gonococci?
    a. Gene mutation
    b. Elaboration of drug destroying enzymes
    c. Pumping out of drug from bacterial cells
    d. All of the above

13. A 37-year-old female sex worker presents with a firm, rounded painless sore (chancre) on labia majora. Serological VDRL is reactive with a titre of 1:16. The patient is diagnosed with early syphilis.
    i. Which of the following is drug of first choice?
        a. Amoxicillin
        b. Benzathine penicillin
        c. Ornidazole
        d. Cotrimoxazole
    ii. Describe the dose and duration of treatment with the chosen drug.

14. Match the sexually transmitted disease with causative organism.
    a. Granuloma inguinale   1. Treponema pallidum
    b. Neurosyphilis   2. Chlamydia trachomatis
    c. Lymphogranuloma
       venereum   3. Hemophilus ducreyi
    d. Chancroid   4. Klebsiella granulomatis

15. Identify the drug used as a single-dose therapy for trichomonal vaginitis.
    a. Azithromycin   b. Ciprofloxacin
    c. Metronidazole   d. Doxycycline

Summary

- Urinary tract infections frequently involve the lower part of the urinary tract. The infection may spread upwards to the kidneys causing upper UTI. It may be acute, chronic, and recurrent.
- Some acute urinary infections may resolve with increased urine flow rate alone, while others require treatment with antispasmodic drugs for symptom relief and urinary antiseptics like **methenamine**, **nitrofurantoin**, and **nalidixic acid** that achieve therapeutic concentration *only in the urine* upon oral administration.

- Nalidixic acid has been superseded by FQs.
- Methenamine requires an acidic urine pH to act. So, mandelic or ascorbic acid must be given with it. Due to their adverse effects and the availability of better alternatives, these drugs are less commonly used nowadays.
- It is important to obtain midstream urine sample for culture sensitivity before starting empirical antibiotic therapy. Amoxicillin, along with clavulanic acid, first- or second-generation cephalosporins and flurquinolones such as ciprofloxacin, ofloxacin and norfloxacin are the drugs of choice for UTI.
- Amoxicillin and cephalosporins act by inhibiting cell wall synthesis, whereas FQs cause inhibition of DNA gyrase enzyme. Cotrimoxazole is a fixed-dose combination of sulphamethoxazole and trimethoprim, which causes sequential blockade of synthesis of DHF and its reduction to THF. Cotrimoxazole is effective, but since many organisms have developed resistance to it, its use in UTI has decreased.
- During pregnancy, recurrent UTIs are common. Hence, antenatal checkups include screening for bacteriuria, so that UTIs are promptly detected and managed.
- Treatment of UTIs in a patient with pre-existing renal dysfunction is challenging. Repeated culture sensitivity and use of specific AMAs that are not contraindicated in renal disease is advocated.
- Sexually transmitted diseases include gonorrhea, syphilis, LI, LGV, chancroid, and trichomonal vaginitis. In addition to appropriate antibiotic therapy, instructions to patients regarding safe sexual practices, adherence to prescribed medications and psychological counseling are very important.

Questions for practice

1. Describe the pharmacotherapy of UTIs.
2. Enumerate AMAs useful in UTIs.
3. Comment on the role of following in UTIs.
   a. Urinary antiseptics
   b. Macrolides
   c. Fosfomycin
   d. Amoxicillin + clavulanic acid
4. Describe important instructions for successful management of UTIs and STDs.

Hints for problem-based questions and MCQs

1. i. a. Methenamine is a urinary antiseptic for chronic, resistant UTIs.
   ii. In acidic urine, methenamine forms formaldehyde → antibacterial action. ADRs of methenamine include gastritis, chemical cystitis, hematuria. Refer to page 691.
2. i. b. Drotaverine
   ii. It is a PDE4 inhibitor that has → smooth muscle relaxant action. ADRs of drotaverine include headache, drowsiness, fall in BP and flushing. Refer to page 691.
3. a. Methenamine
4. a–2; b–5; c–4; d–3; e–1.
5. a–3; b–3; c–2; d–1.
6. i. Patient shows features of UTI. Microbiological testing of urine is indicated to determine the causative organism and its sensitivity to various AMAs. Care should be taken to obtain midstream sample of urine before starting empirical antibiotics.
   ii. Patient should receive flavoxate for symptom relief and empirical antimicrobial therapy. Amoxicillin alone or with clavulanic acid or one of the cephalosporins – cephalexin/cefadroxil/cefuroxime axetil, or flurquinolones like norfloxacin/ciprofloxacin/ofloxacin are the drugs of first choice. Any of the agents may be used considering various factors like patient factors and cost.
   iii. Treatment should be continued for 3–5 days. If patient fails to respond to therapy or if the culture sensitivity report shows insensitivity to prescribed AMA, a change in AMA is indicated. Symptomatic treatment is however continued.
7. Amoxicillin is bactericidal through inhibition of cell wall synthesis. Clavulanic acid causes progressive inhibition of penicillinase enzyme. Thus, their combination re-establishes the sensitivity to amoxicillin in resistant organisms. Refer to page 693.
8. b. Ciprofloxacin
9. b. Amoxicillin
10. d. Azithromycin
11. i. Gonorrhea
    ii. c. Azithromycin
12. b. Elaboration of drug destroying enzymes called penicillinase.
13. i. b. Benzathine penicillin
    ii. Dose is 2.4 MU given intramuscularly as 1–3 weekly injections.
14. a–4; b–1; c–2; d–3.
15. a. Azithromycin

CONCEPT MAP – DRUGS FOR UTI

Drugs for UTI

Urinary Antiseptics

AMAs attaining effective antibacterial concentration only in the urinary tract, used orally as a local therapy

Nitrofurantoin: Reduced by susceptible bacteria to form reactive intermediates that damage bacterial DNA → bacteriostatic (bactericidal at higher concentration in acidic urine) action.

No cross-resistance with any other AMAs.

Indications for use: Uncomplicated lower UTI caused by *E. coli* & prophylaxis of UTI in patients with catheterisation, women with recurrent UTIs

ADRs: Nausea, vomiting, epigastric pain and tenderness Fever, Chills, Leukopenia, hemolysis in G6PD deficiency. Neurological complications, liver damage, pulmonary fibrosis on long-term use.

Methenamine: Urine must be acidified by using mandelic or ascorbic acid to elicit useful antibacterial effect. Effective in chronic resistant UTI but not used much because of adverse effects.

Nalidixic acid: DNA gyrase inhibitor, mainly effective against *E. coli*, *Klebsiella*, *Proteus*, *Shigella*, *Enterobacter*, but not *Pseudomonas*.

Rarely used, as FQs have better efficacy & tolerability.

UTI

Types: Lower UTI: Urethritis, cystitis, cystourethritis, vulvovaginitis, prostatitis

Upper UTI: Acute pyelonephritis

Symptoms: Increased frequency of micturition, dysuria, pyuria, hematuria in lower UTI

Severe constitutional symptoms fever with rigors/chills, headache, nausea, vomiting, pain in loins, flanks, burning micturition in upper UTI

Organisms: *Escherichia coli* is most common. Others include *Proteus*, *Klebsiella*, *Pseudomonas*, *Enterobacteriaceae*, enterococci, *Chlamydia*, and *Gardnerella vaginalis*.

Drugs for Symptomatic Relief

Vesicoselective anticholinergic drugs: Flavoxate, Oxybutynin, Tolterodine, Darifenacin, Solifenacin

Relax ureter and urinary bladder by M_3 blockade → relieve dysuria, frequency and urgency

Anticholinergic antispasmodic drug, **Valethamate** for relieving colic in UTI associated with renal calculi.

ADRs: Dryness of mouth, skin, eyes, blurring of vision, urinary retention especially in elderly males, constipation etc.

Drotaverine, a phosphodiesterase 4 inhibitor, relieves renal colic. Adverse effects are headache, dizziness, flushing and fall in BP.

Phenazopyridine relieves symptoms associated with cystitis.

ADRs: Nausea, vomiting & epigastric pain

Change in Urine pH

Nitrofurantoin, Methenamine, Tetracyclines, Methicillin, Cloxacillin are more effective in acidic urine

Cotrimoxazole, Aminoglycosides, Cephalosporins and FQs work better in alkaline pH.

In patients not responding adequately to antimicrobial therapy, measuring pH of urine and applying corrective measures may be helpful. Acidification is necessary for action of methenamine

Antimicrobials

AMAs used for empirical treatment for *E. coli* infection and for initial treatment of other infections If patient responds adequately → drug continued to complete the course (3–5 days for uncomplicated lower UTIs). Inadequate clinical response → AMA changed as per culture sensitivity report.

Cotrimoxazole used in acute uncomplicated UTIs

FQs: Norfloxacin, Ciprofloxacin, Ofloxacin are drugs of choice for lower uncomplicated UTI caused by *E. coli*. Also used in amoxicillin-resistant UTIs in patients with prostatitis and indwelling catheters, urethritis caused by *Chlamydia* and for chronic UTIs.

Combination of **Amoxicillin + Clavulanic acid** for β-lactamase producing staphylococci, *E. coli*, *Proteus*, *Klebsiella*, etc.

Cephalosporins: Cephalexin, Cefadroxil, Cefuroxime axetil are among drugs of choice for management of UTIs, no cross-resistance with penicillins

Azithromycin is DOC in urethritis caused by *Chlamydia trachomatis* and PPNG.

Fosfomycin: No cross-resistance with other AMAs, used as a reserve drug in treatment of lower UTIs, cystitis & prostate infections.

SECTION 10   Chemotherapeutic Drugs

54   Antitubercular and Antileprotic Drugs

PH 8.5 Explain the types, kinetics, dynamics, therapeutic uses and adverse effects of drugs used in tuberculosis. Devise management plan for tuberculosis treatment in various categories.
PH 8.6 Discuss the types, kinetics, dynamics, adverse effects of drugs used for leprosy and outline the management of lepra reactions.

Learning objectives

A student of MBBS phase II should be able to:

Antitubercular drugs
- Classify antitubercular drugs and describe their mechanisms of action.
- Enumerate first-line antitubercular drugs and detail their uses, adverse effects and contraindications.
- Enumerate drugs for MDR-TB and XDR-TB.
- Describe the mechanisms of action, indications, adverse effects, and contraindications of the drugs used in MDR-TB and XDR-TB.
- Describe steps in the management of ADRs of antitubercular drugs.
- Describe the management of TB in pregnancy and lactation.
- Describe the management of drug-sensitive and drug-resistant TB as per national guidelines.
- Enumerate conditions where chemoprophylaxis with antitubercular drugs is indicated.

Antileprotic drugs
- Differentiate between multibacillary and paucibacillary leprosy (MBL and PBL).
- Classify antileprotic drugs and explain their mechanisms, indications, adverse effects, and contraindications.
- Describe lepra reactions and their management.
- Describe multiple drug therapy (MDT) as per the National Leprosy Eradication Programme (NLEP).

TUBERCULOSIS

Tuberculosis, caused by *Mycobacterium tuberculosis*, is a major public health concern in developing countries. There are many challenges associated with TB treatment, including the emergence of multidrug-resistant strains and increased risk of *Mycobacterium avium* complex (MAC) infection in HIV-positive patients. Based on the responsiveness to first-line drugs, tuberculosis can be of the following types:

- *Mycobacterium tuberculosis* sensitive to high-efficacy, low-toxicity drugs cause **drug- susceptible TB (DS-TB)**.
- **Drug-resistant tuberculosis (DR-TB)** occurs when *Mycobacterium tuberculosis* becomes resistant to one or more anti-TB drugs.

The different types of drug-resistant TB include:

i. **Mono-drug resistant TB**, where the organisms are resistant to one drug out of the first-line drugs, e.g.,
   - resistance to **isoniazid (INH)** alone (called **'H-mono' resistance TB**)
ii. **Rifampicin-resistant TB (RR-TB):** Resistance to rifampicin, with or without resistance to other drugs. Rifampicin resistance is a key indicator of more complex resistance patterns and is often associated with multidrug resistance.
iii. **Multidrug-resistant TB (MDR-TB):** Resistance to both isoniazid (INH) and rifampicin (R), with or without resistance to other first-line drugs. MDR-TB is more difficult to treat than drug-susceptible TB and requires second-line medications.
iv. **Poly-drug resistant TB (Poly DR-TB):** Resistance to more than one first-line drug (other than both INH and R), e.g., resistance to isoniazid and ethambutol, but not rifampicin.
v. **Pre-extensively drug-resistant TB (Pre-XDR TB):** MDR-TB with additional resistance to fluoroquinolones but without resistance to second-line injectable drugs. In terms of severity, this is closer to XDR-TB.
vi. **Extensively drug-resistant TB (XDR-TB):** MDR-TB with additional resistance to more than 3 out of 6 classes of antitubercular drugs. XDR-TB is more difficult to treat due to limited drug options.

Each form of drug-resistant TB requires specialised treatment regimens, longer treatment durations, and close monitoring to prevent further resistance development.

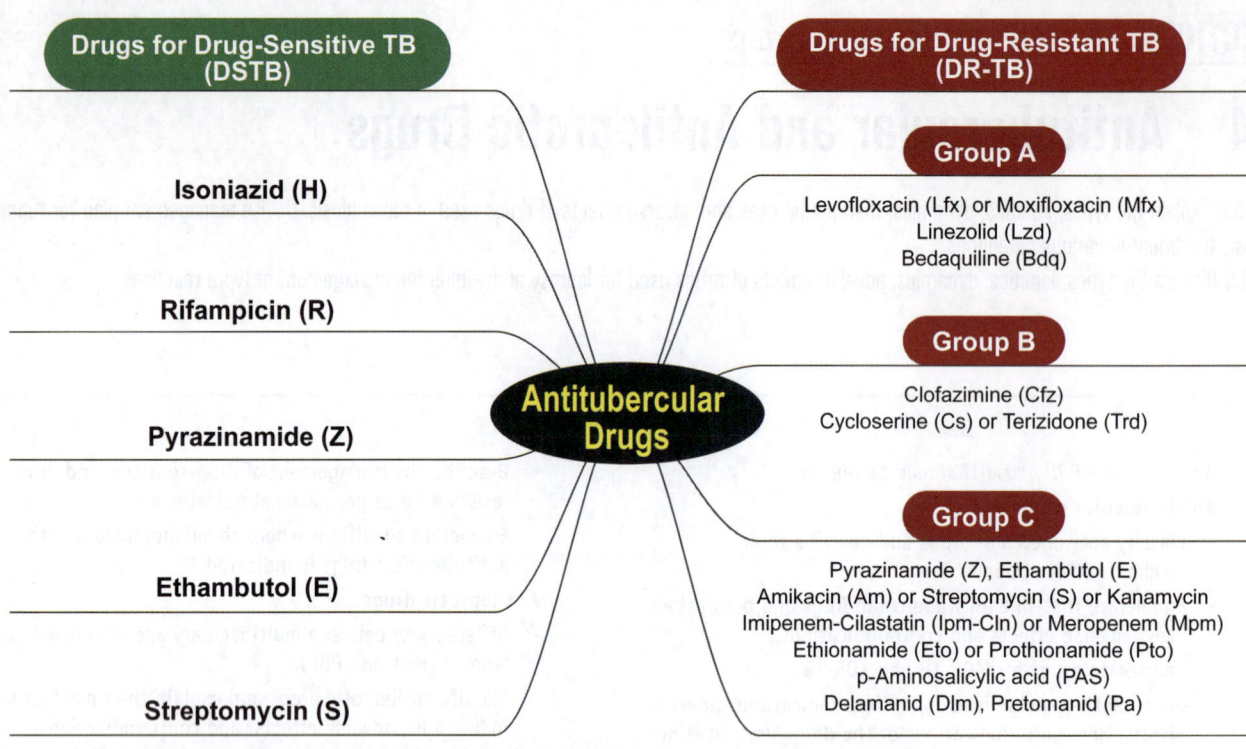

Flowchart 54.1 Classification of antitubercular drugs

ANTITUBERCULAR DRUGS

Classification

Drugs are classified based on whether they are used against drug-sensitive TB (DS-TB) or drug-resistant TB (DR-TB).

Drugs for DS-TB: These drugs have high efficacy and low toxicity and include isoniazid, rifampicin, pyrazinamide, ethambutol and streptomycin.

Drugs for DR-TB: These drugs are categorised into three groups—A, B, and C—based on their drug class, efficacy, and certainty of clinical evidence on effectiveness and safety in longer oral regimens for MDR-TB and XDR-TB (Flowchart 54.1).

DRUGS FOR DS-TB

1. ISONIAZID (INH)

Isoniazid or isonicotinic acid hydrazide (INH) is a high-efficacy tuberculocidal drug. It is represented by letter H in TB treatment regimens.

Mechanism of action

The antitubercular action of INH (Fig. 54.1) involves the inhibition of mycolic acid synthesis and DNA synthesis to exert tuberculocidal effect.

1. INH is a prodrug. After entering the sensitive mycobacterium, it gets converted into a **reactive metabolite INH*** by the action of the enzyme **catalase–peroxidase (KatG)**. [* Indicates active form.]
2. The reactive metabolite **INH* forms adducts with NAD as well as NADP**.

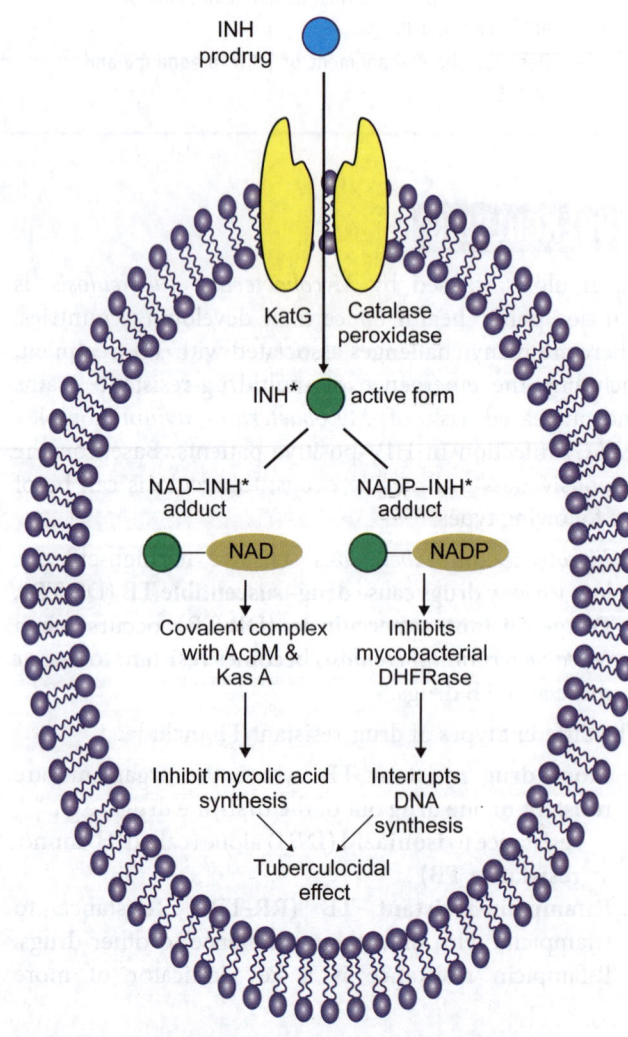

Fig. 54.1 Mechanism of action of isoniazid (INH)

3. The NAD–INH* adduct forms a covalent complex with acyl carrier protein reductase (AcpM) and β-ketoacyl carrier protein synthetase (KasA) and **interferes with mycolic acid synthesis.**
4. The NADP–INH* adduct inhibits mycobacterial dihydrofolate reductase (DHFRase), disrupting DNA synthesis.
5. Both the actions (3, 4 mentioned above) contribute to the tuberculocidal effect of INH.

Mechanism of resistance

The level of **primary resistance** to INH varies across populations, depending on its usage in a given area. On an average, approximately one in 10^6 *Mycobacterium tuberculosis* organisms exhibits resistance to INH.

Acquired resistance to INH can develop by the following mechanisms (Fig. 54.2).

1. The gene coding for catalase–peroxidase enzyme is *katG*. **Mutation of the gene *katG* results in failure to form the reactive metabolite INH*.** This confers a **high level of resistance** to isoniazid, which necessitates the use of alternative drugs. However, there is no cross-resistance with other drugs due to this mutation.
2. The gene coding for acyl carrier protein is *inhA*. Mutation of gene *inhA* causes low level of resistance to isoniazid, which can be overcome by increasing its dose. Cross-resistance with ethionamide can occur due to such a mutation, because ethionamide also has the same mechanism of action as isoniazid.
3. **Increased efflux of isoniazid from the bacterial cell** may also contribute to INH resistance.

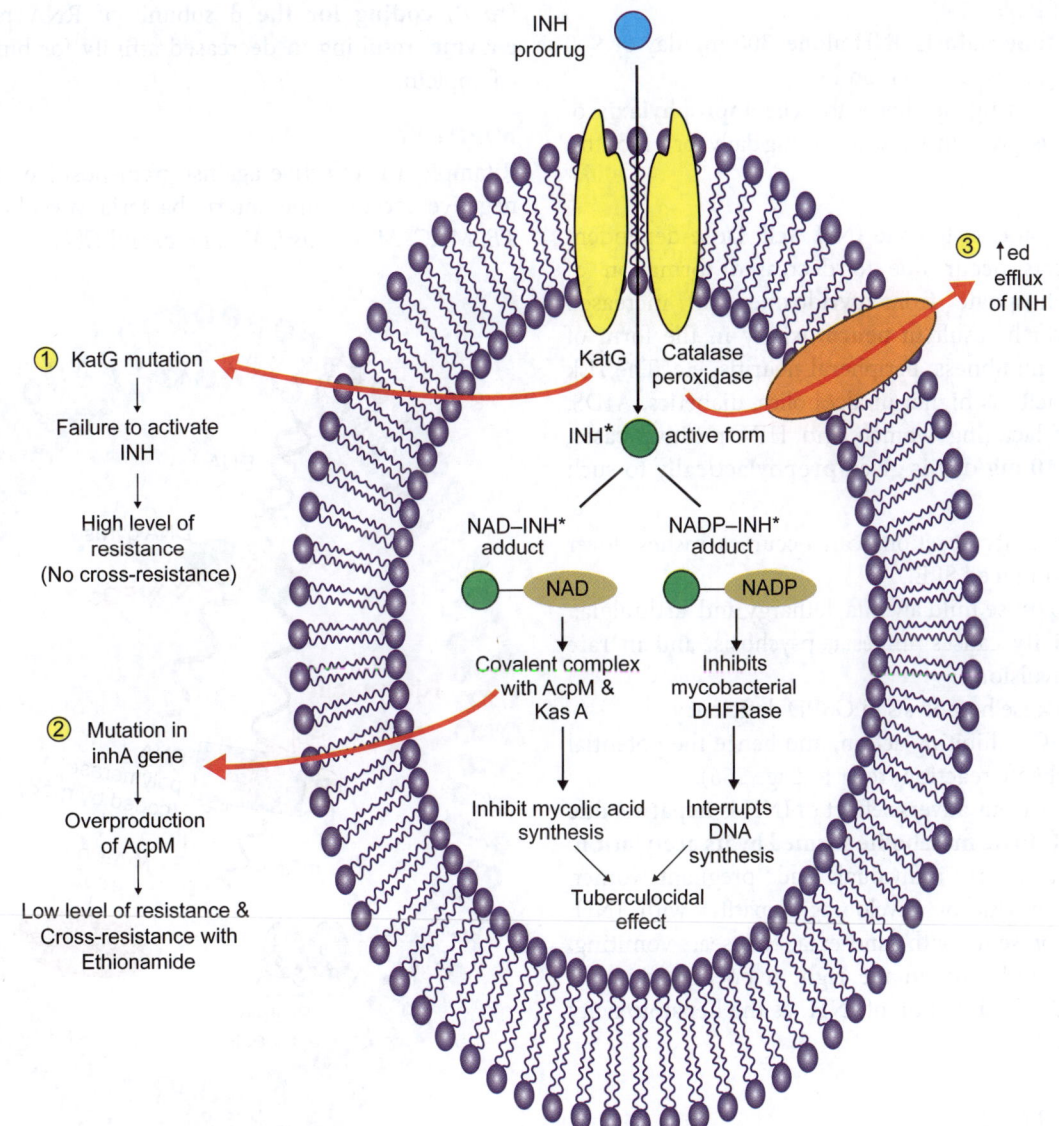

Fig. 54.2 Mechanism of resistance to INH

Pharmacokinetics

INH is **rapidly and completely absorbed** after oral administration. It can **diffuse to reach all body fluids, caseous material in tubercular cavities and meninges.**

Metabolism occurs in the liver through N-acetylation, with the inactivation rate influenced by genetic variations. These differences affect the drug's half-life, resulting in **fast** and **slow acetylators.** The efficacy of the drug decreases in fast acetylators, who are also at greater risk of INH-induced hepatotoxicity due to increased formation of a hepatotoxic metabolite. In contrast, slow acetylators have a higher risk of developing peripheral neuritis.

Therapeutic uses and doses

- For the **treatment of TB,** INH is always combined with other antitubercular drugs. Its dose is 5–10 mg per kg body weight /day. The usual adult dose is 300–600 mg/day in DS-TB, whereas in MDR/RR-TB the dose of INH is higher (Table 54.4).
- In **latent tuberculosis**, INH alone, 300 mg/day or 900 mg weekly, is used for 9 months.
- INH is the drug of choice for **chemoprophylaxis** of tuberculosis, given in a dose of 300 mg daily for 6 months.

ADRs

Most of the patients tolerate INH well. Dose-dependent adverse effects occur due to decreased formation of pyridoxal phosphate from pyridoxine and increased excretion, which result in **neurotoxicity** in the form of paresthesias, numbness, peripheral neuritis, etc. The risk of neurotoxicity is higher in alcoholics, diabetics, AIDS, pregnant or lactating women and HIV positive cases. **Pyridoxine 10 mg/day is given prophylactically** to such patients.

- Hypersensitivity reactions can occur as rashes, fever and drug-induced SLE.
- It can also cause mild anemia, lethargy and arthralgia.
- **CNS toxicity** causes amnesia, psychosis, and in rare cases, convulsions.
- INH can cause hemolysis in G6PD deficiency.
- It has MAO-inhibiting action, and hence the potential to cause cheese reaction (refer to page 266).
- The most serious adverse effect of INH is **hepatitis due to a hepatotoxic metabolite formed by its acetylation.** Alcoholics, elderly individuals and pregnant women are at high risk of developing hepatitis with INH. Patients present with anorexia, nausea, vomiting, jaundice and pain in the right hypochondrium. It requires discontinuation of INH, as the hepatotoxicity could be fatal.

2. RIFAMYCIN (R)

This is a group of drugs that include Rifampicin (represented as R), Rifabutin (Rfb) and Rifapentine (Rpt).

a. Rifampicin (R)

Under the National TB Elimination **Programme (NTEP)**, formerly RNTCP (Revised National TB Control Programme), Rifampicin (R) is one of the **first-line drugs** for the treatment of drug-sensitive tuberculosis (**DS-TB**), similar to isoniazid (H). **Rifabutin (Rfb)** and **Rifapentine (Rpt)** are supplementary first-line drugs.

Mechanism of action and resistance

Rifampicin binds to the β subunit of DNA-dependent RNA polymerase enzyme, resulting in the **inhibition of RNA synthesis** (Fig. 54.3) and bactericidal effect on mycobacteria. It is effective against both intracellular and extracellular organisms. It can penetrate most of the tissues and kill organisms sequestered in cavities and abscesses. Rifampicin has no affinity for human RNA polymerase. Therefore, human RNA synthesis is not affected.

Resistance occurs because of **point mutation in gene (*rpoB*) coding for the β subunit of RNA polymerase enzyme,** resulting in decreased affinity for binding with rifampicin.

Spectrum

Rifampicin is effective against gram-positive and gram-negative cocci, some enteric bacteria, mycobacteria (*M. TB*, MAC, *M. kansasii*, *M. leprae*) and *Chlamydiae*.

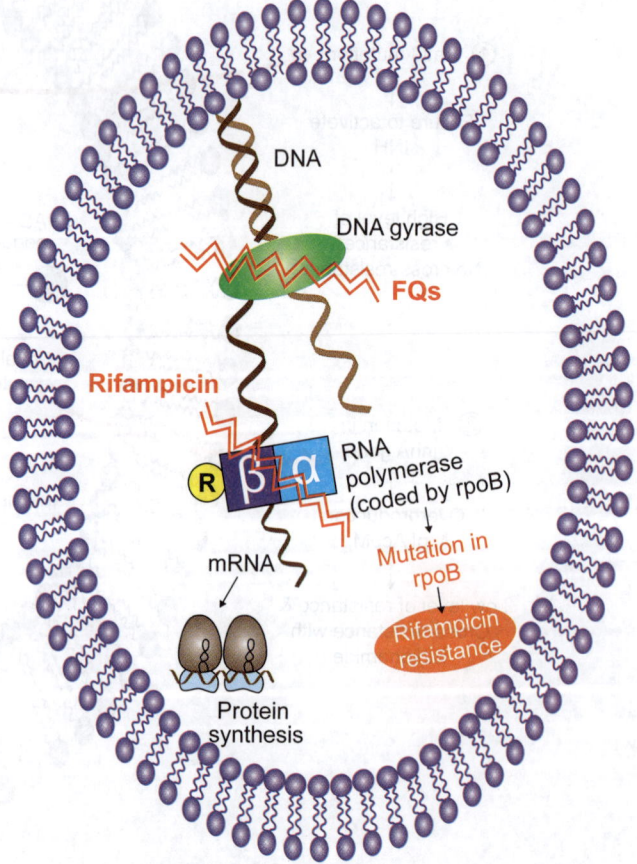

Fig. 54.3 Mechanism of action and resistance to rifampicin and FQs

Pharmacokinetics

Rifampicin is **well absorbed** orally and is **widely distributed** in body fluids and tissues. It penetrates abscesses and tubercular cavities; it kills intracellular organisms as well. It is metabolised in the liver, excreted in bile, and **undergoes enterohepatic circulation.** Excretion occurs in feces. Some part is excreted in urine as well.

Rifampicin is an **enzyme inducer** that accelerates the metabolism of several co-administered drugs, including warfarin, anticonvulsants, contraceptives, and non-nucleoside reverse transcriptase inhibitors (NNRTIs). This increased drug metabolism can lead to significant drug–drug interactions (DDIs).

Therapeutic uses

- It is used **in the treatment of TB** as one of the first-line drugs in combination with other antitubercular drugs. The dose is 10 mg/kg/day or 600 mg/day.
- In **latent tuberculosis**, it can be used in a dose of 600 mg/day for 4 months, as an alternative to INH in patients with INH resistance or adverse effects.
- It is used as a **prophylactic agent in meningococcal and, staphylococcal carriers and close contacts of *H. influenza* type B** patients.
- In **brucellosis**, rifampicin is used in combination with doxycycline.
- It is also useful in **leprosy** as a part of multi-drug-treatment (MDT).

ADRs

Generally, the drug is well tolerated, especially when used in daily regimens. Adverse effects of rifampicin are seen **more with intermittent regimens**. They include:

- Nausea, vomiting, abdominal cramps
- Rashes, thrombocytopenia, nephritis
- Redness and watering of eyes
- Fever, chills, headache, generalised malaise, etc.
- Major adverse effects are **hepatitis and cholestatic jaundice.** The risk is more in patients with chronic liver disease, in alcoholics, and the elderly. Incidence of hepatic dysfunction is more when rifampicin is combined with isoniazid (H) and pyrazinamide (Z).
- Rifampicin gives an **orange-red colour to urine, sweat and tears** (it may cause orange staining of contact lenses)**,** but this is harmless.

b. Rifabutin

Rifabutin has the same mechanism of action and adverse effects as rifampicin. It has cross-resistance with rifampicin. However, rifabutin has **less enzyme-inducing potential** than rifampicin and is **preferred in HIV-positive patients receiving protease inhibitors or NNRTIs**. It is also useful in MAC infection in AIDS patients. It can cause pigmentation of skin, uveitis and neutropenia as adverse effects.

c. Rifapentine

It has the same mechanism of action, adverse reactions and enzyme-inducing potential as rifampicin. There is complete cross-resistance, but it has **longer half-life** than rifampicin. It is used **in latent TB along with isoniazid (H) in once-a-week-dose regimen**. It may be used in the continuation phase of TB treatment.

3. PYRAZINAMIDE (Z)

Pyrazinamide (Z) is also a high-efficacy, first-line antitubercular drug.

Mechanism of action

Pyrazinamide is taken up by macrophages and is converted by mycobacterial pyrazinamidase enzyme (encoded by *pncA* gene) to pyrazinoic acid (Fig. 54.4). Pyrazinoic acid inhibits fatty acid synthase-I and **interferes with mycobacterial cell membrane metabolism and function,** resulting in tuberculocidal action (weaker than INH).

Pyrazinamide remains inactive at neutral pH but becomes **active in an acidic environment, particularly at a pH of 5.5**. This unique property allows it to exert its maximum effect on intracellular *Mycobacterium tuberculosis* residing within the acidic compartments of lysosomes and at inflammatory sites. By targeting these persistent bacteria, pyrazinamide plays a crucial role in **sterilising lesions** and **reducing the risk of relapse**.

Resistance to pyrazinamide develops readily due to

- impaired uptake or
- reduced conversion into active form due to *pncA* mutations

However, there is **no cross-resistance to other first-line anti-TB drugs** such as **isoniazid (H) or rifampicin (R)**.

Therapeutic uses

Pyrazinamide is mainly used as one of the first-line drugs in the **intensive phase of DS-TB** in combination with isoniazid, rifampicin and ethambutol in a dose of 25–35 mg/kg/day. Average daily dose depends on the body weight-band, ranging from 750–2000 mg.

Pyrazinamide is also used in **H-Mono (isoniazid mono-resistant)-TB/poly-DR-TB, MDR/RR-TB in shorter Bdq- or injectable-containing regimens.**

Adverse effects

The major ADR is **hepatotoxicity, which is dose-related**. Pyrazinamide appears to be better tolerated in Indian patients compared to their western counterparts. Nausea, vomiting, fever, rashes, arthralgia, the **hyperuricemia**

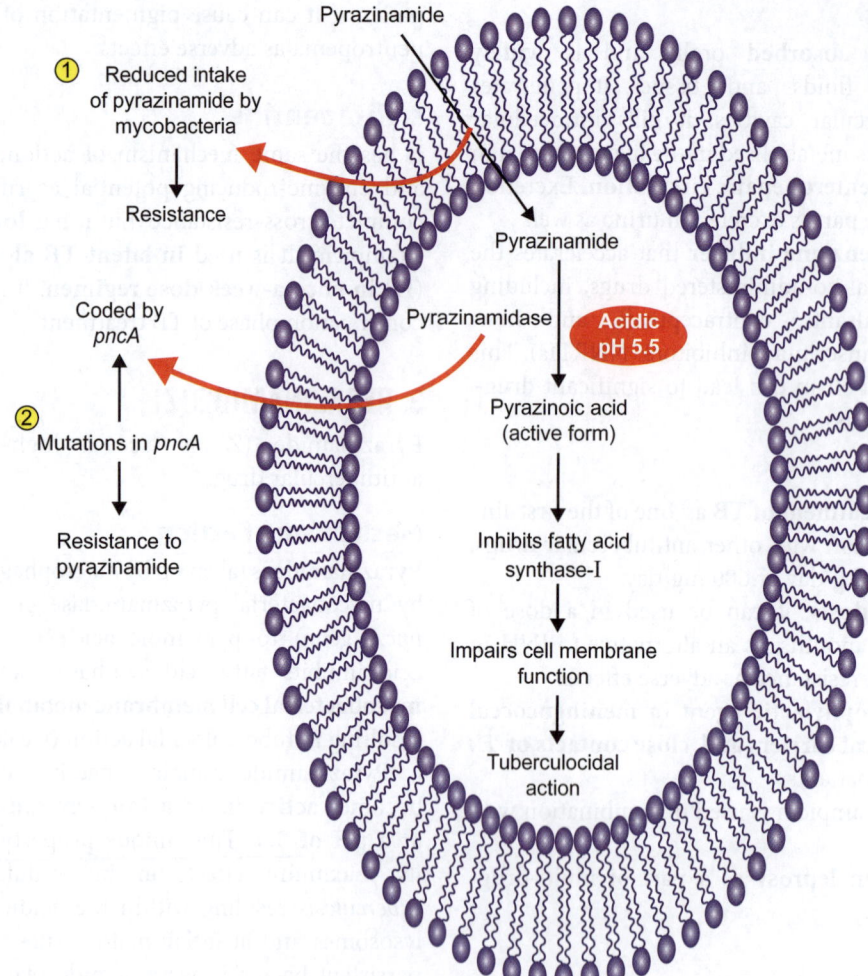

Fig. 54.4 Mechanism of action and resistance to pyrazinamide

are other adverse effects. Hyperuricemia, usually asymptomatic, may precipitate gout; however, the drug should not be stopped if hyperuricemia occurs. It is contraindicated in liver disease but is safe during pregnancy.

4. ETHAMBUTOL (E)

Ethambutol is a **tuberculostatic** drug effective against **mycobacterium TB** and **MAC**.

Mechanism of action

Arabinosyl transferase plays a crucial role in polymerising arabinose into arabinan, which then forms arabinogalactan, an essential component of the mycobacterial cell wall. Ethambutol inhibits arabinosyl transferase, blocking arabinose polymerisation and arabinogalactan synthesis, thereby **disrupting mycolic acid incorporation into the cell wall** of mycobacteria (Fig. 54.5). The gene coding for arabinosyl transferase is *embCAB*. Mutations of the *embCAB* gene causes overproduction of arabinosyl transferase, resulting in the development of resistance to ethambutol.

Therapeutic uses

- Ethambutol is used along with other first-line drugs **in initial** as well as **continuation phase of treatment of DS-TB** in a dose of 15–25 mg/kg/day.
- Like pyrazinamide, ethambutol is also used in H-mono/poly DR-TB, MDR/RR-TB in shorter Bdq- or injectable-containing regimens. The dose depends on the body weight band.

ADRs

It is well tolerated. Important adverse effects are dose-related **retrobulbar optic neuritis**, loss of the ability to distinguish between red and green colours, and decrease in visual acuity. It decreases excretion of uric acid, and hence, it should **used with caution in patients of gout**.

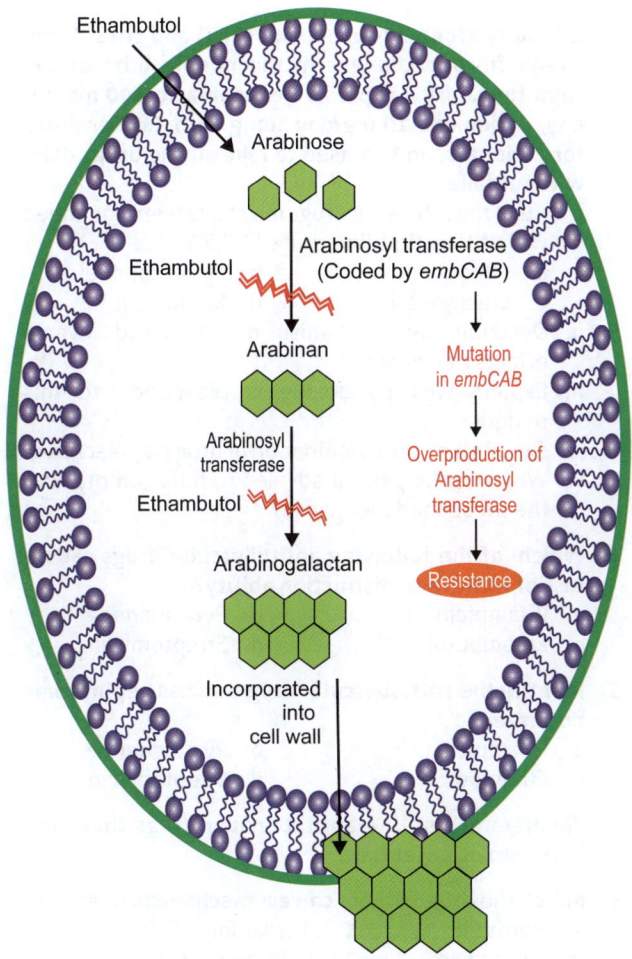

Fig. 54.5 *Mechanism of action and resistance to ethambutol*

5. STREPTOMYCIN

Streptomycin is an aminoglycoside that acts by binding to 30S ribosomal subunit. It **prevents initiation of protein synthesis and polysome formation, and distorts mRNA codon leading to misreading of mRNA** (Fig. 54.6). Secondary changes in cell membrane integrity result **in bactericidal activity**.

Streptomycin is less effective than isoniazid and rifampicin. Being polar in nature, streptomycin has poor penetration into cells. Thus, **it kills only the extracellular bacilli**. It does not cross the blood–brain barrier but can reach tubercular cavities. It is not widely used because of its potential to cause **ototoxicity, nephrotoxicity and neuro-muscular blockade**. Other drawbacks are rapid development of resistance and the **need for IM injection**. Previously, it was considered a **supplementary first-line drug** and was used only during the first two months of the intensive phase in previously treated cases of tuberculosis, with other first-line drugs as a reserve alternative.

REGIMEN FOR DRUG-SENSITIVE TB CASES

In the **intensive phase (IP)** of 8 weeks (2 months) duration, four drugs are used (Table 54.1), whereas in the **continuation phase (CP)** of 16 weeks (4 months) duration, fixed-drug combination of three drugs (HRE) is given. The continuation phase, however, can be extended to 12–24 weeks in certain forms of TB, such as skeletal TB and disseminated TB, as decided by the treating physician.

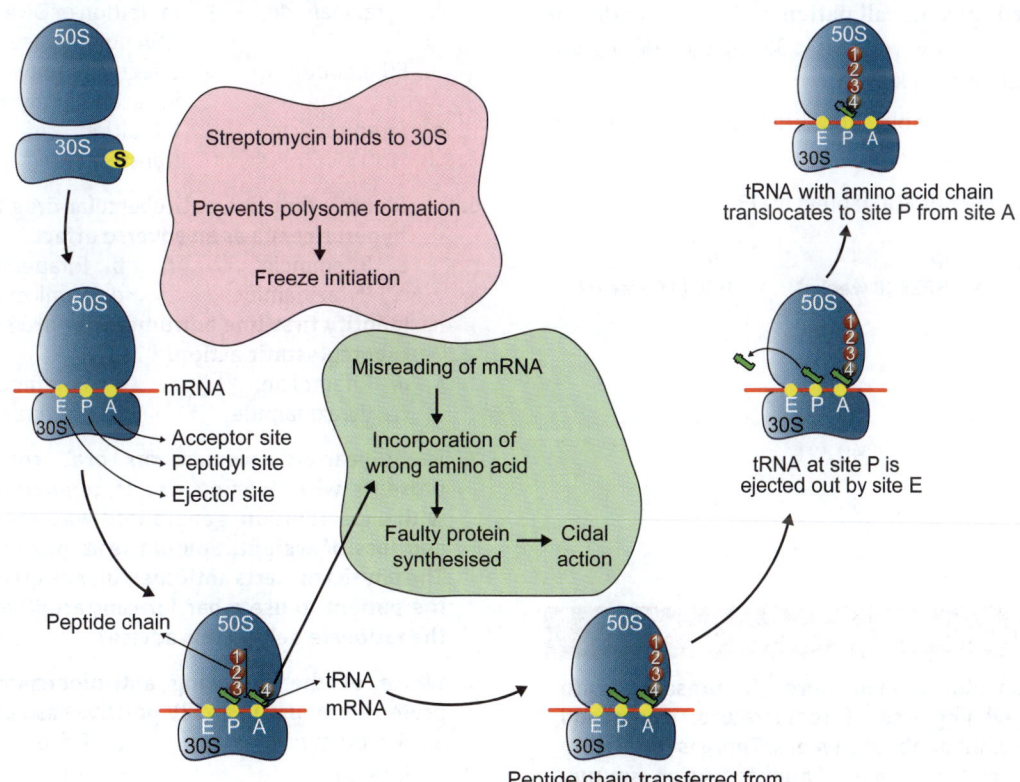

Fig. 54.6 *Mechanism of action of streptomycin*

Table 54.1 Regimen for DS-TB

Intensive Phase (IP; 2 months or 8 weeks)		
Drug	Dose per kg per day	Average daily adult dose
Isoniazid (H)	5–10 mg	300–600 mg
Rifampicin (R)	10 mg/kg	600 mg
Pyrazinamide (Z)	25–35 mg	2000 mg
Ethambutol (E)	15–25 mg/kg	1500 mg
Continuation Phase (CP; 4 months or 16 weeks)		
Isoniazid (H)		
Rifampicin (R)	Dose as in IP	Dose as in IP
Ethambutol (E)		

FDC TABLETS

Under RNTCP and NTEP, separate **FDC tablets** are available for IP and CP for simplification of the treatment regimen. Each tablet contains:

- **For intensive phase:** Isoniazid 75 mg; Rifampicin 150 mg; Pyrazinamide 400 mg; Ethambutol 275 mg
- **For continuation phase:** Only isoniazid, rifampicin and ethambutol combination with same amount as in intensive phase. Pyrazinamide is not added in this tablet.
- **Pyridoxine is given to all patients.** Dose of pyridoxine is 50 mg/day if body weight is < 30 kg, and 100 mg/day for body weight > 30 kg.

The number of FDC tablets for different weight-bands is shown in Table 54.2.

Table 54.2 Number of FDC tablets in DS-TB

Body weight in kg	IP HRZE (8 weeks)	CP HRE (16 weeks)
25–34	2	2
35–49	3	3
50–64	4	4
65–75	5	5
>75	6	6

Clinical problem-based questions and MCQs

1. A 42-year-old woman, Mrs X, presents with fatigue, evening rise of temperature, cough and expectoration for about 2 weeks. There is no history of such symptoms in past. On investigation, sputum is positive for acid-fast bacilli (AFB) and chest X-ray shows fibrotic changes in the middle lobe of the right lung. Mrs X is prescribed isoniazid 300 mg per day, pyridoxine 10 mg/day along with 3 other drugs for 2 months, and advised to take all the drugs daily without fail.
   i. All of the following drugs may have been combined with INH as first-line drugs EXCEPT
      a. Ethionamide b. Pyrazinamide
      c. Ethambutol   d. Rifampicin
   ii. Describe the mechanism of action and adverse effects of isoniazid.
   iii. Explain why pyridoxine is prescribed to this patient.
   iv. Explain why the combination of drugs is prescribed.
   v. Why was the patient advised to fully comply with the prescribed medicines?

2. Which of the following antitubercular drugs causes loss of red–green distinction ability?
   a. Rifampicin   b. Pyrazinamide
   c. Ethambutol   d. Streptomycin

3. Identify the antitubercular drug that has nephrotoxic potential.
   a. Rifampicin   b. Pyrazinamide
   c. Ethambutol   d. Streptomycin

4. Enumerate first-line antitubercular drugs that have hepatotoxic potential.

5. Match the drug with its correct mechanism of action.
   a. Isoniazid   1. Misreading mRNA
   b. Rifampicin   2. Inhibition of mycolic acid synthesis
   c. Pyrazinamide   3. Inhibition of DNA dependent RNA polymerase
   d. Ethambutol   4. Effect only against intracellular mycobacteria
   e. Streptomycin   5. Inhibition of arabinosyl transferase

6. i. Identify first-line antitubercular drug that causes hyperuricemia as an adverse effect.
      a. Rifampicin   b. Rifapentine
      c. Pyrazinamide d. Isoniazid
   ii. Identify first-line antitubercular drug that exerts tuberculostatic action.
      a. Rifampicin   b. Ethambutol
      c. Pyrazinamide d. Isoniazid

7. A 34-year-old woman on oral contraceptives presents with evening rise in temperature, cough with expectoration, generalised weakness, anorexia and loss of weight. Sputum tests positive for AFB. The physician starts antitubercular drugs and advises the patient to use a barrier contraceptive. Describe the rationale behind this advice?

8. Which of the following anti-tubercular drugs is preferred for use in an HIV positive case and why?
   a. Streptomycin   b. Rifapentine
   c. Rifabutin   d. Ethionamide

CONCEPT MAP – DRUGS FOR DS-TB

Isoniazid or INH (H)

Mechanism: Activated by catalase–peroxidase, forms adducts with NAD → inhibits AcpM and KasA → interferes with mycolic acid synthesis → tuberculocidal effect.

INH*-NADP adduct → inhibits mycobacterial DHFRase → inhibit DNA synthesis.

Resistance: Mutation of gene *KatG* → failure to form reactive metabolite → high level of resistance, no cross-resistance.

Mutation in gene inhA → overproduction of acyl carrier protein reductase → low level of resistance & cross-resistance to ethionamide.

Uses: Treatment of DS-TB, RR-TB, chemoprophylaxis, latent tuberculosis.

Dose: 5–10 mg/kg/d or 300–600 mg/day.

ADRs: Neurotoxicity → paresthesias, numbness, peripheral neuritis. Risk is more in alcoholics, diabetics, AIDS, pregnancy & lactation. Pyridoxine 50–100 mg/d combined prophylactically.

Risk of hepatitis due to a hepatotoxic metabolite formed by its acetylation, especially in alcoholics, elderly individuals and pregnant women

Hypersensitivity reactions, amnesia, psychosis, anemia, hemolysis in G6PD deficiency.

Rifampicin (R)

Mechanism: Inhibits DNA-dependent RNA polymerase by binding to its β subunit → inhibits mRNA & protein synthesis → tuberculocidal action.

Resistance: Mutation in *rpoB* gene coding for mycobacterial RNA polymerase.

Uses: Treatment of DSTB, as alternative to INH in latent TB. Dose 10 mg/kg or 600 mg.

Other uses are leprosy, as a prophylactic agent in meningococcal/staphylococcal carries & close contact with *H. influenza* patients, used with doxycycline in brucellosis.

ADRs: Nausea, vomiting, abdominal cramps, rashes, thrombocytopenia, nephritis, redness & watering of eyes, fever, chills, headache, generalised malaise, orange-red discolouration of secretions. Risk of hepatitis & cholestatic jaundice is more when combined with INH and pyrazinamide.

Interactions due to enzyme induction can cause contraceptive failure.

Pyrazinamide (Z)

Mechanism: Converted by mycobacterial pyrazinamidase enzyme to pyrazinoic acid → inhibits fatty acid synthase I → interferes with mycobacterial cell membrane metabolism & function → tuberculocidal action.

Resistance: Due to mutation in *pncA* gene coding for pyrazinamidase.

Uses: Only indication for use is tuberculosis. Mainly used in intensive phase of DS-TB, MDR/R R-TB short Bdq/injectable-containing regimens. Dose: 25–35 mg/kg/day.

ADRs: Dose-related hepatotoxicity, nausea, vomiting, fever, rashes, arthralgia, hyperuricemia. Safe in pregnancy.

Ethambutol (E)

Mechanism: Inhibits arabinosyl transferase → inhibits polymerisation of arabinose → interferes with incorporation of mycolic acid into cell wall of mycobacteria → tuberculostatic action.

Resistance: Mutations of *embCAB* gene → overproduction of arabinosyl transferase.

Uses: In initial phase of treatment of DS-TB, MDR/RR-TB short Bdq/injectable-containing regimens in a dose of 15–25 mg/kg/day.

ADRs: Dose-related retrobulbar optic neuritis, loss of ability for red-green colour distinction, decrease in visual acuity, decreased excretion of uric acid.

DS-TB

Streptomycin (S)

Mechanism: Binds to 30S ribosomal subunit → prevents polysome formation, freeze initiation of protein synthesis, misreading of mRNA → faulty amino acid incorporation→ secondary changes in cell membrane integrity → bactericidal activity.

Uses: Used only for first two months of intensive phase in previously treated cases of DS-TB.

Limitations: Polar nature → poor penetration into cells → kills only the extracellular bacilli, does not cross blood-brain barrier but can reach tubercular cavities, and the need for IM injection.

Potential to cause ototoxicity, nephrotoxicity and neuromuscular blockade.

NTEP Regimen for DSTB (New case)		
Body-weight bands	No. of tablets IP HRZE (8 weeks)	No. of tablets CP HRE (16 weeks)
25–34 kg	2	2
35–49 kg	3	3
50–64 kg	4	4
65–75 kg	5	5
>70 kg	6	6

Each tablet contains :
Isoniazid   75 mg
Rifampicin   150 mg
Pyrazinamide   400 mg
Ethambutol   275 mg

* Indicates active form.

DRUGS FOR DR-TB

Drugs for DRTB are divided into three groups (A, B, and C; see Flowchart 54.1). Group A includes levofloxacin (Lfx), moxifloxacin (Mfx), linezolid (Lzd) and bedaquiline (Bdq). [Mnemonic: LLB, for the first letters of the drug names]

GROUP A

1. Levofloxacin (Lfx) and Moxifloxacin (Mfx)

These are fluoroquinolones, having bactericidal action on *M. tuberculosis*. Moxifloxacin is more active against *M. tuberculosis* than levofloxacin. They are also active against Mycobacterium avium complex (MAC) and *M. fortuitum*.

Mechanism of action

FQs act by **inhibiting DNA gyrase** enzyme (refer to Fig. 52.2). Resistance develops due to mutation of DNA gyrase gene, albeit slowly. FQs can penetrate cells and kill intracellular mycobacteria in macrophages. The main **indication for use is multidrug-resistant tuberculosis**.

Under NTEP, levofloxacin is used in both shorter, longer and oral Bdq-containing regimens. The dose varies from 250 to 1000 mg, based on the weight band. In BPaLM and injectables-containing regimens, moxifloxacin (200–400 mg) is used.

ADRs

These are usually mild, such as
- Anorexia, nausea, vomiting, bad taste
- Headache, dizziness, anxiety, insomnia, restlessness
- Hypersensitivity reactions like rash, itching, urticaria.
- Risk of damage to tendons in patient above 60 years of age or those receiving corticosteroids
- Cartilage damage may occur in children
- Not safe during pregnancy
- Moxifloxacin can cause QT prolongation, increasing the risk of cardiac arrhythmias.

2. Bedaquiline (Bdq)
Mechanism of action

Bedaquiline is a diarylquinoline which inhibits mycobacterial ATP synthase, reducing energy production. It can kill *M. tuberculosis*, *M. leprae* and other non-tubercular mycobacteria. It is effective against both rapidly- multiplying as well as dormant bacilli. Human ATP synthase, however, has very low affinity for Bdq. Resistance to Bdq develops due to genetic mutations, which reduce the affinity of the mycobacterial enzyme for the drug. Increased efflux of drug from mycobacterium cell may also cause resistance. Bedaquiline (Bdq) does not exhibit cross-resistance with other anti-TB drugs.

Pharmacokinetics

Bdq is slowly absorbed and has a prolonged terminal elimination half-life. Bdq persists in the body for > 5 months after stopping its administration. Therefore, other drugs must be continued for the total duration of regimen (24 months) to ensure that surviving bacilli do not get exposed to Bdq alone, as this may favour development of resistance to Bdq.

Therapeutic uses

In NTEP, Bdq is used in shorter as well as longer oral regimens for the management of MDR/RR-TB and XDR-TB in adults. It is administered with meals as 400 mg/day for 2 weeks and then 200 mg 3 times a week for 22 weeks. It is **not continued beyond 24th week.** Other drugs are continued for total 24 months to ensure that surviving bacilli are not exposed to Bdq alone.

In pediatric patients (5–18 years of age) Bdq can be used, if needed, in consultation with a pediatrician. It is not used in patients who weigh less than 15 kg.

ADRs

These include headache, arthralgia, nausea, QTc prolongation and potential to cause hepato-toxicity. Bdq is not to be used for extrapulmonary TB, DS-TB, non-tubercular mycobacterial infections, in pregnant women and patients with cardiac arrhythmias.

3. Linezolid (Lzd)

It is an oxazolidinone derivative.

Mechanism of action

Linezolid exerts bacteriostatic action by inhibiting protein synthesis. It binds to P site of 50S ribosomal sub-unit, distorting the tRNA binding site. Thus, it interferes with the initiation of protein synthesis (refer to Fig. 52.4).

Linezolid is active against many resistant cocci and bacilli, including methicillin-resistant *Staphylococcus aureus* (MRSA), vancomycin-resistant *Staphylococcus aureus* (VRSA), vancomycin-resistant enterococci (VRE), penicillin-resistant streptococci and pneumococci, *Mycobacterium tuberculosis*, *Corynebacterium diphtheriae*, *Bacteroides fragilis*, and *Clostridium* species. Linezolid, though primarily a bacteriostatic drug, may exert cidal action against *Bacteroides fragilis*, streptococci and pneumococci.

Therapeutic uses

In NTEP, linezolid is used in patients suffering from severe MDR-TB, complicated extrapulmonary TB and INH-resistant cases with double gene mutation. Such patients need longer Bdq-containing regimens of 18–20 months. The dose of linezolid varies from 300–600 mg based on the weight band.

Other uses are in complicated skin and soft tissue wound infections, serious hospital acquired pneumonias, febrile neutropenia and other infections caused by drug-resistant gram-positive bacteria. Linezolid is not effective against gram-negative bacteria.

ADRs
Linezolid may cause nausea, abdominal pain, diarrhea, and altered taste. Rarely, it can lead to rashes, itching, thrombocytopenia, anemia, or oral candidiasis. Due to its MAO-inhibiting activity, it poses a risk of interactions with drugs that enhance adrenergic or serotonergic activity.

GROUP B
This group includes three drugs: Cycloserine, Terizidone and Clofazimine [Mnemonic: CTC] (Flowchart 54.1)

1. Cycloserines
Cycloserine is an analogue of D-alanine, a key component of the bacterial cell wall. It exerts a tuberculostatic effect by inhibiting the enzymes L-alanine racemase (which catalyses the racemisation of L-alanine to D-alanine) and D-alanine ligase (which links two D-alanine residues), thereby inhibiting bacterial cell wall synthesis.

Spectrum: Cycloserine is effective against Gram-positive bacteria, *E.coli*, *Chlamydia*, *Mycobacterium tuberculosis* and MAC (mycobacterium avium complex).

Therapeutic uses
It is used only for treatment of **drug-resistant TB,** as it **has no cross- resistance with any other antitubercular drug.** Treatment is initiated with 250 mg BD, which can be increased to a maximum of 750 mg per day in patients weighing > 45 kg.

ADRs
Neuropsychiatric symptoms such as headache, sleepiness, tremors, seizures (rare), slurring of speech, frank psychosis and depression may occur. **Neurotoxicity** can be checked with pyridoxine 100 mg/day.

2. Terizidone (Trd)
Terizidone, composed of two cycloserine molecules, shares its mechanism of action and properties but is reportedly less neurotoxic. It achieves higher and more sustained urinary concentrations, making it a potential **alternative to cycloserine for genitourinary TB.**

3. Clofazimine (Cfz)
Clofazimine is a phenazine derivative that acts by interfering with DNA template function and electron transport chain in mitochondria. It also affects membrane permeability. It exhibits bacteriostatic activity against *M. tuberculosis*, *M. leprae* and atypical mycobacteria.

Therapeutic uses
Under NTEP, clofazimine is part of shorter/longer Bdq-containing regimens as well as injectables-containing regimen for MDR/RR-TB and XDR-TB in a dose 50–200 mg, based on the body weight band. Other uses are in **leprosy and *M. intracellulare*** infection in AIDS patients. It has anti-inflammatory action, and is hence useful in the management of **lepra reactions or ENL.**

ADRs
Red to brown or black discolouration of skin and gastrointestinal adverse effects can occur.

GROUP C
Drugs included in this group are pyrazinamide, ethambutol, injectable drugs such as streptomycin/amikacin/kanamycin (covered earlier), ethionamide or prothionamide, para-aminosalicylic acid (PAS), delamanid, imipenem–cilastatin or meropenem.

1. Ethionamide (Eto)
Ethionamide has **structural similarity to isoniazid** and has the same mechanism of action and resistance. It is activated by mycobacteria and disrupts mycolic acid synthesis and kills both intracellular and extracellular organisms. Low-level INH resistance due to *inhA* mutations, which affect acyl carrier protein (AcpM), leads to cross-resistance with ethionamide.

Therapeutic uses
In NTEP, ethionamide is included in shorter regimens for MDR/RR-TB. It is also used as a reserve drug for MAC infections in AIDS patients and certain leprosy cases. The dosage ranges from 375–1000 mg per day, depending on body weight.

ADRs
It is a **poorly-tolerated** drug. Adverse effects such as anorexia, nausea, vomiting, epigastric pain, metallic taste, and sulfurous belching are commonly reported. Generalised aches and pains and rashes may occur. Prolonged treatment needed in tuberculosis is associated with menstrual irregularities, impotence, goitre, peripheral neuropathy and behavioural changes. Neurotoxicity can be prevented by pyridoxine.

Prothionamide closely resembles ethionamide in chemical structure, mechanism of action, pharmacokinetics and resistance profile, and is used interchangeably with it, particularly in the treatment of MDR-TB and MAC infection.

2. Para-Aminosalicylic Acid (PAS)
It has same mechanism of action as sulphonamides, i.e., it **interferes with folate synthesis only in *Mycobacterium tuberculosis*** (refer to Fig. 52.1). It is **tuberculostatic** and one of the least active drugs. It does not add to efficacy but **only delays development of resistance.** It is a well-absorbed, well-distributed drug. However, it does not enter CSF. Metabolism is partially by acetylation. It can compete with and inhibit the metabolism of isoniazid so that half-life of INH gets prolonged.

It is included in longer regimens for MDR-TB only when the initial drugs need to be replaced due to resistance or adverse effects. The recommended dose is 200 mg/kg per day, administered in divided doses.

ADRs
PAS is a **poorly-tolerated** drug. Gastrointestinal adverse reactions like anorexia, nausea, and epigastric pain are frequent. Fever, rashes, malaise, blood dyscrasias may occur because of hypersensitivity. It may also cause liver and kidney dysfunction, goitre and hypokalemia.

3. Delamanid (Dlm)
It is a dihydro-nitro-imidazooxazole that acts by **inhibiting methoxy mycolic acid and keto mycolic acid** (components of mycobacterial cell wall). It is indicated **only in MDR-pulmonary TB in patients > 14 years of age**, together with other drugs in a dose of 100 mg BD for 6 months. It is effective in **XDR-TB also**.

Adverse effects include nausea, vomiting, dizziness, QT prolongation, and anxiety.

4. Pretomanid (Pa)
Pretomanid is approved for use in combination with bedaquiline and linezolid as part of the BPaLM regimen for MDR- and XDR-TB in patients over 14 years of age. The recommended dose is 200 mg once daily.

Mechanism of action
Its tuberculocidal action against actively replicating mycobacteria is exerted through inhibition of mycolic acid biosynthesis. It is a prodrug which gets activated by a deazaflavin-dependent nitroreductase enzyme (Ddn) to form a des-nitro derivative. This metabolite increases levels of nitric oxide (NO) and acts as a bacterial respiratory poison under anaerobic conditions. Such bactericidal activity against anaerobes shortens the duration of antibiotic treatment in anaerobic infections.

Kinetics
Pretomanid is orally absorbed, with its absorption enhanced when taken with high-calorie, high-fat meals. It exhibits plasma protein binding of 80–90%, undergoes partial metabolism, and is excreted in urine.

ADRs
It has the potential to cause QT prolongation, hepatotoxicity and myelosuppression.

> **Clinical problem-based questions and MCQs**
>
> 9. All of the following antitubercular drugs cause QT prolongation EXCEPT
>   a. Moxifloxacin   b. Bedaquiline
>   c. Delamanid   d. Terizidone
> 10. Which of the following shows cross-resistance with isoniazid – a first-line antitubercular drug?
>   a. Cycloserine   b. Bedaquiline
>   c. Ethionamide   d. Pyrazinamide
> 11. Which antitubercular drug causes neuropsychiatric adverse effects?
>   a. Cycloserine   b. Rifabutin
>   c. Ethambutol   d. Pyrazinamide
> 12. Prescribe for the patient Mrs X (described in question 1) who is a newly diagnosed case of TB as per NTEP guidelines.

MANAGEMENT OF DR-TB

Individualised regimens are sometimes required depending on the results of drug sensitivity tests and adverse effects/contraindications to particular drugs in some cases or in the presence of other patient factors such as pregnancy, HIV positive status, and hepatic/renal impairment, as indicated below.

1. INH Only (H-mono)/Polydrug-resistant TB
When resistance to isoniazid (INH) is detected, it often serves as a surrogate marker for resistance to multiple first-line drugs except rifampicin (R). Under NTEP, the treatment regimen for such patients is for 6–9 months, with no specified intensive or continuation phase. As the bacilli are sensitive to rifampicin, patients receive rifampicin (R), pyrazinamide (Z) and ethambutol (E), along with levofloxacin (Lfx). **Dose of the drugs** depends on the patient's body weight as shown in Table 54.3.

Table 54.3 Drugs regimen for H-mono/Polydrug-resistant TB

Weight band (kg)	Drug dose			
	Rifampicin (R)	Pyrazinamide (Z)	Ethambutol (E)	Levofloxacin (Lfx)
16–29	300 g	750 mg	400 mg	250 mg
30–45	450 mg	1250 mg	800 mg	750 mg
46–70	600 mg	1750 mg	1200 mg	1000 mg
> 70	750 mg	2000 mg	1600 mg	1000 mg

[Mnemonic: **P**ig **R**unning on **ZE**bra **L**ines, i.e **P**olydrug-resistant cases: rifampicin (**R**), pyrazinamide (**Z**), ethambutol (**E**) and levofloxacin (**L**fx).]

2. Rifampicin Only (RR) and INH and Rifampicin-resistant (MDR)TB

According to the most recent guidelines issued in 2024, the first-choice regimen for patients of MDR/RR-TB who are >14 years of age is BPaLM for 6–9 months. Patients <14 years of age receive short oral Bdq-containing regimen of 9–11 months based on various eligibility criteria. The shorter injectable-containing regimen is used only in areas where the availability of Bdq is not adequate.

a. BPaLM regimen

Inclusion criteria for administration of this regimen include:

- Newly confirmed case of MDR/ RR-TB
- Age more than 14 years
- No QTc prolongation in ECG
- History of no exposure/exposure < one month to Bdq, Lzd, and/or Pa. In patients with exposure more than a month, the sensitivity should be documented.

There is no intensive or continuation phase in this regimen. Four drugs (Bdq, Pa, Lzd, Mfx) are given for 26–39 weeks, i.e., 6-9 months duration. Doses are shown in Table 54.4.

b. Shorter, oral Bdq-containing regimen (9–11 Months)

This regimen (Table 54.5) is recommended for MDR/RR-TB patients meeting the following criteria:

- The patient is not eligible for BPaLM regimen (age less than 14 years, documented resistance to Bdq/ Lzd/ Pa, severe hepatic dysfunction, etc.)
- Age > 5 years and body weight > 15 kg.
- INH resistance due to a mutation in *KatG* or *inhA*, but not both.
- No resistance to fluoroquinolones.
- No prior exposure to drugs in this regimen for more than one month.

Patients of MDR-TB who do not fulfil the above-mentioned criteria for shorter regimens of 9–11 months duration are treated with longer Bdq-containing regimens like that of XDR-TB.

Table 54.4 BPaLM regimen: Duration 26–39 weeks (6–9 months)

Drug	Dosage
First-line drug	**Group A drug**
Bedaquiline (Bdq)	400 mg daily for the first 2 weeks, then 200 mg three times per week until 6 months
Pretomanid (Pa)	200 mg once daily
Linezolid (Lzd)	600 mg once daily
Moxifloxacin (Mfx)	400 mg once daily

Note: Pyridoxine is included in all regimens.

Dosage: 50 mg for patients < 30 kg, 100 mg for patients >30 kg

Shorter regimens are not suitable for extensive pulmonary TB, severe extrapulmonary TB, and pregnant or lactating women.

3. Pre - XDR

Pre-XDR TB refers to MDR/RR-TB with additional resistance to fluoroquinolones (FQs). Treatment depends on the level of fluoroquinolone (FQ) resistance.

- **Low-level FQ resistance**: A longer Bdq-containing regimen is recommended, with a high dose of moxifloxacin (Mfx).
- **High-level FQ resistance**: A longer Bdq-containing regimen is used, but moxifloxacin (Mfx) is replaced with delamanid (Dlm).

4. Extensively-resistant TB (XDR-TB)

Multidrug-resistant TB along with resistance to fluoroquinolone and at least one more group A drugs (Bdq or Lzd) or both of them, is labelled as extensively drug-resistant (XDR) TB.

XDR-TB patients as well as MDR-TB not suitable for shorter regimens are managed with longer Bdq-containing oral regimen of 18–20 months duration. There is no distinction between intensive or continuation phase in this regimen. Drugs used in longer Bdq regimen are shown in Table 54.6.

Table 54.5 Shorter Bdq-containing oral regimen for MDR/RR-TB

Intensive phase (IP) – Duration 4–6 months			
1st line	**Group A**	**Group B**	**Group C**
• Isoniazid high dose (Hh) • Pyrazinamide (Z) • Ethambutol (E)	• Levofloxacin (Lfx) • Bedaquiline (Bdq) 400 mg for 2 weeks, then 200 mg thrice in a week till 24 weeks	Clofazimine (Cfz)	Ethionamide (Eto)*
Continuation phase (CP) – Duration 5 months			
• Pyrazinamide (Z) • Ethambutol (E)	Levofloxacin (Lfx)	Clofazimine (Cfz)	
Pyridoxine [50 mg if weight is <30 kg; 100 mg if weight is >30 kg] is continued throughout			

* Linezolid is also recommended instead of ethionamide in recent guidelines.

Table 54.6 Longer Bdq-containing oral regimen (Duration 18–20 months)

Drugs from group A: All three are used:	Drugs from group B: Two drugs are used:
Levofloxacin (Lfx) Linezolid (Lzd) Bedaquiline (Bdq)	Clofazimine (Cfz) Cycloserine (Cs)

These 5 drugs are used for the first 6 months.
At the end of the sixth month, Bdq is discontinued, and the other 4 drugs are given for the next 12 months.

Pyridoxine is always given.

If there is a need to change any of these drugs, other choices available are drugs of group C, i.e., Delamanid, PAS, Z, E, Meropenem, Imipenem–Cilastatin, etc.

NATIONAL HEALTH PROGRAMME FOR TUBERCULOSIS

India's national health programmes for tuberculosis include the **Revised National Tuberculosis Control Programme (RNTCP)** and its successor, the **National Tuberculosis Elimination Programme (NTEP)**.

The RNTCP was launched in 1993, and in 1997, the **directly observed treatment short-course (DOTS)** strategy was officially adopted. By 2005, the program had achieved nationwide coverage. During the **second phase of RNTCP (2006–2011)**, efforts focused on improving the quality and accessibility of TB services to target global case detection and cure. While these targets were met by 2007–08, challenges remained, particularly concerning multidrug-resistant tuberculosis (MDR-TB) and TB-HIV co-infections.

In response, the **National Strategic Plan for TB Control (NSP)** was developed (2012–2017) with the long-term goal of a TB-free India. This plan integrated TB control with general health services and mandated the notification of all TB cases. Additionally, it provided guidelines for diagnostic services, the programmatic management of drug-resistant TB (PMDT), a single-window service for TB-HIV cases, national drug resistance surveillance, and public-private partnerships.

The **National Strategic Plan for TB Elimination (NSP 2017–2025)** aims to control and eliminate TB in India by 2025. This plan is built on four strategic pillars: **Detect, Treat, Prevent, and Build (DTPB)**.

1. Detect

The aim is to **detect** all drug-sensitive TB (DS-TB) and drug-resistant TB (DR-TB) cases. The need to reach TB patients seeking care from private providers and undiagnosed cases in high-risk populations (migrants, prisoners, HIV-positive cases, close contacts, etc.) is emphasised. Notification of all TB cases to district health officer/authorities every month from all healthcare providers, all laboratories and all chemists has been made mandatory.

- **NIKSHAY** is a case-based, web-based TB surveillance system developed by RNTCP to facilitate notification of TB.
- Incentives are provided to private providers for notification and management of disease as per standards for TB care in India (STCI).
- Free antitubercular drugs and diagnostic tests are provided to TB patients seeking treatment from private sector.

2. Treat

This is the next step and involves initiating and sustaining all tubercular patients on anti-TB treatment wherever they seek it, with a patient-friendly system and social support. Free antitubercular drugs in the form of daily fixed-dose combinations (FDCs) are provided for all cases.

Directly observed treatment (DOT) is a specific strategy to improve adherence to treatment by observing the patient taking medications in the real time. This can be done by a relative, friend or lay person working as a treatment supervisor or supporter. Screening of patients for Rifampicin resistance (and for other drugs when indicated) is also done.

3. Prevent

1. **Prevention** is the **third important strategy** in the national MDR-TB elimination plan. It calls for:
   - Airborne infection control measures by early diagnosis and treatment, health education about cough etiquette and sputum disposal.
   - BCG vaccination at birth or as early as possible till one year of age. BCG vaccine protects against meningitis and disseminated TB.
   - Addressing social determinants of TB, such as malnutrition, poverty, urbanisation, and indoor air pollution.
   - Contact tracing of all close contacts of TB patients, especially those with highest susceptibility to infection.
   - **Isoniazid preventive therapy (IPT)** or chemoprophylaxis with isoniazid to reduce the risk of TB in people exposed to infection or with latent infection.

- In India, 71% household contacts (HHC) of patients with pulmonary tuberculosis are reported to have baseline tubercular infection. Eligibility for **tuberculosis preventive therapy (TPT)** involves ruling out active TB and making a risk–benefit assessment of the cases.

The target population for TPT, after ruling out active TB, includes the following.

a. **All household contacts (HHCs)** of pulmonary tuberculosis patients notified in Nikshay, from public as well as private sector, irrespective of age.
b. In **people living with HIV (PLHIV)**, infants under 12 months receive tuberculosis preventive treatment (TPT) after active TB is ruled out. For adults and older children, screening involves assessing four key symptoms: cough, fever, night sweats, and weight loss. If there are no symptoms, TPT is given. If any of the 4 symptoms is present, TPT is given after ruling out active TB.
[Isoniazid 6-months preventive therapy is given, irrespective of the degree of immunosuppression, antiretroviral therapy, pregnancy status, and previous tubercular treatment.]
c. Individuals receiving **immunosuppressive drugs, anti-TNF treatment**, suffering from **silicosis, on dialysis, planning for organ/ hematological transplantation.**
d. For **children (HHCs more than 5 years of age)** and **adults**, all efforts are made to arrange for chest X-ray and TB testing to rule out active disease. However, preventive therapy should not be deferred in absence of these tests.
e. People living in high-TB transmission settings, such as hospitals, prisons, slums, mines, and migrant labourers, should be included in the vulnerability mapping exercise.

> **TPT Drugs:** The standard drug is isoniazid 300 mg for 6 months. Rifapentine 10 mg/kg + isoniazid 15 mg/kg for 3 months is equally effective. Pyridoxine is used along with chemoprophylaxis in a dose of 10 mg/day for children and 25 mg/day for adults.

- **Contraindications to TB preventive treatment (TPT)** include active tubercular disease, active hepatitis, regular/heavy alcohol intake and peripheral neuropathy

4. Build

The strategy to strengthen the health system by making strengthening/enabling policies, empowering institutions and human resources with enhanced capacities is the fourth most important strategy (pillar) of the national TB elimination plan.

TB IN PREGNANCY

Streptomycin is contraindicated. The standard 6-months regimen of DS-TB for 2 months and HRE for 4 months is recommended in DS-TB. All pregnant patients receiving isoniazid should receive pyridoxine 10–25 mg/day. If organisms are drug resistant, care should be taken to design regimens in a way as to avoid ethionamide up to 32 weeks of pregnancy, because animal experiments show the harmful effect of ethionamide on fetus. Well-controlled studies to see teratogenic effects of ethionamide in pregnancy are lacking. Therefore, in pregnant women suffering from DR-TB, the longer oral M/XDR regimen is useful. The Shorter Bdq-containing regimen is avoided, especially before 32 weeks of gestation.

TB IN LACTATION

Standard 6-months regimen is given. In addition, isoniazid prophylaxis for 6 months to infant along with pyridoxine 5 mg/day + BCG vaccination is recommended.

TB WITH AIDS OR HIV POSITIVE CASES

The risk of developing TB is higher in HIV-positive cases. Moreover, there are more chances of extrapulmonary, more severe and serious TB. HIV infection unmasks the latent cases. Risk of adverse reactions to antitubercular drugs also increases. Starting antiretroviral therapy (ART) and an improved CD4 cell count reduces the incidence of TB among HIV patients.

- Anti-TB regimen in HIV patients is the same as in non-HIV cases, i.e., HRZE for 2 months and HRE for 4–7 months
- + Pyridoxine added for prophylaxis of neurological adverse effects (more likely in HIV-positive patients).
- + Cortimoxazole prophylaxis for prevention of *Pneumocystis jirovecii* infection (it can increase mortality in TB + HIV patients)
- Rifampicin is an enzyme inducer. It increases the metabolism of protease inhibitors (PI) and non-nucleoside reverse transcriptase inhibitors (NNRTIs). Instead of rifampicin, **rifabutin** may be used. Nucleoside reverse transcriptase inhibitors (NRTI) are not induced by rifampicin, so NRTIs can be used.
- MDR-TB in HIV positive is treated with standard regimen; however the duration of treatment is prolonged to 24 months.
- In case of DR-TB in HIV positive patients, prompt initiation of second-line antitubercular drugs and ART, infection control measures and sound patient support system are important strategies. As there is a risk of drug–drug interactions in patients on anti-TB+ART regimens, close monitoring is advised.

- Some patients with HIV and TB coinfection develop paradoxical worsening of TB on starting anti-TB drugs. This is called immune restitution (IRIS) syndrome, characterised by high-grade fever, lymphadenopathy, worsening of intrathoracic lesions and radiological findings of TB. This can be managed with prednisolone given in a dose of 1–2 mg/kg body weight for a week or two and then gradually tapering it down.

MANAGING ADVERSE EFFECTS OF ANTITUBERCULAR DRUGS

First-line drugs are well tolerated.

1. Minor adverse effects, e.g., anorexia, nausea, do not warrant stopping or changing dose of drugs. These can be decreased by administering the drugs with meals.
   - rowsiness by administering drugs at bed time.
   - Peripheral neuritis, especially with isoniazid can be prevented by pyridoxine supplementation.
   - For arthralgia, NSAIDs can be used.
2. In severe hypersensitivity reactions such as rash, itching → stop all the drugs so that reaction subsides. Then reintroduce one drug at a time to identify the offending drug. Only the offending drugs is then discontinued.
   If hypersensitivity reaction occurs in the form of thrombocytopenia, hemolysis or renal failure → rifampin should not be reintroduced.
3. Ethambutol is discontinued at the onset of optic neuritis.
4. Hepatotoxicity is a risk with isoniazid, rifampicin and pyrazinamide (H, R, Z). If hepatitis occurs, all drugs are immediately stopped so that the reaction subsides. The treatment is restarted with non-hepatotoxic drugs, i.e., ethambutol, streptomycin and fluoroquinolones. Then resume treatment with rifampicin, followed by isoniazid. Detect the culprit drug and stop using it.
   - If rifampicin and isoniazid are tolerated, do not add pyrazinamide but give isoniazid, rifampicin and ethambutol (HRE) for 9 months.
   - If isoniazid is offending, give rifampicin, ethambutol and pyrazinamide (REZ) for 9 months.
   - If rifampicin is offending, give isoniazid, ethambutol and streptomycin (HES) for 2 months and HE for 10 months.

ROLE OF CORTICOSTEROIDS IN TB

They are used for short term only, under chemotherapy cover for serious conditions such as:
- seriously ill patient with miliary, severe pulmonary TB, to buy time for drugs to act.
- in tubercular meningitis, pericardial/pleural effusions, renal TB.
- patients with AIDS and severe TB.
- patients developing hypersensitivity reactions to antitubercular drugs.

However, corticosteroids should never be used in intestinal TB because of the risk of silent perforation.

Clinical problem-based questions and MCQs

13. Mrs X (described in question 1) continued with her treatment for a period of 3 months, but after that she stopped taking treatment since she experienced relief from most of her symptoms. However, 15 days after stopping treatment, she presented again with fever, cough and expectoration. How should she be managed at this stage?

14. A 54-year-old laborer presented with fever, cough, expectoration, anorexia, and weight loss. He reported experiencing similar symptoms approximately a year ago, for which he underwent treatment for 2–3 months but discontinued the medication once his symptoms improved. Sputum is AFB positive. Chest X-ray shows signs of fibrosis and cavitary lesion in the left lung. Drug sensitivity testing reports showed resistance to both isoniazid and rifampicin.
    i. What is the diagnosis?
    ii. How this case should be managed as per NTEP guidelines?

15. A 35-year-old pregnant woman is diagnosed with pulmonary TB. She has no history of TB or taking treatment for it in the past.
    i. Which of the following first-line drugs is contraindicated in this patient?
       a. Ethambutol
       b. Streptomycin
       c. Isoniazid
       d. Pyrazinamide
    ii. How this case should be managed?

16. A 75-year-old male patient receiving treatment for TB for the last one month develops jaundice. Liver enzymes are raised.
    i. Identify the drug that should be immediately stopped.
       a. Rifampicin
       b. Isoniazid
       c. Pyrazinamide
       d. All the above
    ii. How this patient should be managed?

17. A 45-year-old male, a known HIV +ve case, develops TB. Describe management of TB in this case.

18. The prescription of a 35-year-old female patient, a known case of renal TB, includes corticosteroids in addition to antitubercular drugs. Comment on the rationality of the prescription.

CONCEPT MAP – DRUGS FOR DR-TB

DR-TB

Group A

Levofloxacin (Lfx) or Moxifloxacin (Mfx)
Mechanism: FQs, inhibit DNA gyrase, penetrate cells & kill intracellular mycobacteria in macrophages. Moxifloxacin is more active against *Mycobacterium tuberculosis* than levofloxacin. Active against MAC & M. fortuitum also.
Use: Mainly in MDR/RR-TB. Used in both shorter & longer oral Bdq-containing regimens under NTEP.
ADRs: Anorexia, nausea, vomiting, bad taste, headache, dizziness, anxiety, insomnia, restlessness, hypersensitivity reactions, damage to tendons, cartilage, QTc prolongation with moxifloxacin.

Bedaquiline (Bdq)
Mechanism: Diarylquinoline, reduces energy production in mycobacteria by inhibiting mycobacterial ATP synthase. It inhibits *M. tuberculosis*, *M. leprae* & other non tubercular mycobacteria. However, Human ATP synthase has very low affinity for Bdq.
Uses: Used in shorter as well as longer oral regimens for management of MDR/RR & XDR-TB in patients > 15 kg & children > 5 years of age. Dose is 400 mg/day for 2 weeks & then 200 mg 3 times a week for 22 weeks, with meals. It is not continued beyond 24th week. Persists in body for > 5 months after stopping the drug.
ADRs: Headache, arthralgia, nausea, QTc prolongation, potential to cause hepatotoxicity.
Bdq is not to be used for severe extrapulmonary TB, DS-TB, non-tubercular mycobacterial infections, pregnant women & patients with cardiac arrhythmias.

Linezolid (Lzd)
Mechanism: Oxazolidinone, binds to P site of 50S ribosomal subunit → distorts tRNA binding site → inhibits protein synthesis → bacteristatic action.
Uses: In patients suffering from severe MDR-TB, complicated extrapulmonary TB and INH-resistant cases with double gene mutation, linezolid 600 mg twice a day is given in longer Bdq-containing regimens of 18–20 months.
Complicated skin, soft tissue, wound infections, serious hospital acquired pneumonias, febrile neutropenia.
ADRs: Nausea, abdominal pain, diarrhea, altered taste. Rarely rashes, itching, thrombocytopenia, anemia, oral candidiasis.
MAO-inhibiting activity → potential of interaction with drugs increasing adrenergic or serotonergic activity.

Group B

Cycloserine (Cs)
Mechanism: Inhibits bacterial cell wall synthesis → tuberculostatic. Spectrum- cycloserine is effective against gram-positive bacteria, *E.coli*, *Chlamydia*, *Mycobacterium tuberculosis* & MAC.
Uses: Only for treatment of drug resistant TB in a dose 250–750 mg.
ADRs: Neuropsychiatric symptoms as headache, sleepiness, tremors, seizures, slurring of speech, frank psychosis & depression may occur. Neurotoxicity can be checked by pyridoxine 100 mg/day.

Terizidone
It consists of 2 molecules of cycloserine, same mechanism, used as an alternative to cycloserine for genito urinary TB, less neurotoxic.

Clofazimine (Cfz)
Mechanism: Interferes with DNA template function & electron transport chain in mitochondria → affects membrane permeability → bacteristatic action in *M. leprae*, *M. tuberculosis* and also atypical mycobacteria.
Therapeutic uses: Under NTEP, clofazimine is part of shorter /longer Bdq-containing regimens as well as injectable-containing regimen for MDR/RR & XDR-TB.
Other uses are leprosy and *M. intracellulare* in AIDS patients.
It has anti-inflammatory action → lepra reactions or ENL.
ADRs: Red to brown or black discolouration of skin, GI adverse effects can occur.

Group C

Pyrazinamide, Ethambutol, Streptomycin or Amikacin Imipenem–Cilastatin or Meropenem

Ethionamide (Eto) or Prothionamide (Pto)
Mechanism same as INH.
Uses: In NTEP, ethionamide is used in shorter regimens for MDR/RRTB, MAC, AIDS & in some cases of leprosy, as a reserve drug. Dose is 250–750 mg/day.
ADRs: Frequent like anorexia, nausea, vomiting, epigastric pain, metallic taste, sulfurous belching, generalised aches & pains, rashes may occur. Prolonged treatment causes menstrual irregularity, impotence, goiter, peripheral neuropathy & behavioural changes. Neurotoxicity can be prevented by pyridoxine.

p Aminosalicylic acid (PAS)
Mechanism: Interferes with folate synthesis in *Mycobacterium tuberculosis* only.
Used in longer regimens for MDR TB only when there is need to change initially started drugs because of resistance or adverse effects.
ADRs: Poorly tolerated. Causes anorexia nausea, epigastric pain, fever, rashes, malaise, blood dyscrasias due to hypersensitivity, liver & kidney dysfunction, goiter & hypokalemia.

Delamanid
Mechanism: Inhibits methoxy & keto-mycolic acid which are components of mycobacterial cell wall.
Uses: Only in MDR – pulmonary TB & XDR-TB. dose of 100 mg BD for 6 months.

NTEP Regimens

H-mono/Poly DRTB
R Z E Lfx for 6–9 months.

MDR/RR-TB (No FQ resistance, H resistance by 1 gene mutation
Shorter Bdq-containing regimen (9–11 months)
IP: H ^{h} Z E Lfx Bdq Cfz Eto (4–6 months)
CP: Z E Lfx Cfz (5 months)
Shorter injectable-containing regimen (9–11 months)
IP: H ^{h} Z E Mfx Cfz Eto Km / Am (4–6 months)
CP: Z E Mfx Cfz (5 months)
Pyridoxine 50–100 mg/day

XDR-TB, MDR/RR-TB with FQ resistance, Both gene mutation to H, extensive pulmonary TB, Severe extrapulmonary TB
Longer Bdq-containing regimen (18–20 months)
Lfx Lzd Bdq Cfz Cs
only for 6 months

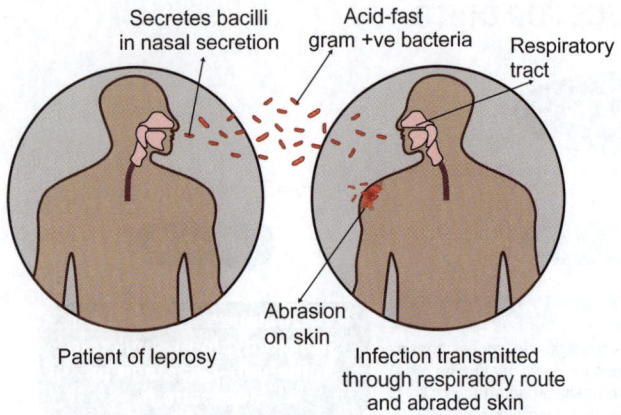

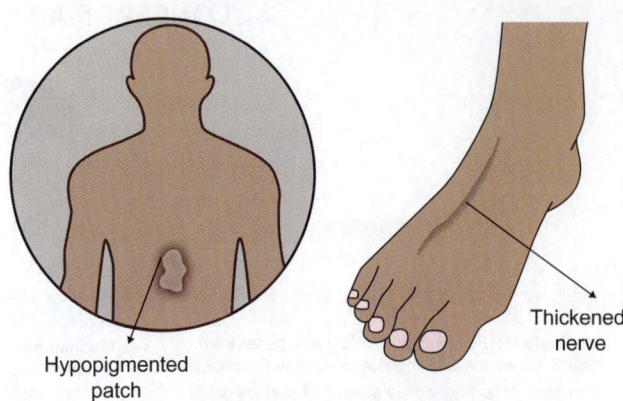

Fig. 54.7 Transmission of *Mycobacterium leprae*

ANTILEPROTIC DRUGS

Leprosy or Hansen's disease is a mycobacterial infective disease that affects skin, cutaneous/peripheral/autonomic nerves, mucous membranes and internal organs. It is caused by **Mycobacterium leprae**, a rod-shaped acid-fast bacilli, which is **shed in the nasal discharge** of patients. The organisms gain entry through skin abrasions or upper respiratory tract mucus membranes (Fig. 54.7). The **incubation period varies** from 2–7 years, but could be as long as 30 years.

DIAGNOSIS OF LEPROSY

A person having one or more of the following features is diagnosed with leprosy (Fig. 54.8).

- Hypopigmented patch or reddish lesions with loss of sensations
- Thickening of peripheral nerves with loss of sensations
- Slit skin smear positive for AFB or histological demonstration of granuloma affecting nerves. The density of bacilli in smear is called **bacterial index(BI)**. If there are 1–10 bacilli in hundred fields, BI is labelled as 1+; if many clumps of bacilli are seen in an average field, BI is labeled as 6+. Relapse rate is shown to be high if bacillary load is high, i.e., a BI > 4+.

TYPES OF LEPROSY

The clinical outcome of *M. leprae* infection is variable and depends on the immune status of the infected person. Leprosy can be of following types, in increasing order of their severity: **indeterminate, tuberculoid, borderline** and **lepromatous types**. For treatment purposes, it is important to differentiate between tuberculoid and lepromatous leprosy. The important differences between these two are given in Table 54.7.

Borderline (BB), borderline tuberculoid (BT) and borderline lepromatous (BL) leprosy have mixed features.

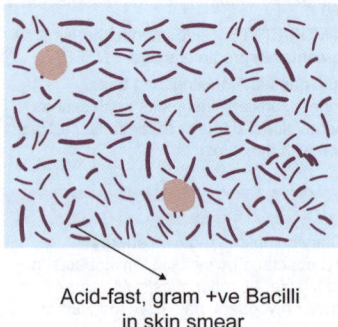

Fig. 54.8 Diagnosis of leprosy

According to the 2025 NLEP guidelines, leprosy is classified into two categories—paucibacillary (PB) and multibacillary (MB)—based on the number of skin lesions, the number of peripheral nerves involved, and the presence or absence of acid-fast bacilli in slit-skin smears (Table 54.8).

MANAGEMENT OF LEPROSY

Leprosy is a chronic granulomatous infectious disease requiring long-term therapy.

1. **Patient and family education** about the nature and course of disease, measures to be taken to prevent the spread of the disease to contacts of the patient, and expected duration and outcome of the treatment is important.
2. **General health** should be improved, co-morbid conditions should be adequately treated.
3. **Antileprotic chemotherapy:** Different regimens have been used in the past for variable durations. However, currently, for mass treatment **in PBL, multiple drug therapy (MDT) is given for 6 months, whereas for MBL multi-drug therapy is continued for 12 months**. If relapse occurs due to dormant bacilli, the same drugs can be used again. The aim is to achieve smear negativity in individual patients.
4. **Preventive measures:** Early diagnosis and treatment is the most effective prevention of leprosy. **Household**

Table 54.7. Differences between tuberculoid and lepromatous leprosy

Features	Tuberculoid leprosy (TT)	Lepromatous leprosy (LL)
Type of lesions	- Hypopigmented or erythematous - May be flat or raised - Surface over the lesion is dry and rough - Sensations of pain and temperature are impaired	- Hypopigmented or coppery red - Flat (later on, papules/nodules are formed) - Smooth and shiny surface over lesion - Early lesions do not show loss of sensation
Slit skin smear	Negative for AFB	Positive for AFB; nasal discharge highly positive for AFB
Nerves	Nerves in the vicinity of skin lesions are palpably thickened	Symmetrical nerve damage occurs late in this type. Nerve trunks are enlarged and soft to feel.
Mucous membranes	Not much affected	Ulceration of mucosa of mouth, nose, larynx and trachea, damage to nasal bones, premaxilla may occur
Face	Sometimes features of facial palsy occur on one or both sides of the face.	Leonine facies due to infiltration and thickening of skin of face
Cell mediated immunity	Normal	Absent
Lepromin test (not done nowadays)	Negative	Positive
Clinical outcome	Prolonged remission and periodic exacerbation of symptoms	Worsens and anesthesia of distal parts, atrophy, ulceration, even absorption of digits may occur.

Table 54.8. Types of leprosy

Types	Number of skin lesions	Number of nerves involved	Bacilli in slit skin smear
Paucibacillary (PB)	1–5	No	Absent
Multibacillary (MB)	>5	one or more	Present

contacts of a leprosy patient **should be screened** for symptoms of the disease **every six months. Chemoprophylaxis is used for rifampicin** in people at high risk of developing the disease.

ANTILEPROTIC DRUGS

Flowchart 54.2 lists the drugs used in treatment of leprosy. These include dapsone, clofazimine, antitubercular drugs as Rifampicin, ethionamide, prothionamide and some antibiotics.

1. Dapsone
Mechanism of action
Dapsone is diamino diphenyl sulfone (DDS). It has **leprostatic** action at very low concentrations. Mechanism of action is the **same as sulphonamides,** i.e., it competes with PABA for folate synthase and inhibits synthesis of dihydrofolate (refer to Fig. 52.1).

Mechanism of resistance
Resistance to dapsone can be primary or secondary. Primary resistance is seen in patients who have never been treated with dapsone whereas secondary resistance occurs in patients who have received dapsone monotherapy in the past. Incidence of secondary dapsone resistance is up to 20% with monotherapy. So, in current practice, monotherapy is not used and dapsone is used as a component of MDT.

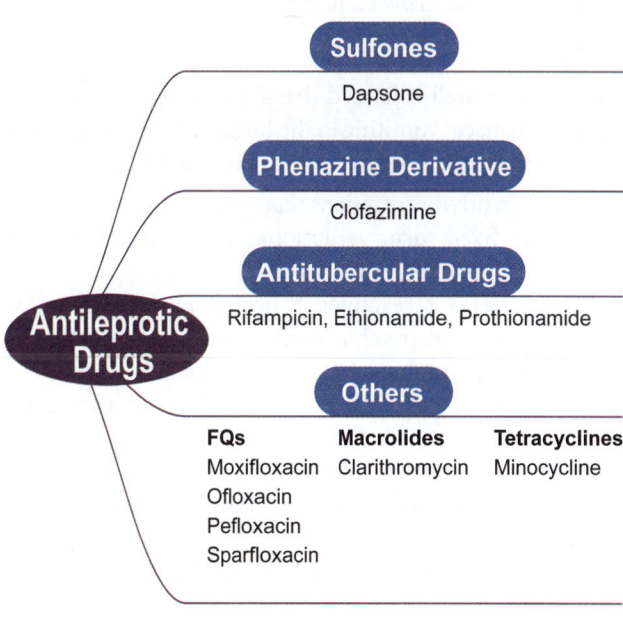

Flowchart. 54.2 Classification of antileprotic drugs

Dapsone resistant *M. leprae* have **mutation in enzyme folate synthase, resulting in low affinity for the drug**. Low-to-moderately-resistant organisms can be inhibited by a high dose of dapsone 100 mg/day. It is because the leprostatic action of dapsone is present at very low concentrations. When dapsone is given in a dose of 100 mg/day, the plasma concentration achieved is about 500 times more than that required for leprostatic action. So, bacilli having mild-to-moderate resistance can be inhibited, and the relapse rate is low (2–3% only). However, some bacilli are sensitive to dapsone but hide themselves, i.e., become dormant in tissues and become inaccessible for drug. These are called **persisters** and may be responsible for relapse.

In addition to antileprotic action, dapsone is effective against *Plasmodium falciparum*, *Toxoplasma gondii* and *Pneumocystis jirovecii*. Dapsone has some anti-inflammatory action also.

Pharmacokinetics

DDS is well absorbed orally, well distributed throughout body fluids and tissues, except CSF where it has poor entry. Plasma protein binding is to the extent of 70%. Dapsone **accumulates in the skin**, particularly in areas infected with *M. leprae*, as well as in the liver, muscles, and kidneys. It undergoes metabolism through acetylation and glucuronide/sulphate conjugation. It is secreted in bile, and undergoes enterohepatic circulation, with a half-life of 1–2 days. Excretion of metabolites occurs in urine, and the dose needs to be adjusted in renal function impairment.

Therapeutic uses

- Dapsone is used **in MDT for leprosy in a dose of 100 mg/day, along with rifampicin and clofazimine.**
- It can be used in combination with pyrimethamine in **chloroquine-resistant malaria, toxoplasmosis** and *Pneumocystis jirovecii* **infection.**

ADRs

Daspone is a well-tolerated drug. However, it can cause anorexia, nausea, vomiting in the beginning of therapy, but these adverse effects decrease with continued treatment.

- Hypersensitivity reactions can occur as rashes and itching, fixed drug eruptions, hypermelanosis and severe exfoliative dermatitis.
- Phototoxic reactions, peripheral neuropathy, paresthesia and psychosis may occur. In rare cases, it can cause agranulocytosis and hepatitis.
- In patients with G6PD deficiency, dapsone can cause hemolysis.
- In severe lepromatous leprosy, dapsone can precipitate erythema nodosum leprosum (ENL), i.e., type 2 lepra reactions.
- Sulfone syndrome can occur with MDT in malnourished patients. It is characterised by generalised malaise, fever, lymph node enlargement, jaundice, anemia and desquamation of skin. Dapsone should be stopped in these patients. Symptoms are controlled with corticosteroids.

Contraindications: It should not be given in G6PD deficiency, patients with history of hypersensitivity reactions, and anemia (Hb < 7 g/dL).

2. Clofazimine

It is a phenazine derivative. It exerts **leprostatic** effect by

- Interfering with DNA template function.
- Disrupting electron transport chain in mitochondria.
- Altering membrane permeability, affecting transport through cell membrane.

Response to clofazimine is slower than dapsone but it **can inhibit dapsone-resistant *M. leprae* after a lag period of 2 months.**

In addition to leprostatic action, clofazimine inhibits atypical mycobacteria and has anti-inflammatory action that is useful in ENL.

Pharmacokinetics

Clofazimine absorption from gut is variable (40–70%). After absorption, it is **stored in reticuloendothelial tissues and subcutaneous fat** as needle shaped crystals, from where it is released slowly overtime. It has a **long half-life of about 70 days,** which allows **intermittent therapy**. It is excreted mainly in feces, but some excretion also occurs in urine or bile.

Therapeutic uses

It is used in MDT for **leprosy** in combination with dapsone and rifampicin.

- Useful in management of **lepra reactions or ENL** owing to its anti-inflammatory effect
- Sometimes it is used in **XDR TB** and *M. intracellulare* **infection** in AIDS patients.

ADRs

Clofazimine can cause **discolouration of skin**. Red to brown or black discolouration may occur, but it clears off after drug is stopped. Gastrointestinal adverse effects can occur.

Antitubercular Drugs

Rifampicin is most potent **cidal drug** against *M. leprae* and is a component of standard MDT. It has **quick response**. Nasal symptoms are relieved in 2–3 weeks and skin lesions also regress in 2 months. However, nerve damage is not improved much. Rifampicin is effective in monotherapy also, but it is **used with dapsone and clofazimine as MDT to prevent emergence of resistance.**

Rifampicin rapidly kills 99.99% of *M. leprae* in 3–7 days when given in a dose of 600 mg/day. Thus, a large quantity of mycobacterial antigens is released, which may cause **type 2 lepra reactions or ENL.** Rifampicin is contraindicated in hepatic and renal dysfunction.

Ethionamide and prothionamide can cause hepatotoxicity. These are considered only when it is very necessary, as in cases of dapsone resistance or patients not tolerating dapsone.

4. Other Drugs: AMAs

Fluoroquinolones

Fluoroquinolones exert **cidal effect** by inhibition of DNA gyrase. Ciprofloxacin has poor activity against *M. leprae*, but **moxifloxacin, ofloxacin, pefloxacin** and **Sparfloxacin** possess good action in leprosy. Moxifloxacin is the most potent fluoroquinolone against *M. leprae*. These have cidal action and ofloxacin, 400 mg once a day, has been shown to kill 99.9% bacilli after 22 days of treatment. Thus, it may be **used as an alternative to rifampicin** for prevention of development of resistance to dapsone and shorten the duration of MDT, but the safety of long-term use is not documented.

Minocycline

It is a tetracycline that is more effective than clarithromycin but less effective than rifampicin. It may be used as **an alternative when really necessary**. Long-term use causes vertigo, which may be disabling.

Clarithromycin

It is the only macrolide antibiotic that is active against *M. leprae*, but its **efficacy is much lower than that of rifampicin and minocycline**. It may be used as alternative if rifampicin is contraindicated or not tolerated.

LEPRA REACTIONS

These are **Jarisch–Herxheimer reaction or Arthus type reactions** associated with the release of mycobacterial antigens from killed bacteria in lepromatous leprosy. It can be mild, severe or a life-threatening type called erythema nodosum leprosum (ENL) In severe lepra reactions, the existing lesions suddenly become large, swollen, red and painful. Several new lesions also appear. Constitutional symptoms like fever, generalised malaise are also present. **In severe cases, dapsone is discontinued**. Clofazimine possesses anti-inflammatory activity that is useful in lepra reactions. It is given in a dose of 200 mg daily for symptom control.

Corticosteroids are very useful in lepra reactions because of their non-specific antiinflammatory and immunosuppressant actions. Prednisolone, 40–60 mg is given daily and continued till reaction subsides. Thereafter it is tapered down over a period of 2–3 months.

Thalidomide is an anti-inflammatory, cytokine-modulating drug that may be used as an alternative to prednisolone. It modulates the effect of TNFα, interferons and interleukins. Dose of thalidomide is 100–300 mg, once a day.

REVERSAL REACTION

It is a delayed hypersensitivity reaction to *M. leprae* antigens that is seen in borderline and tuberculoid leprosy. In this reaction, **cutaneous ulceration, swelling, and tenderness in multiple nerves occur after completion of treatment.** It is managed with **corticosteroids or clofazimine**, but there is no role for thalidomide, probably because cytokines are not involved in the causation of the reversal reaction.

Clinical problem-based questions and MCQs

19. Which of the following macrolides has activity against *M. leprae*?
    a. Erythromycin
    b. Clarithromycin
    c. Azithromycin
    d. Roxithromycin

20. Which of the following is most potent cidal drug against *M. leprae*?
    a. Clofazimine
    b. Rifampicin
    c. Minocycline
    d. Dapsone

21. Which of the following correctly describes the mechanism of action of dapsone?
    a. Inhibition of folic acid synthesis
    b. Inhibition of mycobacterial cell wall synthesis
    c. Inhibition of DNA gyrase enzyme
    d. Inhibition of protein synthesis

22. A 49-year-old male patient is suffering from lepromatous leprosy. Which of the following statements is true?
    a. He has flat or raised skin lesions.
    b. Nerves in vicinity of skin lesions are palpably thickened.
    c. CMI is absent.
    d. Lepromin test is negative.

23. Dapsone is useful in which of the following conditions?
    a. Paucibacillary leprosy
    b. Chloroquine resistant malaria
    c. Toxoplasmosis
    d. All of the above

24. Which of the following drugs has NO role in reversal reaction
    a. Prednisolone
    b. Clofazimine
    c. Thalidomide
    d. All of above

25. A 42-year-old woman, a known case of MBL, is receiving multidrug therapy with dapsone, rifampicin and clofazimine. Patient reports in dermatology OPD with brown discolouration of the skin on face.
    i. Identify the drug responsible for the discolouration of skin.
    ii. How is it managed?

LEPROSY ERADICATION PROGRAMMES

The National Leprosy Control Programme, launched in 1955, was revised in 1982 as the National Leprosy Eradication Programme (NLEP). The **primary objective of NLEP** is to make patients non-contagious, thereby reducing disease transmission.

Monotherapy is not practiced these days. The **approach to NLEP is multidrug therapy (MDT), comprising administration of dapsone, rifampicin and clofazimine**. With MDT, the prevalence rate of leprosy was reduced to <1/10000 population by year 2005, except in few states and union territories (Dadra, Nagar Haveli, Chandigarh, Goa, Lakshadweep, Bihar and Odisha). Current guidelines do not allow monotherapy. All cases of MB and PB are treated with the same MDT. However, the duration of treatment varies.

MDT Regimens under NLEP

As per the guidelines issued in April 2025, the multi-drug therapy (MDT) regimen based on a 3-drug combination is recommended for both PB and MB leprosy cases. The drugs, i.e., dapsone, rifampicin and clofazimine, as well as their doses remain the same in both PB and MB leprosy cases. However, the duration of treatment is shorter for PB (6 months) than in MB (12 months). The doses of drugs for adults, children 10-14 years and < 10 years are shown in Table 54.9.

Advantages of MDT

In leprosy cases with no primary resistance to dapsone, MDT is effective because:

- Use of drug combination prevents the emergence of resistance to dapsone.
- Addition of cidal drug rifampicin allows for quick relief of symptoms, makes patient non-contagious within few days itself, and checks progression of the disease.
- Total duration of therapy is reduced to 6 months in PBL and 12 months in MBL.
- Rate of relapse is reduced to < 1%. Resistance to rifampicin and clofazimine does not occur, and the same drugs can be used to manage the relapse.
- MDT is safe, efficacious and acceptability is excellent.

Alternative Regimens

These are useful in case of **rifampicin resistance** or **when it is not possible to give standard MDT**.

- **Intermittent ROM regimen**: A combination of rifampicin (600 mg), ofloxacin (400 mg), and minocycline (100 mg) is given monthly for **3-6 months** in **PBL** and **12-24 months** in **MBL**.
- **Intermittent** RMMx regimen: A combination of rifampicin (600 mg), minocycline (200 mg), and moxifloxacin (400 mg) is administered once a month for **6 months** in **PBL** and **12 months** in **MBL**.
- Rifampicin (600 mg) + sparfloxacin (200 mg) + clarithromycin (500 mg) + minocycline (100 mg) given daily for 12 weeks.
- Clofazimine (50 mg) + any two of ofloxacin (400 mg)/minocycline (100 mg)/clarithromycin (500 mg) given daily for 6 months. Thereafter, clofazimine (50 mg) + either ofloxacin (400 mg) or minocycline (100 mg) is given daily for 18 months.
- In the **standard regimen**, clofazimine can be replaced by ofloxacin (400 mg) or minocycline (100 mg).

PREVENTIVE MEASURES

1. Early diagnosis and adequate treatment are the best ways to prevent the spread of leprosy and progression of the disease to a disabling stage.
2. BCG vaccination protects against leprosy to a variable extent, ranging from 34-80%.
3. Contacts of leprosy patient should be examined regularly, every 6 months. Close contacts of the patient, who are at a higher risk of getting infected, should receive chemoprophylaxis with rifampicin in a dose of 15 mg/kg body weight, given once in a month for 6 months.
4. Health education of society is an important strategy to reduce the stigma associated with the disease, improve compliance to treatment in mass programmes and prevent spread of the disease.
5. Rehabilitation has a role in management of disabilities caused by leprosy. MDT, surgical correction of disabilities, preventing further injury to disabled limbs, protection from keratitis and social rehabilitative measures are useful.

Table 54.9. Multi-drug therapy (MDT) in PB and MB leprosy

Age Group	Dapsone	Rifampicin	Clofazimine	Duration of Treatment
Adults	100 mg daily	600 mg once monthly	300 mg once monthly and 50 mg daily	PB: 6 months MB: 12 months
10–14 years	50 mg daily	450 mg once monthly	150 mg once monthly and 50 mg on alternate days	Same as above
< 10 years or < 40 kg (typically 20–40 kg)	2 mg/kg daily	10 mg/kg once monthly	100 mg once monthly and 50 mg twice weekly	Same as above

Clinical problem-based questions and MCQs

26. A 60-year-old male patient, Mr L, presents with multiple, diffuse lesions over face and arms. Lesions are raised, hypopigmented and there is no sensations over the lesion. Ulnar nerve is thickened and palpable. The patient has a history of similar symptoms 8 years ago, for which he had received prolonged treatment. Skin smear is negative for AFB.
    i. What is the likely diagnosis?
    ii. Enumerate drugs that may be useful in the management of his condition.
    iii. Describe the MDT regimen for Mr L.

27. Enumerate the advantages of MDT over monotherapy.

28. i. Describe FDT-12 for a patient with MBL.
    ii. Describe the advantages of FDT-12 over longer treatments.

29. A 36-year-old male, diagnosed with lepromatous leprosy, is having G6PD deficiency.
    i. Which of the following drugs can cause hemolysis in G6PD deficiency?
       a. Rifampicin   b. Dapsone
       c. Clofazimine   d. clarithromycin
    ii. Describe alternative regimens for treatment of leprosy in this case.

Summary

ANTITUBERCULAR DRUGS
- First-line antitubercular drugs include isoniazid (H), rifampicin (R), ethambutol (E), pyrazinamide (Z) and streptomycin. **INH** exerts tuberculocidal effect by interfering with mycolic acid and DNA synthesis. Resistance develops due to mutations in *katG* and *inhA* genes causing failure to activate the drug or overproduction of mycolic acid.
  ADRs: It can cause adverse neurotoxic effects like paresthesias, numbness and peripheral neuritis, which can be prevented by adding pyridoxine to the treatment regimen.
  INH is metabolised by acetylation → forms hepatotoxic metabolite. Genetic polymorphism of acetylation is seen.
- **Rifampicin (R)** exerts cidal effects by inhibiting DNA dependent RNA polymerase enzyme. Resistance develops due to a mutation in *rpoB* gene, causing decreased affinity of target enzyme for drug. Rifampicin is useful in treatment of tuberculosis as first-line drug, in latent tuberculosis, leprosy, Prophylaxis of meningococcal/ staphylococcal carriers, and type B *H. influenza*.
  ADRs occur as nausea, vomiting, abdominal cramps, thrombocytopenia (TCP), rashes, nephritis, headache, fever, chills. It causes harmless red discolouration of secretions. Major ADRs are hepatitis and cholestatic jaundice. Many interactions may occur due to its potential to induce microsomal enzymes, notably contraceptive failure.
- **Pyrazinamide (Z)** interferes with mycobacterial cell membrane metabolism and function; it affects only intracellular mycobacteria. Resistance occurs due to mutation in *PncA* gene, resulting in impaired uptake/activation of the drug. ADRs include nausea, vomiting, rashes and arthralgia. It is hepatotoxic and is not used in patients with liver disease.
- **Ethambutol** is tuberculostatic drug which interferes with incorporation of mycolic acid into mycobacterial cell wall. It is used only in initial intense phase of treatment of TB. ADRs: Typical toxicity includes retrobulbar optic neuritis, decreased visual acuity and risk of recipitation of gout.
- **Streptomycin,** an aminoglycoside, is not much in use because of its toxicity, rapid development of resistance and the need for intramuscular injection.
- **Drugs for DR-TB are divided in 3 groups: A, B, C.**
  - **Group A drugs** are Lfx or MFx, linezolid and bedaquiline. Among FQs, moxifloxacin is most active against *M. Tuberculosis*, followed by levofloxacin. Bedaquiline inhibits ATP synthetase enzyme and shows no cross-resistance. Linezolid inhibits protein synthesis and exerts bacteriostatic action.
    ADRs: Headache, arthralgia, nausea, QTc prolongation, potential to cause hepato-toxicity.
  - In **group B drugs,** clofazimine, an antileprotic drug, is part of short- and long-BDQ-containing regimens. Cycloserine inhibits mycobacterial cell wall synthesis, shows no cross-resistance with other drugs but has the potential to cause neuropsychiatric symptoms. **Terizidone** is similar to cycloserine. It has 2 molecules of cycloserine and shares its mechanism of action and properties but is **less neurotoxic**.
  - In **group C drugs,** imipenem–cilastatin or meropenem, amikacin or streptomycin, ethambutol, pyrazinamide, ethionamide or prothionamide, PAS, pretomanid and delamanid are included.
    Ethionamide and prothionamide have the same mechanism of tuberculocidal action as INH and show cross-resistance with it. Ethionamide is not safe in pregnancy.
- **Revised national programme for control of TB (RNTCP), now NTEP,** is based on four strategic pillars of **detect, treat, prevent** and **build.**

- DS-TB cases need treatment with HRZE for 8 weeks in intensive phase and HRE for 16 weeks in continuation phase.
- In isoniazid mono-resistance/poly-resistance: Treatment with RZE, Lfx is given for 6–9 months.
- In MDR/RR TB, in patients > 14 years, BPaLM regimen is the first choice. It includes four drugs, Bdq, Pa, Lzd, and Max given for 6-9 months. In patients < 14 years, shorter oral Bdq or injectable-containing regimen is used. Shorter Bdq regimen involves 7 drugs in IP (H^h, Z, E, Lfx, Bdq, Cfz) for 4–6 months and 4 drugs (Lfx, Cfz, Z,E) for 5 months. The total duration is 9–11 months. The injectable-containing regimen has moxifloxacin instead of Lfx along with Km/Am, Eto, Cfz, Z, H^h and E for 4–6 months, and Mfx, Cfz, Z, E for 5 months. It is used if Bdq is not available.
- MDR-TB cases with additional resistance to FQs and XDR cases are managed with longer (18–20 months) Bdq-containing regimen of 5 drugs comprising Lfx, Bdq, Lzd, Cfz, and Cs.

ANTILEPROTIC DRUGS

- Leprosy is a chronic infectious disease caused by *M. leprae*. Major clinical types are lepromatous leprosy with extensive involvement and tuberculoid leprosy with single or few skin lesions and nerve involvement. Other types are borderline and indeterminate type leprosy. Paucibacillary leprosy (PBL) includes types TT, BT, and multibacillary leprosy (MBL) includes BB, BL, LL types.
- Dapsone, rifampicin and clofazimine are main antileprotic drugs that are part of standard MDT in NLEP.
- Dapsone acts by inhibiting folic acid synthesis. It exerts leprostatic action at very low concentration. Mutations causing reduced affinity of folate synthase for the drug lead to the development of dapsone resistance. It can cause anorexia, nausea, vomiting, hypersensitivity reactions, psychosis, peripheral neuropathy and hemolysis in G6PD deficiency.
- Rifampicin is an antitubercular drug having the most potent cidal action against *M. leprae*. Rapid cidal action may precipitate lepra reaction or ENL in patients with LL, which is managed by corticosteroids, clofazimine or thalidomide. It is contraindicated in renal and hepatic function impairment.
- Clofazimine is a phenazine dye that exerts static action. It has anti-inflammatory action also. It causes red-brown discolouration of skin, which is reversible on stopping the drug.
- Other drugs having antileprotic effect are ethionamide, prothionamide, FQs like moxifloxacin, ofloxacin, pefloxacin, sparfloxacin and minocycline, and clarithromycin. These are used only in cases of rifampicin-resistance or when the standard regimen cannot be given.
- NLEP started in 1982 relies on MDT with dapsone 100 mg daily + rifampicin 600 mg monthly + clofazimine 300 mg monthly and 50 mg daily for 6 months in PBL. MDT for MBL is with all the 3 drugs in the same doses but the treatment is continued for 12 months (FDT- 12). Continuation of therapy beyond 12 weeks does not show additional benefits. So, FDT-12 is advised, which is more cost effective, has less ADRs and a better patient compliance.
- Release of mycobacterial antigens can cause lepra reaction characterised by the existing lesions becoming large, swollen, red and painful. Several new lesions also appear. Constitutional symptoms like fever, generalised malaise is also present. It can be managed with corticosteroids, clofazimine or thalidomide

Practice Questions

1. Describe short-course chemotherapy for a newly diagnosed case of TB.
2. Explain why
   i. Antitubercular drugs are used in combination
   ii. Ethionamide may show cross-resistance with isoniazid
   iii. Pyridoxine is combined with antitubercular drug regimens
   iv. Rifabutin is used in HIV positive tubercular patients.
3. Describe the management of MDR and XDR-TB.
4. Write short notes on
   i. Chemoprophylaxis in TB
   ii. Role of corticosteroids in TB
5. Describe standard MDT regimen as per NLEP for
   a. MBL
   b. PBL
6. Describe features of lepra reaction and its management.
7. Describe alternative regimens for leprosy patients in which standard MDT cannot be given

Hints for problem-based questions and MCQs

1. i. a. Ethionamide is a second line antitubercular drug.
   ii. Mechanism of action of INH: interferes with mycolic acid synthesis and interrupts DNA synthesis. Refer to page 700.
   ADRs: Refer to page 702
   iii. INH prevents formation of pyridoxal phosphate and increased excretion. This causes neurotoxic effects like paresthesias, numbness and peripheral neuritis. Pyridoxine is given 10 mg/day prophylactically to patients like alcoholics, diabetics, AIDS, pregnant and lactating women who are at high risk for neurotoxicity.
   iv. To prevent development of resistance, by reducing selective pressure.
   v. Irregular treatment favours development of resistance. If patient develops resistance to first-line drugs, it becomes necessary to prescribe second-line drugs having lower efficacy and higher risk of adverse effects.

2. c. Ethambutol
3. d. Streptomycin
4. Isoniazid, rifampicin, pyrazinamide
5. a–2   b–3   c–4   d–5   e–1
6. i. c. Pyrazinamide
   ii. b. Ethambutol
7. Rifampicin used as first-line antitubercular drug is an enzyme-inducer that can cause contraceptive failure and unwanted pregnancy. Therefore, the patient is advised to use barrier contraception.
8. c. Rifabutin, because its enzyme-inducing potential is less. Thus, the risk of drug interactions with NNRTIs and protease inhibitors is less.
9. d. Terizidone does not cause QT prolongation.
10. c. Ethionamide shows cross-resistance with isoniazid.
11. a. Cycloserine
12. For newly diagnosed cases, as per RNTCP, in the intensive phase of 8 weeks duration, 4 drugs, HRZE, are used. Then in the continuation phase of 16 weeks duration, Z is discontinued but HRE is continued. Dose of INH is 5 mg/kg/day, rifampicin is 10 mg/kg/day, ethambutol is 15 mg/kg/day and pyrazinamide is 25 mg/kg/day.
13. This is a previously treated case of TB. Therefore, drug sensitivity tests are advisable as there is risk of development of resistance in such cases. Treatment should be resumed based on sensitivity testing results, following guideline recommendations for H-mono, poly-drug resistant, MDR, or RR-TB cases. (Refer to page 710–712).
14. i. The patient is suffering from MDR-TB.
    ii. As the patient has extensive pulmonary lesions, he should be put on longer Bdq-containing regimen. Refer to page 712
15. i. b. Streptomycin is contraindicated in pregnancy.
    ii. Management is the same as in the other newly diagnosed cases. Newborn should be given chemoprophylaxis with isoniazid and BCG vaccination. (Refer to page 713).
16. i. d. All drugs should be stopped.
    ii. The patient is receiving treatment for the past one month, so he is still in the intensive phase of treatment. He shows sign and symptoms of hepatotoxicity with drugs.
    - Firstly, all the drugs should be stopped till hepatotoxic reaction subsides.
    - Treatment is restarted with non-hepatotoxic drugs, i.e., streptomycin + fluoroquinolone + ethambutol.
    - To identify the offending drug, restart rifampicin. If it is tolerated, restart isoniazid. If it is also tolerated, then do not reintroduce pyrazinamide; continue HRE for 9 months.
    - If reaction occurs with isoniazid, give RZE for 9 months.
    - If isoniazid is tolerated but rifampicin is the offending drug, give HES for 2 months and HE for 10 months.
17. Management of HIV + TB remains the same, but
    - Rifabutin is used instead of rifampicin because of reduced risk of enzyme induction with it.
    - Continuation phase may be prolonged up to 7 months.
    - Pyridoxine is given to prevent neurological adverse effects.
    - Cotrimoxazole prophylaxis is indicated to prevent *Pneumocystis jirovecii* infection, which may increase mortality in such patients.
18. Corticosteroids are recommended for short-term use alongside antitubercular therapy in severe TB cases, including miliary TB, renal TB, severe pulmonary TB, tuberculous meningitis, pericardial or pleural effusion, severe TB with AIDS, and hypersensitivity reactions to anti-TB drugs. If a patient presents with any of these conditions, corticosteroid prescription is justified.
19. b. Clarithromycin
20. b. Rifampicin
21. a. Inhibition of folic acid synthesis
22. c. CMI is absent; the remaining 3 options are features of tuberculoid leprosy.
23. d. All of the above
24. c. Thalidomide
25. i. Clofazimine causes skin discolouration.
    ii. It is completely reversible on discontinuation of the drug. So, the patient should be reassured and advised to continue treatment till completion of one year (FDT 12).
26. i. The patient is experiencing a relapse of leprosy, with symptoms indicative of tuberculoid leprosy.
    ii. Dapsone, rifampicin, clofazimine are main antileprotic drugs.
    iii. As tuberculoid leprosy is PBL, it is treated with dapsone 100 mg daily along with rifampicin 600 mg once a month given under supervision. Both the drugs are continued for 6-months. Subsequently, the patient is followed up for 1–2 years.
27. MDT prevents emergence of resistance to dapsone, provides quick relief of symptoms, makes the patient non-contagious within few days itself, and checks the progression of the disease.
    - Total duration of therapy is reduced to 6 months in PBL and rate of relapse brought down to < 1%. Resistance to rifampicin and clofazimine does not occur, and the same drugs can be used to manage relapse.
    - MDT is safe, efficacious and acceptability is excellent
28. i. Fixed-duration therapy of 12 months (FDT-12) is used in MBL. It includes dapsone 100 mg daily combined with clofazimine 50 mg daily + 300 mg once a month and rifampicin 600 mg once a month.
    ii. Reduction in duration of treatment increases the cost-effectiveness of the programme, decreases ADRs, improves patient compliance and acceptability of the treatment. Moreover, organisms responsible for relapse are persisters that remain sensitive to the same drugs. Thus, relapse is successfully managed with the same MDT.
29. i. b. Dapsone
    ii. Refer to page 720 for alternative regimens.

CONCEPT MAP – ANTILEPROTIC DRUGS

Management
- Patient and family education
- Improvement of general health
- Preventive measures

Antileprotic Drugs:
Sulfones: Dapsone
Phenazine derivative: Clofazimine
Antitubercular drugs: Rifampicin, Ethionamide, Prothionamide
Others: Fluoroquinolones – Moxifloxacin, Ofloxacin, Pefloxacin and Sparfloxacin
Macrolides: Clarithromycin
Tetracyclines: Minocycline

Types
Lepromatous (LL), Tuberculoid (TT), Borderline (BT, BB, BL) & Indeterminate.

Paucibacillary leprosy (TT, BT): Non-infectious, 1–5 lesions with few bacilli. No or only one nerve involvement, skin smear is negative.

Multibacillary leprosy (BB, BL, LL): Infectious, 6 or more lesions with heavy load of bacilli, > one nerves involved, skin smear positive at least at one site.

Dapsone
- Inhibits dihydrofolate synthesis, leprostatic
- Resistance due to mutation in enzyme folate synthase, resulting in low affinity for drug
- Well absorbed orally, well distributed throughout body fluids and tissues except CSF, gets concentrated in skin, liver, muscles and kidney. Metabolised by acetylation, glucuronide/sulphate conjugation and shows enterohepatic circulation

Uses: In MDT for leprosy with rifampicin and clofazimine
- With pyrimethamine in chloroquine-resistant malaria, toxoplasmosis and *Pneumocystis jirovecii* infection

ADRs: Anorexia, nausea, vomiting, hypersensitivity reactions, phototoxic reactions, hemolysis in G6PD deficiency, may precipitate erythema nodosum leprosum (ENL) in severe LL cases. It may cause generalised malaise, fever, lymph node enlargement, jaundice, anemia and desquamation of skin (sulfone syndrome) in malnourished cases.

Clofazimine
Leprostatic effect due to interference with DNA template function, disruption of electron transport chain & altered membrane permeability.

Response is slower than dapsone.

Stored in reticuloendothelial tissues and subcutaneous fat → long half-life that allows intermittent therapy.

Uses: MDT for leprosy, lepra reactions or ENL, XDR-TB and *M. intracellulare* infection in AIDS patients.

ADRs: Red to brown or black discolouration of skin, GI adverse effects

Rifampicin
Rifampicin is the most potent cidal drug against *M. leprae*, having quick response, used as a component of standard MDT with dapsone and clofazimine.

It may cause type 2 lepra reactions or ENL and is contraindicated in hepatic and renal dysfunction.

National Leprosy Eradication Programme (2025 Guidelines)

For PBL: MDT with dapsone 100 mg daily + rifampicin 600 mg/month and clofazimine 50 mg/day and 300 mg/month given for 6 months.

For MBL: MDT with dapsone 100 mg/day + rifampicin 600 mg/month and clofazimine 50 mg/day and 300 mg/month given for 12 months.

SECTION 10 Chemotherapeutic Drugs

55 Antifungal Drugs

PH 8.8 Explain the types, kinetics, dynamics and adverse effects of drugs used for fungal infections.

Learning objectives

A student of MBBS phase II should be able to:
- Classify antifungal drugs.
- Describe the mechanism of action of antifungal drugs.
- Explain important pharmacokinetic features of drugs used in fungal infections.
- Enumerate therapeutic uses and ADRs of antifungal drugs.

Fungal infections can cause diseases that range from mild, manageable, superficial mycoses to severe and life-threatening systemic conditions. Important fungal infections in humans include aspergillosis, blastomycosis, candidiasis, cryptococcosis, chromoblastomycosis, histoplasmosis, mucormycosis, coccidioidomycosis, sporotrichosis, onychomycosis, fungal pneumonia, meningitis, and eye infections. The management of superficial, mucocutaneous fungal infections primarily relies on antifungal drugs applied topically at the site of infection, in the form of creams, gels, ointments, and similar formulations. Systemic absorption is negligible upon topical application; therefore, antifungal drugs are safe for topical use. However, for severe, life-threatening systemic fungal infections, systemic administration of antifungal drugs is required, which is associated with many toxic effects and interactions with other simultaneously administered drugs.

CLASSIFICATION

Antifungal drugs are classified (Flowchart 55.1) based on their **use** and **route of administration** into:

- **Systemic antifungal drugs:** Used for both **systemic** and **mucocutaneous fungal infections**.
- **Topical antifungal drugs:** Exclusively used for **mucocutaneous infections**.

Additionally, antifungal drugs can be classified based on their **mechanism of action** as inhibitors of synthesis of ergosterol/cell wall/nucleic acids and those that inhibit mitosis or increase cell membrane permeability (Flowchart 55.2).

A. SYSTEMIC DRUGS FOR SYSTEMIC FUNGAL INFECTIONS

1. Amphotericin B

Amphotericin B is a polyene antibiotic obtained from *Streptomyces nodosus*.

Mechanism of action

Amphotericin B exerts fungicidal effect (Fig. 55.1) by binding to ergosterol (a sterol in the fungal cell membrane), resulting in formation of pores that alter membrane permeability. This causes leakage of ions and macromolecules, ultimately leading to cell death. While high concentrations of the drug produce a fungicidal effect, lower doses exert fungistatic action.

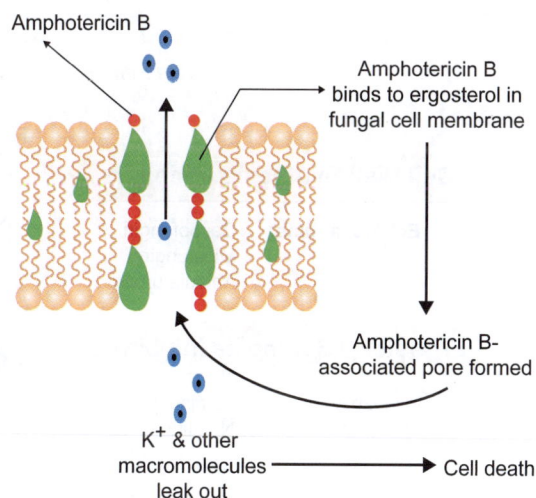

Fig. 55.1 Mechanism of action of amphotericin B

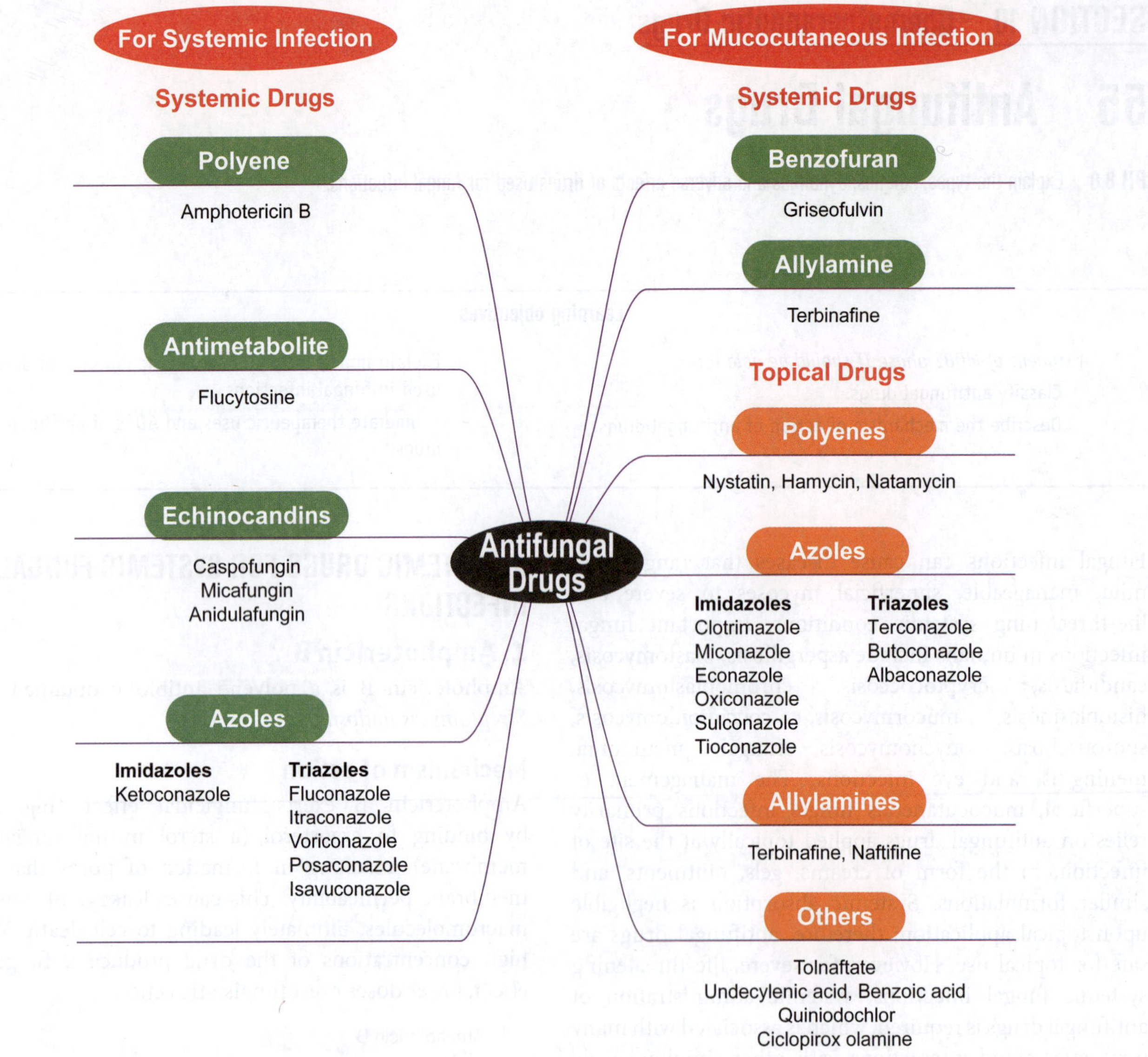

Classification of Antifungal Drugs

For Systemic Infection

Systemic Drugs

- **Polyene**: Amphotericin B
- **Antimetabolite**: Flucytosine
- **Echinocandins**: Caspofungin, Micafungin, Anidulafungin
- **Azoles**:
  - Imidazoles: Ketoconazole
  - Triazoles: Fluconazole, Itraconazole, Voriconazole, Posaconazole, Isavuconazole

For Mucocutaneous Infection

Systemic Drugs

- **Benzofuran**: Griseofulvin
- **Allylamine**: Terbinafine

Topical Drugs

- **Polyenes**: Nystatin, Hamycin, Natamycin
- **Azoles**:
  - Imidazoles: Clotrimazole, Miconazole, Econazole, Oxiconazole, Sulconazole, Tioconazole
  - Triazoles: Terconazole, Butoconazole, Albaconazole
- **Allylamines**: Terbinafine, Naftifine
- **Others**: Tolnaftate, Undecylenic acid, Benzoic acid, Quiniodochlor, Ciclopirox olamine

Flowchart 55.1 Classification of Antifungal Drugs

Classification based on mechanism of action

Antifungal Drugs

- **Cell Wall Synthesis Inhibitors**
  - Echinocandins: Caspofungin, Micafungin, Anidulafungin
- **Ergosterol Synthesis Inhibitors**
  - Imidazoles, Triazoles, Terbinafine, Naftifine
- **↑ed Cell Membrane Permeability**
  - Amphotericin B, Nystatin
- **Nucleic Acid Synthesis Inhibitor**
  - Flucytosine
- **Mitosis Inhibitor**
  - Griseofulvin

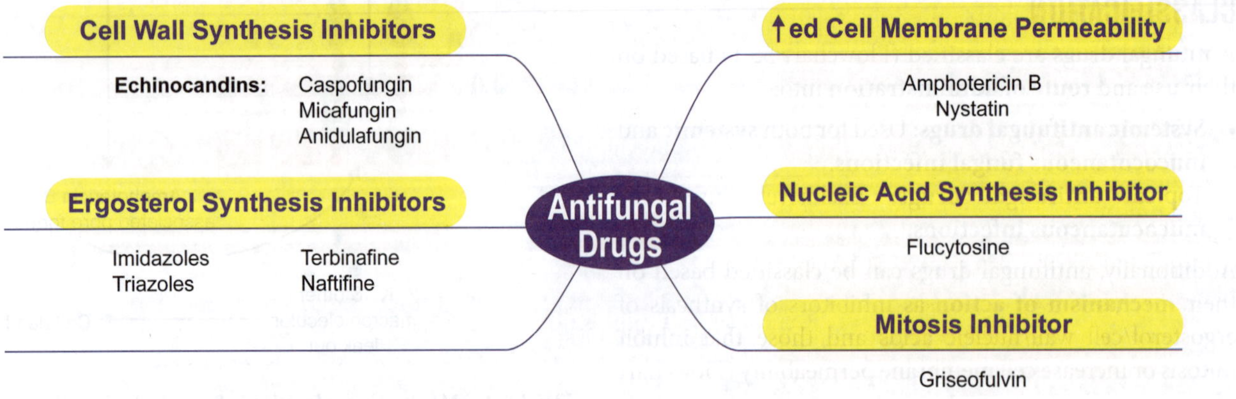

Flowchart 55.2 Classification of antifungal drugs based on mechanism of action

Amphotericin B has a broad spectrum of antifungal action. It is active against:
- Yeasts such as *Candida albicans* and *Cryptococcus neoformans*
- Fungi responsible for endemic mycosis such as *Histoplasma capsulatum*, *Blastomyces dermatitidis*, and *Coccidioides immitis*
- Molds such as *Aspergillus fumigatus* and *Mucor*

Mechanism of resistance: Resistance to amphotericin B develops due to reduced concentration of membrane ergosterol or decreased affinity of fungal ergosterol for the drug. However, resistance is not much of a problem in clinical use of amphotericin B.

Pharmacokinetics

Oral absorption of amphotericin B is poor as it is insoluble in water. Therefore, oral administration can only treat fungal infections within the gut lumen. For systemic fungal infections, intravenous administration is required. Because of its poor water solubility, amphotericin B is prepared as a colloidal suspension with sodium deoxycholate for IV infusion.

The drug is widely distributed in tissues, with up to 90% binding to plasma protein. However, its distribution to the CNS is limited due to high plasma protein binding and only 2–3% of blood levels are reached in CSF. Hence, in fungal meningitis, intrathecal administration is indicated. Approximately 60% of the administered amphotericin B is metabolised by the liver and eliminated in bile; some part is slowly excreted in urine. However, metabolism of amphotericin B is not much affected by hepatobiliary diseases, and therefore, dose adjustment is not required in hepatic function impairment.

Amphotericin B has a long half-life (15 days).

Therapeutic uses

1. Life-threatening mycotic infections: Amphotericin B is the drug of choice for almost all life-threatening mycotic infections. It is used initially as 'induction therapy' in serious fungal infections, especially in immunocompromised patients with fungal pneumonia and cryptococcal meningitis with altered mental status. Amphotericin B is administered by slow IV infusion in a dose of 0.5–1 mg/kg body weight/day. In such cases, maintenance therapy is usually with azoles.
2. Amphotericin B is the preferred drug for invasive **a**spergillosis, **b**lastomycosis, **c**ryptococcosis, **c**andida esophagitis, **c**occidioidomycosis, **p**aracoccidioidomycosis, **m**ucormycosis, **h**istoplasmosis and extracutaneous **s**porotrichosis, etc. [Mnemonic: **ABC** of **P**olicies of **M**inistry of **H**ealth and **S**anitation].
3. Topical administration of amphotericin B is useful in cutaneous, vaginal and oropharyngeal candidiasis. Local administration of amphotericin B is successful as eyedrops in mycotic corneal ulcers/keratitis, intra-articular injection in fungal arthritis and as bladder irrigation in candiduria.
4. Amphotericin B is very effective in the management of visceral as well as mucocutaneous leishmaniasis.

ADRs

- Amphotericin B causes **immediate infusion-related reactions** such as fever, chills, muscular spasm, headache, vomiting, and fall in BP, in nearly all patients. Such adverse effects can be reduced by lowering the dose or slowing the infusion rate. Premedication with antipyretics, antihistamines and corticosteroids is also effective.
- Amphotericin B has some affinity for human cell membrane sterols (mainly cholesterol), which results in toxic effects. The most significant toxic reaction of amphotericin B is renal damage secondary to reduced renal perfusion and renal tubular injury. Renal damage leads to azotemia, acidosis, hypokalemia and inability to concentrate urine. It can be checked by sodium loading, and therefore, normal saline infusion is usually given with daily doses of amphotericin B.
- Intrathecal injection may cause headache, vomiting and nerve palsy.

However, in newer preparations, amphotericin B is packaged in lipid-associated delivery systems called **liposomal amphotericin B,** which is less toxic and achieves targeted delivery, especially in the reticuloendothelial cells of liver and spleen. Incidence of infusion-related reactions and renal damage is lower with liposomal amphotericin B than with colloidal amphotericin. The affinity of the drug for lipids of the vehicle is between that for fungal ergosterol and mammalian cholesterol. Thus, the drug binds preferentially to the fungal membrane ergosterol, reducing the toxicity without compromising efficacy. Reduction in toxicity allows administration of higher dosages. Liposomal amphotericin B is especially useful in kala azar, critically ill patients with deep mycosis, and immunocompromised patients. Although liposomal amphotericin B is equally efficacious and less toxic than the colloidal preparation, it is more expensive.

Clinical problem-based questions and MCQs

1. **Amphotericin B is a broad-spectrum antifungal drug, useful in all the following conditions, EXCEPT:**
   a. Blastomycosis
   b. Paracoccidioidomycosis
   c. Onychomycosis
   d. Cryptococcal meningitis

2. **A 65-year-old patient, diabetic for the last 30 years, presented in OPD with headache, slurring of speech, nasal congestion and swelling on left side of face, since last evening. On examination, there are brownish-black lesions on nose bridge, nasal mucosa**

is congested. KOH staining confirms diagnosis of mucormycosis.
   i. Identify the drug of choice amongst the following:
      a. Clotrimazole   b. Caspofungin
      c. Amphotericin B d. Griseofulvin
   ii. Describe the mechanism of action of the selected drug.
   iii. Enumerate adverse effects of the selected drug, and methods to prevent the same.
3. Identify the advantage of liposomal amphotericin B preparation over colloidal amphotericin B
   a. Better oral absorption
   b. Bypasses hepatic first-pass metabolism
   c. Better penetration into CNS
   d. Lower toxicity

2. Echinocandins

These include semisynthetic cyclic lipopeptides like caspofungin, micafungin and anidulafungin.

Mechanism of action

Echinocandins act by inhibiting the β-glucan synthase enzyme complex in the fungal plasma membrane. This enzyme complex is responsible for the synthesis of a unique component of the fungal cell wall, β-1,3-glucan. The cross-linking of β-1,3-glucan with fibrillar polysaccharide-chitin toughens the fungal cell wall. Echinocandins inhibit the synthesis of β-1,3-glucan and weaken the fungal cell wall, which results in cell death due to osmotic susceptibility (Fig. 55.2). Echinocandins exert fungicidal action against candida species, and are also effective against triazole-resistant organisms. However, they have static action against aspergillus.

a. **Caspofungin** is not absorbed orally and is therefore administered by the IV route. 70 mg is infused over one hour, and then 50 mg is injected daily. It is useful in deep/invasive candidiasis, esophageal candidiasis, invasive aspergillosis, and in immunocompromised patients with non-responding fever.

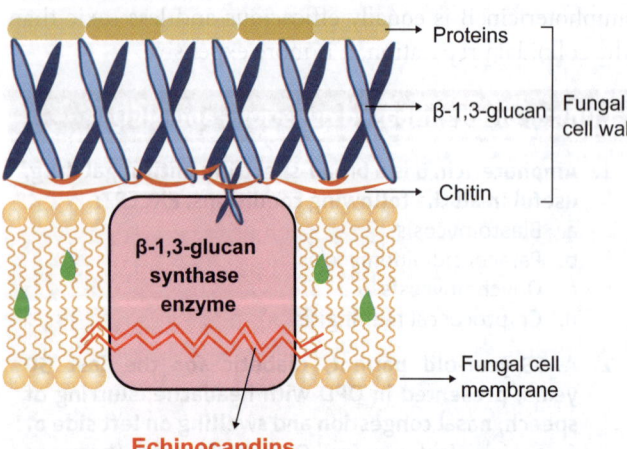

Fig. 55.2 Mechanism of action of echinocandins

ADRs: It is a well-tolerated drug; however, it may cause rashes, vomiting, joint pain, dyspnea, hypokalemia and acute febrile reaction.

b. **Micafungin** is longer acting with a half-life of 12–15 hours. It is effective in esophageal candidiasis, candidemia, and for prophylaxis of candida infection in bone marrow transplant patients.

c. **Anidulafungin** has a half-life of 36 hours.

3. Flucytosine

It is a potent antifungal drug that is chemically related to 5-fluorouracil.

Mechanism of action

Flucytosine enters fungal cells by the action of enzyme cytosine permease. Inside the cell (Fig. 55.3), it is first deaminated by the action of enzyme cytosine deaminase to form 5-fluorouracil (5-FU). 5-FU is then phosphorylated to form 5-fluorouridine monophosphate (FUMP).

- FUMP gets converted to 5-fluoro-deoxyuridinemonophosphate (5-FdUMP) through the action of ribonucleotide reductase and inhibits DNA synthesis.
- FUMP also forms 5-fluoro-uridinetriphosphate (5-FUTP) through the action of kinase and inhibits RNA synthesis. Both actions result in fungicidal activity.

Human cells cannot metabolise flucytosine into these active metabolites. However, flucytosine shows synergistic activity with amphotericin B, owing to enhanced penetration of fungal cells by flucytosine through amphotericin B-associated pores in the fungal cell membrane (Fig. 55.3). Flucytosine also shows synergism with azoles in vitro, but the mechanism is not clearly understood.

Mechanism of resistance: When used alone, resistance develops to flucytosine through alterations in its metabolic pathway.

Spectrum: Flucytosine has narrow antifungal spectrum. It is effective only against *Cryptococcus neoformans*, some *Candida* species and the molds which cause chromoblastomycoses.

Pharmacokinetics

Flucytosine is well absorbed (> 90%) orally. It has poor plasma protein binding and penetrates well into all body fluids and compartments, including CSF. Elimination occurs via the renal route by glomerular filtration, with a half-life of 3–4 hours. There is a narrow therapeutic window for flucytosine, because toxic reactions occur at higher drug levels, while resistance develops rapidly at subtherapeutic levels. Therefore, serum concentration should be monitored periodically to reduce the risk of toxic reactions, especially when it is combined with nephrotoxic agents like amphotericin B.

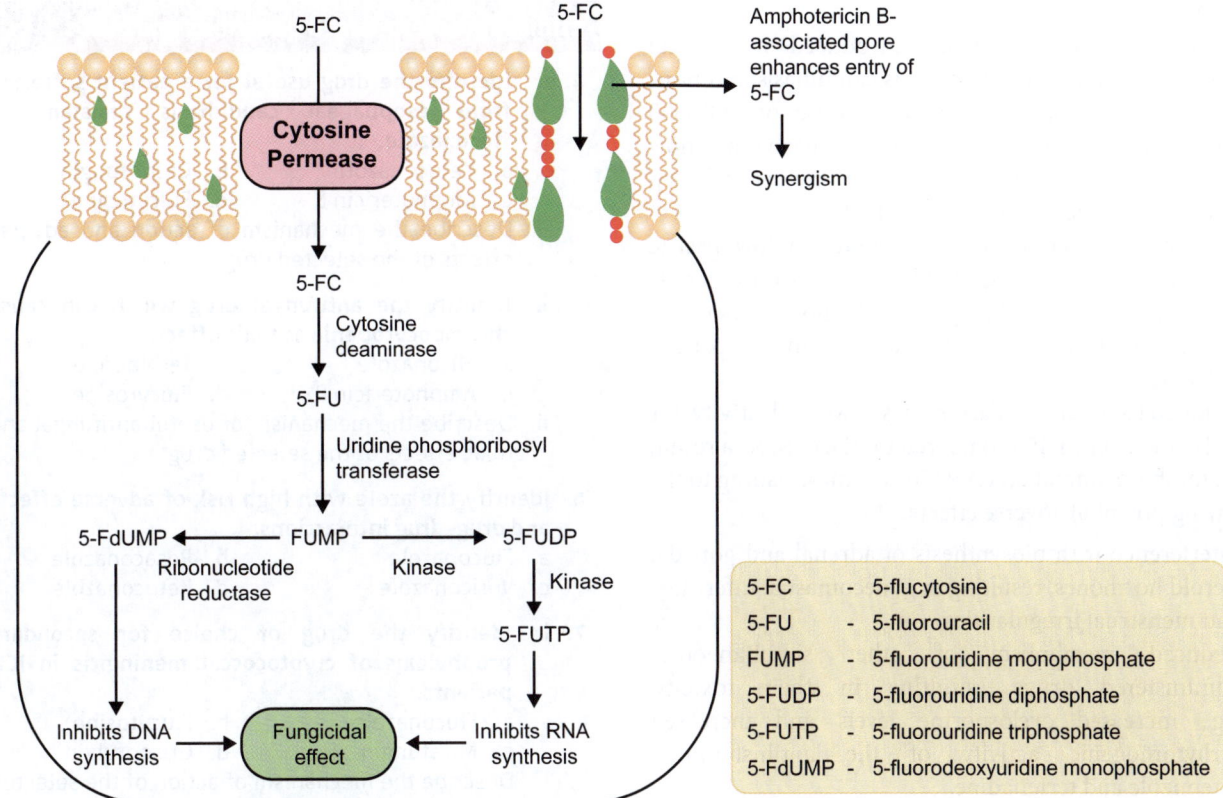

Fig. 55.3 Mechanism of action of flucytosine

Therapeutic uses
Flucytosine is used as combination therapy with amphotericin B for cryptococcal meningitis, and with itraconazole for chromoblastomycosis. It is given in a dose of 150 mg/kg/day by oral route in patients having normal renal function.

ADRs
Toxic effects of flucytosine are more commonly observed in patients with renal function impairment and AIDS. Drug may get metabolised by intestinal flora to form 5-FU, which causes toxic effects. Bone marrow toxicity manifesting as anemia, thrombocytopenia and leukopenia may occur. Liver enzymes are deranged. Toxic enterocolitis may be caused.

4. Azoles
These are synthetic compounds that have a five-membered azole ring in their structure. These include:
- **Imidazoles:** Ketoconazole (oral/topical), clotrimazole, econazole, miconazole and oxiconazole (topical)
- **Triazoles:** Fluconazole, itraconazole, voriconazole, posaconazole, isavuconazole (systemic), terconazole, butoconazole (topical)

Mechanism of action
Azoles exert antifungal effect by inhibiting the fungal cytochrome P450 enzyme, 'lanosterol 14-demethylase', which is responsible for converting lanosterol to ergosterol. This results in reduced ergosterol synthesis (Fig 55.4). The affinity for fungal CYP is much more than that for human CYP enzyme. However, specificity for fungal CYP is lower with imidzoles than triazoles. Therefore, ADRs and drug–drug interactions are more frequently seen with imidazoles.

The **spectrum of antifungal activity of azoles** is broad, including candida species, *Cryptococcus neoformans*, endemic mycosis (histoplasmosis, blastomycosis, coccidioidomycosis), dermatophytes and *Aspergillus*, *Nocardia* and *Leishmania*. However, azoles do not affect *Mucor*.

Resistance to azoles is not a major concern, except for resistance to fluconazole in *Candida*, which causes deep mycosis such as esophageal mycosis. Such organisms, however, respond well to itraconazole and voriconazole.

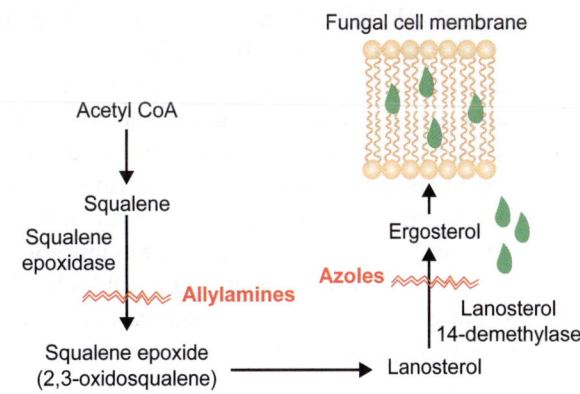

Fig. 55.4 Mechanism of action of allylamines and azoles

a. Ketoconazole

Ketoconazole, the first azole introduced in clinical practice is useful in mucocutaneous candidiasis and non-meningeal coccidioidomycosis, in a dose of 200–600 mg/day. However, itraconazole and fluconazole are now preferred over ketoconazole for their greater efficacy, longer half-life, and fewer adverse effects.

Absorption of ketoconazole is better at low gastric pH. Hence, agents such as H_2 blockers that raise gastric pH interfere with its absorption. Rifampicin increases hepatic metabolism of ketoconazole, resulting in reduced effectiveness.

Ketoconazole, an imidazole, has lower selectivity for fungal cytochrome P450 compared to triazoles. As a result, it can inhibit mammalian CYP450 enzymes, leading to the following potential adverse effects:

- Interference with biosynthesis of adrenal and gonadal steroid hormones, resulting in gynecomastia, infertility, and menstrual irregularities.
- Reduced metabolism of other simultaneously administered drugs, resulting in their toxicity, e.g., increased cyclosporine levels and increased arrhythmogenic activity of the antihistamines, astemizole and terfenadine.

b. Itraconazole

It is the most potent drug among the azoles, used in a daily dose of 100-400 mg orally.

- It is well absorbed at low gastric pH and when given with food. Penetration into CSF is poor.
- It is the drug of choice for dermatophytosis, histoplasmosis, blastomycosis, sporothrix infection and onychomycosis. It is the only azole that has significant effect in aspergillosis.
- It interacts with hepatic microsomal enzymes to a lesser extent compared to ketoconazole. So, steroid hormone synthesis is not much affected and there are fewer interactions with other drugs cleared by liver.

c. Fluconazole

Fluconazole is effective orally in a dose of 100–800 mg/day.

- It has good water solubility, and thus can be used by the IV route.
- It has minimal interaction with human hepatic microsomal enzyme, and therefore, the least risk of drug interactions. Also, it has a wide therapeutic window.
- Fluconazole is the drug of choice for secondary prophylaxis of cryptococcal meningitis, candidemia in ICU patients, and prophylaxis in individuals with AIDS or undergoing bone marrow transplantation. It penetrates well into CSF and is as effective as intrathecal amphotericin B in coccidioidal meningitis. It is also the drug of choice in mucocutaneous candidiasis; however, ketoconazole remains in use for this indication due to its lower cost.

Clinical problem-based questions and MCQs

4. i. Identify the drug useful for a patient suffering from esophageal candidiasis resistant to fluconazole.
   - a. Ketoconazole
   - b. Caspofungin
   - c. Amphotericin B
   - d. Flucytosine
   ii. Describe the mechanism of action and adverse effects of the selected drug.

5. i. Identify the antifungal drug which can cause thrombocytopenia as toxic effect.
   - a. Miconazole
   - b. Terbinafine
   - c. Amphotericin B
   - d. Flucytosine.
   ii. Describe the mechanism of useful antifungal and toxic effects of the selected drug.

6. Identify the azole with high risk of adverse effects and drug–drug interactions.
   - a. Fluconazole
   - b. Posaconazole
   - c. Voriconazole
   - d. Ketoconazole

7. i. Identify the drug of choice for secondary prophylaxis of cryptococcal meningitis in ICU patients.
   - a. Fluconazole
   - b. Flucytosine
   - c. Micafungin
   - d. Griseofulvin
   ii. Describe the mechanism of action of the selected drug.

B. SYSTEMIC DRUGS FOR MUCOCUTANEOUS FUNGAL INFECTIONS

1. Griseofulvin

Mechanism of action

Griseofulvin is a fungistatic drug which gets deposited in newly forming cells, binds to the keratin there, and protects the skin from new infections. Its mechanism of action at the cellular level is not clearly understood. It likely interferes with mitosis, resulting in the formation of stunted, multinucleated hyphae. Since it prevents infection of new cells, it must be administered for at least 2–6 weeks; this allows new infection-resistant skin/hair cells to replace the infected keratin. Nail infections require longer therapy (few months) to allow the growth of new, protected nail.

Therapeutic uses

Griseofulvin is used in a dose of 1 g/day for systemic treatment of dermatophytosis. Griseofulvin is water-insoluble, but its absorption is enhanced by using a microcrystalline formulation and administering it with fatty food. It has largely been replaced by itraconazole and terbinafine for this indication.

ADRs

Griseofulvin can cause serum sickness-like allergic reaction and hepatitis. It induces metabolism of warfarin, whereas phenobarbitone may induce griseofulvin metabolism.

2. Terbinafine

Mechanism of action

Terbinafine is an allylamine, which exerts fungicidal action by interfering with ergosterol synthesis due to inhibition of fungal squalene epoxidase enzyme (Fig 55.4). Thus, squalene accumulates, which is toxic to the organism.

Terbinafine gets concentrated in keratin-containing cells. It is useful in dermatophytosis, especially onychomycosis, in a daily dose of 250 mg administered orally. After administration for 12 weeks, the cure rate in nail infections is 90%, which is higher than that with the fungistatic drug griseofulvin and the oral azole itraconazole.

ADRs

Terbinafine can cause mild adverse effects such as headache and GI upset. It does not show significant drug interactions because of its lack of effect on human cytochrome P450 enzymes.

C. TOPICAL ANTIFUNGAL DRUGS

1. Polyenes

Polyenes **nystatin, hamycin** and **natamycin** have similar mechanism of action as amphotericin B, but are too toxic for systemic administration. Hence, they are used only topically as creams, ointments and suppositories. Because systemic absorption after topical application on skin/mucous membrane is negligible, toxicity is not caused by topical use.

- Nystatin is useful for suppression of local candida infections like oropharyngeal thrush, vaginal candidiasis, and intertriginous candidiasis.
- Hamycin is similar to nystatin, but is more water soluble. It is used topically for oral thrush, cutaneous candidiasis, vaginitis, otomycosis etc.
- Natamycin has a broader spectrum than nystatin. It is mainly used for fungal keratitis, as it is non-irritant to the eyes.

2. Azoles

Clotrimazole: It is effective in topical treatment of tinea infection, oral thrush, athletes foot, and otomycosis. It is particularly preferred for vaginitis because of its residual effect (i.e., ability to remain active at the site of application) following once-a-day application. There are no systemic adverse effects after topical application, although local irritation, stinging and burning sensation have been reported.

Econazole is as effective as clotrimazole in dermatophytosis, otomycosis, and oral thrush, but less effective than clotrimazole in vaginitis.

Miconazole is very effective for tinea, vulvovaginitis and cutaneous candidiasis. However, vaginal irritation is more frequently reported with miconazole than with clotrimazole.

3. Other Topical Agents

- **Tolnaftate:** It is effective against tinea cruris and tinea corporis. However, it is less effective against tinea pedis and not effective against tinea capitis and tinea unguium because of poor penetration. Tolnaftate is not effective in candidiasis as well. It is less irritant than many topical agents, excluding imidazoles.
- **Ciclopirox olamine:** It is useful against tinea, pityriasis, dermal candidiasis, and vaginal infections. It has good local tolerance.
- **Undecylenic acid** is inferior to other topical agents.
- **Benzoic acid** is a fungistatic drug used as an important ingredient in Whitfield ointment.
- **Sodium thiosulphate** is a weak fungistatic agent, useful in pityriasis versicolor.
- **Quiniodochlor** is used in dermatophytosis, eczema, seborrheic dermatitis, etc.

Clinical problem-based questions and MCQs

8. Which antifungal drug gets deposited in newly formed keratin?
   a. Amphotericin B b. Griseofulvin
   c. Undecylenic acid d. All of the above

9. i. Identify the drug that has maximum cure rate in fungal infections of nails.
   a. Itraconazole b. Griseofulvin
   c. Terbinafine d. Flucytosine
   ii. Describe the mechanism of action of the selected drug.

10. All of the following drugs are fungicidal, EXCEPT:
    a. Amphotericin B b. Micafungin
    c. Griseofulvin d. Flucytosine

Summary

- Antifungal drugs include systemic drugs and topical drugs. Systemic antifungals include amphotericin B, echinocandins, flucytosine.
- **Amphotericin B (AMB)** binds to fungal ergosterol and forms pores in the fungal membrane through which macromolecules leak out, resulting in cell death (fungicidal action). It is effective against many fungi that cause serious systemic mycosis. AMB is the drug of choice for invasive aspergillosis, blastomycosis, cryptococcal pneumonia/meningitis, Candida esophagitis, coccidioido-/paracoccidioido-mycosis, etc. It is used as IV infusion. ADRs include infusion-related reactions and renal damage, which can be reduced by using liposomal AMB that has the advantage of targeted delivery and fewer adverse effects than the colloidal preparation.

- **Echinocandins** such as caspofungin, micafungin and anidulafungin inhibit the synthesis of β-1,3-glucan, weakening the fungal cell wall → osmotic susceptibility → fungicidal action; they are effective against *Candida* and triazole-resistant organisms. However, they have static action against aspergillus. Caspofungin is used in deep/invasive candidiasis, esophageal candidiasis, invasive aspergillosis, and in immunocompromised patients with non-responding fever. It is a well-tolerated drug; can cause rashes, vomiting, joint pain, dyspnea, hypokalemia and acute febrile reaction in some cases.
- **Flucytosine** is deaminated and phosphorylated inside the fungal cell to form FUMP, which is then converted to 5-FdUMP and 5-FUTP which inhibit DNA and RNA synthesis, respectively, resulting in cidal action. Effective only against *Cryptococcus neoformans*, some *Candida* species and the molds that cause chromoblastomycoses. It shows synergism with AMB as well as azoles. Toxic effects include bone marrow toxicity, derangement of hepatic enzymes and toxic enterocolitis.
- **Azoles** include **imidazoles** [ketoconazole (oral/topical), clotrimazole, econazole, miconazole and oxiconazole (topical)] and **triazoles** [fluconazole, itraconazole, voriconazole, posaconazole, isavuconazole (systemic), terconazole, butoconazole (topical)]. They act by interfering with the conversion of lanosterol to ergosterol. Imidazoles have lower selectivity for fungal cytochrome P450 compared to triazoles, resulting in greater risk of adverse effects such as gynecomastia, infertility, and menstrual irregularities and drug–drug interactions.
- **Systemic azoles,** e.g., itraconazole, is the drug of choice for dermatophytosis, histoplasmosis, blastomycosis, sporothrix infection and onychomycosis, and fluconazole in secondary prophylaxis of cryptococcal meningitis and candidemia in ICU patients.
- **Systemic drugs for superficial mycosis** include griseofulvin and terbinafine. **Griseofulvin** gets deposited in newly forming cells and interferes with mitosis, resulting in the formation of stunted, multinucleated hyphae and fungistatic action. Long-term treatment is required for weeks, even months, to replace the infected keratin with new, infection-resistant cells. ADRs include serum sickness-like allergic reaction and hepatitis. Itraconazole and terbinafine are preferred over griseofulvin for dermatophytosis and onychomycosis. **Terbinafine** gets concentrated in keratin-containing cells and exerts fungicidal action by inhibition of fungal squalene epoxidase enzyme. It is useful in dermatophytosis, especially onychomycosis, with maximum cure rate (90%) in nail infections.
- **Topical azoles** are useful in tinea infection, oral thrush, athlete's foot, otomycosis, vulvovaginitis, etc. ADRs are mild in the form of local irritation, stinging and burning sensation.
- Ciclopirox olamine, benzoic acid, tolnaftate, and sodium thiosulphate are some other topical antifungal agents.

Questions for Practice

1. Explain why:
   a. Liposomal amphotericin B is preferred over colloidal preparations.
   b. Itraconazole is preferred over ketoconazole in systemic fungal infections.
   c. Terbinafine is preferred over griseofulvin in fungal infection of nails.
   d. Griseofulvin is given with food.
2. Write short notes on:
   a. Topicl antifungal drugs
   b. Azoles
   c. Liposomal amphotericin B

Hints for problem-based questions and MCQs

1. c. Onychomycosis
2. i. c. Amphotericin B
   ii. AMB binds to fungal ergosterol, and forms pores, through which macromolecules leak out, resulting in fungicidal action. Refer to page 725, Fig. 55.1.
   iii Severe infusion-related reactions such as headache, fever, chills, vomiting, muscular pain and fall in BP. Prolonged use is associated with renal damage. Prevention of ADRs by premedication with antihistamines, antipyretics and corticosteroids. Use of liposomal AMB reduces acute infusion-related adverse effects as well as renal damage.
3. d. Lower toxicity, because affinity of the drug for lipids of vehicle is intermediate between that for fungal ergosterol and mammalian cholesterol. Thus, the drug binds preferentially to fungal membrane ergosterol, reducing the toxicity without compromising efficacy of targeted delivery.
4. i. b. Caspofungin
   ii. Acts by interfering with synthesis of β-1,3-glucan, weakening the fungal cell wall, cidal action due to osmotic susceptibility. ADRs include rashes, vomiting, joint pain, dyspnea, hypokalemia and acute febrile reaction.
5. i. d. Flucytosine
   ii. Antifungal effect due to inhibition of DNA, RNA synthesis in fungi. Toxicity due to bone marrow suppression by 5-FU, formed from flucytosine by intestinal flora.
6. d. Ketoconazole
7. i. a. Fluconazole
   ii. Inhibits lanosterol 14-demethylase, thus interfering with the conversion of lanosterol to ergosterol. Refer to page 729.
8. b. Griseofulvin
9. i. c. Terbinafine
   ii. Inhibits squalene epoxidase, causes accumulation of squalene, which is toxic to cell.
10. c. Griseofulvin

CONCEPT MAP – ANTIFUNGAL DRUGS

Amphotericin B

Mechanism: Binds to 'ergosterol' in fungal cell membrane → forms pores → alters membrane permeability → ions/macromolecules leak out, resulting in fungal cell death.

It has the broadest spectrum of antifungal action, including *Candida albicans*, *Cryptococcus neoformans*, *H. capsulatum*, *Blastomyces dermatitis*, *Coccidioides immitis*, *Aspergillus fumigatus* & *Mucor*

Kinetics: Insoluble in water, poor oral absorption, intravenous administration is required for systemic fungal infections.

Uses: Used initially as 'induction therapy' in serious fungal infections, such as fungal pneumonia, meningitis, especially in immunocompromised patients. Maintenance therapy in such cases is with azoles.

ADRs: Immediate infusion-related reactions such as fever, chills, muscular spasm, headache, vomiting and fall in BP. Renal damage → checked by sodium loading. The incidence of infusion-related reactions and renal damage is lower with liposomal amphotericin B.

Echinocandins

Caspofungin, micafungin & anidulafungin

Mechanism: Inhibit β-glucan synthase enzyme complex in the fungal plasma membrane → inhibit synthesis of β-1,3-glucan → weaken the fungal cell wall → osmotic susceptibility→ fungicidal effect.

Kinetics: Not absorbed orally → used by IV route.

Uses: Caspofungin in deep/invasive candidiasis, esophageal candidiasis, invasive aspergillosis, and in immunocompromised patients with non-responding fever.

ADRs: Well tolerated, however may cause rashes, vomiting, joint pain, dyspnea, hypokalemia and acute febrile reaction.

Micafungin and anidulafungin are longer acting than caspofungin.

Azoles

Imidazoles: Ketoconazole (oral), miconazole and clotrimazole (topical)

Triazoles: Itraconazole and fluconazole (oral), terconazole (topical)

Mechanism: Inhibit fungal cytochrome P450 enzyme, resulting in reduced ergosterol synthesis.

Broad spectrum including *Candida species*, *Cryptococcus neoformans*, endemic mycosis (histoplasmosis, blastomycosis, coccidioidomycosis), dermatophytes and *Aspergillus*.

Uses: Fluconazole is the drug of choice for secondary prophylaxis of cryptococcal meningitis, candidemia in ICU patients, & for prophylaxis in AIDS & bone marrow transplant patients & mucocutaneous candidiasis.

Itraconazole is drug of choice for dermatophytoses, histoplasmosis, blastomycosis, sporothrix infection, onychomycosis. It is the only agent possessing significant effect in aspergillosis.

Flucytosine

Taken up by the fungal cells via 'cytosine permease' → forms 5-FU and then 5-fluorouridine monophosphate (FUMP), which forms 5-fluorodeoxyuridine monophosphate (5-FdUMP) → inhibits DNA synthesis & 5-fluorouridine triphosphate (5-FUTP) → inhibits RNA synthesis

Synergistic activity with amphotericin B, owing to enhanced penetration of fungal cell by flucytosine through amphotericin-B-associated pores.

Effective only against *Cryptococcus neoformans*, some *Candida* species and the molds which cause chromoblastomycosis

Uses: Flucytosine is used as combination therapy with amphotericin B for cryptococcal meningitis, and with itraconazole for chromoblastomycosis.

ADRs: Flucytosine may get metabolised by intestinal flora to form 5-FU, which causes bone marrow toxicity → anemia, thrombocytopenia & leukopenia. Liver enzymes are deranged, toxic enterocolitis may occur.

For systemic infections

Antifungal Drugs

For mucocutaneous infections

Systemic Drugs

Griseofulvin

Mechanism: Fungistatic drug, gets deposited in newly forming cells, binds the keratin there, and protects the skin from new infection.

Uses: Is used in a dose of 1 g/day for systemic treatment of dermatophytosis for at least 2–6 weeks so that new, infection-resistant skin/hair cells replace infected keratin. Largely been replaced by itraconazole and terbinafine for this indication.

ADRs: Serum sickness-like allergic reaction, hepatitis and drug interactions due to enzyme induction.

Terbinafine

Mechanism of action: Inhibits fungal squalene epoxidase → interferes with ergosterol synthesis, causes squalene accumulation, which is toxic to the organism.

Terbinafine gets concentrated in keratin containing cells, & is useful in dermatophytosis, especially onychomycosis in a dose of 250 mg daily given by oral route. 90% cure rate after 12 weeks of treatment.

ADRs: Mild, such as headache and GI upset. No effect on human cytochrome P450 enzymes → less risk of drug interactions.

Topical Drugs

Polyenes: Nystatin, hamycin, natamycin have similar mechanism of action as amphotericin B.

Used only topically as creams, ointments, suppositories for suppression of local candida infection like oropharyngeal thrush, vaginal candidiasis, intertriginous candidiasis.

Azoles: Clotrimazole is effective in topical treatment of tinea infection, oral thrush, athlete's foot, otomycosis.

It is particularly preferred for vaginitis because of its residual effect after once-daily application.

Econazole is less effective than clotrimazole in vaginitis.

Miconazole: Vaginal irritation is more frequently reported with it than with clotrimazole.

Tolnaftate: It is effective against tinea cruris and tinea corporis, but due to poor penetration → less effective against tinea pedis and not effective against tinea capitis and tinea unguium.

Ciclopirox olamine: It is useful against tinea, pityriasis, dermal candidiasis, vaginal infection & has good local tolerance.

Benzoic acid: Is fungistatic drug, and is used as an important ingredient in Whitfield ointment.

Sodium thiosulphate: Is a weak fungistatic agent, useful in pityriasis versicolor.

Quiniodochlor: Used in dermatophytosis, eczema, seborrheic dermatitis, etc.

SECTION 10 Chemotherapeutic Drugs

56 Antiviral Drugs

PH 8.10 Discuss the types, kinetics, dynamics, adverse effects, indications and contraindications of drugs used for viral diseases

---

Learning objectives

A student of MBBS phase II should be able to:
- Classify antiviral drugs.
- Describe the mechanism of action of antiviral drugs.
- Enumerate therapeutic uses of antiviral drugs.
- Enlist ADRs and contraindications of antiviral drugs.

INTRODUCTION

Viruses are the most abundant of all biological entities. They are submicroscopic infectious agents that **can replicate only inside the living cells of a host,** which maybe a human, animal, plant or bacterial cell. Viruses exist as independent particles called virions. Each **virion comprises** (Fig. 56.1):

- A nucleic acid core that contains genetic material (either DNA or RNA)
- A protein coat called 'capsid' surrounding the genetic material
- An outer envelope of lipids

The virions of most of virus species are 1/100th the size of bacteria, i.e., submicroscopic, and cannot be seen with an optical microscope.

Viruses can be **transmitted vertically as well as horizontally.** Vertical transmission occurs from mother to fetus, e.g., hepatitis B virus (HBV), human immunodeficiency virus (HIV), and varicella zoster virus (VZV). Horizontal transmission of viral infection occurs through exchange of body fluids, intake of contaminated food, water or aerosols containing the virus, and insect vectors. Most **viral infections have an incubation period** ranging from few days to few weeks, during which the patient remains asymptomatic. The incubation period is followed by or overlaps with a period of communicability, wherein the infected person is contagious, i.e., capable of spreading the infection to others.

An outbreak of a viral infection in a population, community or region is called an epidemic. Outbreaks that spread worldwide are called pandemics, e.g., the ongoing HIV pandemic since the 1980s, the SARS pandemic in 2003, and the 2019 coronavirus pandemic.

Prominent human viral diseases include hepatitis, herpes simplex infection, HIV, influenza and other respiratory infections.

There are **two challenges in antiviral drug development.**

- Drugs which damage the virus can damage the host cell also.
- While the infected person is asymptomatic during the incubation period, they can spread the infection to others.

To reduce the risk of host cell damage, the different steps of viral replication are identified. Drugs are chosen to interfere with these steps such that they check viral multiplication without suppressing the host cell metabolic processes.

The main steps in viral replication include: viral attachment and entry into the host cell; uncoating of viral genetic material; nucleic acid synthesis; early and late protein synthesis; and the packaging, assembly and release of virions. Antiviral drugs interfere with viral replication at different steps (Fig. 56.2), for example:

- Docosanol and interferon block the very first step, i.e., viral attachment and entry into host cells.

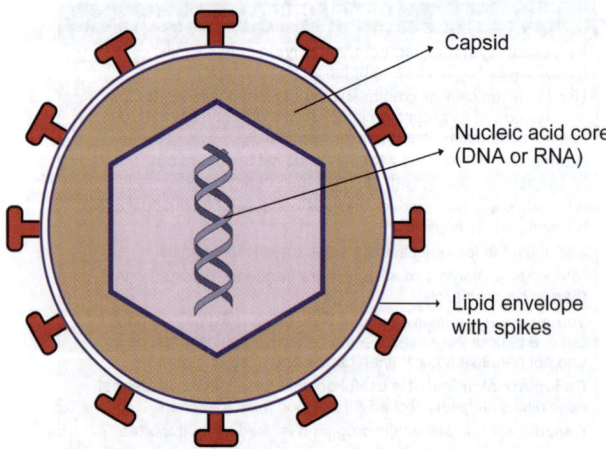

Fig. 56.1 Structure of virion

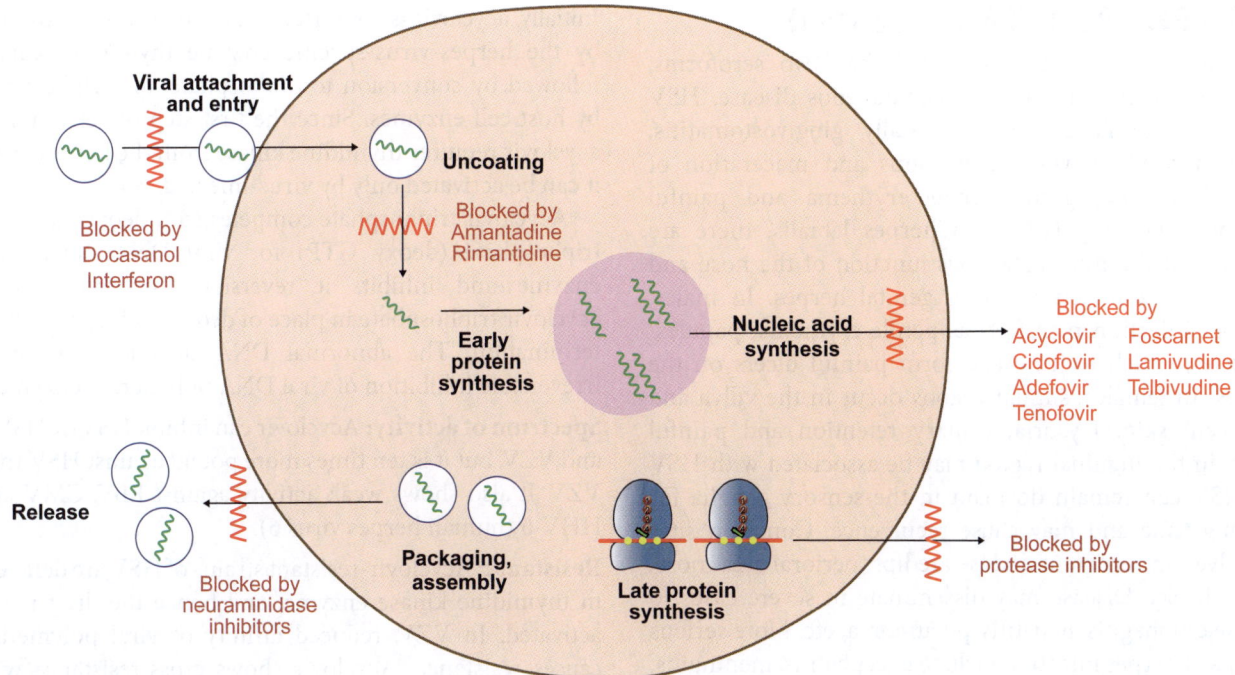

Fig. 56.2 Steps of viral replication and sites of action of antiviral drugs

- Uncoating of viral DNA/RNA inside host cells is blocked by amantadine and rimantadine.
- Drugs such as acyclovir and its analogues, adefovir, tenofovir, cidofovir, foscarnet, lamivudine and telbivudine, inhibit nucleic acid synthesis.
- Protease inhibitors block late protein synthesis.
- Neuraminidase inhibitors such as oseltamivir interfere with the last step of viral replication, i.e., release of virions.

CLASSIFICATION OF ANTIVIRAL DRUGS

All antiviral drugs are virustatic. They are classified based on the viruses against which they are effective, such as drugs for HSV/VZV, CMV, RSV/influenza virus, HBV, and HCV (Flowchart 56.1).

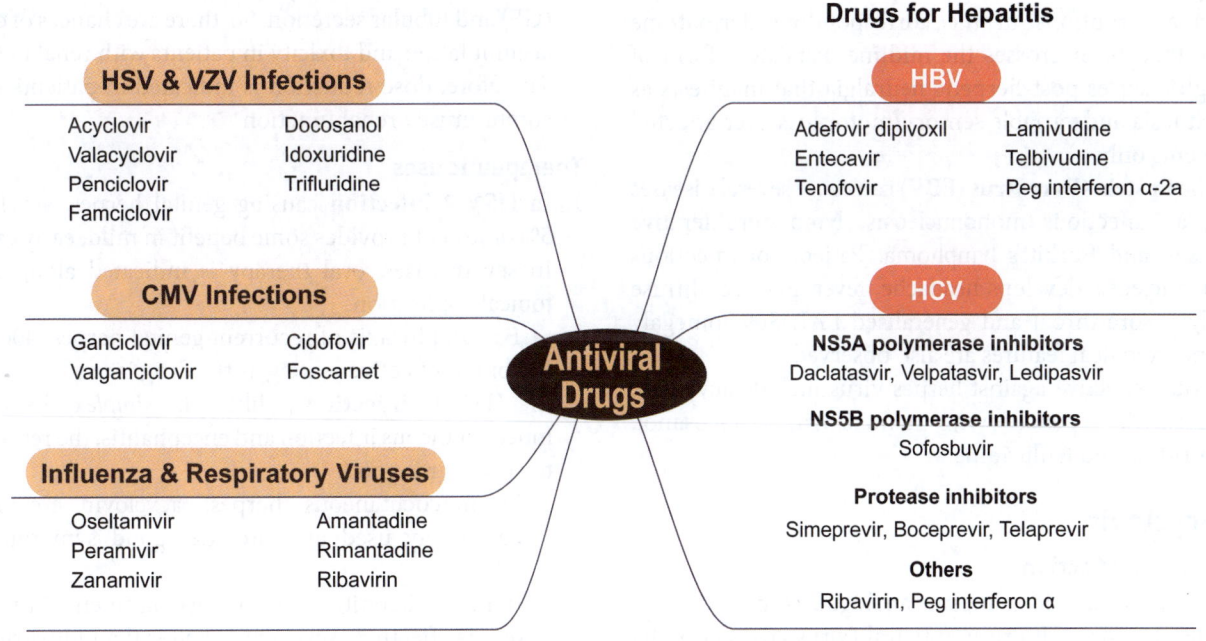

Flowchart 56.1 Classification of antiviral drugs

ANTIVIRAL DRUGS FOR HERPES VIRUS

The herpes simplex virus (HSV) has two seroforms, HSV 1 and 2, that cause mucocutaneous disease. HSV 1 causes orofacial herpes, usually gingivostomatitis, characterised by vesicles, erosions and maceration of buccal mucosa, gum edema/ erythema and painful lymphadenopathy (LAP). In herpes labialis, there are vesicles at the mucocutaneous junction of the nose and lips. HSV 2 infection causes genital herpes. In males, herpes infection manifests as penile erythema, papules/vesicles, which rupture and form painful ulcers on the penis. In females, similar lesions occur in the vulva and adjacent skin. Dysuria, urinary retention and painful LAP in the inguinal region may be associated with HSV 2. HSV can remain dormant in the sensory ganglia for a long time and may cause recurrence. Common sites involved in recurrent disease are lips, perioral area, nose, and cheeks. Disease may disseminate in severe cases to cause esophagitis, hepatitis, pneumonia, etc. More serious forms of herpes infection include encephalitis, meningitis, and disseminated infection.

VZV can cause herpes zoster (shingles) and chickenpox. Chickenpox is a highly contagious disease characterised by disseminated vesicular eruptions. It can have serious complications such as thrombocytopenia, hemorrhages in intestines/conjunctiva, varicella pneumonia, myocarditis, nephritis, arthritis, orchitis, and neurological complications such as meningitis, myelitis and encephalitis. VZV becomes dormant in neural tissue, especially trigeminal ganglia, dorsal root ganglia and cranial nerves. Reactivation of the dormant form may cause shingles and post-herpetic neuralgia. Shingles is characterised by painful radiculitis and vesicular eruptions in the corresponding dermatome alone that never crosses the midline. Persistent form of shingles causes post-herpetic neuralgia that manifests as paresthesia and variable sensory/motor loss over affected segments only.

The **Epstein–Barr virus (EBV)** can cause several diseases such as infectious mononucleosis, lymphoproliferative diseases, and Burkitt's lymphoma. Patients of infectious mononucleosis develops headache, fever, malaise, diffuse myalgia, sore throat and generalised LAP. Splenomegaly and neurological features are also observed.

Drugs effective against herpes virus include acyclovir, valacyclovir, penciclovir, famciclovir, docosanol, idoxuridine and trifluridine.

1. Acyclovir

Mechanism of action

Acyclovir, an acyclic guanosine analogue, is the prototype antiherpetic drug. It exerts antiviral (virustatic) action by interfering with viral nucleic acid synthesis. For this, first, acyclovir needs to be activated by three phosphorylations. Initially, acyclovir is converted to acyclovir monophosphate by the herpes-virus-specific enzyme thymidine kinase, followed by conversion to diphosphate and triphosphate by host cell enzymes. Since the first step of activation of acyclovir requires thymidine kinase from the herpes virus, it can be activated only by virus-infected cells.

Acyclovir triphosphate competes with deoxyguanosine triphosphate (deoxy GTP) for viral DNA polymerase enzyme and inhibits it reversibly. Incorporation of acyclovir triphosphate in place of deoxy GTP causes chain termination. The abnormal DNA thus formed causes irreversible inhibition of viral DNA polymerase enzyme.

Spectrum of activity: Acyclovir can inhibit HSV-1, HSV-2 and VZV, but it is ten times more potent against HSV than VZV. It also shows weak activity against EBV, CMV and HHV-6 (human herpes virus 6).

Resistance: Acyclovir-resistant strains of HSV are deficient in thymidine kinase enzyme, and hence the drug is not activated. In VZV, reduced affinity of viral polymerase causes resistance. Acyclovir shows cross-resistance with other drugs of the same class.

Pharmacokinetics

Oral bioavailability of acyclovir is low; just $1/5^{th}$ of the oral dose gets absorbed. Hence, the oral dose is much higher than parenteral dose. Oral dose is 200 mg, five times a day, whereas the intravenous dose is 5–15 mg/kg given over 1 hour. Absorption from topical application is also minimal, but it can penetrate the cornea.

- Plasma protein binding (PPB) is negligible; therefore, it is well distributed in body fluids including cerebrospinal fluid (CSF).
- Excretion occurs mainly through glomerular filtration (GF) and tubular secretion. So, there are chances of drug accumulation and toxicity in patients with renal failure. Therefore, dose reduction is indicated in patients with compromised renal function.

Therapeutic uses

1. In **HSV-2 infection** causing genital herpes, acyclovir 5% ointment provides some benefit in mild, early cases. In severe cases, oral therapy is indicated along with topical application.

    For prophylaxis of recurrent genital herpes, 400 mg BD oral is effective as long as the drug is used.

2. In **HSV-1 infections**, like *H. simplex* keratitis, mucocutaneous infection and encephalitis, the response to acyclovir is good.
    - In mucocutaneous herpes, acyclovir cream is commonly used and provides good symptomatic relief.
    - In herpes keratitis, acyclovir eye ointment, 5 times a day, is effective. Acyclovir is better than idoxuridine for deep stromal ulcers because of its better corneal penetration.

- Acyclovir is the drug of choice for *H. simplex* encephalitis. It is given as I/V 10–20 mg/kg TDS for about 10 days.
3. The efficacy of acyclovir is lower in **varicella zoster infection** than in HSV infections; however, acyclovir promotes fast healing of lesions and relieves symptoms.
    - For chicken pox in immunodeficient patients and neonates, intravenous acyclovir 15 mg/kg/day for 7 days is the drug of choice.

ADRs

As there is selective activation of acyclovir by the virus-infected cells, non-infected host cells fail to activate the drug. Hence, there is negligible effect on normal host cells.

ADRs of acyclovir depend upon the route of administration.

- Topical application of 5% ointment causes local irritation, burning and tingling sensation.
- On oral administration, nausea, vomiting, diarrhea and headache may occur.
- On I/V administration, it can cause sweating, rashes and hypotension.

The most important toxic effects of acyclovir are dose-dependent fall in GFR, disorientation, hallucinations, convulsions, etc.

2. Valacyclovir

Valacyclovir is a valyl ester of acyclovir. In comparison to acyclovir, it has **high oral bioavailability** as it is actively transported in the intestines through peptide transporters.

During the first pass, esterases convert valacyclovir into acyclovir, which then exerts antiviral actions. Once-daily (OD) dose for prevention of recurrent genital herpes and twice-daily (BD) dose for its treatment make valacyclovir convenient for use and improves patient compliance.

3. Penciclovir

This is another acyclic guanosine analogue with the same mechanism of activation, action, resistance and spectrum of activity as acyclovir. However, penciclovir triphosphate does not cause DNA chain termination and has lower affinity for viral DNA polymerase, even though it persists inside the viral infected cells for a much longer time than acyclovir triphosphate.

Penciclovir is **well tolerated** and causes mild ADRs like nausea and headache. It is used topically as 1% cream for recurrent herpes labialis. ADRs are uncommon and occur in the form of local reactions at the site of application.

4. Famciclovir

It is a diacetyl ester prodrug of penciclovir. It is deacetylated during first-pass metabolism to penciclovir. Its **oral bioavailability is 70%**, so it can be given orally for treatment and prevention of recurrent genital herpes, herpes labialis and acute varicella zoster infections. It is a **well-tolerated drug** with minor ADRs like nausea, diarrhea and headache.

5. Docosanol

Docosanol is an aliphatic alcohol that interferes with the fusion of the HSV envelope with the host cell membrane, thereby preventing the very first step of viral replication, i.e., entry of the virus into the host cell. It is used as topical cream 10% for HSV lesions. ADRs occur as burning/tingling sensation.

6. Idoxuridine and Trifluridine

These get incorporated into viral DNA, which easily breaks down. However, they are very toxic for systemic use because of their low viral selectivity, i.e., they can get incorporated into the host cell DNA as well. The only indication for their use is topical application as eyedrops in superficial herpes simplex keratitis. ADRs include ocular irritation and lid edema.

B. DRUGS FOR CMV INFECTION

Cytomegalovirus (CMV) infection may be asymptomatic in healthy individuals. However, in immunodeficient states, it causes serious illnesses such as retinitis, pneumonia, enteritis, and encephalitis. Hepatitis and Guillain–Barré type neuropathy can also occur in severe cases.

Drugs against CMV include ganciclovir, valganciclovir, cidofovir and foscarnet.

1. Ganciclovir

This has a mechanism of action similar to that of acyclovir. It is active against CMV, HSV, VZV and EBV, but efficacy is maximum against CMV. Oral bioavailability is low and, half-life is just 2–4 hours. However, ganciclovir triphosphate gets accumulated inside virus-infected cells and exerts action for a longer time.

Ganciclovir is used for prophylaxis and treatment of serious CMV infections like colitis, retinitis and pneumonia in immunocompromised patients (e.g., AIDS, transplant recipients and patients on cancer chemotherapy). Because of its low oral bioavailability, it is given as intravenous infusion in a dose of 10 mg/kg/day.

ADRs: Ganciclovir can cause serious systemic toxicity such as **bone marrow suppression**, fever, rashes, vomiting and neuropsychiatric symptoms.

2. Valganciclovir

Valganciclovir is the valyl ester prodrug of ganciclovir, with higher (60%) bioavailability. Hence, it is **effective by the oral route**. It has replaced ganciclovir for treatment and prophylaxis of CMV infection in immunocompromised patients because of the convenience of oral administration in a dose of 900 mg OD or BD. Ganciclovir is reserved for very serious CMV infections and for preventing vision loss in retinitis.

ADRs: These are the same as for ganciclovir. Both ganciclovir and valganciclovir **show cross-resistance** with acyclovir.

3. Cidofovir

Cidofovir is a cytosine monophosphate nucleotide analogue. Since it is already phosphorylated, it does not require activation by viral phosphokinases. Cidofovir diphosphate, the active form of the drug, is formed by host cell enzymes. Cidofovir diphosphate inhibits viral DNA polymerase in the virus-infected cells for a long period. Hence, although the plasma half-life of cidofovir is only 2–3 hours, **weekly or fortnightly administration** in a dose of 5 mg/kg intravenous is adequate for acyclovir-resistant herpes and ganciclovir-resistant CMV infections, especially in immunocompromised patients.

Cidofovir is **nephrotoxic** and hence contraindicated in patients with pre-existing renal disease. Probenecid given with cidofovir can decrease its tubular secretion and nephrotoxicity.

4. Foscarnet

It is a straight-chain pyrophosphate that interferes with viral nucleic acid synthesis by inhibiting viral DNA and RNA polymerase enzymes competitively. It is effective against CMV, HSV and HIV.

Oral bioavailability is low. The advantage of foscarnet is that virus strains resistant to other drugs respond to it. However, it is **highly toxic**. It can cause acute renal failure, anemia, nausea, fever, convulsions, etc. It can chelate divalent cations like Ca^{2+}, Mg^{2+}, causing hypomagnesemia and hypocalcemia. Because of its high toxicity, use is limited to ganciclovir-resistant CMV infections and acyclovir-resistant HSV and VZV infections.

Clinical problem-based questions and MCQs

1. **A 25-year-old woman is diagnosed with genital herpes virus infection.**
   i. Which agent is indicated for use in this case?
      a. Valacyclovir
      b. Cidofovir
      c. Ganciclovir
      d. Zanamivir
   ii. Describe the mechanism of action, uses and adverse effects of the chosen agent.
2. **A 65-year-old patient with recent kidney transplant develops CMV retinitis.**
   i. Suggest drugs that can be given to the patient.
   ii. List the characteristic adverse drug reactions of the chosen drugs.
3. **Identify the antiviral drug that has bone marrow suppressant effect.**
   a. Penciclovir
   b. Famciclovir
   c. Ganciclovir
   d. Cidofovir
4. **Which of the following antiviral drugs is nephrotoxic?**
   a. Valganciclovir
   b. Acyclovir
   c. Cidofovir
   d. Valacyclovir
5. **Identify the drug that interferes with viral entry into the host cell.**
   a. Docosanol
   b. Foscarnet
   c. Cidofovir
   d. Trifluridine

C. HEPATITIS B

Hepatitis B is a permanent infection caused by hepatitis B virus (HBV). It is a DNA virus that can form covalently closed circular (ccc) DNA. It persists inside the host cell for the lifetime of the latter, and can get reactivated, resulting in relapses. Hence, eradication of HBV is not achievable.

The disease begins with a prodromal phase characterised by anorexia, nausea, fatigue, and mild fever for the first few days. This is followed by jaundice and diffuse inflammation of liver. Hepatitis B and C viruses tend to persist, resulting in chronic hepatitis, cirrhosis and carcinoma as late complications.

Aims of treatment in hepatitis B infection

- Non-detectable levels of HBV DNA
- Seroconversion of HBeAg or HBsAg from positive to negative
- Normal serum transaminase levels.

Achievement of these endpoints reduces the risk of hepatic inflammation, necrosis, cirrhosis and hepatocellular carcinoma secondary to HBV infection.

Duration of treatment: Typically, anti-HBV drugs should be continued for at least 6 months after HBeAg becomes negative, unless contraindicated by loss of efficacy or appearance of adverse effects.

ANTI-HBV DRUGS

These include adefovir dipivoxil, entecavir, tenofovir, lamivudine, telbivudine and interferon.

1. Adefovir Dipivoxil

It is a diester of adefovir, which releases adefovir in circulation. Adefovir is an acyclic analogue of the phosphonated adenine nucleotide AMP (adenosine monophosphate). The active form, adefovir diphosphate, is formed by the action of cellular kinases that:

- Inhibit viral DNA polymerase competitively. Its affinity for viral DNA polymerase is higher than that of the host cells.
- Gets incorporated into viral DNA and results in chain termination.

Spectrum

Adefovir is effective against many DNA and RNA viruses including HBV, HIV and herpes viruses.

Pharmacokinetics

Its oral bioavailability is approximately 60%, and plasma protein binding is low. Moreover, adefovir diphosphate persists inside cells for 18 hours, which allows once-daily dosing. Elimination occurs via glomerular filtration and tubular secretion. Therefore, dose reduction is indicated in patients with renal function impairment.

Therapeutic uses

Response to adefovir is **slower** than response to tenofovir and lamivudine. So, it is not the first-choice drug.

Adefovir dipivoxil 10 mg/day is useful orally in:

- Lamivudine-resistant chronic hepatitis B
- HBV in HIV patients.

ADRs

It is a well-tolerated drug.

- ADRs like abdominal pain, diarrhea, headache, sore throat, and flu-like symptoms may occur.
- High doses (30–60 mg/day) can cause dose-dependent nephrotoxicity, especially in patients with pre-existing renal dysfunction.
- Severe acute hepatitis can occur on stopping adefovir therapy in one-fourth of the patients.

2. Tenofovir Disoproxil Fumarate (TDF)

Like adefovir, TDF is also a monophosphate analogue of adenosine nucleotide (AMP). It is a prodrug which improves bioavailability of tenofovir. The mechanism of action is the same as adefovir, but **response is faster**. Cellular kinases convert it into tenofovir diphosphate, which causes inhibition of HBV DNA polymerase and HIV reverse transcriptase. However, its affinity for host cell DNA polymerase is very low. The incorporation of tenofovir diphosphate in DNA results in chain termination.

Therapeutic uses

TDF is one of the **first-line drugs** in the treatment of chronic hepatitis caused by HBV, given orally in a dose of 300 mg/day. It is effective against lamivudine- and entecavir-resistant cases also, but has low efficacy against adefovir-resistant viruses.

ADRs

ADRs are mild and occur as gastrointestinal effects (nausea, abdominal pain, fatigue, dizziness, diarrhea, headache, etc.) Increase in serum creatinine and risk of renal function impairment may occur.

3. Entecavir

It is an analogue of guanosine nucleoside. It is activated through phosphorylation by cellular kinases and inhibits HBV DNA polymerase. Weak anti-HIV activity is also present.

Entecavir exhibits a faster and more profound response than lamivudine. The chances of emergence of resistance are very low up to 5 years of treatment. So, it is one of the **first-line drugs in HBV infection**.

Oral absorption is nearly 100%, but is reduced by presence of food. Hence, entecavir should be given on an empty stomach in a dose of 0.5–1 mg, once daily. Elimination occurs through the renal route.

ADRs

It is a well-tolerated drug with mild ADRs in the form of nausea, headache, fatigue, diarrhea, dizziness, fever, rashes, dyspepsia, insomnia, etc.

4. Lamivudine

This is an analogue of nucleoside deoxycytidine. Like other drugs, it gets activated intracellularly via phosphorylation by cellular kinases and competitively inhibits HBV DNA polymerase and HIV reverse transcriptase, causing chain termination. It has low toxicity because of its low affinity for human DNA polymerase. **Resistance to lamivudine develops rapidly** because of point mutations in target enzymes.

Pharmacokinetics

Lamivudine has good oral bioavailability and persists inside cells for a long time. It persists for up to 19 hours in HBV-infected cells as compared to 15 hours in HIV infected cells This allows once-daily dosing, with a low dose in HBV treatment. It is mainly excreted unchanged by the kidneys.

Therapeutic uses

Lamivudine is an essential component of the first-line triple-drug regimens for HIV treatment.

- It is effective in hepatitis B also but is not preferred due to rapid emergence of resistance in up to 70% of patients. It shows cross-resistance with entecavir and emtricitabine.
- It can decrease transmission of HBV from mother to baby if used in the last month of pregnancy.

ADRs

ADRs are mild and occur as fatigue, anorexia, nausea, diarrhea, rashes, dizziness and headache. In rare cases, it can cause neuropathy and pancreatitis, especially in patients having concomitant HIV and HBV infection.

5. Telbivudine

It is a thymidine nucleoside analogue that gets phosphorylated by cellular kinases inside the cell to form telbivudine triphosphate which:

- Competitively inhibits HBV DNA polymerase.
- Gets incorporated into the viral DNA causing chain termination.

Action of telbivudine is **faster and more intense** than that of lamivudine or adefovir; however, **higher risk of emergence of resistant strains** is a limiting factor, because of which it is not a drug of first choice.

ADRs
ADRs are mild and occur as abdominal pain discomfort, diarrhea, headache, muscular aches and pain, cough, dizziness, etc.

HEPATITIS C (HCV)
Hepatitis C virus is an RNA virus that does not get integrated into the host cell DNA. Therefore, HCV infection is chronic but curable.

The **aim of treatment** in HCV infection is to maintain HCV RNA at undetectable levels in blood for up to 6 months after stopping therapy. This is called 'sustained viral response (SVR)'. Relapse rate is very low in such patients.

ANTI-HCV DRUGS
Several new drugs that specifically inhibit non-structural viral proteins (such as NS5A and NS5B polymerase and NS3/4A protease) are increasingly preferred for hepatitis C. In India, non-selective, conventional drugs, such as ribavirin and peg-IFNα are still widely used.

1. NS5A Polymerase Inhibitors
NS5A polymerase is a non-structural protein in the hepatitis C virus that plays an essential role in viral RNA replication, assembly and packaging of daughter virions. NS5A inhibitors interfere with these key functions.

NS5A polymerase inhibitors include drugs such as **daclatasvir, velpatasvir** and **ledipasvir**.

Daclatasvir and velpatasvir are effective against all 6 genotypes (1–6) of HCV. Ledipasvir is effective only against 1, 4, 5, and 6 genotypes.

- **Pharmacokinetics:** Absorption of velpatasvir and ledipasvir is dependent on gastric pH; it is impaired by acid-lowering drugs like H_2 blockers and proton pump inhibitors.
- NS5A inhibitors are metabolised by microsomal CYP3A enzyme. Hence, dosage adjustments are indicated if enzyme inducers/inhibitors are co-administered.
- These drugs may be pumped out of the cell by P-glycoproteins. Thus, combination with P-gp-inducing drugs should be avoided, or dose should be increased.
- These drugs are used orally in combination with **sofosbuvir** for improving efficacy and preventing emergence of resistant strains. **Ribavirin** can also be added.
- **ADRs** are mild (headache, fatigue, muscular pain, nausea weakness, etc.).

2. NS5B Polymerase Inhibitors
NS5B RNA polymerase is required for HCV replication.
- NS5B inhibitors are of two types:
  - Nucleoside/nucleotide analogues like **sofosbuvir** that compete for the active site of the enzyme.
  - Non-nucleoside analogues like **dasabuvir** that bind to the allosteric site.
- **Sofosbuvir** is a prodrug of a uridine analogue that is activated into a triphosphate nucleotide in liver cells. The active form inhibits NS5B, the HCV RNA polymerase, gets incorporated into viral RNA, causing chain termination. It is effective in all the six genotypes of HCV. It is always used in combination with other non-structural protein inhibitors or with ribavirin and IFNα. Sofosbuvir resistance is not common, but efflux through P-glycoprotein transporter can occur. So, it should be avoided in patients receiving P-gp-inducing drugs like rifampin and phenytoin and those with renal function impairment.
- **ADRs** are fatigue, anemia, joint pain, abdominal pain and agitation.

3. NS3/4A Protease Inhibitors
NS3/4A protease is essential for processing the single polyprotein encoded by the HCV RNA into individually active proteins (NS4A, NS4B, NS5A and NS5B). Thus, inhibition of NS3/4A protease disrupts HCV replication. Drugs in this category include **simeprevir, paritaprevir, grazoprevir, glecaprevir and voxilaprevir**.

- They are metabolised by CYP3A enzyme; hence, many interactions with enzyme inducers may occur.
- The chances of developing resistance are higher when these are used alone. So, these drugs are commonly combined with other drugs like ribavirin.
- ADRs can occur as rashes, pruritus, nausea, anemia and fatigue.

4. Ribavirin
Ribavirin is a **non-selective drug**. It is a guanosine analogue. Ribavirin triphosphate inhibits the synthesis of GTP and viral RNA. The **spectrum of activity** of ribavirin includes many DNA and RNA viruses like respiratory syncytial virus (RSV), influenza A and B, and all six genotypes of HCV. Resistance to ribavirin is uncommon.

Therapeutic uses
It is still extensively used:
- for treatment of chronic hepatitis C. It is usually combined with peg-IFNα. It can be combined with direct-acting antivirals like sofosbuvir in patients with decompensated cirrhosis.
- as nebuliser in the treatment of RSV bronchiolitis in infants and children.

ADRs

It can cause dose-dependent hemolytic anemia, bone marrow suppression, central adverse effects, GI intolerance and bronchospasm with aerosol administration. It also has teratogenic potential.

5. Peg-IFNα

Viral infections, TNFα and interleukin-1 induce production of glycoproteins called interferons (IFNs) in host cells. IFNs act on JAK/STAT tyrosine kinase receptors to phosphorylate cellular proteins that cause synthesis of 'interferon-induced proteins'. These IFN-induced proteins affect viral replication at many steps such as:

- penetration into host cell
- synthesis of mRNA
- direct/indirect suppression of viral protein synthesis
- assembly and release of virion.

IFNs are **non-selective for viruses**. They inhibit many DNA and RNA viruses but are **specific to the host** species, i.e., humans. IFN α, β, and γ have antiviral action. However, for clinical use, only IFNα-2a and IFNα-2b are available. These can be injected I/M or S/C. Polyethylene glycol complexes of IFNs are suitable for weekly administration, as peg-IFN is absorbed slowly from the site of administration. It is useful for the treatment of hepatitis B, hepatitis C, herpes simplex, VZV and CMV. In addition, IFNs are effective in the treatment of HIV-related Kaposi sarcoma, condylomata acuminata caused by human papilloma virus, multiple myeloma, chronic myeloid leukemia (CML) and T-cell lymphomas.

ADRs

- IFNs cause severe ADRs just after injection in the form of flu-like symptoms (fever, malaise, fatigue, anorexia, nausea and disturbances of vision and taste).
- Dose-dependent neutropenia and thrombocytopenia (TCP) can occur.
- Thyroid function is disturbed.
- Hypertension, arrhythmia and hepatic dysfunction may occur.
- Central adverse effects like depression, altered behaviour, sleepiness, tremors, convulsions, numbness and neuropathy are common.

RESPIRATORY VIRAL INFECTIONS

Viruses causing respiratory infection include influenza A and B and RSV. In influenza, there is a sudden onset of symptoms such as fever, myalgia, spasmodic non-productive/dry cough, and conjunctival injection (redness). Infection with respiratory syncytial virus (RSV) manifests as fever and cough with rhinitis. Severe infection may cause otitis media, pneumonia, bronchiolitis, and even respiratory failure. Infection with RSV worsens chronic bronchitis and emphysema.

While immunisation is preferred for influenza viruses, drug treatment is indicated in patients who have allergic reactions to vaccine or during epidemics.

ANTI-INFLUENZA DRUGS

Anti-influenza drugs include:

- Neuraminidase inhibitors: Oseltamivir, panamivir, peramivir
- Amantadine, rimantadine
- Ribavirin

1. Neuraminidase Inhibitors

a. Oseltamivir

Neuraminidase enzyme plays an essential role in viral replication. The influenza viruses insert a specific neuraminidase into the host cell membrane, which assists in the release of daughter virions from the cell. Thus, neuraminidase inhibitor drugs interfere with the last step of viral replication, i.e., release of daughter virions from the cell, thereby controlling the spread of virus in the body. **Resistance to oseltamivir** can occur due to mutation of viral neuraminidase enzyme.

Therapeutic uses

They are effective for prevention as well as symptom control in influenza A including H5N1 (bird flu), H1N1 (swine flu) strains and influenza B.

Treatment with oseltamivir should be started early because viral replication is at its peak during the first 2 days of the onset of symptoms. For prophylactic use also, administration within 2 days of exposure to influenza patients prevents infection. Dose for prophylaxis is 75 mg OD, and for treatment it is 75 mg BD for 5 days.

Pharmacokinetics

Oseltamivir is **effective orally** and has 80% bioavailability. It gets converted into its active form, oseltamivir carboxylate, during first-pass metabolism. It is not metabolised and is excreted unchanged by the kidneys. Therefore, in patients with renal function impairment, dose reduction is indicated.

ADRs

Gastric irritant effects such as nausea, epigastric pain and diarrhea occur, and so, it is preferably given with food. Headache, somnolence, insomnia, weakness are other frequent side effects.

b. Zanamivir

Zanamivir has the same mechanism of action and uses as oseltamivir. It is given by the **inhalational route** because of its very low oral bioavailability. Dose is 10 mg, twice a day, through rotacap or breath-actuated inhaler.

Some oseltamivir-resistant strains respond to zanamivir. So, it is reserved for patients infected with oseltamivir-resistant strains or those who are immunocompromised.

ADRs

Inhalational administration can cause severe bronchospasm, especially in asthma patients. Hence, it is contraindicated in bronchial asthma. Nausea, headache, dizziness and rashes may also occur.

c. Peramivir

Peramivir also has the same mechanism of action, uses and ADRs as oseltamivir but very low oral bioavailability. Therefore, it is administered by the I/V route. Elimination occurs via the renal route, indicating dose adjustment in patients with renal disease. Its half-life is long (20 hours), which allows single daily dosing. It is also effective against oseltamivir-resistant strains.

2. Amantadine and Rimantadine

Amantadine and rimantadine (methyl derivative of amantadine) act by inhibiting the viral ion channel (M2 protein), which prevents uncoating of the viral genome within the infected cell.

Spectrum: Influenza A virus is sensitive, but H1N1 strains of influenza A and influenza B are not affected by these drugs. Due to a mutation in the M2 protein, many other strains of influenza A also have developed resistance. There is complete cross-resistance between the two drugs. So, they are not much used in current clinical practice.

Clinical problem-based questions and MCQs

6. i. Identify the first-line drug for a 28-year-old drug addict with HBV infection.
   - a. Adefovir
   - b. Entecavir
   - c. Cidofovir
   - d. Penciclovir
   ii. Justify your choice.
   iii. Describe the aim of treatment in this patient and mechanism of action of the chosen drug.

7. A 56-year-old patient complains of low-grade fever, anorexia, nausea, fatigue and malaise. There is yellow discolouration of skin and eyes. Serum bilirubin is raised and hepatitis C is positive.
   i. Which of the following drugs is most suitable for this case?
   - a. Interferon α with lamivudine
   - b. Oseltamivir with amantadine
   - c. Cidofovir with IFN
   - d. Sofosbuvir with ribavirin
   ii. Describe the aim of treatment and mechanism of action of the chosen drugs.

8. Which of the following drugs interferes with the processing of the single HCV polyprotein into individual proteins?
   - a. Sofosbuvir
   - b. Peg-IFN
   - c. Simeprevir
   - d. Daclatasvir

9. i. Identify the neuraminidase-inhibiting drug among the following.
   - a. Tenofovir
   - b. Peramivir
   - c. Amantadine
   - d. Ribavirin
   ii. What is the indication for using the chosen drug?

10. i. Identify the antiviral drug used by inhalational route.
    - a. Rimantadine
    - b. Zanamivir
    - c. Sofosbuvir
    - d. Peg-IFN
    ii. What is the adverse effect of inhalational administration of the chosen drug?

Summary

- Antiviral drugs are classified based on viruses against which they are effective.
- **Antiherpes drugs** include acyclovir, its valyl ester valacyclovir, penciclovir, famciclovir, docosanol, and idoxuridine.
- **Acyclovir** interferes with viral nucleic acid synthesis after phosphorylation by virus-specific thymidine kinase (activated only in virus-infected cells). It is useful in genital herpes, *H. simplex* keratitis, encephalitis, mucocutaneous infection, and chicken pox. ADRs are burning and tingling on local application, headache, nausea, vomiting and diarrhea after oral use and sweating, rashes and hypotension after IV administration.
- **Penciclovir** is better tolerated than acyclovir and is mostly used topically in herpes labialis.
- **Famciclovir** is used by the oral route in prevention and treatment of herpes labialis, genital herpes and VZV infections.
- Idoxuridine and trifluridine are too toxic for systemic use, and the only indication for their use is as eyedrops in superficial *Herpes simplex* keratitis.
- **Drugs for CMV** include ganciclovir, valganciclovir, cidofovir and foscarnet.
- **Ganciclovir** resembles acyclovir, but is more effective against CMV. It is used for CMV retinitis, colitis and pneumonia in immunocompromised patients by the IV route. It can cause bone marrow suppression, fever, rashes and neuropsychiatric symptoms as ADRs.
- **Valganciclovir,** a prodrug of ganciclovir, has better oral bioavailability.
- **Cidofovir and foscarnet** are toxic to kidneys and reserved for ganciclovir-resistant CMV and acyclovir-resistant VZV infections.
- **Hepatitis B** eradication is not possible. So, drug therapy is aimed at reducing HBV DNA levels, seroconversion and normalising serum transaminase levels.
- **Adefovir dipivoxil** causes competitive inhibition of viral DNA polymerase enzyme and chain termination. However, response to adefovir is slower than tenofovir and lamivudine, and hence it is used in lamivudine-resistant HBV infection and for HBV in HIV-positive patients. It can cause dose-dependent nephrotoxicity.

- **Tenofovir** is a prodrug with better bioavailability and faster response than adefovir. It is one of the first-line drugs given orally in chronic HBV hepatitis. ADRs are mild but it may cause renal function impairment.
- **Entecavir** is one of the first-line drugs in HBV infection as the response is faster and more profound than with lamivudine. Moreover, the chances of emergence of resistance are very low for up to 5 years of treatment.
- **Lamivudine** is one of the essential components of HIV treatment but is not preferred in HBV infection due to rapid emergence of resistance.
- **Telbivudine** has faster and more intense anti-HBV action than lamivudine and adefovir, but it is not preferred because of rapid development of resistance.
- **Hepatitis C** virus (HCV) infection is chronic but curable. Anti-HCV drugs include NS5A polymerase inhibitors like **daclatasvir, velpatasvir and ledipasvir**. NS5A is a non-structural protein of hepatitis C virus, which plays an essential role in viral RNA replication, assembly and packaging of daughter virions. NS5A-inhibitor drugs interfere with these key functions and are used in combination with sofosbuvir or ribavirin in HCV infection. Interactions can occur with acid-lowering drugs, enzyme inducers/inhibitors and P-glycoprotein-inducing drugs.
- NS5B polymerase inhibitor, **sofosbuvir**, is effective against all six HCV genotypes and is used in combination with other drugs.
- NS3/4A protease inhibitors such as **simeprevir and grazoprevir** interfere with HCV replication as they prevent processing of the single polyprotein into individual proteins. These are usually combined with other drugs as chances of resistance are high with monotherapy.
- Ribavirin and peg-IFN are non-selective drugs. **Ribavirin** is useful against RSV, influenza and HCV. Resistance is uncommon. It causes bone marrow suppression, GI and central adverse effects.
- **Peg-IFN** is non-selective for viruses but specific to human hosts. It is still used in hepatitis B, C, herpes, VZV, CMV infections, Kaposi sarcoma, HPV, etc. However, use of IFN is associated with many ADRs, e.g., immediate flu-like symptoms, neutropenia, TCP, thyroid/hepatic dysfunction, central adverse effects and arrhythmias.
- **Anti-influenza drugs oseltamivir, zanamivir and peramivir** are neuraminidase inhibitors that interfere with the release of daughter virions from the host cell. Oseltamivir is suitable for oral administration, zanamivir for inhalational administration and peramivir for IV administration. Treatment with oseltamivir should be started early because viral replication peaks during the first 2 days of onset of symptoms.
- Amantadine and rimantadine interfere with the uncoating of the influenza virus inside host cells, but clinical use is limited because of many resistant strains.

Questions for practice

1. Classify anti-herpes virus drugs. Describe the mechanism of action, therapeutic uses and ADRs of the most suitable drug for genital herpes.
2. Enumerate drugs useful in:
   a. Influenza   b. CMV retinitis   c. HBV infection
3. Describe the goals of therapy in HBV and HCV infection.
4. Write short notes on:
   a. Interferons
   b. Ribavirin
   c. Direct-acting anti-HCV drugs

Hints for problem-based questions and MCQs

1. i. a. Valacyclovir
   ii. It is a valyl ester of acyclovir, that has good oral bioavailability. It gets converted into acyclovir by esterases. Refer to pages 736, 737.
2. i. Ganciclovir, valganciclovir, cidofovir and foscarnet are used.
   ii. ADRs: Ganciclovir causes serious systemic toxicity by bone marrow suppression. Fever, rashes, vomiting, and neuropsychiatric symptoms are present. Valganciclovir has the same ADRs as ganciclovir. Cidofovir is nephrotoxic. Foscarnet can also cause acute renal failure, anemia, nausea, fever, convulsions, etc. It can chelate divalent cations like Ca^{2+}, Mg^{2+}, causing hypomagnesemia and hypocalcemia.
3. c. Ganciclovir can cause serious systemic toxicity due to bone marrow suppressant action.
4. c. Cidofovir is nephrotoxic, so reserved for ganciclovir-resistant CMV infection.
5. a. Docosanol interferes with fusion of HSV envelop with host cell membrane, so it inhibits viral entry into host cell.
6. i. b. Entecavir
   ii. Adefovir is effective against HBV, but not preferred because of slower action. Cidofovir and penciclovir are not effective against HBV.
   iii. Aim of treatment in HBV is seroconversion, reduction of HBV DNA levels and maintenance of low serum transaminase levels. Eradication of HBV is not possible. Entecavir, a guanosine analogue, acts by causing competitive inhibition of viral DNA polymerase and chain termination.
7. i. d. Sofosbuvir with ribavirin
   ii. Aim of treatment in HCV infection is sustained viral response. Sofosbuvir is a NS5B polymerase inhibitor effective against all 6 genotypes of HCV; it is used in combination with other drugs. HCV RNA polymerase gets incorporated in viral RNA causing chain termination. Ribavarin is a guanosine analogue. Ribavirin triphosphate inhibits synthesis of GTP and Viral RNA.
8. c. Simeprevir
9. i. b. Peramivir
   ii. It is useful in the treatment of influenza A, B, RSV, etc., by IV route.
10. i b. Zanamivir
    ii Inhalational use of zanamivir may cause bronchospasm. So, it is contraindicated in bronchial asthma.

CONCEPT MAP – ANTIVIRAL DRUGS

Antiviral Drugs

Antiherpetic Drugs

Acyclovir
- **Mechanism:** Activated by herpes virus-specific & host cell enzymes → interferes with viral nucleic acid synthesis → virustatic action.
- **Uses:** Treatment and prophylaxis of genital herpes caused by HSV-2. Keratitis, mucocutaneous infection & encephalitis caused by HSV-1.
- **VZV infection:** Chickenpox for fast healing and symptom relief, in immunodeficient patients & neonates given IV route.
- **ADRs:** Well-tolerated drug. Local irritation, burning & tingling sensation on topical application. Nausea, vomiting, diarrhea, headache with oral use. Sweating, rashes, hypotension on I/V use. Dose-dependent fall in GFR, disorientation, hallucination, convulsions.

Docosanol
Prevents entry of virus into host cell. Used topically for HSV lesions. May cause burning / tingling sensation.

Idoxuridine & Trifluridine
Too toxic for systemic use. Only indication is superficial herpes simplex keratitis as eyedrops. May cause ocular irritation & lid edema.

Valacyclovir
Better bioavailability, convenient dosing than acyclovir

Penciclovir
Lower affinity for viral DNA polymerase than acyclovir triphosphate. Used topically as 1% cream for recurrent herpes labialis. Well tolerated.

Famciclovir
Prodrug of penciclovir, used by oral route in recurrent genital herpes, herpes labialis and acute varicella zoster infections. Well tolerated.

Drugs for RSV & Influenza

Oseltamivir
Neuraminidase inhibitors, interfere with release of daughter virions from host cell.
- **Uses:** Prevention & symptom control in influenza A H5N1, H1N1 strains & influenza B. Treatment to be started early, effective orally, dose reduction indicated in impaired renal function.
- **ADRs:** Gastric irritant effects, headache, somnolence, insomnia, weakness.

Zanamivir
Very low oral bioavailability, so used by inhalational route through rotacaps or breath-actuated inhalers, reserved for use in oseltamivir-resistant infection in immunocompromised patients. Contraindicated in BA.

Peramivir
Very low oral bioavailability, used by I/V route. Dose adjustment in patients with renal disease. Effective against oseltamivir-resistant strains also.

Amantadine, Rimatidine
Prevents uncoating of viral genome within the infected cell. Not much used due to resistance.

Drugs for Hepatitis

HBV

Adefovir
- **Mechanism:** Adefovir diphosphate, formed by cellular kinases, competitively inhibits viral DNA polymerase. Drug gets incorporated into viral DNA → chain termination. Effective against HBV, HIV and herpes viruses
- **Uses:** Lamivudine-resistant chronic hepatitis B & HBV in HIV patients. OD dose, dose reduction indicated in renal function impairment.
- **ADRs:** Well tolerated, may cause abdominal pain, diarrhea, headache, sore throat, flu-like symptoms. Dose-dependent nephrotoxicity. Severe acute hepatitis on stopping therapy in 1/4th patients.

Lamivudine, Telbivudine
Effective, but not preferred due to high risk of rapid emergence of resistance.

Tenofovir
Faster response than adefovir, one of the first-line drugs in HBV infection, effective in lamivudine- & entecavir-resistant cases also, but poor efficacy against adefovir-resistant HBV.
- **ADRs:** Mild GI effects, fatigue, dizziness, diarrhea, headache, increased serum creatinine and risk of renal function impairment.

Entecavir
Response is faster and more profound than lamivudine. Very low chances of resistance up to 5 years. Used as first-line drug in HBV as OD dose given on empty stomach. Well tolerated, mild ADRs such as nausea, headache, fatigue, diarrhea, dizziness, fever, rashes, dyspepsia, insomnia, etc.

HCV

NS5A Polymerase Inhibitors
Daclatasvir, Velpatasvir & Ledipasvir.
- **Mechanism:** Interfere with RNA replication, assembly and packaging of daughter virions. Daclatasvir, Velpatasvir effective against all 6 genotypes (1,2,3,4,5,6), but Ledipasvir against 4 genotypes (1,4,5,6) of HCV.
- **Uses:** Orally, with Sofosbuvir & Ribavirin for improving efficacy and preventing resistance
- **Drug interactions** with acid lowering drugs, CYP3A4 inducers/inhibitors & P-gp inducers.

NS3/4A Protease Inhibitors
Simeprevir, Paritaprevir, Grazoprevir, Glecaprevir, Voxilaprevir.
Interfere with processing of polyprotein encoded by HCV RNA into active proteins → disrupt viral replication.
- **Uses:** In combination with other drugs like ribavirin to prevent resistance. Interacts with CYP3A inducers/inhibitors
- **ADRs:** Rashes, pruritus, nausea, anemia, fatigue.

NS5B Polymerase Inhibitor
Sofosbuvir competes for active site of enzyme, effective in all 6 genotypes, always used in combination with other drugs, interacts with P-gp inducers.
- **ADRs:** Fatigue, anemia, joint pain, abdominal pain, agitation.

Peg IFNα
Act on JAK/STAT receptors, interferes with viral penetration, mRNA synthesis, protein synthesis, assembly & release.
- **Uses:** By I/M or S/C injection in HBV, HCV, herpes simplex, VZV, CMV infection, HIV-related Kaposi sarcoma, HPV-induced condyloma acuminata, multiple myeloma, CML & T-cell lymphomas.
- **ADRs:** Severe flu-like symptoms after injection, neutropenia, TCP, hypertension, arrhythmia, central effects, hepatic & thyroid dysfunction

Ribavirin
Active against many DNA & RNA viruses, e.g., RSV, influenza A & B & all 6 genotypes of HCV. Resistance uncommon.
- **Uses:** With peg-IFNα or Sofosbuvir for HCV & as nebuliser for RSV bronchiolitis in infants & children.
- **ADR:** Hemolytic anemia, myelosuppression, central effects, GI intolerance, bronchospasm & teratogenicity

SECTION 10   Chemotherapeutic Drugs

57   Antiretroviral Drugs

PH 8.10 (Continued)   Discuss the types, kinetics, dynamics, adverse effects, indications and contraindications of drugs used for viral diseases including HIV.

Learning objectives

A student of MBBS phase II should be able to:
- Classify antiretroviral drugs.
- Describe mechanism of action of antiretroviral drugs.
- Enumerate therapeutic uses, adverse effects and contraindications of antiretroviral drugs.

HUMAN IMMUNODEFICIENCY VIRUS (HIV)

The **human immunodeficiency virus (HIV)** is a single-stranded RNA retrovirus. A unique feature of this virus is **reverse transcription**: normally, transcription is the formation of RNA from DNA; however, in HIV, proviral DNA is formed from the RNA of the virus. This process occurs under the influence of the enzyme **reverse transcriptase** (Fig. 57.1). The HIV genome, i.e., proviral DNA, gets integrated into the host cell DNA with help of enzyme **integrase.**

Viral polyproteins synthesised thereafter are cleaved into functional viral proteins by the **protease** enzyme.

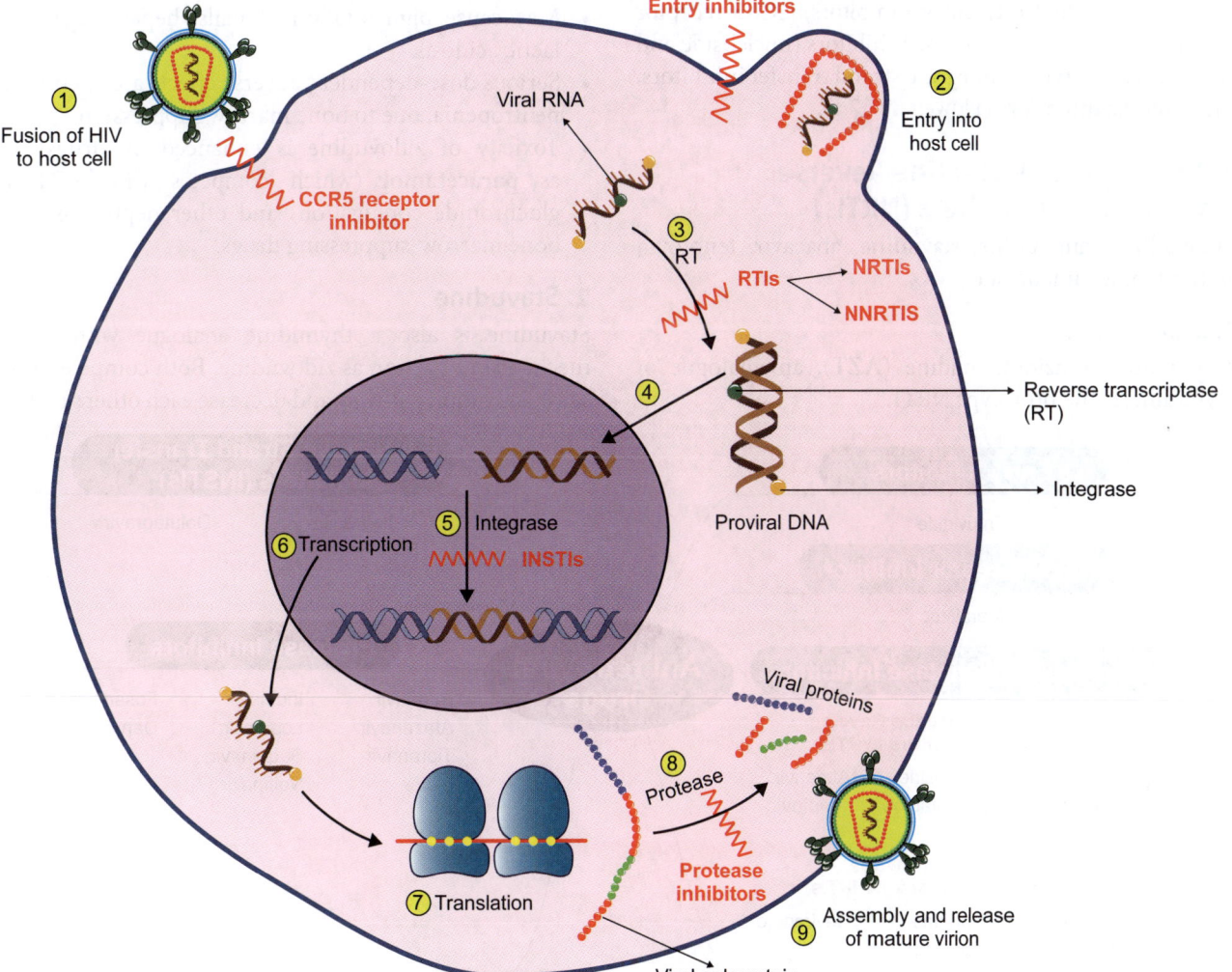

Fig. 57.1   Replication cycle of HIV and site of action of antiretroviral drugs

Therefore, once infected, host cells cannot be cured and eradication of the virus is impossible. The HIV-infected host suffers from **acquired immunodeficiency syndrome** (AIDS), because the virus mainly attacks CD4+ helper T-lymphocytes and macrophages. The decrease in the number of these cells compromises **cell-mediated immunity (CMI)** and the host becomes more susceptible to opportunistic infections.

The **aim of treatment with antiretroviral drugs** is maximal suppression of viral replication for the maximum possible time to prolong life, to delay complications, and improve quality of life. Because HIV infection is permanent, it needs lifelong treatment.

CLASSIFICATION OF ANTIRETROVIRAL DRUGS

The specific targets for drug action include the reverse transcriptase, integrase and protease enzymes. Some drugs exert their antiretroviral effect by interfering with the entry of the virus into host cells either by preventing fusion of the viral envelope with the plasma membrane of host cells, or by blocking chemokine coreceptors (CCR5) on the host cell surface (Fig. 57.1).

Based on their mechanism of action, antiretroviral drugs are classified into entry inhibitors, CCR5 receptor inhibitors, reverse transcriptase inhibitors (nucleoside and non-nucleoside types), integrase strand transfer inhibitors, and protease inhibitors (Flowchart 57.1).

A. Nucleoside/Nucleotide Reverse Transcriptase Inhibitors (NRTIs)

Zidovudine, lamivudine, stavudine, abacavir, tenofovir, emtricitabine, didanosine

1. Zidovudine

Zidovudine or azidothymidine (**AZT**), an analogue of thymidine, is the prototype NRTI.

Mechanism of action

It undergoes phosphorylation inside the host cell (Fig. 57.2) to form zidovudine triphosphate, which **selectively inhibits the viral reverse transcriptase** enzyme competitively, thereby inhibiting the formation of proviral DNA. Zidovudine triphosphate gets incorporated into the proviral DNA and causes chain termination.

Pharmacokinetics

It is well-absorbed orally, metabolised in the liver by glucuronide conjugation, and excreted in urine. Its half-life is 1 hour. It is given in a dose of 300 mg, twice daily.

Mechanism of resistance to zidovudine involves point mutations in viral reverse transcriptase, which reduce its affinity for drug.

Uses

While AZT is not the preferred drug in WHO and NACO regimens, it may be used in **alternative triple-drug regimens** for treatment of HIV infection.

Adverse effects

- Anorexia, nausea, abdominal pain
- Myalgias
- Headache and insomnia
- May cause pigmentation of nails, hepatomegaly and lactic acidosis.
- Serious dose-dependent adverse effects are anemia and neutropenia, due to bone marrow suppression
- Toxicity of zidovudine is enhanced by drugs such as **paracetamol** (which competes with AZT for glucuronide conjugation) and other nephrotoxic and bone marrow-suppressing drugs.

2. Stavudine

Stavudine is also a thymidine analogue with similar mechanism of action as zidovudine. Both compete for the same activation pathway and decrease each other's effect. It

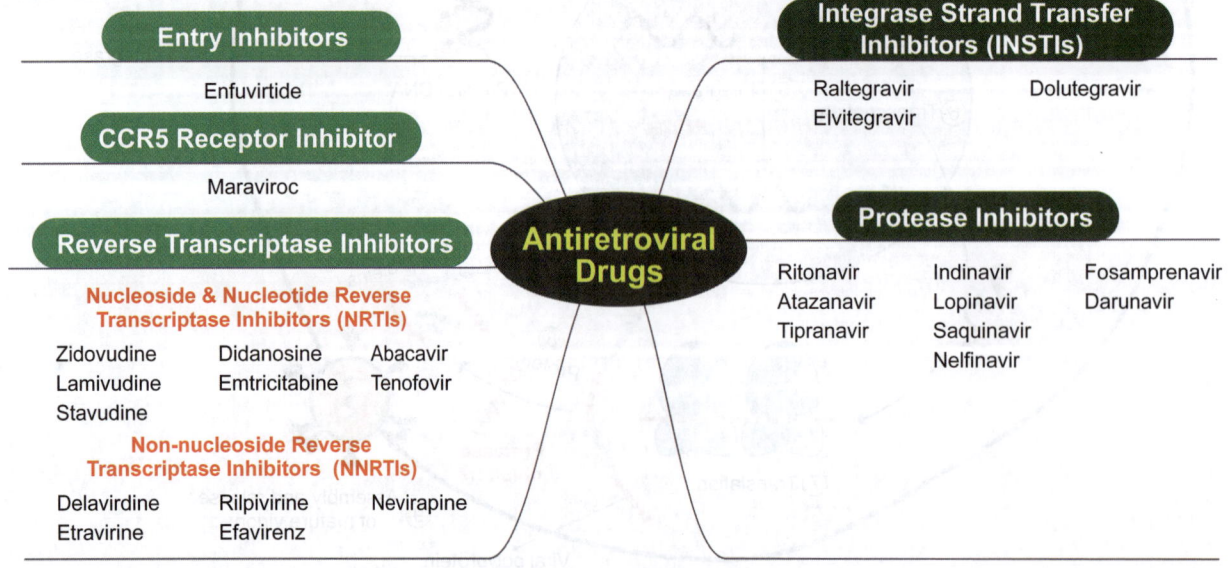

Flowchart 57.1 Classification of antiretroviral drugs based on their mechanism of action

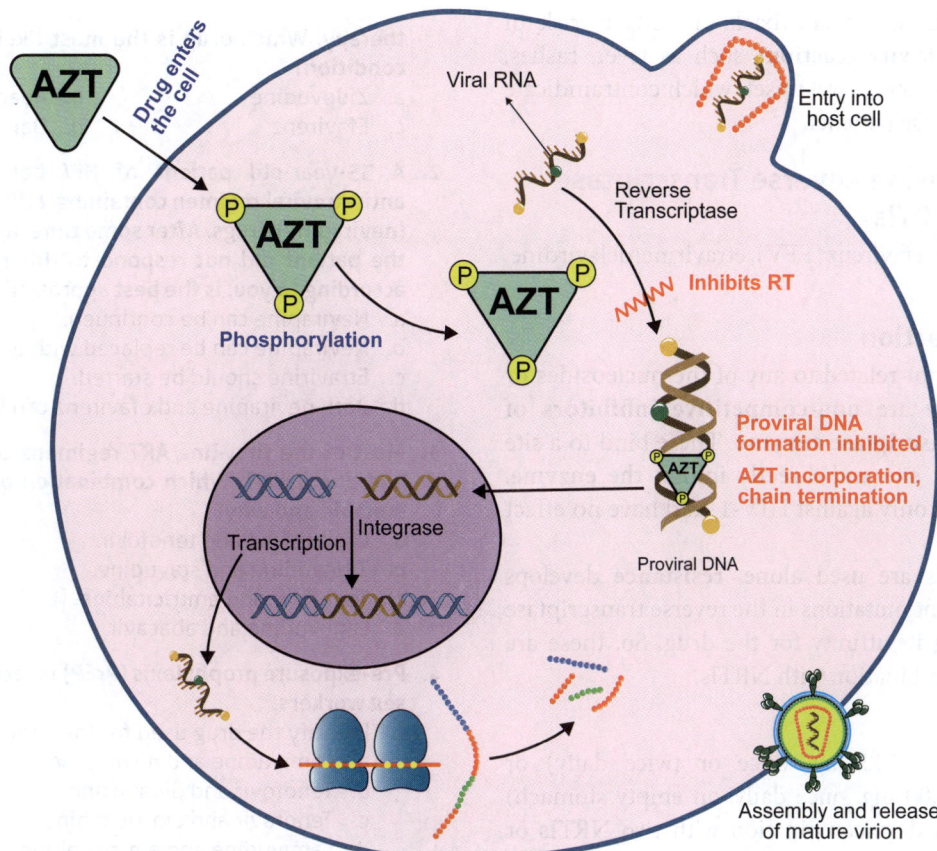

Fig. 57.2 Mechanism of action of zidovudine

is **not used much** because of ADRs such as lactic acidosis, peripheral neuropathy and lipodystrophy.

3. Lamivudine

Lamivudine or 2',3'-dideoxy-3'-thiacytidine (3TC) is a deoxycytidine analogue with the same mechanism of action and resistance as AZT. It is preferred as a **first-line drug in the triple-drug regimen of WHO and NACO**. It is given in a dose of 150 mg, twice daily in combination with another NRTI and an NNRTI/PI. Among NRTIs, lamivudine can be combined with tenofovir, zidovudine, and abacavir. However, it is not combined with didanosine or emtricitabine.

- Lamivudine can inhibit HBV DNA polymerase and has longer intracellular half-life in HBV-infected cells than in HIV-infected cells. Thus, it is **useful in hepatitis B in a lower dose** (100 mg, once a day).
- Lamivudine is suitable in patients with hepatic dysfunction, because it is **excreted unchanged by the kidney**.
- Adverse effects are mild, like anorexia, nausea and abdominal pain.

4. Didanosine

Didanosine is an adenine nucleoside analogue that is **not used much** in current clinical practice because it is more toxic than other NRTIs. Didanosine should not be combined with stavudine (because of increased risk of toxicity), lamivudine (no additive effect) or tenofovir (lower efficacy).

5. Tenofovir (TDF)

Tenofovir is an adenosine monophosphate (AMP) nucleotide analogue (it is the **only nucleotide analogue** drug among antiretroviral drugs) that is effective against HIV as well as HBV (refer to Chapter 56). It is **as efficacious and less toxic than other drugs used in first-line triple-drug regimens** for HIV in adults and adolescents.

6. Emtricitabine (FTC)

Emtricitabine is a fluorinated cytidine analogue with a long intracellular half-life that allows **once-daily dosing**. It is currently in **use as part of the first-line regimen** for HIV. Combination of tenofovir (TDF) 300 mg and emtricitabine (FTC) 200 mg is used as a fixed-dose combination (FDC) for **pre-exposure HIV prophylaxis**. Adverse effects are mild gastrointestinal symptoms, headache and discolouration of exposed skin.

7. Abacavir (ABC)

Abacavir is a guanosine analogue that brings about **quick response** in the form of reduced HIV-RNA and rise in CD4 cell count. Resistance to ABC develops slowly. It is a **preferred drug in triple-drug regimens for HIV-**

positive children. Major drawback of ABC is risk of **severe hypersensitivity reactions** such as fever, rashes, flu-like symptoms, and bowel upset, which contraindicate its future use in these patients.

B. Non-Nucleoside Reverse Transcriptase Inhibitors (NNRTIs)

Nevirapine (NVP), efavirenz (EFV), etravirine, delavirdine, rilpivirine

Mechanism of action

These drugs are not related to any of the nucleosides or nucleotides. They are **non-competitive inhibitors of viral reverse transcriptase enzyme**. These bind to a site near the catalytic site and directly inhibit the enzyme. They are effective only against HIV-1, and have no effect on HIV-2.

When NNRTIs are used alone, **resistance** develops rapidly due to point mutations in the reverse transcriptase enzyme, reducing its affinity for the drug. So, these are always used in combination with NRTIs.

Uses

Nevirapine (NVP; 200 mg, once or twice daily) or **efavirenz** (EFV; 600 mg, once daily, on empty stomach) are commonly used in combination with two NRTIs or one NRTI and one PI.

- Efavirenz-containing regimens are preferred in HIV-positive, pregnant/lactating women.
- There is **cross-resistance between nevirapine and efavirenz**. So, if a regimen that contains nevirapine is not effective, efavirenz should not be tried and vice versa. However, such a patient may respond to the second-generation NNRTI, etravirine.
- **Etravirine is used in cases resistant to other NNRTIs.** It is used in adults and children > 6 years of age, in a dose of 200 mg, twice daily, after meals (food increases its oral absorption).

ADRs

- Nevirapine has the potential to cause **rashes and hepatotoxicity**.
- Efavirenz can cause **neuropsychiatric symptoms** and rashes. Both nevirapine and efavirenz have microsomal enzyme-inducing potential and can induce their own metabolism (**autoinduction**).
- Etravirine can cause rashes, nausea and also causes microsomal enzyme induction; it may result in several drug–drug interactions.

Clinical problem-based questions and MCQs

1. A 30-year-old HIV-positive male patient receiving antiretroviral drugs presents in emergency complaining of fever, rash flu-like symptoms, and bowel and GIT upset, two weeks after starting the therapy. Which drug is the most likely cause of his condition?
   a. Zidovudine   b. Abacavir
   c. Efavirenz   d. Darunavir

2. A 35-year-old patient of HIV has been on the antiretroviral regimen containing 2 NRTIs and 1 NNRTI (nevirapine) drugs. After some time, it was found that the patient did not respond to this regimen. What, according to you, is the best approach?
   a. Nevirapine can be continued.
   b. Nevirapine can be replaced with efavirenz.
   c. Etravirine should be started.
   d. Both nevirapine and efavirenz can be given.

3. Most of the first-line ART regimens contain 2 NRTIs and one NNRTI. Which combination of NRTIs is NOT suitable and why?
   a. Lamivudine and tenofovir.
   b. Zidovudine and stavudine.
   c. Tenofovir and emtricitabine.
   d. Lamivudine and abacavir.

4. Pre-exposure prophylaxis (PrEP) is recommended for sex workers.
   i. Identify the drug used for this indication
      a. Lamivudine and nevirapine.
      b. Tenofovir and didanosine.
      c. Tenofovir and emtricitabine.
      d. Lamivudine and emtricitabine.
   ii. Describe the mechanism of action, dose and adverse effects of each drug used for PrEP.

5. Identify the ARV drug that has hepatotoxic potential.
   a. Nevirapine   b. Lamivudine
   c. Efavirenz   d. Emtricitabine

6. Identify the ARV drug that has the potential to cause neuropsychiatric symptoms
   a. Nevirapine   b. Lamivudine
   c. Efavirenz   d. Dolutegravir

C. Protease Inhibitors (PIs)

Atazanavir (AZV), indinavir (IDV), nelfinavir (NFV), saquinavir (SQV), ritonavir (RNV), amprenavir, lopinavir

Mechanism of action

Production of structural and enzymatic proteins of HIV occurs in two steps (Fig. 57.3): formation of a large viral polyprotein, which is then cleaved by the enzyme aspartic protease into various functional proteins. Protease inhibitor drugs bind to the active site of protease and **interfere with its polyprotein cleaving function**.

- Because the protease enzyme acts at a late step in viral replication, PIs are **effective against newly infected as well as chronically infected cells**.
- Unlike NRTIs, PIs do not need intracellular phosphorylation for activation and are **more effective inhibitors of HIV** than zidovudine.
- PIs cause the formation of noninfectious, immature viral progeny, preventing further rounds of infection.

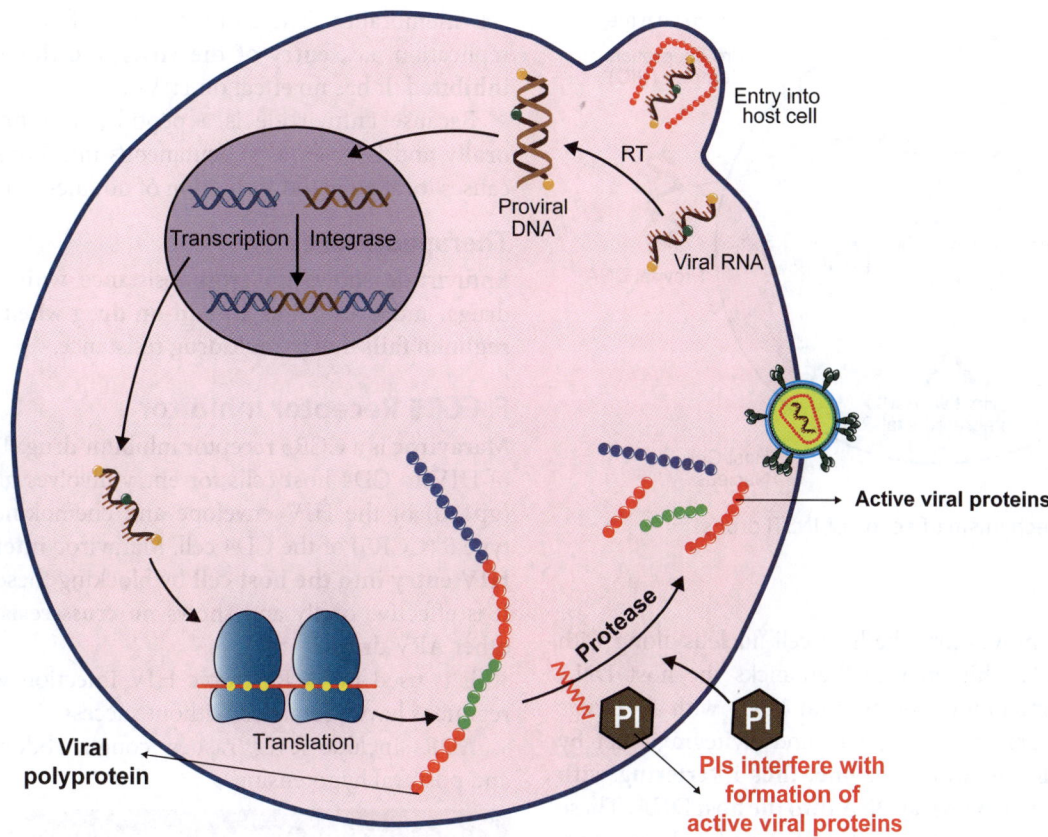

Fig. 57.3 Mechanism of action of protease inhibitors (PIs)

Pharmacokinetics

PIs are extensively metabolised by CYP3A4. Nelfinavir is metabolised by CYP2C19. **Ritonavir and lopinavir can potentially inhibit CYP3A4**. Thus, they reduce metabolism of other PIs (except nelfinavir), reduce their clearance, and hence increase their oral bioavailability. This, in turn, **reduces the required dose and tablet load, and forms the basis for the use of ritonavir in boosted PI regimens.**

- An important shortcoming of PIs is the need to take 6–18 tablets daily, i.e., large tablet load, which reduces patient compliance. Tablet load of PIs (except nelfinavir) is reduced by adding ritonavir 100 mg, which inhibits CYP3A4 and increases oral bioavailability of other PIs. Such ritonavir-containing regimens are called **boosted PI regimens**.
- PIs have the potential to induce some isoforms of CYP. Nelfinavir, lopinavir and ritonavir can induce their own metabolism. Because of this potential to inhibit or induce CYP isoforms, there is **risk of many drug interactions with PIs**. For example, rifampicin induces metabolism of PIs and decreases their efficacy.

Uses

- These are not used as monotherapy, because of the risk of development of resistant strains. They are used in **combinations with two NRTIs or one NRTI and one NNRTI in triple-drug regimens.**

- In WHO and NACO regimens, **PIs are reserved as second-line regimens** if resistance develops to first-line drugs. All PIs, except nelfinavir, are given with ritonavir 100 mg as boosted PI regimens.
- Darunavir is a new PI that is effective against HIV strains resistant to other PIs.
- Fosamprenavir is a prodrug with better bioavailability and is useful in new as well as resistant cases.

ADRs

Protease inhibitors cause GI intolerance, headache, dizziness, asthenia, numbness, tingling sensation, lipodystrophy, hyperlipidemias, hyperglycemia, etc. Indinavir can cause nephrolithiasis, while saquinavir frequently causes photosensitivity reactions, and lopinavir can cause ECG anomalies. Darunavir can cause a rise in hepatic enzymes and hypersensitivity reactions.

D. Integrase Strand Transfer Inhibitors (INSTIs)

Raltegravir, elvitegravir, dolutegravir

Mechanism of action

The HIV virus-specific integrase enzyme gains entry into the host cell along with the viral RNA (Fig. 57.4). Inside the host cell, viral RNA forms proviral DNA, which then moves into the host cell nucleus. The integrase

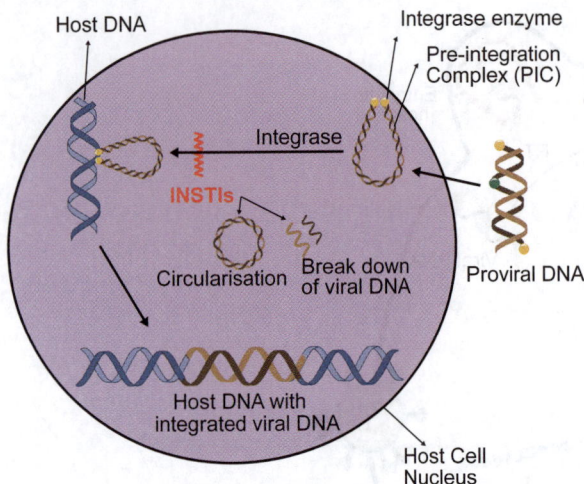

Fig. 57.4 Mechanism of action of INSTI drugs

enzyme also moves into the host cell nucleus along with proviral DNA. This enzyme then nicks the host DNA and causes integration of proviral DNA with it. Drugs such as raltegravir, dolutegravir, and elvitegravir **act by inhibiting the integrase enzyme, thus interfering with incorporation of proviral DNA into the host DNA**. These drugs are effective against both HIV-1 and 2. There is **no cross-resistance with any other group of antiretroviral drugs**

Pharmacokinetics

Raltegravir is rapidly absorbed, but dolutegravir has slow absorption. They are metabolised in the liver by CYP enzymes and glucuronide conjugation. Microsomal enzyme inducers like rifampicin increase their metabolism. Therefore, the dose should be increased in such cases. Cationic medicines such as antacids containing Mg^{2+}/Ca^{2+} salts and iron preparations should be avoided with INSTIs, because of the potential to chelate.

Uses

Dolutegravir may be **combined with 2 NRTIs as a first-line regimen** for treatment of naive patients in a dose of 50 mg, given once a day. In patients with resistance to raltegravir or those receiving enzyme inducers, dose of dolutegravir is doubled.

Adverse effects

Raltegravir can cause headache, nausea, diarrhea, weakness and myopathy. Dolutegravir is better tolerated, but may cause rashes, hypersensitivity and hepatotoxicity.

E. Entry Inhibitors

Enfuvirtide, an entry inhibitor drug, binds to the HIV-1 envelope transmembrane glycoprotein (gp41) and interferes with the fusion of the viral and host cell membranes. Therefore, the very first step of viral replication, i.e., **entry of the virus into the host cell, is inhibited**. It has no effect on HIV-2.

Because enfuvirtide is a peptide, it is **not effective orally** and is given as subcutaneous injections. Injection causes local pain and formation of nodules or cysts.

Therapeutic uses

Enfuvirtide shows no cross-resistance with other ARV drugs, and is useful as an **add-on drug when the initial regimen fails** due to multidrug resistance.

F. CCR5 Receptor Inhibitor

Maraviroc is a CCR5 receptor inhibitor drug. The binding of HIV to CD4 host cells for entry involves glycoprotein (gp120) of the HIV envelope and chemokine receptors type 5 (CCR5) of the CD4 cell. Maraviroc **interferes with HIV entry into the host cell** by blocking these receptors. It is effective orally and shows **no cross-resistance** with other ARV drugs.

It is used in CCR5 tropic HIV infection when other regimens have been tried without success.

ADRs include fever, rashes, cough, abdominal pain, and postural hypotension.

Clinical problem-based questions and MCQs

7. Protease inhibitors are NOT used in first-line regimens of WHO and NACO. What are the limitations of using PIs?

8. Identify the antiretroviral drug that can chelate with polyvalent cations like Ca^{2+} and Mg^{2+}.
   a. Dolutegravir   b. Tenofovir
   c. Enfuvirtide   d. Emtricitabine

9. i. Low-dose ritonavir can be combined with all of the following drugs in boosted PI regimens, EXCEPT:
   a. Nelfinavir   b. Indinavir
   c. Atazanavir   d. Saquinavir
   ii. Explain the pharmacological basis of such boosted PI regimens.

10. Explain why enfuvirtide is used only when multiple drug regimens have already failed.

MANAGEMENT OF HIV INFECTION

HIV infection is not curable, so the treatment is complex and lifelong. The **goal** of the treatment is to inhibit viral replication maximally, for long duration, in order to maintain effective immune response of the patient against infective organisms and limit disease transmission.

General Principles of HIV Treatment

1. Recommendation on ART

In current clinical practice, early institution of antiretroviral therapy (ART) or immediate start is recommended. It provides better outcomes in people living with HIV (PL-HIV), improves prognosis and reduces chances of drug resistance. Disease transmission to uninfected sexual partner is also reduced.

WHO 2016 guidelines recommend starting ART **in all adults** including pregnant/lactating women, adolescents and children **at the earliest** after diagnosis of HIV-positive status, irrespective of the presence or absence of symptoms, CD4 count, and HIV-RNA load.

2. Optimum response

Aggressive therapy is preferred, and at least **3 ARV drugs** are given in combination. It is called highly active antiretroviral therapy **(HAART)**. Monotherapy favours the development of resistant strains and is not used.

Optimum response to ARV drug regimen includes reduction of HIV-RNA to undetectable levels (< 50 copies/µL), and restoration of CD4 count to near normal levels within 6 months of starting treatment. Opportunistic infections and neurological manifestations subside, and the patient gains weight and experiences a feeling of well-being. New Kaposi's lesions do not appear.

3. Anti-HIV regimens

First-line ART regimens

Choice of ARV drugs depends upon consideration of many factors such as efficacy, tolerability, convenience of administration, drug–drug interactions and chances of development of resistance. First-line regimens usually include **2 NRTIs + 1 NNRTI**.

- Preferred NRTIs are lamivudine, tenofovir, emtricitabine, and abacavir.
- Preferred NNRTI is efavirenz.
- For adult and adolescent ARV-naive people Living with HIV (PLHIV) > **10 years** of age:
  - **If body weight > 30 kg:** Lamivudine + tenofovir + efavirenz
  - **If body weight < 30 kg** or **serum creatinine is raised:** Lamivudine + abacavir + efavirenz
- For children **3–10 years** of age:
  - **If Hb > 9 g/dL:** Lamivudine + zidovudine + efavirenz
  - **If Hb < 9 g/dL:** Lamivudine + abacavir + efavirenz

Integrase inhibitor-containing regimens in ARV-naive PLHIV

2 NRTIs + 1 INSTI

For example, lamivudine + abacavir + dolutegravir

- Dolutegravir has better efficacy in lowering the HIV-RNA load. So, it is preferred **in patients with high HIV-RNA load.**
- This regimen has **better tolerability** and is **more convenient** to use than boosted PIs or efavirenz-containing regimens.
- In patients with **metabolic disorders**, regimens containing dolutegravir are better than PI-containing regimens.

PI-containing regimens

PI-containing regimens are used in all women with prior single-dose NVP exposure during pregnancy, in HIV-2 infection, or HIV-1 and HIV-2 infections.

Lamivudine, tenofovir and lopinavir + ritonavir are given.

4. Duration of treatment

Treatment should be continued **lifelong** in all HIV-positive cases, even if HIV-RNA becomes undetectable, CD4 cell counts recover to normal levels, or there are no opportunistic infections or co-morbidities.

5. Compliance factors

Compliance can be improved by **using fixed-dose combinations (FDCs).** It reduces pill burden and cost of treatment. The risk of development of resistance and treatment failure also decreases

- If adverse toxic effects develop, therapy is not discontinued. Even dose reduction is not attempted. The offending drug should be replaced by another drug of the same or different class.
- Therapy with ARV drugs is not discontinued even during acute opportunistic infections, except when there is intolerance, toxicity or interactions with other drugs used for opportunistic infections. Sometimes, in patients with latent or partially treated opportunistic infections, severe inflammatory reactions occur against residual organisms on starting ART. This is due to the improvement of immune response with ART. It is called Immune Reconstitution Inflammatory Syndrome (IRIS).
- Pregnancy is not a contraindication to ART. Drugs safe in pregnant women include zidovudine, lamivudine, tenofovir, emtricitabine and efavirenz.

6. Drug combinations to avoid

Drug combinations to be avoided include those that have similar toxic effects, lower efficacy, and no additive effect. For example:

- Stavudine antagonises the effect of zidovudine.
- Stavudine and didanosine can both cause lactic acidosis and neuropathy.
- Effect of didanosine is not additive with lamivudine as well as with tenofovir.

7. Failure of ART

An ART regimen is considered to have failed, if, in spite of continued therapy:

- Plasma HIV-RNA load does not reduce to < 50 copies/µL in 6 months.
- HIV-RNA load falls initially, but becomes detectable again.
- Clinical deterioration, serious new opportunistic infections, and fall in CD4 count occur.

8. Second-line regimens

Resistance may develop to an ART regimen. In such cases, all three component drugs in the regimen are changed.

However, **lamivudine, if used in the initial regimen, may be continued in the new second-line regimen also**. This is because it can exert residual antiretroviral action and increases the sensitivity of the virus to tenofovir and zidovudine. Drugs that have the potential of cross-resistance with previously used drugs should not be chosen in second-line regimens, e.g., nevirapine for efavirenz, emtricitabine for lamivudine, and stavudine for zidovudine. Boosted PI is mostly included in second-line regimens.

Some **common second-line regimens** include:

- **(2 NRTIs+ PI) or (1 NRTI + 1 NNRTI + PI)**
  - These regimens are useful in patients in whom **earlier regimens have failed**.
  - Boosted PI regimens have low-dose ritonavir, with the advantage of low tablet load.
- Lamivudine + tenofovir + atazanvir, with low-dose ritonavir
- Lamivudine + zidovudine + atazanvir, with low-dose ritonavir
- Raltegravir + lopinavir with low-dose ritonavir

9. Prophylaxis

Prophylaxis may be pre-exposure and post-exposure.

- **Pre-exposure prophylaxis** (PrEP): It protects high risk groups like sex workers, drug addicts using injectable drugs, transgenders, and men having sex with men from acquiring HIV infections. Drugs used for prophylaxis in such high-risk groups are tenofovir 300 mg + emtricitabine 200 mg, daily.
- **Post-exposure prophylaxis** (PEP): Health care workers like doctors, technicians, and nurses who are inadvertently exposed to HIV due to needle stick injuries or contact with body fluids or blood of infected patients, or after sexual contact with HIV-positive persons are given PEP to suppress local viral replication before its dissemination, to abort infection. PEP is started as soon as possible after the exposure, within 1–2 hours. NACO guidelines do not recommend PEP beyond 72 hours of exposure. PEP usually includes:

  Two NRTIs (lamivudine 300 mg + tenofovir 300 mg, once daily) or 2 PIs (lopinavir 200 mg + ritonavir 50 mg, two tablets, twice a day) given for 28 days. Sometimes, a third drug is added to the 2 NRTIs, e.g., lamivudine and tenofovir, 300 mg each + efavirenz 600 mg.
- **Perinatal prophylaxis** to protect the newborn baby of an HIV-positive mother includes continuing ART in the pregnant woman, delivering baby by cesarean section if the viral load is > 1000 copies/μL, and ARV drugs to newborn. Nevirapine 10–15 mg is given as syrup, based on birth weight of baby, for minimum 6 weeks. If mother has already been treated with nevirapine, baby should be given syrup zidovudine 10–15 mg daily instead of nevirapine.

Clinical problem-based questions and MCQs

11. Describe the general principles of ART.
12. WHO and NACO recommend early institution of ART and aggressive therapy with combination of three drugs.
    i. Justify early institution of therapy.
    ii. Why is combination therapy recommended?
    iii. Describe the first-line ART regimens.
13. Who among the following need PEP for HIV infections?
    a. Transgenders
    b. Health care workers
    c. Sex workers
    d. Drug addicts who share syringes
14. For how long is PEP continued?
    a. 1 month
    b. 3 months
    c. 6 months
    d. Lifelong
15. Which ARV drug is used in newborns to decrease vertical transmission?
    a. Lamivudine
    b. Efavirenz
    c. Nevirapine
    d. Ritonavir

Summary

- Replication of HIV involves the formation of proviral DNA under the influence of RT enzyme followed by its integration with host cell DNA by integrase enzyme. The polyprotein formed after translation from infected host cell is then cleaved into structural and functional proteins by protease enzyme.
- These three enzymes are the main targets for antiretroviral drugs. Some drugs inhibit entry of virus into host cell and prevent its replication.
- RTIs can be nucleoside/nucleotide or non-nucleoside types (NRTIs and NNRTIs). **NRTIs** are activated inside the cell by phosphorylations, inhibit RT and cause chain termination. Zidovudine is the first NRTI.
- Lamivudine has synergistic action with most ARV drugs and low toxicity. It is an essential component of most first-line regimens. It is continued in second-line regimens also in case of treatment failure.
- Tenofovir is active against HIV as well as HBV and is part of most first-line regimens.
- Abacavir is used as a first-line drug in children 3–10 years of age and has a high risk of severe hypersensitivity reactions.
- Emtricitabine is used in first-line regimens as well as for pre-exposure prophylaxis along with tenofovir in high risk groups.
- **NNRTIs** are non-competitive inhibitors of RT enzyme. Among NNRTIs (nevirapine, efavirenz, etravirine, etc.),

- Efavirenz is used in most first-line regimens along with two NRTIs. It may cause neuropsychiatric symptoms.
- Nevirapine has hepatotoxic potential and is mostly used in newborns of HIV positive mothers to reduce vertical transmission.
- Etravirine is used in alternative regimens in patients resistant to nevirapine and efavirenz.
- **Protease inhibitors** (atazanvir, lopinavir, ritonavir, etc.) interfere with formation of structural and functional viral proteins. They do not need intracellular phosphorylation for activation and are effective by oral route, although bioavailability is variable.
- Important limitations of PIs are large tablet load and potential for drug interactions because of microsomal enzyme induction or inhibition of some isoforms of CYP.
- Boosted PI regimens have a low dose of ritonavir combined to other PIs for increasing the bioavailability, which in turn reduces tablet burden. They may cause metabolic adverse effects like insulin resistance, dyslipidemia and lipodystrophy. So, PIs are usually reserved for treatment failure cases.
- **Integrase inhibitors** (raltegravir, dolutegravir) may be used in first-line regimens because of better efficacy, low tablet load, once daily dose and good tolerability.
- Drugs may **interfere with entry of virus** into host cell by binding to viral glycoproteins (enfuvirtide) or host cell chemokine receptors CCR5 (maraviroc). These do not show cross-resistance with other groups and are useful as add-on drugs.
- **ART** is started at the earliest irrespective of symptoms, CD4 counts or HIV-RNA load and continued throughout life as once infected HIV eradication is not possible.
- ARV drugs are used as **triple-drug regimens**. Most first-line regimens contain 2 NRTIs and one NRTI or integrase inhibitor. In case of drug toxicity, the offending drug is replaced but dose is not reduced.
- Failure of treatment needs replacing all drugs of previously used regimen. However, lamivudine may be continued.
- Pre-exposure prophylaxis is recommended for high risk groups with tenofovir and emtricitabine.
- Post-exposure prophylaxis for HCWs or uninfected sexual partner should be started as soon as possible after exposure with 2 NRTIs or 2 PIs and is continued for 28 days.
- Nevirapine or zidovudine given just after birth and continued for 6 months can decrease vertical transmission.

Questions for practice

1. Classify antiretroviral drugs.
2. Write short notes on:
    a. Boosted PI regimens
    b. Integrase inhibitors
    c. Pre-exposure prophylaxis of HIV-infection.
    d. First-line antiretroviral regimen for an adult.
3. Explain why:
    a. PIs are not used as first-line drugs.
    b. Efavirenz is preferred over nevirapine.
    c. ART is life long.
    d. Pre-exposure prophylaxis is advocated in selected patient groups only.

Hints for problem-based questions and MCQs

1. b. Abacavir can cause hypersensitivity reaction such as fever, rashes, flu-like symptoms, and GI upset. Drug should be stopped immediately and is contraindicated for future use.
2. c. Etravirine should be started, as there is cross-resistance between nevirapine and efavirenz.
3. b. Zidovudine and stavudine should not be combined as these two use the same activation pathway and decrease each other's effects.
4. i. c. Tenofovir and emtricitabine
   ii. Both these drugs used for PrEP in high-risk groups are NRTIs. They competitively inhibit of viral reverse transcriptase enzyme. FDC of TDF 300 mg and FTC 200 mg is used. ADRs are mild GI upset, headache and discolouration of skin. Tenofovir and emtricitabine. Refer to page 747.
5. a. Nevirapine
6. c. Efavirenz
7. 7. Important limitation of PIs is large tablet load and risk for drug interactions.
8. a. Dolutegravir: Integrase inhibitors can cause chelation with divalent cations.
9. i. a. Nelfinavir
   ii. Ritonavir inhibits the metabolism of other PIs by inhibiting CYP3A4. So, oral bioavailability of other simultaneously used PIs (which are metabolised by CYP3A4) increases. Consequently, oral dose and tablet load is decreased. However, nelfinavir is metabolised by CYP2C19 and its metabolism is not inhibited by ritonavir.
10. Enfuvirtide is fusion inhibitor that is a peptide. Because it is not effective orally, it is administered by subcutaneous injections, which are painful. Moreover, it has no cross-resistance with other antiretroviral drugs. Therefore, it is not suitable for initial use, but valuable as add-on drug when resistance has developed to many other drugs.
11. Refer to page 750.
12. i. Early institution of ART provides better outcomes, improves prognosis and reduces drug resistance.
    ii. Monotherapy favours development of resistance.
    iii. Refer to page 751.
13. b. Healthcare workers need PEP. The others are high-risk groups in which PrEP is given.
14. a. 1 month
15. c. Nevirapine

CONCEPT MAP – ANTIRETROVIRAL DRUGS

NNRTIs

Mechanism: Non-competitive inhibition of viral RT enzyme. Resistance develops rapidly due to point mutations in RT, if used alone. Cross-resistance between Nevirapine & Efavirenz.

Nevirapine BD or **Efavirenz** OD commonly combined with two NRTIs or One NRTI & one PI.

Etravirine is used in resistant cases.

ADRs: Nevirapine: rashes, hepatotoxicity. Efavirenz: neuropsychiatric symptoms Etravirine: rashes, nausea NNRTIs cause autoinduction due to enzyme induction.

NRTIs

Mechanism: Activated inside cell by phosphorylations, inhibit RT competitively & cause chain termination.

Zidovudine: Not preferred, because of many ADRs.

Tenofovir: Active against HIV as well as HBV, part of most 1st-line regimens.

Abacavir: 1st-line drug in children 3-10 years of age. Risk of severe hypersensitivity reactions.

Emtricitabine: Used in 1st-line regimens & pre-exposure prophylaxis with tenofovir in high-risk groups.

ADRs: Anorexia, nausea, abdominal pain, myalgia, headache, insomnia, pigmentation of nails, hepatomegaly, lactic acidosis, anemia, neutropenia with zidovudine. Mild anorexia, nausea & abdominal pain with tenofovir & emtricitabine Severe hypersensitivity with abacavir.

RTIs

Protease Inhibitors (PIs)

Mechanism: No need of intracellular phosphorylations, interfere with polyprotein cleaving function of protease enzyme → active viral proteins not formed.

Effective against new & chronically infected cells More effective than zidovudine.

Ritonavir and **Lopinavir** inhibit CYP3A4 → reduced metabolism of other PIs (except nelfinavir) → reduced required dose & tablet load (**boosted PI regimens**).

Used in combinations with two NRTIs or one NRTI and one NNRTI in 2nd-line regimens.

ADRs: GI intolerance, headache, dizziness, asthenia, numbness, tingling sensation, lipodystrophy, hyperlipidemias, hyperglycemia, nephrolithiasis, photosensitivity reactions, ECG anomalies.

Antiretroviral Drugs

Integrase Strand Transfer Inhibitors (INSTIs)

Mechanism: Interfere with incorporation of proviral DNA into host DNA. No cross-resistance with any other antiretroviral drugs.

Dolutegravir may be combined with 2 NRTIs as first-line regimen for treatment-naïve patients. Double dose used in **Raltegravir** resistance

ADRs: Raltegravir: headache, nausea, diarrhea, weakness and myopathy. Dolutegravir is better tolerated, but may cause rashes, hypersensitivity & hepatotoxicity.

Entry Inhibitor

Enfuvirtide: Interferes with fusion of viral and host cell membrane. Not effective orally, No cross-resistance with other ARV drugs, Used only as add-on drug in patients with failed initial regimens.

CCR5 Receptor Inhibitors

Maraviroc: Interferes with HIV entry into host cell, effective orally, No cross-resistance with other ARV drugs. It is used in CCR5 tropic HIV infection after failure of several other regimens.

ADRs: Fever, rashes, cough, abdominal pain, postural hypotension.

General Principles of HIV Management

- **Anti retroviral Antiretroviraltherapy (ART)** started at the earliest irrespective of symptoms, CD4 counts or HIV-RNA load and continued throughout life.
- **Triple-drug regimens:** First-line regimens: 2 NRTIs + 1 NRTI / Integrase inhibitor. In case of toxicity with drugs, offending drug is replaced but dose is not reduced.
- **Failure of treatment** → replace all drugs of previously used regimen. However, Lamivudine may be continued.
- **Pre-exposure prophylaxis** for high-risk groups with Tenofovir and Emtricitabine.
- **Post-exposure prophylaxis** for HCWs or uninfected sexual partner with 2 NRTIs or 2 PIs and is continued for 28 days.
- **To prevent vertical transmission:** Nevirapine or zidovudine, just after birth and continued for 6 months

SECTION 10   Chemotherapeutic Drugs

58   Antimalarial Drugs

PH8.7 Discuss the types, kinetics, dynamics, adverse effects of drugs used for the following protozoal/ vector-borne diseases: Malaria

---

Learning objectives

A student of MBBS phase II should be able to:
- Classify antimalarial drugs.
- Describe the mechanism of action of antimalarial drugs.
- Enumerate therapeutic uses, adverse effects and contraindications of antimalarial drugs.
- Describe prophylaxis and treatment of malaria as per National Programme.

Malaria is an important parasitic disease **endemic** in most parts of India and other tropical countries. Malaria is caused by 4 species of *Plasmodium*: *P. vivax*, *P. falciparum*, *P. malariae*, and *P. ovale*. Antimalarial drugs can affect the malarial parasite at different stages of its life cycle. The nature of their action determines their role in treatment and/or prophylaxis of disease.

LIFE CYCLE OF MALARIAL PARASITE

Host: In the life cycle of the malarial parasite, there are **two phases—asexual** and **sexual generations—with an alternation of hosts**. The vector for transmission of malaria is the **female *Anopheles* mosquito**. The two phases in the life cycle of the malarial parasite (Fig. 58.1) are described below.

Asexual Phase (Schizogony)

The asexual phase of the malarial parasite's life cycle takes place in humans, who serve as the **intermediate host**. Humans get infected when an infective female *Anopheles* mosquito bites a person, injecting **sporozoites** (from Greek *sporo*, meaning "seed") from its salivary glands into the human bloodstream.

Once inside the bloodstream, many of the sporozoites are destroyed by phagocytes; however, some reach the liver within an hour of being injected into body where they undergo multiplication by a process known as **schizogony** (*schizo*: to split; *gony*: generation), to form **schizonts**. Schizogony occurs at two distinct sites in the human host:

- **Liver cells**: This stage, called **exo-erythrocytic schizogony** (also referred to as **pre-erythrocytic** or **tissue schizogony**), is a mandatory initial step before the parasite can invade RBCs.

- **Red blood cells (RBCs)**: This phase is known as **erythrocytic schizogony**, during which the parasite continues to multiply inside RBCs.

The products of schizogony are called **merozoites** (*mero*: a part; *zoon*: animal). These are released into the bloodstream to infect additional red blood cells, perpetuating the infection cycle.

a. Pre/exo-erythrocytic or tissue phase (Fig. 58.1, steps 1–3)

1. First, the **sporozoites** enter the hepatocytes. Exo-erythrocytic schizogony involves only a very small proportion of the liver cells; so, no significant damage or clinical illness occurs.
2. The elongated sporozoites become rounded, enlarged, and undergo repeated nuclear division to form several daughter nuclei, each of which is surrounded by cytoplasm. These are called **pre- or exo-erythrocytic schizonts**.
3. The enlarged schizont distends the hepatocytes and bursts in 5–15 days, releasing thousands of **merozoites**. The merozoites enter the blood stream and infect RBCs by the process of invagination.

In *P. vivax* and *P. ovale*, the sporozoites are of two types: those which promptly multiply in the hepatocytes to form schizonts, and those which remain dormant inside liver cells as unnucleated forms for long periods, called **hypnozoites** (*hypnos*: sleep). Some of the hypnozoites are activated intermittently to form schizonts, causing relapse of the clinical disease.

In contrast, the hypnozoites are not seen in *P. falciparum* and *P. malariae*, i.e., the parasites do not persist in the exo-erythrocytic phase. However, in the blood stream, a small number of erythrocytic parasites persist. They multiply to reach significant numbers in due course of time and are responsible for short-term relapse or **recrudescence** of the clinical disease.

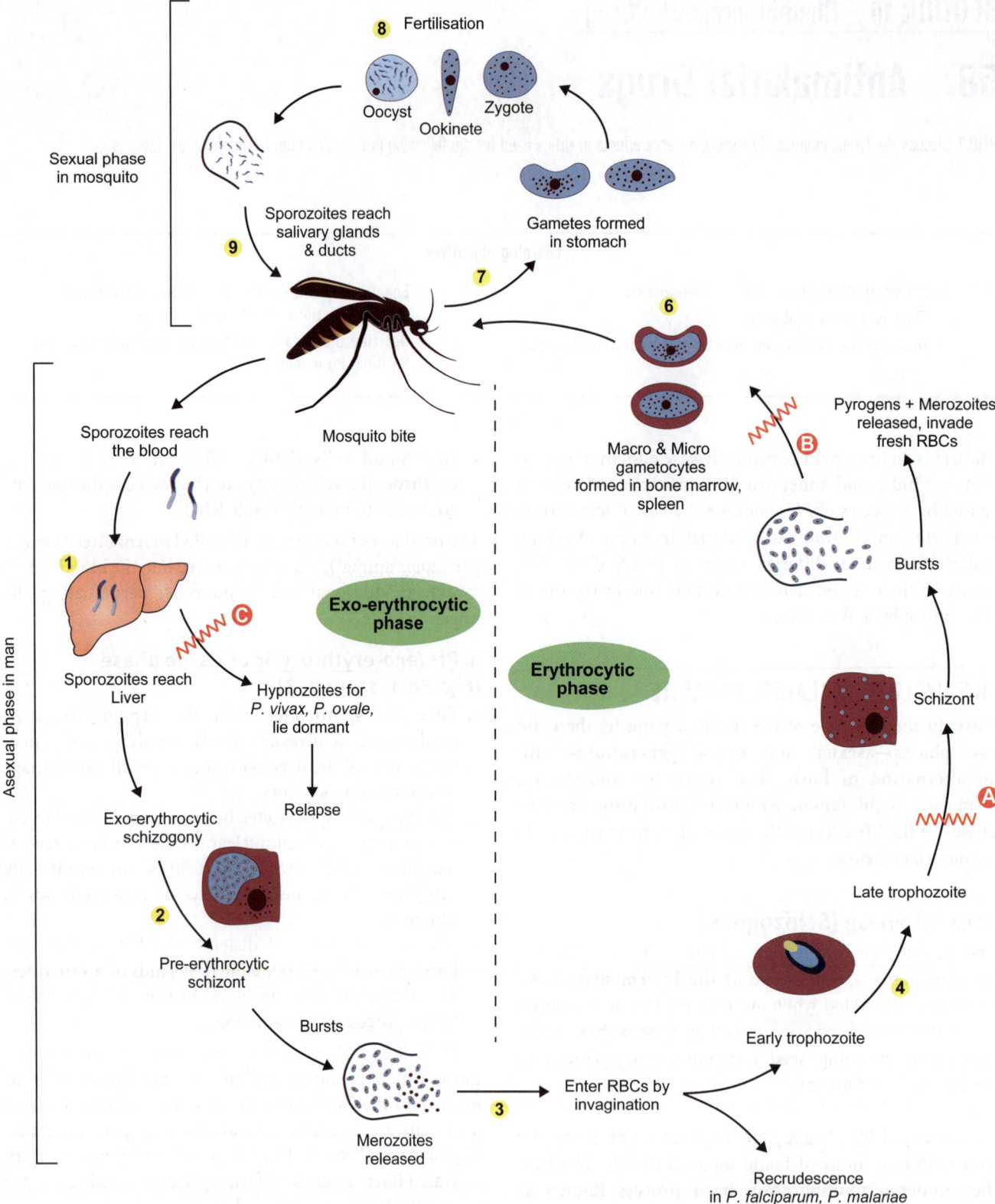

Ⓐ Active against erythrocytic schizonts:
   Fast acting: Artemisinin (fastest), Primaquine, Chloroquine, Quinine, Quinidine, Mefloquine, Amodiaquine,
   Slow acting: Sulphones (Sulfadoxine, Sulphamethopyrazine, Dapsone), Pyrimethamine, Doxycycline, Clindamycin

Ⓑ Active against gametocytes: Primaquine, Artemisinin group,
   Quinine, Quinidine, Chloroquine (active against *vivax/ovale/malariae*, but not *falciparum*)

Ⓒ Active against hypnozoites: Primaquine, Tafenoquine, Atovaquone + Proguanil.
   Drug effective against all stages: Primaquine.

Fig. 58.1 Life cycle of the malarial parasite and the site of action of drugs

b. Erythrocytic phase

The merozoites released by the pre-erythrocytic schizont invade the RBCs by the process of endocytosis within about 30 seconds and the phase of erythrocytic schizogony starts.

4. Inside the RBC, the merozoites round up and assume a ring-form, called the **early trophozoites** (*trophus*: growth, but nucleus has not yet started to divide). The trophozoites feed on Hb in the RBC but do not metabolise Hb completely. The residue accumulates in the parasite as hematin, a globin pigment called the **malaria pigment**. Numerous, fine, golden brown dust like particles in *P. vivax*, coarse dark brown particles in *P. malariae*, blackish brown particles in *P. ovale*, and few solid blocks of black pigment in *P. falciparum* get deposited.

   The ring form enlarges and becomes irregular with amoeboid motility, at which stage it is called a **late trophozoite**.

5. Subsequently, the nucleus undergoes division, and the parasite enters the schizont stage. In the late schizont stage, each daughter nucleus becomes surrounded by a portion of cytoplasm, forming individual merozoites. These mature schizonts rupture periodically, releasing merozoites into the circulation. At the same time large quantities of pyrogens are released, which are responsible for the febrile paroxysms characteristic of malaria.

   This schizogonic periodicity is about 48 hours in *P. vivax/ovale/falciparum*, but 72 hours in *P. malariae*, as a result of which tertian or quartan malaria can occur. The residual mass of unutilised cytoplasm containing malarial pigment is also released into circulation and is phagocytosed by polymorphs and macrophages. Such pigment laden cells in internal organs provide histological evidence of previous malarial infections.

   The released merozoites invade fresh RBCs, and the cycle of erythrocytic schizogony repeats, leading to progressive increase in the intensity of parasitemia.

6. After some cycles of erythrocytic schizogony, a few merozoites develop into sexually differentiated forms the **macro (female) and micro (male) gametocytes** within the internal organs, such as bone marrow and spleen. This is known as 'gametogony'. Gametocytes do not develop or divide further inside the vertebrate host and do not cause any clinical illness in the host.

   A person with gametocytes in circulation is a carrier or reservoir. A gametocyte concentration of 12 or more per cmm of blood in the human host is necessary for a mosquito to become infected.

Sexual Phase (Sporogony)

7. The sexual phase takes place in the mosquito. In its blood meal, the female anopheles mosquito ingests parasitised erythrocytes. Male and female gametocytes are set free in its stomach and mature into male and female gametes.
8. Fertilisation of male and female gametes results in the formation of zygotes. Zygotes elongate to form motile ookinetes, which transform further into oocysts.
9. Once the oocyst matures, its nucleus undergoes multiple divisions and thousands of **sporozoites** are formed, which reach the salivary glands and ducts of the mosquito. Now the mosquito is infective.

ANTIMALARIAL DRUGS

Antimalarial drugs can be classified based on their chemical structure as shown in Flowchart 58.1.

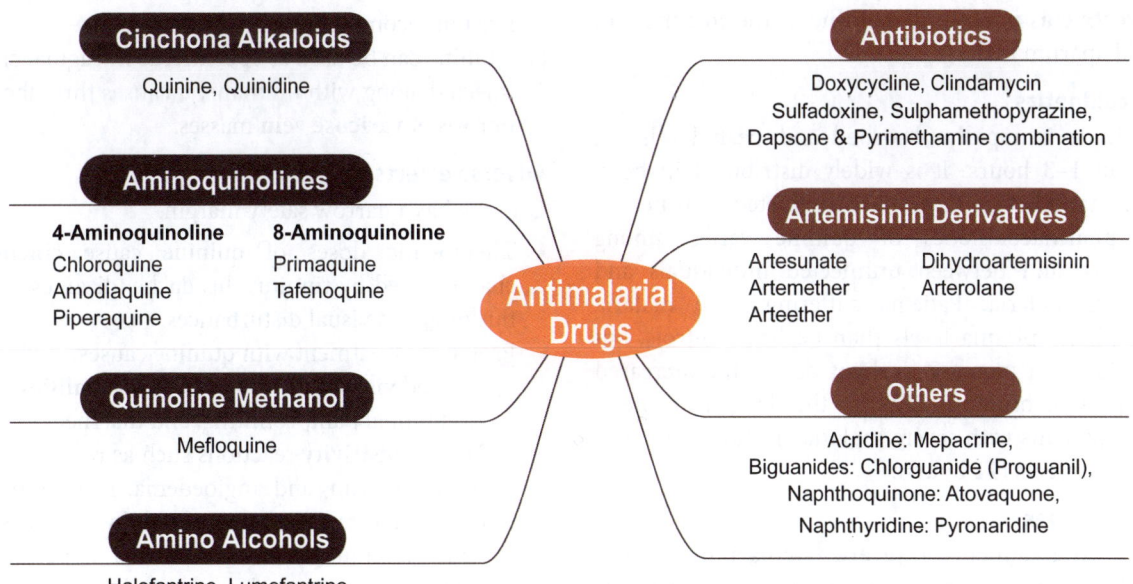

Flowchart 58.1 Classification of antimalarial drugs based on chemical structure

Antimalarial drugs can also be categorised based on their action against different stages of plasmodium. They can target:

- **Erythrocytic schizonts**:
  - **Fast-acting**: Artemisinin (fastest), primaquine, chloroquine, quinine, quinidine, mefloquine, and amodiaquine.
  - **Slow-acting**: Sulphones (sulfadoxine, sulphamethopyrazine, and dapsone), pyrimethamine, doxycycline, and clindamycin.
- **Gametocytes**: Primaquine, artemisinin derivatives, quinine, quinidine, chloroquine (active against *vivax/ovale/malariae*, but not *falciparum*).
- **Hypnozoites**: Primaquine, tafenoquine, atovaquone + proguanil
- **All stages**: Primaquine

1. Cinchona Alkaloids
Quinine
Quinine is an alkaloid obtained from cinchona tree bark. The mechanism of its antimalarial action is unknown—it is likely that quinine, being a weak base, gets concentrated in acidic vacuoles of blood schizonts and **inhibits heme polymerase**.

- It is a **rapidly acting** and highly effective **erythrocytic schizonticide** for all species of *Plasmodium*.
- It is **gametocidal** against *P. vivax*, *P. ovale*, and *P. malariae* but not against *P. falciparum*.
- It has **no action** on hepatic stage parasites.

Resistance
Although resistance is an increasing problem, quinine still provides at least a partial therapeutic effect in most patients

Quinidine, a dextrorotatory stereoisomer of quinine, is **as effective as parenteral quinine** in the treatment of severe falciparum malaria.

Pharmacokinetics
Oral quinine is rapidly absorbed and peak levels are reached in 1–3 hours. It is widely distributed in body tissues, metabolised in the liver, and excreted in urine.

The pharmacokinetics of quinine varies among populations, and between uninfected individuals and those with malaria. Patients suffering from malaria develop higher plasma levels than healthy controls, but toxicity does not increase, perhaps due to the increased plasma protein binding (PPB) of the drug. Half-life is longer in patients with severe malaria (18 hours) than in healthy volunteers (11 hours).

Therapeutic uses
1. Parenteral treatment of **severe falciparum malaria**: Quinine dihydrochloride or gluconate is the treatment of choice for severe falciparum malaria, e.g., cerebral malaria. Quinine 600 mg, diluted with 200–500 mL of 5% glucose is infused slowly over 2–3 hours. Alternatively, it can be used as a diluted solution via the I/M route.

   Nowadays, **quinidine is the standard therapy** for parenteral treatment of severe falciparum malaria. It is given in divided doses or by I/V infusion. I/V quinidine should be administered **with cardiac monitoring** because it has cardiac toxicity and unpredictable pharmacokinetics. When the patient's condition improves sufficiently, oral therapy is started. In addition to antimalarial drugs, cerebral malaria patients need supportive treatment such as maintenance of fluid–electrolyte balance, control of body temperature by external cooling and diazepam for convulsions.

2. For oral treatment of **chloroquine-resistant falciparum malaria**: Quinine sulphate is used **if none of the artemisinin-based combination therapies (ACTs) are suitable** in a patient. However, it is the first-line treatment for uncomplicated falciparum malaria in the **first trimester of pregnancy**. Even multi-drug-resistant strains of *P. falciparum* respond to quinine therapy.

   Quinine is less effective and more toxic than chloroquine against other types of malaria.

3. For **malarial chemoprophylaxis**: Even though quinine 325 mg daily is effective for this indication, it is not used because of its toxicity.

4. **Nocturnal muscle cramps**: A single dose of 300 mg quinine at bed time provides benefit in some patients, but it is not effective in all cases.

5. A single tablet of quinine precipitates weakness in myasthenia gravis; this was previously used as a provocative test for diagnosing myasthenia gravis, but it is not recommended in current practice.

6. Quinine can be used as **spermicide** in vaginal creams.

7. Injected along with urethane, it causes thrombosis and fibrosis of **varicose vein** masses.

Adverse effects
Quinine has a narrow safety margin.

- Therapeutic doses of quinine cause **cinchonism**, characterised by tinnitus, headache, dizziness, nausea, flushing, and visual disturbances.
- Prolonged treatment with quinine causes:
  - Marked **visual and auditory abnormalities**.
  - Abdominal pain, vomiting, and diarrhea.
  - **Hypersensitivity** reactions such as rashes, urticaria, bronchospasm, and angioedema. In rare instances, blackwater fever, characterised by hemolysis and hemoglobinuria, can occur as a hypersensitivity reaction.

- It carries the **risk of**:
  - **Hemolysis** in G6PD deficiency, **leukopenia, thrombocytopenia (TCP),** and **agranulocytosis.**
  - Insulin release: **Hypoglycemia**, especially in pregnancy and severe infection.
  - Uterine **contract**ions in third trimester.
- Rapid IV administration is associated with hypotension and ECG abnormalities.

To reduce toxicity, quinine is commonly used with a second drug (usually doxycycline or sulfadoxine–pyrimethamine) to shorten its duration of use to 3 days.

2. Aminoquinolines
(a) 4-Aminoquinolines
(i) Chloroquine

It is a synthetic 4-aminoquinoline formulated as the phosphate salt for oral use.

Mechanism of action
The mechanism of action of chloroquine is complex (Fig. 58.2) and not fully elucidated. While chloroquine is a weak base, **its accumulation in parasitic lysosomes** is 1000-fold greater than that predicted on this basis, indicating that there are additional parasite-specific drug-concentrating mechanisms at play. One such mechanism is now thought to be a Na^+/H^+ exchange transporter. Inside the lysosome., chloroquine raises the vesicular pH and interferes with the **degradation of Hb,** thereby reducing the supply of amino acids necessary for the parasite's viability. It also **inhibits the heme polymerase enzyme,** inhibiting the conversion of toxic heme to nontoxic pigment hemozoin. Heme can damage parasitic membranes.

Resistance
P. falciparum is mostly resistant to chloroquine due to reduced uptake and/or increased efflux of the drug from parasitic vesicles. *P. vivax* is also developing chloroquine resistance in some geographic areas.

Antimalarial action
- Chloroquine is a rapidly-acting, highly potent, **erythrocytic schizonticidal drug against all species of plasmodia**, even though *P. falciparum* has developed resistance to this drug. Some resistant *P. vivax* strains have also emerged.
- Moderately **effective against gametocytes of *P. vivax*, *P. ovale* and *P. malariae*,** but not *P. falciparum*.
- It has **no activity against hepatic or exo-erythrocytic stage parasites**. Hence, it cannot prevent relapse in vivax and ovale.

Additionally, chloroquine is also effective against *E. histolytica* and *G. lamblia*. It also has anti-inflammatory, local irritant, local anesthetic, weak smooth-muscle relaxant, and antiarrhythmic effects.

Pharmacokinetics
Oral absorption is rapid and almost complete, with PPB up to 50%. It gets concentrated in the **liver, spleen, kidneys, lungs, skin, leukocytes and retina**, because of its affinity for nuclear chromatin and melanin. Chloroquine is partly metabolised in the liver and slowly excreted by the kidney. Half-life is 3–10 days or more; however, because of tight tissue binding, small amounts persist in the body for months.

Therapeutic uses
1. Chloroquine 600 mg stat, 300 mg after 8 hours, and 300 mg daily for 2 days is the **drug of choice for the treatment of non-falciparum and chloroquine-sensitive falciparum malaria.** It rapidly terminates fever (24–48 hours) and clears parasitemia (48–72 hours), but does not eliminate dormant liver forms of *P. vivax* and *P. ovale*. Therefore, primaquine must be added for the radical cure of these species.

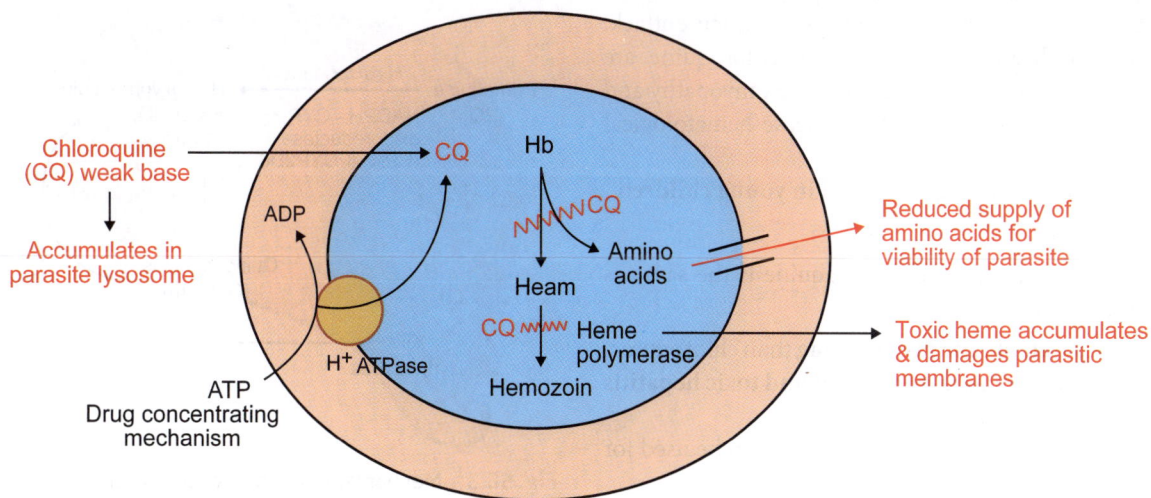

Fig. 58.2 Mechanism of action of chloroquine

2. It is still used to treat falciparum malaria in many areas with widespread resistance owing to:
   - Its safety
   - Low cost
   - Many partially immune individuals responding to chloroquine treatment even when the infecting parasites are partially resistant to chloroquine.
3. Other uses
   - Extra-intestinal amoebiasis
   - Disease modifying agent in rheumatoid arthritis (DMARD)
   - Very effective in discoid lupus erythematosus
   - Lepra reactions
   - Photogenic reactions
   - Symptomatic relief in infectious mononucleosis

Adverse effects

Chloroquine is usually well-tolerated, even with prolonged use.
- Pruritus is common.
- Anorexia, nausea, vomiting, and abdominal pain occurs, but reduces if dose is given after meals.
- Headache and malaise
- Blurring of vision
- Urticaria
- In rare cases, chloroquine can cause **hemolysis** in G6PD deficiency, impaired hearing, confusion, psychosis, seizures, agranulocytosis, exfoliative dermatitis, bleaching of hair, alopecia and ECG changes (QRS widening, T-wave abnormalities).
- Long-term use can cause cumulative toxicity, such as irreversible **ototoxicity, retinopathy, myopathy and peripheral neuropathy.**
- Large I/M, rapid I/V infusion can lead to severe hypotension, cardiac arrest, and respiratory arrest. So, **parenteral administration should be avoided.**

Contraindications

Chloroquine is contraindicated in patients with acute intermittent porphyria, as it may precipitate an acute attack. Other contraindications to the use of chloroquine are psoriasis, retinal/visual field abnormalities, myopathy and history of liver disease/neurological disease/hematological disorders.

It is **safe for use in pregnancy and in young children.**

(ii) Amodiaquine

The mechanism of action of amodiaquine is the same as that of chloroquine.

- It is **more palatable and faster-acting** than chloroquine.
- Some fatal cases of **agranulocytosis and toxic hepatitis** have been reported.
- Not recommended for prophylaxis, but can be used for treatment of clinical attacks.

(iii) Piperaquine

Amodiaquine as well as piperaquine are used in **artemisinin-based combination therapy (ACT).**

Hydroxychloroquine, an antimalarial drug, possesses disease-modifying action in rheumatoid arthritis. It was widely used during the COVID pandemic for prophylaxis against COVID-19 infection; however, evidence of its efficacy is not substantial. With long-term use, retinal damage and corneal opacities may occur due to accumulation in tissue. However, cumulative adverse effects are less with hydroxychloroquine than with chloroquine.

b. 8-Aminoquinolines

(i) Primaquine

The **mechanism of action** is not clearly understood, but it likely generates reactive metabolites that form toxic oxidative species inside the parasites and **disrupts the electron transport chain in mitochondria**.

Primaquine (PQ) is hydroxylated in the liver (Fig. 58.3) by a reaction dependent on NADPH, cytochrome P450 oxidoreductase (CPR), and CYP2D6. The hydroxylated PQ metabolites (OH-PQm) so formed have modest efficacy against hepatic stages and the gametocytes of *P. falciparum*.

Hydroxylated PQm undergoes spontaneous oxidation to form quinoneimine and H_2O_2. Quinoneimine is then reduced by CPR with concomitant and excessive generation of H_2O_2, which results in killing of hypnozoites.

The antimalarial action of primaquine is different from all other drugs because it is **active against**:

- **Hepatic stages of all human malarial parasites**. It is the only available agent active against the dormant hypnozoite stages of *P. vivax* and *ovale*.
- It is also **gametocidal against the 4 human malarial parasite species**.
- It acts against the erythrocytic stage also, but this activity is too weak to play an important role in the treatment.

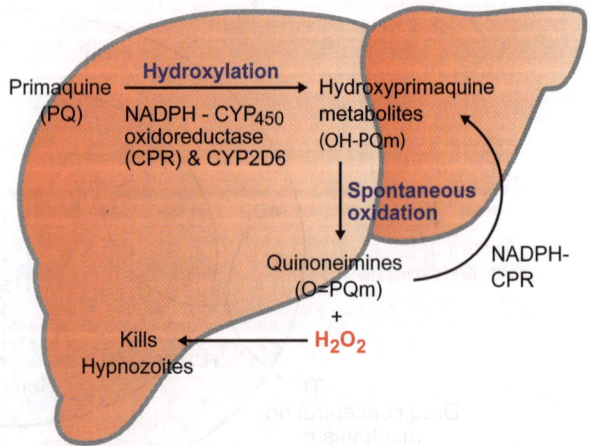

Fig. 58.3 Mechanism of action of primaquine

Resistance

Some strains of **P. vivax** are relatively resistant. Hepatic forms of these strains may not be eradicated by a single standard treatment with primaquine and may **require repeated therapy with increased doses** (30 mg base, daily for 14 days) for radical cure.

Therapeutic uses

1. **Radical cure** of **P. vivax, ovale**: Treatment includes chloroquine to eradicate erythrocytic malarial parasites and primaquine to eradicate hepatic malarial parasites (hyponozoites) to prevent a subsequent relapse.

    It is given in a dose of 15 mg, daily for 2 weeks, with a full curative dose of chloroquine in relapsing malaria. However, before giving this 14-day course, the G6PD status of patient should be tested.

    In India, a **5-day course** is used under NMEP (National Malaria Eradication Programme). An alternative regimen is primaquine 45 mg + chloroquine 300 mg, once a week, for 8–10 weeks. This regimen does not require G6PD testing because it achieves radical cure without inducing significant hemolysis.

2. **In falciparum malaria**, a single 45 mg dose is given with a curative dose of chloroquine to kill the gametes to cut down transmission to mosquitos.

3. A combination of primaquine with clindamycin is an alternative therapy for mild-to-moderate **Pneumocystis carinii pneumonia.**

ADRs

Primaquine is a well-tolerated drug. Sometimes, it can cause nausea, vomiting, epigastric distress, abdominal cramps, uneasiness in chest, and headache. These can be reduced by taking the drug along with meals.

Rarely, serious adverse effects like leukopenia, agranulocytosis, arrhythmia, hemolysis or methemoglobinemia may occur, especially in G6PD deficiency.

Contraindications

- Primaquine is contraindicated in patients with history of granulocytopenia, methemoglobinemia and in patients at high risk of developing myelosuppression (due to other drugs or diseases).
- Primaquine is **never used parenterally,** because severe hypotension can occur.
- It is avoided during pregnancy because the fetus is relatively G6PD deficient and thus at risk of hemolysis.

(ii) Tafenoquine

The actions of tafenoquine are similar to those of primaquine against *P. vivax* hypnozoites. Its half-life is longer (14–19 days) than that of primaquine (6–8 h). So, it acts for weeks after a single dose of 300 mg. It has been approved by FDA in 2018 for the **radical cure of P. vivax in patients older than 18 years**. It is given as a single dose for prevention of relapse. Its adverse effects include gastrointestinal upset and hemolysis in G6PD deficiency. It is better tolerated than the 14-day course of primaquine.

3. Quinoline Methanol
Mefloquine

It is a rapidly acting erythrocytic, schizonticide; however, its action is slower than that of quinine and chloroquine. Mefloquine is effective against chloroquine-sensitive as well as resistant *P. vivax* and *falciparum*. It has **no action on gametocytes or hepatic stages**.

Pharmacokinetics

Mefloquine can be used only **orally**, because parenteral use causes severe local irritation. After oral administration, it is slowly absorbed to a variable extent. It is highly plasma protein bound, and eliminated slowly. So, the treatment regimen is single daily doses, whereas prophylaxis regimen is weekly doses.

Therapeutic uses

1. It is used in **chemoprophylaxis against chloroquine-resistant strains of P. falciparum** (not preferred in areas without chloroquine resistance) in a dose of 250 mg per week, started 1–2 weeks prior to travel.
2. It is effective for the treatment of chloroquine/sulfadoxine–pyrimethamine-resistant falciparum, but not preferred over quinine, which is rapid acting and has lower incidence of resistance. It is recommended to **use mefloquine only in combination with artesunate (ACT) to prevent emergence of mefloquine resistance.**

ADRs

The weekly dose for prophylaxis can cause nausea, vomiting, epigastric pain, diarrhea, headache, dizziness, sleep and behavioural disturbances (depression, confusion, acute psychosis, seizures), and cardiac arrhythmias may occur.

Contraindications

Mefloquine is contraindicated in patients with a history of epilepsy, psychiatric problems, cardiac arrhythmias, and conduction defects. It is **not to be used in combination with quinine, quinidine, and halofantrine** as there is risk of QT prolongation and cardiac arrest.

4. Amino Alcohols
Halofantrine

Its activity against drug-resistant plasmodia is the same as that of mefloquine. It shows cross-resistance with mefloquine and can cause QT prolongation and ventricular arrhythmias at the therapeutic dose. It is not approved in India.

Lumefantrine

Lumefantrine is used along with artemether or arteether in artemisinin-based combined therapy (ACT) for resistant strains of falciparum.

5. Antibiotics

Antibiotics such as doxycycline and clindamycin possess weak erythrocytic schizonticidal activity in resistant *P. falciparum*. Doxycycline is combined with artesunate or quinine for treatment of **chloroquine-resistant falciparum or vivax malaria**. Clindamycin is an alternative to doxycycline in children and pregnant women. Doxycycline is a second-line **prophylactic agent for short-term use** in travellers to areas endemic for multidrug-resistant falciparum.

Sulphonamides/Diaminopyrimidine Combination

Sulphonamides like sulfadoxine, sulphamethopyrazine and dapsone are folic acid synthesis inhibitors. They have effect is weak erythrocytic schizonticidal action in malaria. Pyrimethamine, a diaminopyrimidine, inhibits DHFRase enzyme. It has 2000 times more affinity for plasmodial DHFRase than for the mammalian enzyme. A combination of sulfadoxine/sulphamethopyrazine/dapsone with pyrimethamine shows **supra-additive synergism due to sequential blockade of folic acid synthase and DHFRase enzymes**. The combination acts faster than the component drugs. Each tablet has: Pyrimethamine 25 mg + sulfadoxine 500 mg (OR) sulphamethopyrazine 500 mg (OR) dapsone 100 mg.

Single-dose therapy (3 tablets) of this combination is used for treating **chloroquine-resistant falciparum** malaria, but it is not effective against *P. vivax* and mixed infections. Sulfadoxine–pyrimethamine combination shows **no cross-resistance with other antimalarial drugs**. However, many strains have developed resistance to the sulfadoxine–pyrimethamine combination. Hence, the use of artesunate is recommended along with it to prevent further spread of resistance.

6. Artemisinin Derivatives

Artemisinin (qinghaosu), a compound extracted from the herb *Artemesia annua*, was used traditionally in Chinese medicine to cure fever and malaria. Artemisinin has poor solubility in water as well as oil. Many drugs with different pharmacokinetic properties have been introduced in this group, such as:

- **Artesunate sodium:** Water-soluble derivative suitable for oral/IM/IV use
- **Artemether:** Oil-soluble suitable for oral and IM use
- **Arteether :** Oil-soluble form for IM injection
- **Dihydroartemisinin (DHA):** Suitable for oral use
- **Arterolane :** Synthetic drug suitable for oral use

Mechanism of action

Artemisinins likely act by generating highly reactive free radicals that inactivate the plasmodial sarcoplasmic/endoplasmic calcium ATPase, cause lipid peroxidation, damage the endoplasmic reticulum, and ultimately kill the parasite.

Antimalarial action

These drugs generate an **active metabolite called dihydroartemisinin** (DHA) in the body. It is active against *P. falciparum* (including strains resistant to all other antimalarial drugs) as well as sensitive strains of falciparum and all other plasmodia species.

- It has a potent, **erythrocytic schizonticidal action which is faster than that of chloroquine**. It exerts action against all stages of erythrocytic schizogony (ring-form to early schizonts). Hence, its antimalarial action has a **wide time window**. As a result, parasitemia is cleared quickly within 24–48 hours.
- However, the **duration of action is short and recrudescence may occur with monotherapy.** There are two options to prevent recrudescence: either artemisinin monotherapy is continued even after disappearance of parasitemia, or some long-acting antimalarial drug is combined with artemisinin (ACT). Resistance to artemisinin has not been significant till now. However, as there is always a risk of development of resistance, artemisinin monotherapy is not advocated. There is no cross-resistance with other drugs.
- **The cidal action on early stages of gametes** reduces disease transmission to some extent. However, **mature gametes and hepatic stages are not affected**.

Thus, artemisinins are used in combination with other antimalarial drugs. In **artemisinin-based combination therapy (ACT)**, artemisinin (short-acting) is combined with long-acting antimalarial drugs, to prevent recrudescence and emergence of resistant strains. Artemisinin is given for 3 days, in combination with a long-acting drug.

Therapeutic uses

1. Uncomplicated falciparum malaria (with chloroquine-resistant as well as sensitive strains)
2. *P. vivax* infection: When organisms fail to respond to chloroquine as well as a combination of quinine–doxycycline, **oral artemisinin-based combination therapy (ACT)** is indicated. Artemisinin derivatives can be combined with different antimatarial drugs in 3-day regimens:
   - Artesunate 100 mg (twice a day, for 3 days) with single dose of 3 tablets containing pyrimethamine 25 mg + sulfadoxine 500 mg
   - Artesunate 100 mg (twice a day for 3 days) can be combined with mefloquine 750 mg on day 2 and 500 mg on day 3
   - Artesunate 200 mg + amodiaquine 600 mg (daily for 3 days)
   - DHA 120 mg + piperaquine 960 mg (daily for 3 days)
   - Arterolane 150 mg + piperaquine 750 mg (daily for 3 days)
   - Artemether 80 mg (twice a day) + lumefantrine 480 mg (twice a day for 3 days)

- Artesunate 60 mg + pyronaridine tetraphosphate 180 mg, once daily for 3 days.
3. In severe, **complicated falciparum malaria** with resistant or sensitive strains, parenteral artemisinins are the first choice drugs. Intravenous artesunate is used as it is safer, faster acting, and has higher efficacy and lower mortality than IV quinine in the treatment of complicated falciparum malaria. However, in pregnant patients with severe falciparum malaria, quinine is still used, as the safety of artemisinins is not established.

ADRs

Artesunate and artemether cause mild nausea, vomiting, itching, drug fever, and hemolysis. Rarely, headache, dizziness, tinnitus, leukopenia, and bleeding may occur. However, these are reversible.

7. Other Drugs

a. Mepacrine

Mepacrine is an erythrocytic schizonticide; it is equally effective as chloroquine but is highly toxic. Hence, it is not much in use.

b. Chlorguanide

Chlorguanide (proguanil) is a slow-acting erythrocytic schizonticide, rarely used because of its slow effect. It also possesses tissue schizonticidal action in *P. falciparum*.

c. Atovaquone

It exerts antimalarial effect by inhibiting parasitic mitochondrial electron transport. Atovaquone+ proguanil combination is useful in multiple drug resistant malaria.

d. Pyronaridine

Pyronaridine is an erythrocytic schizonticide, with the same mechanism of antimalarial action as chloroquine. It may be used in combination with artesunate in ACT.

Clinical problem-based questions and MCQs

1. i. Identify the first-choice drug for the radical cure of *P. vivax* malaria?
   a. Chloroquine
   b. Primaquine
   c. Pyrimethamine–sulfadoxine
   d. Quinidine
   ii. Describe the mechanism of action, adverse effects and contraindications for the use of the selected drug.
2. i. Identify the antimalarial drug that can cause cinchonism.
   a. Amodiaquine   b. Primaquine
   c. Pyrimethamine   d. Quinine
   ii. What are the features of cinchonism?
   iii. Describe the indications for use of the selected drug.
3. A 45-year-old male patient presented in the OPD with fever, chills, myalgia, headache and anorexia. He resides in an area where chloroquine resistance of malarial parasite is common. Rapid diagnostic test showed the presence of *Plasmodium falciparum*.
   i. Which of the following drugs is the first-choice treatment for this case?
      a. ACT
      b. Mefloquine
      c. Quinine
      d. Sulfadoxine–pyrimethamine
   ii. Justify your choice.
   iii. Describe the adverse effects of the selected drug(s).
4. i. Which antimalarial drug can be used as a DMARD also?
      a. Chloroquine
      b. Primaquine
      c. Artesunate
      d. Sulfadoxine–pyrimethamine
   ii. Enumerate the adverse effects of long-term use of the selected drug.
5. Identify the drug that can effectively eradicate latent hypnozoites of *P. vivax*.
   a. Doxycycline   b. Primaquine
   c. Chloroquine   d. Mefloquine
6. Which antimalarial drug can cause psychiatric symptoms as an adverse effect?
   a. Atovaquone   b. Mefloquine
   c. Artemisinin   d. Chloroquine
7. All the following antimalarial drugs have the potential to cause hemolysis in a patient with G6PD deficiency, EXCEPT:
   a. Quinine   b. Mefloquine
   c. Tafenoquine   d. Chloroquine
8. A 23-year-old female patient, 6 weeks pregnant, complains of fever with rigors and chills and is diagnosed as having malaria. Which antimalarial is the drug of choice in this patient?
   a. Artemisinin-based combination therapy
   b. Doxycycline
   c. Quinine
   d. Mefloquine

NATIONAL VECTOR-BORNE DISEASE CONTROL PROGRAMME

In 2002, a comprehensive umbrella programme the called the **National Vector-Borne Disease Control Programme (NVBDCP)** was launched for prevention and control of vector borne diseases such as malaria, filaria, kala-azar, Japanese encephalitis, dengue, and chikungunya.

General Strategy of NVBDCP

The strategy followed in general for all vector borne diseases mainly relied on:

1. Disease management by early detection of cases, effective treatment, referral services and surveillance.
2. Epidemic preparedness and rapid response.
3. Integrated vector management by measures such as indoor residual spray (IRS), insecticide-treated bed nets (ITNs), insecticidal nets, larvivorous fish, biolarvicides, and environmental engineering methods.
4. Surveillance to control spread, predict epidemics, investigate epidemics, and ensure rapid response.
5. Entomological surveillance: To collect data about breeding locations, vector density, susceptibility status, etc.
6. Supportive interventions such as behavioural change communication, public–private partnership, intersectoral convergence, and operational research.
7. Vaccination—only against Japanese encephalitis.
8. Annual mass drug administration—only against lymphatic filariasis.

The **National Framework for Malaria Elimination** has been in operation since 2016, followed by the launch of the **National Strategic Plan in 2017**.

Goals

- To achieve zero indigenous cases in the entire country by 2030.
- To maintain malaria-free status in areas where transmission is interrupted and to prevent reintroduction of malaria.

According to the **National Drug Policy on Malaria**, framed in 2013, all cases of fever are suspected to be malaria, once other common causes are ruled out. These are investigated to confirm the diagnosis. Treatment of malaria depends on the species.

1. Monotherapy with artemisinins and presumptive treatment with chloroquine is not advocated.
2. *Plasmodium vivax* **malaria** is treated with:
   - Chloroquine 10 mg per kg body weight on days 1 and 2, followed by 5 mg per kg body weight on day 3.
   - Primaquine 0.25 mg per kg body weight daily for 14 days (primaquine is contraindicated in pregnancy, infants, and patients with G6PD deficiency)

   Treatment of *Plasmodium ovale* is same as *P. vivax*.
3. **Uncomplicated *Plasmodium falciparum* malaria**: As chloroquine resistance among falciparum is widespread, orally given artemisinin-based combination therapy (ACT) is the first line of management.
   - Artesunate (4 mg/kg daily) for 3 days + a single dose of 3 tablets of sulfadoxine–pyrimethamine (25 mg/kg–1.25 mg/kg) combination. This is called **ACT-SP**.
   - On Day 2, a single dose of primaquine 0.75 mg per kg body weight is given.
   - North-eastern states show resistance to sulfadoxine–pyrimethamine combination. In these states, ACT consisting of artemether and lumefantrine is called ACT-AL. The dose of artemether and lumefantrine depends on the age/body weight as shown in Table 58.1.
   - In case of non-response to ACT, treatment is carried out with quinine + doxycycline/clindamycin.
   - In pregnant women, it is managed with quinine [10 mg/kg - 3 times daily for 7 days] in the first trimester and ACT in the second and third trimesters. Treatment of *P. malariae* is same as that for falciparum.
4. **Mixed infections**: Patients with mixed infections are treated as those with uncomplicated falciparum malaria, i.e., ACT-SP in all states except North-Eastern states, where ACT–AL regimen is used. However, in cases of mixed infections, primaquine is given in a dose of 0.25 mg/kg for 14 days.
5. **Complicated severe falciparum malaria** is managed with full dose of parenteral artesunate, followed by full dose of oral ACT. However, quinine is still used in pregnant patients with severe falciparum malaria, as the safety of artemisinins is not established.
6. **Chemoprophylaxis in malaria**: It is indicated only in selected groups in *Plasmodium falciparum*-endemic areas. Use of insecticide-treated bed nets and other

Table 58.1. ACT-AL dosage schedule based on body weight and age

Body weight	Approximate age	Tablets per dose (Artemether 20 mg + Lumefantrine 120 mg)	Total number of doses	Duration
5 – <15 kg	4 months to 3 years	1 tablet	6 doses	3 days
15 – <25 kg	3–7 years	2 tablets	6 doses	3 days
25 – <35 kg	8–11 years	3 tablets	6 doses	3 days
≥35 kg	≥12 years and adults	4 tablets	6 doses	3 days
Face	Sometimes features of facial palsy occur on one or both sides of the face.	Leonine facies due to infiltration and thickening of skin of face		
Clinical outcome	Prolonged remission and periodic exacerbation of symptoms	Worsens and anesthesia of distal parts, atrophy, ulceration, even absorption of digits may occur.		

personal protection measures are advocated for pregnant women and other vulnerable groups. Short-term chemoprophylaxis for up to 6 weeks is given to travellers going to malaria-endemic areas. Longer chemoprophylaxis may be needed for military personnel posted in such areas.

Short-term chemoprophylaxis with doxycycline 100 mg (once a day) is started 2 days before journey, given during stay, and continued for 4 weeks after return. However, doxycycline is contraindicated in pregnancy and children up to 8 years of age.

Longer chemoprophylaxis is required if the stay is longer than **6 weeks.** Mefloquine 250 mg per week is started 2 weeks before the journey and continued for 4 weeks after return from malaria-endemic areas.

Clinical problem-based questions and MCQs

9. A 30-year-old male presented a history of high-grade fever, headache, diarrhea, fatigue, and confusion for the last 3 days. This was followed by an episode of convulsions, after which he appeared semiconscious. There was also a history of recent travel to a tropical, malaria-endemic region with widespread chloroquine resistance. The patient was disoriented and lethargic on admission. Peripheral blood smear was positive for *P. falciparum* malaria with 9.8% parasitemia. Computed tomography scan of the head showed severe cerebral edema with loss of sulci/gyri differentiation.
   i. What is the likely diagnosis?
   ii. Describe the management of this case?

10. Describe the management of uncomplicated falciparum malaria as per National Strategic Plan 2017.

Summary

- Malaria is an endemic parasitic infection caused by *Plasmodium*.
- Its life cycle is completed in two hosts, with an asexual phase in humans and the sexual phase in female *Anopheles* mosquitoes. Infection is transmitted by mosquito bites.
- *P. vivax, ovale, falciparum* and *malariae* are 4 species that usually infect humans. Sporozoites of *P. vivax* and *ovale* can remain dormant in liver cells of host in the form of hypnozoites. These result in relapse of the disease. There are no hypnozoites in *P. falciparum* and *malariae*; however, a few erythrocytic parasites can persist and cause short-term relapse or recrudescence of disease.
- **Quinine** is the first antimalarial drug that has rapid erythrocytic schizonticidal effect against all plasmodium species; it also has gametocidal effect against *vivax* and *ovale* but not *falciparum*. It has no effect on liver stage parasites. It is a toxic drug with narrow safety margin. Hence, it is used only in uncomplicated chloroquine-resistant falciparum malaria in pregnant women. A second drug is usually combined to reduce the duration of treatment to prevent toxic effects. Quinidine is useful in complicated falciparum malaria, e.g., cerebral malaria, administered by parenteral route with cardiac function monitoring. Quinine may be effective in muscle cramps and for thrombosis of varicose veins mass. It can cause cinchonism at therapeutic doses, visual auditory disturbances, hypersensitivity reactions and hemolysis in G6PD deficiency.
- **Chloroquine**, like quinine, has potent and rapid erythrocytic schizonticidal effect against all species of plasmodium, gametocidal effect against vivax, malariae and ovale but not falciparum. It has no effect on liver stage parasites. Many strains of *P. falciparum* have developed resistance to chloroquine. It is accumulated in parasitic lysosomes and interferes with Hb degradation. Inhibition of heme polymerase enzyme causes heme accumulation, which damages parasitic membranes. It is also effective against *E. histolytica* and *G. lamblia*. It is the drug of choice for chloroquine-sensitive falciparum and non-falciparum malaria. Other uses are in DMARDs, lepra reactions, photogenic reactions, extra-intestinal amoebiasis, etc. It can get accumulated in tissues causing retinal damage and corneal opacities upon long-term use. However, tissue damage is less with hydroxychloroquine.
- **Primaquine** is active against the hepatic stages of all human malarial parasites. It is the only available agent that is active against the dormant hypnozoite stages of *P. vivax* and *ovale*. Hence, it is used for radical cure of vivax malaria in a dose of 15 mg/day for 14 days. It is well tolerated with GI adverse effects, but can cause hemolysis in case of G6PD deficiency. **Tafenoquine** has similar activity but long duration of action; therefore, it is approved by FDA for the radical cure of *P. vivax* and relapse prevention in a single dose.
- **Mefloquine** is slower acting than chloroquine and is slowly absorbed. However, it is effective in multidrug-resistant falciparum. Weekly prophylaxis is useful before traveling to malaria-endemic areas; however, for treating chloroquine-resistant *P. falciparum*, quinine is preferred. Mefloquine, is administered with artemisinin derivatives in ACT. It can cause neuropsychiatric problems and cardiac arrhythmias.
- **Artemisinins** are active against falciparum resistant to all other antimalarial drugs. They are rapid erythrocytic schizonticides (quicker action than chloroquine), but are short-acting. As a result,

recrudescence may occur after monotherapy. Hence, they are combined with longer-acting drugs like sulfadoxine–pyrimethamine, lumefantrine, piperaquine, mefloquine, and amodiaquine in ACT to prevent recrudescence and resistance. These, given orally, are well tolerated and are the drugs of choice for uncomplicated falciparum, while IV artesunate is recommended for complicated falciparum malaria. However, in pregnancy, quinine is still preferred.

- The **National Framework for Malaria Elimination** has been operational since 2016, followed by the **National Strategic Plan** launched in 2017. The **goal** of these programmes is to achieve zero indigenous cases in the entire country by 2030, to maintain malaria-free status in areas where transmission is interrupted, and to prevent reintroduction of malaria. According to the **National Drug Policy on Malaria** framed in 2013, all cases of fever are suspected to be malaria once other common causes are ruled out. These are investigated to confirm the diagnosis. Treatment of malaria depends on the vector species. Monotherapy with artemisinins and presumptive treatment with chloroquine is not advocated. *P. vivax* malaria is managed with a 3-day course of chloroquine along with primaquine for 14 days. Uncomplicated falciparum malaria is managed with artemisinin-based combination therapy (ACT), comprising a artesunate + sulfadoxine–pyrimethamine combination. However, in North-Eastern states with resistance to sulfadoxine–pyrimethamine, ACT with combination of artemether and lumefantrine is useful. Complicated falciparum malaria is managed with supportive measures + IV artesunate for 24 hours/or till the patient is able to tolerate oral drugs, followed by a full course of ACT.

Questions for practice

1. Classify antimalarial drugs. Describe the mechanism of action, uses and adverse effects of chloroquine.
2. Comment on role of:
   a. Primaquine in management of malaria.
   b. Quinine in current clinical practice.
   c. Artemisinin-based combination therapies for falciparum malaria.
3. Describe the goals and general strategic measures of NVBDCP.
4. Describe management of the following as per National Drug Policy of 2013.
   a. Chloroquine-resistant uncomplicated falciparum malaria.
   b. Cerebral malaria.
   c. *P. vivax* malaria

5. Explain why:
   a. Primaquine is contraindicated in G6PD deficiency.
   b. Quinine is still used in some cases of malaria.
   c. Artemisinins are not used as monotherapy.

Hints for problem-based questions and MCQs

1. i. b. Primaquine
   ii. It acts by generating reactive metabolites that form toxic oxidative species inside the parasites and disrupt the electron transport chain in mitochondria. Refer to page 761 for ADRs and contraindications
2. i. d. Quinine
   ii. Cinchonism characterised by tinnitus, headache, dizziness, nausea, flushing, and visual disturbances.
   iii. Quinine is indicated for the treatment of chloroquine-resistant falciparum malaria in pregnant women.
3. i. a. ACT
   ii. Artemisinin-based combination therapy is the first-choice treatment in chloroquine-resistant falciparum. Combination prevents recrudescence and development of resistance
   iii. Artesunate and artemether cause mild nausea, vomiting, itching, drug fever, and hemolysis. Rarely headache, dizziness, tinnitus, leukopenia, and bleeding can occur; however, these are reversible.
4. i. a. Chloroquine is useful as a DMARD in rheumatoid arthritis
   ii. Long-term use can cause irreversible ototoxicity, retinopathy, myopathy, peripheral neuropathy
5. b. Primaquine.
6. b. Mefloquine causes psychiatric side effects.
7. b. Mefloquine does not have the risk of hemolysis in the case of G6PD deficiency.
8. c. Quinine is the drug of choice for uncomplicated malaria in the first trimester of pregnancy.
9. i. Cerebral malaria.
   ii. Cerebral malaria patients need supportive treatment, diazepam for convulsions, antimalarial drugs (full dose of parenteral IV artesunate for at least 24 hours), followed by a full dose of oral ACT, when patient is able to tolerate oral medication.
   - Quinine dihydrochloride or gluconate is the treatment of choice for severe falciparum malaria in pregnant women. Refer to page 758.
10. As chloroquine-resistance among falciparum is widespread, artemisinin-based combination therapy (ACT), orally given, is the first line of management.
    - Artesunate 50 mg daily for 3 days is combined with a single dose of 3 tablets of sulfadoxine–pyrimethamine combination. Each tablet contains sulfadoxine 25 mg + pyrimethamine 500 mg.
    - On day 2, a single dose of primaquine 0.75 mg/kg body weight is given.
    North-eastern states show resistance to sulfadoxine–pyrimethamine combination. In these states, ACT consists of artemether 20 mg with lumefantrine 120 mg. In case of non-response to ACT, treatment is carried out with quinine + doxycycline/clindamycin. In pregnant women, it is managed with quinine in the first trimester and ACT in 2nd and 3rd trimesters.

CONCEPT MAP – ANTIMALARIAL DRUGS

Quinine, Quinidine

Mechanism: Inhibit heme polymerase.

Erythrocytic schizonticide for all species of plasmodium.

Gametocidal against *P. vivax*, *P. ovale* but not *P. falciparum*.

Uses: In chloroquine-resistant falciparum malaria, Doxycycline is combined with artesunate or quinine.

Quinidine for parenteral treatment of severe falciparum malaria, e.g., cerebral malaria.

Noctural muscle cramps - single bedtime dose.

As spermicidel in vaginal creams.

Injected with urethane in varicose veins for thrombosis & fibrosis

ADRs: Cinchonism (tinnitus, headache, dizziness, nausea, flushing, visual disturbance.)

Prolonged treatment: Visual and auditory abnormalities.

Abdominal pain, vomiting, diarrhea.

Hypersensitivity reactions

Hemolysis in G6PD deficiency

Leukopenia, TCP, agranulocytosis

Insulin release - hypoglycemia

Hypotension, ECG abnormalities with rapid IV injection

Chloroquine

Mechanism: Accumulates in parasite lysosomes → interferes with Hb degradation → reduced supply of amino acids for parasite's viability.

Inhibits heme polymerase → reduces conversion of heme to non-toxic hemozoin. Heme can damage the parasitic membranes.

Erythrocytic schizonticide for all species.

Gametocidal against *P. vivax*, *ovale, malariae* but not *P. falciparum*.

Uses: Drug of choice for the treatment of non-falciparum & sensitive falciparum malaria. Dose: 600 mg stat, 300 mg after 8 hours & 300 mg daily for 2 days.

Extra-intestinal amoebiasis, DMARD in Rheumatoid arthritis, Discoid lupus erythematosus, Lepra and photogenic reactions.

ADRs: Well tolerated.

Mild ADRs like anorexia, nausea, vomiting, abdominal pain, headache, malaise, and blurring of vision.

Gets concentrated in liver, spleen, kidney, lungs, skin, leukocytes, retina and may cause irreversible ototoxicity, retinopathy, myopathy, peripheral neuropathy on long-term use.

Contraindications: Psoriasis, porphyria, retinal/visual field abnormalities, myopathy, history of liver/neurological/hematological disorders.

Sulphonamides with Pyrimethamine

Mechanism: Sequential blockade of folic acid synthesis & activation → supra-additive synergism, faster action than component drugs.

Uses: Single dose therapy with 3 tablets of Pyrimethamine (25 mg) with sulfadoxine / sulfamethopyrazine (500 mg) or dapsone (100 mg) useful for clinical cure of chloroquine resistant falciparum malaria, but not effective against *P. vivax* & mixed infections.

No cross resistance with other antimalarial drugs.

Mefloquine

Rapidly-acting erythrocytic schizonticide against chloroquinesensitive/resistant *P. vivax, falciparum*. No action on gametocytes or hepatic stages.

Uses: Chemoprophylaxis against resistant *P. falciparum*

Treatment of chloroquine/ sulfadoxine-pyrimethamine resistant falciparum, but not preferred over quinine.

It is recommended to use mefloquine only in combination with artesunate (ACT) to prevent emergence of mefloquine resistance.

Used only orally, because parenteral use causes severe local irritation.

ADRs: Nausea, vomiting, epigastric pain, abdominal pain, diarrhea, headache, dizziness, sleep & behavioural disturbances, seizures and cardiac arrhythmias may occur.

Contraindications: History of epilepsy, psychiatric problems, cardiac arrhythmias, conduction defects.

Not to be used with quinine, quinidine, halofantrine → risk of QT prolongation and cardiac arrest.

Amino alcohols

Halofantrine: Activity against drug resistant Plasmodia, but shows cross resistance with mefloquine. Risk of QT prolongation, ventricular arrhythmias → not approved in India

Lumefantrine: Used with artemether/arteether for resistant strains of falciparum.

ANTI MALARIAL DRUGS

Artemisinin Derivatives

Dihydroartemisinin (DHA), Arterolane for oral use.

Artemether for oral/ IM use, Arteether for IM use.

Artesunate sodium for oral/IM/IV use.

Mechanism: Generates an active metabolite in body called dihydroartemisinin (DHA) that inactivates plasmodial sarcoplasmic endoplasmic calcium ATPase, causes lipid peroxidation, damages endoplasmic reticulum & kills the parasite.

Active against *P. falciparum* resistant to all other drugs and all other Plasmodia species.

Potent, erythrocytic schizonticide action, faster than chloroquine.

Active against all stages of erythrocytic schizogony.

Recrudescence may occur with monotherapy due to short duration of action, thus used as artemisinin-based combination therapy (ACT) in combination with long acting antimalarial drugs.

ADRs: Artesunate and artemether cause mild nausea, vomiting, itching, drug fever, hemolysis.

Rarely headache, dizziness, tinnitus, leukopenia, bleeding can occur, but are reversible.

Primaquine

Mechanism: Involves hydroxylation by CPR & CYP2D6 → forming OH-PQm, which oxidises spontaneously to form O=PQm, H_2O_2. The cidal effect of primaquine on hypnozoites is exerted by H_2O_2 and O=PQm recycled.

Active against hepatic stages & gametocytes of all human malarial parasites. Only drug against hypnozoites of *P. vivax* and *ovale*.

Uses: Radical cure of *P. vivax*, ovale in a dose of 15 mg daily for 2 weeks, with full curative dose of chloroquine in relapsing malaria or a 5 days course under NMEP or primaquine 45 mg + chloroquine 300mg once in a week for 8-10 weeks.

Single 45 mg dose in falciparum malaria with curative dose of chloroquine.

Pneumocystis carinii pneumonia: Primaquine with Clindamycin

ADRs: Well tolerated, may cause nausea, vomiting, epigastric distress, abdominal cramps, uneasiness in chest, headache. Rarely serious adverse effects like leukopenia, agranulocytosis, arrhythmia, hemolysis or methemoglobinemia especially in G6PD deficiency may occur.

Contraindications: History of granulocytopenia, methemoglobinemia, with myelosuppressive drugs/disorders.

Primaquine is never used parenterally because severe hypotension can occur.

Artemisinin-Based Combination Therapy (ACT)

Artesunate 100 mg twice a day for 3 days combined with;
single dose of 3 tablets containing pyrimethamine 25 mg+ sulfadoxine 500 mg
or mefloquine 750 mg on day 2 and 500 mg on day 3
or Artesunate 200 mg with amodiaquine 600 mg daily for 3 days

DHA 120 mg + Piperaquine 960 mg daily for 3 days

Arterolane 150 mg + piperaquine 750 mg daily for 3 days.

Artemether 80 mg twice a day + lumefantrine 480 mg twice a day for 3 days

SECTION 10 Chemotherapeutic Drugs

59 Antiamoebic Drugs

PH 8.7 Discuss the types, kinetics, dynamics, and adverse effects of drugs used for the following protozoal /vector-borne diseases: Amoebiasis, Kala-azar.

Learning objective

A student of MBBS phase II should be able to:
- Classify antiamoebic drugs.
- Describe the mechanism of action of antiamoebic drugs.
- Enumerate therapeutic uses of antiamoebic drugs.
- Enumerate adverse effects and contraindications for the use of antiamoebic drugs.
- Describe drugs used in the treatment of visceral leishmaniasis (kala-azar).

Amoebiasis is an infective disease caused by *Entamoeba histolytica*. Infection occurs upon **ingestion of cysts** of the organism present in water/food contaminated with fecal matter (Fig. 59.1). The **cysts develop into trophozoites** in the lumen of the intestine. The trophozoites have lectin on their membrane; this lectin exhibits structural similarity to host adhesion proteins (selectins and intercellular adhesion molecules (ICAMs)). The trophozoites, thus, have affinity for host proteins, and **persist as commensals on the surface of the colonic mucosa**.

Trophozoites may meet the following fates:

a. They get transformed to cysts that are passed out in stool. Individuals passing cysts in their stools but not having overt disease are called carriers or **chronic cyst passers**. They spread the disease.

b. Trophozoites may invade submucosa and secrete a factor that inhibits INF-γ-activated macrophages. Such patients suffer from **acute intestinal amoebiasis (such as acute colitis) or amoebic ulcers and amoebic dysentery**. They pass blood and mucus in stools. Sometimes, trophozoites may cause **chronic intestinal amoebiasis** with vague abdominal symptoms and form amoebic granuloma called **ameboma. Peritoneum, perianal skin and genitals** may also be involved.

c. From the intestinal submucosa, trophozoites may pass into the blood stream and cause **tissue or extraintestinal amoebiasis**. Trophozoites may reach the liver through portal circulation and cause **hepatic amoebiasis or amoebic liver abscess**. From the liver, infection may spread to the diaphragm, forming **subphrenic abscess** or may reach up to the **lungs**. In rare instances, trophozoites may reach the **lungs, kidney, spleen, suprarenal glands, brain**, etc. via general circulation. **Tissue amoebiasis is always secondary to intestinal amoebiasis**.

ANTIAMOEBIC DRUGS

CLASSIFICATION

The treatment of amoebiasis **depends on the site and type of infection**. Drugs for different types of amoebiasis are shown in Flowchart 59.1. Luminal amoebicide drugs are effective in intestinal amoebiasis. These include amides, 8-hydroxyquinolines and antibiotics such as tetracycline and paromamycin. Tissue amoebicidal drugs include nitroimidazoles, emetine, dehydroemetine and chloroquine.

DRUGS BASED ON SITE OF INFECTION

Luminal Amoebicides

Drugs that posses amoebicidal action in the intestinal lumen include amides (diloxanide furoate, nitazoxanide), 8-hydroxyquinolines (quiniodochlor, diiodohydroxyquin or iodoquinol), and antibiotics such as tetracycline and paromomycin.

1. Amides

Diloxanide furoate

Diloxanide furoate is an effective luminal amoebicide, but is not effective against tissue trophozoites.

- In the lumen of the gut, it splits into diloxanide and furoic acid. About 90% of diloxanide is absorbed, gets conjugated with glucuronide, and is excreted promptly in urine. So, although diloxanide is absorbed, it has negligible activity against tissue trophozoites, and is not effective in invasive amoebic dysentery.
- The remaining unabsorbed 10% diloxanide kills luminal trophozoites of *E. histolytica* by an **unknown mechanism**, before their encystment.

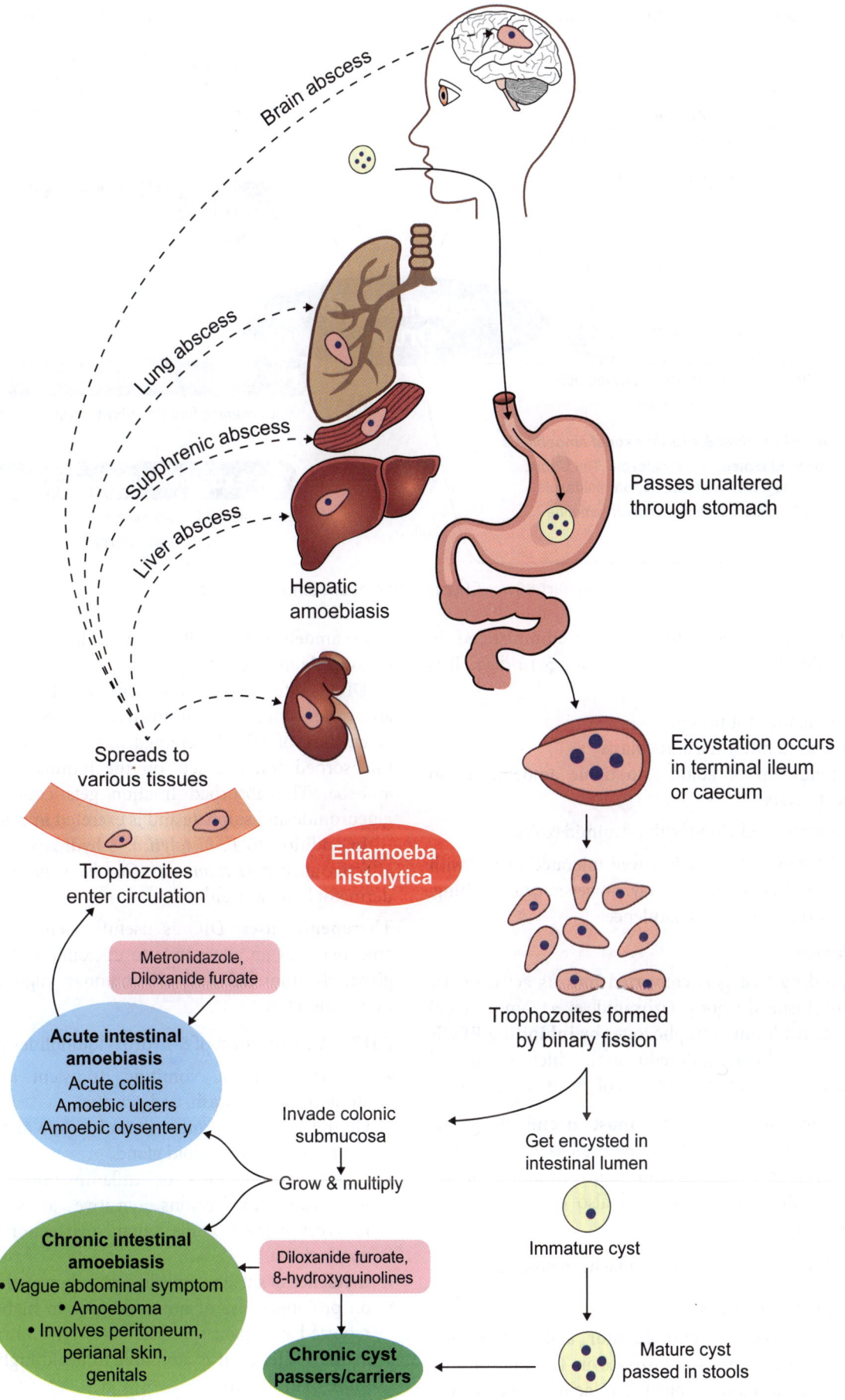

Fig. 59.1 Life cycle of *E. histolytica* and the drugs for amoebiasis

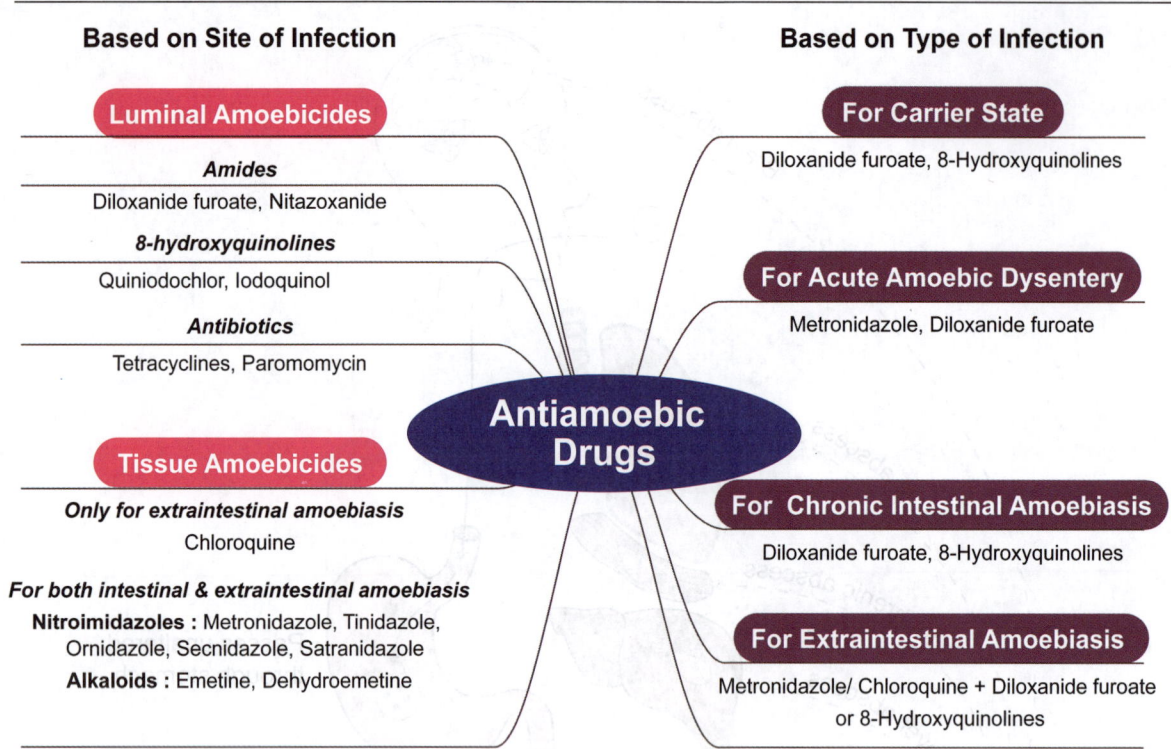

Flowchart 59.1 Classification of antiamoebic drugs

Therapeutic uses: Diloxanide furoate is administered in a dose of 500 mg, three times a day, for 5-10 days. It is indicated in:

- asymptomatic cyst passers
- chronic mild intestinal amoebiasis
- as a follow-up or adjunct to tissue amoebicides to eradicate cysts.

It is commonly used along with nitroimidazoles.

ADRs: Diloxanide furoate is a well tolerated drug, with no serious adverse effects. It may, however, cause itching, rash, urticaria, nausea and flatulence.

Nitazoxanide

It is a prodrug that gets converted into its active form, tizoxanide, inside the body. Tizoxanide exerts amoebicidal activity against luminal trophozoites **by inhibiting PFOR** (pyruvate: ferredoxin oxidoreductase), which is essential for electron transport energy metabolism in anaerobes.

Therapeutic uses: It is the **most useful drug for** *Cryptosporidium parvum*. It can be used as an alternative to diloxanide, as a luminal amoebicide, in a dose of 500 mg, twice daily for 3 days. It is also effective against metronidazole-resistant *Giardia*.

ADRs: Mild abdominal pain, headache, nausea, etc.

8-Hydroxyquinolines

These drugs include **quiniodochlor** and **iodoquinol**. They kill cyst-forming trophozoites in the intestine by an unknown mechanism, but fail to achieve therapeutic concentration at extraintestinal sites; hence, they have no tissue amoebicidal activity. They are **less efficacious than diloxanide** in eradicating cysts.

DIQ is safer than quiniodochlor due to lesser systemic absorption after oral administration. About 90% of the given dose of DIQ is retained in the intestine, and this unabsorbed fraction acts on the luminal cycle of the amoeba. The absorbed fraction gets conjugated with glucuronide and sulphate and is excreted in urine.

In addition to *E. histolytica*, 8-hydroxyquinolines are effective against *Trichomonas, Giardia, Candida* and some dermatophytes as well.

Therapeutic uses: DIQ is useful in chronic intestinal amoebiasis as an alternative to diloxanide. It is used for giardiasis, monilial and trichomonas vaginitis, fungal infections, etc.

ADRs: Adverse effect of 8-hydroxylquinolines include:

- Anorexia, nausea, vomiting, transient loose green stools, headache, rash, and pruritus.
- Goitre: increases protein-bound iodine and decreases iodine uptake by thyroid gland.
- Iodism: furunculosis or inflammation of mucous membrane. In persons sensitive to iodine, DIQ may cause fever, chills, cutaneous hemorrhages and angioedema.
- Incidence of subacute myelo-optic neuropathy (SMON) on prolonged use of quiniodochlor in high doses are reported in Japan; sporadic cases have also occurred in India. Hence, it is advisable to avoid high doses for more than 14 days.

The drug is banned in the pediatric age group.

3. Antibiotics

Tetracyclines
These are **bacteriostatic drugs** that act by inhibiting protein synthesis. Tetracyclines, being incompletely absorbed, reach the colon in large amounts and **exert inhibitory effect on bacterial flora that have symbiotic relationship with E. histolytica.** As a result, proliferation of luminal amoeba is indirectly inhibited. Thus, tetracyclines have an **adjuvant role** with another luminal amoebicide and metronidazole.

Paromomycin
It is an aminoglycoside having **bactericidal** action. Being polar, it is not absorbed significantly upon oral administration. As a result, it is useful against luminal amoeba but has no effect on extraintestinal infections. It is also effective against *Giardia, Trichomonas, Leishmania, Taenia* and *Cryptosporidium.*

Therapeutic uses: It is **as effective as diloxanide furoate in asymptomatic cyst passers** and in chronic amoebic colitis. The dose is 500 mg thrice daily for 7 days. It is also useful as an alternative to metronidazole for giardiasis in the first trimester of pregnancy.

ADRs: Oral paromomycin is not absorbed systemically. Hence, its adverse effects are limited to the GIT, e.g., abdominal cramps, nausea, vomiting, and diarrhea.

Clinical problem-based questions and MCQs

1. Identify the drug that cannot be used as luminal amoebicide.
   a. Paromomycin b. Chloroquine
   c. DIQ d. Diloxanide

2. A 40-year-old male presents with occasional fever, fatigue, mild diarrhea and dull abdominal pain. Microscopic stool examination reveals cysts and trophozoites of *E. histolytica*. The patient is diagnosed with 'chronic intestinal amoebiasis'.
   i. Identify the most suitable drug for this patient.
      a. Emetine b. Dehydroemetine
      c. Diloxanide furoate d. Paromomycin
   ii. Mention the dose of the drug chosen for this patient.
   iii. What are the other indications for use and adverse effects of the chosen drug?

3. i Enumerate luminal amoebicides.
   ii. Identify a luminal amoebicide that inhibits pyruvate: ferredoxin oxidoreductase in luminal trophozoites.
      a. Diloxanide b. Tetracycline
      c. Nitazoxanide d. Diiodoquinol
   iii. Identify a luminal amoebicide that can cause subacute myelo-optic neuropathy (SMON).
      a. Diloxanide b. Tetracycline
      c. Nitazoxanide d. Diiodoquinol

Tissue Amoebicides

a. Drugs for extraintestinal amoebiasis alone

Chloroquine
Chloroquine is an **antimalarial** drug. It gets completely absorbed from small intestine and is highly concentrated in liver, where it kills trophozoites. Hence, it is **effective only for hepatic amoebiasis**. It is as efficacious as **emetine** for amoebic liver abscess. Dose of chloroquine is 600 mg base given orally for first two days, followed by 300 mg daily for about 2–3 weeks. As the duration of treatment with chloroquine is longer (2–3 weeks), it is **used only when metronidazole** (drug for both intestinal and extraintestinal amoebiasis, see below) **is not effective or not tolerated**. Relapses after chloroquine treatment are frequent, so a luminal drug must be combined with it.

b. Drugs for both intestinal and extraintestinal amoebiasis

These include **alkaloids** and **nitroimidazoles**.

1. Alkaloids

Emetine

Emetine is an alkaloid obtained from *Cephaelis ipecacuanha*. It **directly kills trophozoites by interfering with the intra-ribosomal translocation of tRNA–amino acid complex during protein synthesis** (refer to Fig. 52.5). Emetine produces **fast symptomatic relief** in amoebiasis within 1–3 days of starting the therapy, but it is **not curative** as it has no effect on cysts.

A major drawback of emetine is the inconvenience of its administration. It is ineffective orally due to erratic absorption and its irritant nature, which often causes nausea and vomiting. Therefore, it must be administered intramuscularly or subcutaneously. Intravenous use is also not advised because of the risk of cardiac toxicity. As a result, emetine is reserved for cases where metronidazole cannot be used.

ADRs: Pain, tenderness and sterile abscess may occur at the site of injection. Nausea, vomiting, and diarrhea may occur. Muscular weakness is also a common adverse effect of emetine. Cardiac adverse effects like hypotension, ECG changes, cardiac arrhythmias and cardiac failure may occur.

Dehydroemetine

This is a semisynthetic derivative of emetine. It is as efficacious as emetine for symptomatic relief in tissue amoebiasis, but it is less toxic to the heart. So dehydroemetine is preferred over emetine.

2. Nitroimidazoles

These include metronidazole, tinidazole, ornidazole, secnidazole and satranidazole.

Mechanism of action (Fig. 59.2): Once nitroimidazoles enter cells, their **nitro group is reduced by redox proteins**

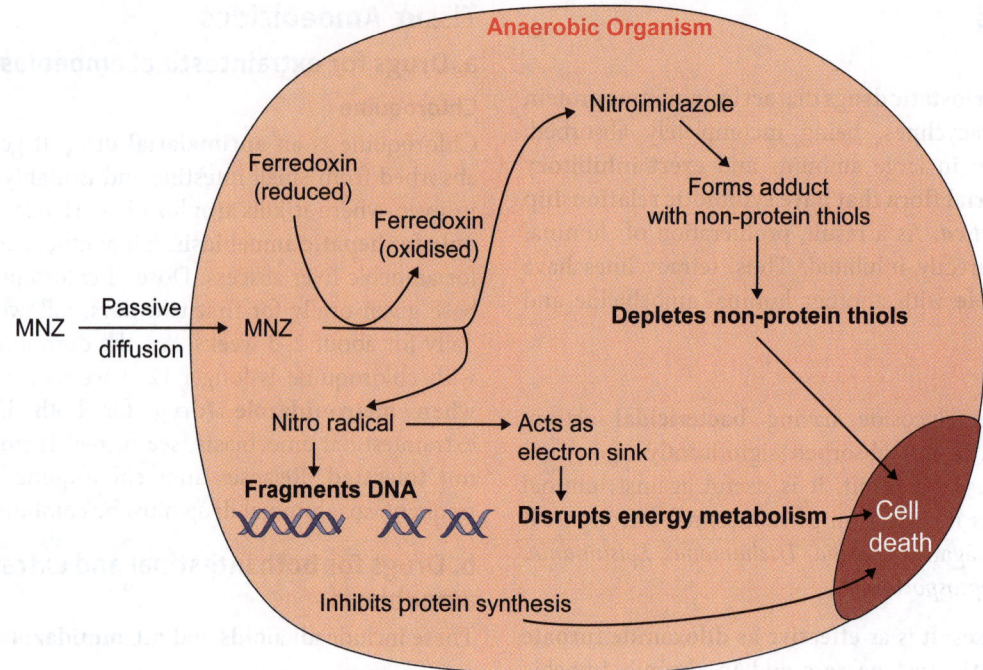

Fig. 59.2 Mechanism of action of metronidazole (MNZ)

(present exclusively in anaerobic organisms), resulting in the formation of nitrosoimidazole and a highly reactive nitro radicals. The nitro radicals acts as **electron sinks** and compete with biological electron acceptors for electrons generated during pyruvate oxidation through the PFOR (pyruvate-ferredoxin oxidoreductase) pathway. As anaerobes are devoid of mitochondria, their energy metabolism gets disrupted. The nitro radical **interacts with DNA**, resulting in loss of its double helix structure, fragmentation of strands and inhibition of protein synthesis, leading to cell death. Anaerobic organisms may acquire resistance to nitroimidazoles due to deficiency of the drug-activating mechanism or due to low levels of PFOR.

Nitrosoimidazole formed during activation depletes non-protein thiols by forming adducts with them. This action contributes to the cidal effect of metronidazole.

Aerobic organisms are not affected by nitroimidazoles because the aerobic environment interferes with formation of nitro radicals, the active form of the drug. Even if nitro radicals are formed, oxygen competes with it for free electrons generated during energy metabolism in aerobes.

a. Metronidazole

This is the prototype nitroimidazole effective against:
- Protozoa: *E. histolytica, G. lamblia, Trichomonas*
- Anaerobes: *Bacteroides fragilis, Fusobacterium, Clostridium perfringens, Helicobacter pylori* and anaerobic streptococci

It facilitates extraction of *Dracunculus medinensis* from under the skin.

Pharmacokinetics: It is nearly completely absorbed from small intestine upon oral administration. After absorption it gets widely distributed, achieving good concentration in CSF, saliva, vaginal secretions, semen, etc. Metabolism occurs in the liver via oxidation and glucuronide conjugation, and excretion occurs through urine. The half-life of metronidazole is 8 hours.

Therapeutic uses:
- *Metronidazole* is the drug of choice for all tissue infections caused by *E. histolytica*, such as **amoebic dysentery** and **amoebic liver abscess.** It is equally effective for invasive intestinal and extraintestinal amoebiasis when given orally in a dose of 800 mg, three times a day, for 7–10 days. However, due to complete absorption, it is not reliable for luminal infection. So, metronidazole is **usually combined with luminal drugs** like diloxanide furoate to eradicate cysts. In severe cases, metronidazole 500 mg can be given by slow IV infusion till oral therapy can be started.
- *Giardiasis:* 400 mg three times a day for 7 days, or 2 g daily for 3 days is very effective.
- *Trichomonal vaginitis and non-specific bacterial vaginosis:* Metronidazole 2 g single dose is the drug of choice. Alternatively, 400 mg three times a day may be given for 7 days. In refractory cases, a repeat course may be needed after a gap of 4–6 weeks. It is important to treat the male partner concurrently.
- *Anaerobic infection occurring after pelvic/colorectal surgery* can be prevented and treated by a combination of metronidazole with gentamicin / cephalosporins, as mixed infection occurs commonly.

- *Trench mouth or acute necrotizsing ulcerative gingivitis*, which is a mixed infection caused by bacteroides, spirochetes, fusobacteria, etc., responds quickly (within few days) to metronidazole 200–400 mg thrice daily, given along with penicillins/ tetracyclines/ erythromycin. Treatment is continued for 5 days.
- *Pseudomembranous enterocolitis:* It is caused by *Clostridium difficile*. Metronidazole given in a dose of 400–800 mg, two to three times daily for 10–14 days is **preferred over vancomycin.** Metronidazole is more effective and less toxic than vancomycin. However, vancomycin is still used in cases that fail to respond to metronidazole.
- *Peptic ulcer:* Nitroimidazoles are an essential component of the **triple-drug regimen for H. pylori eradication.** Metronidazole 400 mg three times a day or tinidazole 500 mg twice a day can be combined with a proton pump inhibitor and an antibiotic (either amoxicillin or clarithromycin).
- Metronidazole also facilitates the *extraction of Dracunculus medinensis* from under skin. Niridazole is the drug of choice for this indication.

ADRs: Common adverse effects of metronidazole include anorexia, nausea, dry mouth, metallic taste, and abdominal cramps. These can be reduced by taking the drug with meals. It can cause headache, dizziness, vertigo, vomiting, neutropenia, dysuria, and dark urine in some cases. Intravenous use may cause thrombophlebitis, seizures, peripheral neuropathy and disulfiram reaction.

Contraindications: Metronidazole is contraindicated in patients with neurological diseases, blood dyscrasia and during pregnancy.

b. Tinidazole
Tinidazole, with a longer half-life of approximately 12 hours, is suitable for once-daily dosing. It is better tolerated than metronidazole, with a lower incidence of adverse effects such as metallic taste, nausea, and rashes. In the treatment of amoebiasis, tinidazole given in a dose of 2 g once daily for 3 days has shown higher cure rates compared to metronidazole.

c. Ornidazole
Ornidazole has a half-life of 12–14 hours. The ADRs, dose and duration of treatment for this drug are the same as those of tinidazole.

d. Secnidazole
This is rapidly and completely absorbed upon oral administration. Its metabolism is comparatively slow. Its half-life is longer (17–29) hours and a single 2 g dose has the same cure rate in amoebiasis as multiple doses of other nitroimidazoles.

e. Satranidazole
This also has a longer half-life (14 hours) and better tolerability. Its dose is 300 mg twice daily for 3–5 days.

Clinical problem-based questions and MCQs

4. A 14-year-old girl presents with history of fever, chills, tenesmus, frequent small stools with passage of blood and mucus along with fecal matter. On microscopic stool examination, cysts and trophozoites of *E. histolytica* are present.
   i. What is the likely diagnosis?
   ii. Which of the following is the first-line drug in this case?
      a. Chloroquine   b. Iodoquinol
      c. Metronidazole   d. Dehydroemetine
   iii. Describe the mechanism of action of chosen drug.
   iv. Enumerate therapeutic uses and adverse effects of the chosen drug.

5. Use of nitroimidazoles in tissue amoebiasis cannot be relied on for eradication of luminal infection.
   i. Explain the inability of nitroimidazoles to eradicate amoebic cysts.
   ii. Which of the following drugs is most suitable after nitroimidazole therapy to ensure cyst eradication?
      a. Chloroquine   b. DIQ
      c. Dehydroemetine   d. Diloxanide furoate

6. Which of the following drugs is suitable for single dose therapy in amoebiasis?
   a. Tinidazole   b. Secnidazole
   c. Ornidazole   d. Satranidazole

7. A 28-year-old pregnant woman patient is diagnosed with invasive amoebiasis. Metronidazole is contraindicated for her.
   i. Identify an alternative drug to nitroimidazoles in this case.
      a. Dehydroemetine   b. Paromomycin
      c. Secnidazole   d. DIQ
   ii. Describe the mechanism of action and adverse effects of the selected drug.

DRUGS FOR VISCERAL LEISHMANIASIS (KALA-AZAR)

Leishmaniasis is an infective disease caused by **Leishmania donovani.** The infection occurs through the bite of female *Phlebotomus* sandfly. Visceral leishmaniasis is the most severe form of the disease, associated with fatal outcomes in the majority of cases if not treated promptly.

Drugs for visceral leishmaniasis include sodium stibogluconate, amphotericin B, paromomycin, and miltefosine.

1. Sodium stibogluconate
It is a pentavalent antimonial compound that was the first-line drug against leishmaniasis. However it is no longer used in India, as there is widespread resistance to it.

2. Amphotericin B
This is a polyene antibiotic that exerts both **antifungal and antiprotozoal** effects It acts by binding to ergosterol

in the cell membrane, leading to formation of micropores, through which water, ions, amino acids, etc., leak out, ultimately resulting in cell death.

Currently, **liposomal amphotericin B (L-AMB)** is the **most effective drug** for treating visceral leishmaniasis (kala-azar). Initially, it was reserved as a secondary treatment in the National Vector Borne Disease Control Programme (NVBDCP) for patients who could not use **miltefosine** (such as pregnant and lactating women). This was due to the limitations of amphotericin B, such as the need for repeated injections, prolonged hospitalisation, and a high incidence of several adverse effects. However, with the increased availability of **L-AMB**, it is now the **first-line treatment for kala-azar**, administered as a single IV infusion at a dose of 10 mg/kg body weight. L-AMB provides sufficient concentration of the drug inside the reticuloendothelial cells in the liver and spleen, where leishmania parasites reside. L-AMB is effective in cutaneous and mucocutaneous leishmaniasis also.

ADRs: The important ADRs of amphotericin B include acute infusion-related reactions such as fever, chills, nausea, vomiting, and dyspnea due to the release of interleukins and TNFα after each infusion. It has the potential to cause dose-dependent **nephrotoxicity**. GFR is reduced, and hypokalemia and azotemia may occur. The renal effects are partially reversible on stopping the treatment. Amphotericin B also has **bone-marrow-suppressant** and **central toxic** effects.

3. Miltefosine

Miltefosine is an **orally active** drug for visceral leishmaniasis. Its action is probably through interference with lipid metabolism, signal transduction and synthesis of anchor proteins in Leishmania. However, the **relapse rate after miltefosine treatment is quite high,** and there are many cases of post-kala-azar dermal leishmaniasis with the use of this drug. Many organisms have developed **resistance** also. So, although it was preferred drug under NVBDCP for some time, it is now an alternative drug used along with paromomycin or amphotericin B.

ADRs: Common adverse effects of miltefosine include anorexia, nausea, vomiting, diarrhea, allergic reactions, **hepatic function impairment** and **reversible renal impairment.**

4. Paromomycin

This is an aminoglycoside used via the IM route in visceral leishmaniasis **in cases resistant to sodium stibogluconate**. It may cause reversible rise in serum transaminase levels, ototoxicity, and pain at the site of injection. In cutaneous leishmania, it is used as a topical application.

5. Combination therapy

Combination of two drugs is more efficacious and decreases chances of development of resistance, reduces the dose, and hence the toxicity of individual drugs, especially amphotericin B.

- Liposomal AMB 5 mg/kg IV single dose can be combined with miltefosine by oral route for 7 days or with paromomycin IM for 10 days.
- Alternatively, miltefosine and paromomycin may be combined for 10 days.

Clinical problem-based questions and MCQs

8. All of the following are useful in visceral leishmaniasis, EXCEPT:
   a. Amphotericin B
   b. Miltefosine
   c. Dehydroemetine
   d. Paromomycin

9. Which of the following correctly describes the mechanism of action of amphotericin B?
   a. Protein synthesis inhibition
   b. Interference with lipid metabolism
   c. Binding to ergosterol, forming micropores
   d. Inhibiting intra-ribosomal translocation of tRNA

10. Which of the following combinations is beneficial in visceral leishmaniasis?
    a. Amphotericin B and paromomycin
    b. Amphotericin B and miltefosine
    c. Sodium stibogluconate and amphotericin B
    d. Sodium stibogluconate and miltefosine

Summary

- Amoebiasis occurs due to ingestion of cysts of *E. histolytica* that develop into trophozoites in the intestine (luminal phase causing chronic intestinal amoebiasis and cyst-passer stage). These trophozoites adhere to and invade the intestinal wall and cause invasive disease (acute intestinal amoebiasis, dysentery and tissue abscess, mainly hepatic amoebiasis and liver abscess).
- Antiamoebic drugs are classified as luminal and tissue amoebicides. Among **luminal amoebicides**, **diloxanide furoate** is the most frequently used drug in chronic cyst passers, chronic intestinal amoebiasis, as well as for eradicating residual cysts following treatment with tissue amoebicides. It is well tolerated with minor adverse effects.
- **Nitazoxanide** is a prodrug having the same indications for use as diloxanide.
- **Iodoquinol** can cause multiple adverse effects, including anorexia, nausea, transient loose stools, furunculosis, goitre and SMON. Hence, it is not preferred.
- **Tetracycline and paromomycin** also possess luminal amoebicide action.
- **Tissue amoebicides** include nitroimidazoles (metronidazole, tinidazole, etc.), emetine, dehydroemetine, and chloroquine.

- **Nitroimidazoles** exert amoebicidal action through an active nitro radical that can gain electrons and disrupt energy metabolism, especially in anerobic organisms. These are useful in invasive amoebiasis, amoebic dysentery, amoebic liver abscess, giardiasis, and trichomonal vaginitis and for the prevention and treatment of anaerobic infections. Important ADRs of metronidazole are anorexia, nausea, dry mouth, metallic taste, abdominal cramps, headache, dizziness, vertigo, vomiting, neutropenia, dysuria, and dark urine in some cases. Intravenous use may cause thrombophlebitis, seizures, peripheral neuropathy and disulfiram reaction.
- **Emetine** directly kills trophozoites by interfering with the intra-ribosomal translocation of tRNA–amino acid complex during protein synthesis. It produces rapid symptomatic relief within 1–3 days of starting therapy, but is not curative as it has no effect on cysts. ADRs include pain, tenderness, sterile abscess at site of injection, nausea, vomiting, diarrhea, and muscular weakness. Cardiac adverse effects such as hypotension, ECG changes, cardiac arrhythmias, cardiac failure can occur.
- **Chloroquine** gets concentrated in liver and has good tissue amoebicidal effect, but it has to be given for 2–3 weeks in hepatic amoebiasis. So, it is not a preferred drug.
- Visceral leishmaniasis or kala-azar is caused by the bite of female *Phlebotomus* sandfly. Currently, liposomal amphotericin B is the first-line drug, given as a single dose 10 mg/kg IV infusion. It can be combined with miltefosine to reduce the dose-related adverse effects. Resistance to sodium stibogluconate has reduced its utility in leishmaniasis. Paromomycin is a good choice for resistant cases.

Questions for practice

1. Describe the mechanism of action, indications and adverse effects of metronidazole.
2. Explain why:
    a. Treatment of tissue amoebiasis needs luminal amoebicidal drugs also.
    b. DIQ is not a preferred antiamoebic drug.
    c. Emetine is used only when metronidazole cannot be given.
    d. Nitroimidazoles are not effective in aerobic organisms.
    e. Chloroquine has good efficacy in hepatic amoebiasis but is not the first-choice drug for this disease.
    f. Combination of two drugs is good for treatment of kala-azar.
    g. Liposomal AMB is the preferred drug for visceral leishmaniasis.

Hints for problem-based questions and MCQs

1. b. Chloroquine
2. i. c. Diloxanide furoate is useful in chronic intestinal amoebiasis
   ii. Dose of diloxanide is 500 mg three times a day for 5–10 days.
   iii. Diloxanide is useful in asymptomatic cyst passers and is also used after tissue amoebicides to cure the disease in invasive amoebiasis. Diloxanide may cause nausea, flatulence, itching, rashes, etc.
3. i. Luminal amoebicides include diloxanide furoate, nitazoxanide, quiniodochlor, iodoquinol, and antibiotics like tetracycline and paromomycin.
   ii. c. Nitazoxanide
   iii. d. Iodoquinol
4. i. The patient has amoebic dysentery.
   ii. c. Metronidazole is the drug of choice in this case.
   iii. Metronidazole forms nitro radicals that act as electron sinks and disrupt energy metabolism in anerobic organisms.
   iv. Uses of metronidazole include acute invasive amoebiasis, amoebic dysentery, amoebic liver abscess, giardiasis, trichomonal vaginitis and for prevention as well as treatment of anaerobic infections after pelvic/colorectal surgery, trench mouth, and pseudomembranous enterocolitis.
   ADRs of metronidazole include anorexia, nausea, dry mouth, metallic taste, abdominal cramps, headache, dizziness, vertigo, vomiting, neutropenia, dysuria, and dark urine in some cases. Intravenous use may cause thrombophlebitis, seizures, peripheral neuropathy and disulfiram reaction.
5. i. Due to complete absorption, nitroimidazoles are not reliable for luminal infection.
   ii. d. Diloxanide furoate
   Metronidazole is usually combined with luminal drugs like diloxanide furoate to eradicate cysts.
6. b. Secnidazole has a longer half life (17–29 hours) and is suitable as a single dose of 2 g in amoebiasis.
7. i. a. Dehydroemetine
   ii. Same as emetine. Refer to page 771.
   Cardiac adverse effects like hypotension, ECG changes, cardiac arrhythmias, cardiac failure are less common than with emetine but may occur.
8. c. Dehydroemetine has no role in visceral leishmaniasis.
9. c. Binding to ergosterol, forming a micropore.
10. b. Amphotericin B and miltefosine.

CONCEPT MAP – ANTIAMOEBIC DRUGS

Antiamoebic Drugs

Luminal Amoebiasis

Nitazoxanide
Prodrug → forms tizoxanide inside body that kills luminal trophozoites by inhibiting PFOR (pyruvate: ferredoxin oxidoreductase), essential for electron transport energy metabolism in anaerobes.
Uses: Alternative to diloxanide as luminal amoebicide.
For *Cryptosporidium parvum* infection
For metronidazole-resistant Giardia.
Dose: 500 mg, BD for 3 days
ADR: Very mild like abdominal pain, headache, nausea

8-Hydroxyquinolines
Quiniodochlor, Iodoquinol
Kills cyst forming trophozoites in intestine by an unknown mechanism. Less efficacious than diloxanide in eradicating cysts.
Poor absorption → no tissue amoebicidal effect
Effective against Trichomonas, Giardia, Candida, dermatophytes also.
Uses: Chronic intestinal amoebiasis as alternative to diloxanide.
Used for giardiasis, monilial & trichomonas vaginitis, fungal infections, etc.
ADRs: Anorexia, nausea, vomiting, transient loose green stools, headache, rash, pruritus, goitre, iodism, Subacute myelo-optic neuropathy (SMON) may occur.

Diloxanide Furoate
Mechanism: 90% gets absorbed, but is promptly conjugated and excreted → not effective against tissue trophozoites. Unabsorbed 10% diloxanide kills luminal trophozoites before encystment by an unknown mechanism.
Uses: Asymptomatic cyst passers
Chronic mild intestinal amoebiasis,
After or with tissue amoebicides to eradicate cysts.
Dose: 500 mg TDS for 5–10 days
ADRs: Well tolerated drug, may cause itching, rash, urticaria, nausea, flatulence.

Antibiotics
Tetracyclines: Indirectly inhibit luminal amoeba by inhibition of bacterial flora having symbiotic relationship with *E. histolytica*
Used as adjuvants with another luminal amoebicide and metronidazole.
Paromomycin: Bactericidal drug, as effective as diloxanide furoate in asymptomatic cyst passers and chronic amoebic colitis.
Also used as alternative to metronidazole for giardiasis in first trimester of pregnancy.
ADRs: Not absorbed after oral use. Limited to GIT as abdominal cramps, nausea, vomiting & diarrhea.

Tissue Amoebicides

Only for Extraintestinal Amoebiasis

Chloroquine
Antimalarial drug.
Highly concentrated in liver, → effective only for hepatic amoebiasis.
Used only when metronidazole is not effective or not tolerated, because of longer duration of treatment with chloroquine & need for adding luminal drug to prevent relapses.

For both Intestinal & Extraintestinal Amoebasis

Alkaloids
Emetine: Kills trophozoites by interfering with protein synthesis. → fast symptomatic relief within 1–3 days of starting therapy, but has no effect on cysts → not curative
Oral absorption is erratic, so needs IM or SC injection. Risk of cardiac toxicity on IV use.
Used only when MNZ cannot be given.
ADRs: Pain, tenderness, sterile abscess at site of injection.
Nausea, vomiting, diarrhea, muscular weakness, hypotension, ECG changes, cardiac arrhythmias, cardiac failure.

Nitroimidazoles
Metronidazole, Tinidazole, Ornidazole
Mechanism: Form highly reactive nitro radicals in anaerobes that act as electron sinks and disrupt energy metabolism. No effect against aerobes as it fails to get activated to nitro radical.
MNZ is effective against Protozoa (*E. histolytica, G.lamblia, Trichomonas*), Anaerobes (*B. fragilis, Fusobacterium, Cl.perfringens H. pylori* & anaerobic streptococci). It also facilitates extraction of *D. medinensis* from under the skin.
Uses: Drug of choice for all tissue infection of *E. histolytica*.
Dose: 800 mg, TDS for 7–10 days. In amoebic dysentery, amoebic liver abscess, MNZ is combined with Diloxanide to eradicate cysts.
Also used in Giardiasis, Trichomonal vaginitis, non-specific bacterial vaginosis, prevention of anaerobic infection occurring after pelvic/colorectal surgery, trench mouth, acute necrotising ulcerative gingivitis, pseudomembranous enterocolitis and as part of triple drug regimen for *H. pylori* eradication.
ADRs: Anorexia, nausea, dry mouth, metallic taste, abdominal cramps, headache, dizziness, vertigo, vomiting, neutropenia, dysuria, dark urine.
Thrombophlebitis, seizures, peripheral neuropathy, disulfiram reaction with IV use
Contraindications: Neurological diseases, blood dyscrasia & pregnancy.

SECTION 10 Chemotherapeutic Drugs

60 Anthelmintics

PH 8.7 Discuss the types, kinetics, dynamics, adverse effects of drugs used for filariasis
PH 8.9 Discuss the types, kinetics, dynamics, adverse effects of drugs used for intestinal helminthiasis.

Learning objectives

A student of MBBS phase II should be able to:
- Classify anthelmintic drugs.
- Describe mechanism of action and pharmacokinetics of anthelmintic drugs.
- Enumerate indications, adverse effects of and contraindications to anthelmintic drugs.

PARASITES

Parasites are living organisms that depend on another living organism for their survival and nutrition, but do not provide any benefit to the host. Parasites that infect humans can be unicellular or multicellular.

- Unicellular parasitic infections, also known as protozoal infections, are caused by organisms such as *E. histolytica, G. lamblia, T. vaginalis, Leishmania, P. vivax, P. falciparum, T. gondii*.
- In contrast, **multicellular parasitic worms** are known as helminths. These are bilaterally symmetrical and can be elongated, flat or rounded in shape.

Helminths belong to 2 phyla:
- Phylum Platyhelminthes (flat)
- Phylum Nematoda or nematodes

Phylum *Platyhelminthes*

Phylum *Platyhelminthes* includes dorsoventrally **flat organisms** without a body cavity. They can be **segmented** (cestodes) or **unsegmented** (trematodes).

- **Cestodes** are **flat, tape-like**, segmented organisms with suckers and often hooks. They do not have an alimentary canal, e.g., *Taenia solium, T. saginata, T. asiatica, Hymenolepis nana, Diphyllobothrium latum*, and *Echinococcus granulosus*.
- **Trematodes** or flukes are **flat, leaf-like**, unsegmented organisms with an incomplete alimentary canal and suckers but no hooks, e.g., *Fasciola hepatica, Schistosoma*.

Phylum *Nematoda*

Nematodes are cylindrical, elongated, unsegmented organisms without suckers and hooks. They have a body cavity and complete alimentary canal, e.g., *Ancylostoma duodenale, Necator americanus, Ascaris lumbricoides, Strongyloides stercoralis, Enterobius vermicularis, Dracunculus medinensis, Trichuris trichiura, Wuchereria bancrofti, Trichinella spiralis*.

Helminthiasis

It is commonly known as **worm infestation**, and is an important cause of chronic ill health. It is especially prevalent in underdeveloped countries due to poor hygiene.

Parasitic infections occur through:
- Contaminated soil and water, undercooked pork, fish, aquatic plants and bites of blood-sucking insects.
- Majority of parasites (*Enterobius, Taenia, Ascaris*) gain entry into the human host through the **feco-oral route** by ingestion of contaminated food, water and through fomites.
- The larval forms of some parasites penetrate **intact skin** (e.g., *Ancylostoma duodenale, Necator americanus, Strongyloides stercoralis*) or enter through insect bites (*Plasmodium*).
- Some parasitic infections may also be acquired through **sexual contact** (*Trichomonas vaginalis*) or from **mother to fetus** (*Toxoplasma*).

The **human host is harmed** by parasitic infections in the following ways:

- Traumatic **damage to the villi** of intestinal walls and bleeding occur at site of attachment of hookworms.
- Intestinal **obstruction and perforation** may be caused by roundworm.
- **Inflammatory response** can occur at the site of parasitic infection.
- **Allergic response** to secretions of growing larvae and dead parasites is harmful, e.g., hydatid fluid released due to rupture of hydatid cyst (*Echinococcus granulosus*) may cause severe allergic reactions like anaphylaxis.
- Penetration of parasites into **extra-intestinal** viscera may damage the tissues, e.g., neurocysticercosis.

COMMON HELMINTHIC DISEASES

1. Cestode Infections

a. *Taenia* (tapeworm) infection

The adult worm is formed in human intestines and attaches to the intestinal wall causing vague abdominal pain and discomfort, chronic indigestion, and anemia. The patient passes eggs or gravid proglottids (egg-bearing segments of adult worms) in feces that are ingested by the intermediate host (pigs/cattle). The oncospheres hatch, penetrate the intestinal wall and reach the muscles of the intermediate hosts, and develop into cysticerci. In humans, infection occurs following the ingestion of raw/undercooked pork (*T. solium*) or beef (*T. saginata*) that contain oncospheres and cysticerci (Fig. 60.1).

Next, the cysticerci may move to extraintestinal tissues like subcutaneous tissues, muscles, and brain, forming nodules at these sites, which may get calcified later on. Epileptic fits may occur in case of neurocysticercosis.

b. *Echinococcus granulosus* (dog tapeworm) infection

In the life cycle of *Echinococcus granulosus* or dog tapeworm, which causes hydatid disease, dogs are the definitive host. The intermediate hosts may be humans, cattle, goats, horses, etc. Infection in humans occurs through contact with infected dogs/cattle or eating raw/undercooked vegetables contaminated with the feces of infected animals.

Larval forms of this parasite cause unilocular hydatid disease called cystic echinococcosis. Hydatid cysts containing a clear, highly toxic and antigenic fluid may develop in the liver, lungs, kidney, spleen, heart, brain muscles, and other organs. However, the most common site is the right hepatic lobe (Fig. 60.2). The growing cysts exert pressure effects, leading to chronic abdominal discomfort. Rupture of the cyst and release of hydatid fluid can cause severe allergic reactions, anaphylaxis, and may even be fatal.

c. *Hymenolepis nana* (dwarf tapeworm) infection

This infection occurs by the feco–oral route and causes abdominal pain, diarrhea, pruritus and allergic reactions.

2. Trematode Infections

Trematodes can cause infection of blood, liver, intestine, and lungs.

a. Schistosomiasis

Schistosomiasis is a waterborne disease. The parasite resides in vesical and pelvic venous plexuses and mesenteric veins of the human host. Its eggs reach the urinary bladder, large intestine and ileocecal region. Schistosomal infection can spread to various tissues and cause acute or chronic schistosomiasis. Various manifestations of schistosomiasis are depicted in Fig. 60.3.

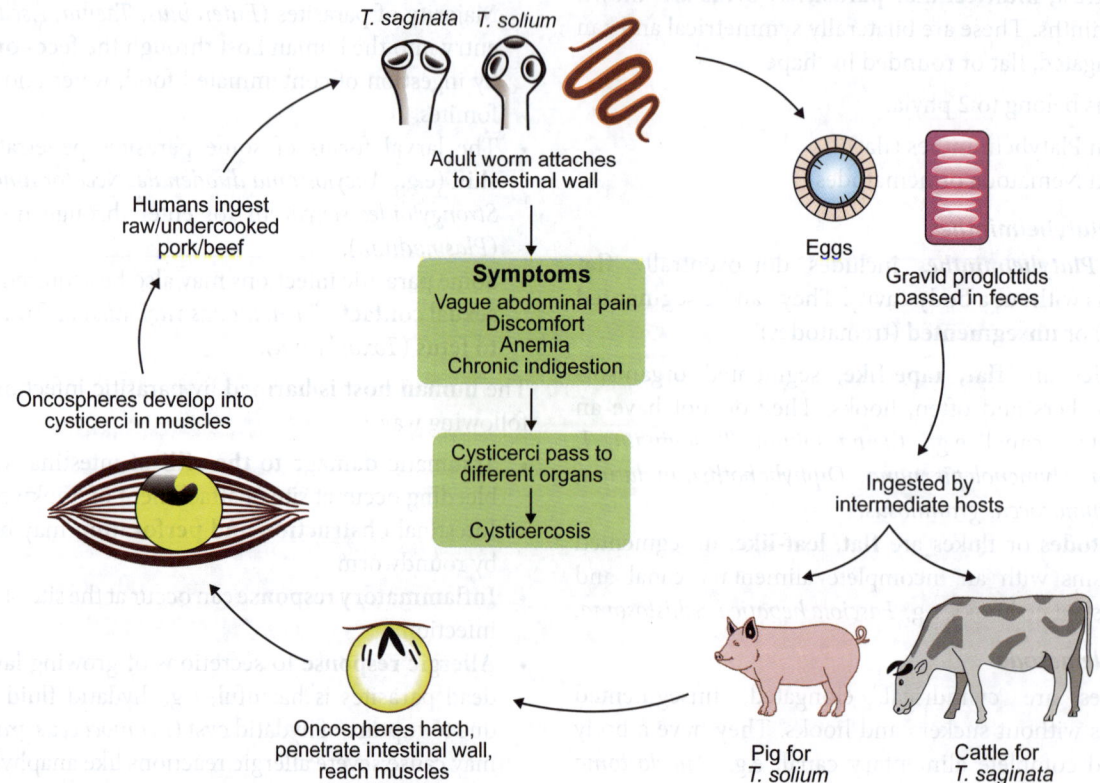

Fig. 60.1 Life cycle of *Taenia*

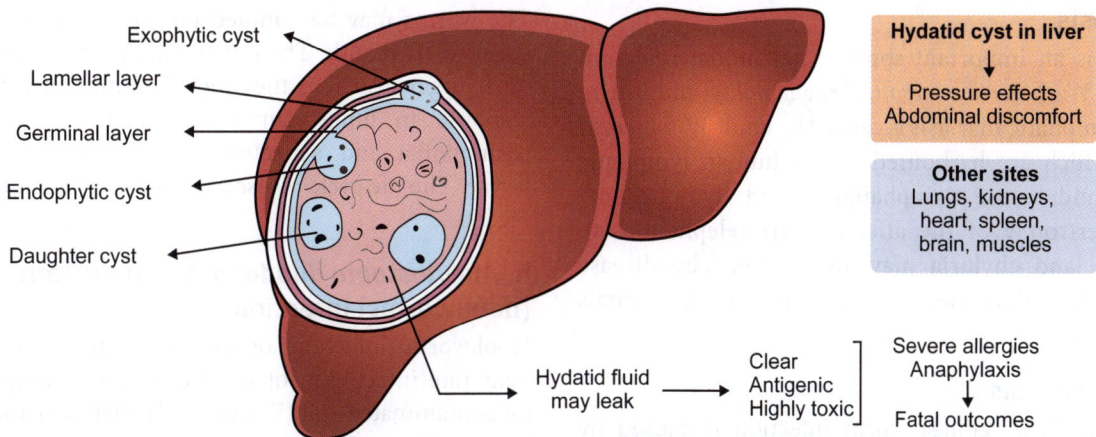

Fig. 60.2 Hydatid cysts in the liver

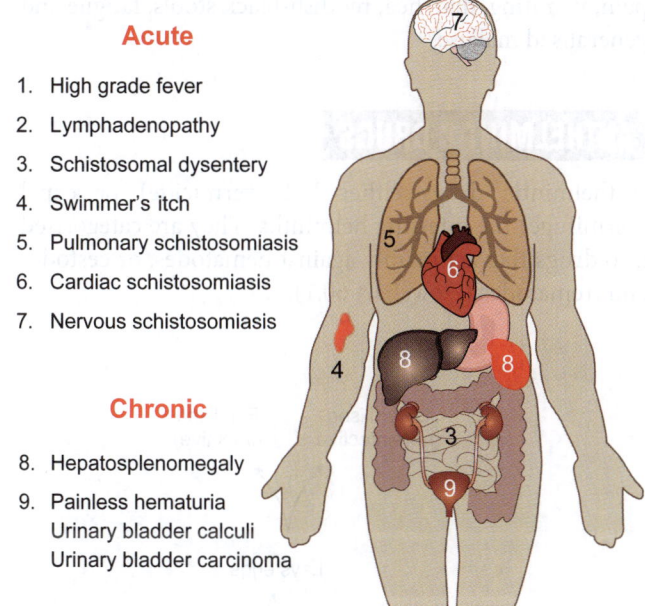

Fig. 60.3 Schistosomiasis

Acute
1. High grade fever
2. Lymphadenopathy
3. Schistosomal dysentery
4. Swimmer's itch
5. Pulmonary schistosomiasis
6. Cardiac schistosomiasis
7. Nervous schistosomiasis

Chronic
8. Hepatosplenomegaly
9. Painless hematuria
   Urinary bladder calculi
   Urinary bladder carcinoma

b. Fasciola hepatica (liver fluke) infection

Liver fluke infection is frequently observed in sheep and cattle herders. This infection causes fever, abdominal pain, liver parenchymal injury and tenderness, hepatomegaly, eosinophil-rich ascitic fluid collection and jaundice.

Fasciolopsis buski, also known as giant intestinal fluke, causes fasciolopsiasis, characterised by mucosal inflammation, ulceration and partial intestinal obstruction. Patients present with abdominal pain, anorexia, nausea, vomiting, and diarrhea along with anemia, asthenia, ascites and generalised toxic symptoms.

c. Trematode infection of the lungs

Infection of the lungs by trematodes results in the formation of granuloma, cystic bronchial dilatation, pneumonitis and lung abscess. The patient presents with cough, hemoptysis (blood in sputum) and chest pain. Parasite eggs may be passed out in sputum.

3. Nematode Infections

Nematodes are thread-like worms. Common nematodal infections include the following.

a. Strongyloidiasis

Strongyloidiasis, an infection by *Strongyloides stercoralis*, can cause cutaneous, pulmonary and intestinal disease. Cutaneous strongyloidiasis manifests as eczema, dermatitis, and itching at the site where the larva enters, especially in perianal, gluteal and abdominal regions. Pulmonary *Strongyloides* infection leads to alveolar hemorrhage, chronic bronchitis, dyspnea, and bronchopneumonia. Intestinal *Strongyloides* infection presents with abdominal pain, distension, alternating diarrhea and constipation, and malabsorption. Hyperinfection usually occurs in AIDS patients and involves repeated infection and increased worm load in lungs, intestines or other organs. Patient may develop meningitis, peritonitis, brain abscess, etc., which may be fatal.

b. Trichinellosis

Trichinellosis is a disease caused by *Trichinella spiralis* infection, which occurs on ingesting raw or undercooked pork containing encysted larvae. In the early intestinal phase, the patient develops nausea, vomiting, diarrhea and abdominal pain. The entry of the larvae into muscles leads to fever, myalgias, muscular weakness, and periorbital edema.

c. Enterobiasis (pinworm infection)

Enterobiasis or pinworm infection usually occurs in children via contaminated foods or beverages. Later on, autoinfection continues through the feco–oral route. It presents as perianal pruritus, perineal eczema and nocturnal enuresis.

d. *Trichuris trichiura* (whipworm)

Trichuris trichiura or whipworm infection results in inflammation of the large intestine, rectal edema, rectal prolapse, bleeding, and abdominal cramps (dysentery-like features). Iron-deficiency anemia may occur in prolonged infection.

e. Filariasis

Filariasis is an important somatic nematodal infection caused by *Wuchereria bancrofti*, *Brugia malayi* and *Brugia timori*. Lymphatic filariasis is caused by adult *W. bancrofti* worms, which are harboured in the human lymphatic system, and cause lymphangitis and lymphedema with hypertrophy of the affected part (elephantiasis). Hydrocele and chyluria may also occur. The disease caused by *B. malayi* does not usually involve the genitals or chyluria.

f. Dracunculiasis

Dracunculiasis or guinea worm infection is caused by *Dracunculus medinensis,* and results in nausea, vomiting, erythema, itching, rash, urticaria, and formation of blisters—usually in the feet, between the metatarsal bones or at the ankles.

g. Ascariasis (roundworm infection)

Ascaris lumbricoides (roundworm) infection in humans occurs upon ingestion of water and food (especially raw vegetables) that are contaminated with its embryonated eggs. Larvae emerge after eggs hatch and invade the intestinal mucosa, resulting in intermittent colicky abdominal pain, anorexia, and nutritional deficiency. The worms may be vomited out or passed out through the nose or mouth. The larvae can also reach and invade other organs, such as the lungs. Inflammatory or allergic response in lungs can cause cough, fever, dyspnea, eosinophilia and expectoration of sputum containing larvae. The life cycle of *Ascaris lumbricoides* is depicted in Fig. 60.4.

h. *Ancylostoma duodenale*, *N. americanus* (hookworms) infection

Hookworm infection occurs when hookworm larvae penetrate intact skin of the feet while walking barefoot on contaminated soil (Fig. 60.5). The larva matures in the intestines into an adult worm that attaches itself to the small intestine mucosa, feeds on blood and causes microcytic, hypochromic anemia. Clinical features include epigastric pain, vomiting, diarrhea, reddish-black stools, fatigue and generalised malaise.

ANTHELMINTIC DRUGS

Anthelmintic drugs either kill (vermicide) or expel (vermifuge) the infesting helminths. They are categorised into drugs that act mainly against nematodes, or cestodes and trematodes (Flowchart 60.1).

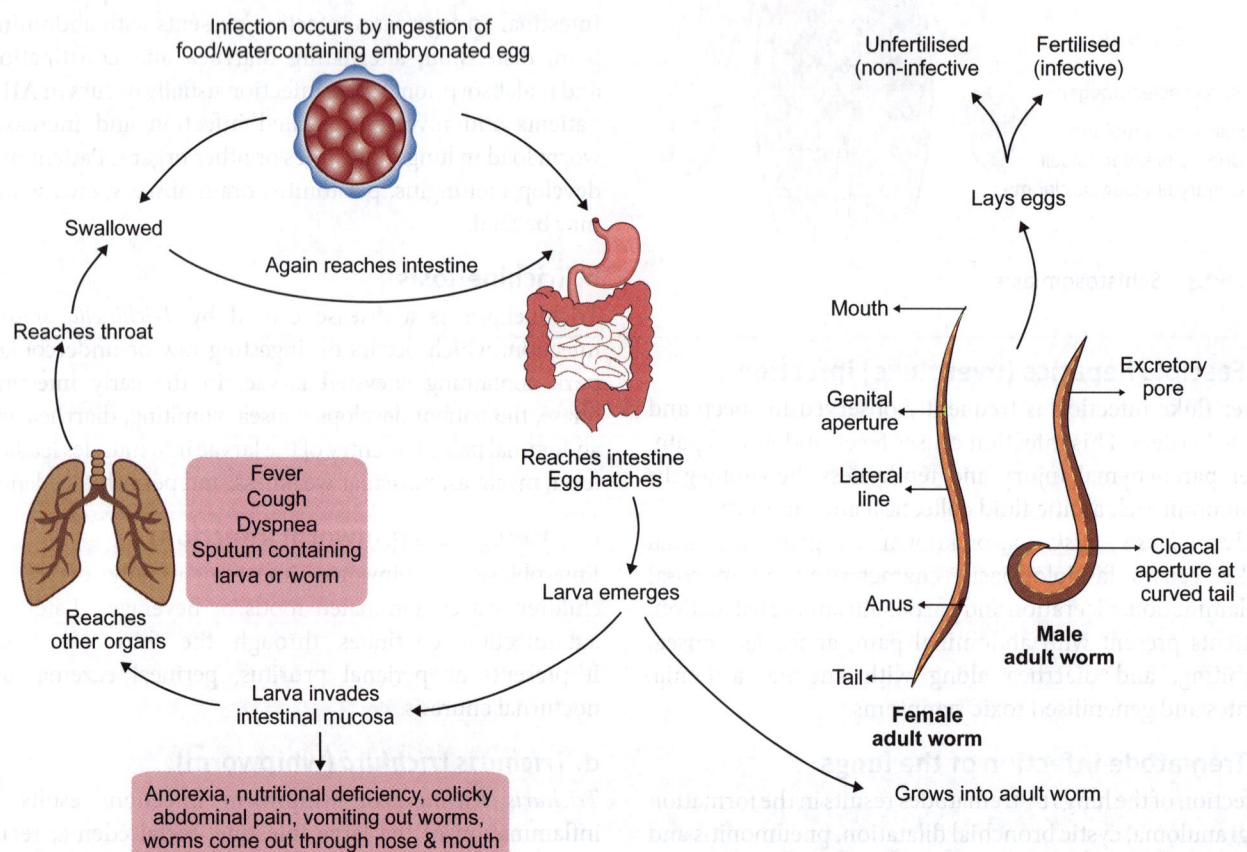

Fig. 60.4 Life cycle of *Ascaris lumbricoides*

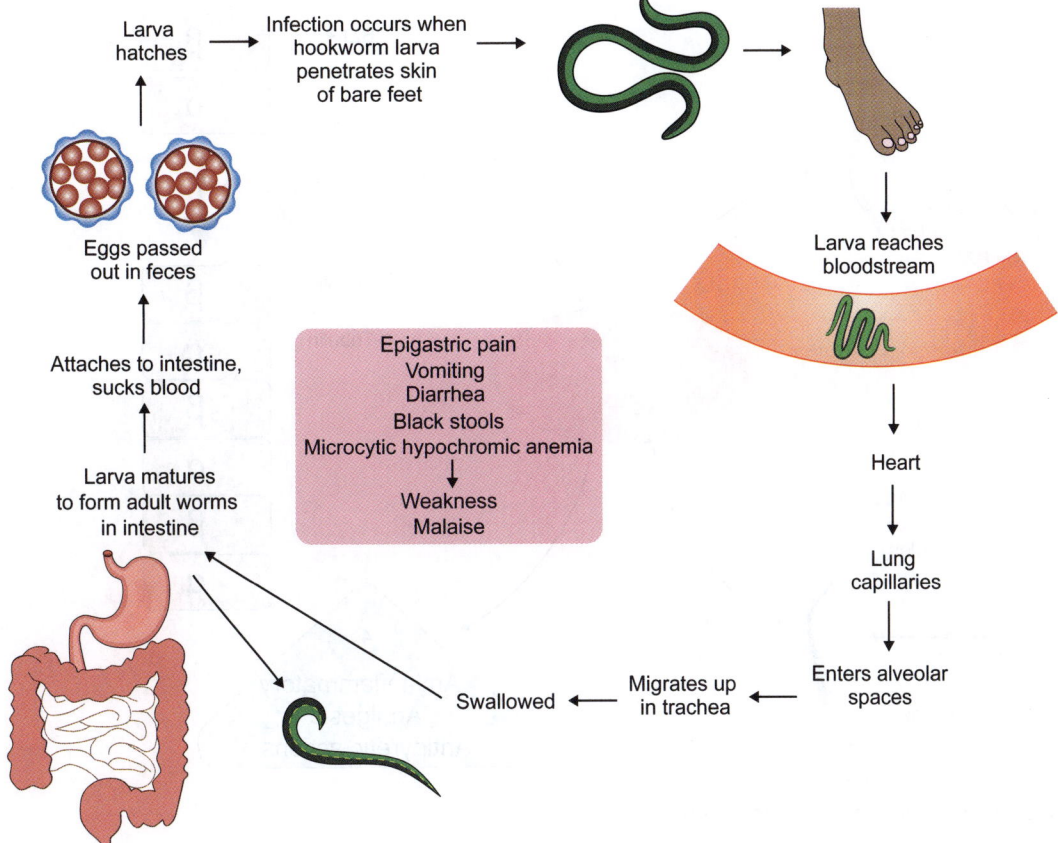

Fig. 60.5 Life cycle of hookworm

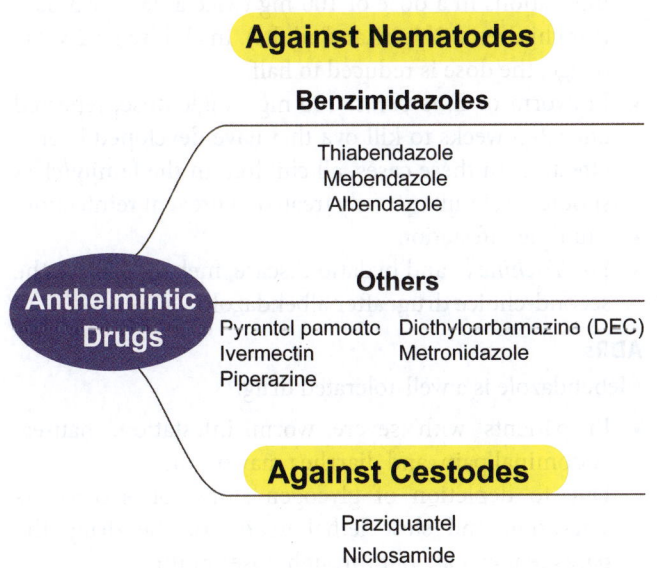

Flowchart 60.1 Classification of anthelmintic drugs

DRUGS AGAINST NEMATODES

1. Benzimidazoles

Thiabendazole, mebendazole, albendazole

Mechanism of action

Benzimidazoles are vermicidal drugs that (see Fig. 60.6):
1. Block glucose uptake in the parasite and deplete its glycogen stores.
2. Inhibit polymerisation of β-tubulin, leading to loss of intracellular microtubules in the worm.
3. Inhibit hatching of nematode eggs and kill *Ascaris* ova.
4. Also have anti-inflammatory, antipyretic and analgesic actions.

a. Thiabendazole

Spectrum of activity

Thiabendazole is practically **effective against all species** of nematodes that infest the GIT, i.e., roundworm (*Ascaris lumbricoides*), hookworm (*Ancylostoma duodenale, Necator americanus*), threadworm (*Enterobius*), whipworm (*Trichuris*), *Trichinella spiralis, Strongyloides*, etc.

It affords symptomatic relief in cutaneous larva migrans, skeletal muscle symptoms resulting from migration of *Trichinella spiralis* larvae to muscles, and guinea worm disease.

Adverse effects

It has good oral absorption; as a result, adverse effects such as nausea, vomiting, loss of appetite, abdominal pain, diarrhea, headache, giddiness, and impaired alertness occur frequently.

Therapeutic uses

Because of **poor patient acceptability,** it is used only when other better-tolerated drugs are ineffective in strongyloidiasis, trichinosis, cutaneous larva migrans, etc.

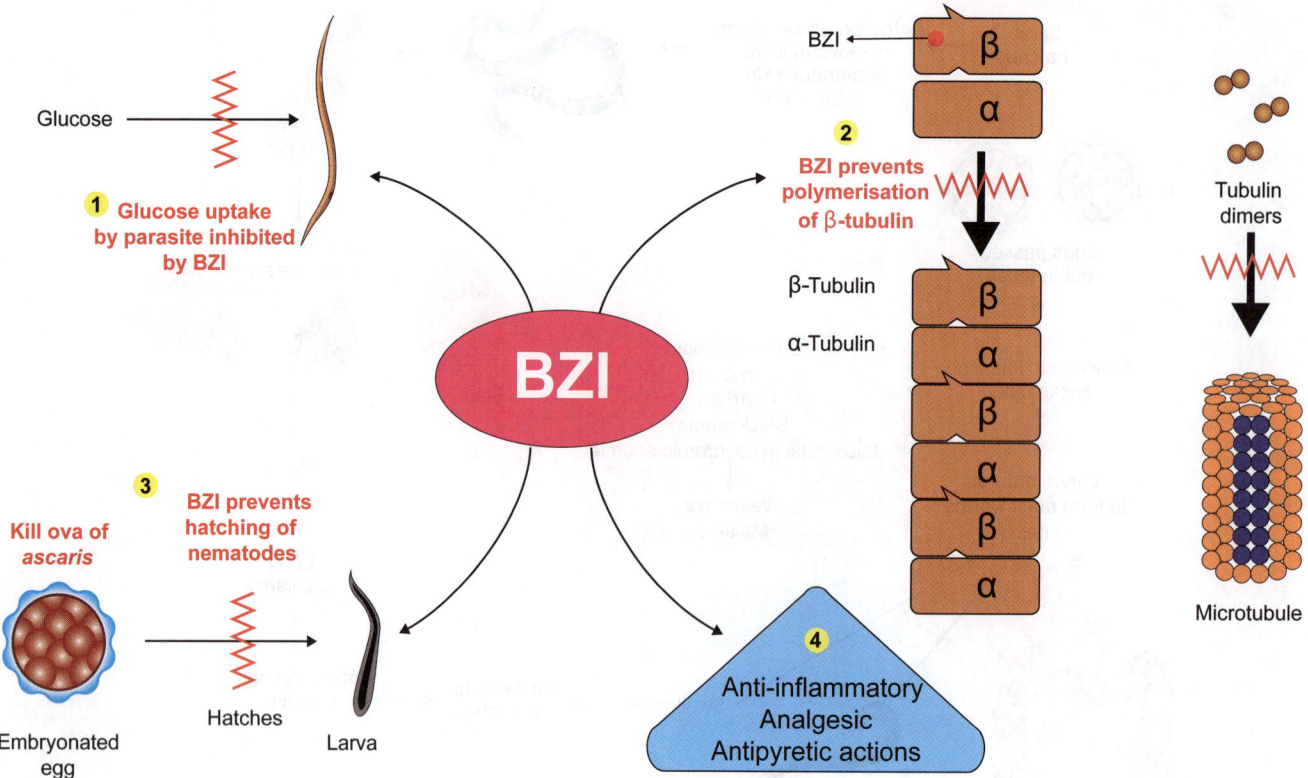

Fig. 60.6 Mechanism of action of benzimidazoles

b. Mebendazole

- It is a thiabendazole congener with the same broad-spectrum anthelmintic activity, but is better tolerated.
- It has the same mechanism of action as thiabendazole. It exerts slowly developing lethal action (in 2–3 days) by inhibiting the polymerisation of β-tubulin, resulting in the slow loss of intracellular microtubules in worms. It also depletes the glycogen stores of parasites by blocking glucose uptake and can inhibit the hatching of nematode eggs and kill *Ascaris* ova.
- Mebendazole is very active against **gastrointestinal nematodes**—roundworm, hookworm, threadworm, and whipworm—but less active against *Strongyloides* than thiabendazole. While it can expel *Trichinella* from the intestine, larvae that have migrated to muscles may not be effectively killed.
- Among the cestodes, **tapeworm may respond**, but it is less effective against *H. nana*. Prolonged treatment is effective for hydatid cysts in the liver caused by *Echinococcus granulosus*.

Pharmacokinetics
Its oral absorption is minimal and about 75–90% of the oral dose is excreted in the feces.

Therapeutic uses
No preparation/fasting/purging is required while using mebendazole

- Used in roundworm, hookworm, and whipworm infestations in a dose of 100 mg twice a day for 3 days (for children > 2 years and adults). In children < 2 years of age, the dose is reduced to half.
- Pinworm or *Enterobius*: 100 mg, single dose, repeated after 2–3 weeks to kill ova that have developed later is effective. In these cases, all children in the family/class should be simultaneously treated to prevent reinfection.
- Multiple infestation
- For *Trichinella* and hydatid disease, mebendazole is the second-choice drug, after albendazole.

ADRs
Mebendazole is a well-tolerated drug.

- In patients with severe worm infestation, nausea, abdominal pain, and diarrhea may occur.
- Due to depletion of glycogen stores of *Ascaris*, its starvation and slow lethal action of the drug, the parasite may pass out through nose/mouth.
- Allergic reactions, alopecia, granulocytopenia may occur with higher doses.
- It is contraindicated in pregnancy as safety is not confirmed.

c. Albendazole
Similar to mebendazole, albendazole has a broad spectrum of anthelmintic action and minor adverse effects. In addition, it has the advantage of single-dose administration in many cases.

Pharmacokinetics

Oral absorption is moderate and increases when the drug is given along with a fatty meal. The absorbed fraction undergoes first-pass metabolism to form an active sulphoxide metabolite that is widely distributed in tissues and enters the brain; as a result, albendazole exerts anthelmintic activity in tissues as well (useful in neurocysticercosis and hydatid disease).

Therapeutic uses

- Roundworm, hookworm, threadworm, and whipworm respond to a single dose (400 mg for children > 2 years and adults; 200 mg for children < 2 years of age).
- In cases of heavy infestation with *Trichuris trichiura*, trichinosis, tapeworm infestation, strongyloidiasis and cutaneous larva migrans, albendazole is given in a dose of 400 mg once daily for 3 days. However, albendazole is not very effective against *Trichinella* larvae that migrate to muscles.
- Cysticercosis of other tissues such as muscles and subcutaneous tissue also responds to albendazole. Albendazole, given in a dose of 400 mg for 8–15 days, is the drug of choice in neurocysticercosis. However, no drug is used in the case of ocular cysticercosis, because of the fear of blindness secondary to allergic reaction to dead cysticerci.
- Longer treatment is required for hydatid disease; albendazole 400 mg, given twice daily for 4 weeks and repeated after 2 weeks is effective. Up to 3 courses may be required.
- In lymphatic filariasis, albendazole (single dose) is used as an adjuvant to diethylcarbamazine (DEC) or ivermectin. These drugs are given yearly to suppress microfilaremia in mass programmes.

ADRs

- While albendazole is usually well-tolerated, it may cause gastrointestinal adverse effects.
- Headache, dizziness, neutropenia, fever, alopecia, and jaundice may occur when it is used for a long time.
- It is contraindicated during pregnancy, and in liver and kidney disease

2. Pyrantel Pamoate

Mechanism of action

Pyrantel pamoate activates nicotinic cholinergic receptors in worms (Fig. 60.7), leading to persistent depolarisation; consequently, the worms slowly develop contracture and spastic paralysis that favours their expulsion. Mammalian skeletal muscle receptors have low affinity for pyrantel. It also has anticholinesterase action. The action of pyrantel pamoate is antagonised by piperazine as it causes hyperpolarisation and flaccid paralysis

Pyrantel pamoate has higher efficacy than mebendazole against:

- *Ascaris* (roundworm)
- *Enterobius* (threadworm)
- *Ancylostoma* (hookworm)

However, its efficacy against *Necator americanus* (hookworm) and *Strongyloides* is lower; it is inactive against *Trichuris* and other worms.

Therapeutic uses

It is used as a single-dose therapy of 11 mg/kg body weight in *Ascaris*, *Ancylostoma*, and *Enterobius* infestations.

However, *Necator americanus* and *Strongyloides* are less affected and a 3-day course is recommended for these infestations. Fasting, purging, or preparation is not required.

ADRs

It is a well-tolerated drug that does not cause any abnormal migration of worms; however, it may occasionally cause GIT symptoms, headache, and dizziness.

Its safety in pregnancy and in children < 2 years age is not established.

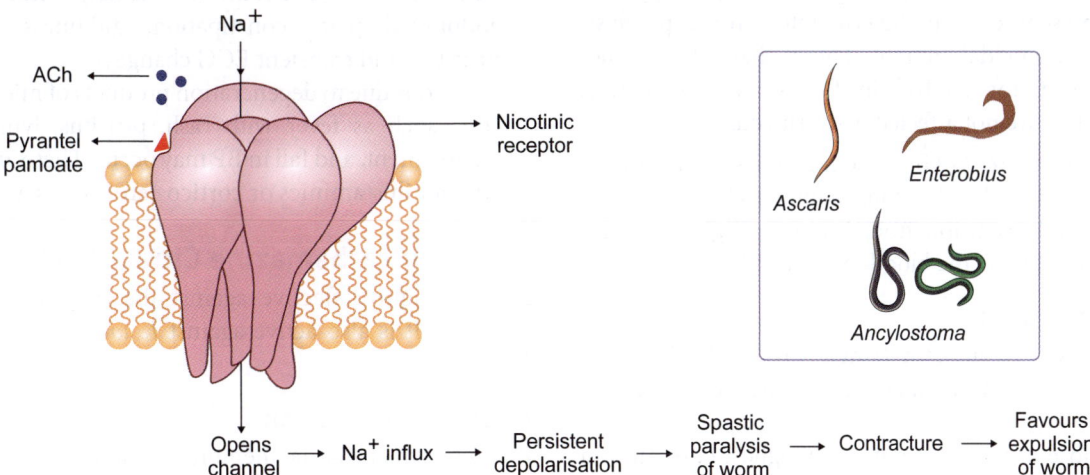

Fig. 60.7 Mechanism of action of pyrantel pamoate

3. Piperazine

Piperazine is highly active against *Ascaris* and *Enterobius*.

Mechanism of action

It acts as an agonist on GABA receptors and causes opening of Cl⁻ channels. This results in **hyperpolarisation and flaccid paralysis** of *Ascaris* muscles (Fig. 60.8). The worm is expelled alive and can be recovered in a piperazine-free medium. No fasting or preparation is required, but **a purgative** is often given along with it. It does not cause any abnormal migration of *Ascaris*, nor does it affect neuromuscular transmission in humans.

Therapeutic uses

Piperazine is a **second-choice drug** for *Ascaris* and *Enterobius* after albendazole/mebendazole. Because it has the capacity to relax the worm, it is of particular value in intestinal obstruction caused by roundworms. Dose is 4 g, once a day, for 2 consecutive days. It can be used during pregnancy, when other drugs are contraindicated.

ADRs

While it is well tolerated, it may occasionally cause nausea, vomiting, abdominal discomfort, and urticaria. High toxic doses may cause excitement, convulsions, respiratory failure, and even death.

4. Ivermectin

Ivermectin is very effective against *Strongyloides stercoralis* and *Onchocerca volvulus*.

- Its efficacy against *Wuchereria bancrofti*, *Brugia malayi*, and cutaneous larva migrans is comparable to that of DEC.
- It has moderate effect on *Enterobius* and *Trichuris*.
- It can also kill some insects such as itch mite (which causes scabies) and head lice.

Mechanism of action

It acts through a special type of glutamate-gated calcium channel, present only in invertebrates. Tonic paralysis results in vermicidal action. These channels are not involved in motor control in flukes and tapeworms; therefore, they are not affected by ivermectin.

- It also potentiates GABAergic transmission in worms.
- It lacks GABA-related actions in humans because of low affinity, and exclusion from brain by P-glycoprotein-mediated efflux at the blood–brain barrier.

Therapeutic uses

- In filariasis, ivermectin (single dose, 10–15 mg) is given along with albendazole 400 mg every year for 5–6 years.
- Single dose of ivermectin has the highest cure rates in strongyloidiasis.
- It has replaced DEC for onchocerciasis.

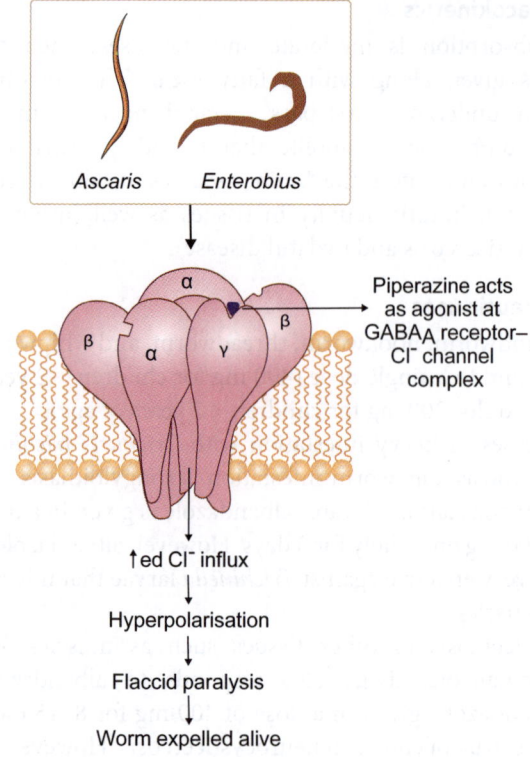

Fig. 60.8 Mechanism of action of piperazine

- It has been used in the river blindness control programme of WHO in Africa and Latin America. One dose every 6–12 months reduces the microfilariae (mf) count in eye and skin and suppresses ocular inflammation/damage and lymphadenopathy (LAP).
- It is the only oral drug for scabies and pediculosis, and is given as a single dose of 0.2 mg/kg for these indications.

Pharmacokinetics

It is well absorbed after oral use, widely distributed (not in CNS), and has a long half-life of 48–60 hours.

ADRs

- Reactions to ivermectin are usually mild (nausea, abdominal pain, constipation, giddiness, lethargy, pruritus, and transient ECG changes).
- Reactions due to degeneration products of microfilariae (mf) such as fever with rash, pruritus, lymph node enlargement, and fall in BP may occur. These are treated with antihistaminics or corticosteroids (if severe).

5. Diethylcarbamazine Citrate (DEC)

DEC is highly effective against the microfilaria of *W. bancrofti*. It is also active against *L. loa*, *O. volvulus*, and *B. malayi*.

Mechanism of action

- It alters microfilarial membranes leading to cidal action.
- The piperazine moiety causes hyperpolarisation, which affects the muscular activity of mf and adult worms; as a

result, these are dislodged and readily phagocytosed by tissue-fixed monocytes.
- Prolonged treatment may kill adult *B. malayi*, *W. bancrofti*, and *L. loa*, but not the adult worm of *O. volvulus*.

Therapeutic uses
- In filariasis, DEC 2 mg/kg, three times a day is the drug of choice. It provides quick symptomatic relief, and the patient becomes noninfective to mosquitoes in 7 days as mf disappear from the blood. However, intermittent microfilaremia and symptoms can occur again, because the adult worm survives in the lymphatics. Therefore, prolonged treatment is required for radical cure. A total dose of 72–126 mg/kg, given over 12 days to 3 weeks is usually required to kill adult worms. A repeat course may be required after 3–4 weeks.
- Elephantiasis caused due to chronic lymphatic obstruction is not relieved by DEC because fibrosis of lymphatics is irreversible.
- Mass treatment with a single dose of DEC 6 mg/kg body weight and albendazole 400 mg can effectively reduce transmission of filariasis.
- For *L. loa* and *O. volvulus*, ivermectin is preferred because DEC can cause a more severe reaction to dying microfilaria.
- Tropical eosinophilia: DEC 2–4 mg/kg, TDS, for 2–3 weeks produces dramatic improvement in signs and symptoms of eosinophilic lung or tropical eosinophilia.

ADRs
- Anorexia, nausea, headache, dizziness, and weakness.
- Reactions due to mass destruction of mf: Fever with rash, pruritus, lymph node enlargement, and fall in BP. This reaction is usually mild; in case of severe reaction, DEC is discontinued and antihistaminics/corticosteroids are given. Subsequent administration of DEC does not cause such reactions.
- Leukocytosis, eosinophilia and mild albuminuria may occur.

Clinical problem-based questions and MCQs

1. A 25-year-old male presents with a 3–4-month history of dull headache, confusion and impaired attention. He experienced a seizure episode one day prior to presentation. A CT scan reveals calcified lesions consistent with neurocysticercosis.
    i. Identify the drug of choice for this case.
        a. Pyrantel pamoate   b. Albendazole
        c. Piperazine   d. DEC
    ii. What is the dosage and duration of use in this case?
    iii. Describe mechanism of action, therapeutic uses and adverse effects of chosen drug.

2. Which of the following drugs is absorbed to a greater extent when consumed along with a fatty meal?
    a. Thiabendazole   b. Albendazole
    b. Pyrantel pamoate   d. Niclosamide

3. Select the appropriate dose schedule of albendazole for a patient with hydatid cyst of liver.
    a. 400 mg, twice daily for 4 weeks
    b. 400 mg, single dose for 8–15 days
    c. 400 mg, twice daily for 3 days
    d. 400 mg, single dose

4. i. Which of the following drugs is more efficacious than mebendazole for ascariasis?
        a. Thiabendazole
        b. Pyrantel pamoate
        c. Diethylcarbamazine
        d. Ivermectin
    ii. Describe the mechanism of anthelmintic action and therapeutic uses of the chosen drug.

5. i. A 32-year-old pregnant woman is suffering from intestinal obstruction due to severe roundworm infestations. Which of the following anthelmintic drugs is safe in pregnancy?
        a. Albendazole   b. Mebendazole
        c. Piperazine   d. Pyrantel pamoate
    ii. Describe the mechanism of action of the selected drug and its dosage.

6. i. A 16-year-old boy complains of constant itching, especially on the trunk and between fingers. Patient gives history of this complaint in his siblings also. He is diagnosed with scabies. Identify an anthelmintic drug that can be given orally to this patient.
        a. Albendazole   b. Pyrantel pamoate
        c. Ivermectin   d. Piperazine
    ii. Describe the mechanism of action, therapeutic uses and adverse effects of the selected drug.

7. A 34-year-old healthy male presents in OPD with sudden onset of chest pain. Transient changes are observed on ECG. On further questioning, he reveals taking a medicine for severe lice infestation. Which is this medicine?
    a. Ivermectin   b. Albendazole
    c. Pyrantel pamoate   d. Mebendazole

8. A 43-year-old male farmer presents to the surgery OPD with painful, chronic, progressive edema of both lower legs in the past 1 year. A night blood smear revealed microfilaria. Diagnosis of lymphatic elephantiasis is made.
    i. Write the causative organism for this condition.
    ii. Which of the following is a first-line drug for microfilariasis?
        a. Ivermectin   b. DEC
        c. Piperazine   d. Albendazole
    iii. Describe the mechanism of action of the chosen drug and its role in this case.

DRUGS AGAINST CESTODES

1. Niclosamide

Spectrum
It is highly effective against cestodes, i.e., *T. solium, T. saginata, H. nana,* and *D. latum.* It is also effective against pinworms (*E. vermicularis*).

Mechanism of action
It interferes with oxidative phosphorylation in mitochondria and anaerobic ATP generation by tapeworms. Such tapeworms get partially digested in the intestines.

ADRs
Niclosamide is a well-tolerated drug.
- It can cause mild abdominal symptoms, light-headedness and malaise.
- It is safe in pregnancy also.
- Ova released after partial digestion of *T. solium* may develop into larva and penetrate the intestinal wall causing tissue cysticercosis. This can be prevented by giving a saline purgative, 2 hours after administering niclosamide, which causes expulsion of worms in feces.

Niclosamide is not preferred now-a-days for the treatment of tapeworms.

2. Praziquantel

Spectrum
It is selectively effective against tapeworms (cestodes, their larval forms) and flukes (trematodes), but lacks activity against nematodes.

Mechanism of action
This drug is quickly taken up by susceptible worms, and causes leakage of calcium through membranes, leading to contracture and paralysis of the worm. Tapeworms, when paralysed, lose their grip on the intestine and are passed out. Flukes and schistosomes get dislodged from tissues and veins upon paralysis. Selectivity of action in cestodes and trematodes is due to the high affinity of Ca^{2+} channel of these organisms for praziquantel. In addition, this drug in high doses can cause release of the contents of the worms, followed by its immune destruction.

Therapeutic uses
- A single dose of 10 mg/kg body weight is highly effective against *T. solium* and *T. saginata*. It can kill the larvae of *T. solium* inside the cysts. Hence, there is almost no chance of systemic cysticercosis after praziquantel therapy.
- Praziquantel, given for 15–30 days, is the second-choice drug after albendazole in cases of neurocysticercosis requiring anthelmintic therapy.
- Single dose (15–25 mg/kg body weight) is as effective as niclosamide against *H. nana* and *D. latum*. A repeat dose after one week is recommended in cases of heavy infestation.
- All flukes and schistosomiasis respond to single-day therapy with praziquantel (40–75 mg/kg body weight). However, *Fasciola hepatica* is not susceptible.

ADRs
It has bitter taste, so it may cause nausea and abdominal pain.
- Headache, generalised malaise and dizziness may occur.
- When used against schistosomes, a reaction to dead flukes can cause itching, rashes, fever, urticaria, etc.
- Use in neurocysticercosis can cause neurological adverse effects due to killing of larvae such as increased ICT, meningeal irritation, and seizures.

DRUG TREATMENT OF NEUROCYSTICERCOSIS

The larvae of *T. solium* tend to migrate to other tissues and the brain through the blood stream, resulting in tissue cysticercosis. Use of anthelmintic drugs in neurocysticercosis is not appropriate in all cases, because the cysts themselves do not cause too many symptoms; however, when the larva dies, intense focal reaction occurs in the form of increased intracranial pressure, meningeal irritation, seizures, etc. Anthelmintic drugs may precipitate this reaction by killing the larvae inside the brain. So, anthelmintic drugs are used only if there are multiple, active, parenchymal or intraventricular cysts, which pose the risk of causing hydrocephalus. Small, silent calcified cysts do not need any treatment.

In these cases, albendazole is preferred over praziquantel because albendazole is cheaper, has higher rates of symptom relief, and cure with shorter duration of therapy (8–15 days only, compared to 15–30 days for praziquantel). Moreover, praziquantel metabolism can be induced by other simultaneously used drugs in these cases like phenytoin, carbamazepine, and dexamethasone. So, bioavailability decreases and therapeutic failure may occur. Albendazole/praziquantel should be given with a fatty meal to enhance their absorption.

It is important to start prior treatment with corticosteroids to suppress reactions to dead larvae. Prednisolone 40–60 mg or dexamethasone 8–12 mg per day is started two days before and continued for up to 2 weeks after the anthelmintic drug.

Anticonvulsant drugs like phenytoin and carbamazepine are given for seizure control; they are started before and continued for 1–6 months after the anthelmintic course.

Tapeworms in the gut must be treated with an anthelmintic to prevent recurrence of neurocysticercosis.

Clinical problem-based questions and MCQs

9. i. Which of the following drugs needs a laxative afterwards for the treatment of taeniasis?
    a. Albendazole
    b. Mebendazole
    c. Niclosamide
    d. Praziquantel
    ii. What is the purpose of laxative use in taeniasis?

10. i. Identify the drug of choice for cestode infestation.
    a. Albendazole
    b. Mebendazole
    c. Niclosamide
    d. Praziquantel
    ii. Describe the mechanism of action, uses and adverse effects of the selected drug.

11. An 18-year-old girl has a single episode of epilepsy at home. There is no relevant past medical history. Her doctor conducts a CT scan of head and neck, which reveals two active cortical parenchymal cysticercoids.
    i. What is the diagnosis and causative agent?
    ii. Which anthelmintic drug is the drug of choice in this case and why?
    iii. Describe the management of this patient.

DRUGS OF CHOICE IN HELMINTHIC INFESTATION

Nematodes	
Ascaris lumbricoides (roundworm)	Albendazole/mebendazole, pyrantel pamoate
Necator americanus (hookworm)	Albendazole/mebendazole, pyrantel pamoate
Ancylostoma duodenale	Pyrantel pamoate, mebendazole/albendazole
Enterobius vermicularis (pinworm)	Pyrantel pamoate, mebendazole/albendazole
Trichinella spiralis	Mebendazole/albendazole
Trichuris trichiura (whipworm)	Mebendazole/albendazole
Strongyloides stercoralis	Ivermectin, albendazole
Wuchereria bancrofti	Diethylcarbamazine citrate, ivermectin

Cestodes	
Taenia solium	Praziquantel
Taenia saginata	Praziquantel
Hymenolepis nana	Praziquantel
Diphyllobothrium latum	Praziquantel
Neurocysticercosis	Albendazole
Echinococcus granulosus	Albendazole/mebendazole

Trematodes	
Schistosoma	Praziquantel

Summary

- Helminths include nematodes, cestodes and trematodes.
- **Nematodal** infestations: **Benzimidazoles** such as **albendazole** and **mebendazole** are the drugs of choice for roundworm, hookworm, whipworm, and trichinella infestations. These drugs deplete glycogen stores in worms, prevent polymerisation of β-tubulin, and cause loss of intracellular microtubules. Albendazole has the advantage of excellent tolerability and single-dose administration.
- **Pyrantel pamoate** has high efficacy against *Ascaris*, *Ancylostoma* and *Enterobius*. It acts by causing activation of N_m receptors in worms, persistent depolarisation, and spastic paralysis. Its effect can be antagonised by **piperazine**, which causes hyperpolarisation and flaccid paralysis, and is the 2nd-choice drug in *Ascaris* and *Enterobius* infections.
- **Ivermectin** is the preferred drug for *Strongyloides*. It acts on glutamate-gated calcium channels, leading to tonic paralysis in the worms. It is given orally for scabies and head lice also. It can cause many adverse effects like nausea, abdominal pain, dizziness, lethargy, and transient ECG changes.
- Filariasis caused by *W. bancrofti* is treated with **diethylcarbamazine citrate**; it clears microfilaremia within a week and the patient becomes noninfective. However, prolonged treatment is needed for killing adult worms. Elephantiasis occurring due to chronic lymphatic involvement, involves fibrosis, and is irreversible.
- For **cestode** (tapeworms) and **trematode** (flukes) infestations, **praziquantel is preferred over niclosamide**. Niclosamide interferes with oxidative phosphorylation in mitochondria and anaerobic ATP generation by tapeworms. Such tapeworms are partially digested in the intestines. The ova released after partial digestion of *T. solium* may develop into larva and penetrate the intestinal wall causing tissue cysticercosis. This can be prevented by giving a saline purgative, 2 hours after administering niclosamide, which causes expulsion of the worms in feces.
- **Praziquantel** is effective against tapeworms and flukes as well as their larval forms. It causes leakage of calcium through membranes leading to contracture and paralysis of the worms. Tapeworms, when paralysed, lose their grip on the intestines and are passed out. Flukes and schistosomes, when paralysed, get dislodged from tissues and veins. A purgative is not required. However, for neurocysticercosis caused by *T. solium*, albendazole

is preferred over praziquantel because of its low cost, shorter duration of therapy, and lack of interaction with anticonvulsant drugs. Pretreatment with corticosteroids can prevent reaction to dead larvae.

Questions for practice

1. Classify anthelmintic drugs.
2. Write short notes on:
   a. Management of filariasis
   b. Management of neurocysticercosis
3. Explain why:
   a. Purgative use is required with niclosamide.
   b. Albendazole is preferred over praziquantel for neurocysticercosis.
4. Enumerate the therapeutic uses and adverse effects of:
   a. Albendazole
   b. DEC
   c. Praziquantel
   d. Ivermectin

Hints for problem-based questions and MCQs

1. i. b. Albendazole
   ii. 400 mg for 8–15 days
   iii. Refer to pages 782, 783.
2. b. Albendazole
3. a. 400 mg, twice daily for 4 weeks, repeated after 2 weeks, up to three courses may be required.
4. i. b. Pyrantel pamoate
   ii. Activation of nicotinic receptors → persistent depolarisation → spastic paralysis. Refer to page 783.
   A single dose therapy of 11 mg/kg body weight is useful in *Ascaris*, *Ancylostoma*, and *Enterobius* infestations. However, for *Necator americanus* and *Strongyloides*, a 3-day course is recommended.
5. i. c. Piperazine
   ii. Piperazine acts as an agonist on GABA receptors, causing opening of Cl⁻ channel resulting in hyperpolarisation and flaccid paralysis of *Ascaris* muscles. Worm is expelled alive. Dose of piperazine is 4 g, once daily, for 2 consecutive days.
6. i. c. Ivermectin
   ii. Refer to pages 784, 785.
   iii. Acts on glutamate-gated calcium channels → tonic paralysis → vermicidal action.
7. a. Ivermectin
8. i. *Wuchereria bancrofti*
   ii. b. DEC is the drug of choice
   iii. Refer to page 785.
9. i. c. Niclosamide
   ii. To prevent tissue cysticercosis. Refer to page 786.
10. i. d. Praziquantel
    ii. Causes leakage of calcium through membranes → contracture → paralysis. Refer to page 786.
11. i. Neurocysticercosis caused by *Taenia solium*.
    ii. Albendazole is the preferred drug for these cases over praziquantel because albendazole is cheaper and has higher rates of symptom relief and cure with shorter duration of therapy (8–15 days only as compared to 15–30 days of praziquantel).
    Moreover, praziquantel metabolism can be induced by other simultaneously used drugs in these cases like phenytoin, carbamazepine, and dexamethasone. So, bioavailability decreases and therapeutic failure may occur. Albendazole/praziquantel should be given along with a fatty meal to enhance their absorption.
    iii. Before starting the anthelmintic drug albendazole, corticosteroids are given to suppress reactions to dead larvae. Prednisolone 40–60 mg or dexamethasone 8–12 mg per day is started two days before and continued for up to 2 weeks after anthelmintic drug.
    - Anticonvulsant drugs like phenytoin and carbamazepine are given for seizure control, started earlier, and continued for 1–6 months after an anthelmintic course.
    - Tapeworms in gut must be treated with anthelmintics.

CONCEPT MAP – ANTHELMINTIC DRUGS

Anthelmintic Drugs

Nematodes

Benzimidazoles

Thiabendazole, Mebendazole, Albendazole

Mechanism: Deplete glycogen stores of parasite by blocking glucose uptake, inhibit β-tubulin polymerisation, inhibit hatching of nematode eggs, kills ascaris ova. Also exert anti-inflammatory, antipyretic & analgesic actions.

Uses: Effective against all species of nematodes infesting GIT i.e., roundworm, hookworm, threadworm, whipworm, *Trichinella spiralis* & *Strongyloides*. Among cestodes, tapeworm may respond to mebendazole.

ADRs: Poor patient tolerability to thiabendazole due to nausea, vomiting, loss of appetite, abdominal pain, diarrhea, headache, giddiness, impaired alertness. With mebendazole, due to slow lethal action, sometimes *Ascaris* passes out through nose/mouth. Allergic reactions, alopecia, granulocytopenia with higher dose.

Albendazole has advantage of excellent tolerability & single dose administration.

Piperazine

Mechanism: Agonist on $GABA_A$ receptors → opens Cl^- channel → hyperpolarisation and flaccid paralysis of worm → worm is expelled alive.

Uses: 2nd choice drug for *Ascaris* & *Enterobius* after albendazole / mebendazole. Safe in pregnancy.

ADRs: Well tolerated, may cause nausea, vomiting, abdominal discomfort, urticaria. Toxic doses → excitement, convulsions, respiratory failure & death.

Pyrantel pamoate

Mechanism: Activates nicotinic receptors in worms → persistent depolarisation, spastic paralysis → favours expulsion of worm.

Uses: Single dose therapy of 11 mg/kg body weight in *Ascaris, Ancylostoma, Enterobius* infestation

ADRs: Well tolerated drug causing no abnormal worm migration. GIT symptoms, headache, dizziness may occur.

Ivermectin

Mechanism: Acts through glutamate-gated calcium channel, present only in invertebrates → tonic paralysis → vermicidal action. These channels not involved in the motor control in flukes & tapeworms → lack of action in flukes and tapeworms. Potentiates GABAergic transmission in worms but not in humans.

Uses: Single yearly dose therapy in filariasis with albendazole for 5–6 years. Single dose therapy for strongyloidiasis. Effective in onchocerciasis, river blindness control program, used orally in scabies & pediculosis.

ADRs: Nausea, abdominal pain, constipation, giddiness, lethargy, pruritus, transient ECG changes. Degeneration products of Mf can cause fever with rash, pruritus, LAP, fall in BP → need antihistaminics or corticosteroids.

Diethylcarbamazine Citrate (DEC)

Mechanism: Alters microfilarial membranes → cidal action. Also causes hyperpolarisation → worms get dislodged & readily phagocytosed by tissue fixed monocytes.

Uses: Drug of first choice in filariasis, 2 mg/kg given TDS

For mass treatment & reducing filaria transmission → DEC 6 mg/kg + albendazole 400 mg single dose.

Controls signs/symptoms of eosinophilic lung or tropical eosinophilia.

ADRs: Anorexia, nausea, headache, dizziness, weakness

Mass destruction of mf → Fever with rash, pruritus, LAP & fall in BP

Cestodes, Trematodes

Niclosamide

Spectrum: Effective against *T. solium/saginata, H. nana, D. latum, E. vermicularis*

Mechanism: interferes with oxidative phosphorylation in mitochondria & anaerobic ATP generation by tapeworms → partial digestion of worms.

ADRs: Well tolerated drug, causes mild abdominal symptoms, lightheadedness & malaise. It is safe in pregnancy also.

Ova released after partial digestion of *T.solium* may develop into larva & penetrate intestinal wall causing tissue cysticercosis → saline purgative should be given 2 hours after niclosamide to expel worms in feces. Not preferred nowadays for taeniasis.

Praziquantel

Mechanism: Quickly taken up by susceptible worms → causes leakage of calcium through membranes → contracture and paralysis of worm. → worms lose their grip on intestine and are passed out.

Flukes and schistosomes get dislodged in tissues & veins after paralysis.

Selective action in cestodes & trematodes due to high affinity of Ca^{2+} channel of these organisms. High doses release contents of worm → its immune destruction.

Uses: Single dose 10 mg/kg is highly effective against *T. solium, T. saginata*. No chance of systemic cysticercosis after praziquantel therapy.

2nd choice drug after albendazole in neurocysticercosis

Also effective against *H. nana* and *D. latum*

All flukes and schistosomiasis respond except *Fasciola hepatica*

ADRs: Bitter taste → nausea, abdominal pain Headache, generalised malaise and dizziness may occur. A reaction to dead flukes can cause itching, rashes, fever, urticaria, etc.

Use in neurocysticercosis can cause neurological adverse effects due to killing of larvae, like increased ICT, meningeal irritation & seizures.

SECTION 10 Chemotherapeutic Drugs

61 Anticancer Drugs

PH 8.11 Describe the types, kinetics, dynamics, adverse effects, indications and contraindications of anticancer drugs. Devise plans for the amelioration of anticancer drug-induced toxicity.

Learning objectives

A student of MBBS phase II should be able to:
- Classify anticancer drugs.
- Explain the principles of cancer chemotherapy.
- Discuss the mechanism of action of commonly used anticancer drugs.
- Describe the indications, adverse effects and contraindications of commonly used anticancer drugs.
- Explain the toxicity amelioration of anticancer drugs with suitable examples

---

CANCER

Cancer is a disease in which **cells lose the mechanisms for control of cell proliferation and differentiation**, resulting in excessive proliferation and lack of differentiation. Consequently, a large number of undifferentiated cells accumulate and form a tumour. These tumours not only compress or invade adjacent normal tissues, but can also spread to distant tissues through the lymph or blood. This spread of tumour/malignant cells to distant sites through the lymph or blood is called metastasis. It occurs at a late stage in cancerous diseases, and usually indicates a poor prognosis.

Treatment Modalities for Malignant Tumours

- **Surgical excision** of a localised tumour is effective when tumour cells have not yet metastasised to distant tissues. Thus, surgery is possible at an early stage in the course of the disease. In many malignant tumours, patients have normal life span and quality of life after surgical treatment.
- **Radiotherapy** is also effective for localised tumours, before their micro or gross metastasis.
- **Chemotherapy** is usually required as an adjuvant to the above-mentioned measures, if tumour cells have already metastasised to distant sites. It involves the administration of anticancer drugs, usually in combination regimens. The aim of chemotherapy is cure, prolonged remission, or palliation, depending upon the type of cancer and stage of disease. Drugs can cause shrinkage of tumours and may alleviate the symptoms.

Anticancer Drugs

Anticancer drugs can be broadly classified as:
- Cytotoxic drugs
- Drugs acting on specific targets—Targeted drugs
- Hormones and related drugs

Cytotoxic drugs include many chemically diverse drugs such as alkylating agents, antimetabolites, antibiotics, topoisomerase I/II inhibitors, platinum coordination complexes, vinca alkaloids and taxanes (Flowchart 61.1). These drugs achieve cell kill by varied mechanisms.

GENERAL PRINCIPLES OF CANCER CHEMOTHERAPY

1. Malignant cells are host cells that exhibit derangement in regulation of growth and differentiation. As a result, drugs that affect malignant cells are toxic to normal host cells also. In other words, anticancer drugs are highly toxic. Efforts are underway to identify tumour antigens and oncogenes and develop drugs that target these specifically, e.g., Philadelphia chromosome, epidermal growth factor, and proteasomes. This would reduce toxic effects on the normal host cells,
2. Interferon α, interleukin-2, and tumour necrosis factor α (TNF-α) can modify the biological response to tumours and are useful as adjuvants in cancer treatment.
3. If a single malignant cell survives chemotherapy or radiation therapy, it can produce daughter cells that lead to recurrence and increased mortality. Thus, in order to achieve cure, the aim of therapy should be '**total cell kill**'.

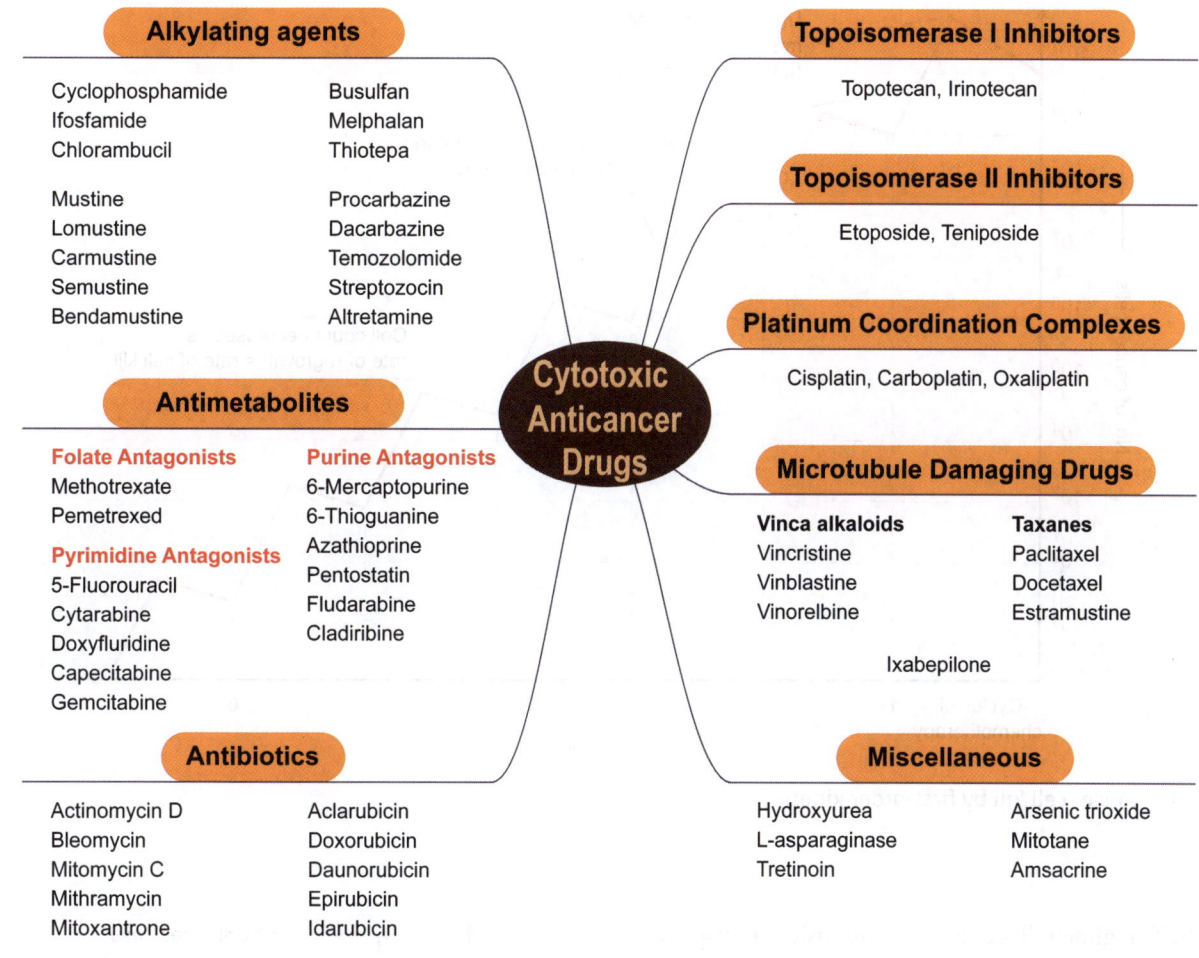

Flowchart 61.1 Classification of cytotoxic anticancer drugs

4. Cytotoxic drugs can be cell-cycle nonspecific (CCNS) or cell-cycle specific (CCS).
   - **CCNS** drugs can kill resting as well as dividing cells, e.g., actinomycin D, busulfan, cyclophosphamide, chlorambucil, carmustine, cisplatin, and dacarbazine. CCNS drugs have greater efficacy in solid tumours with low growth rates.
   - In contrast, **CCS** drugs kill only actively dividing cells. CCS drugs are more effective in cases of hematological malignancy and solid tumours with high growth rates. They also show considerable phase selectivity.
   - The G_0 phase is a non-proliferative phase; cells may remain quiescent for variable periods, but can enter the cell cycle.
   - The G_1 **phase** is the presynthetic interval—vincristine acts in this phase.
   - Synthesis of DNA occurs in the **S phase**. Drugs such as methotrexate, 6-mercaptopurine, 6-thioguanine, 5-fluorouracil, cytarabine, doxorubicin and daunorubicin are S-phase specific.
   - The G_2 **phase** is the postsynthetic interval—bleomycin, and topoisomerase I and II inhibitors act in this phase.
   - Mitosis occurs in the **M phase**, yielding two daughter cells that are in the G_1 phase. These can directly re-enter the next cycle or pass into the nonproliferative G_0 phase. Vinca alkaloids and paclitaxel act in the M phase.
5. CCS drugs are used in short pulses. They are given after a course of CCNS drugs to increase the cell kill.
6. With the goal of total cell kill, **intensive combination regimens** with the **maximum tolerated dose** of drugs are given **at an early stage** to achieve complete remission. Repeated use of any drug can cause resistance because of selection of less responsive cells; such selection is favoured by low doses of a single drug. Therefore, usually, a combination of 2–5 drugs is given in intermittent pulses called 'cycles of chemotherapy' to achieve total cell kill. A time gap is given between chemotherapy cycles for the normal cells to recover.

Examples of combination regimens:
- **VAMP** regimen [vincristine + amethopterin (methotrexate) + 6-mercaptopurine + prednisolone] is used for acute leukemia.
- **MOPP** regimen [mustine + oncovin (vincristine) + procarbazine + prednisolone] used in Hodgkin and non-Hodgkin lymphoma.

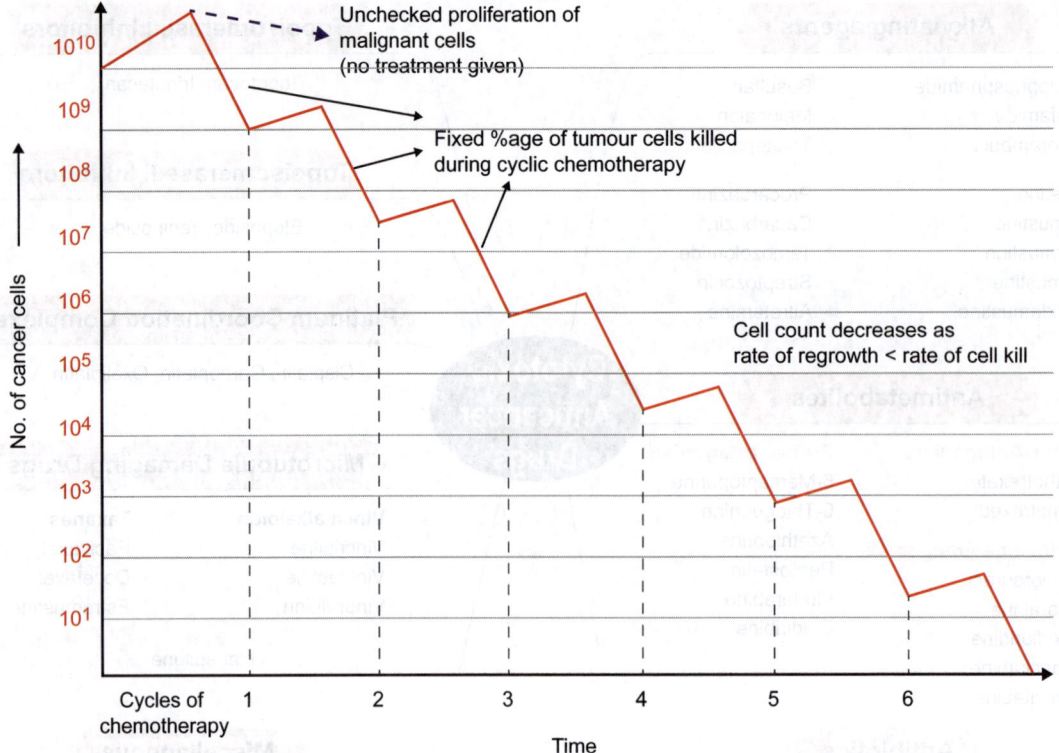

Fig. 61.1 Cancer cell kill by first-order kinetics

- **BEP** regimen (bleomycin + etoposide + cisplatin) used in testis carcinoma.
- **FOLFOX** (5-FU + leucovorin + oxaliplatin) used in colon carcinoma.
- **FOLFIRI** (5-FU + leucovorin + irinotecan) used in colorectal carcinoma.

7. Drugs used in combination must possess anticancer efficacy when used alone, should have different mechanisms of anticancer action, different mechanisms of development of resistance, and different toxic reactions. Moreover, the combination of drugs should have synergistic interaction on cell-cycle specificity/nonspecificity.

8. Subpopulations of the cancer cells have variable susceptibility to drugs. **Drugs kill malignant cells** by **first-order kinetics**, which means that a fixed fraction of cells is killed by the drug. This forms the basis of **cyclic therapy** with anticancer drugs. Usually, 6–11 cycles of treatment are required for optimum response (Fig. 61.1).

9. Combination cyclic treatment, which is palliative for large tumours, may be curative for residual tumours after surgical resection. This justifies the **combined modality approach** for the management of malignant diseases (Fig. 61.2).

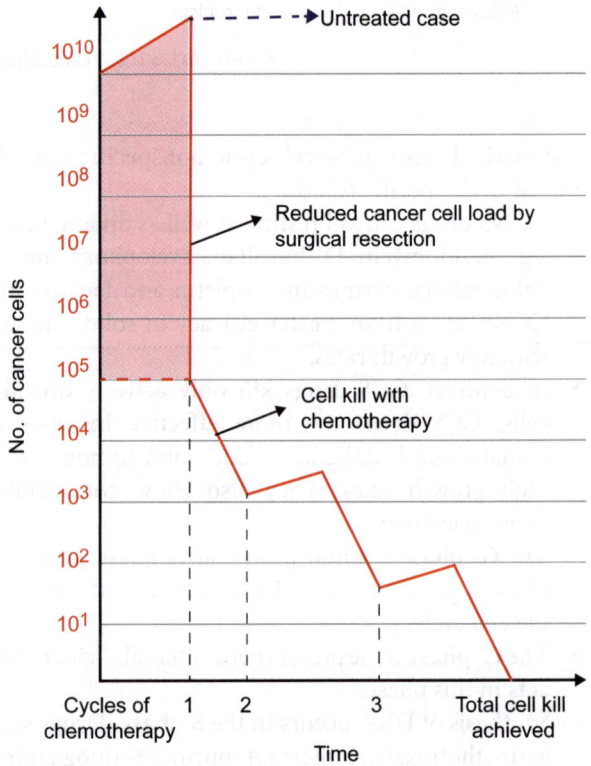

Fig. 61.2 The combined modality approach

Clinical problem-based questions and MCQs

1. The aim of cancer chemotherapy is total cell kill. Justify.
2. Match the drug with the cell-cycle phase that it acts in.

   a. G_1 phase   1. Topotecan
   b. S phase   2. Vincristine
   c. G_2 phase   3. Paclitaxel
   d. M phase   4. 6-Mercaptopurine
3. A 72-year-old female patient diagnosed with Hodgkin lymphoma is put on the MOPP regimen.
   i. Justify use of combination of drugs in this patient.
   ii. Describe the general principles of combining anticancer drugs.

CYTOTOXIC DRUGS

A. Alkylating Agents

Most alkylating agents are cell-cycle nonspecific (CCNS), i.e., they act on dividing as well as resting cells.

Mechanism of action: These agents undergo intermolecular cyclisation, forming highly reactive carbonium ion intermediates that are positively charged; hence, they have affinity for the negatively charged (carboxyl, hydroxyl, thiol, amino, phosphate) groups of DNA, especially guanine residues at position 7 of DNA (Fig. 61.3). This leads to cross-linking with proteins, abnormal base-pairing and scission of DNA strands. Such abnormal DNA is cleaved by nucleases, resulting in cell death. Thus, they exert cytotoxic as well as radiomimetic actions.

Cyclophosphamide

Cyclophosphamide is the most popular agent for many solid tumours such as bronchogenic carcinoma, CA breast, CA bladder, and testicular sarcoma. One of its active metabolites, acrolein, causes hemorrhagic cystitis. Acrolein can be detoxified by SH-containing compounds such as mesna/acetylcystiene. Excess fluid intake and frequent voiding is also helpful. Other ADRs include alopecia, nausea, and vomiting.

Ifosfamide

Ifosfamide is longer acting and causes fewer adverse effects than cyclophosphamide.

Chlorambucil

Chlorambucil is active against lymphoid tissue, but spares myeloid tissue. It is the drug of choice for maintenance therapy in chronic lymphoid leukemia (CLL), and is

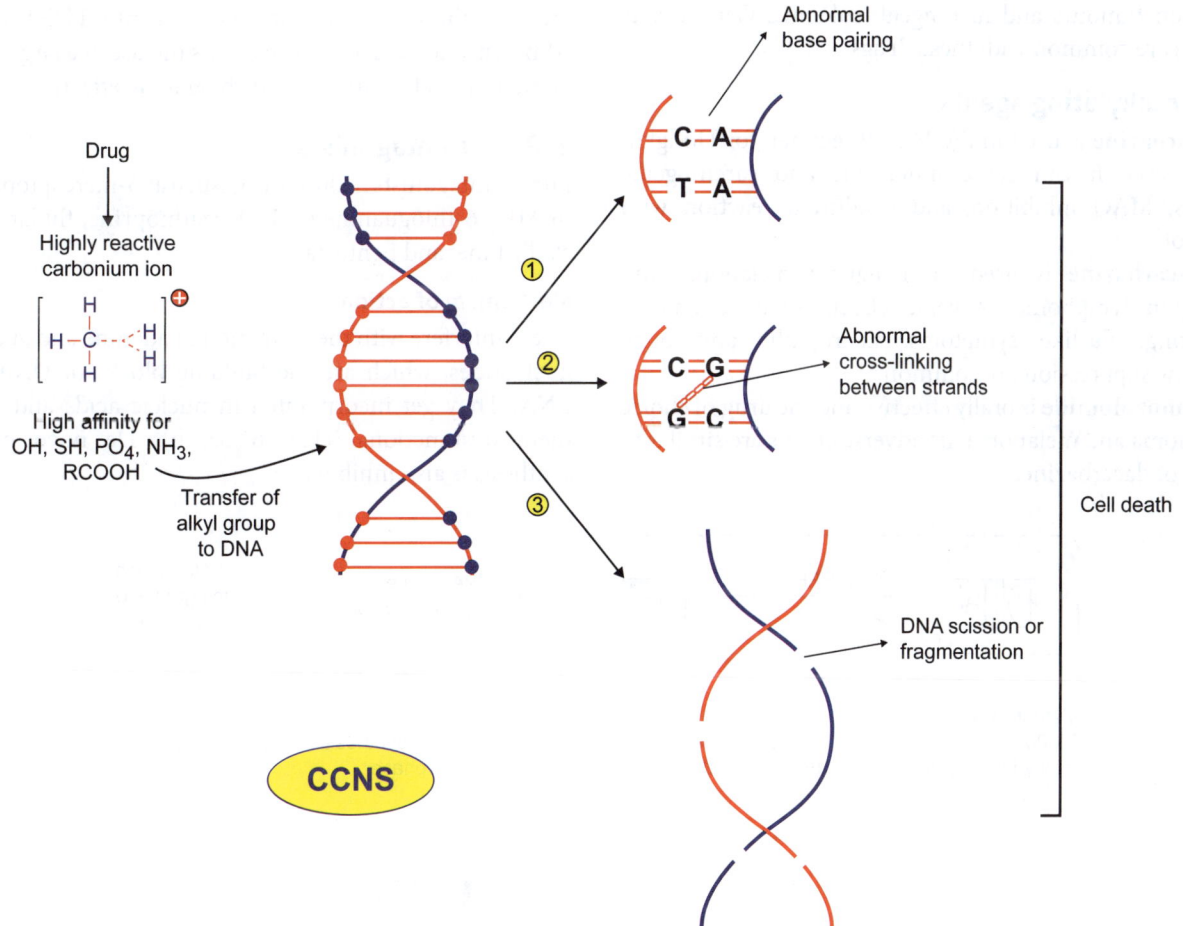

Fig. 61.3 Mechanism of action of alkylating agents

also useful in non-Hodgkin lymphoma. It causes nausea, vomiting and mucositis as adverse effects. In women, menstrual irregularities may be caused.

Busulfan

Busulfan is specifically active against myeloid tissue and is the drug of choice for chronic myeloid leukemia (CML). Important adverse effects include pulmonary fibrosis, hyperuricemia and skin pigmentation.

Melphalan

Mephalan is useful in multiple myeloma. It causes nausea, vomiting, increased risk of infections and pancreatitis as adverse effects.

Mustine

Mustine is indicated as part of the MOPP regimen in Hodgkin and non-Hodgkin lymphomas. The MOPP regimen includes mustine, oncovin (vincristine), procarbazine and prednisolone.

Mustine is highly reactive and has many adverse effects such as nausea, vomiting, hemodynamic changes and sloughing on extravasation.

Carmustine and lomustine

Carmustine and **lomustine** are highly lipid-soluble drugs and can cross the blood–brain barrier; so, these are used in brain tumours and meningeal leukemia. Central side effects are common with these drugs.

Other alkylating agents

Procarbazine is used in the MOPP regimen for Hodgkin lymphoma. It can cause mutagenic and carcinogenic effects, MAO inhibition, and disulfiram reaction with alcohol.

Dacarbazine is used in malignant melanoma and Hodgkin lymphoma. Adverse effects such as nausea, vomiting, flu-like symptoms, neuropathy and bone marrow suppression are common.

Temozolomide is orally effective and the drug of choice for glioma and melanoma. Its adverse effects are similar to those of dacarbazine.

B. Antimetabolites

1. Folate antagonists: Methotrexate

Mechanism of action

Methotrexate enters the cell and forms polyglutamate, which inhibits the enzyme dihydrofolate reductase (DHFRase) and blocks the conversion of dihydrofolate into tetrahydrofolate. Therefore, folates cannot be used for DNA synthesis, resulting in cell death (Fig. 61.4). Methotrexate is cell-cycle specific (CCS), and affects cells in the synthetic **S phase**. Methotrexate has a much higher (50,000 times higher) affinity for DHFRase than DHFA (its normal substrate); so, it causes pseudo-irreversible inhibition.

Therapeutic uses

- Methotrexate is curative in choriocarcinoma and NHL
- Used as a disease-modifying anti-rheumatic drug (DMARD) in rheumatoid arthritis.

ADRs

Myelosuppression: This leads to pancytopenia and megaloblastic anemia. N5-formyl-THFA (folinic acid/leucovorin/citrovorum factor) is useful to curb methotrexate toxicity, because folinic acid can be used for DNA synthesis. Folic acid cannot be used in place of folinic acid because the inhibition of DHFRase by methotrexate prevents the conversion of folic acid into THFA. Thus, administration of leucovorin allows the use of a larger dose of methotrexate, without disturbing toxic effects.

2. Purine antagonists

Purine antagonists include drugs such as 6-mercaptopurine (6-MP), 6-thioguanine (6-TG), azathioprine, fludarabine, cladiribine, and pentostatin.

Mechanism of action

These interfere with the formation of adenine and guanine nucleotides, which are the building blocks of DNA and RNA. They get incorporated in nucleic acids and make them dysfunctional (Fig. 61.5a, b). De novo purine synthesis is also inhibited.

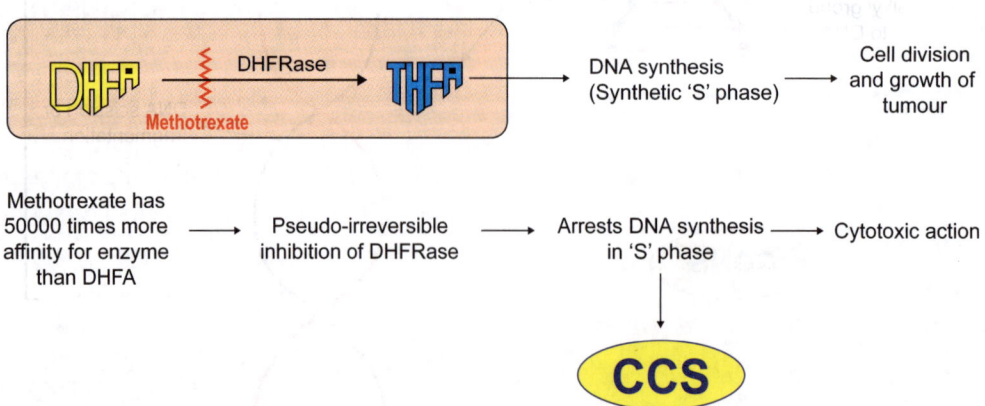

Fig. 61.4 Mechanism of action of methotrexate

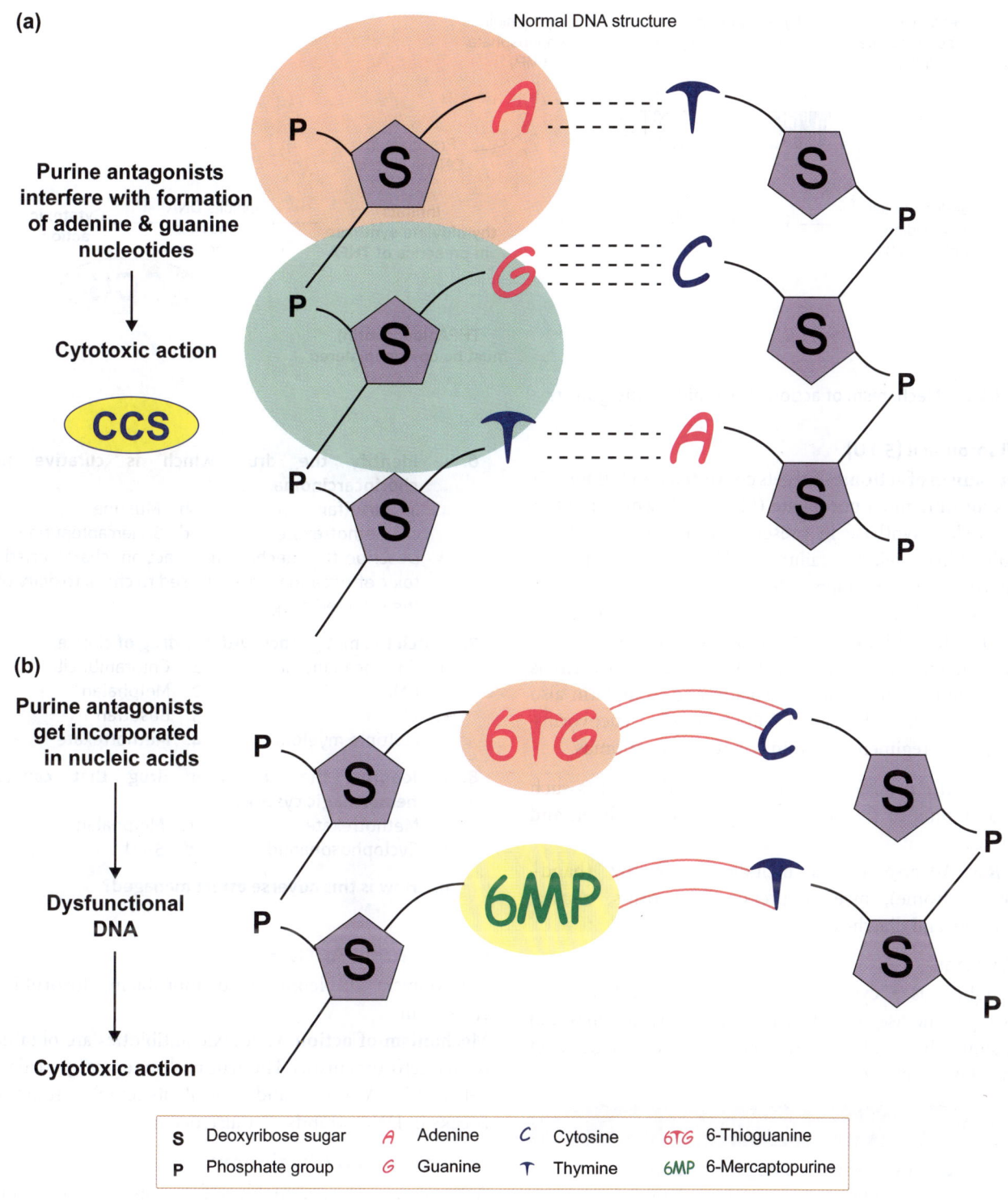

Fig. 61.5a, b Mechanism of action of purine antagonists

Therapeutic uses
Purine antagonists are useful in childhood leukemia, choriocarcinoma and solid tumours. The immunosuppressent effect of azathioprine is more prominent than its anticancer effect.

ADRs
Hyperuricemia is an important adverse effect of these drugs. Allopurinol (a xanthine oxidase inhibitor) is combined to inhibit uric acid synthesis. However, the dose of 6-MP and azathioprine should be reduced when co-administered with allopurinol, because these drugs are also metabolised by xanthine oxidase enzyme.

3. Pyrimidine antagonists
Pyrimidine antagonists include 5-fluorouracil (5-FU), cytarabine, and capecitabine.

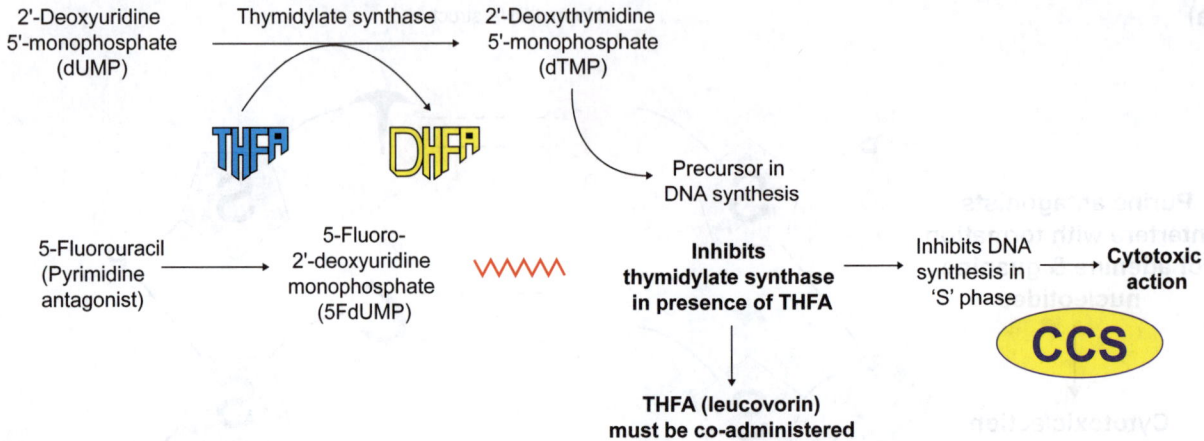

Fig. 61.6 Mechanism of action of pyrimidine antagonists

5-Fluorouracil (5-FU)

Mechanism of action: 5-FU gets converted into 5-fluoro-2-deoxyuridine monophosphate (5FdUMP), which inhibits thymidylate synthase in presence of THFA (Fig. 61.6), resulting in the selective failure of DNA synthesis. 5-fluoro-2-deoxyuridine monophosphate gets incorporated into the RNA and interferes with its synthesis and function. Because the inhibition of thymidylate synthase by 5-FU is dependent on the presence of THFA, leucovorin is administered concurrently. Cisplatin and oxaliplatin also synergise with 5-FU. The FOLFOX (5-FU + leucovorin + oxaliplatin) regimen is used in colorectal carcinomas.

Therapeutic uses: 5-FU is useful in solid tumours such as carcinoma of the colon, rectum, stomach, liver, and pancreas.

ADRs: Adverse effects include neuropathy (hand–foot syndrome), myelosuppression, mucositis, nausea, vomiting, and diarrhea.

Cytarabine

Cytarabine is a cytidine analogue that interferes with DNA polymerase activity. It is useful in lymphomas and leukemias, but not in solid tumours. The major toxic effect is myelosuppression.

Clinical problem-based questions and MCQs

4. i. Identify the purine antagonistic drug.
   a. Azathioprine b. Cytarabine
   c. Doxorubicin d. Methotrexate
   ii. Describe the mechanism of action, uses and adverse effects of the selected drug.
   iii. How does the selected drug interact with allopurinol?

5. A 75-year-old male patient diagnosed with carcinoma of the sigmoid colon with secondaries in the liver was put on the FOLFOX regimen.
   i. Enumerate the drugs included in the FOLFOX regimen.
   ii. Give the pharmacological basis for using this combination.

6. i. Identify the drug which is curative in choriocarcinoma.
   a. Busulfan b. Mustine
   c. Methotrexate d. 6-Mercaptopurine
   ii. Describe the mechanism of action, characteristic toxic effect and measures used to check toxicity of the selected drug.

7. Match the malignancy with the drug of choice.
   a. Choriocarcinoma 1. Chlorambucil
   b. CML 2. Melphalan
   c. CLL 3. Busulfan
   d. Multiple myeloma 4. Methotrexate

8. i. Identify the anticancer drug that causes hemorrhagic cystitis.
   a. Methotrexate c. Melphalan
   b. Cyclophosphamide d. 5-FU
   ii. How is this adverse effect managed?

C. Cytotoxic Antibiotics

Actinomycin D, bleomycin, daunorubicin, doxorubicin, epirubicin

Mechanism of action: Cytotoxic antibiotics are obtained from micro-organisms. The drug molecule gets intercalated between DNA strands and prevents its template function. Breaks in DNA strands may also occur.

Actinomycin D (dactinomycin)

Actinomycin D is a highly efficacious drug in Wilms tumour, rhabdomyosarcoma, Ewing sarcoma and methotrexate-resistant choriocarcinoma. It can cause adverse effects like vomiting, diarrhea, dermatitis, stomatitis, alopecia and bone marrow suppression.

Bleomycin

Bleomycin is a mixture of glycopeptide antibiotics with potent antineoplastic activity. It is highly effective in testicular tumours and squamous cell carcinoma of the skin/oral cavity/esophagus and genito-urinary tract. When administered by intrapleural or intraperitoneal injection, bleomycin can reduce the rate of collection of malignant pleural/peritoneal effusion. The most important adverse effect associated with the use of bleomycin is pulmonary fibrosis.

Daunorubicin/Doxorubicin/Epirubicin

These are all anthracycline derivatives. Daunorubicin is used only in acute myeloid and lymphoid leukemia (AML and ALL), whereas doxorubicin is effective in many solid tumours also, e.g., carcinoma of the breast, bladder, lung, ovary, and thyroid. Epirubicin has the same uses as doxorubicin. These drugs can potentially cause ECG changes, arrhythmias, hypotension, congestive heart failure and cardiomyopathy that may be fatal. They also cause red discolouration of urine. Dexrazoxane, an iron chelator, can prevent the cardiotoxic effects of these drugs, but may itself cause hepatic and renal dysfunction

D. Topoisomerase I Inhibitors
Topotecan, irinotecan

Mechanism of action
These drugs interact with the enzyme topoisomerase I. They allow single strand breaks in DNA, but interfere with resealing after untwisting (Fig. 61.7). Thus, they damage DNA in the S-phase of the cell-cycle and cell death occurs in the G_2 phase.

Therapeutic uses
Topotecan is useful in carcinoma of the ovary and cervix and small cell carcinoma of lung.

Irinotecan is a prodrug that gets activated in the liver. In addition to the same therapeutic indications as topotecan, irinotecan is useful in metastatic colorectal carcinoma also.

ADRs
The major toxicity of these drugs is bone marrow suppression. Irinotecan causes inhibition of cholinesterase enzyme, resulting in symptoms of muscarinic excess that can be prevented by prior atropinisation.

E. Topoisomerase II Inhibitors
Etoposide, teniposide

Etoposide is a semisynthetic derivative of the plant glycoside 'podophyllin' that inhibits topoisomerase. It does not interfere with the cleaving of double-stranded DNA, but prevents subsequent resealing.

Therapeutic uses
It is used in lung and testis carcinoma.

ADRs
The major adverse effects associated with the use of etoposide include alopecia, neutropenia and gastro-intestinal disturbances.

F. Platinum Coordination Complexes
Cisplatin, carboplatin, oxaliplatin

Mechanism of action: These drugs undergo intracellular hydrolysis, and are converted into highly active compounds that cause cross-linking of DNA and interfere with DNA synthesis. Additional radiomimetic activity is also present.

1. Cisplatin

Therapeutic uses
Cisplatin is highly efficacious in metastatic testicular and ovarian carcinoma.

ADRs
- Cisplatin is one of the **most emetic** anticancer drugs. Nausea and vomiting associated with the use of cisplatin can be prevented by the $5\text{-}HT_3$ antagonist, ondansetron.
- It also has nephrotoxic potential that can be reduced by proper hydration and diuresis.
- Deafness and tinnitus due to ototoxic effect and neuropathy has also been reported.
- Sometimes, intravenous infusion can cause shock-like state.

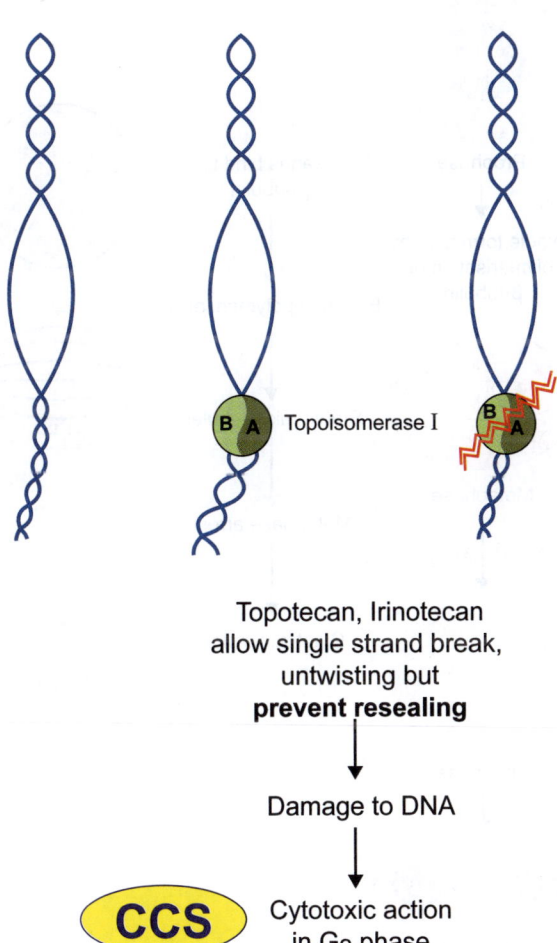

Fig. 61.7 Mechanism of action of topoisomerase I inhibitors

2. Carboplatin

It is a second-generation platinum coordination compound with the same mechanism of action and indications for use as cisplatin. It is preferred over cisplatin in combination chemotherapy because of its **lower potential to induce emesis and renal dysfunction**.

3. Oxaliplatin

Oxaliplatin is a third-generation drug that does not show cross resistance with cisplatin or carboplatin. Therefore, it is effective in **cisplatin/carboplatin-resistant tumours**. It is used along with 5-fluorouracil and leucovorin in metastatic colorectal carcinoma. It can potentially cause peripheral sensory neuropathy that is exaggerated on exposure to cold.

G. Microtubule-Damaging Drugs

Vinca alkaloids, taxanes

1. Vinca alkaloids

Vincristine, vinblastine, vinorelbine

Mechanism of action: These are cell-cycle specific drugs (CCS) acting in the M phase. Vinca alkaloids inhibit mitosis by binding to microtubule protein β-tubulin and preventing the polymerisation and assembly of microtubules (Fig. 61.8). As a result, chromosomes fail to move apart and metaphase arrest occurs.

Vincristine or oncovin is a rapid-acting drug used for inducing remissions in childhood acute lymphocytic leukemia (ALL) and acute myeloid leukemia (AML). However, it is not good for maintenance therapy. It is part of the MOPP regimen used in the treatment of Hodgkin lymphoma and may cause adverse effects such as alopecia, peripheral neuropathy and syndrome of inappropriate ADH secretion (SIADH).

Vinblastine has same mechanism of action as other vinca alkaloids, but is effective in non-Hodgkin lymphoma, neuroblastoma and Kaposi sarcoma. It causes bone marrow suppression as a side effect. The risk of neuropathy and SIADH is lower than for vincristine.

Vinorelbine is useful in non-small cell carcinoma of lung.

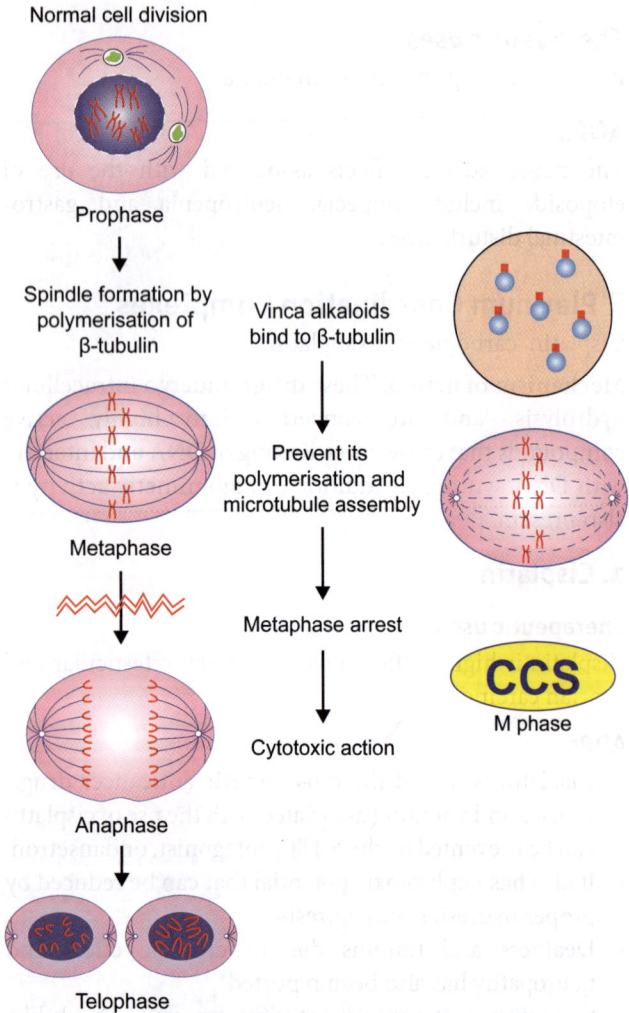

Fig. 61.8 Mechanism of action of vinca alkaloids

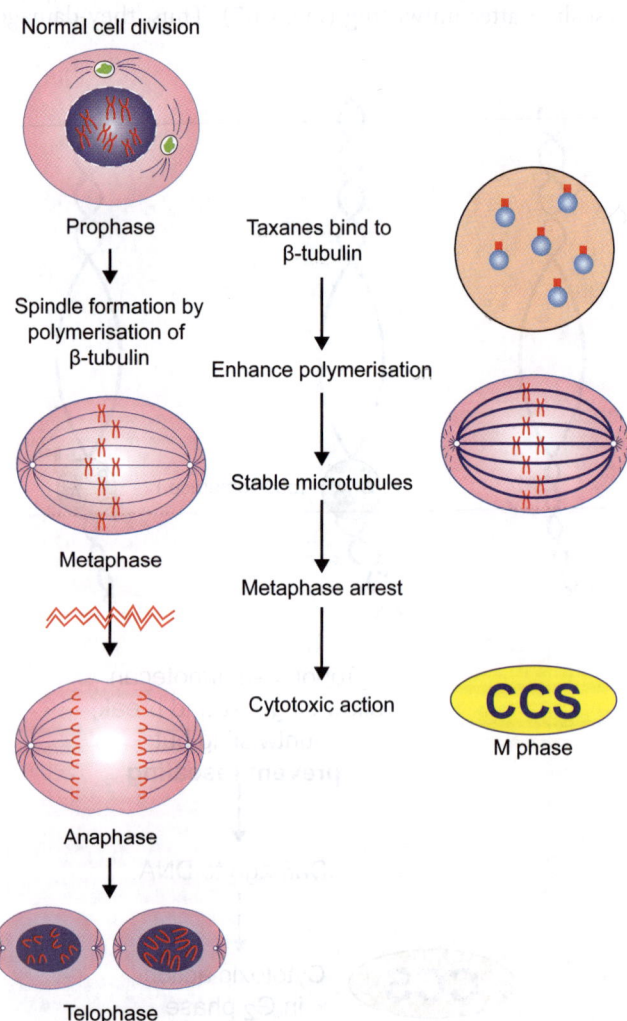

Fig. 61.9 Mechanism of action of taxanes

2. Taxanes

Paclitaxel, docetaxel, estramustine

Their **mechanism of action** is opposite to that of vinca alkaloids, i.e., they bind to β-tubulin and enhance polymerisation, making the microtubules more stable. This hinders the normal dynamic reorganisation of the microtubule network, leading to metaphase arrest (Fig. 61.9).

Paclitaxel is used in carcinoma of the breast and ovary after the failure of first-line drugs or in relapse cases. Its adverse effects include stocking–glove neuropathy and myelosuppression.

Estramustine is a complex of estradiol and normustine. It possesses weak estrogenic activity, no alkylating action, and has same mechanism of action as taxanes. Estramustine gets concentrated in the prostate and is used in metastatic prostate carcinoma, not responding to hormonal treatment. Upon hydrolysis, it releases estradiol and normustine that are responsible for estrogenic side effects (gynecomastia, impotence, fluid retention) and myelosuppression, respectively.

H. Miscellaneous Cytotoxic Drugs

Hydroxyurea, L-asparaginase, tretinoin, arsenic trioxide, mitotane, amsacrine

1. Hydroxyurea

Hydroxyurea is a CCS drug that is effective in the S phase. It acts by inhibiting the enzyme ribonucleoside diphosphate reductase, blocking the conversion of ribonucleotides to deoxyribonucleotides, and thereby blocking DNA synthesis (Fig. 61.10).

Therapeutic uses

It is used in chronic myeloid leukemia (CML), polycythemia vera, psoriasis, sickle cell disease, and as a radiosensitiser, before radiotherapy.

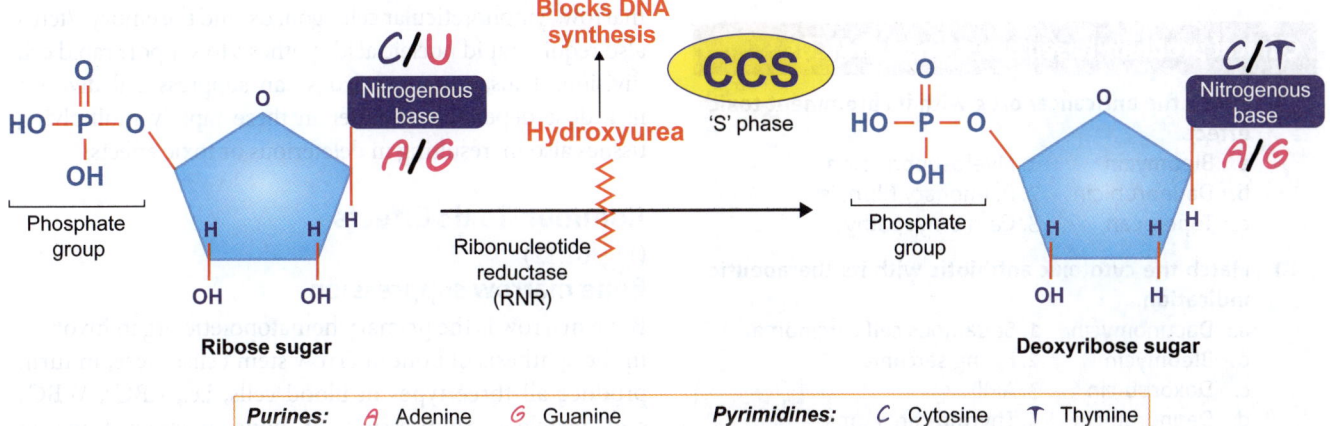

Fig. 61.10 Mechanism of action of hydroxyurea

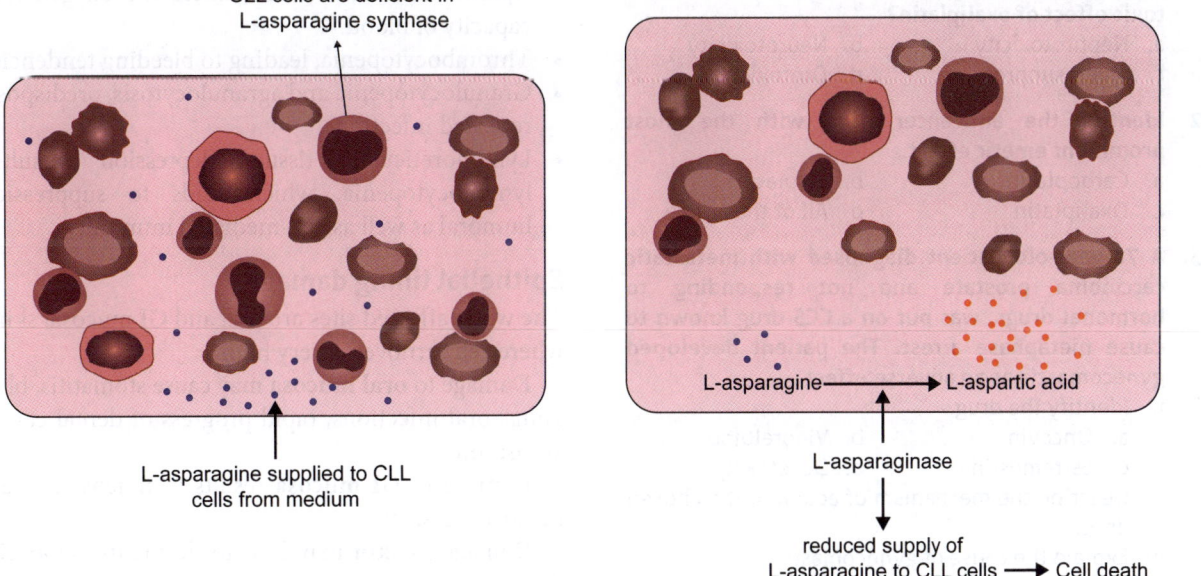

Fig. 61.11 Mechanism of action of L-asparaginase

ADRs

It causes myelosuppression, skin pigmentation and other cutaneous reactions.

2. L-asparaginase

Cells of childhood lymphoid leukemia are deficient in the enzyme asparagine synthetase. So, they depend on the medium for the supply of L-asparagine. The enzyme L-asparaginase converts L-asparagine into L-aspartic acid, depriving the tumour cells of an essential metabolite (Fig. 61.11).

L-asparaginase is useful in acute lymphoblastic leukemia in combination with methotrexate, prednisolone and vincristine. However, resistance develops to its actions.

ADRs

While L-asparaginase lacks typical cytotoxic adverse effects, it can cause hyperglycemia, hypertriglyceridemia, clotting defects and severe allergic reactions.

> **Clinical problem-based questions and MCQs**
>
> 9. Match the anticancer drug with its prominent toxic effect.
>   a. Bleomycin   1. Myelosuppression
>   b. Daunorubicin   2. Pulmonary fibrosis
>   c. Topotecan   3. Cardiomyopathy
>
> 10. Match the cytotoxic antibiotic with its therapeutic indication.
>   a. Dactinomycin   1. Squamous cell carcinoma
>   b. Bleomycin   2. Ewing sarcoma
>   c. Doxorubicin   3. AML
>   d. Daunorubicin   4. Thyroid carcinoma
>
> 11. A 76-year-old male diagnosed with colon carcinoma was prescribed oxaliplatin along with leucovorin and 5-FU. Which of the following is a prominent toxic effect of oxaliplatin?
>   a. Nephrotoxicity   b. Neurotoxicity
>   c. Myelosuppression   d. Ototoxicity
>
> 12. Identify the anticancer drug with the most prominent emetic effect.
>   a. Carboplatin   b. Cisplatin
>   c. Oxaliplatin   d. All of the above
>
> 13. A 78-year-old patient diagnosed with metastatic carcinoma prostate and not responding to hormonal drugs, was put on a CCS drug known to cause metaphase arrest. The patient developed gynecomastia as an adverse effect.
>   i. Identify the drug.
>   a. Oncovin   b. Vinorelbine
>   c. Estramustine   d. Docetaxel
>   ii. Describe the mechanism of action of the chosen drug.
>   iii. Explain the cause of gynecomastia.
>
> 14. A 9-year-old boy diagnosed with acute lymphoblastic leukemia was put on L-asparaginase therapy.
>   i. Describe mechanism of useful action of L-asparaginase in ALL.
>   ii. Enumerate the adverse effects of L-asparaginase.

TOXICITY OF CYTOTOXIC DRUGS AND ITS AMELIORATION

Cancer cells are human cells that have an unregulated rate of cell division and lack of differentiation. A high rate of cell division requires fast synthesis of nucleic acid and its precursors. The beneficial anticancer effect of cytotoxic (*cyto*: cells; *toxic*: having harmful effects) drugs is based on their ability to check this cell division by different mechanisms. Nucleic acids and their precursors are the most important target site for cytotoxic drugs.

Normal rapidly dividing cells in the human body such as epithelial linings (skin, oral mucosa, and GI mucosa), bone marrow, lymphoreticular cells, gonads, and the embryo/fetus also require rapid nucleic acid synthesis to support rapid cell division. Thus, cytotoxic drugs can suppress cell division in a dose-dependent manner in these rapidly multiplying tissues also in, resulting in deleterious or toxic effects.

Common Toxic Effects
(Fig. 61.12)

Bone marrow suppression

Bone marrow is the primary hematopoietic organ involved in the synthesis of bone-marrow stem cells; these, in turn, produce all three types of blood cells, i.e., RBCs, WBCs and platelets. Suppression of bone marrow function by cytotoxic drugs can decrease the blood cell counts, resulting in:

- Aplastic anemia, which reduces the oxygen-carrying capacity of blood.
- Thrombocytopenia, leading to bleeding tendencies.
- Granulocytopenia and agranulocytosis, predisposing to repeated infections.
- Lymphoreticular tissue depression results in lymphocytopenia, which leads to suppression of humoral as well as cell-mediated immunity.

Epithelial lining damage

The worst affected sites are oral and GI mucosa, skin, etc., where cell turnover is very high.

Damage to **oral mucosa** may cause stomatitis, bleeding gums, oral infections, rapid progress of dental caries and xerostomia.

Damage to **GI mucosa** results in mucositis, diarrhea, hemorrhages, etc.

Damage to **skin** may lead to dermatitis, alopecia and delayed wound healing.

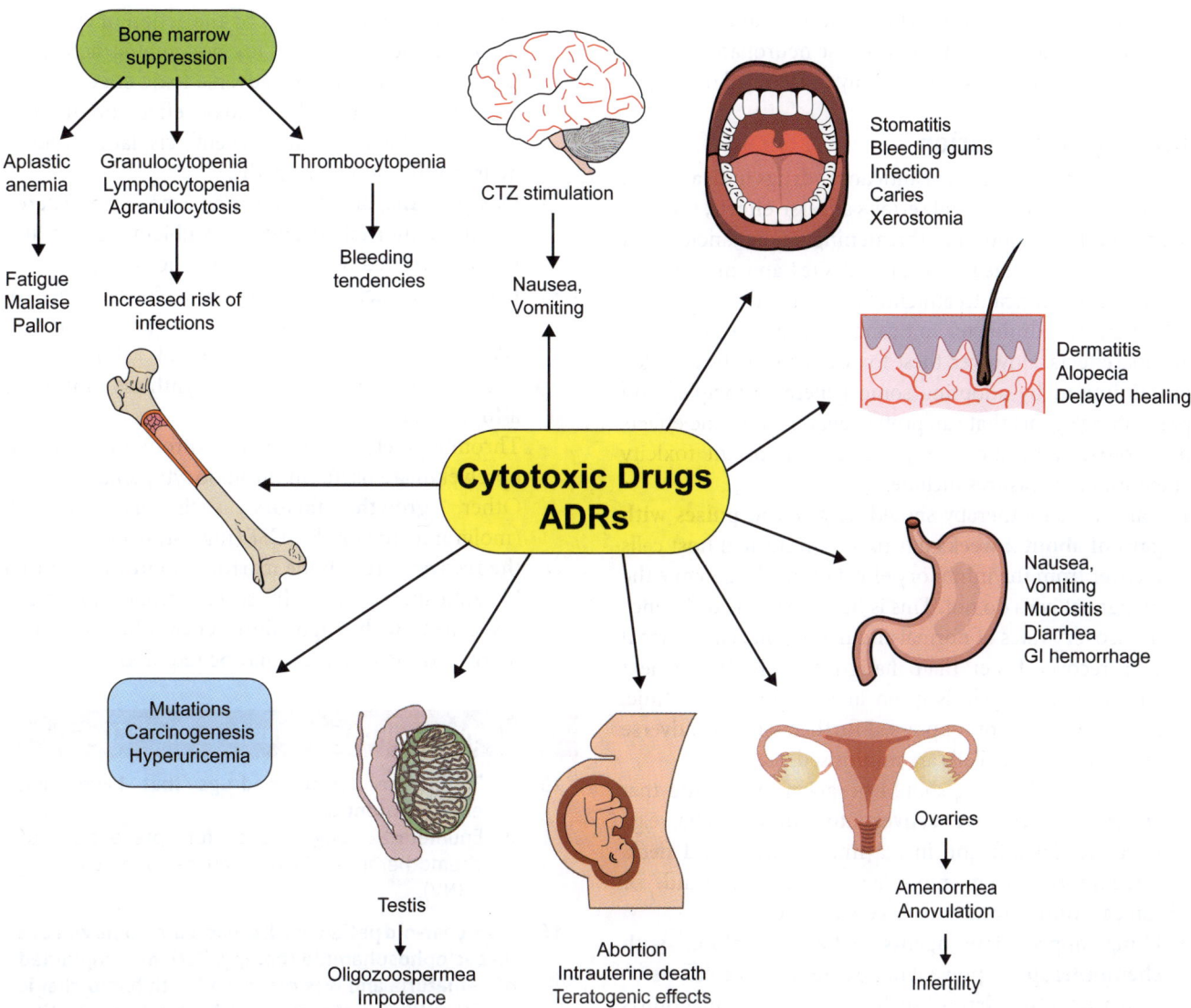

Fig. 61.12 General toxicity of cytotoxic drugs

Infections
Damage of epithelial lining along with lymphocytopenia and agranulocytosis predisposes the patient to **infection**, especially with **opportunistic organisms** such as *Candida*, *Toxoplasma*, Herpes zoster, *Cytomegalovirus*, and *Pneumocystis jirovecii*.

Suppression of gonadal function
Suppression of gonadal function leads to oligozoospermia and impotence in males, while amenorrhea and anovulation occur in females.

Suppression of rapidly dividing cells in the embryo/fetus causes abortion, intrauterine death and teratogenic effects.

Nausea and vomiting
Many cytotoxic drugs cause disturbing nausea and vomiting due to the generation of emetogenic impulses from the upper GIT and stimulation of chemoreceptor trigger zone. The potential to induce emesis is very high with cisplatin, cyclophosphamide, mustine, dacarbazine and actinomycin D.

Raised serum uric acid
Excessive destruction of cells can **raise serum uric acid levels**. It may precipitate gout, formation of urate stones and acute renal failure may occur.

Delayed effects
Delayed effects of cytotoxic drugs include **mutagenesis, carcinogenesis** and secondary tumours/ malignancies, e.g., suppression of CMI and humoral immunity against neoplasia can cause leukemia, lymphoma, etc.

Drug-specific adverse effects
In addition to the above, individual drugs cause **specific adverse effects**, e.g.

- Cyclophosphamide causes severe alopecia and hemorrhagic cystitis.
- Bleomycin may cause pulmonary fibrosis.

- Daunorubicin and doxorubicin cause cardiomyopathy.
- Vincristine and cisplatin may cause neuropathy.
- Cisplatin and streptozotocin may cause renal damage.

Toxicity amelioration

The risk–benefit analysis of anticancer drugs indicates that although they have several serious adverse effects, they are necessary for serious life-threatening malignancies that might have metastasised to distant sites and may not be amenable to surgical treatment. Consequently, it becomes necessary to administer anticancer drugs, despite their adverse effects. However, these toxic effects can be checked or minimised by adopting some general principles and prescribing agents that can protect against the toxic effects of cytotoxic anticancer drugs. These important toxicity amelioration measures include:

1. Cancer chemotherapy should be given in **pulses with gaps of about 2 weeks** during which normal host cells recover from the inhibitory effect of the drug, while the malignant cells do not. This is because of the difference in recovery rates of normal and malignant cells; normal cells recover faster than malignant cells. If the next chemotherapy cycle is given at the appropriate time, malignant cells are suppressed further, whereas adverse effects on normal cells are minimised.
2. If possible, the drug should be given by a route that ensures its **selective delivery to tumour cells**, e.g., intra-arterial infusion into a limb or head and neck, infusing the drug into pleural/peritoneal fluid, or topical administration on accessible sites.
3. Using **appropriate agents before or along with chemotherapy** to prevent or counteract toxic effects:
   - **Antiemetic drugs** such as 5-HT$_3$ antagonists (ondansetron) and neurokinin-1 receptor antagonists (aprepitant, dexamethasone, and metoclopramide) are almost always given before chemotherapy to prevent vomiting. Most anticancer drugs have the potential to induce nausea and vomiting that may otherwise decrease patient acceptability and compliance.
   - **Mesna and acetylcysteine** are thiol (–SH)-containing compounds. These are used to detoxify a toxic metabolite (acrolein) of cyclophosphamide, which can otherwise cause hemorrhagic cystitis. Excess fluid intake and frequent voiding is also helpful in this condition.
   - **Folinic acid** (citrovorum factor or leucovorin) and thymidine can overcome methotrexate toxicity, allowing administration of a higher dose without toxic effects.
   - **Amifostine** is preferentially activated in normal tissues to free thiols and scavenge free radicals and superoxide anions formed by the action of cytotoxic drugs or radiotherapy. This preferential activation in normal cells prevents adverse toxic effects, while preserving the useful cytotoxic effect on tumour cells. Amifostine can prevent cisplatin-induced neuropathy and nephropathy.
   - **Dexrazoxane**, an iron-chelating agent administered before daunorubicin and doxorubicin, can reduce infusion-related reactions and cardiotoxicity.
   - Excess uric acid produced as a consequence of cell kill can be reduced by measures like urinary alkalinisation, excess intake of fluids, and drugs (corticosteroids and synthesis inhibitor **allopurinol**).
   - Thrombopoietic factors such as thrombopoietin and oprelvekin are useful in thrombocytopenia.
   - Other **growth factors** such as GM-CSF (molgramostim) and G-CSF (filgrastim) can speed up the recovery from bone marrow suppression caused by anticancer drugs. In severe myelosuppression associated with high dose chemotherapy, bone marrow transplantation may be required.

Clinical problem-based questions and MCQs

15. i. Enumerate cytotoxic drugs that have high emetic potential
    ii. Enumerate drugs used for prevention of chemotherapy-induced nausea and vomiting (CINV).
16. A 56-year-old patient with breast carcinoma was put on cyclophosphamide therapy. Patient complained of hematuria and was diagnosed with hemorrhagic cystitis. What is the cause of hemorrhagic cystitis and how can it be managed?
17. A patient diagnosed with choriocarcinoma received methotrexate therapy. Leucovorin was prescribed along with methotrexate. Explain the pharmacological basis for prescribing leucovorin in this case.
18. A patient suffering from metastatic testicular tumour, receiving chemotherapy with cisplatin, was prescribed amifostine. Explain why amifostine was given along with cisplatin.
19. Cytotoxic drugs used for cancer chemotherapy are known to cause bone marrow suppression.
    i. Explain causation of myelosuppression with cytotoxic drug.
    ii. Enumerate measures for ameliorating myelosuppression.

The salient features of cytotoxic anticancer drugs are summarised in Table 61.1.

Table 61.1 Salient features of cytotoxic drugs

Drug, mechanism of action	Uses	ADRs
A Alkylating agents		
They form highly reactive carbonium ions upon cyclisation → alkylation of macromolecules results in cross-linking/ abnormal base-pairing, DNA breakdown, and cell death.		
1. Cyclophosphamide	Solid tumours like bronchogenic carcinoma, carcinoma of the bladder, breast, and testicular sarcoma.	Alopecia, nausea, vomiting. Hemorrhagic cystitis because of acrolein; managed with mesna/ acetylcysteine.
Ifosfamide	Longer half-life	Less nausea, vomiting, alopecia
2. Chlorambucil	Drug of choice for chronic lymphoid leukemia (CLL). Also useful in non-Hodgkin lymphoma (NHL)	Nausea, vomiting, mucositis, menstrual irregularities in women.
3. Busulfan	Drug of choice for chronic myeloid leukemia (NML)	Hyperuricemia, pulmonary fibrosis, skin pigmentation
4. Melphalan	Multiple myeloma	Nausea, vomiting, infection, pancreatitis
5. Mustine	Part of MOPP regimen for Hodgkin lymphoma (HL) and non-Hodgkin lymphoma (NHL).	Nausea, vomiting, hemodynamic changes, sloughing of tissue on extravasation
6. Carmustine, Lomustine	Can cross BBB; useful in brain tumours, meningeal leukemia	Nausea, vomiting and central side effects can occur
7. Procarbazine	Part of MOPP regimen for Hodgkin lymphoma	Mutagenic, carcinogenic potential, MAO inhibition, disulfiram reaction
8. Dacarbazine	Malignant melanoma and Hodgkin lymphoma (HL)	Nausea, vomiting, flu-like symptoms, neuropathy, bone marrow suppression
9. Temozolomide	Drug of choice for glioma, melanoma. Orally effective	Nausea, vomiting, flu-like symptoms, bone marrow suppression
B Antimetabolites		
1. **Folate antagonists** Methotrexate causes pseudo-irreversible inhibition of DHFRase → interferes with DNA synthesis → cell death.	Curative in choriocarcinoma, non-Hodgkin lymphoma. Used as disease-modifying agent in rheumatoid arthritis.	Bone marrow suppression leading to pancytopenia, megaloblastic anemia; managed by folinic acid or leucovorin.
2. **Purine antagonists** 6-Mercaptopurine, azathioprine, and thioguanine interfere with formation of adenine and guanine nucleotides, get incorporated in RNA/DNA, inhibit de novo purine synthesis	Choriocarcinoma, childhood leukemias, and solid tumours. With azothioprine, immunosuppressant effect is greater than anticancer effect	Hyperuricemia, which responds to allopurinol. However, dose of 6-MP and azathioprine should be reduced to half or one-fourth if allopurinol is combined.
3. **Pyrimidine antagonists** **5-fluorouracil** inhibits thymidylate synthase enzyme in presence of THFA, also gets incorporated in RNA (Leucovorin increases its efficacy, cisplatin/ oxaliplatin are synergistic)	Solid tumours like carcinoma of rectum, colon, stomach, liver, pancreas FOLFOX regimen is used in colorectal carcinoma.	Hand–foot syndrome due to neuropathy, nausea, vomiting, diarrhea, mucositis, bone marrow suppression
Cytarabine inhibits production of cytidylic acid	Useful in lymphomas, leukemia but not in solid tumours	Myelosuppression

(Continued)

C	**Cytotoxic antibiotics**		
	Drug is intercalated between DNA strands, and interferes with its template function. These can also cause breaks in DNA strands		
1.	Actinomycin D (dactinomycin)	High efficacy in Wilms tumour, rhabdomyosarcoma, Ewing sarcoma	Vomiting, diarrhea, dermatitis, stomatitis, alopecia, and bone marrow suppression
2.	Bleomycin	Testicular carcinoma, squamous cell carcinoma	Pulmonary fibrosis
3.	Daunorubicin	Acute myeloid and lymphoid leukemias	Cardiotoxicity such as ECG changes, arrhythmias, hypotension, CHF, cardiomyopathy
4.	Doxorubicin	Effective in solid tumours also	Dose-related cardiotoxicity like daunorubicin
D	**Topoisomerase I inhibitors**		
	Allows single strand breaks in DNA, but prevents resealing after untwisting		
	Topotecan, irinotecan	Carcinoma of lung, ovary, and cervix	Irinotecan is a cholinesterase inhibitor causing cholinergic adverse effects that may be controlled by atropine
E	**Topoisomerase II inhibitors**		
	Podophyllin derivatives that interfere with the resealing of DNA strand after untwisting; however, they act at a different site than topotecan.		
	Etoposide, teniposide	Carcinoma of lung, testis	Alopecia, neutropenia and gastro-intestinal disturbances
F	**Platinum coordination complexes**		
	They are intracellularly hydrolysed to produce a highly reactive moiety that causes cross-linking of DNA and damages it		
	Cisplatin	Carcinoma of testis, ovary	Most emetic drug, ototoxicity, sensory neuropathy, nephrotoxicity, shock-like state on IV infusion may occur
	Carboplatin	Same as cisplatin	Better tolerated than cisplatin. Nausea, vomiting is mild and delayed. Oto/neuro/nephrotoxic potential is less than with cisplatin
	Oxaliplatin	Effective in cisplatin-resistant tumours, very useful in colorectal carcinoma along with leucovorin and 5-FU.	Peripheral sensory neuropathy, acute allergic reactions
G	**Microtubule-damaging drugs:** vinca alkaloids and taxanes		
	Vinca alkaloids bind to microtubule protein, tubulin, and prevent the polymerisation and assembly of microtubules, resulting in disruption of the mitotic spindle. Thus, chromosomes fail to move apart and metaphase arrest occurs. In contrast, taxanes enhance polymerisation after binding to tubulin, making the microtubules more stable. This again interferes with mitotic function		
	a **Vinca alkaloids** Vincristine (also called oncovin)	It is a rapid-acting drug. Used to induce remission in childhood ALL and AML, but not good for maintenance therapy. It is part of MOPP regimen for Hodgkin lymphoma	Peripheral neuropathy, alopecia, syndrome of inappropriate ADH secretion (SIADH)
	Vinblastin	Kaposi sarcoma, neuroblastoma	Myelosuppression
	b **Taxanes** Paclitaxel, docetaxel	Used in relapse of carcinoma breast and ovary. Also useful in carcinoma head, neck and lungs.	Bone marrow suppression, stocking–glove neuropathy
	Estramustine (a complex of estradiol and mustine)	Estramustine is useful in metastatic carcinoma prostate.	Estramustine causes estrogenic adverse effects
H	**Miscellaneous**		
	a **Hydroxyurea** inhibits conversion of ribonucleotides to deoxyribonucleotides and DNA synthesis	Used in polycythemia vera, sickle cell disease, psoriasis, CML, and as a radiosensitiser before radiotherapy	Cutaneous reactions, skin pigmentation, myelosuppression
	b **L-asparaginase** deprives lymphoid leukemia cells of L-asparagine	Useful in ALL	Hyperglycemia, hyper-triglyceridemia, clotting defects, allergic reactions

TARGETED DRUGS

Studies of cancer biology and molecular mechanisms of carcinogenesis have identified several targets that can be attacked for achieving selective cancer cell kill. These targets include protein tyrosine kinases such as BCR-ABL, EGFR, proteasomes, and VEGFR. Their inhibitors mainly affect cancer cells, sparing normal host cells. Some biological response modifiers like monoclonal antibodies and cytokines. also act selectively against cancer cells. In some malignancies, hormones and related drugs also have beneficial effect. Such targeted and hormonal drugs are shown in Flowchart 61.2.

1. BCR-ABL Kinase Inhibitors

Philadelphia chromosome is formed as a consequence of the fusion of the 'Abelson' (ABL) tyrosine kinase gene at chromosome 9 and 'breakpoint cluster region' (BCR) gene at chromosome 22. Inhibitors of Philadelphia chromosome include imatinib, nilotinib, and dasatinib.

Imatinib

Imatinib inhibits the BCR-ABL kinase expressed by CML cells. However, point mutations in BCR-ABL tyrosine kinase can cause resistance of CML cells to imatinib.

- It can inhibit stem cell receptors and C-KIT receptors that are active in gastrointestinal stromal tumours (GIST).
- It also inhibits related tyrosine kinases such as platelet-derived growth factor receptors (PDGFRs) that are actively involved in dermatofibrosarcoma protuberans.

Therapeutic uses

Imatinib is very useful in inducing remission in CML and C-kit positive GIST, for which it is drug of choice. It is also useful in dermatofibrosarcoma protuberans.

ADRs

Abdominal pain, vomiting, fluid retention, periorbital edema, pleural effusion, congestive heart failure, myalgia and hepatic damage may occur with imatinib.

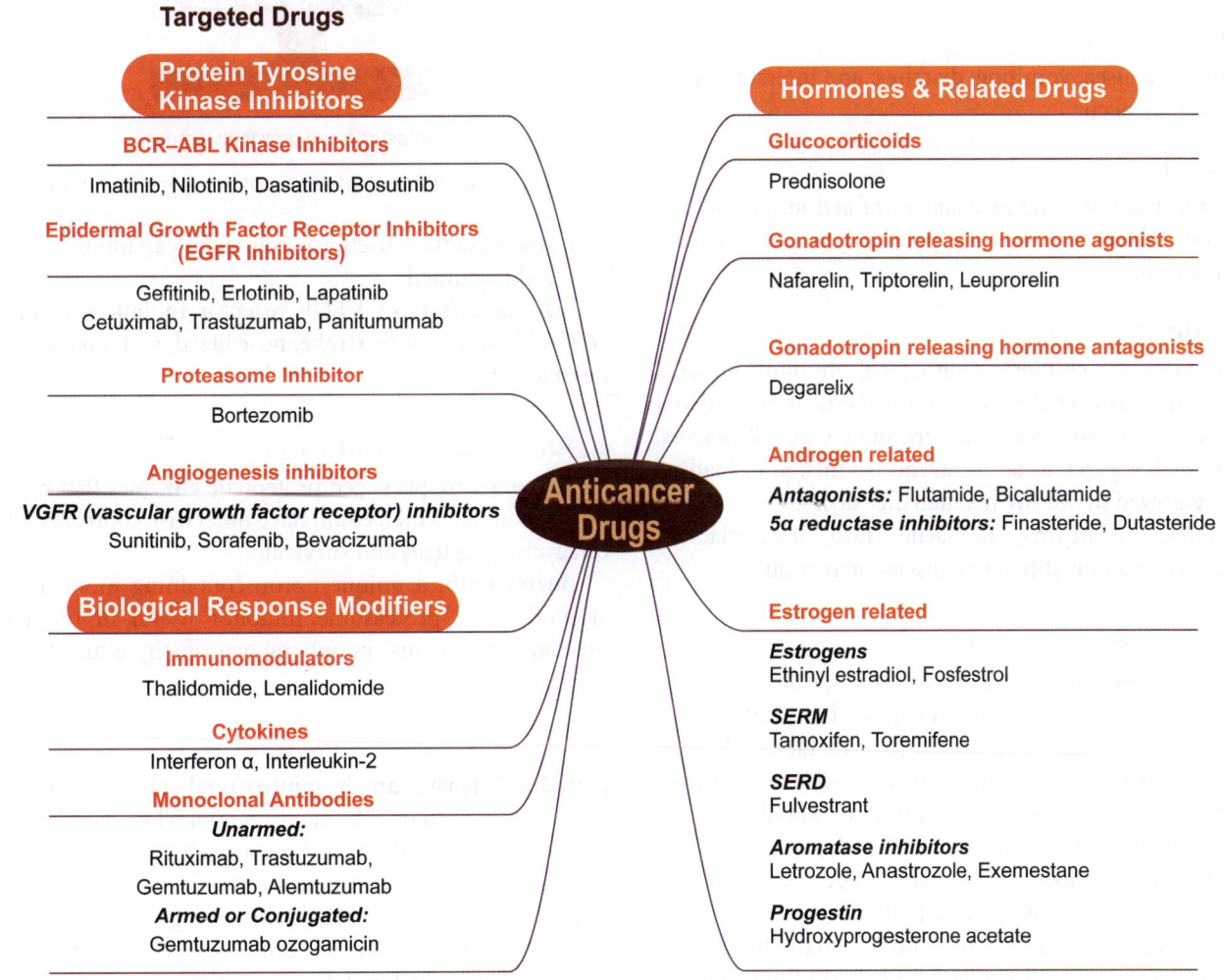

Flowchart 61.2 Targeted and hormonal anticancer drugs

Nilotinib has higher response rates and lower chances of developing resistance than with imatinib.

Dasatinib shows higher and faster cytogenic response than imatinib.

2. Epidermal growth factor receptor inhibitors (EGFR inhibitors)

Gefitinib, erlotinib, cetuximab

EGFR is a transmembrane tyrosine kinase receptor that regulates growth and differentiation of epithelial cells. The growth of some epithelial cell tumours is critically dependent on the activation of this receptor because of its overexpression or mutation. Thus, inhibitors of EGFR exert anticancer activity.

Gefitinib

After entering the cancer cell, the drug binds with tyrosine kinase domain of EGFR and interferes with phosphorylation of regulatory proteins.

Therapeutic uses

Gefitinib is useful in non-small cell carcinoma of lung, which generally affects non-smokers and women.

ADRs

Anorexia, nausea, vomiting, diarrhea, and interstitial lung disease may occur.

Erlotinib

Erlotinib has the same mechanism of action and uses as gefitinib; however, it has the potential to cause hepatic dysfunction.

Cetuximab

Cetuximab is a chimeric monoclonal antibody directed against the extracellular domain of EGFR. It is approved for use in head and neck tumours and colorectal cancers. Cetuximab is given as an intravenous infusion of loading dose, followed by weekly maintenance doses.

ADRs like itching, headache, rash, anaphylactoid reactions, and interstitial lung disease may occur.

3. Angiogenesis Inhibitors

Neovascularisation/angiogenesis, i.e., proliferation of new blood vessels is essential for growth and metastasis of cancers. Vascular endothelial growth factor (VEGF) causes neovascularisation. It can be checked by VEGF receptor inhibitors such as sunitinib, sorafenib, and bevacizumab (Fig. 61.13).

Sunitinib is approved by the FDA for renal cell carcinoma and imatinib-resistant GIST.

Sorafenib is orally effective and less toxic. It is useful in advanced renal cell tumour, and thyroid and hepatic cancers.

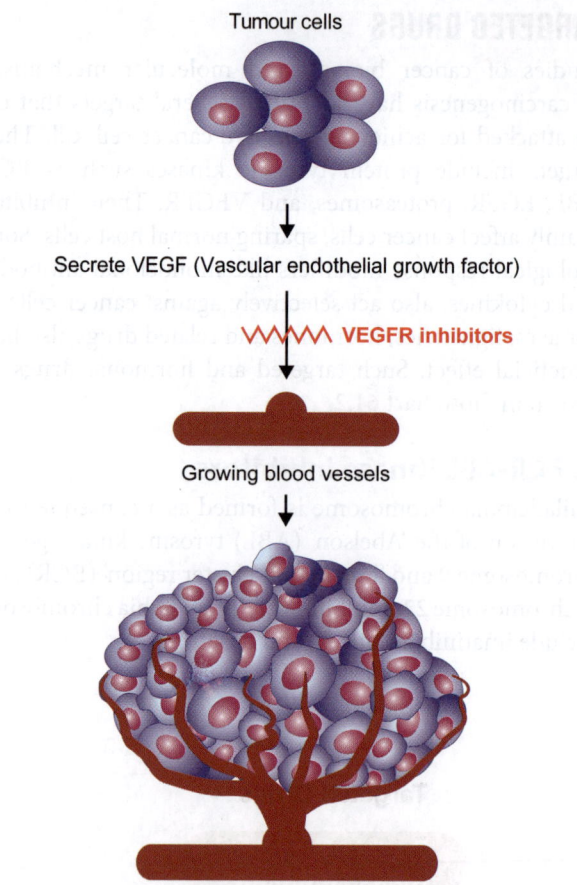

Fig. 61.13 Mechanism of action of angiogenesis inhibitors

Bevacizumab is useful in colorectal carcinoma, along with 5-fluorouracil.

Adverse effects of VEGF receptor inhibitors include rise in blood pressure, stroke, nose bleed, rectal bleed and heart attack.

4. Proteasome Inhibitors

Proteasomes are packaged proteolytic enzymes that break down proteins, which could have otherwise controlled the cell cycle, apoptosis and survival.

Bortezomib, a unique boron-containing monoclonal antibody, is a proteasome inhibitor useful in multiple myeloma. It can cause peripheral neuropathy as an adverse effect.

5. Biological response modifiers

Rituximab, trastuzumab, gemtuzumab, alemtuzumab

These are chimeric, humanised monoclonal antibodies that kill cancer cells by acting against unique antigens present on the surface of cancer cells.

Rituximab is useful in non-Hodgkin lymphoma, chronic lymphoid leukemia, and β-cell lymphoma. ADRs can occur as infusion related reactions as fever, chills, rashes and dyspnea. Neutropenia may occur later on.

Clinical problem-based questions and MCQs

20. Match the drug with its target site present on tumour cells for exerting anticancer action.

a.	Nilotinib	1.	Vascular endothelial growth factor receptor
b.	Erlotinib	2.	Philadelphia chromosome
c.	Sunitinib	3.	Proteasome
d.	Bortezomib	4.	Epidermal growth factor receptor

21. i. Identify the drug effective against imatinib-resistant GIST

    a. Sunitinib   b. Sorafenib
    c. Bortezomib   d. Nilotinib

    ii. Describe mechanism of action of chosen drug.

HORMONAL AND RELATED ANTICANCER DRUGS

These are not cytotoxic, but can be used as palliative therapy in hormone-related malignancies.

They include glucocorticoids, gonadotropin-releasing hormone agonists, and estrogen/progesterone/androgen-related drugs (Flowchart 61.2). The detailed pharmacology of these drugs is described in the respective chapters.

Glucocorticoids have marked lympholytic action because of which they are useful in acute childhood leukemias and lymphomas. They are able to induce quick remission, though relapse occurs in almost all cases. Gradually, the responsiveness of the tumour to glucocorticoids decreases. They have a palliative role in Hodgkin lymphoma and hormone-responsive carcinoma breast. In addition, glucocorticoids play a role in controlling malignancy and chemotherapy-related complications such as hypercalcemia, hemolysis, thrombocytopenia, increased intracranial tension, and mediastinal edema.

Estrogen-related drugs: Estrogens provide symptomatic relief in carcinoma prostate. Gonadotropin-releasing hormone analogues are better for this indication.

Selective estrogen receptor modulators and down-regulators (SERM/SERDs) are important adjuvants in the palliative therapy of breast carcinoma.

Antiandrogens such as **flutamide** and **bicalutamide** have a palliative role in advanced metastatic cases of carcinoma prostate.

5α-reductase inhibitors such as **finasteride** and **dutasteride** prevent the conversion of testosterone to dihydrotestosterone (DHT) and have a palliative role in carcinoma prostate.

Gonadotropin-releasing hormone analogues inhibit the secretion of estrogens/androgens by suppressing the release of FSH and LH from the pituitary. These are useful in carcinoma breast and prostate.

Progesterones have some role in temporary remission in advanced or recurrent endometrial carcinoma

Summary

- For the management of malignant diseases, a combined modality approach is followed.
- Early intensive treatment in maximum tolerated doses is preferred for total cell kill.
- A combination regimen of 2–5 synergistic drugs is given in intermittent pulses.
- Cytotoxic drugs can be cell-cycle specific (CCS) or cell-cycle nonspecific (CCNS).
- Usually CCNS drugs are followed by CCS drugs in pulses to improve cell kill. 6–11 cycles may be needed for optimum effect.
- Cytotoxic drugs have more **deleterious effect** on fast multiplying cells. Myelosuppression, lymphoreticular suppression, epithelial lining damage, gonadal suppression, delayed healing, and fetal toxicity are common.
- Measures taken for toxicity amelioration are the practice of pulse therapy, selective delivery of drug, and bone marrow transplantation.
- Methotrexate toxicity is reduced by folinic acid and thymidine.
- Cyclophosphamide-induced hemorrhagic cystitis is managed with mesna, acetylcysteine, excess fluid intake and frequent voiding.
- Dexrazoxane can prevent doxorubicin- and daunorubicin-induced cardiotoxic effects.
- Amifostine provides thiols to prevent cisplatin-induced nephropathy and neuropathy.
- CINV is managed with ondansetron, aprepitant, dexamethasone and metoclopramide.
- Thrombopoietin, molgramostim and filgrastim are useful to treat bone marrow suppression.
- Hyperuricemia caused by busulfan responds to allopurinol.
- Targeted drugs (such as BCR-ABL, EGFR, VEGFR, and proteasomes inhibitors) inhibit tyrosine kinase and have lower toxicity than cytotoxic drugs.

Questions for practice

1. Classify cytotoxic drugs and enumerate their general toxic effects.
2. Explain why:
    a. Combined modality approach is practiced in cancer management.
    b. Chemotherapeutic drugs are administered in a cyclic manner.
    c. Folinic acid prevents methotrexate toxicity effectively but folic acid does not.
    d. Mesna is used in cyclophosphamide toxicity.
    e. Flutamide has a palliative role in CA prostate.

3. Write short notes on:
   a. Targeted anticancer drugs
   b. Cytotoxic antibiotics
   c. MOPP regimen
   d. Role of corticosteroids in cancer management
   e. Vinca alkaloids

Hints for problem-based questions and MCQs

1. If a single malignant cell survives chemotherapy or radiotherapy, it can produce daughter cells that result in recurrence.
2. a–2; b–4; c–1; d–3.
3. i. To achieve the goal of total cell kill, intensive combination regimens with the maximum tolerated dose of drugs are given at an early stage for achieving complete remission.
   ii. Drugs used in combination must possess anticancer efficacy when used alone, should have different mechanisms of anticancer action, different mechanisms of development of resistance and different toxic reactions. Moreover, combined drugs should have synergistic interaction on cell-cycle specificity/ nonspecificity
4. i. a. Azathioprine
   ii. It is converted into 6-MP; this interferes with formation of guanine nucleotides, which are building blocks of DNA and RNA. It gets incorporated in nucleic acids, making them dysfunctional. De novo purine synthesis is also inhibited. Azathioprine is used in rheumatoid arthritis, IBD, other autoimmune conditions, and for prevention of organ transplant rejection; dose of azathioprine is reduced to half (refer to page 795).
   iii. Allopurinol (a xanthine oxidase inhibitor) is combined to inhibit uric acid synthesis to prevent hyperuricemia, but the dose of azathioprine should be reduced.
5. i. The FOLFOX regimen contains 5-FU, and oxaliplatin.
   ii. 5-FU inhibits thymidylate synthetase in the presence of THFA, so leucovorin is combined. Oxaliplatin exerts a synergistic effect with 5-FU in solid tumours.
6. i. c. Methotrexate is curative in choriocarcinoma.
   ii. Methotrexate forms polyglutamate, which causes pseudo-irreversible inhibition of the enzyme dihydrofolate reductase and blocks the conversion of dihydrofolate into tetrahydrofolate. Therefore, folates cannot be used for DNA synthesis, resulting in cell death. Its typical toxicity is myelosuppression that can be prevented by the use of N5-formyl-THFA or folinic acid (leucovorin).
7. a–4; b–3; c–1; d–2.
8. i. b. Cyclophosphamide causes hemorrhagic cystitis, due to accumulation of acrolein.
   ii. Mesna/acetylcysteine, excess fluid and frequent voiding (refer to page 793).
9. a–2; b–3; c–1.
10. a–2; b–1; c–4; d–3.
11. b. Neurotoxicity
12. b. Cisplatin
13. i. c. Estramustine
    ii. Estramustine gets concentrated in the prostate. It binds to β-tubulin, enhancing its polymerisation and microtubule stability; this hinders the normal dynamic reorganisation of the microtubule network, resulting in metaphase arrest.
    iii. Estramustine gets hydrolysed to form estradiol and mustine. Estradiol is responsible for causing gynecomastia as an adverse effect.
14. i. Cells of childhood leukemias depend on the medium for supply of L-asparagine. L-asparaginase converts L-asparagine into L-aspartic acid; this deprives tumour cells of an essential metabolite, resulting in cell death.
    ii. Important ADRs include hyperglycemia, hypertriglyceridemia, clotting defects and severe allergic reactions.
15. i. Cisplatin, cyclophosphamide, mustine, actinomycin D, dacarbazine
    ii. Ondansetron, metoclopramide, aprepitant, dexamethasone, lorazepam
16. Hemorrhagic cystitis occurs due to a toxic metabolite (acrolein) of cyclophosphamide. Mesna and acetylcysteine are SH-containing compounds that are used to detoxify acrolein. Excess fluid intake and frequent voiding is also helpful in this condition.
17. Folinic acid (citrovorum factor or leucovorin) and thymidine can overcome methotrexate toxicity, allowing administration of a higher dose without toxic effects.
18. In normal tissues, amifostine gets activated to free thiols that scavenge free radicals and superoxide anions formed by the action of cytotoxic drugs or radiotherapy. This prevents adverse toxic effects such as cisplatin-induced neuropathy and nephropathy.
19. i. Cytotoxic drugs suppress cell division in a dose-dependent manner in rapidly multiplying tissues as well as in cancer cells; this results in myelosuppression, which further causes aplastic anemia, TCP, neutropenia, etc.
    ii. Thrombopoietic factors like thrombopoietin and oprelvekin are useful in thrombocytopenia. Other growth factors like GM-CSF (molgramostim) and G-CSF (filgrastim) can expedite the recovery from bone marrow suppression caused by anticancer drugs. In severe myelosuppression associated with high dose chemotherapy, even bone marrow transplantation can be considered.
20. a–2; b–4; c–1; d–3.
21. i. a. Sunitinib
    ii. It acts by preventing angiogenesis or neovascularisation.

CONCEPT MAP – ANTICANCER CYTOTOXIC DRUGS

General Principles
- Combined modality approach with surgery, chemotherapy and radiotherapy.
- Intensive combination regimens with maximum tolerated dose of drugs given at early stage.
- CCS drugs given after a course of CCNS drugs to increase the cell kill.
- Cyclic therapy for 6–11 cycles for achieving total cell kill.

Alkylating Agents
Mechanism: (CCNS) form highly reactive carbonium ion intermediates having affinity for negatively charged groups of DNA, shift alkyl group especially to guanine residues at position 7 of DNA → cross-linking, abnormal base pairing and scission of DNA strands → cytotoxic action.

Uses: Cyclophosphamide: Solid tumours (bronchogenic, breast, bladder)
Chlorambucil: DOC in CLL
Busulfan: DOC in CML
Melphalan: Multiple myeloma
Mustine, Procarbazine: Part of MOPP regimen for Hodgkin lymphoma.

Antimetabolites
Folate antagonist: Methotrexate causes pseudo-irreversible inhibition of DHFRase.
Uses: Curative in choriocarcinoma, non-Hodgkin lymphoma, DMARDs.
Purine antagonists: 6-MP, 6-TG, Azathioprine
Inhibit synthesis of nucleotides of DNA, RNA
Uses: Choriocarcinoma, Childhood leukemias and as immunosuppressants.
Dose reduction indicated with allopurinol
Pyrimidine antagonists: 5 FU: Inhibits thymidylate synthase enzyme in presence of THFA,
Uses: Solid tumours of the rectum, colon, stomach, liver, pancreas.

Microtubule Damaging Drugs
Bind to microtubular protein β tubulin →
Vinca alkaloids prevent its polymerisation and assembly of microtubules → disrupt mitotic spindle → metaphase arrest.
Vincristine: Part of MOPP regimen for Hodgkin lymphoma.
Taxanes enhance polymerisation → form more stable microtubules → metaphase arrest.
Paclitaxel used in relapse of carcinoma of breast, ovary.

Anticancer Cytotoxic Drugs

Platinum Coordination Complexes
Mechanism: Get hydrolysed → form highly reactive moiety → cause cross-linking of DNA.
Uses: Cisplatin, Carboplatin in cancer of testis, ovary
Oxaliplatin in cisplatin-resistant tumours & colorectal carcinoma with 5-FU.

Cytotoxic Antibiotics
Actinomycin D: High efficacy in Wilms tumour, rhabdomyosarcoma, Ewing sarcoma.
Bleomycin: Testicular carcinoma, squamous cell carcinoma.
Daunorubicin: Acute myeloid & lymphoid leukemias.
Doxorubicin: Effective in solid tumours also.

Topoisomerase I inhibitors
Topotecan, Irinotecan used in:
Carcinoma of lung, ovary, cervix

Topoisomerase II inhibitors
Etoposide, Teniposide used in:
Carcinoma of lung, testes

General Toxicity
Myelosuppression (aplastic anemia, TCP, agranulocytosis)
Lymphoreticular suppression (risk of infections),
Epithelial lining damage (stomatitis, mucositis, caries, diarrhea, nausea, vomiting, delayed healing, dermatitis, alopecia),
Gonadal suppression (oligozoospermia, impotence, amenorrhea, infertility)
Fetal toxicity (abortion, IUFD, teratogenicity)

Toxicity Amelioration
Measures: Pulse therapy, selective delivery of drug, bone marrow transplantation.
Drugs: Folinic acid rescue for preventing methotrexate toxicity.
Mesna to prevent Cyclophosphamide-induced hemorrhagic cystitis.
Dextrazoxane to prevent doxo and daunorubicin induced cardiotoxic effects.
Amifostine provides thiols to prevent cisplatin-induced nephropathy and neuropathy.
CINV is managed with ondansetron, aprepitant, dexamethasone and metoclopramide.
Thrombopoietin, molgramostim and filgrastim are useful in bone marrow suppression.
Hyperuricemia caused by busulfan responds to allopurinol

SECTION 11 Drugs Acting on the Gastrointestinal System

62 Drugs for Diarrhea, IBD, and Constipation

PH 6.3 Describe salient pharmacokinetics, pharmacodynamics, therapeutic uses, adverse drug reactions of drugs used for the management of diarrhea and devise pharmacotherapeutic plan to manage acute and chronic diarrhea in adults and children.
PH 6.5 Describe salient pharmacokinetics, pharmacodynamics, adverse drug reactions of drugs used for the management of inflammatory bowel disease and irritable bowel disorders.
PH 6.4 Describe salient pharmacokinetics, pharmacodynamics, adverse drug reactions of drugs used for the management of constipation and devise management plan for a case of constipation.

Learning objectives

A student of MBBS phase II should be able to:
- Classify drugs used as antidiarrheals.
- Describe mechanisms of action of various antidiarrheal drugs.
- Enumerate indications, contraindications and ADRs of antidiarrheal drugs.
- Describe pharmacotherapy of acute and chronic diarrhea.
- Classify the drugs used for IBD.
- Describe mechanisms of action of drugs useful in IBD.
- Enumerate indications for use, doses and ADRs of drugs used in IBD.
- Describe the role of drugs in IBS.
- Classify laxative/purgative drugs.
- Describe the mechanism of action of laxatives/purgatives.
- Enumerate indications for use and ADRs of laxatives.
- Describe management of constipation.

DIARRHEA

Diarrhea is a condition involving **abnormal frequency and consistency of stools.** It is defined as the passage of poorly-formed stools of fluid consistency, more than three times in a period of 24 hours. **Multiple factors** may cause the loss of excess water in stool:

- Hypermotility of intestines
- Increased osmotic load in the GI lumen.
- Reduced absorption of water and electrolytes.
- Increased secretion of water by intestinal mucosa.
- Inflammation of GI mucosa and exudation of fluid into the GI lumen.

Types of Diarrhea

Diarrhea can be acute or chronic. **Acute diarrhea** usually occurs due to infection or irritants, is self-limiting, and subsides within 2 weeks. In contrast, **chronic diarrhea** occurs due to a variety of causes and lasts longer than 2 weeks.

Acute diarrhea can further be classified into 2 types:
- **Noninvasive diarrhea**, in which stools are abundant and watery, causing dehydration. Abdominal pain may be present; however, there is no associated fever or blood or mucus in the stools.
- **Invasive diarrhea** is characterised by slightly loose stools of less volume; blood and mucus are present along with abdominal pain and fever.

Pathophysiology

In normal individuals, the intake and elimination of water are equal, and the osmolality of body fluids is maintained. **Water intake** is regulated by the **thirst mechanism**, which involves the stimulation of osmoreceptors in the medulla oblongata in response to factors such as:

- Increase in plasma osmolality by 3–5 mOsm/kg
- Hypovolemia
- Hypotension

Water elimination from the body occurs mainly through the **skin, lungs and gastrointestinal tract**. The amount of water lost through the skin and lungs depends largely upon the **body temperature, climatic changes**, and **extent of exercise**. The GIT normally eliminates 120–160 mL of water daily.

Salt and water absorption in the GIT occurs by:
- Passive absorption, secondary to the absorption of glucose/amino acids in the jejunum.
- Active salt absorption via Na^+/K^+-ATPase at villus tips in the colon and ileum, along with iso-osmotic absorption of water.

- Glucose-facilitated Na⁺ absorption in the ileum through Na⁺–glucose cotransporter.
- Passive absorption of Cl⁻ and HCO_3^- ions through the paracellular pathway and HCO_3^- ion exchange with Cl⁻ or H⁺.

The volume of water present in stools increases under the following conditions:

- Increased luminal osmotic load due to the presence of nonabsorbable solutes, e.g., disaccharidase deficiency decreases H_2O absorption.
- Structural damage to mucosal cells by viral infections decreases Na⁺/K⁺ ATPase-mediated salt and H_2O absorption.
- Intestinal hypermotility allows less time for absorption of H_2O.
- Secretory activity of GI mucosa is increased by bacterial toxins (enterotoxigenic *E. coli*, *Salmonella*, *Vibrio cholera*, etc.).
- Prostaglandins, increased cAMP or cGMP inside the cell, excess bile acids, carcinoid syndrome etc.

Such **reduced absorption or increased secretion** of water from the GIT causes watery/loose/poorly-formed stools. Water loss leads to dehydration and electrolyte disturbances such as hyponatremia (plasma Na⁺ < 135 mmol/L) and hypokalemia (plasma K⁺ < 3.5 mmol/L). Fluid–electrolyte imbalance can result in clinical features such as dryness of the mouth and skin (due to reduced sweating), poor skin turgor, muscular weakness, decreased urine output, and in severe cases, paralytic ileus.

MANAGEMENT OF DIARRHEA

The management of diarrhea mainly involves **rehydration therapy** to maintain the fluid–electrolyte balance and maintaining adequate nutrition. Specific drug therapy based on the cause of diarrhea is needed in a few cases only.

I. REHYDRATION

Rehydration can be carried out by **oral or parenteral** (intravenous) routes.

Oral rehydration therapy (ORT)

Composition of ORS

The **new** low-osmolarity **Oral Rehydration Solution** (ORS) formula, as recommended by WHO and UNICEF, has a total osmolarity of 245 mOsm/L. Its composition per litre includes: NaCl **2.6 g**; KCl **1.5 g**; Trisodium citrate **2.9 g**; and Glucose **13.5 g**, dissolved in water to make up a final volume of 1 litre.

Role of ingredients

Glucose: The glucose-facilitated absorption of Na⁺ via Na⁺–glucose cotransporter in the ileum remains intact even during severe diarrhea. Thus, glucose **helps in sodium absorption**.

- **Na⁺, K⁺, and Cl⁻** are meant to compensate the ionic loss in stools during diarrhea and **maintain electrolyte balance**.
- **The base** (HCO_3^-/citrate) helps to correct **acidosis** associated with diarrhea. Citrate-based ORS formulas have longer shelf-life than those containing bicarbonate.
- The currently recommended **low-osmolarity ORS formula** offers several advantages over the older formulation, including enhanced fluid absorption, greater reduction in stool output and vomiting, elimination of risk of hypernatremia, and improved cost-effectiveness.
- **Super ORS** is glycine-enriched and allows better absorption of sodium and water.
- Rice water, wheat, maize and cereal-based ORS are also available. These provide more calories but are expensive.
- Home-made lemon water with one fistful of sugar, a pinch of salt, and half a lemon in one litre of water is a good alternative if ORS packets are not available. Rice water, coconut water, buttermilk and fruit juices may also be used if needed.

Indications for use

- In mild-to-moderate fluid loss (5–10% of body weight), oral rehydration therapy (ORT) is the first choice to maintain hydration and fluid–electrolyte balance as well as acid–base balance till diarrhea stops spontaneously. Oral rehydration salts (ORS) solution volume **equivalent to 5–7.5% of body weight** is administered in the **initial 2–4 hours**. Because hypovolemia increases thirst, the patient is encouraged to drink ORS solution at frequent intervals. A rough guide is to **take in as much volume of fluid as is lost in stools**.
- In addition to dehydration due to diarrhea, ORS is useful in heat stroke and for maintaining hydration in postoperative trauma and burn cases.

Advantages

Administration of ORS solution for the prevention and correction of dehydration is a simple, convenient and economical method of replacing lost fluid and electrolytes in comparison to parenteral fluid therapy.

- Stool volume and vomiting is reduced.
- There is no risk of fluid overload and subsequent pulmonary congestion or edema, as intake is mainly driven by dehydration-induced thirst.
- The risk of hypernatremia and hyperkalemia is lower with oral rehydration therapy than with IV administration of fluids.
- No hospitalisation is required for oral administration.

Limitations
Oral rehydration therapy is not possible in patients who are vomiting or are in a shock-like state.

> **Oral rehydration therapy**
> The correct method of preparation and use of ORS solution must be explained to the patient for effective oral rehydration therapy. The contents of the ORS packet are dissolved in 1 litre of drinking water (boiled and cooled, or filtered), and the solution thus prepared should be used within 24 hours. ORS solution should be consumed sip-by-sip and not gulped down quickly. The quantity of ORS solution required varies from patient to patient, based on the presence and degree of dehydration.
> a. If there is **no dehydration**:
>   - The amount of ORS fluid indicated after each loose stool varies with age:
>
> | Age of patient | Amount of ORS solution after each loose stool |
> |---|---|
> | <2 years | 50–100 mL |
> | 2–10 years | 100–200 mL |
> | 10 years or more | As much as desired by patient, driven by thirst |
>
> - In children < 2 years of age → 1–2 tsp of ORS solution should be given every 1–2 minutes. In case vomiting occurs with this frequency of ORS administration, oral fluid therapy should be withheld for about 10 minutes, and then started again with a lower frequency, i.e., 1–2 tsp every 2–3 minutes. Older children should be advised to sip frequently from a cup or glass.
>
> b. If there is **some dehydration**:
>   ORS solution should be given to correct the existing fluid–electrolyte deficit, maintain normal daily fluid requirement, and replace the amount being lost in stools or vomits.

Zinc
Along with ORS, Zn supplementation is useful in pediatric populations to **reduce the severity and duration of diarrhea** episodes.

The mechanism of the beneficial effect of Zn in diarrhea is not well understood. It probably involves reduced secretion of fluid in intestine, enhanced immune response, and faster regeneration of the intestinal epithelium.

WHO recommends the administration of Zn in a dose of 10 mg/day up to 6 months of age, and 20 mg/day for children who are 6 months to 5 years of age. Zn is available as a dispersible tablet for use during acute diarrhea along with ORT. It should be continued for 10–14 days after controlling diarrhea to prevent recurrence of diarrhea within the next few months.

2. Parenteral rehydration therapy
IV fluid therapy is indicated if:
- the patient is not able to take in sufficient fluid orally
- the patient vomits out ORS
- the patient has lost fluid equivalent > 10% body weight
- fluid is being lost at rate of 10 mL/kg/hour
- the patient is unconscious or vomiting.

Dhaka fluid, containing NaCl 5 g, KCl 1 g, and $NaHCO_3$ 4 g in 1 L of 5% glucose is used. An alternative to this is Ringer lactate.

II. MAINTAINING NUTRITION
In current clinical practice, the emphasis is on maintaining good nutritional status in a patient suffering from diarrhea. If the patient skips meals or fasts in recurrent/prolonged diarrhea, it causes nutritional deficiencies. Moreover, **disaccharidase enzyme** in the brush border of GI mucosa **decreases, further reducing the absorption of salt, water and nutrients.** Deficiency of disaccharidase increases the luminal osmotic load.

Allowing **simple, easily digestible foods** such as breast milk for infants, 50% diluted buffalo milk or cow milk, rice water, soft cooked rice and lentils, banana and sago is beneficial. Foods with high fat or fibre content should be avoided.

III. ANTIDIARRHEAL DRUGS
In addition to maintaining adequate rehydration and nutrition, drugs are useful in the treatment of some cases of diarrhea. These include antimicrobial drugs, antimotility and antisecretory drugs, absorbants, and probiotics (Flowchart 62.1).

a. Antimicrobials
Role in management of diarrhea
Although antimicrobials are not needed for the management of all cases of diarrhea, they are **frequently prescribed, irrationally**. This practice must be checked and controlled. Antimicrobials have no beneficial effect in patients presenting with diarrhea due to cardiac diseases, tropical sprue, irritable bowel syndrome, thyrotoxicosis, etc. Diarrhea due to digestive enzyme deficiency or rotavirus infection are also non-responsive to antimicrobial therapy.

Indications for antimicrobial therapy in diarrhea
Diarrhea caused by entero-invasive organisms require treatment with antimicrobial drugs. The preferred drugs for these organisms are:
- Enteropathogenic E. coli (**EPEC**): Fluoroquinolones (FQs)
- Enterotoxigenic E. coli (**ETEC**): Doxycycline, cotrimoxazole

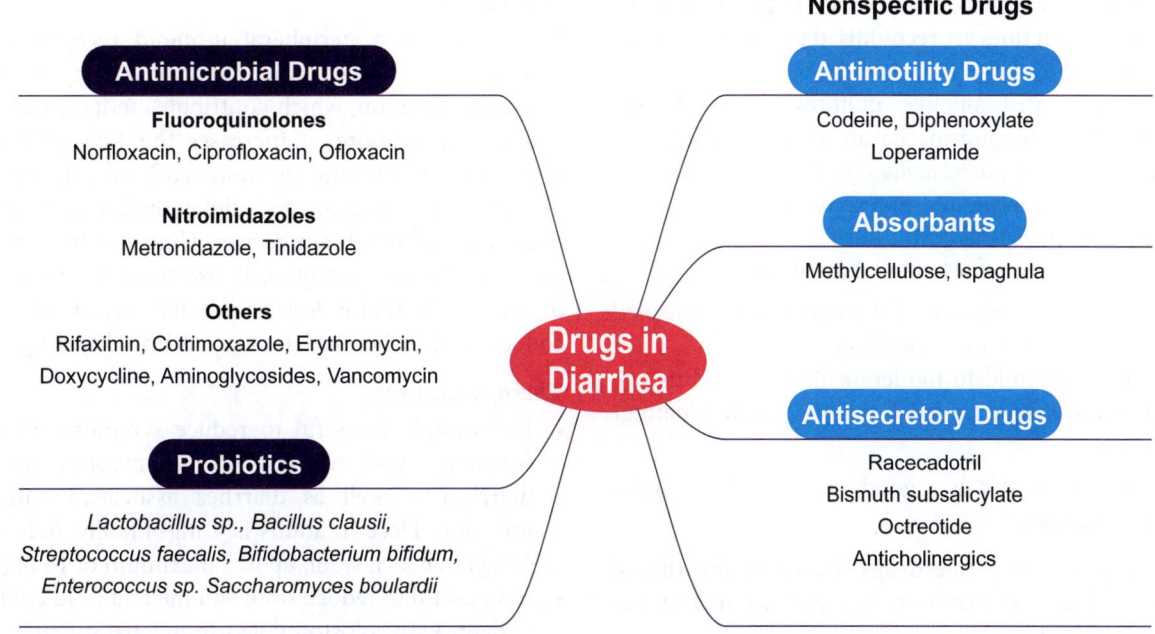

Flowchart 62.1 Classification of antidiarrheal drugs

- *Campylobacter jejuni*: Erythromycin
- *Salmonella*: Restrict the use of antimicrobials to severe cases or immunocompromised patients.
- *Shigella*: FQs and azithromycin are used.
- *Yersinia enterocolitica*: FQs are preferred over cotrimoxazole.
- *Giardia lamblia, Entamoeba histolytica*: Metronidazole 500 mg oral, thrice daily.
- *Clostridium difficile*: Oral vancomycin 125 mg, 6-hourly, for 10–14 days.
- *Vibrio cholera* Along with fluid replacement, tetracyclines are administered in all cases (12.5 mg/kg, 4 times a day for 3 days). Instead, a single dose of doxycycline, 200 mg or 4 mg/kg body weight in patients < 15 years of age may be used to reduce stool volume.

Rifaximin

- It is related to rifamycin. Its **oral absorption is minimal**, resulting in reduced systemic adverse effects and high fecal concentration (about 97% of oral dose); however, it exerts bactericidal effect against many enteric pathogens.
- Its mechanism of action involves irreversible binding to the β-subunit of bacterial DNA-dependent RNA polymerase and **inhibition of bacterial protein synthesis.**
- Rifaximin exerts **bactericidal** action against a wide spectrum of enteric pathogens including **ETEC, Salmonella, Shigella,** and *Campylobacter*. Some enteric antiprotozoal activity is also present.
- Another advantage of rifaximin is **minimal alteration of normal gut flora.**
- Rifaximin is approved by the FDA for the treatment of **travellers' diarrhea**, which is mostly due to enterotoxigenic *E. coli* (ETEC), campylobacter or viruses. The recommended dose for ETEC in patients > 12 years of age is 200 mg, thrice a day, for 3 days.
- However, the efficacy of rifaximin is lower in cases of invasive bacterial diarrhea as its **bactericidal activity is largely restricted to the GI lumen** owing to its poor absorbability.
- Other indications for use include:
  - For the prevention of infection during the perioperative period of gut surgery.
  - For reducing risk of recurrence of hepatic encephalopathy by suppressing NH_3-producing enteric bacteria. Higher doses (up to 550 mg) are used in these cases.
  - 400 mg, given twice/thrice daily, relieves abdominal bloating, flatulence, and flatus by suppressing colonic bacteria.

ADRs

It is a **very well-tolerated** drug with minimal adverse effects because of negligible systemic absorption. However, some patients report ADRs such as **headache, urgency of defecation, and abdominal pain.**

b. Probiotics

Recurrent diarrheal episodes along with irrational and rampant use of antimicrobial agents, even in acute self-limiting diarrhea alters the composition of gut flora. If the nonpathogenic gut flora are recolonised in the gut, balance may be restored.

Probiotics consist of live cultures or lyophilised microbial cells. The organisms that are most frequently used as probiotics include *Lactobacillus sp., Bifidobacterium, St. faecalis, Enterococcus faecalis, Enterococcus faecium*, and a yeast, *Saccharomyces boulardii*.

Probiotics have been reported to be useful in:

- Prevention and treatment of the antibiotics-associated diarrhea and respiratory infections.
- As adjuvants in mild-to-moderate ulcerative colitis.
- Symptomatic subjective relief in patients with bloating/flatulence.

Natural yogurt or curd is a good source of lactic acid-producing organisms.

ADRs: These are very safe drugs. However, the risk of infections and acidosis may be there, especially in immune-compromised individuals.

c. Nonspecific Drugs
1. Antimotility drugs
Codeine, diphenoxylate, loperamide

These are **opioids** that exert their antidiarrheal action through μ- and δ-opioid receptors present on enteric neuronal networks. These drugs also have direct effects on intestinal muscles and mucosa.

Antimotility drugs increase tone, segmentation and reduce propulsive movement → increased resistance to luminal flow → increased transit time → contents remain in the intestinal lumen for longer time → more time is provided for absorption → increased absorption of water from luminal contents + decreased secretion from the intestinal epithelium → constipating effect.

Codeine
It is not used as an antimotility drug because of its abuse potential.

Diphenoxylate
The abuse potential of **diphenoxylate** is much lower than that of codeine; however, it can cross the blood–brain barrier and cause respiratory depression and other central effects. Diphenoxylate is used as an antidiarrheal, exclusively in combination with a **low dose of atropine as a fixed-dose combination**. Although diphenoxylate has good constipating action, the addition of atropine produces disturbing adverse effects such as dry mouth and checks the abuse of diphenoxylate. It is not used in young children as there is risk of paralytic ileus and toxic megacolon.

Loperamide
Loperamide is a peripheral μ-opioid receptor agonist with additional weak anticholinergic activity. It inhibits intestinal secretion, which contributes to its antidiarrheal action. Furthermore, it increases the tone of the anal sphincter, contributing to improved fecal continence. Its advantage over codeine and diphenoxylate is its inability to cross the blood–brain barrier. Thus, it is free of central effects and abuse potential. It also has a longer duration of action. Therefore, loperamide has largely superseded codeine and diphenoxylate as an antimotility drug.

Therapeutic uses

- Loperamide is useful to reduce symptoms like stool frequency and urgency in noninvasive, travellers' diarrhea as well as diarrhea associated with HIV infection. Dose in adults is 4 mg initially, followed by 2 mg after each stool, up to a maximum of 10 mg/day.
- Also useful to reduce stool volume and fluid content in patients with colostomy/ileostomy/anal surgery.
- In chronic diarrhea as in IBS, loperamide is used (2 mg, twice a day) on a short-term basis.

Contraindications

Antimotility drugs are contraindicated in:

- Acute invasive diarrhea caused by EPEC, *Entamoeba histolytica, Shigella*, etc., because of the risk of absorption of toxins from the gut and systemic invasion.
- Severe IBD, because these drugs can raise intraluminal pressure.
- Children < 4 years of age, because of the risk of toxic megacolon, paralytic ileus and absorption of bacterial toxins.

2. Absorbents
Absorbents such as methylcellulose, ispaghula, and carboxymethylcellulose are bulk-forming substances that swell up after absorbing water. Thus, only the frequency and consistency of stool improves, while water/electrolyte loss is not checked. These have limited value in the diarrheal phase of IBS and postileostomy/colostomy cases.

Adsorbants such as pectin, kaolin, and attapulgite are not used currently, as there is no evidence of their efficacy in diarrheal diseases.

3. Antisecretory drugs
Racecadotril, bismuth subsalicylate, octreotide, anticholinergics

- **Racecadotril**, an **inhibitor of the enzyme enkephalinase**, interferes with the metabolism of enkephalins. Enkephalins are endogenous opiates and mainly decrease intestinal secretion through their agonist effect on δ-opioid receptors. However, racecadotril lacks antimotility effect (probably because the antimotility effect of opioids is mediated through μ receptors). Due to this, it is not contraindicated in children (unlike loperamide and diphenoxylate).

It is useful in acute secretory diarrhea (dose: 100 mg, thrice a day, for up to 7 days). Adverse effects include drowsiness, flatulence, nausea and vomiting.

- **Octreotide** is a somatostatin analogue that has antimotility as well as antisecretory effects. It is used for **controlling refractory diarrhea** in cases of carcinoid tumours secreting vasoactive intestinal peptide (VIP) and AIDS patients. It is administered by S/C injection only.
- **Anticholinergic** drugs have some utility in drug-induced diarrhea, diverticulitis and dysentery.

Clinical problem-based questions and MCQs

1. **A 15-year-old boy presents with acute-onset diarrhea characterised by small-volume stools containing blood and mucus, accompanied by cramping abdominal pain. He reports anorexia and a mild fever. There is a history of consuming spicy snacks from a restaurant one day prior to symptom onset. On examination, the patient is febrile, with signs of dehydration including a dry tongue and reduced skin turgor.**
   i. Is this patient suffering from invasive or noninvasive diarrhea?
   ii. Describe the management of this patient.
   iii. Comment on the role of antibiotic treatment in this case.
   iv. Which of the following antibiotics is LEAST effective in this patient?
      a. Ciprofloxacin   c. Doxycycline
      b. Rifaximin   d. Cotrimoxazole

2. **All are advantages of low osmolarity ORS, EXCEPT:**
   a. More reduction in stool volume
   b. Lower risk of hypernatremia
   c. More economical
   d. Slow sustained absorption of water

3. i. Enumerate the constituents of ORS and comment each of their roles.
   ii. What are the various instructions to be given to the patient about safe and effective use of ORS?

4. **IV fluids are indicated in patients of diarrhea if the fluid loss is equivalent to:**
   a. < 5% of body weight
   b. 5–7.5% of body weight
   c. 7.5–10% of body weight
   d. >10% of body weight

5. **Justify the following statements about use of drugs in diarrheal diseases with the pharmacological basis.**
   i. Rifaximin is very beneficial in travellers' diarrhea, but has low efficacy in invasive diarrhea.
   ii. Racecadotril is not contraindicated in children.
   iii. Loperamide has superseded codeine and diphenoxylate as an antimotility drug.

6. **Comment on the use of following in diarrhea.**
   a. Antisecretory drugs
   b. Antimicrobials
   c. Antimotility drugs
   d. Probiotics

INFLAMMATORY BOWEL DISEASE (IBD)

Inflammatory bowel disease (IBD) is an autoimmune disorder characterised by chronic inflammation of the gastrointestinal tract, resulting in damage to the GI mucosa. Genetic, environmental, infectious, and other factors are implicated in the causation of IBD.

Types

Two main inflammatory conditions of the bowel are **ulcerative colitis (UC)** and **Crohn's disease**. Crohn's disease can involve any part of the GI tract from the mouth to anus, whereas ulcerative colitis mainly affects the large intestine or colon. Patients exhibiting features of both ulcerative colitis and Crohn's disease are said to have **indeterminate colitis**.

Clinical Features

IBD symptoms usually manifest following exposure to a gastric irritant (e.g., NSAIDs, antimicrobial agents (AMAs)) or after GI infection. Patients usually complain of abdominal pain (commonly in the epigastric region), cramps, diarrhea, fecal incontinence or urgency, blood in stool, fever, anorexia, weight loss, anemia, other nutritional deficiencies, anxiety and depression. In severe, long-standing forms of IBD, the GI wall may get infected, resulting in the formation of abscesses, fistulas and strictures. Prolonged disease increases the risk of developing colorectal carcinoma. Several extraintestinal features may accompany IBD such as stomatitis, aphthous ulcers, fatty liver, gall stones, sclerosing cholangitis, renal stones, urinary tract infections, joint inflammation, erythema nodosum, and eye inflammations (e.g., episcleritis and uveitis).

Diagnosis

Because the symptoms of IBD overlap with other GI diseases, diagnosis of IBD involves a combination of positive family history, colonoscopy or upper endoscopy with biopsy, imaging (X-rays, CT scan, MRI), stool sample analysis, and biomarkers [erythrocyte sedimentation rate (ESR), C-reactive protein (CRP), anti-saccharomyces cerevisiae antibodies (ASCA) and antineutrophil cytoplasmic antibodies (ANCA)].

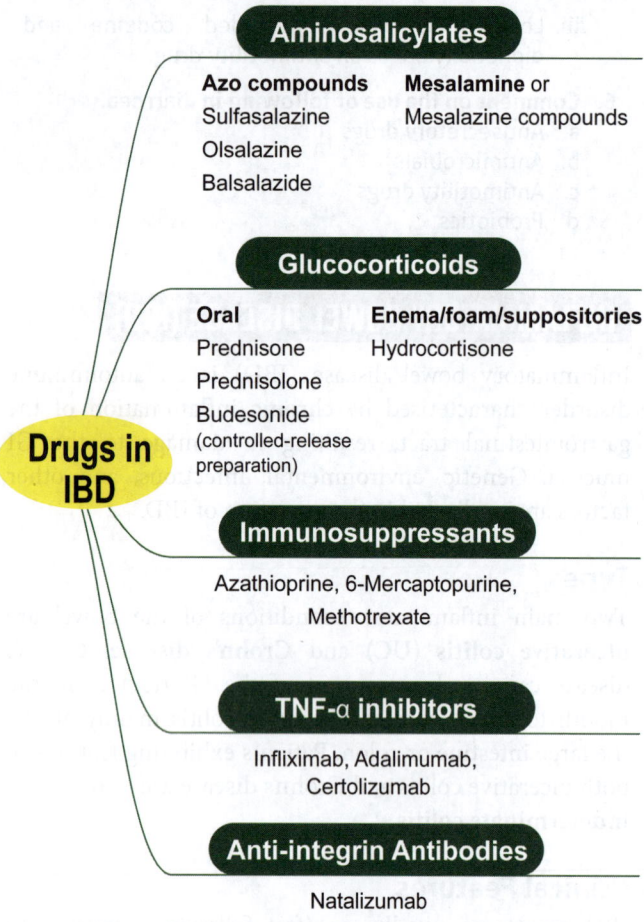

Flowchart 62.2 Drugs for inflammatory bowel disease (IBD)

Management

There is no cure for IBD. The aim of treatment is to control the symptoms, heal inflammation, and maintain remission.

DRUGS USED IN IBD

Drugs useful in IBD can be classified as shown in Flowchart 62.2. These include aminosalicylates. glucocorticoids, immunosuppressants, TNF inhibitors and anti-integrin antibodies.

1. Aminosalicylates

Aminosalicylates include azo compounds such as sulfasalazine, olsalazine, balsalazide and the mesalazine compound mesalamine.

Mechanism of action

5-Aminosalicylic acid (5-ASA) contains an amino group at position 5. Approximately 80% of 5-ASA is absorbed from the small intestine. Delivery of 5-ASA to distal parts of the small intestine and colon can be ensured by decreasing its absorption in the proximal part of small intestine. This is achieved by binding 5-ASA to other molecules by an azo (N=N) bond. 5-ASA is bound to sulphapyridine in sulfasalazine to another 5-ASA molecule in olsalazine, and to 4-aminobenzoyl-β- alanine in balsalazide (Fig. 62.1).

The N=N bond reduces small intestinal absorption of the drug. In the terminal ileum and colon, oxidoreductase enzyme released by commensal bacteria breaks the azo bond, releasing active 5-ASA that exerts topical anti-inflammatory action (Fig. 62.1b). The mechanism of anti-inflammatory action of 5-ASA involves reduced synthesis of prostaglandins and leukotrienes due to inhibition of cyclooxygenase (COX) and lipoxygenase (LOX), respectively. In addition, inhibition of cytokines, TNF-α, PAF, and nuclear transcription factor play an important role in suppressing inflammation.

Mesalamine (or mesalazine) is a controlled-release preparation of 5-ASA coated with pH-sensitive polymers designed to ensure delivery of 5-ASA at specific segments of the small intestine or colon.

Therapeutic uses

The anti-inflammatory effect of 5-ASA released from azo compounds is useful only in ulcerative colitis, and has limited efficacy in Crohn's disease. Sulfasalazine is used in a dose of 3–4 g/day, to induce remission in mild-to-moderate ulcerative colitis exacerbation. The dose for maintenance of remission is 1–2 g/day.

Patients in whom the rectum and distal colon are involved, 5-ASA suppositories or enema (4 g enema given once or twice a day) are effective.

ADRs

- Headache, abdominal pain, nausea and diarrhea are common dose-related ADRs with sulfasalazine.
- Rashes, itching, leukopenia and hypersensitivity reactions have been reported, though rare.
- Sulphapyridine released after degradation of sulfasalazine in the colon gets absorbed and causes many adverse drug reactions such as fever, arthralgia, rashes, blood dyscrasias, hemolysis, oligozoospermia, and male infertility.
- Olsalazine is free of the above ADRs, but it may aggravate diarrhea at the beginning of therapy.
- Balsalazine also has an inert carrier, and is better tolerated than sulfasalazine.
- Mesalazine is also better tolerated but has nephrotoxic potential.

2. Corticosteroids

Corticosteroids play an important role in controlling symptoms and inducing remission in acute exacerbation of both ulcerative colitis as well as Crohn's disease. Corticosteroids are also used in patients who do not respond to aminosalicylates. Prednisolone is used orally in a dose of 40–60 mg. In patients with proctitis and proctosigmoiditis, hydrocortisone foam/enema is useful, although its efficacy is lower than oral prednisolone.

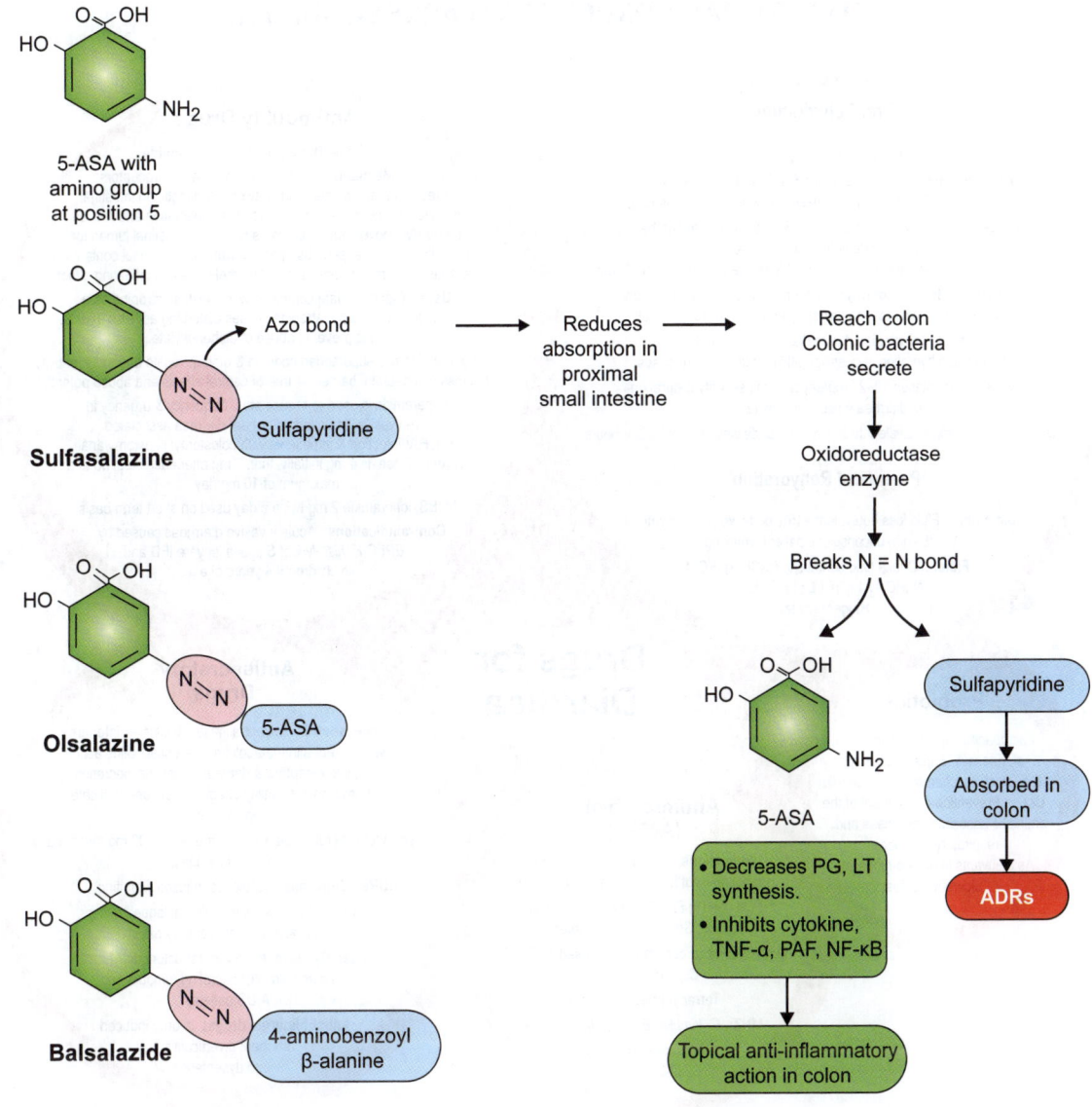

Fig. 62.1 (a) Structure of aminosalicylates, (b) Mechanism of action of sulfasalazine

Treatment with corticosteroids is given for short term only to induce remission, followed by tapering down of dose and stopping therapy. Remission is then maintained with aminosalicylates.

3. Immunosuppressants

Azathioprine and 6-mercaptopurine are purine antagonists. Methotrexate causes pseudo-irreversible inhibition of dihydrofolate reductase enzyme. While immunosuppressants have good efficacy in maintaining remission, they are not dependable for inducing remission.

In steroid-resistant and steroid-dependent cases of severe IBD, however, they are used to induce remission. Steroid-resistant cases fail to respond to steroids, while steroid-dependent cases show flare up of disease upon stopping steroid therapy.

Azathioprine and 6-mercaptopurine are used frequently. Methotrexate given as weekly injections is used in patients of Crohn's disease who do not respond to or tolerate azathioprine.

4. TNF-α inhibitors

Infliximab is a chimeric anti-TNF-α antibody that has several adverse toxic effects such as acute reactions and decreased immunity to infections. Therefore, it is reserved for use in patients suffering from severe refractory Crohn's disease with fistulas and ulcerative colitis that do not respond to corticosteroids or immunosuppressants.

Adalimumab and certolizumab also have anti-TNF-α action, but are used only in refractory cases because of their intolerable adverse effects.

5. Anti-integrin antibody

Natalizumab is a new drug indicated in patients of Crohn's disease not responding to or not tolerating infliximab or other anti-TNF-α antibodies.

CONCEPT MAP – DRUGS FOR DIARRHEA AND IBD

Drugs for Diarrhea

Oral Rehydration

Low Osmolarity ORS

Ingredients: NaCl 2.6 g, KCl 1.5 g, Trisodium citrate 2.9 g, Glucose 13.5 g and Water to make 1 litre (total 245 mOsm/L).

Role: Na^+, K^+, Cl^- make up for ionic loss & maintain electrolyte balance. HCO_3^- / citrate help to correct acidosis. Glucose facilitates absorption of Na^+ via Na^+–glucose co-transporter in ileum.

Advantages of low osmolarity: Faster absorption, more reduction in vomiting & stool volume, no risk of hypernatremia, economical.

Uses: Dehydration due to diarrhea, heat stroke. To maintain hydration in post-operative, trauma & burn cases. Zn supplementation 10–20 mg/day reduces severity & duration of diarrhea episode in children.

Dose: ORS volume equivalent to 5–7.5 % of body weight in initial 2–4 hours

Parenteral Rehydration

Indications: Fluid loss equivalent >10% body weight or at rate of 10 mL/kg/h, unconscious patient, vomiting.

Fluids: Dhaka fluid containing NaCl 5 g, KCl 1 g $NaHCO_3$ 4 g in 1 L of 5% glucose Ringer lactate.

Probiotics

Lactobacillus sp, Bifidobacterium, st. Faecalis, Enterococcus sp. & a yeast *Saccharomyces boulardii.*

Uses: Prevention & treatment of the antibiotic-associated diarrheas and respiratory infections. As adjuvants in mild-to-moderate ulcerative colitis.

Antimicrobials (AMAs)

Indications: Frequently prescribed irrationally, but have role only in following;

FQs used in EPEC, severe *Salmonella* infection, *Shigella, Yersinia* infection.

Doxycycline or cotrimoxazole used in ETEC, *C. jejuni* infection.

Tetracyclines in cholera.

MNZ: *G. lamblia, E. histolytica* infection.

Oral vancomycin in *C. difficile* infection.

Antimotility Drugs

Codeine, Diphenoxylate, Loperamide

Mechanism: Opioids act on µ and δ receptors present on enteric neuronal networks & directly on intestinal muscles & mucosa → increase tone, segmentation and reduce propulsive movement → contents remain in intestinal lumen for longer time → increased absorption of water from luminal contents & decreased secretion from intestinal epithelium → constipating effect.

Uses: Diphenoxylate combined with low dose atropine as a fixed-dose combination. Atropine causes disturbing adverse effects, thus prevents abuse of diphenoxylate.

Loperamide has superseded codeine & diphenoxylate due to its inability to cross blood–brain barrier → free of central effects and abuse potential.

Loperamide is used to reduce stool frequency & urgency in non-invasive, travellers, diarrhea, diarrhea associated with HIV infection & in patients with colostomy/ ileostomy/anal surgery. Dose is 4 mg initially, then 2 mg after each stool up to a maximum of 10 mg/day.

In IBS, loperamide 2 mg twice a day used on short term basis.

Contraindications: Acute invasive diarrheas caused by EPEC/*E. histolytica*/ *Shigella*, severe IBD and in children < 4 years of age.

Antisecretory Drugs

Racecadotril: Enkephalinase inhibitor → interferes with enkephalin metabolism → enkephalins act on δ-opioid receptors & decrease intestinal secretion, but have no antimotility effect, so not contraindicated in children.

Use: Acute secretory diarrheas in a dose of 100 mg thrice a day for up to 7 days.

ADRs: Drowsiness, flatulence, nausea, vomiting.

Octreotide: Somatostatin analogue having antimotility + antisecretory effect.

Use: By SC route only in refractory diarrhea in carcinoid, VIP-secreting tumours and AIDS patients.

Anticholinergic drugs: In drug induced diarrhea, diverticulitis and dysenteries.

Drugs for IBD

Aminosalicylates

Sulfasalazine, Olsalazine, Balsalazide, Mesalazine

Mechanism: Azo N=N bond reduces small intestinal absorption of drug. In terminal ileum and colon, oxidoreductase enzyme breaks the azo bond, releasing active 5-ASA → topical anti-inflammatory action.

Uses: Sulfasalazine 3–4 g/day, to induce remission in mild-to-moderate ulcerative colitis exacerbation. Dose for maintenance is 1–2 g. 5-ASA suppositories or enema in patients having involvement of rectum or distal colon. Limited efficacy in Crohn's disease.

ADRs: Headache, abdominal pain, nausea, diarrhea. Rarely rashes, itching, leukopenia and hypersensitivity reactions. Sulfapyridine released after degradation of sulfasalazine in colon, gets absorbed → fever, arthralgia, rashes, blood dyscrasias, hemolysis, oligozoospermia, male infertility etc. Olsalazine is free of above ADRs, but may aggravate diarrhea at beginning of therapy. Balsalazine is better tolerated than sulfasalazine. Mesalazine is better tolerated, but has nephrotoxic potential.

Others

Glucocorticoids

Control symptoms & induce remission in acute exacerbation of ulcerative colitis and Crohn's disease.

Prednisolone oral 40–60 mg used in patients not responding to aminosalicylates. Hydrocortisone foam/enema used in patients with proctitis and proctosigmoiditis, although its efficacy is less than oral prednisolone.

Corticosteroids given for short term only to induce remission, followed by tapering down of dose and stopping therapy. Remission then maintained with aminosalicylates.

Immunosuppressants

Azathioprine, 6-mercaptopurine, methotrexate have good efficacy in maintaining remission, but are not dependable for inducing remission. Used in steroid-dependent and steroid-resistant cases.

TNF-α inhibitors

Infliximab is reserved for use in patients suffering from severe refractory Crohn's disease with fistulas, ulcerative colitis, not responding to corticosteroids as well as immunosuppressants. Many ADRs like acute reactions, decreased immunity.

Chapter 62 Drugs for Diarrhea, IBD, and Constipation

> **Clinical problem-based questions and MCQs**
>
> 7. A 27-year-old female patient was referred to the surgery department hospital with a 2-months history of severe abdominal pain, persistent diarrhea with passage of > 15 watery stools with mucus and blood, and intense urgency to defecate after every meal. The patient avoided eating much for fear of aggravation of her symptoms and has lost 5–6 kg of body weight. She also complained of tiredness and weakness in her legs. On examination, tenderness is present in the left iliac fossa and hypogastrium. GI infection was ruled out in routine investigations. Colonoscopy revealed friable mucosa, multiple ulcerations, and pseudopolyps extending up to the level of transverse colon. Biopsy shows crypt abscesses, shortening and branching of crypts, and neutrophil infiltration in mucosa and submucosa. A diagnosis of ulcerative colitis was made.
>   i. Enumerate the drugs used for inducing remission in this case.
>   ii. Enumerate the drugs for maintaining remission, once it is achieved.
> 8. Azo compounds do not have much efficacy in Crohn's disease. Explain.
> 9. i. Identify the correct method used for reducing absorption of 5-ASA from the proximal small intestine.
>   a. Binding with sulphapyridine through the N=N bond.
>   b. Adding a carbon moiety at position 5
>   c. Making microfine preparations
>   d. All of the above
>   ii. What is the advantage of reduced absorption of 5-ASA in the proximal small intestine?

does not involve any dysfunction of the pelvic floor is called **colonic inertia** or **slow transit constipation (STC)**. It may be attributed to reduced peristaltic activity in the colon due to endocrine abnormality or disorders of enteric nervous system (ENS).

Secondary constipation is related to some diseases, mechanical obstruction, or drugs.

Management

The initial management of constipation includes disimpaction by manual manoeuvring and transrectal enemas. Chronic constipation is prevented and managed by following the **bowel management pyramid** (Fig. 62.2).

- **Lifestyle modification** and laxative drugs form the wide base of the pyramid. Dietary changes have great impact in preventing constipation. Patients are counselled to increase water intake to stay hydrated, increase fibre intake, correct nutritional deficiencies, and reduce consumption of constipating foods like milk/tea/coffee/alcohol. In addition, aerobic exercises are reported to activate bowel movement. Toilet training and patient education and awareness are other important measures in the management of constipation.
- Pharmacological measures include **laxatives**. Though effective in the short term, long-term use is habit forming and not recommended.
- In patients who do not show adequate response, **nonpharmacological measures** such as biofeedback therapy, suppositories, and acupuncture, are indicated. Bio-feedback therapy involves neuromuscular training, along with visual and verbal feedback in patients having incoordination of abdominal and pelvic floor muscles.

CONSTIPATION

Constipation is a frequent symptom of GIT diseases. According to the Rome IV criteria, a patient is classified as constipated if any two of the following features are present:

- Fewer than 3 spontaneous bowel movements in a week
- Straining at stool
- Passing hard stools or need for manual manoeuvring for at least 25% of defecation attempts
- Feeling of incomplete evacuation
- Pain in anorectal region

Additional symptoms such as abdominal bloating, lower backache, spurious diarrhea, and painful defecation may be present.

Types

Constipation can be primary or secondary.

Primary constipation is functional or idiopathic, and is commonly encountered in elderly people from lower socioeconomic strata. Severe functional constipation that

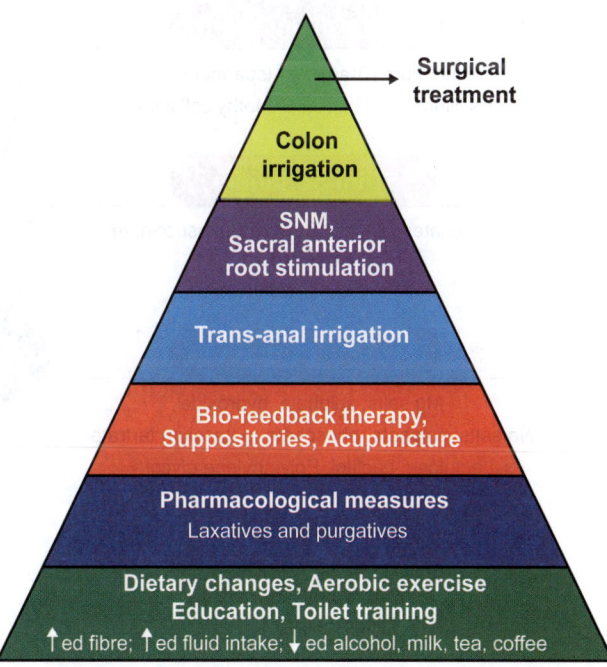

Fig. 62.2 Bowel management pyramid

- In refractory cases, **trans-anal irrigation** (TAI) is advised. It is a simple procedure in which water at body temperature is self-administered into the rectum through a catheter or silicone cone. This results in evacuation of stool from the lower part of the bowel.
- In intractable cases, more **invasive procedures** like sacral nerve modulation (SNM), colon irrigation, sacral anterior root stimulation, and surgery are required.
- The sacral nerve, which supplies the rectal nerve and muscle complex, is electrically stimulated by a small pacemaker-like device implanted under the skin in the upper buttock region. It can be useful for managing intractable constipation or rectal incontinence due to trauma, surgery or congenital abnormalities of the anal canal. Sacral anterior root stimulation may relieve bowel symptoms associated with spinal cord injury.
- In patients suffering from chronic constipation due to diseases like spina bifida, megacolon, and recurrent sigmoid volvulus, surgical treatment is indicated. Procedures such as subtotal colectomy, segmental resections, and loop colostomy may be considered as a last resort to relieve chronic constipation in such patients.

Laxatives and Purgatives

Laxatives and purgatives promote gut evacuation. **Laxatives or aperients have milder action** and cause elimination of soft, formed stools, whereas **purgatives or cathartics have stronger action** and cause more fluid evacuation. Many drugs act as laxative in low dose and purgative in higher dose.

CLASSIFICATION OF LAXATIVES/PURGATIVES

Important drugs used as laxatives/purgatives are shown in the Flowchart 62.3. These include bulk purgatives, stool softeners, osmotic and stimulant purgatives and peripheral opioid antagonist.

Bulk Purgatives

Dietary fibre (Bran)

Bran is a by-product of the flour industry and has ~40% insoluble dietary fibre. Insoluble dietary fibre consists of the cell wall and other constituents of vegetable food that are **not absorbed**, i.e., cellulose, pectins, glycoproteins, and other polysaccharides.

Psyllium/Ispaghula

Psyllium or ispaghula husk is a source of soluble fibre (natural colloidal mucilage), which forms a gelatinous mass by absorbing water.

Methylcellulose/carboxymethylcellulose

These are semisynthetic, colloidal, hydrophilic derivatives of cellulose.

Mechanism of action
- Bran **absorbs water in the intestines** to form a bulky emollient gel that distends the colon and promotes peristalsis. It swells up and increases water content of feces. It softens stool and favours its colonic transit (Fig. 62.3).

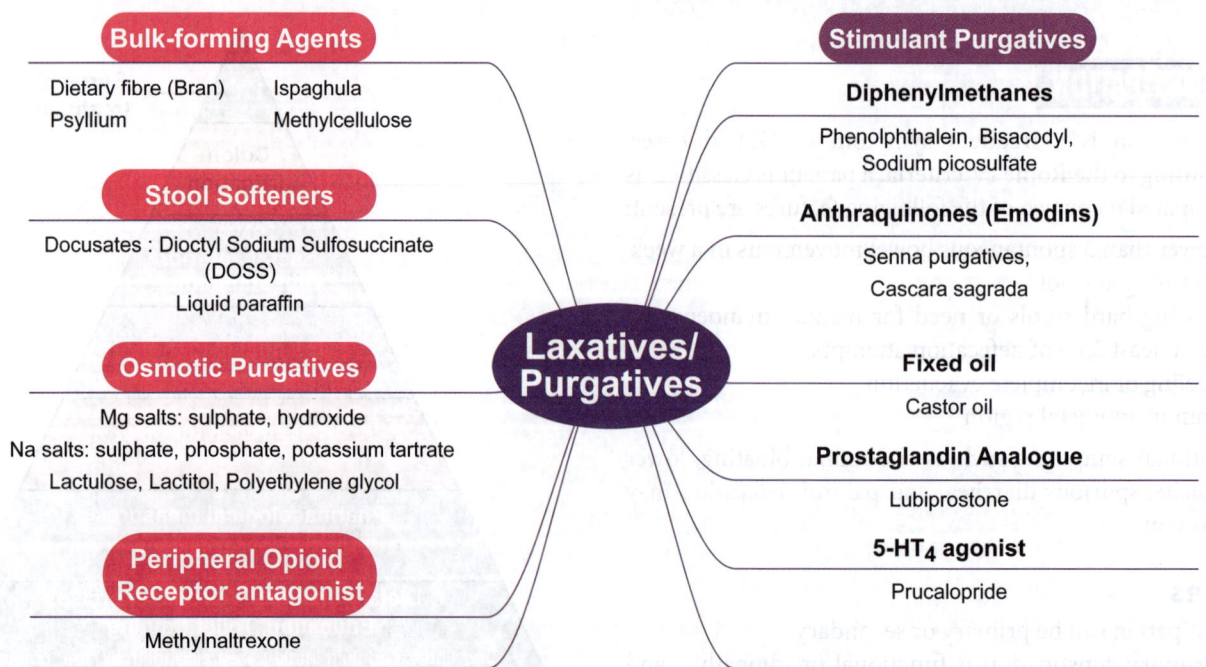

Flowchart 62.3 Classification of laxatives/purgatives

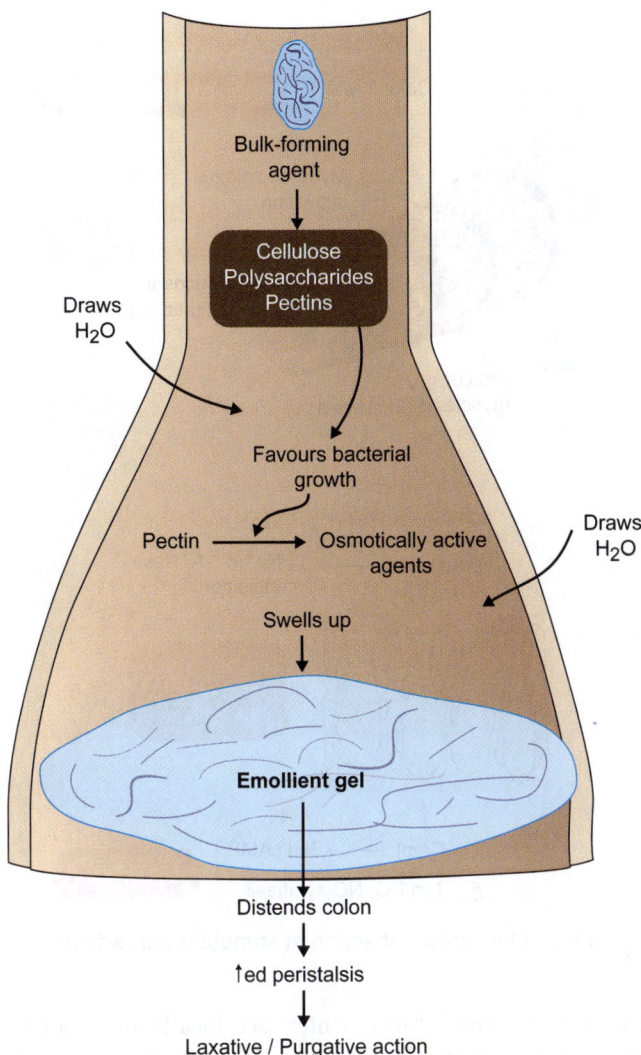

Fig. 62.3 Mechanism of action of bulk purgatives

- Bacterial degradation of pectins, etc., in the colon may form osmotically active products which retain water.
- Prolonged intake of bran or other bulk-forming agents reduces recto-sigmoidal intraluminal pressure → relief of symptoms of IBS, colonic diverticulosis. Their fermentation in the colon increases bacterial content, resulting in softening of feces.

Some dietary fibres such as gums, pectins, and lignins **bind to bile acids** and are excreted in feces. This, in turn, favours cholesterol degradation in the liver, resulting in lowering of plasma LDL cholesterol.

Therapeutic uses
Main use of bulk purgatives is to prevent functional constipation (most appropriate first-line method), especially if the patient's diet is deficient in fibre.

- A large quantity of bran (20–40 g/day) needs to be ingested.
- Psyllium/ ispaghula (3–12 g) is freshly mixed with water or milk and given daily. Action starts in 1–3 days.

However, it should not be swallowed dry for fear of esophageal impaction.
- Methylcellulose is useful when straining at stools has to be avoided (as in cardiac patients and after eye surgery) and to improve consistency of stools in colostomy patients. The dose is 4–6 g/day.
- Water intake must be sufficient with all bulk-forming agents, as these swell up upon absorbing wate.

Limitations
Bulk purgatives are safe and useful for the prevention, but not for treatment of constipation. Moreover, they:

- are unpalatable
- do not soften feces already present in the colon or rectum. Full effect appears after 3–4 days.
- cause flatulence.
- are not to be used in patients with gut ulcerations, adhesions, stenosis, etc., for the fear of fecal impaction.
- may worsen symptoms of IBS.

2. Stool Softeners or Surfactants
Dioctyl sodium sulfosuccinate (DOSS)
Dioctyl sodium sulfosuccinate is an anionic detergent with mild action.

Mechanism of action
DOSS emulsifies colonic contents and increases water and lipid penetration into feces, resulting in softening of stools. It is used in conditions when straining at stools must be avoided (after eye surgery, hernia, cardiac disease, anal fistula, and anal surgery).

ADRs
- It can disrupt the mucosal barrier, **enhancing the absorption** of many nonabsorbable drugs such as **liquid paraffin**. Therefore, DOSS and liquid paraffin should not be combined.
- It may cause **cramps and abdominal pain**.
- Bitter taste can cause **nausea** in liquid preparations.
- Prolonged use may have hepatotoxic effects.

Liquid paraffin
Liquid paraffin is a pharmacologically inert mixture of petroleum hydrocarbons. It lubricates hard scybala by coating them, and softens stools after 2–3 days of use. However, it is **not preferred because of many disadvantages** such as unpalatable taste, risk of formation of foreign body granulomas in intestines, lipid pneumonia, impaired healing of anorectal lesions, and deficiency of fat soluble vitamins associated with long-term use.

Glycerin suppositories may also be used as a stool softener.

3. Stimulant Purgatives
Stimulant purgatives usually have stronger action than other purgatives.

Mechanism of action

Multiple mechanisms contribute to purgative action of stimulant purgatives (Fig 62.4).

- They irritate the intestinal mucosa, stimulating motor activity.
- Some of them primarily increase motility by acting on myenteric plexuses.
- They alter the absorptive and secretory activity of mucosal cells → accumulation of water and electrolytes in the lumen.
- They act by inhibiting Na^+/K^+-ATPase at the basolateral membrane of villous cells → reduced transport of Na^+ and accompanying water into the interstitium.
- Secretion is enhanced by the activation of cAMP in crypt cells.
- Increased NO and PG synthesis also enhances secretion.

The following groups are included in stimulant purgatives.

a. Diphenylmethanes

Phenolphthalein, bisacodyl, sodium picosulfate

- These are partly absorbed and re-excreted in bile. Enterohepatic recirculation is more prominent with phenolphthalein, resulting in protracted action.
- **Bisacodyl** is activated in the intestine by deacetylation. The primary site of action is the colon, where it has **irritant action on colonic mucosa** resulting in **increased fluid secretion and peristaltic activity**. Bowel evacuation occurs in 6–8 hours. Bisacodyl suppositories irritate rectal and anal mucosa → reflex increase in motility and evacuation occurs within 20–40 minutes. However, it can cause inflammation and mucosal damage. Dose of bisacodyl is 5–10 mg, based on patient response.
- Sodium **picosulfate** is hydrolysed by colonic bacteria. It also irritates colonic mucosa, increases secretion, and activates myenteric neurons, resulting in increased peristaltic activity.

ADRs

- Fluid evacuations, cramps, and morphological alterations that make colonic mucosa more leaky.
- Allergic reactions like skin rashes and fixed drug eruptions.
- Stevens–Johnson syndrome may occur.
- **Phenolphthalein** has been withdrawn due to reports of tumours, genetic damages, and cardiac toxicity in mice.

b. Anthraquinones (Emodins)

Senna purgatives (obtained from leaves and pods of certain plants of *Cassia* species), *Cascara sagrada* (prepared from the powdered bark of buckthorn tree)

Mechanism of action

Anthraquinones are glycosides, which are not active as such. These drugs are not absorbed in the small intestine, and pass on to the colon. In the colon, bacteria liberate

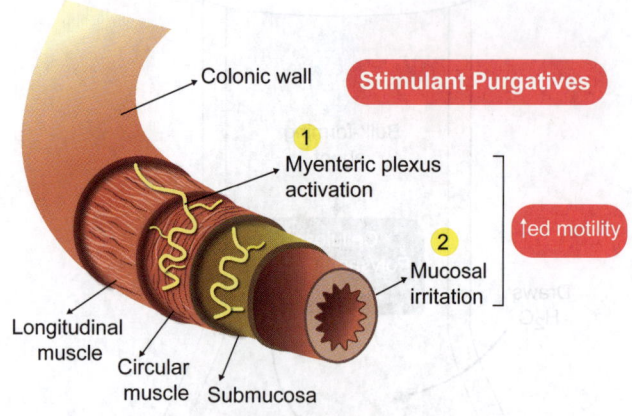
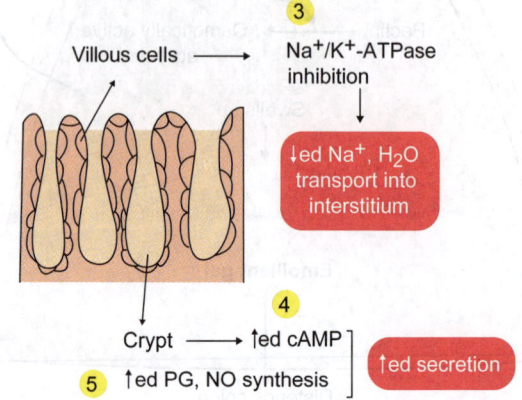

Fig. 62.4 Mechanism of action of stimulant purgatives

the active anthrol form, which act locally on colonic mucosa to **inhibit salt and water absorption**. Some part of the anthrol form gets absorbed and is then secreted in the bile to act on the myenteric plexus in the small intestine, resulting in **increased peristalsis and reduced segmentation**. Therefore, onset of action takes 6–8 hours.

Senna has been shown to stimulate PGE_2 synthesis in rat intestine, which is blocked by indomethacin. Consequently, indomethacin reduces the purgative action of senna.

Adverse effects

- Skin rashes, fixed drug eruptions, cramps, and excess purging.
- Regular use for 4–12 months may cause destruction and dependence of myenteric plexus, leading to colonic atony and dilatation.
- Brown pigmentation of colonic mucosa called melanosis coli.

c. Fixed oils

Castor oil is a bland vegetable oil that contains a triglyceride of ricinoleic acid. It gets hydrolysed in the ileum by lipase to form **ricinoleic acid** and **glycerol**. Ricinoleic acid is polar and hence poorly absorbed. It was believed to **irritate the mucosa** and stimulate intestinal contractions.

However, its primary action is shown to be decreased intestinal absorption, and enhanced secretion of water and electrolytes through a **detergent like action** on the mucosa. **Peristalsis is increased** secondarily.

When taken in a dose of 15–25 mL in the morning, it causes passage of semifluid stool with griping within 2–3 hours.

Adverse effects

It is not frequently used, as it has many adverse effects such as unpalatable taste, violent action with griping, cramping, risk of dehydration, and after-constipation. Regular use may damage intestinal mucosa.

d. Prostaglandin analogues

Lubiprostone acts as an agonist at EP_4 receptors → stimulates guanylyl cyclase C, and activates Cl^- channels in the intestinal mucosa. Thus, intestinal fluid is chloride-rich. Colonic passage of stool is also accelerated. Refractoriness to its action does not occur even with long-term use. However, it can cause nausea, delayed gastric emptying and dyspepsia as adverse effects. Currently, it is recommended only in patients with idiopathic chronic constipation who do not respond to other purgatives, and IBS cases with constipation as the predominant symptom.

e. 5-HT_4 agonist

Prucalopride is an agonist at presynaptic 5-HT_4 receptors present on intrinsic enteric neurons, resulting in increased ACh release. ACh increases propulsive contractions in the ileum and colon, relieving constipation. **Adverse effects** include headache, dizziness, abdominal pain and diarrhea.

4. Osmotic Purgatives

In the colon, fecal water is isotonic. Thus, the colon is unable to dilute or concentrate fecal fluid under normal circumstances.

Mechanism of action: Osmotic purgatives are solutes that are not absorbed in the intestine. These retain water osmotically, resulting in distension of the bowel that indirectly increases peristalsis. These osmotically active solutes include nonabsorbable salts and sugars.

a. Magnesium salts

Magnesium sulphate (5–15 g) is bitter in taste, while magnesium hydroxide (30 mL of 8% w/w suspension) is bland. Mg^{2+} ions release cholecystokinin, which also helps in their purgative action. However, these are contraindicated in renal failure

b. Sodium salts

Sodium sulphate tastes bad; sodium phosphate is not so unpleasant; whereas sodium potassium tartrate has a pleasant taste.

Saline purgatives are contraindicated in CHF. These are used infrequently as they have poor palatability, and cause watery stools, fluid–electrolyte imbalance, and after-constipation.

c. Lactulose

It is a disaccharide containing lactose and fructose that is not digested or absorbed from the small intestine. In the colon, bacteria convert lactulose into osmotically active acidic products that retain water, resulting in the passage of soft, formed stools. Stool pH is lowered, making it unfavourable for the survival of ammonia-producing organisms. Thus, lactulose lowers blood NH_3 concentration. This effect is beneficial in patients with hepatic encephalopathy. It can cause flatulence, flatus, and cramps as adverse effects. Lactulose has a peculiar sweet taste, which is nauseating and unpalatable for some patients.

d. Lactitol

Lactitol is a disaccharide sugar alcohol with the same mechanism of action and uses as lactulose, but with improved taste and patient acceptability.

5. Methylnaltrexone

Methylnaltrexone is an antagonist at peripheral opioid μ-receptors, which is used to reverse opioid-induced constipation in terminally ill patients on opioid therapy. As it does not cross the blood–brain barrier, the analgesic action of opioids is not blocked.

INDICATIONS FOR USE OF PURGATIVES

1. **Functional constipation**: This is a condition where stool frequency is less than once in 2 days, there is straining at stool, and a feeling of incomplete evacuation. While nonpharmacological measures such as increased water and dietary fibre intake, and regular exercise are helpful, drug treatment is indicated when there is inadequate response to these measures.
   - In spastic constipation, characterised by hard/rounded/difficult to pass stools, the drug of choice is ispaghula or bran, which relieves the symptoms over a few weeks. Stimulant purgatives are not to be used in spastic constipation.
   - In sluggish bowel causing atonic constipation, bulk-forming or osmotic purgatives are used. Stimulant purgatives are given only in refractory cases that do not respond to bulk-forming or osmotic purgatives.
2. To avoid straining at stools in conditions such as hernia, hemorrhoids, anal fissures, and after ophthalmic/cardiovascular/anal surgery, bulk-forming, agents or stool softeners like DOSS or lactulose are used frequently.
3. To prevent or treat constipation in chronically sick, bedridden patients (following stroke, fractures, MI, etc.), bulk-forming laxatives such as docusates and lactulose are frequently prescribed.

4. Saline purgatives, senna purgatives, and bisacodyl are used for gut preparation before surgical procedures.
5. Saline purgatives may be used in the case of food or oral drug poisoning to quickly excrete the unabsorbed portion.
6. Saline purgatives are used to flush out tapeworms or other helminths, for example, with piperazine.

ADRs

Self-prescription and overuse of purgatives causes **purgative abuse** that may have adverse consequences such as fluid–electrolyte imbalance, spastic colitis, malabsorption syndrome, steatorrhea, and protein-losing enteropathy.

Clinical problem-based questions and MCQs

10. i. Which of the following purgatives is CONTRAINDICATED in a patient of stroke having functional constipation and chronic renal failure?
    a. Magnesium hydroxide   b. Saline purgatives
    c. Lactitol   d. Ispaghula
    ii. Describe the mechanism of purgative action of the selected drug.

11. A 45-year-old male patient is admitted in the medicine ward with severe alcoholic liver disease and hepatic encephalopathy. Raised blood NH_3 can worsen encephalopathy. All of the following drugs can lower blood NH_3 levels, EXCEPT:
    a. Oral neomycin   b. Lactulose
    c. Lactitol   d. DOSS

12. i. All of the following are stimulant purgatives, EXCEPT:
    a. DOSS   b. Senna purgatives
    c. Lubiprostone   d. Bisacodyl
    ii. Describe the mechanism of purgative action of the selected drug.

13. Match the drug with the correct mechanism of action.

    | a. Bisacodyl | 1. Retains water osmotically |
    | b. Lubiprostone | 2. Agonist at 5-HT_4 presynaptic receptors |
    | c. Prucalopride | 3. Inhibiting Na^+/K^+-ATPase on villous cell |
    | d. Lactitol | 4. Agonist at EP_4 receptors |

IRRITABLE BOWEL SYNDROME (IBS)

Irritable bowel syndrome (IBS) is characterised by altered bowel movements and abdominal discomfort. It is more prevalent in females. IBS may be caused by increased nerve sensitivity or motility problems arising from the incoordination between nerves and GI wall muscles.

- IBS can be constipation-predominant, diarrhea-predominant, mixed type with alternating periods of constipation and diarrhea, or unclassified. Usually, there are complaints of abdominal bloating and cramps, but without any inflammation of the GI tract. Diagnosis is based on complete medical history, physical examination and investigations to rule out other gastrointestinal diseases.
- The Rome criteria for diagnosing IBS are: presence of abdominal pain/discomfort as well as any two of the following three symptoms—pain while defecating, change in consistency, or change in frequency of stools.
- Management of IBS mainly aims at symptomatic control by lifestyle modification, dietary changes, avoidance of factors that trigger symptoms, stress reduction, regular exercise, etc. Drug treatment is symptom-specific, based on predominant symptoms in a particular patient. Constipation-predominant IBS is managed using laxatives, while the diarrhea-predominant type is managed using antisecretory and antispasmodic drugs. In addition, antidepressant drugs are sometimes prescribed to control the associated psychological symptoms.

Summary

Antidiarrheals

- Management of diarrhea involves rehydration therapy (oral or parenteral), maintaining nutritional status, and nonspecific drugs (antimotility, antisecretory, antimicrobials, probiotics, etc.).
- Oral rehydration therapy is used in mild-to-moderate fluid loss (5–10% of body weight) to maintain hydration and fluid–electrolyte and acid–base balance. ORS volume equivalent to 5–7.5% of body weight is given in the initial 2–4 hours. ORS contains NaCl 2.6 g, KCl 1.5 g, trisodium citrate 2.9 g, glucose 13.5 g, and made up to 1 litre using water.
- Low-osmolarity formula is recommended, as it is reported to cause faster absorption, greater reduction in incidence of vomiting and stool volume than the older formula, and is economical. Moreover, the risk of hypernatremia is not seen with it.
- Parenteral rehydration (using NaCl 5 g, KCl 1 g, and $NaHCO_3$ 4 g in 1 L of 5% glucose) is required when fluid loss is > 10% of body weight.
- Simple, easily digestible foods are given to maintain nutritional status; if not, disaccharidase enzyme in the brush border of GI mucosa decreases, which reduces the absorption of salt, water and nutrients, and increases the luminal osmotic load.
- AMAs are used in invasive diarrhea caused by EPEC, ETEC, *Campylobacter jejuni*, *Salmonella*, *Shigella*, *Yersinia enterocolitica*, *Giardia lamblia*, *Entamoeba histolytica* and *Vibrio cholera* infections. FQs are effective against infections caused by EPEC, Yersinia, and Shigella. MNZ is used in the treatment of amebiasis and giardiasis. Doxycycline is effective against Vibrio cholerae and ETEC, while rifaximin is indicated for traveler's diarrhea.

- Among antimotility drugs, loperamide is preferred over codeine and diphenoxylate as it is free of central side effects and abuse potential. These are not used in children for risk of obstruction, paralytic ileus, megacolon, etc.
- Antisecretory drug racecadotril interferes with degradation of enkephalins; so, it affects δ but not μ receptors. It has antisecretory but not antimotility effect, and is not contraindicated in children.

Inflammatory bowel disease (ulcerative colitis, Crohn's disease, and indeterminate colitis)
- Aminosalicylates (sulfasalazine, olsalazine, balsalazide, mesalazine) release 5-ASA in the terminal ileum and colon for topical anti-inflammatory action. These are useful for maintaining remission in ulcerative colitis, but have low efficacy in Crohn's disease. Adverse effects of sulfasalazine (fever, rashes, arthralgia, blood dyscrasia, hemolysis, oligozoospermia, and infertility) are attributed to its sulphapyridine moiety. Olsalazine and balsalazide are better tolerated than sulfasalazine.
- Glucocorticoids such as oral prednisolone are used to induce remission in acute exacerbation of both ulcerative colitis and Crohn's disease. However, systemic use of steroids causes many disturbing adverse effects, and should be limited to short periods. Aminosalicylates are given after tapering down steroids for maintaining remission.
- Immunosuppressants (azathioprine, 6-MP) are given in steroid-dependent and steroid-resistant cases.
- TNF-α inhibitors (e.g., infliximab) are reserve drugs for patients not responding to steroids or immunosuppressants.

Laxatives and purgatives
- Bran is nonabsorbable dietary fibre that absorbs water and swells up; it forms osmotically active substances from pectins, and promotes bacterial growth in the colon. It binds to bile acids and lowers LDL. It is useful in prevention, but not treatment, of constipation. Limitations include bad taste and the resulting flatulence; it may cause fecal impaction in adhesions, and stenosis in ulcer patients, and thus, contraindicated.
- Psyllium and ispaghula are natural colloidal mucilage, while methylcellulose is a semisynthetic derivative; they form a gelatinous mass by absorbing water and relieve symptoms of IBS.
- DOSS emulsifies colonic contents and increases water and lipid penetration into feces, resulting in softening of stools. It is used when straining at stools must be avoided.
- Liquid paraffin can lubricate hard scybala by coating these, but is not used due to its several disadvantages.
- Stimulant purgatives act by inhibiting Na^+/K^+-ATPase at the basolateral membrane of villous cells → reduced transport of Na^+ and accompanying water into the interstitium. Bisacodyl has irritant action on colonic mucosa, resulting in increased fluid secretion and peristaltic activity. Bowel evacuation occurs in 6–8 hours.
- Osmotic purgatives are solutes that are not absorbed from the intestine, and get converted to osmotically active products in the colon; they retain water and help in passing soft, formed stools. Magnesium salts are contraindicated in renal failure and sodium salts in CHF. Lactulose and lactitol are useful in hepatic encephalopathy for reducing blood NH_3 concentration.
- Laxatives or purgatives are useful in functional constipation (spastic/ atonic), prevention of constipation in chronically ill, bedridden patients, to prevent straining at stools, along with some anthelmintics, and for gut preparation before surgery.

Hints for problem-based questions and MCQs

1. i. Invasive diarrhea
   ii. Rehydration and antimicrobial therapy. Refer to pages 811, 812.
   iii. Refer to page 812.
   iv. b. Rifaximin has bactericidal activity but is largely restricted to the GI lumen due to its poor absorbability. So, it is least effective in case of invasive diarrhea.
2. d. Slow, sustained absorption of water
3. i. Refer to page 811.
   ii. Refer to page 812.
4. d. > 10 % of body weight
5. i. Poor absorption of rifaximin
   ii. Action is mainly antisecretory through δ-opioid receptors, but is devoid of antimotility effect (probably due to lack of action on μ-opioid receptors).
   iii. Does not cross blood–brain barrier, so free of central adverse effects and abuse potential.
6. Refer to page pages 812–814.
7. i. Corticosteroids are used to induce remission, while immunosuppressants are used if steroids fail.
   ii. Aminosalicylates are used for maintaining remission
8. 5-ASA is released from azo compounds in the terminal ileum or colon, but Crohn's disease can affect any part of the GIT from mouth to rectum.
9. i. a. Binding with sulphapyridine through N=N bond. Reduced absorption of 5-ASA in the proximal small intestine ensures delivery of more of the drug to the terminal ileum and colon to exert topical anti-inflammatory action in ulcerative colitis.
   ii. Refer to page 816.
10. i. a. Magnesium hydroxide is contraindicated in renal failure
    ii. Osmotic purgative. Refer to page 823.
11. d. DOSS
12. i. a. DOSS is a stool softener.
    ii. Refer to page 822.
13. a–3; b–4; c–2; d–1.

CONCEPT MAP – DRUGS FOR CONSTIPATION

Bulk Purgatives

Bran
Mechanism: Bran contains cellulose, pectins, glycoproteins, polysaccharides that absorb water in the intestines → form bulky emollient gel → distends colon & promotes peristalsis.
Useful for prevention of constipation, not for treatment of constipation.
Drawback: Unpalatable, needed in large quantity (20–40 g/day), effect delayed for 3–4 days, no stool softening effect.
May cause flatulence, worsen IBS.
Not useful in patients with gut ulcerations, adhesions, stenosis, etc. for fear of fecal impaction.

Psyllium/Ispaghula
Natural colloidal mucilage, soluble fibres, used freshly mixed with water or milk.
Not to be swallowed dry for fear of esophageal impaction.

Methylcellulose
4–6 g/day used when straining at stools has to be avoided e.g., cardiac patients, hernia, anal fistula, after anal or eye surgery.
Also used to improve consistency of stools in colostomy patients
Water intake must be sufficient with all bulk-forming agents.

Stool Softeners

Dioctyl sodium sulfosuccinate (DOSS)
anionic detergent, emulsifies colonic contents → increases water and lipid penetration into feces → softening of stools.
Used in conditions when straining at stools must be avoided
ADRs: Cramps, abdominal pain, nausea.
It enhances absorption of many nonabsorbable drugs e.g., liquid paraffin. So, these two should not be combined.
Prolonged use: Hepatotoxic effect.

Liquid paraffin: Pharmacologically inert mixture of petroleum hydrocarbons → coats & lubricates hard scybala → softens stools after 2–3 days of use.
ADRs: Not much in use, because of unpalatable taste, risk of formation of foreign body granulomas in intestines, lipid pneumonia, impaired healing of anorectal lesions and deficiency of fat-soluble vitamins with long term use.

Drugs for Constipation

Osmotic Purgatives

Mg sulphate, Mg Hydroxide, Sodium sulphate, Sodium phosphate, Sodium potassium tartrate
not absorbed in intestine → retain water osmotically in colon → distension of bowel → indirectly increase peristalsis

Lactulose converted by colonic bacteria into osmotically active acidic products → lower stool pH, not favourable for survival of ammonia producing organisms → lowers blood NH_3 concentration → beneficial in hepatic encephalopathy.
ADRs: Flatulence, flatus and cramps.

Stimulant Purgatives

Mechanism: Irritate colonic mucosa, stimulating motor activity by action on myenteric plexuses, alter absorptive and secretory activity of mucosal cells.

Bisacodyl, Sodium picosulfate cause bowel evacuation in 6–8 hours.
ADRs: Fluid evacuations, cramps, more leaky colonic mucosa, allergic reactions (skin rashes, fixed drug eruptions, Stevens–Johnson syndrome).

Anthraquinones: Colonic bacteria liberate active anthrol → inhibit salt and water absorption from colonic mucosa. Absorbed part acts on myenteric plexus → increased peristalsis and reduced segmentation.

Castor oil: Hydrolysed to ricinoleic acid + glycerol having detergent-like action on mucosa.

Lubiprostone: EP_4 receptor agonist recommended only in patients with idiopathic chronic constipation, and constipation-predominant IBS.
ADRs: Nausea, delayed gastric emptying, dyspepsia

Prucalopride: $5\text{-}HT_4$ receptor agonist → increased ACh release → propulsive contractions in ileum & colon
ADRs: Headache, dizziness, abdominal pain and diarrhea.

SECTION 11 Drugs Acting on the Gastrointestinal System

63 Antiemetic and Prokinetic Drugs

PH 6.2 Describe types, salient pharmacokinetics, pharmacodynamics, therapeutic uses, adverse drug reactions of prokinetics and drugs used for emesis and antiemetics.

Learning objectives

A student of MBBS phase II should be able to:
- Describe the mechanism of emesis.
- Enumerate drugs used for inducing emesis and their uses.
- Classify drugs used as antiemetics.
- Describe the different mechanisms of action of antiemetic drugs
- Enumerate the indications for use of antiemetic drugs.
- Enumerate the ADRs of and contraindications to antiemetic drugs.

EMESIS

Emesis or **vomiting** is a physical event, resulting in the forceful evacuation of gastric contents through the mouth. Vomiting is preceded by a feeling of nausea (impending vomiting) and is accompanied by repetitive contraction of abdominal muscles (retching), with or without actual expulsion of vomitus.

Nausea is caused by reduced gastric tone and peristalsis. The fundus and body of the stomach, esophageal sphincter and esophagus are relaxed, but duodenum and pyloric stomach contract in a retrograde manner. The rhythmic contractions of the diaphragm and abdominal muscles compress the stomach and cause expulsion of gastric contents.

Etiology

Vomiting is not a disease; it is a symptom of many conditions such as central nervous system infections, increased intracranial pressure, vestibular dysfunction, pregnancy, hepatobiliary disorders, peritonitis, and gastrointestinal obstruction/infection/dysmotility. It is also an adverse effect associated with many drugs/radiotherapy/chemotherapy.

Mechanism of Emesis

Vomiting occurs due to stimulation of the vomiting centre (VC) situated in the medulla oblongata. The chemoreceptor trigger zone (CTZ) and nucleus tractus solitarius (NTS) are relay centres for afferent impulses from the throat, GIT and other viscera. Emetic signals are relayed at the CTZ and NTS through H_1, D_2, 5-HT_3, muscarinic, and μ-opioid receptors.

Unpleasant sensory stimuli such as bad smells, disturbing scenes, fear, severe pain, recall of unpleasant events, and anticipation of emesis cause nausea and vomiting through higher centres (Fig. 63.1).

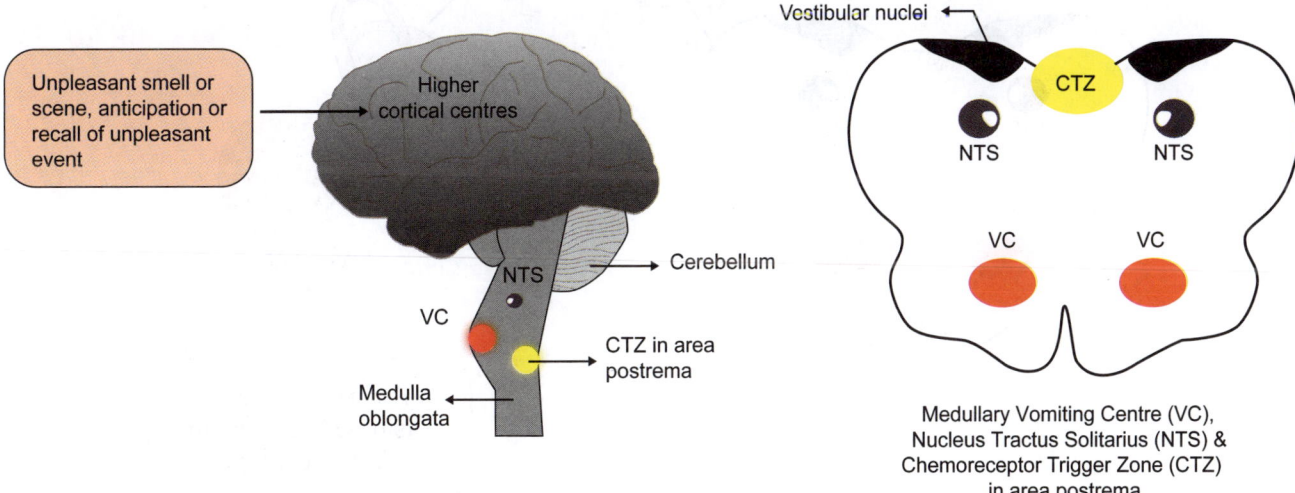

Fig. 63.1 Side view of brain and transverse section at medullary level

Rotation of body, disturbance of equilibrium, and ototoxic drugs (e.g., aminoglycosides) generate impulses from the vestibular apparatus that are mainly relayed from the cerebellum; these reach the vomiting centre and stimulate it through muscarinic and H_1 receptors. Therefore, in such situations, anticholinergic and antihistaminic drugs can effectively control vomiting (Fig. 63.2).

Radiation, chemotherapeutic anticancer drugs, gastrointestinal irritants, toxins, etc., cause serotonin (5-HT) release from enterochromaffin cells. This activates $5-HT_3$ receptors present on the vagal afferents and sends impulses to the CTZ and NTS (Fig. 63.3).

Mediators of inflammation also cause 5-HT release from platelets that reach the CTZ through the blood. The CTZ is not protected by the blood–brain barrier and is therefore accessible to toxins, hormones, mediators, drugs, etc., present in systemic circulation.

Thus, acetylcholine, histamine, dopamine, serotonin and enkephalins are the main neurotransmitters involved in control of the emetic process. In addition, substance P acting at neurokinin-1 receptors in CTZ is also implicated in causing emesis.

EMETIC DRUGS

It is necessary to stimulate vomiting in some situations, e.g., following ingestion of toxic substances. Emetic drugs include **apomorphine** and **ipecacuanha**.

Apomorphine is a semisynthetic derivative of morphine that acts as a dopaminergic agonist in the CTZ. It can induce vomiting within 5 minutes of intramuscular or subcutaneous injection, in a dose of 6 mg. Apomorphine is contraindicated in case of respiratory depression.

Ipecacuanha is used as syrup ipecac in a dose of 15–20 mL in adults and 10–15 mL in children. It irritates the gastric mucosa and stimulates the CTZ, leading to vomiting in about 15 minutes after administration. It is less dependable, but safer than apomorphine.

In addition, powdered mustard suspension and strong salt solution may be used to induce vomiting in emergency situations.

Induction of vomiting **should not be attempted** when:

- The patient is **not fully conscious**, as there is risk of aspirating the vomitus.
- The patient has **ingested a corrosive substance** because there is risk of perforation and injury to esophageal mucosa.

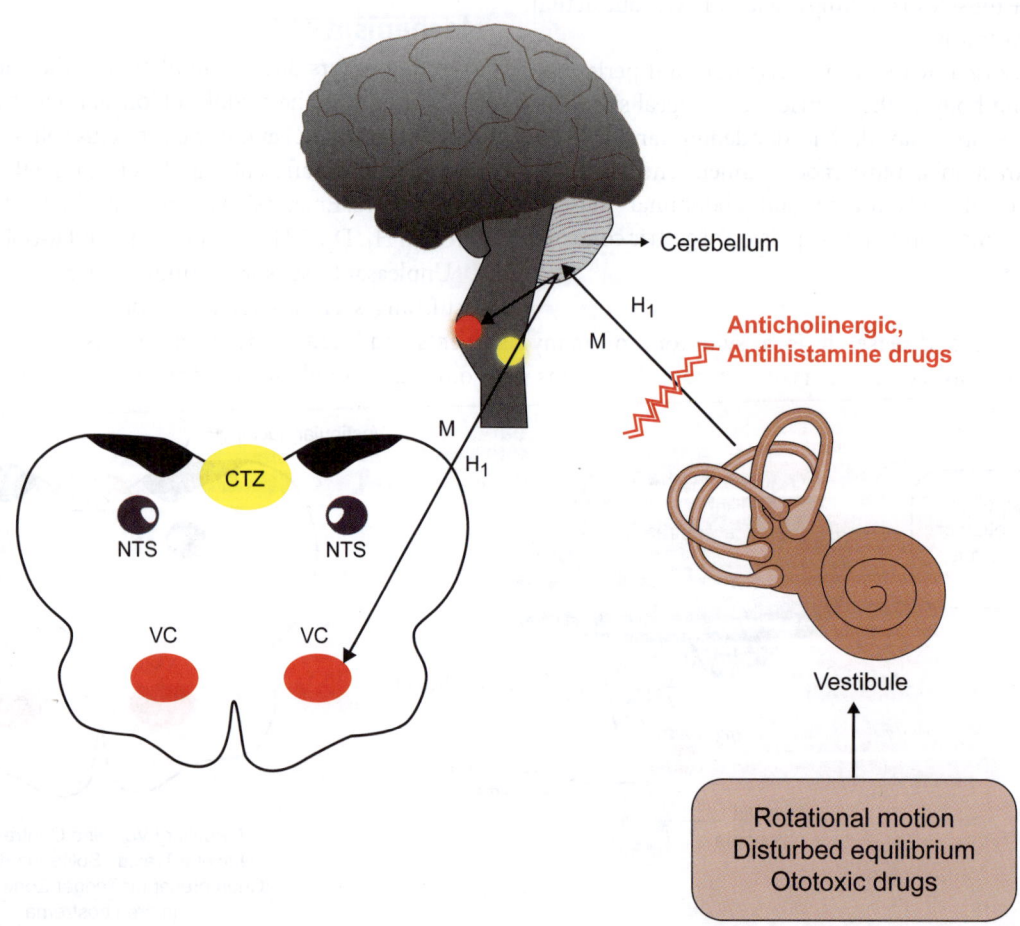

Fig. 63.2 Mechanism of action of anticholinergic and antihistamine drugs in motion sickness

- **Poisoning with CNS stimulant drug**: Use of emetics in these cases may cause convulsions.
- **Kerosene poisoning**: Induction of vomiting is associated with the risk of aspiration of liquid (due to its low viscosity) and chemical pneumonia.
- Poisoning with **morphine and phenothiazines**: emetics are not effective.

ANTIEMETIC DRUGS

Antiemetic drugs can be classified based on their mechanism of action (Flowchart 63.1). These include blockers of M_3, H_1, D_2, $5-HT_3$, and NK-1 receptors along with prokinetic drugs.

1. Anticholinergics

Cholinergic transmission plays important role in vomiting caused by disturbed equilibrium and rotational motion. (Fig. 63.2) Therefore, the anticholinergic drug hyoscine is highly effective for motion sickness. However, it has no role in vomiting due to other causes. Hyoscine has a brief duration of action and sedative effect. To overcome these limitations, it is applied behind the pinna as a transdermal

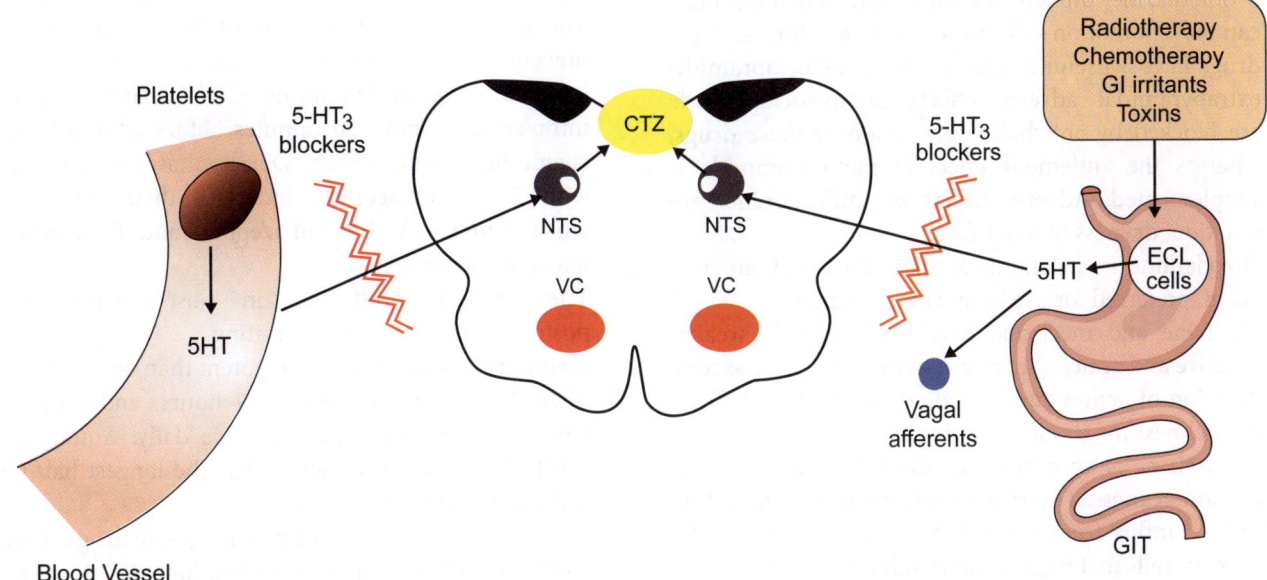

Fig. 63.3 Role of 5-HT in emesis

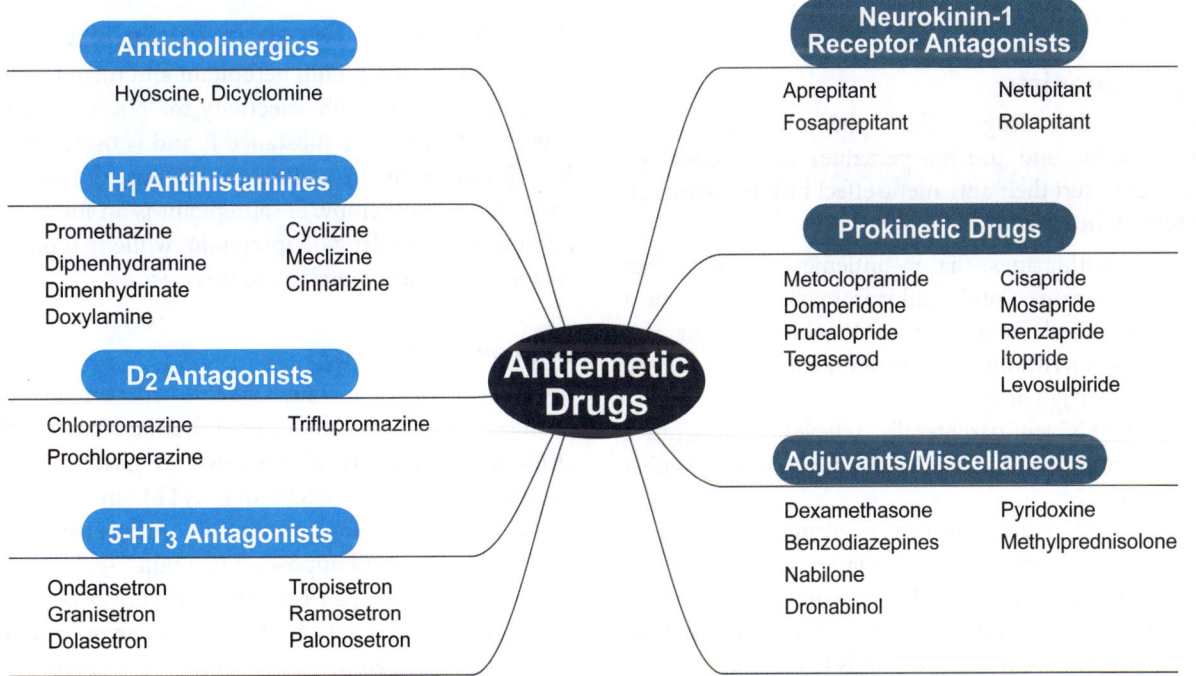

Flowchart 63.1 Classification of antiemetic drugs

patch (1.5 mg), which releases hyoscine in a slow, sustained manner for 3 days. Anticholinergic adverse effects may occur, but are mild.

Dicyclomine (given orally) is also effective in motion sickness. It has no teratogenic potential and is thus useful in morning sickness as well.

2. H_1 Antihistamines

These drugs possess anticholinergic, antihistaminic and sedative actions that contribute to their antiemetic effect. Antihistamines are useful in motion sickness, morning sickness, and postoperative emesis. (Fig. 63.2)

- Promethazine, diphenhydramine and dimenhydrinate can prevent motion sickness for about 4–5 hours. These drugs have a useful interaction with metoclopramide; extrapyramidal adverse effects of metoclopramide are blocked by anticholinergic action of these drugs, whereas the antiemetic effect of metoclopramide is supplemented. Adverse effects of antihistamines are sedation, dryness of mouth, etc.
- Doxylamine is an antihistamine with anticholinergic effect, preferred for use in morning sickness.
- Cyclizine and meclizine have comparatively weaker sedative and anticholinergic activity. Cyclizine has long duration of action and a single dose can protect from sea sickness for about 24 hours.
- Cinnarizine is an antivertigo drug that also prevents motion sickness. It exerts antivertigo action by inhibition of Ca^{2+} influx from the endolymph into the vestibular sensory cells that mediate labyrinthine reflexes.
- For motion sickness, efficacy of antihistamines is higher if given 30 min before starting the journey.
- Antihistamines are suspected to have teratogenicity, and thus avoided in morning sickness.

3. D_2 Antagonists

These include drugs like phenothiazines (e.g., chlorpromazine and prochlorperazine) and droperidol. These drugs exert their antiemetic effect by blockade of D_2 receptors in the CTZ.

- All phenothiazines have antiemetic effect, but prochlorperazine and chlorpromazine are most frequently used for this action. Prochlorperazine also possesses labyrinthine suppressant action and is useful as an antivertigo drug.
- Droperidol given parenterally relieves postoperative nausea and vomiting. Its most disturbing adverse effect is sedation.
- D_2 antagonists are effective in drug-induced (e.g., cancer chemotherapy), radiation-induced, and postoperative vomiting. Disease-induced vomiting caused by gastrointestinal/hepatic disease/malignancy/ uremia and migraine also responds to these drugs.
- These are better avoided in morning sickness, but may be used in severe cases such as hyperemesis gravidarum.

4. $5-HT_3$ Antagonists

Ondansetron, granisetron, dolasetron, tropisetron

The effect of these potent antiemetic drugs is mediated through the blockade of central as well as peripheral $5-HT_3$ receptors. Central $5-HT_3$ receptors are present on the CTZ and NTS, whereas peripheral $5-HT_3$ receptors are present on intestinal vagal afferents (Fig. 63.3; also refer to Table 27.1, page 362).

- These drugs are free of anticholinergic and antidopaminergic actions.
- There is no effect on the motility of the esophagus and stomach. However, colonic transit is slowed down.
- The main indication for use of these drugs is the prevention and treatment of cancer chemotherapy-induced nausea and vomiting (CINV). They are given intravenously about 30 minutes before administering chemotherapeutic drugs. Dexamethasone combined with $5-HT_3$ antagonists increases their antiemetic efficacy in CINV. Benzodiazepines and D_2 blockers may also be combined.
- They are also effective in post-radiation and postoperative nausea and vomiting.
- Granisetron is 10 times more potent than ondansetron.
- Their half-life varies from 4–9 hours, and they are effective when used once or twice daily. Among the $5-HT_3$ blockers, palonosetron has the longest half-life and ondansetron the shortest.
- $5-HT_3$ blockers are well-tolerated and safe drugs. Their ADRs include headache, constipation and dizziness. QT interval is prolonged, but cardiac arrhythmias have not been reported.

5. Neurokinin-1 Receptor Antagonists

Aprepitant, fosaprepitant, netupitant and rolapitant

Aprepitant has high selectivity for NK-1 receptors. It prevents the effect of substance P, and is useful in CINV. It is given orally in a dose of 125 mg, 1 hour before surgery/ chemotherapy. Fosaprepitant is an intravenously administered prodrug of aprepitant, while netupitant and rolapitant are new members of this class.

6. Prokinetic Drugs

Prokinetic (*pro*: favour, *kinetic*: movement) drugs promote gastro-duodenal peristalsis and hasten gastric emptying. These are also known as **gastric hurrying agents**. The major excitatory NTM in the GIT is acetylcholine. Serotonin favours peristalsis through $5-HT_4$ receptors and opposes it through $5-HT_3$ receptors. Dopamine also has an inhibitory effect on GI motility. Thus, drugs which are agonists at cholinergic and $5-HT_4$ receptors or antagonists at D_2 and $5-HT_3$ receptors have prokinetic action, e.g., metoclopramide, domperidone, and cisapride-like drugs.

doses control CINV. It also has a 5-HT$_4$ agonistic effect that contributes to its prokinetic effect.
- Metoclopramide **enhances acetylcholine release from myenteric neurons** in the GIT. This cholinomimetic effect contributes to increased peristalsis, i.e., gastrokinetic effect and raised LES tone.

Uses
Metoclopramide is useful in drug-induced, post-anesthesia, disease-induced, radiation-induced, and cancer chemotherapy-induced nausea and vomiting.
- It increases LES tone and relieves dyspepsia and GERD.
- Its gastrokinetic effect is useful when emergency GA is to be given, e.g., in case of diabetic stasis, postvagotomy stasis, and duodenal intubation.

ADRs
The ADRs of metoclopramide include sedation, dizziness, diarrhea and muscular dystonias. Because metoclopramide can cross the blood–brain barrier, its long-term use is associated with extrapyramidal effects causing drug-induced parkinsonism and hyperprolactinemia that manifests as galactorrhea and gynecomastia.

b. Domperidone
Like metoclopramide, domperidone also has D$_2$ blocking, prokinetic and antiemetic effects; however, it cannot cross the blood–brain barrier, and is thus free of extrapyramidal adverse effects. Its antiemetic efficacy is lower than that of metoclopramide. It causes headache, dryness of mouth and diarrhea as adverse effects.

c. Cisapride
Drugs such as cisapride, mosapride, tegaserod, prucalopride, and renzapride have agonistic effect on 5-HT$_4$ receptors (Fig. 63.4). They also have cholinomimetic effects, due to release of acetylcholine from myenteric plexus neurons. Acetylcholine is responsible for their prokinetic effect that can be blocked by atropine. Diarrhea is a common adverse effect as motility throughout the gut is increased. These are useful in GERD and constipation.

Miscellaneous
- **Pyridoxine** is frequently prescribed in morning sickness, but has no specific antiemetic action.
- **Tetrahydrocannabinoids** (THCs) exert antiemetic effect by acting on the vomiting centre, but are not used routinely due to their hallucinogenic effect and abuse potential. However, they are sometimes required in resistant cases of CINV. **Nabilone** is more effective as an antiemetic than THCs and is less hallucinogenic. It is useful in CINV.
- **Dexamethasone** is used as an adjuvant in CINV.
- **Benzodiazepines** relieve anticipated nausea and vomiting, such as before surgical procedures.

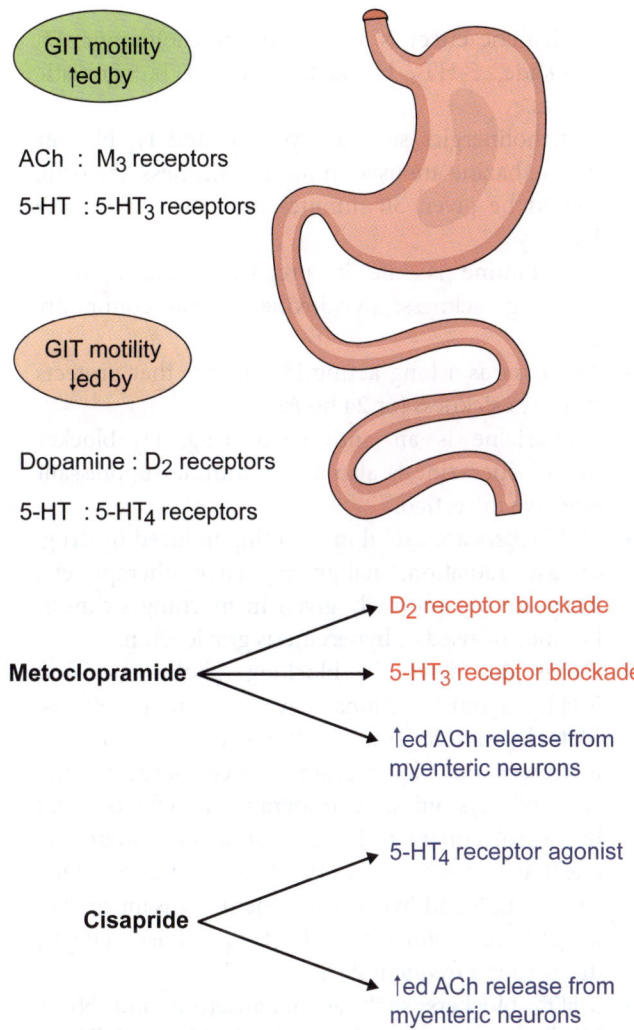

Fig. 63.4 Mechanism of action of prokinetic drugs

a. Metoclopramide

Mechanism of action
Metoclopramide likely acts via three different routes (Fig. 63.1):

In the gastrointestinal tract, dopamine is considered to be an inhibitory transmitter. Acting through D$_2$ receptors, dopamine delays gastric emptying, causes gastric dilatation, and relaxes the lower esophageal sphincter (LES), resulting in nausea. **Metoclopramide blocks this action of dopamine** with the opposite effects, i.e., hastening of gastric emptying (especially if it is slow) and increased tone of LES. Therefore, it prevents gastro-esophageal reflux. It relaxes the pylorus and the first part of the duodenum. These actions result in a prokinetic effect. It also possesses central antiemetic effect, due to D$_2$ blockade in the CTZ. Other antidopaminergic actions include hyperprolactinemia and extrapyramidal adverse effects (however, it has no antipsychotic effect).
- In large doses, metoclopramide **blocks 5-HT$_3$ receptors** on vagal afferents in the GIT, CTZ and NTS. Such large

Clinical problem-based questions and MCQs

1. A patient of carcinoma of sigmoid colon is receiving FOLFOX regimen of chemotherapy, i.e., 5-FU, oxaliplatin and leucovorin. Of these, oxaliplatin has high potential to induce nausea and vomiting.
   i. Which of the following drugs is most useful for the prevention of CINV?
      a. Aprepitant
      b. Cisapride
      c. Hyoscine
      d. Pyridoxine
   ii. Describe the mechanism of antiemetic effect of the selected drug.

2. A 25-year-old primigravida complains of nausea, aversion from some foods and vomiting, especially after waking up in the morning.
   i. Which of the following is most suitable drug for her?
      a. Promethazine
      b. Diphenhydramine
      c. Dicyclomine
      d. Granisetron
   ii. Justify your choice with the pharmacological basis.

3. Which of the following is not used as antiemetic drug
   a. Cinnarizine
   b. Metoclopramide
   c. Palonosetron
   d. Aprepitant

4. Identify a drug that acts on D_2, $5-HT_3$, and $5-HT_4$ receptors.
   a. Metoclopramide
   b. Ondansetron
   c. Prochlorperazine
   d. Droperidol

5. i. Which of these D_2 blockers is free of extrapyramidal adverse effects?
      a. Prochlorperazine
      b. Chlorpromazine
      c. Domperidone
      d. Metoclopramide
   ii. Explain the pharmacological basis for the advantage.

6. Match the drug with its correct receptor action.
   a. Fosaprepitant   1. $5-HT_4$ agonist
   b. Mosapride   2. NK-1 receptor blocker
   c. Palonosetron   3. D-blocker
   d. Domperidone   4. $5-HT_3$ blocker

- Antiemetic effect is a result of anticholinergic, D_2 blockade, $5-HT_3$ blockade, and $5-HT_4$ agonistic effects.
- Anticholinergics such as hyoscine and H_1 blocker promethazine are used in motion sickness; the drug should be given 30 minutes prior to starting the journey.
- Dicyclomine is safe in pregnancy and used in morning sickness; pyridoxine is also commonly used.
- Meclizine is a long-acting H_1 blocker that protects from sea sickness for 24 hours.
- Cinnarizine is an antivertigo drug. D_2 blocker prochlorperazine is also a labyrinthine suppressant effective in vertigo.
- D_2 blockers are useful in vomiting induced by drug, disease, radiation, malignancy, chemotherapy, etc. They are not routinely given in morning sickness, but may be used in hyperemesis gravidarum.
- Drugs that have D_2 blocking, cholinergic, and $5-HT_4$ agonist actions have prokinetic effects. Metoclopramide has all these receptor actions; it crosses the blood–brain barrier increasing the risk of dystonias, extrapyramidal effects, and hyperprolactinemia. Domperidone has prokinetic effect, but does not cross the BBB; it is free of ADRs such as EPS and hyperprolactinemia. Cisapride-like drugs have cholinergic and $5-HT_4$ agonistic effects; diarrhea is a frequent ADR.
- $5-HT_3$ blockers such as ondansetron and NK-1 blockers such as aprepitant are valuable in CINV.

Hints for problem-based questions and MCQs

1. i. a. Aprepitant
   ii. NK-1 receptor blocker.
2. i. c. Dicyclomine
   ii. Free of teratogenic potential
3. a. Cinnarizine is an antivertigo drug
4. a. Metoclopramide.
5. i. c. Domperidone
   ii. Does not cross the blood–brain barrier.
6. a–2; b–1; c–4; d–3.

Summary

- Apomorphine and ipecacuanha are emetic drugs used to induce vomiting in case of ingestion of toxic substances; however, they are contraindicated in unconscious patients and in case of poisoning by corrosives, kerosene, morphine, and CNS stimulants.

CONCEPT MAP – ANTIEMETIC DRUGS

Antihistamines

Promethazine, Diphenhydramine & Dimenhydrinate: Used in motion sickness.
Given with metoclopramide to block its extrapyramidal adverse effects and supplement antiemetic effect.
Cyclizine: Effective in sea sickness
Cinnarizine: inhibits Ca^{2+} influx from endolymph into vestibular sensory cells → antivertigo effect.

Anticholinergics

Hyoscine: Effective only in motion sickness.
No role in vomiting due to other causes.
Short-acting → Transdermal patch given
ADRs: Sedation, mild anticholinergic adverse effects.
Dicyclomine: Used in motion sickness, morning sickness (no teratogenic effect)

D₂ Blockers

Prochlorperazine, Chlorpromazine used for antiemetic effect.
Prochlorperazine has labyrinthine suppressant action → useful as antivertigo drug.
Droperidol: Used P/E in post operative nausea, vomiting
Uses: Drug-induced, radiation-induced, postoperative and disease-induced vomiting.

Miscellaneous

Neurokinin1 receptor antagonists: Aprepitant, Fosaprepitant, Netupitant & rolapitant:
Block NK-1 receptors, preventing effect of substance P. It is useful in CINV.
Tetrahydrocannabinoids not used because of hallucinogenic effect.
Nabilone is less hallucinogenic, useful in CINV
Dexamethasone used as adjuvant in CINV
Benzodiazepines used for relieving anticipated nausea/vomiting.
Pyridoxine used in morning sickness.

Antiemetic Drugs

5-HT₃ Antagonists

Ondansetron, Granisetron, Dolasetron, Tropisetron
Mechanism: Block central 5-HT₃ receptors (CTZ, NTS) and peripheral 5-HT₃ receptors (intestinal vagal afferents).
No anticholinergic, antidopaminergic actions,
Uses: Used once or twice daily for prevention and treatment of cancer chemotherapy-induced nausea, vomiting (CINV). Dexamethasone, Benzodiazepines, D₂ blockers may be combined for increasing efficacy.
Used in post-radiation, post-operative vomiting
ADRs: Headache, constipation, dizziness, QT prolongation, but no cardiac arrhythmias

Prokinetic Drugs

Promote gastro-duodenal peristalsis and hasten gastric emptying.
ACh increases and dopamine reduces GI motility.
5-HT has both actions, 5-HT₄ action increases, but 5-HT₃ action decreases GI motility.
Metoclopramide:
Causes D₂ blocker, 5-HT₃ block & increases ACh release → Prokinetic effect
Uses: Drug/disease/radiation/anesthesia/cancer chemotherapy-induced nausea, vomiting.
It increases LES tone → useful in dyspepsia, GERD.
Gastrokinetic effect is useful, when emergency GA is to be given, in diabetic/post vagotomy stasis & duodenal intubation.
ADRs: Sedation, dizziness, diarrhea & muscular dystonias, extrapyramidal symptoms & hyperprolactinemia manifesting as galactorrhea, gynecomastia.
Domperidone: D₂ blocker, but free of EPS as it cannot cross blood–brain barrier.
ADRs: Headache, dryness of mouth and diarrhea
5-HT₄ agonists: Cisapride, Mosapride, Renzapride, Tegaserod, Prucalopride. Also increase release of acetylcholine from myenteric plexus neurons → prokinetic effect → useful in GERD and constipation.
ADR: Diarrhea.

SECTION 11 Drugs Acting on the Gastrointestinal System

64 Drugs for Acid Peptic Diseases

PH 6.1 Explain types, salient pharmacokinetics, pharmacodynamics, therapeutic uses, and adverse drug reactions of drugs used in acid peptic diseases, including peptic ulcers and GERD, and devise a management plan for a case of peptic ulcer.

Learning objectives

A student of MBBS phase II should be able to:

- Describe the physiology of gastric acid secretion and regulation.
- Classify drugs used for APDs or anti-ulcer drugs.
- Explain mechanisms of action of antacids, H$_2$ blockers and proton pump inhibitors.
- Describe therapeutic uses of antacids, H$_2$ blockers, proton pump inhibitors and their status in current clinical practice.
- Describe triple-drug regimens for *H. pylori* eradication.
- Describe the mechanism of action of ulcer-protective and ulcer-healing drugs.
- Enumerate ADRs and contraindications of anti-ulcer drugs.
- Describe the pharmacotherapy of peptic ulcer.

ACID PEPTIC DISEASES

'Acid peptic diseases' (APDs) is a broad term that includes conditions such as stress- or NSAIDs-induced gastric erosions or ulcers, gastro-esophageal reflux disease (GERD), esophagitis, and gastric and duodenal peptic ulcers.

Etiology

The etiology of APDs is not clearly understood but likely involves an imbalance between aggressive and defensive factors in the gastric mucosa. The **aggressive factors** for erosions/ulceration of gastro-intestinal mucosa are hydrochloric acid (HCl), pepsin, bile and *Helicobacter pylori*. In contrast, mucus, bicarbonate ions (HCO$_3^-$), prostaglandins (PGE$_2$/PGI$_2$), blood flow to mucosa, and the innate resistance or regenerative power of mucosa are mucosal **defensive factors**. In addition, many **psychosomatic**, **vascular** and **humoral derangements** are implicated in the causation of APDs. **External factors** (smoking, alcohol, NSAIDs, stress, foods/drinks that are fatty/spicy/very hot) are also considered to cause mucosal damage.

Clinical Features

Patient of APDs commonly present with epigastric discomfort/burning, heartburn, feeling of fullness, abdominal distension, bloating, belching, nausea, abdominal cramps, etc. The pain of peptic ulcer disease is worsened by gastric acid (as on empty stomach or between meals) and relieved by certain foods or antacids. However, symptoms are usually aggravated by fatty and spicy foods. The diagnosis of peptic ulcer is confirmed by endoscopy. Untreated ulcers can have serious complications such as perforation and bleeding; such patients present with hematemesis, black or tarry stools, reduced appetite, weight loss, etc.

Treatment

The aim of treatment of APDs is the relief of symptoms, healing of ulcers, and prevention of complications/relapses. This can be achieved by suppressing the aggressive factors, especially HCl, and strengthening the mucosal protective factors.

PHYSIOLOGY OF GASTRIC SECRETION

Normally, about 2.5 L of gastric juice is secreted daily. It consists of:

- HCl and intrinsic factor (IF) secreted by parietal cells.
- Pepsinogen secreted by peptic cells. It is activated in the acidic pH of stomach to form pepsin.
- Mucus secreted by **mucus-secreting** cells that are scattered throughout the gastric mucosa.
- Bicarbonate (HCO$_3^-$) ions that form an unstirred gel like protective layer with the mucus. This layer creates a pH gradient between the gastric lumen (pH 1–2) and mucosal surface (pH 6–7).

The mechanism of HCl secretion from parietal cells involves the action of ① carbonic anhydrase enzyme, ② antiporter on the basal surface for exchange of bicarbonate and chloride ions, ③ symporter for movement of potassium and chloride ions into the gastric canaliculi, and ④ proton pump that exchanges potassium ions for protons, as shown in Fig. 64.1.

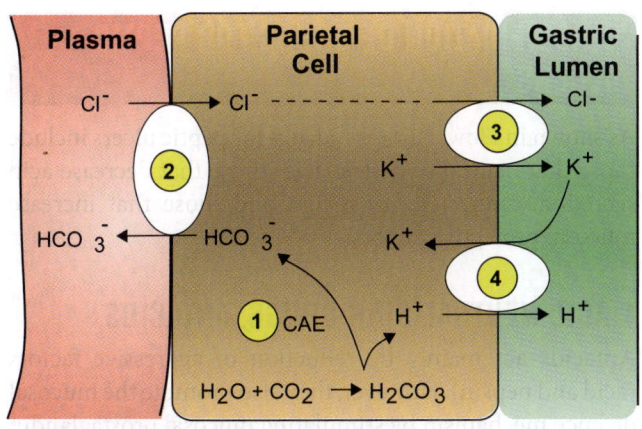

Fig. 64.1 Mechanism of gastric acid secretion

① Carbonic anhydrase enzyme (CAE) catalyses the dissociation of carbonic acid (H_2CO_3) into H^+ and HCO_3^- ions in the parietal cells.
② An antiporter present on the basal surface exchanges HCO_3^- ions with Cl^- ions.
③ Cl^- ions are then actively transported into the gastric canaliculi along with K^+ ions through by a symporter.
④ In the final step, K^+ ions are exchanged for H^+ from within the parietal cell by K^+/H^+ ATPase, also known as proton pump.

Regulation of Acid Secretion

Secretion of HCl by gastric parietal cells is increased by acetylcholine, gastrin, and histamine, and inhibited by prostaglandins E_2 and I_2 (Fig. 64.2).

a. Acetylcholine

The effect of ACh is mediated through histamine and gastrin. However, cholinergic agonists can directly stimulate M_3 receptors present on the parietal cell surface, causing activation of IP_3–DAG pathway → rise in intracellular Ca^{2+} → activation of proton pumps.

b. Gastrin

Release: ACh and other factors such as food, milk, amino acids, calcium and raised antral pH cause gastrin release.

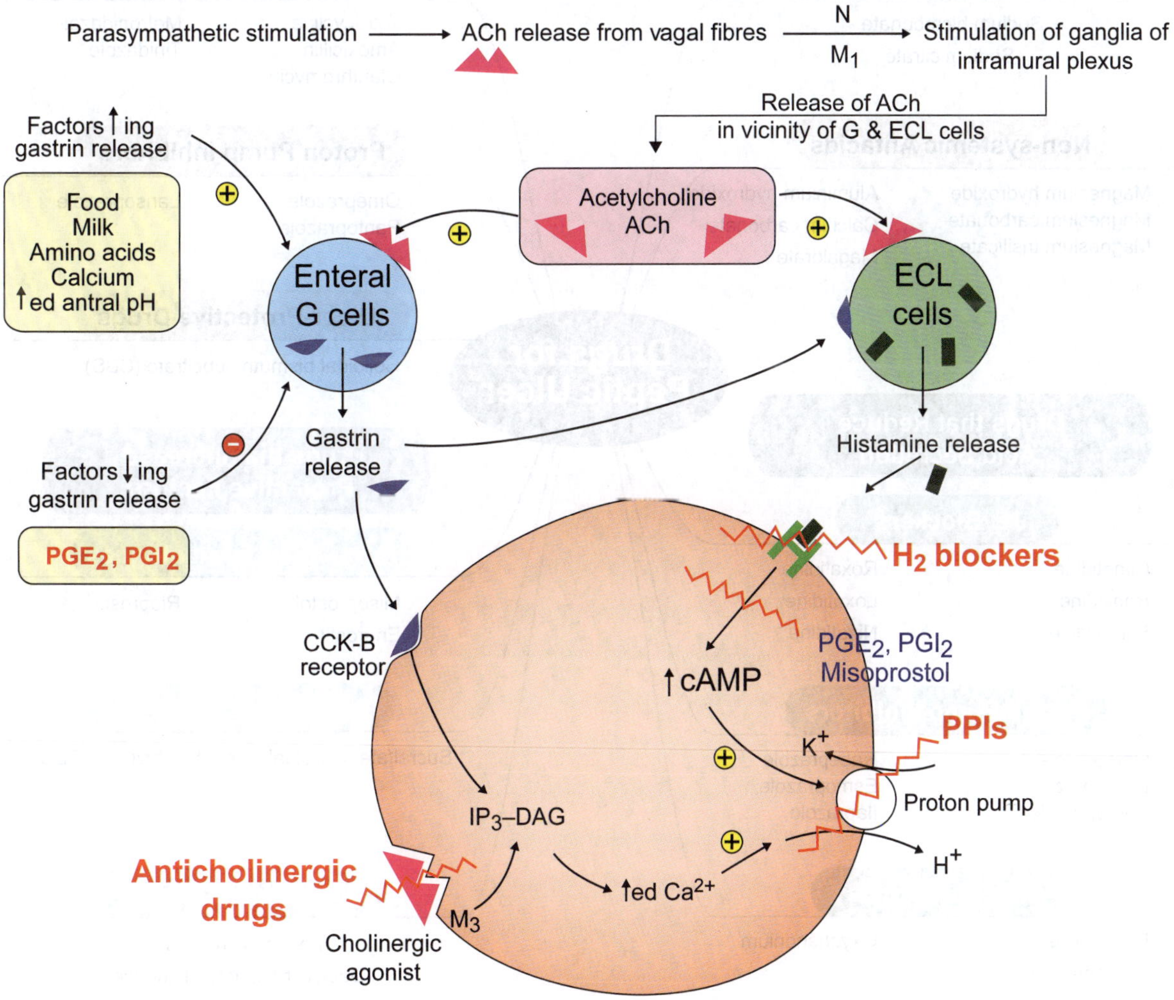

Fig. 64.2 Regulation of gastric acid secretion and site of action of anti-ulcer drugs

Action: Gastrin can act directly on parietal cells causing raised intracellular calcium through the IP_3–DAG pathway, which activates proton pumps to increase acid synthesis. Gastrin acts partly by increasing histamine secretion from ECL cells.

c. Histamine
It acts on H_2 receptors on parietal cells, increasing intracellular cAMP, which activates proton pumps.

d. Prostaglandins E_2 and I_2
They inhibit acid secretion by:
- inhibiting gastrin release from antral cells
- interfere with generation of cAMP inside parietal cell in response to histamine

CLASSIFICATION OF DRUGS FOR PEPTIC ULCERS

As shown in Flowchart 64.1, drugs for peptic ulcers include those that neutralise gastric acid, those that decrease acid secretion, anti-*H. pylori* drugs, and those that increase mucosal protective factors.

1. ACID NEUTRALISING DRUGS: ANTACIDS

Antacids act mainly by reduction of aggressive factors (acid and pepsin). However, they also promote the mucosal defence mechanism by stimulating mucosal prostaglandin synthesis.

Antacids are weakly basic substances → neutralise the gastric acid → salt and water is formed → rise in gastric pH

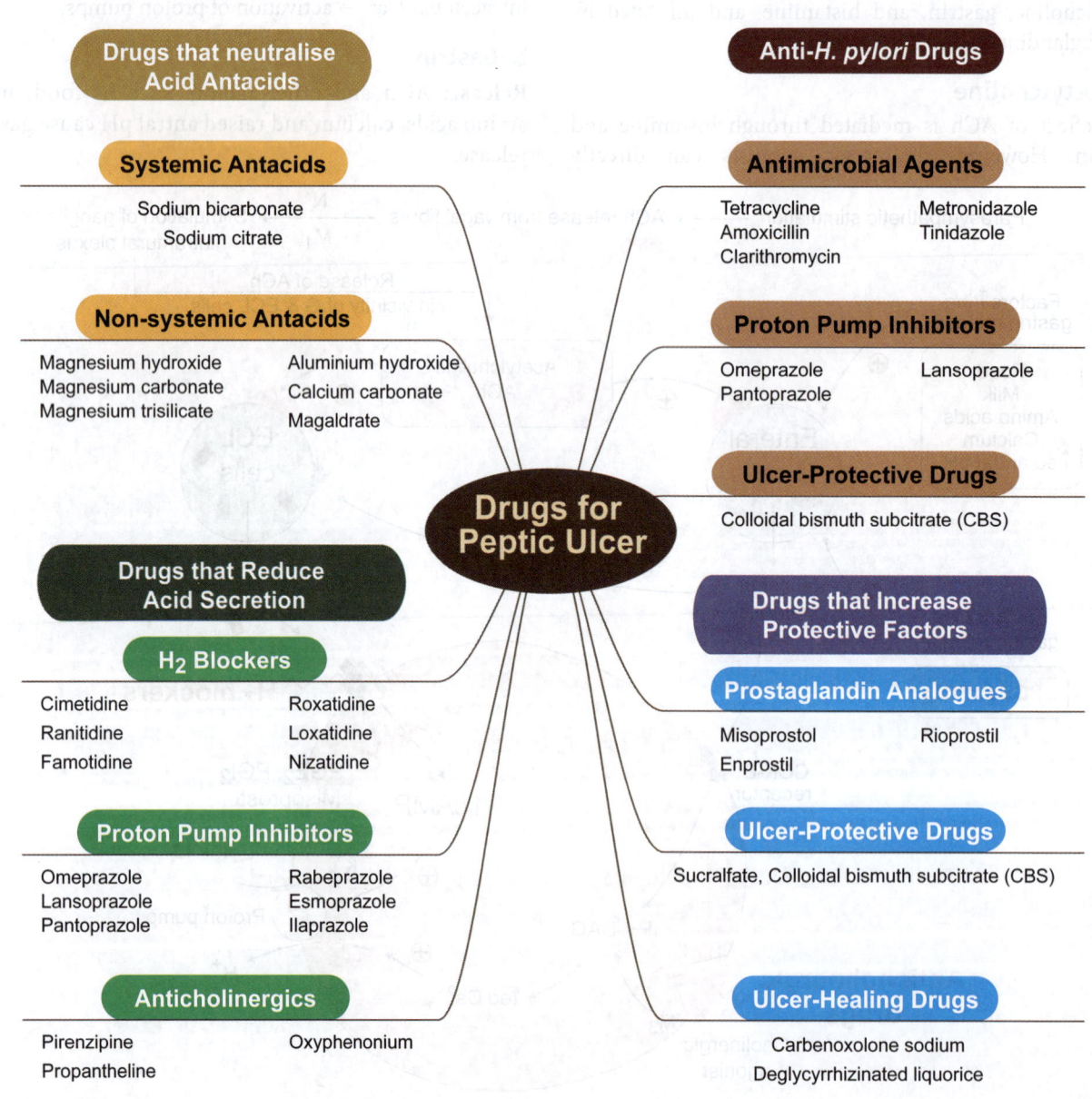

Flowchart 64.1 Classification of drugs for peptic ulcer

→ decreases pepsin activity indirectly (pepsin is secreted as a complex with an inhibitory terminal moiety which dissociates below pH 5. Thus, when pH increases, pepsin activity decreases).

Antacids do not decrease acid production. Rather, they are agents that raise the antral pH. Once the antral pH = 4 → reflex gastrin release → more acid production. This is known as **acid rebound**.

The potency of an antacid is defined in terms of its **acid neutralising capacity** (ANC: the number of milliequivalents of 1 N HCl that are brought to pH 3.5 in 15 minutes by a unit dose of antacid).

Antacids are classified as systemic and non-systemic antacids.

a. Systemic Antacids

Sodium bicarbonate (NaHCO$_3$), sodium citrate.

- **Sodium bicarbonate** is water soluble and reacts instantaneously with HCl.
  $$NaHCO_3 + HCl \longrightarrow NaCl + H_2O + CO_2$$
- The CO$_2$ generated by the chemical reaction may cause gastric discomfort, distension, belching, and increases the risk of ulcer perforation.
- NaCl may get absorbed systemically and exacerbate fluid retention. This is dangerous in patients with hypertension, cardiac disease, edema, etc.
- Unreacted NaHCO$_3$ is also readily absorbed, leading to alkalosis, which is initially compensated by the passage of HCO$_3^-$ ions in urine.
- Sodium bicarbonate is used for management of acidosis, alkalinisation of urine, and only for quick symptomatic relief in heart burn; it is not suitable for healing of peptic ulcers.
- **Sodium citrate** has the same actions as sodium bicarbonate; the only difference is that CO$_2$ is not evolved when it reacts with HCl.

b. Non-systemic Antacids

Non-systemic antacids are insoluble and poorly absorbed into systemic circulation. These include magnesium hydroxide/trisilicate/carbonate, calcium carbonate and aluminum hydroxide gel.

Magnesium hydroxide

Because of its low solubility in water, the aqueous suspension of magnesium hydroxide, called **milk of magnesia,** is used. It **reacts promptly** with HCl to form magnesium chloride and H$_2$O. Unlike sodium bicarbonate, there is **no CO$_2$** generation and **no alkalosis** (the neutralisation reaction consumes most of the alkali and little is left unused for absorption into systemic circulation).

Magnesium trisilicate

Magnesium trisilicate has **low reactivity** and never raises the pH above 3. However, the gelatinous silica produced during its chemical reaction with HCl protects the ulcer base and adsorbs pepsin to decrease its activity.

Magnesium carbonate

It **reacts slowly** with HCl to generate magnesium chloride, CO$_2$ and H$_2$O. While CO$_2$ is formed in this reaction, its rate of formation is much slower than that with sodium bicarbonate. Magnesium chloride formed during these reactions is osmotically active and Mg^{2+} ions induce cholecystokinin release; both these actions have a **laxative effect**. Thus, all antacids containing magnesium cause accelerated gastric emptying and diarrhea as adverse effects.

Calcium carbonate

Calcium carbonate reacts rapidly with HCl to form calcium chloride, CO$_2$ and H$_2$O. While the rate of CO$_2$ generation is slower than that with sodium bicarbonate, it results in belching, bloating sensation, and abdominal distension. Ca^{2+} ions may get absorbed long-term use may result in complications such as hypercalcemia, hypercalciuria, renal stones, and alkalosis. Concomitant administration of milk may cause the milk–alkali syndrome characterised by anorexia, headache, weakness, abdominal discomfort, hypercalcemia, alkalosis, and renal stones. Thus, calcium carbonate is **not a preferred antacid**.

Aluminium hydroxide gel

It is a weak, **slowly reacting** antacid that can adsorb and inactivate pepsin at pH > 3. However, as aluminium hydroxide is a **mild antacid**, it has to be combined with a more potent agent to raise the pH above 3 for pepsin inactivation.

While acid rebound is minimal, aluminium ions relax smooth muscles. Thus, aluminium-containing antacids cause **constipation and delay gastric emptying**. Large doses may cause intestinal obstruction in elderly individuals.

Aluminium hydroxide also possesses **demulcent action**; thus, it coats the ulcer crater and protects it from acid attack.

Binding of aluminium hydroxide to phosphate ions prevents their absorption, resulting in hypophosphatemia upon regular use. Due to this, aluminium hydroxide can be used in treatment of hyperphosphatemia and phosphate stones. It may also cause osteomalacia. A small amount of aluminium ions is absorbed and excreted by the renal route; thus, aluminium hydroxide should be avoided in patients with renal failure.

Antacid combinations

A combination of two or more antacids is better than any single agent. Many antacid preparations contain both magnesium- and aluminium-containing agents. The benefits of such combinations include (Fig. 64.3) the following.

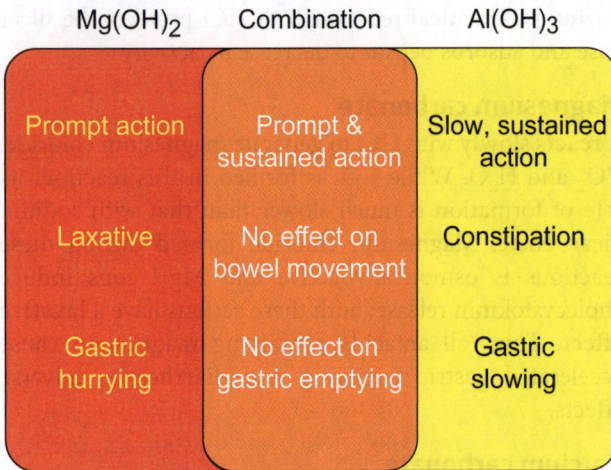

Fig. 64.3 Benefits of Mg(OH)₂–Al(OH)₃ combination

- Magnesium hydroxide acts fast, while aluminium hydroxide has slow but sustained effect. The combination of these two agents thus yields prompt and sustained effect.
- Magnesium has a laxative effect (due to osmotic activity of $MgCl_2$ and Mg^{2+}-induced release of cholecystokinin) while Al^{3+} ions relax smooth muscles and cause constipation. The combination of antacids containing magnesium and aluminium has a minimal effect on bowel movement, i.e., neither diarrhea nor constipation occurs.
- Magnesium and calcium salts cause gastric hurrying, i.e., they hasten gastric emptying, whereas aluminium salts tend to delay gastric emptying. Their combination, however, has negligible effect on gastric emptying.
- When a combination of antacids is used, the dose of individual components gets reduced. So, systemic toxicity of each component is minimised.

Magaldrate

Magaldrate is a hydrated complex of hydroxymagnesium aluminate. This preparation is not just a mixture of magnesium and aluminium hydroxides, but involves chemical bonding between the two components. It offers all the benefits of magnesium and aluminium hydroxide combinations such as prompt and sustained acid-neutralising action along with negligible effect on gastric emptying and bowel movements.

Methylpolysiloxane

- **Methylpolysiloxane** is a surface active agent that is added to many antacid preparations. It causes dispersion of antacid, collapses froth, and reduces gastro-esophageal reflux to relieve heartburn.
- **Simethicone**, an antifoaming agent, reduces the surface tension of gas bubbles, allowing easy expulsion of gases from the GIT by belching or flatus. This relieves bloating and discomfort caused by excessive gas in the stomach.

Drug–Drug Interactions with Antacids

The absorption of several drugs is reduced when given along with non-systemic antacids due to raised gastric pH and formation of complexes. For example, H₂ blockers, iron, tetracyclines, fluoroquinolones, phenothiazines, isoniazid, and ethambutol are absorbed to a lesser extent in the presence of antacids. So, the patient should be advised to maintain a gap of ~2 hours between the intake of antacids and these drugs.

Status of Antacids

In current clinical practice, the use of antacids is restricted to symptom relief in dyspepsia. They have only an adjuvant role in gastro-esophageal reflux disease (GERD) and Zollinger–Ellison syndrome. For healing of gastric and duodenal ulcers, more effective drugs such as proton pump inhibitors and H₂ blockers are preferred over antacids.

Clinical problem-based questions and MCQs

1. **Identify the antacid that has a laxative effect.**
   a. Aluminium hydroxide   b. Calcium carbonate
   c. Magnesium hydroxide   d. Magaldrate

2. **Identify the antacid which produces CO_2.**
   a. Magnesium hydroxide
   b. Sodium bicarbonate
   c. Aluminium hydroxide gel
   d. Magnesium trisilicate

3. **A 55-year-old, overweight woman with occasional dyspepsia was prescribed chewable uncoated tablets containing dried magnesium hydroxide gel 300 mg, magnesium aluminium silicate hydrate 50 mg, aluminium hydroxide 25 mg, and simethicone 25 mg.**
   i. Comment on role of each ingredient in the preparation.
   ii. Describe the rationale behind this combination of ingredients.

---

2. DRUGS THAT REDUCE ACID SECRETION

a. H₂ Blockers

Cimetidine, ranitidine, famotidine, roxatidine, loxatidine, nizatidine

Mechanism of action

All these drugs are **competitive antagonists at H₂ histaminergic receptors** in parietal cells, except loxatidine (which is a non-competitive antagonist) and famotidine (which binds tightly to H₂ receptors).

They are **highly selective** for H₂ receptors, i.e., they have no action on H₁ and H₃ receptors → block H₂ receptors on parietal cells → interfere with binding of histamine released from enterochromaffin-like cells (ECL) with H₂ receptors on parietal cells → reduction in parietal cell cAMP levels → attenuation of parietal cell response to gastrin and acetylcholine → suppression of basal and meal stimulated HCl secretion in a linear, dose-dependent way.

These actions inhibit 60–70% of total 24-hour acid secretion. The **effect on nocturnal acid secretion is more prominent** (as it is mainly histamine-mediated) than on day-time meal-stimulated acid secretion (which is mainly gastrin and ACh-mediated).

- Nocturnal and fasting stage intragastric pH rises to 4–5, owing to the inhibitory effect on acid secretion.
- Acid inhibitory effect lasts for 10 hours, so **twice-daily dose** is sufficient.
- These drugs do not have significant effect on gastrointestinal motility and lower esophageal sphincter tone.

Pharmacokinetics

H_2 blockers are rapidly absorbed after oral administration, but some drugs like cimetidine, ranitidine and famotidine undergo first-pass metabolism resulting in about 50% bioavailability. Nizatidine has low first-pass effect and 100% bioavailability. Elimination from the body occurs through hepatic metabolism, glomerular filtration, and tubular secretion.

Therapeutic uses

- H_2 blockers are commonly used for **intermittent dyspepsia** not caused by peptic ulceration.
- **Uncomplicated gastric or duodenal ulcers**: H_2 blockers, given once daily at bedtime for 6–8 weeks, achieve healing in 80–90% of cases.
- H_2 blockers are administered intravenously for prevention of gastric erosion in **stressful conditions**, e.g., in seriously ill patients in ICU.
- H_2 blockers are sometimes combined with H_1 blockers for patients with severe **unresponsive urticaria**.
- H_2 blockers were used widely for following conditions (though, proton pump inhibitors are now preferred):
  - Bleeding ulcers (prophylactic use of H_2 blockers also reduces risk of rebleeding).
  - Acute ulcers caused by *H. pylori*.
  - NSAID-induced ulcers, particularly when continued NSAID use is necessary.
  - Gastro-esophageal reflux disease
  - Zollinger–Ellison syndrome.

Adverse effects

H_2 blockers are very safe drugs, but may cause **minor** adverse effects like headache, fatigue, myalgias, and diarrhea/constipation.

- Intravenous administration in seriously ill, elderly patients, with hepatic/renal dysfunction may cause **central adverse effects** like restlessness, confusion, agitation and hallucinations. Histamine release may occur, resulting in bradycardia, hypotension, arrhythmia, and even cardiac arrest.

- Cimetidine can cause **endocrine adverse effects** as it interferes with the binding of dihydrotestosterone to receptors and also inhibits estradiol metabolism. Thus, its long-term use may cause impotence and gynecomastia in males and galactorrhea in females. Consequently, cimetidine is not used much in current clinical practice.
- Rarely, H_2 blockers can cause fever, neutropenia, and increased levels of aminotransferases.
- They cross the placental barrier and are secreted in breast milk. As a result, H_2 blockers are **not used in pregnant and lactating women** unless absolutely necessary.

Clinical problem-based questions and MCQs

4. Identify the non-competitive H_2 antagonist.
   a. Cimetidine   b. Ranitidine
   c. Loxatidine   d. Famotidine

5. Cimetidine, the prototype H_2 blocker, is not used much in clinical practice, because:
   a. Long-term use can cause gynecomastia in males
   b. It interferes with the metabolism of many concurrently administered drugs due to CYP450 inhibition.
   c. It inhibits estradiol metabolism
   d. All of the above

6. Which of the following antiulcer drugs has the potential to cause galactorrhea?
   a. Magnesium hydroxide gel   b. Cimetidine
   c. Misoprostol   d. Lansoprazole

7. H_2 blockers are used intravenously to prevent stress-induced ulcers in seriously ill patients. Enumerate the adverse effects associated with intravenous use of H_2 blockers.

b. Proton Pump Inhibitors (PPIs)

Omeprazole, lansoprazole, pantoprazole, rabeprazole, esomeprazole

Mechanism of action

- Proton pump inhibitors are weakly basic prodrugs administered as the inactive form (Fig. 64.4).
- They are acid-labile; their rapid destruction in the acidic gastric lumen can be prevented by use of acid-resistant, enteric-coated formulations.
- PPIs being weakly basic accumulate in the acidic parietal cell canaliculi, where they form active cationic forms (sulfenic acid and sulfenamide).
- Sulfenamide binds to the thiol (SH) group of H^+/K^+-ATPase by a covalent bond, resulting in its irreversible inhibition. The binding of drug with the enzyme is stronger if two molecules of drug react with one molecule of enzyme. These drugs have inhibitory effect on actively acid-secreting pumps, but have no effect on pumps in quiescent, nonsecreting vesicles.

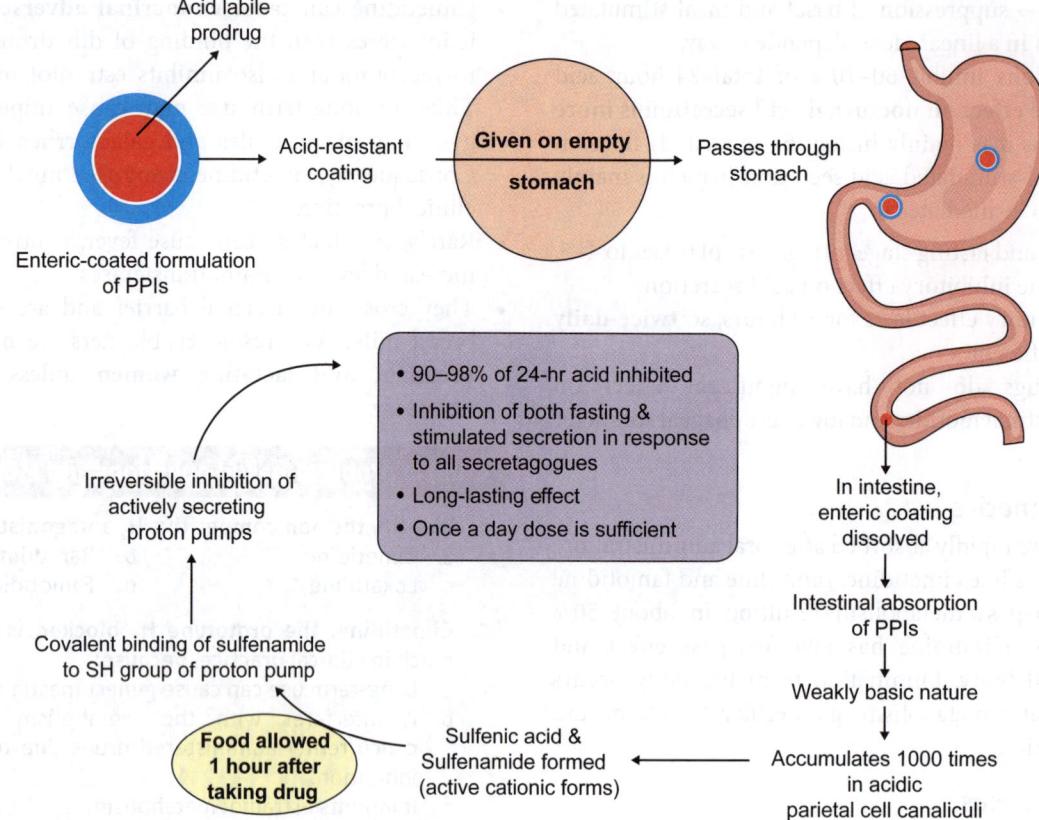

Fig. 64.4 Mechanism of action of PPIs

- Because H^+/K^+-ATPase or the proton pump is the final enzyme involved in gastric HCl synthesis, its inhibition blocks acid secretion in response to all secretagogues.
- Owing to irreversible type of enzyme inhibition by PPIs, proton pump activity is resumed only after synthesis of new enzyme. This may take about 18 hours. Thus, acid inhibitory effect of these drugs lasts longer (maybe up to 24 hours) in spite of their short half-life. Therefore, once-daily administration usually suffices.

Pharmacokinetics

Absorption

PPIs are weakly basic drugs with high lipid solubility; so, these are readily absorbed from the basic medium in the intestine, where they remain unionised. The presence of food decreases their bioavailability by 50%; as a result, **PPIs should always be given orally on an empty stomach.**

PPIs exert inhibitory effect only on actively acid-secreting pumps. While fasting, few proton pumps are actively secreting HCl. When food is allowed **1 hour after giving the drug**, it activates proton pumps for meal-stimulated acid secretion. Thus, the peak concentration of the drug coincides with maximal activity of proton pumps.

The **correct method of use of PPIs** thus involves oral administration of the drug on an empty stomach, i.e., before breakfast or dinner, followed by food after 1 hour. This much time (~1 hour) is required for the drug to reach its site of action and get activated. Food then activates proton pumps and makes them susceptible to inhibition by PPIs.

Metabolism

PPIs undergo rapid first-pass metabolism and systemic hepatic metabolism. Thus, dose reduction is indicated in patients having severe hepatic disease.

Pharmacological actions

- PPIs inhibit the final common pathway of acid secretion. So, they inhibit both fasting and meal-stimulated acid secretion. 90–98% of 24-hour acid secretion is inhibited by PPIs.
- PPIs are **highly selective** drugs, because of their pharmacokinetic characteristics—short half-life, and accumulation and activation of the drug at its site of action, i.e., gastric canaliculi.
- In spite of their short half-life, PPIs have long duration of action due to **irreversible inhibition of proton pumps**.
- PPIs also promote H. pylori eradication. While they have minor direct antimicrobial property, they **oppose H. pylori growth** by raising intragastric pH and lower minimum inhibitory concentrations (MICs) of other antibiotics against H. pylori.

Therapeutic uses

- **Role in peptic ulcer**: PPIs achieve faster symptomatic relief and ulcer healing than H_2 blockers. Notably, duodenal ulcers heal within 2–4 weeks, while gastric ulcers may take 4–8 weeks. More than 90% of duodenal and gastric ulcers are healed by PPIs.
  - High oral dose of PPIs, given for 3–5 days, reduces the incidence of rebleed from ulcers.
  - Anti-*H. pylori* regimens have PPIs as an essential component for ulcer healing and *H. pylori* eradication.
  - In NSAID-induced ulcers, PPIs promote ulcer healing, even if it is not possible to discontinue NSAIDs. PPIs are also used to prevent ulcer disease in patients receiving NSAIDs.
- **Gastro-esophageal reflux disease (GERD)**: PPIs are the most effective drugs in non-erosive and erosive reflux disease, as well as esophageal and extra-esophageal complications of reflux disease. Because there are chances of recurrence, long-term maintenance therapy with PPIs is indicated in erosive GERD.
- In **Zollinger–Ellison syndrome**, PPIs are more efficacious than H_2 blockers.
- In critically ill patients, PPIs can be used to reduce the incidence of stress-induced ulcers; however, H_2 blockers are still preferred for this condition.

ADRs

- In a few patients (1–5%), PPIs can cause headache, dizziness, abdominal pain, and diarrhea.
- PPIs reduce vitamin B_{12} absorption; so, prolonged therapy may cause mild B_{12} deficiency.
- Theoretically, PPIs carry the risk of causing atrophic gastritis, increased bacterial colonisation, intestinal metaplasia and carcinogenic potential..
- Acid suppression caused by PPIs may raise gastrin levels, which theoretically increases the risk of carcinoids. However, despite prolonged use, these complications have not been reported.

c. Anticholinergic Drugs

Pirenzepine, propantheline, oxyphenonium, etc., reduce gastric acid secretion, but have been largely superseded by H_2 blockers and PPIs. This is because anticholinergics reduce pepsin, mucus and volume of gastric secretion along with the acid; the pH is not raised much. Moreover, atropine is contraindicated in gastric ulcers because it delays gastric emptying, which exposes the ulcer bed to acidic contents for longer times.

3. ANTI-*H. pylori* DRUGS

Drugs useful for the eradication of *H. pylori* include PPIs, antimicrobial agents, and colloidal bismuth subcitrate.

Helicobacter pylori is a gram-negative bacillus that exists as a commensal in 20–70% normal persons. *H. pylori* is an aggressive factor in chronic gastritis, dyspepsia, and gastric and duodenal ulcers.

The aim of anti-*H. pylori* treatment is to eradicate the organisms, heal the ulcers and prevent relapse. *H. pylori* eradication is usually achieved using multidrug regimens in 1–2 weeks.

Antimicrobial agents (AMAs) such as tetracyclines, amoxicillin, clarithromycin, metronidazole and tinidazole are effective against *H. pylori*.

PPIs such as omeprazole is lansoprazole, pantoprazole and rabeprazole are given along with AMAs in order to alter the acidic environment and decrease the antral *H. pylori* population. Omeprazole also has minor direct inhibitory effect on these organisms.

Colloidal bismuth subcitrate is an ulcer-protective drug, which coats the ulcer for a few hours and acts as a diffusion barrier for HCl. It detaches *H. pylori* from the surface of mucosa and has direct antibacterial effect as well. Thus, in some regimens, it is added in a dose of 120 mg, four times in a day.

The FDA-approved anti-*H. pylori* regimen consists of:

- **C**larithromycin 500 mg BD + **A**moxicillin 1000 mg BD + **L**ansoprazole 30 mg BD, for 2 weeks [mnemonic: **CAL**]

Other triple drug regimens may include:

- **C**larithromycin 500 mg BD + **A**moxicillin 1 g BD + **R**abeprazole 20 mg BD [mnemonic: **CAR**]
- **C**larithromycin 500 mg BD + **A**moxicillin 1 g BD + **P**antoprazole 40 mg BD [mnemonic: **CAP**]
- **M**etronidazole 400 mg BD + **A**moxicillin 1 g BD + **P**antoprazole 40 mg BD [mnemonic: **MAP**]

Because resistance to metronidazole is quite prevalent in India, regimens containing clarithromycin and amoxicillin along with a PPI are usually preferred. Metronidazole/tinidazole are avoided if the patient has been treated with these in the recent past. Similarly, if the patient has recently received macrolides, clarithromycin is avoided.

The selected regimen is initially given for one week, which eradicates *H. pylori* in about 85% cases. In the remaining patients who fail to achieve complete eradication in one week, the same regimen is continued for another week. PPIs can be continued beyond the triple-drug regimen till complete healing is achieved.

Quadruple therapy is given in case of failure of the triple-drug regimen. It includes four drugs, i.e., clarithromycin, amoxicillin, metronidazole, and PPIs, given twice a day, for two weeks. Another quadruple-drug regimen contains colloidal bismuth subcitrate and tetracycline (given four times a day), along with metronidazole (thrice a day), and PPI (omeprazole) twice a day.

4. DRUGS THAT INCREASE PROTECTIVE FACTORS

These include prostaglandin analogues, ulcer-protective drugs and ulcer-healing drugs.

1. Ulcer-Protective Drugs
Sucralfate, colloidal bismuth subcitrate

Sucralfate
Sucralfate is a salt of sulphated sucrose complexed to aluminium hydroxide.

Mechanism of action

Sucralfate has a viscous consistency and polymerises in water or acidic solutions (pH < 4) by cross-linking of molecules. It forms a sticky gel or tenacious paste upon polymerisation. Electrostatic attraction between negatively charged sucrose sulphate and positively charged proteins in the ulcer/erosion base or crater results in selective binding of this tenacious paste to the ulcer/ erosions. This paste/gel remains bound to the ulcer for up to 6 hours, and forms a **physical barrier** to restrict further exposure of the ulcerated area to acid, pepsin and bile. Dietary proteins bind above sucrose sulphate and form another layer that coats the ulcer. In addition, sucralfate **stimulates the secretion of mucosal prostaglandins and HCO_3^-**. It also enhances **mucosal repair** by binding to epithelial and fibroblast growth factors.

Sucralfate breaks down to form sucrose sulphate and aluminium salts. Intestinal absorption is minimal (< 3%).

Therapeutic uses
- It is used in ICU patients for prevention of bleeding from stress-induced ulcers.
- It can relieve NSAID-induced dyspepsia, but cannot prevent or treat NSAID-induced ulcers.
- Dose is 1 g, four times daily, on empty stomach or an hour before meals.
- Drug–drug interactions: It should never be combined with antacids, because its polymerisation and protective action require an acidic medium.
- It can adsorb many drugs and reduces their absorption and efficacy.

ADRs

Sucralfate has no systemic ADRs, but may cause constipation due to the released aluminium salts. Nausea and dryness of mouth may occur frequently. Released aluminium salts may get absorbed, which is harmful in patients with renal insufficiency.

Colloidal bismuth subcitrate
Colloidal bismuth subcitrate (CBS) is water-soluble, though it precipitates at pH < 5. It probably acts through stimulation of **mucosal PGE_2 production**, which. in turn. increases the secretion of mucus and HCO_3^-. It **adsorbs pepsin**, and reduces pepsin output. CBS forms a glycoprotein bicomplex with mucus, which **coats the ulcer crater** and serves as a diffusion barrier for HCl. In addition, it can **detach H. pylori** from mucosa and has some direct **antimicrobial action**. CBS can bind to enterotoxins and is also useful in travellers' diarrhea. It is widely used by patients for non-specific dyspepsia and acute diarrhea. Dose is 120 mg, four times daily, i.e., with each meal and at night.

ADRs
- While CBS is very safe (bismuth absorption is negligible at < 1%), prolonged treatment is avoided in patients with renal insufficiency.
- It may cause blackening of stools, darkening of tongue, dentures, etc.
- In rare instances, long-term use causes bismuth toxicity characterised by ataxia, confusion, headache, and seizures.

2. Prostaglandin Analogues
Misoprostol is a methyl analogue of PGE_1 that is rapidly absorbed and metabolised to its active form. It has a short half-life of about 30 minutes, which necessitates three or four daily doses.

Mechanism of action

Misoprostol has both mucosal-protective as well as acid-inhibitory actions. It **stimulates secretion of HCO_3^- and mucus**, enhances **mucosal blood flow** and has ill-defined **cytoprotective action**. In addition, it reduces gastrin production and histamine-induced cAMP production in parietal cells, resulting in **modest inhibition of acid secretion**. Prostaglandins also increase fluid and electrolyte secretion from the intestines and increase intestinal motility, resulting in diarrhea as an adverse effect.

Therapeutic uses

Misoprostol decreases incidence of NSAID-induced ulcers and their complications. It is especially valuable in patients who cannot discontinue use of NSAIDs or do not quit smoking.

ADRs

Many adverse effects associated with misoprostol have limited its utility. Cramping abdominal pain and diarrhea are reported in as many as 10–20% patients. It is contraindicated in pregnancy as it causes uterine contractions leading to uterine bleeding and abortion in some cases.

3. Ulcer-Healing Drugs
Carbenoxolone sodium augments mucus production and forms thick viscid mucus, which adheres to the gastric mucosa. In addition, it slows down the destruction of prostaglandins, interferes with pepsinogen activation, and

increases glycoprotein synthesis in the gastric mucosa. Carbenoxolone increases tone of the pyloric sphincter and prevents bile reflux.

ADRs

It has mineralocorticoid effects that can cause sodium and water retention, edema, rise in BP, and hypokalemia. While such ADRs may be prevented by the aldosterone antagonist spironolactone, therapeutic efficacy decreases with this combination.

Deglycyrrhizinated liquorice has the same mechanism of action as carbenoxolone. It is less efficacious than carbenoxolone, but does not cause sodium–water retention.

Clinical problem-based questions and MCQs

8. A 50-year-old obese woman presents with post-meal dyspepsia and bloating sensation. The pain is frequent after spicy, fried food. On examination, epigastric tenderness is present. Her physician prescribes a drug that reduces acid secretion in stomach.
   i. Identify the drug prescribed.
      a. Carbenoxolone sodium
      b. Lansoprazole
      c. Aluminium hydroxide
      d. Colloidal bismuth subcitrate
   ii. Describe the mechanism of action of the prescribed drug.
   iii. What important instructions must be communicated to patient about the use of the drug?

9. *H. pylori*, a species of gram-negative bacteria, is an aggressive factor for dyspepsia and gastric and duodenal peptic ulcers.
   i. All the following drugs are effective in *H. pylori* eradication except:
      a. Rabeprazole
      b. Tinidazole
      c. Sucralfate
      d. Colloidal bismuth subcitrate
   ii. Describe the FDA-approved triple-drug regimen for *H. pylori* eradication.

10. i. Which of the following antiulcer drugs should not be combined with antacids?
       a. Misoprostol   b. Sucralfate
       c. Ranitidine   d. Omeprazole
    ii. Explain why the selected drug cannot be combined with antacids.

11. i. Identify the most suitable drug for the prevention of stress-induced ulcers in critically ill patients.
       a. Intravenous H_2 blockers.
       b. Proton pump inhibitors
       c. Colloidal bismuth subcitrate
       d. Tetracyclines
    ii. Enumerate the adverse effects of the selected drug.

12. i. Identify an antiulcer drug, which shows reduced efficacy on combining spironolactone.
       a. Cimetidine
       b. Colloidal bismuth subcitrate
       c. Misoprostol
       d. Carbenoxolone
    ii. Describe the mechanism of antiulcer effect of the selected drug and its interaction with spironolactone.

MANAGEMENT OF PEPTIC ULCER

Diagnosis

Diagnosis of peptic ulcer is based on clinical features, endoscopic examination of gastric and duodenal mucosa, demonstration of ulcer crater defects by barium swallow studies, and imaging studies (X-ray abdomen erect), and CT scans to detect perforation by presence of air under the diaphragm. *H. pylori* is detected by enzyme-linked immunoassay (ELISA), endoscopic biopsy, and culture tests.

Treatment

The aim of treatment of peptic ulcers is to relieve the symptoms, heal the ulcers, and prevent complications and recurrence. **Treatment** is largely based on lifestyle modifications and drug therapy. Surgical interventions are indicated in complicated cases (bleeding from ulcer and perforated ulcers).

Lifestyle modifications

These measures decrease the severity of symptoms, slow down the worsening of disease, and prevent recurrence. Recommended lifestyle changes include:

- Avoiding very hot, fatty, fried, or spicy foods and caffeinated beverages.
- Reducing alcohol intake.
- Quitting smoking.
- Stress reduction.

Drug therapy

Proton pump inhibitors are the mainstay of drug treatment for healing of peptic ulcers. These achieve better and faster ulcer-healing than other drug groups and have proved to be safe even upon prolonged use. Antacids are useful for quick symptom relief. Anti-*H. pylori* triple drug regimens are very effective for healing ulcers that test positive for *H. pylori*.

Surgical interventions

Surgery is required only for bleeding and perforated ulcers. Bleeding ulcers may be treated by oversewing of the ulcer, vagotomy, and partial gastrectomy. Perforated ulcers need primary repair of the ulcer with an omental patch (Graham patch) and definitive surgery such as a vagotomy with drainage or an antrectomy. Partial gastrectomy may be required in patients with large perforations.

Summary

- Peptic ulcers occur due to increased aggressive factors (acid, pepsin, *H. pylori*) and decreased protective factors (HCO_3^-, mucus).
- Acid in gastric lumen may be neutralised by antacids.
- **Systemic antacids** such as sodium bicarbonate and sodium citrate have many adverse effects and are not preferred. Non-systemic antacids containing magnesium hydroxide and aluminium hydroxide gel are combined to obtain quick onset, long duration of acid neutralising action, and to counteract each other's adverse effect on gut motility.
- Reduction of gastric acid secretion is achieved using H_2 antagonists, proton pump inhibitors (PPIs), anticholinergics, and prostaglandin analogues.
- **Antagonists at H_2 receptors** such as ranitidine and famotidine reduce 24-hour acid secretion by 60–70% and are useful in dyspepsia, peptic ulcer, and GERD. They have been largely superseded by PPIs but are still used IV to prevent ulcers in stressful conditions (seriously ill patients in intensive care units). Adverse effects such as headache, dizziness, and bowel upset may occur. Cimetidine causes CYP450 enzyme inhibition, leading to many DDIs, gynecomastia, and galactorrhea.
- **PPIs** are the most effective antiulcer drugs. They cause irreversible inhibition of the proton pumps, which is the final step of acid secretion from any secretagogue. They decrease 24-hour acid secretion by 80–90%. PPIs are prodrugs used orally in peptic ulcers, bleeding ulcers, stress ulcers, GERD, Zollinger–Ellison syndrome, and aspiration pneumonia. They may cause headache, muscle and joint pain, dizziness, rashes, and atrophic gastritis. PPIs should be given on an empty stomach followed by food after one hour to activate proton pumps, which are more prone to inhibition by the active form of PPIs.
- **Anti-H. pylori** triple-drug regimens include two AMAs along with a PPI; clarithromycin and amoxicillin with omeprazole/lansoprazole/pantoprazole or metronidazole with amoxicillin and a PPI. Quadruple-drug regimens are used when treatment with triple-drug regimen fails.
- **PGE_1 analogue**, misoprostol, acts by stimulating mucus and bicarbonate secretion. It is effective for prevention of NSAID-induced ulcers in patients who cannot stop NSAIDs or quit smoking. It is not preferred because cramps and diarrhea are frequent adverse effects.
- **Ulcer-protective drugs** like sucralfate and colloidal bismuth subcitrate coat the ulcer with a physical barrier to protect it from acid and pepsin exposure. Sucralfate polymerises in acidic pH to form a sticky gel-like substance that adheres to the ulcer base for a few hours.
- Carbenoxolone and deglycyrrhizinated liquorice are ulcer-healing agents.

Hints for problem based questions and MCQs

1. c. Magnesium hydroxide
2. b. Sodium bicarbonate
3. i. Refer to pages 837, 838.
   ii. Refer to page 837.
4. c. Loxatidine
5. d. All of the above
6. b. Cimetidine
7. Central adverse effects, such as restlessness, anxiety, agitation and histamine release, resulting in fall in BP, and arrhythmias.
8. i. b. Lansoprazole
   ii. PPIs. Refer to page 839.
   iii. Drug to be given empty stomach, and food allowed 1 hour after drug. Refer to page 840.
9. i. c. Sucralfate
   ii. Refer to page 841
10. i. b. Sucralfate
    ii. Its activation needs acidic pH. Refer to page 842.
11. i. a. Intravenous H_2 blockers
    ii. Intravenous administration of H_2 blockers may cause central adverse effects such as restlessness, confusion, agitation, and hallucinations. Histamine release may result in bradycardia, hypotension, arrhythmia and even cardiac arrest.
12. i. d. Carbenoxolone
    ii. Refer to page 842.

CONCEPT MAP – DRUGS FOR PEPTIC ULCER

Antacids

Mechanism: Neutralise gastric acid → raise gastric pH → indirectly decrease pepsin activity.

Promote mucosal defense by increasing PG synthesis. Silica produced in reaction of Mg trisilicate with HCl is gelatinous → protects ulcer base & adsorbs pepsin.

But agents raising antral pH to 4 → reflex gastrin release → acid rebound.

Uses: Na bicarbonate: Only for quick symptom relief in heartburn.

Non-systemic antacids: Only for symptom relief in dyspepsia & adjuvant role in GERD, ZE syndrome.

Mg hydroxide/carbonate: Prompt action, forms Mg chloride during reaction → osmotically active, Mg^{2+} ions induce cholecystokinin release → laxative & gastric hurrying effect.

Al hydroxide has slow, sustained action.

Al^{3+} ions relax smooth muscles → constipation & delayed gastric emptying.

Mg and Al containing antacids used in combination for prompt, sustained effect, without any adverse effects on bowel movement & gastric emptying.

H₂ Blockers

Cimetidine, Ranitidine, Famotidine, Roxatidine, Loxatidine, nizatidine.

Mechanism: Competitive H_2 blockers in parietal cells, except Loxatidine & Famotidine → Attenuate parietal cell response to gastrin and ACh → Suppress basal & meal-stimulated HCl secretion, inhibit 60–70% of total 24-hour acid secretion.

Uses: Intermittent dyspepsia not caused by peptic ulceration.

Uncomplicated gastric or duodenal ulcers

Used IV for prevention of gastric erosions in stressful conditions.

Combined with H_1 blockers in severe unresponsive urticaria.

ADRs: Minor as headache, fatigue, myalgia, diarrhea/constipation.

IV use → restlessness, confusion, agitation & hallucinations.

Long-term use of cimetidine may cause impotence, gynecomastia in males & galactorrhea in females.

Rarely fever, neutropenia & increased aminotransferase levels.

Drugs for Peptic Ulcer

Ulcer-protective drugs

Sucralfate

Mechanism: Polymerises at a pH < 4, forms sticky gel that coats ulcers, dietary proteins bind above sucrose sulphate. Also stimulates PG, HCO_3^- secretion & enhances mucosal repair.

Uses: 1 g four times daily on empty stomach or an hour before meals, for prevention of bleeding from stress-induced ulcers, for relieving NSAID-induced dyspepsia.

ADRs: Constipation, nausea, dryness of mouth.

Not to be combined with antacids.

Colloidal bismuth subcitrate

Mechanism: Precipitates at pH < 5, stimulates mucosal PGE_2 production → increased secretion of mucus and HCO_3^-. It forms a glycoprotein bicomplex with mucus that coats the ulcer crater.

Adsorbs pepsin, can detach *H. pylori* from mucosa, has some direct antimicrobial action, binds to enterotoxins.

Uses: In *H. pylori* eradication regimens.

In non-specific dyspepsia and acute diarrhea.

Dose: 120 mg, four times daily

ADRs: Blackening of stools, darkening of tongue, dentures, etc.

Long-term use → ataxia, confusion, headache, seizure

Misoprostol: PGE_1 analogue, stimulates HCO_3^- and mucus secretion, enhances mucosal blood flow and has ill-defined cytoprotective action.

Also reduces gastrin production and histamine-induced cAMP production in parietal cells.

Uses: To decrease incidence of NSAID-induced ulcers and their complications, specially if NSAIDs cannot be discontinued.

ADRs: Many adverse effects, cramping abdominal pain & diarrhea.

Proton Pump Inhibitors (PPIs)

Omeprazole, Lansoprazole, Pantoprazole, Rabeprazole, Esomeprazole

Mechanism: PPIs (enteric-coated formulation) given orally, empty stomach as food reduces bioavailability by 50%.

Food given 1 hour after drug to activate proton pumps

PPIs absorbed in intestine → accumulate in parietal cell canaliculi → form sulfenamide → binds to SH group of active proton pumps → irreversible inhibition of 90–98% of total 24-hour acid secretion due to any secretagogue.

Uses: Peptic ulcer: Essential component of anti-*H. pylori* regimens for ulcer healing, high dose used to reduce incidence of rebleed from ulcers & promote ulcer healing in NSAID-induced ulcers even if NSAID is not discontinued.

Non-erosive/erosive GERD with esophageal or extra-esophageal complications

ZE syndrome

ADRs: Headache, dizziness, abdominal pain, diarrhea, mild B_{12} deficiency.

Anti-*H. pylori* Triple-Drug Regimens

Clarithromycin 500 mg with Amoxicillin 1000 mg and Lansoprazole 30 mg given twice daily for 2 weeks (FDA approved).

Clarithromycin 500 mg BD+ Amoxicillin 1 g BD + Rabeprazole 20 mg BD

Clarithromycin 500 mg BD+ Amoxicillin 1 g BD + Pantoprazole 40 mg BD

Metronidazole 400 mg BD + Amoxicillin 1 g BD + Pantoprazole 40 mg BD

SECTION 12 Miscellaneous Topics

65 Immunomodulator Drugs

PH 9.1 Describe the types, kinetics, dynamics, therapeutic uses, adverse drug reactions of immunomodulators.
PH 9.4 Describe basics of vaccine use and types of vaccines.

Learning objectives

A student of MBBS phase II should be able to:
- Describe normal innate and acquired immune system.
- Describe disorders of abnormal immune functioning.
- Classify immunosuppressant drugs.
- Describe the mechanisms of action of immunosuppressant drugs.
- Enumerate therapeutic uses and adverse effects of immunosuppressant drugs.
- Describe the role of immunosuppression in organ transplantation.
- Classify immunostimulants and describe their role in clinical practice.
- Describe the National Immunisation Schedule.

NORMAL IMMUNE RESPONSE

The **normal immune response** plays an important role in the elimination of pathogens, destruction of malignant cells, and neutralisation of various toxins. It consists of the **innate** and **adaptive** immune systems.

1. Innate Immune System

The innate immune system is the body's first line of defence against infecting organisms (bacteria, fungi, viruses, parasites, etc.), which serve as the antigen (Ag). Innate immunity is conferred by physical, biochemical and cellular barriers.

a. Physical barriers
Physical barriers that contribute to innate immunity consist of **intact skin and mucosa**.

b. Biochemical barriers
- **Lysozymes** that help to dissolve the peptidoglycan cell wall of pathogens.
- **Complement system** comprising nine proteins (C1–C9) that split into fragments during activation.
  - Complements C3a and C5a have chemotactic effect and cause migration of immune cells to the site of inflammation.
  - Complement C3b acts as opsonin, coats the pathogen, and enhances its phagocytosis by macrophages and neutrophils.
  - Complements C5b, C6, C7, C8, and C9 together constitute the **membrane attack complex** (MAC), which creates pores in the pathogen's cell membrane and causes leakage of its components, resulting in cell death.
- **Interferon gamma** (IFN-γ) directly activates macrophages and natural killer (NK) cells and down-regulates T helper type 2 (Th2) cells.

c. Cellular barrier
The cellular barriers consist of polymorphonuclear leukocytes (neutrophils, basophils, eosinophils), monocytes, macrophages, natural killer (NK) cells, and natural killer T (NKT) cells.

The immune response to a pathogenic invasion is described below.

Infection → inflammatory response
↓
Release of chemotactic cytokines*
↓
Migration of neutrophils and monocytes from peripheral circulation to the site of infection
↓
Phagocytosis, degradation of pathogens
↓
Prevention/decreased duration and severity of infective disease

*Chemotactic cytokines [interleukin-8 (IL-8)], macrophage chemotactic protein-1(MCP-1), and macrophage inflammatory protein-1α (MIP-1α) are released from tissue macrophages and activated by endothelial cells.

Natural killer (NK) cells do not kill pathogens but possess a unique ability to kill virus-infected and malignant cells **selectively**, while sparing the normal host cells. This is a result of '**major histocompatibility complex type-1**' (MHC-I) expressed on the surface of normal nucleated

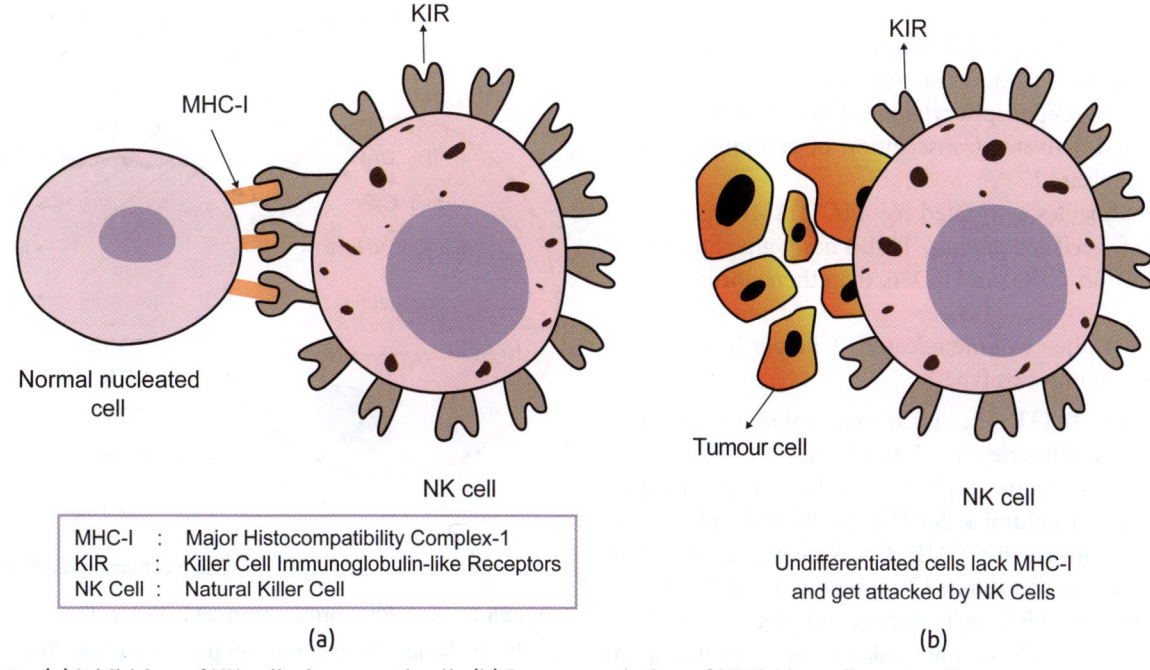

Fig. 65.1 (a) Inhibition of NK cells; by normal cells (b) Down-regulation of MHC-I in malignant cells

cells. MHC-I binds to '**killer cell immunoglobulin-like receptors**' (KIR) present on the surface of NK cells and inhibits them. However, in virus-infected cells and malignant cells, down-regulation of MHC-I expression occurs, making them more prone to attack by NK cells (Fig. 65.1a,b). Natural killer T (NKT) cells possessing T-cell receptors have the ability to recognise lipid antigens. They play an important role in host defence against infections, tumours and autoimmune diseases.

2. Acquired or Adaptive Immune Response

The adaptive or acquired immune system gets activated when the physical, biochemical, and cellular barriers of innate response fail to cope up with infection. The acquired immune response manifests as:

- Humoral immunity through production of antibodies (Ab)
- Cell-mediated immunity (CMI) through activation of T lymphocytes.

The important characteristics of the acquired immune system such as the ability to differentiate between self and non-self antigens, vigorous memory response, and antigen specificity are described below.

a. Ability to differentiate between self-antigen (of the host) and non-self-antigen (foreign particles)

The ability of T-lymphocytes to differentiate between **self-** and **non-self**-antigens develops in the thymus. This occurs through negative selection (apoptosis) of T cells that have higher affinity for self-antigens along with positive selection (retention and expansion) of T cells that recognise foreign antigens in the presence of self-MHC molecules. Similarly, the selection of B lymphocytes occurs in the bone marrow, where B lymphocytes reactive against self-antigens are deleted, whereas those specific for foreign antigens are retained and expanded. Subsequently, these positively selected T and B lymphocytes reach peripheral circulation, lymph nodes, spleen, and lymphoid tissue.

b. Responds to previously encountered antigens through vigorous memory response

The primary antibody response on first exposure is the secretion of IgM antibodies. Subsequent exposure to the same antigen involves **booster response** with secretion of IgA, IgG and IgE antibodies. These antibodies enhance phagocytosis by acting as opsonins, and induce inflammatory response and bacterial lysis by activating the complement system.

c. Antigen specificity

The acquired immune system responds in a specific manner to a wide range of antigens. Antigen specificity is initiated by antigen-presenting cells (APCs) such as B lymphocytes, macrophages, and dendritic cells. These cells phagocytose pathogens and process them into peptides that serve as antigens, generating the first signal.

The **second signal** is the binding of co-stimulatory molecules present on antigen-presenting cells (CD40, CD80 and CD86) with their respective ligands on CD8 T cells (ligand present on T cells for CD40 is CD40L, for CD80 and CD86 it is CD28). Upon activation by both signals, T cells secrete various cytokines (Flowchart 65.1, Fig. 65.2). In absence of the second signal, the T cells become unresponsive and cell anergy or apoptosis occurs.

Peptide antigen loaded on MHC-1 binds to TCR → activates PLC → IP$_3$–DAG pathway → raised intracellular Ca^{2+} → calcium–calmodulin complex formed → activates calcineurin → dephosphorylation of NFAT → moves into nucleus and activates transcription of cytokine genes → cytokines released.

T lymphocytes associated Ag-4 (CTLA-4) regulate the process of T-cell activation. CTLA-4 has higher affinity for co-stimulators CD80 and CD86, than their normal ligand CD28.

Based on the cytokine released, T-helper lymphocytes are classified into two types:

- **T helper-1 (Th1)** cells secrete interferon gamma (IFN-γ) and interleukins 2 and 12 (IL-2, IL-12). These, in turn, activate macrophages, cytotoxic T lymphocytes (CTLs) and natural killer (NK) cells and induce cell-mediated immunity (CMI). Cytokine production from Th1 cells can be inhibited by interleukin-10 (IL-10).
- **T helper-2 (Th2)** cells secrete interleukins 4, 5, 6, 10, and 13. These interleukins cause proliferation and differentiation of B cells into plasma cells, which secrete antibodies (Ab) and induce humoral immunity. Proliferation of Th2 cells is inhibited by IFN-γ.

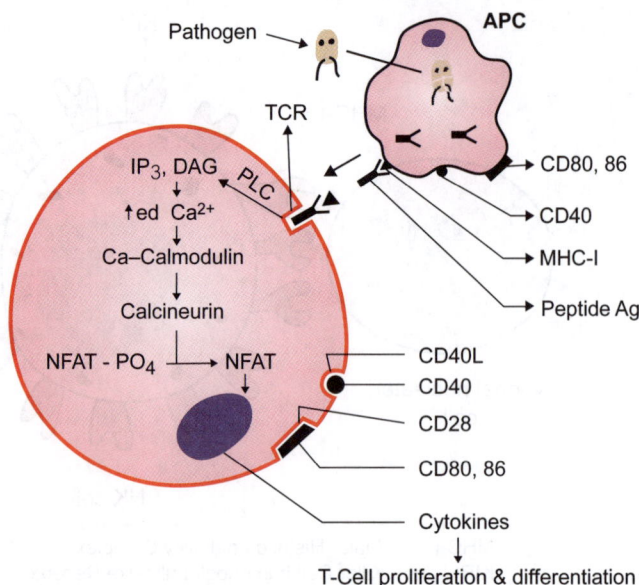

Fig. 65.2 Cytokine production by CD8 T-cells
(MHC-1: Major histocompatibility complex; TCR: T cell receptor; PLC: Phospholipase C; PIP2: Phosphatidylinositol 4,5-biphosphate; IP3: Inositol triphosphate; DAG: Diacyl glycerol; NFAT: Nuclear factor of activated T cells)

> Antigenic stimuli that elicit Th1 or Th2 responses are not clearly understood. However, extracellular bacteria cause cytokine production from Th2 cells, leading to antibody formation that can neutralise the antigen. In contrast, intracellular bacteria trigger a Th1 response, resulting in cytokine production and cell-mediated immunity (CMI). Antigens of virus-infected cells or tumour cells, when processed by APCs and loaded on MHC-I, activate CD8 T-lymphocytes. These cytotoxic T cells induce target cell death via lytic granules, perforin-mediated lysis and apoptosis.

ABNORMAL IMMUNE RESPONSE

Disorders associated with immune response can occur either as inadequate immune response (**immunodeficiency disorders**) or inappropriate immune response, causing **hypersensitivity reactions** and **autoimmune diseases**.

1. Immunodeficiency Disorders

Conditions involving insufficient immune response can be congenital or acquired secondary to bacterial/viral infections or drugs. The patient is more prone to infectious diseases, including opportunistic infections. The disease tends to be more severe, lasts longer, and is often fatal.

a. Congenital immunodeficiency diseases

Congenital immunodeficiency diseases such as X-linked agammaglobulinemia, DiGeorge syndrome, and severe combined immunodeficiency disorder (SCID) occur quite rarely.

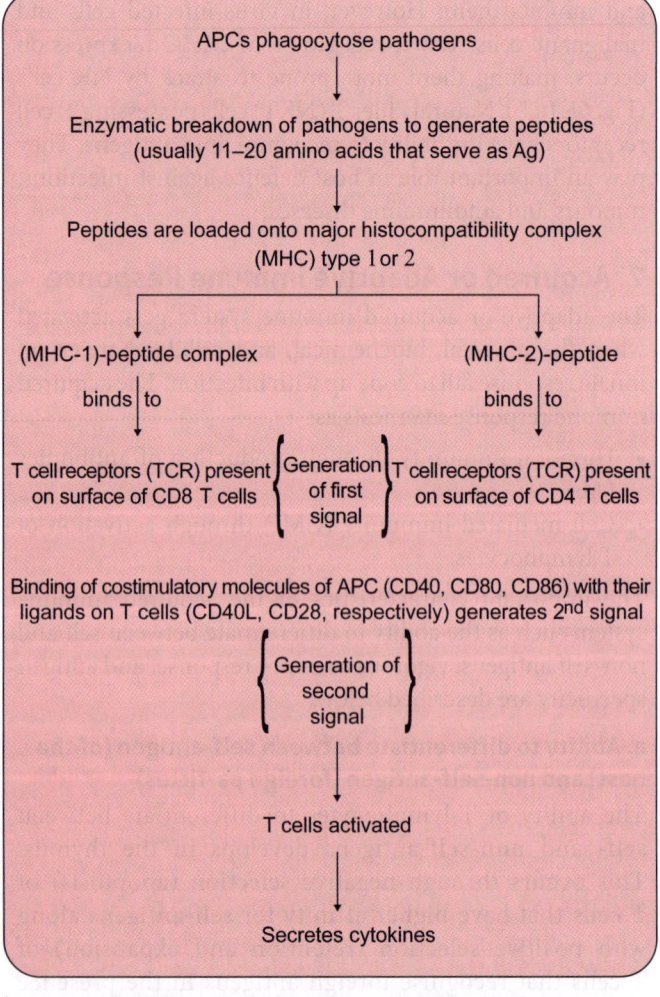

Flowchart 65.1 Cytokine production by T cells

In X-linked agammaglobulinemia, immature B lymphocytes fail to mature into Ab-producing plasma cells. So, in this condition, only humoral immunity is compromised, but CMI is preserved. In contrast, in DiGeorge syndrome the thymus fails to develop; as a result, CMI is deficient and humoral immunity is preserved.

In severe combined immunodeficiency disorder (SCID), both humoral immunity and CMI are compromised by deficiency of the enzyme **adenosine deaminase** (ADA), which is responsible for clearing deoxy ATP. The absence of ADA causes accumulation of deoxy ATP, which damages both T and B lymphocytes.

b. Acquired immunodeficiency conditions

Acquired immunodeficiency conditions include acquired immunodeficiency syndrome (**AIDS**) caused by HIV infection, which leads to deficiency of CD4 T-helper cells. As a result, the risk of opportunistic infections and malignancies increases in AIDS patients. It also causes an imbalance between the activity of Th2 and Th1 cells. Higher Th2 activity causes hypergammaglobulinemia, whereas reduced Th1 activity causes reduced activity of cytotoxic T lymphocytes and delayed hypersensitivity reactions.

2. Inappropriate Immune Function
a. Autoimmune disorders

These are conditions in which the immune system fails to distinguish between **self** and **non-self** or foreign tissue antigens. Activation of self-reactive B and T lymphocytes generates humoral- or cell-mediated immune response, respectively, against self-antigens. Examples of autoimmune diseases include rheumatoid arthritis, multiple sclerosis, systemic lupus erythematosus, and insulin-dependent diabetes mellitus.

Autoimmune processes may involve self-reactive T lymphocyte activity in response to:

- Antigens previously sequestrated from the immune system or pathogenic antigens possessing similar epitopes as normal host tissue.
- Exposure to pathogenic antigens activating the CMI and humoral response, which affects the host tissues as well, e.g., rheumatic fever after *Streptococcus pyogenes* infection.
- Expression of MHC-II on normal host cells causes presentation of self-peptides to T-helper cells, which also results in autoimmune response.

b. Transplant rejections

Transplant rejections can occur due to abnormal immune response against transplanted solid organs. The transplant rejection can be hyperacute, accelerated, acute, or chronic.

Hyperacute transplant rejection occurs within a few hours of the procedure. It is caused by preformed antibodies against the donor organ, e.g., anti-blood group antibodies. Immunosuppressive drugs cannot check this reaction and the transplanted organ gets necrosed rapidly.

Accelerated rejection mediated through CMI and antibodies also cannot be controlled by immunosuppressive drugs.

Acute rejection of the transplanted organ occurs within few days to months of the procedure. It is mainly mediated through the CMI and can be reversed by immunosuppressive drugs.

Chronic transplant rejection may occur months or even years after the procedure. It involves both CMI and humoral immunity and is amenable to immunosuppressive drugs.

c. Graft-versus-host disease

Graft-versus-host disease occurs commonly in patients who receive an allogeneic hematopoietic stem cell transplant. Here, stem cells of an HLA-matched donor are infused after conditioning the recipient with high dose chemo- or radiotherapy. The recipient's immunity is totally suppressed to prevent rejection of the donor stem cells. Slowly, the recipient develops a new immune system from the donor stem cells. Graft-versus-host disease occurs when the donor T cells are unable to recognise the recipient's tissues as self-tissues and attack the recipient tissues such as the skin, liver, and gut. Acute graft-versus-host disease manifests as skin rashes, hepatotoxicity and severe diarrhea within 100 days of allogeneic transplant. Acute reactions may progress to chronic graft-versus-host disease later on. Immunosuppressive drugs are useful both in acute as well as chronic graft-versus-host disease. It usually resolves within a couple of years of the procedure, and the drugs can be discontinued.

d. Hypersensitivity reactions

Hypersensitivity reactions can be Ab-mediated (Types I, II, and III) and CMI-mediated (Type IV). The first exposure to the antigen causes sensitisation, while subsequent exposures cause tissue damage through immunologic memory.

Type I hypersensitivity

This is the immediate reaction mediated through IgE antibodies present on surface of basophils or tissue mast cells. Binding of Ag to surface Abs causes cell degranulation and release of mediators such as histamine, leukotrienes, and eosinophil chemotactic factors that cause asthma, hay fever, urticaria, and anaphylactic shock. It requires immediate treatment.

Type II hypersensitivity

It involves the formation of a complex of surface Ag with preformed IgM or IgG Abs, resulting in the activation of the complement cascade, formation of membrane attack complex, and cell lysis. For instance, when an Rh-negative mother carries an Rh-positive fetus, the IgG anti-Rh antibodies produced by the mother can cross the placenta, bind to Rh antigens on fetal RBCs, and cause hemolytic disease of the newborn.

Such Type II hypersensitivity reactions may also be drug-induced, e.g., with penicillin, which can bind to RBCs and trigger antibody-mediated destruction.

Type III hypersensitivity

These occur due to deposition of antigen–antibody complexes on the basement membrane in blood vessels and tissues. Such deposition activates the C3a, C4a, and C5a components of the complement, causing chemotaxis and increased permeability. The patient develops skin rashes, glomerulonephritis, arthritis, etc., 3–4 days after exposure to the antigen.

Type IV hypersensitivity

These are delayed hypersensitivity reactions involving the CMI. Antigen-specific Th1 cells induce a local inflammatory response resulting in tissue damage, e.g., contact dermatitis and tuberculin positive reaction.

IMMUNOSUPPRESSANT DRUGS

Immunosuppressant drugs include anti-proliferative drugs, corticosteroids, calcineurin inhibitors, mTOR inhibitors, thalidomide and biological agents (Flowchart 65.2).

A. Antiproliferative Drugs
1. Azathioprine

Azathioprine is a prodrug that is selectively taken up by immune cells and activated intracellularly to form mercaptopurine. Mercaptopurine is an antimetabolite, a purine antagonist that **inhibits nucleic acid synthesis** and **de novo purine synthesis**. Hence, azathioprine inhibits

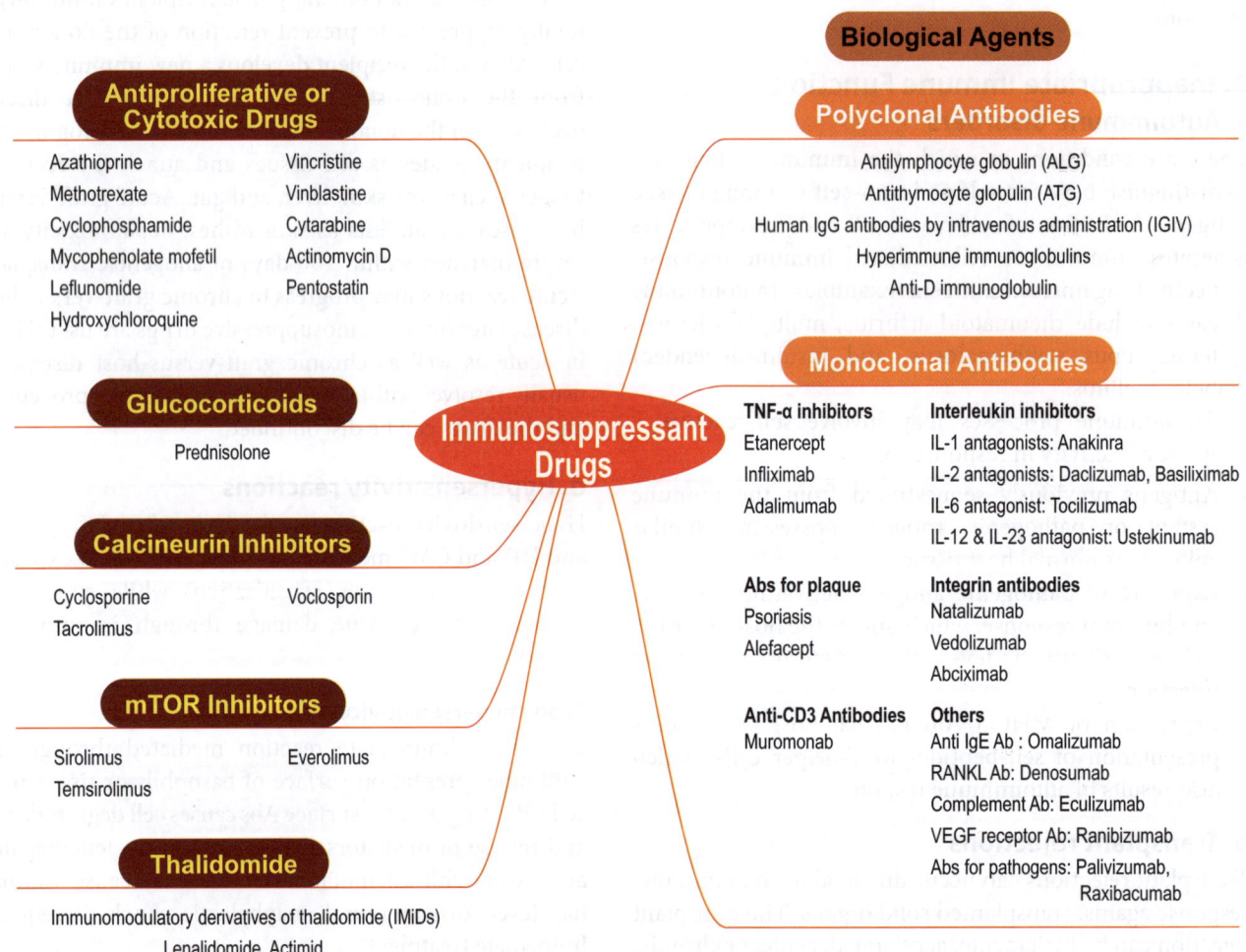

Flowchart 65.2 Classification of immunosuppressant drugs

lymphoid cell proliferation and differentiation, following exposure to antigens. It destroys stimulated lymphoid cells due to its cytotoxic effect; cellular immunity and serum antibody response are blocked. The immunosuppressant effect of azathioprine is more marked than its anticancer effect.

Pharmacokinetics

Azathioprine has good oral absorption. First, it gets converted into the active metabolite mercaptopurine, which exerts immunosuppressive and cytotoxic effect. Mercaptopurine is then metabolised by xanthine oxidase enzyme to form 6-thiouric acid, which is excreted in the urine. Small amounts of azathioprine and mercaptopurine are excreted unchanged by the kidney. Therefore, in patients of chronic gout on allopurinol therapy (xanthine oxidase inhibitor), the dosage of azathioprine should be reduced to one-fourth to one-third of the normal therapeutic dose.

Therapeutic uses

- Azathioprine is less effective than cyclosporine in **preventing graft rejection in renal and other tissue transplants**. So, it is used mainly in patients who develop cyclosporine toxicity.
- Azathioprine is a good alternative to corticosteroids in **autoimmune diseases** such as glomerulonephritis, systemic lupus erythematosus (SLE), multiple sclerosis, Crohn's disease, IBD, autoimmune hemolytic anemia, and idiopathic thrombocytopenia.
- Oral azathioprine combined with topically applied steroids may restore pigmentation in **vitiligo**.
- Low-dose therapy is useful as a disease-modifying antirheumatic drug (**DMARD**).

ADRs

Azathioprine can cause nausea, vomiting, diarrhea, fever, rashes and hepatic dysfunction. Bone marrow suppression may occur, that results in leukopenia, thrombocytopenia, and anemia.

2. Methotrexate

Methotrexate is also an antimetabolite; it is a folate antagonist that inhibits dihydrofolate reductase and interferes with cytokine production. It is a potent inhibitor of CMI and is extensively used as a first-line drug in rheumatoid arthritis (as a DMARD), pemphigus, psoriasis, chronic active hepatitis, uveitis, myasthenia gravis, etc.

Purine antagonists such as azathioprine and MMF are widely used for immunosuppression; however, methotrexate is a good alternative to these drugs in patients who show idiosyncratic reactions.

3. Cyclophosphamide

Cyclophosphamide, an alkylating agent, is considered one of the most effective immunosuppressive drugs. It causes **alkylation and cell death** of proliferating lymphoid cells and has a more marked effect on humoral immunity than on CMI.

Large doses of cyclophosphamide given with or soon after antigen exposure result in the **development of specific tolerance** to the new antigen. This effect is useful in **bone marrow transplantation**. Cyclophosphamide is used as a reserve drug in other transplants.

Small doses are effective in **autoimmune diseases** such as SLE, pemphigus and hemolytic anemia. Cyclophosphamide is effective in patients with acquired factor XIII antibodies, bleeding syndrome, Wegner's granulomatosis and antibody-induced cell aplasia.

ADRs

Large doses of cyclophosphamide may cause nausea, vomiting, electrolyte disturbance, hemorrhagic cystitis, pancytopenia and cardiac toxicity.

4. Mycophenolate mofetil (MMF)

MMF, upon hydrolysis is converted into mycophenolic acid, which **interferes with the de novo synthesis of guanosine nucleotides in T and B cells** and inhibits their response to antigen exposure. Thus, CMI and antibody production in response to antigens is suppressed. Mycophenolic acid is then inactivated by glucuronide conjugation and excreted in the urine.

Therapeutic uses

- MMF is the first-line drug for preventing chronic allograft vasculopathy in **cardiac transplant** recipients.
- It is useful in acute as well as chronic **graft-versus-host reactions** after hematopoietic stem cell transplantation.
- MMF is used orally in a dose of 1.0 g, twice daily as an **add-on drug with corticosteroids and cyclosporine in solid organ transplant rejection** that does not respond adequately to other drugs, or in patients who develop intolerable adverse effects (like nephrotoxicity with cyclosporine). The addition of MMF reduces the dose of cyclosporine, thus reducing nephrotoxicity. The combination of MMF with corticosteroids and sirolimus is not nephrotoxic.
- MMF may be useful in rheumatoid arthritis, IBD, lupus nephritis, etc.

ADRs

MMF is the **least toxic immunosuppressant drug**. ADRs include nausea, vomiting, diarrhea, abdominal pain, gastro-intestinal bleeding, rise in blood pressure, and headache. Reversible myelosuppression that mainly causes neutropenia may also occur.

5. Leflunomide

It is also a prodrug that inhibits pyrimidine synthesis upon activation. It suppresses the proliferation of stimulated lymphocytes and is approved for use as a **DMARD** in rheumatoid arthritis. The active metabolite has a long half-life. Thus, leflunomide is given in a loading dose of 100 mg/day for the first 3 days followed by a maintenance dose of 20 mg, once a day.

ADRs include nausea, diarrhea, alopecia, headache, thrombocytopenia, neutropenia, and hepatic dysfunction.

6. Hydroxychloroquine (HCQ)

HCQ is an antimalarial drug that has low efficacy as an immunosuppressant; it also has lower toxicity than other drugs in this group. HCQ acts by increasing the pH of lysosomes and endosomes and stabilising them. It also causes free radical scavenging. HCQ interferes with the intracellular processing of antigens and loading of peptides onto MHC-II inside Ag-processing cells (APC). Thus, T cell activation is suppressed. It also inhibits B lymphocytes by reducing interleukin-1 secretion from monocytes.

HCQ is useful in some autoimmune disorders such as **nonerosive rheumatoid arthritis, SLE, and after allogeneic stem cell transplantation** for prophylaxis as well as treatment of graft-versus-host reactions.

ADRs

When used for long durations, HCQ can get accumulated in melanin-containing tissues causing retinal damage, corneal opacity, greying of hair etc. It may also cause neuropathy, myopathy, and IBS.

Others

Antiproliferative drugs such as vincristine, vinblastine, cytarabine, actinomycin D and pentostatin also have immunosuppressive effect. Vincristine is used in idiopathic thrombocytopenic purpura that does not respond to corticosteroids. Vinblastine inhibits the release of histamine and other vasoactive peptides from mast cells. Pentostatin is useful to prevent or treat graft-versus-host reaction after allogeneic stem cell transplants.

B. Glucocorticoids

Glucocorticoids possess immunosuppressive as well as non-specific anti-inflammatory activity. They affect the immune response at many steps, as described below.

- Corticosteroids cause a modest increase in the rate of destruction of normal lymphoid cells, but have a marked **lympholytic effect** on malignant lymphoid cells. This differential effect is probably because glucocorticoids interfere with the cell cycle of activated lymphoid cells. The lymphoid content as well as the size of lymph nodes and spleen is reduced. This lympholytic action makes corticosteroids useful in lymphomas.
- Corticosteroids cause sequestration of lymphocytes, eosinophils and basophils in peripheral tissues; this lowers cell counts in circulation (**lymphopenia**), resulting in suppression of CMI response.
- Corticosteroids reduce the ability of antigen presenting cells (APC), especially tissue macrophages, to respond to antigens and mitogens. This **decreases the ability of macrophages** for phagocytosis and killing pathogenic microbes. Secretion of TNF-α, interleukin-1, plasminogen activator, and metalloproteinases from macrophages is also reduced.
- Release of interleukin-12 and IFN-γ from lymphocytes and macrophages decreases, resulting in **reduced activity of T helper-1 cells and CMI response.**

The immunosuppressant action of glucocorticoids is more marked on cell-mediated immunity than on humoral immunity; however, primary antibody response is diminished. Continued use of corticosteroids reduces **previously developed antibody responses**, and increases the rate of breakdown of specific igG Abs.

Therapeutic uses

The immunosuppressant and non-specific anti-inflammatory actions of glucocorticoids have several applications:

- **Autoimmune disorders:** Prednisolone is the **drug of choice** for idiopathic thrombocytopenic purpura, autoimmune hemolytic anemia, and acute glomerulonephritis.
- It is also used in **autoreactive tissue disorders**, e.g., systemic lupus erythematosus, rheumatoid arthritis, multiple sclerosis, chronic active hepatitis, inflammatory bowel disease (IBD), and dermatomyositis.
- **Hypersensitivity reactions**: Glucocorticoids are used in treatment of **allergic reactions** (urticaria, angioneurotic edema, contact dermatitis, serum sickness, etc.) and diseases such as bronchial asthma.
- Corticosteroids are given **prior to blood products or chemotherapy** to prevent undesirable immune reactions.
- **Organ transplants**: Corticosteroids are used as first-line immunosuppressants in recipients of solid organ transplants as well as hematopoietic stem cell transplants.

ADRs

Long-term systemic use of glucocorticoids is associated with a **large number of adverse effects** such as Cushing syndrome, myopathy, psychosis, glaucoma, sodium–water retention, hypertension, risk of cardiac failure, and peptic ulcer. Therefore, the benefits of long-term glucocorticoid therapy should be weighed against these risks.

C. Calcineurin Inhibitors

Cyclosporine, Tacrolimus

Calcineurin is a cytoplasmic phosphatase that is activated by the calcium–calmodulin complex in response to T-cell receptor activation (Fig. 65.2). Calcineurin is necessary for dephosphorylation of NFAT (nuclear factor of activated T cells). NFAT translocates into the nucleus and stimulates transcription of cytokine genes, leading to the production of IL-2 and other cytokines (IL-3, GM-CSF, TNF-α, IFN-γ) that play an important role in T cell proliferation and immune response.

1. Cyclosporine

Mechanism of action

Cyclosporine is a peptide antibiotic that exerts immunosuppressant action by **inhibiting calcineurin**. Cyclosporine binds to an intracellular immunophilin protein called **cyclophilin**. The cyclosporine–cyclophilin complex inhibits calcineurin (Fig. 65.3), resulting in inhibition of gene transcription of IL-2, IL-3, IFN-γ and other factors in antigen-stimulated T cells. Thus, cyclosporine blocks proliferation of T lymphocytes, production of cytokines, and response of inducer T cells to IL-1. It has no effect on suppressor T cells; however, helper T cells fail to respond to antigenic stimulation. Cyclosporine increases the expression of TGF-β (transforming growth factor-β), which attenuates (IL-2)-mediated proliferation of T cells and production of killer lymphocytes. Thus, cyclosporine **selectively suppresses cell-mediated immunity (CMI)**.

Therapeutic uses

As an immunosuppressant cyclosporine may be used alone or along with glucocorticoids, methotrexate, etc. It can be administered orally as well as intravenously.

- Cyclosporine is useful in preventing **graft rejection** reactions in liver, kidney, pancreas and bone marrow transplants. It is also very beneficial in cardiac transplants. Drug is given orally in a dose of 10–15 mg/kg body weight, 12 hours before transplant and continued as long as required. Duration of the treatment is usually 1–2 weeks. However, if graft rejection starts, a dose of 3.5 mg/kg body weight is given intravenously.
- Cyclosporine combined with methotrexate is the standard regimen for prevention of **graft-versus-host disease** in patients undergoing allogeneic stem cell transplantation.
- Cyclosporine is also useful as a **second-line drug** in some **autoimmune diseases** such as asthma, psoriasis, severe rheumatoid arthritis, uveitis, and IBD. For these conditions, cyclosporine is usually combined with methotrexate or corticosteroids.
- The **advantage** of cyclosporine is its selective suppressive effect on the CMI and lack of cytotoxic action. Thus, although rejection of graft is prevented, the patient's ability to defend against infections is intact. Cytotoxic adverse effects such as bone marrow suppression are also not seen with cyclosporine.

ADRs

- Hyperglycemia, hepatic dysfunction, hyperkalemia, hypertension
- Altered mental state and seizures
- Hirsutism
- **Nephrotoxicity**: It is important to monitor plasma drug concentration and renal function.
- It may increase the risk of skin cancer and Kaposi sarcoma in transplant recipients because cyclosporine induces synthesis of TGF-β that enhances tumour invasion and metastasis.

Drug–drug interactions

- Cyclosporine has nephrotoxic potential, which is enhanced by simultaneous use of other nephrotoxic drugs (e.g., amphotericin B, aminoglycosides, vancomycin).
- Enzyme inducers such as rifampicin, phenytoin, and phenobarbitone decrease the efficacy of cyclosporine and graft rejection may occur.
- Enzyme inhibitors (e.g., ketoconazole) increase the risk of cyclosporine toxicity.
- Concomitant use of potassium supplements or potassium-sparing diuretics may cause dangerous hyperkalemia.

2. Tacrolimus

Mechanism of action

Tacrolimus is a macrolide with the same mechanism of action as **cyclosporine**, i.e., inhibitory action on calcineurin. Thus, it prevents dephosphorylation of NFAT and the subsequent production of various cytokines resulting in the prevention of antigen-induced activation and proliferation of T lymphocytes. However, while cyclosporine binds to cyclophilin, tacrolimus binds to another **immunophilin (FK506 binding protein: FKBP)** and inhibits calcineurin.

- Tacrolimus is **more potent** than cyclosporine as an immunosuppressant (10–100 times).

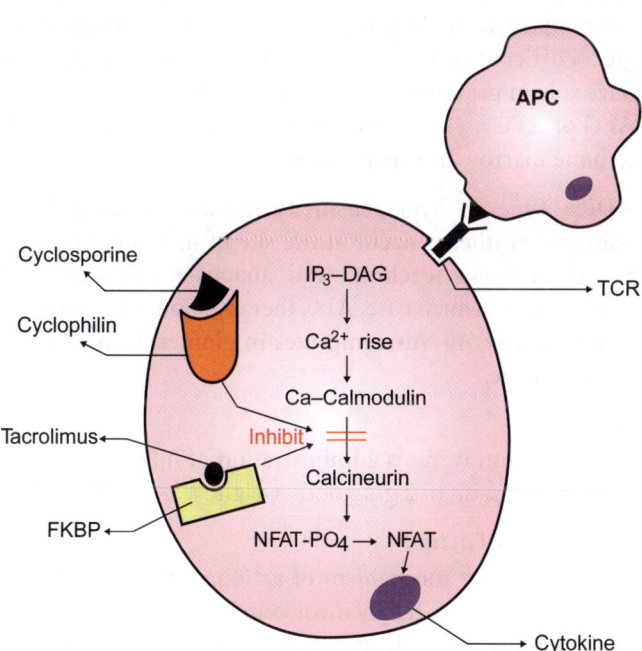

Fig. 65.3 Mechanism of action of calcineurin inhibitors
[TCR: T cell receptor; FKBP: FK506 binding protein; NFAT: Nuclear factor of activated T cells; IP$_3$: Inositol triphosphate; DAG: Diacyl glycerol]

- Similar to cyclosporine, it can be given orally and intravenously. Oral dose is 0.05–0.2 mg/kg body weight, twice daily. Its oral absorption is reduced by food.
- Tacrolimus is metabolised in the liver by CYP3A4.
- **Uses, adverse effects**, and **efficacy** are the same as cyclosporine
- Tacrolimus has higher potency and plasma concentration is easily monitored. Thus, it is preferred for prevention and treatment of organ transplant rejection, especially liver transplant (because its absorption is not affected by bile). It is effective in acute rejection reactions and in patients who do not respond to cyclosporine.
- It is useful to induce remission in **fistulating Crohn's disease**, for which a 10-week course is usually effective.
- Topical application of 0.03–0.1% tacrolimus is effective in **atopic dermatitis**.
- The adverse effects of tacrolimus resemble those of cyclosporine; while hypertension, hyperuricemia, and hirsutism are less likely, the risk of precipitating diabetes, diarrhea, alopecia and nephrotoxicity is higher.

Voclosporin is a new calcineurin inhibitor approved for use in lupus nephritis, along with MMF or glucocorticoids.

D. Proliferation Signal Inhibitors (PSIs) or mTOR Inhibitors

Sirolimus, Everolimus

Proliferation signal inhibitors (PSIs) exert their immunosuppressant action by binding to the immunophilin, FK506 binding protein (FKBP). The drug–FKBP complex blocks mTOR, i.e., mammalian/mechanistic target of rapamycin. mTOR is one of the key components in the intracellular signalling pathway for cell growth, metabolism, proliferation, and angiogenesis. Thus, these drugs are called proliferation signal inhibitors.

mTOR inhibition caused by sirolimus and everolimus leads to:
- Inhibition of interleukin (IL) driven T-cell proliferation.
- Inhibition of B-cell proliferation and immunoglobulin synthesis.

Sirolimus is effective orally and is rapidly absorbed and eliminated by CYP3A4 and CYP3A5. If combined with cyclosporine, plasma concentration of sirolimus can rise to toxic levels. As a result, monitoring of drug levels is indicated.

Therapeutic uses
- Sirolimus is used alone or in combination with other immunosuppressant drugs to prevent solid organ allograft rejection.
- For prophylaxis and treatment of acute graft-versus-host disease that fails to respond to steroid therapy
- It is used topically for skin disorders and uveoretinitis
- Sirolimus-eluting coronary stents are reported to reduce adverse cardiac events in patients suffering from acute coronary artery disease.

ADRs
- Headache, pneumonitis, and hypertriglyceridemia may occur.
- It may cause severe myelosuppression, leading to thrombocytopenia.
- It has hepatotoxic potential.
- However, renal toxicity of sirolimus is less than that of calcineurin inhibitors.
- When combined with tacrolimus, it may cause hemolytic–uremic syndrome.

E. Biological Agents
1. Polyclonal Abs
Antilymphocyte globulins (ALGs)

ALGs act on peripheral lymphocytes that keep circulating between the lymph and blood. However, chronic use of ALG depletes thymus-dependent T lymphocytes in lymphoid follicles also. Thus, delayed hypersensitivity reactions and CMI are suppressed, but humoral immunity is maintained.

Antithymocyte globulins (ATG)

ATG contain antibodies directed against several CD and HLA antigens. It depletes T lymphocytes by cell-mediated and complement-dependent reactions.

Uses: ATG and ALG are used to induce immunosuppression initially in rejection reactions, in solid organ as well as bone marrow transplants. These are also effective in glucocorticoid-resistant transplant rejections. They also have role in prevention of GVHD for which large doses of ALG or ATG are given to the recipient, a week or so prior to bone marrow transplantation.

ADRs: Type III hypersensitivity reactions causing local pain and erythema occur at the site of injection of ALG. Serum sickness reactions and anaphylactoid reactions may occur, in which case, ALG therapy should be stopped. Deposition of Ag–Ab complexes in glomeruli may cause renal damage.

IGIV

It involves intravenous administration of human IgG Abs in high doses, up to 2 g/kg body weight.

Mechanism of action

While the exact mechanism of action of IGIV is not yet clearly understood, it may involve an increase in regulatory T cells, reduction of helper T cells, along with decreased production or increased catabolism of antibodies.

IGIV is effective in autoimmune disorders, HIV disease, bone marrow transplantation and immunoglobulin deficiency states, Kawasaki's disease, SLE, and refractory idiopathic thrombocytopenia.

Hyperimmune immunoglobulins
Hyperimmune immunoglobulins are IGIVs prepared from selected humans with a high titre of antibodies against particular antigens. These are available for treatment of cytomegalovirus (CMV), varicella zoster virus (VZV), hepatitis B virus (HBV), respiratory syncytial virus (RSV), human herpesvirus 3, tetanus, rabies, and digoxin overdose. These are injected intravenously to transfer passive immunity to reduce risk of infection or severity of disease caused by that particular organism. Hyperimmune immunoglobulin for rabies is injected intravenously and also applied at site of dog bite wound. Hyperimmune immunoglobulins are also available for the venoms of rattle snake, coral snake, and scorpions.

Rho(D) immune globulin
This is the human IgG antibody against Rho(D) antigens present on the surface of red blood cells (RBCs). The basic principle underlying the use of Rho(D) immune globulin is that the **primary antibody response** of body to a **foreign antigen** can be **prevented** by giving specific antibodies passively at the time of antigen exposure.

When an Rh-negative mother carries an Rh-positive fetus, fetal blood cells may leak into maternal circulation during childbirth or abortion and antibodies are formed against Rh-positive cells. During a subsequent pregnancy, memory of the maternal immune response causes hemolysis of Rh-positive cells of the fetus leading to **erythroblastosis fetalis** or hemolytic disease of the newborn. This can be prevented by injecting the Rh-negative mother with anti-Rho(D) antibodies 300 mcg intramuscularly within 24–72 hours of birth of an Rh-positive baby. These injected antibodies clear Rh-positive cells from maternal circulation before the generation of B cell response by mother. Thus, there is no memory of this reaction in the maternal immune system and an Rh-positive fetus in subsequent pregnancies is safe.

If an Rh-negative pregnant woman has a past history of abortion or ectopic pregnancy, and the grouping of baby is not known, anti-Rho(D) antibody injection is given before delivery at 26–28 weeks of gestation to prevent hemolytic disease in the newborn.

ADRs to anti-Rho(D) antibody are fever and local pain at the site of intramuscular injection.

2. Monoclonal antibodies
Chimeric and humanised versions of murine monoclonal antibodies against therapeutic targets are prepared by genetic engineering techniques. These are less antigenic than murine monoclonal antibodies. While the suffixes *umab* and *zumab* are used for humanised antibodies, *imab* and *ximab* are used for chimeric antibodies.

Anti-TNF-α antibodies
TNF-α is a cytokine that plays a pro-inflammatory role in many inflammatory diseases such as rheumatoid arthritis. Antibodies directed against TNF-α include **etanercept, adalimumab, golimumab, certolizumab, and infliximab.**

Etanercept or infliximab can be combined with methotrexate in patients of rheumatoid arthritis who do not respond to methotrexate alone. Etanercept is also useful in severe polyarticular juvenile arthritis and ankylosing spondylitis. Infliximab is useful in ankylosing spondylitis, ulcerative colitis, and psoriasis.

Interleukin inhibitors
Anakinra is an IL-1 receptor antagonist used in refractory rheumatoid arthritis, usually in combination with methotrexate and TNF-α inhibitors such as etanercept.

Daclizumab and basiliximab bind to the α-subunit of IL-2 receptors on activated lymphocytes and prevent it from binding to its receptors. These are useful in renal transplant patients along with glucocorticoids and cyclosporine for managing acute rejection reactions. Both daclizumab and basiliximab increase the risk of opportunistic infections and anaphylactic reactions. Fever, dyspnea and edema may occur.

Tocilizumab binds to IL-6 receptors and inhibits (IL-6)-mediated inflammatory processes. It is useful in rheumatoid arthritis.

Ustekinumab prevents the binding of IL-12 and IL-23 to their receptors. It is useful in moderately severe plaque psoriasis. It may be combined with methotrexate. Its advantage over TNF-α inhibitors is faster onset of action and longer-lasting relief of symptoms with less frequent dosing.

Alefacept inhibits T cell activation by preventing CD2/LFA-3 interaction. It is also used in plaque psoriasis. It also reduces the number of circulating CD4 and CD8 T cells, and therefore, the peripheral T cell count should be monitored in patients receiving alefacept therapy.

Integrin antibodies
Natalizumab binds to the $α_4$ subunit of $α_4β_1$ and $α_4β_7$ integrins (expressed on all leukocytic surfaces barring neutrophils) and is used for multiple sclerosis and Crohn's disease. It should not be combined with anti-TNF-α drugs.

Vedolizumab binds to the $α_4β_7$ integrin in the GIT only, and is beneficial in Crohn's disease and ulcerative colitis.

Abciximab is the Fab fragment of a monoclonal antibody that binds with the integrin $GP_{IIb/IIIa}$ receptor present on activated platelets. It exerts antiaggregatory effect by inhibiting the binding of von Willebrand factor, fibrinogen, or other adhesion molecules with activated platelets and preventing platelet aggregation. It is used with aspirin and heparin during PCI to prevent ischemic cardiac complications.

Anti-CD3 antibodies

Muromonab is the oldest murine monoclonal antibody. It binds to CD3 glycoproteins present near T cell receptors (TCR) on helper T cells and prevents the binding of (MHC-II)–antigen complex to TCR. Thus, T cells fail to participate in the immune process. Later on, TCRs are internalised and T cells are shifted to non-lymphoid organs or undergo cytolysis, creating a state of **immune blockade**. It is mainly used for acute transplant rejection, especially in corticosteroid-resistant cases. It is also used before bone marrow transplantation to deplete T cells from the donor's bone marrow. At the beginning of therapy, muromonab can cause release of cytokines (interleukins, interferons, and TNF-α), leading to **cytokine syndrome**, characterised by fever with rigors and chills, generalised body aches, and wheezing. This can be prevented by pretreatment with corticosteroids.

Others

Omalizumab is an anti-IgE monoclonal Ab that prevents the binding of IgE to mast cells and basophils. It therefore interferes with the release of mediators of Type I allergic reactions (histamine and leukotrienes). It is useful in allergic asthma that does not respond to inhalational corticosteroids and in chronic urticaria.

Abatacept consists of the extracellular domain of cytotoxic T-lymphocyte-associated antigen 4 (CTLA-4).

Denosumab binds to RANKL (receptor activator of nuclear factor kappa B ligand) and interferes with osteoclastic maturation. It is useful in post-menopausal women with osteoporosis who have high risk of spontaneous fractures. Calcium and vitamin D supplements are given with denosumab therapy.

Eculizumab binds to the complement component C5 and prevents its activation to form C5a and C5b fragments. This inhibits the pore-forming and lytic activity of complement C5 and intravascular hemolysis is prevented. It is useful in atypical hemolytic uremic syndrome and paroxysmal nocturnal hemoglobinuria. However, in patients on eculizumab treatment, there is an increased risk of meningococcal infection.

Ranibizumab prevents the binding of vascular endothelial growth factor to its receptors and interferes with neovascularisation. It is useful in aged patients with macular edema, degeneration due to diabetes, or vein blockades. It is administered as an intravitreal injection for these conditions. **Pegaptanib** is a peg-complexed oligonucleotide useful in macular degeneration.

Palivizumab binds to respiratory syncytial virus and reduces the frequency and severity of lower respiratory disease caused by this virus in neonates. **Raxibacumab** binds to the PA protein of *Bacillus anthracis*, preventing anthrax toxins from entering the host cell. It is used for prophylaxis of inhalational anthrax.

F. Thalidomide

Thalidomide was initially introduced as an antiemetic, but went into disuse in 1960 owing to severe teratogenic effects. However, now, several **actions** of thalidomide have been recognised:

- It exerts anti-inflammatory and immunosuppressant action.
- Thalidomide inhibits angiogenesis and TNF-α.
- It also decreases phagocytosis by neutrophils.
- It interacts with T cells to increase cell-mediated immune response (CMI).
- Secretion of interleukin-10 is increased.

Therapeutic uses

- Currently, thalidomide is used for treatment of multiple myeloma. Addition of dexamethasone is reported to improve the response rate.
- It is also used for the management of erythema nodosum leprosum (ENL).
- It is useful in the case of skin manifestations of lupus erythematosus.

ADRs

- The most significant adverse effect of thalidomide is teratogenicity.
- Other ADRs include fatigue, rashes, hypothyroidism, and constipation.
- Peripheral neuropathy and deep vein thrombosis (DVT) may occur. The risk of DVT is higher in patients with hematological malignancies. These patients are given anticoagulant therapy with thalidomide.

Immunomodulatory Derivatives of Thalidomide (IMiDs)

Lenalidomide

It has the same efficacy as thalidomide but is less toxic. Teratogenic potential is much lower than that of thalidomide. Lenalidomide is useful in myelodysplastic syndrome and refractory or relapsed cases of multiple myeloma. **Actimid** is a new drug in this class.

Selective Cytokine Inhibitory Drugs (selCIDs)

These are also thalidomide analogues that are potent inhibitors of TNF-α but do not stimulate T cells.

IMMUNOSUPPRESSANTS IN ORGAN TRANSPLANTS

Immunosuppression is essential for successful organ transplantation. The accepted protocol recognises three phases of immunosuppression:

Induction regimen

Induction therapy is started just before the transplant procedure and continued for 2–12 weeks after the procedure, which is when most of the acute rejections occur. The triple-drug regimen used includes:

- Cyclosporine/tacrolimus + MMF/azathioprine + prednisolone
- Sirolimus + MMF + prednisolone; this regimen does not have nephrotoxic potential.

If rejection reaction does not occur after two weeks of use, the doses are gradually reduced.

Maintenance regimen

Triple-drug regimen with maintenance doses is preferred and may be required throughout life. Cyclosporine is usually stopped after one year of the transplant to prevent nephrotoxicity. Long-term steroids also have many systemic adverse effects. If first-line drugs are not tolerated, second-line drugs (daclizumab or basiliximab) and cyclophosphamide are tried.

Anti-rejection regimen

If acute rejection sets in, methylprednisolone 0.5–1.0 g is injected intravenously for three days. For refractory cases that do not respond to this treatment, ATG, muromonab, etc., are tried as **rescue therapy**. Sometimes, tacrolimus, sirolimus, and MMF are also tried out in steroid-resistant rejections.

The most important adverse effects associated with immunosuppressant therapy are an increased risk of opportunistic infections, lymphomas, and related malignancies.

Clinical problem-based questions and MCQs

1. **A known case of diabetic nephropathy is advised to undergo renal transplantation. Comment on the role of immunosuppressant drugs in this patient.**

2. **A 63-year-old patient with severe renal dysfunction underwent renal transplantation one year ago. He is receiving maintenance doses of tacrolimus, prednisone, and mycophenolate mofetil. Suddenly, he develops acute rejection of the transplant.**
   i. Identify the drug given immediately to control the acute rejection.
      a. Omalizumab   b. Prednisolone
      c. Everolimus   d. Ibuprofen
   ii. Mention the dose and duration of treatment with the selected drug.

3. i. Which of the following is the LEAST toxic immunosuppressant?
      a. Tacrolimus   b. Mycophenolate mofetil
      c. Cyclosporine d. Azathioprine
   ii. Describe the mechanism of action and therapeutic uses of selected drug

4. i. All these immunosuppressant drugs inhibit calcineurin in activated T lymphocytes, EXCEPT:
      a. Tacrolimus   b. Cyclosporine
      c. Voclosporin d. Sirolimus
   ii. Describe the mechanism of immunosuppressant action of calcineurin inhibitors with a suitable diagram.

5. i. Which of the following is proliferation signal inhibitor
      a. Sirolimus   b. Tacrolimus
      c. MMF   d. Anakinra
   ii. Enumerate therapeutic uses and adverse effects of selected drug

6. Match the monoclonal antibody with its target site/action
   a. Omalizumab   1. Interleukin-2 receptors
   b. Ustekinumab   2. Mast cells binding with IgE
   c. Basiliximab   3. Interleukin-12 receptors
   d. Adalimumab   4. Tumour necrosis factor-α

7. i. An Rh-negative pregnant woman presents with a history of two previous abortions. It is decided to administer anti-D immune globulin to prevent erythroblastosis fetalis. At what stage of gestation should she be administered anti-D immune globulin?
      a. 12 weeks   b 28 weeks
      c. 32 weeks   d. 38 weeks
   ii. Describe the pharmacological basis for administration of anti-D immune globulin in this case.

8. **A renal transplant patient with onset of acute rejection after 8 weeks of the procedure is given intravenous prednisolone.**
   i. Describe the pharmacological basis for use of prednisolone.
   ii. Enumerate the uses of corticosteroids as immunosuppressants.

IMMUNOSTIMULANTS

Many drugs, vitamins, and immune system components boost the ability of immune system against infections and diseases; these are called **immunostimulants**. Immunostimulants can be **specific**, acting against a particular antigen (e.g., vaccines), or **non-specific**, acting against all antigens (e.g., immunoglobulins).

CLASSIFICATION

Immunostimulants include vaccines, immunoglobulins, antisera and some adjuvants, and miscellaneous drugs (Flowchart 65.3).

A. Vaccines

Vaccines are biological preparations that help to improve immunity against a specific disease. They stimulate the

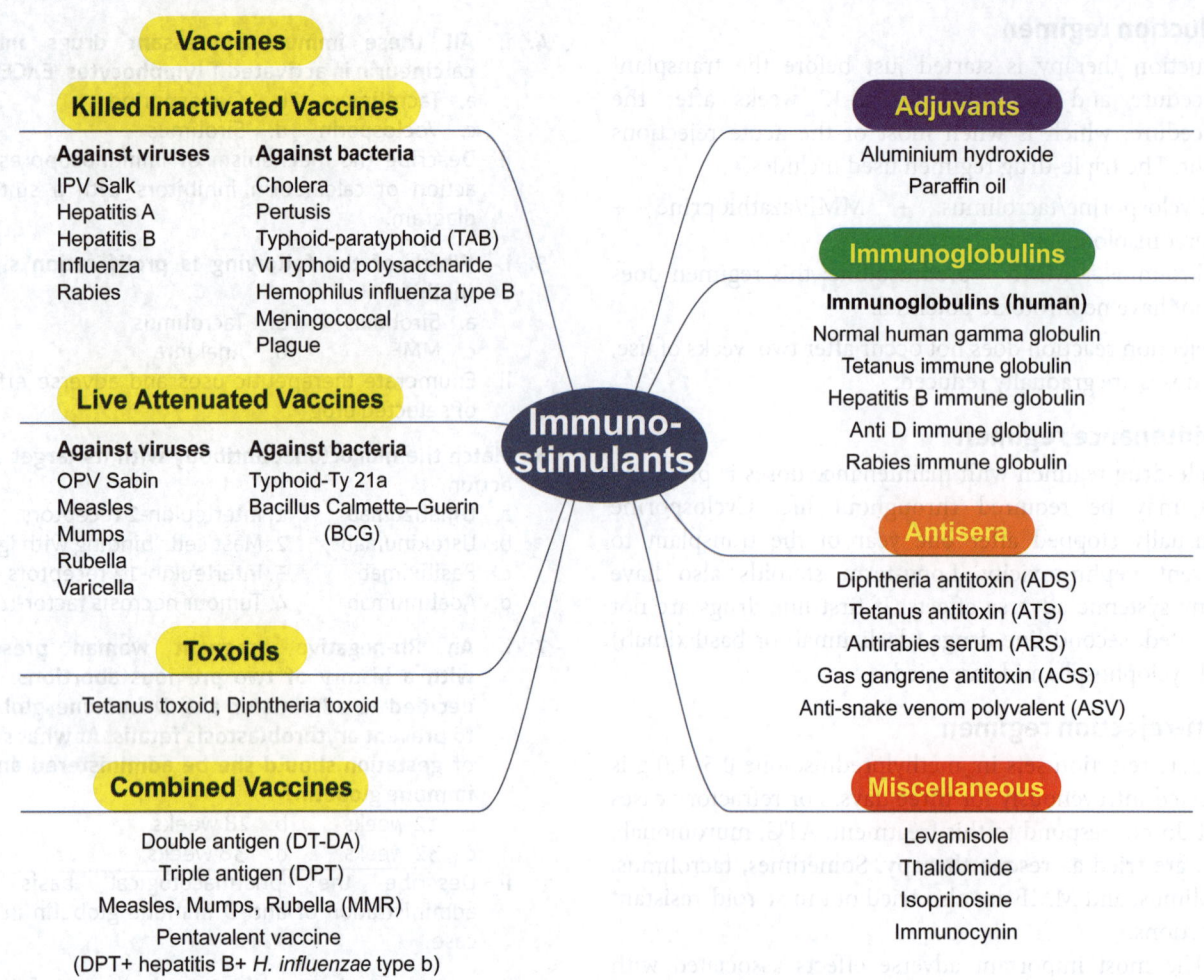

Flowchart 65.3 Classification of immunostimulants

immune system to recognise specific foreign antigens. Vaccines may contain killed, inactivated, or live-but-attenuated microorganisms. The potency of live attenuated vaccines is greater than that of inactivated vaccines. A single dose of live attenuated vaccine may provide lifelong immunity. The immunisation schedule under the National Immunisation Programme of India is described briefly (Table 65.1). Few important vaccines used in national program are described below.

1. Bacillus Calmette–Guerin (BCG) vaccine

This vaccine, contains the attenuated bovine strain of *Mycobacterium tuberculosis* bacillus, and is named after Calmette and Guerin, who developed it. It is dispensed as a dry powder (0.5–1 mg), suspended in sterile water just before injection. BCG vaccine is given to neonates at birth, in a dose of 0.05 mL, by intradermal injection in the deltoid region of the left arm.

The BCG vaccine also has an adjuvant role in cancer immunotherapy.

It may cause fever and regional lymphadenitis. The immunity provided by BCG against tubercular infection is partial, not permanent, and cannot be predicted completely.

Table 65.1 Vaccination schedule under the National Immunisation Programme

	Time	Vaccines given
1	At birth	BCG, OPV, Hepatitis B birth dose
2	6 weeks	OPV-1, fIPV-1, Pentavalent-1, PCV-1, RVV-1
3	10 weeks	OPV-2, Pentavalent-2, RVV-2
4	14 weeks	OPV-3, Pentavalent-3, RVV-3, PCV-2, fIPV-2
5	9–12 months	MR-1, JE-1, PCV booster
6	16–24 months	MR-2, JE-2, OPV booster, DPT booster-1
7	5–6 years	DPT booster-2
8.	10 years	Tetanus and adult diphtheria (Td)
9	16 years	Td
10	Pregnancy	Td-1, Td-2 or Td booster

Contraindications

BCG vaccine is contraindicated in tuberculin-positive and immunocompromised patients.

2. Pentavalent vaccine

The pentavalent vaccine provides combined protection against diphtheria, pertussis, tetanus (DPT), hepatitis B, and *H. influenzae* type b. The DPT component consists of triple antigens against diphtheria, pertussis (whooping cough) and tetanus. The pertussis vaccine is a killed (inactivated) vaccine that reduces β-adrenergic reactivity and enhances sensitisation to other antigens. Along with pertussis, the DPT vaccine includes a modified diphtheria exotoxin and a tetanus toxoid adsorbed onto aluminium hydroxide.

Hepatitis B vaccine is made by the recombinant DNA technique and contains the hepatitis B surface antigen adsorbed onto aluminium hydroxide. It is given to children as part of the pentavalent vaccine and also to individuals exposed to blood/blood products/body fluids such as HCWs, hemophiliacs, dialysis patients, and drug addicts.

The *H. influenzae* type b vaccine contains medium oligosaccharide of *H. influenzae* type b conjugated with the diphtheria toxoid and aluminium hydroxide. It can protect infants and children from *H. influenzae*, meningitis, and pneumonia.

The pentavalent vaccine is given in the Universal Immunisation Programme of India to protect against five diseases, i.e., diphtheria, pertussis, tetanus, hepatitis B and *H. influenzae* meningitis.

ADRs
- Pertussis vaccine can cause pain and induration at site of injection. In rare cases, severe systemic or fatal reactions may occur. High grade fever, convulsions, altered consciousness, and focal neurological deficit are rare, and these contraindicate further dosing.
- Diphtheria and tetanus toxoids can also cause pain, induration, and erythema at the injection site and regional lymphadenitis. Fever, chills, and generalised malaise occur occasionally.
- Hepatitis B vaccine may also cause soreness at injection site, fever, and malaise.

3. Polio vaccines
There are two types of vaccines available against polio infections:
- The Oral Polio Vaccine (OPV, Sabin) is a live attenuated vaccine, given orally in a dose of 2 drops. The OPV produces active immunity and is highly efficacious.
- The fractional-dose Inactivated Polio Vaccine (fIPV, Salk) is preferred over the OPV for adult vaccination and in patients with impaired immune response. It is administered by subcutaneous or intramuscular injections in the deltoid region. Pain at injection site and some allergic reactions are reported.

Polio vaccines are routinely used in the National Immunisation Programme with a gap of 4–6 weeks between the first 2 doses and 12 months between the second and third doses.

Rotavirus vaccine (RVV)
It is a human–bovine reassortant vaccine, given orally as 3 doses at one month intervals. It may cause mild diarrhea and vomiting.

Measles and rubella vaccine (MR)
Both measles and rubella vaccines are live attenuated vaccines, given by deep subcutaneous or intramuscular injections over the deltoid region. Immunity provided by the measles vaccine lasts for about 8 years.

MR vaccine is contraindicated during pregnancy, untreated TB, and in patients with a history of febrile convulsions or epileptic fits.

In addition, the pneumococcal conjugate vaccine (PCV) is given in certain selected states/districts of Bihar, UP, MP, HP, Rajasthan, and Haryana. Japanese encephalitis (JE) vaccine is used only in districts where the infection is endemic.

B. Adjuvants
Adjuvants such as aluminium hydroxide and paraffin oil are substances that are added to various vaccines to increase immune response to foreign antigens. Aluminium hydroxide forms a depot at the injection site which allows slow release of antigens and stimulates antibody-producing plasma cells. It may cause fever and pain at the site of injection.

Paraffin oil prolongs and enhances response to vaccines by forming an oily coating of antigen that forms an antigen depot and protects it.

C. Immunoglobulins
Immunoglobulins are separated human gamma globulins that carry antibodies. Immunoglobulins may be specific for a particular Ag or non-specific, against all antigens.

Immunoglobulins have 2 heavy chains called the Fc region and 2 light chains called the Fab region. The Fab fraction is the antigen binding site, whereas the Fc fragment determines the effector function of Abs and is required for interaction with the complement cascade.

Immunoglobulins obtained from pooled, human adult blood are called **immune serum**, while the more selective gamma globulins against a particular infection, obtained from blood of individuals, is called **hyperimmune serum**.

Therapeutic uses
- Normal human gamma globulin is useful in prophylaxis of viral hepatitis (HAV, HBV). It is also used for prophylaxis and modifies the course of illness in poliomyelitis and chickenpox. It is valuable in treating agammaglobulinemia, burns and leukemia patients.
- Anti-D immunoglobulin has Abs against the Rh(D) antigen. When given to Rho-D-negative women (postpartum/post-abortion of Rho-D positive fetus), it

binds to the Rho antigen and arrests formation of Abs against this Ag. This can prevent hemolytic disease in the fetus in a future pregnancy. Contraindications are Rh-D positive individuals and infants.
- Hepatitis B immune globulin is better than normal human gamma globulin for prophylaxis of HBV infection in persons acutely exposed to HBsAg positive blood/blood products along with the hepatitis B vaccine.
- Rabies immune globulin is better than antirabies serum (ARS) for rabies prophylaxis.

ADRs
Pain, allergic reactions, fever with shivering, nausea, arthralgia.

D. Antisera
- **Antisera** contain the purified, concentrated serum of horses who are actively immunised against a specific antigen.
- Tetanus antitoxin or antitetanic serum (ATS) is used only when human tetanus immune globulin is not available.
- Antidiphtheretic serum (ADS) is given in clinical diphtheria, without waiting for bacteriological confirmation of diagnosis, because it can neutralise only the exotoxin that is released at the site of infection and freely circulating in blood, but not the toxin fixed to tissues. Moreover, it cannot reverse the damage already caused by the toxin.
- Anti-snake venom serum polyvalent can neutralise the venom of cobras, Russell's and saw-scaled vipers, and kraits; it is a life-saving measure in case of snakebite.

ADRs
Hypersensitivity reactions are very common. If time is available, antisera should be given after sensitivity tests. In case of emergencies, adrenaline is given concurrently with antisera, to prevent or control severe hypersensitivity reactions. Steroids and antihistamines are also effective.

E. Miscellaneous
Levamisole restores depressed B cell and T cell functions and modulates the CMI. It is used as an immune-modulating agent in cancer treatment. Adverse effects such as nausea, drowsiness, myalgia, and rashes are common.

Isoprinosine is an analogue of thymus hormones that has immunostimulant and antiviral actions. It increases production of T lymphocytes and their differentiation into T helper cells. It also increases humoral response by increasing the differentiation of B lymphocytes into Ab-producing plasma cells. It suppresses viral RNA synthesis. It is used for a rare complication of measles—**subacute sclerosing panencephalitis**. It may cause headache, nausea, vomiting, diarrhea, abdominal pain, and dizziness.

Clinical problem-based questions and MCQs

9. Polyvalent vaccine is a combined vaccine used in the National Immunisation Programme. It protects against all of the following diseases, except:
   a. Tetanus   b. Whooping cough
   c. Measles   d. Hepatitis B

10. Identify the vaccine given at 9–12 months of age in the National Immunisation Schedule.
    a. DPT   b. MR
    c. fIPV   d. Hepatitis B

11. A 36-year-old primigravida with blood group B negative has given birth to a baby girl with the blood group B positive. The postpartum period is uneventful.
    i. Identify the immunoglobulin to be given to this patient.
       a. Human gamma globulin
       b. Anti-D immunoglobulin
       c. Hyperimmune serum
       d. ADS
    ii. Describe the pharmacological basis for administration of the selected immunoglobulin.

Summary
- Immunity can be innate and acquired. Innate immunity is conferred by physical, biochemical and cellular barriers.
- Acquired immunity manifests as humoral and cell-mediated immune (CMI) response and is characterised by its specificity, ability to differentiate between self and non-self antigens, and vigorous memory response.
- Inappropriate immune response can cause autoimmune diseases, transplant rejections, graft-versus-host disease, and hypersensitivity reactions.
- Immunosuppressant drugs include antiproliferative drugs, corticosteroids, calcineurin inhibitors, mTOR inhibitors, and biological agents. Thalidomide and lenalidomide are immunomodulators.
- Among **antiproliferative** drugs, methotrexate, a folate antagonist, and azathioprine, a purine antagonist, are most commonly used.
- Methotrexate is used as a DMARD in rheumatoid arthritis, pemphigus, psoriasis, chronic active hepatitis, uveitis, and myasthenia gravis. If not effective, it can be combined with TNF-α inhibitors or corticosteroids.
- Azathioprine is useful in graft rejections, rheumatoid arthritis, and IBD. Myelosuppression and hepatotoxicity are its prominent adverse effects. The dose of azathioprine should be reduced when combined with allopurinol.

- Mycophenolate mofetil (MMF) inhibits both the CMI and Ab production in response to antigen exposure and is the least toxic immunosuppressant (ADR: GI upset). It is useful in myasthenia gravis, IBD, graft rejection, and GVHD.
- **Corticosteroids** have lympholytic and lymphopenic action and possess immunosuppressive as well as non-specific anti-inflammatory activity. These are the preferred drugs for idiopathic thrombocytopenic purpura, autoimmune hemolytic anemia, and acute glomerulonephritis. It is also used in hypersensitivity reactions, prevention, and treatment of transplant rejections; however, continued use of corticosteroids has many systemic ill-effects.
- **Calcineurin inhibitors** (cyclosporine and tacrolimus) interfere with the dephosphorylation of NFAT, its transport into the nucleus, and subsequent synthesis and secretion of cytokines. These are useful in graft rejection and GVHD. Tacrolimus is more potent and more toxic than cyclosporine. So, cyclosporine is used initially and tacrolimus is given only if the response is not adequate. ADRs (of both) include hypertension, hyperglycemia, hyperkalemia, neurotoxicity, nephrotoxicity, and hepatotoxicity. Cyclosporine can cause gum hyperplasia, hirsutism, and hyperuricemia.
- **mTOR inhibitors** [sirolimus (rapamycin) and everolimus] are useful in GVHD and graft rejection. ADRs include hypokalemia and thrombocytopenia.
- **Biological inhibitors** include polyclonal and monoclonal antibodies.
- Polyclonal Abs include ALG, ATG, IGIV, hyperimmune immunoglobulin, and anti-Rh$_o$D immunoglobulins.
- Monoclonal antibodies include TNF-α inhibitors, interleukin inhibitors, integrin inhibitors, anti-IgE Abs, etc.
- For a successful organ transplant, induction immunosuppressant therapy with triple-drug regimen is carried out for 2–12 weeks, followed by the maintenance regimen with lower doses, and intensive treatment with intravenous steroids if acute rejection sets in.
- Immunostimulants include vaccines, immunoglobulins, antisera, and some miscellaneous drugs.
- Vaccines can be live attenuated or dead-inactivated. BCG, OPV, fIPV, Pentavalent vaccine, and RVV are administered as part of the National Immunisation Programme.
- Combined vaccines such as double antigen, triple antigen, and Pentavalent vaccines decrease the number of injections.
- Immunoglobulins and antisera provide passive immunity.
- Adjuvants (aluminium hydroxide and paraffin oil) enhance and prolong the response to vaccines.
- Immunoglobulins such as human gamma globulin modify the course of illness in hepatitis, poliomyelitis, and chickenpox. They are also useful in agammaglobulinemia, burns, and leukemia. Anti-D immuneglobulin is used after delivery (or abortion) of an Rh-positive baby to an Rh-negative mother to prevent hemolytic disease in the fetus in a future pregnancy.
- **Antisera** are the concentrated serum of horses that are actively immunised against a specific antigen, e.g., ATS, ADS, ARS, and ASV.

Questions for Practice

1. Classify immunosuppressants. Describe the mechanism of action, uses and adverse effects of cyclosporine.
2. Write short notes on:
   a. mTOR inhibitors
   b. Monoclonal antibodies as immunosuppressants
   c. Graft-versus-host disease
3. Describe the management of organ transplant rejection.
4. Comment on role of:
   a. Corticosteroids as immunosuppressants
   b. Anti D immunoglobulin in neonatal hemolysis.
   c. Methotrexate in autoimmune diseases.
   d. Thalidomide in current clinical practice.
5. Explain why;
   a. Therapeutic drug monitoring is needed in patients on cyclosporine therapy
   b. Dose of azathioprine is reduced in patients on allopurinol therapy.

Hints for problem-based questions and MCQs

1. Immunosuppressant drugs are indicated for prevention of transplant rejection, given as induction and maintenance regimen as well as for treatment of rejection. Refer to page 856.
2. i. b. Prednisolone
   ii. 0.5–1 g IV, for 3 days.
3. i. b. MMF
   ii. Refer to page 851.
4. i. d. Sirolimus is an mTOR inhibitor
   ii. Refer to page 853.
5. i. a. Sirolimus
   ii. Refer to page 854.
6. a-2; b-3; c-4; d-1
7. i. b. 28 weeks of gestation.
   ii. Refer to page 855.
8. a. Refer to page 852.
   b. Refer to page 852.
9. c. Measles
10. b. MR vaccine
11. i. b. Anti-D immunoglobulin
    ii. To prevent hemolytic disease in next pregnancy.

CONCEPT MAP – IMMUNOSUPPRESSANT DRUGS

Antiproliferative Drugs

Azathioprine: Prodrug selectively taken up and activated by immune cells to mercaptopurine that inhibits nucleic acid and de novo purine synthesis.

Inhibits lymphoid cell proliferation and differentiation after Ag exposure

Destroys stimulated lymphoid cells.

Blocks both CMI & serum antibody response.

Uses: To prevent graft rejection in renal & other tissue transplants, in patients developing Cyclosporine toxicity.

Alternative to corticosteroids in autoimmune diseases.

ADRs: Nausea, vomiting, diarrhea, fever, rashes, hepatic dysfunction and bone marrow suppression.

Methotrexate: Folate antagonist, potent inhibitor of CMI.

Uses : First-line drug as DMARD, pemphigus, psoriasis, chronic active hepatitis, uveitis, myasthenia gravis.

Cyclophosphamide: Alkylating agent, having more marked effect on humoral immunity than CMI.

Useful in bone marrow transplantation, but is a graft-versus-host reserve drug in other transplants.

Mycophenolate Mofetil (MMF): Interferes with de novo synthesis of Guanosine nucleotides in T and B cells → suppresses CMI, Ab production in response to Ag.

Uses : DOC for preventing chronic allograft vasculopathy in cardiac transplant recipients, graft-versus-host reactions (acute, chronic) after hematopoietic stem cell transplantation and as **add-on** drug with corticosteroids and cyclosporine in solid organ transplant rejection, not responding to other drugs or in patients developing nephrotoxicity with cyclosporine.

ADRs: Least toxic, may cause nausea, vomiting, diarrhea, abdominal pain, GI bleeding, rise in BP, headache, reversible myelosuppression.

Corticosteroids

Mechanism: More marked immunosuppressant action on CMI than humoral immunity. Their lympholytic effect is modest on normal lymphoid cells & marked on malignant lymphoid cells.

Cause sequestration of lymphocytes, eosinophils and basophils in peripheral tissues → lymphopenia → suppression of CMI.

Reduce ability of Ag-presenting cells (APC) to respond to Ag & mitogens, reduced phagocytosis & secretion of TNF-α, IL-1, IL-12, IFN-γ, PAF, metalloproteinases by macrophages or lymphocytes → reduced CMI.

Uses: Preferred drugs for ITP, hemolytic anemia, acute glomerulonephritis, hypersensitivity reactions, prevention and treatment of transplant rejections.

ADRs: Large number of adverse effects with long-term systemic use like Cushing syndrome, myopathy, psychosis, glaucoma, sodium–water retention, hypertension, risk of cardiac failure, peptic ulcer, etc.

Immunosuppressant Drugs

Calcineurin inhibitors

Cyclosporine:

Mechanism: Selectively suppresses CMI.

Cyclosporine binds to an intracellular protein 'cyclophilin' & inhibits calcineurin → inhibition of gene transcription of IL-2, IL-3, IFN γ and other factors in Ag stimulated T cells → blocks proliferation of T lymphocytes, production of cytokines and response of inducer T cells to IL-1.

No effect on suppressor T cells. Helper T cells fail to respond to Ag stimulation.

Increased expression of TGF-β, which attenuates IL-2 mediated proliferation of T cells and production of killer lymphocytes.

Uses: In preventing graft rejection reaction in liver, kidney, pancreas and bone marrow transplants.

With Methotrexate for prevention of graft-versus-host-disease in allogeneic stem cell transplantation.

2nd line drug in some autoimmune diseases.

Advantage: Ability to defend against infections is intact, no cytotoxic adverse effects.

ADRs: Hyperglycemia, hepatic dysfunction, hyperkalemia, hypertension, altered mental state, seizures, hirsutism & nephrotoxic potential.

Tacrolimus binds to FK506 binding protein(FKBP) and inhibits calcineurin.

More potent than Cyclosporine, but efficacy & ADRs are same.

Biological Inhibitors

Polyclonal Abs: ALG, ATG, IGIV, hyperimmune immunoglobulin and Anti-Rho(D) immunoglobulin.

Monoclonal Abs: TNF-α inhibitors, interleukin inhibitors, integrin inhibitors, Anti IgE Abs etc.

Uses: ATG and ALG used for induction of immunosuppression, initially in rejection reactions in solid organ as well as bone marrow transplants, effective for glucocorticoid resistant transplant rejections also. Larger doses used for GVHD.

IGIV: IgG Abs by IV route given in high doses upto 2 g per kg body weight in autoimmune disorders, HIV disease, bone marrow transplantation and immunoglobulin deficiency states, Kawasaki's disease, SLE, refractory idiopathic thrombocytopenia.

Anti-Rho(D) immunoglobulin: Given before delivery at 26–28 weeks of gestation to prevent hemolytic disease of newborn if Rh-negative pregnant woman gives history of previous abortion, ectopic pregnancy and grouping of baby is not known.

Etanercept or infliximab, Interleukin inhibitors **Anakinra** combined with methotrexate in patients of rheumatoid arthritis.

Abciximab: Fab fragment of monoclonal antibody which binds with integrin GP$_{IIb/IIIa}$ receptor, used with Aspirin and Heparin during PCI to prevent ischemic cardiac complications.

ADRs: Hypersensitivity reactions, local pain and erythema occur at site of injection and renal damage with ALG.

Proliferation Signal or mTOR Inhibitors

Sirolimus, Everolimus: Drug-FKBP complex blocks mTOR i.e. mammalian target of rapamycin → Inhibition of IL-driven T-cell, B-cell proliferation and immunoglobulin synthesis.

Uses: Prevention of solid organ allograft rejection, acute graft-versus-host disease not responding to steroids, topically for skin disorders, uveoretinitis.

ADRs: Headache, pneumonitis, hypertriglyceridemia, severe myelosuppression, TCP, hepatotoxic potential.

SECTION 12 Miscellaneous Topics

66 Toxicology

PH 9.2 Describe management of common drug poisonings, insecticides, common stings and bites.
PH 9.3 Describe chelating agents and make a plan for management of heavy metal poisoning.

Learning objectives

A student of MBBS phase II should be able to:
- Describe the health hazards of common environmental pollutants.
- Describe the prevention/treatment of exposure to common environmental pollutants.
- Discuss management of stings and bites.
- Describe general management of a case of poisoning.
- Describe causes and prominent symptoms of poisoning with heavy metals such as arsenic, mercury, lead, antimony, silver and copper.
- Enumerate chelating agents useful in poisoning with heavy metals – As, Hg, Au, Pb, Sb, Ni, Bi.
- Describe mechanism of action of chelating agents.
- Enumerate uses, dose and adverse effects of different chelating agents.

Humans are exposed to countless chemicals and drugs in the environment, which can pose serious health risks. Additionally, humans are at risk of bites and stings from various animals, including dogs, cats, rats, snakes, bees, and scorpions. Preventive and treatment measures for such exposures are essential in clinical practice. Some common terms associated with environmental/occupational risks are listed below.

Hazard is the subjective estimate of ability of a chemical substance to cause injury in given conditions of use and exposure.

Risk is the expected frequency of occurrence of an undesirable effect after exposure to that agent.

Occupational toxicology involves detection of harmful agents, assessment of the harm from short-term and long-term exposure to these agents, and the conditions for safe use of these agents for minimising health risks.

Environmental toxicology deals with the deleterious effects of environmental pollutants present in soil, air and water. Residues of chemicals used in agriculture (e.g., insecticides and pesticides), and those used in food processing may persist in food as contaminants.

Bioaccumulation refers to the gradual build-up of a contaminant in an organism over time, occurring when the rate of absorption exceeds the rate of elimination. In other words, when the organism's ability to metabolise, inactivate, or excrete the substance is insufficient, the contaminant accumulates in its tissues. Bioaccumulation can occur at different levels of the food chain and may pose health risks to the organisms and those who consume them.

Acute or chronic exposure: A single exposure to a hazardous substance or multiple exposures occurring over a brief period of time (ranging from a few seconds to one or two days) is labelled as acute exposure, e.g., the Bhopal gas tragedy of 1984. On the other hand, multiple exposures occurring over a longer duration are considered as chronic exposure, e.g., exposure to water or air pollutants.

Some common environmental pollutants are described briefly.

1. AIR POLLUTANTS

Carbon monoxide, nitrogen oxides, sulphur oxides, hydrocarbons and particulate matter are major air pollutants. Air pollution is implicated in diseases like bronchial asthma, bronchitis, chronic obstructive pulmonary disease (COPD), emphysema and lung carcinoma.

Carbon monoxide (CO) poisoning

CO generated during incomplete combustion has approximately 200 times more affinity than oxygen for binding to hemoglobin. The resulting carboxyhemoglobin cannot transport oxygen from the lungs to tissues. The presence of carboxyhemoglobin also interferes with the dissociation of oxygen from oxyhemoglobin. By these two mechanisms, carbon monoxide causes tissue hypoxia, which particularly affects the brain and heart.

A patient of carbon monoxide intoxication presents with sign/symptoms of hypoxia, such as psychomotor impairment, headache, confusion, visual disturbances, tachycardia, tachypnea, syncopal attack, convulsions and coma. It can lead to death due to respiratory failure.

Treatment involves stopping further exposure to CO, maintenance of respiration and hyperbaric oxygen.

Sulphur dioxide poisoning

SO_2 is generated by combustion of fossil fuel containing sulphur. On moist surfaces, SO_2 forms sulphurous acid that causes severe irritant effect on the skin, mucus membranes and eyes. Inhaled SO_2 causes bronchoconstriction and increased resistance to airflow. Patients of SO_2 intoxication present with irritation of nose, eyes and throat. Acute, severe asthma may be precipitated in susceptible individuals. Severe cases may develop pulmonary edema. **Treatment** is not specific for SO_2; it is same as for other respiratory irritants and bronchial asthma.

Nitrogen dioxide (NO_2) poisoning

NO_2 is formed in fresh silage. Silage is a moist fermented fodder prepared by storing crops with high moisture content in anaerobic conditions, in a container or structure called a 'silo'. This is fed to domestic animals during dry season. Farmers may get exposed to the NO_2 present in the silo, and the condition is labelled as **'silo-filler's disease'**. Acute NO_2 exposure (50 ppm for about an hour) damages alveolar cells, causing subacute pulmonary lesions and pulmonary edema. Patient presents with irritation of eyes, nose, cough, frothy sputum, dyspnea and chest pain. Symptoms may subside in 2 weeks, but later on, second-stage recurrent pulmonary edema and bronchiolar destruction may occur. Chronic exposure to lower concentrations of NO_2 may cause emphysema. **Treatment** of NO_2 poisoning involves oxygenation, alveolar ventilation, bronchodilators and antimicrobial agents to prevent secondary infections.

Ozone (O_3) poisoning

Ozone may be present around electrical equipment such as high-voltage air purifiers and water purifiers and in polluted air in urban areas. It causes irritation of mucus membranes. O_3 exposure may produce reactive free radicals. Mild exposure to concentration < 0.1 ppm may cause upper respiratory tract irritation and dryness of throat, while exposure to > 0.1 ppm O_3 may cause airway hyper-responsiveness, inflammation, dyspnea, substernal pain, pulmonary edema, visual disturbances, etc. Long-term exposure can cause chronic bronchitis, fibrosis, bronchiolitis and emphysema. Treatment is the same as for NO_2 toxicity.

WATER AND SOIL POLLUTANTS

Common surface water pollutants arise from industrial effluents, agricultural run-off containing pesticides and fertilisers, especially after heavy rains, waste water seepage or spillage with suspended particles, heavy metals, microorganisms, etc. Some soil pollutants penetrate deeper layers and pollute ground water as well. Common pollutants include the following.

Halogenated aliphatic hydrocarbons

Halogenated hydrocarbons like carbon tetrachloride, trichloroethylene, tetrachloroethylene, chloroform, methyl chloroform and freons—used in processes such as solvent degreasing, dry cleaning, and refrigeration—can cause persistent pollution of both surface and groundwater. These compounds have the potential to cause CNS depressant action, resulting in impaired memory and neuropathy. Carbon tetrachloride, chloroform and trichloroethylene have hepatic, renal and cardiotoxic actions. Carcinogenic potential is also reported. Testicular, renal and prostate cancers are reported to have significant association with exposure to halogenated hydrocarbons. Treatment is not specific for the compound, but is based upon the organ toxicity caused.

Aromatic hydrocarbons

Aromatic hydrocarbons like **benzene** may cause CNS depression, presenting as euphoria, drowsiness, headache, vertigo, nausea, etc. On acute exposure to high concentration of benzene (> 3000 ppm), the patient may go into coma. Chronic benzene exposure is myelotoxic and results in aplastic anemia, thrombocytopenia, leukopenia, leukemia, myelodysplastic syndrome and other hematological cancers.

Methyl benzene or toluene has irritant action on the skin and eyes. It also has CNS depressant and fetotoxic actions, but unlike benzene, it is free of bone marrow toxicity. Acute exposure to toluene causes severe fatigue, ataxia and loss of consciousness.

Dimethylbenzene or xylene, while also an irritant and a CNS depressant, is not myelotoxic. Toluene and xylene have practically replaced benzene in most of its commercial applications.

Pesticides

Pesticides include organochlorides, organophosphates, carbamates and botanical pesticides.

Organochlorides are heterocyclic compounds with chlorine substituents. These include dichlorodiphenyltrichloroethane (DDT) and its analogues like methoxychlor and tetrachlorodiphenyl ethane. Benzene hexachloride, lindane, toxaphenes, and cyclodienes such as aldrin, dieldrin, chlordane and heptachlor are some other examples.

Different organochlorides are absorbed from skin, GIT and lungs to variable extents. Organochlorides interfere with the inactivation of sodium channels and transport of calcium ions, thereby enhancing neuronal excitability, causing rapid, repetitive firing of neurons. CNS stimulation, tremors and convulsions may occur in acute intoxication. Chronic exposure is reportedly associated with increased risk of brain tumours, testicular cancers and non-Hodgkin lymphoma.

Organophosphates like malathion, parathion, trichlorfon, diazinon, parathion methyl, and leptophos are widely used as pesticides. Organophosphates get readily absorbed from skin, respiratory tract and GI mucosa. They interfere with acetylcholine metabolism by irreversible inhibition of cholinesterase enzyme (refer to Chapter 7). In addition, some organophosphates may cause progressive demyelination of peripheral nerves, leading to axonal degeneration and paralysis. The lesion is called organophosphorus ester-induced delayed polyneuropathy (OPIDP). Such patients present with tingling and burning sensation in feet, followed by motor weakness and sensory loss in legs and hands. As time progresses, gait is disturbed.

Carbamate pesticides, such as propoxur, carbaryl, and aldicarb, act as inhibitors of the enzyme cholinesterase. In cases of carbamate poisoning, oximes are ineffective because the cholinesterase enzyme's anionic site is not available for oxime binding. Moreover, oximes have weak cholinesterase inhibitory action (refer to Chapter 7).

Botanical pesticides include nicotine, rotenone and pyrethrum. Nicotine causes stimulation followed by blockade of Nn receptors on ganglia (both sympathetic and parasympathetic) and Nm receptors on the motor end plate. Ganglionic stimulation followed by blockade of all ganglia produces widespread effects. Motor end plate shows initial stimulation causing fasciculations, followed by skeletal muscle relaxation and weakness. Rotenone causes conjunctivitis, pharyngitis, rhinitis, dermatitis and GI irritation. Pyrethroids or pyrethrum has central toxic effects, resulting in excitation, convulsions, tetany, paralysis, cutaneous paresthesia, eye irritation, irritant asthma, reactive airway dysfunction syndrome (RADS) and anaphylactic reactions.

Herbicides

Some herbicides (pesticides used for killing unwanted plants) like paraquat are **non-selective** and can kill all plants to which they are applied. Paraquat is a contact herbicide that kills only those parts of the plant that it comes in contact with. Absorption of paraquat from skin and lungs is negligible, but it causes irritation in eyes and skin. If ingested, absorption occurs partially. It generates superoxide free radicals which damage hepatic, renal, pulmonary and cardiac cells.

Patients of paraquat toxicity present with oropharyngeal, esophageal erosions/ulcerations, dysphagia, vomiting, blood in vomit, cough, dyspnea, acute respiratory distress syndrome, renal failure, convulsions, coma and even death. Treatment is mainly supportive, but O_2 therapy should be avoided unless partial pressure of oxygen is below 92%, because oxygen worsens the toxic effects of paraquat. There is no specific antidote; however, cyclophosphamide may be beneficial.

In contrast, **selective herbicides** kill some plants and spare the desired crop, e.g., atrazine, diclofop-methyl and glyphosate.

Glyphosate travels through the xylem and phloem and affects the plant as a whole, and is hence called a systemic herbicide. It causes irritation of skin and has a corrosive effect on the oral mucosa, throat and esophagus, leading to formation of strictures and dysphagia. Severe cases may develop hepatic and renal damage, arrhythmias and fluid–electrolyte disturbances.

Diclofop-methyl persists in surface water and may affect reproduction and development; it has carcinogenic potential.

Insect repellents

These are commonly used for protection against mosquitoes, cockroaches, flies, fleas, etc., and include natural and synthetic repellents.

Natural repellents are lemon–eucalyptus oil, rosemary oil, neem oil and citronella oil. These are less effective and have shorter duration of action than synthetic repellents. However, they are free of neurotoxic actions and are safe for use in pregnancy and children. **Synthetic repellents** include diethyl-m-toluamide (DEET), pyrethroids (prallethrin, transfluthrin), and picaridin. DEET can cause skin irritation, eye irritation, swelling, and rashes. Ingestion may lead to gastric irritant action, nausea and vomiting. No carcinogenic or developmental defect have been reported. Pyrethroids used in vaporisers are the most-frequently used insect repellents. Ingestion of these agents may cause nausea, vomiting, GI ulceration, abdominal pain, dyspepsia, headache, dizziness, blurring of vision, palpitation, chest pain or tightness, convulsions and coma. Picaridin is a good alternative to DEET because it is free of neurotoxic effects.

Food adulterants

Nausea, vomiting, diarrhea, hepatic or renal damage, neurotoxic effects; carcinogenic effects may occur.

- *Claviceps purpurea* or ergot growing on millets like rye and bajra may cause ergotism or **St. Anthony's fire**, vasospastic ischemia, burning sensation, gangrene, abortion in pregnant females, dementia, hallucinations, etc. It can be prevented by removing millets infested with *Claviceps purpurea* by manual picking, air floatation, or floating in 20% salt water.
- **Epidemic dropsy** occurs because of argemone poisoning. It causes vasodilatation, increased permeability, edema, proteinuria, hypoproteinemia, salt/water retention. Headache, diarrhea, dyspnea and right heart failure may occur. To avoid this, growth of wild *Argemone mexicana* shrub along with mustard should be checked and prevented.

- *Aspergillus flavus* growing on food grains stored in hot, humid conditions may cause **aflatoxicosis**. It causes anorexia, nausea, vomiting, hepatotoxicity leading to jaundice, ascites, pedal edema, cirrhosis and hepatic cell carcinoma. To prevent this condition, grains, seeds, and nuts should be stored properly in dry and cool places.
- Kesari dal or *Lathyrus sativus* causes **neurolathyrism** resulting in weakness and paralysis of lower limbs, sclerosis of the spinal motor tracts in the lumbo-sacral region, and UMN type of paralysis of both legs. The cultivation, harvesting and consumption of kesari dal is partially banned in India.

The Food Safety and Standards Authority of India (FSSAI) established in year 2006 supervises the manufacturing, import, storage and sale of food items and to provide license to packaged food items manufacturers.

Clinical problem-based questions and MCQs

1. A 56-year-old woman was brought to the emergency room after being found unconscious in a closed garage with the car engine running. On examination, her heart rate was 120–130 bpm, and her blood pressure was 80/60 mm Hg. Her husband reported a history of anxiety, depression, and previous suicide attempts. Arterial blood gas analysis revealed a pH of 7.32, PCO_2 of 33 mm Hg, PO_2 of 380 mm Hg, bicarbonate level of 16 mEq/L, and a carboxyhemoglobin level of 20% (normal < 2%).
   i. What is the likely diagnosis?
   ii. Explain cause of patient's sign symptoms.
   iii. Describe the management of this case.

2. Which of the following gases is responsible for causing silo filler's disease?
   a. Sulphur dioxide
   b. Carbon monoxide
   c. Nitrogen dioxide
   d. Ozone

3. Identify the aromatic hydrocarbon that has maximum myelotoxic potential.
   a. Toluene
   b. Benzene
   c. Xylene
   d. CCl_4

4. DDT is a commonly used pesticide. Identify the correct mechanism that explains the harmful effects of acute intoxication with DDT.
   a. Interfere with Na channel inactivation
   b. Decrease oxygenation of tissues
   c. Increase ACh levels in blood
   d. Causes ganglionic stimulation

5. Oximes have no role in management of which of the following pesticide poisoning?
   a. Parathion
   b. Trichlorfon
   c. Diazinon
   d. Aldicarb

Key features of important environmental pollutants are presented in the Concept map (page 867).

BITES AND STINGS

Snake Bite

Approximately 70% of snake bites are dry or non-venomous. The toxic components of snake venom are mainly glycopeptides and enzymatic proteins. Elapid venoms secreted by Indian cobra and common krait are neurotoxic, while the viperid venoms secreted by Russell's viper and saw-scaled viper are hemotoxic and vasculotoxic. These four species of snakes are responsible for majority of snake bite cases in India.

Clinical features

- The patient complains of pain at the site of snake bite. Anxiety, panic and phobia is almost always an accompanying initial feature.
- Fang marks are usually visible along with oozing blood, ecchymosis, swelling and formation of blisters. Cellulitis and necrosis may occur with time. These signs are severe in cases of viper bites and minimal in krait bites.
- Viper venom causes coagulopathy and vasculotoxicity. Bleeding can occur from any site, e.g., gum bleed, epistaxis, vaginal bleeding, hematuria, hematemesis, GI bleeds, hemoptysis and intracranial bleeds. In addition, muscular damage of skeletal/smooth/cardiac muscle fibres may occur, resulting in hypotension, tachycardia, arrhythmias, shock, pulmonary edema, etc.
- Cobra venom causes curare-like flaccid paralysis of skeletal muscles, resulting in ptosis, diplopia, facial paralysis, dysphagia, dyspnea, dysphonia, limb weakness, abdominal pain, fall in BP, tachycardia and death due to respiratory failure. Cobra venom effect can be partially reversed by neostigmine.
- Krait venom also causes flaccid paralysis of skeletal muscles by damaging axonal structure of somatic motor nerves. Neostigmine cannot reverse such muscle paralysis.

Management

The patient should be reassured, made to lie in prone position with their head in the left lateral position to protect airways. The affected limb or area should be immobilised to decrease the rate of venom absorption and the patient should be shifted to hospital promptly.

The site of the bite is cleaned with povidone-iodine solution, followed by debridement to remove necrosed tissue, if needed. IV line and ventilator support through a mask or endotracheal tube should be secured. An opioid analgesic is given to relieve pain, anxiety and apprehension associated with snakebite.

In patients with hypotension or shock, hypovolemia should be corrected with IV fluid infusion, along with a dopamine drip administered at a rate of 0.2–0.5 mg per minute. Fresh frozen plasma is infused in viper snakebites to correct coagulopathy.

CONCEPT MAP – TOXICOLOGY

Definitions

Occupational toxicology: Detection of harmful agents, harms of short-term and long-term exposure & conditions for safe use.

Environmental toxicology: Deals with deleterious effects of environmental pollutants, as in soil, air, water.

Hazard: Subjective estimate of ability of a chemical substance to cause injury.

Risk: Expected frequency of occurrence of an undesirable effect after exposure to that agent.

Food adulterant: Any material, addition of which makes food unsafe, substandard, misbranded, or extraneous matter from raw materials/packaging materials, etc. These may cause nausea, vomiting, diarrhea, hepatic or renal damage, neurotoxic effects, carcinogenic effects, ergotism, epidemic dropsy, aflatoxicosis, neurolathyrism, etc.

Acceptable daily intake (ADI): Levels of chemicals from food that appear not to have appreciable risk, if taken during an entire lifetime.

Acute exposure: A single exposure or multiple exposures occurring over a brief period of time from few seconds to one or two days.

Chronic exposure: Multiple exposures occurring over a longer period.

Air Pollutants

Carbon monoxide: Generated during incomplete combustion → binds to Hb → forms carboxyHb → impaired oxygen delivery to tissues → tissue hypoxia → psychomotor impairment, headache, confusion, visual disturbances, tachycardia, tachypnea, syncope, convulsions, coma & death.

Treatment: Stop further exposure, maintenance of respiration & hyperbaric oxygen.

Sulphur dioxide: Generated by combustion of fossil fuel containing sulphur → forms sulphurous acid on moist surfaces → irritant effect on skin, mucus membranes, BC, pulmonary edema.

Treatment: As for other respiratory irritants and bronchial asthma.

Nitrogen dioxide: Formed in moist fermented fodder (silage) → silo filler's disease → subacute pulmonary lesions, pulmonary edema, irritation of eyes, nose, cough, frothy sputum, dyspnea and chest pain.

Treatment: Oxygenation, alveolar ventilation, bronchodilators & antimicrobial agents.

Ozone: present around electrical equipments of high voltage, air purifiers, water purifiers and polluted air in urban areas → upper respiratory tract irritation, dryness, hyper-responsiveness, inflammation, dyspnea, substernal pain, pulmonary edema & visual disturbances → chronic bronchitis, fibrosis, bronchiolitis & emphysema.

Treatment: Same as NO_2 poisoning.

Toxicology
Environmental/Occupational

Water & Soil Pollutants

Halogenated aliphatic hydrocarbons: CCl_4, chloroform, methyl chloroform, freons cause persistent water pollution of surface & ground water → CNS depressant effect, impairment of memory and neuropathy, hepatic, renal and cardiotoxic actions, carcinogenic potential.

Treatment: Based upon the organ toxicity caused.

Aromatic hydrocarbons: Benzene → CNS depression → Euphoria, drowsiness, headache, vertigo, nausea, coma, myelotoxic effects.

Toluene, Xylene: Irritant action on skin, eyes, CNS depressant, fetotoxic actions, but not myelotoxic.

Pesticides

Organochlorides, organophosphates, carbamates and botanical pesticides.

Organochlorides: Dichlorodiphenyltrichloroethane (DDT) & its analogues → enhance neuronal excitability → rapid, repetitive firing of neurons → CNS stimulation, tremors, convulsions.

Organophosphates: Malathion, parathion, trichlorfos, diazinon, parathion methyl, leptophos are irreversible cholinesterase inhibitors, cause progressive demyelination of peripheral nerves → delayed polyneuropathy. Specific antidote for acute toxicity is atropine. Oximes are cholinesterase regenerators.

Carbamate pesticides like propoxur, carbaryl, aldicarb also inhibit cholinesterase.

Botanical: Nicotine causes ganglionic stimulation followed by blockade of all ganglia → widespread effects, fasciculations followed by paralysis of skeletal muscles.

Rotenone: Causes conjunctivitis, pharyngitis, rhinitis, dermatitis and GI irritation

Pyrethrum: Central excitation, convulsions, tetany, paralysis, cutaneous paraesthesia, eye irritation, irritant asthma, reactive airway dysfunction syndrome (RADS) & anaphylaxis.

Herbicides

Pesticides used for killing unwanted plants or weeds. Can be non-selective like Paraquat or selective, e.g., Atrazine, Diclofop-methyl, Glyphosate.

Paraquat: Generates superoxide-free radicals → causes irritation in eyes and skin, hepatic/ renal/pulmonary / cardiac cell damage → oropharyngeal, esophageal erosions/ ulcerations, dysphagia, vomiting, blood in vomit, cough, dyspnoea, ARDS, renal failure, convulsions, coma, and death.

Glyphosate: Causes irritation of skin, corrosive effect in oral mucosa, throat, esophagus → strictures & dysphagia

Neostigmine 1.5 mg is injected intravenously in cobra bites. Muscarinic adverse effects of neostigmine can be prevented or controlled by atropine 0.6 mg IV.

Calcium gluconate 10%, 5 mL, given by slow IV injection can reverse muscle paralysis in krait bites; however, response is partial only.

Polyvalent anti-snake venom (ASV) serum is lifesaving in case of snakebite. Each mL of ASV reconstituted in 10 mL distilled water can neutralise 0.45 mg of standard krait and saw-scaled viper venom and 0.6 mg of standard cobra and Russell's viper venom. For treatment, 8–10 vials of ASV are diluted in 500 mL normal saline or 5% dextrose and infused slowly over 60–100 minutes. Supplemental doses may be required after 1–6 hours, depending upon the severity of coagulopathy or paralysis. Up to 30 vials may be needed in a patient. Allergic reactions to ASV may occur as rashes, urticaria, itching, bronchoconstriction, colic pain and anaphylaxis. This can be prevented by adrenaline 1:1000 injected subcutaneously before ASV infusion.

Dog bite

Dog bites are among the most common animal bites in India. Dog-bite wounds can vary from minor bruises to extensive, life-threatening wounds and lacerations. There is a risk of secondary infection and rabies.

Management of dog bite includes thorough washing of the wound with soap and running water for 10 minutes to remove rabies virus and decrease the risk of rabies.

- Antiseptic like povidone-iodine or cetrimide is applied on wound in all the cases.
- Systemic antibiotic therapy is needed in extensive, contaminated wounds.
- A booster shot of tetanus toxoid is given to patients who have not received TT in the last 5 years.
- *Post-exposure prophylaxis*: Purified chick embryo cell vaccine (PCEV) available as 2.5 IU in a 1 mL ampoule is the most frequently used vaccine in India. It is injected in a dose of 0.1 mL intradermally at 2 sites (over the deltoid in both arms) on days 0, 3 and 7. Then the intradermal injection is given at one site on days 28 and 90 after exposure. Human diploid cell vaccine and purified vero cell rabies vaccines are also available. Protective antibodies against rabies develop in about 10–14 days. Therefore, in cases of severe exposure (single or multiple transdermal bites, scratches which bleed, mucus membrane contamination with dog saliva, licks on broken skin, etc.), rabies immunoglobulin (RIG) is also recommended.

Bee/ Wasp Sting

The venom of bees and wasps contain many active moieties like kinins, histamine, serotonin, neurotoxic proteins and enzymes. A single sting is usually more of an outdoor nuisance and self-treatable, but multiple stings may introduce sufficient quantity of venom to cause systemic effects. Patients complain of burning sensation, sharp pain, redness and swelling at the sting site. Multiple stings by a cluster of wasps or honeybees may cause headache, fever, nausea, dizziness, vertigo and fainting fit. In some cases, hypersensitivity reaction to venom may occur, causing urticaria, itching, angioedema, hypotension, tachycardia, and, in rare cases, anaphylaxis.

Treatment involves cleaning the puncture site with soap and water, removing any stings visible on skin with forceps, and applying an antiseptic solution like povidone-iodine. Pain and swelling can be relieved by cold compress and topical hydrocortisone. In more severe cases, paracetamol or another NSAID is administered orally to reduce pain, swelling and fever. Itching and urticaria may respond to oral antihistaminic drugs like chlorpheniramine. Severe allergic cases with angioedema or anaphylaxis are managed with IV adrenaline injection.

Scorpion Sting

Indian red scorpion is the most poisonous of scorpions; its sting may cause burning and radiating pain at the site of sting. A single hole is visible at the centre of red swollen area; there is paresthesia and hyperesthesia on tapping. In severe cases, 'autonomic storm' occurs due to delay in Na^+ channel closing by the neurotoxin present in scorpion venom. This reaction involves initial transient parasympathetic stimulation, followed by prolonged sympathetic stimulation, leading to the release of large amounts of catecholamines into circulation. Severe cardiovascular symptoms like initial bradycardia, premature beats, followed by high BP, tachycardia and intense cutaneous vasoconstriction leading to cold extremities are seen. Very severe cases may develop pulmonary edema, cardiac arrhythmias and cardiac failure.

Management of a patient with scorpion sting begins with immobilisation of limb for reducing venom absorption. Prazosin, a selective $α_1$ blocker, 1 mg, is given orally as first-line treatment. Supplemental dose of 0.5 mg is given every 3 hours till the effect of the venom subsides. In children, the prazosin dose is half of the adult dose.

Saline infusion is given to correct dehydration. Opioid analgesic is given to reduce pain and anxiety. Inj. Tetanus toxoid booster dose may be needed if the patient has not received it in the last 5 years. Antibiotics are used as per need.

Scorpion antivenom serum (SAV), an equine antivenom, is the specific antidote. It is reconstituted with 10 mL sterile water. One mL of serum can neutralise one mg of red scorpion toxin. 30 mL of SAV diluted in 100 mL saline is infused over 30 minutes, followed by a supplemental dose after 6 hours, as required. Hypersensitivity reactions may occur with SAV, resulting in urticaria, fall in BP, tachycardia, bronchospasm, angioedema, etc. These can be prevented or treated by antihistamines or adrenaline 1:1000.

> **Clinical problem-based questions and MCQs**
>
> 6. Match the venoms/stings with harmful effects in humans.
>   a. Viper venom   1. Autonomic storm
>   b. Cobra venom   2. Coagulopathy
>   c. Red scorpion sting   3. Hypersensitivity
>   d. Wasp sting   4. Skeletal muscle paralysis
>
> 7. A 35-year-old farmer is brought to emergency following a snake bite sustained while working in the fields during rainy season. The patient is anxious and complains of pain at the site of bite. Fang marks are visible, and there is oozing blood, ecchymosis, swelling and blister formation at the site of the bite. Identify the lifesaving measures for this patient.
>   a. Calcium gluconate
>   b. Neostigmine and atropine
>   c. Polyvalent ASV
>   d. Fresh frozen plasma
>
> 8. Indian red scorpion bite causes severe cardiovascular symptoms; initial bradycardia and premature beats, followed by high BP, tachycardia and intense cutaneous vasoconstriction and cold extremities. Identify the first-line drug for control of such features of scorpion sting.
>   a. Prednisolone   b. Adrenaline
>   c. Prazosin   d. Esmolol

HEAVY METAL INTOXICATION AND CHELATING AGENTS

A ligand is a functional group capable of forming a coordinate bond (a type of covalent bond where both shared electrons are donated by the ligand). Typically, atoms such as oxygen (O), nitrogen (N), and sulphur (S) in hydroxy, carboxyl, keto, thiol, disulfide, amino, or phosphate groups function as ligands.

Heavy metal ions combine with and inactivate ligands in enzymes or other critically important biomolecules in the body, resulting in harmful effects. This can be prevented by providing alternative ligands in the form of chelating agents, which bind to heavy metal ions. The term chelating agents is derived from the Greek word '*chele*' which means crab. These agents form complexes with metallic ions, forming a ring structure, i.e., they hold the metal ion like a crab's claw.

Chelating agents usually have 2 or more ligands that can hold the metallic ion from at least 2 sides and form a stable ring-like structure. The chelating agent–metal ion complex is stable, non-toxic, water soluble, and is excreted out easily. However, the efficacy of chelating agents decreases as the interval from exposure to the metal increases, because the metal ions have already formed complexes with body ligands.

A clinically valuable chelating agent is one that:
- Has higher affinity for toxic metals than for Ca^{2+}, because calcium ions are available freely in the plasma as well as extracellular fluid.
- Has higher affinity for metal ions than for body ligands.
- Has the same distribution in the body as that of the metal to be chelated.
- Forms a complex with the metal ions that is stable, water soluble and easily excretable.

Chelating Agents Used for Common Heavy Metal Poisonings

Chelating agents used for common heavy metal poisonings are shown in Flowchart 66.1 and described below.

1. Dimercaprol

It is also known as British anti-Lewisite (BAL) because it was developed by the British as an antidote for the arsenical war gas Lewisite.

Mechanism of action

BAL possesses two thiol (SH) groups that can each donate a lone pair of electrons to form a coordinate bond with metallic ions.

$$\begin{array}{c} CH_2 - CH - CH_2OH \\ | \quad\quad | \\ SH \quad SH \end{array}$$

The complex formed with arsenic ions is non-toxic and water-soluble, allowing it to be rapidly excreted by the kidneys. BAL can form stable complexes with arsenic

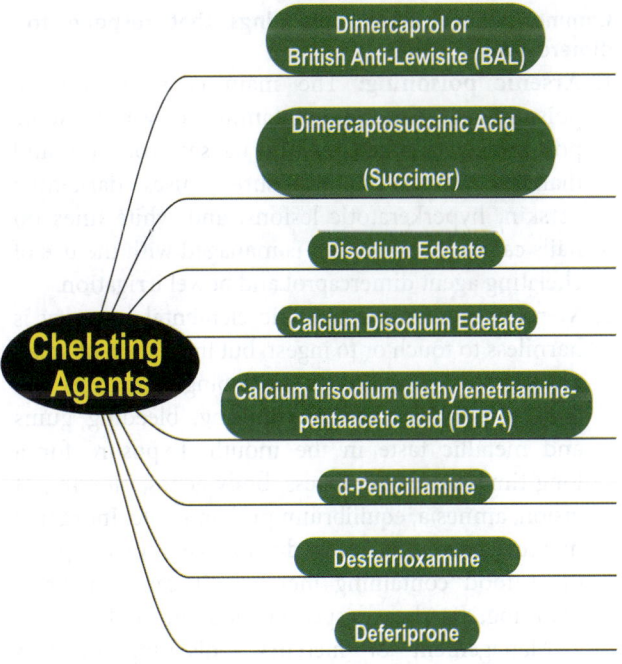

Flowchart 66.1 Chelating agents

as well as with other metals such as mercury (Hg), lead (Pb), antimony (Sb), bismuth (Bi), nickel (Ni), copper (Cu), and gold (Au). The stability of the complex further increases if two molecules of BAL are chelated to each metal ion. This can be achieved by administering BAL in excess to favour the formation of 2:1 complex that can dissociate quickly in acidic urine. The released ions can cause renal damage, so urine must be alkalinised while using dimercaprol.

However, the complex formed by iron and cadmium ions with BAL is toxic. Therefore, BAL is contraindicated in iron and cadmium poisoning.

Therapeutic uses
Dimercaprol is administered in a dose of 5 mg/kg body weight stat intramuscular in As, Hg, Pb, Sb, Cu, Au, Bi, and Ni poisonings. Thereafter, the dose is reduced to 2–3 mg/kg body weight, given 4–8 hourly for 2 days.

ADRs
Dimercaprol causes frequent dose-related adverse effects such as raised BP, tachycardia, headache, vomiting, anxiety, sweating, and cramps. In addition, tingling or burning sensation and inflammation of mucus membrane may occur.

2. Succimer
Succimer or dimercaptosuccinic acid is orally effective in arsenic, mercury, lead, copper, zinc and silver poisoning. Adverse reactions like anorexia, nausea and diarrhea may occur.

> **Common heavy metal poisonings that respond to dimercaprol**
> 1. **Arsenic poisoning:** The main cause of arsenic poisoning is through contaminated water. Acute poisoning is characterised by nausea, vomiting and diarrhea. Long-term exposure causes darkening of skin, hyperkeratotic lesions, and white lines on nails called Mees' lines. It is managed with the use of chelating agent dimercaprol and bowel irrigation.
> 2. **Mercury poisoning:** Organic elemental mercury is harmless to touch or to ingest, but inhalation of small droplets can cause severe disturbing symptoms like cough, dyspnea, nausea, vomiting, bleeding gums and metallic taste in the mouth. Exposure for a long time causes numbness, body aches, blurring of vision, amnesia, equilibrium problems, etc. Inorganic mercury poisoning occurs due to excess consumption of seafood containing mercury. It causes nausea, vomiting, diarrhea, dyspepsia, blood in stool, etc.
>   Management of mercury poisoning involves decontamination, oxygen and chelation therapy with dimercaprol. d-penicillamine is an alternative to dimercaprol in mercury poisoning.
> 3. **Lead poisoning:** Exposure to lead occurs through environmental or occupational hazards. Inhalation of lead particles can occur when lead-containing materials are burned, while ingestion can happen through contaminated food, water, dust, and other sources. Young children are especially vulnerable, as they absorb lead more readily. Lead gets distributed in the liver, kidneys, brain, bones, etc. In children, abdominal pain, constipation, irritability, headache, convulsions, coma, and even death may occur in acute poisoning. Lower levels are not fatal but cause mental retardation and behavioural disturbances. Anemia, renal dysfunction, immunotoxicity and neurological deficit may occur. Treatment mainly involves chelation with dimercaprol or EDTA (edetate disodium – see below).
> 4. **Sb poisoning:** Antimony poisoning is usually associated with occupational exposure. It causes abdominal cramps, nausea, vomiting, irritation of respiratory tract, pneumoconiosis, spots on the skin, etc. Long-term exposure has the risk of carcinogenesis. Antimony used therapeutically in the management of leishmaniasis and schistosomiasis can cause cardiotoxicity and pancreatitis.
> 5. **Silver poisoning:** Exposure to elemental silver or silver dust may cause bluish-grey discolouration of skin called argyrosis. It may be localised to small patches of skin/mucus membrane/conjunctiva or may be generalised, involving large part of visible skin surface. Additional symptoms like nausea, vomiting, diarrhea, and respiratory problems may be occur. Treatment involves chelation with succimer and glutathione.

3. Disodium edetate
It is a potent chelator of calcium and hence may cause tetany on intravenous bolus administration. However, this adverse effect is not seen upon slow intravenous infusion, because with slow administration, calcium is extracted from bones. It is indicated for **emergency control of hypercalcemia**.

$$NaOOCH_2C\!\!>\!\!NCH_2\!-\!CH_2N\!\!<\!\!CH_2COONa$$
$$HOOCH_2C \qquad\qquad\qquad CH_2COOH$$

4. Calcium Disodium Edetate
This is a calcium chelate of disodium edetate that has a higher affinity for metals like **Zn, Mn, Pb, Cd, Cu and radioactive metals** than for calcium. So, calcium disodium edetate can remove these metals from the body in exchange for calcium.

Because calcium disodium edetate is ionised, it is useful only when injected intravenously. Injection given into muscles is very painful. It is polar in nature and gets rapidly excreted in urine by glomerular filtration. Heavy metals bound to calcium disodium edetate get excreted quickly along with it. However, either because of ionisation or its polar nature, calcium disodium edetate fails to cross the blood–brain barrier; so, it can remove metallic ions only from accessible sites.

Therapeutic uses

For treatment of lead poisoning, 1 g of calcium disodium edetate dissolved in 200 mL saline is infused intravenously over a period of 1 hour, twice a day, for 3–5 days. After a gap of 5 days, a second course may be given to facilitate the removal of lead mobilised from deeper or less accessible tissue stores.

Calcium disodium edetate is also useful in Zn, Mn, Cu and Fe poisoning.

ADRs

It may cause fever, chills, tiredness, and malaise. In some cases, anaphylactoid reaction characterised by fall in BP, congestion in eyes and nose may occur. Even though it does not cause tetany, proximal tubular necrosis and renal damage due to partial dissociation of metal from drug in kidneys is a major disadvantage.

Calcium disodium edetate has no role in Hg poisoning because mercury gets distributed in areas where $CaNa_2$ EDTA cannot reach.

5. Calcium trisodium diethylenetriaminepentaacetic acid (DTPA)

- It has more affinity for many metals than EDTA.
- It is used in metal poisonings (especially radioactive metals) that do not respond to EDTA.
- A major drawback of DTPA is its limited distribution in the body.

6. d-Penicillamine

d-Penicillamine is dimethyl cysteine, which is obtained as a degradation product of penicillin. It has high affinity for Cu, Hg, Pb, and Zn ions and is therefore useful only in poisoning by these metals. The dextro (d) isomer is used because the levo (l) isomer and racemic mixtures are more toxic and have the potential to cause optic neuritis.

Therapeutic uses

d-Penicillamine is used in **Wilson's disease**, which is characterised by the genetic deficiency of ceruloplasmin, leading to hepatolenticular degeneration. Ceruloplasmin binds with Cu and facilitates its excretion. Therefore, the deficiency of ceruloplasmin results in raised Cu concentration. Excess Cu gets deposited in liver, substantia nigra and basal ganglia, and causes local degeneration known as hepatolenticular degeneration. Lifelong therapy with d-penicillamine is required. It is given orally in a dose of 0.5–1 g, 1 hour before or 2 hours after meals. Potassium disulphide given with meals decreases the absorption of dietary Cu and is also useful in Wilson's disease.

- d-Penicillamine is the **drug of choice for Cu poisoning**. Acute poisoning due to ingestion can cause severe symptoms like vomiting, dehydration, fall in BP, hematemesis, blood in stool, and jaundice. Mood fluctuations, irritability and anxiety are common. In severe toxicity, there is a risk of cardiac complications, renal dysfunction, and hepatic toxicity; it may even be fatal. Management of Cu toxicity includes chelation therapy with d-penicillamine, while zinc can prevent accumulation of Cu in liver and GIT.
- d-Penicillamine is used as an alternative to dimercaprol in **Hg poisoning.**
- In case of **chronic Pb poisoning**, d-penicillamine is used as adjuvant to calcium disodium edetate.
- d-Penicillamine **prevents formation of renal stones** as it promotes cysteine excretion and prevents its precipitation in the urinary tract.
- It is useful in scleroderma as it increases soluble collagen.
- Previously, d-penicillamine was used as a disease-modifying agent in rheumatoid arthritis, but now more efficacious and better tolerated drugs are available for this indication.

ADRs

d-Penicillamine can cause anorexia, nausea, loss of taste, rashes, itching, fever, etc. Long-term use is associated with risk of renal damage, bone marrow suppression, dermatological, hematological and collagen tissue toxic reactions. Antinuclear antibodies are formed, and SLE or myasthenia gravis may be precipitated.

7. Desferrioxamine

Ferrioxamine is a long-chain iron-containing complex; the removal of iron yields desferrioxamine, which has very high affinity for iron. One gram of desferrioxamine can chelate 85 mg of elemental iron. It is capable of forming complexes with free iron as well as with iron present in hemosiderin and ferritin. However, it cannot extract iron from hemoglobin and cytochrome. It has a low affinity for calcium.

Therapeutic uses

Desferrioxamine is used in cases of **acute iron toxicity**, common in young children who consume iron-containing nutritional supplements. Iron is a gastric irritant. Patient usually develops severe vomiting, abdominal pain, diarrhea and dehydration.

- Desferrioxamine has negligible oral absorption. So, when left in stomach after gastric lavage, desferrioxamine reduces oral iron absorption.
- Desferrioxamine is useful in thalassemia patients who have chronic iron overload and transfusion siderosis.

The dose is 0.5–1.0 g/day by intramuscular route. Alternatively, 2 g of desferrioxamine is administered for each unit of blood transfused.

ADRs

Desferrioxamine can cause histamine release, resulting in vasodilatation, hypotension, flushing, itching and urticaria. Allergic reactions are common. It may cause abdominal pain, loose stools, fever, dysuria, muscular cramps.

8. Deferiprone

It is also an iron chelator, effective by oral route. It is less effective than intramuscular desferrioxamine, but better tolerated and cheaper. It is useful in acute iron poisoning and iron overload in hepatic cirrhosis.

ADRs include anorexia, nausea, vomiting and altered taste. Joint pain, reversible neutropenia and agranulocytosis may occur. Its long-term safety is not yet established.

Clinical problem-based questions and MCQs

9. Which of the following is contraindicated in iron poisoning?
   a. Dimercaprol
   b. Desferrioxamine
   c. Deferiprone
   d. Zinc

10. Dimercaprol or British anti-Lewisite is useful in heavy metal poisoning with all of the following, EXCEPT:
    a. Arsenic
    b. Mercury
    c. Antimony
    d. Cadmium

11. A patient diagnosed with heavy metal poisoning has white lines (Mees' lines) on his nails.
    i. Identify the heavy metal responsible for poisoning in this case.
       a. Arsenic
       b. Lead
       c. Copper
       d. Silver
    ii. Which chelating agent is most useful in this case?
       a. Calcium disodium EDTA
       b. Dimercaprol
       c. Deferiprone
       d. Penicillamine
    iii. Enumerate the adverse effects of the selected drug.

12. A patient suffering from hepatolenticular degeneration is diagnosed with Wilson's disease.
    i. Describe the basic defect in Wilson's disease. How does it cause hepatolenticular degeneration (abnormal copper accumulation in the body)?
    ii. Identify the drug of choice in this case.
       a. BAL
       b. Deferiprone
       c. Calcium disodium EDTA
       d. d-Penicillamine

13. In a patient of lead poisoning, a second course of calcium disodium edetate is given 5 days after the first course.
    i. Explain the pharmacological basis for giving a second course.

    ii. In which of the following heavy metal poisoning is this chelating agent not useful?
       a. Mercury
       b. Lead
       c. Zinc
       d. Manganese

Key features of chelating agents are presented in the Concept map (page 873).

GENERAL MANAGEMENT OF POISONING

Poisoning can occur accidentally or intentionally. Fatal outcomes are more common in cases of intentional poisoning, especially in suicide attempts where individuals may not seek medical help. In contrast, accidental poisoning rarely leads to death if the patient receives timely medical attention and supportive care.

For appropriate management of poisoning cases and reducing fatality rates, a knowledge of the mechanisms responsible for death due to poisoning is crucial.

Major Causes of Death in Poisoning

- CNS stimulation: Central stimulation resulting in seizures, muscular hyperreactivity and rigidity is seen in cases of amphetamine, cocaine, and isoniazid poisoning. Seizures or convulsions may cause brain damage, hypoxia and aspiration, resulting in death. Muscular hyperactivity leads to muscle breakdown, myoglobinuria, hyperthermia, lactic acidosis, hyperkalemia and renal failure that causes death.

- CNS depressant effect shown by opioids and sedative-hypnotics causes unconsciousness and coma. In comatose patients, respiratory drive and protective airway reflexes are lost. Such patients usually die of airway obstruction due to flaccid tongue, aspiration of gastric contents and respiratory arrest.

- In cases of overdose with cardioactive drugs like digoxin, cocaine, amphetamines, or theophylline, cardiovascular suppression and hypovolemia (secondary to nausea, vomiting, diarrhea, and fluid sequestration) can lead to hypotension, peripheral vascular collapse, and rhythm disturbances such as ventricular tachycardia and ventricular fibrillation, which may have fatal outcomes.

- Cellular hypoxia, which impairs oxygen transport/utilisation, leads to tachycardia, hypotension, lactic acidosis, myocardial ischemia, and potentially death in cases of carbon monoxide, cyanide, or hydrogen sulphide (H_2S) poisoning.

- Delayed organ damage can lead to late fatalities in poisoning cases. For example, acetaminophen poisoning can cause centrilobular hepatic necrosis, mushroom poisoning may lead to hepatic encephalopathy, and paraquat exposure can result in pulmonary fibrosis.

CONCEPT MAP – CHELATING AGENTS

Dimercaprol (BAL)

Mechanism: It possesses two SH groups that share electrons to form coordinate bonds with metallic ions → complex formed with metals like As, Hg, Pb, Sb, Bi, Ni, Cu → complex is non-toxic, water soluble → excreted quickly by kidney.

Complex formed by two molecules of BAL with one ion of metal is more stable → administer BAL in excess to favour formation of 2:1 complexes.

Complex can dissociate in acidic urine → released metallic ions can cause renal damage → urine always alkalinised, while using dimercaprol.

Uses: As, Hg, Pb, Sb, Cu, Au, Bi, Ni poisoning, in a dose of 0.5 mg/kg body weight stat IM

ADRs: Rise in BP, tachycardia, headache, vomiting, anxiety, sweating, cramps, tingling or burning sensation and inflammation of mucous membrane.

Contraindications: BAL is contraindicated in Iron and cadmium poisoning as they form toxic complexes with BAL

Succimer: Same mechanism of action, uses
Advantage: Effective by oral route, less toxic.

d-Penicillamine

High affinity for Cu, Hg, Pb, Zn ions, so useful in poisoning with these metals.

Uses: Lifelong therapy is required with d-penicillamine, 0.5–1 g one hour before or 2 hours after meals, orally in Wilson's disease, (characterised by genetic deficiency of ceruloplasmin that plays important role in Cu excretion → leading to raised Cu concentration → hepatolenticular degeneration).

May be used as an alternative to dimercaprol in Hg poisoning, and as adjuvant to calcium disodium edetate in chronic Pb poisoning.

Levo (l) isomer and racemic mixture have potential to cause optic neuritis → not used.

Prevents formation of renal stones, useful in scleroderma & as DMARD.

ADRs: Anorexia, nausea, loss of taste sensation, rashes, itching, fever.

Long term use → Renal damage, bone marrow suppression, dermatological, hematological & collagen tissue disorders, myasthenia gravis.

Chelating Agents

Desferrioxamine

Very high affinity for iron, can form complexes with loose iron & that present in hemosiderin and ferritin. However, iron cannot be extracted from hemoglobin and cytochrome. Affinity for calcium is low. Not absorbed orally.

Uses: Acute iron toxicity, useful in thalassemia patients having chronic iron overload and transfusion siderosis in a Dose 0.5-1.0 g/day IM.

ADRs: Histamine release → vasodilatation, hypotension, flushing, itching and urticaria. Also, fever, dysuria, muscular cramps.

Deferiprone: Orally effective, iron chelator. Less effective than IM desferrioxamine, but better tolerated. Useful in acute iron poisoning, iron overload in hepatic cirrhosis.

ADRs: Anorexia, nausea, vomiting, altered taste. Joint pain, reversible neutropenia and agranulocytosis may occur.

EDTA

Disodium Edetate: A potent chelator of calcium, useful in emergency control of hypercalcemia. Risk of tetany on IV bolus administration, but not with slow IV infusion.

Calcium disodium edetate: Has higher affinity for metals like Zn, Mn, Pb, Cd, Cu and radioactive metals than for calcium → can remove these metals from body in exchange for calcium by renal excretion quickly.

Polar nature → fails to cross blood–brain barrier → removes metallic ions only from accessible sites.

Uses: Useful in Pb, Zn, Mn, Cu and Fe poisoning. Second course given after gap of 5 days, to remove metal mobilised from inaccessible sites. No role in Hg poisoning as mercury gets distributed in areas, where calcium disodium edetate cannot reach.

ADRs: Proximal tubular necrosis, renal damage due to partial dissociation of metal from drug in kidney, fever, chills, tiredness, malaise, anaphylactoid reaction.

Calcium trisodium diethylenetriaminepenta acetic acid (DTPA)
More affinity for metals (especially radioactive metals), Used in metal poisonings not responding to EDTA, but distribution in body is limited

- The behavioural effects of drugs and toxins, such as alcohol, phencyclidine (PCP), and LSD, can include agitation, restlessness, impaired judgment, and hallucinations. These effects may lead to life-threatening or fatal injuries, particularly through falls or traffic accidents.

Thus, appropriate and timely management of poisoning cases are crucial for reducing the number of deaths by poisoning. Appropriate maintenance of airways, breathing, circulation, body temperature and control of seizures improves survival rates dramatically.

Toxicokinetics and Toxicodynamics

These are aspects that must be kept in mind while handling poisoning cases.

Toxicokinetics deals with the absorption, distribution, metabolism and excretion (ADME) of toxins, therapeutic agents at toxic doses, and their metabolites. Two important kinetic parameters to consider in poisoning cases are the **volume of distribution** and **clearance of drug/toxin**.

- A large volume of distribution ($V_d > 5$ L/kg) of toxin/drug (e.g., antipsychotics, antidepressants, opioids) indicates that it cannot be removed easily from blood by hemodialysis. In contrast, drugs with low volume of distribution ($V_d < 1$ L/kg) of toxin (e.g., salicylates, ethanol, phenytoin, lithium) are easily removable from circulation.
- The total clearance for a drug/toxin is the sum of its excretion via different routes, such as hepatic (inactivation), renal (excretion), lungs, skin, and saliva. Overdosage can alter the kinetics of drugs such as the extent of absorption/first-pass metabolism/plasma protein binding and saturation of the drug elimination process. Therefore, while deciding detoxification measures for a drug, the contribution of different organs in drug elimination as well as the possibilities of alteration in ADME at toxic doses must be considered

Toxicodynamics considers quantal dose–response relationships, therapeutic index, and the overlap between dose–response curves (DRCs) for therapeutic and toxic effects. The toxic effect is an extension of the therapeutic effect; drugs with linear DRC exert toxic effects at a dose closer to the therapeutic dose than those with flat DRCs. Drugs which suppress cardiac function affect all other functions dependent on blood flow, like renal/hepatic elimination of drug.

Management of Poisoning

As soon as a patient of poisoning reports, initial supportive treatment is given to **stabilise the vitals**. Once the patient is stable, **detailed evaluation** is carried out (patient history, physical examination and lab investigations). **Decontamination** is performed simultaneously. As specific antidotes are not available for all poisonings, supportive management becomes all the more important.

1. **Supportive measures or ABCD of poisoning case**

In a patient of poisoning with altered mental status, convulsions and coma, it is important to:

- Maintain patent **airways** by keeping the patient in left lateral position, clearing off any vomitus or secretions and endotracheal intubation.
- If the patient has respiratory insufficiency, as assessed by pulse oximetry and arterial blood gas analysis, **breathing** is maintained and supported by intubation and mechanical ventilation.
- **Circulation** is assessed continuously by pulse rate, blood pressure, urine output and peripheral perfusion. Intravenous line is secured.
- If facility for rapid bedside blood glucose testing is available, hypoglycemia is ruled out. If such facility is not available, 50 mL of 50% **dextrose** solution is injected in all patients having altered mental status.
- Initial management also involves administration of thiamine 100 mg, intramuscular to prevent Wernicke's syndrome. Opioid antagonist naloxone is given to reverse respiratory depression caused by all opioids. Flumazenil is used in benzodiazepine toxicity, taking care not to use it in cases of TCA overdose or in epileptics, as there is risk of precipitating seizures.

2. **Evaluation**

a. A **detailed history** is taken in an attempt to ascertain the type and amount of intoxicant consumed. The syringes, empty bottles and other drugs present in the close vicinity of poisoning case are also examined.

b. **Physical examination** of poisoning cases is required in order to monitor the vitals and look for signs suggestive of specific intoxication.
   - **Vitals** (BP, PR, RR and body temperature) are carefully evaluated and monitored continuously.
   - Hypertension and tachycardia indicate poisoning by anticholinergics, cocaine, amphetamines.
   - Hypotension and bradycardia are caused by β blockers, calcium channel blockers and sedative hypnotics.
   - Hypotension and tachycardia are caused by TCAs, vasodilators and β agonists.
   - Respiratory rate (RR) is increased by drugs that cause cellular hypoxia and acidosis, e.g., salicylates and carbon monoxide.
   - Body temperature is increased by drugs that increase muscular hyperactivity, sympathomimetics, anticholinergics, salicylates, etc,. and decreased by CNS depressants.

c. **Neurological examination:** Ataxia, nystagmus and dysarthria is caused by phenytoin, carbamazepine, alcohol and sedative-hypnotics. CNS depressant drugs cause coma and reduced reflexes. Drugs like atropine, cocaine and sympathomimetics cause twitching, hyperactivity of muscles and convulsions. Rigidity occurs in haloperidol and strychnine overdose, and hypertonicity and clonus in the case of serotonin syndrome.

d. **Skin:** In case of atropine poisoning, skin is hot, flushed and dry, whereas in OPC and nicotine toxicity, the patient has excessive sweating. Skin colour is cyanosed due to hypoxia and methemoglobinemia. Hepatic necrosis as seen in acetaminophen/paracetamol poisoning; mushroom poisoning with *Amanita phalloides* causes icterus (yellowish skin).

e. **Eye examination:** Pupil size is of diagnostic importance in poisoning cases. Pinpoint pupils are characteristic of opioid, OPC and clonidine poisoning. In contrast, cocaine, LSD, amphetamine and atropine poisoning causes mydriasis.
   - Presence of nystagmus in horizontal direction indicates possibility of alcohol, barbiturate and phenytoin poisoning. Horizontal as well as vertical nystagmus is seen in phencyclidine poisoning.
   - Ptosis and ophthalmoplegia is seen in botulism.

f. **Mouth:** In cases of alcohol, ammonia and other hydrocarbon solvents, there is typical odour from mouth. Cyanide poisoning causes bitter-almonds-like odour. Burnt areas in mouth may be seen in corrosive poisoning.

g. **Abdominal examination:** Anticholinergic drugs and opioids cause ileus. In contrast, OPCs, mushrooms of *Amantia muscaria* species, theophylline, arsenic, etc., cause abdominal cramps, increased bowel sounds and diarrhea.

3. **Lab investigations**

Important investigations for a poisoning case include:
- Arterial blood gas analysis to note partial pressure of carbon dioxide and oxygen (PCO_2 and PO_2)
- Serum electrolytes: Na^+, K^+, Cl^-, HCO_3^- levels and anion gap [anion gap is $(Na^+ + K^+) - (Cl^- + HCO_3^-)$]

   If the anion gap is greater than normal, it indicates metabolic acidosis such as diabetic ketoacidosis, renal failure and lactic acidosis. Lactic acidosis is caused by metformin and aspirin.

   Serum K^+ levels are raised by KCl, β blockers, digoxin, K^+-sparing diuretics, fluorides, etc., and lowered by loop diuretics, thiazides, β agonists, theophylline, etc.

   Osmolar gap, which is the difference between measured and calculated osmolality, indicates toxicity caused by ethanol, methanol, ethylene glycol and isopropanol.

- Urine analysis, blood urea, and serum creatinine levels are important to assess renal function. Raised serum creatinine kinase levels and myoglobinuria indicate muscle damage as seen during convulsions. Oxalate crystals present in urine indicate ethylene glycol poisoning.

4. **Electrocardiography**
   - Wide QRS complex > 100 milliseconds is seen in TCA and quinidine toxicity.
   - Increased QTc > 440 milliseconds is seen in antidepressant, antipsychotics, lithium and arsenic toxicity.
   - AV blocks and arrhythmias are caused by digoxin.

5. **Toxicological screening**

Toxicological screening is not done routinely, but may be done to confirm or rule out the suspected poison as a cause of brain death.

6. **Decontamination**

This is done simultaneously with evaluation. For decontamination of skin, contaminated cloths are removed and double bagged. Skin is washed with soap and water.
- To reduce further absorption of ingested drug/poison from GIT, activated charcoal is given, which checks further absorption by adsorbing drug/toxin onto its molecules. Dose of activated charcoal should be 10 times the estimated amount of drug/toxin consumed. Emesis can be induced by ipecac syrup, but is contraindicated in corrosive poisoning. Gastric lavage can be done with 0.9% saline solution at body temperature after protecting the airways. Laxatives like polyethylene glycol solution is given orally as 1–2 L per hour in iron poisoning for removing enteric-coated tablets and foreign bodies.

7. **Specific therapy**

Antidotes are available only for few poisons as shown in Table 66.1.

Table 66.1 Antidotes for various drugs and poisons

Name of drug/poison	Name of antidote
Organophosphate compounds	Atropine, Pralidoxime
Rapid mushroom poisoning	Atropine, Pralidoxime
Paracetamol / Acetaminophen	N-acetylcysteine
Benzodiazepines	Flumazenil
β blockers	Glucagon
Calcium channel blockers	Calcium
Iron	Desferrioxamine
Digoxin	Digibind
Methanol	Ethanol, Fomepizole
Cyanide	Hydroxocobalamin
Opioids	Naloxone
Carbon monoxide	Oxygen
Theophylline/ caffeine	Esmolol

All the above-mentioned measures, when used appropriately and adequately, play a crucial role in saving lives in cases of poisoning.

Clinical problem-based questions and MCQs

14. A patient emanates the smell of bitter almonds from his mouth. Identify the poison.
    a. Alcohol
    b. Benzene
    c. Cyanide
    d. DDT

15. Eye examination in a poisoned patient shows pinpoint pupils. Identify the possible cause of poisoning.
    a. Nicotine
    b. Opioids
    c. Malathion
    d. Phenytoin

Hints for problem-based questions and MCQs

1. i CO poisoning
   ii Tissue hypoxia because of impaired oxygen carrying capacity of blood
   iii Maintenance of respiration and hyperbaric oxygen
2. c. Nitrogen dioxide
3. b. Benzene
4. a. Interfere with Na channel inactivation
5. d. Aldicarb
6. a–2; b–4; c–1; d–3.
7. c. Polyvalent ASV
8. c. Prazosin
9. a. Dimercaprol.
10. d. Cadmium
11. i a. Arsenic
    ii b. Dimercaprol
    iii Refer to page 870.
12. i Refer to page 871.
    ii d. d-Penicillamine
13. i To remove heavy metal from inaccessible sites
    ii a. Mercury, as it gets distributed to sites where calcium disodium edetate cannot reach due to its polar nature.
14. c. Cyanide
15. b. Opioids

SECTION 12 Miscellaneous Topics

67 Drugs Used in Dermatological Conditions and Germicidal Drugs

PH 9.6 Describe drugs used in various skin disorders like acne vulgaris, scabies, pediculosis, psoriasis including sunscreens.
PH 9.5 Describe types, precautions and uses of antiseptics and disinfectants.

Leaning objectives

A student of MBBS phase II should be able to:
- Describe pharmacokinetics of topically applied drugs.
- Describe astringents, sunscreens, keratolytic agents, and protectives.
- Enumerate topical steroids.
- Describe general principles for use of topical steroids.
- Enumerate uses and adverse effects of topical steroids.
- Describe drugs used in the management of acne vulgaris.
- Describe drugs used in the treatment of psoriasis.
- Describe drugs used for ectoparasites, e.g., scabies and pediculosis.
- Differentiate between antiseptics and disinfectants.
- Classify germicidal drugs based on their chemical nature.
- Describe the mechanism of action of germicides.

PHARMACOKINETICS OF TOPICALLY APPLIED DRUGS

Drugs are commonly applied topically for treatment of dermatological conditions.

- Pharmacokinetics of topical drugs describes the **time-dependent concentration** of the drug applied on the skin surface, its passage through the skin barrier into underlying layers, and the extent of absorption into systemic circulation.
- Drugs applied topically on the skin surface **diffuse along the concentration gradient** over short distances. A water molecule can migrate up to 10 µm, which is roughly equal to the width of the stratum corneum. (Stratum corneum is a thin layer (~10–20 µm) that acts as a barrier to the diffusion of drugs across skin. It is a highly differentiated structure made up of water insoluble proteins and intercellular lipids.)
- For percutaneous absorption, a topically applied drug molecule must be released from the formulation and penetrate the stratum corneum. Drugs can penetrate the stratum corneum barrier through intercellular, intracellular, follicular and eccrine pathways (Fig. 67.1).
- After crossing the stratum corneum, the drug diffuses through the epidermis to reach dermis, from where it gets absorbed into systemic circulation. Some drugs may diffuse through the dermal and hypodermal layers to get distributed into subcutaneous tissue.

Factors affecting diffusion of drug across skin surface

1. **Evaporation from skin surface:** Water- or alcohol-based topical preparations evaporate rapidly from the skin surface, creating a cooling effect and leaving a supersaturated solution of non-volatile substances. This may lead to the precipitation of active ingredients on the skin.
2. **Physicochemical properties of formulations:** Certain formulations, such as cosmetics and sunscreens, are specifically designed to remain on the skin surface for extended periods, while others are developed to facilitate drug delivery into specific layers or compartments of the skin. In contrast, transdermal formulations are intended to transport the drug across the skin, into systemic circulation.
    - **Vehicles used** for drug delivery should not be good solvents, as the drug molecules will be retained on the skin surface for longer periods, delaying its diffusion across skin layers.
    - **Liposome-based topical preparations** are widely used. Liposomes are microscopic spherical structures consisting of an inner aqueous core enclosed by a lipid bilayer. The application of liposomes provides a mild occlusive effect and helps maintain hydration of the stratum corneum. Liposomal preparations ensure better penetration of the drug across skin

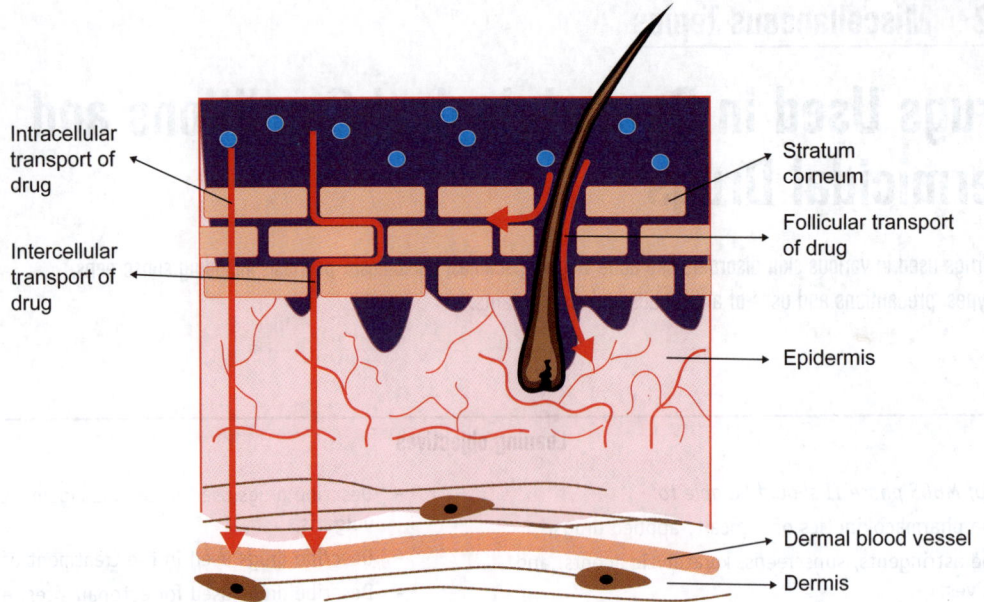

Fig. 67.1 Percutaneous drug absorption

surface. Deep in stratum corneum, the liposomal bilayer releases active drug molecules, which then cross the last cell layer of the stratum corneum to reach viable cells. Liposomal preparations are also useful for delivery of drug into hair follicles and sebaceous glands.

3. **Alterations in composition** of applied formulation over time.
4. Thickness of the layer of topical preparation and the area of skin surface covered.
5. Rubbing or massaging of topical preparation on skin surface.
6. Amount of drug adhering to skin surface, residing in upper layers of stratum corneum (called **drug reservoir**) also alters its bioavailability. Hair follicles, eczematous/scaly skin surfaces serve as efficient reservoirs for topically applied drugs.
7. There are inter-individual and intra-individual variations in the barrier activity of skin. A higher **rate of division of keratinocytes** can disrupt the barrier properties of skin. **Appendages** like hair follicles are potential sites of discontinuity in the skin barrier. The variable density of hair follicles at different body sites alters the extent of drug absorption across skin. The barrier function of skin is reduced in many **disease conditions** such as contact dermatitis, atopic dermatitis, ichthyoses and psoriasis.
8. After crossing the stratum corneum, the drug has to diffuse through viable tissue to reach systemic circulation.
   - The drug may **bind to various proteins** in viable tissues. This alters the extent of drug absorption.
   - Drugs may be **metabolised to varying extent** (up to 2–5%) during this passage through viable tissue by oxidation, reduction, hydrolysis and conjugation reactions. Some skin diseases like acne and hirsutism may alter rate of these metabolic reactions. Some topical preparations contain prodrugs so as to bypass the metabolic reactions on the skin surface and in the stratum corneum/epidermis/dermis.
   - Some part of the drug may be taken up by cutaneous microvasculature. This is called **drug resorption**. The extent of drug resorption varies depending on the application site, individual characteristics, species differences, environmental conditions (such as temperature and humidity), and the presence of certain diseases.

DRUGS ACTING ON SKIN AND MUCOUS MEMBRANE

Drugs acting on the skin include astringents, protectives (such as adsorbents, demulcents, and emollients), irritants, counter-irritants, sunscreens, and caustics/escharotics, each with its specific effects.

1. ASTRINGENTS

Astringents are substances that cause **denaturing and precipitation of proteins,** making the surface mechanically tough and strong. These agents decrease exudation. Tannic acid, tannins, alcohols (ethanol, methanol 50–90%), minerals like alum, and salts of aluminum/zinc/zirconium have astringent activity. These drugs cannot penetrate cells; therefore, after topical application their effect is restricted to the superficial layer of skin and mucous membrane.

Tannic acid obtained from oak, and **tannins** present in tea, nutmeg and betel nut, form protein tannates. These are useful in alkaloidal poisoning, bleeding gums and bleeding piles.

Alcohol
Alcohol possesses astringent activity at a concentration of 50–90%. Spirit is rubbed on skin to prevent formation of bedsores in bedridden patients, and as an aftershave for minor cuts.

Alum
Alum is also used as an aftershave. **Salts of zinc, aluminum and zirconium** can diffuse to reach sweat ducts, causing their blockade and leading to a reduction in sweat gland secretion. They also have antimicrobial action which prevents bacterial decomposition of sweat. So, these mineral astringents are used as antiperspirants to reduce body odour.

2. PROTECTIVES
Adsorbents, demulcents and **emollients** provide protection to skin and mucous membrane.

a. Adsorbents
These are insoluble, inert solids in finely powdered form that can adsorb (bind) irritant/noxious substances on to their surface. They protect skin and mucous membrane from the effect of harmful or irritant substances by their adsorption property.

Drugs that have adsorbent action:

- **Magnesium stearate** and **zinc stearate** particles have an un-wettable, very smooth surface. When applied on exuding surfaces, these agents allow evaporation of water. No crust is formed.
- **Starch**, on the other hand, can absorb moisture and form crust. Hence, it is not indicated for use on exuding surface. However, it is commonly used as a dusting powder and on surgical gloves.
- Hydrous **magnesium silicate**, which spreads easily, is used as talcum powder or face powder. However, it cannot be used on wounds or surgical gloves as it can form granulomas.
- **Boric acid** is also a very smooth, fine powder used in prickly heat powders owing to its deodorant, astringent and mild antimicrobial actions.
- **Calamine** is zinc carbonate with ferric oxide or zinc oxide (called calcined calamine). It possesses soothing, astringent, antiseptic and protective action. It is used as calamine lotion in urticaria, contact dermatitis and sunburns.
- **Aloe vera** gel, obtained from the fleshy leaves of aloe vera plant, has moisturising and soothing effect. It is claimed to be effective in many skin conditions such as acne and psoriasis.
- **Polyvinyl polymer** solution forms an occlusive coating on abraded skin upon drying. It protects minor cuts and abrasions from dust and microbes. It is used along with benzocaine as a spray in aerosol wound dressing.
- **Feracrylyum** forms gel-like complexes when it comes in contact with blood. A thin film of 1–3% feracrylyum gel when applied on cuts and wounds effectively stops bleeding, serving as a physical barrier with protective action.
- **Simethicone** is an inert, non-irritant silicone polymer available as a viscous liquid with froth-collapsing and water-repelling properties. It reduces surface tension to break down froth. When formulated as a 15% cream, it adheres to and protects the skin, prevents excoriation and provides relief from conditions like urine-soiled skin, bedsores, ulcers, and burns.
- **Sucralfate** is an aluminum salt of sulphated sucrose used as 10% gel on bedsores, diabetic/radiation/aphthous ulcers, aburns, and excoriated skin to cover and protect damaged tissue and aid in healing.

b. Demulcents
Demulcents are thick, colloidal or viscous solutions made from high molecular weight substances, such as gum acacia and gum tragacanth. They have the ability to produce foam and collapse froth by reducing surface tension, and are hence used as suspending agents in formulations.

- **Liquorice** or **glycyrrhiza** is used as a soothing agent in cough lozenges or as a flavouring agent in mixtures.
- **Methylcellulose** is used in contact lens solutions and nasal drops. Orally used methylcellulose acts as a bulk purgative.
- **Propylene glycol** is used in occlusive dressings.
- **Glycerin** is a viscous, sweet-tasting liquid with dehydrating properties, which can produce a sensation of warmth upon application. It is commonly used as a vehicle in gum paints and throat paints due to its adhesive and soothing nature. It is also used in anal canal suppositories to promote evacuation of the bowel.

c. Emollients
Emollients such as **olive** oil, **sesame** oil, **arachis** oil, **cocoa butter**, hard, soft, and **liquid paraffin**, **wool fat**, and **beeswax** are soothing and softening agents that form an occlusive film on the skin surface. These are used in ointment bases to prevent moisture loss and help restore the elasticity of dry, cracked skin. Wool fat may, however, cause severe allergic reactions in some people.

d. Sunscreens
Excessive exposure to sunlight is associated with many harmful effects on skin. UVB rays of shorter wavelength (280–320 nm) are mostly responsible for causing tanning and erythema. Chronic exposure to UVB radiation is widely recognised as a key factor in the development of both skin aging and photo-carcinogenesis, whereas, UVA

rays [of longer wavelength (320-400 nm)] are implicated in causation of tanning, drug-induced photosensitivity reactions, cutaneous lupus erythematosus and polymorphous light eruptions in sensitive individuals.

Sunscreens are agents that protect skin from the harms of excessive sunlight exposure. Based on their major effect on light rays, sunscreens are classified as two types:

- **Physical sunscreens** or **sunshades** are opaque substances that can stop (block) and scatter visible as well as ultraviolet light rays. They can block light waves of longer wavelengths responsible for tanning. **Calamine, zinc oxide, titanium oxide** and **heavy petroleum jelly**, when applied as thick lotion or cream, function as sunblock to prevent tanning, sunburn and photoallergic reactions.
- **Chemical sunscreens** act by absorbing UV rays. These include
    - Benzophenones: Oxybenzone, dioxybenzone, sulisobenzone
    - Octylmethoxy cinnamate
    - Para-aminobenzoic acid (PABA) and its esters: Glyceryl-mono-p-aminobenzoate, dibenzoyl methanes (parasol, eusolex)
    - Terephthalylidene dicamphor sulfonic acid

Chemical sunscreens act by absorbing and scattering the UV rays that are the cause of sunburn and phototoxic reactions. **PABA and its esters** can absorb UVB rays and prevent their harmful effects like ageing, tanning, and erythema. **Benzophenones** are more capable of absorbing light rays over a broader wavelengths range (250-360 nm) compared to PABA, but they are less effective in UVB protection. Since these agents do not absorb the longer wavelengths primarily responsible for tanning, they are useful as adjuvants in the treatment of vitiligo, where they prevent sunburn while still allowing tanning. These are also useful in drug-induced phototoxic reactions. **Terephthalylidene dicamphor sulfonic acid** provides better protection against UVA rays than **dibenzoylmethanes** such as **parasol** and **eusolex**.

The effectiveness of sunscreens against erythema caused by UV rays is measured as **sun protection factor (SPF)**, calculated as the ratio of minimal erythema-producing dose of UVB radiations with and without the application of a sunscreen agent. Value of SPF varies for different preparations. Commonly, an SPF of 15 or more is recommended in fair-skinned individuals, who are more prone to sunburn.

3. KERATOLYTICS

Some dermatological conditions like corns, warts, psoriasis, ringworm, athlete's foot and chronic dermatitis are characterised by hyperkeratotic lesions. Keratolytic agents are useful in these conditions, as their **major action is desquamation of epidermal cells**.

Important keratolytic agents include
- Salicylic acid 3-6% concentration, other NSAIDs
- Propylene glycol 40-70% concentration
- Urea 20%
- Resorcinol 3-10%
- Podophyllum resin and podofilox
- Phenol 80%
- Glacial acetic acid, trichloroacetic acid
- Silver nitrate pencils/sticks

a. Salicylic acid

The exact mechanism of salicylic acid's keratolytic action is not fully understood, but it is believed to involve the solubilisation of cell surface proteins that normally maintain the integrity of the stratum corneum. This leads to desquamation and facilitates the sloughing of hyperkeratotic lesions.

Adverse reactions like urticaria, erythema multiforme, local irritation, infiltration and ulceration may occur with higher concentration. Risk of such lesions is higher upon use of salicylic acid on extremities of patients with diabetes mellitus and peripheral vascular disease. Salicylism may occur rarely, especially in children.

Diclofenac gel 3% also has keratolytic action in patients with actinic keratoses.

b. Propylene glycol

It possesses hygroscopic, mild antifungal, and antiseptic properties. At a concentration of 40-70%, it causes skin maceration and keratolytic effect. It is used with salicylic acid in occlusive polyethylene dressing for palmar/plantar keratodermas, corns, hypertrophic lichen planus, pityriasis rubra pilaris, keratosis pilaris, psoriasis and ichthyosis.In Whitfield's ointment, propylene glycol is used in a concentration of 3-5%. It acts as a vehicle for organic compounds. Due to its hygroscopic nature, it draws water from inner layers of the skin and hydrates outermost layers. Thus, propylene glycol is also effective as humectant to increase water content of the stratum corneum.

Adverse reactions of propylene glycol include allergic contact dermatitis. It has irritant action, especially in patients with eczema.

c. Urea

It is a white crystalline powder that has hygroscopic, water-retaining property, resulting in humectant effect. Urea in 5-20% concentration causes keratin solubilisation, softening, and moisturisation of stratum corneum. In a concentration > 20%, it can cause desquamation of hyperkeratotic lesions. It is used as an ointment base or cream vehicle, as its feel is less greasy than other oils.

It is used under occlusive dressing in hyperkeratosis of soles/palms, xerosis, keratosis pilaris and ichthyosis vulgaris. Still higher concentration (30-50%) is used on nail plate before nail avulsion. Topical use of urea causes no systemic toxicity.

d. Resorcinol
3–10% resorcinol is useful as a keratolytic agent in ringworm infection, seborrheic dermatitis and eczema.

e. Fluorouracil (5-FU)
Fluorouracil, applied topically in concentrations of 0.5, 1, 2, and 5%, exerts cytotoxic effect by inhibiting thymidylate synthase enzyme. It is useful in multiple actinic keratosis. Topical application causes erythema followed by vesiculation, erosion, ulceration, necrosis and re-epithelisation. Treatment with 5-FU should be stopped when necrosis occurs (usually after 3–4 weeks of topical 5-FU application). Healing of necrosed area occurs in 1–2 months after stopping the drug application.

Adverse reactions associated with use of topical 5-FU include burning sensation, pruritus, local pain and hyperpigmentation. Allergic contact dermatitis may occur. These adverse reactions flare up on exposure to sunlight. Hence, sun exposure should be avoided as far as possible.

4. TOPICAL STEROIDS FOR DERMATOLOGICAL CONDITIONS
Glucocorticoids possess non-specific anti-inflammatory, antiproliferative and immunosuppressant actions. These effects are beneficial in a variety of dermatological conditions. However, systemic use of steroids is associated with numerous adverse effects, and therefore, topical application is preferred for skin diseases.

Classification
Topical steroids are classified based on their lipid solubility and ability to pass into deeper layers of skin. They steroids may be high/moderate/mild in potency.
- **Potent drugs** include betamethasone, beclomethasone dipropionate, betamethasone valerate/benzoate, dexamethasone sodium phosphate/trimethyl acetate, clobetasol propionate, halcinonide, triamcinolone acetonide, fluocinolone acetonide and fluocortolone.
- **Moderate potency drugs** are fluticasone propionate, hydrocortisone + urea, hydrocortisone acetate, and prednicarbate.
- **Mild potency drugs** are hydrocortisone acetate/butyrate.

Indications for use
- Topical steroids produce good response in some dermatological conditions, like allergic dermatitis, primary irritant dermatitis, seborrheic dermatitis, atopic or varicose eczema, lichen simplex and psoriasis of face and flexures.
- In some dermatological conditions, the beneficial effect of steroids develops slowly, e.g., lichen planus, alopecia areata, keloids, nail disorders, psoriasis of palm/sole/knee/elbow and cystic acne. In these conditions more potent drugs are used.

Adverse effects
Use of topical steroids is associated with following epidermal and dermal changes:
- Thinning of epidermis
- Dermal atrophy called cigarette paper skin
- Telangiectasia
- Striae
- Hypopigmentation of skin
- Easy bruising
- Impaired/delayed wound healing
- Secondary fungal or bacterial infections

In rare instances, systemic adverse effects are reported with topically used steroids, especially in infants and children after repeated or prolonged use.

General Principles for Topical Use of Steroids
1. The extent of penetration of topically applied corticosteroids varies with the site of application. Areas such as the face, scalp, groin, scrotum, and axilla exhibit higher absorption, and therefore, potent steroids should be avoided at these sites due to a greater risk of local and systemic adverse effects. In contrast, areas with thicker skin, such as the soles, palms, elbows, and knees, show lower penetration, and higher potency preparations may be required, for effective treatment of lesions in such regions.
2. Penetration of topically applied steroids is less at hyperkeratinised, plaque-forming lesions, and more at atopic, exfoliative lesions.
3. Milder drugs are preferred for acute conditions, and more potent ones for chronic lesions.
4. Topical steroids are given as cream or lotion in patients having exudative lesions. Cream/lotion allows evaporation, resulting in drying, cooling and antipruritic effect.
5. For lesions in hairy regions, gels or sprays are the preferred preparations.
6. Use of occlusive dressing retains moisture, increasing steroid absorption. However, maceration of horny layer occurs. Therefore, in scaly, chronic lesions, ointments are the preferred preparation because they form an occlusive film. Continuous application of occlusive dressing in hypertrophied lesions increases the risk of secondary infection. So, occlusive dressing is applied intermittently.
7. Potent preparations are reserved for severe, unresponsive eczema, psoriasis, etc., and are administered for short durations or intermittently. These should not be stopped

abruptly. Once symptoms start improving, potent preparations are substituted with drugs of low potency for some time. Then, steroids are alternated with emollients till complete healing of lesion occurs.
8. The frequency of application of topical steroids should be twice a day.
9. Topical steroids are combined with AMAs in secondarily-infected dermatosis, furunculosis, impetigo, otitis externa, intertrigo, etc.

DRUGS FOR ACNE

Acne vulgaris commonly affects young adolescents. Pathophysiology involves excess secretion of sebum from the sebaceous glands and secondary infection by organisms like *Staphylococcus epidermidis* and *Propionibacterium acnes*. The lipase enzyme secreted by the bacteria causes formation of fatty acids that block follicular ducts, leading to retention of secretion, hyperkeratosis and formation of horny impactions in follicles called comedones. The comedones open up into dermis, resulting in inflammation and formation of pustules.

Drugs used in acne are (i) topical drugs and (ii) systemic drugs.

Topical Drugs

Topical drugs commonly used for acne treatment include benzoyl peroxide, retinoids (retinoic acid, adapalene, tazarotene), azelaic acid, and antibiotics.

Benzoyl peroxide

Benzoyl peroxide is one of the most frequently used drug, applied topically as 5–10% cream/gel/lotion. It is very effective against *P. acnes*. Benzoyl peroxide generates oxygen in the presence of water, leading to bactericidal effect, especially against microaerophilic and anaerobic organisms. In addition to its bactericidal effect, benzoyl peroxide also causes shedding of comedone caps by mild desquamating action. So, retention of sebum is reduced.

ADRs: It has mild irritant effect after topical application, leading to burning, stinging sensation, erythema, edema, dryness and scaling, etc., at the beginning of therapy. However, later on tolerance develops to these actions. If the patient has severe adverse effects, the drug is stopped.

Retinoids

Retinoids are classified as first-, second-, and third-generation drugs (Box 67.1). Clinically important retinoids include retinoic acid, adapalene, and tazarotene.

Tretinoin or **all-trans retinoic acid** as 0.025–0.05% gel/cream alternated with benzoyl peroxide (one drug applied in the morning, the other at night) is very effective. Although tretinoin has no antibacterial effect, it helps in lysing keratinocytes, preventing formation of comedones.

It increases epidermal cell turnover causing peeling. Beneficial effect of tretinoin manifests in 6–10 weeks after starting therapy. In addition to acne, tretinoin has beneficial effect of preventing age related changes in skin due to excessive exposure to sun. **Adverse effects** include skin irritation, stinging sensation, warmth, redness, edema, crusting and teratogenic potential.

Adapalene is a synthetic retinoid, equally efficacious as tretinoin, with lesser irritant effect. It can be safely combined with benzoyl peroxide because, unlike tretinoin, adapalene is not degraded when exposed to benzoyl peroxide.

Tazarotene, also a retinoid, is useful in acne as well as psoriasis.

Box 67.1   First-, second- and third-generation retinoids

1st generation: Retinol, tretinoin, isotretinoin, alitretinoin
Tretinoin: Acne vulgaris, photoaging
Isotretinoin: Severe nodulocystic acne
Alitretinoin: Dermatological manifestations of Kaposi sarcoma

2nd generation
Acitretin: Psoriasis

3rd generation
Tazarotene: Acne, psoriasis
Bexarotene : Cutaneous T-cell lymphoma
Adapalene: Acne

ADRs: Many adverse effects such as dryness of skin, nose bleed, conjunctivitis, hair loss, myalgias, pseudotumor cerebri and mood alterations.

Azelaic acid

Azelaic acid used as 10%/20% cream, and has same the efficacy as benzoyl peroxide in topical treatment of acne. It is also useful in melasma. Azelaic acid possesses antibacterial effect and reduces density of cutaneous bacteria, free fatty acids and keratinocyte proliferation. Response to azelaic acid is also delayed.

Antibiotics

Antibiotics like clindamycin, erythromycin, tetracyclines and nadifloxacin should be used only in patients with inflamed papules and folliculitis. These are not as efficacious as benzoyl peroxide, but are free of irritant effects. They may, however, cause sensitisation.

Systemic drugs
Isotretinoin

Isotretinoin (13-cis retinoic acid) is used orally in a dose of 0.5–1 mg for 20 weeks. It checks sebum production, keratinisation of follicles and brings about dramatic improvement in acne. However, as isotretinoin has severe adverse effects, it is reserved only for refractory cases of severe acne vulgaris. Other indications for its use include prevention of skin cancers, actinic keratoses and leukoplakia.

Adverse reactions

ADRs are severe, like dryness of skin/mouth/nose/eyes, cheilitis, epistaxis, pruritus, conjunctivitis, increased serum lipids, muscular aches and pains, raised intracranial tension and high risk of teratogenicity. Up to one-fourth of exposed fetuses develop structural defects like craniofacial/cardiac/central defects. Therefore, isotretinoin is contraindicated in pregnant women or women likely to become pregnant within a month of acne treatment.

Antibiotics

Antibiotics may be administered systemically in severe cases for initial control of pustules and cysts. Doxycycline and minocycline are commonly used systemic antimicrobial agents. AMAs should preferably be used for short durations only, as long-term maintenance therapy is associated with many adverse effects.

DRUGS FOR PSORIASIS

Psoriasis is an immunological skin disorder characterised by excessive epidermal proliferation and dermal inflammation, resulting in erythematous scaling lesions or plaques. It is not curable, but drug therapy can control the severity of lesions. Drugs are used for prolonged periods of time.

The mainstay of treatment of psoriasis is **topical steroids**. Most of the cases respond within few weeks, especially when the drug is used with occlusive dressing. In severe cases, treatment is **initiated with more potent steroids, then substituted by less potent drugs** and followed by emollients, keratolytics, and antifungal drugs. However, use of topical steroids is associated with risk of numerous topical and systemic adverse effects, and the responsiveness of lesions to topical steroids declines progressively.

Many other drugs are tried topically in psoriasis, like calcipotriol, coaltar and synthetic retinoid tazarotene. Acitretin is an oral synthetic retinoic acid.

Calcipotriol

Calcipotriol is a vitamin D analogue that binds to intracellular vitamin D receptors, checks proliferation, and favours differentiation of keratinocytes. The beneficial effect of calcipotriol in psoriasis manifests slowly over 1–2 months, and is maintained as long as the therapy is continued. Efficacy is increased on combining with topical steroids.

ADRs include itching, irritation, erythema, and scaling. However, the risk of hypercalcemia is negligible as calcipotriol is rapidly metabolised after absorption through skin.

Coaltar

Coal tar, applied topically on psoriatic lesions as an alcoholic solution or ointment, exerts a phototoxic effect on exposure to UVA rays in sunlight and reduces epidermal cell turnover. However, it is rarely used because it is cosmetically unacceptable, has an unpleasant smell and carries the risk of allergic, photosensitivity reactions.

Synthetic retinoids

Synthetic retinoids like tazarotene (used topically) and acitretin (used orally) exert antiproliferative and anti-inflammatory action through intracellular retinoic acid receptors. These drugs are usually reserved for severe, refractory, recalcitrant and pustular types of psoriatic lesions, because retinoids cause severe adverse effects. Topical tazarotene can cause burning sensation, irritation and peeling, so, it should be carefully applied only on the lesions, protecting normal healthy skin. Oral acitretin can cause dry skin, erythema, scaling, alopecia, muscle and joint pains, hepatic damage and abnormal lipid profile. It has high teratogenic potential; therefore, female patients on acitretin therapy should ideally not plan pregnancy during and up to 3 years after discontinuation of its use.

PUVA (Psoralen UVA) or photochemotherapy

PUVA therapy combines the use of a class of light-sensitising medications called psoralens (P), with exposure to **UVA radiation**. This is useful in severe, debilitating type of psoriasis involving extensive areas of skin. Exposure to UVA rays after 1–2 hours of oral **methoxasalen** (a psoralen) interferes with DNA synthesis and reduces turnover of epithelial cells. Other uses of psoralen include accelerating tanning and treating conditions such as urticaria pigmentosa, lichen planus, atopic dermatitis, and cutaneous T-cell lymphoma. Use is restricted because of the serious adverse effects like erythema, burning sensation, blistering, premature ageing of skin, insomnia, nervousness, risk of cataract, immune damage and skin cancers.

Calcineurin inhibitors

Calcineurin inhibitors such as **cyclosporine** are useful in many dermatological conditions like psoriasis, atopic dermatitis, bullous pemphigoid, lichen planus and pyoderma gangrenosum.

Biological agents

Biological agents such as **etanercept, infliximab** and **alefacept** are advanced therapies used to target specific components of the immune system in autoimmune and inflammatory diseases. They are useful in severe psoriasis.

DRUGS FOR ECTOPARASITES

Parasites that inhabit the body surface are called 'ectoparasites.' Common ectoparasitic infections in humans include **scabies** and **pediculosis**.

Scabies

It is an infection caused by *Sarcoptes scabiei/Acarus scabiei*, commonly called 'itch mite'. Itch mite lay eggs while burrowing through the epidermal lining of finger webs. The patient presents with intense itching and papules over finger webs, forearms, trunk, genitals and lower legs. Severe itching may result in secondary bacterial infection. Scabies is a highly contagious condition that spreads through direct contact and shared personal items such as towels, bedsheets, handkerchiefs, and clothing. It commonly affects all or most of the family members and close contacts of patients. Therefore, concurrent treatment of patients and their families/ close contacts is advised.

Pediculosis (Lice Infestation)

Pediculosis is caused by species of *Pediculus*. *Pediculus capitis* infests the scalp hair, *Pediculus corporis* affects body hair, and *Pediculus pubis* targets pubic hair. The eggs of *Pediculus* species, known as "nits," are coated with a chitin-like cement, allowing them to adhere firmly to hair and clothing.

Transmission occurs through shared personal items such as combs, clothing, bedsheets, and towels. Lice feed on human blood, leading to itching and an increased risk of secondary infections. In some cases, lice may also transmit diseases such as relapsing fever and typhus.

Drug for Scabies and Pediculosis

Drugs useful in scabies and pediculosis include permethrin, gamma hexachlorocyclohexane (BHC or lindane), benzyl benzoate, sulphur, crotamiton, dicophane (DDT) and ivermectin. Systemic antibiotic therapy is needed in secondarily infected cases.

1. Permethrin

It can kill lice and itch mites by causing neurological paralysis. It is the drug of first choice for both scabies and pediculosis because of its high potency, broad spectrum action, high cure rates after single application, lack of resistance and negligible toxicity.

Dose and method of application: In scabies, 5% permethrin cream or lotion is applied on the whole body with exception of face and head, and washed with water after about 12 hours.

In head lice infestation, 30 g of 1% permethrin cream rinse is massaged into scalp, and is washed after about 10 minutes.

Permethrin is effective even in ectoparasites not responding to lindane.

ADRs: Permethrin is a well-tolerated drug. Some patients may complain of transient burning, tingling sensation and erythema. Systemic absorption and toxicity are negligible.

2. Gamma benzene hexachloride (BHC or lindane)

It is also a broad spectrum ectoparasitic-cidal drug which penetrates through the chitinous cover of the parasite and causes neurological damage. A single application is effective against most cases of scabies and head lice. Repeat treatment, however if needed, should be given after a week. The method of use is the same as for permethrin. Combination of lindane and benzyl benzoate achieves almost 100% cure rates.

ADRs: As lindane is highly lipid soluble, systemic absorption can cause central stimulation and cardiac arrhythmias, especially in children.

3. Benzyl benzoate

It is used as an oily emulsion, applied to the entire body below the neck after bathing, reapplied the next day, and washed off after 24 hours. It may cause skin irritation and contact dermatitis in children; however, systemic absorption and toxicity are rare.

4. Sulphur

It exhibits ectoparasiticidal, fungicidal, antiseptic, and keratolytic properties. Upon application, it generates hydrogen sulphide (H_2S), sulphur dioxide (SO_2), and pentathionic acid, which disrupt the cuticular layer of the itch mite. However, it is less effective against lice.

Traditionally used as a 10% ointment applied after a warm bath for three consecutive days, sulphur ointment is economical. However, its strong odour, inconvenient application schedule, and messy nature have led to a decline in its use.

5. Crotamiton

Crotamiton has lesser efficacy but is preferred in children because of its low systemic adverse effects.

6. Dicophane (DDT)

DDT is rarely used for treating scabies and lice due to the risk of systemic absorption that can lead to adverse effects such as muscular weakness, tremors, and convulsions. However, it is widely used as an insecticide against mosquitoes, pests, and flies.

7. Ivermectin

It is an anthelmintic drug and the only orally effective ectoparasiticidal agent. It achieves good cure rate in scabies and head lice but is not much used for this indication as other safe and efficacious topical drugs are available.

Clinical problem-based questions and MCQs

1. A teenaged boy presented in skin OPD with severe nodulocystic acne. He reported a three-year history of using various topical treatments, which provided only temporary relief.
   i. Identify the most suitable drug in this case.
      a. Isotretinoin   b. PUVA
      c. Azithromycin cream   d. Calcipotriol
   ii. Describe the mechanism of beneficial effect of the selected drug.

2. i. What are astringents?
   ii. Which of the following agents has astringent action?
      a. Tannic acid   b. Isotretinoin
      c. Calcipotriol   d. All of the above
   iii. Enumerate the indications for use of astringents.

3. i Identify the agent below which has keratolytic action.
      a. Menthol   b. Glacial acetic acid
      c. Salicylic acid   d. Tannic acid
   ii. Describe the mechanism of keratolytic effect and its uses.

4. i. Which of the following dermatological condition responds to PUVA?
      a. Nodulocystic acne   b. Psoriasis
      c. Impetigo   d. Allergic dermatitis
   ii. Describe pharmacological basis for using PUVA in the selected condition.

5. i. Which of the following topical steroids is the least potent?
      a. Beclomethasone   b. Betamethasone
      c. Hydrocortisone   d. Triamcinolone
   ii. Enumerate the therapeutic uses and adverse effects of topical steroids.
   iii. Describe the general principles for use of topical steroids.

GERMICIDAL DRUGS

ANTISEPTICS AND DISINFECTANTS

Germicide is a broad term that includes both the disinfectants and antiseptics. **Disinfectants** are used to **sterilise non-living objects** like water tanks and surgical instruments. **Antiseptics** are used on living surfaces like skin and mucous membranes. However, many drugs have antiseptic and disinfectant effect at different concentrations.

The term **sterilisation** is more absolute than disinfection. Sterilisation is a complete killing of all organisms, including spores. **Disinfection** aims to reduce the number of pathogenic organisms to such a low level that they do not pose a hazard in individuals having normal host defence mechanism.

Germicides classified based on their chemical nature	
- Acids	- Boric acid
- Alcohols	- Ethanol, isopropanol
- Aldehydes	- Formaldehyde, glutaraldehyde
- Phenol	- Cresol, chloroxylenol (Dettol)
- Halogens	- Iodine, iodophors
- Chlorine	- Chlorophores
- Metallic salts	- Zinc oxide, zinc sulphate, silver sulfadiazine, silver nitrate, calamine
- Oxidising agents	- Hydrogen peroxide, potassium permanganate, benzoyl peroxide
- Biguanide	- Chlorhexidine
- Dyes	- Gentian violet, Acriflavine/Proflavine
- Furan	- Nitrofurazone

Mechanism of Action

Germicides either exert detergent-like action on membrane permeability or cause oxidation of protoplasm or denaturation of proteins. Germicidal drugs are not used systemically, as these are non-selective and too toxic for systemic use.

The **potency** of a germicide is referred to as the **Phenol or Rideal-Walker coefficient**, which measures its effectiveness compared to phenol. However, this metric has limited applicability for agents tested on living surfaces, such as antiseptics, because the conditions in these environments differ significantly from those in controlled tests. A better criterion is the **therapeutic index**, which is the ratio of the concentration of the antiseptic drug required to achieve an antimicrobial effect to the concentration that causes adverse effects, such as local irritation, tissue damage, or impaired healing.

Desirable properties of a good antiseptic or disinfectant are chemical stability, wide spectrum of action, non-offensive colour and odour, cidal effect on microorganisms and spores, good penetration into crevices, folds, and a low cost. In addition, an antiseptic should have rapid onset, long duration of action, should be non-irritant to living tissues, non-sensitising and devoid of systemic adverse effects.

Acids

Boric acid is a non-irritant. Saturated 4% aqueous solution of boric acid is used as mouthwash, eye irrigation and douching. 10% ointment is used on abrasions or minor cuts and 30% paint boroglycerate is effective in glossitis and stomatitis. However, systemic absorption may occur after application on burnt surfaces or on more extensive wounds.

Alcohols

Alcohols like ethanol and isopropanol act by causing precipitation of microbial proteins, killing up to 90% of microbes on skin surface. These are used as cleansing agents, hand scrubs, etc. However, due to their irritant effect, alcohols cannot be used on delicate skin or mucous membranes.

Aldehydes
Formaldehyde is a slow-acting protoplasmic poison that denatures proteins, causing hardening and preservation of tissues. In its gaseous form, it has a pungent smell and is commonly used for fumigation. Its aqueous solution, **formalin**, is is used for the preservation of cadavers in dissection halls.

Glutaraldehyde is less pungent, has lesser irritant action, broader spectrum and better sterilising efficacy than formaldehyde.

Phenol
Phenol exerts static action at 0.2% concentration and cidal action at 1% concentration. However, it affects both microorganisms and tissues, resulting in caustic effect that result in skin burns. Hence, it is not used for antisepsis on living tissue. The main use of phenol is to disinfect sputum, pus, urine, feces, etc. **Chloroxylenol (Dettol)** is non-irritant to intact skin, and is used widely for surgical antisepsis and in creams, soaps, mouthwash, etc. However, it cannot be used in burn cases because it is non-irritant only on intact skin.

Iodine and iodophors
Iodine 1:20000 solution causes iodination and oxidation of protoplasm of microbes like bacteria, viruses, fungi, etc., within a brief exposure of one minute. However, for killing spores a higher concentration and longer exposure is needed.

Tincture iodine is 2% iodine in alcohol. It is useful in ringworm infestation and as antiseptic on surgical sites. **Mandl's paint,** a preparation containing 1.25% iodine dissolved in potassium iodide, is used for topical application in sore throat.

Iodophors like povidone-iodine contain iodine complexed with an organic compound (polyvinyl pyrrolidine). It is non-irritant, non-staining and has a long-lasting germicidal effect. It is widely used for burns, ulcers, boils, furuncles, non-specific vaginitis, etc., and also as a surgical scrub.

Chlorine and chlorophores
Chlorine is primarily used for water disinfection. Chlorophores include bleaching powder (used for water disinfection) and sodium hypochlorite solution (used in dairies to sterilise milk cans). In dental practice, sodium hypochlorite solution is commonly used in root canal therapy.

Metallic salts
Silver nitrate is used in hypertrophied tonsils and aphthous ulcers. 1% solution is useful in ophthalmic gonococcal infection in neonates. It causes black staining of tissues. **Silver sulfadiazine** is mainly used in burns cases. **Zinc sulphate** is useful as eyedrops, ear drops, antiperspirant, and in acne, impetigo, etc. **Zinc oxide** is useful as a protective and an adsorbent.

Oxidising agents
Oxidising agents include hydrogen peroxide, potassium permanganate and benzoyl peroxide. H_2O_2 releases nascent oxygen that acts on microbes and necrosed tissues. It helps in removing ear wax, slough, etc. When dissolved in water, potassium **permanganate** liberates oxygen, which oxidises microbial protoplasm. Condy's solution, containing potassium permanganate ($KMnO_4$) in a dilution of 1:40,000 to 1:10,000, is used as an antiseptic for irrigating cavities and wounds, as well as for douching, mouthwashes, and gargles. Higher concentration may cause blistering. **Benzoyl peroxide** is mainly indicated in acne management.

Biguanide
Chlorhexidine acts by causing disruption of bacterial cell membrane and precipitation of proteins. It is widely used as surgical scrub, mouthwash, and as antiseptic in dental practice. It is also an ingredient in toothpastes, oral rinses, etc.

Dyes
Gentian violet solution is more effective on gram-positive organisms and fungi; it is used in chronic ulcer, bedsores, thrush, eczema, ringworm, etc. However, it causes deep staining. **Acridine dyes,** such as acriflavine and proflavine, are active against gram-positive organisms and gonococci. They are non-irritating, hence suitable for use in the treatment of chronic ulcers, wounds and burns.

Furan
The furan derivative **nitrofurazone** is very effective for dressing skin grafts and burns.

Clinical problem-based questions and MCQs

6. i. Which of the following is an iodophor?
   a. Mandl's paint b. Tincture Iodine
   c. Povidone-iodine d. Potassium iodide
   ii. Describe the advantages of the iodophor selected over iodine.
   iii. Describe the use of agent selected in clinical practice.

7. All of the following drugs are suitable for burn dressing except
   a. Silver sulfadiazine b. Acriflavine
   c. Nitrofurazone d. Chloroxylenol

8. Which of the following antiseptic is frequently employed in dental practice?
   a. Potassium permanganate
   b. Chlorhexidine
   c. Benzoyl peroxide
   d. Nitrofurazone

Summary

- Topically used drugs are classified based on their action into the following categories: protectives (demulcents, emollients, adsorbents, sunscreens), astringents, counterirritants/irritants, and keratolytics.
- Astringents (tannic acid, tannins, 50–90% ethanol, methanol) precipitate proteins without entering cells and affect superficial cells only. They decrease exudation, toughen surfaces, and are used for bleeding gums, bleeding piles, minor cuts and as aftershave creams. They have irritant action, especially on raw surfaces.
- Sunscreens protect skin from UVA and UVB rays. SPF is defined as the ratio of minimal erythema-producing dose of UVB radiations with and without sunscreen.
- Adsorbents, demulcents and emollients provide protection to skin and mucous membranes. They protect skin and mucous membranes from the effect of harmful or irritant substances,
- Topical steroids have anti-inflammatory, immunosuppressive and antiproliferative actions. They are used in conditions such as allergic dermatitis, primary irritant dermatitis, seborrheic dermatitis, atopic or varicose eczema, lichen simplex and psoriasis of face and flexures. (The most potent topical steroid is betamethasone dipropionate and the least potent one is hydrocortisone.) Their use under occlusive dressing enhances absorption and and is therefore beneficial in the treatment of chronic hypertrophied lesions. Adverse effects include striae, thinning of epidermis, hypopigmentation, delayed wound healing, fungal and bacterial infections.
- Retinoids (first-, second-, third- generations) are useful in conditions like acne, psoriasis, Kaposi sarcoma, and cutaneous T cell lymphoma.
- Drugs useful in acne include topical drugs (benzoyl peroxide, tretinoin, adapalene, topical antibiotics, azelaic acid, etc.), and systemic drugs (isotretinoin and AMAs). Retinoids have high teratogenic potential and many other adverse effects.
- Management of psoriasis involves topical steroids, PUVA, calcipotriol, tazarotene and immunosuppressive drugs.
- Ectoparasiticidal drugs used in scabies and pediculosis include permethrin (drug of first choice), lindane, benzyl benzoate, and crotamiton. Sulphur, DDT and ivermectin are effective, but not preferred for these indications.

Hints for problem-based questions and MCQs

1. i a. Isotretinoin. It is an oral retinoid possessing keratolytic properties, used in severe cases of acne not responding to topical treatments.
   ii Refer to page 882.
2. i Astringents precipitate proteins without entering cells and affect only the superficial cells.
   ii a. Tannic acid
   iii Used in bleeding gums, bleeding piles, minor cuts and in aftershave creams.
3. i c. Salicylic acid
   ii Refer to page 880.
4. i b. Psoriasis
   ii Refer to page 883.
5. i c. Hydrocortisone
   ii Refer to page 881.
   iii Refer to page 881.
6. i c. Povidone-iodine
   ii Refer to page 886.
   iii Refer to page 886.
7. d. Chloroxylenol is non-irritant only on intact skin; cannot be used in burns case.
8. b. Chlorhexidine

CONCEPT MAP – DRUGS ACTING ON SKIN

Pharmacokinetics of Topical Drugs

Absorption: Drugs applied topically on the skin surface are released from the formulation, diffuse along concentration gradient through stratum corneum by inter/intra cellular, follicular routes. Then, drugs diffuse through the epidermis to reach the dermis, from where they get absorbed.

Factors altering absorption through skin: Water- or alcohol- containing topical preparations evaporate quickly, but supersaturated solution of non-volatile substance remains on skin surface.

Vehicles used for drug delivery should not be good solvents. **Liposomes** are microscopic spherical structures, provide mild occlusive role and maintain hydration of stratum corneum → ensure better penetration of drug across skin surface.

Thickness of layer of topical preparation, area of skin surface covered and rubbing or massaging affect absorption.

Amount of drug adhering to skin surface, residing in upper layers of stratum corneum (called 'drug reservoir'), binding of drug to various proteins and metabolism to varying extent during passage in viable tissues, alters the extent of drug absorption.

Variable extent of drug resorption by cutaneous microvasculature, based on site of application, among individuals, among species, environment and diseases can also affect topical absorption of drugs.

Barrier function of skin is reduced in contact dermatitis, atopic dermatitis, ichthyoses, psoriasis.

Protectives

Adsorbents: Protect skin and mucous membrane from the effect of harmful or irritant substances by their physical property of 'adsorption', e.g., Magnesium stearate, Magnesium silicate, Boric acid, Calamine, Starch, Zinc stearate, Simethicone, Sucralfate.

Demulcents: Produce foam, collapse froth by reducing surface tension and act as suspending agents. They have soothing effect on inflamed skin, e.g., Liquorice or Glycyrrhiza, Methyl cellulose, Propylene glycol, Glycerin, Gum acacia, Gum tragacanth, etc.

Emollients: Soothing, softening oils that form occlusive film on surface like olive/ sesame / arachis oil, cocoa butter, hard/ soft/ liquid paraffin, wool fat, beeswax, etc.
Used to prevent evaporation and restore elasticity of dry, cracked skin and as ointment bases.

Astringents

Substances that cause denaturation and precipitation of proteins → surface becomes mechanically tough and strong.

Examples: Tannic acid, Tannins, Alcohols (ethanol, methanol 50–90%), Minerals like alum, salts of aluminium/zinc, zirconium. These cannot penetrate cells → effect restricted to superficial layer of skin and mucous membrane.

Uses: Tannic acid in alkaloidal poisoning, bleeding gums and bleeding piles.

Alcohol 50–90% used to prevent formation of bedsores in bedridden patients and as aftershave for minor cuts.

Alum used as aftershave.

Salts of zinc, aluminium and zirconium as antiperspirants to reduce body odour.

Drugs Acting on Skin

Topical Steroids

High potentcy: Betamethasone and Beclomethasone dipropionate, Betamethasone valerate/ benzoate, Dexamethasone sodium phosphate/trimethyl acetate, Clobetasol propionate, Triamcinolone acetonide, Fluocinolone acetonide & Fluocortolone.

Moderate potency: Fluticasone propionate, Hydrocortisone + urea, Hydrocortisone acetate, Prednicarbate.

Mild potency: Hydrocortisone acetate/ butyrate.

Uses: Good response in allergic dermatitis, primary irritant dermatitis, seborrheic dermatitis, atopic or varicose eczema, lichen simplex and psoriasis of face and flexures.

Slowly developing effect in lichen planus, alopecia areata, keloids, nail disorders, psoriasis of palm/sole/knee/elbow and cystic acne, etc. → more potent drugs are used.

ADRs: Thinning of epidermis, dermal atrophy (cigarette paper skin), telangiectasia, striae, hypopigmentation, easy bruising, impaired/delayed wound healing, secondary fungal or bacterial infections.

Rarely, systemic adverse effects are reported with topically used steroids, especially in infants, children with repeated or prolonged use.

Keratolytics

Cause desquamation of epidermal cells → used in hyperkeratotic conditions like corns, warts, psoriasis, ringworm, athlete's foot and chronic dermatitis.

Examples: 3–6% Salicylic acid, 40–70% Propylene glycol, Urea 20%, Resorcinol 3–10%, Phenol 80%, Podophyllum resin / podofilox, Silver nitrate pencils/sticks, Glacial/Trichloro acetic acid.

Drugs for Acne

Acne: Excess secretion of sebum from the sebaceous glands → secondary infection → secretion of lipase → formation of fatty acids → blockade of follicular ducts → retention of secretion, hyperkeratosis and formation of horny impactions in follicles called comedones → comedones open up into dermis → inflammation and formation of pustules.

Topical drugs: Benzoyl peroxide is most frequently used. Retinoids (Retinoic acid, Adapalene, Tazarotene) may be alternated with benzoyl peroxide for better effect. Azelaic acid has same efficacy as benzoyl peroxide. Antibiotics (Clindamycin, Erythromycin, Tetracyclines and Nadifloxacin) used only in patients with inflamed papules and folliculitis.

Systemic drugs: Isotretinoin has severe adverse effects → reserved only for severe refractory cases, used for prevention of skin cancers, actinic keratoses, leukoplakia. Antibiotics Doxycycline, Minocycline administered systemically for short term in severe cases for initial control of pustules and cysts.

Drugs for Psoriasis

Excessive epidermal proliferation and dermal inflammation resulting in erythematous scaling lesions or plaques.

Mainstay of treatment is topical steroids → therapy initiated with more potent steroids, then substituted by less potent drugs and followed by emollients, keratolytics, antifungal drugs.

Other treatment options are PUVA, Calcipotriol, Tazarotene and immunosuppressive drugs.

SECTION 12 Miscellaneous Topics

68 Evidence-Based Medicine and New Drug Development

PH 1.2 Describe evidence-based medicine and relevance to therapeutics.
PH 10.7 Describe pharmacoeconomics and manage economic issues in drug use and find out the price of given medication(s).
PH 10.12 Describe overview of drug development including phases of clinical trials and good clinical practice (GCP) and reflect on the role of research in developing new drugs.

Learning objectives

A student of MBBS phase II should be able to:
- Discuss the concept of evidence-based medicine (EBM).
- Justify the need for practice of EBM.
- Describe various study designs and the power of generated evidence.
- Describe the steps in clinical decision-making process.
- Describe various methods used in pharmacoeconomic.
- Describe clinical significance of pharmacoeconomics.
- Describe drug discovery, screening, development, preclinical testing and evaluation in humans.
- Describe the different phases of clinical trials.
- Describe the principles of ICH-GCP.

EVIDENCE-BASED MEDICINE

The practice of medicine is gradually shifting from an **experience-based** approach, where clinical decisions rely primarily on the physician's personal experience, to an **evidence-based** approach, in which scientifically credible evidence forms the basis of clinical decision-making. David Sackett defines evidence-based medicine (EBM) as "the integration of the best research evidence with clinical expertise and patient values to guide decisions tailored to the needs of individual patients" (Fig. 68.1).

EBM emphasises self-directed, problem-based lifelong learning. Its practice involves explicit, judicious and conscientious use of current medical research findings to make decisions about management of patients. Evidence-based healthcare integrates clinical expertise (gained through experience) and skill with systematically obtained research evidence to ensure that decisions are patient-centred and grounded in the best available knowledge.

A knowledge of EBM is essential because ongoing scientific research continually generates new evidence, often prompting revisions in treatment strategies. A large number of research articles are being published in medical journals, but due to time constraints, physicians often find it difficult to stay updated with the latest developments. Studies suggest that physicians' clinical performance may decline over time if they do not consistently update their knowledge and skills, despite gaining more experience.

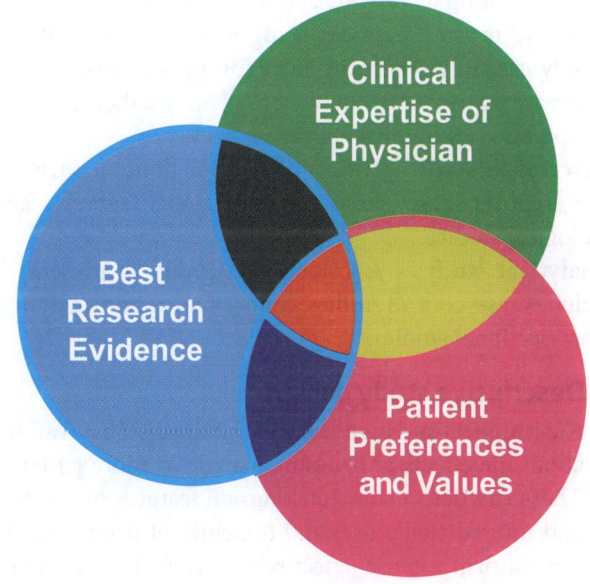

Fig. 68.1 Evidence-based medicine

In the current era of consumer activism, patients are increasingly accessing the same medical literature as clinicians, making them better informed about healthcare options. Therefore, it is essential for healthcare professionals to stay current with advancements in diagnostic techniques and emerging therapies in order to recommend the most appropriate course of action from among the available alternatives.

TYPES OF CLINICAL EVIDENCE

Drugs and other therapeutic/preventive interventions are evaluated using various study designs, which are ranked according to a widely accepted hierarchy of evidence. It is important to understand that not all evidence holds the same weight. Clinical evidence generated from different study designs is ranked according to the strength and reliability they provide. Each design has its own strengths and limitations.

BASIC RESEARCH

Basic research aims at answering a specific, single question under tightly controlled laboratory conditions, e.g., does a particular drug inhibit a particular enzyme, or what is the concentration–response relationship for enzyme inhibition by this drug. The results are reproducible and indicate towards the mechanism of drug action.

HUMAN STUDIES

Human studies can be **observational** or **interventional**.

1. Observational Studies

In observational research, the investigator does not intervene in the treatment being given to a patient. He is only carefully observing the exposures and outcomes. These are further of two types, based on whether there is a comparative group or not, i.e.,

Descriptive study – No comparison is done. It includes case reports, case series, cross-sectional surveys and ecological studies.

Analytical study – A comparison group is present. It includes case-control studies, cohort studies and analytical cross-sectional studies.

a. Descriptive study design

- **Case reports and case series** are clinicians' observations about the effects of drugs in a single or more patients. These can detect some uncommon features of diseases and unpredictable uses and toxicities of drugs, but do not confirm a cause–effect relationship. They generate the least reliable (grade IV) type of evidence for therapeutic/preventive efficacy and toxicity of the given drug or intervention.
  - **Cross-sectional surveys** are the most common study design of the descriptive kind. It involves observing a cross-section of a population at a single point in time. The unit of observation is an individual. They are useful to estimate prevalence of disease, risk factors and their distribution by time, place and person. Multiple exposures and multiple outcomes can be observed. These surveys are easy to conduct, are not very expensive and consume little time.
  - **Ecological Studies** – These are population-based studies. The unit of observation is a group, rather than an individual. These studies are less resource-intensive and help determine whether populations with a high frequency of disease also have a higher rate of exposure to specific risk factors. This study design is useful for investigating rare diseases. But a limitation of ecological studies is that individual level information is not available. In other words, association observed between disease and risk factors at group level may not necessarily represent the same at the individual level. This is known as **ecological fallacy**.

b. Analytical study design

- **Case-control study** is an observational analytical study useful for establishing association between **some suspected rare adverse event and particular drug use**. Patients with a suspected adverse event and a matched control group without this event are selected. Drug history of both groups is then traced backward. However, the evidence generated by this study design is considered less reliable because of the retrospective design, non-random selection of participants, bias and inability to elicit unsuspected adverse effects associated with a drug.

  Odds ratio (OR) is a statistical measure that quantifies the association between an exposure and an outcome in case-control studies by comparing the odds of exposure in cases (those with the outcome) to the odds of exposure in controls (those without the outcome).

	Cases	Control	Total
Exposed	a	b	a+b
Unexposed	c	d	c+d
	a+c	b+d	a+b+c+d

Probability that a case was exposed = $a/(a+c)$

Probability that a case was not exposed = $c/(a+c)$

Odds that the case was exposed =

$$\frac{\text{Probability that the case was exposed}}{\text{Probability that the case was not exposed}}$$

$$= \frac{a}{a+c} \div \frac{c}{a+c} = \frac{a}{c}$$

Similarly, odds that the control was exposed = b/d

$$\text{Odds ratio (OR)} = \frac{\text{Odds that the case was exposed}}{\text{Odds that the control was exposed}}$$

$$= \frac{a}{c} \div \frac{b}{d} = \frac{ab}{bc}$$

An OR of 1 suggests no association, greater than 1 indicates increased odds of the outcome with exposure, and less than 1 suggests a protective effect.

- **Cohort study** is also an observational analytical study. It involves examining a specific group (or cohort) of individuals exposed to a particular drug. The outcomes, such as benefits or adverse effects, are compared with those in individuals not exposed to the drug.

  Cohort studies can be conducted prospectively, such as through prescription event monitoring. In this approach, patients receiving the drug are followed over a defined period to assess their response to the treatment and identify any adverse effects. This method is particularly useful in detecting unexpected or unpredicted adverse drug reactions.

  Alternatively, cohort studies can be retrospective, analysing data where both the exposure to the drug and the outcomes have already occurred before the study begins. This approach relies on historical data to establish associations between drug exposure and observed effects.

  Relative risk (RR) is the ratio of incidence of the disease in the exposed to incidence in the unexposed.

	Outcome present	Outcome not present	Total
Exposed	a	b	a+b
Unexposed	c	d	c+d
	a+c	b+d	a+b+c+d

  Incidence in exposed = a/(a+b)

  Incidence in unexposed = c/(c+d)

  $$\text{Relative risk (RR)} = \frac{\text{Incidence of disease in exposed}}{\text{Incidence in unexposed}} = \frac{a}{a+b} \div \frac{c}{c+d}$$

  An RR = 1 implies no association (risk is equal in exposed and unexposed groups); RR > 1 implies positive association (exposure increases disease risk) and an RR < 1 implies negative association (exposure reduces disease risk, indicating a protective effect).

  The evidence from cohort study also needs further investigation.

- **Analytical cross-sectional study**: It is designed to measure the exposure and outcome simultaneously, to identify association of risk factors with existing disease, i.e., in prevalent cases. It is commonly employed to identify association of permanent characteristics with chronic diseases, e.g., human leukocyte antigen (HLA) types and conditions like diabetes.

  A limitation of cross-sectional design is that although it can be used as preliminary analysis to understand risk factors for a disease, it cannot establish disease etiology. For example, in a study of diabetes and obesity, a cross-sectional survey investigating both conditions simultaneously cannot establish whether diabetes is due to obesity or is the cause of obesity.

2. Interventional Studies

In this study design, the investigator assigns the intervention (diagnostic, preventive, therapeutic) and measures the response. It includes **randomised** or **non-randomised controlled clinical trials.** Quasi-experimental study design is adopted when random allocation of subjects into test arm or control arm is not possible due to ethical or procedural constraints.

Phases of clinical trials

The initial phases of clinical trial, **Phase 1** to **Phase 3**, occur in the pre-marketing phase. Once the drug gets FDA (Food and Drug Administration) approval and is marketed, **Phase 4** of clinical trials, also known as **post-marketing surveillance,** monitor the drug's long-term safety and effectiveness in a broader population and detect any rare adverse effects.

Randomised controlled trials (RCTs)

RCTs are the most rigorous approach for generating evidence. They are the gold standard for interventional studies that generate reliable (Grade II) data regarding safety, efficacy and comparative value of a given drug or therapeutic/preventive intervention. They answer precisely framed questions about effects of medication on clinical end points. Clinical trials for determination of pharmacokinetics and tolerability may be conducted in healthy volunteers, but therapeutic efficacy for most drugs should be assessed only in patients.

In controlled trials, there are always two or more groups. The 'control group' is for comparison, and participants allotted in control group receive either a 'placebo' or 'standard treatment'. A placebo is an inert substance in the guise of medicine, whereas standard treatment is the best therapy for that particular condition at the time of conducting research. The other group is the 'test/ experimental group' which receives the intervention being studied, such as a new drug/ treatment regimen/ procedure.

The test and control groups should be similar in all aspects except the intervention in question. In **parallel group design,** the test group receives the test drug in predetermined dose and regimen, whereas the control group receives placebo or a standard treatment drug; thereafter, the results are compared. In **crossover design,** the same patients receive the test drug and then the placebo/standard drug, one after the other. Thus, the patient serves as their own control.

Randomisation is the process of allotting the study subjects into the test or control arm/group randomly by using computer generated numbers or random number tables in such a way that each subject has an equal chance of being allocated to the test group or control group.

The design of controlled clinical trials can be **open label, single blind, double blind,** or **triple blind**. In case of **open-label** trials, the participant, investigator and data analyst know which treatment is given (trial drug or standard drug/placebo). In other words, everyone is aware to which arm of the trial (test or control) a particular patient is allotted. In **single-blind** design, the study subjects are unaware of treatment given to them. In **double-blind** design, both the subject and investigator are unaware of treatment given, whereas in **triple-blind** design, the data analyst is also not aware of the details. The test and control medication should look alike in colour, weight, number, etc. The blinding process helps to eliminate bias.

The treatment outcomes of the test and control groups are compared using appropriate statistical tests to identify any statistically significant differences between them.

Multicentric trials

These are large trials conducted simultaneously at many centres by multiple researchers. Thus, a larger number of patients can be studied in a shorter span of time. This increases the strength of evidence generated and the results are applicable to a wider population. Results obtained from well designed and well conducted multicentric trials help in framing guidelines for disease management.

Meta-analysis and systematic reviews

They generate the most reliable (Grade I) evidence to form the basis of clinical decisions (Fig. 68.2). In a systematic review, all possible studies related to a particular topic are collected, reviewed and their results are analysed. In meta-analysis, the data obtained from carefully selected, randomised controlled trials using the same class of drugs with similar end points is pooled and statistically analysed. Thus, meta-analysis is an objective and valid method for analysing and combining the results of different studies. This increases the number of subjects (in test as well as control group) and thereby increases the significance and strength of conclusions.

THE EVIDENCE PYRAMID

All evidences generated are not equivalent. Different study designs generate evidence of varying strength or power. The evidence pyramid (Fig. 68.2) shows different study designs in the order of increasing power of evidence from the base to apex.

However, the **study design best suited for answering a question depends on the question itself.** For example, some study designs are more suitable for answering queries related to diagnosis and others for queries related to prognosis, as shown in Fig. 68.3.

For queries related to causation (i.e., etiology), prevention and therapy/treatment, the best study design is the randomised controlled trial (RCT), followed by cohort, case control and case series, in that order. For answering questions related to prognosis, RCTs are not used, but cohort, case control and case series are useful. Diagnostic and clinical examination related queries need prospective study design with blind comparison to gold standard. Economic analysis is done for studies related to cost factors.

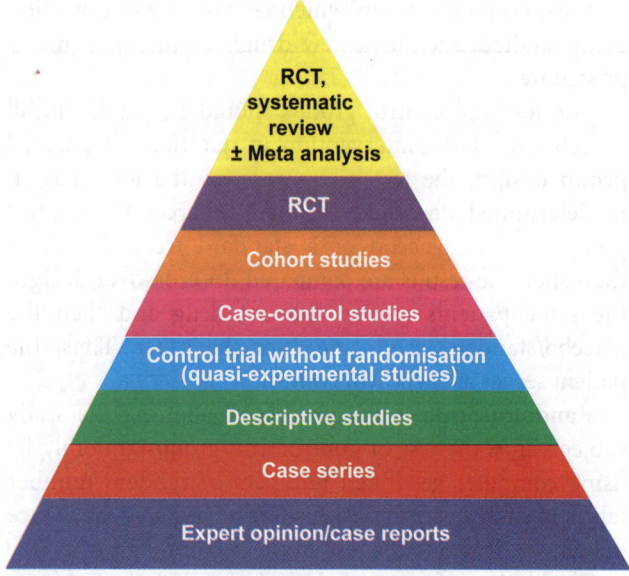

Fig. 68.2 The evidence pyramid

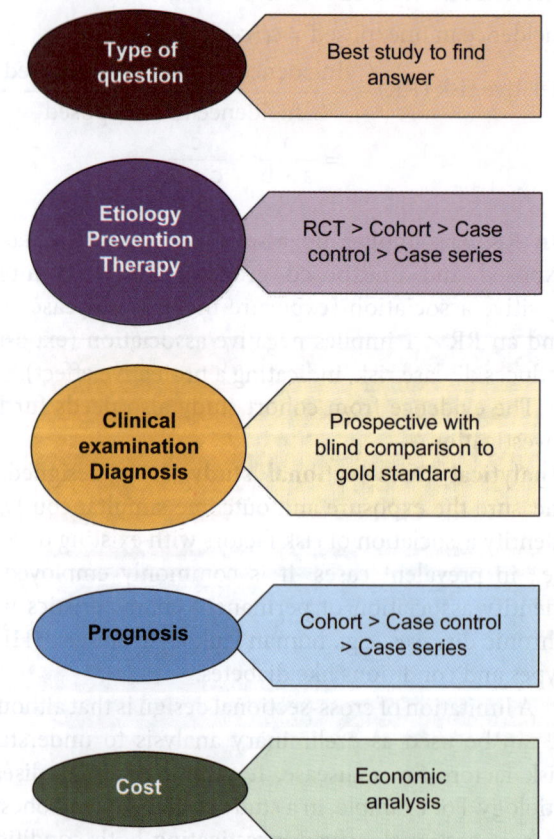

Fig. 68.3 Choice of study designs based on type of questions

CLINICAL DECISION MAKING

Clinical decision making is a stepwise cognitive process of making more deliberate, thoughtful decisions by organising relevant information and defining alternatives. Evidence-based medicine (EBM) plays a crucial role in improving patient care by reducing errors. For clinicians, EBM supports continuous, self-directed learning, helping them stay updated with scientific advancements. Figure 68.4 depicts the stepwise process of clinical decision making.

1. The first and foremost step in practicing evidence-based medicine is to **frame a focused, pertinent and answerable question**. The well-framed question should give the description of the patient or the population (P), intervention (I), explicit comparison or control (C) and relevant outcomes (O). That is, the effectiveness of a question for EBM is judged by PICO. The common clinical questions are about etiology, risk factors, diagnosis, intervention, prognosis and cost-effectiveness of the intervention
2. The next step is an extensive **literature survey** carried out via traditional printed resources as well as online content. Ideally, this source of information should be relevant, of high quality, comprehensive, and contain data on benefits and risks associated with all the interventions possible for that particular condition and their user friendliness. The most popularly searched databases for getting reliable and authoritative information about specific health related queries are the Cochrane Library, Pubmed Central, Scopus, and Map of Medicine.
3. The literature is **critically appraised** for determining its relevance, intent and validity and applicability. It requires reading and analysing the articles carefully for methodology used and conclusions drawn.
4. The evidence gained by literature research is then integrated with clinical acumen or expertise and patient's preferences to arrive at a well-informed decision about choosing one strategy out of the many available alternatives. All patient-related factors (e.g., existence of contraindications, acceptability, economic condition) and intervention-related potential benefits, risks and harm must be carefully considered before **choosing the most appropriate strategy** for a particular situation.
5. The whole process is **evaluated continuously** to make space for further improvement.

BIOSTATISTICS IN HEALTH RESEARCH

The results of biomedical research are expressed using various statistical terms. Few of the frequently used terms and salient features of biostatistics are mentioned here briefly.

Descriptive statistics refers to the use of statistical methods to summarise and describe the main features of a dataset in a clear and understandable manner. It helps make sense of large volumes of data by converting them into meaningful representations, such as single values or visualisations, rather than long lists of numbers or words.

Inferential statistics involves using data from a sample to make generalisations, predictions, or inferences about a larger population (i.e., beyond the sample size). Normally, it is not possible to include each subject or individual of a population in a study. Therefore, a representative sample is used and the results obtained are applied to the larger population.

- **Population** is a group of individuals that share at least one characteristic in common. A statistical value that is calculated from all the values in from sample the whole population is termed a 'parameter'.
- A **sample** is a selection of members within the population. A statistical value calculated from all the values in a sample is called a '**statistic**'.

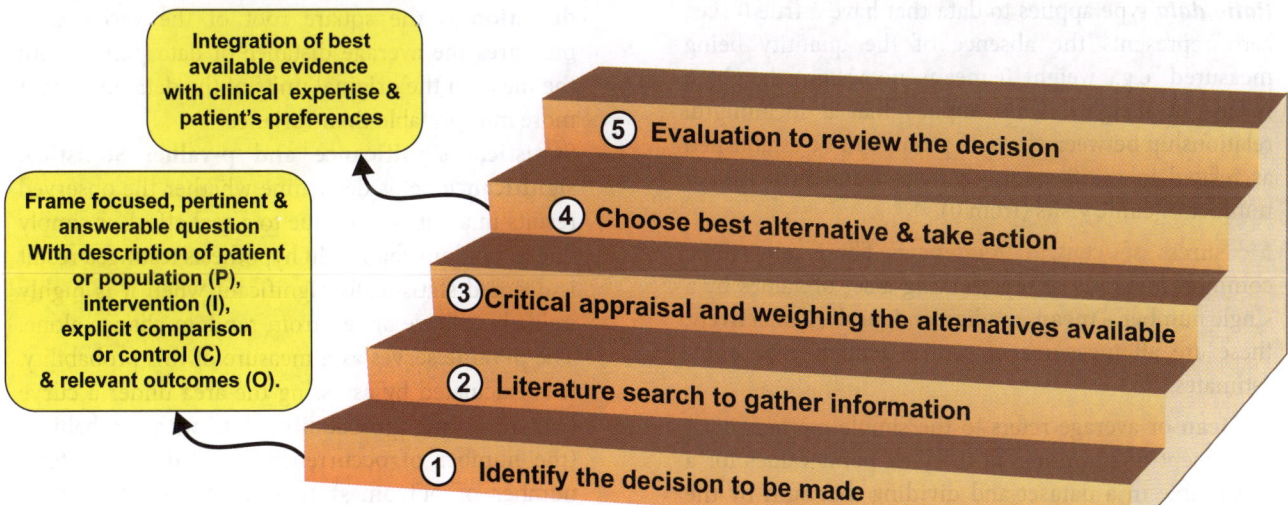

Fig. 68.4 Steps of clinical decision making

- **Variable** is a group name for any data values collected for a study. In a data spreadsheet, each row represents the findings for an individual in a study, and each column name is a variable. A single example value for a variable is called a 'data point'.

Types of data: Different statistical tests are used for different types of data. Data can be **categorical** or **numerical**, each of which has two sub-divisions.

- **Categorical data** refers to categories or things, not mathematical values. It can be further of two types: **nominal** or **ordinal**. Nominal data is described by names, e.g., male/female, while ordinal data refers to a type of data that has a natural order or ranking but the difference between adjacent values is not consistent or meaningful. For examples, the five-point, Likert scale (used in surveys where the responses might be ranked as strongly disagree, disagree, neutral, agree, strongly agree from 1 to 5), pain scores (often rated on a scale such as 0 (no pain) to 10 (worst pain), etc.
- **Numerical data** refers to data which is about measurement and counting, further classified as **interval data** and **ratio data**.

Interval data is a type of quantitative data characterised by ordered values where the differences between values are meaningful and consistent. However, interval data lacks a true zero point, meaning 'zero' does not represent the total absence of the quantity being measured. For example, the difference between 1°C and 2°C is the same as the difference between 3°C and 4°C. However, temperatures expressed in degrees Celsius (or Fahrenheit) do not have a 'true zero' because 0°C is not a true zero. Thus, a numerical *interval data* (like temperature) can be arranged in order, be added or subtracted but cannot be divided or multiplied.

Ratio data type applies to data that have a true 0 (i.e., zero represents the absence of the quantity being measured, e.g., weight 0 means no weight; height 0 means no height). This implies that a meaningful relationship between the data points can be established as related to the 0 value, e.g., age from birth (0), or number of clinic visits (from 0).

Measures of central tendency: There are three common methods of representing a set of values by a single number – **mean, median** and **mode**. Collectively, these are all measures of central tendency or point estimates.

- **Mean** or average refers to the simple mathematical concept of summing all the data point values for a variable in a dataset and dividing that sum by the number of values in the set. It is a meaningful way to represent a set of numbers that do not have outliers (values that are way different from the large majority of numbers).
- **Median** is a calculated value that falls right in the middle of a data set when it is arranged in order (either ascending or descending). That means half of the values are higher than this value and the other half are lower. It is a useful measure when a few of the values are very much different from the majority, thereby skewing the data.
- **Mode** is the most frequently appearing data value, usually used to describe categorical values.
- *Measures of dispersion:* Dispersion is the actual size of the spread of the data points, such as range, quartiles, percentiles, variance, and standard deviation (SD).
- **Range** refers to the difference between the minimum and maximum values and is expressed by noting both the values.
- **Quartiles** divide the group of values into four equal quarters. First quartile (Q1) represents the value below which 25% of the data falls, meaning a quarter of the values are smaller, and three-quarters (75%) are larger. Second quartile (Q2) is the same as median value. The third quartile (Q3) is the value below which 75% of the data falls, meaning three-quarters of the values are smaller and one-quarter (25%) are larger.

The zeroth value is the same as the minimum value and the fourth quartile value is the same as the maximum value. The interquartile range (IQR) is the difference between the values of the first and third quartiles.

- **Variance and standard deviation:** Variance measures the average of the squared differences between each data point and the mean. It quantifies the overall spread of the data. The **standard deviation** is the square root of the variance. It measures the average distance of data points from the mean in the original units of the data, making it more interpretable than variance.
- **Statistical significance and p-value:** Statistical **significance** helps determine whether the observed results in a dataset are due to a real effect or simply due to random chance. In hypothesis testing, a result is deemed statistically significant when it is highly unlikely to have arisen from random chance alone. The **p-value** serves as a measure of this probability. It is calculated by assessing the area under a curve known as the probability plot, with probability (the number of occurrences divided by the total number of outcomes) represented on the y-axis. A p-value of less than 0.05 is taken as statistically significant.

Multiple-choice questions

1. A study is planned to compare the effectiveness of a new antibiotic with the standard treatment drug by selecting 120 patients and randomly assigning 60 of them to receive the new antibiotic and 60 to receive the standard treatment. Both the patients and the medical personnel (including those who evaluate the treatment and collect the data) will not know which antibiotic a particular patient has received, until after the results of the analysis are available.
   What is this type of study?
   a. Cohort study
   b. Case-control study
   c. Randomised, self-controlled trial
   d. Randomised, double-blinded, controlled trial

2. In above mentioned study, data point values were collected pertaining to the variable length of hospital stay. These values were captured in terms of days. Identify the type of data.
   a. Ratio-type numerical
   b. Interval-type numerical
   c. Ordinal categorical
   d. Nominal categorical

3. In the above-mentioned study, standard deviation is used to describe the spread in the data point values for age. What does this represent?
   a. It represents the upper and lower limits within which 95% of the values fall.
   b. It represents the minimum and maximum values in the data set of age values.
   c. It represents the square of the difference between each individual age and the mean (average) age.
   d. It represents the square root of the average of the squared differences of all the values from the mean age.

4. In a questionnaire, patients are asked to rate their opinion to the statement "Use of audio-visual aids during lectures helps in better recall of content" on a scale from 1 to 5, with 1 referring to not agreeing at all, to 5 referring to total agreement.
   What is an appropriate data type for this variable?
   a. Ratio numerical   b. Nominal categorical
   c. Ordinal categorical   d. Interval numerical

NEW DRUG DEVELOPMENT

Development of a new drug is a costly and time-consuming process. It is carried out in a stepwise manner, the major steps being drug discovery, drug development, drug screening, preclinical testing for safety, toxicity and human experimentation. These are described below.

A. Drug Discovery or Synthesis

The discovery or synthesis of a potential new drug compound involves the following:

1. A new drug should not simply mimic the structure and pharmacological actions of a previously available drug but needs elucidation of a new target (which can be a pathophysiological process or a substrate of a disease amenable to modification by the new compound).
2. New molecules are designed rationally, based on an understanding of biological mechanisms and drug–receptor structures. Research on and discoveries of novel pathophysiological processes and molecules modifying them are usually carried out by educational and research institutions.
3. Sometimes 'me-too' analogues are prepared by chemical modification of known drugs. (They may offer advantages like fewer side effects and better dosing regimens, which allow them to compete in the same market.)
4. Natural products, large libraries of organic molecules, nucleic acids, peptides, etc., are screened for biological activity in the pharmaceutical industry. The process of synthesis or isolation of a new compound usually takes about 1–2 years.

B. Drug Development

The development of a new lead or promising compound in laboratories of pharmaceutical industry involves studies for understanding the interaction of the drug with its biological target, its efficacy, potency, selectivity and safety. Such studies are quite resource (time and cost) intensive. Before a drug can be marketed, its efficacy and safety must be established through in vitro and in vivo studies in experimental animals as well as through human **clinical trials**. Once the drug is approved for marketing, safety monitoring is continued for detection of rare and delayed adverse effects.

C. Drug Screening

After obtaining a '**lead compound**' or a promising molecule, translational research involving preclinical and clinical studies is carried out. The **pharmacological profile of the lead compound** is defined by carrying out 'drug screening'. This involves conducting molecular, cellular, and organ system assays, whole animal studies and animal models of the human disease. The mechanism of actions, selectivity, expected as well as unexpected therapeutic and toxic effects are studied. Detection of unexpected therapeutic action is called **serendipity**.

Screening at the **molecular level** determines activity of the new compound on the target, such as affinity for binding to receptors, the effect of cytochrome P450 (CYP450) enzyme on the new compound, and enzyme-inducing/inhibiting potential of new compound. Screening at the **cellular level** looks for pharmacological activity and selectivity (agonist/partial agonist/inverse agonist/antagonist effects) of the new compound on relevant receptors as compared to reference compounds on isolated tissues and in vivo studies.

Screening at the **organ system level** involves determination of the drug's effect in whole animals (normal animals as well as animal models of human disease). Evidence for useful effects of the drug after administration by different routes and duration of action is gathered. Possible adverse effects on major organ systems are also studied.

Animal testing suggests the need for **compound optimisation**, so that the compound is modified for achieving desirable pharmacokinetic and pharmacodynamic properties. Thus, screening tests are repeated with congeners of the original molecule to get a compound which is a leading candidate for a successful new drug called 'lead compound'. At this stage, a patent application for the lead compound is filed. If it is a novel compound, a '**matter patent**' application is filed, but if it is a previously known chemical entity with new therapeutic use, a '**use patent**' application is filed.

D. Preclinical Testing for Safety and Toxicity

Molecules that clear the initial screening procedures are evaluated carefully for potential risks in **preclinical toxicity testing**. It involves estimating the risks associated with exposure to the potential drug in the context of therapeutic needs and expected duration of use. Tests are conducted to assess acute, subacute, and chronic toxicity, as well as mutagenic and carcinogenic potential, and effects on reproductive performance. Such preclinical toxicity testing helps in identifying the relevant potential human toxicities that need monitoring in clinical trials.

In addition, **quantitative studies** to estimate the no-effect dose, maximum-tolerated dose, minimum lethal dose and median lethal dose, etc., are also carried out.

The limitations of preclinical testing, such as cost, time needed, concerns of animal safety, and the uncertain predictive value of animal data for humans necessitate human experimentation, i.e., clinical trials.

E. Evaluation in Humans (Clinical Trials)

For the lead compounds that clear preclinical safety and toxicity testing, and are ready to be studied in humans, a '**Notice of claimed investigational exemption for a new drug' (IND)** is filed. This claim includes information about the composition of the drug, its source, chemical structure, manufacturing details, compilation of data of preclinical testing in animal experimentation, proposed plan for clinical testing and details of investigators.

Human studies are initiated only after completion of sufficient 'acute and subacute animal toxicity' studies. Chronic toxicity, carcinogenic studies in animals are continued alongside the clinical trials.

Clinical trials are carried out in **four phases**. In each phase of the trial, the protocol for conduct of clinical trial must be reviewed for scientific and ethical aspects and approved by a regulating authority (Drug Controller General of India DCGI) as well as by the Institutional Ethics Committee (IEC) or Institutional Review Board (IRB). It is essential to obtain and document the informed consent of all human subjects (both healthy volunteers and patients) after clearly explaining the investigational status of the drug and the potential risks associated with its use.

Phases of Clinical Trials

There are 4 phases of clinical trials: Phases 1, 2, 3, and 4. Recently, Phase 0 or microdosing studies, involving administration of sub-pharmacological doses in healthy volunteers, has been introduced. The objectives of each phase, the subjects used, number of subjects and study designs used in each phase of clinical trial are described below.

Phase 1

Objectives of phase I clinical trials: To establish drug effects as a function of dose, to determine limits of safe dosage range, to help detect predictable toxic effects, and pharmacokinetic parameters such as absorption/half-life/metabolism.

Subjects: Healthy volunteers or patient volunteers (if significant toxicity is expected, like in cancer, HIV infection).

Number: 20–80

Design: Design may be open label, i.e., non-blind. In such trials, investigators as well as subjects know to which arm of the study they belong. Sometimes, single- or double-blinded design is used and usually, a placebo control group is used.

Site: Phase 1 trials are done in research centres by trained pharmacologists.

Phase 2

Objectives of phase 2 clinical trials: To determine efficacy and doses to be used in any follow-on trials and ceiling effect (i.e., where a drug or treatment reaches a maximum level of efficacy, beyond which increasing the dose does not produce a greater therapeutic effect). These may also help to detect broader range of toxicities.

Subjects: Patients with target disease

Number: 100–500

Design: Single blind; placebo control group may be used.

Site: Special clinical centres.

Only one-fourth of INDs cross this phase to reach Phase 3 trials.

Phase 3

Objectives of phase 3 clinical trials: To establish and confirm safety and efficacy. Certain immunological adverse effects are detected. Indications of the drug and guidelines for its therapeutic use are finalised.

Subjects: Patients with target disease.

Numbers: 500–3000

Design: Double blind and cross-over designs are commonly used.

Site: Similar to those anticipated for ultimate use of drug. Phase 3 trials are done by specialists in the disease being treated.

The studies are usually costly, as large number of participants are involved and more data needs to be collected and analysed. Moreover, for phase 3 studies, the investigational drug is formulated as intended for market.

If the IND gives favourable toxicity and efficacy results in the Phase 3 trials, a **'New drug application' (NDA)** seeking marketing approval is filed. All details of preclinical and clinical data are submitted with the NDA.

In urgent situations, such as serious diseases, the processes of preclinical testing, clinical testing, reviews and approvals by the regulating agencies are put on a fast track or are accelerated, as was the case for the development of COVID-19 vaccines during the recent pandemic.

Phase 4

This involves post-marketing surveillance and includes continued monitoring for safety, efficacy and acceptability of the new drug in a larger number of patients in real-life conditions. This is important for detecting rare adverse effects, especially those associated with chronic long-term use of the drug. Duration of the phase 4 trials is not fixed.

The usual time interval between filing a patent application and getting market approval is around 5 years or even longer. Total lifetime of a patent is 20 years, during which the patent owner has exclusive rights of manufacturing and marketing the product. Once the patent expires, other pharmaceutical companies can also file an **'abbreviated new drug application' (ANDA)**, demonstrate equivalence and get approval for marketing the drug as a generic product.

Multiple-choice questions

5. Identify the right time for filing 'matter patent' application.
   a. After completion of initial screening procedure
   b. After preclinical testing
   c. After phase 2 of clinical trials
   d. After phase 4 of clinical trials.

6. Which phase of clinical trials involves healthy volunteers?
   a. Phase 1   b. Phase 2
   c. Phase 3   d. Phase 4

7. Identify a setting suitable for phase 1 clinical trials.
   a. Superspeciality hospitals
   b. Research centres
   c. Special clinical centres
   d. Centres using drug in real-life situation

8. Identify the right time for filing a 'New drug application'.
   a. After discovery of a molecule
   b. At the end of preclinical safety testing
   c. At the end of phase 3 clinical trials
   d. At the end of phase 4 clinical trials

9. Which phase of clinical trials helps in detecting adverse effects of drug associated with its long-term use?
   a. Phase 1   b. Phase 2
   c. Phase 3   d. Phase 4

PHARMACOECONOMICS

This is a branch of health economics vital for promoting rational prescribing. It deals with costs and benefits of drug therapy. The focus of economic evaluation of a new intervention (new drug) is mainly the costs and benefits offered by it over and above those of interventions (drugs) used in current clinical practice.

Pharmacoeconomic Evaluations

These require measurements of inputs (costs) and outcomes (benefits) from the drug use. The **cost of drug therapy** includes direct, indirect and intangible costs.

- Direct cost includes capital cost, staff cost and drug acquisition costs.
- Indirect costs may include loss of earnings, loss of leisure time, loss of productivity, and cost of travelling to healthcare facility.
- Intangible costs include pain, distress suffered by patients and their families. These are difficult to measure in terms of money, but must be considered. The quality of life (QOL) parameters included in the economic analysis may cover intangible costs to some extent.

Benefits of drug therapy include all its favourable consequences, such as:

- Natural units like number of life years saved, number of wounds or ulcers healed, number of acute MI/ strokes prevented
- Utility includes change in patients' sense of well-being or satisfaction. This is based on QOL in terms of physical, emotional and social aspects of well-being. Thus, the main elements of QOL measurements are physical and psychosocial. The physical dimensions measure the presence or absence of physical symptoms, whereas the psychosocial dimensions relate to level of anxiety or depression and capability to cope with problems.
- Quality-adjusted life years (QALY) is a summary of the quantity and quality of life.
- Associated economic benefit measured in monetary terms is also important, e.g., economic benefits to society as a consequence of improved health of a patient returning to work.

Types of economic evaluations: Commonly, four types of evaluations are done.

- Cost-minimisation analysis (CMA) focuses mainly on the costs to health services. It is applied to programmes that achieve the same results, e.g., costs of generic versus branded prescribing.

- Cost-effectiveness analysis (CEA) involves the measurement of costs in monetary units, and measurement of health benefit in natural units. In such studies, it is important to note from whose point of view the study is being conducted.
- Cost–utility analysis (CUA) is similar to CEA, but outcomes are measured in terms of utility, i.e., patient well-being. Such analysis is useful to compare interventions over more than one area of medicine; QOL and QALY are proposed as measures of utility.
- Cost–benefit analysis (CBA) includes associated economic benefits of the intervention. Both the costs and benefits are expressed as monetary equivalents. However, many intangible benefits might get ignored in such analyses.

GOOD CLINICAL PRACTICE

Terms used

- **Good clinical practice (GCP)** is an international ethical standard for designing, conducting, recording and reporting trials that involve the participation of human subjects.
- **ICH:** The International Council for Harmonisation of Technical Requirements for Pharmaceuticals for Human Use issued the ICH guidelines in an effort to overcome inconsistencies in GCP guidelines across countries. ICH GCP guidelines provide a unified standard for the European Union (EU), Japan and United States to facilitate mutual acceptance of clinical data by the regulatory authorities in these jurisdictions, as well as those of Australia, Canada, the Nordic countries and World Health Organisation.

  Original ICH E6(R1): Clinical trials were performed in a largely paper-based process.

  E6(R2): With advances in use of electronic data, standards regarding electronic records and essential documents have been updated.

Principles of ICH GCP

1. **Ethical principles**: Clinical trials should be conducted in accordance with the ethical principles laid down in the Declaration of Helsinki, which binds the physician with the words, 'The health of my patient will be my first consideration', as well as the International Code of Medical Ethics, which declares that 'A physician shall act in the patient's best interest when providing medical care.'
2. **Risk versus benefits**: Before a trial is initiated, risks should be weighed against the anticipated benefit. A trial to be initiated only if the anticipated benefits justify the risks.
3. The **rights, safety, and well-being** of the trial subjects are the most important considerations and should prevail over interests of science and society.
4. The available **information on an investigational product** should be adequate to support the clinical trial.
5. Clinical trials should be **scientifically sound.**
6. A trial should be conducted **as approved by the IRB/IEC.**
7. The medical care and medical decisions made on behalf of subjects should always be the responsibility of a **qualified physician.**
8. Freely given **informed consent** should be obtained from every subject prior to clinical trial participation.
9. All clinical trial information should be recorded, handled, and stored to allow its **accurate reporting, interpretation and verification.**
10. The **confidentiality of records** that could identify subjects should be protected.
11. Investigational products to be manufactured, handled, and stored in accordance with applicable **good manufacturing practice** (GMP).
12. Systems with procedures that assure the **quality of every aspect** of the trial should be implemented.

The Stakeholders in Clinical Trials

Sponsor: An individual or a company or an institution that takes the responsibility for the initiation, management/or financing of a clinical study.

Investigator: The medical doctor/dentist, responsible for the conduct of the study at the trial site.

Institutional ethics committee: An institutional review board/independent ethics committee responsible for verifying protection of the rights, safety and well-being of human subjects involved in the study.

Study subject: An individual who participates in a clinical trial, either as a recipient of the investigational product(s) or as a control.

Multiple-choice question

10. **Identify the stakeholder responsible for verifying the protection of rights of human participants in clinical trials.**
    a. Principal investigator
    b. Institutional ethics committee
    c. Non-governmental organisation
    d. Head of the institution

Hints/solutions for MCQs

1. d. Randomised, double-blinded, controlled trial
2. a. Ratio-type numerical
3. d. It represents the square root of the average of the squared differences of all the values from the mean age.
4. c. Ordinal, categorical
5. a. After completion of initial screening procedure
6. a. Phase 1
7. b. Research centres
8. c. At the end of phase 3 clinical trials
9. d. Phase 4
10. b. Institutional ethics committee

CONCEPT MAP – EVIDENCE-BASED MEDICINE AND NEW DRUG DEVELOPMENT

Evidence-based Medicine

EBM
It the integration of the best research evidence with clinical expertise & patient values in the process of decision making for benefit of individual patient.
Different study designs generate evidence of varying strength or power. But the study design best suited to answer a question depends on the question itself.

Clinical Decision Making
EBM plays a critical role in clinical decision making for optimum patient care by minimising errors. It is a stepwise cognitive process of making more deliberate, thoughtful decision by organising the relevant information and defining the alternatives.

- **Step 1:** To frame focused, pertinent & answerable question.
- **Step 2:** Extensive literature research.
- **Step 3:** Critical appraisal of literature for relevance, intent, validity and applicability.
- **Step 4:** Integration of evidence generated by literature search with clinical expertise & patient's preferences to reach at a well informed decision about choosing one strategy out of many alternatives available.
- **Step 5:** Evaluation

New Drug Development

New Drug Development
Costly and time consuming process, done in a stepwise manner.
- **A.** Drug discovery and synthesis of lead or promising compounds.
- **B.** Translational research involving preclinical & clinical studies.
- **C.** Defining pharmacological profile of lead compounds by doing 'drug screening' by conducting molecular, cellular, organ system assays, whole animal studies & animal models of human disease.
- **D.** Application for patent is filed
- **E.** Evaluation for potential risks in 'preclinical toxicity testing' by conducting tests for acute, subacute, chronic toxicity, mutagenic, carcinogenic potential and effects on reproductive performance & also quantitative studies to estimate no-effect dose, maximum tolerated dose, minimum lethal dose and median lethal dose, etc.

Limitations of preclinical testing: Cost, time needed, concerns of animal safety, uncertain predictive value of animal data for humans.
- **F.** 'Notice of claimed investigational exemption for a new drug' (IND) is filed
- **G.** Clinical trials are done in four phases.

Phases of Clinical Trials

Phase 1 Clinical Trials:
Done in 20–80 healthy volunteers or patient volunteers, to establish drug effects as a function of dose, safe dosage range & detecting predictable toxic effects, pharmacokinetic parameters.
Usually open-label design, done in research centres by trained pharmacologists.

Phase 2 Clinical Trials:
Done in 100–500 patients with target disease in special clinical centres to determine efficacy and doses to be used in any follow-on trials & ceiling effect & help to detect broader range of toxicities.
Design: Single blind, placebo controlled

Phase 3 Clinical Trials:
Done on 500–3000 patients with target disease by specialists for the said disease at sites similar to those anticipated for ultimate use of drug. Phase 3 trials done to establish & confirm safety & efficacy & finalise indications of the drug & formulate guidelines for its therapeutic use.
Double blind, cross-over design is commonly used.

Phase 4 Clinical Trials:
Post-marketing surveillance for continued monitoring of safety, efficacy & acceptability of new drug in large number of patients under real-life conditions. This is important for detecting rare adverse effects, especially those associated with chronic long-term use of drug.

Good Clinical Practice (GCP)

GCP: An international ethical standard for designing, conducting, recording & reporting trials that involve the participation of human subjects.

ICH: International Council for Harmonization of technical requirements for pharmaceuticals for human use.

Principles of ICH GCP
- Clinical trials should be conducted in accordance with the ethical principles laid down in the Declaration of Helsinki.
- Trial to be initiated only if the anticipated benefits justify the risks.
- Rights, safety, and well-being of the trial subjects must be protected.
- Available information on an investigational product should be adequate.
- Trials should be scientifically sound & approved by the IRB/IEC.
- Freely given informed consent should be obtained.
- Data should be recorded, handled, & stored to allow its accurate reporting, interpretation, verification & confidentiality.
- Investigational products should be manufactured, handled & stored in accordance with applicable good manufacturing practice (GMP).
- Systems with procedures that assure the quality of every aspect of the trial should be implemented.

SECTION 13 Applied Pharmacology

69 Pharmacovigilance

PH 1.12 Define pharmacovigilance, its principles, and demonstrate ADR reporting.

Learning objectives

A student of MBBS phase II should be able to:
- Define pharmacovigilance and its importance.
- Explain the Pharmacovigilance Pprogramme of India (PvPI).
- Explain the methods of ADR reporting.
- Fill in the suspected adverse drug reaction form, version 1.4.
- Describe the importance of the mandatory fields of suspected ADR reporting form in causality assessment.

The World Health Organisation (WHO) **defines** pharmacovigilance as **'the science and activities relating to detection, assessment, understanding and prevention of adverse effects or any other drug-related problems'.**

Pharmacovigilance focuses on identifying adverse events or reactions related to drug use and ensuring they are promptly documented and reported to regulatory authorities. This enables necessary actions such as banning drugs, updating package inserts, revising labels by adding usage restrictions or safety warnings, and disseminating information through drug alerts/medical letters/advisories to enhance medication safety.

IMPORTANCE OF PHARMACOVIGILANCE

In Greek, the term *'pharmakon'* signifies both 'remedy' and 'poison', emphasising the inherent quality of drugs to cure and to cause harm, depending on context and dosage.

Interestingly, even the word pharmacology carries within it a hidden reminder: 'harm'. None of the drugs in current use can claim to be completely free of adverse effects.

Each drug undergoes extensive testing on animals and human subjects before marketing. Acute, subacute, chronic and specialised toxicity studies are conducted on animals for each drug that is a potential candidate for the status of 'medicine'. A drug that clears all the animal studies undergoes further clinical trials in humans in a phased manner (Phases I, II, III, IV). In spite of such extensive testing, **adverse events associated with drug use are a common occurrence** because of the following factors.

- Results obtained from **animal experiments are not sufficient to predict human safety**. Human response to a substance (drug) can be quite different from that of experimental animals (rats, mice, etc.).
- Pre-marketing clinical trials (Phases I, II, III) are done on selected study populations, for a limited time period. The frequency of ADRs and safety data generated by these trials are **not sufficient to comment on the safety of the drug in special populations** (pregnant/lactating women, pediatric and geriatric patients, etc.), because such groups were not included in clinical trials. Moreover, the long-term safety of a drug cannot be predicted from trials of limited duration involving a small number of subjects.
- Nowadays, new drugs are launched simultaneously in India and developed countries. As a result, **post-marketing safety data from other countries is not available at the time of launch.** Therefore, it is important to continue to monitor patients receiving the drug in the post-marketing phase as well.
- Numerous **environmental, drug-related and patient-related factors further escalate the risk** of developing adverse reactions. Undergoing drug treatment over a long term as in chronic diseases, simultaneous use of more than one drug, presence of comorbidities, and use of alternative systems of medication (AYUSH, i.e., Ayurveda, Yoga, Unani, Siddha, Homeopathy) along with allopathic medicines may contribute to the risk of unforeseen adverse reactions.

Adverse drug reactions not only increase morbidity, hospitalisation rate and healthcare costs, but are also a threat to patient life/safety and quality of life. ADRs reduce the compliance to drug treatment and have a negative impact on disease prognosis and outcome. However, majority of ADRs are predictable and preventable, provided one suspects adverse effects and the patients receiving the drug therapy are closely observed. Vigilance towards adverse effects in order to detect and manage them is an indispensable aspect of rational drug use.

Early detection of 'signals' of drug safety problems, hence, is of utmost importance. A **'signal'** is **'reported** information' about the **causal relation between an adverse drug event (ADE) and the drug,** which was previously undocumented or incompletely documented. **Sources for ADE reporting** include spontaneous reports from healthcare professionals or patients, patient support programmes, reports of clinical studies, medical literature, and reports provided by companies to regulatory authorities. All healthcare professionals, including doctors, nurses and paramedics, must be trained in recognising and reporting ADRs to safeguard the population from potential harm by drugs.

BENEFITS OF ADR MONITORING

i. The safety of new as well as existing therapies is assessed. ADR monitoring has led to the ban or withdrawal of several drugs worldwide due to safety concerns. For some drugs, package inserts are modified to improve safety. (Package inserts are the set of usage instructions provided with each medicine by the manufacturer. These can be modified according to the observed ADRs in the post-marketing phase.)
ii. It allows detection of preventable ADRs.
iii. ADR monitoring improves the drug safety knowledge of professionals.
iv. It provides quality assurance for use in drug evaluation programmes.

Pharmacovigilance Programme of India (PvPI)

The National Pharmacovigilance Programme was launched by the Central Drug Standard Control Organisation (CDSCO) in 2004. It was a highly participative programme aimed at collection, analysis and archiving of ADR data towards making regulatory decisions. In 2010, the CDSCO, under the Ministry of Health and Family Welfare, launched the nationwide Pharmacovigilance Programme of India (PvPI) in collaboration with the WHO Programme for International Drug Monitoring (WHO PIDM) through the Uppsala Monitoring Centre (UMC), Sweden.

Aim of PvPI

The aim of PvPI is to generate ADR data from the Indian population to ensure safety of drugs available in the Indian market.

The immediate aim was to develop a culture of detecting and reporting ADRs among healthcare workers (HCWs), because **spontaneous reporting of ADRs is the backbone of PvPI**. Healthcare professionals report detected ADRs on individual case safety reports (**ICSRs**). These forms are submitted to the nearest ADR Monitoring Centres (**AMCs**), which are set up in various medical colleges and hospitals across the country. The AMCs then forward the collected data to the National Coordinating Centre (NCC) located at the Indian Pharmacopoeia Commission, Ghaziabad. This information is subsequently shared with the Uppsala Monitoring Centre through **VigiFlow**, a web-based system (http://vigiflow.who.umc.org) developed by UMC for managing the ICSRs of ADEs and ADRs to facilitate the collection, processing, analysis and sharing of data.

Consumers can also report directly to NCC, Ghaziabad, or to the nearest AMC.

What Should Be Reported?

- Reporting of all suspected adverse effects of drugs as well as other medicinal substances including herbal, AYUSH and traditional remedies is encouraged.
- For new drugs (up to five years after the market launch), reporting of all types of ADRs (mild, moderate, severe and serious/life-threatening), including seemingly common/insignificant reactions, is encouraged and practiced to identify widespread errors in prescription writing.
- Even for well-established drugs, all serious or unusual ADRs should be reported.
- All suspected ADRs due to interactions with other simultaneously used drugs, foods, herbal products, environmental pollutants, etc., should also be reported.
- Reactions associated with drug overdose, vaccination, and prescription errors should also be reported.
- Adverse reactions to blood/blood products (Hemovigilance Programme of India, HvPI 2012) and Medical Devices (Materiovigilance Programme of India, MvPI 2015) are also monitored by the Indian Pharmacopoeia Commission (IPC), Ghaziabad.

How to Detect ADEs

For detecting adverse drug events (ADEs), one should **maintain a high index of suspicion** and observe the patient on drug treatment in a step-wise manner.

- **Special populations** like pediatric and geriatric patients, pregnant/lactating women, substance abusers, immunocompromised patients or those with comorbid conditions receiving drug therapy should be closely monitored to detect adverse drug reactions (ADRs).
- It is important to **monitor patients for compliance** to the prescription, to ensure that they have received and taken the prescribed drug correctly, while observing the suggested precautions if any (e.g., drug to be taken on empty stomach, at bedtime.)
- The **time difference** between the beginning of drug therapy and onset of the adverse event should be recorded.
- The **outcome of an adverse event** after discontinuing/decreasing the dose of the offending drug/drugs should be closely tracked. This is called **dechallenge**.

- Sometimes, it may be required to **rechallenge** the patient by giving same drug again and observing for recurrence of reaction. However, utmost care should be taken to first ensure safety of the patient. **Rechallenging just to confirm the cause of suspected ADR is not done, as it is unethical**. However, in some situations the treatment of initial condition warrants its reuse, e.g., cancer chemotherapy is given in a cyclic manner, with a time gap of a week or so. Patient gets rechallenged with the same drug in each chemotherapy cycle. Response of the patient to such accidental rechallenge should be closely monitored and recorded.
- One must **evaluate other causes** (the disease process itself/other drugs, foods, etc.) that may be responsible for the reaction.
- Review of relevant literature, discussions with peers or healthcare experts and the drug manufacturer may be of great assistance in recognising ADRs.

How to Report ADEs

Awareness and training of all healthcare workers, including doctors, dentists, nurses, pharmacists and paramedical workers, towards suspecting/recognising ADRs, filling of suspected ADR reporting form, and reporting to nearby AMCs is of prime importance in developing a successful pharmacovigilance programme. Flowchart 69.1 shows the suspected ADR form (Version 1.4) currently used in PvPI.

While reporting ADRs, it is important to remember that:

- Patient's identity is kept confidential. The staff members involved in recording and reporting ADRs must not disclose identity of patient to anyone. Even in the Suspected ADR Reporting form, **only the patient's initials** are to be mentioned, such as SS for Surjan Singh.
- HCWs involved in filling the Suspected ADR Reporting should **fill the form completely and clearly,** in legible writing, providing all the necessary details as required for causality assessment (CA).
- The **AMC Report number** is filled by AMC. A **worldwide unique number** is generated on Vigiflow after the report is filled.

The suspected ADR reporting form of PvPI has **four mandatory fields** or sections as shown in Flowchart 69.1. On the top right side of the form is the space for the patient's registration/IPD/OPD number.

Section A collects the **patient information.**
1. Initials of name, 2. Age, 3. Gender, 4. Weight, in kg

Section B, regarding the **suspected adverse reaction**, collects the **dates** of:
5. Start of event or reaction
6. End/Stopping of reaction and (6a) **lag time** between administration of suspected drug and onset of reaction
7. The reporter must provide a detailed description of the event in the form of a **brief case history**, ensuring that even a third party, unfamiliar with the patient, can clearly understand the situation. The report should include the **diagnosis, signs or symptoms, abnormal laboratory test results indicating an adverse event, actions taken**, and **the patient's response to those actions**. All details should be documented meticulously to ensure accuracy and clarity.

Section C provides details of **suspected medications.**

8. **All the drugs** taken by the patient should be mentioned. Care should be taken to specify the brand/generic name of drugs, manufacturers, batch number/lot number, expiry date of every drug along with dose, frequency and route used.
    - **Date** of starting, stopping (if done) of each drug and **indication** for use should be mentioned.
    - Last column in the table against Sr. No. 8 of **causality assessment**, is to be filled by AMC after discussion with the causality assessment committee.
9. It is also crucial to enter the **action taken** in response to the adverse reaction at Sr. No. 9, to record whether the suspected drug/drugs were discontinued or dose was altered.
10. The effect of reintroducing the suspected drug **(rechallenge)**, if done, should be mentioned at Sr. No. 10. If rechallenge was not done (as in majority of cases) this column is either left blank or 'not applicable' can be written.
11. Details of **other therapies** such as medicinal products taken concomitantly, including herbals, AYUSH, home remedies and indications for their use, etc., are to be mentioned at Sr. No. 11.
12. Only details of **investigations relevant to the event** are filled. All the investigations done on the patient need not be mentioned.
13. Medical history/history of medication, if any, must be mentioned, e.g., history of any such reactions, allergies, addictions, pregnancy/lactation, etc.
14. **Seriousness of reaction and outcomes** are ticked against appropriate choice at Sr. Nos. 14 and 15, respectively.

Section D collects the **reporter's details** comprising the reporter's name, occupation, contact details, signature and date of reporting. These are required for verifying any of the details, if needed later. The details of treatment of the event and any other information can be mentioned in the 'additional information column' at the bottom left corner of the form, but it is not mandatory.

Following the Coronavirus (COVID-19) pandemic, another suspected ADR reporting form has been issued by the NCC PvPI for drugs used in prophylaxis and treatment of COVID-19. In addition to details collected in the Suspected ADR form, the COVID ADR form requires necessary details of the patient category (confirmed case/HCW or /household contact of patient

SUSPECTED ADVERSE DRUG REACTION REPORTING FORM

Version 1.4

For VOLUNTARY reporting of ADRs by Healthcare Professionals

INDIAN PHARMACOPOEIA COMMISSION   (National Coordination Centre- Pharmacovigilance Programme of India)

Ministry of Health & Family Welfare, Government of India, Sector-23, Raj Nagar, Ghaziabad-201002

PvPI Helpline (Toll free) : 1800-180-3024   (9:00 AM to 5:30 PM, Monday-Friday)

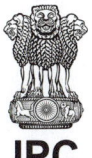

Initial Case ☐   Follow-up Case ☐

A. PATIENT INFORMATION*

1. Patient Initials :
2. Age or date of birth :
3. Gender M ☐   F ☐   other ☐
4. Weight (in kg.) :

B. SUSPECTED ADVERSE REACTION*

5. Event/Reaction start date (dd/mm/yyyy)
6. Event/Reaction stop date (dd/mm/yyyy)
7. Describe Event/ Reaction management with details, if any

FOR AMC /NCC USE ONLY

Reg. No. / IPD No. / OPD No. / CR No. :

AMC Report No. :

Worldwide Unique No. :

12. Relevant investigations with dates

13. Relevant medical/medication history (e.g. allergies, pregnancy, addiction, hepatic, renal dysfunction, etc.)

14. Seriousness of the reaction : No ☐   if Yes ☐   (please tick anyone)
☐ Death (dd/mm/yyyy)   ☐ Congenital – anomaly
☐ Life-threatening   ☐ Disability
☐ Hospitalisation –Initial/ Prolonged   ☐ Other Medically important

15. Outcome:
☐ Recovered   ☐ Recovering   ☐ Not Recovered
☐ Fatal   ☐ Recovered with sequelae ☐ Unknown

C. SUSPECTED MEDICATION(S) *

S. No.	8. Name (Brand/ Generic)	Manufacturer (if known)	Batch No. /Lot No.	Expiry date (if known)	Dose	Route	Frequency	Therapy dates Date started	Therapy dates Date stopped	Indication	Causality Assessment
i											
ii											
iii											
iv#											

9. Action taken after reaction (please tick)

10. Reaction reappeared after reintroduction of suspected medication (please tick)

S. No. as per C	Drug withdrawn	Dose increased	Dose reduced	Dose not changed	Not applicable	Unknown	Yes	No	Effect Unknown	Dose (if re-introduced
i										
ii										
iii										
iv										

11. Concomitant medical product including self-medication and herbal remedies with therapy dates (Exclude those used to treat reaction)

S. No.	Name (Brand/Generic)	Dose	Route	Frequency (OD, BD, etc.)	Therapy dates Date started	Therapy dates Date stopped	Indication
i							
ii							
iii#							

Additional Information :

D. REPORTER'S DETAILS*

16. Name & Address : _____

_____

Pin : _____   Email : _____

Contact No. : _____

Occupation : _____   Signature : _____

17. Date of this report (dd / mm / yyyy)

Signature and Name of receiving personnel:

Confidentiality : The patient's identity is held in strict confidence and protected to the fullest extent. Submission of a report does not constitute an admission that medical personnel or manufacturer or the product caused or contributed to the reaction. Submission of an ADR report does not have any legal implication on the reporter.

\# Use separate page for more information

* Mandatory fields for Suspected ADR reporting form

ADVICE ABOUT REPORTING

A. What to report?

All adverse events should be reported

Report non-serious, known or unknown, frequent or rare adverse drug reactions due to Medicines, Vaccines, & Herbal Products.

Report every serious adverse drug reactions. A reaction is serious when the patient outcome is:

- Death
- Life-threatening
- Hospitalisation (initial or prolonged)
- Disability (significant, persistent or permanent)
- Congenital anomaly
- Report intervention to prevent permanent impairment or damage

NOTE: Serious / Adverse Event following immunization can also be reported in Serious AEFI case Notification Form available on http://www.ipc.gov.in

B. Who can report?

All healthcare professionals (Clinicians, Dentists, Pharmacists and Nurse etc.) can report adverse drug reactions.

C. Where to report?

Duly filled in suspected Adverse Drug Reaction Reporting Form can be sent to the nearest Adverse Drug Reaction Monitoring Centre (AMC) or directly to the National Coordination Centre (NCC0 for PvPI.

Call on Helpline (Toll Free) 1800 180 3024 to report ADRs or directly mail this filled form to pvpi.ipc@gov.in

A list o nationwide AMCs is available at : http://www.ipc.gov.in, http://www.ipc.gov.in/PvPI/Pv_home.html

D. What happens to the submitted information?

- Information provided in this form is handled in strict confidence. The casuality assessment is carried out at AMCs by using WHO-UMC scale. The analyzed forms are forwarded to the NCC-PvPI through ADR database. Finally the data is analyzed and forwarded to the Global Pharmacovigilance Database managed by WHO Uppasala Monitoring Centre in Sweden.
- The reports are periodically reviewed by the NCC-PvPI. The information generated on the basis of these reports helps in continuous assessment of the benefit-risk ratio of medicines.
- The Signal Review Panel of PvPI reviews the data and suggests any interventions that may be required.

E. Mandatory fields for suspected ADR Reporting Form (*)

Patient initials, age at onset of reaction, reaction term(s), date of onset of reaction, suspected medication(s) & reporter information.

For Adverse Drug Reaction Reporting Tools
- E-mail: pvpi.ipc@gov.in
- PvPI Helpline (Toll Free) 1800 180 3024 (9:00 AM to 5:30 PM, Monday-Friday)
- ADR Mobile App : "ADRPvPI"

Flowchart 69.1. Suspected ADR reporting form version 1.4 in PvPI

(The form can be downloaded from https://cdsco.gov.in/opencms/export/sites/CDSCO_WEB/Pdf-documents/Consumer_Section_PDFs/ADRRF_2.pdf)

and pregnancy/lactational status for female patients) in Section A. Section B requires information relating to COVID-19 investigations (rapid test, RT PCR and any other radiological/ biochemical tests done), travel history within/outside country and relevant medical history.

Where to report

The filled form can be sent to the nearest AMC or directly to NCC, Ghaziabad. It can also be sent by email to pvpi@ipcindia.net or pvpi.ipcindia@gmail.com. The list of AMCs can be checked at http://www.ipcgov.in or via the toll free number 1800 180 3024.

Causality Assessment

A causality assessment is carried out **to study the cause–effect relationship** between the drug and reported adverse event based on various criteria. While there are many scales available for causality assessment, PvPI uses the WHO-Uppsala Monitoring Centre (UMC) scale. Criteria for causality assessment include:

- **Temporal (time) relationship** between drug administration and event onset, e.g., if the event occurs immediately after drug intake, it has a strong temporal relationship.

- **Pharmacological acceptability:** The ADE can be explained by knowledge of the **pharmacological characteristics** of the drug such as kinetics, mechanism of action, known actions, any similar reports from literature (case reports/ case series, etc.) and reports in Vigiflow.
- **Medical acceptability/plausibility** of the ADE as assessed from signs, symptoms, investigations and pathological findings (if any), which provide evidence of existence of the event.
- **Exclusion of other causes** that might have caused this event, such as disease and co-administered drugs.
- Response of event to **dechallenge** (drug withdrawal/dose reduction).
- Response to **rechallenge** (if done accidently, as per medical need of patients).

Categories of the WHO-UMC Scale

Based on the above-mentioned assessment criteria, there are six categories of association between a drug and the reported event, as given below.

1. **Certain** (clearly related) **event:** Time relation between the drug use and event is **plausible**, i.e., reasonable, acceptable or believable (2–6 weeks is usually considered plausible). Event is pharmacologically and medically **acceptable**. Response to **dechallenge is positive**. Response to rechallenge (if necessary) is positive.

    It is important to note that **pharmacological and phenomenological events** can be labelled as 'certain' without conducting a rechallenge. A pharmacological event is one that can be explained by the pharmacology of the drug, e.g., dryness of mouth with anticholinergics and hypoglycemia with anti-diabetic drugs.

    A phenomenological event is one that can occur only because of the drugs (e.g., fixed-drug eruptions, anaphylaxis, and acute dystonia) and is labelled as 'certain' without a rechallenge.

    For events like nausea, vomiting, epigastric pain, pancreatitis, and hepatotoxicity, which are not pharmacological or phenomenological, rechallenge is needed before they are labelled as 'certain'. However, exposing a patient again to the risk of an adverse effect just to prove association with the drug is unethical, and hence rechallenge can be accidental but never purposive.

2. **Probable** (likely related) **event:** The association between the drug and event is labelled as 'probable' even without rechallenge if:
    - There is reasonable temporal relation with therapy.
    - Event is not explainable by other drugs or diseases.
    - Dechallenge is positive.

3. **Possible** (may be related) **event:** The association between the drug and event may be described as 'possible' if temporal relation exists, but the event is explainable by other concomitant drugs or diseases. Dechallenge is either not done or information is not available (e.g., OPD cases).

4. **Unlikely** (not related) **event:** When time gap between drug administration and event makes the association doubtful or questionable but not impossible. Event could be explained by other co-administered drugs or doses.

5. **Conditional event:** This requires some more data, obtainable from the reporter.

6. **Unclassifiable events** require more data that is not possible to obtain.

The last 2 categories are not filled in Vigiflow.

Thus, the data collected from all ADR monitoring centers helps in detecting '**drug safety alerts**' that are circulated through various media for dissemination. These activities have played crucial role in modification of package inserts and ban on some drugs.

> **Problem-based questions**
>
> 1. **Define pharmacovigilance. Cite reasons to justify the need for pharmacovigilance.**
> 2. **Describe various categories of WHO-UMC causality assessment scale.**
> 3. **Answer following questions after studying the given case history.**
>   i. A 53-years old woman named Mrs. Daljeet Kaur, weighing 92 kg visited medicine OPD vide OPD registration number PIMS – 0882 on 23 January 2023. She was diagnosed with stage 1 hypertension. Tab Ramipril 5 mg, manufactured by 'X' was prescribed. There was no history of alcoholism, smoking, any concurrent illness or drug intake. The patient started taking the medicine as prescribed. She reported in medicine OPD on 20 February 2023 with complaint of dry, brassy, irritating cough. Patient could not show batch number and expiry date of preparation used. There was no history suggestive of or signs of tuberculosis, any allergic/ asthmatic reaction, respiratory infection, gastroesophageal reflux disease. All basic investigations and X-ray chest were normal on this visit. The patient was advised to stop ramipril and prescribed Tab. Amlodipine 2.5 mg. No specific treatment was given to suppress cough. During a follow-up visit on 3 March, 2023, the patient reported that the cough had disappeared and BP was adequately controlled with amlodipine. The current case has been reported by Dr Surjeet Walia of Department of Medicine in PIMS, Jalandhar, to ADR monitoring centre PIMS. Phone number of reporting doctor is 0999991666. Causality assessment committee of ADR monitoring centre labelled it as 'certain' on WHO-UMC scale.
>   a. Fill the suspected adverse drug reaction form of PvPI.
>   b. Why is this ADR labelled as 'certain'?

c. What is the effect of dechallenge and rechallenge in this case?

ii. A 76-year-old, male patient, Mr Surjan Singh, a resident of Jalandhar, was diagnosed with carcinoma sigmoid colon, stage 4, with secondaries in all seven hepatic segments. Surgical treatment was not possible and the patient was admitted to Oncology vide IPD number 90366 on 10 March 2023. He was put on palliative chemotherapy with the FOLFOX regimen consisting of 5-FU 500 mg/m^2 IV infusion over 3 hours, oxaliplatin 85 mg/m^2 intravenous and injection leucovorin 10 mg intravenous. Six such cycles were to be given at an interval of 15 days. Each cycle was to be preceded by dexamethasone, aprepitant and domperidone. The patient complained of disturbing nausea and 2–3 episodes of vomiting two days after the first chemotherapy cycle. There was bluish discoloration and tenderness at the site of injection after the 4th cycle. The patient was reassured and treated with injection pantoprazole 40 mg for three days, along with Thrombophob ointment for application at the injection site. The adverse effects gradually subsided over a few weeks. Similar effects were observed after each of the six chemotherapy cycles. All routine investigations were within normal limits. The patient suffered severe gastritis approximately 8–9 months ago, for which an endoscopy was performed and treatment provided for 8 weeks. No other medications were administered during this time. The case was reported by Dr. Raghbir Singh (mobile number 1212121212) of Oncology department PIMS, Jalandhar, to ADR monitoring centre PIMS on 8th June 2023. Literature reports indicate that 5-fluorouracil (5-FU) and oxaliplatin are associated with nausea, vomiting, and irritation at the injection site.

a. Fill the suspected ADR reporting form version 1.4 of PvPI.
b. Categorise the ADR using WHO-UMC scale.

Hints for problem-based questions and MCQs

1. Refer to page 900.
2. Refer to page 905.
3. i. a. Form 1.4 to be filled in.
      a. It is 'certain' because of –plausible temporal relation; no other drug/disease explains event/ positive dechallenge/ event is pharmacologically acceptable. So, it is labeled 'Certain' even without rechallenge.
      b. Dechallenge is positive, Rechallenge not done.
   ii. a. Form 1.4 to be filled in.
       b. Category: 'Possible' for nausea, vomiting (as history suggestive of other disease-causing gastric symptoms is present); 'Probable' for injection site irritant effect with oxaliplatin.

SECTION 13 Applied Pharmacology

70 Practical Pharmacology: Essential Drugs, DPL, Legal Aspects

PH 10.8 Describe essential medicines, fixed-dose combination, over-the-counter drugs and explain steps in choosing essential medicines.
PH 10.5 Identify and apply the legal and ethical regulation of prescribing drugs, especially when prescribing for controlled drugs, off-label medicines, and prescribing for self, close family and friends.
PH 10.2 Perform a critical evaluation of the drug promotional literature and interpret the package insert information contained in the drug package.
PH 10.1 Compare and contrast different sources of drug information and update on latest information on drugs.

Learning objectives

A student of MBBS phase II should be able to:
- Define essential medicines and describe the NLEM of India.
- Demonstrate the steps towards selecting essential medicines for a healthcare facility.
- Describe the characteristics of a rational fixed-dose combination.
- Describe implications of irrational FDCs.
- Enumerate the advantages of OTC drugs and the risks associated with their use.
- Describe the importance of various schedules under the Drugs and Cosmetics act.
- Describe schedules C-I to C-V of the US FDA.
- Critically evaluate a provided DPL as per WHO criteria.
- Enumerate and compare different sources of drug information including the latest updates on drugs.

ESSENTIAL MEDICINES

The concept of essential medicines aims at carefully selecting a limited range of essential drugs that **satisfy the priority healthcare needs of the population based on safety, efficacy, quality, and total cost, at all times**. It helps in providing:
- better healthcare.
- better drug management (including the procurement, storage, distribution and quality of the drug).

The intention is that essential medicines should be available at functioning healthcare systems:
- in adequate amounts.
- in appropriate dosage forms.
- with assured quality and adequate information.
- at a price affordable by individuals and the community.
- at all times.

Essential Drugs List (EDL)

The concept of essential medicines dates back to 1977 when WHO published the first model list containing 200 active substances. The list is revised by a WHO expert committee every 2 years. In 2003, there were 315 substances in this list. A separate list for patients of pediatric age group (up to 12 years of age) was published in 2007. The 18th edition of the list was released in 2013.

There is flexibility in implementation of the concept of essential medicines. It is each nation's responsibility to decide the status of 'essential' for a particular drug based on certain criteria. So far, 156 countries have prepared essential drugs lists (EDL) as per their requirements.

India released its first **National List of Essential Medicines (NLEM)** in 1996, which included **279 drugs**. Since then, the list has undergone five revisions (in 2003, 2011, 2015, 2018, and 2022) to incorporate advancements in the medical field and healthcare needs.

The NLEM released in September 2022 is the most recent version, available on the CDSCO website (http://cdsco.gov.in/opencms/opencms/en/consumer/Essential-Medicines/). The new list has 384 medicines; 34 new drugs have been added to the previous list of 2015 (which contained 376 drugs), while 26 drugs have been deleted. These 384 medicines are categorised into 27 therapeutic categories (e.g., general anesthetics, opioid analgesics, antidotes, anti-infective medicines). Only 22 fixed-drug combinations (FDCs) are included, of which 9 are HIV medicines. Among the antibiotics included in the WHO AWaRe classification, 16 antibiotics from the access category, 11 from the watch category, and one belonging to the reserve category have been included in the NLEM.

Based on the level of healthcare delivery system at which a medicine should be made available, the letters P (for primary), S (secondary), and/or T (tertiary) are also indicated in the list.

Core list
This contains the minimum drugs needed for a basic healthcare system; it lists the most safe, efficacious and cost-effective drugs for priority conditions.

Complementary list
Contains essential drugs for priority diseases, which are cost effective but for which specialised healthcare facilities may be needed. The list also includes essential drugs for less frequent diseases.

Selection of Essential Medicines
Before incorporating a drug in the essential list, its comparative effectiveness, safety in real life situations, relative cost-effectiveness and relevance to public health are reviewed.
The selection of content of EDL is a two-step process.
- Market approval, which is based on safety, efficacy and quality.
- Evaluation, which is based on comparison for forming a list for different levels of care.

For each drug included in the **NLEM**, the name of the drug, its category (P/S/T), route of administration, and strength are mentioned.

The NLEM helps in safe, effective treatment of priority diseases, promotes rational use of drugs, and allows optimum use of available health care resources.

State governments prepare their own lists from the NLEM for different levels of healthcare.

Preparing the EML for a Healthcare Facility
The selection of drugs for inclusion in the essential medicine list is based on several factors such as prevalence pattern of diseases, good evidence of efficacy and safety of drugs, comparison of their cost-effectiveness, level of healthcare facility for which EML is to be prepared, and facilities available for drug storage in the healthcare facility.

The process of preparing the EML comprises the following steps.
a. Study the pattern of prevalence of diseases in the area served by the particular healthcare facility.
b. Consider the level and size of healthcare facility, as the number of drugs stored should be appropriate. Storing too many drugs may cause wastage, while storing too few may cause interruption in supplies.
c. Before including a medicine in the EML of a facility, it must be assessed whether equipment/expertise for its administration is available or not. The availability of proper storage facilities should also be assessed.
d. The WHO EML and NLEM should be referred to while preparing list for a healthcare facility.
e. To decide between two medicines possessing similar properties, other factors such as their comparative efficacy, safety, cost and availability should be considered.
f. As far as possible, medicines in the list should be single-drug preparations. FDCs should be included only if there is proven evidence of their advantage over single-drug preparations.
g. Medicine selected should be such that adequate quality and bioavailability can be verified.

FIXED-DOSE COMBINATIONS (FDCs)
An FDC is a formulation that contains two or more active ingredients in fixed doses. To be rational, an FDC should offer proven advantage in safety, efficacy or compliance over the constituent drugs given separately.

Characteristics of rational FDCs
1. The components of FDCs should have comparable pharmacokinetic properties.
2. The adverse effects of ingredients in FDC should not be additive or supra-additive, e.g., combination of NSAIDs with cough and cold remedies increases the adverse effects.
3. The therapeutically useful effects of ingredients in a rational FDC should be additive, e.g., paracetamol and aspirin have additive analgesic effect. Similarly, sulphamethoxazole and trimethoprim combined in a 5:1 ratio produces sequential blockade of folic acid synthesis, making the combination bactericidal, even though the components are bacteriostatic. Another example is the FDC of antitubercular drugs, isoniazid, rifampicin, pyrazinamide and ethambutol, which is therapeutically beneficial as chances of emergence resistance are decreased by their combined use. FDCs also improve compliance of patients in long-term treatments.
4. In a rational FDC, one ingredient increases the therapeutic effect of the other as well as decreases its adverse effects, e.g., levodopa + carbidopa combined in a ratio of 1:1 produces this double benefit. Carbidopa, a peripheral dopa decarboxylase inhibitor, decreases the conversion of levodopa to dopamine in the periphery, whereby more of levodopa is available to cross blood–brain barrier and produce therapeutic benefit in parkinsonism. At the same time, systemic adverse effects decrease because of the formation of less dopamine in the periphery.
5. The drugs in combination formulations should act by different mechanisms.

Implications of irrational FDCs
FDCs are very popular in India due to their perceived convenience and ability to address multiple symptoms

or conditions simultaneously. However, a majority of them are deemed irrational, cause unnecessary exposure to drugs, and are hence unsafe and even dangerous. The following are the implications of irrational FDCs.

1. Patients are unnecessarily exposed to adverse drug reactions. Moreover, it becomes difficult to identify the ingredient in the FDC (e.g., combination of nimesulide with paracetamol, diclofenac with serratiopeptidase) that is responsible for the ADR.
2. It becomes difficult to adjust the dose of individual component drug, even if it is identified as the cause of harmful effects.
3. Some FDCs containing multiple drugs from the same therapeutic group, especially centrally acting drugs (e.g., FDCs of sedatives, antiepileptics, antipsychotics), are particularly dangerous.
4. Some FDCs are used to cover up for the inability to confirm diagnosis due to limited laboratory facilities. This is especially important for antibiotic combinations that can lead to the emergence and spread of resistant bacterial strains, which further escalates the cost of treatment. This is a matter of serious concern in a country like India with poor resources.
5. Irrational FDCs are misleading and increase the chances of medication errors.
6. Different pharmacokinetic properties of ingredients in an FDC raise the problem of deciding the frequency of dosage. There is increased financial burden on consumers without any additional benefit.
7. FDCs that contain dextropropoxyphene, corticosteroids, etc., have abuse potential.
8. Pharmaceutical industry uses FDCs merely as a means to prolong the patent of a product without any advantage to the patient.

Considering these aspects, the Government bans irrational FDCs occasionally, but these efforts are far from satisfactory. The authorities should take stringent action to check the manufacturing and marketing of irrational FDCs to optimise the use of meagre resources.

OVER-THE-COUNTER DRUGS (OTC)

Self-medication drugs or over-the-counter drugs (OTCs) are drugs that can be purchased without a prescription. These are used for self-management of common mild medical conditions such as pain, common cold, diarrhea, constipation and gastritis, which do not need clinical overseeing.

Advantages of OTCs

Due to improved educational status, general knowledge and socio-economic status, the practice of self-medication is successfully integrated into healthcare systems in many countries throughout world. They offer the following advantages:

- Empowers patients by providing them decision-making opportunities about minor ailments.
- Facilitates optimum use of clinical skills.
- Self-medication and the availability of OTC drugs increases patient access to medication and decreases the workload of medical services, especially if these are limited.

Risks of OTCs

Over-the-counter (OTC) medications, while convenient and widely accessible, carry certain risks, such as:

- Inappropriate dose of drug (under-dosage or over-dosage).
- Inappropriate (less or more) duration of drug use.
- Misdiagnosis leading to wrong medication.
- Risk of polypharmacy (the use of multiple medications by a patient) and drug interactions.
- Risk of serious adverse reactions, due to lack of knowledge about contraindications.

Substances like analgesics (e.g., aspirin and paracetamol), dietary supplements, skincare products containing acid-based active ingredients, ointments containing anti-inflammatory agents or antibiotics, medicated toothpastes, mouthwashes, wart removers, and anti-dandruff shampoos are commonly available as OTC drugs. Some drugs were initially used as prescription drugs, but after many years of safe use, they were approved by FDA as OTCs, e.g., ibuprofen and ranitidine.

For the safe use of OTC drugs, consumers should read and understand the labelling and package inserts (which provide a set of usage directions, warnings against unsafe use, and early signs of adverse effects to stop using the product). In case of any doubts, it is advisable to ask the pharmacist. However, the use of OTCs depends on self-diagnosis by the patient based on symptoms, which increases the chances of error. For example, gastritis symptoms may be a signal of impending angina or infarction, and a headache may be a sign of intracranial hemorrhage or other neurological emergencies. Misinterpreting such symptoms as harmless can delay appropriate treatment, which may be dangerous in some critical situations.

Thus, although self-medication with OTC drugs facilitates access to medicine without incurring the cost of a visit to healthcare centre and also reduces the workload on healthcare professionals, more studies are needed to assess the impact of self-medication in diverse healthcare settings. Regulators and manufacturers need to put in combined efforts to ensure the availability of products that are safe and effective along with complete and relevant information about the product. The quality of information as well as the mode of communication used for patient education play a key role in the safe use of OTC drugs.

DRUG SCHEDULES AND ACTS

The most important legal document for regulating the manufacturing, import, sale and distribution of drugs and cosmetics is the **Drugs and Cosmetics Act** (D&C Act), 1940, amended in 2001 and 2017. The supporting legislation, D&C rules, was framed in 1945.

Important Drug Schedules in India

In India there are schedules for each letter of the alphabet, excepting K,L,M, S,T,U,V and Z. The most important ones are:

- **Schedule H drugs** that are to be sold on prescription by a registered medical practitioner. These are labelled 'Schedule H prescription drug – Caution: Not to be sold by retail without the prescription of a registered medical practitioner'. Most pharmaceutical drugs are listed in this schedule.
- **Schedule H1 drugs** are also prescription-only medications considered potentially dangerous if taken without proper medical supervision. These drugs require stricter regulations compared to Schedule H drugs. They must carry the warning: 'Schedule H1 Prescription Drug – Warning: It is dangerous to take this preparation except in accordance with the medical advice. Not to be sold by retail without the prescription of a registered medical practitioner'. Record of their supply is to be maintained separately and record is maintained for up to 3 years. Antitubercular drugs, tramadol, pentazocine, etc., are examples of drugs of this category.
- **Schedule G** drugs include anticancer, diuretics and antiepileptic drugs. They must carry the warning 'Dangerous to take except under medical supervision'.
- **Schedule X drugs** are psychotropic drugs that need special license for their manufacturing and sale. They can be sold by retail on prescription of a registered medical practitioner only, and the retailers are required to save the prescriptions for a period of 2 years.
- **Schedule K** drugs include drugs listed as 'household remedies' such as pain balms, paracetamol, and antacids.
- **Schedule Y** previously regulated the requirements and guidelines for clinical trials and approval of new drugs in India. However, it has now been superseded by the "New Drugs and Clinical Trials Rules, 2019" (NDCT 2019).
- **Schedule C** refer to biological and special products such as vaccines, sera, insulin, toxins, and antitoxins.
- **Schedule F** mentions the requirements for functioning of blood banks.
- **Schedule E1** includes poisonous substances used in Ayurvedic, Siddha, and Unani (ASU) systems of medicine, such as opium, cannabis and snake venom.

Schedules C-I to C-V of the US FDA (Controlled Substances Act)

In the United States, controlled substances are classified into five schedules (C-I to C-V) under the **Controlled Substances Act** (CSA), which is regulated by the Drug Enforcement Administration (DEA) and the FDA. The classification is based on medical use, potential for abuse, and risk of dependence.

- **Schedule C-I:** Drugs like heroine, LSD and marijuana, which have no accepted medical use.
- **Schedule C-II:** Narcotics with high abuse potential and severe physical and psychological dependence, such as morphine, methadone, oxycodone, meperidine, barbiturates and amphetamines.
- **Schedule C-III:** Drugs that have moderate potential for physical, psychological dependence and an lower abuse potential than C-II drugs. Examples are sedatives other than barbiturate and stimulants other than amphetamines.
- **Schedule C-IV:** Limited potential for dependence and still lower abuse potential than C-III drugs, e.g., non-narcotic analgesics, antianxiety drugs.
- **Schedule C-V:** Drugs with lowest potential for abuse among controlled substances, e.g., cough syrups with low doses of codeine and cannabidiol products with very low THC content.

CRITICAL EVALUATION OF THE DRUG PROMOTIONAL LITERATURE

The term 'drug promotion' is used for informational and persuasive activities of drug manufacturers and distributors for inducing prescription, supply and purchase of medicinal drugs. It impacts rationality of drug use, manufacturing, price control mechanisms and overall cost of healthcare.

Prescribing doctors rely on various sources for information regarding the introduction of new drugs, formulations, and combinations, as well as new indications for existing drugs, newly identified adverse effects or interactions, and drug bans or restrictions. Important sources for such information are articles published in journals, verbal interaction with medical representatives of pharmaceutical companies and drug promotional literature (DPL). Due to time constraints, many physicians do not frequently read medical journals and, instead, rely heavily on medical representatives and drug promotional literature (DPL) from the pharmaceutical industry to stay updated. Thus, it is crucial for DPL to be factual, unambiguous, and compliant with established norms. Claims regarding the efficacy and safety of pharmaceutical products should be supported by substantial evidence.

However, DPL is often inaccurate, incomplete, and exaggerated, with efficacy and toxicity claims based on studies with poor methodology. This can lead to inappropriate prescriptions, suboptimal treatment outcomes, and increased healthcare costs. Therefore, physicians must be equipped with the knowledge and skills to critically evaluate the information provided by medical representatives and pharmaceutical industry in DPL to ensure evidence-based prescribing.

The International Code on Pharmaceuticals is developed by Health Action International (HAI). In India, for pharmaceutical marketing practices, the Organisation of Pharmaceutical Producers of India (OPPI) has established a self-regulatory code, with the WHO criteria being widely used for critically evaluating drug promotional literature (DPL). The **WHO criteria for drug promotional literature** include the following:

1. Names of the active ingredients (international non-proprietary name (INN) or approved generic name of the drug)
2. The brand name
3. Pharmacological data: Mechanism of action, brief description of main pharmacological actions
4. Clinical information about intended clinical uses, dosage regimens, relevant pharmacokinetic parameters, dose, frequency, duration of treatment, comments for use in hepatic and renal dysfunction, cardiac conditions, nutritional insufficiencies that may require dose adjustment, adverse effects, therapeutic index, contraindications/precautions/warnings for use, risk of clinically relevant drug–drug interactions, clinical description of symptoms of overdose and its management, comments for use in special populations like pediatric, geriatric patients, pregnant and lactating females.
5. Pharmaceutic information regarding dosage form, strength, excipients, shelf-life, storage conditions required, pack size, legal category, name and address of manufacturer.
6. References of publications to support the claims made about efficacy and safety, promotional matter to reflect superiority over other preparations available, such as pictures, graphs, figures, tables, and pharmaceutical package inserts.

A doctor should carefully examine the relative prominence of the brand name, generic name, efficacy claims, and adverse effects in drug promotional literature (DPL). It is essential to critically evaluate the scientific claims made, the accuracy and relevance of the provided scientific information, the credibility of references, the appropriateness of illustrations, and the methodology of studies supporting the drug's efficacy or safety. If any of these parameters are unclear or not explicitly stated, the necessary information should be requested to ensure that choosing a particular drug over others is well justified.

SOURCES OF DRUG INFORMATION

Drug informatics involves the discovery, utilisation, and management of information related to drug use and medications. It encompasses all aspects, including drug identification, pharmacodynamics, pharmacokinetics, dosing, adverse effects, and cost considerations.

Sources of drug information are categorised into three types: primary, secondary and tertiary sources.

1. **Primary sources** – Original research articles and clinical studies.
2. **Secondary sources** – Indexing and abstracting databases that summarise primary literature.
3. **Tertiary sources** – Reference books, guidelines, and review articles that compile and interpret existing data.

1. Primary sources

These consist of original research articles and clinical studies, providing the most up-to-date and detailed drug-related information. They serve as the foundation for secondary and tertiary sources. Among them, randomised controlled trials (RCTs) are considered to be the most reliable for evaluating drug efficacy and safety. However, review articles, editorials, and commentaries published in journals do not qualify as primary sources of drug information.

Interpreting research findings requires critical appraisal skills and experience. An understanding of the study design, statistical analysis, and potential biases is essential for drawing accurate conclusions.

2. Secondary sources

Secondary sources consist of tools such as *indexes* and *abstracts* that help readers quickly locate relevant research articles from the vast amount of drug-related research. They help in identifying high-quality primary sources that are available for further analysis.

- *Indexing systems* provide only bibliographic details (e.g., author, title, journal, and publication date).
- *Abstracting systems* offer bibliographic information along with abstracts and links to full-text articles when available.

Examples of secondary sources are:

- Electronic databases such as EMBASE, Index Medicus, MEDLINE, and International Pharmaceutical Abstracts (IPA)
- Review articles in journals which summarise and analyse findings from multiple primary sources.

3. Tertiary sources

These provide a concise and easily accessible summary of information derived from primary sources. These sources compile, interpret, and organise established drug-related data, making them useful for quick reference.

Examples of tertiary sources:
- Reference books and textbooks
- Drug compendia, including drug formularies, pharmacopoeias, Annual Physician's Desk Reference (PDR), Monthly Index of Medical Specialities (MIMS)
- Drug bulletins
- National, international, and WHO treatment guidelines
- Essential drug lists
- Medical literature databases, such as PubMed, DOAJ (Directory of Open Access Journals), and the Cochrane Database.

While tertiary sources provide well-established and validated information, they often have a **time lag** and may not reflect the most recent updates in drug research and clinical practice. Therefore, they should be supplemented with primary and secondary sources when seeking the latest data.

Drug compendia

These are tertiary sources of drug information that list the drugs available in the market for use as medicines. The information provided in drug compendia includes chemical composition, generic/brand names, indications, dosage recommendations, adverse effects, and cautions/contraindications in the use of drugs.

Drug compendia can be official or non-official.

- **Official compendia** include formularies and pharmacopoeias of different countries, e.g., National Formulary of India (NFI), Indian Pharmacopoeia (IP), British Pharmacopoeia (BP), US Pharmacopoeia (USP), etc. These are compilations of drugs legally approved for use in a country by their non-proprietary name.

  Formularies contain clinically-oriented pharmacology and regulatory information for prescribing and dispensing drugs.

  Pharmacopoeias contain information about the physical/chemical properties of drugs, identification, assay methods, standards and quality specifications for medicines, such as list of appropriate tests for confirmation of identity, purity, strength, and potency.

- **Non-official compendia,** such as Current Index of Medical Specialities (CIMS) and Monthly Index of Medical Specialities (MIMS), are re-published by professional bodies. They provide information about trade names as well and are reliable sources for drug information.

Questions for Practice

1. Demonstrate the stepwise process for preparing the EML for a given healthcare facility.
2. Enumerate characteristics of rational fixed-dose combinations.
3. Comment on the rationality of fixed-dose combination of:
   a. First-line antitubercular drugs
   b. Any of the NSAIDs with paracetamol
   c. Sedatives with antipsychotics
   d. Atropine and diphenoxylate
   e. Sulphamethoxazole and trimethoprim
   f. Sedatives with antispasmodics
   g. Amoxicillin and cloxacillin
   h. Amoxicillin and clavulanic acid
4. Enumerate the advantages and risks of using OTCs.
5. Describe the meaning of
   a. Schedule H drugs
   b. Schedule X drugs
   c. Schedules of the FDA Controlled Substances Act.

SECTION 13 Applied Pharmacology

71 Practical Pharmacology – Prescriptions, Prescription Errors, P-Drug, Dosage Calculation and Drug Interactions

PH 10.4 Describe parts of a correct, rational and legible prescription and write rational prescriptions for the provided condition (Examples of conditions to be used are given with other relevant competencies).
PH 10.6 Perform a critical appraisal of a given prescription and suggest ways to improve it.
PH 10.3 To prepare and explain a list of P-drugs for a given case/condition.
PH 1.13 Identify and describe the management of drug interactions.
PH 2.3 Explain the rationale and demonstrate the emergency use of various sympathetic and parasympathetic drug agonists/antagonists (like noradrenaline, adrenaline, dopamine, atropine) in case-based scenarios.

Learning objectives

A student of MBBS phase II should be able to:

- Enumerate the parts of a correct, complete and legible prescription.
- Write a rational prescription for a given condition.
- Critically evaluate the provided prescription.
- Identify errors in a prescription, and rewrite it in the correct form.
- Describe the criteria used for drug comparison.
- Describe the methods of ranking drugs.
- Select P-drug for a given condition or clinical problem, demonstrating the stepwise process.
- Calculate the appropriate dose of a drug for an individual patient.
- Enumerate types of drug interactions.
- Explain the various types and basis of interactions with suitable examples.
- Describe clinical significance of drug–drug interactions
- Calculate the dose/infusion rate/flow rate of a drug in a given clinical condition.

PRESCRIPTIONS

A prescription is a written communication that serves as a direct link between the physician, pharmacist and patient. It is a medico-legal document issued by a licensed medical or dental practitioner to guide a pharmacist in dispensing specific medications tailored to an individual patient's needs. While traditional compounding of drugs by pharmacists has largely been replaced by pharmaceutical manufacturing, their role now focuses on accurately dispensing medications and counselling patients on their proper use. Prescriptions are primarily written in English, often including standard Latin abbreviations.

Parts of a Prescription

A prescription has the following parts (Box 71.1).

1. **Date**: It helps pharmacist to ascertain when the prescription was written. This is important for preventing misuse, particularly of controlled substances like narcotics or Schedule H1 drugs.
2. **Patient information**, i.e., OPD number, name, age, sex, address and diagnosis, is important for accurate identification to avoid mix-ups when multiple patients have similar names, and to reconfirm specific needs such as dose for children considering age, weight, etc.
3. **Superscription**: The symbol ℞, found at the beginning of a prescription, is derived from the Latin word *recipere*, meaning "to take." (The symbol is considered as the sign of Jupiter, the Greek god of healing.) While traditionally ℞ was interpreted as a directive ("you take"), in the modern context it symbolises the start of a medical prescription. The pharmacist interprets this as an indication to dispense the prescribed medications, while the patient takes it as an instruction for use.
4. **Inscription**: It is the main body of prescription. It contains the name of drug, dosage form, strength or amount, route by which the medicine should be taken, and number of doses. Name of each medication is written in a separate line. (Previously, physicians used to mention the base or active ingredient, adjuvant and vehicle separately for compounding the medication.)
5. **Subscription**: It is a direction to the pharmacist for preparing the prescription and the number of doses to be dispensed. However, as most of the drugs prescribed are available in suitable formulation nowadays, this part of prescription is now eliminated or considered synonymous with the next part, i.e., the signa.

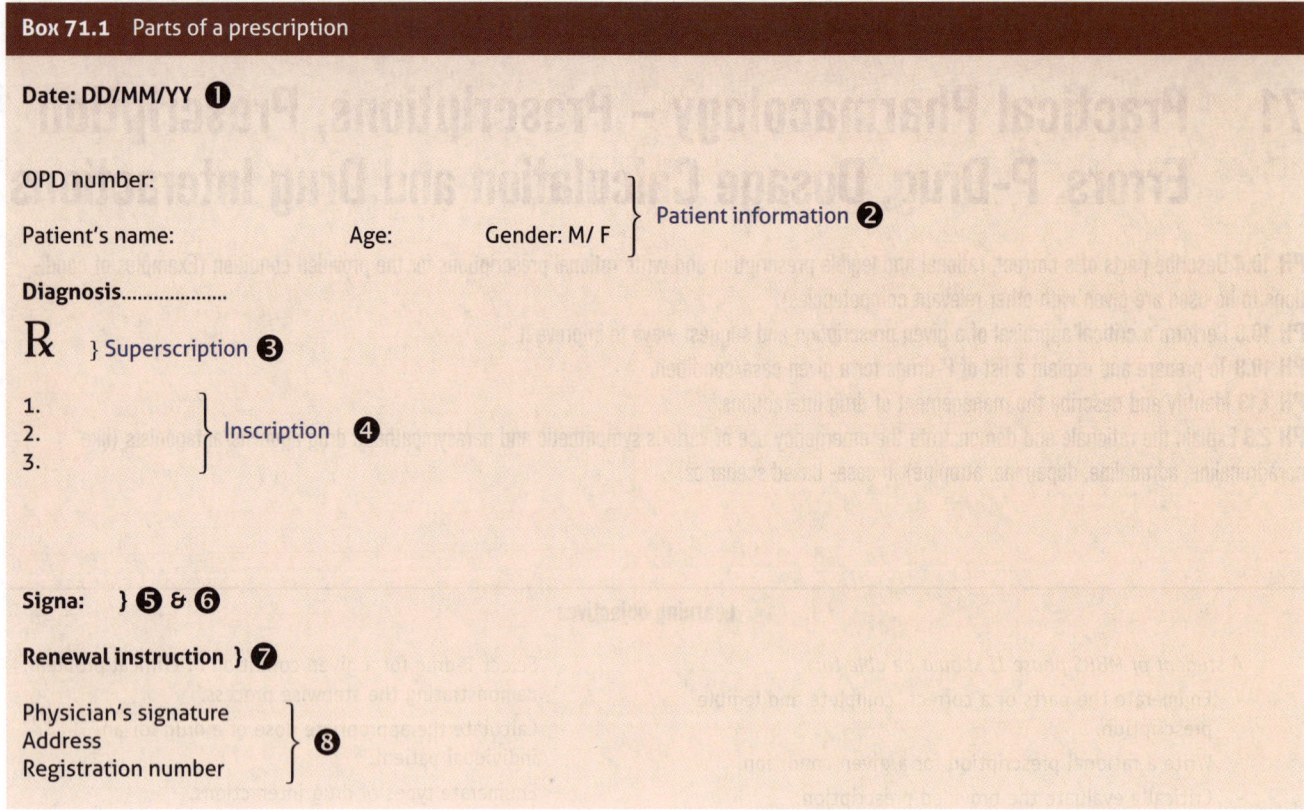

Box 71.1 Parts of a prescription

6. **Signa or Signatura:** This refers to the specific instructions provided by the physician to patients on how to use the prescribed medication such as dosage (e.g., 1 tablet), frequency (e.g., twice daily), route of administration (e.g., oral, topical, injection), duration (e.g., for 7 days) and special instructions (e.g., dilution, if needed). This is interpreted and further explained by the pharmacist to the patient and transferred onto the prescription label if needed.
7. **Renewal instruction:** It indicates whether the older prescription is to be refilled or not. If yes, for how many times. This is especially important for prescriptions containing narcotics and other habit-forming or Schedule H1 drugs.
8. **Signature, address and registration number** of the prescribing doctor is the last part of the prescription. A sample prescription is shown in Box 71.2.

Common Prescription Errors

1. **Abbreviations:** These pose a major problem in understanding the prescription. Prescribers should avoid acronyms like CPZ for chlorpromazine, CBZ for carbamazepine, 5ASA for 5-aminosalicylic acid, and PCM for paracetamol. These are not standard abbreviations and are liable to be interpreted differently by different individuals. To avoid errors due to misinterpretation of abbreviations, it is a good practice to write the full generic name of the drug, preferably in capital letters. Instead of OD, write once daily, and so on.
2. **Look-alike, sound-alike drugs** (LASA): Names of many drugs sound alike or appear similar to some other drugs. Confusion between non-proprietary and proprietary drug names can occur due to their similar appearances or pronunciations, e.g., Lasix (furosemide, a loop diuretic) and Lorax (lorazepam, a benzodiazepine), or Glynase (glyburide, an antidiabetic) and Zinase (a combination of diclofenac and serratiopeptidase). Illegible writing and incomplete knowledge of drugs compound the errors in dispensing. Some drugs have similar packaging, which may cause error while taking the drug.
3. **Strength of preparation:** When a product is marketed in multiple strengths, such as amoxicillin capsules (250 mg and 500 mg) or the amoxicillin–clavulanic acid combination (e.g., Augmentin 375 mg and 625 mg), and H_1 blocker ranitidine (150 mg and 300 mg), specifying the exact strength after the drug's name is crucial to prevent overdosing or underdosing errors. Utmost care should be taken to write the strength of formulation clearly and legibly. One should avoid writing decimals if the digit after the decimal is a zero alone to avoid misreading mishaps, e.g., 1.0 mg could be misread as 10 mg. Likewise, the use of mcg and µg for microgram should be avoided as one may misread mcg as mg (missing the c in between); or µg may be misread as mg, resulting in incorrect dosing.

> **Box 71.2 Sample prescription**
>
> Prescribe for a 50-year-old old male patient suffering from essential hypertension.
>
> Date 13.01.2025
>
> OPD NO: CR1234/13.1.25
> Name: ABC   Age: 50 years   Gender: Male
> Address: 366, Mota Singh Nagar, Jalandhar city
>
> **Diagnosis:** Moderate hypertension
>
> ℞:
> 1. Tab. Olmisartan 20 mg, once daily for 15 days
>
>   Reduce added salt, oily food in diet.
>   Do regular exercise for at least 20 minutes daily.
>   Come for follow-up on 28.01.25.
>
>   Refill: as advised after follow up on 28.01.25
>
>   Signature;
>   Name: Dr XYZ
>   Registration NO: 12345
>   Mob- 1234567890
>   Dept of Pharmacology
>   PIMS, Jalandhar

4. **Errors due to mix-up of words and figures,** etc: Illegible writing can lead to confusion between letters or numbers that resemble each other, such as Z and 2, l and 1, 1 and 7, V and 0, or H and 0. Therefore, while mentioning strength, the unit should always be mentioned and extra care should be taken to write it clearly and legibly.
5. **Dosage form:** Some drugs are available in more than one dosage forms, e.g., tablet/dispersible tablet/capsule. This detail must be clearly mentioned.
6. **Polypharmacy:** Prescription of more than one medication at a time is called polypharmacy. The chances of drug–drug interactions increase with the number of drugs prescribed; hence, it is essential to ensure that the minimum number of **necessary medicines** is prescribed. Special care should be taken to restrict unnecessary prescription of antibiotics, nutritional supplements, proton pump inhibitors, etc., as they not only increase economic burden on the patient but also cause other problems like development of resistance and alteration of the kinetics of prescribed drugs.
7. **Signa or instructions to the patient are incomplete or missing altogether:** They are an essential part of a prescription and have enormous impact on the safe and effective use of drugs. It is essential to communicate treatment instructions to patients clearly and effectively to prevent medication errors. This includes specifying the route, time, dose, and duration of treatment. Additionally, writing these instructions in the patient's vernacular language ensures better understanding and compliance.

Practice prescriptions for commonly encountered conditions

Prescribe for managing the following cases and provide pharmacological basis to justify the drugs prescribed.

Autonomic nervous system

1. A 50-year-old farmer experienced sudden profuse sweating, salivation, lacrimation, and a runny nose while spraying insecticide in his fields. On examination, BP was found low, PR = 60 bpm, and pupils were markedly constricted (pinpoint). He was diagnosed with **organophosphate poisoning**.
2. A 13-year-old boy was brought to emergency with complaints of dryness of mouth and difficulty in talking and swallowing. The boy had a high-grade fever, flushed skin, dilated pupils, and photophobia. PR = 114 bpm. Careful history-taking revealed that he had consumed berries of the **datura plant**.
3. A 40-year-old female patient suffering from SABE was administered injection penicillin G. Within a few minutes the patient complained of breathlessness and sinking sensation. On examination, BP was 84/50. The patient was diagnosed with **anaphylactic shock**.
4. A 70-year-old male patient complained of difficulty in starting micturition, urgency and frequency of micturition, especially during night, weak urinary

stream and sensation of incomplete emptying of bladder. Digital per rectal examination revealed a moderately enlarged prostate, smooth and firm with no nodules. On investigation, prostate-specific Ag (PSA) was found slightly elevated (3.5 ng/mL). A diagnosis of **benign prostatic hypertrophy Grade II** was made.

5. A 48-year-old male patient complained of blurring of vision and headache. On ophthalmological examination, his intraocular pressure was found high and papilledema was present. The patient was diagnosed with **open-angle glaucoma**.

Autacoids

6. A 36-year-old female patient presented with severe throbbing headache on the left side, accompanied by nausea, vomiting, photophobia and phonophobia. A diagnosis of acute **migraine** was made.

7. A 58-year-old female patient complained of morning stiffness and symmetrical pain in small joints of both hands. Rheumatoid factor was positive. A diagnosis of **rheumatoid arthritis** was made.
   i. Prescribe for immediate relief of symptoms
   ii. Prescribe for long-term management of this case.

8. A 69-year-old male patient has pain in right toe. On examination, his metatarsophalangeal (MTP) joints were red, warm and swollen. Investigation revealed raised serum uric acid levels. A diagnosis of **acute gout** is made.
   i. Prescribe for relief of symptoms.
   ii. Prescribe for long-term management of this case.

9. A 24-year-old male patient presented with body aches, cough, sneezing, running nose after travelling by road on a windy night. On examination, conjunctival injection was present. No other abnormality was detected. Patient was diagnosed as suffering from **common cold**.

Central nervous system and NSAIDs

10. A 35-year-old female patient of generalised tonic–clonic epilepsy was brought to emergency in an acute convulsive state. It was diagnosed as **status epilepticus**.

11. A 60-year-old female patient with severe osteoarthritis worries constantly about her decreased ability to walk. Her family members reveal that she remains isolated in her room, and does not talk much to anyone. At times, she starts crying for no reason. A diagnosis of **minor depression** is made.

12. A 19-year-old boy is brought to psychiatry OPD by his parents with complaints of auditory hallucinations and somatic delusions for about 2 months. His behaviour and expressions are also inappropriate. There is history of such symptoms in his maternal uncle also. Patient is diagnosed with **schizophrenia**.

13. A 72-year-old male patient presented with rigidity, tremors and bradykinesia. He exhibited a waddling gait, took small steps (baby steps), and had an expressionless face. A diagnosis of **parkinsonism** was made.

14. A 34-year-old male patient, a known case of schizophrenia on haloperidol therapy, presented with rigidity, mask-like face and baby steps. Patient is diagnosed with **drug-induced parkinsonism**.

15. A 55-year-old male complained of headache, blurring of vision, epigastric pain, vomiting and dyspnea after consuming locally-made alcohol. On examination, BP = 86/58, PR = 48 bpm. Diagnosis of **methanol poisoning** was made. Prescribe for the management of this case.

16. A 17-year-old boy presented with dyspnea and blurring of vision. Examination revealed cyanosis, pinpoint pupils, needlestick marks on both arms and a BP of 80/60. The patient had a history of opioid addiction. A diagnosis of **morphine poisoning** was made.

Cardiovascular system

17. A 65-year-old woman, a known case of hypertension for more than 20 years, presents with peripheral edema, dyspnea, fatigue and reduced exercise tolerance. On examination, JVP was raised and liver enlarged. A diagnosis of low-output **congestive right heart failure** was made.

18. A 40-year-old male visited OPD for routine check-up and investigations prior to joining a new job. His BP was 150/90. There were no other symptoms or findings. A diagnosis of **essential hypertension** was made.

19. A 30-year-old patient with a history of hypertension presented with features of cerebrovascular accident and was diagnosed with **hypertensive crisis**. Prescribe for immediate management of this case.

20. A 75-year-old woman complains of pain in the left chest radiating to jaw and left arm. The pain increased with activity and subsided on resting. ECG showed ST depression and T wave inversion. A diagnosis of **angina pectoris** was made.

21. A 65-year-old male presented with severe chest pain, profuse sweating, anxiety and restlessness. ECG showed appearance of Q wave, ST elevation and T wave inversion. A diagnosis of acute myocardial infarction was made.

Respiratory system

22. A 26-year-old woman complained of some difficulty in breathing on exposure to dust. On auscultation, bilateral rhonchi are found. A diagnosis of **bronchial asthma** is made.

23. A 45-year-old male patient presented with severe breathlessness and wheezing. Examination revealed laboured breathing, exhaustion, and the inability to complete sentences, with speech limited to monosyllables. PR= 124/minute; chest auscultation

revealed bilateral rhonchi. The patient was diagnosed with acute **severe asthma**.

24. Prescribe for a patient complaining of **dry cough**.
25. Prescribe for a patient complaining of **cough with expectoration**.

Endocrinology

26. A 55-year-old obese female patient complains of nocturnal polyuria, polydipsia and polyphagia. On investigation, FBS is 210 mg/dL, urine is positive for glucose and HbA1c is 9.2%. Patient was diagnosed with **non-insulin-dependent diabetes mellitus (NIDDM)**.
27. A 26-year-old patient of IDDM was brought to hospital in semiconscious state. Examination revealed dehydration, low BP, and fruity smell in breath. Investigations showed RBS =490 mg/dL and positive ketone bodies. The diagnosis was **diabetic ketoacidosis**.
28. A 40-year-old woman presented with weight gain, constipation, excessive fatigue, lethargy, and menorrhagia. On investigation, Hb = 10 g/dL, T_3 and T_4 low and TSH raised. A diagnosis of **hypothyroidism** was made.
29. A 38-year-old multigravida had excessive vaginal bleeding with passage of clots after full-term normal vaginal delivery. Diagnosis of **atonic post-partum hemorrhage (PPH)** was made.
30. A 10-year-old boy presented with generalised weakness and pallor. He has a history of delayed milestones and delayed teeth eruption. On examination, costochondral junctions were found swollen. A diagnosis of **rickets** was made.
31. Prescribe for a 65-year-old female patient with **bone pains** and **reduced bone density**.

Chemotherapy

32. A 44-year-old female patient presented in OPD with complaints of anorexia, weight loss, rise of temperature in evening, and cough with expectoration. Investigations showed sputum positive for acid fast bacilli (AFB), and opacity in left lung upper lobe in chest X-ray. A diagnosis of **pulmonary tuberculosis** was made.
33. A 28-year-old male presented with bouts of high-grade fever and shivering on alternate days. Fever was followed by excessive perspiration and gradual drop in temperature to normal. Blood film was positive for malarial parasite. A diagnosis of acute **malaria** was made.
34. A 26-year-old woman presented with frequent grumbling pain in abdomen, frequent passage of watery stools with blood and mucus. On examination, there was tenderness along the line of colon and in the right iliac region. Stool examination confirmed an diagnosis of **amoebic dysentery**.
35. A 40-year-old male had a few asymmetrical, hypopigmented macular lesions accompanied by sensory loss. Ulnar nerve was thickened and enlarged. A diagnosis of paucibacillary **leprosy** was made.
36. A 60-year-old patient had disseminated, symmetrical, hypopigmented patches with smooth shiny surface. Leonine facies were present. A diagnosis of **multibacillary leprosy** was made.
37. A 50-year-old nurse was accidently exposed to needlestick injury from an **HIV-positive patient**. Prescribe **post-exposure prophylaxis** for this healthcare worker.

GIT

38. A 32-year-old male driver presented with pain in epigastrium, nausea, bloating sensation and belching. The symptoms are pronounced after a heavy meal. On endoscopy, a **duodenal ulcer** was seen.

Blood

39. A 6-year-old boy with a habit of eating paper, mud, etc., presented with fatigue, pallor and failure to thrive. Hb was 7 g/dL; PBF showed a microcytic hypochromic picture. Stool was positive for hookworm ova. A diagnosis of **iron deficiency anemia** with **hookworm infestation** was made.
40. A pregnant woman on routine examination had Hb level 5.6 g/dL. PBF showed a macrocytic picture. A diagnosis of folic acid deficiency **megaloblastic anemia** was made.

PRESCRIPTION AUDIT

Prescription audit or critical appraisal of prescription is a tool for systematic evaluation of the quality of prescriptions for improving the quality of healthcare. The intention is not to find fault with healthcare professionals; rather, it promotes discussion of the prescription, with the motive of providing suggestions for improvement. Prescription audits should be carried out at every level of healthcare services—primary, secondary and tertiary. Problems arising from prescription errors may range from mild discomforts to disease aggravation, treatment failure, toxicity, adverse effects, etc. A prescription audit can help prevent such problems with timely detection and corrections to ensure patient safety.

Criteria for Prescription Audit

1. **Format of prescription** should be checked for all components, namely date, patient name/age/sex/weight/contact details, diagnosis, superscription, inscription, subscription, signa, renewal instruction and doctor's signature, name, registration number, and

contact details. Comments should indicate whether the format is adhered to, with respect to each detail.

2. **Details of prescription:** The following parameters should be checked and commented upon:
   a. Diagnosis: provisional or definitive, is mentioned or not
   b. Drugs prescribed: number of drugs, rationality of each drug to detect underprescription or overprescription, whether the prescribed drug is the drug of choice (DOC) for the diagnosed condition based on efficacy and safety
   c. Drugs prescribed by generic or brand names
   d. Name of drug written legibly or in capitals
   e. Mention of dosage form, dose, frequency, route and duration of each drug
   f. Are any of the prescribed drugs banned/irrational/FDC/hazardous
   g. Number of injectables prescribed and rationality of using parenteral preparations
   h. Explanation of correct use of prescribed drugs to the patient.
   i. Cost of treatment

After checking all these details, the prescription is categorised as rational, partially rational or irrational. Changes required for rational therapeutics should also be mentioned, or the prescription is rewritten in the correct form.

LIST OF P-DRUGS FOR A GIVEN CONDITION

Definition of P-Drugs

P-drugs are medications that a **physician prefers to prescribe** most frequently, based on personal experience, familiarity, and individual judgment. These are drugs that the physician has gained confidence and trust in, due to their effectiveness, safety profile and overall clinical experience (drug of choice) for a particular condition. In other words, P-drug is a prescribing **doctor's "personal drug" for a particular disease** and not for any particular patient.

P-drugs can vary from one doctor to another and amongst regions and countries due to differences in the essential drugs list, cost factor, availability, etc.

Selection of P-Drug

The selection of a P-drug is a systematic, stepwise process that includes defining the diagnosis, specifying the therapeutic objective, making an inventory of effective groups of drugs, identifying the second-choice drug group (in case the first choice is not suitable), choosing an active substance, dosage form, dosage schedule and duration of treatment.

Steps in the selection of a P-drug

1. First, the patient's complaint should be clearly defined and the signs, symptoms and investigations should be thoroughly analysed to make a final diagnosis.
2. Then, therapeutic objectives or desired outcome of treatment (e.g., symptom relief, disease resolution, reversal of pathophysiological changes, prevention of complications) are identified.
3. A list of effective groups of drugs for each objective is prepared.
4. An effective group is selected by comparing and ranking drug groups based on 4 important criteria: efficacy, safety, cost, and suitability (Box 71.1).
5. A drug is selected from the group selected in step 4, using the same criteria for comparison and ranking as mentioned in Box 71.1.
6. The pharmacological name of the selected drug, dosage form, dosage schedule and duration of treatment, and information to patient about correct use and warnings (if any) are mentioned in the prescription.

Box 71.1 Ranking of drug groups/drugs

Criteria for drug comparison

Four important criteria recommended for comparison of drugs in *Guide to Good Prescribing* are their efficacy, safety, cost, and suitability.

1. **Efficacy** is defined as maximal response produced by a drug. In the context of prescribing/prescription, the term 'effectiveness' is more appropriate as it is a wider term that includes pharmacokinetic and pharmacodynamic characteristics of the drug.
2. **Comparison of safety** is based on acute, chronic adverse effects of available choices.
3. **Cost:** 'Total cost' of treatment is a more useful criteria as compared to 'unit cost'. For conditions requiring lifelong treatment, it is more meaningful to compare 'per day cost' of treatment using different drug options available.
4. **Suitability:** Refers to the suitability of a specific drug for a given patient/population. It encompasses the above three criteria, i.e. effectiveness, safety, and cost. In addition, other factors requiring consideration are dosage schedule, route of administration, and convenience of dosage form, cautions/contraindications for use and drug–drug or drug–food interactions.

Ranking of drug groups/drugs

There are different methods for ranking drugs based on above four criteria (effectiveness, safety, cost and suitability).

A. The most commonly employed method for drug ranking is the modified multi-attributive utility analysis (MAUA), described below.
   i. A score ranging from 0–1 is given for each criterion such that the total score for all four criteria adds up to one. This depends on the importance of that criteria (called **weight**) for a given disease. For example, a 0.4 weight score for effectiveness, 0.3 for safety, 0.1 for cost and 0.2 for suitability totals to 1 (0.4 + 0.3 + 0.1 + 0.2 = 1). (See Table 71.1.)

ii. A group of drugs is selected based on their classification.
iii. Using a scale of 0–10, numbers are allocated to each drug for all the four criteria, e.g., effectiveness score for a drug 'A' is 8, safety score is 3, cost score is 6 and suitability score is 5.
iv. Scores allocated for particular criteria are multiplied by its weight.
v. Finally, all scores are added to get the final rank for each drug.

Table 71.1 Drug ranking

Criteria	Effectiveness	Safety	Cost	Suitability
Weight (0–1)	(0.4)	(0.3)	(0.1)	(0.2)
Score on the (0–10) scale	8	3	6	5
Weight × Score	3.2	0.9	0.6	1
Total score for drug A	3.2 + 0.9 + 0.6 + 1= 5.7			

In similar manner, the total score is calculated for all drug options available and a score-based ranking is obtained.

B. In some cases, comparisons are based on scores assigned as + or – signs against each criterion, for different drugs as shown in Table 71.2.

Table 71.2

Drug options	Effectiveness	Safety	Cost	Suitability
Drug A	+++	++	--	++
Drug B	+++	-	-	+
Drug C	++	++	+	+++

C. Recently, artificial intelligence techniques like DRUML (Drug Ranking Using Machine Learning) have been used to select the most suitable drug (e.g., anticancer drug) through ordered rankings.

Any of the above methods may be used based on personal choice and ease of use. Prescribing physicians can refer to journal articles, original clinical studies, review articles, newsletters, published books, national formularies and national and international treatment guidelines while preparing lists of available drug groups/drugs for a given condition.

Advantages of P-Drug Concept

1. With repeated use, physicians become more proficient and confident in the procedure.
2. The effectiveness, safety and suitability of the drug for a particular patient is thoroughly considered in the process of selecting the P-drug. Therefore, the chances of therapeutic failures, adverse effects and interactions are lower.
3. The practice of selecting P-drugs increases rationality of prescriptions.
4. It is a simple, convenient and easy way of healthcare delivery.

Practical exercises in P-drug selection

41. A 46-year-old female patient complains of pain and stiffness in small joints of her hands and feet. The pain is worse in the morning and decreases with physical activity. On investigations, ESR and CRP is found raised and RA factor is positive.
   i. What is the diagnosis in this case?
   ii. Select a P-drug for the patient.

42. A 38-year-old male presented with occasional headaches. On general physical examination, his heart rate was 78 bpm, and BP was 150/90 mmHg. Renal function tests (RFT), fasting blood sugar (FBS) and liver function tests (LFT) were within normal limits. He was diagnosed with essential hypertension. Select an appropriate P-drug for this case.

DRUG INTERACTIONS

Sometimes, the combined use of several drugs is essential for achieving desired therapeutic objectives. Multiple drug therapy is the rule rather than exception in conditions like tuberculosis, leprosy, acquired immunodeficiency disease, malignancy, and cardiac failure.

The term **potential drug interaction** refers to the possibility that combined use of two drugs may:

- alter (enhance or diminish) the intensity of pharmacological effects of one or both drugs.
- cause appearance of new effects, not seen with either of drugs used alone.

The drugs prescribed together can interact with each other or with over-the-counter drugs, herbal drugs, and nutritional supplements. Chances of interactions rise with increase in the number of prescribed drugs.

TYPES OF DRUG–DRUG INTERACTIONS (DDIs)

I. Based on Outcome

Based on the outcome, drug interactions can be useful or desirable or harmful or undesirable.

A. Useful or desirable interactions

Such interactions occur when:
- the beneficial effect of the drug is enhanced.
- detrimental or adverse effect of one drug is mitigated by concomitant use of another drug.

The mechanisms responsible include the following:

Additive effect: The resultant effect upon combined use of drugs is equivalent to the sum total of individual drug effects. Drugs with different physiological mechanisms can work together to enhance therapeutic effects and allow lower doses of each drug. Examples include cardiac glycosides and diuretics in CHF, β blockers and diuretics in hypertension, and levodopa with anticholinergic drugs in parkinsonism, where their actions complement each other.

Synergistic effect: The effect produced by the combination of drugs is greater than the sum of the effects produced by individual drugs. For example, sulphamethoxazole and trimethoprim, which target sequential steps in folic acid metabolism, are individually bacteriostatic, but their combination (cotrimoxazole) becomes bactericidal.

Augmentative effect: One drug of the pair induces an increase in the concentration or prolongs the presence of the other drug in body fluids. For example, peripheral dopa decarboxylase inhibitors like carbidopa and benserazide increase levodopa concentration in the brain and augment its antiparkinsonian effect.

Facilitative effect: In this case, one drug facilitates or makes it possible for the other drug to produce its desirable effect. For example, the intact cell wall of enterococci is relatively impermeable to aminoglycosides. Penicillins inhibit cell wall synthesis and facilitate the entry of aminoglycosides into organisms, thereby exerting bactericidal effect.

Reparative effect: In a pair exhibiting such an effect, one drug counteracts the undesirable effect of other drug. For example, in antacid combinations, the laxative effect of magnesium hydroxide counteracts the constipating effect of aluminium hydroxide.

Thus, beneficial or desirable interactions form the pharmacological basis for the combined use of drugs in many clinical conditions like infections, malignant disorders, cardiovascular disorders, contraception, and analgesia.

B. Harmful or undesirable interactions

These occur when the:

- therapeutic effect of one drug is reduced or opposed by the other drug. For example, the hypoglycemic effect of oral antidiabetic drugs is reduced by glucocorticoids.
- adverse effects of simultaneously used drugs are enhanced. For example, propranolol and verapamil are not given together because of the risk of AV blocks.

The concurrent use of multiple drugs for a condition demonstrates the approach of a clinical problem from more than one pharmacological angle. At the same time, it is important to realise that risk of adverse interactions rises with the number of drugs administered to a patient. In clinical practice, the frequency and clinical implications of harmful interactions is so important that beneficial effects of combined drug use are often overlooked.

II. Based on Time of Occurrence

Interactions can occur before administration or after administration, i.e., in vitro or in vivo.

A. Interactions occurring before administration

In vitro interactions occur because of the physical or chemical incompatibility of drugs. Mixing 2 drugs in the same syringe or infusion bottle can result in the following:

- Physical changes like precipitation, colour change and effervescence.
- Change in pH may occur when drugs are added to intravenous fluids. Dextrose 5% as well as normal saline (0.9% NaCl solution) are acidic. pH of dextrose 5% is 3.5–6.5, while that of normal saline is 4.5–7. Thus, their buffering capacity is very low and addition of drugs can readily change the pH of IV infusion fluids. For example, heparin is stable in NaCl 0.9% for up to 24 hours, but loses activity if added to dextrose 5%. In contrast, noradrenaline retains 80% potency in dextrose for about 5 hours but gets rapidly oxidised in blood or 0.9% NaCl.
- Chemical reaction between the drugs: Majority of drugs are weak acids or bases. To make them soluble, their salts are prepared. Mixing solutions of these salts may cause precipitation, e.g.,
  - Succinyl choline chloride and thiopentone sodium interact chemically when mixed in the same syringe.
  - Excess of protamine present in 'protamine-zinc insulin' (PZI) interacts with soluble insulin when filled in the same syringe.

Such interactions are usually mentioned on package inserts as caution regarding 'drugs that cannot be mixed in the same syringe before administration'. Thus, such interactions are easily preventable if the healthcare personnel read the package insert of medications carefully. Moreover, addition of drugs to blood, amino acid solutions, and fat emulsions should be avoided. Drugs should be added to simple solutions as far as possible. Addition of a single drug to simple solutions like NS or dextrose 5% is safer than adding 2 or more drugs to it.

B. Interactions occurring after administration

In vivo interactions happening after administration of two drugs simultaneously or one closely following the other, given by same or different routes, are very common. These interactions are of **two types based on the underlying mechanism.**

a. Pharmacokinetic interactions that involve alteration in drug concentration in body fluids.
b. Pharmacodynamic interactions that occur without any change in drug concentration in body fluids.

a. Pharmacokinetic interactions

Pharmacokinetic interactions occur when one drug alters the ADME (absorption, distribution, metabolism, excretion) of the other drug.

1. Changes in absorption

The rate and extent of absorption of drugs, especially after oral administration, can be altered by food or other simultaneously administered drugs. Changes in the rate of drug absorption usually do not have significant clinical impact, but changes in extent of absorption may cause either sub-therapeutic or toxic levels with serious clinical implications.

- **Presence of food**
  - Fatty food can increase absorption of some drugs like griseofulvin, itraconazole, posaconazole (antifungal drugs).
  - Food decreases absorption of drugs like ampicillin, tetracycline, and erythromycin (antimicrobial agents). Oral absorption of antifungal drug voriconazole is reduced with fatty meal.
  - Dairy products can form complexes with drugs such as tetracyclines, fluoroquinolones, and iron preparations, reducing their absorption.
  - Some drugs interfere with absorption and use of nutrients, e.g., patients taking antacids and metformin develop vitamin B_{12} deficiency as its absorption decreases.
- **Formation of unabsorbable complexes:** Some drugs can form unabsorbable complexes with other concurrently used drugs, e.g., tetracyclines with calcium and iron salts, sucralfate with phenytoin, and cholestyramine with thyroxine, digoxin, warfarin, etc. In such cases, the interaction can be easily prevented by maintaining a gap of 2–3 hours between ingestion of the two drugs.
- **Reduced gastric lumen acidity** due to proton pump inhibitors, H_2 blockers and antacids interferes with absorption of antifungal drugs such as ketoconazole, itraconazole, and posaconazole, and antiviral drugs such as zalcitabine, tipranavir, and amprenavir.
- **Change in gastrointestinal motility:** Prokinetic drugs such as cisapride and metoclopramide cause gastrointestinal hurrying and decrease the transit time through intestines. This reduces the absorption of simultaneously given poorly soluble drugs like digoxin and adrenal steroids. Drugs with anticholinergic effect and opioids have the opposite effect on GI motility, e.g., anticholinergics reduce the rate of absorption of levodopa, paracetamol, etc.
- **Reduced gut flora** associated with the use of broad-spectrum antimicrobial agents like tetracyclines, cotrimoxazole, and ampicillin interferes with the enterohepatic circulation of oral contraceptives and may cause contraceptive failure.
- Drugs with large surface area can adsorb other drugs and reduce their absorption, e.g., activated charcoal suspension is used as antidote for decreasing absorption of many drugs/poisons.

Changes in absorption at sites other than GIT may also be responsible for drug interactions, e.g., hyaluronic acid is a component of connective tissue that prevents the spread of foreign substances. Hyaluronidase depolymerises hyaluronic acid and increases the rate of absorption from subcutaneous and intramuscular injection sites.

- Hyaluronidase is also useful for spreading the irritant drug over a larger area to dilute it and aid absorption if there is perivenous spillage of the latter during IV injection.
- Vasoconstrictors like adrenaline are added to local anesthetics to reduce their systemic absorption, resulting in prolonged effect at the local site.

2. Changes in distribution

Competition at the plasma protein binding site is considered as an important mechanism for drug–drug interactions. Acidic drugs have affinity for plasma albumin and basic drugs for α-glycoprotein. Theoretically, when two highly bound drugs are given together, one drug (the drug with higher affinity or the one given first) displaces the other from the plasma protein binding site, resulting in increased concentration of free drug and toxic effects. Such interactions are called **displacement reactions**. However, these are not of much clinical relevance, because most of the drugs exert therapeutic actions at concentrations at which the plasma protein binding sites are far more than that are required. So, a competition between drugs for binding sites has been overemphasised in the past. Secondly, unbound drug concentration rises only transiently as the free drug gets rapidly distributed, inactivated and eliminated. Some clinically important displacement interactions are:

- Warfarin, an oral anticoagulant, is displaced from the plasma protein binding site by aspirin, indomethacin, clofibrate, etc., resulting in enhanced anticoagulant action and bleeding tendency.
- Tolbutamide, an oral antidiabetic drug, is displaced from plasma protein binding sites by sulphonamides, dicoumarol, salicylates and increases the risk of hypoglycemia.
- Sulphonamides and vitamin K displace bilirubin from binding sites and may cause kernicterus in newborns.

A clinically significant impact of displacement reactions occurs only when a drug is displaced from tissue binding sites, and at the same time its metabolism and/or excretion is also reduced, e.g., quinidine reduces tissue protein binding as well as clearance of digoxin, resulting in digoxin toxicity.

Pharmacokinetic drug interactions can also occur in the plasma itself by **direct chemical reactions**. For example:

- Protamine is strongly basic. It can neutralise heparin, which is acidic. 1 mg of protamine can neutralise 100

units of heparin. This may be useful during heparin overdose.
- Desferrioxamine, a straight-chain compound, twines around ferric ions in plasma and forms a stable, non-toxic complex that can be easily excreted in urine. This interaction has clinical utility in iron overloading.

3. Changes in metabolism

The **induction or inhibition of metabolising enzymes** is the mechanism most frequently responsible for drug–drug interactions.

Enzyme inducers like antiepileptics (phenobarbitone, phenytoin, carbamazepine, primidone), rifampicin, rifabutin, corticosteroids, chronic alcoholism, cigarette smoking, chlorinated hydrocarbon insecticides (DDT), and food additives increase the synthesis of microsomal cytochrome P450 enzymes. This, in turn, increases enzyme activity. These drugs can increase their own metabolism (autoinduction, e.g., carbamazepine) and that of other simultaneously administered drugs.

- This could be troublesome in situations when an enzyme inducer is given to a patient already using a drug requiring precise control of its levels in blood, e.g., warfarin.
- Enzyme inducers can cause contraceptive failure by increasing metabolism of estrogen and progesterone. Before prescribing any enzyme inducer drug to women of the reproductive age group, it should be ascertained that they are not on oral contraceptives. If that is the case, an alternative method of contraception should be advised.

Enzyme inhibitors, in contrast, decrease the metabolism of other concurrently administered drugs and potentiate their effect. Effects of inhibition of metabolising enzymes are generally more predictable and quicker than those of enzyme induction. Few examples of DDIs due to enzyme inhibition are described below.

- CYP450 is inhibited by azole antifungal drugs, macrolides, HIV protease inhibitors, metronidazole, ciprofloxacin, proton pump inhibitors, isoniazid, fluvoxamine, etc.
- Warfarin can inhibit metabolism of phenytoin, tolbutamide, etc., resulting in their toxicity.
- All broad-spectrum antimicrobial agents can inhibit metabolism of warfarin, resulting in bleeding tendencies.
- Allopurinol, a xanthine oxidase inhibitor, decreases metabolism of 6-mercaptopurine (6-MP) and azathioprine and potentiates their effects.
- Erythromycin inhibits metabolism of cyclosporine, calcium channel blockers and statins.
- Many drugs like disulfiram, sulphonylureas and metronidazole inhibit aldehyde dehydrogenase enzyme. This interferes with alcohol metabolism and causes accumulation of acetaldehyde, resulting in unpleasant symptoms. This is called the disulfiram reaction with alcohol.
- Grapefruit juice inhibits metabolism of cyclosporine and terfenadine.
- Metabolism of some drugs depends on hepatic blood flow. For example, reduced hepatic blood flow by propranolol decreases lignocaine metabolism and prolongs its half-life.

4. Changes in excretion

Drugs may compete for the same excretory sites in the kidneys. One drug may interfere with the excretion of the other drug, resulting in prolonged half-life and risk of toxicity. For example, tolbutamide excretion is inhibited by sulfinpyrazone, increasing the chances of hypoglycemia due to increased effect of tolbutamide.

Inhibition of tubular secretion at active transport sites: Many drugs are eliminated by active tubular secretion in the kidneys. Simultaneous administration of another drug may interfere with tubular secretion. Examples include:

Acidic drugs:
- Tubular secretion of penicillins and cephalosporins is inhibited by uricosuric drugs like probenecid, increasing their duration of action.
- Aspirin and probenecid reduce tubular secretion of methotrexate.

Basic drugs:
- Tubular secretion of procainamide is inhibited by amiodarone.

Promotion of tubular reabsorption: Thiazide diuretics, ACE inhibitors, tetracyclines, and certain NSAIDs increase lithium reabsorption in the proximal convoluted tubule (PCT), reducing its excretion and predisposing to lithium toxicity.

Changes in urinary pH: The pH of urine varies widely from 4.6 to 8.2. This can affect the extent of tubular reabsorption of drugs, especially those excreted unchanged in urine. $NaHCO_3$ increases urinary pH so that acidic drugs like aspirin and phenobarbitone get ionised in the tubular lumen, decreasing their reabsorption. This is useful in acidic drug toxicity. Similarly, acidification of urine by ascorbic acid enhances excretion of basic drugs like amphetamines.

Thus, one has to be cautious while prescribing drugs to patients on **chronic therapy** with other enzyme inducers/inhibitors or uricosuric drugs. Appropriate dosage adjustment can prevent many serious drug–drug interactions.

Many pharmacokinetic interactions can be easily prevented by advising the patient about whether a particular drug is to be taken before or after food, whether two drugs can be ingested together or with a gap of 30–60 minutes between them.

b. Pharmacodynamic interactions

These interactions occur due to the effect of simultaneously given drugs on a physiological system in the same or opposite direction, resulting in enhanced or decreased response, respectively. For example:

- Cardiac depressant effects of propranolol and verapamil add up and cause serious conduction and atrio-ventricular blocks.
- The effect of CNS depressant drugs is enhanced by alcohol but decreased by caffeine, theophylline, etc.
- Glucocorticoids decrease the hypoglycemic response of oral antidiabetic drugs.
- Propranolol can mask peripheral symptoms of hypoglycemia caused by antidiabetics, leading to serious hypoglycemic shock.
- NSAIDs blunt the BP-lowering effect of antihypertensives by causing sodium and water retention.
- Dangerous hyperkalemia can occur with concurrent use of ACE inhibitors and K^+-sparing diuretics.
- Anticoagulant warfarin given along with antiplatelet drugs increases the risk of hemorrhagic complications.
- Dopamine antagonists such as neuroleptics reduce the antiparkinsonian effect of levodopa.

c. Combined toxicity

If two or more drugs having toxic effects on the same organ are used concomitantly, extensive organ damage can occur. For example:

- Aminoglycosides and loop diuretics—both are ototoxic.
- Aminoglycosides, vancomycin, some cephalosporins, amphotericin B—all are nephrotoxic.

The list of such interactions is very long, exhaustive and almost impossible to remember. However, clinically significant interactions are mentioned with the pharmacology of specific drugs. Many such harmful pharmacodynamic interactions can be prevented if the prescriber knows the drug actions thoroughly.

III. Based on Severity

DDIs can be mild, moderate, and severe.

Mild: The efficacy is slightly limited or frequency of minor adverse effects (sedation, fatigue, gastrointestinal disturbances, nausea, malaise) increases. No action is usually required.

Moderate: DDIs can cause exacerbation of disease or adverse effects that are distressing or intolerable, but not life-threatening.

Severe DDIs are life-threatening and require stoppage of the offending drugs, hospitalisation and active management of the patient in case of conditions such as liver failure and cardiac arrhythmias. Patient is closely monitored. Change in drug or dosage is needed to control this.

CLINICAL RELEVANCE OF DRUG–DRUG INTERACTIONS

The **incidence of clinically significant drug–drug interactions (DDIs)** ranges from 3–5% in patients receiving few drugs, to up to 20% in patients receiving more than ten drugs. Most hospitalised patients receive at least 6 or more drugs. Thus, the risk of DDIs is much higher in hospitalised patients receiving multiple drug therapy.

Consequences of DDIs can be beneficial or harmful for the patient. Addition of therapeutic/useful effects is beneficial but that of toxic/adverse effects is harmful. In contrast, antagonism of therapeutic effects is harmful and antagonism of adverse effects is useful, as shown in Table 71.3.

PREVENTION OF DDIS

1. The best way to prevent DDIs is to keep the possibility of their occurrence in mind while prescribing.
2. **Patients particularly susceptible** to developing or getting affected by drug–drug interactions include:
   - Elderly patients suffering from multiple diseases, those receiving multiple drugs for various illnesses and those with compromised functioning of drug-

Table 71.3 Consequences of DDIs

	Synergism	Antagonism
Therapeutic effect	Beneficial: - Codeine + paracetamol - Amoxicillin + clavulanic acid - Trimethoprim + sulphamethoxazole	Harmful: - NSAIDs + antihypertensives - Corticosteroids + antidiabetic drugs
Adverse effect	Harmful: - Alcohol + CNS depressants - Propranolol + verapamil - Aminoglycosides + cephalosporins - Furosemide + gentamicin	Beneficial: - Hydrochlorothiazide + spironolactone - Misoprostol + NSAIDs

eliminating systems are at an increased risk of developing DDIs, especially those acting on CNS or CVS.
- Patients with acute illness such as left ventricular failure, pneumonia and status epilepticus usually receive several drugs. At times, it may be difficult to distinguish iatrogenic symptoms from those of the underlying disease in such cases.
- Patients with unstable disease, e.g., diabetes mellitus, epilepsy, cardiac arrhythmias, and dementia may have exacerbation of the disease secondary to adverse drug interactions.
- Patients dependent on drug treatment such as transplant recipients and those with connective tissue disorders are more severely affected by interactions that alter plasma concentration of the drug on which the patient is dependent.
- Patients with severe renal or hepatic impairment, such as in cirrhosis, CHF and uremia, are more prone to develop drug interactions because the liver and kidney are mainly responsible for drug elimination.
- Patients getting treatment from more than one doctor are more prone to develop interactions because each doctor is unaware of the totality of the patient's treatment details.

3. **Drugs with greater potential** to cause DDIs.
   - Drugs with a major effect on a vital process, e.g., antiarrhythmic drugs, warfarin, CNS depressants
   - Drugs with steep dose–response curve, e.g., verapamil, loop diuretics
   - Drugs causing concentration-dependent toxicity, e.g., digoxin, lithium, aminoglycosides, methotrexate
   - Drugs whose loss of effect leads to breakthrough disease, e.g., prednisolone, antianginals, valproate
   - Prophylactic drugs, on whose action the patient depends, e.g., cyclosporin, oral contraceptives
   - Drugs with saturable hepatic metabolism, e.g., phenytoin, ethanol, theophylline

Hence, the need for utmost caution while prescribing drugs that cause DDIs cannot be overemphasised. Care should be taken to individualise doses as needed and plan frequent follow-up visits to regularly monitor therapeutic response, lab values and presence of any adverse toxic effects.

Commonly asked DDI-based practice questions

43. Comment on the following drug combinations.
    a. Atropine and diphenoxylate
    b. Neostigmine and atropine
    c. Enalapril and spironolactone
    d. Furosemide and spironolactone
    e. Diuretics and digoxin
    f. Amlodipine and atenolol
    g. Levodopa and carbidopa
    h. Sulphamethoxazole and trimethoprim
    i. Sulfadoxine and pyrimethamine
    j. Amoxicillin and clavulanic acid
    k. Isoniazid and pyridoxine
    l. Imipenem and cilastatin

44. Comment on following drug combinations.
    a. Propranolol and insulin
    b. Succinylcholine and thiopentone
    c. Phenytoin and oral contraceptives
    d. Levodopa and pyridoxine
    e. Alcohol and cefoperazone
    f. Alcohol and metronidazole
    g. MAO inhibitors and tyramine
    h. Propranolol and verapamil
    i. Nitrates and sildenafil
    j. Diuretics and digoxin
    k. Diuretics and lithium
    l. Diuretics and indomethacin
    m. Furosemide and aminoglycosides
    n. Phenytoin and tolbutamide
    o. Aspirin and warfarin
    p. Tetracycline and iron
    q. Rifampicin and oral contraceptives
    r. 6-Mercaptopurine and allopurinol
    s. 5-FU and folinic acid

EMERGENCY USE OF AUTONOMIC DRUGS

Sympathetic agonists such as adrenaline, noradrenaline, dopamine, and dobutamine are lifesaving drugs in certain emergency situations, as listed below.

- Adrenaline is a physiological antagonist of histamine (the most important mediator in immediate type hypersensitivity reactions). Adrenaline 0.5 mg given intravenously quickly reverses bronchoconstriction and vasodilatation caused by histamine and is lifesaving in anaphylactic shock.
- Intravenous adrenaline 1:10,000 is administered in the central vein along with other emergency life-saving measures like cardiac massage in cardiac arrest secondary to drowning, electrocution, or Stokes–Adam syndrome
- A cotton swab soaked in 1:10,000 adrenaline or 1% phenylephrine can be inserted into the nasal cavity for control of epistaxis. α_1-mediated vasoconstriction arrests bleeding from the nasal mucosa. Such use can control local bleeding in surgery, trauma, and even gastric erosions.
- Noradrenaline is a pressor agent used in shock, However, in cases of hypovolemic shock, dopamine infusion (2–3 mcg/kg/minute) is preferred over noradrenaline as it maintains renal perfusion.
- In patients with acute cardiac decompensation due to severe resistant congestive heart failure (CHF) or

myocardial infarction (MI) or patients undergoing cardiac surgery, short-term intravenous infusion of drugs having β_1 agonistic action like dopamine or dobutamine helps to tide over the crisis. Dose of dopamine is 4–5 mcg/kg/minute. The initial dose of dobutamine is 0.5–1 mcg/kg/minute and then 2–20 mcg/kg/minute, but should not exceed 40 mcg/kg/minute.

- Anticholinergic drug atropine is lifesaving in organophosphate insecticide poisoning as it blocks muscarinic receptors and can reverse central as well as peripheral actions of organophosphates. Atropine is administered in a dose of 2 mg intravenously and can be repeated after 10 minutes.

In most emergency situations, drugs are given intravenously. The dose should be carefully calculated and administered at the correct flowrate, as mistakes can have disastrous outcomes.

Dose, Infusion Rate and Flowrate Calculations

For administration of the correct dose, body weight of the patient, strength of the solution and type of infusion set must be known.

a. *Body weight of patient* is used to calculate the total dose of drug to be administered, e.g., dose of dopamine in acute decompensated heart failure is 4–5 mcg/kg/minute. For a patient weighing 60 kg, infusion rate will be 60 × 4–5 = 240–300 mcg/minute. The rate will be higher for a heavier patient and vice-versa.

b. *Strength of solution*: Most drugs to be used by intravenous route are dispensed as solutions in ampoules or vials. In weight by volume (W/V) solutions, when solids are mixed with liquids, 1 g of solid is mixed with liquid ingredient to make a total of 100 mL of 1% formulation.

Thus, 1% W/V solution contains 1 gram of substance dissolved in 100 mL of solution. Since 1 gram = 1000 milligrams, a 1% solution contains: 1000 mg in 100 mL → 10 mg/mL.

Adrenaline 1:1000 solution implies that it contains 1 g in 1000 mL, i.e., 1000 mg in 1000 mL = 1 mg/mL.

c. *Type of infusion set*: The main types of infusion sets available are regular/macro and micro infusion sets. Drop factor of an infusion set refers to the 'number of drops that make 1 mL', and depends on the type of infusion set.

- Drop factor of a **regular/macro** infusion set = 15 drops per mL
- Drop factor of **blood transfusion set** = 15 drops per mL
- Drop factor of **micro infusion set** = 60 drops per mL

Formulae used

1. Volume (mL) = Rate of infusion (mL/minute) × Time
2. Rate of infusion = Volume (mL) / Time (minute)
3. Flow rate = Infusion rate (mL/minute) × Drop factor (gtts/minute)

Gtts stands for the Latin word 'guttae', meaning drops. So, gtts/minute means drops/minute.

Examples

1. Adrenaline is available as 1:1000 solution. Calculate the volume required to administer 0.5 mg dose in a patient suffering from anaphylactic shock.
   Ans: 1:1000 solution contains 1 g in 1000 mL, i.e., 1 mg per mL. So, 0.5 mL of this solution will contain 0.5 mg.

2. A drug 'X' is to be injected in a dose of 0.8 mg/kg bodyweight in a patient weighing 50 kg. It is available as a 10% solution. Calculate the required volume for the correct dose.
   Ans. Dose = 0.8 mg/kg = 0.8 × 50 = 40 mg
   Strength of solution = 10% = 10 g in 100 mL, i.e., 10 × 1000 mg in 100 mL
   = 1 mg in 0.01 mL.
   So, the required dose is 40 mg in 40 × 0.01 mL = 0.4 mL.

3. Calculate the IV flow rate for 1200 mL normal saline (NS) solution to be infused in 6 hours using a regular infusion set.
   Ans. Infusion rate = Volume (mL)/ Time (minutes) = 1200 mL /6 × 60 minute = 3.33 mL/minute.
   Flow rate = Infusion rate × Drop factor = 3.33 (mL/minute) × 15 gtts/mL) = 45 gtts/minute.

4. Calculate the flow rate of dopamine in a patient of shock, given that the weight of the patient = 60 kg, dose of dopamine 4 mcg/kg/minute, using a macro infusion set with drop factor 15 drops/mL and strength of dopamine injection = 40 mg/mL.
   Ans. Dose = 4 mcg/kg/minute = 4 × 60 = 240 mcg/minute.
   Strength of injection = 40 mg/mL = 40 × 1000 mcg/mL.
   Dissolve 1 mL of dopamine injection in 500 mL infusion fluid so that infusion fluid has dopamine = 40000 mcg in 500 mL = 80 mcg/mL.
   Infusion rate = 80 mcg/mL × 240 mcg/minute = 3 mL/minute.
   Flow rate = infusion rate × drop factor = 3 mL/minute × 15 gtts/mL = 45 gtts/minute.

Questions for practice: Dose calculation

45. Calculate the IV flow rate for infusing 200 mL NS over 2 hours, using an infusion set with drop factor = 60 gtts/minute.

46. Calculate the flow rate required to infuse 1 litre of normal saline over 5 hours, using a regular infusion set with a drop factor of 15 gtts/mL.

47. Quinine sulphate, available as 600 mg/mL ampoule is to be infused at a dose of 10 mg/kg body weight in an adult patient weighing 60 kg, over 4 hours in 200 mL of 5% dextrose. Calculate the infusion rate.

48. How much adrenaline is present in 1 mL of 1:10000 adrenaline solution used for nasal packing in a young boy to control epistaxis?

49. Rate of infusion for aminophylline is 0.8 mg/kg/hour. Calculate the dose to be given for a 70 kg man.

50. 2.5 litres of NS is to be infused at a rate of 200 mL per hour. Calculate the time required for infusion.

Hint for solutions

(Refer to respective chapters for doses and pharmacological basis.)

1. Atropine, pralidoxime
2. Mainly supportive, paracetamol, diazepam, physostigmine (sometimes)
3. Adrenaline, hydrocortisone, chlorpheniramine
4. Tamsulosin, finasteride
5. Timolol eyedrops, latanoprost eyedrops
6. Naproxen, sumatriptan, metoclopramide
7. i. Diclofenac
   ii. Methotrexate, folic acid
8. i. Diclofenac
   ii. Allopurinol
9. Paracetamol, levocetirizine
10. Inj. lorazepam, fosphenytoin, midazolam, supportive
11. Fluoxetine
12. Haloperidol
13. Levodopa, carbidopa (FDC)
14. Trihexyphenidyl
15. Gastric lavage, Inj. Na bicarbonate, KCl, fomepizole, calcium leucovorin, ethanol via nasogastric tube.
16. Supportive, naloxone
17. Bed rest, oxygen, furosemide, ramipril
18. Lifestyle modification, salt restriction, ramipril
19. Esmolol, nitrates or sodium nitroprusside
20. Nitroglycerine, sublingual
21. Inj. morphine, Inj. streptokinase, Inj. heparin, promethazine, supportive.
22. Formoterol and inhalational corticosteroids
23. Nebulise with ipratropium, salbutamol/formoterol, oxygen, Inj. hydrocortisone, Inj. salbutamol, intubation/mechanical ventilation as per need, antibiotics.
24. Antitussive drug
25. Antitussive and mucolytic drugs
26. Weight control, exercise, blood sugar monitoring, metformin
27. IV fluid therapy, insulin, KCl, Na bicarbonate, supportive
28. Levothyroxine, monitor T3, T4, TSH
29. Inj. methylergometrine, 15-methyl PGF
30. Vitamin D, calcium
31. Alendronate, calcium
32. Isoniazid, rifampicin, pyrazinamide, ethambutol, pyridoxine
33. Chloroquine, primaquine, paracetamol
34. Metronidazole, diloxanide furoate
35. Dapsone, rifampicin
36. Dapsone, rifampicin, clofazimine
37. Zidovudine
38. Lansoprazole, amoxicillin, tinidazole
39. Albendazole, ferrous sulphate
40. Folic acid, methylcobalamin, ferrous sulphate
41. i. Rheumatoid arthritis
    ii. Naproxen, methotrexate
42. Telmisartan
43. All are useful interactions. Refer to respective chapters for details.
44. All are harmful interactions. Refer to respective chapters for details.
45. Infusion rate (200/ 2 × 60) × Flow rate (60 gtts/minute) = 100 gtts/minute
46. Infusion rate (1000 mL / 5 × 60 min) × Drop factor (15 drops / minute) = 50 gtts/minute
47. Dose = 60 × 10 = 600 mg, volume 200 mL, flow rate = 200 / 4 × 60 = 0.83 mL/minute.
48. 1 g in 10000 mL = 1000 mg in 10000 mL = 0.1 mg per mL
49. Dose = 0.8 × 70 / 60= 0.93 mg/minute, nearly equals 1 mg/minute.
50. Time = volume/infusion rate = 2500 × 60 / 200 = 750 minutes = 12.5 hours.

SECTION 14 AETCOM

72 Attitude, Ethics, and Communication

Module 2.2 The Foundations of Bioethics

Learning objectives

Describe and discuss the role of:
- Non-maleficence as a guiding principle in patient care.
- Autonomy and shared responsibility as a guiding principle in patient care.
- Beneficence as a guiding principle in patient care.
- Justice as a guiding principle in patient care.
- Role of a physician in healthcare system.

EVOLUTION OF MEDICAL ETHICS

The history of medical ethics traces its roots to early civilisations, where health concerns gave rise to diverse healing traditions and ethical guidelines. In ancient Egypt and Mesopotamia, codes governed medical conduct, often blending medicine with religion and magic. Healers included priests, seers, and physicians, each playing distinct roles. A major shift in this approach occurred in ancient Greece, where Hippocratic medicine separated empirical observation from superstition. The **Hippocratic oath**, though its origin is unclear, emphasised moral duty, integrity, and protection of patients from harm and injustice, laying the groundwork for ethical practice.

In ancient India, medical texts like the *Charaka Samhita* and *Susruta Samhita* outlined causes and treatments of diseases, along with directives for the conduct of physicians. 'The oath of initiation' practiced in ancient Indian Ayurvedic medicine was quite similar to the 'Hippocratic oath'. Chinese medicine promoted a holistic approach, valuing both book learning and apprenticeship. In the eastern world, medical morality was rooted in beliefs of religion, philosophy, and polite, gracious behaviour.

During the early Christian era, thinkers like Galen emphasised the integration of principled behaviour, philosophy, logic, bedside manners, and scientific knowledge. In the Islamic world, medical writings highlighted the importance of justice, compassion, and service of all individuals equally. Similarly, Judaism contributed principles for guiding responsible and altruistic practice.

By the Middle Ages, European medical guilds began balancing professional interests with public service and formulated 'public health regulations' to prevent malpractice and negligence. In the 19th century, the establishment of medical associations in North America led to the development of written codes of ethics. These codes were periodically updated to address evolving concerns such as patient autonomy, care of the elderly, the physician–pharmaceutical industry relationship, and end-of-life dignity. Fundamental ethical principles of beneficence, non-maleficence, respect for person and justice were recognised for the first time in the code of ethics issued by the Canadian Medical Association in 1996.

After World War II, global outrage over unethical medical experiments on war prisoners led to the development of key ethical frameworks, including the **Nuremberg Code**, the **Declaration of Helsinki**, and the **Belmont Report**. Good Clinical Practice (GCP) guidelines were developed by the International Council for Harmonization of Technical Requirements for Pharmaceuticals for Human Use (ICH), with contributions from regulatory authorities such as the US FDA. In India, the Indian Council of Medical Research (ICMR), founded in 1911, remains the key body overseeing biomedical research.

These frameworks, along with guidelines from international bodies, continue to shape ethical standards in clinical care, medical education, and research practices across the world.

FUNDAMENTAL PRINCIPLES OF BIOETHICS

The four principles that form the core of modern bioethics are **non-maleficence, beneficence, autonomy** and **justice**. The central themes of each of these principles are described here.

1. Non-maleficence

Non-maleficence is a fundamental principle of medical ethics, meaning *"first, do no harm"* (*primum non nocere*). It requires that physicians avoid causing harm to patients and carefully weigh the potential benefits and risks of any treatment/diagnostic test/surgical procedure. It also implies that only qualified and experienced professionals should provide medical care.

Non-maleficence, though closely linked to beneficence—which focuses on actively enhancing patient well-being—differs from it in two important ways:

- **Non-maleficence** sets a minimum standard—if a treatment poses more harm than benefit, it should be avoided.
- **Non-maleficence** is a constant obligation to avoid harm, while **beneficence** is context-specific, focusing on choosing the best possible option for each patient.

2. Beneficence

Beneficence is a core principle of bioethics that goes beyond the obligation to "do no harm" (non-maleficence), by encouraging healthcare providers to act in the best interest of patients. It requires physicians to evaluate all available treatment options by considering:

- Their ability to resolve the patient's current medical issue
- Proportionality to the severity of the condition
- Suitability to the individual patient circumstances
- Alignment with the patient expectations and values

After thorough consideration, the most appropriate course of action should be chosen based on what serves the patient best in that specific situation.

Beneficence underpins a patient-centred approach to care, emphasising the need to tailor decisions to each patient's unique needs, concerns and expectations. It recognises that what benefits one patient may not necessarily be beneficial for another.

According to prominent American bioethicists Beauchamp and Childress, beneficence includes two aspects: **positive beneficence**—the duty to provide benefit—and **utility**—balancing benefits against risks to achieve the best possible outcome. This framework forms the basis of risk–benefit analysis in clinical decision-making.

However, beneficence can sometimes come into conflict with **patient autonomy**—the right of individuals to make their own healthcare choices. A patient's preferred decision may differ from what the physician believes is best. To resolve this, clinicians must ensure patients are well-informed about all options, including potential risks and benefits, so they can make decisions in their best interests.

3. Autonomy

This core principle of 'respect for person' refers to a patient's right to self-determination in making healthcare decisions, including the choice to accept or refuse treatment. Healthcare professionals are ethically obligated to respect a patient's decisions, even when those decisions do not align with what the practitioner believes is in the patient's best interest.

For autonomy to be practiced, the patient must have the **capacity** to understand the available options, evaluate their risks and benefits, and make a voluntary decision free from coercion or undue influence. Most conscious, mentally sound adults are considered competent to decide for themselves. Challenges arise when dealing with unconscious, mentally impaired, or vulnerable individuals (e.g., minors, elderly with cognitive decline, prisoners, migrants). In such cases, consent must be obtained from a **legally authorised representative (LAR)**.

Informed consent is the practical application of autonomy in clinical and research settings. It has three key components:

1. **Disclosure:** Providing clear, relevant information about the medical condition, treatment options, and associated risks/benefits.
2. **Comprehension:** Ensuring the patient understands the information. Ideally, information should be provided in simple language, avoiding technical words, allowing time for the patient to process the information and express their concerns. A Patient Information Sheet (PIS) is provided to potential participants in clinical research.
3. **Voluntariness:** Confirming that the decision to choose a particular treatment option or participate in research is made freely, without pressure or manipulation.

The process is documented using an **Informed Consent Document (ICD)**, which comprises an '**Informed Consent Form (ICF)** and a Patient Information Sheet (PIS) that contains all the necessary information for each patient. If the patient or LAR is illiterate, an impartial witness must be present during informed consent documentation. In some clinical trials, audio or video recording of the consent process is required by regulatory bodies such as CDSCO (Central Drugs Standard Control Organisation). Importantly, informed consent is an ongoing process—patients have the right to ask questions and withdraw consent at any time without impact on their care.

Conflicts may arise between autonomy and other ethical principles like beneficence or non-maleficence—for example, a severely anemic patient refusing a lifesaving blood transfusion due to religious beliefs. In such cases, the model of **shared decision-making**—which balances patient preferences with clinical expertise—offers a constructive path forward.

Respect for autonomy also includes ensuring **privacy and confidentiality**:

- **Privacy:** Privacy refers to the patient's right to control how, when, to whom and how much of their personal or medical information is shared. The patient's wish for provision of appropriate private environment during clinical examination/procedure should be respected.

- **Confidentiality:** It is the duty of healthcare providers to safeguard patient information and share it only with authorised personnel. In research, data anonymity is maintained through coding; in pharmacovigilance, only initials may be used on adverse drug reaction (ADR) forms.

However, in some situations, confidentiality can be breached, such as:

- Reporting notifiable communicable diseases to public health authorities.
- Disclosing a minor's or incapacitated patient's condition to a guardian or LAR.
- Legal requirements (e.g., court orders, risk of harm to self or others, certain conditions like HIV).
- Scientific or legal needs in research, where ethics committee approval is required.

In all cases, protecting patient rights and dignity remains the guiding principle.

4. Justice

This is the most challenging of the core medical ethics principles to put into practice. In healthcare, justice primarily concerns **fair access to medical services** and the **equitable distribution of limited resources**. The core ethical dilemma is whether **healthcare should be considered a universal right**. Answering "yes" raises further questions: What level of care should be universally provided? How can fairness in allocation be ensured? And who will bear the cost? Conversely, if healthcare is **not** a universal right, it becomes difficult to address the needs of those who cannot afford care.

Among the four recognised types of justice—**distributive, procedural, restorative, and retributive**—distributive justice is the most relevant to healthcare. It emphasises the **fair distribution of resources, benefits, and opportunities** across society. In practice, this means allocating more resources to those with greater needs.

In the context of **medical research**, distributive justice involves ensuring that the risks and benefits of research are distributed fairly across all groups, with particular attention to protecting vulnerable populations and avoiding the reinforcement of existing social, racial, or ethnic disparities. Achieving this requires careful study design, rigorous ethical oversight (the process of ensuring that clinical trials are conducted in accordance with established ethical principles, legal standards, and moral responsibilities), and a strong awareness of the broader social implications of the research.

Ultimately, justice in healthcare requires **balancing individual needs with societal fairness**, and ensuring that policies and practices do not exclude or disadvantage those who are already marginalised.

THE ROLE OF A PHYSICIAN IN THE HEALTHCARE SYSTEM

The role of a physician extends far beyond examining patients and prescribing medication. The medical profession, often regarded as one of the noblest, involves caring for individuals when they are most vulnerable—during illness, pain, anxiety, and dependence. In such moments, patients seek not only treatment but also compassion, empathy, and emotional support. Hence, a doctor is more than just a prescriber; they are a caregiver, guide, and advocate.

The National Medical Commission (NMC) outlines the key roles of a physician in its Competency-Based Medical Education (CBME) guidelines. An Indian Medical Graduate (IMG) is trained to acquire a defined set of competencies, to function effectively as a **clinician, communicator, leader, professional, researcher, teacher, and lifelong learner**. Each role entails specific responsibilities.

1. Clinician

The physician's primary responsibility is the diagnosis, treatment, and prevention of disease, as well as the promotion of overall health. A competent clinician provides preventive, promotive, curative, palliative, and holistic care with empathy and compassion. This role demands thorough knowledge of human anatomy, physiology, disease mechanisms, diagnostic methods, and therapeutic options—along with an understanding of their risks and benefits. Additionally, clinicians must uphold medicolegal, ethical, societal, and humanitarian principles in their practice.

2. Communicator

Effective communication, coupled with genuine empathy is central to the physician–patient relationship. A doctor must be able to communicate clearly, respectfully, and empathetically with patients, families, colleagues and the wider community. Communication should be in a language the patient understands and in a manner that promotes patient participation in shared decision-making. Physicians must also respect the patient values, preferences, beliefs, privacy, and confidentiality, thereby fostering trust and improving health outcomes.

For example, when prescribing **oral contraceptives**, physicians must clearly explain the correct method of use, potential side effects, and address concerns related to missed dose, risk of contraceptive failure, and fertility after discontinuation of use. This requires sensitivity and the ability to tailor information to the patient's individual needs and values. Similarly, in the case of **anti-tuberculosis (TB) treatment**, which often involves multiple drugs given for long durations, physicians must communicate the importance of adherence to prevent drug resistance and relapse. They must also recognise and address issues such as fear of social stigma or consequences of non-compliance, potential adverse effects and protection of close contacts with empathy and support.

3. Leader

Physicians often serve as leaders and active members of multidisciplinary healthcare teams. They are expected to collaborate efficiently with professionals from various disciplines, recognising and respecting the roles and responsibilities of each team member. Leadership also involves advocating for health promotion, disease prevention, and a comprehensive approach to patient care across primary and secondary healthcare settings.

4. Professional

Medical practitioners are viewed by society as professionals committed to excellence and ethical conduct. Core values include selflessness, integrity, accountability, respect for professional boundaries, and adherence to legal and ethical standards. Physicians are expected to demonstrate responsiveness to patient needs and to contribute to the continuous advancement of the medical profession.

5. Lifelong Learner

Medicine is a constantly evolving field, and a physician must commit to ongoing learning and skill development. This includes staying updated with current evidence, evaluating emerging research, and applying novel techniques for better patient outcomes. Reflection, critical thinking, and the ability to adapt are essential for continuous professional growth.

6. Teacher and Researcher

Physicians who take on the role of educators bear a significant responsibility in shaping future healthcare professionals. As teachers and researchers, they must foster innovation, uphold the highest standards of ethical research, and contribute to knowledge that enhances future healthcare delivery. Their dual role strengthens the foundations of medical education and evidence-based practice.

Module 2.3 Healthcare as A Right

Learning objectives

Describe and discuss the role of justice as a guiding principle with focus on:
- Healthcare a right, implications of healthcare as a right for society, economics and doctors.
- Missing links in healthcare as a right.
- Barriers in the implementation of healthcare as a right.

Healthcare as a Right

Health is not merely the absence of disease but a state of complete physical, mental, and social well-being. It depends on adequate nutrition, clean water, sanitation, housing, a safe environment, access to education, healthcare and opportunities for recreation.

Healthcare, one of the indicators of health, refers to the services provided by medical, nursing, and allied health professionals to prevent and manage illness and promote physical as well as mental well-being. It includes diagnostics, consultations, medication, surgical and non-surgical interventions, emergency services, and rehabilitation.

Health is a fundamental human right, and equitable access to healthcare is essential for realising it. A just and inclusive health system must provide quality medical services as well as address broader social determinants. Governments have a moral and constitutional obligation to ensure that every individual can live a healthy, dignified life—free from discrimination, financial hardship, and systemic barriers.

International recognition of the right to health

The Universal Declaration of Human Rights (UDHR, 1948), adopted by the United Nations, affirms in its Article 25 that everyone has the right to a standard of living adequate for health and well-being, including access to medical care, particularly during illness, disability, and old age. It also entitles motherhood and childhood to special care and protection.

The World Health Organisation (WHO) upholds health as a human right, stating in its constitution that "the enjoyment of the highest attainable standard of health is one of the fundamental rights of every human being without distinction of race, religion, political belief, economic or social condition." WHO promotes *people-centered care*, that is the Embodiment of human rights in the practice of healthcare.

According to WHO's 2017 Human Rights Day statement, the *right to health* means:

- Access to necessary health services, when and where needed without financial hardship
- Control over one's health and body, including right of access to sexual and reproductive information and services
- Protection of privacy and the right to be treated with dignity

These principles support **Universal Health Coverage (UHC)** as a global priority.

India's constitutional and policy framework

India, as a signatory to the UDHR and a member of WHO, reflects these commitments in its national framework.

- **Article 21** of the Indian Constitution guarantees the *right to life with dignity*, and personal liberty as a fundamental right, which is interpreted to include access to healthcare, food, clean air, shelter, education, and privacy.
- The **Directive Principles of State Policy (DPSP)** guide the state to:
  - Improve nutrition and public health (Article 47)
  - Minimise social and economic inequalities and equitable distribution of resources (Articles 38 and 39)
  - Ensure fair working conditions and maternity relief (Article 42)

Though not enforceable by law, these principles serve as a foundation for health policies and welfare programs.

Implications of Healthcare as a Universal Right

Implications for the state

When health is recognised as a universal right, the state has a legal obligation to ensure accessible, affordable, and quality healthcare for all. It must also guarantee essential health determinants like clean water, food, housing, and sanitation—free from discrimination. Universal health coverage not only improves public well-being but also strengthens the nation's human capital, its greatest asset.

Socio-economic implications of health as a universal right

- **Reducing inequality:** Universal access to healthcare can help bridge disparities in health outcomes across demographic groups, fostering social equality and collective responsibility for public well-being.
- **Improved public health:** When healthcare is accessible to all, preventive care and early diagnosis become widespread, reducing the burden of chronic and infectious diseases.
- **Economic benefits:** A healthier population boosts workforce productivity, reduces absenteeism, and lowers healthcare-related financial hardships, contributing to poverty reduction and economic growth.
- **Support for vulnerable groups**
  - Women benefit from better work conditions, maternity relief, and free postnatal care, reducing gender-based discrimination.
  - Children gain access to essential services like nutrition, vaccination, and treatment.
  - People with disabilities are ensured equal rights, including healthcare.
  - Migrant workers and their families are entitled to emergency medical care.

Implications for doctors

- An expanded patient base increases the workload on healthcare providers.
- Physicians must take a more active role in public health advocacy and resource optimisation.
- Adapting to evolving healthcare policies and ensuring quality care amidst rising demand become essential responsibilities.

Challenges/Barriers to Implementation

While universal healthcare coverage (UHC) offers immense benefits for individuals and society, its implementation in India faces several hurdles.

1. **Financial barriers:** With a large population and limited resources, securing sustainable healthcare funding is a major challenge. Even when public funds are allocated, inefficiencies due to low administrative capacity and lack of accountability often lead to underutilisation or mismanagement.
2. **Infrastructure limitations:** Inadequate health infrastructure, a shortage of trained personnel, and time constraints hinder consistent delivery of quality care. Public healthcare suffers from under-provision and poor patient satisfaction, while the private sector often provides excessive and overpriced services. Substantial investment is needed for infrastructure development and workforce training.
3. **Organisational barriers:** Fragmentation between the public and private healthcare sectors, as well as poor coordination across primary, secondary, and tertiary levels of care leads to gaps in service delivery and disrupts continuity of care. Additionally, India's health system still follows a vertical, programme-based approach (e.g., TB control, maternal health) rather than an integrated, comprehensive model required by UHC.

4. **Political constraints:** UHC demands financial reallocation and policy reform, which may be obstructed by political opposition and differing priorities. Lack of political consensus and will slows progress at all levels of government.
5. **Legal barriers:** Outdated or restrictive laws impede the establishment of cohesive health systems. Legal reforms are often delayed by lengthy legislative processes and bureaucratic hurdles.
6. **Socio-cultural constraints:** Public awareness, trust, and cultural attitudes significantly influence healthcare utilisation. Traditional beliefs, stigma, and discrimination often lead to underuse of available services, particularly by those who need them most. Despite availability, the state cannot compel individuals to access healthcare, posing a challenge to equity.

Achieving universal healthcare in India requires a multifaceted strategy involving robust political commitment, systemic reforms, public engagement, and targeted investment in infrastructure and human resources. Success lies in ensuring that no one, especially in rural, tribal, or marginalised communities, is left behind.

Missing Links in Universal Healthcare

Despite various policy initiatives, India's progress toward Universal Health Coverage (UHC) lags behind. Key gaps in planning and implementation include:

1. **Misconception regarding UHC:** UHC aims to ensure financial protection through access to high-quality, integrated, and affordable care. It has to be differentiated from universally available health insurance.
2. **Overemphasis on hospitals:** Current systems prioritise hospital-based care, though only about 2.5% of patients require it. Strengthening primary care for prevention, health promotion, and early detection—with a robust referral system—can optimise resource utilisation
3. **Narrow targeting:** UHC should cover the entire population, not just low-income groups. Including the middle class enhances equity and broadens the resource pool.
4. **Lack of role clarity:** Determinants of health (like food, water, and sanitation) must be addressed separately from healthcare delivery to improve accountability, resource allocation, and policy formulation.

Module 2.5 Patient Autonomy and Decision Making

Learning objectives

- Identify, discuss and defend medico-legal, socio-cultural and ethical issues.
- Contrast autonomy and paternalism.
- Describe responsibilities of patients and doctor in shared decision making.
- Discuss full and reasonable disclosure.

Paternalism vs. Autonomy in Healthcare

Paternalism in healthcare refers to situations where medical professionals make decisions on behalf of patients, assuming that, based on their knowledge, skills, and experience, they know what is best for the patient—even if it contradicts the patient's own wishes. This approach is often criticised as it undermines the ethical principle of autonomy.

Autonomy, on the other hand, upholds a patient's right to make informed choices about their care, even when those choices differ from the recommendations of their healthcare providers. It emphasises respect for individual values, preferences, and self-determination.

Paternalism and autonomy lie at opposite ends of the decision-making spectrum—one excludes the patient, while the other places full responsibility on them. Both extremes carry the risk of flawed decisions. A more balanced and ethical approach is **Shared Decision Making (SDM)**, where patients and healthcare professionals collaborate to make informed decisions that align with both clinical evidence and patient values.

Shared Decision Making (SDM)

Shared decision making is a collaborative process that involves active participation from both the doctor and the patient. It requires a two-way exchange of information—doctors provide medical insights, while patients share their values, preferences, and concerns. In this model, the patient makes the final decision with the guidance of the doctor, ensuring that autonomy is respected without compromising on clinical accuracy.

SDM reduces the risk of poor choices by allowing patients to make informed decisions with professional support. It also strengthens trust and satisfaction in the patient–provider relationship. Promoting SDM often benefits from a **multidisciplinary team approach**, where various healthcare professionals contribute to holistic and patient-centered care.

Physician's role in SDM

It is the physician's responsibility to present all available treatment options, including their potential risks, benefits, and likely outcomes. This also includes explaining the consequences of opting for no treatment or adopting a "wait and watch" approach, based on clinical experience. The physician should guide the patient towards the best course of action while facilitating a joint decision-making process.

Patients should be encouraged to consult with family or friends if they wish, and involve them in the process. The physician must ensure that the patient has understood the information, provide opportunities to clarify doubts, and respect patient values, concerns, and beliefs when comparing different options.

To support informed decision-making, physicians must continually update their knowledge and clinical skills through continued medical education (CME) and self-directed learning (SDL), ensuring they offer the most appropriate and up-to-date treatment options.

Patient's responsibilities

SDM upholds a patient's right to autonomy and informed choice, but it also entails certain responsibilities.

- Patients must provide complete and honest information regarding their symptoms, allergies, medical and family history.
- They are expected to actively engage in the process (by understanding the information shared, asking questions or requesting clarification, voicing their concerns, and discussing personal preferences with their healthcare providers) to help determine the most suitable course of treatment.

Outcomes of shared decision making

SDM enhances the patient's understanding of their condition and treatment, encouraging active participation in the therapeutic process. It fosters trust between patients and healthcare providers, reducing anxiety and uncertainty about the treatment outcomes. When the treatment aligns with the patient's beliefs and preferences, adherence to the treatment and follow-up plan improves significantly.

Full and Reasonable Disclosure

The core bioethical principle of autonomy is put into practice by the process of **informed consent**. It is the process of communication between the doctor and patient, resulting in documentation of the patient's voluntary consent to undergo a specific intervention. This process not only reinforces patient autonomy but also improves patient satisfaction, builds trust, reduces the risk of litigation, and upholds ethical standards in medical practice. Failure to obtain documented informed consent is considered medical negligence and malpractice.

A critical element of informed consent is **enabling patient decision-making** through clear, accessible information. This includes the nature of the illness, proposed treatment or procedure, expected benefits, potential risks, alternative options, chance of success, recovery time, costs, prognosis without treatment, and implications of refusal. To enhance patient comprehension, visual aids such as charts, diagrams, or videos may be employed.

Doctors should actively listen to understand patient concerns, expectations, and values, and respond to their queries with clarity and empathy. The emotional and psychological impact of the information—on both the patient and family—must also be taken into account. Communication should always be supportive, empowering the patient to make an informed choice.

Even after consent is given, patients have a right to continuous updates regarding their treatment progress and follow-up. Transparent disclosure of any medical errors—including corrective actions is essential to maintaining trust, minimising harm and preventing recurrence.

Ethical dilemmas and exceptions to full disclosure

Informed consent requires full and reasonable disclosure of sufficient, relevant information regarding diagnosis, treatment options, risks, benefits, and outcomes to support patient decision-making. However, certain situations may pose ethical dilemmas and justify exceptions to full disclosure:

- *Determining sufficiency of information:* There is often uncertainty about how much information should be disclosed. Excessive detail may overwhelm the patient, while insufficient information can undermine autonomy and hinder trust in the physician.
- *Conflicts with family or legal representatives (LAR):* When a legal guardian or family member consents on behalf of the patient, there may be a conflict with the patient's own wishes or a lack of opportunity to express them, compromising patient autonomy.
- *Emergency situations:* In emergencies where immediate intervention is critical, healthcare professionals may initiate treatment without full disclosure to avoid delays. While this challenges autonomy, it is ethically justified under the principle of beneficence.
- *Voluntary waiver of autonomy:* Some patients may choose to delegate decision-making authority to their physician or another trusted individual, thereby waiving their right to self-determination.
- *Therapeutic privilege:* In rare cases, a physician may withhold specific information if disclosure is believed to cause significant psychological harm. However, this must be approached with caution, justified clearly, and applied narrowly.
- *Requests from family to withhold information:* Family members may urge physicians not to disclose certain details to the patient out of concern for their well-being. Despite these requests, respect for patient autonomy takes precedence unless the patient lacks decision-making capacity.

- *Court-mandated treatment:* In cases where a patient is deemed legally incompetent or poses a threat to self or others, the court may mandate treatment without the patient's consent.

Barriers to full and reasonable disclosure

Gaps in communication skills, language barriers, socio-cultural differences, low patient literacy, the emotional impact of bad news on patients and families, and an organisational culture driven by fear of blame or litigation are significant obstacles to achieving full and reasonable disclosure in clinical practice.

COMMUNICATION SKILLS IN MEDICAL PRACTICE

Successful medical practice requires a combination of appropriate knowledge, practical skills, and the right attitude. A key aspect of ethical practice is respecting patient autonomy, which includes obtaining informed consent through full and reasonable disclosure. As such, communication skills are an indispensable part of medical training.

Essential Elements of Communication in Medical Encounters

The **Kalamazoo Consensus Statement** (1999) identified seven key components of effective communication in doctor–patient interactions. These are:

1. **Building a doctor–patient relationship:** A patient-centred approach to care with emphasis on eliciting patient's history of illness while guiding the interview with diagnostic reasoning. The relationship is viewed as a partnership, where patient participation in decision-making is to be ensured.
2. **Opening of the discussion:** The patient should be allowed to express their concerns fully at the start. Their complete set of issues should be elicited. A personal connection should be established and maintained throughout the encounter.
3. **Gathering information:** The physician should ask open-ended or close-ended questions as appropriate, and the patient's responses should be organised, clarified, and summarised. Active listening should be demonstrated through verbal and non-verbal cues—such as nodding, making eye contact, and encouraging remarks—so the patient feels heard and understood.
4. **Understanding the patient's perspective:** It is important to explore contextual factors such as the patient's culture, family background, social situation, economic status, and spiritual beliefs. The physician should acknowledge and respond to the patient's ideas, values, and emotions.
5. **Sharing information:** Relevant information should be communicated clearly, using simple, non-technical language in terms that the patient can understand. Comprehension should be confirmed, and patients should be encouraged to ask questions or seek clarification.
6. **Reaching agreement on problems and plans:** Patients should be supported to participate in decisions to the extent they are comfortable. Their ability and willingness to follow the proposed plan should be assessed, and available resources or support systems should be identified.
7. **Providing closure:** At the end of the encounter, the patient should be invited to raise any remaining questions or concerns. The treatment plan should be summarised and confirmed, and follow-up arrangements—including steps to take in case of unexpected outcomes—should be clearly communicated.

These seven steps provide a structured framework for doctor–patient encounters, enabling **effective exchange of information and mutual understanding**. Strong communication skills not only enhance the therapeutic relationship but also reduce the risk of conflict and litigation in medical practice.

Interaction between the doctor and pharmaceutical representative

When engaging with pharmaceutical representatives, physicians should prioritise clarity, ethical responsibility, and patient welfare. The interactions should be structured, time-bound, and guided by professional standards.

To use time effectively, doctors should clearly communicate their specific areas of interest and the type of information they are seeking. The emphasis should be on clinically significant data—such as a drug's safety, effectiveness, and evidence base—rather than on promotional messaging. Physicians are encouraged to request and critically evaluate supporting studies or independent research that substantiate the claims made.

Physicians should remain mindful of potential commercial biases, as pharmaceutical representatives are often incentivised to promote their own products. It is important to question how a drug compares to existing alternatives—evaluating aspects such as therapeutic benefit, safety profile, dosage form, ease of use, storage requirements, and appropriateness for different patient groups (e.g., children or older adults).

For drugs that are similar to existing ones, often referred to as follow-on or "me-too" drugs, any increase in cost should be justified by clear clinical advantages. When discussing newer medications, doctors should ask about the drug's intended place in the treatment algorithms and the benefits it offers in that context.

Throughout all interactions, ethical principles and professional communication should guide the conduct.

Doctors are encouraged to provide respectful, constructive feedback and engage meaningfully, with the ultimate goal of improving care and outcomes for patients.

Interacting with the media to share information about drugs

When engaging with the media to share information about a new drug or dosage form, it is important to choose journalists and media platforms with a proven track record of accurate and responsible reporting. The goal should be to ensure that the public receives reliable, balanced, and evidence-based information.

Any information shared should be current, scientifically validated, and supported by credible research. Physicians should focus on communicating key aspects such as the drug's safety, effectiveness, and potential impact on public health. Additionally, promoting scientific literacy and encouraging critical thinking among the audience can help counter misinformation and build public trust.

While interacting with the media, doctors must uphold ethical standards, particularly in safeguarding patient confidentiality. No identifiable patient information should be disclosed, and all communications should be handled with sensitivity and professionalism.

Further reading
1. A review of the four principles of bioethics.
   http://archive.journalchirohumanities.com/vol%2014/JChiroHumanit2007v14_34.
2. Universal Declaration of Human Rights.
   https://www.un.org/sites/un2.un.org/files/2021/03/udhr.pdf
3. Missing links in universal health care.
   https://www.thehindu.com/opinion/lead/Missing-links-in-universal-health-care/article59784065.ece

Index

1,25-Dihydroxy calcitriol 650
5-Fluorouracil (5-FU) 796
5-HT$_3$ antagonists 830
5α-Reductase inhibitors 636
6-Mercaptopurine 794
6-Thioguanine 794
8-Hydroxyquinolines 770
α Blockers 134
α$_1$-Blockers 424
α-Glucosidase inhibitors 581
β Blockers 423, 439
β-Lactamase inhibitors 679
β-Lactams 659

A
Abacavir (ABC) 747
Abaloparatide 653
Abarelix 552
Abatacept 344, 856
Abciximab 518, 855
Absence seizures 224
Absorbents 814
Absorption 4, 34
Abstracting systems 911
Abuse 665
Acamprosate 281
Acarbose 581
Acebutolol 147
Aceclofenac 322
ACE Inhibitors 418
Acenocoumarol 510
Acetazolamide 386
Acetylcholine 93
Acetylcysteine 370, 802
Acetyl-L-carnitine 230
Acipimox 529
Acne 882
Acquired immunodeficiency conditions 849
Acquired immunodeficiency syndrome 746
Acridine 97
Acridine dyes 886
Actinomycin D 796
Actin–troponin–tropomyosin complex 437
Active transport 32
Acute salicylate poisoning 320
Acyclovir 736
Adalimumab 344, 855
Adapalene 882
Adaptation 662
Additive effect 919
Adefovir dipivoxil 738
Adenosine 394, 492
Adenylyl cyclase 56
ADH antagonists 440
Adrenaline 125
Adrenochrome monosemicarbazone 501
Adsorbents 879
Adverse drug event 66
Adverse drug reaction 6, 66

Affinity 55
Aflatoxicosis 866
Afrezza 575
Afterload 436
Agonist 5, 55
Albendazole 782
Albiglutide 579
Alcohol 879
Aldosterone 599
Aldosterone antagonists 422
Alefacept 883, 855
Alemtuzumab 806
Alendronate 650
Alfentanil 306
Aliglitazar 582
Aliskiren 406, 420
Alkylating agents 793
Allopurinol 333, 802
Almorexant 205
Almotriptan 359
Aloe vera 879
Alogliptin 579
Alprenolol 147
Alprostadil 644
Alteplase 519
Alum 501, 879
Aluminum 879
Aluminium hydroxide gel 837
Alzheimer's disease 99
Amantadine 238, 742
Ambenonium 98
Ambroxol 370
Amifostine 802
Amikacin 684
Amiloride 392
Aminoglycosides 659, 684
Aminophylline 377
Aminorex (Ice) 289
Aminosalicylates 816
Amiodarone 491
Amisulpride 256
Amlodipine 413
Ammonium carbonate 370
Ammonium chloride 370
Amodiaquine 760
Amoxicillin 676
Amphotericin B 725, 773
Ampicillin 676
Anabolic steroids 635
Anakinra 332, 855
Analeptics 293
Analytical study 6, 890
Anaphylactic reactions 68
Anastrozole 608
Angel dust 290
Angiotensin-converting enzyme inhibitors 403
Angiotensin II 400
Angiotensin receptor antagonists 405

Angiotensin receptor blockers 405, 420
Anidulafungin 728
Anion gap 875
Anorectics 126
Antagonism 5, 923
Antagonists 5, 55
Anthraquinones 822
Antibiotics 658
Antibiotic stewardship 666
Anti-CD$_3$ antibodies 856
Anticholinergic drugs 841
Anticholinergics 829
Antidiphtheritic serum (ADS) 860
Antidotes 875
Antifibrinolytics 500
Antihemophilic 500
Antihistamines 369
Anti-integrin antibody 817
Antilymphocyte globulins 854
Antimicrobial 812, 841
Antimicrobial agents (AMA) 658
Antimicrobial drug resistance 661
Antimotility drugs 814
Antiproliferative drugs 852
Antiseptics 885
Anti-snake venom serum polyvalent 860
Antitetanic serum (ATS) 860
Antithymocyte globulins 854
Anti-TNF-α antibodies 855
APD 443
Apixaban 508
Apomorphine 644, 828
Apraclonidine 150
Aprepitant 369, 802, 830
Ardeparin 504
Argatroban 508
Aripiprazole 256
Aromatase inhibitors 608
Aromatic hydrocarbons 864
Arsenic poisoning 870
Artemisinin 762
Arthus reactions 68
Arthus type reactions 719
ART regimens 751
Aspirin 323, 515
Astringents 878
ASV 868
Atenolol 147
Atomoxetine 293
Atonic seizures 224
Atopaxar 518
Atorvastatin 526
Atosiban 629
Atovaquone 763
Atrial natriuretic peptide 394
Atropine 105
Augmentative effect 920
Augmented reactions 66
Autoimmune disorders 849

Autonomy 928
Aversion therapy 292
Avibactam 680
Aviptadil 645
AWaRe classification 666
Azapirones 206
Azathioprine 342, 794, 850
Azelaic acid 882
Azithromycin 685
Azoles 731
Aztreonam 679

B
Bacitracin 680
Baclofen 241
Bacteriuria 694
Balsalazide 816
Bambuterol 376
Bapineuzumab 230
Barbiturates 190, 200
Baricitinib 344
Baroreceptor pathway 401
Basiliximab 855
BCG vaccine 858
Beclomethasone 374
Beclomethasone dipropionate 881
Bedaquiline (Bdq) 708
Bee sting 868
Bendroflumethiazide 390
Beneficence 928
Benign prostatic hypertrophy (BPH) 135
Benralizumab 379
Benserazide 236
Benzapril 403
Benzathine penicillin G 676
Benzbromarone 335
Benzene 864
Benzhexol 105
Benzimidazoles 781
Benzodiazepines 191, 202, 831
Benzoic acid 731
Benzoyl peroxide 882
Benzthiazide 390
Benztropine 105
Benzyl benzoate 884
BEP 792
Betamethasone 591, 595, 881
Betaxolol 147, 150
Bethanechol 93
Bevacizumab 806
Bezafibrate 530
Bhang 290
Bicalutamide 807
Bicalutamide 636
Bicuculline 293
Bier's block 176
Biguanide 580, 886
Bimatoprost 149
Bioaccumulation 863
bioavailability 4
Bioavailability 4, 35
Bioequivalence 4, 36
Biotransformation 4
Biperiden 105, 238
Bipolar disorders (BPD) 260
Bisacodyl 822

Bisoprolol 147
Bisphosphonates 650
Bivalirudin 507
Bizarre reactions 68
Bleomycin 796
Blood–brain barrier 4, 39
Blood:gas partition coefficient 185
Blood transfusion set 925
Bolus dose 508
Boosted PI regimens 749
Boric acid 879, 885
Bortezomib 806
Botanical pesticides 865
Botulism 92
Brain natriuretic peptide 394
Brand 3
Brimonidine 150
Brinzolamide 386
British anti-Lewisite (BAL) 869
British Pharmacopoeia (BP) 912
Bromhexine 370
Bromocriptine 553, 582, 641, 644
Bronchodilators 126, 375
Buccal route 17
Bucricaine 178
Budesonide 374
Bumetanide 389
Bupivacaine 177
Buprenorphine 306
Bupropion 96, 267
Buserelin 552
Buspirone 206
Busulfan 794
Butorphanol 306

C
Cabergoline 553, 641
Caffeine 293, 361
Calamine 879
Calcineurin inhibitors 883, 852
Calcipotriol 883
Calcitonin 653
Calcium 649
Calcium carbonate 837
Calcium channel blockers 421, 492, 629
Calcium disodium edetate 870
Calcium trisodium
    diethylenetriaminepentaacetic acid
    (DTPA) 871
Canagliflozin 581
Canakinumab 332
Candesartan 405
Cannabinoids 290
Capecitabine 795
Capreomycin 684
Capsules 16
Captopril 403
Carbachol 93
Carbamate pesticides 865
Carbamazepine 216
Carbenoxolone sodium 842
Carbetocin 626
Carbidopa 236
Carbimazole 562
Carbocisteine 370
Carbon monoxide 863

Carboplatin 798
Carboprost 627
Carboxymethylcellulose 820
Carcinogenicity 69
Cardiac glycosides 442
Cardiac performance 435
Cardiac stimulants 125
Cardiogenic shock 471
Carmustine 794
Carperitide 394
Carrier-mediated transport 32
Carvedilol 148, 423, 425
Cascara sagrada 822
Case-control study 890
Case reports and case series 890
Caspofungin 728
Categorical data 894
Cauda equina syndrome 175
Causality assessment 904
CCNS drugs 791
CCS drugs 791
Cefaclor, cefuroxime 678
Cefadroxil 678
Cefazolin 678
Cefepime 678
Cefoperazone 678
Cefotaxime 678
Cefpirome 678
Cefpodoxime proxetil 678
Ceftaroline 678
Ceftazidime 678
Ceftizoxime 678
Ceftobiprole 678
Ceftriaxone 678
Ceftriaxone 241, 678
Cefuroxime 678
Cefuroxime axetil 678
Cefuroxime, cefoxitin 678
Celecoxib 322
Celiprolol 147
Cell-mediated immunity (CMI) 746
Centchroman 620
Cephalexin 678
Cephalexin 678
Cephalosporinase enzyme 678
Cephalosporins 678
Certain event 905
Certolizumab 855
Ceruloplasmin 871
CETP inhibitors 531
Cetrorelix 552
Cetuximab 806
CGRP antagonists 361
Chancroid 695
Charaka Samhita 927
Charas 290
Chelating agents 869
Chemical antagonism 81
Chemotherapeutic agents 658
Chemotherapeutic index 658
Chemotherapy 9, 658
Chlorambucil 342, 793
Chloramphenicol 659, 683
Chlorguanide 763
Chlorhexidine 886
Chlorine 886

Chlorophores 886
Chloroquine 343, 759, 771
Chlorpromazine 255, 830
Chlorpropamide 577
Chlortetracycline 682
Chlorthalidone 390, 422
Cholestyramine 530
Choline esters 93
Choriogonadotropin 552
Ciclopirox olamine 731
Cidofovir 738
Cilastin 679
Cilostazol 468, 518
Cimetropium bromide 110
Cinnarizine 830
Ciprofloxacin 672
Circulating RAAS 399
Cisapride 831
Cisplatin 797
Citalopram 267
Citicoline 294
Citrovorum factor 802
Cladribine 242
Clarithromycin 685, 719
Clavulanic acid 679
Clearance 44
Clidinium 110
Clindamycin binds 685
Clinical decision making 893
Clinical pharmacology 6
Clinical trials 896
Clobazam 223
Clofazimine 718
Clofazimine (Cfz) 709
Clofibrate 529
Clomiphene citrate 607, 640
Clonazepam 223
Clonidine 128, 425
Clonidine withdrawal syndrome 135, 425
Clopamide 390
Clophedianol 369
Clopidogrel 517
Clotrimazole 696, 731
Cloxacillin 676
Clozapine 255
CNS stimulants 126
Coagulants 499
Coaltar 883
Cocaine 173, 288
Codeine 306, 368
Cohort study 891
Colchicine 331
Colesevelam 530, 582
Colestipol 530
Colloidal bismuth subcitrate 841, 842
Colloidal PVEs 473
Combined pills 616
Combined toxicity 923
Competitive antagonist 55
Compound optimisation 896
Compressed tablets 16
Computerised miniature pumps 26
Concentration-dependent killing 670
Conditional event 905
Conduction block 174
Confidentiality 929

Congenital immunodeficiency diseases 848
Conivaptan 394, 440
Conjugases 42
Conjugation 662
Conscious sedation 182
Continuous reactions 69
Contractility 435
Controlled Substances Act 910
Convulsants 293
Corticosteroids 332, 595, 816
Cost–benefit analysis 898
Cost-effectiveness analysis 898
Cost-minimisation analysis 897
Cost–utility analysis 898
Cotrimoxazole 671, 672
Coumarins 509
Creams 12
Cross-dependence 286
Crossover design 891
Cross-resistance 663
Cross-sectional study 891
Cross-sectional surveys 890
Cross-tolerance 80
Crotamiton 884
Cryoprecipitate 500
Crystalline penicillin G 676
Crystalloids 475
CSII 575
C-type natriuretic peptide 394
Cu poisoning 871
Cumulative toxicity 80
curing dose (CD) 658
Current Index of Medical Specialities (CIMS) 912
Cushing syndrome 596
Cutaneous route 23
Cyclandelate 468
Cyclizine 830
Cyclopentolate 109
Cyclophosphamide 342, 793, 851
Cycloplegia 106
Cycloserine 680, 709
Cyclosporine 853
Cyproheptadine 361
Cyproterone acetate 636
Cytarabine 796
Cytochrome P450 42
Cytolytic reactions 68
Cytosolic 58
Cytotoxic antibiotics 796

D

D_2 antagonists 830
Dabigatran etexilate 508
Daclatasvir 740
Daclizumab 855
Dactinomycin 796
Dalbavancin 680
Dale's reversal phenomenon 121
Dalfampridine 241
Dalfopristin 686
Dalteparin 504
Danazol 635, 642
Dapagliflozin 581
Dapoxetine 267

Dapsone 717
Darbepoetin alfa 544
Daridorexant 205
Darifenacin 110
Data point 894
Daunorubicin 797
DCGI 896
De-addiction 291
Decontamination 67, 875
Deferasirox 539
Deferiprone 872
Deflazacort 591
Degarelix 552
Deglycyrrhizinated liquorice 843
Dehydroemetine 771
Dehydroepiandrosterone 632
Dehydroepiandrosterone sulphate (DHEAS) 632
Delamanid (Dlm) 710
Delayed hypersensitivity 68
Delayed reactions 69
Demeclocycline 683
Demulcents 879
Denosumab 653, 856
Dental cone 13
Depot medroxyprogesterone acetate 618
Desamino oxytocin 626
Descriptive statistics 893
Descriptive study 6, 890
Desensitisation 80
Desferrioxamine 539, 871
Desirudin 507
Desmopressin 395
Desmopressin acetate 501
Desoxycorticosterone acetate 599
Desquamation 880
Desvenlafaxine 267
Dexamethasone 591, 595, 802, 831, 881
Dexmedetomidine 192
Dexrazoxane 802
Dextran 40, 70, 474
Dextromethorphan 369
Dextrose 5% 475
Dhaka fluid 812
DHPs 421
Diabetic nephropathy 404
Diacetylmonoxime 100
Diacetyl morphine 304
Diaminopyrimidines 671
Diastolic dysfunction 434
Diazepam 223
Diazinon 99
Diazoxide 426, 427
Dibenamine 133
Dichlorphenamide 386
Diclofenac 322
Diclofop-methyl 865
Dicloxacillin 676
Dicophane (DDT) 884
Dicoumarol 510
Dicyclomine 110
Didanosine 747
Dietary fibre (bran) 820
Diethylcarbamazine citrate 784
Diffusion 30
Diffusion hypoxia 186

Diflunisal 323
Digitalis 442
Digoxin 442
Dihydralazine 426
Diloxanide furoate 768
Diltiazem 410, 421, 492
Dimercaprol 869
Dimethylbenzene (xylene) 864
Dioctyl sodium sulphosuccinate (DOSS) 821
Diphenhydramine 830
Diphenoxylate 306, 814
Dipivefrine 150
Dipyridamole 518
Direct renin inhibitors 420
DiSalvo syndrome 511
Disinfectants 885
Disintegration 37
Disodium edetate 870
Dissolution 37
Distribution 4, 37
Distributive shock 470
Disulfiram 281
Diuretics 385, 390
Divalproex 218
DMARDs 341
DNA gyrase 672
Dobutamine 125, 446
Docosanol 737
Dofetilide 492
Dog bite 868
Dolasetron 830
Dolutegravir 749
Domperidone 831
Donepezil 229
Donovanosis 695
Dopamine 124, 446
Doripenem 679
Dorzolamide 386
Dosage form 915
Dose–response curve 6, 59
Double-blind design 892
Douches 13
Down-regulation 58
Doxapram 293
Doxophylline 377
Doxorubicin 797
Doxycycline 683
d-Penicillamine 343, 871
DPP-4 inhibitors 579
Dronedarone 491
Droperidol 255, 830
Drop factor 925
Drops 12
Drotaverine 110
DR-TB 700
Drug 1
Drug abuse 285
Drug bulletins 912
Drug categories 70
Drug compendia 912
Drug dependence 286
Drug–drug interactions (DDIs) 919, 923
Drug habituation 285
Drug metabolism 40
Drug misuse 285

Drug promotion 910
Drug promotional literature 911
Drug-releasing implants 25
Drug schedules 910
DS-TB 700
Dulaglutide 579
Duloxetine 267
Dupilumab 379
Dusting powders 12
Dutasteride 636, 807
Dynorphins 308

E
Echinocandins 728
Econazole 731
Ecothiophate 149
Ectoparasites 884
Eculizumab 856
Edaravone 241
Edrophonium 97, 98
Efavirenz 748
Efficacy 60
Elixir 17
Eluxadoline 307
Emetine 771
Emodins 822
Emollients 879
Empagliflozin 581
Emtricitabine (FTC) 747
Emulsions 17
Enalapril 403
Endocervicitis 695
Endorphins derived from pro-opiomelanocortin 307
Enema 13
Enfuvirtide 750
Enkephalins 308
Enoxaparin 504
Enoximone 445
Entacapone 237
Entecavir 739
Enteral routes 15
Environmental toxicology 863
Enzymatic receptors 57
Enzyme induction 42
Enzyme inhibition 51
Enzyme stimulation 51
EPEC 812
Epidemic dropsy 865
Epidural anesthesia 176
Epirubicin 797
Eplerenone 392
Eplivanserin 205
Epoetin alfa 544
Epoetin beta 544
Eprosartan 405
Epsilon-aminocaproic acid 500
Eptifibatide 518
Erectile function 135
Ergometrine 626
Ergonovine 626
Ergot alkaloids 359
Erlotinib 806
Ertapenem 679
Erythromycin 685

Erythropoiesis-stimulating agents (ESAs) 543
Erythropoietin 543
Escitalopram 267
Eslicarbazepine 217
Esmolol 147, 423, 491
Essential drugs list (EDL) 907
Essential medicines 907
Estramustine 799
Estrogen 653, 807
Etanercept 344, 855, 883
ETEC 812
Ethacridine 627
Ethambutol (E) 704
Ethamsylate 501
Ethanol 277, 885
Ether 189
Ethical dilemmas 933
Ethical principles 898
Ethionamide (Eto) 709
Ethosuximide 221
Ethotoin 216
Ethyl biscoumacetate 510
Ethylmorphine 369
Etidocaine 178
Etidronate 650
Etizolam 205
Etodolac 322
Etomidate 192
Etoposide 797
Etoricoxib 322
Etravirine 748
Everolimus 854
Evidence-based medicine 6, 889
Evidence pyramid 892
Excretion 4, 42
Exemestane 608
Exenatide 579
Expectorants 370
Extraction ratio 35
Exubera 575
Ezetimibe 530

F
Facilitated diffusion 32
Facilitative effect 920
Famciclovir 737
Fanconi syndrome 683
Faropenem 679
Febuxostat 334
Felbamate 221
Fenofibrate 530
Fentanyl 305
Feracrylyum 879
Ferric carboxymaltose 538
Ferrous sucrose 538
Fesoterodine 110
Fetal warfarin syndrome (Di Sala syndrome) 511
Fibrin 501
Field block 174
Filgrastim 544, 802
Finasteride 136, 636, 807
Fingolimod 241
fIPV 859
First-dose phenomenon 424

First-order kinetics 44
First-pass metabolism 35
Fixed-dose combinations (FDCs) 908
Fixed oils 822
Flavoxate 110
Flecainide 490
Floppy iris syndrome 137
Flow rate 925
Fluconazole 730
Fludrocortisone 599
Flumazenil 204
Fluocinolone 881
Fluoroquinolones 672, 719
Fluorouracil 881
Fluoxetine 267
Fluoxymesterone 634
Fluphenazine 255
Flurbiprofen 323
flutamide 807
Flutamide 636
Fluticasone 374
Fluvoxamine 267
Foam 501
FOLFIRI regimen 792
FOLFOX regimen 792
Folic ACID 542
Folinic acid 802
Follitropin α 552
Follitropin β 552
Fomepizole 282
Fondaparinux 505
Food adulterants 865
Formaldehyde 886
Formoterol 376
Fosaprepitant 830
Foscarnet 738
Fosfomycin 680, 693
Fosinopril 403
Fosphenytoin 216
Framycetin 684
Frovatriptan 359
Full and reasonable disclosure 933
Fulvestrant 608
Furan 886
Furosemide 389, 422

G
Gabapentin 220, 369
Galantamine 229
Gamma benzene hexachloride 884
Gamma-hydroxybutyric acid (GHB) 289
Ganciclovir 737
Ganirelix 552
Ganja 290
Gargles 12
G-CSF 544
Gefitinib 806
Gelatin 475, 501
Gels 12
Gemeprost 627
Gemfibrozil 530
Gemifloxacin 672
Gemtuzumab 806
Generic 3

Gentamicin 684
Gentian violet 886
Gepants 360
Gepirone 206
Germicide 885
Gestrinone 611, 641
GH antagonists 550
GINA guidelines 380
Ginkgo biloba 294
Glatiramer acetate 241
Glecaprevir 740
Glibenclamide 577
Gliclazide 577
Glimepiride 577
Glipizide 577
Globulin 500
GLP-I receptor agonists 579
Glucocorticoids 241, 852
Glutaraldehyde 886
Glycerin 370, 879
Glycerol 822
Glycopeptides 680
Glycopyrrolate 110
Glycopyrronium 376
Glycyrrhiza 879
Glyphosate 865
GM-CSF 544
Gold 343
Golimumab 855
GnRH agonists 552
GnRH antagonists 552
Gonadotropins 552
Gonorrhea 695
Good clinical practice (GCP) 898
Goserelin 552
Gossypol 620
G protein-coupled receptors 56
Graded DRC 62
Graft-versus-host disease 849
Granisetron 830
Granuloma inguinale 695
Grazoprevir 740
Grey baby syndrome 683
Griseofulvin 730
Guaiphenesin 370
Gugulipid 531

H
H-mono TB 710
H_1 antihistamines 830
H_2 blockers 838
H_2O_2 886
Halcinonide 881
Half-life 45
Halofantrine 761
Halogenated aliphatic hydrocarbons 864
Haloperidol 255
Halothane 189
Hamycin 731
Hazard 863
Healthcare as a universal right 931
Heart rate 435
Hepatolenticular degeneration 871
Herbicides 865

Heroin 304
Highly active antiretroviral therapy (HAART) 751
High-output failure 434
Hippocratic oath 927
Hirudin 507
Histrelin 552
Hog 290
Human albumin 473
Hydralazine 426, 440
Hydrochlorothiazide 390, 422
Hydrocortisone 594
Hydroflumethiazide 390
Hydroxychloroquine 343, 852
Hydroxyethyl starch (hetastarch) 474
Hydroxyurea 799
Hyoscine 105, 109
Hyperimmune immunoglobulins 855
Hyperimmune serum 859
Hypersensitivity reaction 68, 849
Hypertensive emergency 430
Hypertensive urgency 430
Hyperthyroidism 560
Hypothyroidism 560
Hypovolemic shock 470

I
Iatrogenic diseases 72
Ibuprofen 323
Ibutilide 492
ICH GCP 898
Idoxuridine 737
Idraparinux 506
Imatinib 805
Imidazoles 729
IMiDs 856
Imipenem 679
Immune serum 859
Immunoglobulins 859
Immunostimulants 857
Immunosuppressants 817
Inamrinone 445
Indacaterol 376
Indapamide 390, 422
Indexes 911
Indexing systems 911
Indian Pharmacopoeia (IP) 912
Indinavir 748
Indirect costs 897
individual case safety reports (ICSRs) 901
Infantile spasms 224
Inferential statistics 893
Infiltration anesthesia 174
Infliximab 344, 817, 855, 883
Infusion rate 925
Inhalational corticosteroids (ICS) 374, 595
Inhalational route 13
Inscription 913
Insect repellents 865
INSTIs 749
Institutional ethics committee 896, 898
Institutional review board 896
insulin aspart 573
Insulin degludec 574

Insulin detemir 574
Insulin glargine 574
insulin glulisine 573
Insulin lispro 573
Insulin pumps 575
Insulin syringes 575
Intangible costs 897
Integrase 745
Integrin antibodies 855
Interferon β 241
Interleukin inhibitors 332, 855
Intermittent RMMx regimen 720
Intermittent ROM regimen 720
International normalised ratio (INR) 510
Interquartile range 894
Interval data 894
Interventional studies 6, 891
Intolerance 69
Intradermal route 22
Intramuscular route 21
Intrauterine devices 13, 618
Intravenous route 19
Intrinsic activity 55
Intrinsic sympathomimetic action 143
Inverse agonist 5, 55
Investigator 898
Iodine 886
Iodophors 886
Iodoquinol 770
Ion trapping 31
Ipecacuanha 828
Ipratropium 107, 376
Ipratropium bromide 109
Ipsapirone 206
Irbesartan 405
Irinotecan 797
Iron dextran (Imferon) 538
Iron isomaltoside 1000 539
Iron sorbitol–citric acid 539
Irrational FDCs 909
Irrigations 13
Isoflurane 189
Isolated diastolic hypertension 418
Isolated systolic hypertension 418
Isoniazid (INH) 700
Isophane insulin 574
Isoprinosine 860
Isopropamide 110
Isopropanol 885
Isotretinoin 882
Isoxsuprine 628
Ispaghula 820
Itraconazole 730
Ivermectin 784, 884
IVRA 176

J
Jarisch–Herxheimer reaction 678, 719
Jet injections 575
Juxtaglomerular (JG) cells 399

K
K^+-sparing diuretics 422
K^+ supplementation 445

K2 290
Kalamazoo consensus statement 934
Kappa analgesics 306
Kanamycin 684
Keratolytics 880
Ketamine 192, 290
Ketoconazole 730
Ketolides 685
Ketoprofen 323
Ketorolac 323
Ketotifen 379

L
LABAs 376
Labetalol 148, 425
Lacis cells 399
Lacosamide 220
Lactitol 823
Lactulose 823
Lamivudine 739, 747
Lamotrigine 217
Lanreotide 551
Lasmiditan 359
L-asparaginase 800
LAST 177
Latanoprost 149
Latent or hidden syphilis 695
Laxatives 820
Lead compound 895
Lead poisoning 870
Ledipasvir 740
Lefamulin 684
Leflunomide 343, 851
Lemborexant 205
Lenalidomide 856
Lennox–Gastaut syndrome 224
Lenograstim 544
Lente insulin 574
Lepirudin 507
Lepra reactions 719
Lesinurad 334
Lethal dose (LD) 0.1 658
Letrozole 608
Leucovorin 802
Leukotriene receptor antagonists 378
Leuprolide 552
Levamisole 860
Levetiracetam 221
Levobetaxolol 150
Levodopa 233
Levofloxacin (Lfx) 708
Levonorgestrel 617
Levopropoxyphene 369
Levosimendan 445
LHF 434
Ligands 54
Lignocaine 177, 488
Linagliptin 579
Lincosamides 685
Lindane 884
Linezolid (Lzd) 686, 708
Liniments 12
Liposomal amphotericin B 727, 774
Liposomes 26, 877

Liquid paraffin 821
Liquorice 370, 879
Liraglutide 579
Lisinopril 403
Literature survey 893
Lithium 268
Li toxicity 272
Lixivaptan 394
Loading dose 85
Local RAAS 399
Lomustine 794
Long-loop negative feedback 402
Look-alike, sound-alike drugs (LASA) 914
Loop diuretics 389, 422
Loperamide 814
Lopinavir 748
Lorazepam 223
Lornoxicam 323
Losartan 405
Lotions 12
Lovastatin 526
Low molecular-weight heparins 504
Low-output failure 434
Lozenges 13
LSD 289
L-type Ca^{2+} channel 437
L-type calcium channels 421
Lubiprostone 823
Lumefantrine 761
Lutropin 552
Lymphogranuloma 695
Lypressin 395

M
Macrolides 659
Macro infusion set / 925
Macula densa 399
Mafenide 672
Magaldrate 838
Magnesium carbonate 837
Magnesium hydroxide 837
Magnesium stearate 879
Magnesium sulphate 629, 823
Magnesium trisilicate 837
Maintenance dose 85
Major depressive disorders (MDD) 260
Malathion 99
Malignant hyperthermia 189
Mandl's paint 886
Manic depressive psychosis (MDP) 260
Mannitol 388
Maraviroc 750
Margin of safety 61
Marijuana 290
Mean, median and mode 894
Measles vaccine 859
Mebendazole 782
Mecasermin 550
Mecasermin rinfabate 550
Meclizine 830
Medical guilds 927
Medical literature databases 912
Mefenamic acid 323
Mefloquine 761

Meglitinides 578
Melagatran 508
Meloxicam 322
Melphalan 794
Memantine 230
Menadiones 499
Menaquinone 499
Menotropin 552
Mepacrine 763
Meperidine 305
Mercury poisoning 870
Meropenem 679
Mesalazine 816
Mescaline 289
Mesna 802
Mesterolone 637, 641
Meta-analysis 892
Metabolism 4
Metformin 580
Methacholine 93
Methacycline 682
Methadone 292, 305
Methandienone 635
Methanol poisoning 281
Methazolamide 386
Methenamine 691
Methicillin 678
Methimazole 562
Methotrexate 342, 794, 851
Methoxyflurane 189
Methoxy polyethylene glycol-epoetin beta 544
Methsuximide 222
Methyl benzene or toluene 864
Methylcellulose 820, 879
Methylcysteine 370
Methyldopa 425
Methylenedioxymethamphetamine (MDMA) 288
Methylergometrine 626
Methylnaltrexone 307, 823
Methylphenidate 293
Methylpolysiloxane 838
Methylprednisolone 591
Methyl salicylate 323
Methyltestosterone 634
Methylxanthines 377
Methysergide 361
Metoclopramide 802, 831
Metolazone 390
'me-too' analogues 895
Metoprolol 147
Metronidazole 661, 696, 772
Metyrosine 116
Mexiletine 488
MDR-TB 711
Mianserin 268
Micafungin 728
Miconazole 731
Micro infusion set 925
Microsomal enzymes 41
Mifepristone 611, 627
Miglitol 581
Milnacipran 267

Milrinone 445
Miltefosine 774
Minimum alveolar concentration 186
Minimum bactericidal concentration (MBC) 659
Minimum inhibitory concentration 658
Minocycline 344, 683, 719
Minoxidil 426, 427
Mirtazapine 267
Misoprostol 627
Misoprostol 842
Missing links 932
Misuse 665
Mitiglinide 578
Mitoxantrone 242
Modafinil 293
Molded tablets 16
Molgramostim 544, 802
Monitored anesthesia care (MAC) 181
Monoclonal Antibodies (MAbs) 26, 855
Montelukast 378
Monthly Index of Medical Specialities (MIMS) 912
MOPP 791
moricizine 490
Morphine 299, 304
Moxifloxacin (Mfx) 672, 673, 708
MSA 143
mTOR inhibitors 854
Mucokinetics 370
Multicentric trials 892
Multidrug therapy (MDT) 720
Muromonab 856
Mustine 794
Mutagenicity 69
Mutation 662
Mycophenolate mofetil (MMF) 851
Myoclonic seizures 224
Myxedema coma 561

N
N_2O 189
Na^+/Ca^{2+} exchanger 437
Na^+/K^+-ATPase 437
Nabilone 831
N-acetyl cysteine 324
Nadroparin 504
Nafarelin 552, 641
Naldemedine 307
Nalidixic acid 692
Nalmefene 307
Naloxegol 307
Naltrexone 281, 307
Nandrolone 635
Naproxen 323
Naratriptan 359
Nasal Decongestants 125
Nasal route 24
Natalizumab 241, 817, 855
Natamycin 731
National Formulary of India (NFI) 912
National List of Essential Medicines (NLEM) 907
N-bomb 290

N-BOMe 290
Nebivolol 147, 423
Nebulisers 14
Nedocromil 379
Nelfinavir 748
Neomycin 684
Neostigmine 98
Neprilysin inhibitor 440
Nerve block 174
Nesiritide 394, 440
Neuraminidase inhibitors 741
Neurocysticercosis 786
Neurokinin-1 receptor antagonists 830
Neurolathyrism 866
Nevirapine 748
NEW DRUG DEVELOPMENT 895
Niacin 528
Niclosamide 786
Nicotine 96, 289
Nicotinic acid 528
Nifedipine 412
Nimesulide 322
Nitazoxanide 770
Nitrates 440
Nitrofurantoin 691
Nitrogen dioxide (NO2) 864
Nitroglycerine 440
Nitroimidazoles 771
NLEP 720
NNRTIs 748
Non-maleficence 927
Non-proprietary name 2
Non-receptor-mediated mechanisms 51
Non-systemic antacids 837
Nootropic drugs 294
Norethindrone enanthate 618
Norfloxacin 673
Normal saline 475
Norpethidine 305
NPH 574
NRTIs 746
NSAIDs 311, 331, 340, 358
NTEP 712
Nuclear receptors 58
Numerical data 894
NYHA 434
Nystatin 731

O
Obidoxime 100
Observational study 6, 890
Obstructive shock 471
Occupational toxicology 863
Octreotide 551, 815
Official compendia 912
Ofloxacin 673
Ointments 12
Olanzapine 256
Olodaterol 376
Olsalazine 816
Omalizumab 379, 856
Omega-3 fatty acids 531
Ondansetron 802, 830
Open label 891

Opiates 304
Opioid analgesics 191
Opioid antagonists 307
Oprelvekin 544, 802
OPV 859
Oral rehydration solution 811
Oral rehydration therapy 812
Oral route 15
Organochlorides 864
Organophosphates 99, 865
Oritavancin 680
Ormeloxifene 620
Ornidazole 773
Orthonovum 617
Oseltamivir 741
Osmotic diuretics 388
Osmotic purgatives 823
Over-the-counter drugs 909
Overuse 8, 665
Overuse of drugs 8
Oxacillin 678
Oxaliplatin 798
Oxandrolone 634
Oxazolidinones 686
Oxcarbazepine 217
Oxetacaine 178
Oxethazaine 178
Oxidised cellulose 501
Oxidising agents 886
Oxybenzone 880
Oxybutynin 110
Oxymetholone 635
Oxytetracycline 682
Oxytocin 624
Oxytocin antagonists 629
Ozone 864

P

Package inserts 909
Paclitaxel 799
Paints 12
Palivizumab 856
pamidronate 650
papaverine/phentolamine-induced penile erection 135
Para-aminobenzoic acid (PABA) 880
Para-Aminosalicylic Acid (PAS) 709
Paracetamol 323
Parallel group design 891
Paramethasone 591
Parathion 99
Parathormone 652
Parecoxib 322
Parenteral Routes 19
Paritaprevir 740
Parnaparin 504
Paromomycin 684, 771, 774
Paroxetine 267
Partial agonist 5, 55
Partial cross-resistance 663
Passive mydriasis 106
Pastes 12
Pastilles 13
Paternalism vs. autonomy 932

Patient autonomy 928
PDE5 inhibitors 643
P-Drugs 918
Pediculosis 884
Pegaptanib 856
Pegfilgrastim 544
Peg-IFNα 741
Pegloticase 335
Pegvisomant 551
Pelvic sepsis 679
Penbutalol 147
Penciclovir 737
Pen devices 575
Pendred syndrome 558
Penfluridol 255
Pentavalent vaccine 858
Pentazocine 306
Pentoxifylline 468
Pentylenetetrazol 293
Peramivir 742
Perampanel 221
Perinatal prophylaxis 752
Potassium permanganate 886
Permethrin 884
Pessaries 13
Pesticides 864
Pethidine 305
P-glycoprotein 79
Pharmaceutical factors 36
Pharmacodynamics 5
Pharmacoeconomics 6, 897
Pharmacoepidemiology 6
Pharmacogenetics 7, 76
Pharmacogenomics 7, 76
Pharmacokinetics 3
Pharmacopoeias 912
Pharmacotherapeutics 7
Pharmacovigilance 6, 900
Pharmacovigilance Programme of India 901
Pharmacy 7
Pharyngeal demulcents 370
Phase I reactions 40
Phase II reactions 40
Phased pills 616
Phases of clinical trials 891, 896
Phencyclidine 290
Phenformin 580
Phenol 886
Phenolphthalein 822
Phenomenological events 905
Phenothiazines 830
Phenothiazines 255
Phenoxybenzamine 133
Phensuximide 222
Phentolamine 133
Phentolamine 134
Phenytoin 215
Pheochromocytoma 134
Pholcodine 306, 369
Phosphodiesterase 3 Inhibitors 445
Phospholipase C 56
Photo-allergic reaction 69
Photochemotherapy 883

Photosensitivity 69
Phototoxic reactions 69
pH partition 31
Physical antagonism 81
Physiological antagonism 81
Physostigmine 149
Phytonadione 499
PICO 893
Picrotoxin 293
Pilocarpine 96, 149
Pimozide 255
Pindolol 147
Pioglitazone 581
Piperacillin 676
Piperazine 784
PIPE therapy 135, 137, 644
Piracetam 294
Pirenzepine 110
Piribedil 294
Piroxicam 323
Pitavastatin 526
Placental barrier 4, 39
Plasma fractions 500
Plasma protein binding 38
Plasminogen activator inhibitor-1 (PAI-1) 399
Plausibility 905
Pleuromutilins 683
PMDI 13
Poisoning 67
Poisons 6
Polidocanol 501
Polycystic ovary disease 642
Polydrug-resistant TB 710
Polyenes 731
Polygeline 474
Polypharmacy 71, 915
Polyvalent anti-snake venom (ASV) 868
Polyvinyl polymer 879
Polyvinyl pyrrolidine 475
Population 893
Positive beneficence 928
Possible event 905
Post-antibiotic effect (PAE) 659, 670
Post-coital contraceptive pills 617
Post-exposure prophylaxis (PEP) 752
Potassium citrate 370
Potassium iodide 370, 563
Potency 60
Potentiation 81
Povidone-iodine 886
PPIs 841
Pralidoxime 100
Pramipexole 241
Pramlintide 582
Prasugrel 517
Pravastatin 526
Praziquantel 786
Prazosin 133, 424
Pre-anesthetic medication 109, 193
Preclinical testing 896
Prednisolone 332, 591
Prednisone 341, 591
Pre-eclampsia 402

Pre-exposure prophylaxis 752
Preferential COX-2 Inhibitors 321
Pregabalin 221, 369
Pregnancy-induced hypertension 426
Preload 435
Prescription audit 917
Prescription drugs abuse 291
Pressor agents 124
Pretomanid (Pa) 710
Pre-XDR 711
Priapism 137
Prilocaine 177
Primaquine 760
Privacy 928
Probable event 905
Probenecid 334
Probiotics 813
Procainamide 488
Procaine penicillin G 676
Prochlorperazine 830
Procyclidine 105, 238
Prodrug 25
Progestasert 618
Progesterone 609, 807
Progestin-only pills 617
Prokinetic drugs 830
Prolactin 553
Proliferation signal inhibitors 854
Promethazine 830
Propafenone 490
Propofol 191
Propoxyphene 306
Propranolol 361, 423, 491
Proprietary name 2
Propylene glycol 879, 880
Propylthiouracil 562
Protease 745
Protease inhibitors (PIs) 748
PROTECTIVES 879
Proton pump inhibitors 839
Prucalopride 823
Psilocybin 289
Psoralen UVA 883
Psoriasis 883
Psychostimulants 293
Psyllium 820
Purified chick embryo cell vaccine (PCEV) 868
Purgatives 820
PUVA 883
p-Value 894
Pyrantel pamoate 783
Pyrazinamide (Z) 703
Pyridostigmine 98
Pyridoxine 831
Pyrimethamine 762
Pyritinol 294
Pyronaridine 763

Q

Quality of life 897
quantal DRCs 62
Quartiles 894
Quetiapine 256

Quinagolide 553
Quinidine 487
Quinine 627, 758
Quiniodochlor 731, 770
Quinolones 672
Quinupristin 686

R

RAAS Inhibitors 438
Racecadotril 814
Radioactive Iodine 563
Raloxifene 608
Raltegravir 749
Ramelteon 205
Ramipril 403
Randomisation 891
Randomised controlled trials (RCTs) 891
Range 894
Ranibizumab 856
Rasagiline 237
Rasburicase 336
Ratio data 894
Rational Prescribing 8
Raxibacumab 856
Rebound reactions 70
Receptor antagonism 81
Receptor-mediated mechanism of action 53
Receptor regulation 58
Rectal route 18
Redistribution 38
Regular insulin 573
Regular infusion set 925
Remifentanil 306
Renewal instruction 914
Repaglinide 578
Reparative effect 920
Resistance 70
Resorcinol 881
Resting membrane potential (RMP) 443
Retapamulin 683
Reteplase 519
Retigabine 221
Retinoids 882
Reversal reaction 719
Reverse transcriptase 745
Reviparin 504
rHCG 641
RHF 434
Rho(D) immune globulin 855
Ribavirin 740
Ricinoleic acid 822
Rideal-Walker coefficient 885
Rifabutin 703
Rifampicin (R) 702, 718
Rifampicin only (RR) TB 711
Rifapentine 703
Rifaximin 813
Rilonacept 332
Riluzole 241
Rimantadine 742
Ringer lactate 475
Risedronate 650
Risk versus benefits 898

Risperidone 256
Ritodrine 628
Ritonavir 748
Rituximab 806
Rivaroxaban 508
Rivastigmine 229
Rizatriptan 359
RNTCP 712
Rolofylline 394
Romosozumab 654
Rosiglitazone 581
Rosuvastatin 526
Rotahaler 13
Rotavirus vaccine 859
Rubella vaccine 859
Rufinamide 220
Rutin 501
Ryanodine 437

S

SABAs 376
Sacubitril 440
Safinamide 238
Salbutamol 376, 628
Salicylic acid 323, 880
Salicylism 320
Salmeterol 376
Sample 893
Sarecycline 683
Sargramostim 544
Saroglitazar 530, 582
Satavaptan 394
Satranidazole 773
Saxagliptin 579
Sb poisoning 870
Scabies 884
Schedules C-I to C-V 910
Scleroderma crisis 404
Scorpion sting 135, 868
Secnidazole 773
Secondary effects 67
Secondary syphilis 695
Second gas effect 186
Selective Cox-2 inhibitors 322
Selective estrogen receptor down-regulators 608
Selective estrogen receptor modulators (SERMs) 607
Selective herbicides 865
Selective toxicity 658
Selective β_2-agonists 129, 628
Selegiline 237
Self-medication 909
Semilente insulin 573
Senna purgatives 822
Serious ADR 66
SERM/SERD 807
Serratiopeptidase 325
Sertraline 267
Sevoflurane 190
SGLT-2 inhibitors 581
Shared decision making 932
Short-loop negative feedback 402
Side effects 67

Signa 914, 915
Sildenafil 643
Silodosin 136
Silver nitrate 886
Silver poisoning 870
Silver sulfadiazine 672, 886
Simeprevir 740
Simethicone 838, 879
Simvastatin 526
Single-blind design 892
Sirolimus 854
Sitagliptin 579
Sjogren's syndrome 96
Slope of the DRC 61
Smoking cessation 96
SNRIs 267
Sodium citrate 370
Sodium cromoglycate 379
Sodium depletion theory 422
Sodium iodide 563
Sodium nitroprusside 427, 440
Sodium picosulphate 822
Sodium stibogluconate 773
Sodium sulphate 823
Sodium tetradecyl sulphate 501
Sodium thiosulphate 731
Sofosbuvir 740
Solid dosage forms 16
Solifenacin 110
Solithromycin 685
Solutions 17
Somatostatin analogues 551
Somatropin 550
Sorafenib 806
Sotalol 147, 492
Spacers 14
Spare receptors 59
Sparfloxacin 673
Special K 290
Spike 290
Spinal anesthesia 174
Spironolactone 392, 422
Sponsor 898
SSRIs 267
Stakeholders 898
Standard deviation 894
Stanozolol 634
St. Anthony's fire 865
Starch 879
Statistic 893
Status asthmaticus 381
Status epilepticus 225
Stavudine 746
Stimulant purgatives 821
Stiripentol 221
Stool softeners 821
Strength of preparation 914
Strength of solution 925
Streptogramins 686
Streptokinase 519
Streptomycin 684, 705
Strontium ranelate 653
Strychnine 293
Styptics 501

Subcutaneous route 22
Sublingual route 17
Subscription 913
Sucralfate 842, 879
Sufentanil 306
Sulbactam 679
Sulfacetamide sodium 672
Sulfadiazine–pyrimethamine 672
Sulfadoxine 762
Sulfadoxine–pyrimethamine 672
Sulfasalazine 343, 672, 816
Sulfinpyrazone 334
Sulphur 884
Sulphamethoxazole 672
Sulphate 886
Sulphonamides 660, 671
Sulphonylureas 577
Sulphur dioxide 864
Sumatriptan 359
Sunitinib 806
Sunscreens 879
Superinfection 661
Super ORS 811
Superscription 913
Suppository 13
Supra-additive synergism 81
Surface anesthesia 173
Suspensions 17
Susruta Samhita 927
Sustained viral response (SVR) 740
Sutezolid 686
Suvorexant 205
Synergism 80, 923
Synergistic effect 920
Synthetic cathinones 289
Synthetic progestins 610
Systematic reviews 892
Systemic antacids 837
Systolic dysfunction 434

T
Tablets 16
Tachyphylaxis 80
Tacrine 229
Tacrolimus 853
Tadalafil 644
Tafenoquine 761
Tamoxifen 241
Tamoxifen citrate 607
Tamsulosin 136
Tannic acid 501, 878
Tannins 878
Tapentadol 307
Taxanes 799
Tazarotene 882, 883
Tazobactam 680
TCAs 261
Tedizolid 686
Teicoplanin 680
Telavancin 680
Telbivudine 739
Telenzepine 110
Telithromycin 685
Telmisartan 405

Temporal (time) relationship 904
Tenecteplase 519
Teniposide 797
Tenofovir disoproxil fumarate 739
Tenofovir (TDF) 747
Teratogenicity 70
Terbinafine 731
Terbutaline 376, 628
Terephthalylidene dicamphor sulfonic acid 880
Teriparatide 652
Terizidone (Trd) 709
Terlipressin 396
Tertiary or late syphilis 695
Testosterone 632
Tetrabenazine 239
Tetracyclines 659, 682, 771
Tetrahydrocannabinoids 831
Tetrahydrocannabinol (THC) 290
Tezepelumab 379
Thalidomide 856
Theophylline 377
Therapeutic drug monitoring 85
Therapeutic index 61
Therapeutic window 62
Thiabendazole 781
Thiazide 390
Thiazide diuretics 422
Thiazolidinediones 581
Thioridazine 255
Thrombin 501
Thrombopoietin 544, 802
Thymoxamine 468, 645
Thyroid hormones 559
Thyroid storm 561
Thyrotoxicosis crisis 561
Tiagabine 221
Tibolone 606
Ticagrelor 517
Ticarcillin 676
Ticlopidine 517
Tigecycline 683
Time-dependent killing 670
Timolol 150
Tincture iodine 886
Tinidazole 773
Tinzaparin 504
Tiotropium 376
Tiotropium bromide 109
Tirofiban 518
TNF-α inhibitors 817
Tocilizumab 855
Tofacitinib 344
Tolazoline 468
Tolbutamide 577
Tolcapone 237
Tolerance 80
Tolnaftate 731
Tolterodine 110
Tolvaptan 394
Topical routes 12
Topical steroids 881
Topiramate 220
Topotecan 797

Torcetrapib 531
Toremifene 608
Torsemide 389
Toxic effects 67
Toxicity amelioration 802
Toxicodynamics 874
Toxicokinetics 874
Toxins 6
Tramadol 307
Tranexamic acid 500
Transdermal therapeutic systems 23
Transduction 662
Transduction mechanisms 5
Transduction systems 55
Transformation 662
Transplant rejections 849
Trastuzumab 806
Trazodone 267, 644
Treatment guidelines 912
Triamcinolone 332, 591, 881
Triamterene 392
Triazoles 729
Trichomonas vaginitis 696
trifluoperazine 255
Triflupromazine 255
Trifluridine 737
Trihexyphenidyl 238
Trimethadione 223
trimethoprim 672
Triple-blind design 892
Triptorelin 552, 641
Triquilar 616
Tropicamide 109
Tropisetron 830
Trospium 110

U
Udenafil 644
Ularitide 394
Ulipristal 611, 617
Ultralente insulin 574
Unclassifiable events 905
Undecylenic acid 731
Unfractionated heparin 504

Unlikely event 905
Unoprostone 149
Upadacitinib 344
Up-regulation 58
Urate excretion 316
Urea 880
Urethritis 673, 695
Uricosuric drugs 334
Urinary antiseptics 691
Urodilatin 394
Urofollitropin 552
Urokinase 519
US Pharmacopoeia (USP) 912
Ustekinumab 855
Uterine Relaxants 126
Utility 928

V
VABAs 376
Valacyclovir 737
Valdecoxib 322
Valethamate 110
Valganciclovir 737
Valsartan 405
VAMP 791
Vancomycin 680
Vardenafil 644
Varenicline 96
Variable 894
Variance 894
Vasodilators 426, 440
Vasopressin 395
Vedolizumab 855
Velpatasvir 740
Venereum 696
Venlafaxine 267
Verapamil 410, 421, 492
Vigabatrin 221
Vilanterol 376
Vildagliptin 579, 580
Vinblastine 798
Vinca alkaloids 798
Vincristine 798
Vinorelbine 798

Vitamin B 540
Vitamin D 649
Vitamin K 500
Voglibose 581
Volinanserin 205
Volume of distribution 4, 38
Vorapaxar 518
Voxilaprevir 740

W
Warfarin 510
Wasp sting 868
Weight by volume (W/V) solutions 925
WHO-UMC scale 905
Wilson's disease 871
Wintergreen 323

X
Xanthinol nicotinate 468
XDR-TB 711
Ximelagatran 508
Xipamide 390
Xylene 864

Y
Yohimbine 644

Z
Zafirlukast 378
Zaleplon 205
Zanamivir 741
Z drugs 204
Zero-order kinetics 44
Zidovudine 746
Zileuton 378
Zinc 812, 879, 886
Zinc oxide 886
Zinc stearate 879
Ziprasidone 256
Zirconium 879
Zolpidem 204
Zonisamide 220
Zopiclone 204